Veterinary Hematology, Clinical Chemistry, and Cytology

Third Edition

About the cover

From left: Nala was rescued by Ross University veterinary students in 2016 on the island of St. Kitts, where she was found covered with ticks and ill with ehrlichiosis. Nala adopted Dr. Clarissa Freemyer and now lives in Raleigh, North Carolina. **Middle top:** Bone marrow aspirate from a cat with systemic histoplasmosis. Macrophages have phagocytized numerous *Histoplasma* organisms. **Middle middle:** Cerobrospinal fluid from a dog with Large Granular Lymphocyte lymphoma. Note the azurophilic granules in the large lymphoid cells. **Middle bottom:** A Hyacinth Macaw photographed by Dr. Robin W. Allison in the wilds of the Pantanal, Brazil- the world's largest tropical wetland. **Right:** Imprint of an ulcerative lesion on a cat's paw showing numerous *Cryptococcus* organism. This was Mary Anna Thrall's first attempt at taking a cytologic sample, and the inspiration for her to become a clinical pathologist (circa 1974, new methylene blue stain).

Veterinary Hematology, Clinical Chemistry, and Cytology

THIRD EDITION

EDITED BY

Mary Anna Thrall, BA, DVM, MS, DACVP

Professor Emerita, Colorado State University
Professor of Clinical Pathology
Department of Biomedical Sciences
Ross University School of Veterinary Medicine
Basseterre, St. Kitts, West Indies

Glade Weiser, DVM, DACVP

Clinical Pathologist, ACVP Emeritus member
Loveland, Colorado

Robin W. Allison, DVM, PhD, DACVP

Adjunct Professor of Clinical Pathology
Department of Veterinary Pathobiology
Oklahoma State University College of Veterinary Medicine
Stillwater, Oklahoma

Terry W. Campbell, MS, DVM, PhD

Professor Emeritus
Department of Clinical Sciences
College of Veterinary Medicine and Biomedical Sciences
Colorado State University
Fort Collins, Colorado

WILEY Blackwell

This edition first published 2022

Edition History
First Edition © 2005 Lippincott Williams & Wilkins; Second Edition © 2012 John Wiley & Sons, Inc.

Registered Office
John Wiley & Sons, Inc., 111 River Street, Hoboken, NJ 07030, USA

Editorial Office
111 River Street, Hoboken, NJ 07030, USA

For details of our global editorial offices, customer services, and more information about Wiley products visit us at www.wiley.com.

Wiley also publishes its books in a variety of electronic formats and by print-on-demand. Some content that appears in standard print versions of this book may not be available in other formats.

Library of Congress Cataloging-in-Publication Data Applied for

[HB]: 9781119286400

Cover Design: Wiley
Cover Images: © Mary Anna Thrall, © Robin W. Allison

Set in 9/12pt MeridienLTStd by Straive, Chennai, India

Printed in Singapore
M067821_100122

Dr. Mary Anna Thrall dedicates the third edition of this book to her veterinary students, interns, residents, graduate students, and other trainees at Colorado State University and Ross University School of Veterinary Medicine who have made the profession of veterinary medicine and the specialty of clinical pathology extremely rewarding and enjoyable for many years. I also dedicate this edition to my adult children Joseph Bammer, Dr. Anna Freemyer-Brown, Sarah Freemyer, and Dr. Clarissa Freemyer, all of whom are happy, wonderful, and productive people who excelled in spite of my somewhat neglectful parenting.

Dr. Glade Weiser dedicates this edition to Dr. Gary Kociba for his mentorship and willingness to risk hiring a faculty member as an untrained clinical pathologist coming out of internal medicine. Soon after, Drs. Bob Hall and Don Meuten joined the section as trainees. Truth be known the three of us jointly contributed to each other's training. In addition, I treasure the numerous mentorship and working relationships over the years with faculty, staff, and colleagues at the University of California Davis, the Ohio State University, Colorado State University, Coulter Electronics Inc., Heska Corporation, and the American College of Veterinary Pathologists. Lastly, working with many clinical pathologists in training over the years was a most rewarding renewable source of inspiration.

Dr. Robin W. Allison dedicates this edition to Dr. Mary Anna Thrall, who was my inspiration to become a clinical pathologist somewhat late in life. As a veterinary technician in mixed animal practice taking continuing education classes at Colorado State University, I marveled at her knowledge of cytology and vowed to "become her." I may not have entirely succeeded, but not for lack of trying. I will always treasure the wonderful relationships with so many talented clinical pathologists I've become friends with over the years. Additionally, this edition is dedicated to the trainees and veterinary students that made sure I never stopped learning by asking great questions; you are the future of clinical pathology.

As someone trained in clinical pathology but having a career in clinical exotic animal medicine, Dr. Terry W. Campbell dedicates this edition to his animal patients who have been the fountainhead of his education. It has been a joyfully inspirational experience working with clinical pathologists at Kansas State University and Colorado State University and exploring the world of comparative clinical pathology throughout the many years.

Contents

Editors

Mary Anna Thrall, **BA, DVM, MS, DACVP**
Professor Emerita, Colorado State University
Professor of Clinical Pathology
Department of Biomedical Sciences
Ross University School of Veterinary Medicine
Basseterre, St. Kitts, West Indies

Robin W. Allison, **DVM, PhD, DACVP**
Adjunct Professor of Clinical Pathology
Department of Veterinary Pathobiology
Oklahoma State University College of Veterinary Medicine
Stillwater, Oklahoma, USA

Terry W. Campbell, **MS, DVM, PhD**
Professor Emeritus
Department of Clinical Sciences
College of Veterinary Medicine and Biomedical Sciences
Colorado State University
Fort Collins, Colorado, USA

Glade Weiser, **DVM, DACVP**
Clinical Pathologist, ACVP Emeritus member
Loveland, Colorado, USA

Section VII Guest Editor

Alex Mau, **DVM**
Pathology Intern
Department of Biomedical Sciences
Ross University School of Veterinary Medicine
Basseterre, Saint Kitts and Nevis

Chapter Contributors

Anne Avery, **BA, VMD, PhD**
Professor of Immunology and the Director of the Clinical Immunology Laboratory
Department of Microbiology, Immunology, and Pathology
College of Veterinary Medicine and Biomedical Sciences
Colorado State University
Fort Collins, Colorado, USA

Andrea A. Bohn, **DVM, PhD, DACVP**
Associate Professor of Clinical Pathology
Department of Microbiology, Immunology, and Pathology
College of Veterinary Medicine and Biomedical Sciences
Colorado State University
Fort Collins, Colorado, USA

Karl E. Jandrey, **DVM, MAS, DACVECC**
Associate Dean, Admissions and Student Programs
Professor, Clinical Small Animal Emergency and Critical Care
University of California, Davis, School of Veterinary Medicine
Veterinary Medicine Student Services and Administration Center
Davis, California, USA

Wayne A. Jensen, **DVM, PhD, MBA**
Professor and Head
Department of Clinical Sciences
College of Veterinary Medicine and Biomedical Sciences
Colorado State University
Fort Collins, Colorado, USA

Kristina Meichner, **DVM, DECVIM-CA (oncology), DACVP**
Assistant Professor of Clinical Pathology
Department of Pathology
University of Georgia College of Veterinary Medicine
Athens, Georgia, USA

Jim Meinkoth, **DVM, MS, PhD, DACVP**
Professor, Clinical Pathology
Department of Veterinary Pathobiology
College of Veterinary Medicine
Oklahoma State University
Stillwater, Oklahoma, USA

Donald Meuten, **DVM, PhD, DACVP**
Professor Emeritus
North Carolina State University
Raleigh, North Carolina, USA

M. Judith Radin, DVM, PhD, DACVP
Professor Emerita
Department of Veterinary Biosciences
The Ohio State University College of Veterinary Medicine
Columbus, Ohio, USA

Sreekumari Rajeev, BVSc, PhD, DACVM, DACVP
Professor of Infectious Diseases
Biomedical and Diagnostic Sciences
University of Tennessee, College of Veterinary Medicine
Knoxville, Tennessee, USA

Emily D. Rout, DVM, PhD, DACVP
Research Scientist
Department of Microbiology, Immunology, and Pathology
College of Veterinary Medicine and Biomedical Sciences
Colorado State University
Fort Collins, Colorado, USA

Saundra Sample, DVM, DACVP
Assistant Professor of Veterinary Clinical Pathology
Department of Veterinary Pathobiology
University of Missouri College of Veterinary Medicine
Columbia, Missouri, USA

dawn Seddon, BVSc, MSc Vet Path, DACVP (Clin Path), NHD Microbiol, MRCVS
Professor of Clinical Pathology
Director of Lab Services (Clinical Pathology)
Department of Pathobiology
School of Veterinary Medicine
St. George's University, True Blue Campus
Grenada, West Indies

Linda M. Vap, DVM, Diplomate ACVP
Associate Professor, Clinical Pathology Section Chief
Department of Microbiology, Immunology, and Pathology
Colorado State University
Fort Collins, Colorado, USA

Section VII New Case Contributors

Patrice Bernier, BSBA
Senior Laboratory Technician
Lab Services
Ross University School of Veterinary Medicine
Basseterre, St. Kitts, West Indies

Pedro Bittencourt, DVM, MSc, PhD
Assistant Professor of Immunology
Department of Biomedical Sciences
Ross University School of Veterinary Medicine
Basseterre, St. Kitts, West Indies

Pompei Bolfa, DVM, MSC, PhD, DACVP
Professor of Anatomic Pathology
Biomedical Sciences Department
Ross University School of Veterinary Medicine
Basseterre St. Kitts, West Indies

Clarissa Freemyer, BS, DVM
Radiation Oncology Resident
College of Veterinary Medicine
North Carolina State University
Raleigh, North Carolina, USA

Allan Kessell, BVSc, Mast.Vet.Clin.Stud, MANZCVS, DACVP
Pathologist
6A Vernon Cresent
Maslin Beach 5170
South Australia
Australia

Crystal Lindaberry, BA, DVM
FYGVE Clinical Instructor
US Army Veterinary Corps
Fort Benning, Georgia, USA

Ananda Muller, DVM, MS, PhD
Associate Professor of Veterinary Bacteriology
Department of Biomedical Sciences
Ross University School of Veterinary Medicine
Basseterre St. Kitts, West Indies

Donald E. Thrall, DVM, PhD, DACVR
Professor Emeritus
College of Veterinary Medicine
North Carolina State University
Raleigh, North Carolina, USA
Radiologist/Quality Control
IDEXX Telemedicine
Clackamas, Oregon, USA

Judit Wulcan, DVM, MSc
Resident, Veterinary Anatomic Pathology
Veterinary Medical Teaching Hospital
University of California, Davis
Davis, California, USA

Preface

On behalf of the contributing authors and Wiley-Blackwell, we are pleased to introduce the Third Edition of *Veterinary Hematology and Clinical Chemistry*, now titled *Veterinary Hematology, Clinical Chemistry, and Cytology*. Our goal is to provide an image-rich, readable resource addressing routine laboratory diagnostics in veterinary practice. The theme of the presentation is applied clinical pathology for veterinary students and veterinary health professional teams in the practice setting. We aimed to maintain our intended target audience and original organizational structure. We believe that the addition of cytology to the textbook makes it a complete and valuable reference for anyone interested in clinical pathology.

Audience

A continuing trend in frontline veterinary medicine is the movement of laboratory diagnostics into the veterinary facility. Evolving technological advancements in point-of-care diagnostic capability drive this trend, which increases the need for education in veterinary clinical pathology. Although this book was written primarily for veterinary students and practitioners, it has applications for a broader audience, serving as a useful adjunct for the educational and reference needs of a variety of other users. The following audiences may benefit from this resource:

- Students in professional veterinary medical education programs.
- Health professional teams in veterinary care facilities.
- Clinical pathologists and clinical pathologists in training.
- Product development groups using veterinary clinical pathology.

Organization

Veterinary Hematology, Clinical Chemistry and Cytology is organized into seven sections, arranged as follows:

I: Presents principles of laboratory technology and test procedures used in veterinary laboratories to generate laboratory results. It also presents perspectives on how laboratory data interpretation is used in diagnosis and overall clinical case management.

II: Presents hematology and hemopathology of common domestic species. This includes all aspects of the hemogram or complete blood count, bone marrow, hemostasis, and transfusion medicine.

III: Presents hematology of common nondomestic species encountered in veterinary practice.

IV: Presents clinical chemistry of common domestic species and is organized primarily by organ system.

V: Presents clinical chemistry of common nondomestic species.

VI: Presents cytology of common domestic species and includes cytology of inflammation, neoplasia, skin and subcutaneous tissue, body cavity effusions, joint fluid, internal organs, and lymph nodes.

VII: Provides a compilation of clinical cases. Each case includes a signalment, brief history, and pertinent physical examination findings. Then, relevant laboratory data are presented in tables followed by a narrative interpretation of the data.

Comments, Revisions, and Addition Highlights

Development of data interpretation skills by veterinary students, clinical pathologists in training, and practitioners continues to be the primary focus in this edition. While rules for interpreting diagnostic tests assume homogeneity of pathophysiologic responses, we realize that not all of our animal friends have "read the book," although most do, as seen in Figure P.1.

Revisions of chapters have been made throughout where needed. Chapters that have been extensively revised are the following:

- Glade Weiser updates Chapter 2 to include a section on cytology, with details on fluid and tissue sample collection, preparation, staining, and approach to specimen examination.

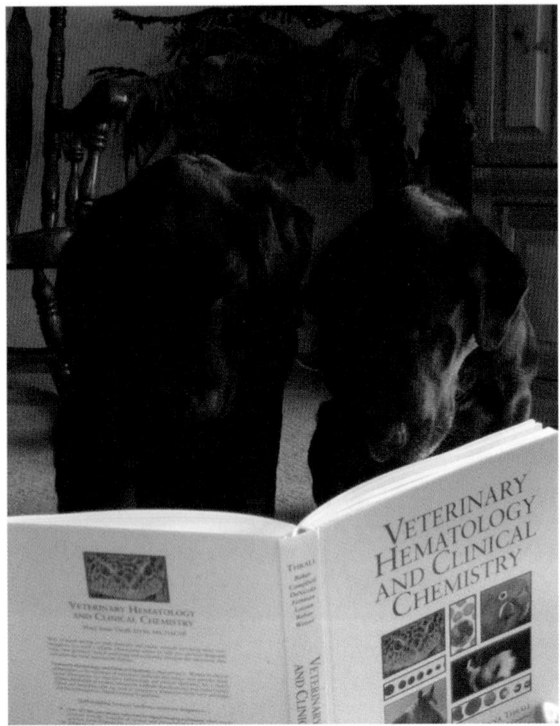

Figure P.1 Dogs caught "reading the book" in an attempt to make their disease responses predictable. Not all will read the book. Source: Courtesy of Dr. Sara Hill.

- Jim Meinkoth, Oklahoma State University, provides a complete revision of the chapter on diagnosis of hemostasis disorders.
- Karl E. Jandrey, University of California, who is board certified in veterinary emergency and critical care, provides new information from a criticalist viewpoint as a coauthor of the chapter on blood transfusion and cross-matching.
- Saundra Sample, University of Missouri, is a new coauthor of two chapters on laboratory evaluation of the kidney and laboratory evaluation of the thyroid, adrenal, and pituitary glands.

Additions include the following: Sreekumari Rajeev, who is board certified in both anatomic pathology and microbiology and is a professor of infectious disease at the University of Tennessee, provides a new chapter on laboratory diagnosis of infectious disease, which discusses a logical approach to the use of modern tools that are available to diagnose infectious disease, a topic of increasing importance particularly as it relates to zoonotic diseases.

Another very important addition is a new cytology section, with seven new chapters. Contributors of new chapters include the following:

- Robin W. Allison from Oklahoma State University is the author of two of the new chapters, one on inflammation and infectious agents and one on body cavity effusions.
- Jim Meinkoth, co-author of *Diagnostic Cytology and Hematology of the Dog and Cat,* 3rd edition, is the author of a chapter on cytology of joint fluid.
- Donald Meuten, who is board certified in both clinical and anatomical pathology, and the editor of the 5th edition of *Tumors in Domestic Animals*, brings years of experience and expertise to the chapters discussing cytology of neoplasia, skin masses, and lymph nodes.
- Kristina Meichner, who is board certified in both clinical pathology and internal medicine (oncology), brings her expertise in cytology and oncology to three of the new chapters.
- Mary Anna Thrall is the coauthor of three of the new chapters on cytology, including cytology of abdominal organs, and cytology of lymph nodes.
- Andrea Bohn is the coauthor of two of the new chapters, cytology of abdominal organs and cytology of lymph nodes.

The clinical case presentations in what is now Section VII, edited by Dr. Alex Mau, are intended to provide readers "practice" to develop interpretive skills by seeing examples of how data are interpreted into pathologic processes and how pathologic processes may culminate in a diagnostic scenario, not unlike reading and solving a mystery in a novel. The original cases are retained because their classical usefulness does not change. Forty-three new cases have been added to this edition by several contributors, to whom we are grateful for sharing.

It is our wish that readers not only learn principles and skills from this work but also enjoy interacting with it. As veterinarians and specialists in bioanalytical pathology, we share our passion for the art and science of laboratory diagnostics applied to animal health.

Respectfully submitted,

Glade Weiser
Mary Anna Thrall
Robin W. Allison
Terry W. Campbell

About the Companion Website

This book is accompanied by a website containing:

- Case studies
- Figures
- References and Suggested Reading

www.wiley.com/go/thrall/veterinary 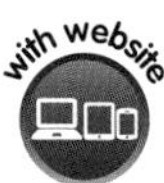

I

General Principles of Laboratory Testing and Diagnosis

1 Laboratory Technology for Veterinary Medicine

Glade Weiser
Loveland, CO, USA

This chapter presents an overview of the laboratory technology used to generate data for hematology and clinical biochemistry. For the procedures and technologies likely to be employed within veterinary hospitals, general instructions and descriptions provide a review of the principles previously learned in laboratory courses. This, in conjunction with the instructions accompanying different devices and consumables, should enable users to reproduce the procedures to a satisfactory performance standard. For technologies more likely to be used only in large commercial or research laboratories, the overview provides familiarity with the basic measuring principles.

Hematologic techniques

Basic techniques applicable for any veterinary hospital

The procedures outlined here are most appropriate for the in-house veterinary laboratory in most practice settings. These procedures, with the exception of a cell-counting hematology system, require minimal investment in instrumentation and technical training. These basic hematologic procedures include:

- Blood mixing – for all hematologic measurements.
- Packed cell volume or hematocrit by centrifugation.
- Plasma protein estimation by refractometry.
- Cell-counting instrumentation.
- Microscopic differential leukocyte count and assessment of blood film pathology.

Blood mixing

The blood sample is assumed to have been freshly and properly collected into an ethylenediaminetetraacetic acid (EDTA) tube (as described in Chapter 2). When performing any hematologic procedure, it is important that the blood is thoroughly mixed. Cellular components may settle rapidly while the tube sits on a counter or in a tube rack (Figure 1.1).

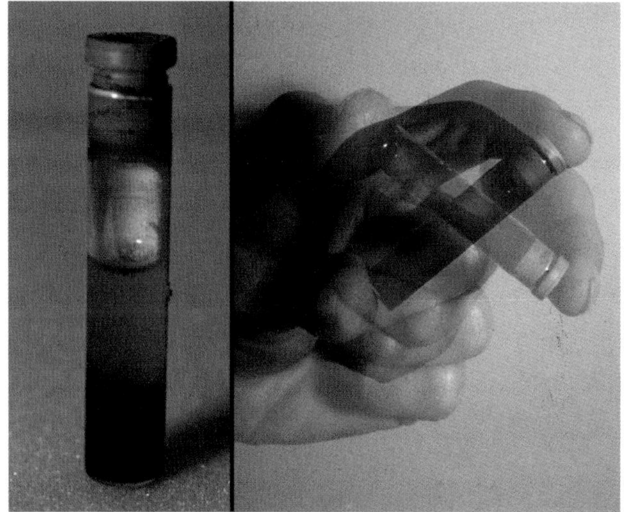

Figure 1.1 Left. Gravity sedimentation of whole blood. Right. A gentle, repetitive, back-and-forth tube inversion technique used to manually mix blood before removing aliquots for hematologic procedures.

As a result, failure to mix the sample before removing an aliquot for hematologic measurement may result in a serious error. Mixing can be performed by manually tipping the tube back and forth a minimum of 10–15 times (Figure 1.1). Alternatively, the tube may be placed on a rotating wheel or tilting rack designed specifically to mix blood (Figure 1.2).

Packed cell volume

The packed cell volume value is the percentage of whole blood composed of erythrocytes. It is measured in a column of blood after centrifugation that results in maximal packing of the erythrocytes. Tools for performing the packed cell volume include 75 × 1.5 mm tubes (i.e., microhematocrit tubes), tube sealant, a microhematocrit centrifuge, and a tube-reading device.

The procedure is performed using the following steps. First, the microhematocrit tube is filled via capillary action

Veterinary Hematology, Clinical Chemistry, and Cytology, Third Edition. Edited by Mary Anna Thrall, Glade Weiser, Robin W. Allison and Terry W. Campbell.

Companion website: www.wiley.com/go/thrall/veterinary

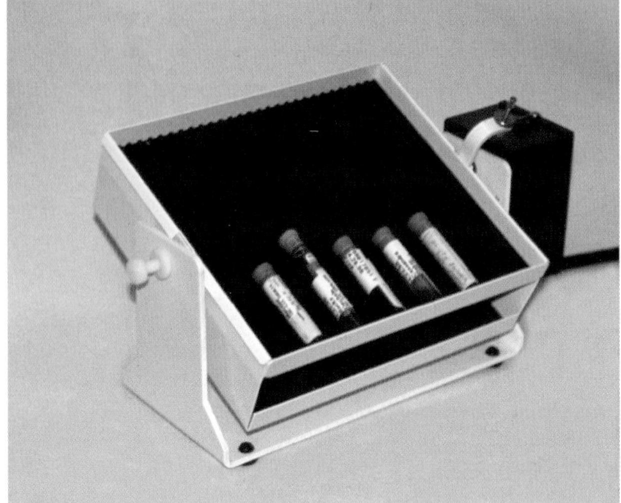

Figure 1.2 Representative mechanical blood-mixing table. The surface holds several tubes on a ribbed rubber surface and tilts back and forth at the rate of 20–30 oscillations per minute.

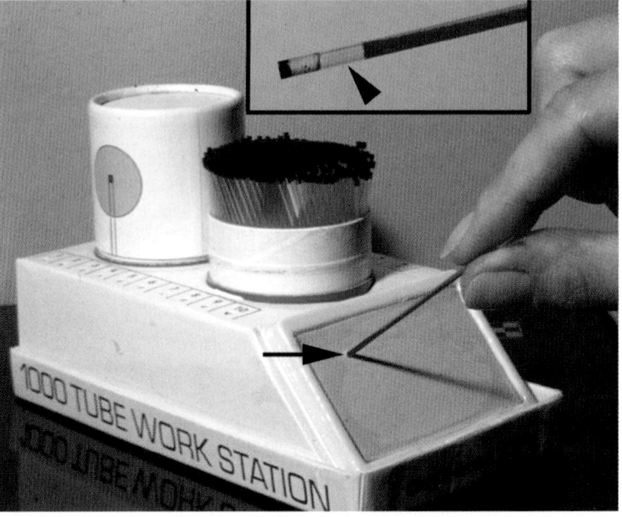

Figure 1.4 A microhematocrit tube is sealed by pressing two to three times into the clay sealant (arrow). Note that a small amount of air trapped between the blood and white clay is not a problem (arrowhead in the inset).

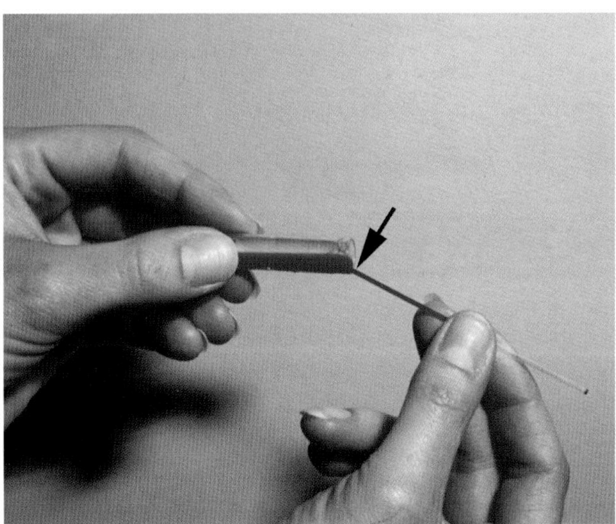

Figure 1.3 Proper technique for filling a microhematocrit tube. The tube should be positioned horizontally or tilted slightly downward to facilitate filling by capillary action. Capillary action is established by touching the upper end of the tube to the blood (arrow).

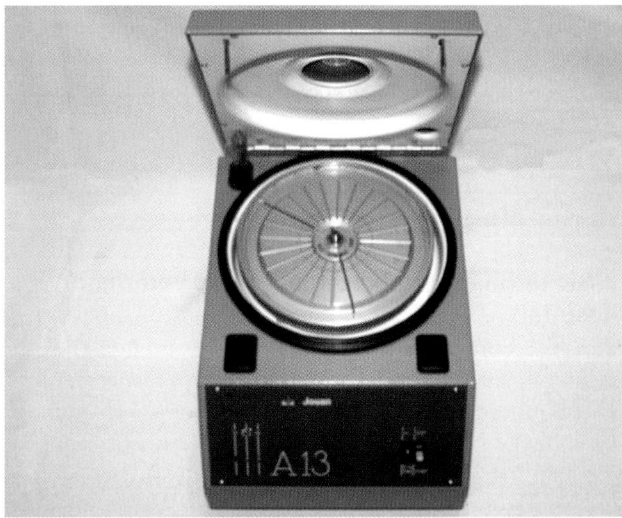

Figure 1.5 Representative microhematocrit centrifuge. The head and motor are designed to spin the tubes at very high speeds to achieve maximal erythrocyte packing.

by holding it horizontally or slightly downward and then touching the upper end to the blood of the opened EDTA tube (Figure 1.3).

Next, allow the tube to fill to approximately 70–90% of its length. Hold the tube horizontally to prevent blood from dripping out of the tube, and seal one end by pressing the tube into the tube sealant once or twice (Figure 1.4). Note that air may be present between the sealant and the blood (Figure 1.4). This is not a problem, however, because the trapped air is removed during centrifugation.

The tube is then loaded into the microhematocrit centrifuge according to the manufacturer's instructions (Figures 1.5 and 1.6). The microhematocrit centrifuge is designed to spin the lightweight tube at very high speeds to generate sufficient centrifugal force to completely pack the red cells within 2–3 minutes. With such centrifugal force, most (or all) of the plasma is removed from the layers of packed cells.

Three distinct layers may be observed in the tube after removal from the centrifuge: the plasma column at the top, the packed erythrocytes at the bottom, and a small, middle white band known as the buffy coat (Figure 1.7). The buffy coat consists of nucleated cells (predominantly leukocytes) and platelets, and it may be discolored red when the nucleated erythrocyte concentration is prominently

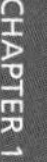

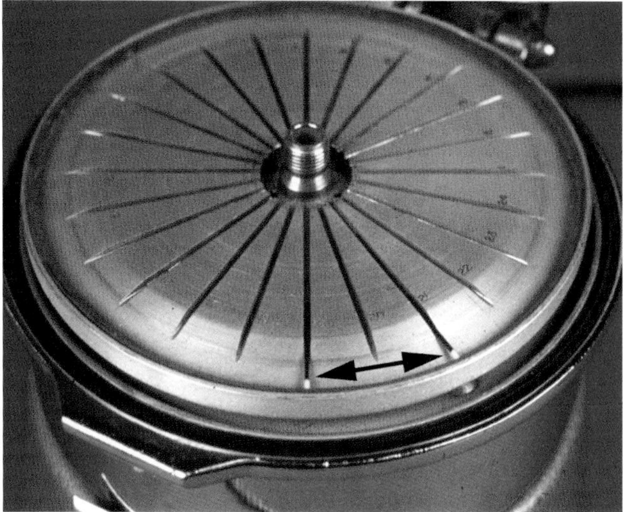

Figure 1.6 Placement of microhematocrit tubes on a microhematocrit centrifuge head. Note the proper orientation of two microhematocrit tubes, with the clay-sealed end positioned at the outer ring of the centrifuge head (double arrow).

increased. Observations of any abnormalities in the plasma column above the red cells should be recorded. Common abnormalities such as icterus, lipemia, and hemolysis are shown in Figure 1.7. Icterus is excessively yellow pigmentation of the plasma column that suggests hyperbilirubinemia; the magnitude of this hyperbilirubinemia should be confirmed by a biochemical determination of serum bilirubin concentration (see Chapter 27). The observation of an icteric coloration to the plasma is diagnostically useful in small animals. It is not reliable in large animal species, however, because their serum usually has a yellow coloration from the normal carotene pigments associated with their herbivorous diet. Lipemia is a white, opaque coloration of the plasma column because of the presence of chylomicrons. Lipemia most commonly is associated with the postprandial collection of blood, but it also may be associated with disorders involving lipid metabolism (see Chapter 32). Hemolysis is a red discoloration of the plasma column, which usually results from artifactual lysis of red cells induced during the collection of blood. A small quantity of lysed erythrocytes is sufficient to impart visual hemolysis. Therefore, if the hematocrit is normal, one may assume it is an artifact. Less commonly, causes of anemia that result in intravascular hemolysis give rise to observable hemolysis in the plasma fraction, which also is known as hemoglobinemia (see Chapter 9). This will typically also be associated with hemoglobinuria.

The packed cell volume is measured on a reading device, such as a microhematocrit card reader (Figure 1.8). The procedure is performed by positioning the erythrocyte–clay interface on the 0 line and the top of the plasma column on the 100 line. The position of the top of the erythrocyte column is then read on the scale as the packed cell volume.

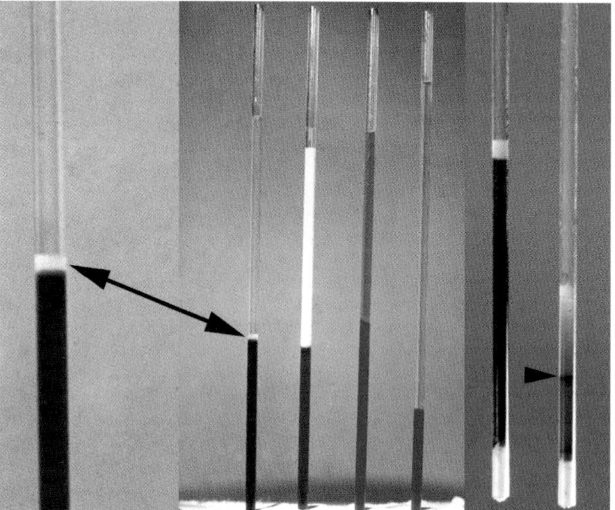

Figure 1.7 Normal and abnormal spun microhematocrit tubes (four tubes in middle panel). The tube on the left is normal. Note the packed erythrocytes at the bottom, plasma layer at the top, and buffy coat in the middle (arrow; enlarged at left). The second tube illustrates lipemia, the third hemolysis, and the fourth icterus. Note also that the hematocrit is considerably decreased in the fourth tube. Two additional tubes illustrate buffy-coat abnormalities (enlarged at right). The first of these tubes has an increased buffy coat that correlates with an increased leukocyte concentration. The second (right) is from a sheep with leukemia and has a dramatically increased buffy coat. The leukocyte concentration was greater than 400,000 cells/μL. There is also severe anemia. With such major abnormalities in cell concentration, separation of erythrocytes and leukocytes is not complete, and division may be blurred. What is interpreted as being the "top" of the erythrocyte column is indicated by the arrowhead. The red discoloration of the buffy coat may be caused by a prominent increase in nucleated erythrocytes.

Plasma proteins by refractometry

After measurement and observation of the microhematocrit tube, the plasma column may be used to estimate the plasma protein concentration on the refractometer (Figure 1.9). This instrument may be used to estimate the concentration of any solute in fluid according to the principle that the solute refracts (or bends) light passing through the fluid to a degree that is proportional to the solute concentration. The principle or property being measured is the refractive index relative to distilled water. The scale for a particular solute can be developed from refractive index measurements calibrated to solutions with known solute concentrations. In clinical diagnostics, refractometry is used to estimate the plasma protein concentration and urine specific gravity.

Plasma protein is measured using the plasma column in the microhematocrit tube. The tube is broken above the buffy-coat layer (Figure 1.10), and the portion of the tube containing the plasma is used to load the refractometer (Figure 1.11). The instrument then is held so that an ambient light source can pass through the prism wetted with

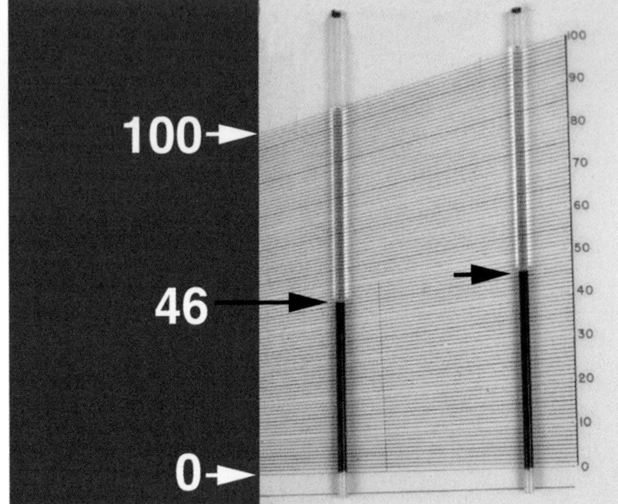

Figure 1.8 Determination of packed cell volume on a microhematocrit tube card reader using two tubes of blood from the same patient sample. Note that the scale allows the tube to be read over a considerable range of filling levels. The steps are to line up the erythrocyte–clay interface with the 0 line, line up the top of the plasma column with the 100 line, and then read the top of the erythrocyte column on the scale. The positions of these steps are indicated by the arrows. Note in this example that the packed cell volume is 46%.

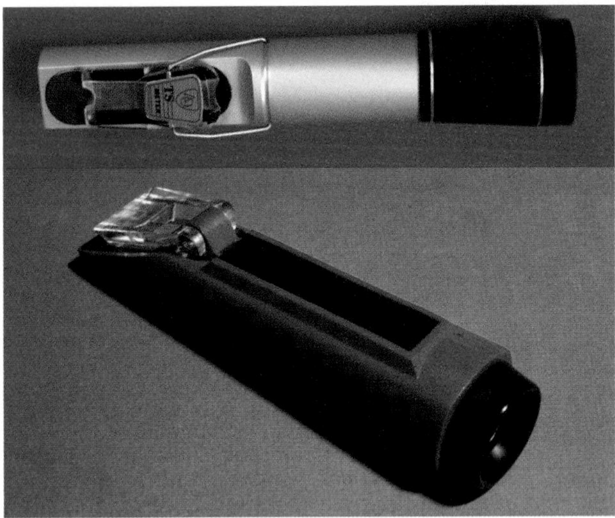

Figure 1.9 Refractometers. The lower refractometer is more rugged, because it is encased in rubber. It is known as a veterinary refractometer, and it has a canine and feline urine specific gravity scale that calibrates for minor differences between species during this determination.

plasma, and the light refraction is read on a scale through an eyepiece (Figure 1.12).

The protein measurement is regarded as being an estimate based on calibration, assuming that other solutes in the serum are present in normal concentrations. The measurement may be influenced by alterations in other solutes. Most notably, lipemia may artificially increase the protein

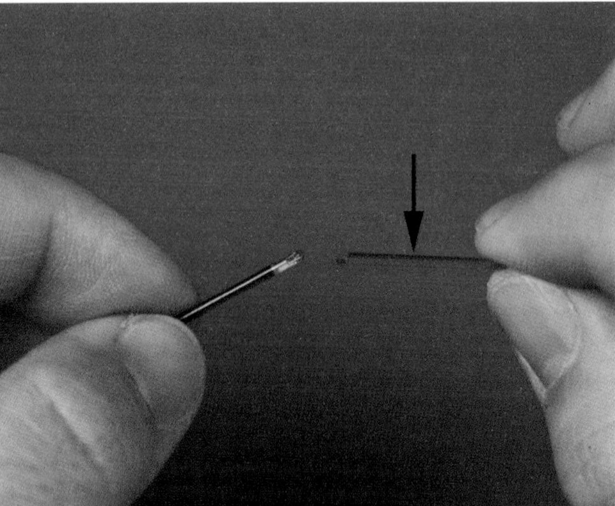

Figure 1.10 Preparation of the microhematocrit tube for measuring plasma protein concentration. The tube is broken just above the buffy coat to yield a column of plasma (arrow).

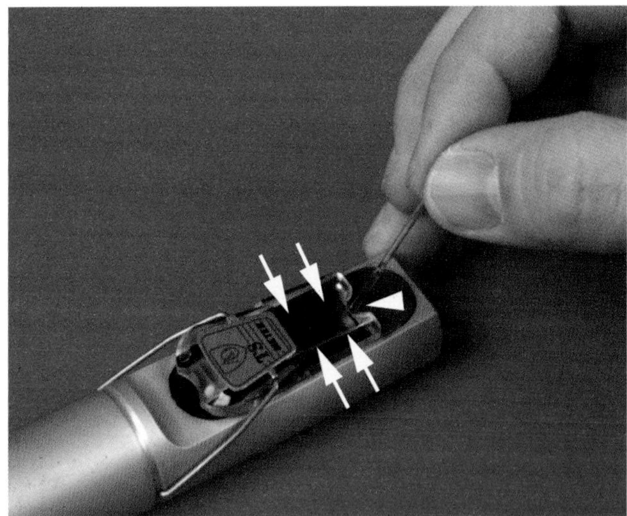

Figure 1.11 Loading plasma from the microhematocrit tube to the refractometer. To wick plasma onto the refractometer, capillary action is established by touching the end of the plasma tube at the notch of the prism cover (arrowhead). Flow should establish a thin layer of plasma under the plastic cover to fill the area delineated by arrows. After reading, the plastic cover is flipped back and wiped clean with a laboratory tissue.

estimate by as much as 2 g/dL. Other alterations of solutes such as urea and glucose influence the protein estimate to a much lesser, and usually negligible, degree.

Determination of total leukocyte concentration

Two general approaches are available to determine the leukocyte concentration. Historically, cell concentrations were measured manually using a blood dilution placed onto a hemocytometer and counted while observing by

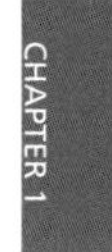

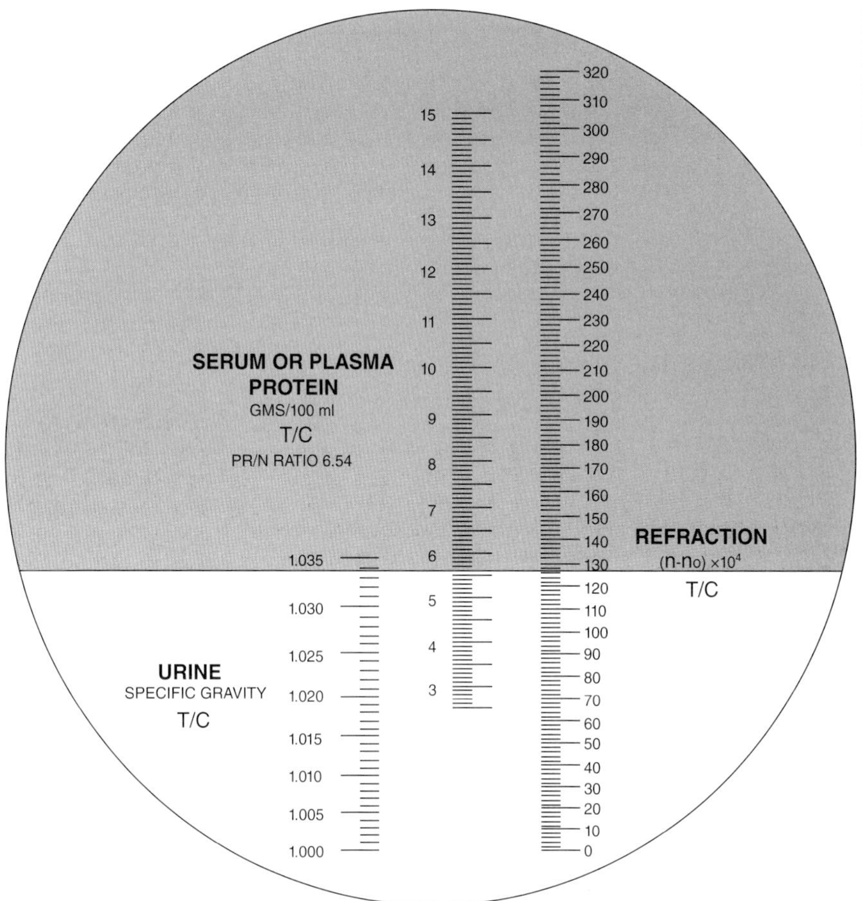

Figure 1.12 Representative refractometer scale as seen through the eyepiece. Light refraction creates a shadow–bright area interface that is read on the appropriate scale.

microscopy. This procedure, and associated consumables, is regarded as obsolete for the veterinary practice setting. This procedure has been replaced by automated hematology cell-counting systems or alternatively expanded buffy-coat analysis technology in which cellular estimates are made from layers in a specialized hematocrit tube. The total leukocyte count is the concentration of nucleated cells, because the techniques detect all the nuclei in solutions from which erythrocytes have been removed by lysis or centrifugation. Therefore, nucleated erythrocytes typically are included in this count. In most cases the concentration of NRBC is negligible, but on rare occasion they may make up an appreciable fraction of the total nucleated cell concentration.

A variety of electronic cell counters operate by enumerating nuclear particles in an isotonic dilution in which a detergent is used to lyse the erythrocytes. These systems must be engineered for animal blood, however, to generate accurate measurements of cell concentrations. There are also continued advances in these hematology systems for performing leukocyte differentiation. Three-, four-, and five-part differential systems exist. The differential capability works best with normal blood, but there are individual exceptions. All systems may produce questionable results when there is leukocyte pathology, and none properly detect abnormalities such as left shift, toxic change, and cell types outside the routine five normal cell types (see below). (For principles of hematology system operation, see the discussion of advanced hematologic procedures later in this chapter.) The quantitative buffy-coat analysis system (Idexx Autoread™, Idexx Laboratories) estimates the leukocyte concentration by measurement of the buffy-coat layer in a specialized microhematocrit tube, in which a float is present to expand the buffy-coat region for optical scanning.

In isolation, the total leukocyte count is not particularly useful for interpretive purposes; this measurement is used to determine the concentration of various leukocyte types that make up the differential count. The concentration of individual leukocyte types is the most useful value for the interpretation of disease processes. This information is determined by evaluating the stained blood film. Because of the limitations in automated leukocyte differentiation described above, it is important to utilize blood film examination in conjunction with automated hematology systems when blood is abnormal. This is essential not only for leukocyte characterization but also for evaluation of erythrocytes in cases of anemia and platelets when the instrument produces a decreased platelet concentration value. See further detail in the next section.

CHAPTER 1

Microscopic differential count and assessment of morphology

The microscopic differential count and blood film examination is not necessarily required for all complete blood count (CBC) samples. Many samples can be classified as normal when analyzed by modern hematology instruments, especially when the CBC is part of a wellness examination. When all the data are normal, it is very unlikely to find additional useful information from the blood film examination. The need for blood film examination may be determined by examination of the instrumentation data output. The examples of data abnormalities that should prompt blood film evaluation include anemia, any data abnormality in the automated total leukocyte count or automated differential, and any concern about platelet concentration. Almost all automated instrument measurements are highly reliable on well-maintained systems. The measurement most likely to have inaccuracies is the automated differential count. This is because these systems are less likely to recognize and/or properly classify all of the nucleated cell types that do not belong in normal blood. Examples include nucleated erythrocytes, immature and blast forms of any cell lineage, and left shifted neutrophils. Therefore, it is important to perform a microscopic differential whenever the total leukocyte concentration is abnormal and/or when the distribution of cells determined by the instrument differential is abnormal. The next most likely problem is instrument counting of platelets. This is because platelet microclots are common in animal blood samples, especially from cats. The hematology instrument system will not count platelets in microclots. The blood film is helpful for identifying platelet microclots, qualitatively assessing their impact on an instrument platelet measurement value that is abnormally decreased. The examination procedures are described below.

Preparation of blood films and initial approach to blood film examination is detailed in Chapter 2, under "Collection, Preparation, and Examination Techniques for Clinical Microscopy Samples." Using the blood film monolayer area (aka counting area), the microscope should be adjusted to 100× objective oil immersion or high magnification observation for these procedures. The observer will then perform a systematic evaluation of the three major cell lines. This includes a differential count for leukocytes with notation about any abnormal cells, evaluation of erythrocyte morphology, and evaluation of platelets.

Within the counting area, the observer will move across fields and obtain the differential leukocyte count by classifying a minimum of 100 consecutively encountered cells. Cells are classified into a minimum of five to six categories, with the presence of abnormal cells being recorded into a category of "other." The specification of "other" is described or defined for the sample being examined. The common six categories of normal cells – neutrophil, band neutrophil, lymphocyte, monocyte, eosinophil, and basophil – are shown in Figure 1.13. (See Chapter 11 for additional visual details regarding leukocyte identification that may be helpful in differential counts.)

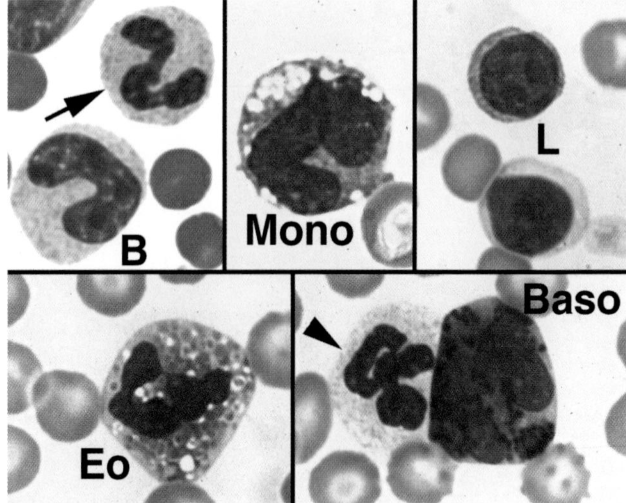

Figure 1.13 Basic leukocytes encountered in the differential count. Upper left. Neutrophils. Note the segmented neutrophil (arrow) and the constrictions in the nuclear contour. The band neutrophil (B) has smooth, parallel nuclear contours. Upper middle. Monocyte (Mono). The nucleus may have any shape, from round to bean-shaped to ameboid and band-shaped, as in this example. The cytoplasm is blue-gray and may variably contain vacuoles. Upper right. Two lymphocytes (L). Lower left. An eosinophil (Eo). Note that granules stain similar to the surrounding erythrocytes. Occasionally, granules may wash out in the staining procedure, leaving vacuoles. Lower right. Basophil (Baso) with dark granules that stain similar to nuclear chromatin. Note the adjacent neutrophil (arrowhead) and that neutrophils may have small, poorly staining granules that are much smaller than those of eosinophils or basophils.

The result of counting 100 cells is that the number of each leukocyte type is a fraction of 100, or a percentage of the leukocyte population. Once cells are categorized into percentages, they must be converted to absolute numbers for interpretation purposes. This is done by multiplying the total leukocyte concentration by the percentage of each leukocyte type, which yields the absolute number or concentration of each leukocyte in the blood sample. The following example illustrates the conversion of percentages to absolute numbers: (See Example 1.1, next page)

Any abnormalities in leukocyte morphology also should be noted. Important morphologic abnormalities are detailed in Chapter 13.

Erythrocyte morphology is then systematically evaluated. The observer should note any important erythrocyte shape or color abnormalities; this is particularly important for evaluating anemias. (See Chapter 6 for a review of morphologic erythrocyte abnormalities.)

The presence of platelet adequacy may be interpreted from a properly prepared blood film. A minimum of 8–12 platelets per oil immersion high-power (1000×) field may

Example 1.1. Conversion of percentage counts to absolute concentrations

Total white-blood-cell count = 10,000/μL
Differential white-blood-cell count:

	Percentages	Absolute numbers/μL
Neutrophils	60%	(6000)
Lymphocytes	30%	(3000)
Monocytes	5%	(500)
Eosinophils	5%	(500)

be interpreted as adequate. The number seen may be considerably greater than described, however, because of the wide range of normal platelet concentrations. This number is only a guideline for most microscopes with a wide field of view. It should be adjusted downward when using a microscope with a narrow field of view and upward if using one with a superwide field of view. If the platelets appear to be decreased, a search for platelet clumps on a low-power setting at the feathered edge should be performed. The ability to look for platelet clumps is also important when a cell counter produces a decreased platelet concentration value; this is a frequent problem in cats. Morphology of platelets also may be noted. Platelets that approach the diameter of erythrocytes or larger are referred to as macroplatelets or giant platelets. In dogs, these suggest accelerated platelet regeneration, but this interpretation usually is not applied to macroplatelets in cats.

Advanced hematologic techniques

Historically, these capabilities were limited to central laboratories. Over the past 20 years, there has been rapid technological evolution resulting in reduced cost and complexity such that these capabilities are now available to the common veterinary facility. Currently, the predominant differences of the larger, more expensive systems used by commercial laboratories are higher throughput rate, automated tube handling, and more sophisticated differential counting technology. (See Chapter 2 for additional discussion of equipment and laboratories.) Hemograms performed on modern hematologic instrumentation provide the following additional measurements.

Items determined by spectrophotometry or calculation:

- Hemoglobin concentration of blood, g/dL.
- Mean cell hemoglobin content, pg.
- Mean cell hemoglobin concentration (MCHC), g/dL.

Items determined by cell (particle) counting and sizing:

- Erythrocyte concentration of blood, $\times 10^6$ cells/μL.
- Mean cell volume (MCV; the average size of erythrocytes), fl.
- Hematocrit (equivalent to the packed cell volume), %.
- Platelet concentration of blood, $\times 10^3$ cells/μL.
- Mean platelet volume (MPV), fl.
- Total and differential leukocyte concentrations, $\times 10^3$ cells/μL.
- Reticulocyte concentration, $\times 10^3$ cells/μL.

The method and applicability for each of these measurements are now described.

Items determined by spectrophotometry or calculation

Hemoglobin concentration

This measurement of the quantity of hemoglobin per unit volume, expressed as g/dL, is performed in conjunction with the total leukocyte count. Briefly, a blood sample is diluted, and a chemical agent is added to rapidly lyse cells, thereby liberating hemoglobin into the fluid phase. Nucleated cells remain present in the form of a nucleus with organelles collapsed around it. The absorbance of light at a specific wavelength then may be measured by spectrophotometry in a small flow cell known as a hemoglobinometer. The absorbance of light is proportional to the concentration of hemoglobin. The system is calibrated with material of known hemoglobin concentration using reference techniques.

Interpretation of the hemoglobin concentration is the same as that of the packed cell volume, or hematocrit. It is an index of the red cell mass per unit volume of blood in the patient. Because it is roughly equivalent to the packed cell volume, however, it is not particularly useful for clinical interpretations. Most clinicians are more familiar or experienced with interpreting packed cell volumes. The hemoglobin value is always proportional to hematocrit and is a separate, independent measurement. Therefore, the hemoglobin value may serve as a quality-control adjunct for laboratory personnel when used to calculate the MCHC.

Mean cell hemoglobin

The mean cell hemoglobin is calculated from the hemoglobin concentration and erythrocyte concentration. It is regarded as being redundant to other measurements and, therefore, is not useful.

Mean cell hemoglobin concentration

The MCHC is calculated from the hemoglobin concentration and the hematocrit. It provides an index for the quantity of hemoglobin (HGB) relative to the volume of packed erythrocytes (expressed as g/dL):

$$\frac{\text{HGB (g/dL)}}{\text{PCV (\%)}} \times 100 = \text{MCHC (g/dL)}$$

where PCV is the packed cell volume. An example calculation is

$$\frac{10\ \text{g/dL}}{30\%} \times 100 = 33.3\ \text{g/dL}$$

A universal relationship among mammalian species, other than the camel family, is that the hemoglobin value normally is approximately one-third of the hematocrit value. Thus, from the relationship described, the MCHC for all mammalian species ranges from approximately 33–38 g/dL. Because members of the camel family (camel, llama, alpaca, vicuna) have relatively more hemoglobin within their cells, their MCHCs are expected to range from 41 to 45 g/dL.

The MCHC is not particularly useful for clinical interpretations; however, it is useful to laboratorians for monitoring instrument performance. The rationale is that the hematocrit and hemoglobin are determined on different blood aliquots, which are diluted in two different subsystems of the instrument. A malfunction in either of these subsystems may result in a mismatch between the hemoglobin and the packed cell volume, which is reflected by a deviation from the reference interval. In addition, some abnormalities of blood can result in an artifactually increased MCHC, and these can include any factor that causes a false increase in the spectrophotometric determination of hemoglobin relative to the hematocrit. Severe hemolysis in the sample is a common cause of an increased MCHC. Alternatively, common examples of increased turbidity that interfere with light transmittance are lipemia and a very large number of Heinz bodies (see Chapter 9) in cats. Erythrocyte agglutination, as may occur in immune-mediated hemolytic anemia, may result in a false-high MCHC. In this situation, the hemoglobin measurement is accurate, but the hematocrit is falsely low because the agglutinated erythrocytes are out of the system's measuring range and are therefore not counted or sized in derivation of hematocrit.

Two erythrocyte responses related to anemia may be associated with a slightly decreased MCHC. The first is marked regenerative anemia. Reticulocytes or polychromatophilic cells are still synthesizing hemoglobin and, therefore, have not yet attained the cellular hemoglobin concentration of a mature erythrocyte. A very high fraction of reticulocytes is required, however – such as greater than 20% – to develop a detectable decrease in MCHC. The second is severe iron deficiency, in which cells have a reduction in hemoglobin content because they are smaller (i.e., microcytic) but also may have a minor reduction in cellular hemoglobin concentration. There are no causes of a dramatically decreased MCHC (<28 g/dL) other than an analytic instrument error.

Items determined by cell (particle) counting and sizing

Cell-counting and sizing technologies

A brief overview of cell-counting and sizing technology common to all of these measurements is appropriate. One of two technologies is used by most hematology instrument systems.

The first is light-scatter measurement of cells passing through a light source. Cells are passed through a flow cell that is intersected by a focused laser beam. The physical properties of the cell scatter light to different degrees and at different angles relative to the light source. Cell passages eliciting scatter events may be counted to derive the cell concentration. The degree of scatter in the direction of the light beam, which is known as forward-angle scatter, is proportional to the size of the cell. In addition, measurement of light scattered to different angles may be correlated with cellular properties, which leads to the ability to differentiate nucleated cell types.

The second is more common and incorporated into a wider range of instrument designs and may also be used as a second measuring principle in light-scatter systems. This is electronic cell counting, which is also known as impedance technology or Coulter technology (after the original inventor). It is based on the principle that cells are suspended in an electrolyte medium, such as saline, that is a good conductor of electricity. The suspended cells, however, are relatively poor conductors of electricity. Thus, these cells impede the ability of the medium to conduct current in a sensing zone known as an aperture. By simultaneously passing current and cells through a small space or aperture, deflections in current can be measured (Figure 1.14). In addition, the size of the cell is proportional to the resultant deflection in current. This volumetric size discrimination may be used to measure the size distribution of erythrocytes, to discriminate platelets from erythrocytes, and to partially differentiate leukocytes. Cells within a given population are counted and assigned to a size distribution by particle-size-analyzer circuitry (Figure 1.15). The particle-size analyzer assigns each cell to a size scale that is divided into a large number of discrete size "bins" of equal size. The size scale is calibrated with particles of known size. By rapidly accumulating several thousand cells, a frequency distribution of the sizes of the cell population may be constructed (Figure 1.16).

The size distribution curve is most useful for the evaluation of erythrocytes in the laboratory. It also may be used to derive leukocyte differential and platelet information.

The following measurements derive from the described cell-counting and sizing technology. Because of the considerable differences in erythrocyte and platelet sizes between species, instrument systems require careful design and/or adjustment to accurately obtain the various measurements. For example, instruments manufactured for the analysis of human blood do not perform accurately for most animal species without modification.

Erythrocyte concentration

The erythrocyte concentration is measured directly by counting the erythrocyte particles in an isotonic dilution of blood.

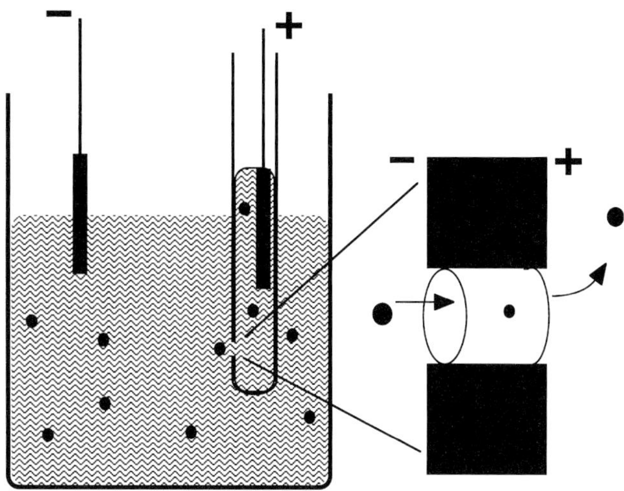

Figure 1.14 Principle of electronic impedance cell counting. Left. Overview of the fluidic chamber. Cells (dots) are diluted in an isotonic fluid (wavy lines). Two electrodes (+ and −) are separated by a glass tube containing a small opening or aperture. Electric current is conducted by the isotonic fluid across the electrodes via the aperture. Vacuum is applied to move the fluid and cells through the aperture. Right. Magnified, diagrammatic view of the aperture. Cells flow through the aperture (arrows). The aperture is a cylindric shape with a volume called the sensing zone. While occupying space within the aperture, cells transiently impede the flow of current. Cell passages are counted as deflections in the current voltage. In addition, the magnitude of voltage deflection is proportional to the volume of the cell.

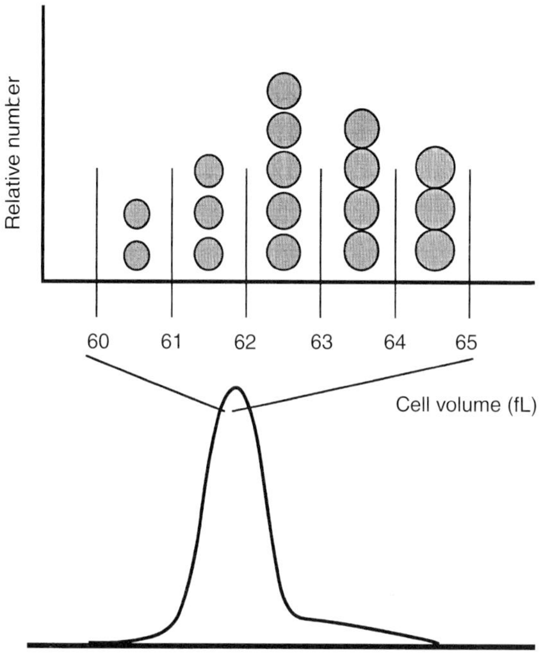

Figure 1.15 Cell volumes assigned to size bins. In the case of erythrocytes, a cell volume scale of approximately 30–250 fl is divided into a large number of discrete size bins (e.g., 60–61 fl, 61–62 fl). As the cells are counted, they are assigned to size bins (circles). Accumulation of many cells allows the construction of a size distribution histogram on the cell-volume scale (curve tracing at bottom). The drawing of bins at the top would represent a small area of the total curve.

This value is not useful for purposes of clinical interpretation. It generally parallels the packed cell volume and hemoglobin concentration, but the packed cell volume is the preferred value for the interpretation of erythrocyte mass. The erythrocyte concentration is used by the instrument to calculate the packed cell volume (described later).

Mean cell volume, erythrocyte histogram, and red cell distribution width

As the erythrocytes are counted, their size distribution is simultaneously constructed (Figure 1.16), and from this size distribution, the MCV is easily calculated. The red cell distribution width (RDW) is a mathematic index describing the relative width of the size distribution curve. It is the standard deviation of most of the erythrocytes divided by the MCV. The tails of the erythrocyte distribution usually are excluded from this mathematic treatment.

These values are useful for the evaluation of anemia. Iron deficiency results in the production of microcytic erythrocytes, and accelerated erythrocyte regeneration results in the production of macrocytic erythrocytes. Early in these responses, a widening of the erythrocyte size distribution and RDW value may be observed (Figure 1.16). As a larger proportion of these cells accumulate during the response, the curve shifts in the respective direction, and eventually, the MCV may fall out of the reference interval. The RDW

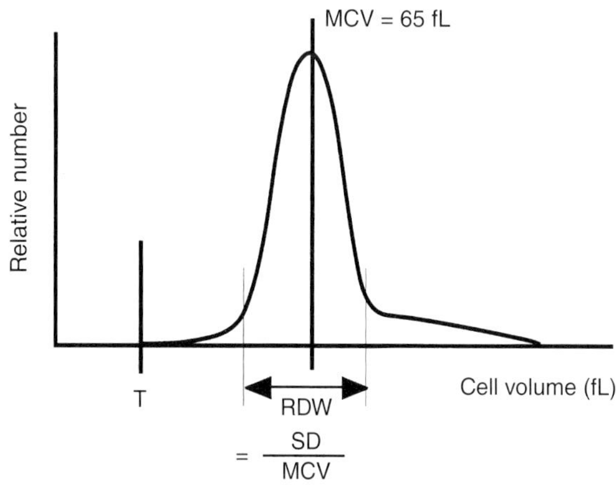

Figure 1.16 Histogram of erythrocyte size distribution. The *x* axis is the cell volume, and the *y* axis is the relative number of cells at each volume. Only cells above a specified volume or threshold are included in the analysis; this is indicated by the vertical bar (T). The mean cell volume (MCV) is indicated by the large vertical bar. The RDW (red-cell distribution width) value, an index of volume heterogeneity, is the standard deviation (SD) divided by the MCV, with the SD being that of the volumes of erythrocytes within the region indicated by the fine lines marked by the double arrow.

is more useful in the laboratory, in conjunction with the examination of blood films, whereas the laboratorian and the clinician both may interpret the MCV. Examples of interspecies variation and representative reference intervals for MCV are

Humans	80–100 fl
Dogs	60–72 fl
Cats, horses, and cows	39–50 fl
Sheep	25–35 fl
Llama	21–29 fl
Goat	15–25 fl

For additional detail on microcytic and macrocytic anemias and other breed-specific information regarding erythrocyte size, see Chapter 7.

Hematocrit

One of the advantages of hematology instrumentation is that the hematocrit may be determined by calculation, thereby avoiding the need for microhematocrit centrifugation. The instrument calculates hematocrit (HCT) using the erythrocyte concentration (RBC) and the MCV:

$$(\text{MCV} \times 10^{-15}\ \text{L}) \times (\text{RBC} \times 10^{12}\ \text{L}) = \text{HCT}$$

Or, simplified:

$$\frac{\text{MCV} \times \text{RBC}}{10} = \text{HCT}$$

Thus, for example:

$$\frac{\text{MCV 70 fL} \times 7.00\ \ \text{RBC}}{10} = \text{HCT 49\%}$$

Platelet concentration

Platelets may be counted simultaneously with erythrocytes. Because platelets are considerably smaller than erythrocytes, however, they are analyzed in a separate area of the particle-size-analyzer scale. Most species have little or no overlap between platelet and erythrocyte volume, thereby making such analysis both simple and accurate. Cats are an exception, in that their platelets are approximately twice the volume of those in other domestic species. In addition, macroplatelet production is a frequent response during most hematologic disturbances in cats. This response is not specific for any specific disease pattern, but it results in considerable overlap between erythrocyte and platelet size distributions, thus making determination of accurate counts difficult. Therefore, feline platelet counts should be regarded as being estimates only. Because large platelets tend to get counted as erythrocytes, the platelet concentration frequently may be artifactually low. Microclots are also a common contributor to some fraction of platelets not being counted. In general, if the platelet concentration falls in the reference interval, it may be regarded as being adequate. If the platelet concentration is decreased, however, the blood film should be examined by a laboratorian as described above to confirm this finding.

White blood cell and differential leukocyte concentrations

To analyze leukocytes, a lytic agent is first added to a dilution of blood. This agent rapidly lyses or dissolves cytoplasmic membranes, thereby making the erythrocytes and platelets "invisible" to the detection technologies. Only nuclear particles of nucleated cells remain, around which is found a "collapse" or condensation of cytoskeletal elements and any attached organelles. These particles are measured by one of the detection technologies previously described to obtain the total leukocyte concentration. Using specially formulated lytic reagents, the degree of collapse may be controlled to different degrees in different leukocyte types. The result is a differential size that can be measured by a particle-size analyzer or light-scatter technology. Automated differential leukocyte counting is not as perfected in domestic animals as in humans; however, the procedure is reasonably accurate for normal blood and, therefore, is very useful in situations such as safety assessment trials, in which most (or all) of the blood samples to be analyzed are normal. When blood is abnormal, however, the frequency of analytic error in the differential count increases considerably. Analytic errors are handled by using the blood film for comparison and the visual differential count whenever an instrument analytic error is either present or suspected. It is essential to monitor instrument performance by visual inspection of the histogram or cytogram display for each sample to know when analytic failure occurs. It is very difficult, if not impossible, to determine this simply by monitoring numeric data from the instrument. Therefore, use of this technology requires considerable training and expertise by the operator to monitor the instrument performance and appropriately intervene with visual inspection of the blood film.

Summary of blood analysis by automated or semiautomated instrumentation

The flow of dilutions, analysis, and calculations within an automated hematology instrument is summarized in Figure 1.17. This flow has two main pathways. In one, an isotonic dilution of blood is made for erythrocyte and platelet analysis. In the other, a dilution is made, into which a lytic agent is added; in this pathway, leukocytes and hemoglobin are measured.

Reticulocyte concentration

Reticulocyte enumeration

The reticulocyte concentration is very useful in the evaluation of anemias. The rate of release of reticulocytes from the

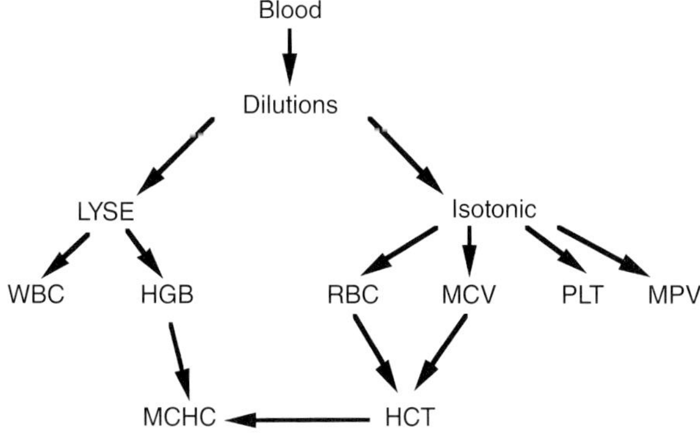

Figure 1.17 Summary of blood analysis pathways in an automated instrument. Two major dilutions are made (see text). In the left pathway, a lytic agent is added, and leukocytes are counted and the hemoglobin concentration measured. In the right pathway, erythrocytes and platelets are counted and sized. From the direct measurements, the hematocrit is calculated. A cross-check between the two pathways is provided by calculation of the mean cell hemoglobin concentration (MCHC).

bone marrow is the best assessment regarding the function of the erythroid component of bone marrow. (See Chapters 7–9 for a more detailed discussion of the anemias.)

The basis for the reticulocyte count involves the events in the maturation of erythroid cells. The developing erythroid cell is heavily involved in aerobic metabolism and protein (i.e., hemoglobin) synthesis. As it nears the final stages of maturity, the nucleus undergoes degeneration and is extruded from the cell, and the organelles supporting the synthetic and metabolic events are removed. After denucleation of the metarubricyte, the remaining erythrocyte undergoes its final maturation, which involves the loss of ribosomes and mitochondria during a period of 1–2 days. To enumerate reticulocytes, a stain is applied to erythrocytes, thereby causing aggregation of these residual organelles. This results in visible, clumped granular material that can be seen microscopically (Figure 1.18). The aggregation is referred to as reticulum, hence the name reticulocyte. Reticulocytes are equivalent to the polychromatophilic cells observed on the Wright-stained blood films (Figure 1.18). Evaluation of polychromatophilic cells on the Wright-stained blood film can provide an assessment of the bone marrow response to anemia. The appearance of these cells, however, is more subjective, and they are more difficult to quantitate than counting the corresponding cells on the reticulocyte stain.

Stains that can be used are new methylene blue (liquid) and brilliant cresyl blue, which is available in disposable tubes that facilitate the procedure (Figure 1.19). First, several drops of blood are added to the stain in a tube. The tube then is mixed and incubated for 10 minutes. From this mixture, a conventional blood film is made and air-dried. A total of 1000 erythrocytes are counted and categorized as either reticulocytes or normal cells. From this, the percentage

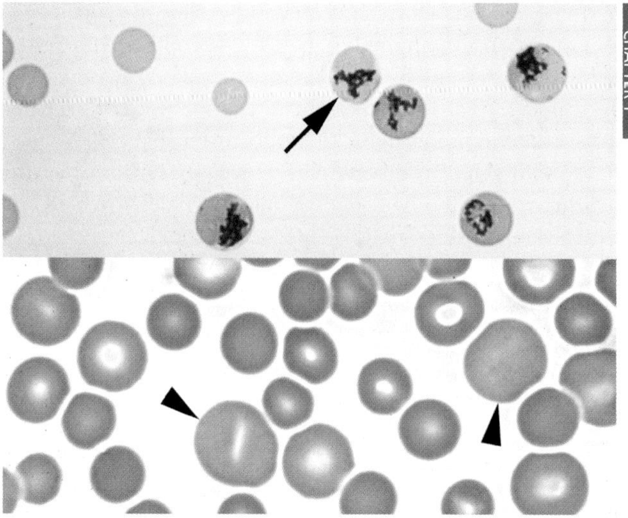

Figure 1.18 Reticulocytes. Top. Representative reticulocyte (arrow) using new methylene blue stain. Note the dark-staining, aggregated organelles in several reticulocytes. Bottom. Blood film stained with Wright-Giemsa stain. Polychromatophilic cells (arrowheads) are roughly equivalent to reticulocytes on the counterpart stain.

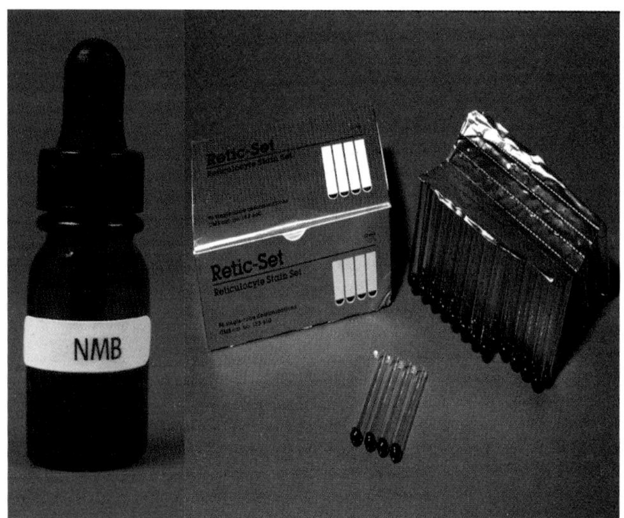

Figure 1.19 Examples of reticulocyte stains. Left. New methylene blue in a liquid dropper bottle. Right. Commercial preparation of brilliant cresyl blue. The stain is coated on the bottom of disposable tubes.

of reticulocytes is derived. Interpretation of the percentage reticulocytes is somewhat misleading, however, because it does not account for the degree of anemia. Thus, for purposes of interpretation, the absolute reticulocyte concentration should be calculated by multiplying the erythrocyte concentration (RBC) by the percentage of erythrocytes that are reticulocytes:

$$\text{RBC}/\mu\text{L} \times \% \text{ Reticulocyte} = \text{Reticulocytes}/\mu\text{L}$$

Some instrument systems are also capable of reticulocyte enumeration. The method involves staining erythrocytes with a fluorescent dye that binds to residual RNA in the reticulocyte that is not present in the mature erythrocyte. RNA content, proportional to fluorochrome per cell, is measured and gated to differentiate reticulocytes from mature erythrocytes and other nonerythroid cell types. The percent and absolute values are presented as described above.

Interpretation of the Reticulocyte Concentration

The reticulocyte concentration is most useful in dogs and cats, and it also has some application in cows. It is not used in horses, however. Reticulocyte maturation is confined to the marrow space in the horse, and reticulocytes almost never are released into their circulation. Reticulocyte concentration guidelines for domestic mammals are the concentrations to be expected when the hematocrit is normal:

Dogs and cats	0–60,000 cells/μL
Cows	0 cells/μL
Horses	Do not release reticulocytes

When anemia is present, a greater degree of release from the marrow is to be expected if the marrow can respond to the anemia. This gives rise to the following guidelines for the interpretation of reticulocyte concentrations with respect to the type of anemia present:

Nonregenerative anemia to very poor regeneration	0–10,000 cells/μL
Nonregenerative to poorly regenerative anemia	10,000–60,000 cells/μL
Regenerative anemia with mild to moderate output	60,000–200,000 cells/μL
Maximal regeneration	200,000–500,000 cells/μL

Reticulocyte maturation

In dogs, reticulocyte maturation occurs in 24–48 hours. Maturation involves a continuum of progressive loss of the visible organelles (Figure 1.20).

Cats are unique in that more than one kind of reticulocyte may be present. These reticulocytes are of the aggregate and the punctate forms (Figure 1.21). The aggregate reticulocyte has a clumped reticulum that appears to be identical to that of other species. In the punctate reticulocyte, discrete dots are seen without any clumping; other species do not have this reticulocyte counterpart. Only aggregate reticulocytes appear to be polychromatophilic with Wright stain. Punctate reticulocytes are indistinguishable from normal, mature erythrocytes with Wright stain.

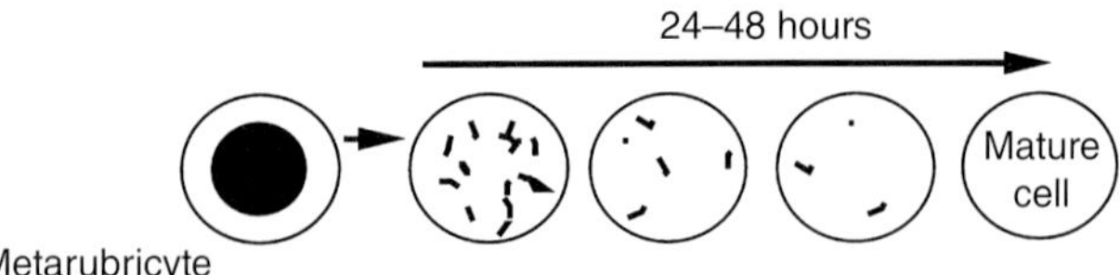

Figure 1.20 Sequential erythroid maturation as related to the reticulocyte stain and interpreted in dogs. The metarubricyte denucleates on leaving the reticulocyte. Reticulum is progressively lost during a 24–48-hour period, resulting in a mature erythrocyte.

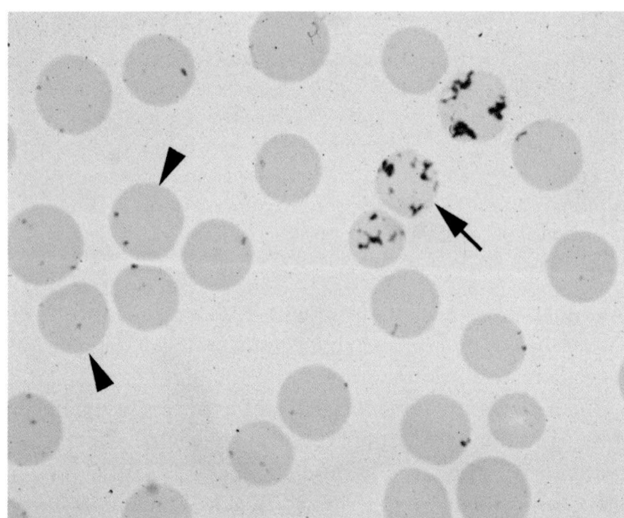

Figure 1.21 Feline reticulocyte morphology with new methylene blue stain. Three aggregate reticulocytes are in the field; note the representative one (arrow). The remainder of the cells are punctate reticulocytes; note the representative cells (arrowheads).

Reticulocyte maturation in cats also may be viewed as a continuum (Figure 1.22). Aggregate reticulocytes mature to the punctate form in approximately 12 hours; the punctate cells may continue to mature for another 10–12 days. Because of the short maturation time of aggregate reticulocytes, these cells are the best indicator of active marrow release. Therefore, only aggregate cells are counted in cats, and interpretive guidelines apply to this cell type only. Experience is required to exclude punctate cells when performing the reticulocyte count.

Organization of the complete blood count (hemogram)

It is useful to summarize the described basic and advanced determinations in a way that shows the organization of how they are performed and interpreted. This provides a mental framework for simplifying the complexity of this information into an everyday, intuitive tool: the hemogram. The techniques for generating data may be organized conceptually as

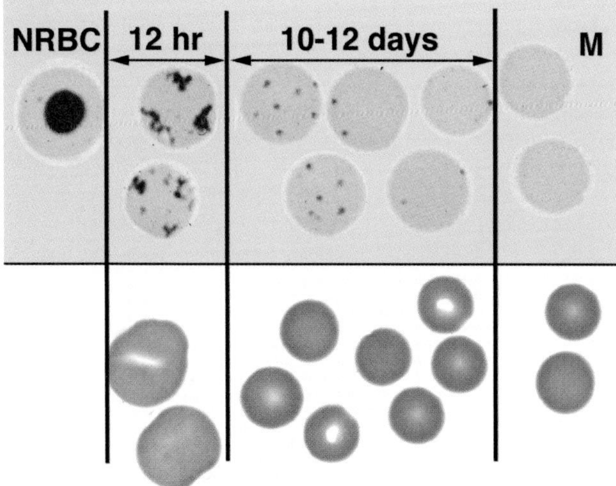

Figure 1.22 Feline reticulocyte maturation, progressing from left to right. Top. Cells stained with new methylene blue. After denucleation of the metarubricyte (NRBC), an aggregate reticulocyte is formed. This cell matures to the punctate form in approximately 12 hours. The punctate forms continue to mature by slow loss of punctate granules during a 10–12-day period. Mature cells (M) on the right have no granularity. Bottom. Corresponding cells stained with Wright-Giemsa stain. Note that polychromatophilic cells correspond to aggregate reticulocytes. Punctate and mature cells are indistinguishable with Wright-Giemsa stain.

direct measurements, microscopic procedures, and calculations. The CBC may include:

Direct measurements:

- Packed cell volume (by microhematocrit centrifugation).
- Hemoglobin concentration.
- Red cell concentration (RBC).
- Mean cell volume (MCV).
- White cell concentration.
- Plasma proteins (by refractometer).
- Platelet concentration.
- Mean platelet volume (MPV).

Microscopic procedures:

- Differential white cell count.
- Red cell morphology.
- Platelet morphology and assessment of adequacy.
- Microscopic reticulocyte enumeration in patients with anemia.

Calculations:

- Hematocrit, when instrument derived.
- Erythrocyte indices (e.g., MCHC, MCH, and RDW).
- Absolute white blood cell differential values.
- Absolute reticulocyte count.

These determinations are organized into a report form that aids the clinician in efficiently interpreting the information. The best way for this information to be organized is into banks of data that relate to the three major cell lines (i.e., erythrocytes, leukocytes, and platelets). For each cell line, all pieces of relevant information are organized in one place on the form.

Laboratory tests useful in the diagnosis of immune-mediated hemolytic anemia

Coombs or antiglobulin test

The Coombs or antiglobulin test is used as an aid in establishing the diagnosis of immune-mediated hemolytic anemia by detecting species-specific immunoglobulin that is adsorbed or attached to the surface of erythrocytes. The test uses the Coombs reagent, which is a polyclonal serum (usually prepared in rabbits) to the immunoglobulins of the species of interest. Some reagent manufacturers claim their reagent also detects complement. The procedure involves washing the erythrocytes in saline to remove plasma proteins and immunoglobulin that may be nonspecifically associated with erythrocytes. An aliquot of washed cells then is incubated with the Coombs serum. If appreciable patient immunoglobulin is attached to the erythrocytes, the Coombs serum induces erythrocyte agglutination. By means of two binding sites per molecule, the Coombs reagent immunoglobulin binds the patient immunoglobulin attached to the erythrocytes. The two binding sites result in progressive bridging of erythrocytes, which is visualized as agglutination. The absence of agglutination is interpreted as being a negative result, whereas the presence of agglutination is interpreted as being a positive result. Appropriate controls are performed as well.

False-negative reactions are a common problem with the Coombs test, likely because of the elution of pathologically adsorbed immunoglobulin or immune complexes during washing of the erythrocytes in preparation for the test. The best evidence for this is that prominent autoagglutination may disappear with washing. Autoagglutination, if confirmed microscopically, may be interpreted as being equivalent to a positive Coombs test. False-positive reactions also may occur, but are less well documented because the test is typically only performed when one suspects the disease.

Saline fragility test

Resistance of patient erythrocytes to hemolysis is measured in decreasing concentrations of saline. This test is not commonly used because of its complexity and labor intensity. It remains a useful diagnostic aid, however, in occasional cases of immune-mediated hemolytic anemia in which other hallmark pieces of information are not clearly interpretable. An equal aliquot of erythrocytes is added to a series of tubes containing decreasing concentrations of saline. After incubation, the tubes undergo centrifugation, and the hemoglobin concentration then is measured on the supernatant. A tube with distilled water serves as an index for 100% hemolysis. A plot of the percentage hemolysis and the concentration of saline facilitates interpretation, as shown in Figure 1.23.

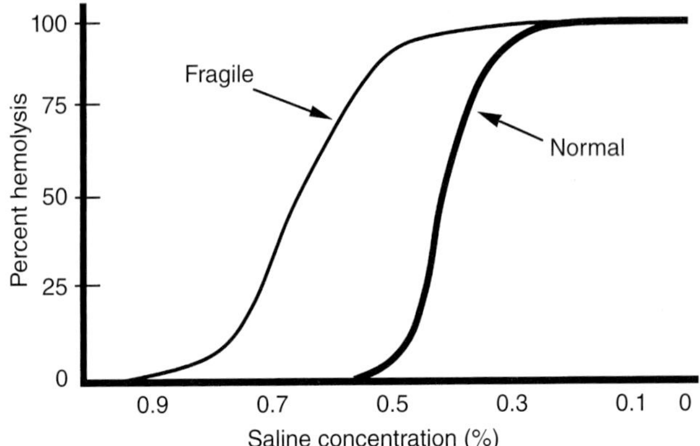

Figure 1.23 Erythrocyte fragility curve. Percentage hemolysis is plotted against decreasing saline concentration. Note the normal curve (arrow marked Normal). Increased erythrocyte fragility is recognized by a shift of the curve to the left (arrow marked Fragile).

These tests must not be used or interpreted in isolation. They are to be used in conjunction with analysis of other hematologic data and morphologic evaluation of the blood film by the laboratorian. Because of the frequency of false-negative and -positive results with the Coombs test, interpreting the results of this test in the light of the other available hematologic information is important. (See Chapter 9 for a detailed discussion of the strategy for diagnosing immune-mediated hemolytic anemia.)

Chemistry techniques

A wide variety of techniques, which have been incorporated into many different instrument designs, are used in veterinary clinical chemistry. No attempt is made here to discuss all of these techniques and instruments, but the basic information on a variety of chemistry techniques used in analyzing samples from animals is provided. A complete understanding of these techniques is not necessary for veterinarians who send clinical chemistry samples to a reference laboratory; however, an increasing number of chemistry instruments are being marketed to veterinarians for in-practice use. Therefore, an understanding of how these instruments work is important for understanding the advantages and disadvantages of the various instruments, the laboratory techniques necessary for their use, the problems that might arise during their use, and the basic principles underlying their variations in design.

The chemistry techniques discussed in this chapter and the substances that may be measured with them are listed in Table 1.1. Absorbance or reflectance photometry is used to measure most of the substances in clinical chemistry profiles. Fluorometry also is used to measure certain analytes in some clinical chemistry analyzers. Blood pH, partial pressures of carbon dioxide and oxygen, and concentrations of electrolytes such as sodium, potassium, and chloride most commonly are measured by electrochemical methods. Atomic absorption spectrophotometers are not commonly used in clinical chemistry laboratories; rather, they are more common in laboratories testing for elements considered nutrients and/or toxicants. Osmometers are common in clinical chemistry laboratories and are used to measure blood and urine osmolality or osmolarity. Protein electrophoresis is used to measure concentrations of the various protein fractions comprising the total serum protein, especially in samples with either decreased or increased protein concentrations. Light-scatter techniques that quantitate

Table 1.1 Techniques in veterinary clinical chemistry and substances measured with those techniques.

Technique	Substances measured
Photometry	
Absorbance photometry	Glucose, BUN, creatine, calcium, phosphorus, magnesium, protein, albumin, bilirubin, bile acids, ammonia, cholesterol, bicarbonate, total CO_2, enzymes
Reflectance photometry	Similar to those measured by absorbance photometry
Atomic absorption spectrophotometry	Many elements including nutrients and toxicants (e.g., calcium,[a] magnesium,[a] lead, arsenic)
Fluorometry	Glucose, bilirubin, bile acids, calcium, magnesium, enzymes, antithrombin III, heparin, plasminogen, hormones, drugs
Light-scatter techniques	
Turbidimetry	Immunoglobulins, antigen–antibody complexes, other large proteins, drugs
Nephalometry	Immunoglobulins, antigen–antibody complexes, other large proteins, drugs
Electrochemical methods	
Potentiometry	Blood pH, PCO_2, sodium,[b] potassium,[b] chloride[b]
Amperometry	PO_2
Coulometry and conductometry[c]	BUN
Osmometry	Osmolality or osmolarity
Protein electrophoresis	Albumin, α-globulin, β-globulin, γ-globulin

BUN, blood urea nitrogen.
[a]May be used to measure the concentration of these substances in solid tissues that have been ashed or digested. Absorbance photometry is more commonly used to measure concentrations of these substances in serum or plasma.
[b]Electrodes used to measure concentrations of these electrolytes are called ion-selective electrodes.
[c]Conductometry also is used to perform cell counts in some hematology analyzers.

turbidity are used less commonly to measure the concentrations of substances such as large protein molecules.

Photometry

Photometry is a general term used to describe an analytical chemistry technique in which the concentrations of substances and the activities of enzymes are determined by measuring the intensity of light passing through or emitted from a test chamber. This test chamber contains the substance to be detected and, in most cases, reagents intended to react with that substance to produce a color reaction. Strictly speaking, the term spectrophotometry should be applied when the instrument being used has the ability to produce light of a variety of wavelengths through some type of light-fractionating device, such as filters, prisms, or diffraction gratings.

Absorbance spectrophotometry

Absorbance spectrophotometry is an analytic technique in which concentrations of substances are determined by directing a beam of light through a solution containing the substance to be detected (or a product of that substance) and then measuring the amount of light that either of these absorb. The principles described here are incorporated into automated and semiautomated processes on today's chemistry analyzers. Automation, from sample and reagent addition management to calculation of test results to generation of a patient diagnostic report, is made possible by computer control and information processing integral to these systems.

To understand absorbance spectrophotometry, some basic knowledge regarding light is necessary. Typically, light is classified by its wavelength, which is measured in nanometers (nm). Light with the shortest wavelengths (<380 nm) is termed ultraviolet (UV) light (Table 1.2). Light in the visible spectrum has wavelengths of 380–750 nm. Light with the longest wavelengths (>750–2000 nm) is termed infrared (IR) light. The energy of light is inversely proportional to its wavelength; therefore, UV light has the highest energy and IR light the lowest.

Table 1.2 Wavelengths resulting in ultraviolet light, various colors of visible light, and infrared light.

Wavelength (nm)	Color
<380	None (ultraviolet)
380–440	Violet
440–500	Blue
500–580	Green
580–600	Yellow
600–620	Orange
620–750	Red
750–2000	None (infrared)

The visible spectrum includes a variety of wavelengths that represent the colors with which we are familiar. It is important to remember that color results from the transmittance or reflectance of light. In other words, a green object is that color because it reflects the green area of the visible spectrum and has absorbed the other wavelengths of light in that spectrum. Likewise, a green solution is green because it allows light in the green area of the visible spectrum to be transmitted through it and has absorbed the visible light of other wavelengths. These same principles also apply to light outside the visible spectrum. Different substances absorb and reflect different wavelengths in a pattern that is typical for that substance. The pattern in which a substance absorbs light at various wavelengths is known as its absorption spectrum, and each substance has its own unique absorption spectrum.

A basic absorbance spectrophotometer is diagrammed in Figure 1.24. Various sources of light can be used, with the choice being based on the portion of the spectrum desired plus issues such as longevity of the bulb and the basic instrument design. In the application of absorbance spectrophotometry for measuring the concentration of a substance, a wavelength of light that is absorbed by that substance (or by a product of that substance) is used. This wavelength is determined by examining the absorption spectrum of the substance of interest. Usually, the wavelength chosen is the one at which the maximum absorbance occurs. Occasionally, however, some other wavelength may be chosen to avoid interference with substances such as hemoglobin and bilirubin, which may be present in serum samples secondary to hemolysis (*in vitro* or *in vivo*) or disease leading to high bilirubin concentration. Hemoglobin and bilirubin have their own absorption spectrums, and methods attempt to avoid using the wavelengths that these substances strongly absorb.

A monochromator is an optical device between the light source and the measuring cuvette. It will narrow the spectrum of light that passes to and through the cuvette. Monochromators can be filters, prisms, or diffraction gratings. When attempting to produce light of a specific wavelength, the actual range of wavelengths produced by a monochromator is called the spectral bandwidth. Each type of monochromator can produce rays of light at certain spectral bandwidths. Monochromators capable of producing light of a narrow spectral bandwidth have more spectral purity. The importance of spectral purity varies with the type of spectrophotometry, however, and with the substance being analyzed. Filters may be a thin layer of colored glass that transmits light at wavelengths corresponding to the filter's color, or they may be more complex structures, with a layer of dielectric material sandwiched between two pieces of glass coated with a thin layer of silver. The latter type of

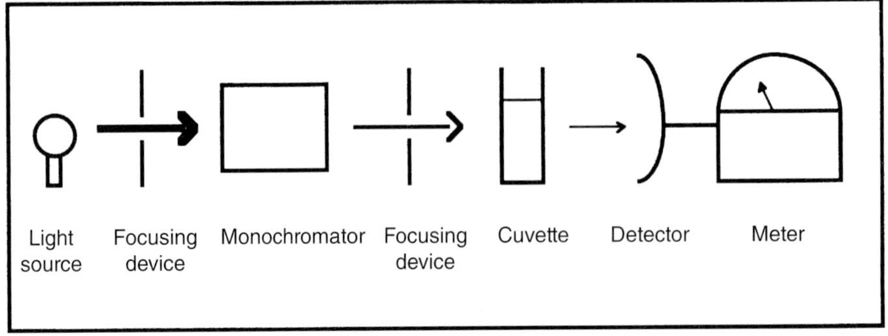

Figure 1.24 Components of a simple absorbance spectrophotometer. Arrows represent light.

filter transmits light at wavelengths equal to or at multiples of the thickness of the dielectric layer. In some cases, multiple filters may be placed in series to produce light of greater spectral purity. Prisms separate the wavelengths of white light by refracting this light. As light passes through a prism, shorter wavelengths are bent more than longer wavelengths, thus separating them. The desired wavelength then can be selected from this spectrum for transmission. Diffraction gratings are a metal or glass plate covered with a layer of metal alloy into which multiple parallel grooves have been etched. When the grating is illuminated, each groove separates the light into a spectrum, and light of specific wavelengths is produced as wavelengths that are in phase are reinforced and those that are not in phase are canceled.

The focusing devices usually are lenses or slits that are inserted before and/or after the monochromator. This placement varies with the instrument. Focusing devices are used to narrow the light beam, to produce parallel light rays, and/or to regulate the intensity of the light reaching the photodetector. In some modern instruments, application of fiber optics has eliminated some of the lens and slits used for narrowing and directing the light beams.

Cuvettes are also known as absorption cells. They have constant dimensions for a given instrument, and they can be made of various materials (e.g., glass, quartz, or plastic) and be of various shapes (e.g., round, square, or rectangular). The materials or shapes used depend on the instrument design and on the portion of the light spectrum being used. During analysis, a solution containing the absorbing substance is placed in the cuvette, and the light rays that have been produced pass through the cuvette walls and the solution. If the correct wavelength has been chosen, the substance absorbs this light in direct proportion to its concentration. In addition to the absorbing substance, the cuvette walls and the solution in which the substance is suspended also absorb small amounts of light. It is, therefore, necessary to "zero" spectrophotometers in order to eliminate the effect of these other factors, and this typically is accomplished by taking an absorbance reading on a cuvette containing only the solution in which the substance is suspended (i.e., the solution contains none of the absorbing substance). The absorbance reading of the instrument typically is set to zero while reading the absorbance of this "blank." Some spectrophotometers are designed to read the absorbance of the test solution and the blank solution simultaneously, which requires splitting the light beam and then shining each beam through either the test or the blank cuvette.

Photodetectors collect the light that has passed through the cuvette (i.e., the light that has not been absorbed). Several different technologies can be used in photodetectors. Factors such as cost, sensitivity, speed of response to changes in light intensity, propensity to fatigue (i.e., decreased response over time despite constant light intensity), and heat sensitivity help to determine which technology is used in a given application. Regardless of the type of photodetector, the underlying mechanism involves the production of electrons and, therefore, an electrical current in response to light striking the detector. This electrical current then is transmitted to a readout device or meter.

Readout devices or meters measure the electrical current produced by the photodetector. This current can be read out directly, but more commonly, this information is converted to a readout that gives either the absorbance or the actual concentration of the substance being measured. This conversion usually requires some type of microprocessor, which can store and use calibration information (discussed later) and also automatically adjust for the reading of the blank sample. The actual readout might be presented as some type of digital display, but it more commonly is printed.

Modern readout devices also incorporate recorders for obtaining multiple absorbance readings on the same sample over time. This is most useful in kinetic assays. In such assays, a reaction is allowed to occur over a period of time, and the production or disappearance of the absorbing substance is evaluated at multiple time points by measuring the absorbance of light normally absorbed by that substance. The change in absorbance over the time period is proportional to the activity of an enzyme or to the concentration of a substance, depending on which is being assayed. Such an assay obviously requires a device that can record and use data produced over time.

In addition to the basic instrumentation of absorbance spectrophotometry, the basic physical chemistry principles used in obtaining measurements via this technology also should be understood. When a light beam of a certain wavelength is projected through a solution containing a substance that absorbs light at that wavelength, the light is absorbed in direct proportion to the concentration of that substance. The intensity of the light leaving the solution, therefore, is less than the intensity of the light entering the solution. If these two intensities are known, the percentage transmittance of light (%T) can be calculated. For instance, if the intensity of light entering the cuvette is designated as I_1 and the intensity of light leaving the cuvette as I_2, then %T is calculated as

$$\%T = \frac{I_2}{I_1}$$

The intensity of light entering the cuvette is measured by projecting light of the appropriate wavelength through a cuvette containing the solution in which the substance to be measured is suspended. In this case, however, the solution contains none of the substance. Therefore, %T is set at 100% for this "blank" solution. The solution containing the substance to be measured is then placed in a similar cuvette, and the light is intensity measured, after which the %T can be assessed.

In the described situation, transmittance varies inversely and logarithmically with the concentration of the substance being measured. If %T versus the concentration of such a substance is plotted, a curved line results (Figure 1.25). Light that is not transmitted is absorbed; therefore, transmittance and absorbance are inversely related, as described by the formula

$$\text{Absorbance} = 2 - \log \%T$$

Because of this relationship, absorbance of light increases linearly with increasing concentration of the substance being measured (Figure 1.25). This linear relationship between absorbance and concentration makes it more convenient to deal with absorbance than with transmittance during spectrophotometric analysis. Modern spectrophotometers measure transmittance but then convert transmittance to absorbance. In addition, microprocessors in most spectrophotometers convert absorbance results to concentrations or activities and then report these in a final diagnostic test result format.

The concentration of a substance can be calculated from the absorbance by use of Beer's law:

$$A = abc$$

where A is the absorbance measured, a is the molar absorptivity (also known as the proportionality constant), b is the light path in centimeters (the diameter or width of the cuvette through which the light passes), and c is the concentration of the substance in question. The concentration (c) then can be calculated as

$$\text{Concentration} = \frac{A}{ab}$$

For Beer's law to apply, a linear relationship must exist between concentration and absorbance. In some cases, this might be true only up to certain concentrations or absorbance levels. To assure that Beer's law applies to a given assay, calibration solutions (also known as calibrators), which contain known concentrations of the substance to be measured, are used. The ranges of concentrations used as calibrators should include those that might be measured in samples from patients. Absorbance results for each calibrator are plotted against the concentrations of these calibrators to establish a calibration curve. Ideally, this curve is a straight line rather than an actual curve, showing that a linear relationship exists between absorbance and concentration (Figure 1.26). In most applications, one or more calibrators are included with each series of sample measurements. It is

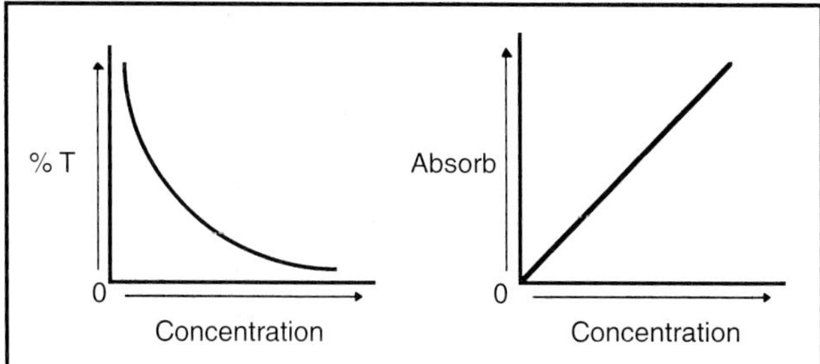

Figure 1.25 The relationships between percentage transmittance (%T), absorbance (Absorb), and concentration of a substance being measured. Note that as the concentration increases, %T decreases logarithmically or nonlinearly and absorbance increases linearly.

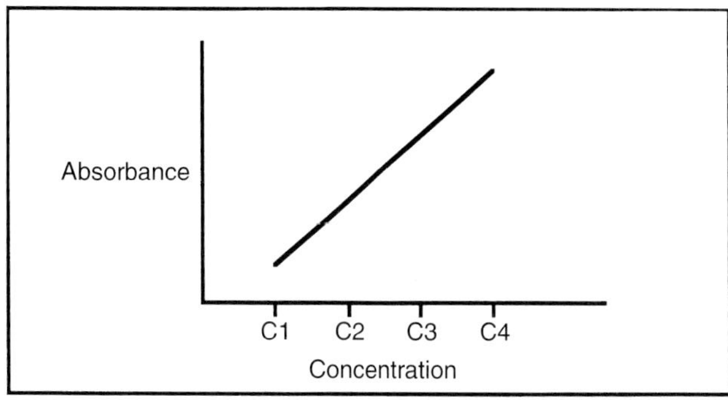

Figure 1.26 Use of calibrators to establish a calibration curve. In this case, four calibrators (C1, C2, C3, C4) were used. Note the linear relationship between concentration of the substance being measured and resulting absorbance.

best, however, to reestablish the calibration curve at frequent intervals (at least daily), because many slight day-to-day changes in the conditions of the test can affect this curve. These changes (e.g., light intensity, temperature, condition of reagents) can occur even in situations when instruments and reagents have been designed to minimize such variation. If a linear relationship does exist between the concentrations of the calibrators and the resulting absorbances, the solutions are said to obey Beer's law, and the calibrators can be used to establish a calibration constant (K):

$$K = \frac{\text{Concentration of the calibration solution}}{\text{Absorbance of the calibration solution}}$$

If K is known, then the concentration of an unknown solution can be calculated as

$$\text{Concentration of unknown} = (\text{Absorbance of unknown}) \times K$$

Microprocessors in instruments can plot absorbance results from calibrators, assure that a linear relationship exists, and calculate the calibration constant. These results are stored, and the concentrations of unknowns are calculated by measuring their absorbances and calibration constant.

A linear relationship between concentration and absorbance over the possible range of unknown concentrations is highly desirable, but a nonlinear calibration curve also can be used to derive unknown concentrations. In such a case, enough calibrators must be used to define the shape of the calibration curve, and as with a linear calibration curve, the range of calibrator concentrations should include the possible range of concentrations that might be found in samples from patients.

In absorbance spectrophotometry, two types of assay methods – endpoint or kinetic – may be used. In both types, the same principles of spectrophotometry described earlier apply. Endpoint assays usually are applied when measuring the concentration of some preexisting substance in serum or plasma. In such an assay, reagent(s) is added to a quantity of serum, and a chemical reaction occurs. The product resulting from this reaction then is measured by spectrophotometry. In other words, the solution in which the reaction has occurred is placed in a cuvette (or the reaction itself might have occurred in the cuvette), a light beam of a wavelength absorbed by the product is projected through a cuvette, and the absorbance is measured. By using a calibration curve and/or a calibration constant, the concentration of the substance being measured then is calculated. An example of an endpoint assay is a method for measuring the concentration of serum calcium:

$$\text{calcium} + \text{o-cresolphthalein complexone} \rightarrow \text{calcium–cresolphthalein complexone}$$

In this assay, the substance of interest (i.e., calcium) is complexed with cresolphthalein complex one, which has a purple color and absorbs light at a wavelength of 570 nm. This reaction is allowed to occur long enough to allow nearly all of the calcium in the sample to be complexed. More calcium–cresolphthalein complex one results in more light being absorbed and a higher concentration of calcium reported by the instrument. After the absorbance is determined, it is compared with the absorbance of a calibration solution, and the absorbance of the unknown then is calculated as

$$\text{Concentration of the unknown} = \text{Absorbance of the unknown} \times \frac{\text{Concentration of the calibration solution}}{\text{Absorbance of the calibration solution}}$$

Note that the second portion of this formula is the calibration constant (K).

Kinetic assays typically have been used to measure enzyme activities but also have been adapted to measure the concentrations of many analytes in blood. Typically, enzyme concentrations are not measured directly in clinical chemistry. Rather, the amount of enzyme in the serum usually is gauged indirectly, by the activity of that enzyme. Enzymes are proteins that catalyze (i.e., speed-up) chemical reactions, with the result that substrate is converted to product more quickly:

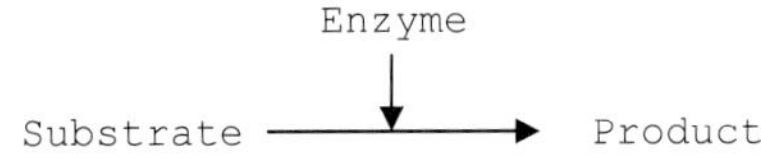

To measure an enzyme's activity, the rate at which it converts a substrate to a product must be assessed. The more quickly conversion occurs, the higher the enzyme activity is assumed to be. To measure the rate of conversion from substrate to product, the rate at which the product is being produced must be assessed, and this requires multiple measurements of the product concentration over time. Because this type of assay is a dynamic process, it is termed a kinetic assay. In a kinetic assay of enzyme activity, a solution containing the substrate of the enzyme of interest is added to the sample serum in a cuvette that already is in a spectrophotometer. When enzyme in this serum begins to convert substrate to product, absorbance is measured periodically by the same methods and using the same principles of spectrophotometry described previously (i.e., using a light beam of a wavelength absorbed by the product). In this process, the conversion rate of substrate to product is monitored. This rate can be converted to enzyme activity by using a formula involving the rate of absorbance change and several constants related to the absorptivity of the product as well as to test characteristics such as sample volume, total sample volume, and light path.

An example of a kinetic enzyme assay is an assay of alanine aminotransferase (ALT) activity:

$$\alpha\text{-Ketogluterate} + \text{L-alanine} \xrightarrow{\text{ALT}} \text{L-Glutamate} + \text{Pyruvate}$$

$$\text{Pyruvate} + \text{NADH} + \text{H}^+ \xrightarrow{\text{LDH}} \text{L-Lactate} + \text{NAD}^+$$

where LDH is lactate dehydrogenase. In this assay, NADH is converted to NAD^+ at a rate proportional to the activity of ALT in the sample. The NADH absorbs light at 340 nm, and its rate of disappearance is measured by periodically assessing the absorbance of the reaction mixture. The rate of absorbance change in this mixture can be converted to units of ALT activity.

As previously noted, kinetic assays also are used for measuring the concentrations of preexisting substances in the blood. In these assays, the rate of appearance or disappearance of an absorbing substance is monitored by periodically measuring the absorbance of the reaction mixture. An example of a kinetic assay for measuring the concentration of a preexisting substance is an assay of the blood urea nitrogen (BUN) concentration, which uses the chemical reaction

$$\text{Urea} + H_2O + 2H^+ \xrightarrow{\text{Urease}} CO_2 + 2\,NH_4^+$$

$$NH_4^+ + \alpha\text{-Ketogluterate} + \text{NADH} \xrightarrow{\text{GLDH}} \text{L-Glutamate} + \text{NAD}^+ + H_2O$$

where GLDH is glutamate dehydrogenase. In this reaction, the disappearance rate of NADH is monitored by periodically assessing the absorbance of the reaction mixture at a wavelength of 340 nm. The disappearance rate is proportional to the urea nitrogen concentration in the serum being tested. The BUN concentration is calculated by relating the rate of change in the absorbance of the sample with that of a calibrator.

Enzyme activity also can be measured by endpoint methods, which involve mixing serum with reagent containing substrate for the enzyme and then allowing the conversion of substrate to product to proceed for a specific period of time. At the end of that period, the concentration of substrate or product is measured. The more substrate used or product produced during the time period, the higher the enzyme activity is assumed to be.

Reflectance photometry

The principle of reflectance photometry is used in a few large, automated clinical chemistry analyzers and in several of the smaller clinical chemistry analyzers designed for in-practice use. Most of these instruments use "dry chemistry" systems, in which the fluid to be analyzed is placed on a carrier that contains the reagents for the assay. This carrier can take different forms, including a dry fiber pad or a multilayer of film. After the sample is applied, the chemical reaction occurs in this carrier, and a product is formed in a concentration proportional to that of the substance being measured. The carrier then is illuminated with diffused light, and the intensity of the light reflected from the carrier is measured and compared with that of either the original illuminating light or the intensity of light reflected off a reference surface. Reflectance photometry, therefore, is analogous to absorbance photometry in that the chemical reaction occurring in the carrier results in a product that absorbs a portion of the illuminating light. The remaining light is reflected, analogous to transmittance in absorbance spectrophotometry, to a photodetector that measures its intensity. The intensity of the reflected light is not related linearly to the concentration of the substance being produced. As a result, formulas are required to convert the reflectance results to concentrations. These formulas vary with the type of instrument being used.

Atomic absorption spectrophotometry

Atomic absorption spectrophotometry (AA) is used for measuring the concentrations of many elements. Advantages of AA include its superior sensitivity (i.e., it can detect smaller concentrations) and its ability to measure the concentrations of various elements. AA is typically limited to toxicology laboratories for clinical purposes. Applications include measurement of concentrations of elements such as lead, copper, and selenium in fluids or tissues. As the name implies, AA involves measuring absorption of energy by atoms. This technique involves heating a sample in a flame that is hot enough to cause the element in question to dissociate from its chemical bonds and form neutral atoms – but not hot enough to cause large numbers of electrons to jump to the excited state. These atoms then are in a low-energy (i.e., ground) state and can absorb light of a narrow wavelength that is specific for that element. If a light of this wavelength is projected through the flame, the amount of light absorbed is proportional to the concentration of the element in the sample. Measurement of the amount of light absorbed, therefore, allows the concentration of that element in the sample to be calculated. Focusing devices, photodetectors, meters, and readout devices serve the same purposes in AA as in other types of spectrophotometry.

Fluorometry

Fluorometric techniques can be used in a wide variety of applications, ranging from measurement of the concentrations of substances to assessment of the numbers and other characteristics of larger particles, including cells. This section discusses use of these techniques in measuring concentrations of various substances in body fluids.

Among the substances that can be measured by these techniques are some that commonly are measured in clinical chemistry analysis (e.g., bilirubin, bile acids, glucose, calcium, magnesium, and various enzymes), substances related to coagulation (e.g., antithrombin III, heparin, and plasminogen), drugs, and hormones. Some of these substances are fluorescent; in other cases, measurement of these substances is possible by linking other fluorescent substances to the analyte of interest, either directly or indirectly, as the result of a series of chemical reactions.

The basic principle underlying use of fluorometry is that certain substances, when exposed to light of the proper wavelength, will fluoresce. Fluorescence results when a substance absorbs light at one wavelength and then emits light at a longer (i.e., lower energy) wavelength. The ability to fluoresce varies with a compound's chemical structure; therefore, not all compounds can be readily measured by fluorometry.

The basic design of a fluorometer is shown in Figure 1.27. A variety of light sources, including various types of bulbs and lasers, can be used. Most fluorescent compounds absorb light at 300–550 nm; therefore, light sources must produce light at these wavelengths. The primary monochromator isolates light at the proper wavelength to produce fluorescence in the substance being analyzed. Each compound can best be caused to fluoresce at specific wavelengths, and these wavelengths are known as the apparent excitation spectrum of the compound. Of these wavelengths, a narrow band at which peak fluorescence is caused usually is chosen to be isolated by the primary monochromator and, from there, transmitted to the cuvette. When light strikes the solution in the cuvette, it produces fluorescence in the substance being measured. The detector of this fluorescent energy usually is placed at a 90° angle from the projected (i.e., the exciting) light beam. This placement means that light from the exciting light beam continues straight through the cuvette and does not need to be dealt with by the secondary monochromator or the detector. Because fluorescent energy is projected in all directions, this energy can be measured at 90° without measuring the energy from the exciting light beam. Some fluorometers incorporated into absorbance spectrophotometers measure fluorescence directly in the path of exciting light (i.e., an end-on design), because this is the typical light path for absorbance spectrophotometers. In such cases, mechanisms must be incorporated to exclude excitation light that has passed through the cuvette.

The secondary monochromator excludes light from sources other than the fluorescence itself and allows only a narrow band of wavelengths to pass to the photodetector. Just as each fluorescent compound has an apparent excitation spectrum of light in which optimum fluorescence occurs, each compound also has an emission spectrum, which is the spectrum of wavelengths in which most of the emitted fluorescent energy from that compound is found. To develop a fluorescent assay, the emission spectrum of the compound of interest must be determined. Then, the narrow band of wavelengths in which maximum emission occurs is isolated by the secondary monochromator. Light passing from the monochromator is collected by a photodetector, measured, and processed in a manner similar to that described for spectrophotometry. Various lenses, slits, and, in some cases, polarizing devices are included in fluorometers

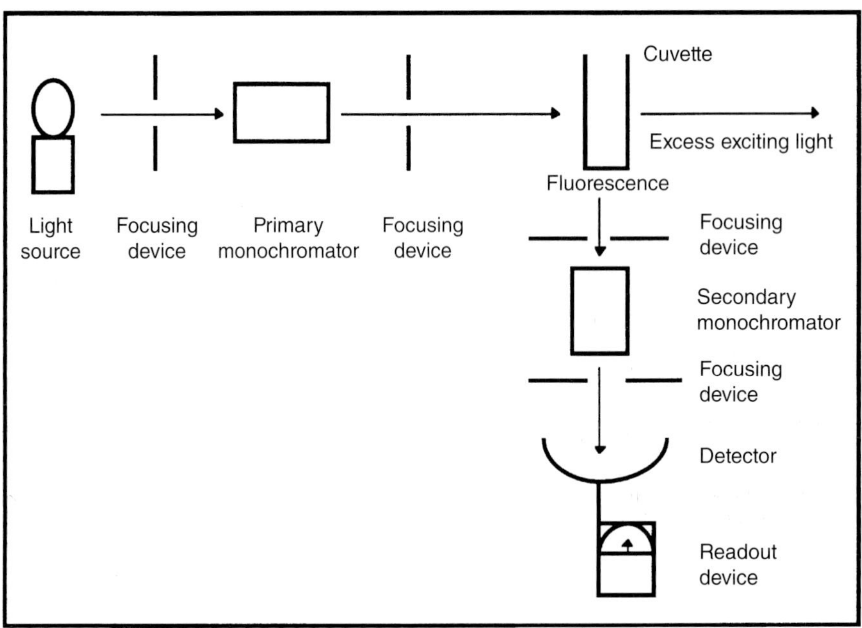

Figure 1.27 The basic design of a fluorometer. Arrows represent light.

to help direct and/or polarize light as well as to reduce stray light in the system.

A wide variety of fluorometer designs are available. Strictly speaking, fluorometers are instruments that can produce light at only a few wavelengths, because their primary monochromator is a filter. Many instruments that use fluorometry have primary monochromators that are diffraction gratings or prisms. These instruments can produce a spectrum of excitation wavelengths and are known as spectrofluorometers. Some fluorometers are designed to compensate for variations in the intensity of the light source and, therefore, decrease the frequency with which calibration is required. Fluorometers also might use a pulsed light source and measure fluorescence only during those periods of time when the source is off. This technique, which is known as time-resolved fluorometry, eliminates the effects of light scatter.

Interference by other molecules is a potential problem when biologic fluids are being analyzed by fluorometry. Some of these molecules fluoresce (e.g., bilirubin and some proteins), whereas others scatter light (e.g., proteins and lipids). When developing assays on biologic fluids, adjustments must be made to minimize the effects of these molecules.

Although the mechanism of measuring concentrations is different, the basic procedure for performing fluorometry is similar to that for absorbance spectrophotometry. Calibrators are used to establish a calibration curve, and blanks are used to negate any effects other than those attributable to the substance of interest. At low concentrations of fluorescing substances (e.g., resulting in an absorbance of <2% of the exciting light), a direct, linear relationship usually exists between fluorescence and concentration. If the concentration of the fluorescing substance is high (e.g., >2% of the exciting light is absorbed), the relationship between fluorescence and concentration might be nonlinear.

Light-scatter techniques

Light-scatter techniques can be used to measure the concentrations of larger molecules in fluids. When light is projected through solutions containing large molecules such as immunoglobulins and other large proteins, antigen–antibody complexes, and some drugs, these molecules cause light to scatter in all directions. These techniques, therefore, are potentially useful in measuring the concentrations of these substances. With light scattering, the wavelength of the light being scattered is the same as that of the light being projected into the solution. By assessing the degree of light scattering, the concentration of the substance of interest can be measured. Two techniques, turbidimetry and nephelometry, use the principles of light scattering to make such measurements.

In turbidimetry, the decreased intensity of a light beam passing through a turbid solution is measured. The intensity of light decreases, because a portion of it has been scattered by the large molecules of interest. A basic turbidimeter is diagrammed in Figure 1.28. In a turbidimeter, light rays are projected through a cuvette containing the analyte in solution, and the intensity of light leaving the solution (i.e., the transmitted light) is measured in a straight line from the transmitted light. The decrease in transmitted light intensity is proportional to the concentration of the analyte. A turbidimeter, therefore, is similar in principle to an absorbance spectrophotometer.

In nephelometry, a beam of light also is projected through a solution containing the analyte, but the photodetector is placed at a 90° angle to the cuvette (Figure 1.29). In addition, scattered rather than transmitted light is measured. The intensity of the scattered light is proportional to the concentration of the analyte. Nephelometry, therefore, is analogous to fluorometry in terms of configuration of the light path. If a solution is not visibly turbid, nephelometry is a somewhat better technique than turbidimetry.

A direct relationship exists between the concentrations of light-scattering molecules and the degree of light scattering. A direct relationship also exists between the sizes of the light-scattering molecules and the degree of light scattering. When developing light-scatter techniques, the size of the particles being measured must be considered, because larger particles (e.g., immunoglobulin M, chylomicrons,

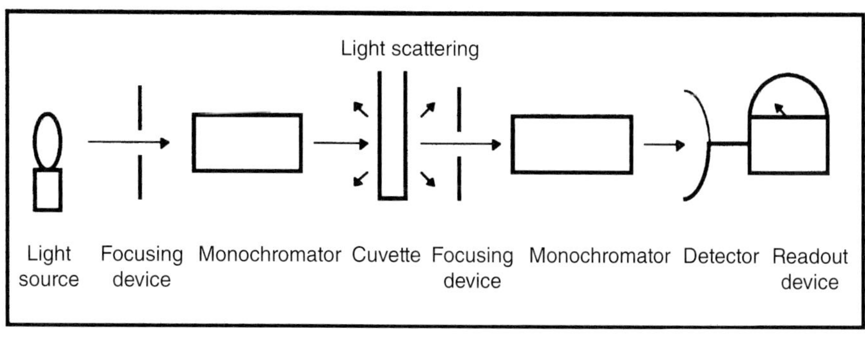

Figure 1.28 A basic turbidimeter. Arrows represent light.

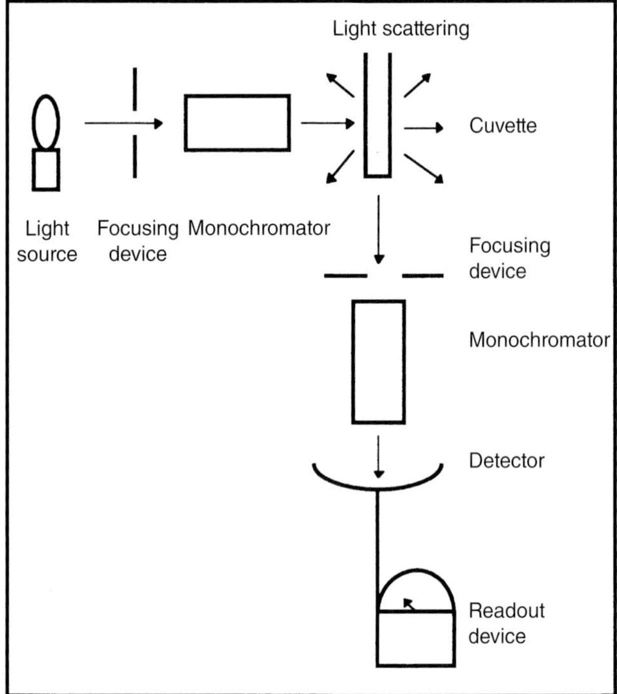

Figure 1.29 A basic nephalometer. Arrows represent light.

and antigen–antibody complexes) cause an asymmetric distribution of scattered light. In some cases, the position of the photodetector must be altered to adjust for this. Large molecules or particles other than those of interest can interfere with light-scatter techniques as well.

With light-scatter techniques, the analytic procedures are similar to those of absorbance spectrophotometry. Calibrators are used to establish a calibration curve, and blanks are used to negate the effects of reagents and other light-scattering molecules.

Electrochemical techniques

A variety of electrochemical techniques are used in clinical chemistry and most often are applied in measurements of electrolytes and acid-base status. This includes electrolytes such as sodium (Na^+), potassium (K^+), chloride (Cl^-), ionized calcium (Ca^{+2}), pH (H^+), and partial pressures of oxygen (pO_2) and carbon dioxide (pCO_2) in whole blood. These techniques also can be used to measure other substances if the chemical reactions used in the assay system result in production or consumption of an ion. For example, such reactions exist for determination of glucose, urea, and creatinine concentrations. Basic electrochemical techniques and examples of some of their applications are described in this section. Electrochemical methods are applied through a wide variety of electrode and instrument configurations. In recent years, several electrochemical systems have had complexity, cost, and applications reduced to practice in point-of-care formats. These systems have rendered blood gas, electrolyte, and selected chemistry capability both affordable and practical in the typical veterinary facility. Some of these devices utilize microfabricated disposable cartridges in which these measurements are made on whole blood. Other systems use small volumes of blood injected into a port leading to sample flow-through fluidics within the analyzer. Regardless of design, these instrument systems typically combine potentiometry, amperometry, and conductometry to provide acid-base and electrolyte panels, as described below.

Potentiometry

Potentiometry is commonly used for measurement of pH (i.e., hydrogen ion concentration), partial pressures of carbon dioxide and oxygen, and concentrations of electrolytes in whole blood or serum. In potentiometry, the electrical potential between two electrodes is measured, thereby giving a value that can be used to calculate the concentrations of various electrolytes.

Potentiometry involves the development and measurement of the potential difference between two electrodes. This technique is used to measure electrolyte concentrations using ion-selective membrane electrodes, also known as ion-specific electrodes (ISEs). The technique is used to measure ion concentrations in whole blood, plasma, serum, and occasionally other body fluids. The ISE is the variable electrode sensor immersed in the sample of measurement interest; see Figure 1.30. The ISE has a barrier or membrane that isolates the internal electrode from the body fluid. Only the specific ion being measured is allowed to cross or interact

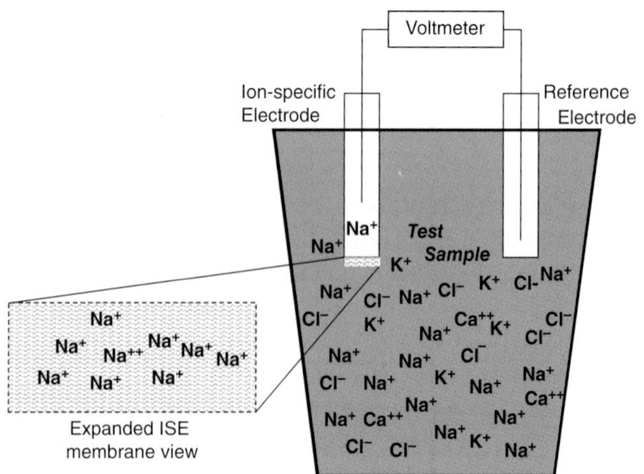

Figure 1.30 Schematic drawing of an ion-selective electrode (ISE) for potentiometric measurement; see text for further explanation. There is a reference electrode, chemically saturated to have fixed potential. The test sample contains differing concentrations of various ions. The ISE selectively allows movement of the ion of interest (e.g., Na^+) into or across the membrane, resulting in a potential difference between the two electrodes (expanded view). The potential difference is proportional to the concentration of specific analyte being measured.

with the barrier, leading to accumulation of charge on the internal electrode. At equilibrium, the potential in the ISE will vary depending on the concentration of ionic interaction with the sample. The second electrode is a reference electrode that has constant, fixed potential. The basic principle is that contact of the ion-selective membrane with the body fluid results in ion-selective passage or interaction with the ISE membrane leading to development of a potential difference from a reference electrode. A sensitive voltmeter is used to measure the potential difference when the ISE has come to equilibrium with the sample. The potential difference that develops is due to the activity of the ion being measured. The potential difference is used to calculate the concentration of ion in the sample. The ISE system is calibrated with solution containing known concentration of the ion of interest.

ISEs are the core technology in most or all modern blood gas and electrolyte analyzers, including those recommended for in-clinic applications. The design and materials used to manufacture these electrodes vary considerably. An important component of each electrode is a membrane that is selective for the ion that the electrode measures. The membrane may be composed of thin glass specially formulated to allow diffusion of a specific ion; glass is used in ISEs for pH and Na^+ measurement. A second type of membrane involves a water insoluble ion exchange chemistry coupled with a barrier membrane matrix. This type of electrode may be used to measure K^+, NH_4^+, and Ca^{2+}. There are also solid-state electrodes consisting of a single crystal of some ion-selective material or salt imbedded in an inert matrix membrane. This type of electrode is typically used to measure chloride (Cl^-).

The partial pressure of carbon dioxide (PCO_2) in the blood also is measured by potentiometry. This method is used in blood-gas analyzers. Whereas CO_2 is not an ion, the CO_2 electrode is designed to produce an ion in proportion to the PCO_2 in the blood. The design of such an electrode is shown in Figure 1.31 as a modified pH electrode. In this electrode, a chamber containing sodium bicarbonate solution is separated from the blood sample by a thin membrane. The CO_2 diffuses through the membrane into the sodium bicarbonate solution, and the following chemical reaction occurs:

$$CO_2 + H_2O \rightarrow H_2CO_3$$

$$H_2CO_3 \rightarrow H^+ + HCO_3^-$$

The amount of CO_2 that diffuses through the membrane affects the H^+ concentration in the sodium bicarbonate solution in direct proportion to the PCO_2. The remainder of this electrode is a pH electrode that senses the change in H^+ concentration of the sodium bicarbonate solution. These changes alter the electrical potential of this electrode, and the instrument then calculates the PCO_2 from these changes.

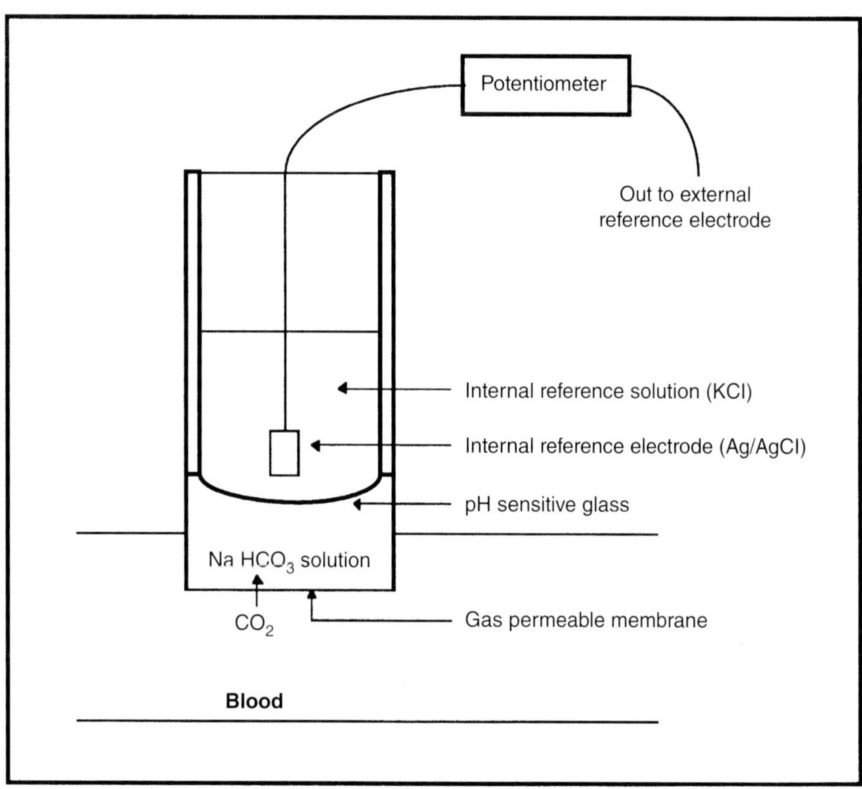

Figure 1.31 An electrode designed to measure the partial pressure of carbon dioxide in the blood.

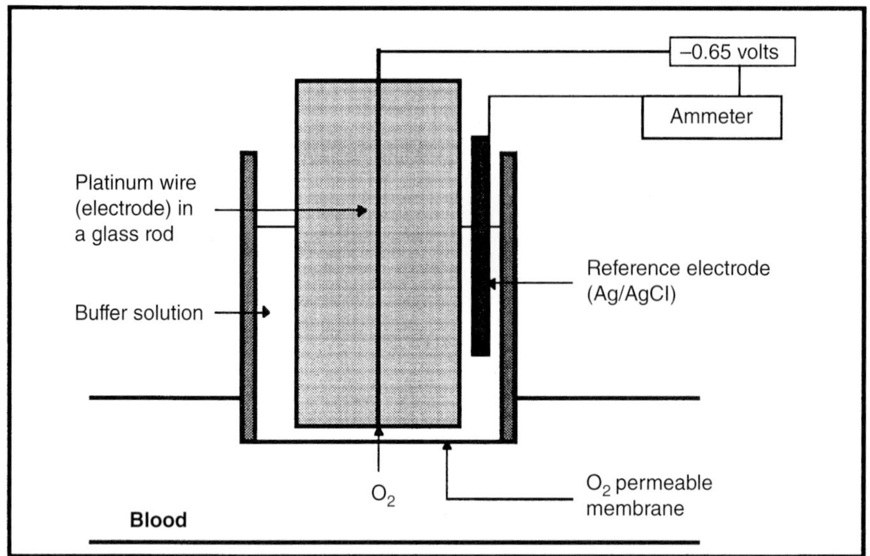

Figure 1.32 An electrochemical cell designed to measure the partial pressure of oxygen in the blood.

Amperometry

Amperometry is a technique that measures the electrical current passing between two electrodes in a chemical cell while a constant voltage is applied. This differentiates the technique from potentiometry, in which no electrical current flows and no voltage is applied. The most common application of amperometry in clinical chemistry is electrochemical measurement of the partial pressure of oxygen (PO_2) in blood.

The technique is most easily understood by considering how this electrochemical cell operates. A typical PO_2 electrode is diagrammed in Figure 1.32. An electrical potential of −0.65 V is applied to this electrode, and almost no current passes through this electrode if no oxygen is present. When this electrode is submersed in blood, O_2 from the blood diffuses through the O_2-permeable membrane and comes into contact with the tip of the platinum electrode. The O_2 then is reduced by the reaction:

$$O_2 + 2H_2O + 4\ \text{electrons} \rightarrow 4\ OH^-$$

This process consumes electrons and, therefore, produces an electrical current under these conditions. An ammeter is used to measure this current as amperage. The amount of current produced is proportional to the PO_2 of the blood. Calibration solutions are used to relate the amperage to the PO_2 of the unknown.

Coulometry and conductometry

Coulometry and conductometry are two other electrochemical methods that occasionally are used to measure the concentrations of substances. Coulometry involves measurement of the amount of electrical energy passing between two electrodes in an electrochemical cell. This electrical current is produced by chemical reactions occurring at the surfaces of each of two electrodes, resulting in the loss or gain of electrons by these electrodes. The amount of electrical current produced is directly proportional to the concentration of the substance being measured. This substance is consumed in an electron-using or electron-producing process. Unlike potentiometry, the actual current rather than the potential between two electrodes is measured, and unlike amperometry, no outside voltage is applied to the system. This method has been applied to the measurement of serum chloride concentrations.

Conductometry involves measurement of a fluid's ability to conduct an electrical current between two electrodes when a voltage is applied to the sample in the system. This property, which is known as electrolytic conductance, occurs via movement of ions in the fluid. The conductivity of an aqueous fluid depends on the concentration and ionic strength of the electrolytes in that fluid: the higher the electrolyte concentration, the higher the conductivity. Conductometry can be used to measure the production of ions by chemical reactions. Therefore, it is possible to measure the concentration of a substance in a fluid if it is used in a chemical reaction producing ions in numbers proportional to the substance of interest. The increased conductivity resulting from the production of these ions would then be proportional to the original concentration of the substance being measured. It is also possible to measure hematocrit by conductometry on some clinical systems. The plasma fraction readily conducts current while cellular mass acts as an insulator, impeding current. As the hematocrit increases, the ability of the sample to conduct current decreases. This measurement can be calibrated. The calculation factors in electrolyte concentrations simultaneously measured in the same sample.

Osmometry

Osmometry involves measurement of the concentrations of particles in a fluid. The clinical significance of these concentrations, which are reported as osmolality (particles per kilogram of solvent [osmol/kg]) or osmolarity (particles per liter of solvent [osmol/L]), is discussed in Chapter 25. To understand osmometry, the changes that occur in a solution when concentrations of particles (i.e., solute) dissolved in a fluid (i.e., solvent) increase must be understood. These changes, which are known as colligative properties, are increased osmotic pressure, decreased vapor pressure, increased boiling point (because of decreased vapor pressure), and decreased freezing point. Any of these colligative properties could be used to measure osmolality or osmolarity. Among those properties that actually are used to make these measurements are freezing-point depression and decreased vapor pressure.

The freezing-point depression technique is the most commonly used. As the name implies, this type of osmometer measures the freezing point of a solution through a number of steps involving freezing, thawing, and freezing again. This process is monitored by a thermistor, which measures temperature, and it determines the freezing point by determining the temperature at equilibrium between freezing and thawing. The osmolality or osmolarity of the fluid then is determined by comparing this temperature with those of various calibration fluids with known osmolality or osmolarity.

Vapor pressure osmometers are less commonly used. These instruments measure the osmolality or osmolarity of a fluid by determining the dew point (i.e., the temperature at the point of equilibrium between vaporization and condensation) of that fluid. The dew point is a gauge of vapor pressure: the higher the osmolality or osmolarity of a fluid, the lower its dew point. In general, vapor pressure osmometers are not considered to be as precise as freezing-point osmometers. In addition, volatile substances such as ethanol are not detected by vapor pressure osmometers, whereas they are detected by the freezing-point depression technique.

Protein electrophoresis

Electrophoresis is an analytic technique based on the movement of charged particles through a solution under the influence of an electrical field. In clinical chemistry, electrophoretic techniques most commonly are used to separate and analyze serum proteins. When serum is placed on or in a supporting substance that allows migration of these proteins and can carry an electrical charge, these proteins move through this material just as other charged particles do. The movement of proteins through such a substance depends on the net charge on the protein molecule, the size and shape of the protein molecule, the strength of the electrical field applied, the type of supporting medium, and the temperature. In a given electrophoresis application, the latter three items are held constant. Therefore, the migration of protein molecules depends on the net charge and on the size and shape of the molecules. As a result, different serum proteins migrate at different rates and, possibly, in different directions in the supporting substance.

A simple electrophoresis chamber is demonstrated in Figure 1.33. Small amounts of serum are placed in specific areas on the surface of the supporting substance or in small depressions cut at one end. Supporting substances commonly used include agarose gel and cellulose acetate. Starch gel is less commonly used in clinical applications. Polyacrylamide gel also can be used for protein electrophoresis and separates more serum protein fractions than the other supporting substances. Polyacrylamide electrophoresis does produce interesting information, but the clinical applications of this information in veterinary medicine are not understood. The common supporting substances usually are in the form of a sheet, and they either have buffer incorporated into them when they are produced or are soaked in buffer before use. The buffer determines the pH at which the

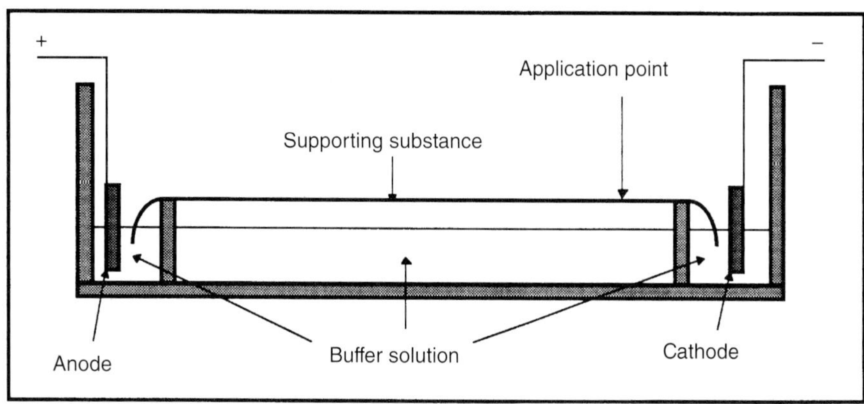

Figure 1.33 A simple electrophoresis chamber.

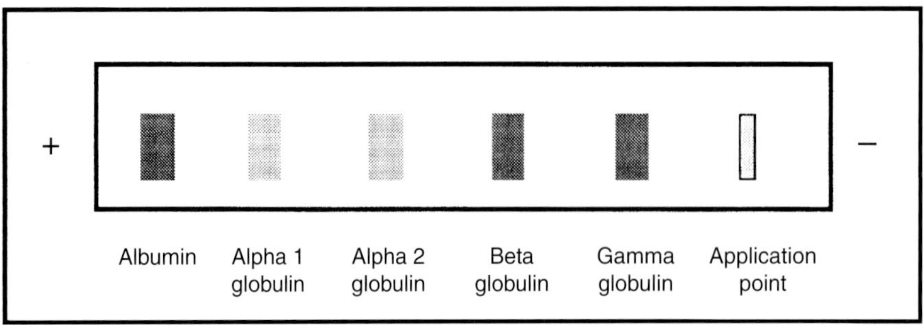

Figure 1.34 Typical electrophoretic separation of serum proteins in a sheet of supporting substance. The type and number of fractions actually separated depends on the type of electrophoresis application and on the species from which the serum was sampled.

process occurs, and the pH determines the type of charge as well as the net charge on each type of protein molecule. Both ends of the supporting substance are in contact with buffer solution in an adjacent well. These buffer solutions are not in contact with each other, however, or with the buffer solution in the center well. The electrical current is applied to the system by electrodes placed into each of these wells. A negatively charged cathode is placed in the well at one end, and a positively charged anode is placed in the well at the other end. The serum sample typically is applied at the end near the cathode, because most proteins are negatively charged and migrate toward the anode. When an electrical current is applied to this system, proteins migrate toward either the anode or the cathode, depending on whether they are negatively charged (i.e., toward the anode) or positively charged (i.e., toward the cathode). As noted, the rate of this migration depends on both the net charge of the molecule and its size and shape, and because these vary with the different types of proteins, different proteins migrate at different rates. If this migration is allowed to occur for a fixed period of time, various protein fractions are isolated along a straight line in the supporting substance.

A typical distribution of serum protein fractions in a sheet of supporting substance after electrophoretic separation is shown in Figure 1.34. Albumin is the smallest of the serum proteins and has the highest net negative charge relative to its size. Albumin, therefore, migrates faster than the other proteins, and it advances further toward the anode during the time allowed for separation. The globulins are larger than albumin and therefore do not migrate as far toward the anode. The relative migration distances of the globulins depend on the relationship of their size to their net negative charge. The gamma globulins have the smallest net negative charge relative to their size and, therefore, migrate the shortest distance toward the anode. In some techniques, the application point actually might lie in the gamma-globulin region, with some gamma globulins migrating to the cathode side of this point. The number of fractions separated depends on the electrophoretic technique used and the species being analyzed. (These separations are discussed in more detail in Chapter 30.)

Once electrophoretic separation is completed, the protein fractions usually are identified and quantified. Staining these fractions aids in this process. Various types of dye that stain protein can be used, including amido black, bromphenol blue, Coomassie brilliant blue, nigrosin, and ponceaus. After staining, it is possible, with experience, to visually identify the various protein fractions based on their order of migration. Visual examination also sometimes reveals apparently increased quantities of some protein fractions. This quantitation is more easily accomplished using a densitometer to scan the protein pattern and calculate the percentages and absolute quantities of protein in each fraction. A densitometer measures the amount of protein in each fraction by projecting light through these fractions as these are mechanically passed over the light source. A photodetector determines the width and density of each fraction. Results are reported as a densitometer scan, which more commonly is known as an electrophoretic pattern or electrophoretogram, as shown in Figure 1.35 and as both a percentage and an absolute value for each protein fraction. The absolute value for each fraction is calculated by the microprocessor in the instrument using the total protein concentration,

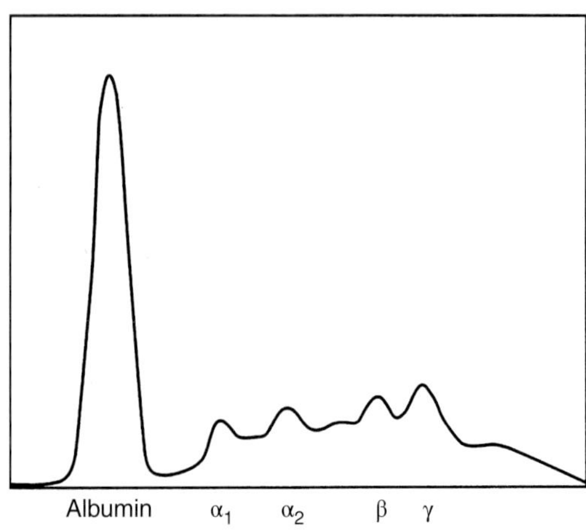

Figure 1.35 A densitometer scan (electrophoretic scan) of a serum protein electrophoresis separation.

which is entered by the operator, and the percentage of each fraction as determined by the densitometer:

$$\text{Absolute quantity of each fraction} = \frac{\text{Percentage of each fraction} \times \text{Total serum protein}}{100}$$

Most densitometers automatically identify each fraction as well as the boundaries between these fractions. The operator can and should change these in some cases.

Once the absolute quantities in the various fractions are determined, they can be compared with known reference intervals for that species, and any abnormalities can be identified. Use of such data in clinical chemistry of proteins is discussed in Chapter 30.

2 Sample Collection and Processing, Preparations for Clinical Microscopy, and Analysis of Laboratory Service Options

Glade Weiser
Loveland, CO, USA

In the previous chapter, laboratory technology was reviewed. To take advantage of this technology and its medical diagnostic capability, however, samples for the respective procedures must be properly collected and prepared. In particular, the use of clinical microscopy for blood and cytology has steadily grown over the last 30 years. Proper technique for preparing material for microscopic examination would benefit considerably from improvement and is an emphasis in this chapter.

The veterinarian must make laboratory diagnostics choices from a vast array of in-clinic and centralized service options. Although there is continual growth and improvement in in-clinic diagnostic instrumentation, this capability is not for all facilities. The choices may be influenced by several factors. The important factors include the type of practice (e.g., general, outpatient clinic, emergency facility, specialty referral center), geographic location, expertise of paraprofessional employees, and practice style of the individuals involved. This chapter presents rules for proper sample processing and guidelines for selecting laboratory diagnostics options.

Blood sample collection and processing

Regardless of the technique or laboratory used for any diagnostic test, obtaining reliable results starts with proper collection and handling of the sample. Sample collection, processing, testing, and interpretation all must be properly performed as a complete, sequential chain of events for a diagnostic result to have its intended value. For example, even the most reliable test, performed in the most reliable facility and interpreted by the most skilled diagnostician, cannot overcome the error introduced by an inappropriate technique used in sample collection or handling. This section provides guidelines for sample collection and handling that will ensure the initial sequence of events are properly performed.

Containers for sample collection

A variety of commercially available tubes are used for blood collection. These tubes contain the appropriate anticoagulant for the various diagnostic procedures and a vacuum for drawing in the appropriate volume of blood. These tubes are commonly known as vacutainer tubes (after the trademark of Becton Dickinson). The following commonly used vacuum tubes are described in the approximate order of their frequency of use. Tubes are commonly referred to by their stopper color, which is used to identify the type of anticoagulation system the tube contains (Figure 2.1).

Red-top or serum collection tube

The red-top or serum collection tube contains no anticoagulant. Blood that is placed in this tube is expected to clot so that serum may be harvested. This tube is used to collect serum for common biochemical determinations, such as those tests used in creating biochemical profiles.

Lavender-top tube

The lavender-top tube contains the anticoagulant ethylenediaminetetraacetic acid (EDTA) salt. This tube is used to collect blood for hematologic determinations. The EDTA anticoagulant results in the most consistent preservation of cell volume and morphologic features on stained films. The liquid tripotassium (K3) salt has the most commonly used form of EDTA. A newer formulation is dipotassium (K2) salt that is spray dried into plastic tubes. The tubes are larger and have a recommended visual fill line. Either of these formulations is preferred for use in preservation of cell volumes as measured on automated hematology analyzers. The plastic K2 tubes may be more forgiving of underfilling. It is anticipated that plastic K2 tubes may eventually make

Veterinary Hematology, Clinical Chemistry, and Cytology, Third Edition. Edited by Mary Anna Thrall, Glade Weiser, Robin W. Allison and Terry W. Campbell.

Companion website: www.wiley.com/go/thrall/veterinary

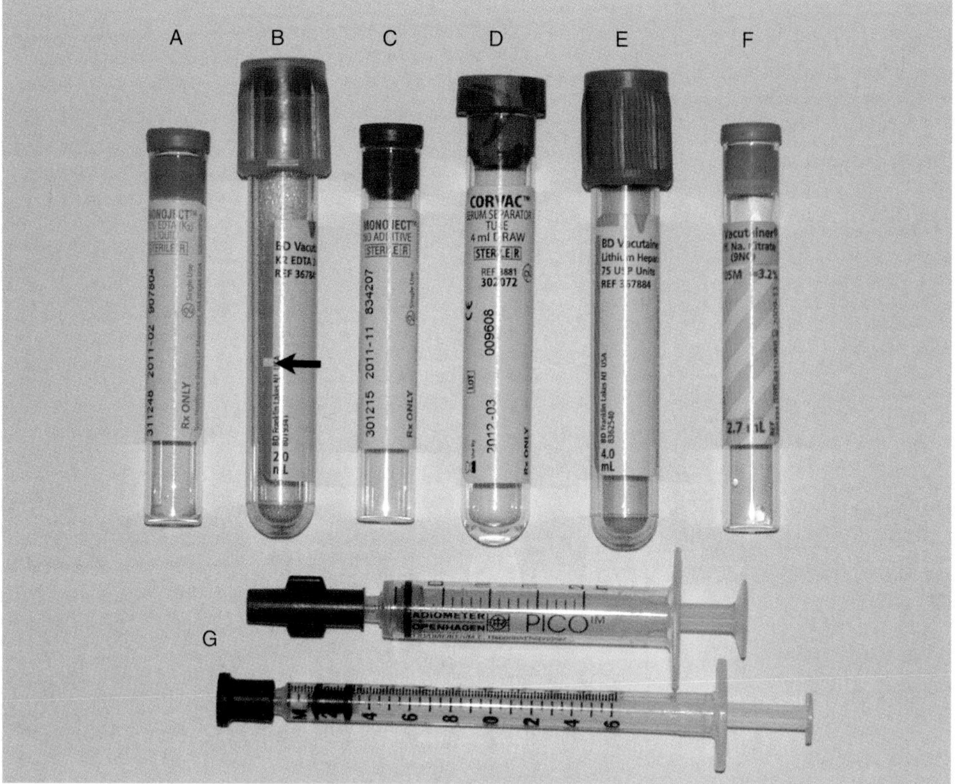

Figure 2.1 Representative collection devices for blood samples submitted for diagnostic tests. A: 3 mL glass lavender-top K3-EDTA tube; B: 2 mL plastic lavender-top K2-EDTA tube, note subtle white fill line indicated by arrow; C: a red-top tube without anticoagulant; D: a serum-separation tube; E: a lithium heparin green-top tube; F: a blue-top citrate tube; G: example balanced heparin syringes with caps for electrochemical diagnostic test collection.

the K3 liquid in glass tubes obsolete. Powdered forms are not recommended because of slower, inconsistent mixing with blood that is added to the tube.

Green-top or heparin tube

The green-top tube contains lithium heparin. This anticoagulant is used for certain special biochemistry tests, particularly those that require a whole-blood aliquot for determination and that might be influenced by the presence of other chemical anticoagulation systems.

Some in-house systems also recommend use of lithium heparin for all common clinical chemistry determinations. The advantage is that time is not required for clotting to completion to yield serum. The plasma may be separated immediately for testing, and results for most analytes are equivalent for serum and plasma. There are two exceptions. Total protein will be slightly higher for plasma because it includes fibrinogen. Potassium averages about 0.5 mmol/L higher for serum because of platelet release during clotting.

Lithium heparin is also used for electrochemical determinations. A common sample handling error is overheparinization inherent in manual addition of heparin to collection syringes. The various heparin salts will cause errors to most electrochemical measurements including blood gases, electrolytes, and hematocrit by conductometry. Various in-house electrochemical acid-base and electrolyte analyzers are now available. It is highly recommended that special collection syringes containing "balanced" or "saturated" heparin be used. These are manufactured to contain the minimal amount of heparin. Heparin has the ability to weakly bind calcium and cause false-low ionized calcium measurement. Balanced heparin is a formulation that has the binding sites saturated with calcium so that binding in the patient sample does not occur. Use of these syringes will minimize sample handling errors for electrochemical measurements.

Blue-top or citrate tube

The blue-top tube contains sodium citrate. It is used for coagulation biochemistry determinations.

Sure-Sep tube

The Sure-Sep tube is a variation of the red-top tube containing no anticoagulant. The stopper is red with black mottling. The tube contains a gel that separates packed cell fractions from serum when it undergoes centrifugation. It is convenient for use in situations when centrifugation at the site of collection and transport to the laboratory without the transfer of serum to a separate tube are desirable. The gel physically separates cells from the serum fluid, thus preventing analyte metabolism from occurring at the cell/fluid interface.

Gray-top or fluoride tube

The gray-top tube contains sodium fluoride. Fluoride is not an anticoagulant, however. Rather, it inhibits enzymes in the glycolytic pathway and prevents erythrocytes from metabolizing glucose while whole blood is transported to the laboratory. It is not commonly used.

Microtainers

Very small volume tubes are available for special applications such as very small laboratory animals. These may range from 0.25 to 1 mL. These should be avoided in general veterinary practice because of sample handling error potential. For example, it is very difficult to achieve proper mixing of blood in a 0.5 mL EDTA tube because of surface tension within a very small tube.

Tips for filling vacuum tubes

A few simple habits must be developed for appropriately filling tubes:

1. The ratio of blood to anticoagulant volume is important for hematology and blood coagulation biochemistry tests; therefore, a tube with anticoagulant should be filled to the volume specified for that tube. The amount of vacuum in the tube facilitates this, but the user should watch to ensure that this consistently occurs.

2. Recommendations for the tube filling order after venipuncture vary. Animal applications are different from the human setting because of differences in collection. When collecting blood for several diagnostic procedures, fill the tube(s) containing anticoagulant first and the tube containing no anticoagulant last. The most commonly used combination of tubes is an EDTA and clot/serum tube. The EDTA tube should be filled first so that platelet aggregation and clot formation is minimized. This is unimportant in the tube without anticoagulant because the blood is expected to clot in that tube. This deviates from the recommendation for humans. When filling the EDTA tube first, there is potential to contaminate the blood remaining in the syringe with EDTA. This can severely alter chemistry measurements such as calcium and potassium. Therefore, it is critical when filling an EDTA tube to avoid backflow of blood from the tube to the needle or connected syringe.

3. Vacuum tubes should be filled using minimal positive force, because forceful passage of blood through the needle may cause hemolysis, which in turn may cause an error in the biochemical measurements. Smaller-gauge needles are more likely to cause hemolysis. In particular, use of a 25-G needle, advocated by some, should be avoided because of inherent slow draw and hemolysis in tube transfer. An 18- to 20-G needle is best for most collection procedures.

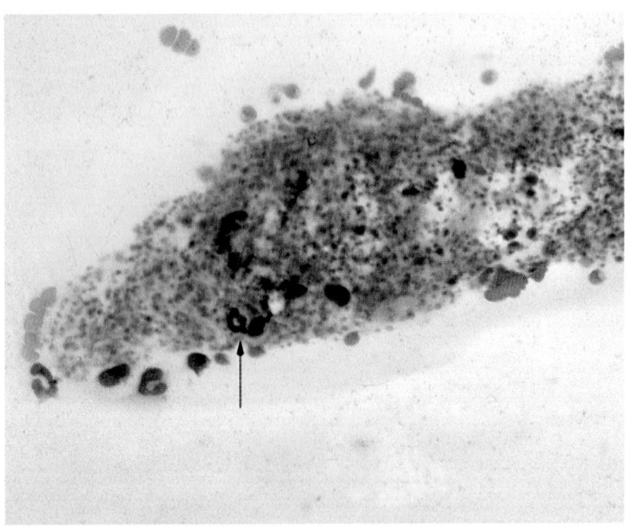

Figure 2.2 Platelet aggregation observed on a stained blood film. Tissue contamination may result in microclots that consist of hundreds of platelets, which falsely decrease the platelet concentration. Microclots also may trap leukocytes. Note the representative leukocyte (arrow); low magnification.

4. Clean venipunctures with no tissue contamination are important. Tissue contamination may result in unwanted platelet aggregation and clotting in samples collected using anticoagulants (Figure 2.2). As a result, select venipuncture sites (e.g., the jugular vein) that likely will yield the appropriate volume of blood needed for the diagnostic tests being ordered for a given patient.

5. Select a venipuncture site that will yield the desired amount of blood easily. This means being able to draw the blood with little or no collapse of the vein so that blood may be transferred to the anticoagulant tubes as rapidly as possible. Recommended venipuncture sites for diagnostic screening procedures such as a hemogram and biochemical profile include the jugular vein for small dogs, cats, horses, and cows; and the cephalic or jugular vein in medium to large dogs. These procedures generally require 4–12 mL of blood depending on the laboratory and the complexity of the screening procedures.

General sample handling procedures

Hematologic procedures

Blood collected for a complete blood count (CBC) should be analyzed within 1 hour or be prepared in the proper way for analysis at a later time. If the blood is not analyzed within one hour, a blood film should be prepared (see below) and the tube refrigerated. Morphologic features of cells may deteriorate rapidly on storage of blood in an EDTA tube; an air-dried blood film preserves the morphology of such cells for later examination. Refrigeration of the blood tube also helps to preserve the cell components that are measured by automated cell-counting systems. For example, cell swelling that could produce artifactual increases in mean cell volume

(MCV) and hematocrit will occur, as blood is stored in a tube at room or higher temperature. For some analytical systems with differential capability, it is recommended by the laboratory that blood be held at room temperature. Blood should never be frozen, however, because this will result in lysis of the cells. In addition, blood films should not be refrigerated, because water condensation on the glass may damage the cellular morphology.

For hematologic measurements, the EDTA tube should be filled to the specified volume, and tissue contamination during venipuncture should be avoided. Underfilling the EDTA tube results in excess EDTA, which osmotically shrinks erythrocytes. In turn, this results in falsely decreased packed cell volume and calculated MCV when the microhematocrit procedure is used.

Clinical biochemistry procedures

Blood collected in the red-top tube is allowed to clot for 15–30 minutes and then centrifuged to separate the cellular components from the resultant serum. The fluid phase of the blood should be separated from the cellular elements, because cells metabolize certain chemical components in the serum. The most notable example is glucose. If left in contact with cellular elements, glucose is metabolized at a rate of approximately 10% per hour. After centrifugation, serum is harvested by a transfer pipette to a second tube or is dispensed directly to devices for biochemical determinations (Figure 2.3). Harvested serum should be analyzed quickly; otherwise, it can be refrigerated for as long as 24–48 hours. If serum is to be held for longer than 24–48 hours, it should be frozen, and serum that is to be held frozen indefinitely (e.g., for archival purposes) should be stored at −70 °C. Most chemical constituents are stable under these conditions. If serum is frozen and then thawed for analysis, the thawed aliquot should be thoroughly mixed before testing.

Serum enzymes require separate consideration regarding storage. A general rule is that for best reliability, serum enzyme activities should be determined within 24 hours of collection. Long-term archival storage of samples for determination of serum enzyme activity is not advised. Data on the exact stability of serum enzyme activity under various storage conditions are difficult to interpret. Knowledge regarding this subject has not been updated in any systematic way in recent years, and historical data were not collected in any consistent manner. Thus, our current understanding of enzyme stability during storage may be summarized as follows: Commonly measured enzymes, including alanine aminotransferase (ALT), aspartate aminotransferase, and alkaline phosphatase, and amylase activities are satisfactorily stable (>70% activity) when stored at 4 °C. Freezing, however, may result in considerably accelerated loss of ALT activity. Creatine kinase activity should be measured as soon as possible, because considerable activity is lost after 24 hours regardless of the storage conditions.

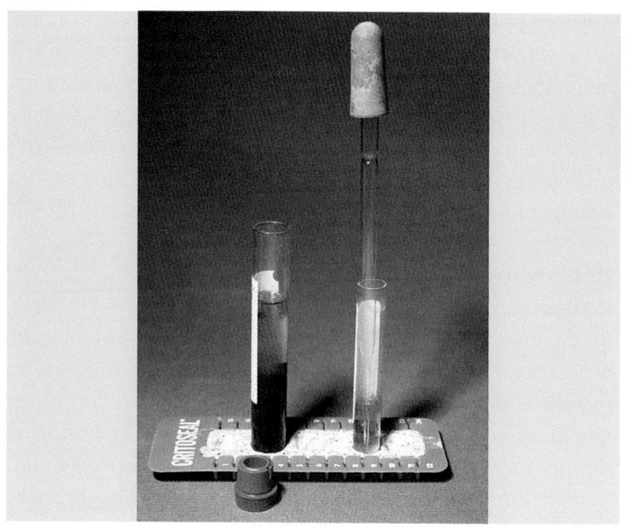

Figure 2.3 Serum preparation for biochemical tests. The tube on the left was allowed to clot and then centrifuged to pack the cells below the serum layer. A transfer pipette is used to transfer serum from the centrifuged sample to the tube on the right.

Special procedures

Special laboratory diagnostic procedures are usually performed by centralized or commercial laboratories because of the complexity or specialized instrumentation involved. These procedures are performed less frequently, and they are more dependent on unique requirements of the technology employed by the laboratory undertaking the procedure. For example, endocrine assays may vary in measuring principle and reagents used, resulting in considerable sample handling and results interpretation differences. As a result, the laboratory protocol for special procedures should be rigorously followed rather than committing these requirements to memory.

Collection, preparation, and examination techniques for clinical microscopy samples

The purpose of this section is to provide guidance on slide preparation for hematologic and cytologic samples. Sample handling techniques that limit interpretability will also be illustrated.

Ability to maximize blood and cytology sample microscopic diagnostic yield involves considerable skill and experience. One skill is pattern recognition. Pattern recognition in microscopy is the ability to (i) identify features such as cellularity, individual cellular detail, and any organization present between cells, and (ii) interpret the integrated findings into a pattern consistent with a specific diagnostic interpretation. See Chapter 3 for discussion about perspective on pattern recognition skill. Another, perhaps more important skill involves a sequence of collection and processing procedures. These sample handling procedures include ability to properly collect, prepare, stain, and utilize a microscope to extract diagnostic information from slides. A defect in any of these sample handling procedures may introduce compromising artifacts and/or render the cytology nondiagnostic.

Hematology – blood films

Collection

Blood collection in an EDTA tube for the CBC or hemogram is described above. It is important that a "clean stick" occur to collect blood for hematology. This means insertion of the needle directly into the sampling vein before aspiration of sample to avoid any tissue contamination. Tissue contamination during venipuncture results in platelet aggregation (Figure 2.2). Platelet aggregation artifactually decreases the platelet concentration measurement determined by cell-counting systems and may contribute to fluidic obstruction in hematology instruments. The blood film may be made immediately following venipuncture by transfer of blood directly from the needle to the slide(s) but is most often made from a small aliquot removed from the EDTA tube.

Blood film preparation

The stained blood film is an essential tool for determining the concentrations of individual leukocyte types (i.e., differential count) and for evaluating important pathologic abnormalities involving leukocytes, erythrocytes, and platelets. Successful derivation of information from the blood film requires a proper technique, which both creates a monolayer of individually dispersed cells and a minimal disturbance of relative cell distributions that reflect the cell concentrations in mixed blood. A poorly prepared film presents confusing artifacts and may result in cell distributions on the slide that lead to serious errors in the differential count. Preparation of a good-quality blood film requires mastery of a specific technique (Figures 2.4–2.6). The most common procedure is known as the wedge or push technique and uses two glass microscope slides. A drop of blood is placed near one end of the first slide supported on the counter. The second slide is placed on the first in a way that forms a "wedge" consisting of a 30–45° angle in front of the drop of blood. The second slide, which is known as the pusher slide, then is backed into the drop of blood and advanced forward to the end. This should be accomplished in one rapid motion that involves a flip of the wrist holding the pusher slide. Downward pressure on the pusher slide should be minimal.

Learning this technique in the presence of someone experienced with making good films is helpful, and considerable practice is advised. A common poor technique is to push the pusher slide too slowly, thereby creating a film that is too thin. This results in very poor distribution of leukocytes at the end of the film and artifacts in the evaluation of erythrocytes.

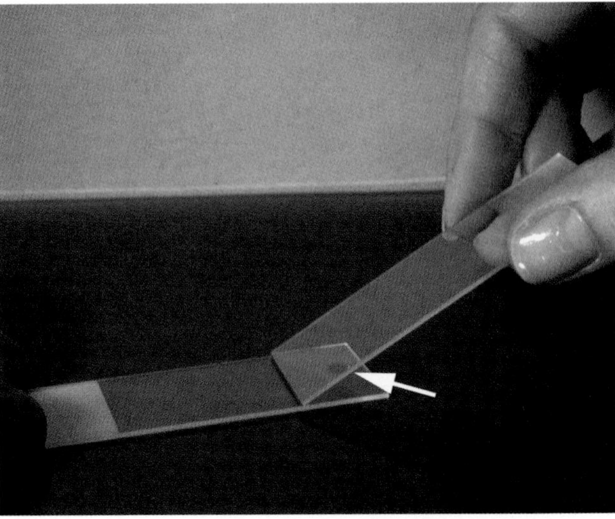

Figure 2.4 Blood film preparation. The blood slide is held on a firm surface, and a drop of blood is placed near the end (arrow). The pusher slide then is placed on the blood slide in front of the drop of blood to form an angle of approximately 30°.

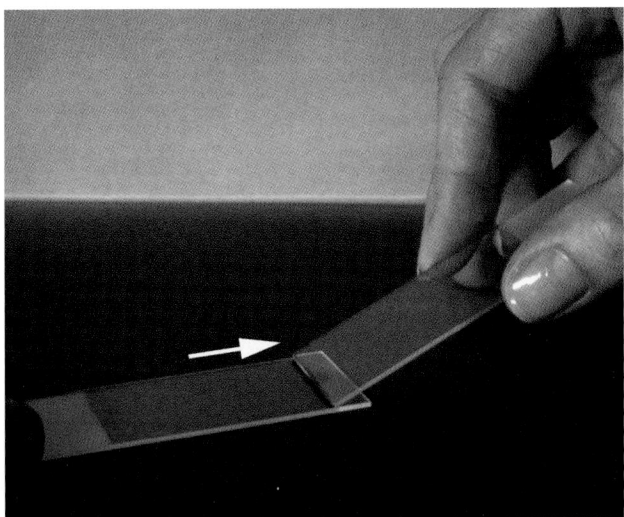

Figure 2.5 Blood film preparation. The pusher slide is backed into the drop of blood with a directional movement (arrow).

In blood with reduced viscosity, such as that from patients with severe anemia, increasing the angle to avoid a slide that is too thin is useful.

Diagnostic cytology – fluid and tissue samples

Collection

Tissue aspirates

Required materials used for aspiration are typically a 5–12 mL syringe and a needle ranging from 18 to 20-G having adequate length for the site being sampled. Very small needle diameter such as a 25-G is discouraged. For superficial tissue aspirates such as lymph nodes and cutaneous or

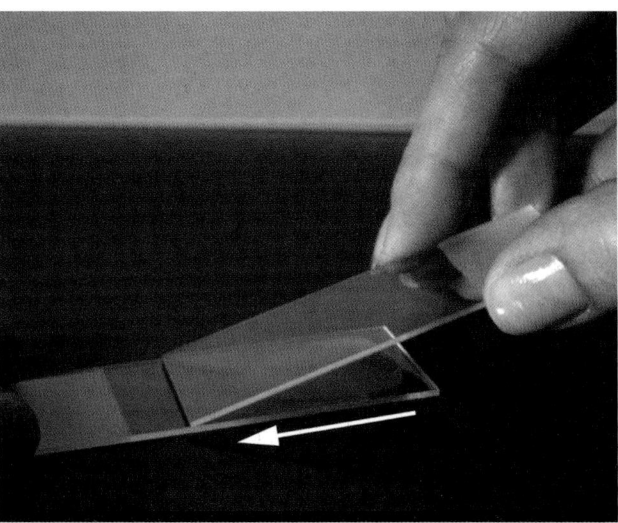

Figure 2.6 Blood film preparation. The pusher slide is pushed forward with a rapid directional movement (arrow). It is important that the movements shown in Figures 2.4–2.6 are a single, rapid procedure involving a flip of the wrist. Considerable practice is required to develop this skill. The result should be a uniform film of blood that gets progressively thinner (see Figure 2.16).

subcutaneous lesions, the mass or area of interest should be moderately isolated by digital manipulation. This will facilitate needle insertion and associated potential movement of the mass away from the insertion force. For body cavity organ or mass lesions physical isolation is not feasible, and the aspiration may typically be ultrasound guided.

There are varying techniques promoted for the physical process of aspiration. The technique recommended here is to apply aspiration negative pressure with the syringe as soon as the needle is placed in the desired location. Aspiration negative pressure may be progressively increased until one to two drops of material appear in the hub of the syringe. If blood is initially obtained, negative pressure should immediately be released. Additional aspiration is likely to yield only a blood sample. Slides should be made of this initial sample to determine if diagnostic tissue cells other than blood are present. If no material is obtained in this initial attempt, the needle may be redirected in adjacent tissue in the area of interest followed by another attempt at aspiration.

Once the sample is aspirated, slides should be made as soon as possible to avoid possible sample clotting. Material is transferred from the syringe and needle directly to slides using the preparation procedure described below.

Body cavity fluid aspirates

Examples of commonly sampled fluids are abdominal, thoracic, synovial, cerebrospinal fluid (CSF), and large abnormal encapsulated tissue fluid spaces. Cavity fluid aspiration is intuitive once the needle is placed in the fluid-containing space. Typically, only a few milliliters of fluid are needed for analysis and cytology. The aspirated fluid is transferred to an appropriately sized EDTA tube to prevent clotting. Aliquots of fluid are then available for various analysis procedures and for preparation of air-dried slides. Additional fluid should also be placed in a red-top tube if there is possibly a reason for biochemical analysis procedures.

Bone marrow aspirates

Marrow samples are unique in that cortical bone must be accessed and penetrated with a special needle to prevent plugging while accessing the marrow space. The sites that most commonly are used for bone marrow aspiration in dogs are the proximal end of the femur at the trochanteric fossa, the iliac crest, and the proximal humerus (Figure 2.7). The trochanteric fossa and humerus are the preferred sites in cats, and the ilium, ribs, or sternum usually are aspirated in horses, cattle, and camelids. If general anesthesia or sedation is not used, a local anesthetic is indicated. Both the subcutis and periosteum should be infiltrated with anesthetic. Bone marrow biopsy needles (16–22-G) are commercially available (Figures 2.7 and 2.8); conventional hypodermic needles without stylets tend to plug with bone and are not suitable. After surgical preparation of the skin, the needle is introduced. In thick-skinned animals, the skin may be incised to facilitate introduction of the needle. Once the needle is against cortical bone, it should be rotated until firmly seated in the bone and then advanced a few more millimeters, all while keeping pressure on the stylet to prevent any backward movement and subsequent bone plugging (Figure 2.8). The stylet then is removed, the syringe attached, and negative pressure applied, but only until marrow becomes visible in the syringe barrel. Aspiration of a larger volume results in contamination of marrow

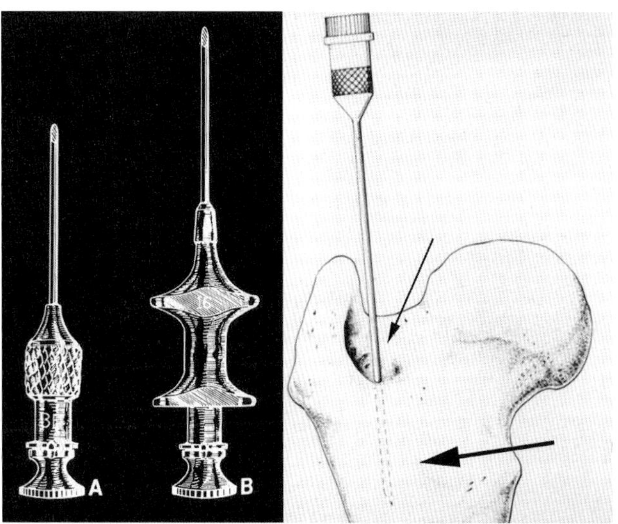

Figure 2.7 Left. Examples of commercially available bone marrow needles with stylets. Right. Correct placement of bone marrow needle in the trochanteric fossa.

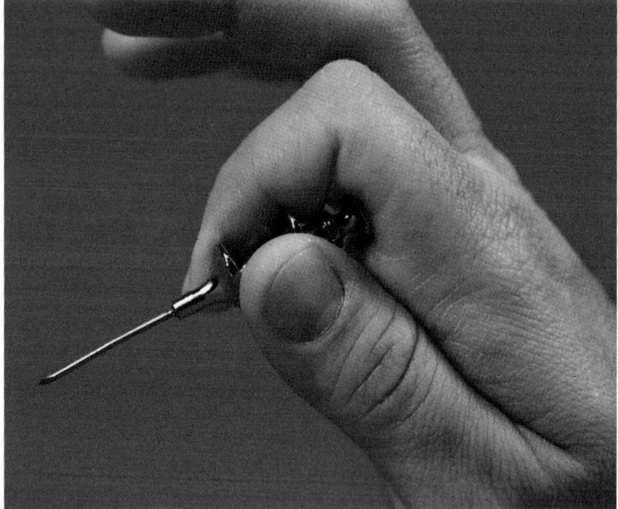

Figure 2.8 The bone marrow needle must be held with pressure against the stylet to keep the stylet in place within the needle, thus preventing bone plugs.

with blood. Once the marrow is collected, it should be placed in an EDTA (disodium ethylenediaminetetraacetate) tube, or slides made very quickly, because clotted samples are nondiagnostic. Alternatively, two or three drops of 10% EDTA solution can be placed in the syringe before aspiration. Pull films are prepared as indicated below by the pull film technique described under slide preparation.

If marrow elements cannot be obtained by aspiration even though multiple sites may be attempted, a core biopsy is indicated. Core biopsies are collected using a Jamshidi marrow biopsy needle. An infant- or pediatric-sized needle should be used for small animals. After collection, the core of marrow can be gently rolled onto the surface of a glass slide for cytologic evaluation before placing the core in formalin solution for fixation.

Tissue imprint

Imprint cytology has become relatively uncommon. However, some may use it occasionally for samples of tissue taken during exploratory surgery or in the postmortem examination setting. The key to making a monolayer imprint is to utilize a small amount of tissue and minimize the tissue fluid present. If a large tissue mass is excised, a small (less than 1 cm square) area should be cleanly cut for imprinting. The imprint surface should then be gently blotted on a paper towel or other absorbent surface to remove excess surface tissue fluid. The blotted surface is then gently touched to the glass slide in several places. Avoid "painting" the slide with the tissue or moving it laterally while touching down to the glass. If the imprints look wet and dry slowly, blot again and repeat the procedure.

Imprints are also occasionally made of ulcerated dermal lesions. The same principles apply, although trimming of the tissue is not done. The lesion should be gently cleaned of contaminant debris as much as practical and then blotted as above before making an imprint to the glass slide.

Slide preparation of fluid and tissue aspirate samples, including bone marrow

Perspective

An observed obstacle to diagnostic yield is the fraction of cytologic preparations with varying degrees of less than desirable quality, from compromised by excess artifact to being uninterpretable. A large part of success in pattern recognition is ability to navigate various artifacts. Artifacts are present on well-prepared cytologic samples, but they dramatically increase in suboptimally prepared samples. Additional artifacts or complications in the general practice setting can be related to inadequate stain maintenance and a maladjusted microscope. Experience at pathology laboratories indicates that cytologic slide preparation is the major weak link in all of the steps leading to the procedure's ability to provide useful diagnostic information. The fraction of uninterpretable or compromised samples is surprising.

The objective of preparing diagnostic samples of tissue or fluid aspirates is to create a monolayer of cellular material from the sample. This is more difficult to achieve for cytology than for making blood films because of the variation in viscosity and texture across various sample types. Body cavity fluid samples tend to be the least viscous, usually much less than blood. Tissue aspirates are much more variable and may have small particulate tissue aggregates.

Body cavity fluid samples may be directly used to make slides when there is adequate cell concentration. An adequate cellularity guideline is greater than 10,000/µL. With lower cell concentrations, such as occurs in transudates and CSF, it is desirable to concentrate an aliquot of sample for slide preparation. This may be done by sample centrifugation, removing most of the supernatent, mixing the pellet with residual supernatent, and then making slides as described below. Central laboratories may use a cytocentrifuge designed to make concentrated slide preparations. This is typically required for CSF samples.

Recommended technique

The recommended technique involves use of as little fluid material as possible to allow spreading of material into a reasonable monolayer between two glass slides. In the laboratory, this is often called the "pull film" technique. The described steps are as follows:

- Pull films are made using a pair of slides. Multiple pairs may be prepared. (See Figure 2.9.)
- Using the syringe, transfer a small amount of material to one end of the first slide. This is typically one drop.
  - In the case of a body cavity fluid, the transfer may be made with a small laboratory pipette.

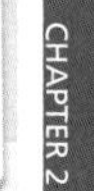

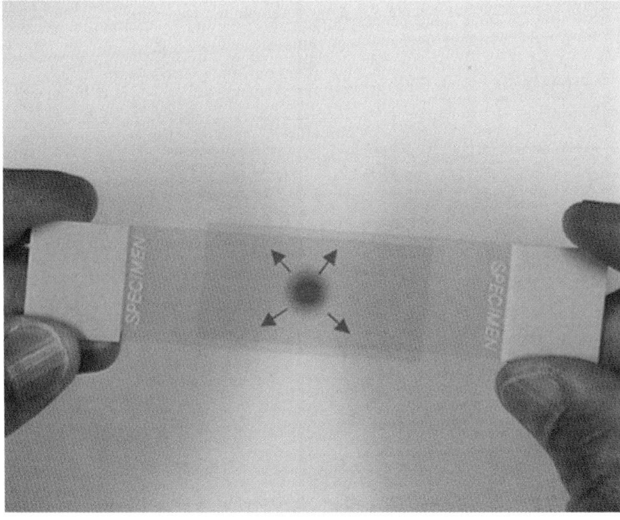

Figure 2.9 Two-slide technique for preparing pull films for cytology samples. The drop of material is allowed to spread slightly before pulling the two glass slides apart parallel from one another.

- In the case of a tissue aspirate, material may be transferred from the syringe or syringe and needle directly to slides.
- If a very small amount of tissue aspirate is obtained, it may be sprayed onto the same area and followed by the next step.
- Bone marrow aspirate is often placed in an EDTA tube. Material is transferred from the tube to the slide using an appropriate applicator such as a microhematocrit tube.

• Position the second slide to overlap the first, with the amount of overlap being about equal. Then, place the second slide onto the first and watch the material spread between the slides.

• As soon as the spreading slows, pull the two slides apart, making sure the slides remain parallel to each other.

• The result should show some feathering of the edges of the spreading (Figure 2.10). If the material covers all of the area of the slide overlap, too much fluid or material has been applied. Make another attempt with less material.

• If there is considerable friction in pulling the slides apart, then the material has spread too far. This will result in more broken cells due to shearing force on the glass.

• Air-dry the slides as rapidly as convenient and label them appropriately.

Sample slides are then ready for staining to confirm that cells other than blood are present. (See "Perspective on Use of Cytopathology" in Chapter 3.) Slides sent to a commercial laboratory should be labeled and placed in a suitable holder. Ideally some unstained slides are included. A plastic slotted slide holder is recommended. Cardboard slide holders are satisfactory but are associated with smashed slides more frequently. To avoid damaging water condensation on slides, do not refrigerate the slides or holder containing slides.

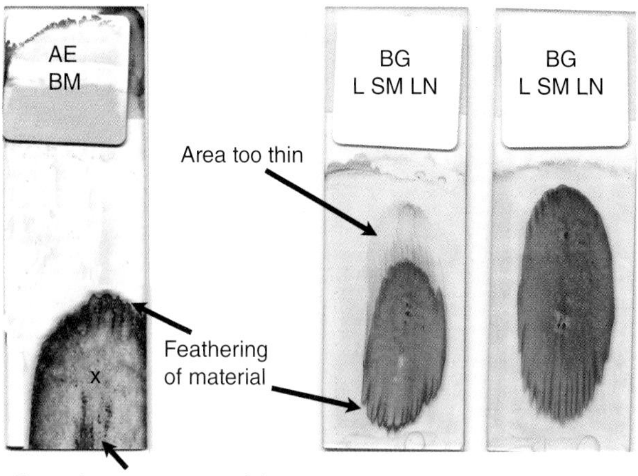

Figure 2.10 Examples of recommended "pull film" technique. The stained slide on the left is from a bone marrow sample. The "x," near the end of the glass slide, indicates the approximate location of the drop placed for spreading between two slides. The violet area indicates an area of marrow particle cellularity that is spread out. The two stained slides on the right are from a lymph node aspirate. Note that the droplet of material was placed more in the center of the first slide. This results in spreading over a larger area. An area indicated as too thin will consist of mostly broken cells. Both samples have feathering of material at the end or edge of material spreading. This indicates a desirable degree of spreading occurred and that good monolayers of intact cells will be present.

Examples of compromised to uninterpretable cytologic slide preparation

Examples of slide preparations that limit the diagnostic usefulness of cytology are illustrated here. Pathologists in the receiving laboratory setting commonly encounter these examples.

Slides that are too thick

There are a few techniques that result in thickness that prevents visualization of cells at worst and evaluation of cellular detail at best. A rule is: if one cannot see through material on the slide with the naked eye, it will be too thick to visualize cells with the microscope.

Too much material placed on slide. This is the most common cause of nondiagnostic slide preparations. This is usually seen with tissue aspirates having appreciable tissue fluid volume and bone marrow aspirates. Figure 2.11 shows example slides. So much material was applied that there is no area on the slide for spreading into a monolayer to occur. The result is a very thick background and complete lack of individual cellular detail. This is due to severe rounding up of cells and/or cells being superimposed in multiple layers, especially when there is background blood. On preparations like these, the thickness obscures light transmittance much more than on the thick part of a blood film.

Spray droplet and splatter techniques. Figure 2.12. This happens when the syringe is used to spray material onto the

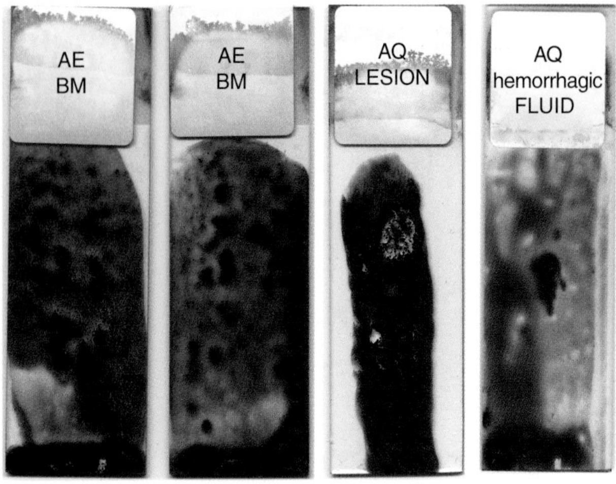

Figure 2.11 Three examples of very thick sample preparations. The two slides on the left are from bone marrow. The other two are bloody tissue aspirates. The problem is that too much material was placed on the slides. This prevents ability to spread material into a monolayer. Grossly, light transmittance is very poor. The result is inability to identify cells in almost all areas and marked rounding up of cells obscuring individual cell detail in the less thick areas. Samples such as these are usually not diagnostic.

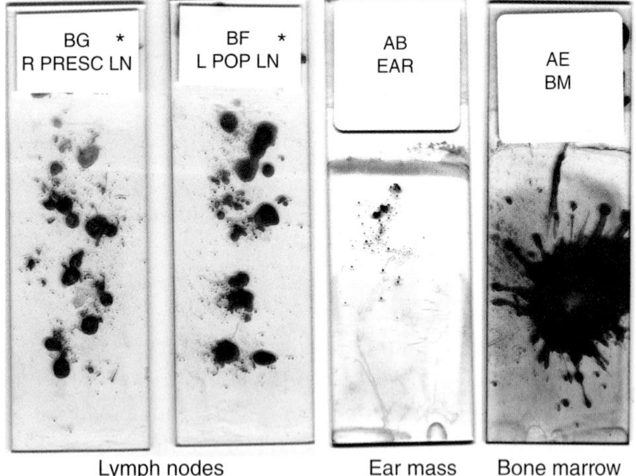

Figure 2.12 Examples of droplet, spray droplet, and splatter techniques. Note that in all of these slides there was no attempt to spread the applied material. Even the smallest droplets will be dark with thick background and very rounded up cells. How the bone marrow slide was prepared is beyond imagination.

slide, with no attempt to spread the material between two slides. This may happen when a very small amount of material is present, perhaps only in the needle hub. Alternatively, volume is present but there is no attempt to spread the material into a monolayer. The result is a background multiple cell layers thick and inability to visualize cellular detail.

Miscellaneous techniques. The "pull apart" technique is illustrated in Figure 2.13a. The technique involves placing a drop (usually large) of material between two slides and then pulling the slides apart perpendicular to each other. There is some spreading between the slides, but there is minimal filming into a monolayer. The result is a characteristic pattern of suction created by perpendicular slide separation. The appearance is like an image of tree branches. There will likely be areas thin enough for evaluation. However, this increases the skill required to navigate the slide to avoid the thicker material and concentrate on areas of better cellular detail. A bone marrow technique is shown in Figure 2.13b. A relatively large sample volume is loaded at one end of the slide. The slides are then positioned upright to allow the sample to flow down the slide by gravity. The objective is to not disrupt marrow particles of architecture as they separate from the fluid. Cellularity of particles may be evaluated this way on low power, but the sample is too thick for proper evaluation of individual cellular detail.

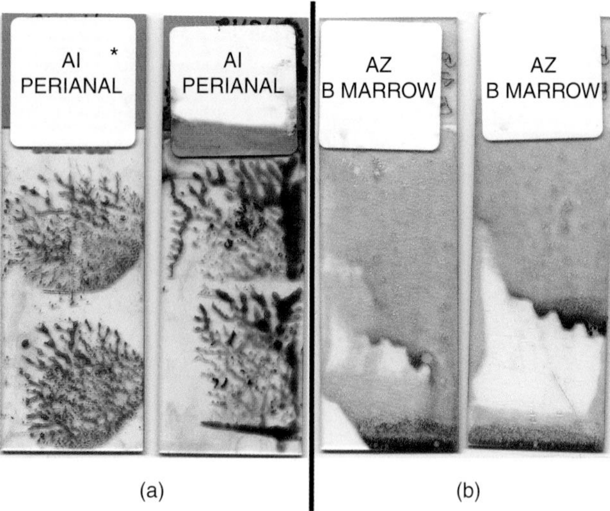

Figure 2.13 Two stained slides marked (a) are made by the pull-apart technique giving the characteristic arboreal appearance. Much of the material is too thick for evaluation. The observer must carefully navigate to find suitable monolayer material. The two unstained slides (b) are made from a bone marrow sample. Too much material was placed on the slides and then allowed to flow by gravity. Particles, indicated by the fatty droplet areas, are present. However, most of the material will be too thick for proper evaluation of individual cellular detail.

Procedures that may rupture more cells than desirable

Broken cells are present on almost all cytology preparations, but some techniques result in an undesirable fraction of broken cells making interpretation more challenging.

The painting technique. Some have an artistic urge to paint the sample onto the slide, as shown in Figure 2.14. The result will likely be a combination of thin areas in which most or all of the cells are broken. There may also be thick areas that are not spread properly. There will likely be interpretable areas, but navigation around the artifacts makes interpretation more challenging.

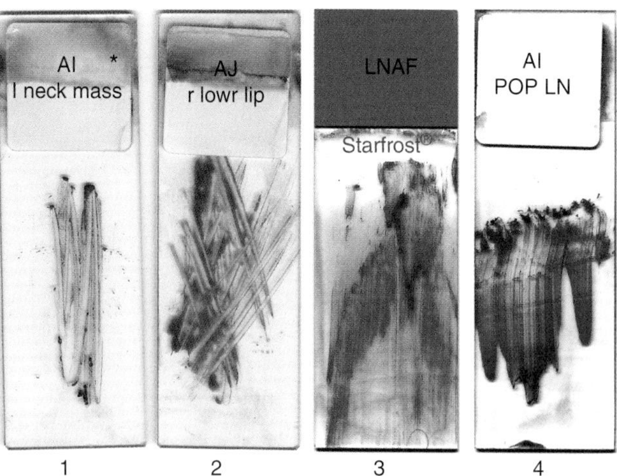

Figure 2.14 Stained slides marked 1 and 2 are examples of painting the cytology material on the slide. Stained slides marked 3 and 4 are examples of shearing the material on glass, as indicated by the long shear line pattern in the material. Both sample types will have many broken cells in the thin areas and variable areas of thickness.

The shearing technique. This involves spreading the material over a long distance of glass, creating a glacier effect. As the material gets thin there is a shearing force that ruptures the cells. This is seen grossly by long linear streaking of the material as seen in Figure 2.14. There may be interpretable areas, but navigation around the artifacts makes interpretation more challenging.

Staining, use of microscope, and examination of blood and cytology samples

Staining

After preparation, the blood film is usually stained within minutes. However, it may be stained within hours to days if it is being sent to a diagnostic laboratory. The staining system used for microscopic evaluation of cellular elements is the Wright stain, or a Wright stain modified by the addition of Giemsa. This is a relatively complex procedure that requires care and maintenance, thus often being limited to larger laboratory facilities. Quick-stain procedures that mimic the classical Wright stain are available, however, and for convenience, these are the most commonly used stains in the veterinary practice setting. The best-known stain kit is Diff-Quick (various online suppliers). Quick stains may result in nuclear over-staining and smudging of chromatin detail, but they provide sufficient quality for differential leukocyte counting and screening for morphologic abnormalities. Experience indicates that quick stains may suffer from inadequate maintenance in the veterinary practice setting. In particular, the basophilic dyes can be depleted as use of the stain progresses over time. This is seen as an insidious loss of nuclear staining and paleness of other basophilic organelles. It is important to regularly change the stain containers to prevent dye depletion. Examples of manual to automated staining systems are shown in Figure 2.15.

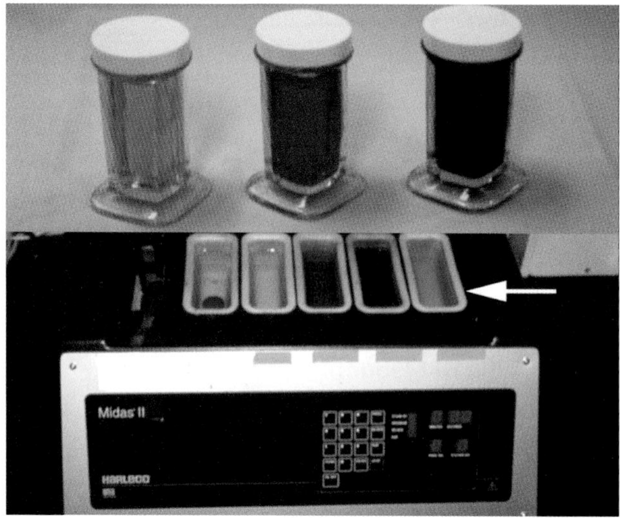

Figure 2.15 Blood film and cytology staining apparatus. Top. Manual staining jars containing Diff-Quick stain. Slides are manually moved from one jar to the next according to the manufacturer's instructions. Bottom. An automated stainer used for higher-throughput situations. Note the mechanical arm that moves a rack of slides (not shown) through the sequence of staining procedure baths (arrow). The stainer may be programmed to control the timing in each bath. Most such machines provide the ability to stain as many as 20–25 slides per cycle.

Use of the microscope

The microscope should be of good quality and optimally adjusted to minimize optically induced artifact on air-dried blood and cytology preparations. The good-quality microscope ideally has bright halogen or LED illumination at high magnifications, a flat field (plan) high-power objective, wide field of view optics, and an adjustable substage condenser. Oil immersion is typically required for cytology and hematology. Even with a quality microscope, a common problem is condenser maladjustment, especially when there are multiple users. When wet mounts are examined, it is necessary to dial the condenser's iris diaphragm down to increase contrast. An alternative to diaphragm adjustment is to lower the condenser. Either of these adjustments are a problem for the next user looking at an air-dried cytology of blood film sample. The increased contrast of a maladjusted condenser will obscure fine cellular detail important to pattern recognition in cytology. The user must be aware of the problem and adept at adjusting the condenser back to Kohler illumination. Kohler illumination involves raising the condenser to a proper height under the stage and ensuring the iris is opened. This adjustment optimizes optical performance by creating a light beam of relatively parallel rays passing through the specimen. Another more desirable solution is to employ two microscopes. One of lesser quality is sufficient for wet mount preparations (e.g., fecal floatation, urine sediment, and skin scraping preparations). The second-quality microscope maintained by routine maintenance and proper condenser adjustment for Kohler illumination is reserved for air-dried preparations. The Kohler illumination adjustment procedure may be found in the microscope's documentation. The procedure may also be found in online tutorials such as https://www.microscopyu.com/tutorials/kohler or https://www.olympus-lifescience.com/en/microscope-resource/primer/anatomy/kohler.

Examination of blood films

Once stained, the anatomy of a blood film must be known to properly orient the slide for microscopic viewing (Figure 2.16). The largest part of the film is the thick area or body, in which cells are superimposed and leukocytes are rounded up, thereby making microscopic evaluation of all components difficult. The feathered edge occurs at the end of the film. Artifacts in this area include broken leukocytes and the inability to evaluate the erythrocyte morphology. The counting area is a small area between the thick portion and the feathered edge, and it consists of the best monolayer of cells in which microscopy is optimal. Leukocytes are flattened out so that the internal detail is most evident.

The amount of interpretive disease relevance that can be gained from examination of the blood film is proportional to the expertise available for the examination. Success in dealing with all components of such examination depends on the quality of film making, stain maintenance, ability to look in the correct place, ability to differentiate preparation artifacts from morphologic abnormalities, and experience with interpretive blood film pathology. To the extent that the user cannot make these distinctions, abnormal blood films should be referred to a specialist for examination and/or second opinion. This is especially important when the numerical data indicate a major hematologic abnormality such as anemia, abnormal leukocyte concentrations, or suspected thrombocytopenia.

It is important to examine the gross appearance of blood films as a correlate to artifact recognition. Improper preparation can be recognized, thereby alerting the observer to artifacts that can be avoided and preventing any associated, errant interpretations. Common abnormalities that may be recognized grossly are presented in Figure 2.17. The most common and important abnormality is a slide that is too thin, which can be recognized by streaks progressing toward the feathered edge. This results in a leukocyte distribution that presents major errors in the differential count. In addition,

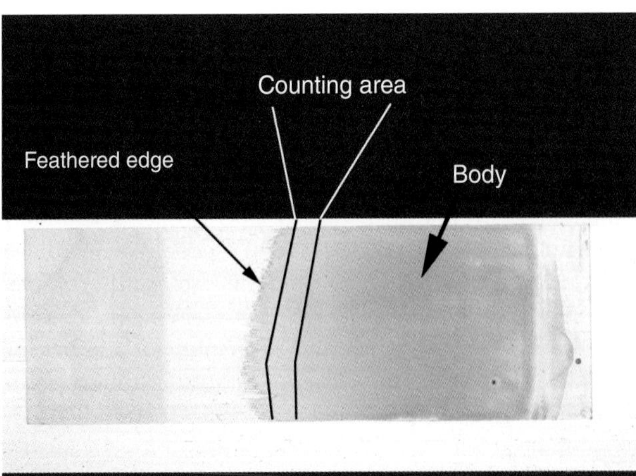

Figure 2.16 Anatomy of a stained blood film. Note the feathered edge (thin arrow) and the thick area or body of the slide (thick arrow). The counting area containing a monolayer of cells is present in a relatively small area, which is delineated approximately by the lines across the slide. This gross examination of the slide is very helpful in orienting the observer before placing the slide on the microscope stage. This facilitates alignment of the optics over the proper area of the slide, making it easier and faster to perform low-magnification observations and to find the counting area.

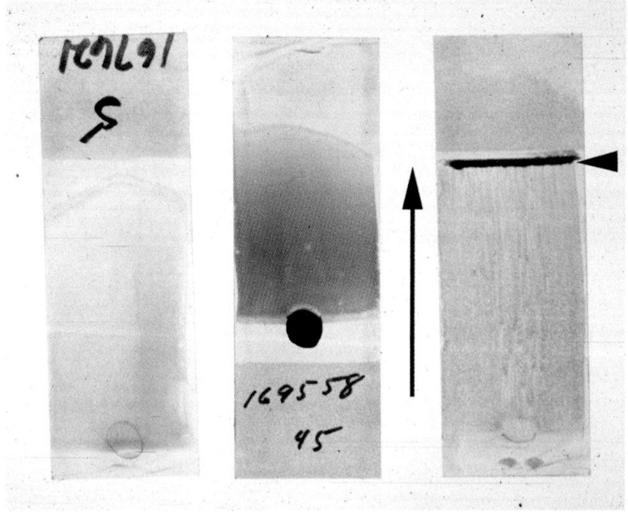

Figure 2.17 Gross appearance of blood films. All three of these films are oriented the same way. The drop of blood was placed near the bottom of the picture, and the film was made by pushing in the direction of the arrow. The middle film has a normal appearance and intensity of color. The appearance is homogeneous but gets progressively thinner as one approaches the feathered edge. The film on the left is very pale; this is the appearance when severe anemia is present. With severe anemia, blood viscosity is reduced, resulting in a much thinner film. The film on the right is made improperly and does not yield accurate information. The pusher slide was pushed too slowly, making a thin film with streaks. Note the streaking and irregularity over most of the slide. Blood was still present at the end of the slide as well, resulting in a line of densely concentrated cells (arrowhead). It is not possible to find a good monolayer for evaluation of erythrocyte morphology on this slide. In addition, the leukocytes are disproportionately concentrated at the end of the slide, which ordinarily has a feathered edge. Performing a differential count will be difficult in this case – and likely not accurate. A thin slide as a result of pushing too slowly is the most common problem in technique found at veterinary facilities.

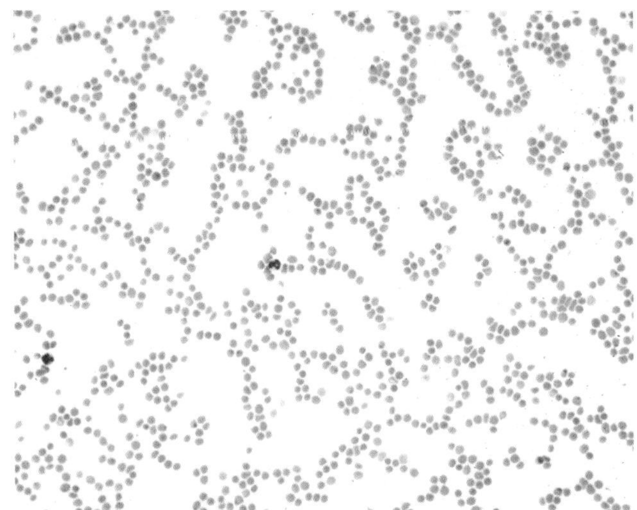

Figure 2.18 Low-magnification appearance of the feathered edge. Note the reticulated pattern of erythrocyte distribution. Artifactual loss of central pallor makes evaluation of erythrocyte morphology difficult, and false interpretation of pathologic abnormalities is likely to occur in this area.

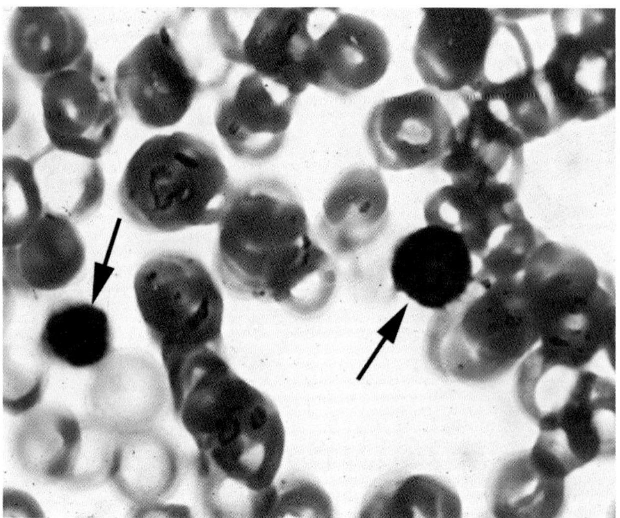

Figure 2.20 High-magnification appearance of cells in the thick area or body of slide. Note the superimposition of erythrocytes, thus making evaluation of erythrocyte morphology difficult. In addition, specifically identifying leukocytes (arrows) is difficult to impossible. In this area, leukocytes are spherical or rounded up rather than flattened. It is not possible to see intracellular detail or even the delineation between the cytoplasm and the nucleus. This makes cell identification very difficult, especially in cytology samples.

there is not an area adequate for the evaluation of erythrocyte abnormalities.

The observer should locate the counting area using the 10× objective. The feathered edge is recognized by a loss of erythrocyte central pallor and a reticulated pattern of erythrocyte distribution on the film (Figure 2.18). Quick, low-power examination of the feathered edge is useful for the detection and identification of abnormalities such as microfilaria, platelet clumps, and unusual large cells that are preferentially deposited here (Figure 2.19). The thick area is recognized by a progressive superimposition of erythrocytes as the observer moves further into the thick area of the slide. In very thick areas, the evaluation of cells is severely compromised (Figure 2.20). The counting area is recognized by a monolayer of evenly dispersed cells (Figures 2.21 and 2.22).

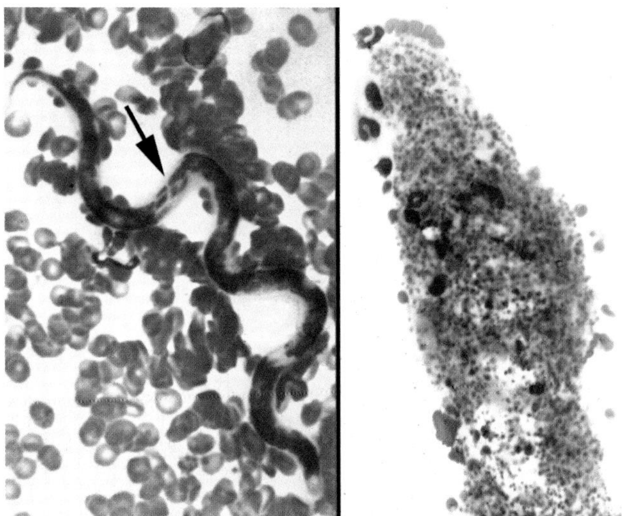

Figure 2.19 Large items pushed to the feathered edge. Left. Microfilaria (arrow) in an animal with heartworm disease. Right. A large clump of platelets with trapped leukocytes. Several hundred platelets are contained in this microclot.

Once the counting area is located, the experienced observer can estimate the leukocyte concentration on a well-prepared blood film. This is useful as a gross quality-control measure, and it is recommended that the observer gain experience at this by repetitive comparison of leukocyte density on well-prepared blood films with total leukocyte counts from a cell counter. The low-power appearances of a leukocyte count in the normal range, marked leukopenia, marked leukocytosis, and high magnification leukocyte detail are shown in Figures 2.23–2.25, respectively.

Once these assessments are completed in the counting area, the microscope should be set to 100× for oil immersion, high-magnification observation. The observer will then perform a systematic evaluation of the three major cell lines. This includes a differential count for leukocytes with notation about any abnormal cells, evaluation of erythrocyte morphology, and evaluation of platelets. These procedures are defined in detail in Chapter 1.

Examination of cytology slides

Tissue aspirates including bone marrow

As indicated above, blood film evaluation involves seeking a specific area of the slide. The area is specified by the best probability of finding a monolayer of cells. Within that

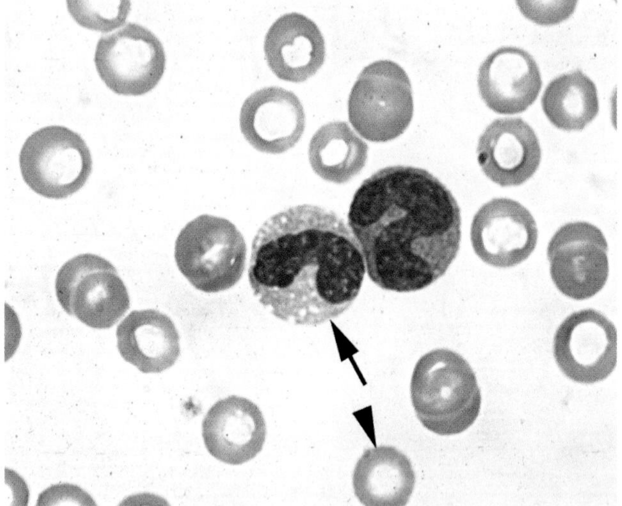

Figure 2.21 High-magnification appearance of cells in the counting area or monolayer. Note the minimal superimposition of erythrocytes, which facilitates evaluation of erythrocyte morphology (arrowhead). Leukocytes (arrow) are flattened on the slide, which makes it possible to see details of the cytoplasm and nucleus. Note that the nuclear borders are sharply delineated from the surrounding cytoplasm.

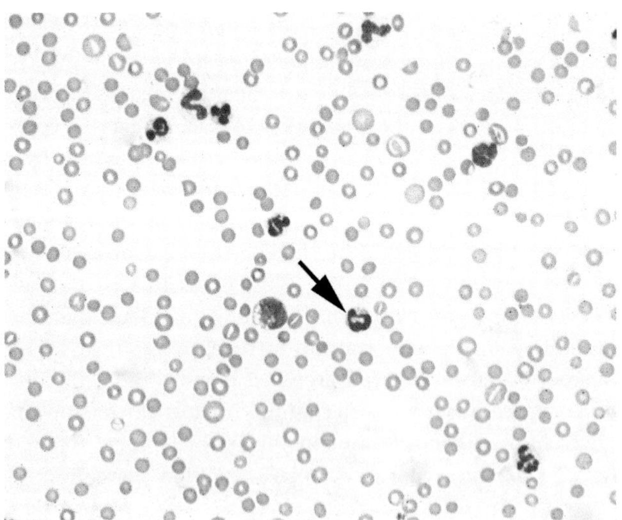

Figure 2.22 Low-magnification appearance of the counting area. Note the evenly dispersed cells and the ability to visualize the erythrocyte central pallor. The density of leukocytes (arrow) is that expected with a leukocyte concentration in the normal range.

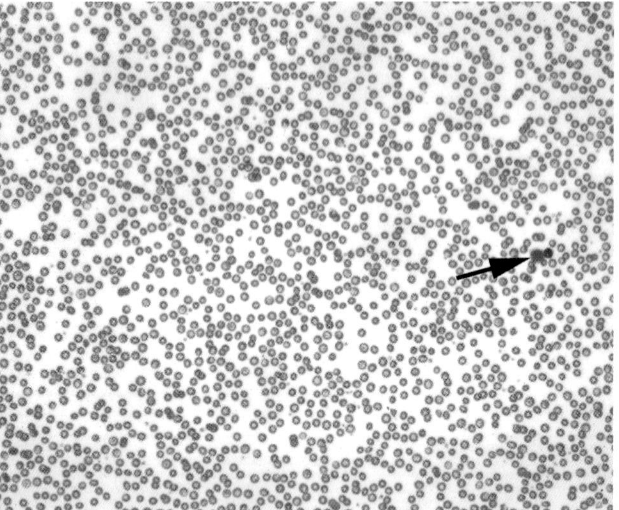

Figure 2.23 Low-magnification appearance of the counting area with a marked decrease in the leukocyte concentration. A rare leukocyte per field is present (arrow).

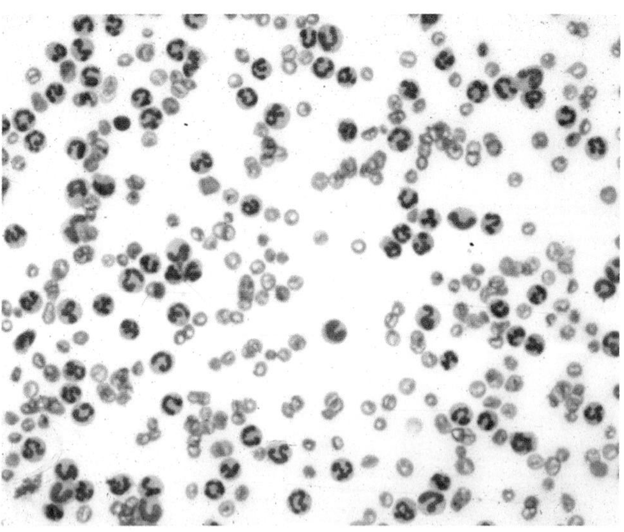

Figure 2.24 Low-magnification appearance of the counting area with a marked increase in leukocyte concentration. The density of leukocytes is considerably greater than that seen in Figure 2.22.

area, the sample is homogeneous in that cells are somewhat evenly dispersed per unit area because of sample mixing. In contrast, evaluation of cytology slides is very different. This is because the sample is likely very heterogenous in terms of distribution of elements on the slide(s). The findings that will be of interest may be completely unpredictable in terms of location on the slide. There is little to no fluid phase in which the cellular elements may be evenly mixed. The approach required is somewhat like a search and rescue mission. The procedure starts with using low power. For most, this is the 10× objective. Some will use the 4× objective, particularly on samples with low cellularity. Low power is used to scan the slide area primarily for cellular areas and secondarily to navigate to avoid areas of broken cells (thin areas) and areas of rounded up cells (thick areas). See Figure 2.20 for an example of rounded up cells in blood. Once a sense of the best areas of the slide is obtained, high magnification is used to evaluate individual cellular detail and make searches for other relevant findings. The presence of organisms is an example of an additional relevant finding in a lesion

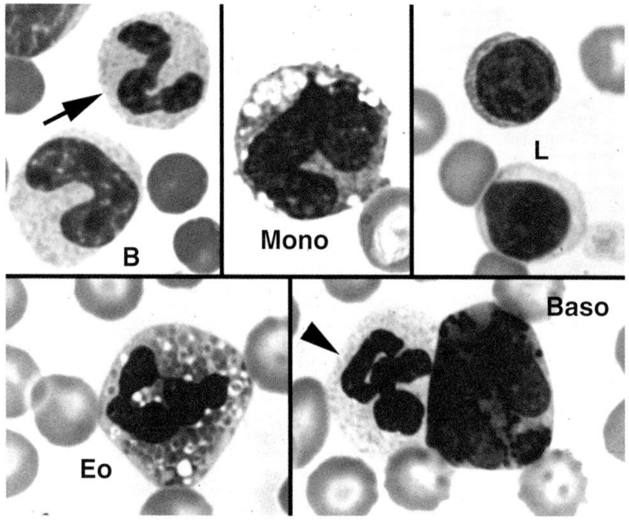

Figure 2.25 Basic leukocytes encountered in the differential count. Upper left. Neutrophils. Note the segmented neutrophil (arrow) and the constrictions in the nuclear contour. The band neutrophil (B) has smooth, parallel nuclear contours. Upper middle. Monocyte (Mono). The nucleus may have any shape, from round to bean-shaped to ameboid and band-shaped, as in this example. The cytoplasm is blue-gray and may variably contain vacuoles. Upper right. Two lymphocytes (L). Lower left. An eosinophil (Eo). Note that granules stain similar to the surrounding erythrocytes. Occasionally, granules may wash out in the staining procedure, leaving vacuoles. Lower right. Basophil (Baso) with dark granules that stain similar to nuclear chromatin. Note the adjacent neutrophil (arrowhead) and that neutrophils may have small, poorly staining granules that are much smaller than those of eosinophils or basophils.

characterized as inflammatory based on the cellular pattern present. In straightforward diagnoses, this scanning process is completed rapidly by examination of multiple fields. This is because the low-power findings appear consistent across multiple examined areas. In more complicated cases, the process of going back and forth between low and high magnification is used to assess many different areas, and sometimes multiple slides. During this process, experience is required to not be misled by confusing artifacts.

During the examination process, a cumulative description of the findings is made mentally or on paper. The findings become the basis of the diagnostic report and will support the concluding interpretation or diagnosis. Additional factors specific to examination of bone marrow aspirates are detailed in Chapter 15.

Body cavity fluids

Fluid samples are more like blood in that the distribution of elements on the slide is more homogeneous. This is because the cell population is usually evenly mixed and suspended in the background fluid. Therefore, the approach is similar to the above but can be limited to evaluation of less area. The recommended approach is to seek an area in which the cells are least rounded up. Then, use high magnification for identification of cell types present and evaluation of any morphologic abnormalities. Often, a differential count is performed to accompany a cell concentration measurement.

Analysis of diagnostic service implementation options

The veterinary facility has several options for obtaining laboratory diagnostic data. These may be generally considered as falling into three categories:

1. In-house (performed on the premises).
2. Commercial veterinary laboratory.
3. Human laboratory or community hospital.

Several factors should be considered when formulating a strategy for using one (or more) of these options. The veterinary facility should self-assess the following:

1. Type of practice (e.g., general practice, outpatient clinic, emergency facility, specialty referral center).
2. Geographic location (proximity to reliable service options).
3. Practice style of the individuals involved.
4. Willingness to implement and evaluate quality-assurance programs.
5. Willingness to invest the time to evaluate and troubleshoot diagnostics systems that have varying degrees of complexity.
6. Willingness to invest in a good microscope and training of personnel regarding basic clinical microscopy.
7. Desired turnaround times.
8. Ability to invest in instrumentation and training for the operators.

Advantages and disadvantages of in-house laboratory testing

It is known that approximately 85% of veterinary facilities utilize instrumentation for hematology and clinical chemistry to some degree. The available instrumentation has been rapidly evolving to increase sophistication and capability that approaches that of the central laboratory [1]. Modern information management allows integration of diagnostic system results into client reports as well as the electronic medical record.

Advantages of in-house laboratory testing include rapid turnaround time and control over when testing is performed relative to when samples are collected in a particular practice setting. In-house testing may also have economic advantages in certain situations.

Disadvantages of in-house laboratory testing include the issue of technical operator expertise for basic laboratory technology, which may not be available or affordable in many veterinary facilities. Attention to detail and quality assurance also must be managed by someone on site, and the investment in instrumentation is required. In addition, access to a clinical pathologist to help with the characterization of abnormal screening tests, particularly blood film analysis for hematology, must be cultivated, and arrangements for specialized testing to supplement in-clinic diagnostic tests must be procured.

Advantages and disadvantages of commercial veterinary laboratories

The major advantages of commercial veterinary laboratories are the cost leveraging of automated instrumentation and centralized testing volume, a complete menu of testing services, professional oversight of technical performance, and pathology support. Because the automated instrumentation is dedicated to animal-specific diagnostics, it is usually already adapted for the proper analysis of animal samples. Quality-control programs are usually implemented as well, but these may be variable.

The major disadvantages of commercial veterinary laboratories include relatively fixed turnaround times, which are dictated by local sample transportation logistics. In addition, sample transportation is a major part of the cost of the service.

Advantages and disadvantages of human laboratory facilities

The advantage of human laboratory facilities is that they may be the only available option in less populated areas. The disadvantages, however, are considerable. The instrumentation, particularly for hematology, is usually not modified for animal-specific diagnostics, and knowledge about the consequences is often lacking. Animal-specific pathology support is usually nonexistent or minimal. The technologists do not have training in veterinary hematology, and nobody on site can provide that training. In addition, turnaround times for animal testing may not receive the appropriate priority relative to the primary purpose of the laboratory.

Factors to consider when committing to in-house testing

Investment in instrumentation

Acquiring diagnostic capability in chemistry and hematology requires an investment of approximately $10,000–$25,000 – or more. The cost of instrumentation has somewhat stabilized in this range, but the technical capability for this investment continues to improve. For example, advanced diagnostic capability in hematology that cost in excess of $80,000 during the 1980s now has greater capability and can be obtained for $10,000–$15,000. The useful technical life span of most instrumentation should be viewed as being from 5 to 7 years. Lease plans may facilitate the acquisition of instrumentation in ways that involve planned replacement at 3–7-year intervals. Such plans may involve both the system and consumables. These plans generally pay for themselves during use by their flow of diagnostics revenue generation per month.

Commitment to personnel

Commitment to personnel requires hiring – and retaining – a technologist who is capable of reliable performance in diagnostics. Essential elements include an understanding of the basic laboratory technology, an ability to perform these procedures, a willingness to implement quality control, and a mindset that allows the technologist to seek consultation when he or she is confronted with uncertainty.

Commitment to quality assurance

A commitment to quality assurance involves a willingness to invest in periodic training regarding diagnostic technology for the personnel who perform these procedures as well as in the oversight of a regular quality assurance program [2]. The latter involves regular monitoring of instrumentation accuracy and precision using commercial control materials with known target values. This may cost from $100 to $300 per month for materials.

Establishing a pathology consultation relationship

A working relationship with a veterinary clinical pathologist to provide help with data interpretations and morphologic assessments in difficult cases, as well as microscopy support, is highly desirable. A relationship with an anatomic pathologist is also required for interpretations of surgical biopsy specimens.

The business plan

Veterinarians who are considering in-house testing must have a mindset that allows them to use diagnostics liberally as part of their practice style. Instrument salespersons may make a compelling case for how one or two CBCs per day will pay for the cost of an instrument system. The same occurs for chemistry as well. First and foremost, these schemes are profitable for the seller, but this may or may not be true for the buyer. One should not make this investment without first analyzing the costs of various alternatives, such as the use of external laboratories. Veterinarians who perform only occasional diagnostic workups likely are better off using an external laboratory. Alternatively, diagnostics may be viewed as a source of revenue if the practice style calls for a combination of frequent diagnostic workups, preanesthetic testing, and wellness testing programs. Thus, a business plan should be created that projects the number of diagnostic tests to be performed across the practice caseload. Multiplying these numbers by the projected internal charge for laboratory tests will yield the gross revenue of the proposed in-house testing effort. Recommended target values are the charges for similar tests imposed by a veterinary commercial laboratory in the region. The projected gross revenue then should be compared with the projected costs, including instrumentation amortization, consumable supplies, personnel, training, quality assurance, and time for supervision.

For chemistry, one must recognize that most of the currently available systems are not economically favorable for performing complete biochemical profiles in-house. For example, the cost of consumables per test with an in-house system may easily exceed $1–$3 per test. This cost can be higher with plans that consolidate instrument placement with a consumable use plan. By comparison, a complete biochemical profile may be obtained from a commercial laboratory for approximately $16–$20. With these circumstances, one is paying a premium for the convenience of in-house profile results, often while the client waits. In-house chemistry is more economically favorable for monitoring single tests or mini-panels after a diagnosis and treatment plan have been implemented.

Factors to consider when selecting external laboratory services

Instrument adaptation

Instrumentation must be suitably adjusted for animal blood testing. This is particularly important regarding hematologic analyses. Such adaptation is most likely to occur in veterinary commercial laboratories, and it is much less likely to be found in human hospital laboratories that analyze animal samples as a secondary priority.

Sample pickup service

Many veterinary laboratories offer once or twice daily sample pickup service to facilitate the shortest possible time from sample collection to the return of results. The tradeoff is that courier services represent a considerable fraction of the cost of the laboratory service. Human laboratory facilities usually rely on users to transport samples to the facility.

Appropriate turnaround time

In general, the rate-limiting step is transporting the sample to the laboratory. The trend toward consolidation of laboratory services, however, often results in very large transportation distances, thus extending the turnaround time. Once a sample arrives at the laboratory, most facilities perform the analyses as rapidly as possible and then electronically report the results. Laboratories that prioritize animal samples behind a busy human diagnostics schedule may not provide convenient timing for the delivery of results.

Species-specific ability

The laboratory should have the ability to recognize and interpret species-specific morphologic and pathologic abnormalities. In addition, the laboratory should be able to provide knowledgeable evaluation of abnormalities in data and morphology on blood films and cytology.

Consultation

The veterinary user must be able to consult with laboratory staff and pathologists regarding abnormal or unusual data generated by the laboratory. This may involve a combination of telephone and email.

Decision process

The analysis of one's diagnostic options may be summarized as follows: The decision process for implementing diagnostic support is complex, and this complexity is enhanced by rapidly changing technologies and services. It is advisable to run some experiments to facilitate this analysis. To maintain flexibility when uncertainty exists, it is advisable to avoid entering long-term purchase or service agreements.

3 Perspectives in Laboratory Data Interpretation and Disease Diagnosis

Glade Weiser[1] and Robin W. Allison[2]

[1]Loveland, CO, USA
[2]Department of Veterinary Pathobiology, Oklahoma State University College of Veterinary Medicine, Stillwater, OK, USA

The ability to interpret laboratory data is based on knowledge regarding the normal physiologic mechanisms underlying each laboratory test and recognition of the effects of diseases on these normal physiologic mechanisms and, therefore, on the test results themselves. With these perspectives, one can assess possible explanations for an alteration in a laboratory test result, and one can sort through these possibilities to identify the most likely explanations. If performed properly, laboratory testing and interpretation of laboratory data can provide significant insights regarding diseases and respective therapeutic options. Most chapters in this book discuss normal physiologic mechanisms and the effects of disease processes on these mechanisms as well as on laboratory test results; this chapter provides basic information that applies to the interpretation of all types of laboratory data.

Introduction

The typical laboratory diagnostic workup may consist of 30–50 different parameters or pieces of information. Laboratory reports could be more simplified. For example, about half of the values in a routine hematology report are either redundant calculations or are used solely for calculation of more important parameters. These unimportant values are not diagnostically useful and cause time-consuming clutter. However, both instrument manufacturers and laboratory service providers are reluctant to remove those parameters for fear of appearing to offer less information than competitors.

The busy clinician is faced with distilling this complex body of information into a summary that, when combined with other historical and physical findings, may diagnose health or potential disease. The veterinary clinician in training often learns this process by trial and error. The purpose here is to provide some basic background and perspective to facilitate that process. This includes an understanding of reference intervals, sensitivity/specificity of laboratory tests, knowledge of factors that may introduce errors in laboratory results, the role of laboratory quality control, and a discussion of how to develop a skilled approach to interpreting laboratory data.

Reference interval background

To recognize laboratory results as being abnormal, the values expected to be obtained from healthy animals must be known. These normal values are correctly termed reference intervals; although they may also be referred to as reference ranges, this is technically incorrect since the term "range" refers to a single number describing the difference between two values. A reference interval is typically defined as values encompassing the median 95% of a tested population of apparently healthy animals. Inherent in this definition is that 2.5% of the healthy population will have values outside either side of the median 95%, suggesting they are abnormal.

When interpreting patient data, the first interpretive step is to sort data into normal and abnormal values. Flagging each abnormal value on the laboratory report form often starts this process. Information systems can do this by comparing the value against the defined reference interval. However, determination of abnormal is not as simple as it may seem for a couple of reasons. First, reference intervals are usually based on limited population testing and do not account for variation within subpopulations defined by age, sex, breed, or other factors. Second, one must think probabilistically about values that are near the reference limit. An abnormal flag does not necessarily mean the value is abnormal for that animal.

Veterinary Hematology, Clinical Chemistry, and Cytology, Third Edition. Edited by Mary Anna Thrall, Glade Weiser, Robin W. Allison and Terry W. Campbell.

Companion website: www.wiley.com/go/thrall/veterinary

Different statistical methods can be used to establish reference intervals, but all of them begin with the sampling of animals from an apparently healthy population. In most cases, healthy animals are those that have no apparent illness and have no detectable abnormality in cursory examination. Reference intervals must be established for each species being tested, but such intervals would ideally also be established for subdivisions within that species when some characteristic of a subgroup results in significantly different reference intervals compared with those for the species as a whole. These subdivisions might occur on the basis of age, breed, gender, pregnancy status, or type of husbandry. Because establishing reference intervals is an expensive, time-consuming task, intervals for such subdivisions are usually not established, and veterinarians generally use a single reference interval for all animals of a given species. When this is the case, it is important to consider variations in those test results that could relate to the previously mentioned characteristics (e.g., age, breed, gender) and to consider these characteristics when evaluating the possible causes of values falling outside the reference interval (especially mildly abnormal values). For example, the hematocrit (HCT) reference interval for dogs is usually regarded to be approximately 36–55%. However, it is known that some small breeds, notably the poodle, typically have HCT values in the 50s. A poodle dog with an HCT of 42 may be anemic. Another example is the serum enzyme alkaline phosphatase (ALP). Because bone remodeling is a potential source for this enzyme, serum ALP activity is considerably greater in young growing animals than in adults of the same species. Many such interpretive nuances are developed from experience. Refinement of population subset reference intervals may someday be performed in veterinary medicine, but this will require compilation of a huge database.

Adequate numbers of normal animals must be sampled to develop intervals that are valid for healthy animals from the defined population. In general, the more animals that are sampled, the more likely the reference intervals will truly reflect the range of values to be expected from healthy animals. Sampling large numbers of animals to make the results most reflective of the healthy population is desirable, but practical constraints (e.g., availability of apparently healthy animals, costs of obtaining samples and of performing large numbers of tests) dictate limits on the number of animals that can actually be tested. For best reliability, at least 120 samples should be analyzed when establishing reference intervals. The minimum number of samples to establish a crude reference interval is generally considered to be 40.

Several statistical methods exist for establishing reference intervals. The method of using mean ±2 SD was historically used to define the median 95% of the tested population, but this is only valid if the test results have a normal or Gaussian distribution (Figure 3.1a). This approach is flawed if the test results are not normally distributed (Figure 3.1b).

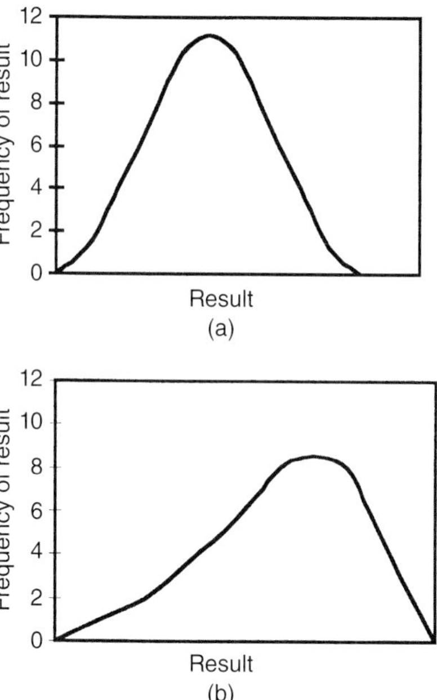

Figure 3.1 Two distributions of values resulting from sampling a large number of apparently healthy animals. (a) Plotted by their frequency of occurrence, these values form a symmetric, bell-shaped curve. This is known as a normal or Gaussian distribution. (b) Plotted by their frequency of occurrence, these values form an asymmetric distribution that is skewed toward the higher values. This is not a normal distribution (a non-Gaussian distribution).

It is now thought that most laboratory test data are not normally distributed. A simple solution is to derive reference intervals using a nonparametric technique. With nonparametric methods, all of the test values are rank ordered, any outliers are removed, and then the middle 95% of test results define the reference interval. As an example, for a population of 120 rank-ordered results, the lowest 3 and highest 3 ($2.5\% \times 120 = 3$) are removed, and the remaining results define the median 95% of the population. A few values from the apparently healthy sample population might be markedly higher or lower than most of the other values. These extreme values are known as outliers and are likely indicative of occult disease. If outliers are included in the sampled values when the intervals are calculated, they will widen the reference intervals, thus making the test less sensitive for the detection of unhealthy animals. One relatively simple rule of thumb for defining an outlier is to calculate the difference between the highest (or lowest) value and the second-highest (or lowest) value. If this difference exceeds one-third of the range of all values, then consider the highest (or lowest) value to be an outlier, and eliminate it when calculating the reference intervals. Once this value has been eliminated, the same test can be applied to the next highest (or lowest) value. For example, Figure 3.2 presents the blood glucose values obtained from a population of 120 apparently healthy animals plotted in

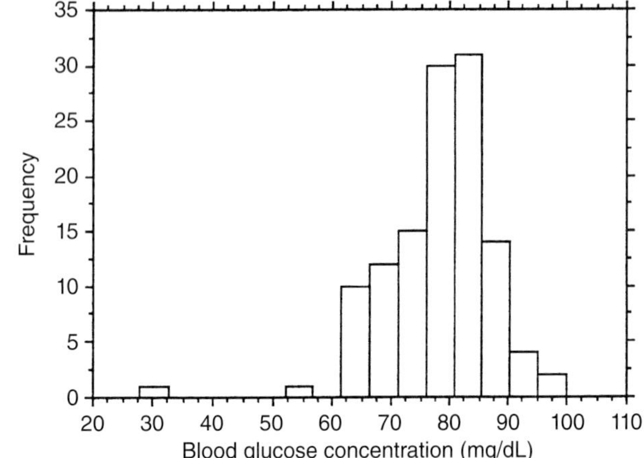

Figure 3.2 Blood glucose values obtained from a population of 120 apparently healthy animals and plotted in a frequency distribution histogram. Frequency represents the total number of samples with that blood glucose concentration.

a frequency distribution histogram. One value (30 mg/dl) is obviously much lower than the others. The difference between this value and the next lowest value is 25 mg/dl, and the range of all values is 70 mg/dl (100–30 mg/dl). Because 25 mg/dl is greater than one-third of the range of all values (70 ÷ 3 = 23.3), the lowest value (30 mg/dl) is eliminated as an outlier. If this value is eliminated, the difference between the remaining lowest value (55 mg/dl) and the next lowest value is then 10 mg/dl. This is less than one-third of the range of all remaining values (45 ÷ 3 = 15) and, therefore, should not be eliminated as an outlier.

An example of establishing a reference interval by the rank order nonparametric method is presented in Table 3.1, which uses the data as presented in Figure 3.2. As noted earlier, one value (30 mg/dl) has been eliminated as an outlier; therefore, the range of the remaining 119 values is 55–100 mg/dl. Identifying and eliminating those values in the lowest 2.5% and in the highest 2.5% then determines the central 95% of these ranked values.

The statistical method just described is applicable when the sampled population includes 40 or more animals. If fewer than 40 animals are sampled, the lower and upper 2.5% of values cannot be reliably determined. In such a case, the reference interval is considered to be the observed range of values that remains after the outliers have been eliminated. Such a reference interval is less reliable than those determined from a larger population.

Limiting reference intervals to 95% rather than 100% of values obtained from healthy animals is an attempt to maximize detection of diseased animals. As defined by reference intervals, approximately 5% of healthy animals will have values considered to be abnormal for any given test.

Table 3.1 An example of nonparametric determination of a reference interval.[a]

Lowest 10 values and their ranks										
Value	30	55	65	65	65	65	65	65	65	65
Rank	1	2	3	4	5	6	7	8	9	10
Highest 10 values and their ranks										
Value	90	90	90	90	95	95	95	95	100	100
Rank	110	111	112	113	114	115	116	117	118	119
Highest value of the lower 2.5% = 0.025 × (number of values + 1)										
Highest value of the lower 2.5% = 0.025 × (119 + 1) = **3**										
Lowest value of the upper 2.5% = 0.975 × (number of values + 1)										
Lowest value of the upper 2.5% = 0.975 × (119 + 1) = **117**										
Lower values eliminated from reference interval										
Value	30	55	65							
Rank	1	2	3							
Upper values eliminated from reference interval										
Value	95	100	100							
Rank	117	118	119							
Resulting reference interval = 65–95										

[a] Blood glucose concentrations were obtained from 120 apparently healthy animals, and one of these values was eliminated as an outlier (see Figure 3.2). The method involves ranking values from lowest to highest, calculation of ranks representing the highest rank of the lower 2.5% of values and the lowest rank of the upper 2.5% of values, and eliminating values corresponding to these ranks as well as values corresponding to lower and higher ranks, respectively. The remaining values are the central 95% and are used as the reference interval.

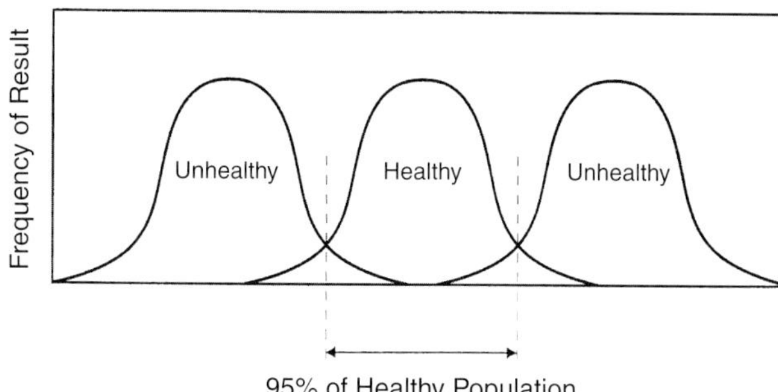

Figure 3.3 The overlap of laboratory values that can be expected from healthy and unhealthy populations (populations with diseases that cause either decreases or increases in the values for a given test). Note that defining the reference interval at 95% of the healthy population excludes the values from some healthy animals, but it also excludes the values from most unhealthy ones (i.e., it allows one to recognize these animals as being potentially unhealthy). If the reference interval were broadened to include more of the potential values from healthy animals, it would also recognize more values from unhealthy animals as being normal (i.e., the unhealthy animal might not be detected). Using a reference interval based on 95% of the healthy population is a compromise that increases the sensitivity of the test for recognizing unhealthy animals while causing only a few healthy animals to be recognized as being potentially unhealthy.

By extension, if many tests are performed on an individual animal (as is common in biochemical profiles), the likelihood of that individual having at least one abnormal test result increases dramatically. For example, in a 20-test biochemical profile, approximately 64% of healthy animals will have at least one abnormal value. It is also possible that animals with disease may have respective laboratory values just within the reference interval. One must recognize the reality that healthy and unhealthy animals overlap at each end of the reference interval (Figure 3.3). Thus, the concept of a black-and-white delineation between normal and abnormal does not exist. The clinician must learn to think probabilistically about laboratory data, particularly for values close to reference limits. Therefore, laboratory values that are close to the reference limits need to be more closely correlated with the patient history, clinical signs, or other laboratory data to assess the likelihood that they represent disease. Test results that are markedly above or below the reference limits, however, are more easily recognized as representing disease.

An adjunct to population reference intervals is the individual health database. Ideally, a laboratory value database is established for young adult companion animals or other animals of value. This data may serve to identify more precisely where that animal's values reside relative to the more broad range of the general species population. For example, a dog has an HCT value of 52% defined in its health database. If sometime later the HCT is measured at 39%, there is a high probability of an underlying disease resulting in anemia, even though the laboratory report may not flag the value as abnormal.

Sensitivity, specificity, and predictive values

When interpreting laboratory abnormalities, the concepts of sensitivity, specificity, and predictive values must be considered. Sensitivity is a measure of the frequency with which the test result will be positive or abnormal in animals with the respective disease process. The following formula is used to determine sensitivity:

$$\text{Sensitivity}(\%) = \frac{\text{TP}}{\text{TP} + \text{FN}} \times 100$$

where TP (true positive) is the total number of animals that tested positive and actually have the disease process, and FN (false negative) is the total number of animals that tested negative but actually have the disease. For instance, if the sensitivity of a test for a disease is 99%, then 99 of 100 animals with that disease will have a positive (i.e., abnormal) result. One percent of the animals with the disease will have a negative (i.e., normal) result; that is, 1% of the tests would have false-negative results. Specificity is a measure of the frequency with which the test result will be negative or normal in animals without the disease one wishes to detect. The following formula is used to determine specificity:

$$\text{Specificity}(\%) = \frac{\text{TN}}{\text{TN} + \text{FP}} \times 100$$

where TN (true negative) is the total number of animals that tested negative and actually do not have the disease, and FP (false positive) is the total number of animals that tested positive but actually do not have the disease. For instance, if the specificity of a test for a disease is 99%, then 99 of 100 nonaffected animals will have negative (i.e., normal) results. One percent of nonaffected animals will have a positive (i.e., abnormal) result; that is, 1% of the tests would have false-positive results.

Sensitivity and specificity are established by applying the test in question to animals with known disease status (i.e., animals known to have or not have the disease in question). Another diagnostic procedure, often termed the "gold standard," is used to establish which animals do or do not have the disease. This gold standard is often another laboratory test known to be reliable for detecting the disease. Sensitivity and specificity, therefore, do not apply directly to animals of unknown disease status, but they do provide information regarding the reliability of the test in question for detecting that disease.

In practice, one needs to know the reliability of a test for detecting a certain disease in animals with unknown disease status. In other words, how reliable is an abnormal or a normal test result for predicting whether the animal does or does not have the disease in question? In this situation, predictive values define the chances that abnormal or normal test results are reliable indicators of disease status. Predictive values depend on the sensitivity and specificity of a test, but the prevalence or likelihood of the disease in the population being tested affects predictive values as well. Such prevalence or likelihood of disease is established before performing the test, based on the judgment of the veterinarian of the chance (expressed as a percentage) that the animal has the disease in question. This judgment can be based on several other observations, including patient history, clinical signs, other test results, and epidemiologic data. Both positive (i.e., abnormal) and negative (i.e., normal) test results have predictive values. The predictive value of a positive test (positive predictive value) is the probability that a positive (abnormal) test result truly indicates the animal has the disease:

$$\text{Positive Predictive Value} = \frac{\text{TP}}{\text{TP} + \text{FP}} \times 100$$

where TP is the total number of animals that tested positive and actually have the disease, and FP is the total number of animals that tested positive but actually do not have the disease. The higher the predictive value of a positive test, the more likely it is that an animal with a positive (i.e., abnormal) test result actually has the disease in question. Tests with high positive predictive values will produce few false-positive results; thus confidence is high in a positive test result.

The predictive value of a negative test (negative predictive value) is the probability that a negative (normal) test result truly indicates the animal does not have the disease:

$$\text{Negative Predictive value} = \frac{\text{TN}}{\text{TN} + \text{FN}} \times 100$$

where TN is the total number of animals that tested negative and actually do not have the disease, and FN is the total number of animals that tested negative but actually do have the disease. The higher the predictive value of a negative test, the more likely it is that an animal with a negative test result does not have the disease in question. Tests with high negative predictive values will produce few false-negative results; thus confidence is high in a negative test result. As stated previously, predictive values are determined from a combination of the sensitivity and specificity of the test and the veterinarian's pretest judgment regarding the likelihood of the disease in that animal. A rather complex formula to estimate predictive values based on these factors does exist, but the roles of sensitivity, specificity, and disease prevalence or likelihood in the interpretation of diagnostic test results can be understood without it. The roles of these three factors are best understood by considering a hypothetic situation in which an excellent diagnostic test is used to detect a specific disease. The heartworm antigen test is a good example of such a diagnostic for which there is abundant data. This test has a sensitivity of 99% (i.e., it will be positive or abnormal in 99 of 100 animals with the disease) and specificity of 99% (i.e., it will be negative or normal in 99 of 100 animals without the disease). This test has excellent performance when applied in areas with reasonable prevalence of heartworm infection. However, if this test is used for screening a population of animals in which you, as the veterinarian, judge there is a 1% chance of the disease being present, the following predictive values result:

$$\text{Predictive value of a positive test} = 50\%$$

$$\text{Predictive value of a negative test} = 100\%$$

In other words, a positive or abnormal test is correct 50% of the time and incorrect 50% of the time. This is equivalent in reliability to flipping a coin, and it might lead one to question the wisdom of performing such a test in a population with a low likelihood of disease. In this situation, however, a negative or normal test result is almost 100% reliable in ruling out the possibility that an animal has the disease (i.e., the predictive value of a negative test is approximately 100%). This combination of excellent test sensitivity and specificity with low prevalence or likelihood of disease is quite common when using serologic tests to screen for various infectious diseases.

Because most diagnostic tests have an inherent sensitivity and specificity, the most easily altered factor that affects the predictive value is the pretest likelihood of the disease. Veterinarians can use this to enhance the predictive values. For instance, in the previous example, a test with excellent sensitivity and specificity was used to screen for a disease in a population with a low prevalence of that disease. This resulted in a low positive predictive value. If, however, a veterinarian were presented with an animal that had a history, clinical signs, and other features suggesting that disease, such an animal would represent a different population, and the veterinarian would establish a different, higher pretest likelihood for that disease. In such a case, the veterinarian would, perhaps, be 75% certain that the animal had the disease in question. Therefore, the predictive value of a positive test result would be nearly 100%, and the predictive value of a negative test result would be approximately 97%. The test result in this scenario would, in fact, be very reliable for predicting the presence or absence of the disease in question.

In summary, the more likely that an animal has a certain disease before the test is performed, the more reliable a positive or abnormal test result suggesting the presence of that disease will be. The effects of the pretest likelihood of disease on the positive and negative predictive values of a test are demonstrated in Figures 3.4 and 3.5. In practice, most veterinarians incorporate this approach to diagnostic testing instinctively. If the test result is compatible with the disease the veterinarian suspected before conducting the test, this result is considered to be supportive evidence that the

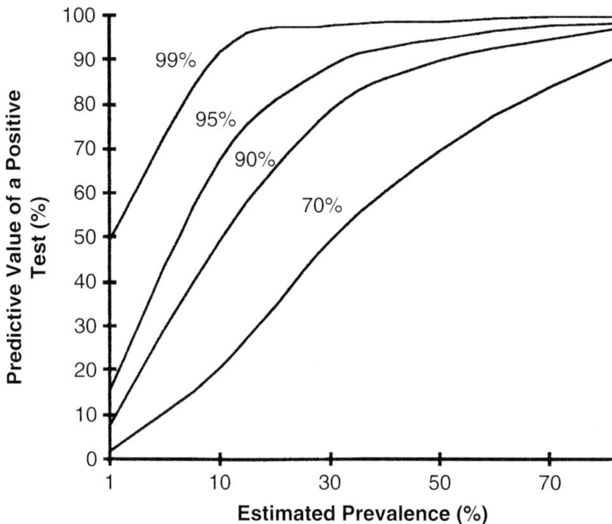

Figure 3.4 The effect of various pretest estimates of disease likelihood on the predictive value of a positive test. Each line represents a different level of sensitivity and specificity (99% = 99% sensitivity and specificity, 95% = 95% sensitivity and specificity, and so on). The predictive value of a positive test decreases as the pretest estimate of disease likelihood decreases.

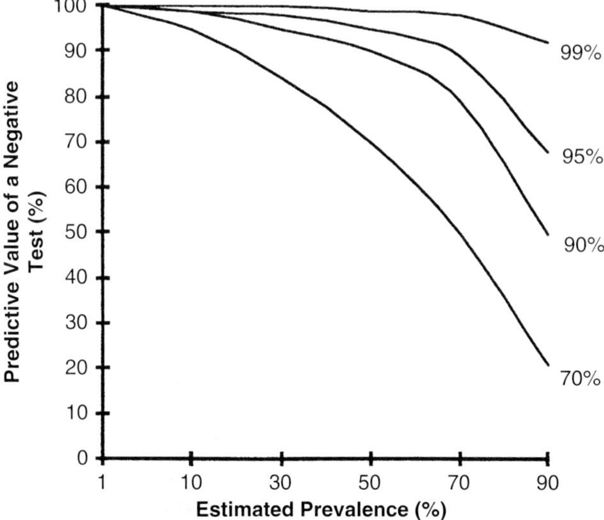

Figure 3.5 The effect of various pretest estimates of disease likelihood on the predictive value of a negative test. Each line represents a different level of sensitivity and specificity (99% = 99% sensitivity and specificity, 95% = 95% sensitivity and specificity, and so on). The predictive value of a negative test increases as the pretest estimate of disease likelihood decreases.

animal has the disease; if the result is not compatible with the suspected disease, the veterinarian does not completely rule out that disease but does begin to consider other options more seriously. Biochemical abnormalities that suggest a disease that was not strongly suspected before the profile was completed will occasionally be detected, and in this situation, these abnormalities are not as reliable in predicting that disease as they would be had the disease been previously suspected.

Most routine clinical pathology tests (i.e., hematology, biochemistry, and urinalysis) have sensitivities and specificities for detecting any given disease that are considerably less than the 99% in the previous example. This makes the pretest likelihood of disease an even more important factor in this type of testing. For instance, both the sensitivity and specificity of the pancreatic enzyme amylase for detecting pancreatitis are quite low. Serum amylase activity is routinely measured on some biochemical profiles. Thus, an increased serum amylase activity on a biochemical screen from a dog in which pancreatitis was not previously suspected would have a very low positive predictive value, because the sensitivity, specificity, and pretest likelihood of pancreatitis are all low. On the other hand, an increased serum amylase activity on a biochemical profile from a dog with clinical signs that suggest pancreatitis would have a much higher positive predictive value. This concept is important to remember whenever unexpected abnormalities are detected on any routine clinical pathology test.

Quality control

To obtain reliable laboratory test results, the quality of the results being produced must be monitored so that they are both accurate and precise. Accuracy is a gauge of how close the result is to the true value for that test, and precision is a gauge of how repeatable the result is when assaying the same sample. A single result might be accurate, for instance, but if a similar result cannot be obtained repeatedly using the same sample (i.e., if the test is not precise), then the results for that assay are not reliable. Conversely, one may obtain the same result repeatedly using the same sample, but if that result does not reflect the true value for the substance being measured (i.e., if the test is not accurate), then the results again are not reliable.

Reputable laboratories maintain quality-control programs to ensure the accuracy and precision of their results. This is accomplished by assaying control samples at previously determined intervals along with the samples from patients. These intervals might be daily or several times per day, depending on the workload of the laboratory. The control samples are similar to those from patients (e.g., blood or serum) and are usually obtained from a commercial source. Control samples can be categorized as either assayed (i.e., the probable accurate value for the test in that control sample has been previously determined) or unassayed (i.e., the probable accurate value for the test in that control sample has not been previously determined). If unassayed control samples are obtained, the laboratory then establishes the probable accurate value for that sample using methods similar to those summarized earlier for determining reference intervals. Because establishing such probable accurate values is both time-consuming and expensive, most laboratories today use assayed control samples. Only assayed controls are suitable for in-clinic quality control.

During routine laboratory operation, the result from each control sample is compared with what is documented to be the accurate result for that sample. This tests the accuracy of the assay. In addition, results obtained from the control sample over time are analyzed to determine if the value obtained changes over time, thus establishing the precision of the test. Both accuracy and precision usually are assessed by graphing the values obtained from the control sample on a quality-control chart (Figure 3.6). Some instrumentation will have onboard software for automated analysis and management of quality-control data. If the results obtained from the control sample are outside the previously established acceptable range, which is also known as the control limit (usually ±2–3 SD from the mean), or if the results drift either up or down over time, then a problem with the analytic instrument, reagents, or operator may exist. Results obtained from patient samples during these "out-of-control" periods are rejected, and the analytic methods used are carefully reviewed to correct the problem.

Quality-control programs are common in large reference laboratories, but they are also important for in-clinic laboratories. Manufacturers may supply quality-control materials with laboratory instruments. These programs should be followed in detail to have some assurance that the results produced by the in-clinic laboratory are reliable.

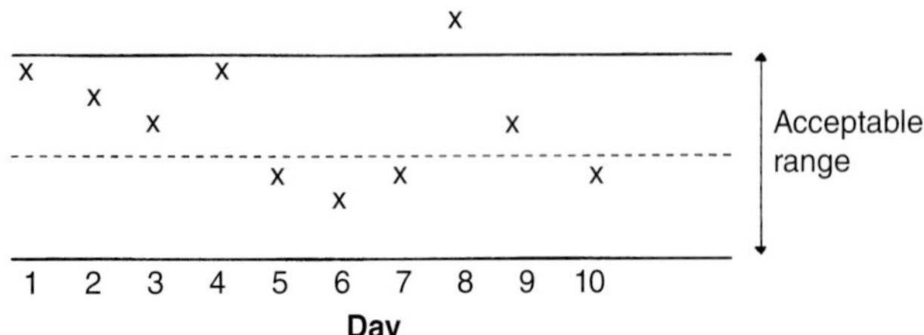

Figure 3.6 An example of a quality-control chart used to monitor the accuracy and precision of a laboratory test. To produce this chart, a control sample was analyzed each day along with the patient samples. Daily results from the control sample are plotted (X). The dashed line (- - -) represents the expected mean value for this sample. Solid lines (—) represent acceptable positive and negative variation from the mean value. Note that the result on Day 8 was outside the acceptable range of variation. This would trigger rejection of the results for the test on that day until completion of an assessment of the instrument, reagents, and operator to identify and correct the problem. The chart indicates problem resolution on Day 9 with acceptable control performance.

Common factors that introduce error in laboratory values

There are a number of factors that can cause laboratory test result errors that may affect interpretation of the patient status. These should be considered whenever a laboratory result(s) is either nonsensical or does not match the patient's condition. These factors can be classified as preanalytical, analytical, and postanalytical errors. Preanalytical errors are the most common and may be introduced by a number of problems related to sample collection and handling. Analytical errors occur at the level of the test methodology and may be due to either an interfering substance or phenomenon within the sample or a problem with the test method performance. The latter is now relatively rare and is typically recognized and prevented with a quality-control program. Postanalytical errors may be due to transcription or other errors related to report generation and distribution. Postanalytical errors are also relatively rare with the current use of automated laboratory information systems and report generation.

Sample handling errors

A number of preanalytical factors may result in laboratory test errors. Improper handling of samples is the most common cause of gross errors in laboratory test values. These are procedural errors that violate handling rules related to sample stability or other processing variables. Some common sample handling errors in veterinary facilities include:

- Sample labeling and transcription errors, leading to data assigned to the wrong patient.
- Use of wrong anticoagulant
- Inappropriate anticoagulant contamination of the sample.
- Improper ratio of anticoagulant to sample.
- Traumatic transfer of blood to tubes causing hemolysis (see below).
- Improper storage conditions during transportation to a laboratory.
- Improper sample storage conditions before analysis.
- Lack of or insufficient mixing of blood for hematology measurements.

There are specific sample handling procedures that must be followed to ensure sample quality, and these may vary depending upon the laboratory test being requested. Central laboratories provide these procedures for proper sample submission. Suppliers of in-clinic diagnostic instrumentation also provide these procedures. Failures related to these procedures occur because the person(s) involved are either not aware of them or are not paying attention to detail. It is the responsibility of the veterinary facility to ensure that the respective procedures be followed exactly to minimize associated errors in laboratory results. The various personnel in the

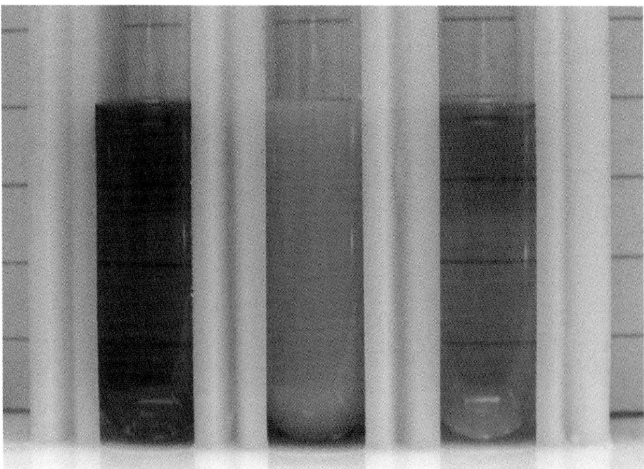

Figure 3.7 Hemolysis, lipemia, and hyperbilirubinemia (left to right) in serum samples. Lipemic serum here is tinged pink as a result of concurrent hemolysis; it may appear white to red-tinged.

veterinary facility often have limited training in laboratory technology. For this reason, it is recommended that facilities designate a lead person or key laboratory operator to educate others about and monitor laboratory-related procedures.

Interfering substances: lipemia, hemolysis, and hyperbilirubinemia

An interfering substance is a common source of analytical error that is present in the sample. Hemolysis, lipemia, and increased serum bilirubin (Figure 3.7) can potentially affect the results of biochemical assays. Hemolysis refers to the lysis of erythrocytes and liberation of hemoglobin and may occur either in the circulating blood (*in vivo*) or during or after blood collection (*in vitro*). Hemolysis in the sample is usually due to improper sample collection or handling. Hemolysis may interfere with assay results by color interference with spectrophotometric assays. Less commonly, hemolysis may cause a false increase in analyte being measured as a result of marked differential concentrations or enzyme activities between serum and erythrocytes. For instance, horses and cattle have high concentrations of potassium within erythrocytes, whereas dogs (with some exceptions) and cats do not. Therefore, marked hemolysis may result in a falsely increased serum potassium concentration in horses and cattle, but not in most dogs or in cats.

Lipemia causes visible turbidity of the serum, often making it opaque to transmitted light. It is expected to occur in small animals when they have not been fasted before blood collection. It may also occur in hyperlipidemic syndromes. This interference with light transmission can interfere with spectrophotometric assays, particularly in liquid or cuvette chemistry systems. It can also result in apparent dilution of normal substances (e.g., electrolytes) in the aqueous component of serum, resulting in falsely decreased concentrations (ion exclusion effect).

Increased serum bilirubin concentrations result in a serum with a darker-yellow color than normal for that species. This increased color can interfere with the results of spectrophotometric assays.

The potential alterations in biochemistry results caused by hemolysis, lipemia, and hyperbilirubinemia vary with the substance being assayed and with the method being used for the assay itself. Reference laboratories usually can provide specific information regarding the effects of hemolysis, lipemia, or hyperbilirubinemia on test results. Likewise, manufacturers may provide this information for in-house diagnostic laboratory instrumentation.

It is also conceivable that drugs and other chemicals may alter laboratory test reactions. Known interferents are typically outlined in reagent application sheets. This information is usually available from the laboratory or in the form of technical briefs from diagnostics suppliers.

Approach to interpreting laboratory data

Comments on general approach

It is important to appreciate that individual diagnostic test results are rarely interpretable into a clinical diagnosis. Abnormal test results typically indicate a relatively nonspecific pathologic process. Grouping of several abnormal results may improve the specificity of the process or processes. It is usually only after integration of history, physical findings, and other diagnostic procedures with laboratory data abnormalities that a more defined clinical diagnosis is achieved. Most laboratory abnormalities have multiple potential causes, and the history and physical examination results should be used to determine which of these potential causes is most likely. Using a combination of history, physical examination results, and the pattern of laboratory abnormalities, the veterinarian should attempt to summarize the likely operative pathologic processes present. This summary can often be translated into a working clinical diagnosis or diagnoses. Patterns of abnormal test results often suggest which tissue or organ systems are affected, which pathologic processes are occurring, or both. For example, a combination of an increased concentration of blood urea nitrogen (BUN; a test of kidney function) with a urine specific gravity indicative of inadequate urine concentration is very suggestive of renal failure, whereas an increased BUN with concentrated urine (high specific gravity) is more suggestive of conditions such as dehydration or shock.

Of course, not every abnormality will fit neatly into one disease process, nor will every laboratory profile result in a specific diagnosis. In some cases, more than one disease process may be occurring, thereby producing a confusing combination of abnormalities. These are considered difficult cases that may require analysis over time to unravel and may benefit from consultation or second opinion interaction with associates.

Analysis of sequential changes in laboratory values over time is sometimes helpful in establishing a diagnosis and is important for monitoring progress of the disease or case management. For instance, periodic determinations of BUN in an animal with renal failure may indicate whether treatment to reestablish renal function is succeeding (i.e., BUN should be decreasing) or not. Negative findings in the form of normal test results also have value. These can rule out tentative differential diagnoses that were considered on the basis of history or physical examination findings.

Expectations and skilled diagnostics interpretation

Behind the scenes of the general approach described above, there are a number of nuances that may be described as expectations related to diagnostics. Sometimes clinicians are handicapped by unrealistic expectations for laboratory data. The discussion here is aimed at clarifying some of the more common expectations to aid the clinician-in-training to be more adept at data interpretation. Important considerations include the following:

- How measurement reproducibility affects data interpretation.
- Magnitude of change associated with disease(s).
- Relationships or interdependency between diagnostic tests.
- Reference intervals and the elusive determination of what is normal vs. abnormal.
- Laboratory test results that are inconsistent with preconceived notions.

Measurement reproducibility

This is discussed first because it influences other expectations and is important for interpretation of sequential laboratory data. A common misconception is that the numbers on a laboratory report are definitive numbers. The reality is that if an individual test is repeated multiple times on the same sample by the same method in the same laboratory, a range of results will be obtained. If results are produced by two different laboratory methods, even more variation may be encountered. Actual reproducibility will vary, but some guidelines for satisfactory analytical performance for a single method are:

- Most hematology results – ±10% of value.
- Platelets – ±20% of value.
- Most clinical chemistry results – ±10% of value.
- Enzyme activities in clinical chemistry – ±15% of value.

When comparing results between laboratories or methods, even greater variation should be expected.

A practical understanding of the expected reproducibility results in the following interpretive guidelines:

- Data must be interpreted with some latitude, especially when test results are near reference limits. This is discussed further under "Interpreting Normal Versus Abnormal."
- When two different laboratories or methods generate results for the same sample, relatively large differences in "numbers" may occur, but usually the interpretation of those numbers is the same. This often occurs when comparing in-house results with commercial laboratory results.
- When a new sample is analyzed to evaluate patient change, only relatively large change should be interpreted as conclusive change in the patient.

Magnitude of change associated with disease

Considerable experience is required to understand the relationship between the *magnitude* of a given laboratory test abnormality and the *severity* of the associated disease condition. It is not practical to communicate detailed guidelines for all laboratory tests in this chapter. Small numerical changes or abnormalities indicate important or severe disease for some laboratory tests. Examples might include pH, potassium (K^+), creatinine, calcium, phosphorus, albumin, and endocrine assays. For most other laboratory tests, it takes a considerably larger numerical change or abnormality to indicate important or severe disease. Examples include enzyme activities, BUN, glucose, and most hematologic measurements.

The desired interpretive experience comes from repeated analysis of clinical case material. A starting point for veterinarians-in-training includes case discussions in various classes. This is narrated to some degree in various chapters in this textbook, and case presentations at the end of this textbook provide some representative examples. This knowledge is then expanded upon with the clinical cases encountered during the first several years of practice.

Relationships between diagnostic tests

Laboratory tests are more meaningful when interpreted in groupings that are interrelated with respect to pathophysiology. For example, a moderately abnormal increased BUN interpreted in isolation may define the relatively nonspecific process of decreased glomerular filtration rate. However, when grouped with hematocrit, total protein, creatinine, phosphorus, and urinalysis findings, the integrated interpretation is likely to be much more specific as to the probable cause of decreased glomerular filtration rate. In addition, the other values may corroborate each other when there is a question about the validity of a given value. Ideally, laboratory reports are organized in a way to provide some initial grouping that facilitates this relationship in interpretation. This is often organized by organ system, realizing that some analytes may have secondary relationships with more than one organ system. However, chemistry, hematology, and urinalysis reports are almost always segregated. The user must learn how to cross-interpret sections of the report to

Table 3.2 Grouping of laboratory tests for interpretation. Hematology is interpreted separately, but abnormalities may be referable to chemical abnormalities in the groups below.

Kidney	Liver	Metabolic	Specialty
BUN	Bilirubin	Glucose	CK
Creatinine	ALT	Calcium	Amylase
Phosphorus	AST	Total protein	Lipase
Urinalysis:	ALP	Albumin	Endocrine tests
Specific gravity	GGT	Cholesterol	Immunoassays
Chemistry	Bile acids	Sodium	Other special tests
Microscopic		Chloride	
		Potassium	
		pH	
		HCO_3	
		pO_2 (arterial)	

BUN, blood urea nitrogen; ALT, alanine aminotransferase; AST, aspartate aminotransferase; ALP, alkaline phosphatase; GGT, gamma glutamyltransferase; CK, creatine kinase.

achieve all of the useful groupings. Table 3.2 shows one method of grouping laboratory tests that achieves most of the primary relationships for integrated interpretation. This is a place to start, realizing that secondary relationships will become more apparent with experience.

Interpreting normal versus abnormal

As discussed in the section "Reference Interval Background," laboratory data is often not conclusively interpretable as normal or abnormal, particularly when values are near the limits of the reference interval. Laboratory reports may contain flags, usually H for high or L for low. This flagging conditions the user to think too strictly about normal versus abnormal. Clinicians should be encouraged to interpret borderline and mildly abnormal values more loosely, in a probabilistic manner. When a laboratory test result is suspiciously abnormal, look for corroboration in other findings. Also factor in possible age and known breed considerations for suspect values.

Laboratory test results that are inconsistent with preconceived notions

Occasionally the clinician is surprised by an unexpected lab test value that is moderately or markedly abnormal. A common first reaction is to not believe the result is possible. A more appropriate reaction is to reanalyze the clinical situation. One should look for other laboratory values or undetected clinical abnormalities that may corroborate the value(s) in question. The history and physical should be reevaluated for findings that may corroborate the abnormal value; additional questions may need to be asked of the owner. Next, the possibility of a sample or sample handling error should be considered. Last, if no corroboration or errors can be found, it may be appropriate to repeat the test in question.

Summary of interpretive considerations

When interpreting laboratory data in conjunction with all other clinical and physical findings, remain aware of the following interpretive factors. With practice, these become habit of the astute clinician:

- Interpret laboratory values in related groups, organized by organ system.
- Interpret laboratory values probabilistically for abnormality, particularly when values are borderline with respect to the reference interval limits.
- Develop a sense of the expected magnitude of change in a value that is associated with important disease.
- Consider that analytical reproducibility is such that only relatively large changes in sequential values are indicative of true change.
- When laboratory values initially do not seemingly fit the clinical condition(s), evaluate for corroborating laboratory and clinical data.
- Train staff to prevent improper sample handling and interfering substances that may lead to erroneous laboratory data. Consider these possibilities when laboratory data is seemingly nonsensical.

Perspective on use of cytopathology

Pattern recognition is often portrayed in classrooms and textbooks as "easy." This is done using optimally prepared samples and then selecting images that are most representative of a specific diagnosis or interpretation. It is not so easy given the complexity of diagnostic expectations in place today. As a result, maximizing diagnostic yield usually requires the experience of an accomplished clinical pathologist.

By way of historical background, the teaching of diagnostic cytology for use in the veterinary practice setting was started by limited application to superficial swellings or growth lesions. Cytology was largely a screening procedure to determine if the process was inflammatory or neoplastic. If inflammation such as an abscess was ruled out, biopsy with histology was utilized for diagnosis. Body cavity effusions were relatively easy to evaluate. The practice progressed to evaluation of superficial enlarged lymph nodes and round cell tumors. Histology was utilized if the aspirate findings were difficult to interpret. This limited spectrum of processes was taught in veterinary school as easy to do by the general practitioner.

The evolution of cytology over the last 30 years has resulted in a marked increase in interpretive complexity. Examples contributing to this outlook include:

- Lesions such as lymphadenopathy and other swellings are recognized and sampled earlier in the disease progression.

- The degree of variation in morphologic manifestations in common cytological lesions has grown with accumulated years of practice experience.
- Both earlier sampling and degree of variation in morphology have necessitated special staining or molecular procedures to clarify diagnosis.
- Almost all organs and internal growth abnormalities are now sampled.
- In the cultural shift to minimize invasive procedures, expectations are that cytology provide as much definitive information as possible.

These changes in the practice of cytopathology have made interpretive complexity a specialty considerably beyond the ability of the general practitioner. The specialty has grown to be the predominant activity of clinical pathologists certified by the American College of Veterinary Pathologists. However, this evolution has not sufficiently influenced how cytopathology is taught in veterinary schools. There is still a trend to teach that general practitioners can be proficient in cytopathology, utilizing the traditional textbook samples in teaching laboratories. Most graduates independently discover that submission of samples to a diagnostic laboratory is best practice for cytopathology. This realization is perhaps counter to what is learned in clinical pathology courses.

A perspective offered for veterinary education would be to change the emphasis in clinical microscopy education. Important emphases offered are:

- Examine example case material in the classroom and teaching laboratory (slides) with emphasis on types of disease processes in which cytology best contributes to case management. De-emphasize the expectation that general practitioners can master cytology without a special interest in developing the expertise.
- Most important is how to prepare slides with minimal artifact. See Chapter 2.
- Examine at least one slide to make sure cells other than blood are present. Avoid nondiagnostic sample submissions that are acellular.
- Visualize what pathologists do in clinical microscopy in order to optimize future interaction with pathologists on case material.
- Prepare a good history along with submission of unstained slides to a diagnostic laboratory with a veterinary clinical pathologist. Experience how clinical history, or lack of, influences interpretation of cytopathology.
- Understand the diagnostic capability differences between cytology and histopathology in case management. These are highlighted in Chapter 40.

Comments on some current trends

In recent years, there has been a marked increase in fine needle aspiration of abdominal organs. The cultural shift toward less invasive procedures has been a major driver. Advances in radiographic and ultrasonographic capabilities coupled with the trend to use cytologic sampling of overt and suspicious imaging abnormalities has moved to the forefront of practice and subordinated exploratory laparotomy and thoracotomy. This has been challenging for pathologists. This is because there may be a gap in clinician expectations for diagnostic yield of body cavity organ cytology and what is feasibly deliverable. Certain practices that are now very common have questionable return on investment. Some of the more common samples received by laboratories are splenic and liver aspirates. Some examples of cytologic procedures that would benefit by qualification include the following.

Liver aspirates. The history accompanying many liver aspirate samples is limited to "increased liver enzymes." Without extensive further study, we propose this clinical finding in isolation is not an indication for liver aspiration. Almost always the cytologic findings are not specific and shed no light on why there are increased liver enzymes. Our experience is that liver aspirates are most helpful in documentation of either hepatic infiltrative disease or the suspicion that a mass is tissue that does not belong in normal liver. These examinations are prompted by other collective clinical findings suggestive of infiltrative disease or a definitive mass. Increased liver enzymes may be associated with those other more compelling clinical findings indicating cytologic sampling.

Splenic aspirates. The best part about retirement is no more splenic aspirates. Aspirates are often performed with the history that a nodule or suspicious echogenicity pattern was found on a routine abdominal ultrasound examination. Most adult to aged dogs may have incidental splenic nodular hyperplasia. These almost always yield cytologic findings consistent with nodular hyperplasia, or extramedullary hematopoisis, or no abnormalities because the sample consists of only blood. The above should not be an indication for splenic aspirate unless there is other clinical suspicion of more important splenic involvement of an infiltrative disease.

Another misconception is that splenic aspirates will confirm diagnosis of splenic hemangiosarcoma. The typical hemangiosarcoma is composed of mostly vascular sinus space. Aspiration yields only blood. It is uncommon for the aspirate to yield confirmatory sarcoma cells. The diagnosis is often suggested based mostly on signalment, presence of a splenic mass, history of hemoabdomen, and possibly the presence of a rare mesenchymal cell. All findings other than the rare cell make the diagnosis more likely.

In summary, the best indication for splenic aspirate is the presence of generalized splenomegaly in conjunction with suspicion of infiltrative disease such as lymphoma, myeloproliferative disease, mastocytosis, or malignant histiocytosis.

Diagnosis of specific organ neoplasia. Textbooks specializing in cytology may show cytologic examples of specific organ neoplasia. An example might be pancreatic carcinoma. This may lead the clinician to believe that aspiration of a mass in the region of the pancreas can yield a specific diagnosis of pancreatic carcinoma. However, at best the cytology showed features of neoplasia. The textbook discussion indicates the lesion was confirmed by architecture seen by histopathology. The location is the better suggestion of pancreatic specificity than the cytologic findings. For most organ neoplasms, cytology suggests the presence of neoplasia based on general features of neoplasia. Then, location, location, location is often highly utilized in cytologic interpretation to suggest tissue of origin specificity. See Chapter 40 for additional perspective.

CHAPTER 4

4 Immunodiagnostics: Current Use and Future Trends in Veterinary Medicine

Wayne A. Jensen

Colorado State University, Fort Collins, CO, USA

Introduction

Immunodiagnostics are tests that use antibody–antigen binding to generate a measurable result that assists in the diagnosis of disease. As such, immunodiagnostics are also "immunoassays" (although the reverse is not always true). Antibodies are plasma glycoproteins, called gamma globulins or immunoglobulins (Ig), generated in response to exposure of the immune system to an antigen. Simply defined, an antigen is any substance that stimulates the immune system to produce antibodies. Antigens are usually proteins or polysaccharides. Immunodiagnostics were initially used in the diagnosis of infectious diseases, either indirectly by detection of antibody or directly by detection of antigen. Detection of antibody indicates previous exposure and not necessarily the active presence of the antigen.

Immunodiagnostics take advantage of the specific binding of an antibody to its antigen. An epitope is the portion of an antigen bound by an antibody. Binding between an antibody and its epitope is dependent on noncovalent interactions including ionic interactions, hydrogen bonds, and hydrophobic interactions. The strength of the interaction between a single antigen-binding site on the antibody and its epitope is called its affinity. Most antigens (e.g., viral capsid proteins) have multiple epitopes. Epitopes to which the greatest amount of antibody is produced are called immunodominant epitopes.

Immunodiagnostics are capable of detecting the presence (qualitative tests) or amount (quantitative tests) of an analyte (either antibody or antigen) present in the sample at concentrations below what can be accurately determined by other routine testing methodologies. Detection is usually accomplished by "labeling" either antigen or antibody and then using the labeled reagent to probe samples for the presence of antibody or antigen, respectively. Common labels used in immunoassays include enzymes (e.g., horseradish peroxidase, alkaline phosphatase, glucose oxidase, luciferase), fluorochromes (e.g., fluorescein, phycoerythrin), radioisotopes (e.g., I-125), or microparticles (e.g., colloidal gold, latex beads). For quantitative results, the signal measured from the sample is compared to the signal obtained from standards containing known concentrations of the analyte.

In addition to detection of antibodies or antigens associated with infectious disease, immunodiagnostic tests are also used for measurement of many other analytes including drugs, hormones, tumor markers, and markers of cardiac injury. In the case of drugs and hormones, the analytes measured are frequently haptens. A hapten can only elicit production of antibodies when combined with an antigenic carrier molecule. However, once formed, haptens can react with antibodies in the absence of association with the carrier.

Antibody structure

Antibodies or immunoglobulins are proteins produced by differentiated B lymphocytes. There are five classes of antibodies, namely, immunoglobulin A (IgA), immunoglobulin D (IgD), immunoglobulin E (IgE), immunoglobulin G (IgG), and immunoglobulin M (IgM). Each antibody consists of four polypeptides – two heavy chains and two light chains held together by interchain disulfide bonds to form a "Y"-shaped molecule (Figure 4.1). The IgD, IgE, and IgG antibody classes are found as a single structural unit, whereas IgA antibodies may contain either one or two units, and IgM antibodies consist of five disulfide-linked units (Figure 4.2).

Intrachain disulfide bonds support structural "domains" of approximately 110 amino acid residues in length each. Heavy chains are composed of either three (IgA, IgD, IgE) or four (IgE, IgM) constant domains and a single amino-terminal variable domain. The constant domains of the heavy chain define the class of each antibody and are responsible for the biological activity of the antibody. Light chains are composed

Veterinary Hematology, Clinical Chemistry, and Cytology, Third Edition. Edited by Mary Anna Thrall, Glade Weiser, Robin W. Allison and Terry W. Campbell.

Companion website: www.wiley.com/go/thrall/veterinary

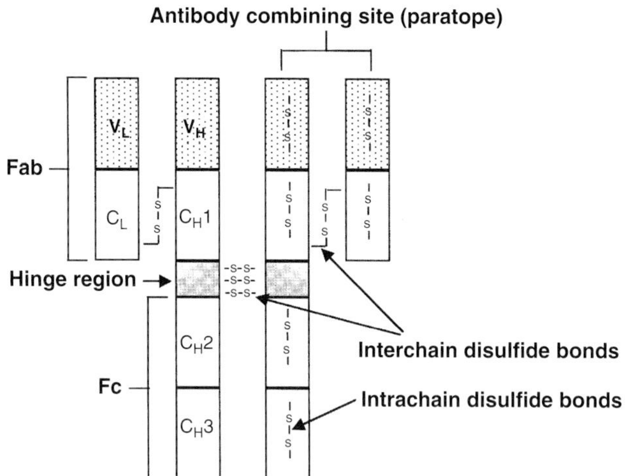

Figure 4.1 Schematic of an antibody molecule illustrating the heavy (H) and light (L) chains held together by interchain disulfide bonds. Intrachain disulfide bonds create structural "domains," each approximately 110 amino acid residues in length. The variable (V) domains of the heavy and light chains form the antigen binding site. The constant (C) domains define the class of the heavy (A, D, E, G, and M) and light (kappa or lambda) chains. Fab fragments contain the entire light chain and the variable and amino-terminal most constant domain of the heavy chain. Fc fragments contain the remaining constant domains of the heavy chain.

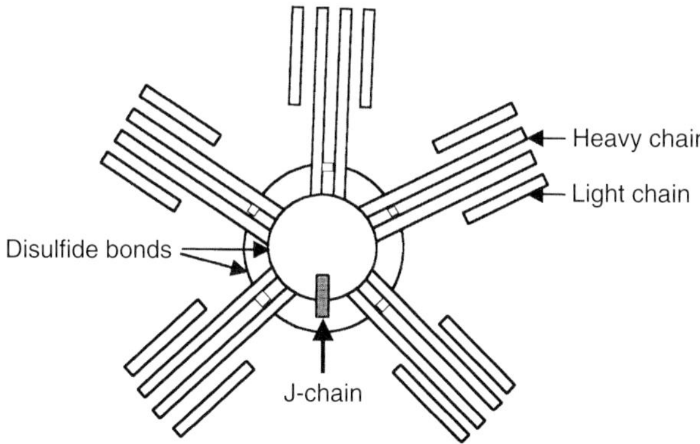

Figure 4.2 Schematic of IgM illustrating its pentameric structure, interchain disulfide bonds, and the J-chain.

of a single constant domain and a single amino-terminal variable domain. The constant domain of the light chain defines the type of light chain as either kappa or lambda. The combined variable regions of the heavy and light chains form the antigen binding site and are responsible for the specificity of antibody–antigen interaction. The presence of two heavy and two light chains results in two antigen binding sites for each antibody molecule (Figure 4.1).

Historically, proteolytic enzymes (proteases) have been used to cleave antibody molecules into functional fragments. Antibody molecules are cleaved into three fragments by limited digestion with the protease papain. Two of the fragments are identical and represent the two "arms" of the "Y." These fragments contain the antigen-binding activity and are termed Fab fragments (Fragment antigen binding). Fab fragments contain a complete light chain and the variable and amino-terminal most constant domain of the heavy chain (Figure 4.1).

The third fragment obtained from digestion with papain contains the remaining constant domains of the heavy chains and does not bind antigen. This fragment is referred to as the Fc fragment (Figure 4.1) because it was found to be readily "crystallizable." The Fc fragment is the part of the antibody molecule that interacts with effector molecules and cells. An example of this is the interaction of IgE with the FcERI receptor on mast cells. Relative to immunodiagnostics, Fc fragments are used to raise species- and class-specific antibodies for the detection of antibody responses to many infectious diseases. For example, anti-cat IgM and anti-cat IgG are used to differentially detect an IgM versus IgG immune response, respectively, which has been reported to be useful in the diagnosis of acute *Toxoplasma gondii* infection in clinically ill cats [1].

Another protease, pepsin, cleaves on the carboxy-terminal side of the disulfide bonds, generating a fragment, referred to as the $F(ab')_2$ fragment, that contains both "arms" of the "Y" (Figure 4.1). Pepsin cleaves the remaining portion of the heavy chain into several smaller fragments. Because the $F(ab')_2$ fragment contains both antigen-binding sites, it has the same antigen–cross-linking capabilities as the original antibody molecule. $F(ab')_2$ fragments are occasionally used in diagnostic assays because they maintain the specificity of the original antibody but lack the Fc fragment, which is sometimes associated with nonspecific binding.

Generation of antibodies used in immunoassays

Immunodiagnostics use antibodies to detect both antigens (e.g., proteins from infectious agents) and antibodies generated in response to foreign proteins. Antibodies used as reagents in immunodiagnostic tests can be either polyclonal or monoclonal. Antibodies are named by the species from which they were obtained and the antigen to which they were produced. For example, rabbit anti-canine γ chain is rabbit antibody specific for γ chain of dog IgG. Unless otherwise specified, antibodies are assumed to be polyclonal.

Polyclonal antibodies

Polyclonal antibodies are generated via hyperimmunization of an animal (e.g., rabbit, sheep, goat) with the antigen of interest. The animal's immune response to the antigen produces antiserum, a heterogeneous mixture of antibodies. Polyclonal antibodies therefore represent a mixture of antibodies derived from many different B lymphocyte clones, each with a unique B cell receptor and each capable

CHAPTER 4

of binding the antigen. As a result, within each pool of polyclonal antibodies will be antibodies that bind to the numerous epitopes present on the antigen. Some of these antibodies will bind to their respective epitope with high affinity and some will have lower affinities.

Monoclonal antibodies

In 1975, Georges Köhler and César Milstein [2] demonstrated that fusion of antibody-producing B cells with myeloma cells that had lost their ability to secrete antibodies resulted in an immortal cell line or "hybridoma" that secreted a single monospecific antibody. In the fused hybridoma cell, the B cell supplies the ability to secrete a specific antibody, and the myeloma cell gives it immortality. The generation and use of monoclonal antibodies has been an important tool in research and medicine (in 1984, Köhler and Milstein received the Nobel Prize in Physiology or Medicine for their discovery of monoclonal antibodies).

Monoclonal antibodies are typically made using polyethylene glycol to fuse myeloma cells with spleen cells from a mouse that has been immunized with the antigen of interest. The success rate of fusion is low, so a selective medium is used that only allows the growth of hybridoma cells. After fusion, the mixture of cells is diluted and aliquoted into 96-well microtiter plates so that only approximately one-third of the wells will contain cells. This increases the chance that each resultant "clone" of cells was generated from a single parent cell.

Cell culture supernatants are then tested for the presence of antibody with the ability to bind to the antigen of interest (usually the same antigen that was used for immunization of the B cell donor mouse). Immunodiagnostic assays used for the screening process are typically high-throughput assays (e.g., ELISA or immunodot blot) to allow for the screening of hundreds of hybridoma clones. The subcloning process is repeated at least three times to ensure that the final clone was generated from a single parent cell. The most productive and stable clone (some hybridomas lose the ability to produce antibody over time) is then grown in culture medium to a high volume for large-scale production of monoclonal antibody.

Immunoassay formats

Immunoassays can be either competitive or noncompetitive. In competitive immunoassays, the analyte (antigen or antibody) in the sample competes with labeled antigen or antibody, and the signal generated is inversely proportional to the concentration of analyte in the sample (Figures 4.3 and 4.4). In noncompetitive immunoassays, the amount of analyte (antigen or antibody) in the sample is directly proportional to the signal generated (Figure 4.5).

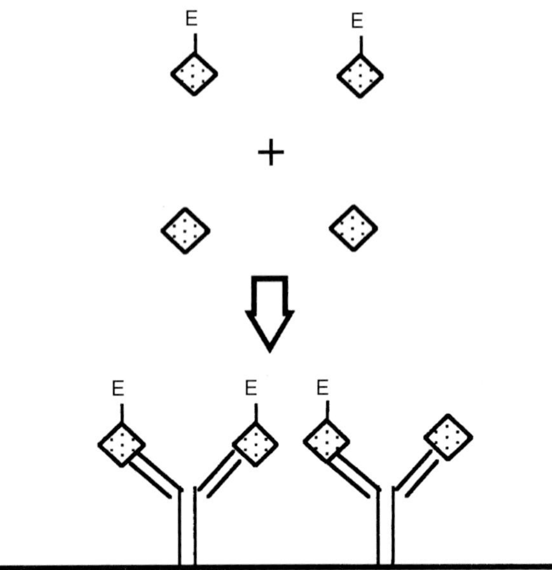

Figure 4.3 Illustration of a competitive immunoassay for the detection of antigen. In this example, antigen in the patient's sample competes with enzyme-labeled antigen for antibody bound to a solid phase. After a wash step to remove unbound enzyme-labeled antigen, addition of chromogenic substrate results in a color change that is inversely proportional to the quantity of antigen in the patient's sample.

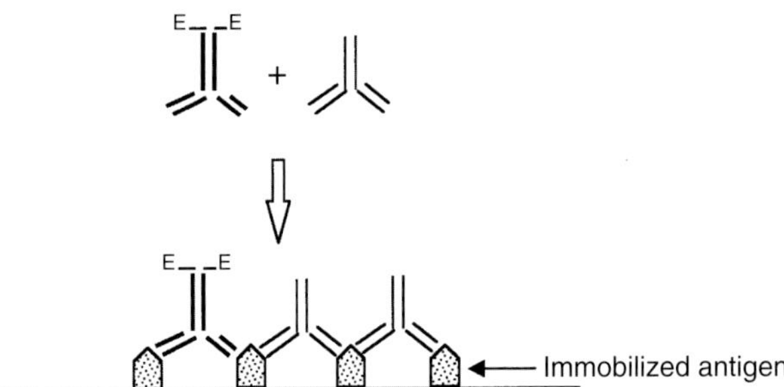

Figure 4.4 Illustration of a competitive immunoassay for the detection of antibody. In this example, antibody in the patient's sample competes with enzyme-labeled antibody for antigen bound to a solid phase. After a wash step to remove unbound enzyme-labeled antibody, addition of chromogenic substrate results in a color change that is inversely proportional to the quantity of antibody in the patient's sample.

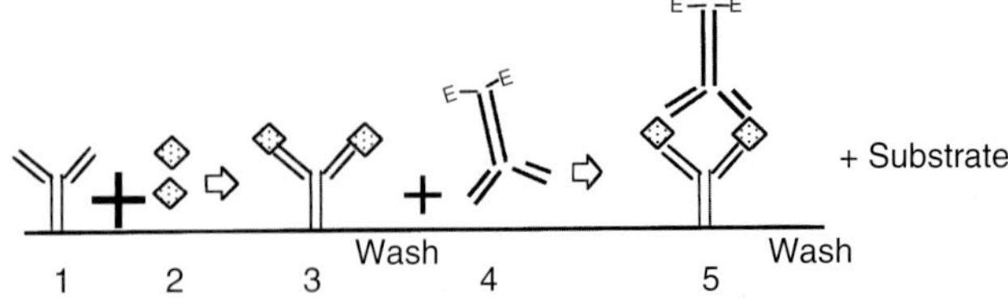

Figure 4.5 Illustration of a noncompetitive immunoassay for the detection of antigen. In this example, antigen in the sample is captured by antibody bound to a solid phase. After a wash step, enzyme-labeled antigen-specific antibody binds to the captured antigen. After another wash to remove unbound enzyme-labeled antibody, addition of chromogenic substrate results in a color change that is proportional to the quantity of antigen in the patient's sample.

Immunodiagnostic assays can also be either homogeneous or heterogeneous. Homogeneous immunoassays are performed simply by mixing the sample with reagents and measuring the signal generated (or a decrease in signal for competitive immunoassays) by the reaction chemistry that results from antigen–antibody binding. As such, homogeneous immunoassays do not require the separation of bound antigen–antibody from free antigen (or antibody). For this reason, homogeneous immunoassays tend to be easier and faster to perform; however, they are generally less sensitive. An example of a homogeneous immunoassay is the detection of antigen–antibody complex formation by measuring the resultant decrease in light transmission through the sample (turbidimetry); see Chapter 2.

Newer homogeneous immunoassay technologies utilize enzyme donor and enzyme acceptor pairs that readily associate to generate active enzyme. In these assays, antibody binding to an antigenic epitope or hapten incorporated into either the enzyme donor or acceptor subunit blocks the association (and, therefore, activity) of the enzyme. Analyte present in the sample binds the antibody and prevents it from binding to the enzyme subunit, thereby allowing the formation of active enzyme. As such, these assays are considered to be competitive immunoassays because the analyte–antibody binding reaction competes with the binding of antibody to the hapten-conjugated enzyme. Another example of a newer competitive homogeneous immunoassay technology utilizes fluorescence energy transfer where a "fluorescer" is conjugated to the hapten and the "quencher" is conjugated to the antibody. In the absence of analyte in the sample, the quencher-conjugated antibody binds the hapten-conjugated fluorescer and extinguishes the signal. In the presence of analyte in the sample, a portion of the quencher-conjugated antibodies bind the analyte and are therefore no longer available to bind the hapten-conjugated fluorescer and quench the fluorescence signal.

Unlike homogeneous immunoassays, heterogeneous immunoassays require the separation of antigen–antibody complexes from unbound antigen (or antibody) because the label is not affected by the antigen–antibody binding event. Using enzyme immunoassays (EIAs) as an example, unbound enzyme-conjugated reagent must be physically removed from bound enzyme-conjugated reagent prior to the addition of the enzyme substrate. This removal step is usually accomplished by "washing." Another characteristic of heterogeneous immunoassays is the requirement for unconjugated reagent to be fixed to a solid phase (Figures 4.3–4.5) to allow for removal of unbound enzyme-conjugated reagent without removal of the bound enzyme-conjugated reagent. Examples of solid phases commonly used in immunoassays include microtiter wells, nitrocellulose, and latex or magnetic beads.

Similar to homogeneous immunoassays, heterogeneous immunoassays can also be formatted as either competitive or noncompetitive assays. With competitive assay formats, the presence of analyte in the sample decreases the amount of signal generated. Common competitive immunoassay formats include:

1. Antigen in the sample competing with free labeled antigen for a limited quantity of bound unlabeled antibody (Figure 4.3).

2. Antigen in the sample competing with bound unlabeled antigen for a limited quantity of free labeled antibody.

In both of these formats, the binding of antigen in the sample to antibody (either bound or free) blocks binding of the labeled reagent to the solid phase and thus allows the removal of the labeled reagent in the subsequent wash step. Sensitivity can be improved in the first competitive immunoassay format by adding the sample to the bound unlabeled antibody prior to addition of the labeled antigen. Similarly, sensitivity can be improved in the second competitive assay format by adding the sample to the free labeled antibody prior to incubation with the bound unlabeled antigen.

In contrast to competitive immunoassays, noncompetitive immunoassays rely on direct measurement of antibody binding sites occupied by analyte. Another difference between competitive and noncompetitive immunoassays is in the relative concentration of reagents. As mentioned previously, competitive assays require limiting the quantities of antigen, antibody, or both. In contrast, reagents are applied in excess for noncompetitive heterogeneous immunoassays to maximize sensitivity.

A common noncompetitive heterogeneous immunoassay format for antigen is the capture or sandwich immunoassay (Figure 4.5). In this format, bound antibody (either polyclonal or monoclonal) specific for the antigen of interest is incubated with sample, washed, then incubated with another labeled antibody (either polyclonal or monoclonal) specific for the antigen of interest. Antigen present in the sample is "captured" (i.e. sandwiched) between the bound antibody and the labeled antibody with the amount of signal generated dependent on the amount of antigen in the sample. Examples of an antigen capture immunoassay frequently utilized in veterinary clinics are heartworm antigen tests manufactured by Heska (Solo Step® CH), IDEXX Laboratories (SNAP® RT and 4Dx), Zoetis (Vetscan® and Witness®), and others [3]. Noncompetitive immunoassay formats for the detection of antibody frequently use bound antigen to "capture" specific antibody and anti-Fc labeled antibodies for detection of captured antibody.

Factors influencing immunoassay design

Considerations in the selection of an immunoassay format include analyte characteristics and concentration, desired endpoint (qualitative or quantitative), and the environment in which the test will be used.

Analyte characteristics and concentration

Small nonprotein analytes and haptens (e.g., thyroxine) are not readily detected in noncompetitive immunoassays due to the inability to "sandwich" the analyte because of a lack of a sufficient number of binding sites (epitopes). These analytes are best measured in heterogeneous competitive immunoassay or homogeneous immunoassay formats. Homogeneous immunoassay formats are most appropriate for antigens or haptens whose concentrations are relatively high (nmol/L) (e.g., total serum thyroxine), whereas heterogeneous competitive immunoassay formats are capable of detection limits in the picomolar range (e.g., free serum thyroxine). Noncompetitive heterogeneous assays in which reagents are applied in excess are capable of detection limits approaching 1 fmol/L [4].

Desired endpoint

All immunoassay formats can be used to report a qualitative result simply by identifying an assay "cutoff" (usually arbitrarily determined as three standard deviations above the mean of the negative controls) and reporting results as either positive or negative. Visual read test results are usually qualitative, but some test formats allow for semi-quantitative results without the need for instrumentation by comparing the intensity of the signal generated from the patient's sample to an internal reference (e.g., IDEXX SNAP tests for equine IgG, canine and feline pancreatic lipase, and feline pro-brain natriuetic peptide) [5]. Most immunoassay formats can also be used to report quantitative results as long as the signal recognition technology is capable of detecting differences in signal magnitudes. Quantitative results usually require the use of calibrators containing known concentrations of analyte to establish a standard curve from which the sample analyte concentration is determined.

Environment

The environment in which the immunoassay is performed has important implications for format selection. As discussed previously, homogeneous immunoassays tend to be easier to perform because there are no washing steps involved. For this reason, homogeneous immunoassay formats are well suited for automation on high-throughput clinical analyzers. Due to the requirement for washing between reagents, heterogeneous immunoassays tend to require greater technical skill of the operator. Quantitative immunoassays (both homogeneous and heterogeneous) have historically required sophisticated equipment (e.g., spectrophotometer, spectrofluorometer, luminometer) for detection and quantitation of generated signals and are, therefore, usually performed in centralized laboratories.

Simple-to-use qualitative heterogeneous immunoassays have been available for use in veterinary practice for many years. These single-use, "in-clinic" tests (sometimes referred to as "point-of-care tests" or POCTs) either have built-in wash buffer that is manually activated (e.g., IDEXX SNAP), require the addition of wash buffer after application of sample (e.g., Zoetis VetScan and Witness), or do not require wash buffer (Heska Solo Step). The IDEXX SNAP tests are sandwich ELISA formatted tests for the detection of either antigen or antibody. The Zoetis VetScan and Witness tests and the Heska Solo Step test are lateral flow immunoassays (LFIAs). LFIAs are sandwich immunoassays that do not use enzyme/substrate for signal amplification but rather use antibody (or antigen) conjugated to particles (sometimes referred to as microspheres or beads) made of latex, gold, carbon, or metal for detection of antigen–antibody binding (Figure 4.6).

In LFIAs, the microsphere-labeled reagent (e.g., antibody) reacts with the analyte (e.g., antigen) as the sample wicks through the pads and membranes making up the test strip. As the mixture migrates through the "test window," antigen–antibody–microsphere complexes are captured at a "test" line by immobilized antibody (either antibody specific for the antigen of interest or an anti-Fc antibody). Excess and antigen-free complexes (e.g., in the case of a negative sample) continue migrating beyond the test line. Both the ELISA and LFIA in-clinic tests have built-in procedural controls. These are not true "positive" controls but rather

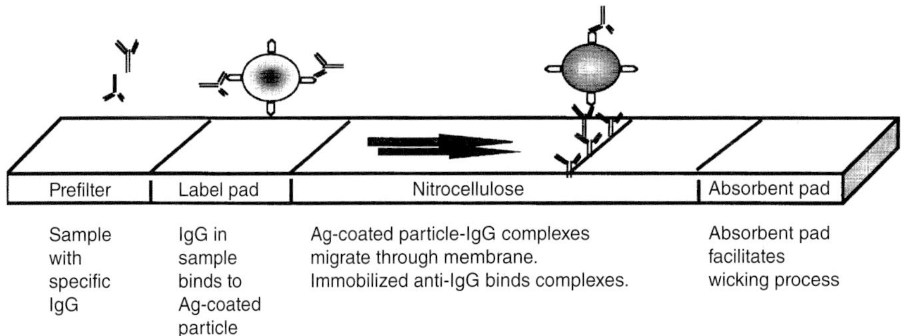

Figure 4.6 Illustration of a lateral flow immunoassay (not drawn to scale).

ensure that the enzyme was active and the sample flowed correctly for ELISA and LFIA tests, respectively.

Factors influencing immunoassay performance

As discussed earlier, immunoassay format can impact performance. In addition, both the reagents and samples used in immunoassays play a fundamental role in the quality of results provided.

Reagent considerations

Immunoassays for the detection of allergen-specific IgE serve as an example of the impact reagents can have on immunoassay performance. The ideal immunoassay would use high-affinity antibodies that are minimally cross-reactive. The specificity of early immunoassays for the detection of allergen-specific IgE was questioned due to the potential cross-reactivity of polyclonal anti-IgE antibodies with IgG [6, 7]. Allergen-specific IgG is found in sera from both atopic and nonatopic animals. Therefore, any cross-reactivity of the anti-IgE antibodies will decrease immunoassay specificity. For this reason, specific monoclonal anti-IgE antibodies and Fc epsilon receptor have been used as IgE detection reagents in allergen-specific IgE immunoassays [6, 8].

In addition to cross-reactivity of antibody, antigen cross-reactivity can also impact immunoassay specificity. In allergen-specific IgE immunoassays, it was found that taxonomically unrelated allergens contained cross-reacting carbohydrate epitopes. Specific IgE binding to these cross-reacting carbohydrate epitopes results in false positives relative to intradermal skin test results or immunoassay results using deglycosylated allergens [9, 10]. Importantly, cross-reacting carbohydrate epitopes are also found on horseradish peroxidase, an enzyme frequently used as a label in immunoassays. Under these conditions, non-IgE antibody (e.g., IgG) can simultaneously bind the carbohydrate epitopes found on both the allergen and horseradish peroxidase, generating a false-positive result for allergen-specific IgE [9, 11, 12]. For this reason, many allergen-specific IgE immunoassays now use alkaline phosphatase as the reporter enzyme rather than horseradish peroxidase [13].

Sample considerations

Relative concentrations of analyte in the sample can impact the quality of immunoassay results. In homogeneous immunoassays that measure antigen–antibody complex formation, excess antigen can saturate antibody binding sites and thereby prevent complex formation. The interference of excess analyte, resulting in a lower-than-actual measurement of analyte concentration, is referred to as the prozone effect or prozone phenomenon. Similarly, in immunoassays measuring a specific antibody class, excess antibody of a different class can bind the antigen and prevent binding by the antibody class of interest. Examples include interference due to excess IgG in allergen-specific IgE immunoassays resulting in an underestimation of IgE concentration (in atopic animals, the amount of IgG is frequently in great excess relative to the amount of IgE) [14].

Interference in immunoassays can also be caused by the presence of endogenous immunoglobulins that bind to antibodies from other species (heterophilic antibodies). Because mouse antibodies are frequently used as reagents for immunoassays, the detection of interference due to heterophilic antibodies specific for mouse immunoglobulin is not uncommon [15, 16]. In people these antibodies are termed human anti-mouse antibodies (HAMA), and they are thought to originate from either environmental exposure to mice or medical agents containing antibodies derived from mice [15]. Heterophilic antibodies have also been reported in dogs and cats [17, 18]. Heterophilic dog anti-mouse antibodies cause occasional false-positive results in some in-clinic heartworm antigen capture assays. In heartworm antigen tests, false positives can be differentiated from true positives by denaturing the antibodies (using heat or acid treatment of the sample) prior to performing the immunoassay (fortunately, heartworm antigen survives these denaturation processes). For this reason, it is important to verify positive heartworm antigen test results obtained from nondenatured samples prior to treatment for heartworms. Last, the presence of excess quantities of antigen-specific immunoglobulins in the sample can block capture immunoassays, resulting in false-negative results. The presence of blocking antibody is one cause of occasional false-negative heartworm antigen test results in *Dirofilaria immitis* microfilaria-positive dogs and cats [19, 20]. Similar to false-positive results, false-negative heartworm test results due to blocking antibody can be differentiated from true negatives by heat or acid treatment of the sample prior to performing the immunoassay.

Future trends for use of immunodiagnostics in veterinary medicine

In addition to development of new immunodiagnostic tests for both infectious and metabolic diseases of animals, future immunodiagnostics technology will provide quantitative immunoassays in the in-clinic environment. These instruments will be smaller and less expensive than the current quantitative instruments found in central immunodiagnostic laboratories. Benefits will include improved patient care due to the decreased time to obtain results, lower costs, and alleviation of concerns with shipping of samples to outside laboratories.

The first quantitative in-clinic immunoassay for thyroxine designed for use in veterinary medicine was developed using an EIA format in a single-use cartridge with results measured by a benchtop reader. Initial studies indicated that reproducibility and correlation with the reference standard laboratory-based test were inadequate [21]. However, more recent comparisons demonstrated acceptable reproducibility and better correlation of in-clinic and laboratory-based thyroxine immunoassays [22, 23]. Quantitative immunoassays for bile acids and cortisol using an EIA-based cartridge and reader system are also available. Studies indicate that there is very good agreement between the in-clinic and laboratory-based assays for bile acids and less so for the in-clinic and laboratory-based assays for cortisol [24, 25].

Quantitative immunoassay formats that do not use enzyme-dependent signal amplification would have the advantage of not requiring special handling (e.g., refrigeration) to prevent deterioration of the enzyme and substrate. However, current non-EIA-based qualitative tests (e.g., LFIAs) lack sufficient sensitivity for routine use in quantitative tests [26, 27].

Efforts are under way to develop quantitative immunoassays that retain the simplicity of non-EIA-based qualitative tests (e.g., LFIAs) with improved sensitivity. Following are examples of quantitative immunoassay technologies based on single-use cassettes that have potential for in-clinic use in veterinary medicine.

1. LFIAs that use a fluorescent dye instead of immunogold particles or latex beads result in 100–1000-fold increase in sensitivity [27–29]. Use of an LED light source and a CCD-camera-based instrument with densitometric analysis software would allow quantitation of the signal.

2. The Rapid Analyte Measurement Platform (RAMP™) produced by Response Biomedical Corporation (Vancouver, BC, Canada) uses fluorescent-dyed latex particles in an LFIA cassette. Antibody-conjugated latex particles bind to the analyte and are captured at the test line. Unbound antibody-conjugated latex particles are captured at the control line and serve as an internal calibrator. Fluorescence measured at the test and control lines is converted into a ratio that allows for correction of test-to-test variation. The RAMP immunoassay system has been shown to provide results comparable to a central laboratory immunoassay platform [30].

3. Magnetic particles have also been incorporated into LFIAs to increase sensitivity and provide quantitative results [31–33]. To function in LFIAs, the particles must be superparamagnetic, becoming magnetic only when placed in a strong magnetic field. Under these conditions, the magnitude of the change in the magnetic field is directly proportional to the amount of magnetic particles captured at the test line, which is proportional to the analyte quantity in the initial sample. Magnetic-particle-based immunoassays have a distinct advantage in that the signal is very stable over time.

4. The use of piezofilm in quantitative immunoassays was initially described in 2008 [34]. Piezofilm is a polymer film with piezoelectric properties that generates an electric charge when the film is exposed to heat or mechanical strain. In piezofilm-based immunoassays, capture antibody is attached to the surface of the film, and the detection antibody is conjugated to carbon colloids that absorb light. In the presence of antigen, the capture antibody–antigen-detection antibody complex is localized on the surface of the piezofilm. Upon stimulation with light, the generated heat is transferred to the piezofilm, eliciting an electric charge. An advantage of this technology is the lack of necessity for removal of the unbound carbon-conjugated antibody because heat generated by unbound conjugates is dissipated into the assay medium. The piezofilm immunoassay technology was developed as a point-of-care system by Vivacta Ltd. [34], acquired by Novartis in 2012 and then recently sold to Psyros Diagnostics.

5 Laboratory Diagnosis of Infectious Diseases of Animals

Sreekumari Rajeev
The University of Tennessee, Knoxville, TN, USA

CHAPTER 5

The laboratory confirmation of infectious diseases complements veterinarians' clinical judgment through accurate identification of an etiologic agent. This improves patient care by enhancing the ability to implement appropriate treatment and preventive measures. To undertake an effective approach to diagnose infectious diseases, a veterinary practitioner must have basic knowledge of infectious agents observed in clinical syndromes. Regular submission of clinical specimens for diagnostic workup will advance a veterinarian's knowledge and interpretation skills, and in due course, the diagnostic process will become less cumbersome and more cost-effective. Veterinary practitioners must acquire adequate skills in pursuing a presumptive diagnostic strategy and reaching a differential diagnosis of clinical conditions based on history, symptoms, and direct examination of clinical samples. To improve efficiency, it is imperative that veterinary practitioners exercise evidence-based medicine and appraise the necessity of pursuing laboratory diagnosis of clinical cases they come across. During the diagnostic process, if laboratory confirmation is pursued, selection of appropriate sample type, sample collection and transport methods, diagnostic tests, and a laboratory that can offer these services are necessary. Preparation of a complete submission form, including all relevant patient information, is required to obtain meaningful test results. Finally, knowledge and experience in the interpretation of results and awareness of inherent issues associated with individual diagnostic tests are also needed.

Laboratory diagnosis of infectious diseases in animals is achieved mainly by two approaches: (i) the detection of the infecting agent or its components, and/or (ii) the detection of the host immune response to the infecting agents. The method of choice will be largely determined by the nature of infecting agents, the disease suspected, the stage of infection, the species of animals affected, and the availability of diagnostic tests. Although the use of diagnostic tests is not always required to establish the cause of an infectious disease, it is beneficial to attain a conceptual understanding of the usefulness of diagnostic tests and will prospectively help the practitioner save time and resources. The emergence, occurrence, and transmission of infectious diseases are dynamic processes. Evidence-based medicine can be better practiced by using the data obtained from routine diagnostic testing and developing diagnostic algorithms based on clinicians' experience in the geographic area of their practice. When interpreting diagnostic test results, consideration must also be given to sensitivity, specificity, and predictive values of the diagnostic tests used.

The processes involved in the diagnosis of an infectious disease can be categorized into three stages: preanalytic stage, analytic stage, and postanalytic stage, and each of these stages will ultimately support the accurate diagnosis of infectious diseases and optimal patient care [1]. The preanalytic stage involves steps taken by the veterinarian and the testing laboratory for specimen collection, transport and storage, and any other processing that occurs before the testing process happens. During the analytic stage, laboratory testing is done and procedures performed provide results. Laboratories must have strict quality-control and quality-assurance procedures in place to comply with testing protocols and reduce errors in testing. The postanalytic stage includes the final result preparation, entry of the data, reporting, and to some extent laboratory interpretation of results. All of these stages are prone to human error and may affect patient management. When an infectious disease process is suspected, a veterinarian must evaluate all of the possibilities of selecting a cost-effective and expedient diagnostic approach. To achieve this, a practitioner should not hesitate to consult with a pathologist and a clinical microbiologist. This chapter provides an overview of the general approaches used in the laboratory diagnosis of infectious diseases in animals.

Veterinary Hematology, Clinical Chemistry, and Cytology, Third Edition. Edited by Mary Anna Thrall, Glade Weiser, Robin W. Allison and Terry W. Campbell.

Companion website: www.wiley.com/go/thrall/veterinary

Sample collection and shipping

Specimens suitable for diagnostic workup must be collected from the site of infection with minimal contamination, as soon as possible after the onset of disease, and before the initiation of therapy. Good specimen collection includes procedures in place to avoid introduction of contaminant bacteria from the surrounding skin or mucous membranes. To achieve this, disinfection or collection using specialized devices must be used as indicated for various body sites. Disinfection of the sample collection site using 70% ethyl alcohol, tincture of iodine, or chlorhexidine is recommended. Swabs are appropriate and commonly used collection devices; however, when a larger volume of a sample is necessary or when multiple diagnostic methods are to be applied, tissue affected or tissue aspirates may be submitted in lieu of a swab. There are many commercially available transport media to ensure the integrity of the specimen during transportation to the diagnostic laboratory. A variety of transport media are available and discussed at this manufacturer-sponsored site: www.bd.com/ds/productCenter/CT-Systems.asp. Appropriate sample storage is also critical in maintaining the integrity of the infectious agents in question. If delivered within 24–48 hours and collected in appropriate transport media, refrigeration is not generally required but advised to protect the sample in the event of any unforeseen delays in shipping.

Transportation of biological samples

Veterinary clinics and diagnostic laboratories must be vigilant in preventing exposure of individuals to zoonotic infectious agents. Leak-proof containers placed in a secure outer packaging are recommended for routine transportation of biological materials. Federal regulations apply to the transport of potentially infectious biological material, and veterinary staff must be familiar with packaging and transport requirements including preparation of shipping documents and potential changes to these guidelines.

Direct examination of clinical specimens

Macroscopic and microscopic examination of the clinical specimens may offer valuable clues about the ongoing infectious processes. For example, an abnormal macroscopic appearance of a clinical sample such as cloudiness in a urine sample, joint fluid, or cerebrospinal fluid (CSF) may indicate a possible inflammatory and a likely infectious process. Gross examination for the presence of external parasites such as ticks may direct the clinician to choose appropriate diagnostic tests targeting vector-borne diseases, especially in cases of diseases manifesting with broad clinical signs. Direct detection and identification of an infectious agent benefits improved patient care through the timely and appropriate choice of therapy before confirmation by downstream diagnostic procedures. Examination of unstained wet mounts is a simple but useful technique where a clinician examines a specimen directly placed on a glass slide under a coverslip by light microscopic examination. For example, detection of yeast cells with a halo representing the mucopolysaccharide capsule of *Cryptococcus neoformans* in an India ink stained wet mount preparation from the cerebrospinal fluid of cats with neurological signs or smears from skin lesions is diagnostic for *Cryptococcus* infection (Figure 5.1A). Use of 5% Lugol's iodine added as a nonspecific contrast dye to a fresh unpreserved fecal specimen enhances the detection of parasitic eggs and larvae parasitic cysts (Figure 5.1B). Examination of KOH-treated hair specimens for the diagnosis of dermatophyte infection is another useful technique.

Microscopic examination of stained clinical specimens provides useful information on the likelihood of an infection, likely pathogens, and predominant organisms if present. Immediate information on the number, morphologic characteristics of the microorganisms, and the host cellular response may provide useful information to the nature of infectious disease process. For example, observation of bacteria, fungal structures (hyphae, yeasts, and spores), and viral inclusions may render an immediate presumptive diagnosis and helps in making rational choices for therapy. Romanowsky staining methods used in cytology, such as Giemsa and Wright stains and their modification, quick stains such as Diff-Quik, are simple staining procedures and often may also have value in detecting infectious agents (Figure 5.2).

These stains are very helpful in demonstrating pathogenic yeasts (*Blastomyces, Cryptococcus, Histoplasma, Sporothrix schenkii*) and protozoan parasites (*Leishmania* and *Trypanosoma*) and occasionally inclusions resulting from viral infections caused by certain viruses, *Chlamydia*, and *Anaplasma*. Advanced and more specific techniques such as direct fluorescent antibody (DFA) staining are also available for a few agents. The need for a specific fluorescent

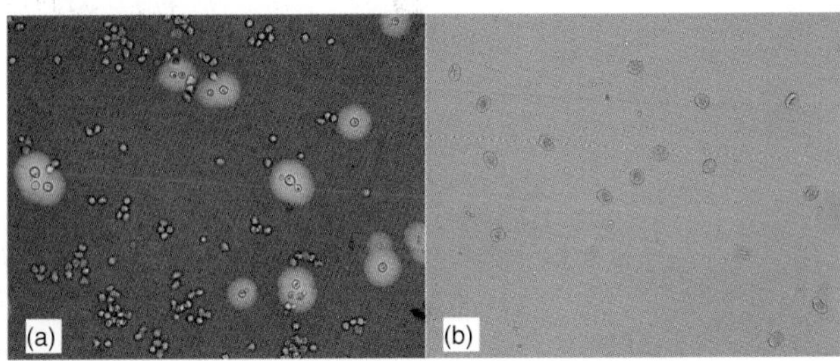

Figure 5.1 A: India ink stained preparation of cerebrospinal fluid from a horse infected with *Cryptococcus gattii*. B: Lugol's iodine stained fecal preparation from a canine feces showing *Giardia* cysts.

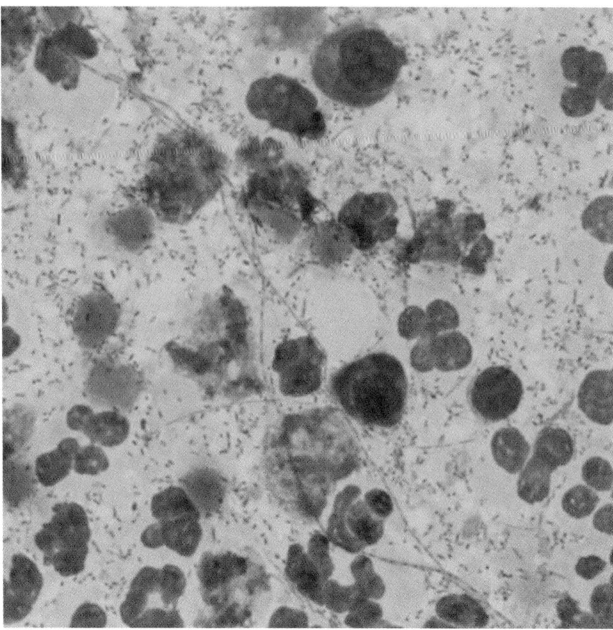

Figure 5.2 Bronchoalveolar lavage from a dog with aspiration pneumonia, Diff-Quik stain. Numerous mixed-type bacteria admixed with numerous neutrophils.

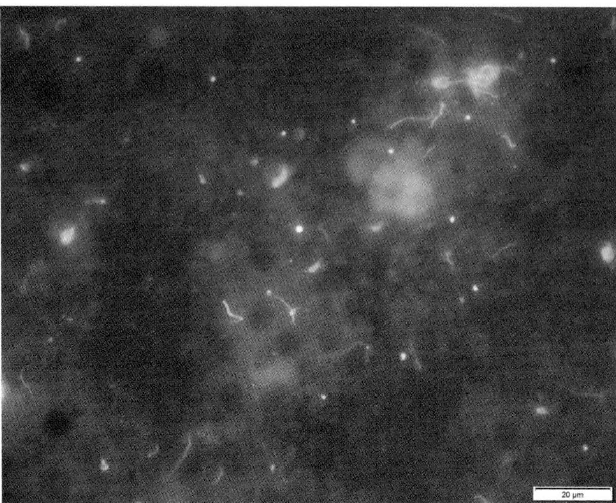

Figure 5.3 Direct fluorescent antibody staining from a urine sample from a suspected leptospirosis case; see intact spirochetes with morphology compatible with *Leptospira* sp.

tagged antibody and a fluorescent microscope precludes its application at point-of-care facilities. This technique is effective when organism-specific antibodies are used to stain morphologically distinct organisms such as *Leptospira* (Figure 5.3).

Detection of antigens and microbial toxins through immunological techniques such as ELISA, agglutination tests, and precipitation tests is used for the detection of some pathogens; however, when interpreting the results, consideration must be given to published or manufacturer-supplied test parameters such as sensitivity, specificity, and predictive values of individual tests used.

Diagnostic approaches for bacterial infections

Direct microscopic examination

The presence of bacterial pathogens and any associated inflammatory components can be visualized by direct microscopic examination of stained smears. Gram, Wright, Giemsa, Diff-Quik, and acid-fast stains are used for the detection of bacterial pathogens from clinical specimens. Gram staining will allow the observer to differentiate between Gram-positive and Gram-negative bacteria; nevertheless, recognition of the host cell response is not optimal by this method (Figure 5.4).

Gram staining is a moderate to highly complex procedure, and the observer should have optimal training in differentiating bacterial pathogens and artifacts. The staining performance and interpretation can be challenging due to the complexity of the methodology, which is often underappreciated. Training and experience in interpretation are needed to achieve proficiency in this technique. An experienced microbiologist's skills are superior to veterinary clinical staff, and it is advisable that a veterinary practice seeks help from laboratories that routinely perform Gram staining. Size, shape, and Gram staining reactions of microorganisms may change in different environments as clinical samples are far more diverse than the material cultured in the laboratory and described in textbooks. The sensitivity of detection of bacteria by direct microscopy is low, and at least 10^4 bacteria must be present per milliliter of the sample to be visualized

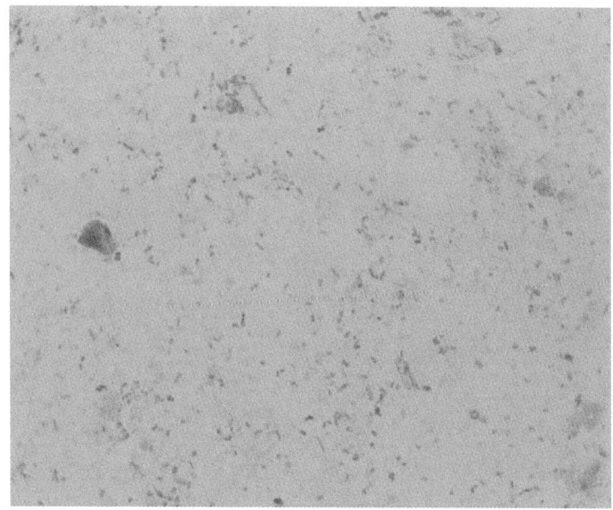

Figure 5.4 Gram stain of a canine ear swab. Mixed population of Gram-positive and Gram-negative bacteria are present.

by examination under a 100× oil immersion objective. Another drawback is that samples such as blood and CSF often yield the suboptimal sensitivity, resulting in false negatives. Direct smears routinely performed and examined in the diagnostic laboratory are quality-control indicators of outcomes of collection, transport, and downstream culture procedures.

Culture and isolation

Culture and isolation of bacterial pathogens followed by their identification is a relatively easy, sensitive, and specific method routinely used for reaching an etiological diagnosis of bacterial diseases. Isolation of a microbial pathogen supports its further characterization through genotypic and phenotypic analysis and antimicrobial susceptibility testing (AST) and can facilitate further epidemiologic studies. There are different types of culture methods, and the appropriate method or a combination of methods must be chosen based on pathogens in question. For example, fecal samples contain a variety of bacteria that are deemed as normal flora, and requesting a selective enrichment culture is necessary to improve the sensitivity of recovery of enteric pathogens *Salmonella, Listeria,* and *Escherichia coli*. Consultation with a clinical microbiologist is paramount in these situations for proper sample collection and selection of the appropriate culture method. General guidelines for microbiology test selection are given in Table 5.1.

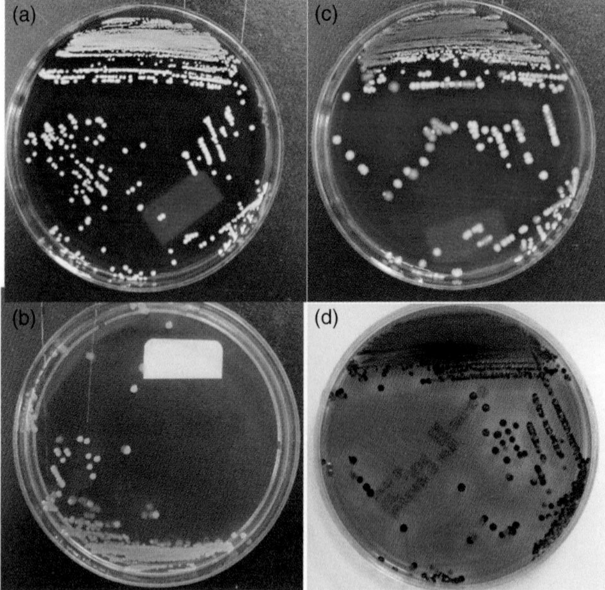

Figure 5.5 Primary culture media used for the growth of bacteria in aerobic cultures. (a) Trypticase soy agar with sheep blood allows the growth of a wide variety of bacteria. (b) MacConkey agar allows the growth of Gram-negative bacteria and can differentiate between a lactose positive and a lactose negative organism. (c) Phenylethyl alcohol agar allows the growth of Gram-positive bacteria. (d) Chromogenic agar specific for *Salmonella* allows the differentiation of *Salmonella* from other members of Enterobacteriaceae.

Aerobic culture

Aerobic culture is routinely requested for fast-growing bacterial organisms that have aerobic or facultative anaerobic metabolism. This culture method utilizes a combination of nonselective media (Trypticase soy agar with sheep blood) and selective media that can recover Gram-negative organisms (MacConkey agar) and Gram-positive organisms (phenylethyl alcohol agar). Diagnostic laboratories are increasingly using chromogenic agars, which allow faster, selective, and presumptive detection of specific bacterial pathogens. Figure 5.5 shows microbial growth in various types of media used in a microbiology laboratory.

Routine aerobic culture procedures take approximately 24–72 hours to complete. The isolation of fastidious bacteria may have additional nutrient requirements (e.g., *Mycobacteria*), and the recovery of these may take longer and need special media or culture procedures. Fastidious *Mycobacteria*, including *M. bovis* and *M. avium* subsp. *paratuberculosis*, are routinely cultured in automated and continuously monitored culture systems, of which many are commercially available. The samples with positive signals from the machine must be confirmed by a combination of staining and polymerase chain reaction (PCR).

Table 5.1 General guidelines for microbiology test selection.

Clinical samples	Tests
Skin and superficial lesions	Aerobic culture
Wounds and abscesses	Aerobic culture, anaerobic culture, fungal culture
Tracheal and bronchial washes	Aerobic culture/anaerobic, fungal cultures
Eye, ear	Aerobic culture
Body fluids (pleural, peritoneal, joint spinal)	Aerobic culture and anaerobic culture
Milk	Aerobic culture
Blood	Aerobic culture, anaerobic culture
Feces	Aerobic, anaerobic, *Salmonella* culture

Anaerobic bacterial culture

Anaerobic bacterial infections are not uncommon in clinical conditions such as pneumonia, pleuritis, peritonitis, wounds, and abscesses. When mixed infections with aerobic and anaerobic bacteria are suspected, an anaerobic culture must be pursued along with routine aerobic cultures. Anaerobic bacteria do not tolerate atmospheric oxygen, and an anaerobic transport medium must be used for shipping. As anaerobic commensal bacteria are present in the mucous

Table 5.2 List of common anaerobic bacterial agents and choice of diagnostic tests.

Organism	Disease and species affected	Tests of choice
Clostridium perfringens	Wound infections, enteric infections, enterotoxaemia	Enterotoxin ELISA, PCR, anaerobic culture
Clostridium difficile	Enteric infections	Toxin ELISA, PCR, anaerobic culture
Clostridium chauvoei, *Clostridium novyi*, *Clostridium septicum*	Myositis in food animals (malignant edema, blackleg, gas gangrene)[a]	Direct fluorescent antibody staining
Fusobacterium sp., *Bacteroides* sp., *Dichelobacter* sp., *Prevotella* sp., *Porphyromonas* sp.	Abscess, various soft-tissue and bone infections, diarrhea	Anaerobic culture, PCR

[a]Anaerobic culture is often unrewarding in these cases.

membranes of animals, extreme care must be taken to avoid contamination. Culture may not be the appropriate method for some anaerobic agents. Table 5.2 lists common anaerobic bacterial agents and common choices of diagnostic tests.

Limitations of routine culture

Understanding the limitations of routine aerobic cultures and requesting special culture protocols or other suitable diagnostic procedures are required when infections with *Salmonella, Listeria, Mycoplasma, Brucella, Chlamydia,* and *Leptospira* are suspected. In *Salmonella* enteric infections, a selective enrichment culture is more sensitive in isolating *Salmonella* from other enteric bacteria than routine cultures. *Listeria* is a fastidious bacteria, and an enrichment culture is needed for the isolation of the bacteria from suspected neurologic cases from ruminants. *Mycoplasma* and some *Brucella* species need specific growth factors and incubation conditions. *Rickettsia* and *Chlamydia* will not grow in *in vitro* culture media, and cumbersome cell cultures are needed to cultivate them. Therefore, the choice of diagnostic test is critical in obtaining accurate and timely results. Similarly, attempts to culture for disease diagnosis can be barely rewarding in the decision-making process for some fastidious bacteria. For example, *Leptospira* culture needs prolonged incubation and special media, and alternative procedures such as serology, DFA test, or PCR or a combination of these tests will provide timely results. Interpretation of results should also account for differentiating normal flora from potential pathogens because many body sites harbor microbial flora. Correlation of the results with clinical signs and the presence of quantity and the type of organisms can assist the practitioner in the decision-making process. A heavy growth of a pure culture of a bacteria is indicative of infection, while multiple types of organisms (three or more types) isolated from a single sample in the absence of the growth of an obligate or primary pathogenic bacteria should be interpreted as contamination. When a negative result is obtained in the presence of obvious clinical signs or in a nonresolving illness, factors such as special bacterial growth requirements, prior treatment, sample collection and transport methods, and information from direct staining must be considered, and the process must be reevaluated.

Antimicrobial susceptibility testing

Antimicrobial therapy plays a vital role in controlling infections. AST routinely performed in conjunction with a bacterial culture determines whether a bacteria is susceptible to a particular antimicrobial agent; use this information for selecting an antimicrobial agent for treatment. A disk diffusion test (Kirby–Bauer test) and broth dilution test are commonly available; the broth dilution test is quantitative and provides the minimum inhibitory concentration (MIC) of an antimicrobial agent. MIC is the minimum concentration of the drug required to inhibit bacterial growth, and the availability of these data improves the selection of antimicrobial agents and dosage to optimize a favorable treatment outcome. In addition to the MIC value, several factors including pharmacokinetics, pharmacodynamics, and concerns of resistance emergence have to be considered while choosing the antimicrobial agents. Routine AST may also allow the building of an antibiogram to guide veterinarians in selecting the empiric therapy for future patients and will also help to monitor the evolution of drug resistance. Practitioners' awareness of the intrinsic resistance observed in certain bacterial pathogens will avoid inappropriate and ineffective therapies. A typical example is the use of aminoglycosides in treating anaerobic infections.

Diagnostic approaches for fungal infections

Fungi are eukaryotic organisms with complex and diverse morphological structures and as such, precise identification of a fungal species can be challenging. Only a limited number of fungi are known pathogens that can cause disease in a healthy animal, yet a large number of them are emerging as opportunistic and invasive infections in animals and humans. Frequent antimicrobial use and alterations in normal flora may predispose the colonization of fungi such as *Candida* in the skin and mucous membranes and may lead to clinical disease. Proper collection, handling, and transport of samples are required, as in the case of bacterial infections. Transportation and storage of clinical materials at room temperature are recommended because some of the fungal agents such as dermatophytes are known to be sensitive to cold temperatures. Direct microscopic examination of clinical samples used in conjunction with culturing is a routine option for the diagnosis of fungal infections. By microscopic examination of these smears, arthrospores of dermatophytes can be observed within the hair shaft (endothrix) and outside of the hair shaft (ectothrix). Geographic location and travel history are important components of a diagnostic investigation because some fungal pathogens are endemic to certain geographic locations; *Coccidiodomyces* in the southwestern states of the United States and *Cryptococcus gattii* in the northwestern United States and western Canada are a few examples. The presence and characteristics of certain fungal organisms such as size, morphological features, and cellular location in clinical specimens may offer diagnostic clues.

Fungal culture and isolation are done using a specialized media (Sabouraud's dextrose agar) and low incubation temperature (29 °C), and so a specific laboratory request is necessary. Because prolonged incubation facilitates the growth of contaminant bacteria and saprophytic fungus, the addition of antibiotics or inhibitory chemical agents such as chlorhexidine in the media is necessary to isolate fungal organisms. Dermatophyte test media (DTM) is widely used by veterinary practitioners at the point of care for the diagnosis of ringworm infection. If dermatophytes are present, the media will change color due to the change in pH. However, color change itself should not be considered as diagnostic for dermatophytes, as other saprophytic fungal contaminants can cause a similar change in pH. Microscopic examination and identification of unique fungal species-specific structures such as hyphae, macroconidia, and microconidia must be performed for definitive identification.

Interpretation of fungal culture results must be pursued with caution because some body sites, especially the nasal cavity, skin, and mucous membranes, can easily be contaminated with fast-growing saprophytic fungal spores. Correlation of culture results with cytological and histopathologic evidence of fungal structures along with compatible host inflammatory response is required to make a confirmatory diagnosis. A negative result should also be interpreted with caution because some fungal agents may not grow in a routine fungal culture media.

Antifungal susceptibility tests

Antifungal susceptibility tests are not widely available, and service from reference laboratories must be sought for pursuing this. Choice of antifungal agents and the availability of AST interpretive criteria are limited. An accredited laboratory following Clinical and Laboratory Standards Institute (CLSI) or European Committee on Antimicrobial Susceptibility Testing (EUCAST) guidelines must be selected to assure appropriate quality control and quality assurance of testing.

Fungal antigen detection

Antigen detection methods are available for some systemic and invasive infections (galactomannan detection for *Aspergillus*). Antigen detection for dimorphic fungal infections (*Blastomyces, Coccidioides, Cryptococcus,* and *Histoplasma*) and a few others are available through commercial laboratories (MiraVista Diagnostics, Indianapolis, IN). A serum-based β-d-glucan assay is also available for the presumptive diagnosis of invasive fungal infections for which there is difficulty in obtaining clinical samples.

Diagnostic approaches for viral infections

Accurate and timely diagnosis of viral diseases in animals allows applicable clinical management, determination of prognosis, and prevention of transmission by enhancing biosecurity protocols and strategic use of vaccination protocols and management practices. In addition, an accurate diagnosis of a viral infection avoids unnecessary use of antibiotics and thereby minimizes the potential emergence of antimicrobial resistance. Viral diagnostics are challenging because virus growth requires sophisticated cell culture systems that are available only in reference diagnostic laboratories. Direct detection of viral pathogens includes detection of inclusion bodies by light microscopy in cytology and histopathology specimens, observing viral particles by electron microscopy, or by the detection of the agent or its components using immunological methods such as DFA test. The rapidity of these tests is useful for early diagnosis. Conventional techniques routinely used for the diagnosis of viral infections are time-consuming and often not practical for patient management. Developments in technology including the generation of specific monoclonal antibodies and improvements in enzyme immunoassays, shell vial cultures for virus isolations, and nucleic acid amplification methods have tremendously improved the timely detection of viral pathogens. Preanalytical steps, including specimen selection, collection transport, and processing methods, are as important as the selection of laboratory tests. Understanding of the viral pathogenesis and target organs affected is essential for the selection of clinical specimens for testing. Sample collection devices also have a significant effect on detection. For example, wooden shaft swabs may contain toxic compounds such as formaldehyde and are not suitable for virus isolation procedures. Calcium alginate-aluminum shaft swabs may also have inhibitory effects on PCR.

Rapid point-of-care tests

A variety of rapid point-of-care tests targeting viral antigens are available for detection in clinical specimens. In these tests, antibodies targeting specific viral antigens are either immobilized on a membrane or coated on plastic wells, and the viral antigens can be detected by various detection systems. These tests are fast and easy to use in clinics. Immunoassays for viral antigen detection are commercially available for the diagnosis of a few viral infections (canine parvovirus, feline leukemia virus) and can be performed at the point of care. Specific attention should be given to the manufacturer's guidelines for proper running and interpretation.

Direct fluorescent antibody testing

DFA testing is a common method for detecting viral infection. When infecting cells, the virus localizes either within the cytoplasm or the nucleus depending on the type of virus and can be detected by use of FITC labeled, virus-specific polyclonal or monoclonal antibodies and observation through a fluorescent microscope.

Electron microscopy

Electron microscopy allows visualization of viral particles in clinical specimens with a highly specialized microscope that uses electron beams for detection. Electron microscopy is useful in diagnosing enteric viral infections such as parvovirus, coronavirus, and rotavirus infections. There are two types of electron microscopes, a transmission electron microscope and a scanning electron microscope; the former is the most often used for the diagnosis of infectious diseases. Negative staining using phosphotungstic acid is used for the detection of viral particles in clinical specimens. Specific morphology observed in these preparations allows the diagnostician to identify viruses to the genus level (Figure 5.6A,B). When inclusion bodies are suspected in lesions observed in H&E stained tissue histopathology preparations, a transmission electron microscope can reveal viral particles (Figure 5.6C,D).

Electron microscopy is especially useful in diagnosing emerging infectious diseases and unusual infections where etiology is completely unknown. Once the general morphologic characteristics of the virus are known, confirmation can be done by virus isolation, PCR, and sequencing. Electron microscopy offers excellent specificity due to the characteristic morphology of virus families but low sensitivity as a

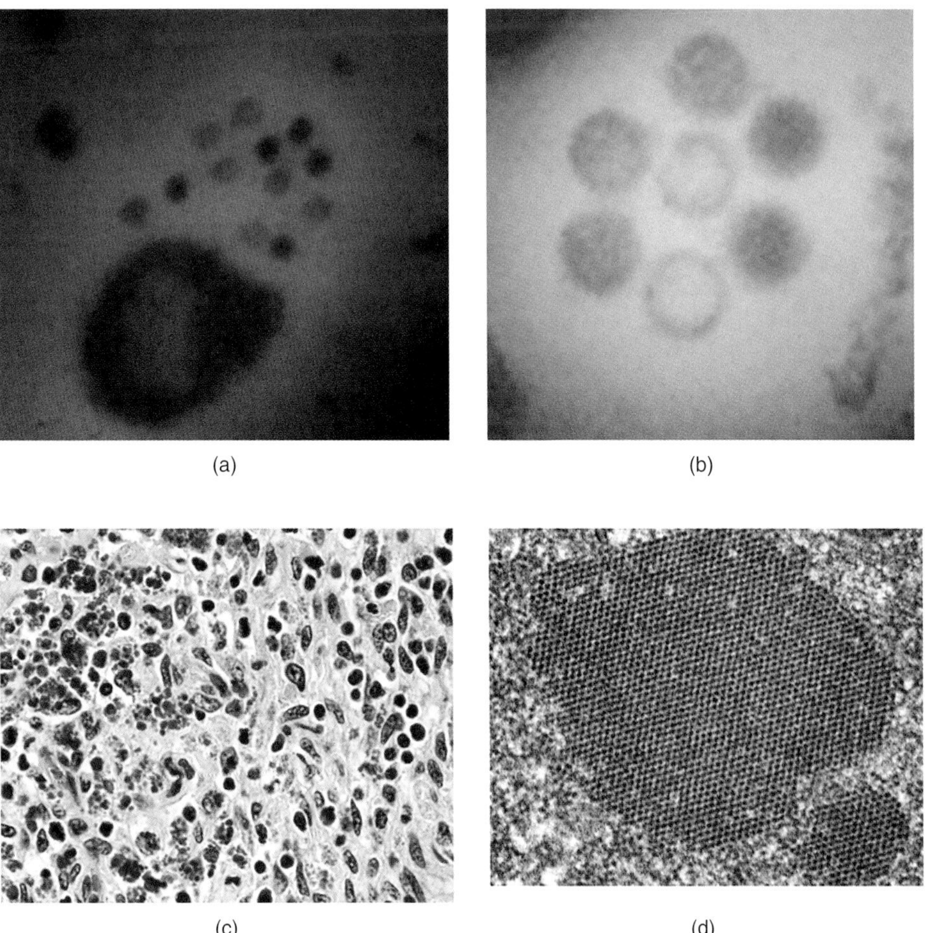

Figure 5.6 Electron microscopy is a valuable tool for the diagnosis of viral infections. A: Transmission electron microscopy (TEM) image of a negative stained feces containing parvovirus. B: TEM image of a negative stained feces containing rotavirus. C: H&E stained image of a lymph node containing cirocovirus inclusion bodies. D: TEM micrograph of the above section showing paracrystalline array of circovirus.

large number of viral particles are needed for visualization under the electron microscope. This technique is also useful for screening cell cultures when there are no detectable cytopathic effects (CPEs) as a result of virus growth

Virus isolation

Virus isolation in cell cultures, the gold standard test for the confirmation of viral infection, is a laborious process and requires growth of virus from clinical specimens in permissible cell lines. Processing of clinical specimens involves homogenization of samples in the cell culture media, removal of contaminant bacteria by filtration, and addition of antibiotics before inoculation. The growth of virus is detected by the presence of characteristic changes in the infected cells called CPEs. This is followed by confirmation using fluorescent antibody staining, PCR, or electron microscopy. Animal inoculations and isolation in embryonated chicken eggs are needed for growing a few viruses. The advantage of this technique is that a viable virus isolate, when obtained through cell culture or animal/egg inoculation, will allow further characterization of its properties, including virulence and antigenic variations, which can lead to development of vaccines, diagnostics, and antiviral drugs. Virus isolations are expensive, time-consuming, and need facilities for maintaining cell culture. This technique is not desirable for making quick and timely clinical decisions, and recently has increasingly been replaced by molecular techniques.

Antibody detection

Detection of antiviral antibodies is a widely used and reliable practice for the diagnosis of viral infections. The collection of serum is an easy, noninvasive procedure. Viral agents may not be present in the body during the entire duration of infection, but exposure to the virus can be confirmed by the presence of serum antibodies. Tests commonly used include virus neutralization (VN), agar gel immunodiffusion (AGID), hemagglutination inhibition (HI) assay, immunofluorescence assay (IFA), Western blots, complement fixation tests, and enzyme-linked immunosorbent assay (ELISA).

Virus neutralization

VN is a highly sensitive and specific detection procedure where virus neutralizing antibodies prevent the growth of the virus in cell culture. The antibody present in the serum can be quantitated, and the highest dilution of the serum that inhibits the neutralization is recorded as the antibody titer. Another variation of this test is the plaque reduction neutralization test (PRNT), which is used for plaque-forming viruses such as arboviruses. Paired serum antibody titer determination is often needed for confirmation of an active infection vs. exposure or a vaccine response. A paired serum testing of the acute and convalescent serum samples and the observation of a fourfold increase in antibody titer should confirm an active infection. This is achieved by testing a serum sample collected from an acutely ill animal and a sample collected after 2–4 weeks (convalescent serum sample) side by side. VN or PRNT assays are not widely available as these methods are laborious, time-consuming, and expensive. They also require maintenance of cell cultures, preparation and storage of titered virus stocks, trained personnel, and stringent quality-control measures.

ELISAs

One of the most common commercially available serology tests is ELISAs. These tests use plastic wells coated with viral antigens, and when the test serum is added, antiviral antibodies, if present in the test sera, will bind to the antigen. A secondary species-specific antibody conjugated with an enzyme such as horseradish peroxidase will allow the detection of the antibodies. Differentiation of antibody class IgM or IgG can facilitate the diagnosis of recent antibodies from ongoing infections or exposure. Interpretation of serology results can be complex and confounding. The nature of the disease, the pathogen, and the test parameters influence the outcome. A single positive or negative result is informative for only a few infectious diseases. For example, for diseases caused by retroviruses such as equine infectious anemia in horses, a single antibody positive test (a widely used AGID, or Coggins, test) can confirm infection. It is important to understand that in a patient with an infection, false-negative test results could still be observed in the early stage of an infection. Serology tests are beneficial in herd situations, where seronegative status provides a reasonable evidence of the absence of infection in a population.

Diagnostic approaches for parasitic infections

"Parasite" is a broad term and refers here mainly to eukaryotic organisms belonging to protozoa (single cell) and metazoa (arthropods and helminths, including nematodes, trematodes, and cestodes). Unlike bacterial and viral infections, historical diagnosis of parasitic infections was by identification of organisms using morphological criteria utilizing gross or light microscopical examination. Recently, many of these techniques have been replaced by molecular methods (PCR and sequencing) and antigen detection through immunoassays. Commercial and in-house kits for antibody detection are also increasingly available.

The most common specimen submitted for parasitology examination is the fecal sample for the detection of ova and parasites. Preservation of stool (5–10% formalin) is often practiced to retain the morphology of certain protozoan parasites and to prevent continued development of helminth eggs and larvae if there is a delay in transport of materials. Three common methods available are direct wet mount, concentration, and permanently stained smears. Fresh feces is required for direct wet mounts to identify motile trophozoites. Wet mounts are not attempted in preserved specimens. The concentration of fecal samples using flotation or sedimentation is commonly used, and the concentrated samples are examined under the light microscope. Both surface film and the sediment must be examined in order to detect some of the heavy helminth and operculated eggs. Samples should be collected in clean screw cap and wide mouth containers without any water or urine contamination because the presence of urine will destroy the motile organisms. Permanently stained smears can be used for the detection of intestinal protozoa, and two common methods used are Gomori tissue trichrome–Wheatley modification and iron hematoxylin stains. These stains can be used for the confirmation of structures observed in wet smears (> than 300 fields must be examined).

Molecular methods

The golden era of molecular diagnostics originated after Dr. Kary Mullis's 1983 Nobel Prize–winning invention, the PCR, and has undergone remarkable advancements since then. In the diagnosis of infectious diseases, PCR applies to the amplification of pathogen-specific target nucleic acids, DNA or RNA using specific enzymes called DNA polymerases. For the detection of RNA as in RNA viruses, an additional step of conversion of RNA to DNA (reverse transcription) is carried out using an enzyme called reverse transcriptase. Primers specific to the target DNA fragment are designed for specific amplification of the pathogens. Automated machines called thermocyclers are used in the amplification of the nucleic acid. PCR allows sensitive and specific detection of pathogen-specific nucleic acid in a shorter turnaround time compared to conventional bacterial cultures or virus isolation. Challenges include false-positive reactions due the extremely sensitive nature of the assay, often arising due to contamination. False-negative results occur as a result of the inherent inhibition of the PCR assays due to the presence of PCR inhibitors in the sample and the quantity of DNA below the detection threshold. Interpreting the PCR results in the relevant clinical context may overcome some of these challenges. Depending upon the nature of agents sought, DNA, RNA, or total nucleic acid can be extracted using appropriate in-house techniques or commercially available nucleic acid extraction kits. In a conventional PCR, the amplified DNA fragment is detected using agarose gel electrophoresis and then visualized under ultraviolet (UV) light (Figure 5.7a). In a real-time PCR, DNA binding fluorescence dyes such as SYBR green or a DNA probe labeled with a fluorescent dye are used. The amplification of DNA is measured and observed real time using computer software (Figure 5.7b).

The real-time PCR assay can also be modified to quantify the pathogen load in a clinical sample. There are many design variations of PCRs; however, discussion of them is not within the scope of this chapter. One should discuss the advantages and disadvantages of these techniques with the laboratory provider. Recent advances such as the development of reagents with superior amplification efficiency, discriminatory target development to improve specificity, automated high-throughput platforms, the ability to multiplex and detect multiple pathogens at the same time, and a high potential for standardization have reduced the cost and improved the efficiency of PCR testing. PCR combined with sequencing of various targets as in multilocus sequence typing (MLST) allows the classification of strains and the detection of changes or mutation in virulence factors in

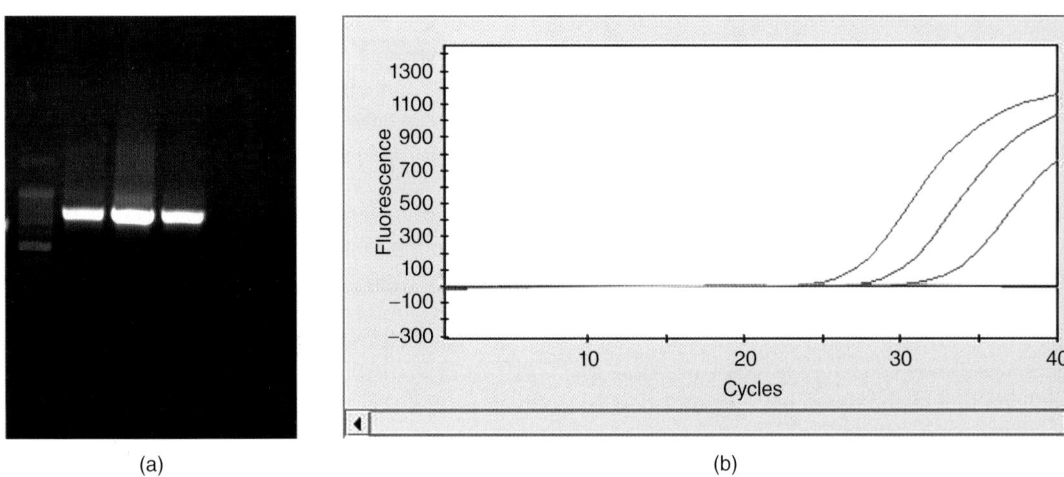

Figure 5.7 (a) DNA is amplified by a conventional PCR using pathogen-specific primers and a validated thermocycling protocol. The amplified product is subjected to agar gel electrophoresis and visualized under the UV light. (b) For real-time PCR, fluorescent dye that binds to the amplified DNA or a hydrolysis probe is used for the detection of the product. The product can be quantified in relation to pathogen load using optimized and well-validated protocols.

microbial pathogens. A repertoire of PCR-based diagnostic tests are available for veterinary infectious disease diagnosis through state veterinary diagnostic laboratories or other commercial labs.

Next-generation sequencing

One of the latest technologies, next-generation sequencing (NGS), is increasingly becoming accessible for the diagnosis of infectious diseases [2]. Also referred to as "deep sequencing," "massively parallel sequencing," or "high-throughput sequencing," this procedure can be successfully implemented in clinical specimens where an infectious agent is suspected but cannot be detected by commonly available techniques. NGS is increasingly being used in human medicine and is especially beneficial in identifying novel and emerging pathogens.

Role of postmortem investigation in infectious disease diagnosis

Postmortem examination for understanding the cause of mortality is more commonly performed in veterinary medicine than in human medicine. The value of postmortem histopathology and microbiology is well recognized in the veterinary field in diagnosing infectious diseases during outbreaks of economically important diseases among food animal populations, uncovering emerging infectious diseases, and identifying those diseases for which the diagnosis might have been missed using other approaches. Accurate identification of infectious agents, tracking of antimicrobial resistance in organisms isolated, understanding the changes in pathogen virulence due to mutations, and epidemiological patterns of diseases will benefit future investigations. There is disagreement among clinicians about the value and usefulness of postmortem microbiology testing, as postmortem invasion and contamination can influence the interpretation of results. Correlation with patient history and the gross and microscopic findings is required for meaningful interpretation. Certain infectious diseases present with pathognomonic or characteristic lesions that can be used for the presumptive diagnosis and for the selection of follow-up tests. Storage of the carcass in a cooler and completion of the postmortem examination soon after death may reduce the postmortem overgrowth and increase the likelihood of accurately identifying the pathogens in question. Examination of the carcass soon after death is not practical in veterinary medicine due to the time taken for transport to reference veterinary diagnostic laboratories that are often not available closer to the patient location. Tissues with gross signs of infection must be collected carefully following sterile precautions using sterile equipment. Adequate size of tissue should be collected to allow proper searing to remove surface contaminants. Swabs are also acceptable for microbial culture; however, multiple swabs must be collected for multiple procedures. Fluids collected in nonleaking sterile screw-cap containers are preferable over those transported in syringes.

Role of biopsy and histopathology in infectious disease diagnosis

Routine biopsy and histopathology can provide strong evidence of the presence of an infectious agent, and associated inflammation that can help in the selection of downstream diagnostic tests required for confirmation. The knowledge of the presence and the location of bacterial organisms, their differential staining properties, and the nature of inflammation can help in the diagnostic process. Certain infectious diseases are easily diagnosed by histopathological evaluation of samples. The pathological changes in the tissue and the morphology of certain pathogens can definitively diagnose few infections. This is especially valuable for certain fungal infections where characteristic morphology of fungal organisms can be observed [1]. The typical examples include large spherules containing endospores in the tissue in *Coccidioides immitis* infection, broad-based budding yeasts in *Blastomyces dermatitidis* infections, and round to oval yeast cells surrounded by a large halo representative of a capsule in *C. neoformans* infections [1]. In addition, histopathology examination may reveal the evidence of coinfections that would have been missed by a single targeted microbiologic testing.

In viral infections, observation of inclusion bodies in the cytoplasm or nucleus, the formation of syncytia, and the nature of cellular infiltration can be significant findings. Characteristic intranuclear inclusion bodies in tissues of animals with herpesvirus infections, intracytoplasmic inclusion bodies in cases of canine distemper in dogs, and formation of a syncytium in respiratory syncytial virus infections in cattle can be diagnostic. Special staining of histopathology sections using Gram stains (Brown–Hopps or Brown and Brenn), acid-fast stains (Fite's acid-fast stain, Ziehl–Neelsen stain), Giemsa stains, and silver stains (Warthin–Starry stain, Grocott–Gomori's stain) is useful for the detection and differentiation of pathogens.

Immunohistochemistry techniques using pathogen-specific antibodies can reveal additional information that is not generally obtained by the examination of routine hematoxylin and eosin stained tissue sections (Figure 5.8) [3]. The examination of H&E stained specimens may be the best choice to diagnose conditions caused by those agents that may not grow in laboratory cultures. Examples include finding bacilli with haystack-like appearance in the hepatocytes in Tyzzer's disease caused by *Clostridium piliforme*, large sporangium containing spores in nasal polyps caused by *Rhinosporidium*

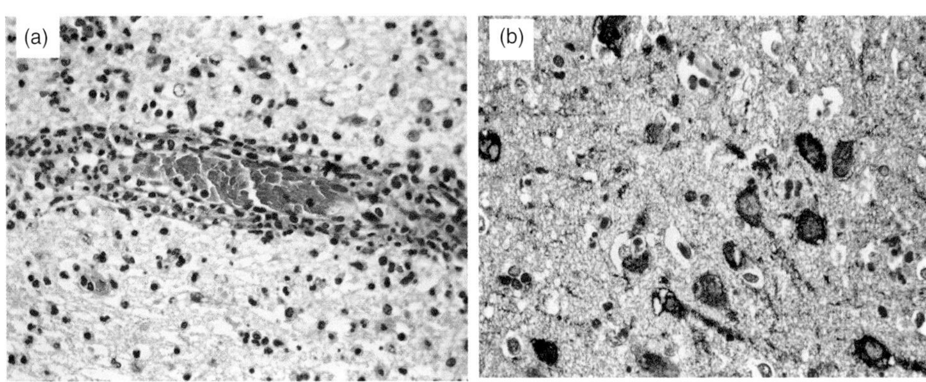

Figure 5.8 Perivascular cuffing is a feature of CNS infections. To identify the viral etiology an immunohistochemistry (IHC) was applied to detect eastern equine encephalitis (EEE) antigen in the brain. A: H&E stained brain section showing perivascular cuffing. B: IHC using anti-EEE antibodies was used to detect EEE antigen in the neuronal cytoplasm.

seeberi, and the presence of spiral bacteria in the intestinal epithelium in *Lawsonia intracellularis* infection.

Laboratory diagnosis of infections affecting various body systems

Certain infectious agents have predilections toward a particular body system, whereas some others may infect and alter multiple body systems. The outcome of infections depends on the pathogen, host, and conditions where infections were acquired. Opportunistic infections are on the rise in animals and humans due to changes in immunocompetency of the host and ecology. Diagnostic strategies for infectious diseases affecting various body systems are briefly discussed below. A list of selected pathogens, infectious diseases, the species of animals, and the recommended diagnostic tests are given in the Appendix 5.A.

Skin and soft-tissue infections

Skin, the major barrier in the body against microbial invasion, constantly interacts with the environment and is normally colonized with microbial organisms such as *Staphylococcus*, *Streptococcus*, and *Corynebacterium*. Infections of the skin and underlying tissues may have varying clinical presentations, and severity may range from superficial pyoderma to deep cellulitis and occasionally life-threatening conditions such as necrotizing fasciitis. *Staphylococcus*, *Streptococcus*, and rarely Gram-negative anaerobes are generally involved in these conditions. When deciding on the diagnostic approach, practitioners must be aware of those infectious and noninfectious systemic diseases that have cutaneous manifestations. For example, submitting a skin sample is required for diagnosing greasy pig disease caused by *Staphylococcus hyicus*, but submitting a skin sample for diamond skin disease, a systemic disease caused by *Erysipelothrix rhusiopathiae*, will result in false-negative results. Traumatic injuries to the skin and underlying tissue may allow invasion of anaerobic organisms leading to deep-seated infections resulting in an abscess, draining tracts, and myositis. In these situations, a delay in the identification of the cause and treatment lead to invasion of infection into deeper structures and blood and can be detrimental to the host. Cytological examination, skin biopsy, and bacterial and fungal culture are the common methods used for diagnosing skin infections. Samples must be collected after cleaning and debridement of the affected tissue. Because the majority of skin conditions are secondary to other predisposing factors such as allergy, ectoparasitism, and trauma, identifying and removing the predisposing factor and then addressing the infections will enhance the therapeutic success. A full-thickness biopsy is preferred over punch or wedge biopsy for histopathologic assessment of nonresolving skin lesions. Systemic viral infections including pox and vesicular diseases induce skin lesions. Many systemic infections caused by fungal organisms *B. dermatitidis*, *Histoplasma capsulatum*, *C. immitis*, and *C. neoformans* can have cutaneous manifestations. As skin may harbor normal flora, interpretation and differentiation of pathogens from colonizers is imperative to avoid initiating unnecessary antimicrobial therapy.

Gastrointestinal infections

A wide variety of microorganisms inhabit the gastrointestinal tract including aerobic, facultative anaerobic, and obligate anaerobic organisms, and the identity of many of them is unknown. The consortium of microorganisms termed as the intestinal "microbiome" is essential for the health and well-being of the host. Any imbalance in the composition of the microbiome may induce a disease state.

Oral cavity infections including gingivitis and periodontitis are common in dogs and cats, and the polymicrobial nature of these conditions can be confounding when trying to identify a precise etiology. Primary oral lesions occur with viral infections such as canine distemper virus, canine herpesvirus, feline calicivirus, and viral vesicular diseases along with other systemic manifestations. The pursuit of diagnostic testing for pharyngitis and tonsillitis can be unrewarding due to the presence of a multitude of organisms in these locations unless a specific etiology is suspected (e.g., *Fusobacterium necrophorum* or *Histophilus somni* in calves causing necrotizing laryngitis). Low pH of the stomach inhibits the survival of many bacteria, but members of the species *Helicobacter* can colonize the stomach and cause ulcers and gastritis. Primary enteropathogenic organisms such as *E. coli, Salmonella, Clostridium perfringens, Clostridium difficile,* and *Campylobacter* spp. can be diagnosed by fecal cultures. Special selective enrichment cultures for these pathogens are often necessary to improve the detection sensitivity in the presence of normal microflora.

Detection of relevant toxins is more significant in cases of infections caused by *C. perfringens* and *C. difficile* because these organisms can be a part of the normal gastrointestinal flora. A freshly voided fecal specimen collected in sterile screw-cap containers and transported under refrigeration conditions is ideal for the recovery of enteric pathogens. A transport media such as Cary-Blair is recommended. If fresh feces is not available, a rectal swab may be collected after cleaning the anus with 70% alcohol. Multiple swabs must be collected for different tests such as culture, PCR, toxin testing, etc.

Respiratory tract infections

Primary viral and bacterial pathogens as well as commensal microbes present in the nasal cavity and oropharynx are capable of causing respiratory disease. Viral infections can destabilize the innate immune response mechanisms and make the host susceptible to secondary respiratory bacterial infections. In addition, several sporadically occurring systemic diseases such as anthrax, plague, and tularemia, though rare in animals, often have respiratory manifestations. Culture is one of the most common methods used for the diagnosis of respiratory tract bacterial infections. Interpretation of results can be perplexing due to the presence of normal microflora, which is abundant in the upper respiratory tract and nasal cavity. Therefore, the culture of nasal cavity, pharynx, and larynx is usually unrewarding, unless selected pathogens are sought. Infections of the lower respiratory tract, such as pneumonia and pyothorax, may induce systemic abnormalities; leukograms, blood gas analysis, and blood chemistry findings may provide further clues to the nature of the infectious process. Fecal testing is advised to rule out respiratory tract infections of parasitic origin. Imaging using radiography, ultrasonography, and endoscopic examination may also be pursued to obtain a better understanding of the location and severity of infections. Samples collected by fine-needle aspiration and properly collected transtracheal and bronchoalveolar lavage can be submitted for aerobic, anaerobic, or fungal cultures if indicated. Members of the genus *Mycoplasma* are involved in respiratory tract infections of many animal species and often occur as coinfection with other bacterial and viral agents; a mycoplasma culture or PCR must be requested. Direct staining (Gram's and acid-fast) will differentiate Gram-positive vs. Gram-negative bacteria and infections caused by organisms such as *Mycobacteria* and *Nocardia*.

Urogenital tract infections

The lower urogenital tract is normally colonized by bacteria. Bacterial infections of the urinary system affecting the urethra, bladder, ureters, and sometimes renal pelvis are common among companion animals. Asymptomatic colonization and bacteriuria may be observed in some animals. Gram-negative organisms *E. coli, Proteus, Klebsiella, Pseudomonas,* and *Enterobacter* and Gram-positive organisms *Staphylococcus, Streptococcus,* and *Enterococcus* are the most common isolates in canine urinary tract infections. Method of urine collection is a significant factor in interpreting urine culture results. Collection through cystocentesis is preferred over catheterization or midstream urine collection. Catheterization and midstream collection introduce commensal bacteria in the urine sample and are not preferable collection methods. A small volume of urine aseptically collected is useful for quantitative cultures. The culture results must be interpreted in conjunction with urine analysis results.

Infections of the reproductive tract may result in abortion or early embryonic death in pregnant animals. Fetal internal organs and stomach or abomasal fluid are ideal for testing if available. Fetal serum and paired serum samples (acute and convalescent) from the dam are also valuable resources for diagnostic testing.

Nervous system infections

Infectious diseases affecting the nervous system are often fatal, and the antemortem diagnoses can be challenging. Accurate and timely diagnosis is critical in therapy implementation. Developing a list of differential diagnoses through history and clinical examination, a complete blood count, serum biochemical profile, imaging, and serology in conjunction with CSF analysis imparts valuable information about the potential pathogen involved and will help the clinician in ruling in or out potential infectious agents. CSF analysis should be performed as quickly as possible after collection to avoid cell lysis. Refrigeration and the addition of bovine serum albumin or fetal calf serum to CSF can slow down the degeneration of the cells. Cloudiness due to increased cells, red discoloration due to either blood contamination or hemorrhage, and increased nucleated cell count in CSF (pleocytosis), and the presence of microbes may be observed in infections of the central nervous system (CNS).

Systemic infections

Systemic infections can be caused by a wide variety of infectious agents including bacterial, viral, fungal, and parasitic organisms. Colonization of various body systems may occur depending on the portal of entry before dissemination of the agent or its toxins. In the case of tetanus or botulism, the systemic effects are due to the local infection and the production of toxins or ingestion of food contaminated with the toxin. A quick determination of the type of organism, potential entry and dissemination sites, and pathogenesis will result in a better prognosis. Although many infectious agents have a tissue tropism, almost all infectious agents can spread systemically in immunocompromised patients.

Conclusion

The basic approaches in the laboratory diagnosis of infections remain the same despite the changes in technology and the discovery of new and emerging infectious diseases. The diagnostic approach for each suspected infectious disease is dependent on availability of assays, assay performance, turnaround time, and the affordability of testing. Preanalytic steps strictly followed by the submitting clinician and the testing laboratory have a profound effect on the outcome. Infectious disease and clinical manifestations are a result of interactions between host, pathogen, and the environment, and each of these impact the nature of the disease and its manifestations. In view of all of the possibilities of infectious disease outcomes, including transient disease followed by recovery, subclinical or chronic disease and recovery, severe debilitating clinical disease, or persistent infections, a judicious yet pragmatic diagnostic approach and interpretation of the laboratory results are critical for management of the patient. Many pathogens can be seen as a part of normal flora, and an evaluation of the role of microbial agents or host response detected as a part of the disease process, although challenging, may be necessary for accurate interpretation.

5.A. List of Selected Pathogens/Major Infectious Diseases, Species of Animals, and the Recommended Diagnostic Tests

Steps involved in the laboratory diagnosis of infectious diseases:

1. Evaluate the objective of the diagnostic testing (patient management, herd screening, etc.).
2. Evaluate the benefits of the chosen testing process.
3. Identify a suitable laboratory and discuss the sample and test selection, transportation methods, turnaround time, cost, test parameters, and interpretation guidelines.
4. Collect and ship samples using proper guidelines for the sample and suspected infectious agent.
5. Interpret the test results and use the results based on the objective of the diagnostic testing process.

Bacterial pathogens

Organism: *Actinomyces* spp. (*A. viscosus, A. israelii, A. hordeovulneris*)
Diseases and species affected: Abscess, osteomyelitis, pleuritis, pyothorax, in dogs, cats, and other animals; pyogranulomatous osteomyelitis or lumpy jaw (caused by *A. bovis*) in cattle.
Preferred diagnostic tests: Aerobic and anaerobic cultures are required because there are aerobic and anaerobic members in this genus.
Comments: Opportunistic pathogens present in the mucosa; presence of sulfur granules in the lesion is suggestive of infection.

Organism: *Anaplasma* spp.
Diseases and species affected: *A. phagocytophilium* causes canine granulocytic anaplasmosis and infects neutrophils; *A. platys* causes canine cyclic thrombocytopenia and infects platelets; *A. marginale* causes tick fever in cattle and infects RBCs.
Preferred diagnostic tests: Complete blood count and visualization of the organisms in infected cells, serology, PCR.
Comments: Obligate intracellular pathogens, vector-borne infection.

Organism: *Bacillus* spp.
Diseases and species affected: *Bacillus anthracis* causes anthrax in domestic animals and human; *Bacillus cereus* and *Bacillus subtilis* are involved in wound infections, abortions, and food poisoning.
Preferred diagnostic tests: Aerobic culture, PCR.
Comments: *B. anthracis* can be presumptively diagnosed by detecting large rod-shaped bacteria with a capsule using the polychromatic methylene blue staining; anthrax is a reportable disease; zoonosis.

Organism: *Bartonella* spp.
Diseases and species affected: *Bartonella henslae* causes cat scratch fever in humans and a variety of nonspecific manifestations in cats, the reservoir host.
Preferred diagnostic tests: Peripheral blood smear evaluation, PCR, *Bartonella* culture, serology.
Comments: *Bartonella* spp. are host-adapted bacteria and are vector borne. They cause chronic and prolonged intraerythrocytic bacteremia; there are multiple species of *Bartonella* colonizing animals and their vectors.

Organism: *Bordetella bronchiseptica*
Diseases and species affected: Infectious tracheobronchitis in dogs and cats; atrophic rhinitis in swine.
Preferred diagnostic tests: Aerobic culture and PCR.
Comments: *B. bronchiseptica* is one of the pathogens involved in infectious respiratory disease complex in dogs.

Organism: *Borrelia* spp.
Diseases and species affected: There are many *Borrelia* species involved in Lyme disease and relapsing fevers in different host species.
Preferred diagnostic tests: Serology, PCR, *Borrelia* culture (rarely used).
Comments: Spirochete bacteria, vector-borne infection.

Organism: *Brachyspira hyodysentriae*
Diseases and species affected: Causes swine dysentery.
Preferred diagnostic tests: Anaerobic culture, PCR.
Comments: Spirochete bacteria.

Organism: *Brucella* spp.
Diseases and species affected: *Brucella abortus* (cattle), *Brucella melitensis* (sheep and goats), *Brucella suis* (pigs), *Brucella canis* (dogs) can cause reproductive tract and systemic diseases in various species of animals.
Preferred diagnostic tests: Serology, *Brucella* culture, PCR.
Comments: Reportable disease, zoonosis.

Organism: *Campylobacter* spp.
Diseases and species affected: *Campylobacter jejuni* is involved in enteric disease in animals. *C. fetus subsp. fetus* and *C. fetus subsp. venerealis* are involved in reproductive diseases in cattle, sheep, and goats.
Preferred diagnostic tests: Campylobacter culture, PCR.
Comments: *Campylobacter jejuni* is a major foodborne pathogen. They are microaerophilic and need specific specimen transport conditions.

Organism: *Chlamydia* spp.
Diseases and species affected: *C. abortus* causes ruminant abortion, *C. felis* causes pneumonia and conjunctivitis in cats, *C. psittaci* causes systemic disease in birds and is zoonotic.
Preferred diagnostic tests: Cytology (for the detection of inclusion bodies), PCR, isolations in cell culture.
Comments: Obligate intracellular bacteria, zoonosis.

Organism: *Clostridium* spp.
Diseases and species affected: *C. perfringens* and *C. difficile* are involved in enteric disease in animals. *C. chauvoei, C. novyi, C. septicum* cause myositis and systemic disease in food animals. *C. perfringens* is involved in enterotoxemia in animals. Several clostridial species are involved in abscess and wound infections. *C. tetani, C. botulinum* belong to a neurotoxic group.
Preferred diagnostic tests: Direct immunofluorescence testing, anaerobic culture, PCR, toxin screening.
Comments: The choice of diagnostic test is varied and depends on the condition of the animal species and infecting clostridial species.

Organism: *Corynebacterium* spp.
Diseases and species affected: *C. pseudotuberculosis* causes caseous lymphadenitis in sheep and goats, ulcerative lymphangitis in horses. *C. renale* group causes pyelonephritis in cattle. Numerous species can cause opportunistic infections.
Preferred diagnostic tests: Aerobic culture, PCR serology (synergetic hemolysin inhibition assay) to detect internal forms of disease.
Comments: Commensals in the skin and mucosa.

Organism: *Coxiella burnetii*
Diseases and species affected: Q fever, cattle, sheep, goats, dogs, cats.
Preferred diagnostic tests: PCR, serology, isolations in cell culture, serology using microimmunofluorescence tests (rarely performed).
Comments: Obligate intracellular bacteria, zoonosis.

Organism: *Dermatophilus congolensis*
Diseases and species affected: Skin infection in cattle, horses, and other mammals.
Preferred diagnostic tests: Cytology, aerobic culture, PCR.
Comments: Tram track-like appearance of bacteria in stained cytology preparations is diagnostic.
Organism: *Ehrlichia*
Diseases and species affected: *E. canis* causes canine monocytotropic ehrlichiosis, *E. ruminantium* causes heart water in ruminants.
Preferred diagnostic tests: Serology, PCR. *E. ruminantium* morula can be detected within the endothelial cells in stained brain squash preparations.
Comments: Obligate intracellular pathogen, vector-borne infection.

Organism: *Escherichia coli*
Diseases and species affected: Enteric and systemic infections in all animals.
Preferred diagnostic tests: Aerobic culture, PCR.
Comments: Pathogenicity varies with the virulence factors present. Presence or absence of a virulence factor can be screened through PCR.

Organism: *Francisella tularensis*
Diseases and species affected: Causes tularemia in dogs, cats, and other mammals.
Preferred diagnostic tests: Culture, PCR.
Comments: Tick-borne infection, zoonosis.

Organism: *Fusobacterium* spp.
Diseases and species affected: Causes abscess and wound infections in animals; *F. necrophorum* is involved in calf diphtheria, foot rot, and liver abscess in cattle.
Preferred diagnostic tests: Anaerobic culture, PCR.
Comments: Normal inhabitants of the mucosa.

Organism: *Helicobacter* spp.
Diseases and species affected: Multiple species of *Helicobacter* can cause gastric disease in animals. *H. hepaticus* and *H. bilis* are rodent pathogens.
Preferred diagnostic tests: PCR, *Helicobacter* culture.
Comments: *H. pylori* is involved in human gastric ulcers and neoplasms.

Organism: *Histophilus somni*
Diseases and species affected: Thromboembolic meningoencephalitis, pneumonia myocarditis, necrotic laryngitis in cattle.
Preferred diagnostic tests: Aerobic culture, PCR.
Comments: Involved in shipping fever pneumonia complex in cattle.

Organism: *Leptospira* spp.
Diseases and species affected: multiple species/serovars cause systemic, renal, hepatic, and reproductive disease in animals.
Preferred diagnostic tests: Serology (microscopic agglutination test), PCR, direct fluorescent antibody staining.
Comments: Numerous serovars are maintained in kidneys of many mammalian hosts; zoonosis.

Organism: *Listeria monocytogenes*
Diseases and species affected: Febrile and systemic illness in monogastric animals, meningoencephalitis in ruminants.
Preferred diagnostic tests: *Listeria* enrichment culture, PCR.
Comments: Food safety pathogen; organism survives and grows under refrigeration conditions.

Organism: *Mannheimia hemolytica*
Diseases and species affected: Causes pneumonia in ruminants.
Preferred diagnostic tests: Aerobic culture, PCR.
Comments: Involved in shipping fever pneumonia complex in cattle.

Organism: *Mycobacterium* spp.
Diseases and species affected: There are numerous pathogenic and saprophytic members in this group. *M. bovis* is a broad host range pathogen, causes tuberculosis in a variety of hosts. *M. avium subsp. paratuberculosis* causes chronic granulomatous enteritis (Johne's disease).
Preferred diagnostic tests: Test choice must be based on the suspected *Mycobacterium* spp.; for tuberculosis and paratuberculosis, specific cultures and PCRs are available; serology used for screening herds for paratuberculosis; mycobacterial culture or genus-specific PCR for other species; biopsy and acid-fast staining of the lesion.
Comments: Intradermal tests and interferon-gamma test available for screening herds for *M. bovis* infection.

Organism: *Mycoplasma* spp.
Diseases and species affected: Numerous species causing mainly respiratory diseases in animals and birds
Preferred diagnostic tests: *Mycoplasma* culture, PCR, serology.
Comments: Cell wall deficient bacteria.

Organism: *Nocardia* spp.
Diseases and species affected: Granulomatous inflammation of skin and internal organs, pleuritis, mastitis.
Preferred diagnostic tests: Biopsy and acid-fast staining, aerobic culture, PCR.
Comments: Sulfur granules may be present in the lesion, and the bacteria are partial acid-fast positive.

Organism: *Pasteurella* spp.
Diseases and species affected: *Pasteurella multocida* causes hemorrhagic septicemia and pneumonia in cattle, pneumonia and atrophic rhinitis in pigs, and fowl cholera. Other *Pasteurella* species can cause respiratory infections and bite wound infections.
Preferred diagnostic tests: Aerobic culture, PCR.
Comments: Opportunistic pathogens; *P. multocida* is a part of shipping fever pneumonia complex in cattle.

Organism: *Pseudomonas* spp.
Diseases and species affected: Multiple species involved in opportunistic infections of various body system. Major bacteria involved in canine otitis externa.
Preferred diagnostic tests: Aerobic culture.
Comments: Antibiotic resistance is common in this group.

Organism: *Rickettsia* spp.
Diseases and species affected: *R. rickettsia* causes Rocky Mountain spotted fever in dogs and cats.
Preferred diagnostic tests: Serology, PCR.
Comments: Vector-borne disease, infects endothelium, zoonosis.

Organism: *Rhodococcus equi*
Diseases and species affected: Causes foal pneumonia, ulcerative colitis, mesenteric lymphadenitis in horses.
Preferred diagnostic tests: Cytology of bronchoalveolar lavage fluid, aerobic culture, PCR.
Comments: Facultative intracellular bacteria.

Organism: *Staphylococcus* spp.
Diseases and species affected: Coagulase-positive species cause pyogenic infection of skin, bacteremia.
Preferred diagnostic tests: Aerobic culture, PCR.
Comments: Commensals on the skin and mucous membranes, can infect multiple body systems.

Organism: *Streptococcus* spp.
Diseases and species affected: Many species cause pyogenic infection in a broad range of hosts; *S. equi subsp. equi* causes strangles in horses.
Preferred diagnostic tests: Aerobic culture, PCR.
Comments: Commensals of the mucous membranes, can infect multiple body systems.

Organism: *Salmonella* spp.
Diseases and species affected: Enteric and systemic infections in animals.
Preferred diagnostic tests: *Salmonella* culture, PCR.
Comments: There are host-adapted and host-specific (*S. gallinarum and S. pullorum*) species. A major food safety pathogen.

Organism: *Shigella* spp.
Diseases and species affected: Causes gastroenteritis in nonhuman primates.
Preferred diagnostic tests: *Shigella* culture, PCR.
Comments: Causes dysentery in humans.

Organism: *Trueperella pyogenes*
Diseases and species affected: *T. pyogenes* causes abscess in internal organs in cattle.
Preferred diagnostic tests: Aerobic culture and PCR.
Comments: A secondary invader in shipping fever pneumonia complex in cattle.

Organism: *Yersinia* spp.
Diseases and species affected: *Yersinia pestis* causes plague,
Y. enterocolitica and *Y. pseudotuberculosis* cause gastrointestinal infections.
Preferred diagnostic tests: *Yersinia* culture, PCR.
Comments: Plague is a vector-borne disease transmitted through rat fleas; zoonosis.

Fungus and fungus-like pathogens

Organism: *Aspergillus* spp.

Diseases and species affected: Rhinosinusitis, systemic infections in dogs and cats, abortion in cattle.

Preferred diagnostic tests: Cytology (presumptive), biopsy and histopathology, fungal culture, serology for antibody and antigen detection (galactomannan EIA, beta-D-glucan test).

Comments: *Aspergillus* spp. are saprophytic fungi ubiquitous in the environment. Disseminated aspergillosis occurs in dogs and cats.

Organism: *Blastomyces dermatitidis*

Diseases and species affected: *B. dermatitidis* causes systemic fungal infection with cutaneous manifestations (pyogranulomatous inflammation of skin and organs) in dogs, cats, horses, and humans.

Preferred diagnostic tests: Cytology, biopsy and histopathology, serology for antigen and antibody detection, fungal culture (not required).

Comments: Dimorphic fungus, environmental origin, large broad-based budding yeast in tissues, infections geographically restricted to Ohio and Mississippi River valley.

Organism: *Candida* spp.

Diseases and species affected: Local and systemic infections in animals, urinary tract infections in dogs and cats, thrush in birds.

Preferred diagnostic tests: Aerobic or fungal culture and PCR.

Comments: Commensals on the mucous membrane, antibiotic treatment predisposes animals to infection.

Organism: *Cryptococcus* spp.

Diseases and species affected: *Cryptococcus neoformans* and *C. gattii* cause chronic mycosis in dogs, cats, and rarely other animals. The most common systemic mycosis in cats.

Preferred diagnostic tests: Cytology, biopsy and histopathology, fungal culture, *Cryptococcus* latex agglutination test for antigen detection, PCR.

Comments: Environmental transmission; CNS infections are common in cats; a distinct mucopolysaccharide capsule that can be detected in wet smears stained with India ink.

Organism: *Coccidioides immitis*

Diseases and species affected: Pulmonary and disseminated coccidioidomycosis in animals.

Preferred diagnostic tests: Cytology, biopsy and histopathology, fungal culture, serology for antigen detection, PCR.

Comments: Dimorphic fungus, environmental transmission, geographically endemic in southwestern and western United States. Large spherules containing endospores can be detected in cytology or histopathology specimens.

Organism: Dermatophytes

Diseases and species affected: *Microsporum* and *Trichophyton* species cause ringworm in animals (dogs, cats, horses, cattle) and humans.

Preferred diagnostic tests: Direct examination for the detection of spores, dermatophyte culture, histopathology.

Comments: Zoonosis.

Organism: *Histoplasma capsulatum*

Diseases and species affected: Causes systemic fungal infection (pyogranulomatous inflammation of lungs and gastrointestinal tract and other organs) in dogs, cats, horses, and humans.

Preferred diagnostic tests: Cytology, biopsy and histopathology, serology, fungal culture (not required).

Comments: Dimorphic fungus, environmental transmission, small intracytoplasmic yeast cells in macrophages by cytology or histopathology.

Organism: *Malassezia* spp.

Diseases and species affected: Causes dermatitis, otitis externa in dogs.

Preferred diagnostic tests: Cytology, culture (fungal and aerobic).

Comments: Yeast cells with characteristic morphology can be observed in cytology; some species require special media to grow.

Organism: *Prototheca* spp.

Diseases and species affected: *P. wickerhamii* and *P. zopfii* cause cutaneous, gastrointestinal, CNS, eye, and rarely disseminated infections in dogs and cats and mastitis in cattle.

Preferred diagnostic tests: Cytology, biopsy and histopathology, aerobic and fungal culture, PCR.

Comments: A saprophytic achlorophyllus algae.

Organism: *Sporothix schenckii*

Diseases and species affected: Cutaneous, lymphocutaneous, and rarely systemic disease is seen in dogs and cats.

Preferred diagnostic tests: Cytology, biopsy and histopathology, fungal culture.

Comments: Dimorphic fungus, small cigar-shaped yeast cells are observed in direct smear examination.

Organism: Zygomycets

Diseases and species affected: This group of fungi (*Rhizopus, Absidia, Mucur, Conidiobolus, Basidiobolus*) can cause systemic and subcutaneous infection in dogs and cats and abortion in cattle.

Preferred diagnostic tests: Biopsy and histopathology, fungal culture.

Comments: Saprophytic fast-growing contaminant; careful interpretation of laboratory results is needed.

Viral pathogens

Organism: Adenoviridae
Diseases and species affected: Canine adenovirus 1 causes infectious canine hepatitis in young dogs, canine adenovirus 2 causes respiratory disease.
Preferred diagnostic tests: PCR, direct fluorescent antibody staining, virus isolation, serology (IgM detection), electron microscopy.
Comments: DNA virus; intranuclear inclusion bodies in affected cells can be detected on histopathology evaluation of lesions.

Organism: Arteriviridae
Diseases and species affected: Equine arteritis virus (EAV) infection in horses causes systemic disease, arteritis, and pneumonia(foals); porcine reproductive and respiratory syndrome (PRRS) virus causes reproductive and respiratory disease in swine.
Preferred diagnostic tests: RT-PCR, virus isolations, serology (virus neutralization assays, ELISA).
Comments: Enveloped RNA virus, may cause asymptomatic infections.

Organism: Bunyaviridae
Diseases and species affected: Akabane virus causes congenital disorders in animals, Rift Valley fever virus causes systemic disease and abortion in animals.
Preferred diagnostic tests: Serology, RT-PCR, virus isolation.
Comments: RNA virus, arbovirus (vector-borne virus).

Organism: Circoviridae
Diseases and species affected: Porcine circovirus 2 (PCV 2) is associated with postweaning multisystemic wasting syndrome in pigs; psittacine beak and feather disease virus causes a debilitating disease in psittacine birds; chicken anemia virus causes acute immunosuppressive disease in young chicken.
Preferred diagnostic tests: Histopathology, PCR.
Comments: Nonenveloped DNA virus, presence of intracytoplasmic botryoid inclusions in the lesions on histopathology.

Organism: Calciviridae
Diseases and species affected: Feline calicivirus is a major cause of feline respiratory disease; rabbit hemorrhagic disease virus causes hemorrhagic disease with high mortality in lagomorphs.
Preferred diagnostic tests: RT-PCR, direct immunofluorescence assay, virus isolation, electron microscopy.
Comments: Nonenveloped RNA virus.

Organism: Coronaviridae
Diseases and species affected: Transmissible gastroenteritis virus (TGEV) causes gastroenteritis in pigs; feline infectious peritonitis virus (FIPV) causes multisystemic disease in cats; avian infectious bronchitis virus causes tracheobronchitis in poultry.
Preferred diagnostic tests: FIPV, serology (antibody titers), histopathology, RT-PCR; TGEV direct immunofluorescence, antigen capture ELISA, RT-PCR.
Comments: Enveloped RNA virus; members of this family are many and can cause enteric and respiratory disease in animals.

Organism: Flaviviridae
Diseases and species affected: Bovine viral diarrhea virus (BVDV) causes a respiratory, gastrointestinal, and reproductive disease in cattle; border disease virus causes congenital defects in sheep; classical swine fever virus causes systemic disease in swine; West Nile virus (WNV) causes neurologic disease in animals and humans.
Preferred diagnostic tests: BVDV antigen capture ELISA and ear notch immunohistochemistry for the detection of persistently infected animals, serum neutralization assay, RT-PCR, ELISA for routine testing. WNV infection is diagnosed by IgM ELISA
RT-PCR, virus neutralization assay.
Comments: Many members are vector borne and zoonotic.

Organism: Herpesviridae
Diseases and species affected: Canine herpesvirus causes systemic disease in neonatal puppies with hemorrhage and necrosis of various organs, respiratory disease in adults. Bovine herpesvirus 1, equine herpesvirus 1, and porcine herpesvirus 1 can cause respiratory, reproductive, or neurologic disease in their hosts; alcelaphine herpesvirus causes malignant catarrhal fever.
Preferred diagnostic tests: PCR, direct fluorescent antibody staining, virus isolation, serology (IgM detection).
Comments: DNA virus, intranuclear inclusion bodies in affected cells can be detected on cytology or histopathology evaluation.

Organism: Orthomyxoviridae
Diseases and species affected: Influenza virus (equine influenza virus, swine influenza virus, avian influenza virus, and canine influenza virus) causes respiratory illness in the respective host species.
Preferred diagnostic tests: RT-PCR, virus isolation, serology (hemagglutination inhibition assay, ELISA, AGID).
Comments: Enveloped RNA virus, zoonosis.

Organism: Paramyxoviridae
Diseases and species affected: Parainfluenza virus in animals causes respiratory illness; avian paramyxovirus 1 (APMV1) causes Newcastle disease, a severe multisystemic including CNS disease in birds; canine distemper virus (CDV) causes multisystemic and neurologic disease in dogs.
Preferred diagnostic tests: APMV1-RT-PCR, serology (ELISA, hemagglutination inhibition); CDV-RT-PCR, direct fluorescent antibody staining, virus isolation, serology (IgM detection).
Comments: Enveloped RNA virus. There are several members in this group that cause respiratory and neurologic disease in animals. Intracytoplasmic and intranuclear inclusion bodies in affected cells can be detected on cytology or histopathology evaluation.

Organism: Papillomaviridae
Diseases and species affected: Causes papilloma in animal hosts (bovine papilloma, canine papilloma, equine papilloma).
Preferred diagnostic tests: PCR, electron microscopy.
Comments: Nonenveloped DNA virus. Papilloma virus causes preneoplastic and neoplastic conditions and is generally host specific.
Organism: Picornaviridae
Diseases and species affected: Foot and mouth disease virus (FMDV) causes a contagious vesicular disease, encephalomyocarditis virus cause encephalomyelitis and myocarditis in swine and elephants.
Preferred diagnostic tests: RT-PCR, virus isolation.
Comments: Nonenveloped RNA virus. There are several other members of the family causing respiratory and gastrointestinal diseases.

Organism: Polyomaviridae
Diseases and species affected: Avian polyomavirus causes budgerigar fledgling disease. Simian polyomavirus (SV40) causes CNS disorders in immunocompromised nonhuman primates.
Preferred diagnostic tests: PCR, electron microscopy.
Comments: Nonenveloped DNA virus. Large glassy, intranuclear inclusion bodies are typical in histopathology lesions.

Organism: Poxviridae
Diseases and species affected: Several species-specific pox viruses cause pox in animal species, general systemic disease, or local infections.
Preferred diagnostic tests: PCR, electron microscopy, virus isolation.
Comments: DNA virus enveloped, intracytoplasmic inclusions in affected epithelium.

Organism: Parvoviridae
Diseases and species affected: Canine parvovirus 2 generalized disease and enteritis in puppies; feline panleukopenia virus causes generalized illness and congenital lesions in cats. Porcine parvovirus causes reproductive disease and abortion in pigs.
Preferred diagnostic tests: PCR, electron microscopy, virus isolation, serology (hemagglutination inhibition assay).
Comments: Nonenveloped DNA virus, intranuclear inclusion bodies are typical in histopathology lesions.

Organism: Reoviridae
Diseases and species affected: Members of the orbivirus group, bluetongue virus (BTV), African horse sickness, and epizootic hemorrhagic disease virus can cause multisystemic disease in animals.
Preferred diagnostic tests: RT-PCR and serology (ELISA).
Comments: RNA virus, arbovirus (vector borne).

Organism: Rhabdoviridae
Diseases and species affected: Rabies virus cause rabies in animals and humans; bovine ephemeral fever virus causes febrile illness in cattle; vesicular stomatitis virus (VSV0) causes vesicular disease in cattle, pigs, and horses.
Preferred diagnostic tests: Postmortem diagnostics for rabies virus include histopathology, direct immunofluorescence, RT-PCR.
Comments: Enveloped RNA virus. VSV can be confused with foot and mouth disease so laboratory confirmation is essential.

Organism: Retroviridae
Diseases and species affected: Numerous species-specific (mammalian and avian) members. Feline leukemia virus (FeLV), feline immunodeficiency virus, bovine leukemia virus (BLV), caprine arthritis and encephalitis virus, visna-maedi virus.
Preferred diagnostic tests: Depending on the virus and the animal species affected, tests for antibody and antigen screening are available.
Comments: Retroviral genome integrates into the host genome.

Organism: Togaviridae
Diseases and species affected: Eastern equine encephalitis, Western equine encephalitis, Venezuelan equine encephalitis cause neurologic disease in equines, humans, and other animals.
Preferred diagnostic tests: RT-PCR, serology (IgM ELISA, serum virus neutralization, hemagglutination inhibition), virus isolation.
Comments: RNA virus, arbovirus (vector borne).

Parasitic infections

Organism: *Babesia* spp.
Diseases and species affected: Causes babesiosis characterized by hemolytic anemia in dogs, cattle, horses, and other mammals.
Preferred diagnostic tests: Blood smear examination, serology, PCR.
Comments: Protozoan parasite, vector borne, infects erythrocytes.

Organism: *Cytauxzoon felis*
Diseases and species affected: Cytauxzoonosis a nonspecific acute illness with broad manifestations in cats.
Preferred diagnostic tests: Peripheral blood smears, followed by PCR confirmation.
Comments: Protozoan parasite, vector borne (ingestion of infected ticks), infects erythrocytes and macrophages.

Organism: *Cryptosporidium* spp.
Diseases and species affected: *C. parvum* causes gastroenteric illness in a variety of animal species.
Preferred diagnostic tests: Acid-fast staining, fecal floatation, direct immunofluorescence assay, PCR.
Comments: Protozoan parasite, zoonosis.

Organism: *Hepatozoan* spp.
Diseases and species affected: *H. canis* and *H. americanum* cause asymptomatic to debilitating illness in dogs.
Preferred diagnostic tests: Peripheral blood smear evaluation, biopsy and histopathology of affected muscles, serology, PCR.
Comments: Protozoan parasite, vector borne, infects neutrophils and macrophages, myositis is a common lesion.

Organism: *Leishmania* spp.
Diseases and species affected: *L. infantum*, the main cause of canine and human leishmaniasis, causes cutaneous and visceral lesions (granulomatous inflammation) in dogs, humans, and other animals.
Preferred diagnostic tests: Cytology, biopsy and histopathology, serology, PCR.
Comments: Protozoan parasite, vector borne.

Organism: *Toxoplasma gondii*
Diseases and species affected: Multisystemic disease in animals; cats are reservoirs; abortion in sheep and pigs.
Preferred diagnostic tests: Serology (antibody detection), histopathology, PCR.
Comments: Zoonotic disease.

Organism: *Trypanosoma* spp.
Diseases and species affected: A variety of domestic and wild animals are affected. *T. cruzi* causes American trypanosomiasis (Chagas disease). *T. congolensis*, *T. vivax* cause African trypanosomiasis in domestic and wild animals.
Preferred diagnostic tests: Peripheral blood smear evaluation, serology, PCR.
Comments: Protozoan parasite, vector borne, zoonotic.

II

Hematology of Common Domestic Species

6 Erythrocyte Production, Function, and Morphology

Mary Anna Thrall

Department of Biomedical Sciences, Ross University School of Veterinary Medicine, Basseterre, Saint Kitts and Nevis

Erythrocyte production

Erythrocytes are primarily produced in the bone marrow (see Chapter 15) by a process called erythropoiesis, which is regulated by an oxygen-sensing mechanism. Erythropoietin, a cytokine produced in the kidney, is produced in response to low blood oxygen tension. Erythropoietin then binds to erythropoietin receptors on erythrocyte precursor cells; receptor activation then signals various pathways that allow the precursors to differentiate into mature erythrocytes (see Chapter 10). The maturation process includes cell divisions, decreased cell size, loss of organelles and, in mammals, loss of the nucleus, development of a membrane that is capable of moving through the microcirculation, and production and accumulation of hemoglobin for oxygen transport.

Erythrocyte function

The primary function of the erythrocyte is to transport hemoglobin, which carries oxygen from the lungs to the tissues to support oxidative metabolism. Hemoglobin is made of alpha- and beta-globin molecules associated with a heme molecule that contains an iron atom (Fe) in the reduced state. One coordination site on Fe binds reversibly with oxygen. A wide range of animals, vertebrate and invertebrate, use hemoglobins to transport oxygen. Comparative studies of hemoglobin are numerous, and differences exist between hemoglobins of mammalian species.

Erythrocyte morphology

The deformable, permeable membrane that encloses the red-cell components is made of lipids including phospholipids, cholesterol, and glycolipids, proteins, and carbohydrates. Alterations in the lipid or protein composition of the membrane may result in abnormal red-cell shapes. Membrane proteins form the cytoskeleton of the membrane and are attached to the cytoplasmic surface of the membrane. These proteins play key roles in maintaining both cell shape and integrity and have been named according to their relative location from the place of migration when solubilized and subjected to electrophoresis. Bands 1 and 2 (i.e., spectrin) and band 5 (i.e., actin), protein 4.1, paladin, and ankyrin are the major cytoskeletal proteins. The protein skeleton is coupled to the lipid membrane by ankyrin, which binds to band 3, and is strengthened by band 4.2. Proteins that are embedded in and span the lipid membrane are called integral proteins, and they play a role in tethering the protein skeleton to the lipid membrane. The anion bicarbonate/chloride exchanger band 3 is the most abundant protein in the erythrocyte membrane. It plays a role in gas exchange and maintaining erythrocyte hydration and also has a structural role by binding the lipid component of the membrane with ankyrin and protein band 4.2, 4.1, and other proteins. Even after shearing, the structure of the membrane can remain intact, resulting in erythrocyte fragments. Glycophorins are sialoglycoproteins that span the erythrocyte membrane and help prevent erythrocyte to erythrocyte and erythrocyte to endothelial cell association.

Normal erythrocyte morphology varies among different species (Figure 6.1). Mammalian erythrocytes are anucleate, unlike those of all other vertebrates, which have nuclei. Erythrocytes are round and somewhat biconcave in most mammalian species, except in members of the family Camellidae (e.g., llamas, camels, and alpacas), which have elliptical (oval) erythrocytes. The biconcavity causes stained red blood cells to appear to have a central, pale area, because the observer is looking through less hemoglobin in this area of the cell. This central pallor is most apparent in canine erythrocytes. Species with smaller erythrocytes, such as the cat, horse, cow, sheep, and goat, have less concavity and, thus, little to no central pallor. The biconcave disc shape is

Veterinary Hematology, Clinical Chemistry, and Cytology, Third Edition. Edited by Mary Anna Thrall, Glade Weiser, Robin W. Allison and Terry W. Campbell.

Companion website: www.wiley.com/go/thrall/veterinary

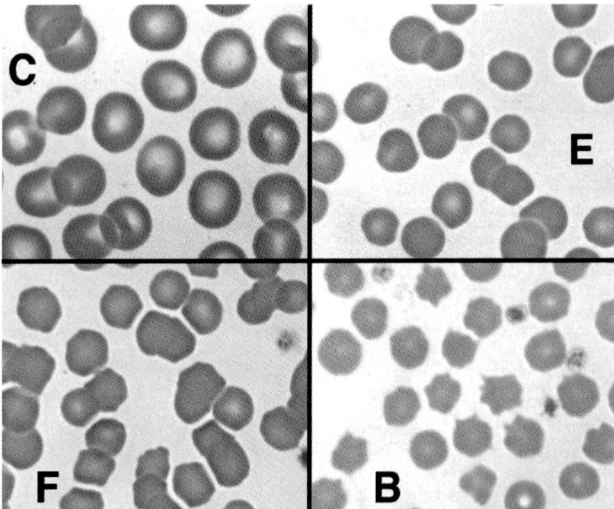

Figure 6.1 Normal canine (C), equine (E), feline (F), and bovine (B) erythrocytes. Note the larger size and marked central pallor of the canine erythrocytes compared to those of the other species. Wright stain.

efficient for oxygen exchange, and it allows the cell to be deformable as it moves through vasculature with a smaller diameter than that of the erythrocyte. Briefly, the significant differences between species are size, shape, amount of central pallor, tendency to form rouleaux, presence of basophilic stippling in regenerative response to anemia, and the presence of reticulocytes in response to anemia (Table 6.1).

Erythrocyte morphology often is an important aid in establishing a diagnosis regarding the cause of anemia, and it sometimes is helpful in establishing the diagnosis of other disorders as well. Critical to blood cell evaluation is adequate preparation of a blood film (see Chapter 1). The observer should examine the leukocyte counting area to evaluate erythrocyte morphology, because the red blood cells are neither too dense nor too flattened in this area. The interpretation of red-blood-cell morphology should be made in conjunction with other quantitative data from the complete blood count. For example, the degree of polychromasia in erythrocytes usually is more significant when the red-cell mass is decreased.

This chapter concentrates primarily on those morphologic characteristics that are most diagnostically useful. Morphology of erythrocytes is categorized here according to color, size, shape, structures in or on the erythrocytes, and the arrangement of cells on blood films.

Erythrocyte color

Polychromasia

Polychromatophilic cells are young erythrocytes that have been released early. Usually, they are large and more blue in color than mature erythrocytes (Figure 6.2). The blue color results from organelles (i.e., ribosomes, mitochondria) that are still present in the immature cells. The presence or absence of polychromatophilic erythrocytes is very important when determining the cause of anemia. If immature cells are released, the likely cause of the anemia is blood loss or blood destruction, with the bone marrow attempting to compensate by the early release of cells (see Chapter 9). If the anemia is caused by erythroid hypoplasia or aplasia within the marrow, then the level of polychromatophilic cells will not be increased (see Chapter 8). Horses are unique, however, in that they do not release significant numbers of polychromatophilic cells in the face of anemia.

The degree of polychromasia correlates well with the reticulocyte concentration, but it is more objective to quantify the regenerative response by counting reticulocytes (see Chapter 1). The reticulocyte is analogous to the polychromatophilic erythrocyte, but it is stained with a vital stain (e.g., new methylene blue or brilliant cresyl blue), which causes the ribosomes and other organelles to clump into visible granules (see Figure 1.18).

Hypochromasia

Hypochromic red blood cells are pale and have increased central pallor as a result of decreased hemoglobin concentration

Table 6.1 Significant differences in erythrocytes between species.

Species	Diameter (μm)	Rouleaux	Central pallor	Basophilic stippling	Reticulocytes (%)[a]	MCV (fl)
Dog	7.0	+	++++	–	1	60–72
Pig	6.0	++	±	–	1	50–68
Cat	5.8	++	+	±	0.5	39–50
Horse	7	++++	–	–	0[b]	36–52
Cow	5.5	–	+	+++	0	37–53
Sheep	4.5	±	+	+++	0	23–48
Goat	3.2	–	–	++	0	15–30

[a]With normal packed cell volume.
[b]Does not increase in response to anemia.

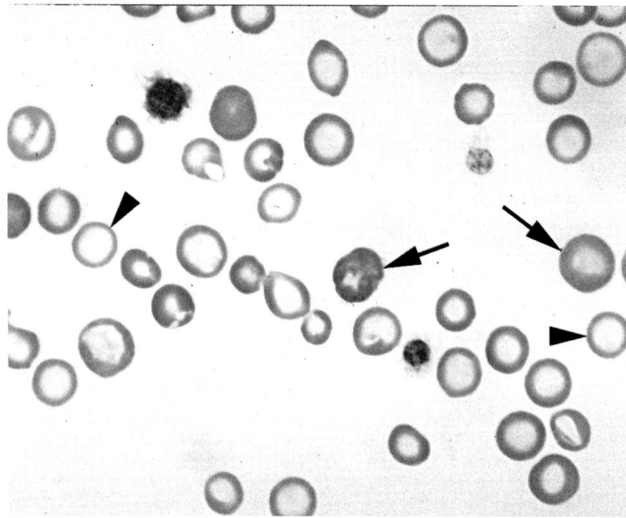

Figure 6.2 Blood film from a dog with iron-deficiency anemia. Note the lack of density of the blood film, suggesting marked anemia. Most of the erythrocytes are small and hypochromic (arrowheads). The anemia is regenerative, and numerous polychromatophilic erythrocytes are present (arrows). Wright stain.

from iron deficiency (Figure 6.2). Erythrocytes of iron-deficient dogs have more obvious hypochromasia than erythrocytes of other species with iron deficiency; erythrocytes of iron-deficient cats usually are not hypochromic. One needs to distinguish hypochromic cells from bowl-shaped (i.e., torocytes) or "punched-out" cells, which are insignificant (Figure 6.3). Bowl-shaped cells have a sharply defined, central clear area, and they also have a thicker rim of hemoglobin than is seen in true hypochromic

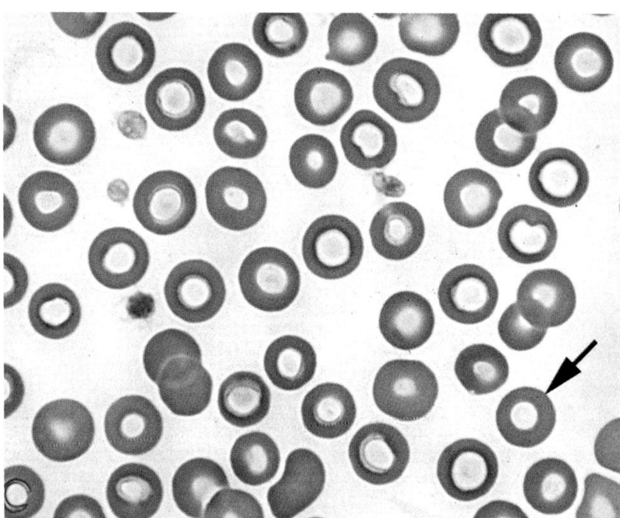

Figure 6.3 Blood film from a dog showing numerous torocytes ("punched-out" erythrocytes). Note the wide rim of hemoglobin and lack of hemoglobinization in the center of the cells (arrow). Torocytes can be mistaken for true hypochromasia. Wright stain.

cells. Immature polychromatophilic erythrocytes also may appear to be hypochromic, because their hemoglobin concentration is less than normal due to their increased volume. Although hyperchromic states do not exist, spherocytes appear to have increased color intensity because of their lack of concavity.

Erythrocyte size

Variation in erythrocyte size is termed anisocytosis. This variation may result from the presence of large cells (i.e., macrocytes), small cells (i.e., microcytes), or both. In itself, the term does not provide any meaningful information. Red blood cells may appear to be small on the blood film because of decreased diameter, but the cell volume is the true measurement of red-cell size and is determined electronically (see Chapter 1). The best example of this is the spherocyte, which appears to be small because of its spheric shape and subsequent decreased diameter; however, the red-cell volume of spherocytes is almost always within the reference interval. Conversely, hypochromic microcytic iron-deficient red blood cells with an electronically determined decreased volume may have a normal diameter and, thus, not appear to be small on the blood film.

Microcytic erythrocytes

Cells must be markedly small before their decreased diameter can be visually detected (Figure 6.2). Mean corpuscular volume (MCV) is more valuable than blood film examination in assessing the true size of erythrocytes. Using automated cell-counting systems, a histogram or volume–distribution curve of the erythrocyte population can be generated. Mean cell volume is determined by analysis of the volume–distribution curve, and the hematocrit is then calculated by multiplying the MCV by the erythrocyte concentration (see Chapter 1). The most common cause of microcytosis is iron-deficiency anemia; a decreased MCV is the hallmark of such anemia. In some iron-deficient patients, the MCV may be normal even though the animal has a microcytic population of cells. In these cases, examination of the volume–distribution curve is helpful (see Chapter 1). The pathophysiology of the microcytosis is theorized to involve erythroid precursors continuing to divide until a near-normal complement of hemoglobin concentration is reached, resulting in small erythrocytes. Cells cannot obtain a normal hemoglobin concentration because iron is required to make hemoglobin. If the iron deficiency is severe, microcytosis and hypochromia may be observed on the blood film. In addition, membrane defects are present, which often lead to specific abnormalities in shape and fragmentation (discussed below).

Dogs and cats with portocaval shunts (portosystemic vascular anomalies) may have microcytosis that usually is related to abnormal iron metabolism. Many of these animals, especially cats, are not anemic; microcytosis without anemia should trigger evaluation for a portosystemic shunt. Some breeds of dogs (e.g., Akitas and Shiba Inus) and cats (Abyssinian) may have smaller erythrocytes. Microcytosis, usually mild, can also be seen with other causes of iron-restricted hematopoiesis, such as anemia of inflammatory disease. Mild microcytosis has been reported in approximately 25% of cats with hyperthyroidism; the cause is unknown but may be due to iron-restricted hematopoiesis.

Excessive ethylenediaminetetraacetic acid (EDTA) in a blood sample can result in erythrocyte dehydration, shrinkage, and spurious microcytosis. Hyponatremia can also result in *in vitro* microcytosis with certain instruments as a result of erythrocyte shrinkage when put into the diluent; these erythrocytes had previously adjusted *in vivo* to being in a hyponatremic environment by increasing cytoplasmic water. Storing blood at room temperature for more than 24 hours before analysis may result in a falsely increased MCV, thus masking microcytosis caused by iron deficiency or portosystemic shunts.

Macrocytic erythrocytes

Macrocytic erythrocytes are large and have an increased MCV (see Figure 1.18, bottom). The most common cause of macrocytosis is increased numbers of immature erythrocytes that are polychromatophilic on Wright-stained blood films. Unlike other domestic species, horses release macrocytes that are not polychromatophilic. The associated increase in MCV usually is the only evidence of erythroid regeneration in horses. During regeneration, species other than dogs tend to produce regenerative macrocytes that are approximately twice the size of normal erythrocytes, resulting in a marked change in the MCV. Dogs, however, release macrocytes that usually are only slightly larger than normal erythrocytes. Macrocytosis without polychromasia or other evidence of an appropriate regenerative response is a common finding in anemic cats with myelodysplasia and myeloproliferative disease (see Chapter 16). This macrocytosis may be associated with feline leukemia virus (FeLV) or feline immunodeficiency virus (FIV) infection, and it also may be seen in FeLV-infected cats that are not anemic.

Other, more infrequent causes of macrocytosis include macrocytosis of miniature and toy poodles and hereditary stomatocytosis. Macrocytosis of miniature or toy poodles is rare, is thought to be hereditary, and is usually an incidental finding. Affected dogs are not anemic, but their erythrocyte count may be decreased. The MCV is usually 90–100 fL. Other findings include increased nucleated erythrocytes, increased Howell-Jolly bodies (often multiple), and hypersegmented neutrophils. Numerous abnormalities are seen in erythroid precursors on bone marrow film examination, including megaloblasts with nuclear and cytoplasmic asynchrony of maturation. The cause of the defect is unknown, and no clinical signs are associated with the disorder. Finally, stomatocytes in Alaskan malamutes and miniature schnauzers with hereditary stomatocytosis are macrocytic (discussed later).

Some anticonvulsant drugs, such as phenobarbital, phenytoin, and primidone, have been thought to induce macrocytosis, but macrocytosis was not experimentally reproduced in dogs receiving long-term anticonvulsant drugs. Vitamin B_{12} (i.e., cobalamin) and folate deficiency do not cause macrocytosis in domestic animals, but these deficiencies are a common cause of macrocytosis in humans. Giant schnauzers with hereditary cobalamin malabsorption are anemic, but this anemia is normocytic rather than macrocytic. Inherited cobalamin deficiency has also been reported in border collies and beagles and is commonly seen in animals with chronic enteropathies.

Spurious macrocytosis can be a result of erythrocyte swelling associated with storing blood at room temperature prior to analysis. Falsely increased MCV can also be seen in blood with agglutinated erythrocytes in patients with immune mediated hemolytic anemia when analyzed with an impedance-type analyzer, because agglutinated cells (doublets and triplets) may be recognized as one large cell. Agglutination can be recognized by examining the erythrocyte histogram. Hypernatremia results in erythrocytes being dehydrated *in vivo*, and with certain types of electronic cell counters, a spurious increase in MCV will be seen due to erythrocyte swelling *in vitro* after being placed in the diluent.

Erythrocyte shape

Abnormally shaped erythrocytes are termed poikilocytes. This terminology is not helpful, however, because it does not suggest a specific change in shape. Thus, no specific interpretation is possible. The most important shape changes include various types of spiculated erythrocytes, spherocytes, and eccentrocytes. Spiculated erythrocytes have one or more surface spicules and include echinocytes, acanthocytes, keratocytes, and schistocytes. One should be as specific as possible when describing shape changes, because certain types of abnormal red-cell shapes are associated with certain diseases. Less significant abnormally shaped red blood cells include leptocytes (i.e., folded or target cells), codocytes (i.e., target cells), dacryocytes (i.e., teardrop-shaped erythrocytes), and torocytes (i.e., bowl-shaped erythrocytes).

A few inherited abnormalities associated with red-cell shape change have been described in animals and include hereditary stomatocytosis in dogs, hereditary elliptocytosis resulting from band 4.1 deficiency in dogs reported in 1983, and more recently in a dog, elliptocytosis caused by a mutation in beta-spectrin was reported. Hereditary spherocytosis has been reported in Japanese black cattle resulting from band 3 deficiency and has also been reported in mice. Heriditary spherocytosis in people is usually a result of a spectrin defect. Hereditary spectrin deficiency has been reported in Dutch golden retrievers, and some of these dogs had spherocytosis and hemolytic anemia.

Most inherited abnormalities of red blood cell shape are associated with abnormalities of cytoskeletal protein, or plasma or red-cell membrane cholesterol or phospholipid concentration. Hereditary high potassium and reduced glutathione concentrations in erythrocytes of some dogs of certain Asian breeds (e.g., Akita, Shiba, and Jindo) lead to greater susceptibility to onion-induced oxidative damage.

Hemoglobinopathies have not yet been described in domestic animals, although they are reported frequently in humans. A relatively common hemoglobinopathy in humans is sickle cell anemia, which results from a single amino acid substitute in the adult beta-globin protein. Sickle cells (drepanocytes) from numerous deer species as well as some sheep and goat breeds have been reported, as shown in Figure 9.18. They were first described in 1840 and occur when the blood comes into contact with atmospheric oxygen or an alkaline pH. Most authors believe deer erythrocyte sickling is exclusively an *in vitro* shape change, and the sickling does not cause any pathologic traits.

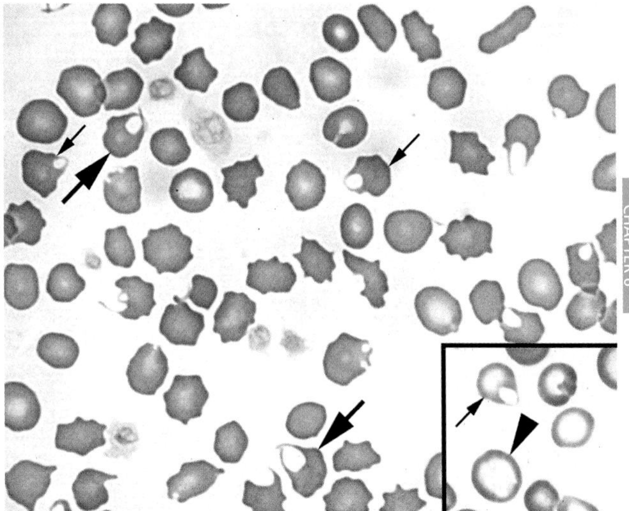

Figure 6.5 Blood film from a cat with iron-deficiency anemia. Note the erythrocyte membrane abnormalities. Lack of hypochromasia is typical for feline iron-deficient erythrocytes. Blister cells (small arrows) and keratocytes (large arrows) also are present. Inset. Blood film from an iron-deficient dog. Note the blister cell (small arrow) and hypochromic erythrocyte (arrowhead). Wright stain.

Schistocytes and keratocytes

Erythrocyte fragments, also termed schistocytes, usually result from shearing of the red cell by intravascular trauma. This may be observed in animals with disseminated intravascular coagulopathy (DIC) as a result of erythrocytes being broken by fibrin strands, with vascular neoplasms (e.g., hemangiosarcoma), and with iron deficiency. Animals with DIC also may have a concurrent thrombocytopenia (Figure 6.4). When erythrocyte fragments are observed in blood films from dogs with hemangiosarcoma, acanthocytes usually are present as well. Fragmentation in iron-deficient erythrocytes apparently results from oxidative injury, leading to membrane lesions or increased susceptibility to intravascular trauma. Iron-deficient erythrocytes initially develop an apparent blister or vacuole, which is thought to represent an oxidative injury and in which inner membrane surfaces are cross-linked across the cell. Exclusion of hemoglobin may account for the colorless area. These lesions subsequently enlarge and break open to form cells with one or more spicules. When one spicule is present, these cells are commonly termed apple-stem cells; when two or more spicules are present, they are termed keratocytes (Figure 6.5). The projections from the keratocytes then fragment from the erythrocytes, thereby forming schistocytes.

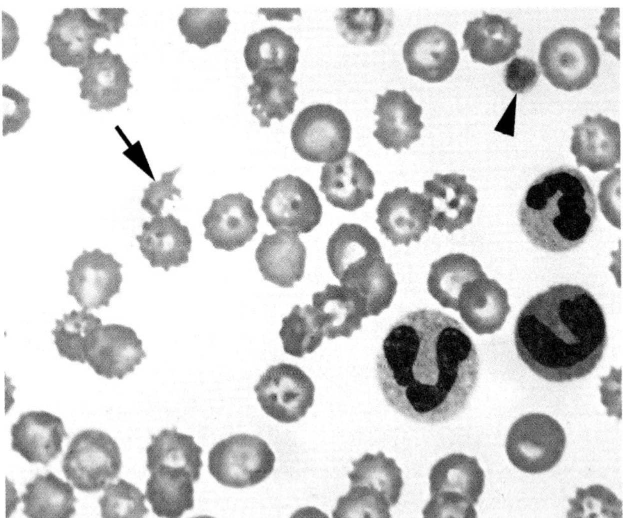

Figure 6.4 Blood film from a dog with splenic hemangiosarcoma and disseminated intravascular coagulopathy. Note the schistocyte (arrow) and single platelet in the field (arrowhead). Wright stain.

Acanthocytes

Acanthocytes, or spur cells, are irregular, spiculated erythrocytes with few, unevenly distributed surface projections of variable length and diameter (Figure 6.6). Acanthocytes occur through two mechanisms. They may result from changes in cholesterol or phospholipid concentrations in the red-cell membrane and commonly are seen on blood films from humans with altered lipid metabolism, such as may occur with liver disease; they are occasionally observed on blood films from dogs with liver disease. Acanthocytes, however, are commonly observed on blood films from cats with hepatic lipidosis. Approximately 25% of cats with hyperthryoidism were reported to have acanthocytes on the blood films.

They are also associated with mechanical injury such as may result from vascular trauma and are seen in approximately 25% of dogs with hemangiosarcoma. Although the

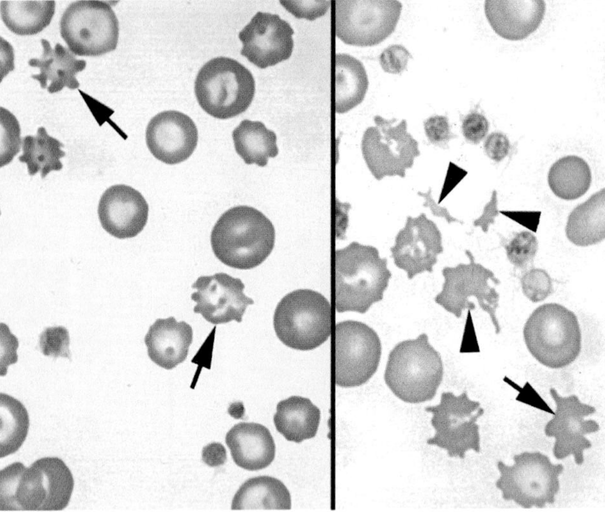

Figure 6.6 Blood film from an anemic dog with a ruptured hemangiosarcoma of the spleen. Left. Numerous acanthocytes are present (arrows). Note the large polychromatophilic cells in the same field, indicating that the anemia is regenerative. Right. Acanthocytes (arrow) and schistocytes (arrowheads) are typical findings in dogs with hemangiosarcoma. Wright stain.

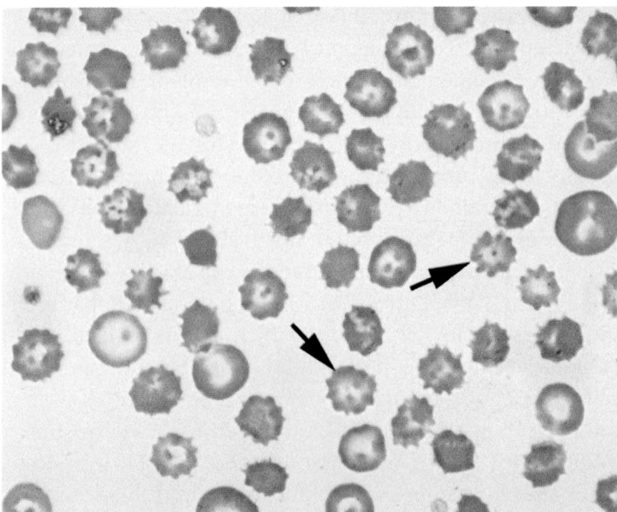

Figure 6.7 Blood film from a dog with lymphoma. Numerous echinocytes are present (arrows). Wright stain.

presence of acanthocytes in middle-aged to old large-breed dogs with a concurrent regenerative anemia may be suggestive of hemangiosarcoma, acanthocytes may also be observed in dogs with other types of neoplastic disease such as osteosarcoma and lymphoma, and they are also seen on blood films from dogs with non-neoplastic diseases including gastrointestinal, musculoskeletal, renal, immune-mediated disorders, DIC, and iron-deficiency anemia.

Echinocytes

Echinocytes (i.e., burr cells) are spiculated cells with numerous short, evenly spaced, blunt to sharp surface projections that are quite uniform in size and shape (Figure 6.7). Echinocyte formation can be an artifactual result (i.e., crenation) of a change in pH from slow drying of blood films, but it also has been associated with renal disease, lymphoma, snake envenomation, and chemotherapy in dogs and after exercise in horses. The echinocytes seen with snake envenomation are termed type 3 echinocytes, and they are quite characteristic, with numerous very fine spicules on all erythrocytes, except in cells that are polychromatophilic (Figure 6.8). In some instances of rattlesnake and bee envenomation, spheroechinocytes are formed. These erythrocytes appear to be spherocytes with fine spicules, usually present from 24 to 48 hours after envenomation, and are a reliable indication that envenomation has occurred.

Elliptocytes

Elliptocytes (ovalocytes) are elliptical or oval erythrocytes. Elliptocytosis is normal in members of the camel family,

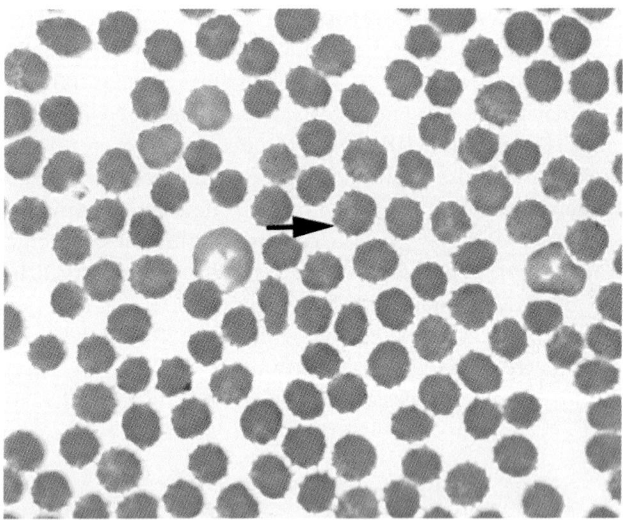

Figure 6.8 Blood film from a dog that was bitten by a rattlesnake approximately 24 hours previously. Almost all of the erythrocytes are echinospherocytes (arrow). Note that the polychromatophilic erythrocytes are not affected. Wright stain.

but in other mammals is either a hereditary (Figure 6.9) or acquired defect. Acquired elliptocytosis has been reported in dogs with myelofibrosis and myelodysplastic syndromes, in cats with portosystemic shunts and liver disease, and in cats that were given doxorubicin.

Spherocytes

Spherocytes are darkly staining erythrocytes that lack central pallor (Figure 6.10). They appear to be small, but their volume is normal. Spherocytes are not easily detected in species other than dogs because of the small size and lack of central pallor in the normal erythrocytes of most other domestic

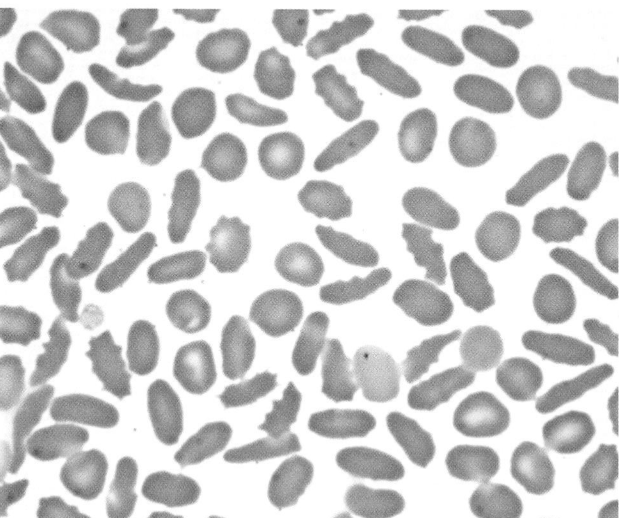

Figure 6.9 Blood film from a dog with elliptocytosis caused by a mutant beta-spectrin. Wright stain. Source: Courtesy of Drs. Melinda Wilkerson, Roberta Di Terlizzi, Steve Stockham, and Karen Dolce, Kansas State University.

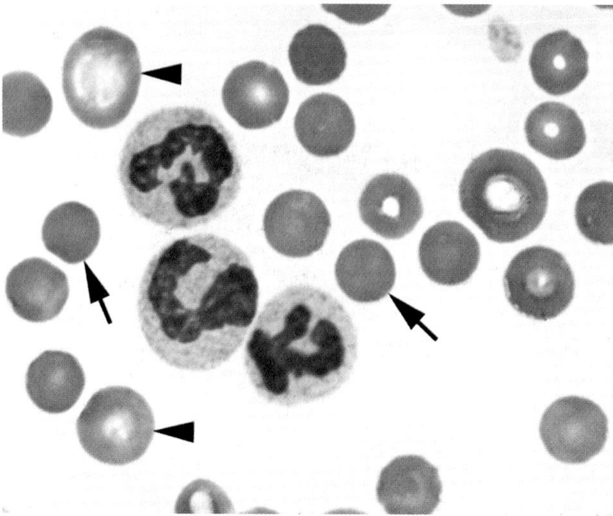

Figure 6.10 Blood film from dog with immune-mediated hemolytic anemia. Note the numerous spherocytes (arrows). The anemia is regenerative, as indicated by the polychromatophilic erythrocytes (arrowheads). Wright stain.

animals. Spherocytes have a reduced amount of membrane as a result of partial phagocytosis, which occurs because antibody or complement is on the surface of the erythrocyte. Spherocytes are very significant, in that their presence suggests immune-mediated hemolytic anemia (see Chapter 9). They also, however, may be seen after blood transfusion with mismatched blood.

Spherocyte formation has been reported in dogs with bee and snake envenomation and zinc toxicosis, and zinc toxicosis also may cause Heinz-body anemia. The mechanism of spherocyte formation with bee and snake envenomation

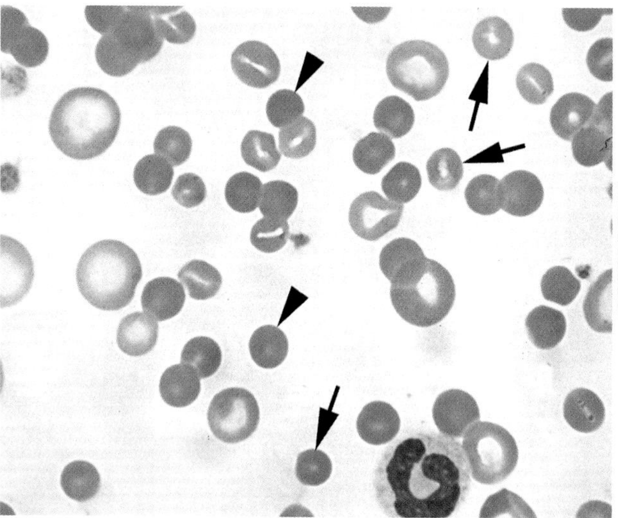

Figure 6.11 Blood film from a dog with immune-mediated hemolytic anemia. Many of the erythrocytes are spherocytes (arrowheads), and several incomplete spheres are present (arrows). Wright stain.

is a result of venom-containing enzymes and proteins. Melittin in bee venom induces pore formation in erythrocyte membranes, binds and stiffens spectrin, and stimulates phospholipase. Phospholipase A2 in bee and snake venom is an enzyme that alters phospholipid in the erythrocyte membrane.

Sometimes, a small amount of central pallor will remain in a spherocyte, and it then is termed an incomplete spherocyte (Figure 6.11). These spherocytes likely represent a continuum of membrane removal that finally results in a complete sphere.

Eccentrocytes

Features of eccentrocytes include shifting of hemoglobin toward one side of the cell, loss of normal central pallor, and a clear zone outlined by a membrane (Figure 6.12). They are associated with oxidative damage, especially in dogs that have ingested onions and other *Allium* family plants, and may be found in conjunction with Heinz bodies (discussed later). Eccentrocytosis and hemolytic anemia in horses have been associated with the ingestion of wilted red maple leaves and wilted leaves of trees of the *Pistacia* species. Animals with an inherited erythrocyte enzyme deficiency, glucose-6-phosphate dehydrogenase deficiency, may show increased susceptibility to oxidant-induced erythrocyte injury, resulting in eccentrocyte formation or increased incidence of Heinz bodies.

Leptocytes and codocytes

Leptocytes are erythrocytes that have undergone a surface-to-volume ratio change in which there is excess membrane relative to the internal contents, resulting in membrane folding and target-cell formation (Figure 6.13). They have

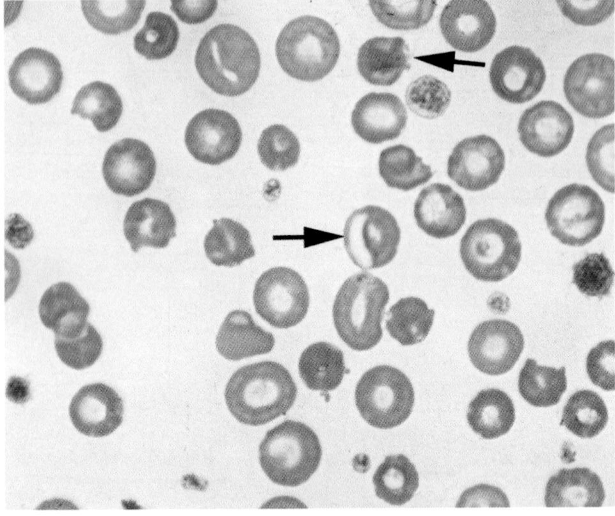

Figure 6.12 Blood film from a dog with Heinz-body anemia after ingestion of onions. Eccentrocytes are present (arrows). Wright stain.

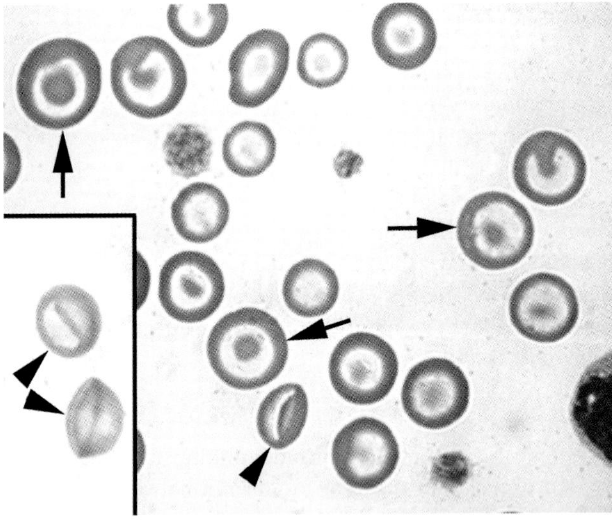

Figure 6.13 Blood film from a dog with numerous leptocytes. Note the numerous target cells (arrows) and folded cells (arrowheads). Wright stain.

little diagnostic significance, however, and may form *in vitro* secondary to contact with excess EDTA as a result of improperly filling the blood-collection tubes. Target cells also are referred to as codocytes and are thin, bowl-shaped erythrocytes with a dense, central area of hemoglobin that is separated from the peripheral hemoglobinized region by a pale zone. Target cells may be seen in dogs with increased serum cholesterol concentration, but they also are seen in a variety of other conditions and have little significance.

Stomatocytes

Stomatocytes are uniconcave erythrocytes with a mouth-like, clear area near the cell center (Figure 6.14). A few stomatocytes on the blood film usually are insignificant.

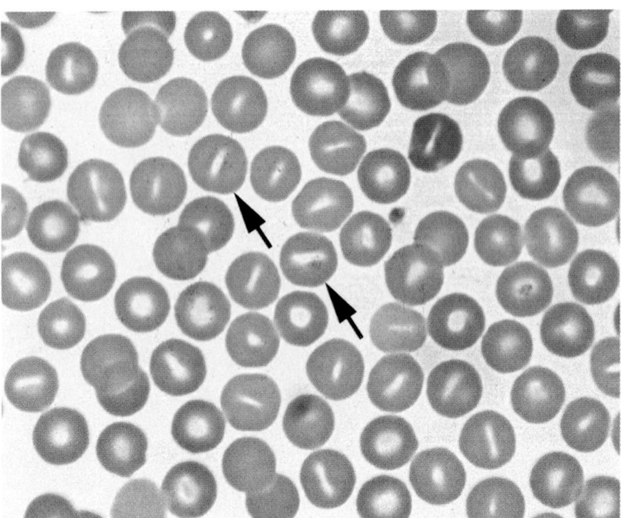

Figure 6.14 Blood film from a miniature schnauzer mix breed dog with hereditary spherocytosis. Note the numerous slit or mouth-shaped clear areas in the stomatocytes (arrows). Wright stain.

Hereditary stomatocytosis has been reported in several dog breeds, including Alaskan malamutes, miniature schnauzers, standard schnauzers, and the Drentse partrijshond. All of the disorders are inherited in an autosomal-recessive manner, but stomatocyte formation is caused by different defects in different breeds, involving either cell membranes or regulation of cell volume. Alaskan malamutes with hereditary stomatocytosis also have chondrodysplasia, and only a small percentage of the erythrocytes are stomatocytes. These stomatocytes are thought to form secondary to a membrane defect that allows increased sodium and water content of erythrocytes. Drentse partrijshond dogs with stomatocytosis also have hypertrophic gastritis, retarded growth, diarrhea, renal cysts, and polyneuropathy, and in this breed, the erythrocyte defect is thought to result from an abnormal concentration of phospholipids in the erythrocyte membrane. Miniature and standard schnauzers with stomatocytosis are asymptomatic; the cause of the erythrocyte defect in these breeds has not been described.

Structures in or on erythrocytes

Heinz bodies

Oxidative denaturation of hemoglobin results in Heinz body formation. Approximately 1–2% of erythrocytes from normal cats contain Heinz bodies, presumably because of an unusual propensity for hemoglobin denaturation due to feline hemoglobin molecules containing at least twice the number of reactive cysteine sulfhydryl groups as are in hemoglobin molecules of other species. Heinz bodies appear as small, eccentric, pale structures within the red cell, and they commonly seem to protrude slightly from the red-cell margin on Wright-stained blood films (Figure 6.14). Heinz bodies usually are 0.5–1.0 µm in diameter but may

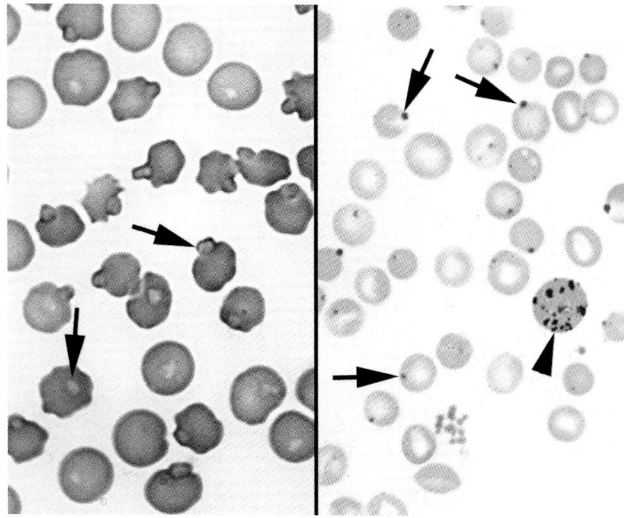

Figure 6.15 Blood films from a cat with acetaminophen toxicosis. Left. Heinz bodies appear as pale, light-blue structures (arrows). Wright stain. Right. Heinz bodies appear as blue structures (arrows). Note the reticulocyte (arrowhead). Brilliant cresyl blue stain.

be larger. They usually occur as single, large structures in feline erythrocytes, but in canine erythrocytes, they more commonly are small and multiple. Heinz bodies are difficult to see on Wright-stained blood films, particularly with canine erythrocytes, in which eccentrocyte formation may be more apparent. When stained with vital stains (e.g., new methylene blue or brilliant cresyl blue), Heinz bodies appear as blue structures (Figure 6.15). The presence of Heinz bodies reduces the deformability of the cell, making it more susceptible to both intravascular and extravascular hemolysis, and in some instances may change the antigenicity of the red cell membrane, resulting in immune mediated destruction. If large numbers of erythrocytes are affected, severe hemolytic anemia may result. Oxidative drugs and compounds known to induce Heinz-body formation include onions, garlic, leeks, chives, *Brassica* species of plants, wilted or dried leaves from red maple (*Acer rubrum*), benzocaine, zinc, copper, acetaminophen, propofol, phenazopyridine, phenothiazine, phenylhydrazine, naphthalene, vitamin K, methylene blue, propylene glycol, and skunk musk. Ill cats may develop a high concentration of Heinz bodies without being exposed to oxidant chemicals or drugs. The most common disorders associated with an increased concentration of Heinz bodies in cats are diabetes mellitus, lymphoma, and hyperthyroidism, but increased concentrations also may be seen in association with a wide variety of other diseases (see Chapter 9). The presence of Heinz bodies may result in falsely increased hemoglobin concentration readings, and subsequently an abnormally high mean corpuscular hemoglobin concentration (MCHC), as well as other spurious findings, such as leukocytosis and abnormal automated reticulocyte counts that have been observed with flow-based automated cell counters.

Basophilic stippling

In vivo aggregation of ribosomes into small basophilic granules is termed basophilic stippling (Figure 6.15). Normally, basophilic stippling is associated with immature erythrocytes in ruminants, and it may be seen to a lesser extent in cats and dogs with intensely regenerative anemia. Basophilic stippling not associated with severe anemia is suggestive of lead poisoning, but not all animals with lead poisoning have basophilic stippling. The enzyme pyrimidine 5′-nucleotidase, which is present in reticulocytes, normally catabolizes ribosomes; the activity of this enzyme is reduced in lead toxicosis and normally is low in ruminants.

Nucleated erythrocytes

Increased numbers of erythrocytes in which the nucleus remains (Figure 6.16) are associated with regenerative anemias and early release of these cells in response to hypoxia. Increased concentrations of nucleated erythrocytes also may be seen in animals with a nonfunctioning spleen and with increased levels of endogenous or exogenous corticosteroids. An increase in nucleated erythrocytes out of proportion to the degree of anemia frequently is associated with lead poisoning, but not all animals with lead poisoning have increased nucleated erythrocytes. In cats, the presence of nucleated erythrocytes in the absence of significant polychromasia is usually an indication of myelodysplasia or myeloproliferative disease.

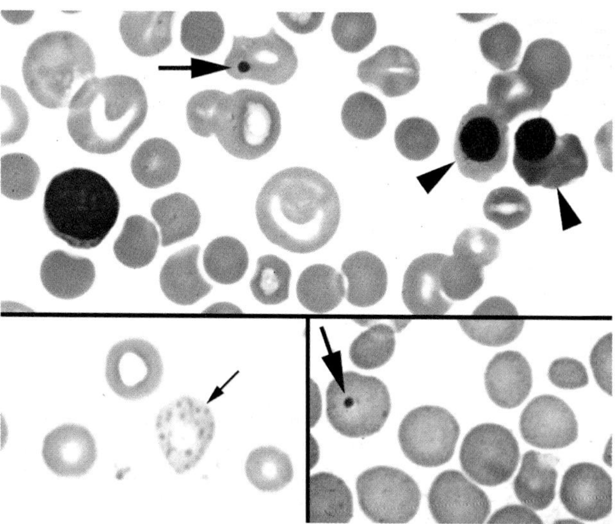

Figure 6.16 Top. Blood film from dog with immune-mediated hemolytic anemia. The anemia is very regenerative, and polychromatophilic erythrocytes, nucleated erythrocytes (arrowheads), and a Howell-Jolly body (arrow) are present. Note that the nucleated erythrocytes (metarubricytes) have variably colored cytoplasm. The one on the left has mature cytoplasm, whereas the one on the right has polychromatophilic cytoplasm. Lower right. A nuclear remnant, or Howell-Jolly body, is indicated by the arrow. Lower left. Basophilic stippling (small arrow) in a blood film from a dog with lead poisoning. Wright stain.

Howell-Jolly bodies

Nuclear remnants in erythrocytes are termed Howell-Jolly bodies. An increased concentration of Howell-Jolly bodies is associated with regenerative anemia, splenectomy, and suppressed splenic function. These bodies are small, round, dark-blue inclusions of variable size (Figure 6.16).

Siderotic granules

Siderotic granules are stainable iron granules within mitochondria and lysosomes. These siderotic inclusions are also referred to as Pappenheimer bodies, and their presence is thought to be associated with impaired heme synthesis. Erythrocytes containing these inclusions are termed siderocytes (Figure 6.17). Siderocytes in domestic animals are rare, but they have been associated with chloramphenicol therapy, myelodysplasia, and ineffective erythropoiesis of unknown cause.

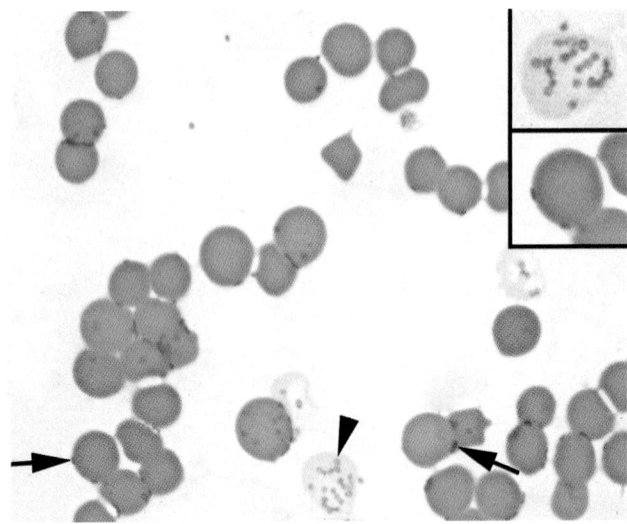

Figure 6.18 Blood film from an anemic cat. Note the numerous *Mycoplasma haemofelis* organisms. Some of these appear as small, ring-shaped organisms on the surface of a "ghost" erythrocyte that has lysed (arrowhead). Others appear as rod-shaped structures on the edge of erythrocytes (arrows). Insets. Higher magnification of both the ring and the rod-shaped forms. Wright stain.

Parasites

Erythrocyte parasites are discussed in more detail in Chapter 9. Spherocyte formation and agglutination may be observed on blood films from animals with erythrocyte parasites, because the organisms induce an immune-mediated anemia.

The primary parasitic disease of feline erythrocytes is infection with *Mycoplasma haemofelis* (Figure 6.18), which is a hemotropic mycoplasma organism that is the causative agent of feline infectious anemia. These organisms are attached to the external erythrocyte membrane and appear as rod-shaped organisms on the periphery of the erythrocyte or as a delicate, basophilic ring on the cell. A less common erythrocyte parasite in cats is the protozoan *Cytauxzoon felis*, which appears as a ring (diameter, 0.5–1.5 μm) and contains a small, basophilic nucleus (Figure 6.19).

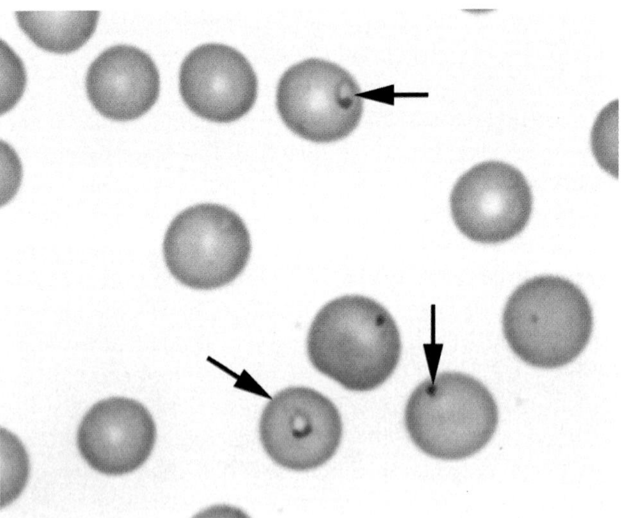

Figure 6.19 Blood film from a cat with *Cytauxzoon* organisms (arrows). Wright stain.

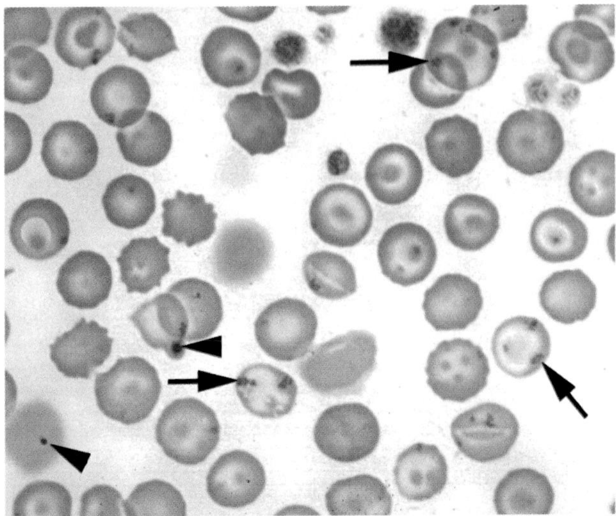

Figure 6.17 Blood film from a dog. Numerous erythrocytes (siderocytes) containing siderotic granules are present (arrows). Note the Howell-Jolly bodies (arrowheads). Wright stain.

In dogs, erythrocyte parasites are rare in most parts of the United States. *Mycoplasma haemocanis* usually only occurs in dogs that have been splenectomized or that have nonfunctional spleens. The organisms appear as small dots that chain across the surface of the erythrocyte (Figure 6.20). *Babesia canis, Babesia vogeli,* and *Babesia gibsoni* are protozoal red-cell parasites in the dog that produce severe hemolytic anemia. Usually, *B. canis*, and *B. vogeli* appear as a

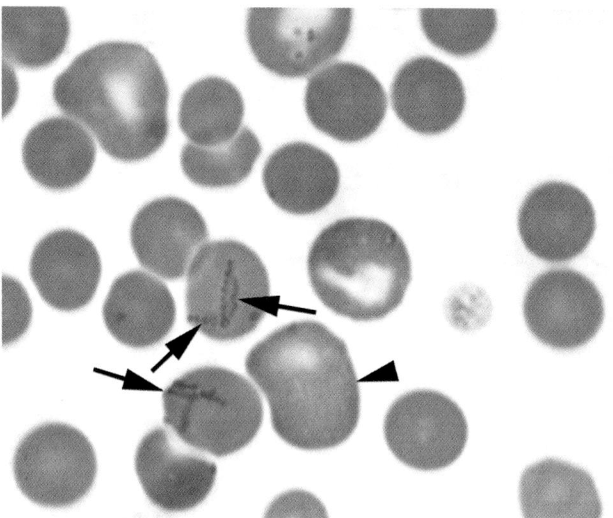

Figure 6.20 Blood film from a splenectomized dog with *Mycoplasma hemocanis*. Note the dot-like organisms that chain across the surface of the erythrocyte (arrows). The anemia is regenerative, as indicated by the polychromatophilic cell (arrowhead). Wright stain.

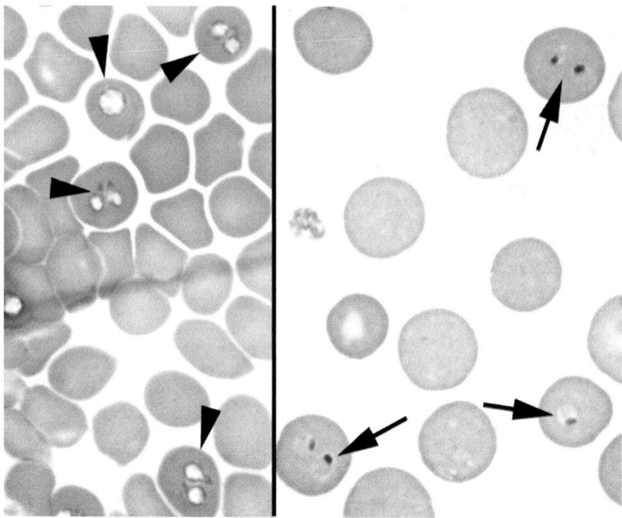

Figure 6.21 Blood film from dogs with babesiosis. Left. *Babesia canis* organisms appear as poorly staining, teardrop-shaped structures (arrowheads). Right. Blood film from a dog with *Babesia gibsoni* (arrows). Wright stain.

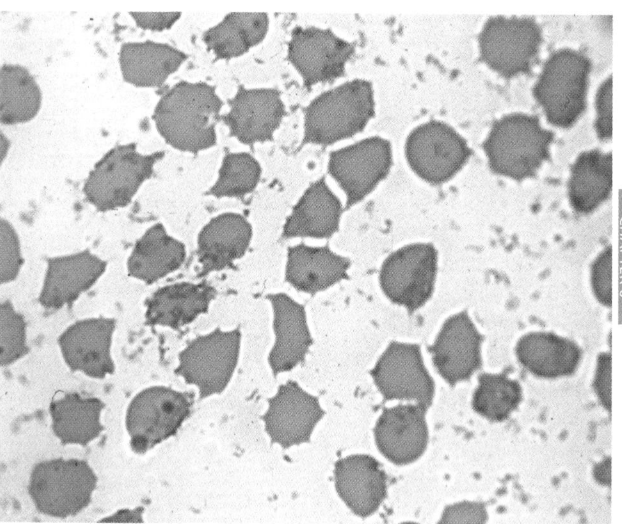

Figure 6.22 Blood film from a cow with *Mycoplasma wenyoni*. Note the many free organisms in the plasma. Wright stain.

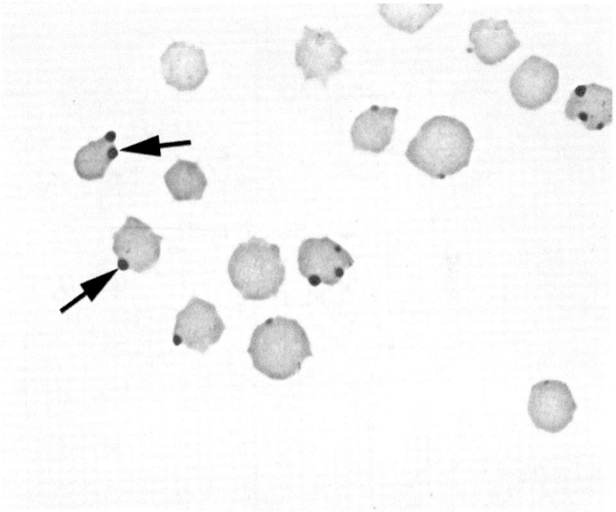

Figure 6.23 Blood film from an anemic cow with anaplasmosis. Note the numerous *Anaplasma marginale* organisms on the periphery of the erythrocytes (arrows). Wright stain.

teardrop-shaped structure (Figure 6.20, left), but *B. gibsoni* is smaller and varies considerably in both size and shape (Figure 6.21, right). Other examples of erythrocyte parasites include, *Mycoplasma wenyoni* (Figure 6.22), and *Anaplasma* sp. (Figure 6.23).

Viral inclusions

Viral inclusions are occasionally seen in erythrocytes from dogs with distemper. Distemper inclusions, also sometimes referred to as Lentz bodies, are variable in size (~1.0–2.0 µm), number, and color (faint blue to magenta) and are more frequently seen in polychromatophilic erythrocytes (Figure 6.24). Staining is typically more intense when using one of the quick Romanowsky stains.

Erythrocyte arrangement on blood films

Rouleaux formation

Rouleaux formation is the spontaneous association of erythrocytes in linear stacks, and its appearance is similar to a stack of coins (Figure 6.25). Marked rouleaux formation is normal in horses, a moderate amount is normal in cats, and a slight amount is normal in dogs. Rouleaux formation is enhanced, however, when the concentration of plasma proteins such as fibrinogen or immunoglobulins is increased.

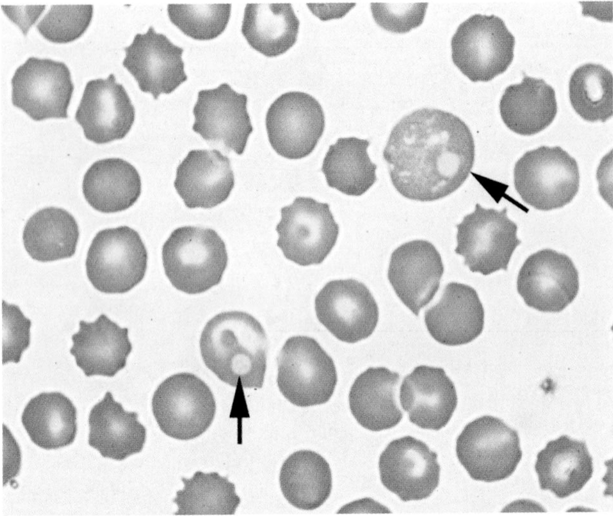

Figure 6.24 Blood film from a dog with distemper. Note the pale-blue viral inclusions of distemper with the erythrocytes (arrows). These inclusions may stain pale blue to dark magenta in color. Wright stain.

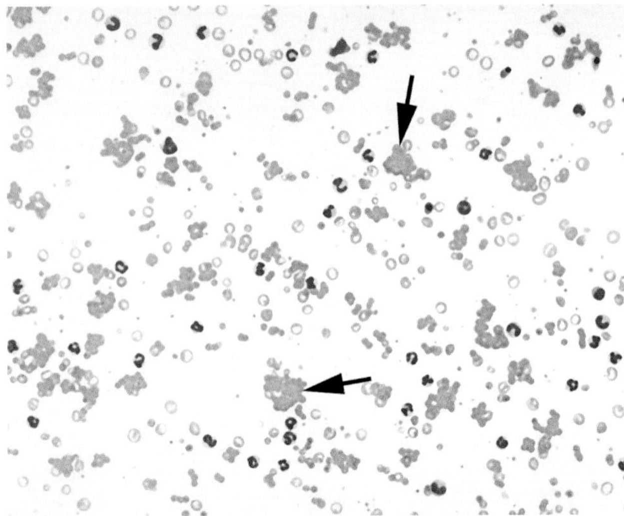

Figure 6.26 Blood film from an anemic dog with immune-mediated hemolytic anemia and marked agglutination. Note the large aggregates of spherocytes (arrows). Wright stain, low magnification.

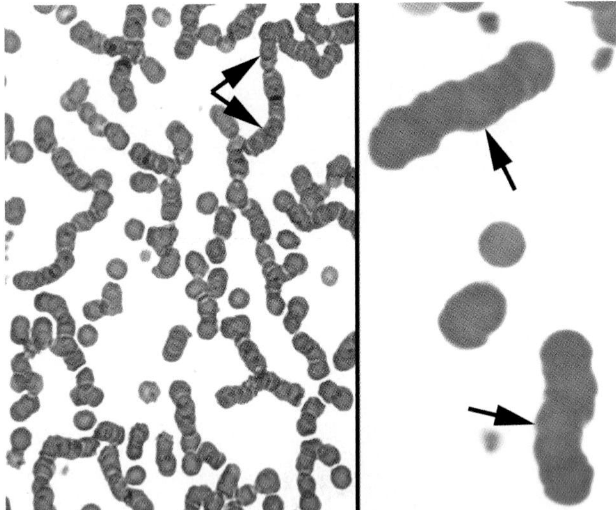

Figure 6.25 Blood film from a normal horse, illustrating rouleaux formation (arrows). Wright stain.

Increased rouleaux formation often is suggestive of a gammopathy; animals with multiple myeloma and canine ehrlichiosis almost always have increased rouleaux formation.

Agglutination

Agglutination of erythrocytes results in irregular, spheric clumps of cells because of antibody-related bridging (Figure 6.26). Agglutination is very suggestive of immune-mediated hemolytic anemia, but it also may be seen after a mismatched blood transfusion. To confirm that agglutination is present, mix several drops of isotonic saline with a drop of blood. This procedure is commonly referred to as a saline agglutination test. The recommended procedure of mixing one drop of saline with one drop of blood often results in false positives, especially if rouleaux is marked. Agglutination will persist in the presence of saline (Figure 6.26, left), whereas rouleaux formation will disperse. Agglutination may be so marked that it can be seen grossly on blood films and on the side of EDTA tubes (Figure 6.27, right). Agglutination may result in a falsely increased MCV and a falsely decreased red-blood-cell count, because agglutinated red cells (i.e., doublets and triplets) may be counted as large cells (see Chapter 1).

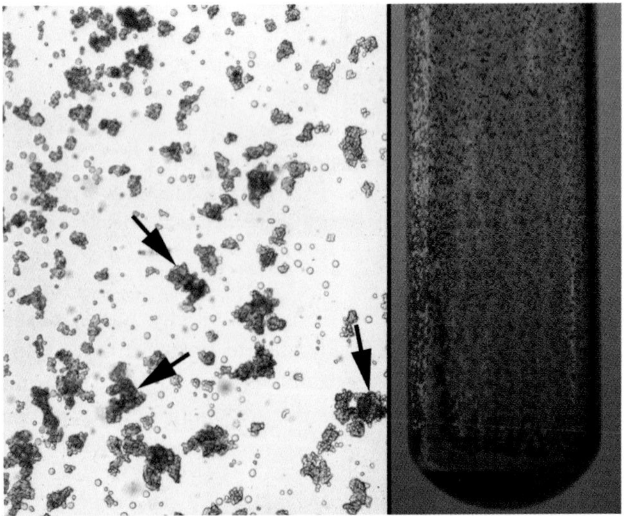

Figure 6.27 Blood from a dog with immune-mediated hemolytic anemia. Left. Blood has been mixed with isotonic saline, and agglutination persists (arrows). Right. Agglutination is so severe that it can be visualized grossly on the side of the EDTA blood-collection tube.

Erythroid dysplasia and neoplasia

Dysplasia and leukemia of red blood cells is covered in more detail in Chapter 16. Briefly, erythroid dysplasia, which is commonly seen in cats associated with FeLV, is characterized by a nonregenerative anemia in conjunction with macrocytosis and megaloblastic erythroid precursors, in which there is advanced cell hemoglobinization with incomplete nuclear maturation. Red-cell leukemia (M6) is relatively rare in dogs, but in cats, it usually is associated with FeLV. In these patients, an increased concentration of quite immature nucleated erythrocytes typically is present in the face of a severe, nonregenerative anemia (see Chapter 16).

CHAPTER 7

7 Classification of and Diagnostic Approach to Anemia

Mary Anna Thrall

Department of Biomedical Sciences, Ross University School of Veterinary Medicine, Basseterre, Saint Kitts and Nevis

Anemia is a decrease in the red blood cell (RBC) mass that results in decreased oxygenation of tissues. The RBC mass is determined by measuring the packed cell volume (PCV; i.e., hematocrit), the amount of hemoglobin in the blood, and the erythrocyte count (see Chapter 1). Of these three, PCV is used most commonly as the primary value for interpretation in North America, although when the hematocrit is calculated by automated cell counters, hemoglobin concentration is more accurate.

Anemia is a manifestation of an underlying disease that has produced increased erythrocyte destruction, increased erythrocyte loss through hemorrhage, decreased production of erythrocytes, or some combination of these events. Clinical signs usually relate to decreased oxygenation or associated compensatory mechanisms and may include pale mucous membranes, lethargy, reduced exercise tolerance, increased respiratory rate or dyspnea, increased heart rate, and murmurs caused by increased blood turbulence. Nonspecific clinical signs, such as weight loss, anorexia, fever, or lymphadenopathy, may be present if the animal has an underlying systemic illness. Specific clinical signs that are associated with blood destruction may include splenomegaly, icterus, and darkly pigmented urine resulting from hemoglobinuria or bilirubinuria.

The severity of clinical signs usually relates to the duration of onset, because animals with a slow onset, resulting from chronic blood loss or bone marrow dysfunction, usually compensate to some extent for the hypoxemia. Compensatory mechanisms include increased concentration of erythrocyte 2,3-diphosphoglycerate, which decreases the oxygen–hemoglobin affinity and, thus, enhances the delivery of oxygen to tissues, increases cardiac output, and aids in the redistribution of blood flow to vital organs. Death may occur in animals that experience severe acute blood loss or blood destruction. Appropriate therapy and prognosis is facilitated by determining whether the anemia is a result of erythrocyte destruction, blood loss, or lack of erythrocyte production, followed by establishing the diagnosis of the underlying disease. This chapter addresses the classification of and diagnostic approach to anemia.

Classification of anemia

Three general schemes are used to classify anemia: erythrocyte size and hemoglobin concentration, bone marrow response, and classification by pathophysiologic mechanism. The classification by erythrocyte size and bone marrow response are the most useful for clinical purposes, because they are tools that allow veterinarians to follow a mental pathway to a differential diagnosis. The pathophysiologic classification merely provides a conceptual framework for a diagnostic library of disorders that cause anemia.

Erythrocyte size and hemoglobin concentration

Traditionally, anemia has been classified by erythrocyte volume (i.e., mean cell volume [MCV]) and the amount of hemoglobin within erythrocytes (i.e., mean corpuscular hemoglobin concentration [MCHC]). An anemia is referred to as being microcytic when the erythrocytes are small, normocytic when they are of normal volume, and macrocytic when they are larger than the reference interval. Moreover, anemia is referred to as being hypochromic when the cells contain a less-than-normal hemoglobin concentration and as normochromic when they contain a normal hemoglobin concentration. Hyperchromic anemias do not occur, but the MCHC is falsely increased when the hemoglobin determination is falsely increased because of intravascular hemolysis, lipemia, or the presence of Heinz bodies. The MCHC is also falsely increased if the erythrocyte size falls below the threshold of RBC detection in the hematology analyzer. This will effectively reduce the hematocrit and increase the MCHC. Although spherocytes appear to be hyperchromic on blood films because of their shape, the hemoglobin concentration

Veterinary Hematology, Clinical Chemistry, and Cytology, Third Edition. Edited by Mary Anna Thrall, Glade Weiser, Robin W. Allison and Terry W. Campbell.

Companion website: www.wiley.com/go/thrall/veterinary

is normal in these erythrocytes. The MCHC, however, may be falsely increased in patients with immune-mediated hemolytic anemia because of intravascular hemolysis or agglutination, which causes errors in measurement of the RBC mass.

This classification system is useful, particularly as it relates to cell volume, in that microcytic anemias almost always result from iron deficiency. Other causes of microcytosis include hepatic portocaval vascular shunts in dogs and cats, some cases of anemia of inflammatory disease, and normal variations in certain breeds of dogs such as Akitas and Shiba Inus. A macrocytic anemia usually indicates that the marrow is functional and is releasing immature cells that are larger than normal in size. Macrocytosis without polychromasia or reticulocytosis should be evaluated further, because a regenerative response likely is not the cause in these patients. The MCV is of particular value in horses, because reticulocytes are almost never released into the circulation in significant numbers. Other causes of macrocytosis include feline leukemia virus, myelodysplasia, poodle macrocytosis, and hereditary stomatocytosis (see Chapter 6). Animals with a normocytic anemia usually have a nonregenerative or a preregenerative anemia. Preregenerative refers to anemia in animals with blood loss or blood destruction, but in which evidence of regeneration in the blood is not yet evident. Animals with a regenerative anemia, however, may have an MCV within the reference interval and, thus, be classified as having a normocytic anemia. The generated histogram or computer graphic is valuable in these patients, in that the subpopulation of macrocytic cells can be observed even though the MCV is normal (discussed later).

The MCHC is less useful in the classification of anemia, in that hypochromia usually is simply associated with an increased concentration of large, immature cells (i.e., regenerative anemia). Reticulocytes are still synthesizing hemoglobin; therefore, their hemoglobin concentration is less than that of mature erythrocytes. Occasionally, animals with iron deficiency may have a hypochromic as well as a microcytic anemia, but in most iron-deficient animals, the MCHC is within the reference interval.

Historically, MCV and MCHC were derived by calculations based on the PCV, hemoglobin concentration, and erythrocyte count. The MCV was calculated by dividing the PCV by the erythrocyte (RBC) count. For example, if the patient's PCV is 42% and its RBC count is 6.0×10^6, then the PCV divided by the RBC count is 70 fL (i.e., 42/6 = 7). In terms of mathematical logic, 1 μL = 10^9 fL, and 42% of 10^9 fL is 420,000,000 fL. Therefore, the MCV = 70 fL (i.e., 420,000,000 ÷ 6,000,000). The MCHC, which is the ratio of the weight of hemoglobin to the volume of erythrocytes in grams per deciliter, can be calculated by the following equation:

$$\text{MCHC(g/dL)} = \frac{\text{HGB}}{\text{HCT}} \times 100$$

For example, if the hemoglobin is 14 g/dL and the PCV is 42%, then the MCHC is 33.3 g/dL.

Electronic cell counters have made calculation of the MCV obsolete, because the cell volume can be measured electronically. Thus, the MCV and RBC are used to calculate the hematocrit (see Chapter 1). This technology has improved the usefulness of this classification of anemia, because subpopulations of microcytic or macrocytic erythrocytes can be observed in histograms or computer graphics, even when the MCV is within the reference interval (Figure 7.1). The RBC distribution width, which describes the width of the RBC size distribution, increases when subpopulations of either microcytic or macrocytic erythrocytes are present and often is increased before the MCV value falls out of the reference interval. The MCHC is still derived using the hemoglobin and PCV determinations; however, laser-detection technology using light scatter now allows for direct determination of the amount of hemoglobin within cells. Hemoglobin concentration using this type of technology is reported as corpuscular hemoglobin concentration mean (CHCM). Using this detection system, lipemia or hemolysis will not falsely increase the CHCM. Heinz bodies, however, may, because erythrocytes containing Heinz bodies are more optically dense. Electronic cell counters with flow cytometry capability calculate the indices of reticulocytes, which is very useful in detecting iron-deficiency anemia at an early stage (see Chapter 9).

Bone marrow response

Classification of anemia based on responsiveness of the bone marrow is very useful diagnostically. An anemia is classified as either regenerative or nonregenerative based on the number of immature erythrocytes that are circulating. Early release of immature erythrocytes is a normal marrow response to increased erythropoietin production, primarily by renal tissue, secondary to hypoxia. Increased numbers of immature erythrocytes are released into the circulation after blood loss or blood destruction, and they are indicative of a regenerative anemia. An increased concentration of immature erythrocytes usually is seen within 2–4 days after blood loss or destruction. A lack of circulating immature erythrocytes in the face of anemia indicates a nonregenerative anemia and should be considered as evidence of marrow dysfunction.

Immature erythrocytes observed using a Wright-stained blood film are polychromatophilic, and they have a blue-staining reticulum (i.e., reticulocyte) when new methylene blue or brilliant cresyl blue stains are used (see Chapters 1 and 6). In general, an anemia is considered to be regenerative if the reticulocyte concentration is greater than 60,000 cells/μL (see Chapter 1), or if there is increased polychromasia on the blood film. Reticulocytosis or increased polychromasia is a better indication of bone marrow responsiveness than is an increased MCV (see

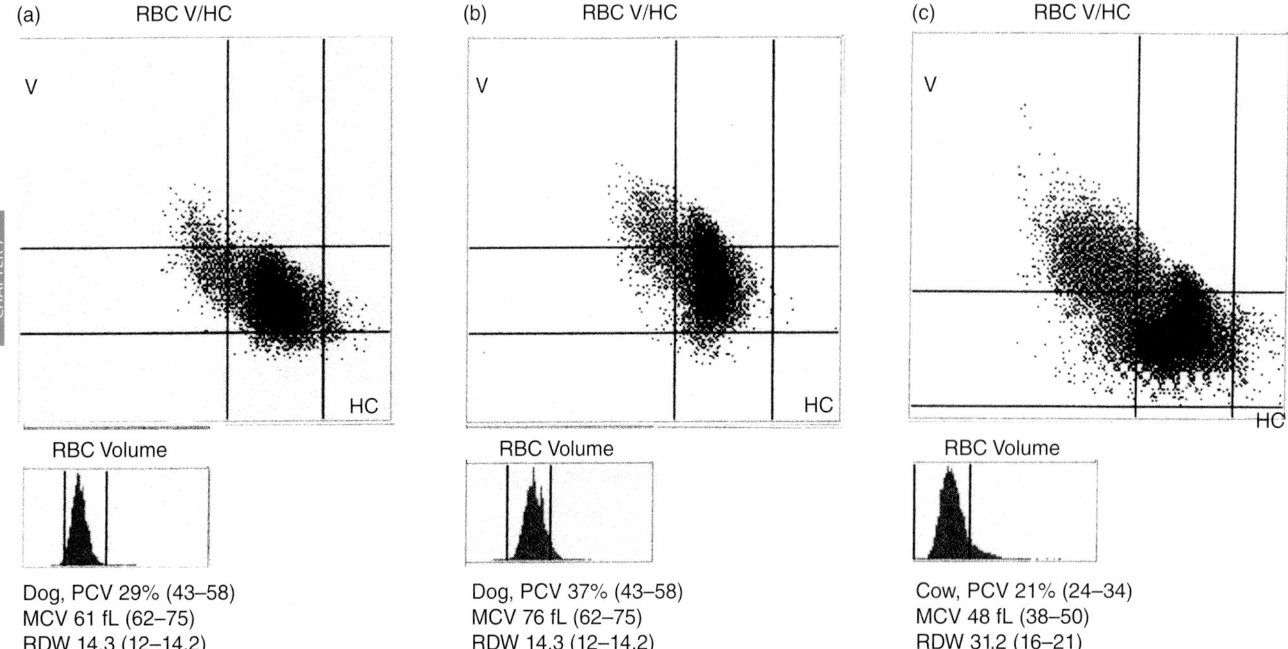

Figure 7.1 Red-blood-cell volume/hemoglobin concentration (RBC V/HC) cytograms and RBC volume histograms from six anemic animals generated by a Bayer Advia 120 (Bayer Corporation, Tarrytown, NY). On the RBC V/HC cytogram, hemoglobin (Hgb) concentration is plotted along the *x* (i.e., horizontal) axis, and cell volume is plotted along the *y* (i.e., vertical) axis. Each RBC is displayed based on volume and Hgb concentration, and normocytic normochromic cells are in the center box of each nine-box cytogram. Larger cells are displayed toward the top of the cytogram and hypochromic cells toward the left; thus, macrocytic hypochromic cells are displayed to the upper left of the cluster of normal erythrocytes. The RBC volume histogram represents the distribution of the RBCs by cell volume; normal samples have a bell-shaped curve. The mean corpuscular volume (MCV) and RBC distribution width (RDW) are determined from this histogram. The MCV is the mean of the RBC volume histogram, and the RDW is the coefficient of variation of the population. Each animal's species, packed cell volume (PCV), MCV, and RDW are provided beneath the RBC V/HC cytogram and RBC volume histogram. Reference intervals are in parentheses. (a) A 12-year-old mixed-breed dog with a mild anemia, mildly decreased MCV, and mildly increased RDW. The RBC V/HC cytogram shows that many of the erythrocytes are toward the bottom of the middle square, indicating they are microcytic. In addition, a population of hypochromic cells is present, some of which are normocytic and some of which are macrocytic. The RBC volume histogram is shifted toward the left, also indicating that many of the erythrocytes are slightly small. Iron-deficiency anemia was suspected in this patient and was confirmed by decreased serum iron concentration. The dog had a 3-month history of epistaxis associated with a nasal passage chondrosarcoma. (b) A 12-year-old miniature schnauzer with a very mild anemia, mildly increased MCV, and mildly increased RDW. The RBC V/HC cytogram shows a population of cells above the middle square that represents large cells. A population of macrocytic hypochromic cells is present as well. The RBC volume histogram is shifted slightly toward the right, and a population of macrocytic cells is evident. This is indicative of a regenerative anemia. (c) A 1-week-old anemic calf. Note the population of macrocytic hypochromic cells, even though the MCV is within the reference interval. The RDW is markedly increased. The reticulocyte count is 90,000 cells/μL (2%). The presence of macrocytic cells and reticulocytes indicates that the anemia is regenerative. The calf's umbilical stump had been bleeding since birth, and it also had blood in the feces for three days. The PCV on the previous day was 9%, and the calf received a blood transfusion at that time. Many of the normocytic cells probably are donor erythrocytes. The calf responded well to supportive therapy and 1 week later, the PCV was 27%. (d) A 13-year-old cat with a mildly decreased MCV. The RBC V/HC cytogram and RBC volume histogram are similar to those of the dog in panel a, suggesting iron-deficiency anemia. The cat had blood in the feces, as a result of intestinal (primarily colonic) lymphoma, for several weeks before this CBC was performed. The reticulocyte count is 108,000 cells/μL, indicating that the anemia is regenerative, but the immature erythrocytes are also small because of iron deficiency. (e) A 6-year-old cat with a slightly increased RDW. Note that most of the cells are macrocytic and hypochromic. The RBC volume histogram is shifted far toward the right because of numerous large erythrocytes, and the reticulocyte count is 233,260 cells/μL (10.7%), indicating a very regenerative anemia. The cat was Coombs positive, and a diagnosis of immune-mediated hemolytic anemia was made. No *Haemobartonella* organisms were observed on blood films taken during various days, but polymerase chain reaction for *Haemobartonella felis* was not performed. The cat was negative for feline leukemia virus. (f) A 12-year-old horse with a macrocytic anemia. Note the population of large cells, some of which are hypochromic. The RBC volume histogram is shifted toward the right, indicating a subpopulation of large cells. Reticulocytes are not released in horses, but the presence of macrocytic erythrocytes suggests that the anemia is regenerative. The horse was dehydrated, so it likely was more anemic than would be indicated by the PCV. Blood loss or blood destruction should be suspected in this case.

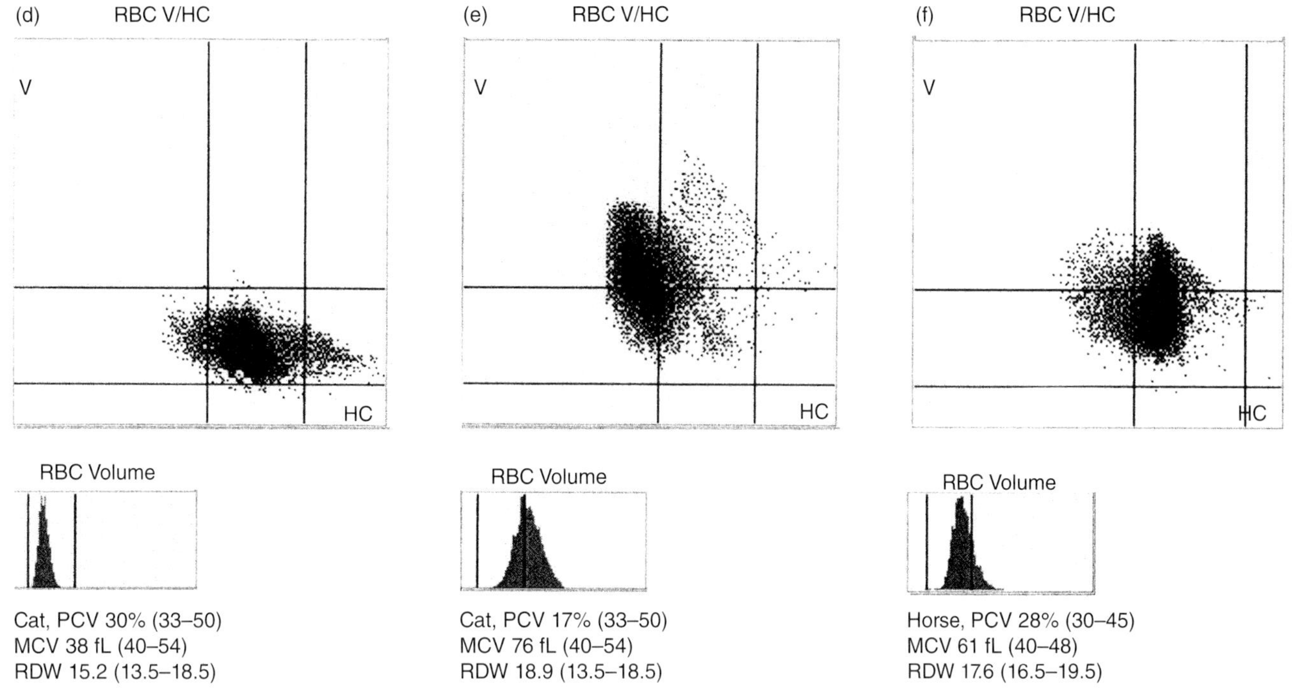

Figure 7.1 (*Continued*)

Chapter 6). Horses almost never release significant numbers of reticulocytes into the circulation.

Pathophysiologic classification

The pathophysiologic classification of anemia essentially is a categorization based on the underlying disorder. Nonregenerative anemia results from defective or decreased erythropoiesis (see Chapter 8). Decreased erythropoiesis usually is classified according to whether neutrophil and platelet production are also decreased (i.e., aplastic anemia) and whether RBC production is simply decreased (i.e., hypoplasia) or is completely absent (i.e., aplasia). Moreover, impaired erythrocyte production may be caused by an intrinsic (i.e., primary) marrow disorder, such as myelofibrosis, myelodysplasia, or myeloproliferative disorder, or it may be caused by an extrinsic (i.e., secondary) disorder. Secondary disorders include chronic renal disease; some endocrine disorders; inflammatory diseases; infectious agents, such as *Ehrlichia* sp., equine infectious anemia virus, and feline leukemia virus; immune-mediated destruction of erythrocyte precursors; and drug- or chemical-induced damage (see Chapter 15).

Regenerative anemia is caused by blood loss or erythrocyte destruction (see Chapter 9). Blood loss may be external or internal, and it may be acute or chronic. Causes of acute blood loss include trauma, bleeding lesions (e.g., tumors or large ulcers), and hemostatic disorders (e.g., thrombocytopenia or an inherited or acquired coagulopathy such as warfarin toxicosis or disseminated vascular coagulopathy). Common causes of chronic blood loss include bleeding lesions, particularly within the gastrointestinal tract, and gastrointestinal or external parasites. Erythrocyte destruction (i.e., hemolysis) may be either intravascular or extravascular, and it may result from intrinsic (i.e., primary) defects, such as hereditary membrane defects or enzyme deficiencies, or from extrinsic (i.e., secondary) causes, such as erythrocyte parasites or immune-mediated destruction. Intravascular hemolysis is the actual lysis of erythrocytes within the vascular system. Extravascular hemolysis occurs when abnormal erythrocytes are phagocytized by macrophages, usually within the spleen or liver. Common causes of erythrocyte destruction include immune-mediated mechanisms, erythrocyte parasites, and drugs and chemicals that produce oxidative damage, resulting in Heinz body formation. Less common causes of hemolysis include hypophosphatemia, water intoxication in young ruminants, bacteria (e.g., *Leptospira* and *Clostridium* sp.), heparin overdose, and hereditary erythrocyte enzyme deficiencies and membrane defects.

Diagnostic approach

When presented with an anemic patient, the ultimate goal is to establish a definitive diagnosis of the underlying disorder so that appropriate therapy can be initiated and a prognosis established. Information can be obtained from the laboratory evaluation, the patient history, and the physical examination. The most clinically useful approach to anemia is based on the classification schemes involving a combination of bone marrow response and erythrocyte size.

Laboratory evaluation

The classification of an anemia based on erythrocyte size and marrow response (discussed earlier) is very important. Essential laboratory data include PCV, MCV, and reticulocyte count. Either blood loss or destruction will result in a regenerative anemia, and marrow dysfunction will result in a nonregenerative anemia. Furthermore, microcytosis usually is evidence of iron-deficiency anemia, and macrocytosis usually is evidence of regeneration. Additional information may be obtained from examination of the blood film; erythrocyte morphology may even reveal a definitive diagnosis (see Chapter 6).

Other laboratory procedures that may provide helpful information include plasma protein estimation by refractometry (see Chapter 1). Blood loss usually results not only in a loss of erythrocytes but also in a loss of other blood components, including protein. Thus, patients with blood loss may be hypoproteinemic. Other causes of hypoproteinemia, however, still must be considered (see Chapter 30). If blood is lost internally, such as within a body cavity, the protein usually is reabsorbed within hours.

Other components of the complete blood count (CBC) also may provide useful information. For example, if a patient is severely thrombocytopenic, anemia may be caused by blood loss secondary to impaired clot formation. On the other hand, if the leukocyte concentration, platelet concentration, and PCV are all decreased and the anemia is nonregenerative, then complete bone marrow failure is the likely cause of the anemia. An animal with a mild, nonregenerative anemia and increased immature neutrophils likely has an anemia of inflammatory disease (see Chapter 8).

Specific laboratory tests can be performed to help confirm or exclude a suspected diagnosis. If spherocytes are observed on the blood film of an anemic patient, then a Coombs test or a saline fragility test (see Chapter 1) can help to confirm immune-mediated hemolytic anemia. In patients with microcytic anemia, serum iron should be measured to determine if the microcytosis is caused by iron deficiency. In addition, the feces should be examined for blood, because chronic blood loss from the gastrointestinal tract is a common cause of iron-deficiency anemia (see Chapter 9). Anemic dogs, particularly those with a concurrent thrombocytopenia and hyperglobulinemia, should be tested for ehrlichiosis, and anemic cats should be tested for feline leukemia virus and feline immunodeficiency virus. Anemic horses should be tested for equine infectious anemia.

The biochemical profile also may provide essential information. Patients with mild to moderate, nonregenerative anemia may have disorders that are extrinsic to the marrow but that affect the marrow function. For example, animals with a nonregenerative anemia that are also azotemic because of kidney dysfunction likely have decreased erythropoietin production. All patients with an unexplained nonregenerative anemia should undergo bone marrow aspiration and examination (see Chapter 15).

Signalment and history

A complete and accurate patient history from the owner may provide valuable information. In some cases, the signalment is also helpful, because certain disorders are more common in certain breeds. For example, immune-mediated hemolytic anemia is relatively common in cocker spaniels. Acute blood loss results in acute onset of clinical signs, whereas both chronic blood loss and marrow dysfunction result in chronic onset of clinical signs. Therefore, determining if the onset of clinical signs was acute or chronic may be helpful. Asking the owner if other clinical signs are present may be useful as well. For example, a dog that is also experiencing polyuria and polydipsia may be anemic as a consequence of renal dysfunction. Alternatively, a dog that is experiencing periodic episodes of weakness may have recurring, intermittent, intra-abdominal hemorrhage secondary to a bleeding lesion (e.g., hemangiosarcoma). One should also determine any history of trauma or recent surgery and if the owner has observed any evidence of blood loss, such as hematuria or epistaxis. Melena, on the other hand, must be very severe to be obvious by visual examination of feces. Finally, one should inquire if the patient has had any possible exposure to plants, drugs, or chemicals that might induce blood destruction, marrow dysfunction, or gastrointestinal ulceration and associated blood loss.

Physical examination

A careful, routine physical examination may reveal additional information. For example, if bruising, petechiae, or ecchymoses are present in an anemic patient, the anemia may be secondary to decreased or dysfunctional platelets or to a coagulation disorder (see Chapter 17). If abdominal distension is present, intra-abdominal hemorrhage should be suspected, and an abdominal paracentesis and fluid evaluation should be performed. If the mucous membranes are icteric as well as pale, erythrocyte destruction should be suspected. If the mucous membranes are cyanotic or brown as well as pale, methemoglobinemia, which may accompany Heinz-body anemia, may be present.

Summary

In summary, the clinical signs, laboratory evaluation, signalment, history, and physical examination are all important in establishing a diagnosis for the underlying cause of anemia. Chronic external blood loss usually results in iron-deficiency anemia, which can be diagnosed on the basis of decreased MCV and serum iron. Acute external blood loss usually can be diagnosed during the physical examination; however, internal blood loss may initially be difficult to differentiate from blood destruction. Significant internal blood loss usually occurs within a body cavity, so careful physical examination, body cavity aspiration, or other methods of visualization usually are diagnostic. Furthermore, many causes of blood destruction, such as immune-mediated destruction, Heinz bodies, or erythrocyte parasites, can be detected based on examination of blood films and erythrocyte morphology. Diagnostic procedures for specific causes of anemia are discussed in more detail in Chapters 8 and 9.

8 Nonregenerative Anemia

Mary Anna Thrall

Department of Biomedical Sciences, Ross University School of Veterinary Medicine, Basseterre, Saint Kitts and Nevis

Anemia is classified as either regenerative or nonregenerative based on the number of circulating immature erythrocytes (polychromatophilic erythrocytes or reticulocytes). A lack of circulating immature erythrocytes indicates a nonregenerative anemia and provides evidence of marrow dysfunction. Most nonregenerative anemias are normocytic. Because the marrow takes approximately 2 days to respond to anemia (see "Reticulocyte Maturation," Chapter 1), patients with acute blood loss or blood destruction may appear to have a nonregenerative anemia, but it is actually preregenerative.

Nonregenerative anemia is further subclassified based on whether granulopoiesis (neutrophil production) and thrombopoiesis (platelet production) are also affected. Animals with nonregenerative anemia in conjunction with neutropenia and thrombocytopenia (pancytopenia) have either reversible or irreversible stem cell injury. Irreversible stem cell injuries are discussed in Chapter 15 and represent an intrinsic defect in proliferative behavior and/or regulation of stem cell entry into differentiated hematopoiesis. Some irreversible injuries may be induced by drugs, chemicals, viruses (e.g., feline leukemia virus [FeLV]), radiation, and immune-mediated stem cell injury, but the cause often is never discovered. Manifestations of stem cell injury range from dysplasia to lack of cell production (aplastic anemia) to uncontrolled neoplastic proliferation. Reversible stem cell injury is transient but also may be caused by drugs, chemicals, viruses, radiation, and immune-mediated destruction of stem cells. Reversible stem cell injury does not progress to neoplasia; however, both reversible and irreversible stem cell damage may be associated with myelofibrosis or myelonecrosis in response to the injury.

Pancytopenia also may result from myelophthisic disorders in which nonhematopoietic neoplasms, such as lymphoma and malignant histiocytosis, either metastasize to or originate in the marrow. In addition, pancytopenia may be seen with hemophagocytic syndrome, a rare condition that occurs secondary to infectious, neoplastic, or metabolic diseases and is characterized by the proliferation of benign histiocytic cells that phagocytize hematopoietic precursors.

Animals with nonregenerative anemia in conjunction with normal neutrophil and platelet concentrations may have an intrinsic marrow defect (pure red cell hypoplasia, aplasia, or apparent erythroid maturation defect), or they may have a disorder that is extrinsic to the bone marrow but results in defective or decreased erythropoiesis. Pure red cell aplasia also may be either reversible or irreversible, and it usually is immune mediated or caused by viral (FeLV) damage. Extrinsic causes of nonregenerative anemia include anemia of inflammatory disease, anemia of renal failure, anemias associated with endocrine disorders, and, rarely, nutritional deficiencies.

Aplastic anemia (aplastic pancytopenia)

Drugs, chemicals, toxins, and estrogen

Antineoplastic and immunosuppressive drugs, such as doxorubicin, cyclophosphamide, cytosine arabinoside, vincristine, hydroxyurea, and azathioprine, probably are the most commonly used agents that cause reversible stem cell damage in dogs. These drugs are used for brief periods of time, however, and usually result in a neutropenia and thrombocytopenia rather than a significant nonregenerative anemia. Drugs that have been associated with stem cell injury in animals include estrogen (dogs and ferrets), phenylbutazone (dogs and possibly horses), meclofenamic acid (dogs), griseofulvin (cats), phenobarbital (dogs and cats), phenytoin (dogs), colchicine (dogs), azidothymidine (a reverse transcriptase inhibitor; cats), chloramphenicol (dogs and cats), thiacetarsamide (dogs), and albendazole (a broad-spectrum anthelmintic; dogs and cats). Some drugs may induce stem cell destruction by immune-mediated mechanisms. In dogs, trimethoprim-sulfadiazine, cephalosporin, and phenobarbital have been associated with pancytopenia that may be immune-mediated. Drug-induced

Veterinary Hematology, Clinical Chemistry, and Cytology, Third Edition. Edited by Mary Anna Thrall, Glade Weiser, Robin W. Allison and Terry W. Campbell.

Companion website: www.wiley.com/go/thrall/veterinary

Table 8.1 Drugs, chemicals, plants, and hormones associated with nonregenerative anemia in domestic animals.

Dogs
Albendazole
Estrogen
Cephalosporins
Chemotherapeutic agents
Colchicine
Meclofenamic acid
Phenobarbital
Phenylbutazone
Phenytoin
Quinidine
Thiacetarsamide
Cats
Albendazole
Azidothymidine
Griseofulvin
Cattle
Bracken fern
Mycotoxins
Trichlorethylene
Horses
Mycotoxins
Phenylbutazone

immune-mediated stem cell injury usually responds to discontinuation of the drug. Idiopathic immune-mediated stem cell injury often responds to immunosuppressive therapy, but these injuries may take several weeks to respond and often require long-term treatment for resolution. Table 8.1 summarizes drugs and chemicals that may cause aplastic anemia in domestic animals.

Estrogen toxicosis may occur in bitches given exogenous estrogen for mismating, termination of pseudopregnancy, or urinary incontinence. Myelosuppression may result from the administration of excessive amounts of estrogen or from an idiosyncratic sensitivity to estrogen. Endogenous estrogen, resulting either from Sertoli cell tumors in male dogs or from cystic ovaries or granulosa cell tumors in female dogs, also may result in bone marrow suppression. Because ferrets are induced ovulators, marrow suppression from endogenous estrogen is a common – and potentially fatal – disorder in this species. The mechanism of estrogen toxicosis is unclear, but it is thought to result from the secretion (by thymic stromal cells) of an estrogen-induced substance that inhibits stem cells. Marrow suppression is preceded by an initial thrombocytosis and neutrophilia.

Aplastic anemia in cattle has been associated with grazing on bracken fern and ingestion of soybean meal contaminated with the solvent trichloroethylene. Benzene, a commonly used solvent, may cause aplastic anemia as well as leukemia. Mycotoxins have been associated with bone marrow suppression in horses and cattle, and experimental aflatoxin B_1 toxicity has been reported to cause aplastic anemia in pigs.

Infectious agents

FeLV can result in anemia by many mechanisms, one of which is induction of aplastic anemia. In addition, FeLV is associated with anemia that manifests as pure red cell aplasia or hypoplasia, myeloproliferative disorders (see Chapter 16), anemia of inflammatory disease, and hemolysis. Hemolytic anemias that may be associated with FeLV infection include Heinz-body anemia, immune-mediated hemolytic anemia, and feline infectious anemia (see Chapter 9). Before widespread use of the FeLV vaccine, approximately 70% of anemic cats were infected with FeLV. Anemia caused by FeLV often is macrocytic, or a subpopulation of the erythrocytes is macrocytic in the absence of reticulocytosis. This may be caused by prolonged dysplastic erythrocyte production resulting from FeLV-induced myelodysplasia (see Chapter 16).

Ehrlichia canis may result in pancytopenia by two mechanisms: immune-mediated destruction of circulating cells, or aplastic anemia (which also may be an immune-mediated mechanism). In addition, dogs with ehrlichiosis may present with only one decreased cell line (e.g., thrombocytopenia), may have a lymphocytosis, and commonly have hyperglobulinemia. The organism rarely is seen on blood films.

Equine infectious anemia virus (a lentivirus) causes anemia by a number of mechanisms, one of which is bone marrow suppression (possibly immune mediated). Parvovirus infection in dogs and cats causes acute bone marrow necrosis, but these animals usually recover or die before the anemia becomes significant.

Other infectious agents, such as systemic fungal or protozoal infections, have been reported to result in pancytopenia. The mechanism may be immune mediated.

Pure red cell aplasia/nonregenerative immune mediated anemia

Pure red cell aplasia is characterized by a markedly decreased concentration of erythroid precursors in the bone marrow in the face of normal granulopoiesis and thrombopoiesis, resulting in a severe nonregenerative anemia with normal neutrophil and platelet concentrations. Congenital pure red cell aplasia (Diamond-Blackfan anemia) is very rare in people, and has only been reported, but not proven, in one dog. Acquired pure red cell aplasia almost always is caused by immune-mediated destruction of erythroid precursors, and it often responds to immunosuppressive therapy. Spherocytes and agglutination are occasionally present, hemolysis is variable but is sometimes present, and approximately half the affected dogs in some studies were Coombs' positive. Bone marrow examination usually reveals an apparent arrest at some stage of erythroid precursor maturation, ranging from the rubriblast to the metarubricyte stage. Phagocytosis of rubricytes or metarubricytes (rubriphagocytosis) is commonly seen in bone marrow aspirates, and some degree of myelofibrosis is seen in approximately half of affected dogs. Erythropoiesis is usually expanded (erythroid hyperplasia) up to the stage of the erythrocyte precursor that is being phagocytized. Occasionally, however, erythroid precursors are completely absent. Nonregenerative immune-mediated anemia is also referred to as precursor-targeted immune-mediated anemia (PIMA). While most affected dogs and cats respond to immunosuppressive therapy, the time from onset to a regenerative response (reticulocytosis) is usually several weeks, and may be months.

Some dogs and horses treated with recombinant human erythropoietin developed an immune response against the recombinant as well as endogenous erythropoietin, resulting in a reversible pure red cell aplasia. Recombinant, species-specific erythropoietin does not produce this syndrome. In one retrospective study, only 6% of dogs developed pure red cell aplasia associated with the administration of darbepoetin, a long-acting glycosolated synthetic recombinant human erythropoietin analog. Darbepoetin is thought to be less likely to produce pure red cell aplasia in dogs and cats than was epoetin, the first recombinant erythropoietin developed.

Finally, certain strains of FeLV virus (subgroup C) cause pure red cell aplasia.

Red cell hypoplasia

Nonregenerative anemia may result from abnormalities that are extrinsic to the marrow, including anemia of inflammatory disease, anemia of chronic renal failure, and anemia associated with endocrine disease, and rarely, anemia associated with nutritional deficiencies. Other laboratory findings such as an inflammatory leukogram, azotemia, other biochemical profile abnormalities or endocrine panel abnormalities usually are key to establishing the diagnosis of these types of anemias.

Anemia of inflammation

Anemia of inflammation (anemia of chronic disease) is probably the most common anemia in domestic animals, but it usually is mild and clinically insignificant. This type of anemia is associated with various types of inflammatory processes, including infections, trauma, kidney disease, neoplasia, heart failure, and obesity, and usually is mild to moderate, nonregenerative, and usually normocytic but occasionally microcytic. The pathogenesis of anemia of inflammatory disease is multifactorial, including changes in iron homeostasis, altered proliferation of erythroid progenitor cells and production of erythropoietin, and decreased RBC life span. Immune stimulation results in activation of T cells and monocytes that produce cytokines, such as interferon-γ (IFN-γ), tumor necrosis factor-α (TNF-α), interleukin (IL)-1, IL-6, and IL-10 that affect iron metabolism. Lipopolysaccharide (LPS) and IL-6 induce hepatic production of hepcidin, which regulates iron homeostasis by repressing intestinal iron absorption as well as iron release from ferritin stores and by mediating other regulators of iron. Specifically, hepcidin inactivates ferroportin, which is responsible for transporting iron out of cells, and LPS can also downregulate divalent metal transporter 1 (DMT1) and ferroportin expression. These events result in inhibition of duodenal iron absorption and also decrease iron release from stores in macrophages and hepatocytes. Moreover, inflammatory cytokines up-regulate DMT1 expression on macrophages with a resultant increased uptake of iron into these cells. Additionally, IL-10 increases transferrin receptor expression, resulting in increased uptake of iron into cells, and TNF-α, IL-1, IL-6, and IL-10 also up-regulate ferritin expression, promoting intracellular storage and retention of iron. The combined effect of these changes is a relative iron deficiency in both the transport and functional pools, which limits availability of iron for erythropoiesis [see more on iron metabolism under "Chronic Blood Loss (Iron Deficiency Anemia)" in Chapter 9]. Independent of hepcidin and iron impairment of erythropoiesis, cytokines such as IL-1 and TNF also inhibit hypoxia-mediated stimulation of erythropoietin production in the kidney.

Laboratory findings include a decreased serum iron concentration, normal or decreased total iron-binding capacity (transferrin), normal or increased serum ferritin, and normal or increased stainable iron stores in the bone marrow. An inflammatory leukogram may be present as well. Occasionally animals with anemia of inflammation may have a microcytic anemia, and that along with the decreased serum iron concentration, makes anemia of inflammation sometimes difficult to distinguish from iron-deficiency anemia; in these cases, serum ferritin or bone marrow stainable iron (hemosiderin) may be helpful in differentiating the two disorders. However, transferrin is down-regulated with inflammation (a negative acute-phase protein), and ferritin is up-regulated with inflammation (a positive acute-phase protein), which may confound the differentiation. In humans with concurrent anemia of inflammation and iron deficiency anemia, the anemia is less microcytic and hypochromic than in patients with simple iron deficiency anemia, and this may be true in animals as well. Hepcidin measurement may become useful in distinguishing anemia of inflammation from iron deficiency anemia, since hepcidin is typically increased in patients with anemia of inflammation, and decreased in iron deficiency anemia. However, in humans with renal disease, serum hepcidin is increased since it is eliminated through the kidney, rendering the test nondiagnostic for differentiating iron deficiency anemia from anemia of inflammation. In addition to iron metabolism parameters, other laboratory tests such as reticulocyte hemoglobin content and red cell distribution width (RDW) may be helpful in differentiating iron deficiency anemia and anemia of inflammation. Reticulocyte hemoglobin content has been shown to be decreased in dogs and cats with iron restricted hematopoiesis but has not yet proven to be very useful in differentiating true iron deficiency from functional iron deficiency such as is seen with anemia of inflammation and portosystemic shunts.

A decreased serum iron concentration presumably is advantageous to patients with inflammatory disease, because it reduces the availability of iron for bacterial growth. Treatment is aimed at alleviating the underlying disease. Parenteral iron supplementation may have some benefit, and treatment with recombinant erythropoietin may result in an increased hematocrit. Inhibitors of hepcidin and inflammatory modulators show promise for the future.

Anemia of chronic renal disease

Anemia associated with chronic renal disease usually is moderate to severe, nonregenerative, and normocytic. The severity of the anemia usually correlates with the severity of the renal failure as evidenced by the degree of azotemia. The primary cause for this anemia is lack of production of erythropoietin by the kidney, and treatment with recombinant canine erythropoietin or the more recently developed darbepoetin, a long-acting recombinant human erythropoietin analog, effectively increases the hematocrit in most dogs and cats. Other factors, such as increased bleeding tendencies, also may play a role in this type of anemia. Increases in serum parathyroid hormone and phosphorus concentrations and increased erythrocyte osmotic fragility have not been found to correlate significantly with the degree of anemia. Some patients with anemia of renal disease have concurrent anemia of inflammatory disease. Inflammation and oxidative stress are thought to play a role in the progression of chronic kidney disease, and increases in acute-phase proteins such as hepciden are associated with decreased serum iron, total iron binding capacity, and hematocrit in cats with chronic renal disease. It is likely that anemia of inflammatory disease, a functional iron deficiency, also plays a role in the development of anemia of chronic renal disease in dogs and cats, just as it does in humans.

Anemia associated with endocrine disease

Hypothyroid dogs almost always have a mild, nonregenerative, normocytic anemia, usually with a hematocrit of approximately 30%. This anemia responds to therapy for hypothyroidism and may simply be a manifestation of the lowered metabolic rate. Some dogs with hypoadrenocorticism, particularly those with glucocorticoid deficiency, have a mild, nonregenerative, normocytic anemia that often is masked by dehydration.

Anemia associated with nutritional deficiencies

Iron-deficiency anemia is the most common anemia associated with a nutritional deficiency, and while common in people, lack of nutritional iron is rarely seen in adult domestic animals. This type of anemia usually is regenerative until the late stages (unless complicated by anemia of inflammatory disease) and is discussed in Chapter 9. Other types of anemia related to nutritional deficiency are diagnosed very infrequently.

Cobalamin and folate are water soluble B vitamins that are cofactors of enzymes that are required for normal DNA synthesis, hematopoiesis, and neuron myelination. In humans, cobalamin and folate deficiencies result in nonregenerative macrocytic anemias as a result of defective DNA synthesis, ineffective hematopoiesis, and erythrocyte precursor maturation arrest. Macrocytosis is a result of asynchronous development of the erythrocyte cytoplasm and nucleus. Cobalamin deficiency is observed in dogs and cats as a result of a hereditary absence of intrinsic factor cobalamin receptors in ileal enterocytes, which is inherited as an autosomal recessive trait. This anemia is nonregenerative and usually normocytic, unlike the human counterpart, and has been reported in border collies, a beagle, giant schnauzers, and cats. Affected puppies fail to thrive. Other findings include neutropenia with hypersegmentation, anemia with anisocytosis and poikilocytosis, megaloblastic changes of the bone marrow, decreased serum cobalamin concentrations, methylmalonic aciduria, and homocystinemia. Parenteral, but not oral, cyanocobalamin administration eliminates all abnormalities except the decreased serum cobalamin concentration. Chinese Shar Peis have a high prevalence of cobalamin deficiency compared to other breeds and healthy Shar Peis may have subclinical cobalamin deficiency. The disorder is suspected to be hereditary; the hematologic findings have not been reported to date.

Hematologic findings in animals with acquired cobalamin deficiency as a result of gastrointestinal or pancreatic disease have not been well characterized, although some animals with acquired cobalamin deficiency have been reported to have a mild normocytic anemia. A recent retrospective study in dogs showed no association between cobalamin or folate deficiency and the nonregenerative macrocytic anemia that is seen in humans. Some cats with hyperthyroidism are hypocobalaminemic but not anemic. Cobalt deficiency in ruminants results in a normocytic, nonregenerative anemia and is caused by grazing on cobalt-deficient soil. Cobalt is required for synthesis of cobalamin by rumen bacteria.

9 Regenerative Anemia

Mary Anna Thrall
Department of Biomedical Sciences, Ross University School of Veterinary Medicine, Basseterre, Saint Kitts and Nevis

The term "regenerative anemia" implies that the bone marrow is attempting to compensate for the anemia by increased erythrocyte production, as well as early release of immature red cells. This response is primarily due to increased erythropoietin production by hypoxia-sensing cells in the kidney (see discussions of erythrocyte production in Chapters 6 and 10). Indications that the anemia is regenerative are increased polychromasia on the Wright-stained blood film and increased reticulocyte concentration (other than in equine species, which do not release many immature erythrocytes). Mean cell volume (MCV) may be increased but is a less reliable indication of early release of cells than is the presence of reticulocytes or polychromasia. Regenerative anemia is caused by either blood loss or blood destruction or may be seen in the recovery phase of marrow dysfunction. Blood loss may be external or internal and may be acute or chronic. Causes of acute blood loss include trauma; bleeding lesions, such as tumors or large ulcers; and hemostatic disorders. Examples of hemostatic disorders include thrombocytopenia, inherited coagulopathies, and acquired coagulopathies, such as warfarin toxicosis or disseminated intravascular coagulopathy (DIC). Common causes of chronic blood loss include bleeding lesions, particularly within the gastrointestinal (GI) tract, and gastrointestinal or external parasites.

Blood destruction (hemolysis) may be either intravascular or extravascular and may be due to intrinsic (primary) defects, such as hereditary membrane defects or enzyme deficiencies, or extrinsic (secondary) causes, such as erythrocyte parasites or immune-mediated destruction. Intravascular hemolysis is the actual lysis of erythrocytes within the vascular system. Extravascular hemolysis occurs when abnormal erythrocytes are phagocytized by macrophages, usually within the spleen or liver. Common causes of erythrocyte destruction include immune-mediated mechanisms, erythrocyte parasites, and drugs and chemicals that produce oxidative damage resulting in Heinz body formation. Less common causes include hypophosphosphatemia, water intoxication in young ruminants, bacteria (*Leptospira, Clostridium*), heparin overdose, and hereditary erythrocyte enzyme deficiencies and membrane defects.

Blood loss

If blood is lost outside of the body, including loss into the GI tract, components of the blood such as iron and plasma protein are lost. On the other hand, if bleeding occurs within a body cavity, the protein is reabsorbed within hours, and most of the erythrocytes are reabsorbed by lymphatics within a few days. The remaining cells are lysed or phagocytized, and iron is reutilized.

Acute blood loss

If blood loss is acute, the packed cell volume (PCV) initially remains normal because both cells and plasma are lost. However, within a few hours both the PCV and plasma protein decrease as a result of dilution, as interstitial fluid is added to blood. By 72 hours post-bleed, polychromatophilic erythrocytes (reticulocytes) should begin to appear in blood, and their concentration usually peaks within approximately 1 week. Plasma protein should return to normal within about 1 week, unless blood loss is recurrent or ongoing. Examples of disorders causing acute blood loss include trauma and surgical procedures, coagulation disorders, thrombocytopenia, and bleeding tumors.

Thrombocytopenia may result in bleeding when the platelet concentration is less than 20,000–30,000 μL; however, in the author's experience, spontaneous bleeding does not usually occur until the platelet concentration is less than 5000 μL. Blood loss does not usually cause platelet concentrations to drop below 90,000 μL, although platelet function defects have been reported following acute blood loss. Electronic platelet cell count may be erroneously decreased due to platelet clumping but can then be estimated from the blood film (see Chapter 17). The combination of anemia,

Veterinary Hematology, Clinical Chemistry, and Cytology, Third Edition. Edited by Mary Anna Thrall, Glade Weiser, Robin W. Allison and Terry W. Campbell.

Companion website: www.wiley.com/go/thrall/veterinary

reticulocytosis (or increased polychromasia), and hypoproteinemia is suggestive of blood loss, unless hypoproteinemia is coincidental to the blood loss. Causes of hypoproteinemia other than blood loss include decreased intake (malabsorption, maldigestion, starvation), decreased production (liver failure), or other types of protein loss (glomerulonephropathy, protein losing enteropathy).

Blood loss outside of the body is usually easy to diagnose, since the source of blood loss is apparent, unless it is being lost via the gastrointestinal tract. Blood loss within a body cavity is more difficult to diagnose, and thoracic or abdominal fluid evaluation may be necessary to confirm the diagnosis.

Erythrocyte morphology is usually normal with acute blood loss, with the exception of blood loss from hemangiosarcoma, one of the most common tumors of middle-aged to older dogs, especially large breeds such as German shepherds and golden retrievers. Hemangiosarcomas have been reported in cats but are rare. They are malignant vascular tumors typically found in the spleen, liver, and right atrium of the heart, and most have metastasized to the lungs or other organs by the time the diagnosis is made. Many dogs present due to acute signs associated with anemia as a result of rupture of the tumor, with blood loss into the abdominal cavity. Some affected dogs have a history of intermittent weakness, as a result of multiple events involving tumor rupturing and bleeding, followed by absorption of blood from the abdominal cavity.

Acanthocytes and schistocytes are seen in some dogs with hemangiosarcoma (Figure 9.1); these morphologic changes are helpful in making the diagnosis, although acanthocytes are seen in numerous disorders other than hemangiosarcoma (see Chapter 6). Acanthocytes may also be observed in blood aspirated from the abdominal cavity (Figure 9.2),

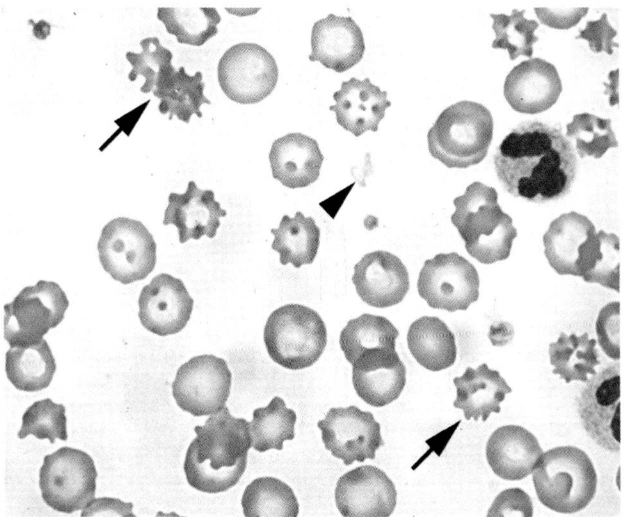

Figure 9.1 Blood film from a dog with hemangiosarcoma of the spleen. Note the acanthocytes (arrows) and schistocyte (arrowhead). Wright stain.

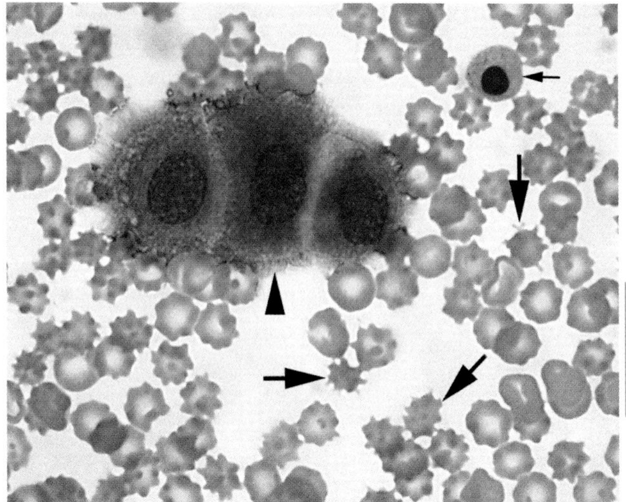

Figure 9.2 Abdominal fluid from a dog with ruptured splenic hemangiosarcoma and resultant hemoabdomen. Although morphology of erythrocytes is usually insignificant in body cavity effusions, animals with hemoabdomen resulting from hemangiosarcoma may have acanthocytes (large arrows) that are diagnostically useful. Mesothelial cells (arrowhead) and a nucleated erythrocyte are also present (small arrow). Wright stain.

although the diagnostic usefulness of this is controversial since erythrocyte shape abnormalities are commonly seen in body cavity effusions. Other common laboratory findings in dogs with hemangiosarcoma include reticulocytosis (increased polychromasia), transient hypoproteinemia, and thrombocytopenia, usually mild to moderate, as a result of localized microangiopathy within the tumor, or disseminated intravascular coagulation. Dogs with intra-abdominal bleeding hemangiosarcomas that are treated with surgical resection alone have a mean survival time of approximately 2–3 months, and dogs that are treated with a combination of surgical resection and chemotherapy have a mean survival time of approximately 4–10 months, depending on the protocol used.

Acute blood loss does not typically result in iron deficiency since iron stores are usually adequate for increased erythropoiesis. However, chronic blood loss over weeks to months is almost always associated with iron deficiency.

Chronic blood loss (iron deficiency anemia)

Iron is a critical component of the hemoglobin molecule, which is made up of four heme groups surrounding a globin polypeptide group, forming a tetrahedral structure. Heme accounts for 4% of the weight of the molecule, and is composed of a ringlike organic compound known as a porphyrin to which an iron atom is attached. Iron is the site of the attachment with oxygen (O_2). Iron must be in the reduced ferrous state (Fe^{2+}) to bind with O_2, forming oxyhemoglobin. The hemoglobin carrying iron in the ferric state (Fe^{3+}) cannot carry oxygen, and is referred to as methemoglobin. Methemoglobinemia can be inherited due to a reductase defect, or can be acquired. Many of the oxidant drugs and chemicals that cause Heinz body anemia can also cause methemoglobinemia, and are discussed later.

Dietary iron is absorbed primarily in the duodenum in the form of ferrous iron, is transported across intestinal epithelial cells by divalent metal transporter 1 (DMT1), is exported by ferroportin, then bound to transferrin in the plasma where it is available for use or storage. Storage iron is primarily in the form of ferritin, which is soluble, and hemosiderin, which has more iron than protein, is insoluble, and stainable within macrophages of the liver, spleen, lymph nodes, and bone marrow. To prevent excessive iron in the body, which can be hepatotoxic, iron uptake from the intestine is regulated by the hormone hepcidin, which is produced by the liver. When iron stores are adequate or high, hepcidin binds to ferroportin and decreases its production or destroys it. The iron then remains in the intestinal epithelial cell when it is shed into the gut lumen. When iron stores are low, hepcidin production and secretion are decreased, thus increasing iron uptake from the intestine into the plasma. Inflammatory cytokines upregulate hepcidin production. Ferroportin is also present in the membranes of hepatocytes and macrophages. Hepcidin, therefore, not only affects serum iron concentration through its effects on intestinal epithelial cells but also causes sequestration of iron within macrophages and hepatocytes, preventing efflux of iron into plasma. This role of hepcidin in anemia of inflammation is discussed in Chapter 8. Upregulation of intestinal iron absorption in patients with iron deficiency is often not sufficient to restore adequate plasma iron, therefore oral iron supplementation as therapy is often not adequate (see "Therapy" below).

Chronic blood loss results in iron deficiency anemia, and in adult animals is the most common cause of iron deficiency anemia. Inadequate dietary iron does not occur in adult animals that are fed a commercial pet food diet but may be seen in dogs and cats that are fed a vegetarian diet without appropriate iron supplementation. The dietary iron requirement for adult dogs and cats is estimated at 80 mg/kg dry matter and is even higher in puppies and kittens. Iron deficiency anemia commonly occurs in neonates of all domestic animal species due to inadequate dietary iron intake, since milk contains little iron and growth rates are high. This anemia is often referred to as the "physiologic anemia of neonates." Anemia is particularly severe in baby pigs that have no access to iron-containing soil but also occurs in kittens, puppies, foals, and calves. When blood loss is ongoing, iron stores are depleted relatively quickly. One milliliter of blood contains 0.5 mg of iron; normally 1 mg of iron is absorbed and excreted daily but iron intake must be much higher, since animals absorb only a very small fraction of available dietary iron. Iron deficiency anemia is quite common in dogs, less common in ruminants, and relatively rare in cats and horses.

Gastrointestinal bleeding is the most common cause of chronic blood loss. Causes of chronic gastrointestinal blood loss include neoplasms such as lymphoma, leiomyomas, leiomysarcomas, and carcinomas; gastrointestinal ulcers, usually as a result of the use of ulcerogenic drugs such as glucocorticoids, nonsteroidal anti-inflammatory drugs, and salicylates; hypoadrenocorticism; inflammatory bowel disease; and intestinal parasites such as hookworms. Heavy infestations of ectoparasites that utilize blood, such as fleas and some lice, can also lead to iron deficiency anemia. Overuse of blood donors may also lead to manifestations of iron deficiency, although the degree of anemia may be very mild. Rarely, thrombocytopenia or inherited hemostatic defects can lead to chronic blood loss. Iron deficiency is usually categorized into three stages: storage iron deficiency, iron deficient erythropoiesis, and iron deficiency anemia. Once anemia occurs, clinical signs include pallor, lethargy, and weakness, and are somewhat variable, depending on the underlying cause of the blood loss and the severity of the anemia. Pica, particularly eating dirt (geophagia), has been observed in dogs with iron deficiency anemia. Iron deficient humans also exhibit pica, including pagophagia, the compulsive eating of ice.

Laboratory findings

The hallmark of iron deficiency anemia is a decreased MCV or a subpopulation of microcytic cells (see Chapters 1 and 6). Microcytosis occurs because erythrocyte precursors continue to divide in an attempt to reach their full hemoglobin content. Additional divisions result in smaller than normal erythrocytes. Examination of the erythrocyte histogram or computer graphic generated by the electronic cell counter is often useful, because subpopulations of microcytic erythrocytes can be observed, even when the MCV is within the reference interval (see Chapter 6). The MCV of reticulocytes is also decreased, since even immature iron deficient erythrocytes are smaller than normal. The red cell distribution width (RDW), which describes the width of the size distribution, is usually increased when subpopulations of microcytic erythrocytes are present, and will often be increased before the MCV decreases below the reference interval. Although one might expect the Mean cell hemoglobin concentration (MCHC) to be decreased in these patients, since the cells contain less hemoglobin than normal, it is commonly within the reference interval.

The anemia is usually regenerative with reticulocytosis but may become nonregenerative in the late stages. Quite commonly, the bone marrow response may be inadequate due to underlying anemia of inflammation, since many of these animals have concurrent inflammation related to their bleeding lesions. Reticulocyte indices can be determined with flow-cytometry type electronic cell counters. These indices, especially average reticulocyte hemoglobin content (CHr, also known as RETIC-HGB when determined by certain analyzers) and reticulocyte volume (MCVr) are good indicators of iron deficiency anemia, as both are decreased quite early in patients with iron deficiency, usually before changes in conventional indices. However, reticulocyte hemoglobin content and other reticulocyte indices are also decreased with other types of functional iron deficiency such as is seen with anemia of inflammatory disease or portosystemic shunts, although the decreases are usually not of the same magnitude as is seen with iron deficiency anemia. It may be of more value to use diagnostic cutoffs based on the magnitude of abnormality, rather than the reference interval, when differentiating true iron deficiency from functional iron deficiency. Other useful reticulocyte indices for detecting iron deficient erythropoiesis include reticulocyte hemoglobin concentration (CHCMr), percentage of reticulocytes with decreased CHCMr (%Hypo-r), variability in reticulocyte size (RDWr), and variability in CHCMr (HDWr).

Blood film examination is diagnostically useful, particularly in the late stages of iron deficiency anemia. Erythrocytes of most species, other than cats, may appear pale, with increased central pallor, and sometimes only a thin rim of hemoglobin is present (Figure 9.3). Membrane abnormalities are common, including keratocyte and schistocyte formation, presumably due to increased susceptibility to oxidative damage (see Chapter 6). Initially the erythrocyte develops what appears to be a blister or vacuole where inner membrane surfaces are crosslinked across the cell. These lesions subsequently enlarge, break open to form "apple-stem cells" and keratocytes, spiculated red cells with

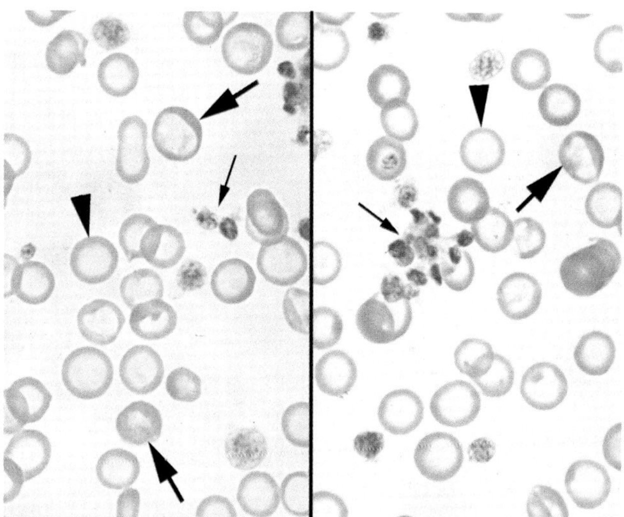

Figure 9.3 Blood film from a dog with iron deficiency anemia and hypochromic erythrocytes (arrowheads). Note the presence of polychromatophilic erythrocytes (large arrows), indicating that the anemia is regenerative. Animals with iron deficiency anemia commonly have increased platelets (small arrows), some of which may be large. Wright stain.

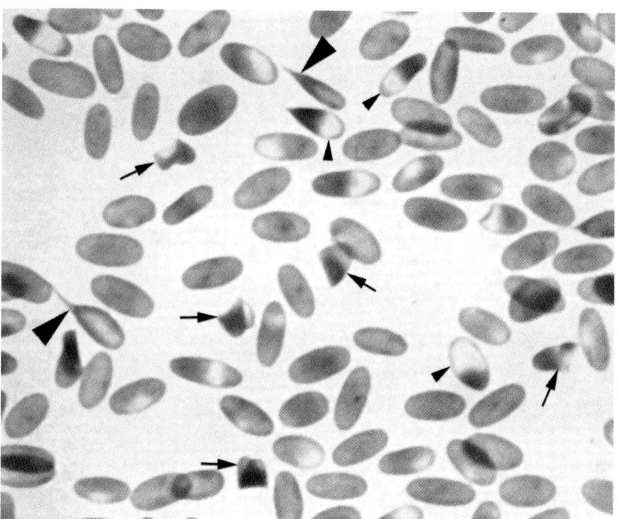

Figure 9.4 Blood film from a llama with iron deficiency anemia. Typical morphologic abnormalities associated with iron deficiency in llamas include dacryocytes (large arrowhead), folded erythrocytes (arrows), and eccentric pallor (small arrowheads). Wright stain.

two or more pointed projections. The projections from the keratocytes may then fragment from the cell, forming schistocytes. Erythrocytes are thin, and folded cells may be seen, particularly in llamas (Figure 9.4).

Thrombocytosis is present in approximately 50% of iron deficient patients, and many have increased platelet size and increased platelet aggregation. The mechanism for the increased platelet concentration is not well understood but may be due to increased erythropoietin or other cytokines. While inflammation can cause thrombocytosis, the thrombocytosis seen with iron deficiency will occur independent of inflammation. Megakaryopoiesis in iron deficient rats has been shown to be altered, with increased megakaryocyte ploidy and size and accelerated megakaryocyte differentiation. Studies in mice have shown that iron deficiency causes megakaryocyte/erythroid precursor cells to selectively differentiate into megakaryocytes rather than erythroid cells. It has been theorized that iron deficient thrombocytosis may have evolved to maintain or increase the coagulation capacity in patients with chronic bleeding. Another theory is that by making megakaryocytes rather than erythrocytes, iron is conserved for more important functions.

Other laboratory findings in patients with iron deficiency include decreased serum iron concentration, decreased transferrin (a glycoprotein in plasma that transports iron between compartments) saturation, and low storage iron. Serum iron concentration is usually lower in animals with iron deficiency than it is in animals with anemia of inflammation. Total iron binding capacity, a test for measuring the amount of transferrin available to transport iron, is usually normal in iron deficient dogs and cats, although it is usually increased in other species with iron deficiency.

Iron is stored as either ferritin or hemosiderin. Although ferritin is primarily an intracellular iron storage compound, it can be detected in serum. Hemosiderin, on the other hand, is insoluble, and can only be detected by staining cells and tissues. Thus, storage iron can be evaluated by measuring serum ferritin, or by examining a bone marrow aspirate and noting lack of hemosiderin in macrophages. Disadvantages of serum ferritin are that it is available from few laboratories, is species-specific, and since it is an acute phase reactant protein, tends to increase whenever inflammation or liver disease are present. Special iron stains, such as Prussian blue, are not necessary in order to visualize hemosiderin in the bone marrow (see Chapter 15). The absence of hemosiderin in feline bone marrow aspirates is not significant, since hemosiderin is rarely seen in aspirates of bone marrow from normal cats. Hypoproteinemia is seen in approximately one-third of animals with chronic blood loss, as protein production sometimes cannot keep pace with loss.

For practical purposes, the combination of low serum iron in a patient with a decreased MCV and anemia is usually adequate to diagnose iron deficiency anemia, and should trigger additional diagnostic procedures to determine the source of blood loss, such as testing the feces for occult blood. An excellent review of diagnosis of iron metabolism disorders in dogs and cats has been published [1].

Therapy

Treatment consists of finding and treating the source of blood loss. Iron supplementation with intramuscular injectable iron dextran in iron-deficient neonates is useful, especially baby pigs, which are usually given 200 mg iron. Iron dextran is absorbed by the lymphatic system within days. Iron dextran can be given at a dose of 10 mg elemental iron per kg body weight weekly to dogs, and at a dose of 50 mg per cat once every 3–4 weeks. An initial small dose of intramuscular iron is recommended in case a hypersensitivity reaction were to occur. Although oral iron supplementation is commonly used to treat iron deficiency, it is often of little value, particularly in dogs and cats, because commercial pet food usually contains more iron than can be absorbed by the intestine. However, intestinal absorption of iron increases dramatically when animals are iron deficient. Oral iron should not be given to neonatal animals, especially kittens, since it can be toxic. If oral iron is administered, it should be in the ferrous state, such as ferrous sulfate or ferrous gluconate. Ferrous sulfate can be administered at a dose of 15 mg iron salt per kg body weight (5 mg elemental iron per kg) divided every 8–12 hours. Side effects are gastric irritation.

Differential diagnoses

Other causes of microcytosis include portosystemic shunts, which are vascular connections between the portal and systemic circulation that divert portal blood around the liver. The cause of the microcytosis in these animals is not well understood but is associated with abnormal iron metabolism, perhaps similar to anemia of inflammatory disease and possibly related to decreased hepatic production of proteins involved in iron metabolism; a few of these patients may actually have iron deficiency anemia secondary to chronic blood loss. The anemia, if present, is usually mild, and although serum iron may be decreased, storage iron is usually normal to slightly increased. Approximately two-thirds of dogs and one-third of cats with portosystemic shunts have microcytosis.

Animals with anemia of inflammation usually have normocytic anemias, but occasionally the MCV will fall below the reference interval. While serum iron is decreased in these animals, storage iron is normal to increased (see "Anemia of Inflammation," Chapter 8).

Finally, some dogs of the Asian breeds such as Shiba Inus, Akitas, chow chows, and Shar Peis normally have microcytosis without anemia. The microcytosis is apparently not associated with the high red cell potassium content seen in some Akitas.

Blood destruction (intravascular or extravascular hemolysis)

Immune-mediated hemolytic anemia

Immune-mediated hemolytic anemia (IMHA) is a consequence of increased red cell destruction, either as a result of antibody directed against erythrocytes, or immune complexes attaching to erythrocytes. IMHA is usually a markedly regenerative anemia, with increased polychromasia (reticulocytosis). However, in some instances, the anemia is nonregenerative as a result of antibody formation against RBC precursors, with destruction of polychromatophilic erythrocytes or earlier red cell precursors. Nonregenerative immune-mediated anemia is also referred to as precursor-targeted immune-mediated anemia (PIMA) and is discussed in Chapter 8. While most affected dogs and cats with PIMA eventually respond to immunosuppressive therapy, the time from onset to a regenerative response is usually several weeks to months. Other potential causes of a lack of regenerative response may include underlying anemia of inflammation with iron sequestration, and functional iron deficiency, in which the rate of iron release may not keep up with the increased rate of erythropoiesis.

The onset may be acute or gradual. IMHA is often classified as primary (idiopathic), or secondary, if concurrent disease is present. Often the cause is never determined, but in some instances it can be related to other disorders or events, such as infections, other immune-mediated disorders, modified live virus vaccination, neoplasia, particularly of the lymphoid system, bee stings, snake envenomation, zinc toxicosis, and administration of drugs. Whether snake and bee venoms actually induce immune-mediated destruction or simply cause erythrocytes to become sphere-shaped is controversial (see "Differential Diagnoses" below). Drugs that have been associated with IMHA are numerous and include penicillin, cephalosporins, trimethoprim-sulfamethoxazole, levamisole, and amiodarone; in these cases, immune-mediated destruction occurs due to either the drug binding directly to erythrocytes (penicillin), or by the formation of drug-antibody immune complexes, which also may bind to red blood cells. Red cell parasites such as large or small forms of *Babesia* and *Mycoplasma haemocanis* may induce IMHA in dogs (see "Erythrocyte Parasites" below).

RNA sequencing of whole blood from IMHA-affected untreated dogs found overexpressed genes in pathways related to neutrophil function, coagulation, and hematopoiesis. The most highly overexpressed gene was a phospholipase scramblase, which mediates the externalization of phosphatidylserine from the inner to the outer leaflet of cell membranes. This family of genes has been shown to be important for programmed cell death of erythrocytes as well as the initiation of the clotting cascade. However, some of the changes in gene expression that were observed may possibly be found in dogs with any type of regenerative anemia or inflammatory response. Interestingly, no genes for infectious agents were found in this study [2]. Future studies will likely be performed to further evaluate the role of phospholipase scramblases in the pathogenesis of canine IMHA.

IMHA is the most common cause of hemolytic anemia in the dog in the United States, and has been described in horses, cattle, and cats. Breeds of dogs more commonly affected include cocker spaniels, springer spaniels, poodles, Old English sheepdogs, flat-coated retrievers, and collies, and the disorder is slightly more common in females than in males. In horses, IMHA has been associated with penicillin and other antibiotic administration, clostridial infections, and neoplasia, but primary IMHA has been reported, sometimes in conjunction with immune-mediated thrombocytopenia. In cats, IMHA has been most commonly associated with *Mycoplasma haemofelis* infection, feline leukemia virus, and lymphoproliferative and myeloproliferative disease. IMHA has been reported in cattle with theileriosis and anaplasmosis, which is not surprising, since antibody is likely to be directed against the erythrocyte parasite. However, primary IMHA has been reported in a few cattle.

Mechanisms of red cell destruction can be due to either erythrophagocytosis or intravascular hemolysis. Macrophages have receptors for antibody as well as complement (C_3b), and removal of erythrocytes by macrophages occurs in multiple organs, including the spleen, bone marrow, and liver. Rarely, monocytes that have phagocytized erythrocytes may be observed on blood films (Figure 9.5). Partial erythrophagocytosis by macrophages results in the formation of spherocytes, the hallmark of IMHA. Spherocytes appear small, although their volume is normal, because they are sphere-shaped, lack central pallor, and appear to be dense (Figure 9.6). They have a shortened half-life because they are not as deformable as normal biconcave disk-shaped erythrocytes. They exhibit increased saline fragility, which may be diagnostically useful. Spherocytes are difficult to detect in species in which the red cells normally lack central pallor. They are, however, readily detectable in dogs, although imperfect spherocytes, which have a small amount of central pallor, are sometimes missed. If complement fixation goes to completion, resulting in membrane attack complex formation, intravascular lysis occurs. In these

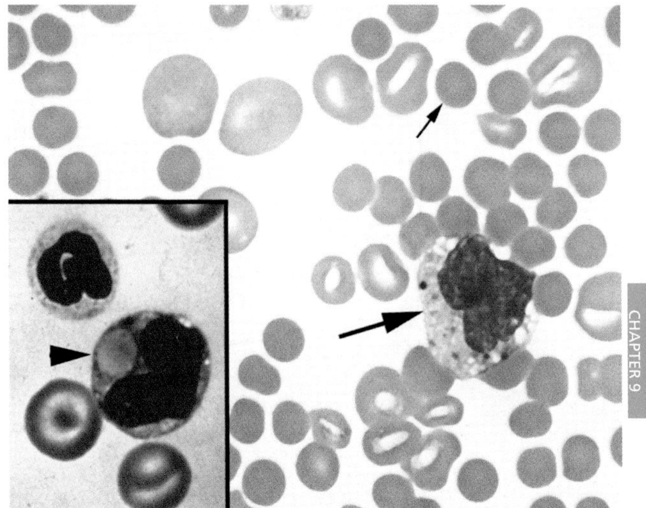

Figure 9.5 Blood film from a dog with immune-mediated hemolytic anemia. Numerous spherocytes (small arrow) are present. Rarely, monocytes may be observed that contain hemosiderin (large arrow) or phagocytized erythrocytes (inset, arrowhead). Wright stain.

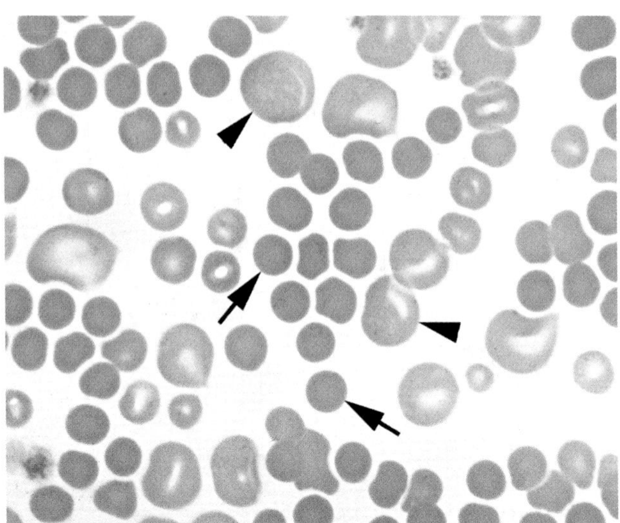

Figure 9.6 Blood film from a dog with immune-mediated hemolytic anemia. The polychromatophilic erythrocytes (arrowheads) indicate that the anemia is regenerative; numerous spherocytes (arrows) are present, as is agglutination. Wright stain.

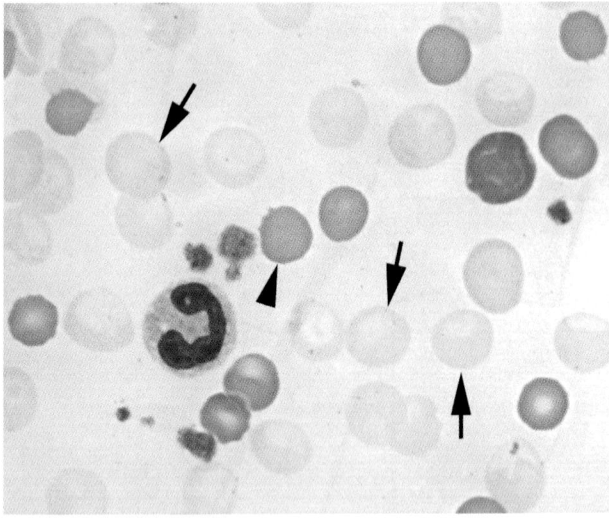

Figure 9.7 Blood film from dog with intravascular hemolysis secondary to immune-mediated hemolytic anemia. Numerous spherocytes (arrowhead) and lysed "ghost" erythrocytes (arrows) are present. Wright stain.

instances, ghost erythrocytes are occasionally observed on blood films (Figure 9.7). Hemoglobinemia, hemoglobinuria, hyperbilirubinemia, and bilirubinuria are often present.

Antibodies associated with IMHA are usually IgG or IgM, but IgA has also been reported to bind to erythrocytes. Usually the antibody is attached to erythrocyte membrane glycoproteins. If IgM is involved, agglutination of erythrocytes can usually be observed on the blood film, and may be grossly evident in the blood tube. IgG is sometimes referred to as an incomplete antibody, since it usually does not result in intravascular hemolysis or agglutination, but rather predisposes to erythrocyte phagocytosis by macrophages. The presence of antibody can be detected by performing a Coombs test (see Chapter 1 and below). Antibodies against erythrocytes are sometimes classified as either warm, which is common, or cold reactive, which is rare. Warm antibodies react most strongly at body temperature, and cold antibodies react more strongly at cold temperatures. Cold agglutinin disease may result in red blood cell agglutination in distal extremities such as the tips of the ear pinnae, tail tip, nose, and digits, with subsequent obstruction of small vessels and necrosis. Hemolytic anemia is sometimes associated with this syndrome, which has been described in the dog and cat.

Clinical signs and laboratory findings

Clinical signs are variable and often include lethargy, splenomegaly, fever, and icterus, as well as other general signs associated with anemia, such as pale mucous membranes, dyspnea, tachycardia, and systolic heart murmur if the anemia is severe. If the anemia is acute, animals may present in a state of collapse, whereas animals with a more chronic onset may accommodate to the anemia, and show much less severe clinical signs.

Laboratory findings vary but always include a decreased packed cell volume, red blood cell count, and hemoglobin concentration indicative of anemia. If intravascular hemolysis is present, hemoglobinemia, hemoglobinuria, hyperbilirubinemia, and bilirubinuria may be present. Additionally, the hemoglobin concentration may be falsely increased relative to the packed cell volume, thus falsely increasing the MCHC.

Blood film examination almost always reveals spherocytosis, which is the most diagnostically useful laboratory finding in these patients. Blood films should be evaluated for spherocytes in the counting area, since erythrocyte flattening at the feathered edge can appear similar to spherocytosis (see "Spherocytes," Chapter 6). More than three spherocytes/oil immersion field is suggestive of IMHA.

Agglutination may be present and can be differentiated from rouleaux formation by mixing one drop of blood with four drops of isotonic saline; agglutination will persist in the presence of saline while rouleaux formation will disperse (see "Agglutination," Chapter 6). Agglutination can be confirmed in samples with equivocal results (due to marked rouleaux formation) by washing erythrocytes three times in a 1 : 4 ratio with room temperature saline. Agglutination may be so marked that it can be seen grossly on the blood film or on the side of the ethylenediaminetetraacetic acid (EDTA) tube. If agglutination is present, the MCV may be falsely increased, since agglutinated red cells (doublets and triplets) may be counted as large cells by impedance electronic cell counters (see Chapter 1). The MCV will also be increased if reticulocytosis is present but often does not exceed the reference interval.

The leukogram is almost always inflammatory, with a mature neutrophilia, increased bands, and monocytosis. This inflammatory response was once thought to be due to release of colony stimulating factors from activated macrophages. More recently, the degree of neutrophilia, as well as increased immature neutrophils, has been thought to correlate with the amount of tissue damage secondary to hypoxia and thromboembolic disease.

Platelet concentration may be decreased because of concurrent immune-mediated destruction (Evans syndrome) or secondary DIC. Because both subclinical and clinical DIC are commonly associated with IMHA, other laboratory tests that may be abnormal are those that are used to diagnose DIC, including a prolonged activated partial thromboplastin time, prolonged one-stage prothrombin time, decreased antithrombin activity, increased fibrin(ogen) degradation products concentration, and increased D-dimer concentration.

Bone marrow aspiration is usually not indicated in IMHA but is commonly performed in patients in which the anemia is nonregenerative. In these cases, an apparent maturation arrest of the erythroid series, often at the rubricyte stage, may be present, due to destruction of more mature forms of erythrocytes. Metarubricytes and polychromatophilic erythrocytes are often decreased to absent in the marrow from such patients, and occasionally, increased erythrophagocytosis and phagocytosis of nucleated erythrocytes may be observed.

A Coombs test may be useful for diagnosis. A species-specific antiglobulin reagent (Coombs serum) is added to a saline-washed suspension of the patient's erythrocytes. Agglutination results if the red cells are coated with autoantibody. However, if agglutination is already present, a Coombs test is not indicated. In some cases in which agglutination is observed, the Coombs test is falsely negative, presumably because the IgM antibody is eluted from the erythrocytes during the washing process. The Coombs test was first developed for use in humans in 1945 by R.R.A. Coombs, a veterinary immunologist in the Department of Pathology at Cambridge University, who hypothesized that antibody to human globulin could be synthesized by rabbits inoculated with human globulin, and this sera could then attach to globulin binding to erythrocytes, resulting in agglutination. This test is also known as the direct antiglobulin test (DAT). The Coombs test has numerous limitations in domestic animals because of false-negative and false-positive results, both of which are common. False-negative results occur due to the following: low concentration of antibody bound to erythrocytes, improper antiglobulin to antibody ratio, not incorporating the drug that is suspected of inducing the antibody response, and improper temperature. False-positive results occur when various types of disease cause immune complexes or complement to bind to erythrocytes, without resulting in anemia. False positives are particularly common in cats. Previous treatment with glucocorticosteroids may cause a negative result, and previous blood transfusion may cause a positive result. A more sensitive enzyme linked immunosorbent assay (ELISA) to detect immunoglobulins bound to erythrocytes has fewer false-negative results. However, this direct enzyme-linked antiglobulin test (DELAT) may also be falsely positive, is laborious, and not available in most laboratories. Direct immunofluorescence (DIF) flow cytometry is more sensitive (but less specific) than the Coombs test, can be used to determine the class of antibody present, detects the percentage of erythrocytes bound with antibody, and can thus be used to monitor response to therapy.

Azotemia may be present, either prerenal or renal, if intravascular hemolysis is severe. Free hemoglobin binds to haptoglobin, but when the available haptoglobin is saturated, hemoglobinuria secondary to hemoglobinemia occurs. Acute renal failure may be due to either erythrocyte membrane antigen-antibody complex deposition or direct toxicity of free hemoglobin to renal tubular cells.

Differential diagnoses

IMHA can usually be easily differentiated from other types of hemolytic anemia by the presence of spherocytes on blood film from patients with IMHA. However, spherocytes occasionally may be seen in dogs with rattlesnake envenomation (Figure 9.8) and bee envenomation (see Section VII, Case 18). Spheroechinocytes and type III echinocytes are seen commonly in dogs with rattlesnake envenomation (see Chapter 6); spherocytes may be present after the echinocytic changes have disappeared. It is likely that spherocyte formation is simply a result of membrane alterations induced by phospholipase A_2 (PLA_2) present in the snake venom. Bee venom contains melittin and a PLA_2 that is very similar to that found in snake venom, both of which have been shown to induce hemolysis, both *in vivo* and *in vitro*, through a chemical mechanism associated with echinocyte formation at low doses and spherocyte formation at higher doses. Melittin also induces band 3 clustering, and delayed hemolytic anemia could be due to antibody formation against altered erythrocyte membranes.

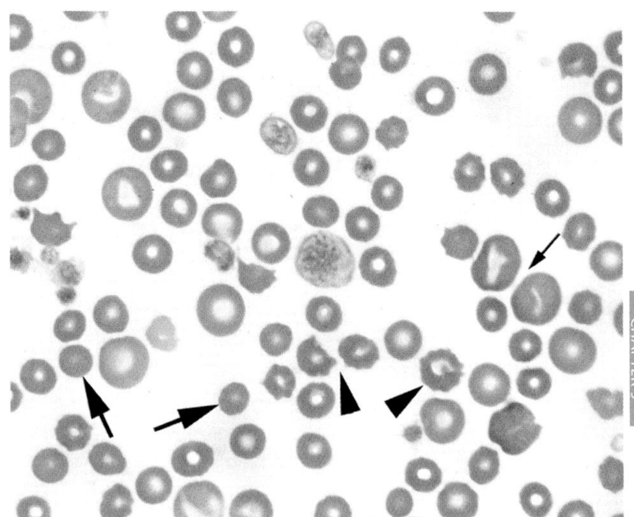

Figure 9.8 Spherocytes (large arrows) in a blood film taken from a dog several days following rattlesnake envenomation. The dog previously had echinospherocytes, and some spiculated erythrocytes remain (arrowheads). The anemia is regenerative, as indicated by the polychromatophilic erythrocytes (small arrow). The dog is recovering from thrombocytopenia; a giant "young" platelet is in the center of the field. Wright stain.

Spherocytes, along with spheroechinocytes and type III echinocytes, may also be observed in horses with clostridial infections presumably as a result of the bacterial phospholipase hydrolyzing erythrocyte membrane phospholipids (sphingomyelin and lecithin), producing lysolecithin, an echinogenic agent. These cases may be confusing, as clostridial infections in horses have been associated with IMHA, diagnosed by the presence of spherocytes, autoagglutination, and positive Coombs test. However, clostridial organisms also can directly induce hemolysis through the release of toxins. It is also possible that phospholipases may be able to induce immune-mediated hemolysis, likely as a result of attachment of antibody to altered erythrocyte membranes.

IMHA may be mistakenly diagnosed in horses with Heinz body anemia, possibly because collapse of the erythrocyte membrane following eccentrocyte formation results in erythrocytes that appear similar to spherocytes. However, an alternative explanation is that immune-mediated destruction of erythrocytes with spherocyte formation occurs, since Heinz body formation may result in band-3 clustering with secondary antibody attachment. Spherocyte formation secondary to band-3 clustering is also seen in dogs with zinc toxicosis. Interestingly, dogs with zinc toxicosis are Coombs negative, and it has been hypothesized that during the erythrocyte washing process, zinc is removed, band 3 is returned to a dispersed distribution, and antibodies are eluted, resulting in a negative test. Finally, animals that have had incompatible blood transfusions may develop some degree of IMHA and spherocytosis, and animals that have fragmentation of erythrocytes may have spherocytosis, as the fragments may "round-up" and appear to be small spherocytes. Spectrin deficiency has been reported in Dutch golden retrievers; some, but not all, affected dogs had spherocytosis.

Prognosis

Mortality rates vary, and are reported to range from 25% to 50%. Although some reports suggest that dogs that are autoagglutinating or have intravascular hemolysis have the highest mortality, this is controversial. Thromboembolism is a common finding in dogs that die. Recurrence of IMHA or other immune-mediated disorders such as immune-mediated thrombocytopenia is relatively common.

Therapy

Differentiation of spontaneous (primary) IMHA from secondary IMHA associated with a trigger factor is an important component of treatment and prognosis. Initial treatment of dogs consists of glucocorticosteroids (usually prednisone, 2–3 mg/kg per os every 12 hours), which decreases antibody production, T cell activity, and diminishes macrophage function. Dexamethasone is often used in horses, and has been reported to be effective in cattle. Disadvantages of glucocorticoids include predisposing patients to infection, thromboembolic disease, and polyuria and polydipsia. Combination treatment may be warranted in dogs that are not responsive to or are intolerant of glucocorticoids; other immunosuppressive drugs may allow tapering of the glucocorticoid. Therapeutic modalities may include azathioprine, danazol, cyclosporine, cyclophosphamide, bovine hemoglobin solution, or human immunoglobulin. However, in one retrospective study, no difference in mortality was detected between the use of multiple immunosuppressive agents and the use of glucocorticoids alone, and in fact the risk of death was slightly lower (30%) with glucocorticoids alone than the overall mortality rate of 50%. In addition, the use of cyclophosphamide and bovine hemoglobin solution has been associated with increased risk of death, and are currently not recommended. Danzol, a synthetic androgen, and cyclosporine, an immune response inhibitor, have been reported to be of no benefit with respect to reducing mortality. Some immunosuppressive drugs, other than the glucocorticoids, may injure marrow, resulting in a transient loss of regenerative response, and some drugs may not be effectively metabolized with severe anemia, making them more toxic than usual. Dogs usually respond to glucocorticoid therapy within 1 week, although dogs with antibody directed against erythrocyte precursors usually take longer to respond. The dosage of glucocorticoids is gradually decreased once the PCV increases, and can sometimes be discontinued 2 or 3 months after the PCV returns to normal. In some cases, however, low dose therapy (0.5 mg/kg per os every other day) with prednisone or prednisolone may be required indefinitely.

Fluid therapy is indicated, particularly in patients with intravascular hemolysis, and lactic acidosis secondary to anemia should be corrected. In addition, therapy is recommended to inhibit thrombosis, particularly pulmonary thromboembolism, a common cause of death in dogs with IMHA. The American College of Veterinary Internal Medicine has published a consensus statement of guidelines for therapy of IMHA in dogs [3]. A very brief summary of their guidelines follows.

1. Packed red cells or whole blood transfusions should be given to dogs that have severe clinical signs of decreased tissue oxygen delivery. Even if dogs have no clinical signs, transfusion should be given when the PCV decreases to 12% or less. Bovine hemoglobin solutions and frozen plasma are not recommended.

2. Predinisone or prednisolone at a dose >2 mg/kg is strongly recommended. Dose should be decreased to <2 mg/kg d if the PCV is stabilizing. Once the patient is stable, the dose should be decreased by 25% every 3 weeks. A typical duration of 3–6 months of prednisone or prednisolone should be anticipated. Monitoring for iatrogenic Cushing's syndrome and infections secondary to immunosuppression should be done.

3. A second immunosuppressive drug should be given if the dog is not responding to glucocorticoids or is experiencing serious glucocorticoid side effects. Recommended second immunosuppressive drugs are azathioprine, cyclosporine, or mycophenolate mofetil. Cyclophosphamide should not be given.

4. Heparin is recommended to prevent thromboembolism, and therapy should be monitored. If antiplatelet drugs are administered, clopidogrel is recommended over aspirin.

5. If gastroprotectant therapy is given to prevent ulceration secondary to glucocorticoids, a proton pump inhibitor is recommended.

In summary, IMHA is a very important cause of morbidity and mortality in dogs and occurs much more frequently in dogs than in other species. The American College of

Veterinary Internal Medicine has published a consensus statement on the diagnosis of IMHA in dogs and cats that emphasizes recognition of triggering factors [4].

Neonatal isoerythrolysis

Neonatal isoerythrolysis (NI) is a form of IMHA that occurs in newborn animals secondary to maternal antibodies against the neonate's bloodgroup antigen attaching to the neonate's erythrocytes, with subsequent erythrocyte hemolysis. The maternal antibodies are usually produced after sensitization of the mother with blood group-incompatible erythrocytes, usually from the blood of a previous fetus gaining access to maternal circulation but sometimes from vaccinations that contain erythrocytes or from mismatched blood transfusions. The disorder is most common in horse and mule foals but occurs in less than 1% of thoroughbreds. The disorder rarely occurs in puppies, kittens, piglets, and calves. Cats are unique, in that antibodies against kitten erythrocytes can be produced with no previous exposure of the queen to incompatible erythrocytes. In domestic animals, the maternal antibody gains access to the neonate's blood following ingestion of colostrum containing antibody. Hemolytic anemia has been reported in lambs fed bovine colostrum during the first few days of life, and the anemia appears to be immune-mediated.

Affected animals are normal at birth, but within 24–48 hours they become weak, lethargic, pale, and anemic, with icterus and dyspnea. Hemoglobinemia and hemoglobinuria may be present, as well as splenomegaly and hepatomegaly. Thrombocytopenia and DIC may also occur. Immune-mediated neutropenia in conjunction with IMHA has also been reported in a foal. In foals, approximately 90% of all cases of NI are attributable to the Aa or Qa antigen, but other antigens may be involved. The occurrence in mule foals may be due to a xenoantigen. It is possible that all mule pregnancies (donkey sire × horse dam) are incompatible with regard to this factor and a potential for NI exists in all cases.

Laboratory diagnosis

Diagnosis is usually made by confirming the presence of maternal antibodies on the neonate's erythrocytes by a Coombs or a hemolytic test. Blood from pregnant mares can be tested 2 weeks prior to foaling for the presence of antibodies in order to predict the likelihood of NI in the foal. If the dam is sensitized, then her colostrum can be withheld from the foal for the first 48 hours of life, substituting another mare's colostrum.

Treatment

Treatment consists of blood transfusion if the animal is severely anemic. If the mare's blood is used, the erythrocytes must be washed extensively to remove antibody-containing plasma. Glucocorticoids may be helpful in reducing the rate of clearance of antibody coated erythrocytes.

Erythrocyte parasites

Microorganisms that directly infect erythrocytes may result in intravascular hemolysis or extravascular hemolysis, and some may not cause hemolytic anemia. Traditionally, hemoparasites have been detected by examination of blood films. However, the development of highly sensitive and specific polymerase chain reaction (PCR) assays to detect small quantities of organisms has made diagnosis much more accurate for many of these diseases, in some cases even before the onset of clinical signs. The majority of the hemoparasites cause anemia by immune-mediated extravascular hemolysis. Antibody against the organism, immune complexes, or complement bound to erythrocytes results in phagocytosis by macrophages. However, *Babesia* and *Theileria* species cause intravascular hemolysis. Specific hemoparasites are discussed below.

Hemotropic mycoplasmas

Hemotropic mycoplasmas are pleomorphic bacteria that parasitize erythrocytes of many domestic animal species. These organisms are small (approximately 0.3 µm in diameter), lack a cell wall, and stain gram-negatively. They adhere loosely to the surface of the erythrocyte membrane, and in many species, fall off easily, therefore appearing in the plasma. They were originally discovered in laboratory rodents in the 1920s and assigned to the *Bartonella* genus. Approximately one decade later they were reclassified into the order Rickettsiales in the family Anaplasmataceae, and either to the genus *Haemobartonella* or *Eperythrozoon* on the basis of whether they occurred more commonly as "ring forms," and whether they were found free in the plasma. If they fulfilled both of the previous criteria, they were assigned to the genus *Eperythrozoon*. These characteristics are now considered insignificant. With the advent of DNA sequencing and phylogenetic analysis based on ribosome gene sequence comparisons, these organisms have been reclassified as members of the genera *Mycoplasma*.

The first description of such bacteria in an anemic cat was published in 1942, and was initially named *Eperythrozoon felis* and shortly thereafter renamed *Haemobartonella felis*. Three strains of the organisms previously called *H. felis* have been recognized. The "large" or Ohio strain has been renamed *M. haemofelis*, and the "small" California strain has been named *Candidatus Mycoplasma haemominutum*. A third strain, *Candidatus Mycoplasma turicensis*, was originally identified in a Swiss cat but is now known to also have a worldwide distribution. Assays based on PCR technology are the most sensitive and specific diagnostic tests available for these organisms. Of the feline mycoplasmas, *M. haemofelis* is the most pathogenic species, and causes hemolytic anemia in immunocompetent cats. The presence of *Candidatus Mycoplasma turicensis* and *Candidatus Mycoplasma haemominutum* is not always associated with anemia. However, *Candidatus Mycoplasma haemominutum* has been associated with fever, anorexia, lethargy, and anemia and is likely a primary pathogen. *Candidatus Mycoplasma turicensis* has reportedly not been seen by light microscopy, likely due to the small numbers of parasites present but possibly due to its smaller size (0.25 µm). It has been morphologically characterized using electron microscopy. Two other species, *Candidatus Mycoplasma haematoparvum* and *Candidatus Mycoplasma haematoparvum*-like, have been detected in cats using ribosomal gene analysis, but their pathogenicity is not known.

Haemobartonella canis has been renamed *M. haemocanis*. *Eperythrozoon suis*, *Eperythrozoon wenyoni*, and *Eperythrozoon ovis* have been renamed *Mycoplasma haemosuis*, *Mycoplasma wenyonii*, and *Candidatus Mycoplasma ovis*, respectively. The eperythrozoon in alpacas and llamas, previously not named, has been named *Candidatus Mycoplasma haemolamae*. The designation *Candidatus* is reserved for incompletely described members of taxa, to give them provisional status, and is eventually dropped.

Mycoplasma haemofelis

Mycoplasma haemofelis appears as small (0.3 µm) dark blue rods or ring forms on the surface of erythrocytes; it is more easily seen at the feathered edge of the blood film where the erythrocytes are flattened (Figure 9.9). Agglutination of erythrocytes may be present, as the presence of the organism on erythrocytes results in an IMHA. *M. haemofelis* is quite pathogenic, and can cause severe, sometimes fatal, hemolytic anemia. It is transmitted through infected blood, presumably by blood feeding arthropods such as fleas and ticks, cat bites, and iatrogenic exposure, and is present throughout the world. The organism is also transmitted from queens to kittens, either in utero, at birth, or by nursing. The parasitemia is intermittent, making diagnosis by blood film examination sometimes difficult. A PCR assay is much more diagnostically sensitive than blood film examination.

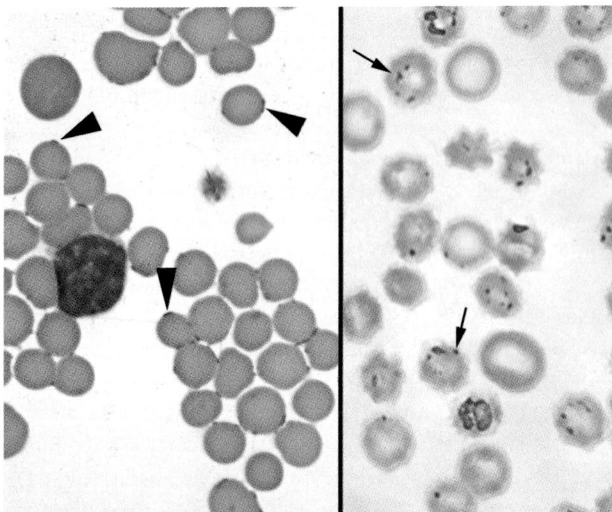

Figure 9.9 Left. Blood film from an anemic cat with *Mycoplasma haemofelis* (arrowheads), previously known as *Haemobartonella felis*. Right. Erythrocyte parasites are sometimes mistakenly diagnosed when artifacts are on erythrocytes (arrows). Artifacts may be caused by stain precipitate or staining the blood film before it is dry. Wright stain.

Clinical signs include those of anemia, including splenomegaly, fever, lethargy, and sometimes icterus. Concurrent disease, immunosuppression, or splenectomy may predispose animals to acute infection. The anemia is regenerative unless underlying disease, sometimes related to feline leukemia virus, is present that would inhibit erythropoiesis. Infected cats should be examined for the presence of feline leukemia virus and feline immunodeficiency virus.

Treatment consists of blood transfusion if the anemia is severe. Prednisone (2 mg/kg per os every 12 hours) will suppress the immune-mediated destruction of erythrocytes, but its use is controversial. Doxycycline (5 mg/kg per os every 12 hours for 4 weeks) is effective against the organism, but cats that recover may become latent carriers. Toxicity of doxycycline may include fever, gastrointestinal disturbances, and rarely, esophageal stricture formation. Enrofloxacin (5–10 mg/kg per os every 24 hours) a fluoroquinolone anti-Mycoplasma antibiotic, has been shown to be effective against *M. haemofelis*, but a rare complication is acute blindness. An excellent update on therapy of feline hemoplasmosis has been published [5].

Mycoplasma haemocanis

Mycoplasma haemocanis, formerly known as *Haemobartonella canis*, is an opportunistic organism, usually causing disease only in splenectomized or severely immunosuppressed dogs. It is closely related phylogenetically to *M. haemofelis*, with 99% homology of the 16SrRNA gene. Dogs that are splenectomized develop active infections if they are transfused with infected blood, or if they have latent infections. Active infection may manifest days to weeks after splenectomy. The microorganism appears somewhat different than *M. haemofelis*, in that they appear as small chains of cocci across the surface of the erythrocyte. The chain commonly branches, and appears Y-shaped (Figure 9.10). Clinical signs include those of anemia, and icterus is rarely present. Treatment consists of 5 mg/kg doxycycline orally twice daily for 3 weeks. *Candidatus Mycoplasma haemominutum* and *Candidatus Mycoplasma haematoparvum* have been reported in dogs, as well. *M. haemocanis* has also been shown to be transmitted vertically.

Haemoplasmas of ruminants

Mycoplasma wenyonii also occurs worldwide, and similar to *M. haemocanis* in dogs, usually only causes severe anemia in immunosuppressed or splenectomized cattle. The organism may be transmitted iatrogenically, by using the same syringe and needle in multiple animals in feedlot situations. Very large numbers of organisms can be seen on blood films, many

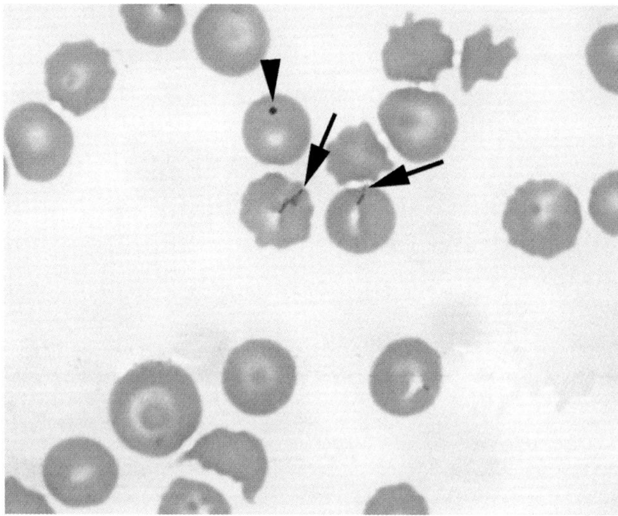

Figure 9.10 Blood film from an anemic splenectomized dog. Note the presence of *Mycoplasma haemocanis* (arrows) (previously *Haemobartonella canis*). Howell-Jolly bodies (arrowhead) are usually increased in splenectomized animals. Wright stain.

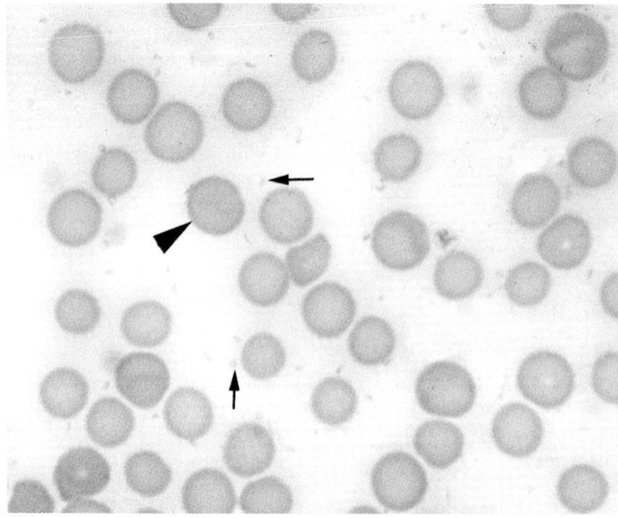

Figure 9.11 Blood film from a cow with hind limb and teat edema. Many *Mycoplasma wenyonii* (previously *Eperythrozoon wenyonii*) organisms are present in the background (small arrows). *Polychromasia* (arrowhead) is present, indicating regeneration. Wright stain.

of which are free in the plasma, in cattle that are not anemic (Figure 9.11). However, a syndrome has been recognized in cattle that are heavily parasitized, which includes dependent edema and lymphadenopathy. Although the haemoplasma of sheep and goats, formerly known as *E. ovis* (Figure 9.12) is generally considered nonpathogenic in adults, its role as a cause of anemia in lambs is controversial. It has been renamed *Mycoplasma ovis*. There is considerable genetic diversity in haemoplasmas of ruminants, and additional

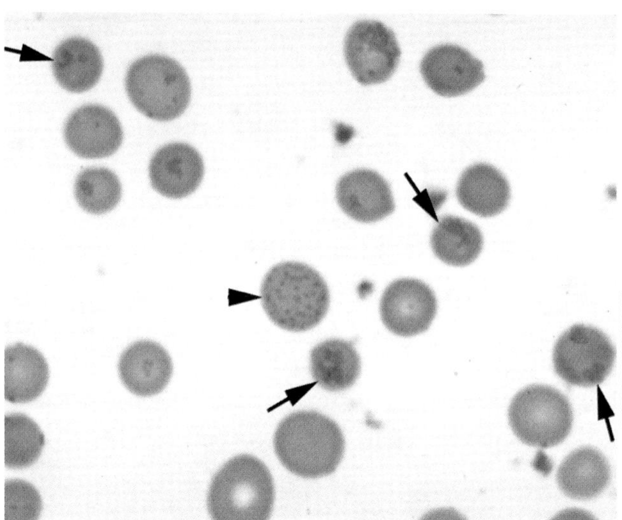

Figure 9.12 Blood film from a sheep with *Eperythrozoon ovis* (arrows). This organism will be renamed *Mycoplasma ovis*. Wright stain.

ones have been described, such as *Candidatus Mycoplasma haemobos*.

Mycoplasma suis

At least three species of *Mycoplasma* have been described in pigs: *Mycoplasma suis*, *Mycoplasma parvum*, and *M. haemosuis*. *M. suis* is associated with porcine hemoplasmosis and is pathogenic in very young pigs, as well as pigs that have been splenectomized, causing severe hemolytic anemia and sometimes death. In older animals, infection is associated with poor weight gain. The organisms appear similar to those in cattle, with many free organisms present on blood films (Figure 9.13). Baby pigs are usually treated with a single

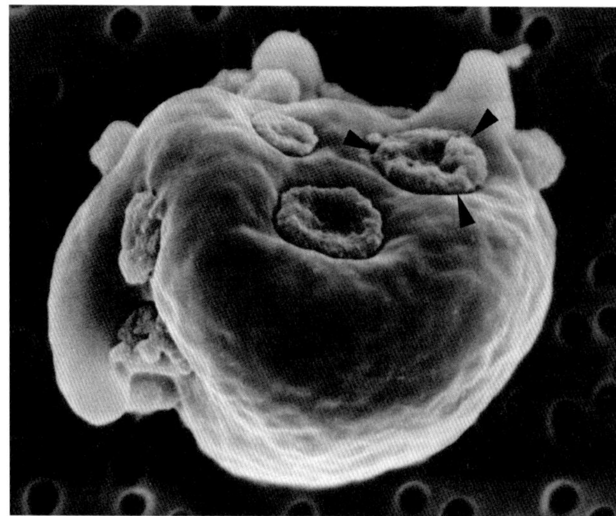

Figure 9.13 Electron micrograph of *Mycoplasma haemosuis* (arrowheads), formerly *Eperythrozoon suis*. Source: Photograph provided by Dr. Joanne Messick.

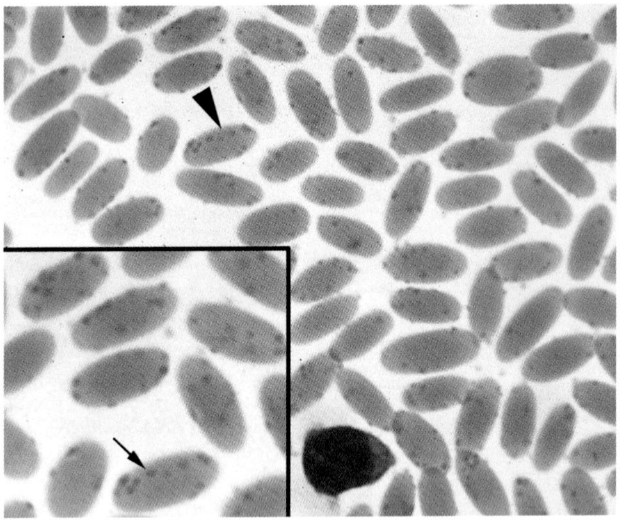

Figure 9.14 Blood film from a poor-doing llama with *Candidatus Mycoplasma haemolamae* (arrowhead), formerly *Eperythrozoon* spp. Higher magnification of the organisms (arrow) is shown in inset. Wright stain.

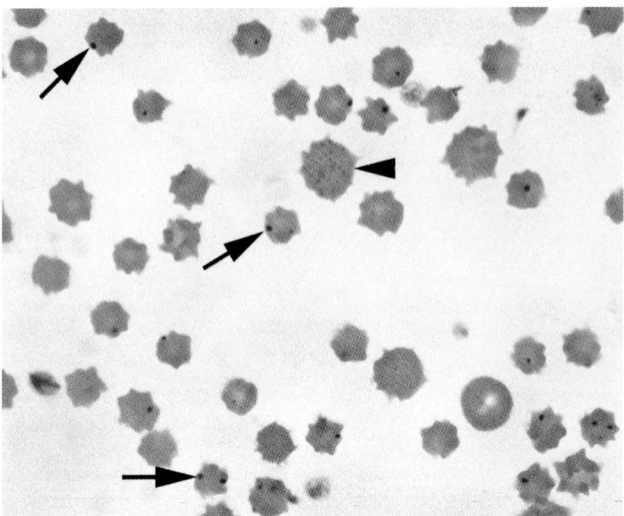

Figure 9.15 Blood film from an anemic cow with *Anaplasma marginale* (arrows). Note the basophilic stippling in the large polychromatophilic erythrocyte (arrowhead). Wright stain.

dose of long acting oxytetracycline (25 mg). Tetracycline is sometimes added to hog food to prevent the acute form of the disease.

Mycoplasma haemolamae

Haemoplasmas in llamas and alpacas appear to be opportunists that proliferate in animals doing poorly, and usually only cause a mild anemia. The organism appears similar to that in cattle (Figure 9.14).

Anaplasmosis

Bovine anaplasmosis, first characterized by Sir Arnold Theiler in 1910, and caused by the intraerythrocytic rickettsia *Anaplasma marginale*, is the most prevalent tickborne disease of cattle and occurs worldwide. *Anaplasma centrale* causes a milder less virulent form of disease, and occurs in south America, the Middle East, and South Africa. *A. marginale* has also been reported in deer, elk, and bison. *Anaplasma ovis* has been reported in goats and sheep, and causes hemolytic anemia. The organism appears similar to *A. marginale*. The organisms are transmitted by ticks, biting flies, and iatrogenically. *A. marginale* appears as a small (0.5–1 μm) dark blue inclusion on the margin of erythrocytes (Figure 9.15). *A. centrale* appears similar but is in a more central appearing location on erythrocytes. Infection with the organism can cause a fatal hemolytic anemia; older animals are usually more severely affected. The mechanism of anemia may be immune mediated. Untreated cattle that survive may become chronic carriers. Diagnosis can be made by PCR assays, as well as examination of blood films. Therapy consists of long acting oxytetracycline, but the most efficient method to control anaplasmosis is by vaccination using live *A. centrale*, which is capable of inducing significant protection against the more virulent *A. marginale*. However, these methods of control have numerous limitations and improved approaches are needed. Inactivated or subunit vaccines and alternative pharmacological interventions are being developed. The *Anaplasma* genus has been expanded to also include *Anaplasma phagocytophilum* (formerly known as *Ehrlichia phagocytophila*, *Ehrlichia equi*, and the agent of human granulocytic ehrlichiosis), Anaplasma *bovis* (formerly *Ehrlichia bovis*), and *Anaplasma platys* (formerly *Ehrlichia platys*).

Piroplasmosis

The order Piroplasmida are obligate intracellular hemoprotozoan parasites that are transmitted by ticks. They are classified into three families based on the type of vertebrate cells in which they develop. Theileriidae infect mammals, first developing in leukocytes, then erythrocytes; Babesiidae infect mammals and some birds but develop only in erythrocytes; Hemohormidiidae infect fish and reptiles, where they develop in nucleated red blood cells. The word piroplasm comes from Latin pirum, meaning pear, as the organisms are often pear-shaped. Two piroplasmid genera, *Babesia* and *Theileria*, are responsible for some of the most important diseases of domestic and wild animals and are discussed below. The genus *Cytauxzoon* is closely related to *Theileria* and is also discussed below. The piroplasm stages in the erythrocytes are morphologically very similar. *Theileria* and *Cytauxzoon* were originally thought to differ from one another by the location of schizogony within the host cells. Schizogony of *Cytauxzoon* spp. occurs in macrophages, whereas *Theileria* schizogony was thought to take place exclusively in lymphocytes. It is now known that *Theileria* species can also infect and transform macrophages. The mechanism of anemia is primarily immune mediated, with antibodies directed against the organisms. However, damage to and alteration of the erythrocyte membrane likely also triggers immune-mediated erythrocyte destruction.

Babesiosis

Babesia spp are tick-borne protozoan parasites that infect erythrocytes of domestic and wild animals, as well as humans, often causing a potentially lethal hemolytic anemia. The disease is named after the Romanian biologist, Victor Babes, who isolated the organism from cattle in 1888. In 1893 it was discovered that the organism was transmitted by ticks and was the cause of Texas cattle fever. Babesiosis was considered an animal disease until it was discovered in a Yugoslavian cattle farmer in 1957.

Canine babesiosis is associated with hemolytic anemia, thrombocytopenia, and other manifestations of systemic inflammation, including liver, lung, pancreas, kidney, heart, and brain dysfunction, and is caused by numerous species that were previously identified by their morphologic appearance and size. Classification by size is thought by some to be problematic, because piroplasms undergo marked morphological changes during their development in erythrocytes. Large forms were classified as *Babesia canis,* and small forms were classified as *Babesia gibsoni*. Large forms (2–5 μm) appear as single, paired, or tetrad oval erythrocyte inclusions that stain lightly basophilic with an eccentric nucleus (Figure 9.16). Small forms (1–3 μm) of *Babesia* appear as round organisms (Figures 9.17 and 9.18). Usually only a few erythrocytes on blood films contain organisms, and they tend to be concentrated at the feathered edge of the blood film. While babesiosis may be diagnosed by blood film or buffy coat film examination, PCR is much more sensitive and specific. In areas where PCR is not available, acridine orange fluorescent dye staining method has been shown to be more sensitive and specific than Wrights-Giemsa stains.

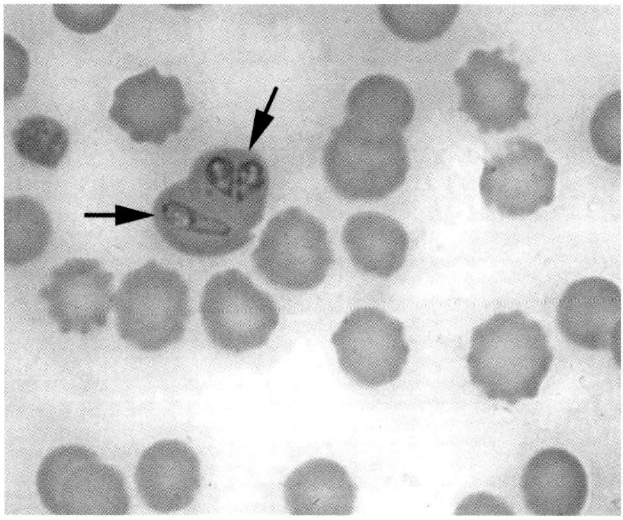

Figure 9.16 Blood film from an anemic dog with *Babesia vogeli* (arrows). Wright stain.

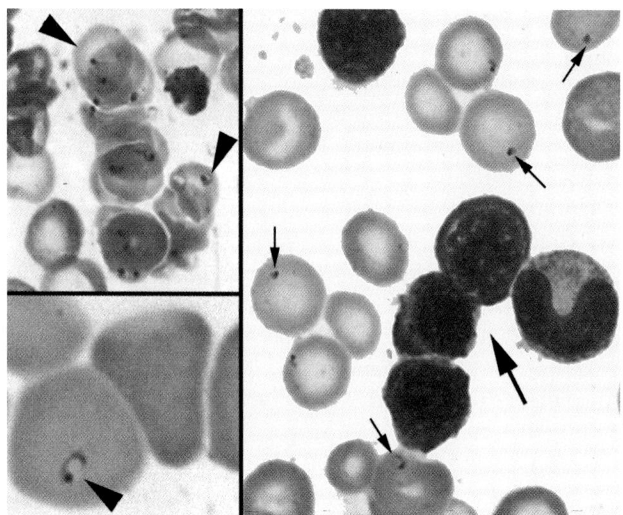

Figure 9.17 *Babesia gibsoni* in a bone marrow aspirate from a severely anemic pit bull terrier from Kentucky. Aspirate provided by Antech Diagnostics, Inc. Wright stain.

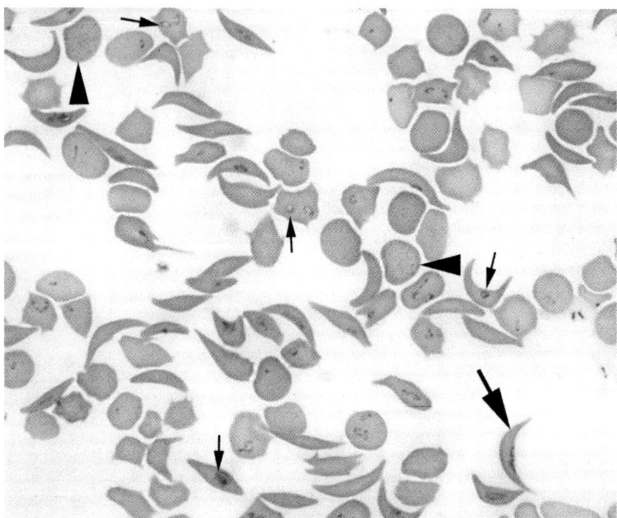

Figure 9.18 *Babesia* or *Theileria* organisms in a deer (small arrows). Note that the erythrocytes have become sickle-shaped, which occurs *in vitro* (large arrow). Basophilic stippling is also present (arrowhead). Wright stain.

Using molecular methods, it has now been shown that several genetically distinct species cause disease in dogs, including *B. canis, Babesia vogeli, Babesia rossi, B. gibsoni, Babesia conradae,* and *Babesia vulpes*. These various species have been shown to have different susceptibility to anti-protozoal drugs, thus identification by PCR should be done. Large forms (*B. canis, B. vogeli, B. rossi*) are susceptible to imidocarb dipropionate (Imizol, Merck Animal Health) and diminazine aceturate; the latter has serious side effects and is not available in the United States. The small forms

(*B. gibsoni, B. conradae, B. vulpes*) are relatively resistant to imidocarb dipropionate but are sensitive to a combination of the hydroxynaphthoquinone atovaquone and the antibiotic azithromycin, although they may remain carriers. A thorough discussion of therapy for canine babesiosis has been published [6].

Canine babesiosis is becoming increasingly common in the United States. *B. vogeli* is transmitted by *Rhipicephalus sanguineus*, the brown dog tick, and is pandemic in the southeastern United States, particularly in greyhounds, and is also found in the Caribbean, South and Central America, the Mediterranean, the Middle East, Asia, and Australia. It usually only causes severe hemolytic anemia and life-threatening disease in young dogs or dogs that are heavily parasitized, although adult greyhounds have more serious clinical signs. Infected dogs are often co-infected with *Ehrlichia canis, A. platys*, and *Hepatozoon canis*, since the same species of tick is responsible for transmission of all four diseases. Another species, *B. rossi*, is more pathogenic, and is in South Africa. A third species, *B. canis* is found in Europe, the United Kingdom, and parts of Asia, and is intermediate in pathogenicity.

B. gibsoni, a small form of *Babesia*, also can inflict severe disease, and is endemic in northern Africa, the Middle East, southern Asia, and parts of the Caribbean, and is increasingly observed in the United States, particularly in the Southeast and Midwest. Since 1999 *B. gibsoni* has been reported in numerous states east of the Mississippi River. The disease is primarily seen in American pit bull terriers and Staffordshire terriers. Many dogs survive the acute phase and become chronic carriers. Prevention includes aggressive tick control. The high prevalence in the pit bull breed is now thought to be due to direct blood transmission. *B. conradae*, a small *Babesia* originally thought to be *B. gibsoni*, was described in California dogs in 1991. This organism causes severe disease, including hemolytic anemia, icterus, vasculitis, thrombocytopenia, hepatitis, glomerulonephritis, and reactive lymphadenopathy. *B. vulpes* (also known as *Babesia microti, Babesia annae* and *Theileria annae* (see "Theileriosis" below) is found in dogs in Europe and North America and is a common infection in wild red foxes. *B. vulpes* appears to be more resistant to therapy. Because many dogs with babesiosis are Coombs positive and exhibit erythrocyte agglutination, a differential diagnosis is IMHA. Hyperglobulinemia, thrombocytopenia, and neutropenia are commonly observed, therefore canine monocytic ehrlichiosis must also be considered as a differential diagnosis, as these are common laboratory findings in that disease as well.

Feline babesiosis is rare compared to canine babesiosis, and occurs in numerous regions of the world. Small *Babesia* species infecting cats include *B. felis, B. cati*, and *B. leo*. Large *Babesia* species including *B. herpailuri* and *B. pantherae* have been reported in wild felids. Numerous species of both large and small *Babesia* normally occurring in dogs have also been reported in cats, many of which are clinically healthy. For example, 13% and 4% of clinically healthy cats tested on the Caribbean island of St. Kitts, West Indies were positive for *B. vogeli* and *B. gibsoni*, respectively. Severe disease is seen in cats infected with *B. felis* in South Africa. In contrast, disease caused by other *Babesia* species is usually mild and chronic.

Bovine babesiosis is mainly caused by *Babesia bovis* and *Babesia bigemina* in tropical and sub-tropical regions of the world. *B. bovis* is usually considered more virulent than *B. bigemina*, and has a higher mortality. Cause of death is usually hemolytic anemia. Adults are usually more severely affected than calves. *Babesia divergens* is primarily responsible for bovine babesiosis in Europe and may also infect immunocompromised humans. Other *Babesia* species have been infrequently reported in cattle. Bovine babesiosis if of economic importance in both the beef and dairy cattle industries, and remains poorly controlled in many parts of the world. *B. bovis* can be transmitted transplacentally, and should be considered as a differential diagnosis of fetal loss, stillbirth, and neonatal death in cattle where babesiosis occurs. Babesiosis in small ruminants such as sheep and goats is also of economic importance in tropical and subtropical areas. *Babesia motasi* and *B. ovis* are pathogenic, while *Babesia crassa, Babesia foliata*, and *Babesia taylori* are mild to nonpathogenic.

Equine babesiosis (piroplasmosis) is caused by two species, *B. equi* (more recently referred to as *Thelieria equi*) and *Babesia caballi*, and occurs in many parts of the world. Placental transmission has been documented, and is a cause of fetal death or neonatal infection. Horses commonly recover but become persistently infected carriers.

Theileriosis

Theileriosis is probably the most significant tick-borne disease to affect domestic ruminants in Africa. Although hemolytic anemia is common, piroplasm parasitemia does not correlate with disease severity. Many clinical and pathologic manifestations are related to proliferation of transformed leukocytes, with associated necrosis, thromboembolism, body cavity effusions, and lung edema. When infected ticks feed on their mammalian host, sporozoites enter mammalian leukocytes and divide to form multinucleated schizonts (Figure 9.19). These may be seen within leukocytes on blood films, as well as aspirates of lymph node and other tissue. Some schizonts undergo asexual reproduction (merogony) to form merozoites that undergo maturation; they then induce leukocytolysis and subsequently infect erythrocytes to form piroplasms, which are small (1 μm) and appear signet-ring- or comma-shaped. Schizonts can also induce pseudo-neoplastic proliferation of leukocytes, usually lymphocytes but likely also monocytes/macrophages, that disseminate to various organs. *Theileria* species are classified as pathogenic (schizont "transforming" leukocytes)

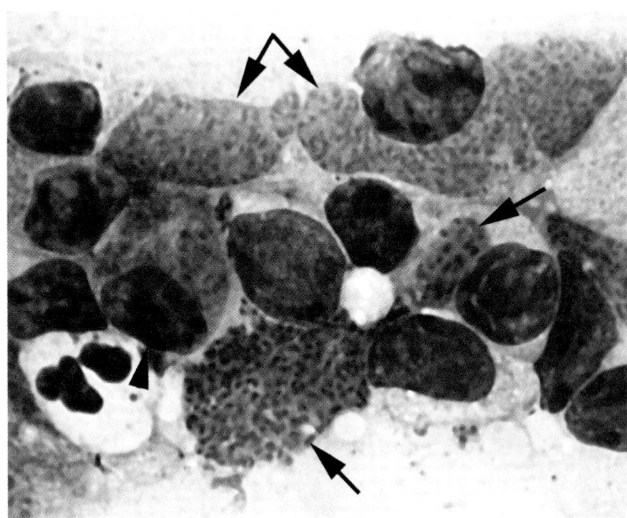

Figure 9.19 Lymph node aspirate from a cow with theileriosis. Lymphocytes are filled with schizonts (arrows). Wright stain.

or benign to mildly pathogenic ("nontransforming"). The pathogenic theilerias cause disease via transformation of host leukocytes to induce blastogenesis, uncontrolled proliferation, and widespread leukocyte dissemination. Transformed leukocytes appear atypical and are difficult to distinguish from neoplastic cells. Nuclei are indented, lobed, sometimes multiple, with prominent nucleoli, and abundant often vacuolated cytoplasm. Numerous cells in mitosis may be seen in aspirates or imprints of lymph nodes or other tissue.

Theileria parva, the cause of East Coast fever in eastern, central, and southern Africa, is responsible for the deaths of more than a million cattle per year, as well as reductions in growth rate and productivity. *Theileria annulata* causes bovine tropical theileriosis in North Africa, southern Europe, and large parts of Asia. Numerous "benign" typically leukocyte nontransforming species have been described in cattle, such as *Theileria taurotragi*, *Theileria mutans*, and *Theileria buffeli/orientalis*, but these can occasionally become leukocyte transforming. For example, *T. taurotragi* can cause an atypical fatal disease characterized by significant leukocyte transformation, proliferation, and invasion of the brain and spinal cord. Theileriosis also impacts wildlife in Africa. Although most *Theileria* species are nonpathogenic in wild ungulates, including deer and elk in North America, they may have pathogenic theileriosis with significant death rates that seriously impact endangered species, particularly in Africa. Small domestic ruminants such as sheep and goats also contract theileriosis. *Theileria ovis*, *Theileria lestoquardi, and Theileria annulate* have been reported, with *T. lestoquardi* causing the most significant disease.

Equine theileriosis, usually referred to as equine piroplasmosis, is caused by *T. equi*; this organism was formerly named *Babesia equi* (see earlier discussion under "Babesiosis"). The clinical signs of equine babesiosis and theileriosis are similar and include fever, anemia, inappetence, edema, icterus, hepatomegaly, splenomegaly, and occasionally abortion and death. *T. equi* appears smaller in erythrocytes than does *B. caballi*.

The literature on canine theileriosis is quite contradictory, and it seems that the species infecting dogs are nonleukocyte transforming. As mentioned previously, *B. vulpes*, also known as *B. microti*, *B. annae* and *T. annae*, is now considered a *Theileria* by numerous parasitologists; red foxes are considered the primary intermediate host of this organism. *T. annulata* was detected in an asymptomatic dog, and *T. equi* was identified in dogs in various countries.

Rangeliosis

Rangelia vitalli is a piroplasm for which there are conflicting reports as to whether it is in the family Theileriidae or Babesiidae, but since it infects leukocytes and endothelial cells, as well as erythrocytes, it is most likely from the family Theileriidae, if that distinction between the two families remains valid. *R. vitalli* causes severe anemia and thrombocytopenia in dogs and is transmitted by the tick *Amblyomma aureolatum*. Canine rangeliosis has been reported in Argentina, Uruguay, and Brazil. Common clinical signs include splenomegaly, hepatomegaly, lymphadenopathy, icterus, hematochezia, and pinnal bleeding. The organism appears similar to *B. vogeli* on blood films.

Feline cytauxzoonosis (bobcat fever)

Cytauxzoon felis is a protozoan piroplasm within the same family as *Theileria*. Like *Theileria*, merozoites (piroplasms) infect erythrocytes, while a tissue phase, the schizonts, infect and fill leukocytes, primarily monocytes/macrophages, within and surrounding blood vessels throughout the body. While cytauxzoonosis was first described in 1948 in African wild ungulates, the organism was likely a *Theileria* species. Cytauxzoonosis was initially reported in cats from Missouri in 1976 and is primarily in the southeastern and central United States but has been more recently reported in South America, and a less virulent species of *Cytauxzoon* has been reported in Europe. The organism is transmitted by the ticks *Amblyomma americanum* and *Dermacentor variabilis* in America. Although erythroparasitemia may occur following blood inoculation such as with a blood transfusion, the tissue phase of the organism and disease do not develop. Bobcats, Florida panthers, and Texas cougars, which serve as natural reservoirs, usually have persistent asymptomatic infections, although bobcats occasionally have fatal disease. Fatal cytauxzoonosis has also been described in a Bengal tiger and white tiger. The disease is often fatal in untreated domestic cats, although they too can have subclinical infections and act as reservoirs. Pathologic findings include thrombosis of numerous vessels as a result of distended macrophages occluding vessels. Clinical findings include acute lethargy, anorexia, fever, and icterus. Although the organism causes a

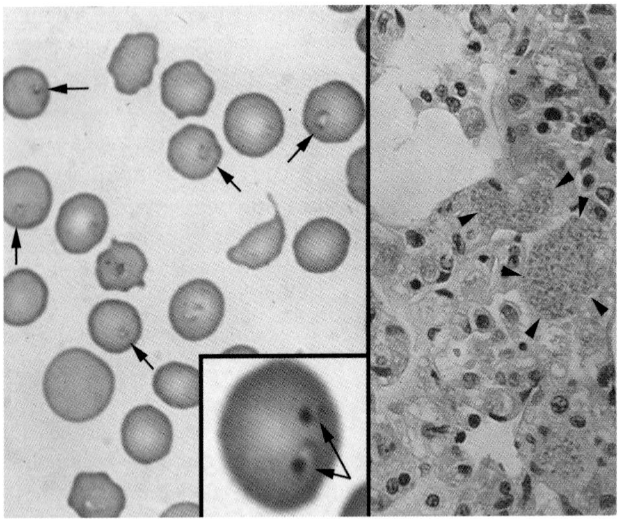

Figure 9.20 Left. Feline blood film with *Cytauxzoon* piroplasms in erythrocytes (arrows). Wright stain. Right. *Cytauxzoon* schizonts in macrophages of the same cat. H&E stain.

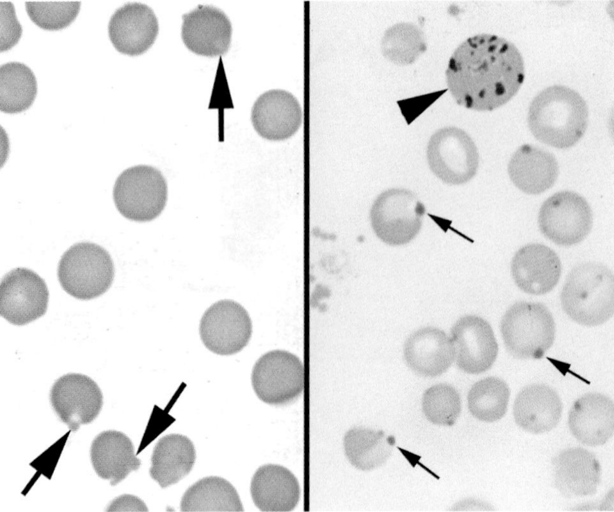

Figure 9.21 Left. Blood film from a cat with Heinz body anemia. Heinz bodies appear pale and are more apparent when they protrude from the edges of the erythrocytes (arrows). Wright stain. Right. Brilliant cresyl blue-stained blood film. Heinz bodies appear as medium-blue structures on the edges of the erythrocytes (arrows). A reticulocyte is also present (arrowhead).

hemolytic anemia, the anemia may be nonregenerative and is sometimes accompanied by leukopenia and thrombocytopenia. Diagnosis is made by finding the signet-ring-shaped piroplasms in erythrocytes in blood films relatively late in the course of the disease or by finding the schizonts in macrophages by cytologic or histopathologic examination of spleen, liver, lymph node, or bone marrow (Figure 9.20), or by PCR assay, which is very sensitive and specific. Historically, cytauxzoonosis was considered a fatal disease in domestic cats, but with recent advancements in therapy, and possibly less virulent strains of the virus, survival rates have markedly improved. Survival rates of 60% have been reported in cats treated with the combination of atovaquone (15 mg/kg PO q 8 hours) and azithromycin (10 mg/kg PO q 24 hours) in conjunction with supportive therapy to prevent clot formation.

Heinz body anemia

Erythrocytes are particularly susceptible to oxidative damage, both because they carry oxygen and because they may be exposed to various chemicals in plasma. Oxidants that are constantly generated include hydrogen peroxide (H_2O_2), superoxide free radical (O_2^-), and hydroxyl radicals (OH). When oxyhemoglobin is converted to methemoglobin (ferric state to ferrous state), superoxide radicals react with hydrogen peroxide, producing hydroxyl radicals. Formation of reversible and irreversible hemichromes then occurs. Reversible hemichromes include hemoglobin hydroxide and dihistidine ferrihemochrome. These reversible hemichromes can be converted back to methemoglobin and reduced hemoglobin. If irreversible hemichromes are formed, the hemoglobin denaturation continues, and aggregates of irreversible hemichromes are formed. These aggregates are called Heinz bodies, first recognized by Heinz in 1890 in humans and animals exposed to coal-tar drugs. Heinz bodies appear as small eccentric pale structures within the red cell and may protrude slightly from the red cell margin on Wright-stained blood films (Figure 9.21). They are usually large and single in cat erythrocytes (Figure 9.22) and small and multiple in dogs. When stained with vital stains such as new methylene blue or brilliant cresyl blue, Heinz bodies appear as blue structures (see Chapter 6).

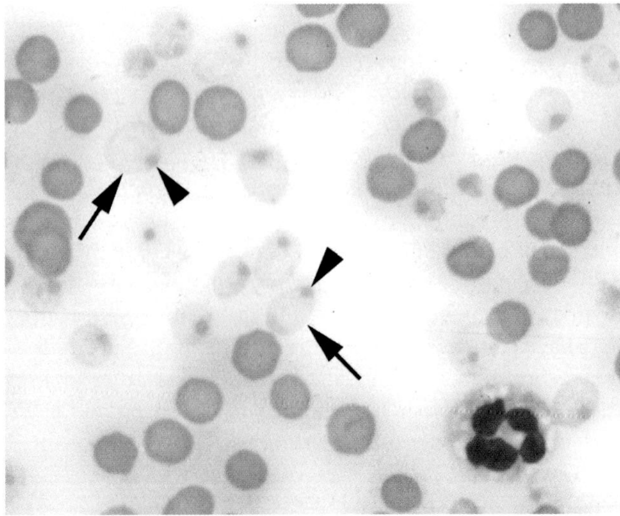

Figure 9.22 Blood film from an anemic cat with acetaminophen toxicosis. Note the lysed "ghost" erythrocytes (arrows). The Heinz bodies (arrowheads) are very apparent in the ghost cells. The pink background is due to hemoglobinemia. Wright stain.

The sulfhydryl groups on the globin portion of the molecule are also susceptible to oxidative damage, and although Heinz bodies may form by oxidation of these sulfhydryl groups, hemichrome formation is likely more important. Hemichromes have an affinity for membrane protein band 3. The protein band 3-hemichrome complex causes membrane protein band 3 to form clusters, both on the inside and outside of the erythrocyte membrane. This external clustering of protein band 3 creates a recognition site for autoantibodies. Erythrocytes with attached antibody are then phagocytized by macrophages. The clustering of protein band 3 and associated autoantibodies may be the best explanation for why animals with Heinz body formation may also have spherocyte formation and agglutination, such as has been described in zinc toxicosis and methylene blue toxicosis in dogs, and red maple leaf toxicosis in horses. Alternately, erythrocytes may have a spherocyte-like appearance because of collapse of the erythrocyte membrane following eccentrocyte formation. Some oxidants may affect the erythrocyte cytoskeleton, resulting in eccentrocyte formation without Heinz body formation. Features of eccentrocytes include shifting of hemoglobin to one side of the cell, loss of normal central pallor, and a clear zone outlined by a membrane (Figure 9.23).

In addition to formation of protein band 3-hemichrome complexes, spectrin-hemoglobin crosslinking also occurs, increasing erythrocyte membrane rigidity and decreasing deformability, ultimately making the erythrocyte more susceptible to removal. Heinz bodies may also be removed by the spleen, with the remaining portion of the erythrocyte returning to circulation. Hemichrome binding to the erythrocyte membrane also may stimulate proteolysis, contributing to breakdown of erythrocyte membrane integrity.

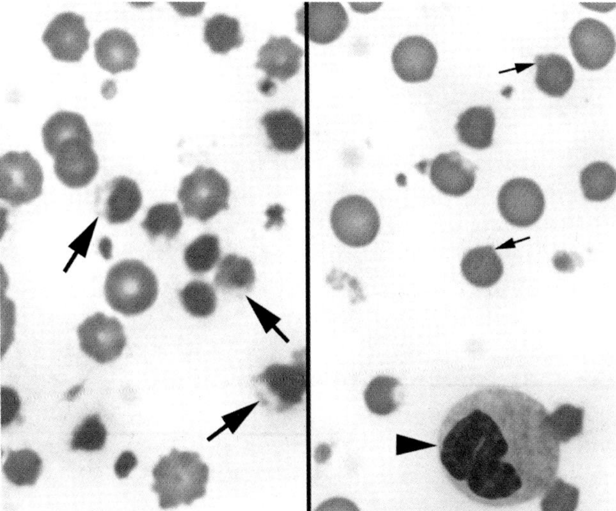

Figure 9.23 Blood film from a cow with oxidant-induced anemia. Note the eccentrocytes (large arrows) and Heinz bodies (small arrows). A neutrophil is present (arrowhead).

Oxidative injury occurs when enzymes and substrates used in the pathway to reverse oxidative processes are depleted, absent, or inhibited. Normally approximately 3 % of the hemoglobin is oxidized to methemoglobin daily, but even that small amount is constantly being reduced back to hemoglobin by a reduced nicotinamide-adenine dinucleotide (NADH)-dependent methemoglobin reductase enzyme within erythrocytes. Methemoglobin forms at higher concentrations when oxidative compounds are increased. Other enzymes also protect against oxidative damage to erythrocytes. These include superoxide dismutase (SOD), a zinc and copper containing enzyme that converts superoxide to hydrogen peroxide and water. Nicotinamide-adenine dinucleotide phosphate (NADPH) maintains glutathione in the reduced state, and glucose-6-phosphate dehydrogenase (G6PD) plays an important role in the initial steps of the pathway. Glutathione has an easily oxidizable sulfhydryl group that acts as a free-radical acceptor to counteract oxidant damage. Glutathione peroxidase catalyzes the conversion of hydrogen peroxide to water, producing oxidized glutathione, which is in turn reduced by glutathione reductase. Selenium is an important component of glutathione peroxidase. Finally, catalase is an enzyme that converts hydrogen peroxide to water and O_2 and may be more important than glutathione peroxidase.

Cats are considered to be more susceptible to Heinz body formation than other domestic species for a number of reasons, including differences in their hemoglobin structure, and normal cats commonly have a small percentage of circulating erythrocytes that contain Heinz bodies. Feline hemoglobin has eight sulfhydryl groups, compared with four in dogs and two in most other species. Many causes of oxidative damage to erythrocytes resulting in Heinz body or eccentrocyte formation have been reported, including oxidant drugs and chemicals, oxidant-containing plants, inherited enzyme deficiencies, and nutritional deficiencies. Treatment depends on predisposing cause of Heinz body formation. Many of the oxidative compounds that result in Heinz body formation also cause methemoglobinemia, which when severe is characterized by brown discoloration of blood and cyanosis. These oxidants are discussed in more detail below.

Plants

Allium family (onions, chives, leeks, and garlic)

Onion, chive, leek, and garlic ingestion may result in Heinz body anemia and eccentrocyte formation in most species of domestic animals. Sources of onions and garlic include the feeding of cull onions to cattle and sheep, ingestion of wild onions by horses, and ingestion of raw, cooked, dehydrated onions, and baby food containing onion or garlic powder, by dogs and cats. The oxidative compounds in onions and garlic are aliphatic sulfides, specifically allyl and propyl di-, tri-, and tetrasulfides, with the allyl compounds being more potent than the propyl. These compounds decrease G6PD activity in erythrocytes, which in turn curtails the regeneration of reduced glutathione needed to prevent oxidative denaturation of hemoglobin. Interestingly, the allyl derivatives are also thought to be effective in increasing tissue activities of cancer-protective enzymes such as quinone reductase (QR) and glutathione S-transferase (GST), thus decreasing the risk of cancer in humans who ingest these vegetables. Moreover, aged garlic extract is sometimes used to treat sickle cell anemia, because the extract is thought to contain antioxidants that prolong the life of sickle red blood cells.

Although the feeding of cull domestic onions (*Allium cepa*) appears to be reasonably safe in sheep, cattle may develop onion toxicosis. Sheep have been fed an exclusive onion diet, and although they initially developed a Heinz body hemolytic anemia with approximately 25% reduction in packed cell volume, there was no significant decrease in pregnancy or lambing rate, body condition, or fleece weight. Adaptation to an exclusive onion diet in sheep is thought to be due to a strong marrow response to the anemia, as well as modification of rumen metabolism of sulfoxides; one study showed that there was a marked increase in the number of sulfide-metabolizing bacteria (*Desulfovibrio* spp). Conversely, rumen microorganisms that convert sulfur containing amino acids to oxidants have been reported to exacerbate onion- and brassica-induced Heinz body anemia. One study showed that sheep fed onions (50 g/kg body weight/day) for 15 days developed more severe Heinz body hemolytic anemia than did the sheep fed the equivalent amount of onions with 5 g/d ampicillin sodium salt.

Feedlot cattle, on the other hand, can be fed a diet containing up to 25% cull onions on a dry-matter (DM) basis. Although a decrease in PCV occurs due to Heinz body-related hemolysis, the PCV returns to normal within 30 days after onion feeding is discontinued. Average daily gain and feed conversion ratios are not affected. It is thought, however, that the 25% (DM) probably approaches the toxic threshold for onion consumption in cattle. Onions should be mixed in a balanced ration, and cattle should not be allowed free access to the onions, as they may eat them preferentially.

Onion ingestion is the most common cause of Heinz body and eccentrocyte formation in dogs, and is a relatively common cause of clinical and subclinical anemia. In one study in which dogs were fed 5.5 g/kg body weight dehydrated onions, 70% of the erythrocytes contained Heinz bodies at 24 hours, and eccentrocytes were also common. Packed cell volume dropped approximately 20% by day 5. There appears to be some variation in individual susceptibility to the effects of onion ingestion in dogs. Erythrocytes with high concentrations of reduced glutathione, such as is seen in some Japanese Shiba dogs, may be more susceptible to oxidative damage produced by onions. Garlic will also induce Heinz body and eccentrocyte formation in dogs.

Ingestion of onion soup and baby food containing onion powder has also been shown to produce Heinz body anemia in cats. In one study, as little as 0.3% onion powder significantly increased Heinz body formation; some commercial baby food may contain up to 1.8% onion powder on a dry weight basis.

Brassica (cabbage, kale, rape)

Ingestion of plants belonging to *Brassica* species may result in Heinz body anemia in ruminants. These plants contain S-methyl-L-cysteine sulfoxide, which is metabolized to the oxidant dimethyl disulfide by rumen bacteria. *Brassica* species not only have a high sulfur content, which reduces copper availability, but also are low in copper and zinc concentration. While this copper deficiency may play a role in oxidative hemoglobin damage, copper deficiency has not been shown to exacerbate susceptibility of lambs to brassica anemia. As with onion toxicosis, the severity of the Heinz body anemia is proportional to the quantity of brassica in the diet. A maximum concentration of 30% DM for *Brassica* species consumption is recommended to avoid significant anemia.

Wilted red maple leaves (Acer rubrum)

Severe Heinz body anemia and possibly death in horses, ponies, llamas, and zebras may be caused by ingestion of wilted or dried (not fresh) red maple leaves. Eccentrocyte formation and hemolysis may occur without concurrent Heinz body formation. Other findings commonly include methemoglobinemia, hemoglobinuria, hemoglobinuric nephrosis, and hepatic necrosis. The oxidative compound, thought to be gallic acid, causes a rapid depletion of glutathione; leaves are toxic when administered at doses of 1.5 g/kg of body weight or more. Therapy consists of ascorbic acid, fluids, and blood transfusions, if necessary.

Drugs and chemicals

Acetaminophen (paracetamol)

Acetaminophen (Tylenol; paracetamol) ingestion is probably the most common cause of Heinz body anemia in cats. Owners, unaware of its toxic effects, often give the anti-inflammatory human drug to cats. Acetaminophen is metabolized in part by glucuronide conjugation; cats have limited ability to form acetaminophen glucuronides, probably due to very low activity of the liver enzyme acetaminophen UDP-glucuronosyltransferase, thus resulting in increased oxidant metabolites of acetaminophen. As a result, glutathione concentration is decreased and oxidative damage to erythrocytes occurs. Other findings commonly include methemoglobinemia, with associated brown discoloration of blood and cyanosis, and hepatic necrosis. The toxic dose of acetaminophen in cats is 50–60 mg/kg body weight. (One Extra Strength Tylenol Gelcap contains 500 mg acetaminophen, and one Extra Strength Excedrin contains 250 mg acetaminophen.) To confirm the diagnosis, acetaminophen concentrations can be determined on serum. Treatment consists of providing glutathione donors, such as N-acetylcysteine, orally. Acetaminophen-induced Heinz body anemia also occurs in dogs; the toxic dose is approximately 150 mg/kg body weight.

Propylene glycol

Propylene glycol, sometimes used as an additive in semi-moist pet food, causes Heinz body formation in cats but does not cause an anemia when ingested in those small quantities. However, cats eating such diets may be more susceptible to other additional causes of oxidative injury. Even though overt anemia may not occur, red cells with Heinz bodies have a reduced life span.

Zinc

Ingestion of zinc-containing materials, including United States Lincoln pennies produced since 1983 that are 98% zinc by weight, other metal objects such as nuts and bolts in animal carriers, zinc toys, and zinc oxide containing ointments have been reported to cause Heinz body anemia in dogs. The mechanisms by which zinc results in oxidative damage and Heinz body formation are unclear but are thought to be due to zinc interference with glutathione reductase. Zinc is known to play a role in band-3 clustering, thus directly damaging the erythrocyte membrane. As a result of this clustering, opsonization of antibody and spherocyte formation may occur. Zinc also damages other organs, including the liver, kidneys, and pancreas (see Section VII, Case 22).

Copper

Copper toxicosis in ruminants, especially sheep, results in Heinz body hemolytic anemia (Figure 9.24). Copper accumulates in the liver of animals ingesting high concentrations of copper. This copper is released following stress, resulting in a hemolytic crisis. Copper deficiency has also been associated with Heinz body formation.

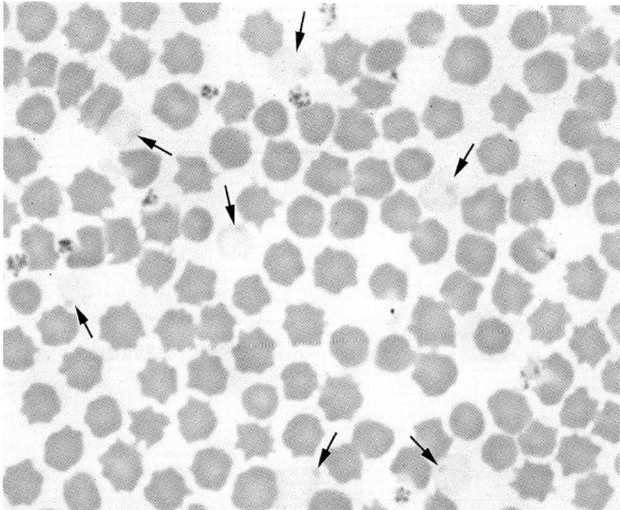

Figure 9.24 Blood film from a sheep with copper toxicosis. Note the Heinz bodies (arrows), which can be seen within "ghost" erythrocytes.

Selenium deficiency

Selenium deficiency in ruminants, associated with grazing on selenium deficient soils in certain parts of the world, including New Zealand and the Florida Everglades, has been associated with Heinz body anemia. Selenium deficiency has also been associated with reduced activity of glutathione peroxidase in erythrocytes of humans that live in selenium deficient areas, including New Zealand and Finland. It is speculated that reduced glutathione peroxidase activity may be the mechanism of the Heinz body anemia in selenium-deficient cattle.

Methylene blue

Methylene blue was historically used as a urinary antiseptic in cats, and commonly resulted in Heinz body anemia with chronic administration. More recently, it has been associated with Heinz body anemia in river otters that were fed bait fish that had been kept in water containing methylene blue, which is used to detoxify ammonia in fish tanks. Interestingly, methylene blue is the drug of choice in the treatment of methemoglobinemia in humans and most domestic animals. There is no evidence to suggest that single therapeutic doses of methylene blue cause hemolytic anemia, even in cats.

Crude oil

Ingestion of crude oil by marine birds results in Heinz body anemia, one of the primary mechanisms of toxicity associated with the ingestion of crude oil by birds.

Other chemicals

Multiple other chemicals, such as naphthalene, a mothball ingredient; propofol, an intravenous anesthetic; phenazopyridine, a urinary analgesic; phenothiazine, an anthelmintic; ecabapide, a gastroprokinetic drug; benzocaine, a local anesthetic; and phenylhydrazine, an oxidative compound commonly used to experimentally induce hemolytic anemia, have been reported to cause Heinz body anemia. Skunk spray, which contains thiols and other oxidizing agents, can also cause Heinz body anemia in dogs.

Diseases

Heinz body formation is increased in specific disease states in cats and may contribute to anemia. Diabetes mellitus, hyperthyroidism, and lymphoma have been correlated with Heinz body formation. Diabetic cats in particular may have marked Heinz body formation. In one study, these diseases together accounted for nearly 40% of cats with Heinz body formation. Ketoacidotic cats had significantly more Heinz bodies than nonketotic diabetic cats. Percentage of Heinz bodies in diabetic cats is directly correlated with plasma beta-hydroxy-butyrate concentration, indicating that ketones are associated with oxidative hemoglobin damage in cats. This is likely a potential source of *in vivo* oxygen radical generation in animals with ketosis, such as may be seen in postparturient cattle.

Hypophosphatemia-induced hemolysis

Severe hypophosphatemia, usually less than 1 mg/dL, has been reported to induce hemolysis in several species of animals, as well as humans. Erythrocyte glycolysis is inhibited by hypophosphatemia, primarily by decreasing intracellular phosphorus that is required for the enzyme glyceraldehyde phosphate dehydrogenase. This results in decreased glycolysis, leading to decreased erythrocyte adenosine triphosphate (ATP) concentrations, and subsequent hemolysis. In some cases, this appears to be due to decreased glutathione, and increased susceptibility to oxidative injury. The most well-recognized syndrome of hypophosphatemia-induced hemolysis is postparturient hemoglobinuria in cattle. Causes in small animals include hypophosphatemia related to diabetes, and enteral alimentation (refeeding syndrome). Severe hypophosphatemia can be life-threatening, not only because of hemolysis but also owing to depression of myocardial function, rhabdomyopathy, seizures, coma, and acute respiratory failure.

Postparturient hemoglobinuria

Postparturient hemoglobinuria in cattle is a sporadic disease of multiparous, high-producing dairy cows characterized by intravascular hemolysis, anemia, and hemoglobinuria. It usually occurs within 4 weeks of calving. Most, but not all, cows with this syndrome are hypophosphatemic at the time of anemia. It is theorized that previous hypophosphatemia predisposes erythrocytes to injury and oxidative damage, primarily by decreasing ATP and glutathione. Experimental hypophosphatemia (1 mg/dL) in postparturient cattle results in a decrease in erythrocyte ATP by 50% and a decrease in glutathione by 30%. The syndrome is complex, because some of the postparturient cattle with hemolytic anemia have Heinz body anemia, and some have ketoacidosis due to their nutritional status prior to and immediately following calving. Ketones are associated with oxidative hemoglobin damage, and may be a potential source of *in vivo* oxygen radical generation.

Hypophosphatemia in diabetic cats

Hypophosphatemia is sometimes present in diabetic animals due to phosphorus loss in the urine of polyuric animals. Several instances of hypophosphatemia-induced hemolysis have been reported in cats. Similar to the situation in cows with postparturient hemoglobinuria, diabetic cats may also be ketotic and have Heinz body anemia; in those cases, the hemolysis may be due to hypophosphatemia, ketosis, or a combination, since ketosis predisposes to Heinz body formation. Hypophosphatemia resulting in hemolytic anemia has also been reported in cats with hepatic lipidosis.

Enteral alimentation in cats – refeeding syndrome

A retrospective study of cats with hypophosphatemia revealed that hypophosphatemia can occur 12–72 hours after initiation of enteral alimentation. In this study, the nadir for phosphorus concentrations ranged from 0.4 to 2.4 mg/dL. Hemolysis occurred in six of the nine cats that were hypophosphatemic. In a more recent retrospective study, 100% of 11 cats developed anemia following refeeding, and 7 required blood transfusions. Many of the affected cats had hepatic lipidosis. Refeeding syndrome with accompanying hypophosphatemia is well documented in human medicine. In response to insulin release following refeeding, phosphorus is taken up by cells, resulting in decreased serum phosphorus. Hypokalemia, hypomagnesemia, and hypoglycemia are also commonly associated with refeeding syndrome.

Microorganisms (other than erythrocyte parasites)

Bacteria

Clostridial and leptospiral infections may result in hemolytic anemia. *Clostridium perfringens* Type A (and rarely D) infections results in a hemolytic anemia in lambs and calves, sometimes referred to as "yellow lamb disease" or "enterotoxemic jaundice." The bacteria produces a phospholipase, which hydrolyses cell membrane phospholipids of erythrocytes, as well as those of other cells. Clinical signs include lethargy, fever, pale mucous membranes, anemia, hemoglobinuria, and icterus. Necropsy findings include evidence of intravascular hemolysis, renal hemoglobin casts, intestinal mucosal necrosis, hepatic necrosis, and petechial and ecchymotic hemorrhages. *C. perfringens* has been associated with IMHA in horses.

Clostridium haemolyticum, an anaerobic motile, sporulating, rod-shaped bacterium, causes hemolytic anemia in cattle and occasionally sheep that is sometimes referred to as "bacillary hemoglobinuria" or "red water disease," which is acutely fatal. The disease, first described in 1916, occurs in summer and early fall, is commonly associated with liver fluke migration, and is endemic in swampy areas of numerous countries, including the United States. Other causes of decreased liver perfusion, including other bacterial infections or liver biopsy, may also predispose to the growth of the clostridial organism. Clinical signs include those of anemia, lethargy, arched back, bloody diarrhea, fever, dyspnea, and occasionally hemoglobinuria. The organisms is mainly found in soil of areas with poorly drained pastures and alkaline pH, where viable spores can survive for years. Bacterial spores are ingested and reside in macrophages of the liver. Anaerobic conditions within the liver, usually resulting from liver fluke migration, result in growth of the bacteria and production of toxic enzymes, including lecithinase, that metabolize lipids and protein in cell walls. Hemolysis and necrosis of other cells, including endothelial cells and hepatocytes, result in death. Necropsy findings include pale and icteric mucous membranes, foci of hepatic necrosis, hemorrhages, thoracic and abdominal effusion, hemoglobinuria, renal hemoglobin casts, and edema.

Leptospirosis (*Leptospira pomona*) may cause hemolytic anemia in young calves and lambs but is almost never a feature of the disease in adult animals; leptospirosis very rarely causes hemolytic anemia in dogs, although thrombocytopenia is common. The mechanism of the anemia may be toxins produced by the bacteria that act as hemolysins, but it is more likely an IMHA, probably IgM mediated. Necropsy findings in lambs include icterus, hemoglobinuria, renal tubular necrosis with hemoglobin casts, and hepatocellular necrosis.

Viruses

The equine infectious anemia (EIA) virus may result in hemolytic anemia in the acute stage of the disease. The anemia is likely immune mediated as a result of the virus binding with the erythrocyte membrane and activating complement. Later in the disease the anemia is nonregenerative, possibly similar to anemia of inflammatory disease. EIA was first described in 1843, and in 1904 was shown to be caused by a filterable agent (a virus) that was transmitted by blood, usually by insect vectors such as horse flies and deer flies. It is also referred to as "swamp fever." Diagnosis is made by detecting antibody against the EIA virus, using a Coggins test or a competitive ELISA test.

Water intoxication-induced hemolysis in calves

Water intoxication resulting in hemolysis, hemoglobinuria, pulmonary edema, brain edema, convulsions, coma, and death may occur in calves that have unlimited access to water following its unavailability. Water intoxication may cause death within 2 hours, but most calves survive with no permanent ill effects. Cause of hemolysis is decreased osmolality of plasma. It has been theorized that water intoxication-induced hemolysis occurs in calves from 4 to 5 months of age because osmotic fragility of their erythrocytes is greatest at that age, possibly related to the residual presence of iron deficient erythrocytes. The disorder is rare in adult cattle; severe dilutional hyponatremia resulting in cerebral edema is usually the cause of death, rather than hemolysis.

Hereditary membrane defects and metabolic disorders

Either inherited membrane defects or enzyme deficiencies leading to metabolic disorders may result in hemolytic anemia. Inherited erythrocyte membrane defects reported in domestic animals include hereditary spherocytosis, hereditary elliptocytosis, hereditary stomatocytosis, and membrane transport defects. However, hereditary elliptocytosis in dogs, which is caused by a hereditary protein 4.1 deficiency, results in increased osmotic fragility, elliptocytosis, membrane fragmentation, microcytosis, and poikilocytosis but does not result in anemia (see Chapter 6).

Membrane defects

Hereditary spherocytosis (HS) results in hemolytic anemia, spherocytosis, and splenomegaly. Hereditary spherocytosis has been reported in people, mice, dogs, and cattle. In cattle, HS is due to hereditary band 3 deficiency, an autosomal dominant trait that has been reported in Japanese black cattle. Band 3 protein is the most abundant protein in mammalian erythrocyte membranes, and functions include anion exchange across the membrane, as well as maintenance of normal erythrocyte shape. Cattle homozygous for the trait lack band 3 protein in their erythrocyte membranes, have a mild anemia, spherocytosis, hyperbilirubinemia, splenomegaly, and growth impairment. The disease is more severe in calves; adults are relatively normal. Heterozygotes have a partial deficiency of band 3, mild spherocytosis, and compensate for their hemolytic anemia with increased erythrocyte regeneration. Hereditary spherocytosis may also be due to spectrin deficiency. Spectrin is the major constituent of the cytoskeletal network underlying the erythrocyte plasma membrane. It associates with band 4.1 and actin to form the cytoskeletal superstructure of the erythrocyte plasma membrane. This complex is anchored to the cytoplasmic face of the plasma membrane via another protein, ankyrin, which binds to beta-spectrin and mediates the binding of the whole complex to the transmembrane protein band 3. The interaction of erythrocyte spectrin with other proteins through specific binding domains lead to the formation of an extensive subplasmalemmal meshwork that is thought to be responsible for the maintenance of the biconcave shape of erythrocytes, for the regulation of plasma membrane components and for the maintenance of the lipid asymmetry of the plasma membrane. Spectrin deficiency has been reported in a family of Dutch golden retrievers.

Hereditary stomatocytosis has been reported in miniature schnauzers, chondrodysplastic Alaskan malamutes, and in the Drentse patrijshond breed of dogs that also have hypertrophic gastritis (see Chapter 6). These disorders have different underlying causes in these three breeds, and the schnauzers do not have anemia, although their red cell survival time is slightly shortened.

A Coombs negative chronic intermittent hemolytic anemia has been reported in Abyssinian and Somali cats. Clinical signs and laboratory findings include mild to severe anemia, splenomegaly, increased MCV, and the presence of a few stomatocytes. Osmotic fragility of erythrocytes is markedly increased. Some of the cats improved following splenectomy. The specific cause of the hemolytic anemia is not known, but a membrane defect is suspected.

Animals with erythrocyte membrane transport defects, especially those with defects in transport of amino acids involved in glutathione metabolism, may develop hemolytic anemia (Heinz body anemia) when exposed to oxidants. Some Finnish Landrace sheep have red cell glutathione deficiency, inherited as autosomal recessive. Cysteine uptake and glutathione synthesis are impaired, and glutathione concentration in erythrocytes is only 30% of normal. A similar defect is thought to be common in thoroughbred horses but does not cause anemia. Some Japanese Shiba and Akita dogs have erythrocytes with high potassium, low sodium concentrations, due to retention of Na,K-ATPase in mature erythrocytes, inherited as an autosomal recessive trait. Some of these dogs have an increased concentration of reduced glutathione in their erythrocytes, which protects the cells against oxidative damage by acetylphenylhydrazine, but increases the risk of oxidative damage by onions (see "Heinz Body Anemia").

Metabolic disorders

Inherited erythrocyte enzyme defects result in abnormalities in metabolic pathways, often resulting in hemolytic anemia. Energy in mature mammalian erythrocytes is generated exclusively by anaerobic glycolysis, also known as the Embden-Meyerhof (EM) pathway, since they have lost their mitochondria, and thus their oxidative phosphorylation capabilities. Briefly, metabolism of glucose produces ATP, which is used to maintain erythrocyte shape, deformability, membrane transport, and synthesis of purines, pyrimidines, and glutathione. Many enzymes are involved in anaerobic glycolysis, including phosphofructokinase (PFK) and pyruvate kinase (PK). Deficiencies of both of these enzymes have been described in domestic animals. Erythrocyte enzyme deficiencies do not usually lead to a shortened life expectancy, other than PK deficiency in dogs, and occasionally PFK deficiency in dogs having a hemolytic crisis. These hemolytic anemias are usually very regenerative and must be differentiated from more common causes of hemolytic anemia such as IMHA, hemotrophic parasites, or Heinz body anemia.

Pyruvate kinase deficiency

PK deficiency is the most common enzymopathy in humans and dogs, and was first recognized in Basenji dogs in 1971. Since that time, it has been reported in beagles, West Highland white terriers, Cairn terriers, miniature poodles, pugs, Labrador retrievers, and various other breeds. Clinical signs include those of anemia, such as exercise intolerance. The anemia is very regenerative, and half or more of the erythrocytes on the blood film may be reticulocytes. The MCV may be markedly increased due to the reticulocytosis. Hepatosplenomegaly may be present. Affected dogs die of myelofibrosis, secondary hemochromatosis, or hepatic failure by 3–5 years of age. Myelofibrosis and osteosclerosis are a consistent finding in PK-deficient dogs but do not develop in PK deficient people or cats. In certain breeds (basenjis, West Highland white terriers) in which the mutation is specific, diagnosis can be made by PCR-based tests. Bone marrow transplantation has been shown to correct the disorder and prevent the development of osteosclerosis. PK deficiency in cats has been described in various breeds, including Abyssinian, Somali, and domestic short hair cats. The hemolytic anemia is mild to moderate, slightly to strongly regenerative, and intermittent. Splenectomy has been reported to reduce the severity of hemolytic anemia. Additional signs include lethargy, weakness, weight loss, jaundice, and occasionally splenomegaly. Laboratory findings in addition to anemia may include hyperglobulinemia, hyperbilirubinemia, and increased serum liver enzymes activity. Osteosclerosis does not develop in cats.

Phosphofructokinase deficiency

PFK deficiency is a rare genetic disorder in humans, and has been described in English springer spaniels, American cocker spaniels, whippets, Wachtelhunds, and mixed-breed dogs. The cocker spaniel had an ancestor that was bred in a kennel that also had English springer spaniels, and the mixed-breed dog was thought to be part English springer spaniel. The mutation in the first described dogs was identical. Other missense mutations have been described in Wachtelhunds. It is inherited as an autosomal recessive trait, and is also referred to as glycogen storage disease type VII, since the enzyme deficiency also results in a lack of lactate production and accumulation of sugar phosphates and glycogen in muscle. Intermittent severe intravascular hemolysis is triggered by mild alkalemia; even mild respiratory alkalosis caused by hyperventilation and panting may precipitate a hemolytic crisis. Moreover 2,3-diphosphoglycerate (2,3-DPG), a compound that decreases the oxygen affinity for hemoglobin, thus making oxygen more available to tissues, is generated in the EM pathway. PFK deficiency results in a deficiency of 2,3-DPG, which results in tissue hypoxia of affected dogs. However, this tissue hypoxia stimulates erythropoietin production, and thus, except when in hemolytic crisis, these dogs are not anemic. Clinical signs include excitement or exercise-induced hemolytic anemia and occasional mild muscle cramping. Life expectancy can be normal if hemolytic crises are avoided. The disorder can be identified in affected dogs, as well as carriers, by a PCR-based DNA test that is specific for the English springer spaniel mutation.

Glucose-6-phosphate dehydrogenase deficiency

The pentose phosphate pathway (PPP) generates reduced nicotine adenine dinucleotide phosphate (NADPG), which is protective against mechanical and metabolic insults, particularly oxidants. G6PD is the rate-limiting enzyme in the

PPP. In humans, G6PD deficiency is inherited as an X-linked disorder, which causes hemolytic anemia, particularly following exposure to oxidants. Hemolytic anemia caused by G6PD deficiency has been described in an American saddle bred colt, as well as a dog. Morphologic abnormalities in the colt included eccentrocytosis, and the colt's dam, which was a heterozygote for the disorder, also had eccentrocytes on her blood film.

Hereditary methemoglobinemia

Methemoglobin is not able to bind oxygen because the iron moiety of the heme group has been oxidized to the ferric state (see "Heinz Body Anemia"). Approximately 3% of hemoglobin is oxidized to methemoglobin each day, but this methemoglobin is reduced back to hemoglobin, primarily by the enzyme NADH-methemoglobin reductase. Inherited deficiencies of this enzyme have been described in numerous breeds of dogs and cats. This disorder does not cause significant problems in dogs and cats, other than increased risk associated with anesthesia. Glutathione reductase deficiency has been described in horses, and even in the absence of oxidants, resulted in a mild hemolytic anemia with eccentrocyte formation and methemoglobinemia. Horses in one report had normal methemoglobin reductase activity, but activity was reduced in a separate case.

Porphyrias

Hemoglobin synthesis occurs in erythroid precursors, where protoporphyrin, iron, and globin molecules are brought together and assembled into functional hemoglobin. Synthesis of the heme portion of the molecule is complex, and requires numerous enzymes. Inherited deficiencies of these enzymes result in an accumulation of porphyrin precursors, as well as a failure to adequately synthesize hemoglobin, and the disorders are known as erythropoietic porphyrias, which have been described in humans, cattle, swine, and cats. Some of the erythropoietic porphyrias result in hemolytic anemia. Hepatic porphyrias are caused by different enzyme deficiencies, and to date have been discovered only in humans; the liver is the site of synthesis for enzymes containing heme, such as catalase, cytochromes, and peroxidase.

Another inherited disorder, erythropoietic protoporphyria, is due to a defect of the enzyme heme synthetase (ferrochelatase). This disorder has been described in Limousin and Blonde d'Aquitaine cattle, and the only clinical manifestation is severe photosensitivity with intense pruritus. Anemia, porphyrinuria, and discolored teeth are not observed. Inheritance of erythropoietic protoporphyria is recessive in cattle and only occurs in homozygotes, unlike in humans in whom the heterozygous condition results in clinical signs.

Toxins, especially lead, may destroy many of the enzymes involved in the synthesis of heme. These toxicoses lead to a decrease in heme synthesis, as well as an excess of heme precursors, which are eliminated in increased concentration in the urine. These toxicoses are referred to as porphyrinurias.

Clinical signs associated with porphyrias vary, depending on the specific enzyme abnormality, and the amount of residual activity of the affected enzyme. Porphyrins are reddish-brown in color, have a characteristic red fluorescence when exposed to ultraviolet light, and stain various tissues, including teeth and bones; congenital erythropoietic porphyria in cattle was called "pink tooth" at one time. The porphyrins in these animals are excreted excessively in all body fluids, including urine, feces, saliva, sweat, and tears. One of the most common abnormalities is photosensitivity resulting in photodermatitis, particularly evident on light colored areas of the skin. This is due to excitation of porphyrins by ultraviolet light, and subsequent transfer of oxygen to tissues, causing oxidation of cellular lipids, proteins, and organelles.

Bovine congenital erythropoietic porphyria

Bovine congenital erythropoietic porphyria has been reported in Holsteins and Shorthorns, and is caused by a partial deficiency of uroporphyrinogen III cosynthetase (UROgenIII Cosyn), resulting in an accumulation of uroporphyrin I and coproporphyrin I, which accumulate in tissues, and are excreted in urine and feces in increased quantities. Clinical signs include pigmentation of tissues including teeth, anemia, and photosensitization. The disorder is inherited as an autosomal recessive trait. Affected animals have hemolytic anemia that is regenerative, and blood film findings are those of a regenerative anemia in cattle, including polychromasia, macrocytosis, anisocytosis, basophilic stippling, and increased nucleated erythrocytes. Affected calves have a particularly striking regenerative response, with many nucleated erythrocytes present. Erythrocyte life span is shortened, due to both the heme synthesis disorder, as well as the porphyrin-related damage to erythrocyte membrane lipids. Ultraviolet light may increase severity of hemolysis, due to exposure of erythrocytes while in surface capillaries. The disease has been almost completely eliminated in cattle.

Porphyria of cats

Two forms of porphyria have been described in cats. One type, described in a family of Siamese cats, is due to a partial deficiency of UROgenIII Cosyn, and is similar to the disorder in humans and cattle. Affected cats had photosensitivity and severe hemolytic anemia, as well as renal disease. The renal disease was characterized by mesangial hypercellularity and proliferation and ischemic tubular injury. Membrane-enclosed lamellar bodies were present in cytoplasmic and extracellular locations of various tissues, similar to those seen in lysosomal storage disorders.

A second type of porphyria has been described in domestic cats in which the clinical signs are only discoloration of teeth and urine due to the presence of uroporphyrin, coproporphyrin, and porphobilinogen. Anemia and photosensitization are not present. The disorder in domestic cats is inherited as autosomal dominant.

Porphyria of swine

Porphyria has been described in affected swine, which have discoloration of teeth and excessive uroporphyrin in the urine. Affected swine are not anemic and photosensitization is not present. The specific defect is not known, and no animals are currently available for study. The disorder is inherited as autosomal dominant.

10 Classification of and Diagnostic Approach to Erythrocytosis

Mary Anna Thrall

Department of Biomedical Sciences, Ross University School of Veterinary Medicine, Basseterre, Saint Kitts and Nevis

Erythrocytosis, sometimes referred to as polycythemia, is an increase in the concentration of erythrocytes in the blood as evidenced by an increased packed cell volume (PCV) or hematocrit, red blood cell count, or hemoglobin concentration. Because the term polycythemia implies that all blood cells, including platelets and leukocytes, are increased in concentration, the term erythrocytosis is more accurately descriptive. In domestic animals with primary or true erythrocytosis (polycythemia vera), usually only the erythrocytes are increased in concentration, unlike in humans in whom platelet and leukocyte concentrations are typically also increased.

Erythrocytosis may be either relative or absolute. Relative erythrocytosis may occur due to decreased plasma volume or erythrocyte redistribution. Examples of the former include dehydration and body fluid shifts. The latter is the result of splenic contraction seen most commonly in excitable animals such as cats and horses. Absolute erythrocytosis is caused by an actual increase in the red cell mass and may be primary or secondary. Secondary absolute erythrocytosis results from overproduction of erythrocytes secondary to increased erythropoietin (EPO) concentration, which in turn is secondary to either generalized hypoxia, localized renal hypoxia due to a renal lesion resulting in inappropriate erythropoietin increase, or overproduction of erythropoietin by a tumor. Absolute primary erythrocytosis (polycythemia vera) is a disorder in which erythropoiesis occurs independent of the EPO concentration. Primary erythrocytosis is a well-differentiated myeloproliferative disorder that is usually diagnosed in domestic animals by excluding relative and secondary erythrocytosis.

Erythrocyte production (erythropoiesis) is regulated by the glycoprotein cytokine EPO, which was discovered in 1977. Erythropoietin production occurs primarily in peritubular fibroblast-like interstitial cells in the kidney that are regulated by an elaborate oxygen-sensing mechanism that was discovered in the early 1990s. The erythropoietin receptor (EPOR) was discovered in 1989. Erythropoietin drives erythropoiesis by stimulating this receptor on the surface of erythrocyte precursors. The EPOR is bound to an intracytoplasmic essential partner, Janus kinase 2 (JAK2) tyrosine kinase. Following activation of JAK2, signaling molecules enter the nucleus of the erythroid precursor to activate numerous target genes that promote erythroid precursor expansion and survival, regulate maturation, mediate iron uptake, and regulate feedback inhibition of EPOR signaling to prevent excessive red-cell production. Erythropoiesis is reviewed in detail by Bhoopalan et al. (see "Suggested Reading").

Relative erythrocytosis

Relative erythrocytosis caused by fluid shifts or dehydration

Patients with relative erythrocytosis caused by a reduction in plasma volume usually have a concurrent increase in plasma protein. In addition, clinical evidence of dehydration usually is present. Some dehydrated animals, however, may have normal or decreased plasma protein concentration resulting from decreased protein intake, decreased protein production by the liver, or increased protein loss via the kidney, gastrointestinal tract, or cutaneous lesions (see Chapter 30). Moreover, fluid shifts may occur so rapidly, such as in patients with acute gastrointestinal disease or severe acute hyperthermia, that the classic clinical signs of dehydration may not be apparent. Relative polycythemia is treated by diagnosis of and therapy for the underlying disease and by replacement of fluids and electrolytes.

Veterinary Hematology, Clinical Chemistry, and Cytology, Third Edition. Edited by Mary Anna Thrall, Glade Weiser, Robin W. Allison and Terry W. Campbell.

Companion website: www.wiley.com/go/thrall/veterinary

Relative erythrocytosis caused by transient increase in red cell mass secondary to splenic contraction

Splenic contraction causes only a modest increase in PCV, usually to no greater than 60%. Erythrocytosis as a result of splenic contraction typically is seen only in animals that normally have a high PCV, such as some poodles, greyhounds, and dachshunds. Splenic contraction may occur secondary to exercise, or it may be a response to epinephrine release in animals that are excited or in pain. Plasma protein concentration is not increased, and the presence of fear, pain, or excitement at the time of blood collection usually is apparent. An excitement leukogram also may be present, as evidenced by a mature neutrophilia and lymphocytosis; occasionally, mild thrombocytosis also is noted. Transient erythrocytosis has no clinical significance, and the red cell concentration reverts to normal in a short period of time.

Absolute erythrocytosis

Absolute erythrocytosis can be either secondary or primary.

Secondary absolute erythrocytosis

Secondary absolute erythrocytosis caused by generalized hypoxia or hypoxemia (physiologically appropriate erythrocytosis)

Physiologically appropriate polycythemia is observed when inadequate tissue oxygenation triggers an increase in erythropoietin production, which in turn stimulates erythrocyte production and release so that more oxygen can be carried to the tissues. Generalized hypoxia and hypoxemia (reduced PaO_2) may be seen in animals with severe chronic heart or lung disease. Congenital heart disorders that result in shunting of blood away from the lungs are associated more often with erythrocytosis than in acquired heart disease. Severe lung disease also may result in hypoxemia, but it must be of chronic duration to induce polycythemia. Other causes of hypoxemia include living at very high altitude, alveolar hypoventilation, and severe obesity. Polycythemia associated with hypoxia without hypoxemia occurs in people with certain rare inherited hemoglobinopathies, but hemoglobinopathies have not been reported in domestic animals. Acquired chronic hemoglobinopathies (e.g., carboxyhemoglobinemia secondary to carbon monoxide poisoning or methemoglobinemia) may induce polycythemia as well.

Secondary absolute polycythemia caused by hypoxemia is diagnosed by detecting decreased PaO_2 and oxygen saturation. The reference interval for PaO_2 varies somewhat with the altitude. At sea level, the lower end of the reference interval is 80 mmHg, and oxygen saturation is 92%; at approximately 6000 ft above sea level, the lower end of the reference interval is 74 mmHg. Usually, the PaO_2 must be less than 60 mmHg to induce polycythemia. Imaging of the heart and lungs as well as other diagnostic procedures to detect cardiopulmonary disease can then be used to establish a more definitive diagnosis.

Secondary absolute erythrocytosis caused by increased erythropoietin production (physiologically inappropriate polycythemia)

Physiologically inappropriate erythrocytosis occurs when erythropoietin production is increased in the absence of generalized tissue hypoxia. In dogs, hematocrits as high as 82% have been reported with secondary erythrocytosis. Erythropoietin production may be increased in patients with renal lesions such as tumors that induce localized renal hypoxia. Increased production of erythropoietin or of an erythropoietin-like substance by nonrenal tumors such as hepatoblastomas in horses, nasal fibrosarcoma, lymphoma, intestinal leiomyosarcoma and schwannoma in dogs, and hemangiosarcoma in a cat have been reported, but paraneoplastic erythropoietin production is rare. Animals with physiologically inappropriate polycythemia have normal to slightly decreased PaO_2 and oxygen saturation. Mild hypoxemia may be present as a result of poor perfusion, and patients usually have increased serum erythropoietin concentration. Other diagnostic procedures to evaluate the kidneys, such as imaging, renal aspiration cytology or biopsy, and urinalysis, should be performed.

Primary absolute erythrocytosis

Familial primary erythrocytosis

Familial primary erythrocytosis is very rare and has been described in humans and cattle. In humans, the autosomal dominant disorder is associated with various mutations in the gene encoding the EPOR that result in truncation of the intracellular domain of the receptor with subsequent hypersensitivity to erythropoietin. The disorder is autosomal recessive in cattle.

Acquired (neoplastic) primary erythrocytosis (polycythemia vera)

Acquired primary absolute erythrocytosis (polycythemia vera) is a well-differentiated clonal myeloproliferative disorder in which erythrocytes proliferate uncontrollably, producing an increased hematocrit. Median PCV was 70% in one series of 18 cats with primary erythrocytosis, and ranges from 65% to 85% have been reported in dogs. Unlike most other types of hematopoietic neoplasia, the neoplastic erythroid cells are morphologically normal and have a normal maturation sequence. In humans with polycythemia vera, an abnormal proliferation of neutrophils and platelets often accompanies erythrocyte proliferation, resulting in leukocytosis and thrombocytosis. An abnormal proliferation of cells other than red blood cells is rarely observed in domestic animals; thus, in dogs and cats, the disorder is now referred to as primary erythrocytosis, rather than as primary polycythemia or polycythemia vera.

Humans with polycythemia vera have an increased risk of thrombosis and eventual marrow fibrosis or transformation into acute myeloid leukemia. The median age at diagnosis is 60 years, and the disorder is more common in males. The presence of an acquired recurrent mutation within the JAK2 gene has been identified in more than 97% of human patients with polycythemia vera. This mutation (V617F) results from a somatic G to T mutation and the resultant amino acid substitution of valine to phenylalanine in the pseudokinase domain of JAK2 that is known to have an inhibitory role, resulting in hyperactivation of erythropoietin-induced cell signaling. Detection of the mutation is a major diagnostic tool in humans for polycythemia vera diagnosis. Identical mutations of the JAK2 gene giving rise to active JAK2 kinase have been shown in dogs with polycythemia vera, suggesting a common mechanism for the human and canine disease.

While the disorder continues to be diagnosed by excluding other causes of erythrocytosis, it is likely that detection of the mutation may soon be used for diagnosis. Most cases of primary erythrocytosis in domestic animals have been reported in dogs and cats, but a few have been reported in horses, cattle, a ferret, and a llama.

Clinical findings

Clinical findings may be secondary to the underlying cause of the erythrocytosis or may result from the increased number of erythrocytes per se. In animals with relative erythrocytosis, dehydration or excitement may be clinically evident. In animals with secondary absolute erythrocytosis caused by hypoxia, clinical signs associated with congenital heart disease (e.g., murmurs, cyanosis) or with pulmonary disease (e.g., cyanosis, dyspnea, abnormal lung sounds) may be observed. In animals with secondary absolute erythrocytosis caused by inappropriate erythropoietin production, clinical signs associated with renal disease often are not apparent.

Clinical signs associated with erythrocytosis are secondary to increased blood volume and viscosity. They include deep-red mucous membranes, sometimes with slight cyanosis. Increased blood viscosity may result in sluggish blood flow and subsequent decreased tissue perfusion and oxygen transport as well as hemorrhage and thrombosis. Mild to severe central nervous system signs associated with decreased oxygen transport, such as lethargy, ataxia, blindness, or seizures, also may be observed. In a series of 18 cats with primary erythrocytosis, seizures and mentation changes were the most common presenting signs (10 of 18).

Polyuria and polydipsia occasionally are reported and are thought to result from impaired release of vasopressin. Splenomegaly rarely is observed in domestic animals. However, human patients commonly have splenomegaly, may have generalized pruritis, and eventually may develop marrow fibrosis and lymphoid neoplasia.

Diagnostic approach

When PCV is increased, one should consider if the patient is excited or dehydrated and then perform a second complete blood count to confirm that the finding is repeatable. If the total protein concentration also is increased, the erythrocytosis likely is relative, secondary to dehydration and decreased plasma volume. Sometimes, however, animals with rapid fluid shifts, such as those with gastrointestinal disease, may not have an increased total protein. Moreover, total protein may be decreased or normal in dehydrated animals that have decreased protein intake, production, or increased loss.

If relative erythrocytosis is excluded, secondary absolute polycythemia due to hypoxemia from congenital heart disease or pulmonary disease should be considered. Hypoxemia is best diagnosed by performing an arterial blood gas analysis to determine the PaO_2 and oxygen saturation. If the PaO_2 is less than 60 mmHg, then hypoxemia likely is the cause of erythrocytosis. Pulse oximetry can also be used to estimate oxygenation, and if oxygen saturation is below 92%, arterial blood gas should be performed. Imaging using thoracic radiographic and ultrasonic examination will provide additional information.

If hypoxemia is excluded, secondary absolute erythrocytosis caused by increased erythropoietin production should be considered. Tumors of the kidney are the most common cause of increased erythropoietin production. In these cases, imaging with renal ultrasonography or intravenous urography is indicated. Serum erythropoietin concentration usually is increased in animals with hypoxemia or inappropriate erythropoietin production and is normal to decreased in animals with primary erythrocytosis (Table 10.1). Erythropoietin concentrations appear to be more useful in dogs than in cats. If secondary erythrocytosis caused by inappropriate erythropoietin production is excluded, then the likely diagnosis is primary erythrocytosis.

Table 10.1 PaO_2 and erythropoietin in animals with erythrocytosis.

Erythrocytosis	PaO_2	Erythropoietin
Relative	Normal	Normal
Secondary		
Caused by hypoxemia	Decreased	Increased
Caused by inappropriate erythropoietin production	Normal	Increased
Primary	Normal	Normal or decreased

Other laboratory findings are not particularly helpful. Affected humans commonly have neutrophilia and thrombocytosis, but these findings are rare in domestic animals. Neutrophilia associated with stress or inflammation is a more likely finding. Other than mild increased cellularity and mild erythroid hyperplasia, bone marrow aspirates usually are normal in appearance. Measuring total red cell mass with a dye technique or radioisotope-labeled erythrocytes, though infrequently performed, can help to establish a more definitive diagnosis. Due to the abnormally high PCV in patients with erythrocytosis from any cause, hypoglycemia may be erroneously diagnosed if using a point-of-care blood glucose meter.

Therapy

Relative erythrocytosis is treated by therapy for the underlying disease and correction of dehydration with fluid therapy. The underlying disorder also is treated in animals with secondary erythrocytosis caused by hypoxemia or inappropriate erythropoietin production. Phlebotomy may be contraindicated in animals with hypoxemia, because the erythrocytosis is physiologic. If the PCV is very high in these patients, however, then tissue perfusion may be impaired, and phlebotomy may be helpful.

Primary erythrocytosis is commonly treated – and often with long-term success – by performing repeated phlebotomy to maintain the PCV in the high-normal range. Injectable iron may need to be given to avoid iron deficiency anemia. Chemotherapy to decrease red cell production is usually useful; oral hydroxyurea is the most common such treatment. Dose and frequency are variable, depending on the response. A reported complication in cats is methemoglobinemia and Heinz body anemia. While radioactive phosphorus has been used with success in some cases, it is now very rarely used. Survival time in cats with primary erythrocytosis managed with a combination of phlebotomy and hydroxyurea has been reported to be greater than 17 months, with some cats living more than 5 years after diagnosis. JAK2 inhibitors have been developed and used with some success in humans. A veterinary oncologist should be consulted for up-to-date treatment options.

11 Introduction to Leukocytes and the Leukogram

Glade Weiser
Loveland, CO, USA

Interpretation of leukocyte concentrations in blood provides insight regarding potential processes that may be occurring in the patient. The complete set of numeric data in the leukocyte profile, along with any noted morphologic abnormalities, is known as the leukogram. The leukogram consists of about half of the numerical data in the complete blood count (CBC). An abnormal leukogram usually leads to identification of a pathologic process (e.g., inflammation) but not to establishment of a specific diagnosis. Interpretation of leukocyte abnormalities into a process coupled with clinical findings, however, may lead toward a diagnosis.

To interpret leukocyte patterns in disease, one must first learn the normal characteristics of the leukogram as a basis for recognizing abnormal patterns. This chapter presents background information regarding the normal leukogram that is necessary for building skills in its interpretation.

Common blood leukocytes: general functions and morphology

This section reviews pertinent characteristics of blood leukocytes, such as general functions and morphologic features, including species variations in morphology.

Neutrophils

Neutrophils participate in inflammatory responses by means of chemoattraction into tissue sites of inflammation and phagocytosis of organisms and other foreign material. After phagocytosis, lysosomal granules fuse with phagosomes to kill organisms and then degrade the material by enzymatic digestion.

Neutrophil morphology is introduced in Figure 11.1. The neutrophilic metamyelocyte is not present in normal blood. It has a bean-shaped nucleus that, as it matures, changes to the horseshoe shape that is characteristic of the band neutrophil. The band nucleus has smooth, parallel sides and no constrictions in the nuclear membrane. The band neutrophil may be present in normal blood in small concentrations. Segmented neutrophils are normally the nearly exclusive circulating form and have a horseshoe-shaped nucleus with variable degrees of indentation and constriction along its perimeter (Figure 11.1). As the nucleus develops constrictions, it may fold into various shapes (Figure 11.2). Neutrophils have numerous small, very poorly stained granules. These vary among individual animals from colorless, invisible granules to lightly staining granules. Neutrophilic granules of the cow often stain faintly pink, giving the cytoplasm a slightly orange-pink tint overall (Figure 11.3). Neutrophils observed in cytologic samples may on occasion have altered staining of the neutrophilic granules. The granules may appear more prominent and stain pink. This change is most likely to be observed in neutrophils exudated in airway samples.

Lymphocytes

Blood lymphocytes represent a diverse set of lymphocyte subpopulations, but these subpopulations cannot be distinguished by blood-film examination or by techniques routinely used in clinical veterinary laboratories. The subpopulations include B lymphocytes, which are responsible for humoral immunity, and T lymphocytes, which are responsible for cell-mediated immunity and cytokine responses. T lymphocytes may be further classified as T-inducer (i.e., helper; CD4-bearing) cells and T-cytotoxic/suppressor (CD8-bearing) cells. Null cells are a third population present at small concentrations. Null cells consist of at least several lymphocyte subtypes, including large granular lymphocytes, natural killer cells, and other cells with killer activity. Lymphocyte subtypes may be differentiated by surface immunoglobulin and cluster designation (i.e., CD) markers; however, this technology is not yet part of the routine hemogram. These measurements are currently made in specialized laboratories, usually in cases of leukemia

Veterinary Hematology, Clinical Chemistry, and Cytology, Third Edition. Edited by Mary Anna Thrall, Glade Weiser, Robin W. Allison and Terry W. Campbell.

Companion website: www.wiley.com/go/thrall/veterinary

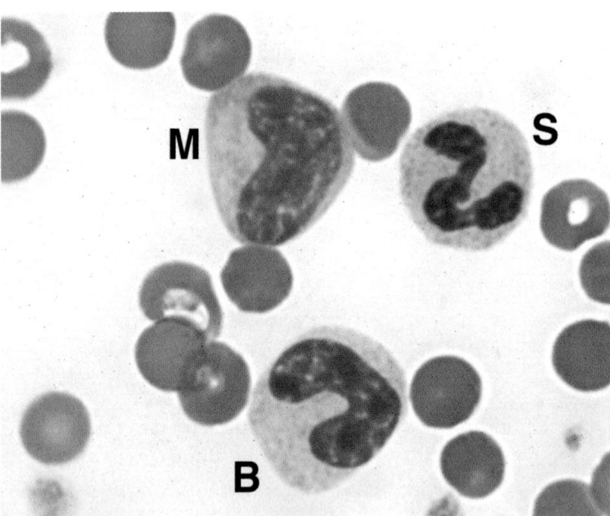

Figure 11.1 Neutrophil maturation sequence commonly seen in blood. The segmented or mature neutrophil (S) has an irregular nuclear membrane, with one or more constrictions. Note the small, faintly staining neutrophilic granules in the cytoplasm. The neutrophilic granules vary in prominence from animal to animal. The band neutrophil (B) has a horseshoe-shaped nucleus with smooth, parallel sides. The metamyelocyte (M) has a bean-shaped nucleus. Wright-Giemsa stain, high magnification.

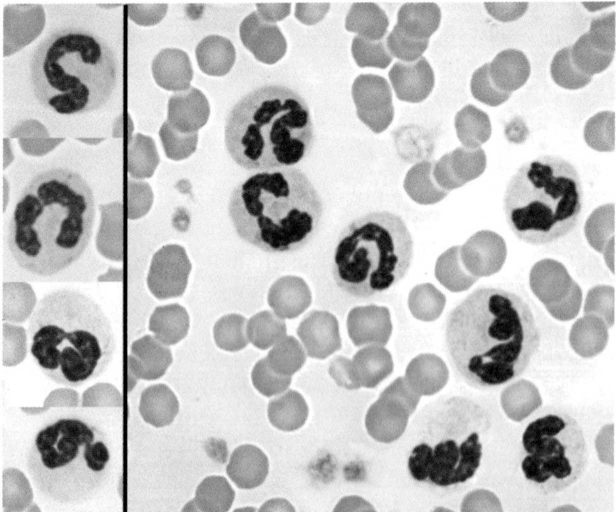

Figure 11.2 Representative segmented neutrophils illustrating variation in nuclear shape. Segmented neutrophils start with the horseshoe-shaped nucleus of the band cell. As the neutrophil nucleus develops more constrictions, it may more easily fold into various shapes. Note the "S"-shaped and horseshoe-shaped nuclei in the upper left. Then, note the various nuclear shapes that result from folding and superimposition of the folded nucleus on itself. Cells are arranged in this figure with greater degrees of folding moving toward the bottom. Wright-Giemsa stain, high magnification.

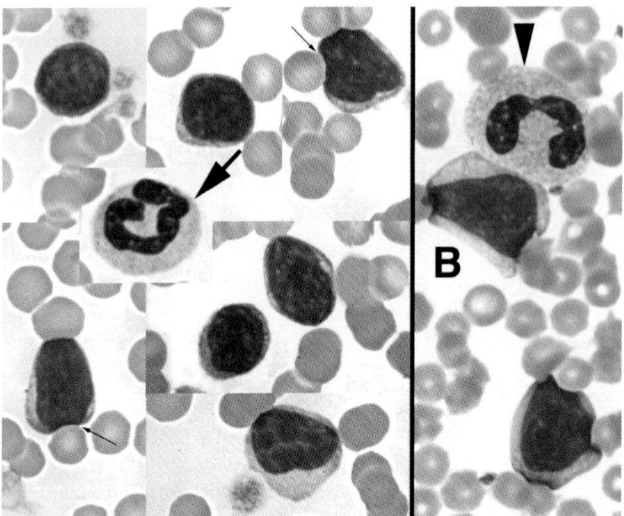

Figure 11.3 Variation in normal lymphocyte morphology in comparison to neutrophils. In the left panel, note that the lymphocyte nucleus may vary from round to oval. The cell shape, including the nucleus, may be indented by adjacent erythrocytes (thin arrows). The amount of cytoplasm varies from virtually none to a modest amount. Lymphocytes in most species have smaller diameter than adjacent neutrophils (thick arrow). An exception is indicated in the right panel: bovine lymphocytes (B) may be larger in diameter than lymphocytes of other common species and may have the same diameter as that of adjacent neutrophils (arrowhead). Note that the bovine neutrophil has slightly pink neutrophilic granules. Wright-Giemsa stain, high magnification.

(see Chapter 14). Such laboratories may provide special procedures for quantitation of certain subpopulations (e.g., B- and T-cell concentrations).

Lymphocytes are recognized by a round to oval nucleus and a minimal amount of clear, almost colorless cytoplasm. The amount of cytoplasm may be variable, as illustrated in Figure 11.3. Normal circulating lymphocytes have smaller diameters than those of neutrophils. In ruminants, lymphocytes may be more irregular in size and have diameters equal to those of neutrophils (Figure 11.3). Less common forms of lymphocytes include reactive lymphocytes and granular lymphocytes (Figure 11.4). Reactive forms likely are B cells capable of producing immunoglobulin. They have intensely basophilic cytoplasm, and the nucleus may be more irregularly shaped. In addition, the nucleus may have a cleft or an amoeboid shape. Large reactive lymphocytes are observed normally in juveniles of most species. Granular lymphocytes have a small number of pink-purple granules. These are large granular lymphocytes, some of which are thought to be natural killer or T cells. Large granular lymphocytes are most commonly observed in normal ruminant blood.

Monocytes

Monocytes also participate in inflammatory responses. Monocytes in blood are regarded as intermediate on a continuum of maturation. Monocytes migrate into tissues, where

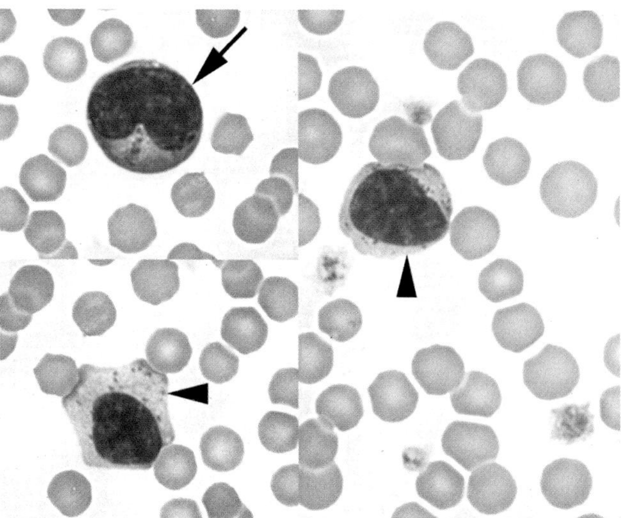

Figure 11.4 Variations in lymphocytes less commonly seen in blood. The reactive lymphocyte (arrow) is characterized by royal-blue cytoplasm. Its nuclear shape may be irregular, often with an indentation or cleft. Large granular lymphocytes (arrowheads) have an increased amount of light-staining cytoplasm, with a sparse sprinkling of azurophilic granules. The granules may vary in size. Large granular lymphocytes are most frequently seen in normal ruminants. Wright-Giemsa stain, high magnification.

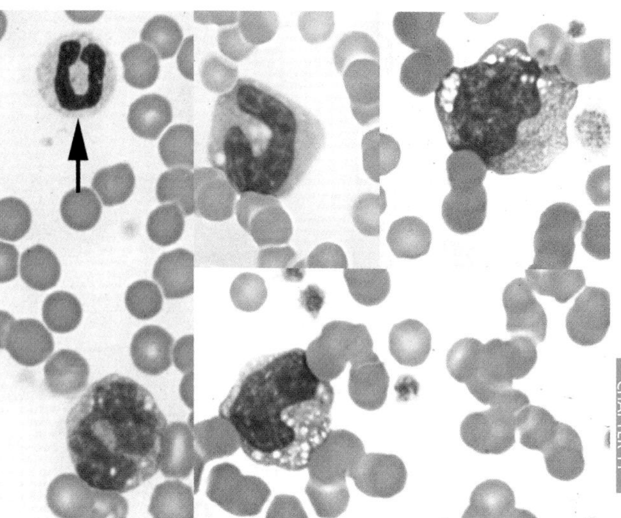

Figure 11.5 Variation in blood monocyte morphology; note the cells not marked by an arrow. Monocytes are typically larger than neutrophils (arrow). Monocytes may have cytoplasmic vacuoles, but this is not consistent. The monocyte nucleus is highly variable in shape: it may be round to bean-shaped to amoeboid-shaped, or it may be horseshoe-shaped and even segmented (like the nuclei of neutrophils). Inexperienced observers frequently confuse monocytes with horseshoe-shaped nuclei for neutrophils. The consistent features of monocytes are larger diameter than an adjacent neutrophil (arrow) and darker blue-gray cytoplasm compared with neutrophils. Wright-Giemsa stain, high magnification.

they continue to develop into macrophages. Mononuclear phagocytes may phagocytize bacteria, larger complex organisms (e.g., yeast and protozoa), injured cells, cellular debris, and foreign particulate debris. These cells play an important immunoregulatory function by presenting processed antigen to T lymphocytes. These cells are also responsible for normal erythrocyte destruction, associated metabolic iron recycling, and some mechanisms of pathologic erythrocyte destruction.

Monocytes are the most misidentified cell on blood films, particularly in the veterinary hospital laboratory. The nucleus may be of almost any shape, including oval-, bean-, ameboid-, or horseshoe-shaped (like that of neutrophils). The chromatin pattern may be slightly less condensed than that of neutrophils. The key distinguishing features are a larger diameter and more grayish coloration to the cytoplasm compared with adjacent neutrophils (Figure 11.5). The cytoplasm may contain extremely fine, light-purple granules. When uncertainty exists regarding monocyte identification, view at low power to make cell-to-cell comparisons (Figure 11.6). At low power, monocytes will stand out as larger cells. Species differences in monocyte morphology are not remarkable.

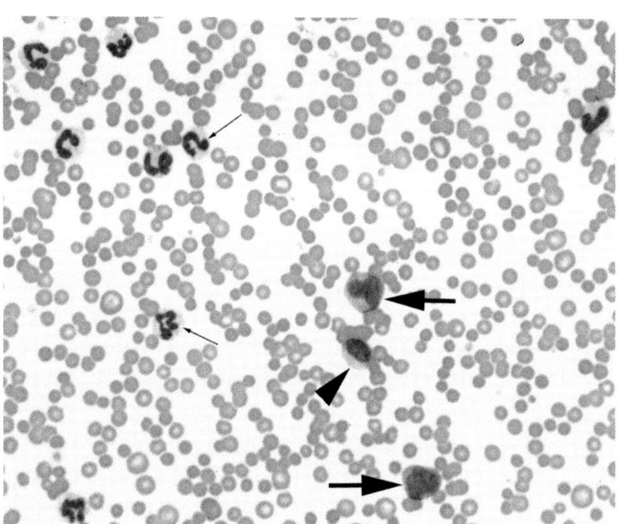

Figure 11.6 Low-magnification comparison of neutrophils and monocytes. When in doubt regarding identification of monocytes, use a lower magnification to make cell-to-cell comparisons that may be difficult at higher magnification. Note that the two monocytes (thick arrows) have larger diameters than the representative neutrophils indicated by thin arrows. A lymphocyte (arrowhead) is smaller than the adjacent neutrophils. Wright-Giemsa stain, low magnification.

Eosinophils

The functions of eosinophils are not well understood, even though a considerable number of studies and observations have been reported. Eosinophils contain proteins that bind to and damage parasite membranes, and they are responsible for providing a defense mechanism against larval

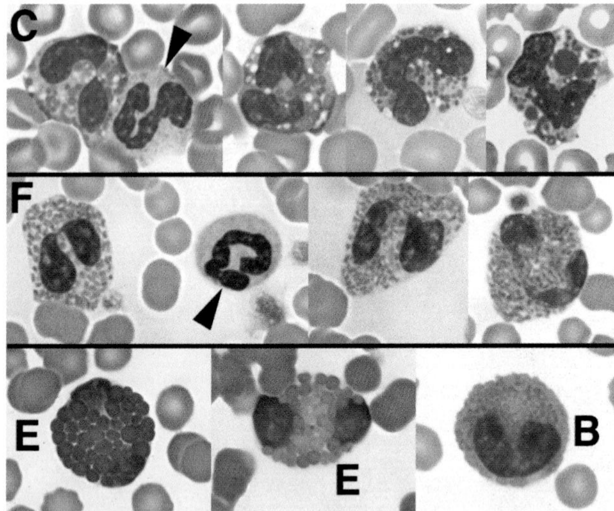

Figure 11.7 Species variation in eosinophil morphology. Representative neutrophils are shown for comparison (arrowheads). Eosinophils are typically larger in diameter than neutrophils. Canine eosinophils are shown in the top band (C). Note the variation in eosinophil granule size in dogs, which also may have eosinophil granules that appear to dissolve during the staining process, leaving a clear space that resembles a cytoplasmic vacuole. Feline eosinophils are shown in the middle band (F). Eosinophil granules of the cat are shaped like barrels or short rods. The density of the granularity may vary as shown. Large animal eosinophils are indicated in the bottom band. Equine eosinophils (E) have large, brightly staining granules that may obscure the nucleus, whereas bovine eosinophils (B) have smaller, brightly staining granules that are densely packed within the cytoplasm. Wright-Giemsa stain, high magnification.

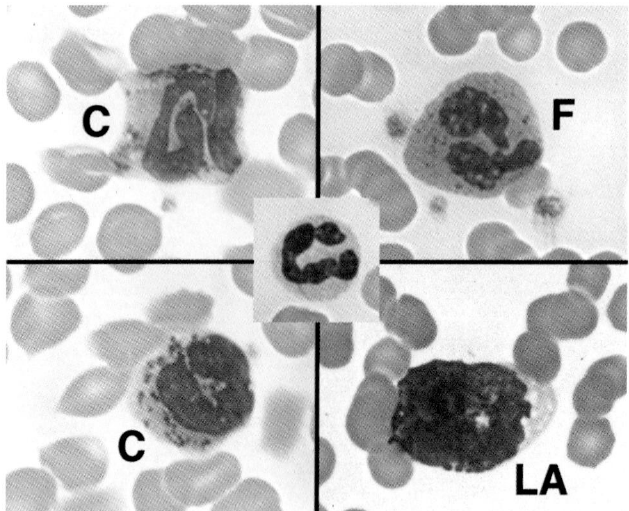

Figure 11.8 Species variation in basophil morphology. A representative neutrophil is shown in the center for comparison. Basophils are larger in diameter than neutrophils. Canine basophils (C) are poorly granulated. Note the sprinkling of basophilic granules in the cytoplasm. Feline basophils (F) have cytoplasm packed with large, poorly staining gray granules that are arranged like pavement stones. Large animal basophils (LA) have numerous dark-staining granules that often obscure the nucleus. Wright-Giemsa stain, high magnification.

stages of parasitic infestation. They are also involved in the modulation of allergic inflammation and immune-complex reactions.

Eosinophils vary in morphology among species (Figure 11.7). The nucleus is segmented (like that of neutrophils). The hallmark feature of eosinophils is prominent, red-orange granules that are tinctorially similar to erythrocytes. Canine eosinophils have highly variable granule size and number per cell. On rare occasions, a few large granules the size of erythrocytes may be present. Eosinophil granules also may wash out during the staining process, leaving what appears to be an empty vacuole; this observation is most pronounced in greyhound dogs. Feline eosinophils are densely packed, with uniform, rod- or barrel-shaped granules. Equine eosinophils have a raspberry appearance because of numerous round, large granules that may obscure the nucleus. Ruminant eosinophils have uniform, numerous round granules.

Basophils

The function of basophils is, basically, unknown. Basophils contain histamine and heparin. The cytoplasmic membrane has bound immunoglobulin E, like mast cells; however, their pathophysiologic role in the circulation is unknown. No convincing evidence has been reported that blood basophils migrate into tissues and become tissue mast cells. Concentrations of basophils in the circulation are very low, and they usually are not encountered in the routine differential count.

Basophils are larger in diameter than neutrophils. The nucleus is segmented (like those of other granulocytes). The granule morphology varies among species (Figure 11.8). Dogs have a small number of dark-violet granules. Cats have large, faint-gray granules that form a pavement-stone arrangement. Large animal basophils are packed with dark-violet granules that are so numerous they often obscure portions of the nucleus.

Reference values: the normal leukogram

The approach to interpretation of the leukogram involves a series of steps to arrive at a conclusion regarding what is normal or abnormal. Interpretive attention should focus only on the absolute values within the differential count data (see Chapter 1). When examining the hematology report, one should look first at the total leukocyte concentration. The total leukocyte concentration is only used to calculate absolute differential concentrations; it is not directly interpreted. For interpretation purposes, the total concentration only provides some gross guidance for what to anticipate when interpreting the differential concentrations. If the total count is decreased, examine the absolute concentration of each

Table 11.1 Reference intervals for absolute leukocyte concentrations of common domestic animal species.

Leukocyte	Dog	Cat	Horse	Cow	Sheep	Pig
Total WBC (cells/μL)	6 000–17 000	5 500–19 500	5 500–12 500	4 000–12 000	4 000–12 000	11 000–22 000
Differential WBC: band neutrophils (cells/μL)	0–300	0–300	0–100	0–100	0–100	0–800
Segmented neutrophils (cells/μL)	3000–11,500	2500–12,500	2700–6700	600–4000	700–6000	3200–10,000
Lymphocytes (cells/μL)	1000–5000	1500–7000	1500–5500	2500–7000	2000–9000	4500–13,000
Monocytes (cells/μL)	0–1200	0–800	0–800	0–800	0–800	200–2000
Eosinophils (cells/μL)	100–1200	0–1500	0–900	0–2400	0–1000	100–2000
Basophils (cells/μL)	Rare, 0–100	Rare, 0–100	0–200	0–200	0–300	0–400

WBC, white blood cell.

cell type to determine which are deficient. If the total count is increased, examine the absolute concentration of each cell type to determine which are present in excess. Even if the total concentration is normal, examine the absolute concentration of each cell type to determine if any abnormalities in distribution are present. Identified abnormalities in the absolute concentrations of individual leukocyte types are then interpreted into processes (see Chapter 13).

Reference values are given in Table 11.1. These values are patterned after general guidelines that have been used for decades (from the original work of Schalm) and are similar to those used by most veterinary laboratories. A more comprehensive, population-based set of reference intervals generated by newer technology for automated cell counting is needed. This has been done in some teaching hospital laboratories for specific automated systems used in the respective settings. Improved precision of automated cell counting as well as improved procedures for statistical analysis may provide more useful interpretive guidelines in the future.

The clinician interprets leukocyte abnormalities by learning to examine the individual differential leukocyte concentrations and then noting any morphologic abnormalities or abnormal cell types present that should not be present in normal blood. Differential leukocyte concentrations are reported in cells per microliter for each cell type. Abnormal nucleated cells include blasts, nucleated erythrocytes, mast cells, and immature granulocytes. Morphologic abnormalities include inherited and transiently acquired morphologic changes. Abnormal morphology is presented in Chapter 13.

12 Neutrophil Production, Trafficking, and Kinetics

Glade Weiser
Loveland, CO, USA

CHAPTER 12

General trends regarding the trafficking and kinetics of neutrophils in blood have been observed. Although species differences are not well studied, there are notable kinetic differences that affect interpretation of concentration changes in response to inflammatory disease. It is important to appreciate that rapid and dramatic changes in blood neutrophil concentration can occur. An understanding of neutrophil production and kinetic behaviors is useful to interpret the timing of responses to disease and the possible sequential changes between hemograms.

Production of granulocytes

Neutrophils are produced almost exclusively in the active bone marrow of healthy, adult domestic animals. Some production may be found in extramedullary sites, most notably the spleen, in juvenile animals. With long-standing increased demand for neutrophils (e.g., in chronic inflammatory disease), extramedullary production may be observed in adult animals. This will be most prominent in the spleen, but it may also be seen in the liver and lymph nodes in extreme cases.

Neutrophils originate from the pluripotential stem cell system, which gives rise to a more differentiated stem cell that has the capacity to create granulocytes and monocytes (GM stem cells). A subpopulation of these GM stem cells enters a pathway of committed differentiation of blood granulocytes, consisting of neutrophils, eosinophils, and basophils. The stem cells are not morphologically distinct, because they are present in small numbers and are probably morphologically indistinguishable from small lymphocytes. Once a cell makes this entry commitment, it undergoes both proliferative and maturational events to propagate blood granulocytes. These proliferative and maturational events are associated with morphologically recognized stages of granulocytes. Recognition of the general progression of these stages is important in the evaluation of bone marrow samples and the identification of cells in blood in response to disease. The morphologic stages of granulocytes are indicated in Figure 12.1.

The myeloblast is the first recognizable cell that is committed to granulocyte production. Myeloblasts are difficult to distinguish morphologically from primitive blasts of other cell lineages. Once committed, the myeloblast produces primary (i.e., azurophilic) granules, the presence of which identifies the progranulocyte stage. At subsequent stages of maturation, the primary granules change their staining character and become indistinguishable in conventional blood stains. In the next stage, the myelocyte begins to produce secondary (i.e., specific) granules that identify whether the cell will be a neutrophil, eosinophil, or basophil. Historically, the naming of the specific granules and the cell type has related to the dye component of the polychrome blood stains taken up by the specific granule. Neutrophil granules have neutral staining affinity; because of poor dye affinity, the granules are very faint or not visible. Eosinophil granules have an affinity for the orange-red dye and stain intensely orange-red. Basophil granules have affinity for basic dyes and stain intensely dark violet. Myeloblasts, progranulocytes, and myelocytes have the ability to undergo cell division as well as to mature from one stage to the next. These stages are relatively rich in ribosomes, giving the cytoplasm a bluish tint. Nuclear features include round to oval shape and relatively fine chromatin pattern.

More mature stages are characterized by the loss of ability to undergo cell division and include metamyelocytes, bands, and segmented granulocytes. Maturation consists mostly of progressive nuclear condensation and change in nuclear shape. The cytoplasm loses most or all of its bluish tint as the ribosome content decreases. The metamyelocyte has a nucleus that has developed an indentation. The band cell nucleus forms a horseshoe shape and has smooth, parallel

Veterinary Hematology, Clinical Chemistry, and Cytology, Third Edition. Edited by Mary Anna Thrall, Glade Weiser, Robin W. Allison and Terry W. Campbell.

Companion website: www.wiley.com/go/thrall/veterinary

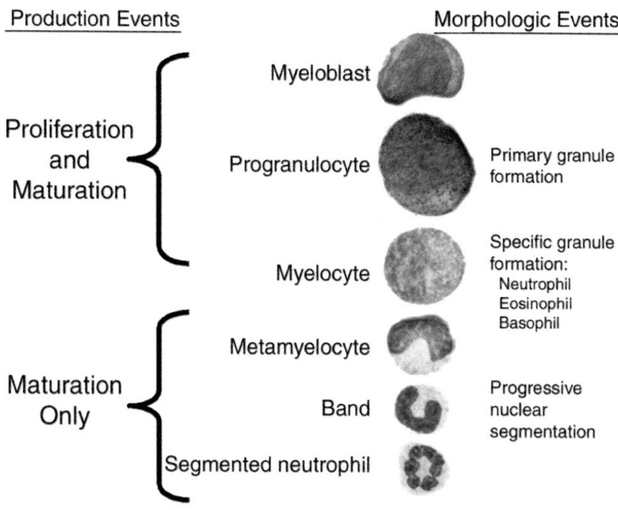

Figure 12.1 Morphologic features of stages of neutrophil maturation. Six morphologic stages are identified on a continuum of maturation, as indicated by the named cells. Cells capable of both cell division and maturation are at the top; cells capable of maturation only are at the bottom. Major changes associated with maturation are indicated on the right. (See text for a more complete description.)

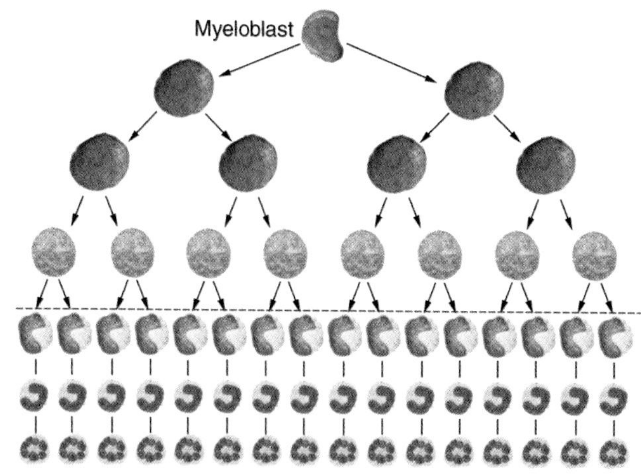

Figure 12.2 Orderly production of neutrophils in bone marrow. Note the progressive increase in relative cell numbers as maturation progresses. The myeloblast may give rise to approximately 16–32 cells before proliferative ability is lost. Cell stages above the dashed line are capable of cell division; cell stages below the dashed line are only capable of maturation. Please refer to Figure 12.1 for reference to cell stages.

nuclear membranes. The segmented or mature neutrophil progressively develops indentations or constrictions in the nuclear membrane. The progressive nuclear condensation results in a coarser chromatin with a darker, irregular staining pattern. See Chapter 11.

Maturation and orderly production

Production normally results in a progressive increase in the relative numbers of more mature stages, as indicated in Figure 12.2. This results from the combined events of proliferating early forms, which amplify both the number of cells and the progress toward more mature stages. In the process, each myeloblast may produce approximately 16–32 segmented neutrophils. The pattern of production seen in the marrow is a mixture of a relatively small number of primitive cells, a larger number of intermediate stages, and even more numerous later mature stages. This progression of a few immature cells to many more mature cells is described as orderly production. Both normal production and accelerated production in response to increased granulocyte demand have this orderly appearance. Cells are also delivered to the blood in this orderly fashion (see the discussion of left shift in Chapter 13). Disorderly production is characterized by a disproportionate relative number of primitive forms and a relative decrease or absence of more mature forms. Disorderly production is one of the features used to identify certain pathologic patterns (e.g., myeloproliferative disorders).

Neutrophil pools and trafficking

To understand neutrophil responses in disease, it is helpful to visualize a set of compartments and pools consisting of bone marrow, blood, and tissues, as depicted in Figure 12.3. The bone marrow compartment may be conceptually divided into a stem cell pool, a proliferative pool, and a maturation and storage pool. The proliferative pool consists of neutrophils at stages during which they still have the ability to undergo cell division and is largely responsible for the amplification of cell numbers. The maturation and storage pool consists of cells having lost the ability to divide and that are completing morphologic maturation. These cells may accumulate to create a modest storage reserve that is variable in size, which depends on the species. The storage capacity is greatest in dogs, least in ruminants, and intermediate in cats and horses.

Neutrophils make a unidirectional migration to the blood compartment, which is divided into the circulating and margination pools. The circulating pool is located in large vessels in which no interaction normally occurs between neutrophils and the endothelial lining of the vessel. Blood samples taken by venipuncture are from the circulating pool. The margination pool consists of the microcirculation. Cells may move bidirectionally between the circulating and margination pools. Neutrophils interact with the endothelial lining of small vessels and capillaries by their property of stickiness. Neutrophils may then unidirectionally migrate into adjacent tissue spaces (i.e., the tissue compartment). It is in the tissue compartment that neutrophils participate in their host-defense purposes.

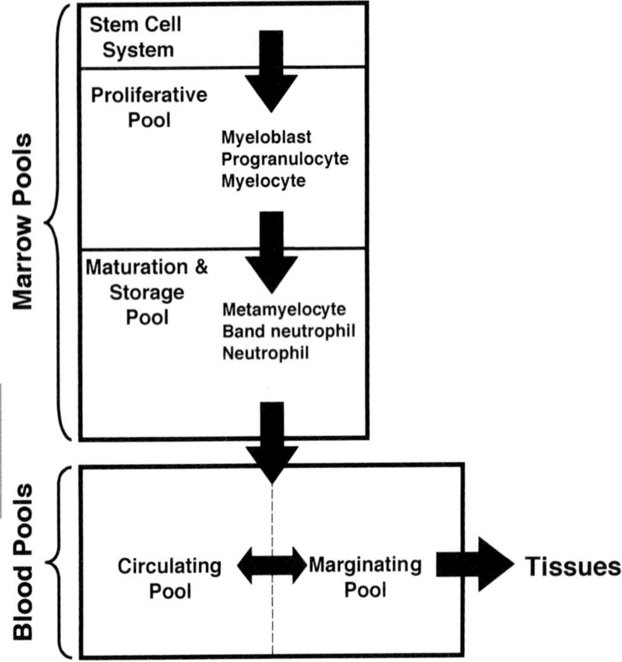

Figure 12.3 Bone marrow and blood neutrophil pools. Single arrows indicate unidirectional movement of cells; double arrow indicates bidirectional movement of cells. (See text for description of various compartments and progress through them.)

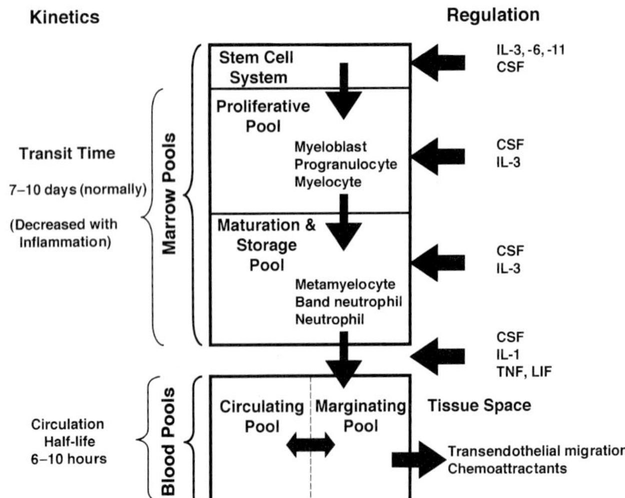

Figure 12.4 Bone marrow and blood neutrophil pools. Kinetic information is given on the left and regulation information on the right. Neutrophil production is regulated by a concert of growth factors and cytokines that act at multiple sites. The transit time is normally 7–10 days but may be shortened with increased demand. The circulation half-life is approximately 6–10 hours.

All neutrophil responses in disease may be understood as being mechanisms and disturbances occurring in this set of pools. They are discussed in detail in Chapter 13.

Growth factors and regulation of production and blood concentration

In health, the concentration of neutrophils in the blood is regulated to stay within a relatively narrow concentration range compared with the range that is possible in disease. Regulation of production is mediated by a complicated set of cytokines and growth factors, a simplified version of which is shown in Figure 12.4. The family of cytokines and growth factors depicted in Figure 12.4 work in concert at various stages to regulate neutrophil production. Colony-stimulating factor (CSF) is a group of characterized molecules; most notable are granulocyte-CSF and GM-CSF. These factors originate from numerous and diverse sites, including mononuclear cells, endothelium, fibroblasts, and other cell types. Mononuclear cells at sites of inflammation are probably the most important source of CSF and may modulate the release of CSFs from the other cell types. Interleukins (ILs) also participate in stimulation of production. The release of neutrophils from the marrow space to blood may be accelerated by IL-1, tumor necrosis factor (TNF), and leukocytosis-inducing factor (LIF). Because of variation in experimental conditions and methods, LIF may be the same as IL-1 and TNF.

In the normal steady state, production is balanced by the transendothelial migration of neutrophils into tissues. This balance yields blood neutrophil concentrations in the normal range. Increased levels of growth factors and cytokines are responsible for marked acceleration of the events to produce neutrophils in response to inflammation. This may result in a dramatic increase in neutrophil production and delivery to blood. Migration into the site of inflammation is accelerated and focused by chemoattractants that are released in the inflammatory lesion. The net result is an increase in the flux of neutrophils from the bone marrow to the inflammatory lesion. After resolution of the inflammatory lesion, blood neutrophil concentrations return to normal over a period of time likely measured in days. This suggests the presence of some negative-feedback mechanism, but its nature is currently unknown.

Neutrophil kinetics

Some basic information about the kinetics of neutrophils in various pools is helpful in the interpretation of sequential changes in the leukogram. The transit time for production and the circulation time in blood are the two key benchmarks for neutrophil kinetics.

The transit time is the amount of time needed for the myeloblast to complete the maturational events and become a segmented neutrophil in blood (see Figure 12.4). In the normal steady state, the transit time is approximately 7 days. When the bone marrow is stimulated by the inflammatory response, the transit time may become as short as 2–3 days.

The circulation time is the amount of time between release of the neutrophil to the blood and its subsequent egress into tissues. Neutrophils randomly migrate into tissues, so their circulation time is variable and not related to cell age. The circulation time is approximately 6–10 hours, encompassing some species variation. This means that the blood neutrophil pools are renewed approximately 2–3 times per day. The circulation time may be shortened considerably when neutrophils are consumed at a more rapid rate (e.g., at a site of inflammation). Given the rapid rate of blood neutrophil renewal in blood, marked changes in the blood neutrophil concentration may occur very rapidly in response to disease. The magnitude of these changes in the cell concentration that may be observed on hemograms sampled only hours apart is often dramatic and surprising. Application of neutrophil kinetics and trafficking knowledge is important and further developed in principles of leukocyte response interpretations in Chapter 13.

13 Interpretation of Leukocyte Responses in Disease

Glade Weiser
Loveland, CO, USA

CHAPTER 13

To communicate about leukocyte responses, one must first become familiar with the descriptive terminology associated with abnormal patterns of cell concentrations in blood. To identify and interpret leukocyte responses, the rules for interpreting abnormal concentration patterns as indicators of disease processes must be learned. This chapter presents terminology, abnormal morphologic features encountered in the laboratory, and guidelines for interpretation of leukocyte patterns.

Terminology of abnormal leukocyte concentration patterns

Suffixes

Abnormal concentrations are described using a variety of suffixes attached to the name of the cell type(s) involved.

The suffix -penia refers to a decreased concentration of the cell type in blood. A general term, cytopenia, refers to a decrease in leukocyte concentration in a nonspecific manner. Cytopenias that are important for interpretation include neutropenia, lymphopenia, and eosinopenia. Cytopenia does not apply to monocytes, because a decreased concentration of this cell type is not important. It also does not apply to band neutrophils, metamyelocytes, basophils, metarubricytes, and other abnormal cells because the absence of these cells in blood is normal.

The suffixes -philia or -cytosis refer to an increased concentration of the cell type in blood. Examples include:

- Neutrophilia or neutrophilic leukocytosis
- Eosinophilia
- Basophilia
- Monocytosis
- Lymphocytosis
- Metarubricytosis.

Left shift

Left shift refers to an increased concentration of immature neutrophils in blood. This usually indicates band neutrophils, but metamyelocytes and earlier forms may accompany increased bands. (See Figure 11.1 for neutrophil and left-shift morphology.) A left shift may occur with neutrophilia. A left shift also may occur with neutropenia; this indicates a more severe consumption of neutrophils by a more aggressive inflammatory lesion or an early repopulation of blood following a reversible stem cell injury. An orderly left shift suggests an inflammatory stimulus; in this case, the term orderly means that the concentration of each cell stage decreases with the degree of immaturity of the cell stage.

Leukemia

Leukemia refers to the presence of neoplastic cells in the circulation. The neoplastic cell type that is present more specifically designates the classification of the leukemia present. The classification may be determined by a combination of cell population morphologic differentiation features seen on the blood film, surface marker cytometry panels, and immunocytochemistry reactions (see Chapter 14). Examples include myelomonocytic leukemia and lymphocytic leukemia. The concentration of neoplastic cells may vary from detectable on blood film scanning to extremely high.

Proliferative disorder

Proliferative disorder is a nonspecific term for a hematopoietic cell neoplasm that is distributed in blood, bone marrow, other tissues, or a combination of these and other sites. Proliferative disorders are classified into lymphoproliferative and myeloproliferative categories. The distinction between the lymphoid and bone marrow stem cell systems is somewhat artificial, but these two classes of proliferative disorders

Veterinary Hematology, Clinical Chemistry, and Cytology, Third Edition. Edited by Mary Anna Thrall, Glade Weiser, Robin W. Allison and Terry W. Campbell.

Companion website: www.wiley.com/go/thrall/veterinary

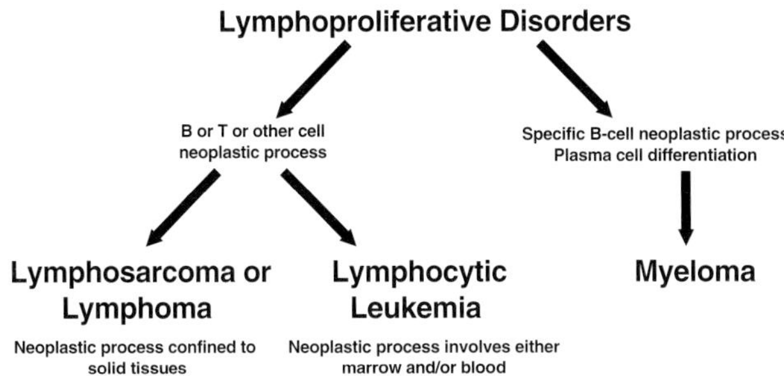

Figure 13.1 Organization and general terminology for lymphoproliferative disorders. See text for discussion.

have different biologic behavior, case management protocols, and prognosis. Proliferative disorders are discussed separately in Chapters 15 and 16.

Lymphoproliferative disorders

Lymphoproliferative disorders, which are characterized in Figure 13.1, are neoplastic processes with lymphoid cell differentiation. If the neoplasm is confined to solid tissues, it is termed lymphosarcoma or lymphoma. If it involves blood and/or bone marrow, it is termed lymphocytic leukemia. A specific form with plasma cell differentiation is termed myeloma, which is usually associated with production of a monoclonal immunoglobulin that may be detected in blood. Immunoglobulin light chains also may be detected in urine. More extensive and detailed classifications of lymphoproliferative disorders based on cellular morphology and immunophenotyping are available (see Chapters 14–16 and "Suggested Reading").

Myeloproliferative disorders

Myeloproliferative disorders arise from the bone marrow stem cell system. More extensive and detailed classifications of myeloproliferative disorders based on cellular morphology and surface markers are available (see Chapters 14–16 and "Suggested Reading"). The recognized lines of differentiation and associated terminology for specific myeloproliferative disorders are detailed in Figure 13.2. Note that more differentiation pathways are recognized for myeloproliferative disorders than for lymphoproliferative disorders. Granulocytic, monocytic, and erythroid differentiations are the most common myeloproliferative disorders; the others are rare.

In recent years, it has become apparent that confirmation of lymphoproliferative disorders or identification of cell lineage in proliferative disorders is limited with morphology. Occasionally, the distinction between reactive and neoplastic lymphoid proliferation is difficult. Primitive blasts having no specific differentiating morphologic features may be difficult to impossible to classify by morphology alone.

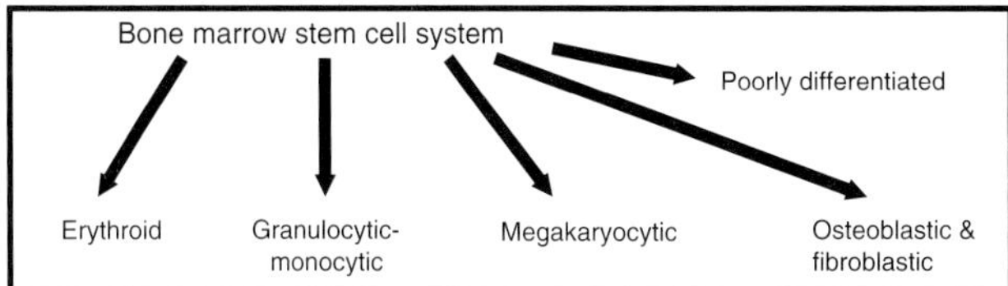

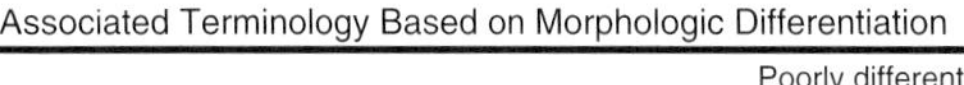

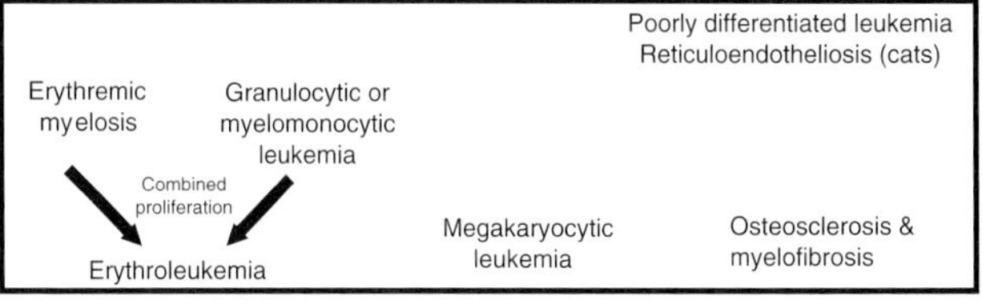

Figure 13.2 Organization and general terminology for myeloproliferative disorders. The top box shows general differentiation pathways based on morphologically recognized cell lineages. The bottom box shows historical and commonly applied terminology for the myeloproliferative disorders based on morphologic identity. See text for discussion.

These are often called lymphoid on initial examination. It has been learned that lymphoid, monocytic, granulocytic, and megakaryocytic blasts can be morphologically indistinguishable. Immunocytochemistry and flow cytometry are now used to identify cell lineage when it is important for treatment considerations. These procedures use panels of chemistry reactions and/or antibody labeling to identify either cytoplasmic activities or surface markers to aid in classification. Furthermore, these tools may be used to determine lymphocytic subpopulation identification. This is the subject of Chapter 14.

Acquired changes in leukocyte morphology

Neutrophil toxic change

Neutrophil toxic change may be observed in association with inflammatory responses. The term toxic change is unfortunate, because it originated from early observations that these alterations in cell morphology were associated with toxemia in human patients. The term implies that the cells are injured or impaired. We now understand that the morphologic change is attributable to altered bone marrow production and that the cells have normal function. When an inflammatory stimulus is delivered to the bone marrow (see Figure 12.4), neutrophils are produced at an accelerated rate. As a result, the cells may have increased amounts of certain organelles that are present during early development. The principal manifestation is cytoplasmic basophilia (Figure 13.3). This is attributable to a larger-than-normal

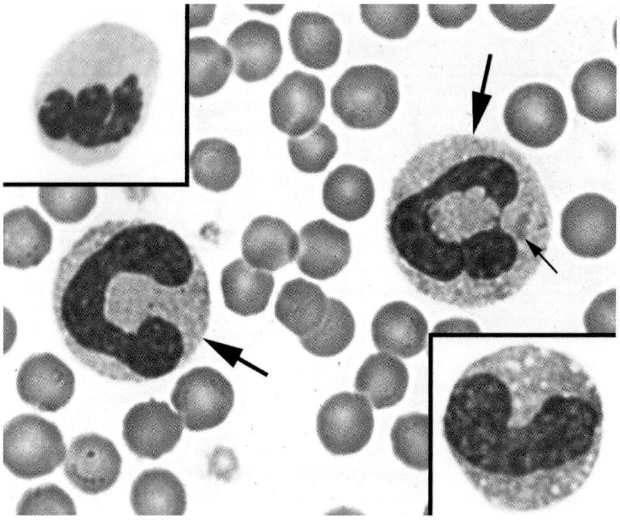

Figure 13.3 Neutrophils with marked toxic change (arrows). Note prominent cytoplasmic basophilia. A Döhle body is indicated by the thin arrow. A toxic neutrophil with fine cytoplasmic vacuolation is shown in the lower right inset. For comparison, a normal neutrophil is shown in the upper left inset. Wright-Giemsa stain, high magnification.

complement of ribosomes. Other, less common manifestations accompanying cytoplasmic basophilia include Döhle bodies and cytoplasmic vacuolation. Döhle bodies are aggregates of endoplasmic reticulum and appear as gray-blue cytoplasmic precipitates. Döhle bodies are seen more commonly in cats (Figure 13.3).

The interpretation of toxic change is that neutrophils are made under conditions of accelerated production that occurs as part of the inflammatory response. As a result, toxic change often accompanies other quantitative changes in the inflammatory leukogram presented later in this chapter.

Neutrophil hypersegmentation

Neutrophil hypersegmentation is the normal progression of nuclear maturation in the neutrophil. The progression from band shape to segmentation to hypersegmentation is a continuum that occurs in a matter of hours. Normally, the process of continued segmentation and, finally, pyknosis occurs in neutrophils after egression to tissues. Hypersegmentation observed on the blood film results from longer than normal retention of neutrophils in the circulation (Figure 13.4). The interpretation of hypersegmentation is relatively unimportant (it is usually associated with steroid effect on the leukogram presented in this chapter).

Neutrophil degeneration

Neutrophil degeneration is a description ordinarily applied to neutrophils from samples other than blood (e.g., cytopathologic specimens). Neutrophils exposed to an unhealthy environment outside of blood may rapidly degenerate. This is accelerated in cytopathologic specimens, which

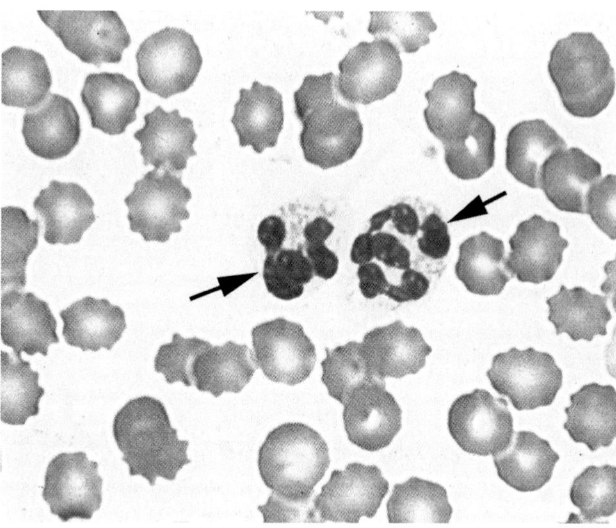

Figure 13.4 Neutrophils with hypersegmentation (arrows). Note the nuclear constrictions to a filament of chromatin that separates approximately 5–7 chromatin lobes. Wright-Giemsa stain, high magnification.

either have a bacterial component or are from epithelial surfaces such as skin, airways, or the gastrointestinal tract (Figure 13.5). Features include cytoplasmic vacuolation and nuclear swelling seen as a loss of chromatin pattern and light staining. These changes may progress to cell lysis. It

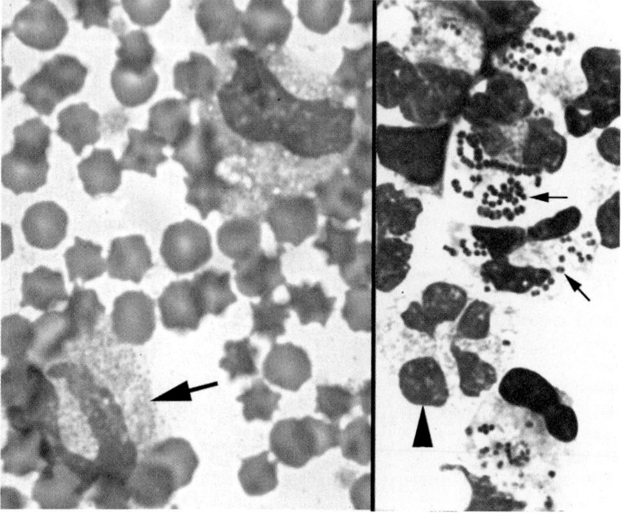

Figure 13.5 Neutrophil degeneration. The left panel shows neutrophil (arrow) degeneration on a blood film that is an artifact of aging in the collection tube before blood-film preparation. Note the swollen chromatin that results in lighter staining and loss of chromatin detail. The right panel shows neutrophils in various stages of degeneration in a cytologic preparation. This results from an unhealthy environment that is created, in part, by numerous bacteria (thin arrows). A neutrophil with chromatin swelling and loss of detail is indicated by the arrowhead. Wright-Giemsa stain, high magnification.

is an artifact in blood seen on the blood film if that film is made from blood that has aged for 12 hours or longer after collection from the animal (Figure 13.5). In blood, it therefore is interpreted as an artifact of improper sample handling.

Leukocyte agglutination

Leukocyte agglutination is an immunoglobulin-mediated agglutination of leukocytes *in vitro*. It may affect either neutrophils or lymphocytes. This phenomenon does not occur in the animal at body temperature, and it likely has no pathologic consequence *in vivo*. It is thought to be attributable to a cold-reacting immunoglobulin that acts at temperatures well below body temperature. When the blood cools to room temperature or below, this abnormal immunoglobulin binds to its leukocyte target and bridges cells into agglutinated particles. It therefore occurs in the blood tube after collection from the patient. Its importance is that it may result in a falsely low total white-blood-cell concentration, because agglutinated leukocytes may not be counted properly by instruments. It is observed on scanning the blood film (Figure 13.6).

Lymphocyte vacuolation

Lymphocyte vacuolation may be an acquired change associated with ingestion of certain plants containing the toxic substance swainsonine. An example is locoweed ingestion in horses or cattle. The appearance is similar to that of lymphocyte vacuolation associated with inherited storage disorders (discussed later; see Figure 13.11).

Inherited abnormalities of leukocyte morphology and function

Inherited abnormalities of neutrophil morphology and/or function

Inherited abnormalities of neutrophil morphology include Pelger-Huët anomaly, Birman cat neutrophil granulation anomaly, mucopolysaccharidoses, and Chédiak-Higashi syndrome.

Pelger-Huët anomaly

Mature, hyposegmented neutrophils are seen in heterozygotes for Pelger-Huët anomaly. These cells have an immaturely shaped nucleus (i.e., band or myelocyte form) but a coarse, mature chromatin pattern (Figure 13.7). Neutrophils function normally, and affected animals are healthy. Typically, no segmented neutrophils are seen in blood films from these animals. Eosinophils are also affected and appear as band forms. The importance of recognizing Pelger-Huët anomaly is to prevent misidentification of a major left shift and misinterpretation as an inflammatory response in an otherwise apparently healthy, affected individual.

Birman cat neutrophil granulation anomaly

Neutrophils from affected cats contain fine eosinophilic to magenta-colored granules (Figure 13.8). This anomaly is inherited in an autosomal recessive manner. Neutrophil function is normal, and cats are healthy. This granulation must be distinguished from toxic granulation, which is

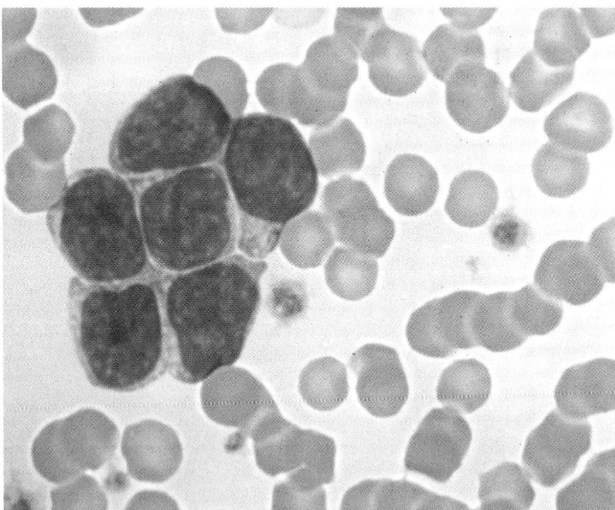

Figure 13.6 Leukoagglutination involving lymphocytes. Note the tight adherence of cells in a cluster. Multiple clusters are observable at low magnification. These cell clusters result in falsely low white-blood-cell counts when present in the counting fluid diluent (see text). Wright-Giemsa stain, high magnification.

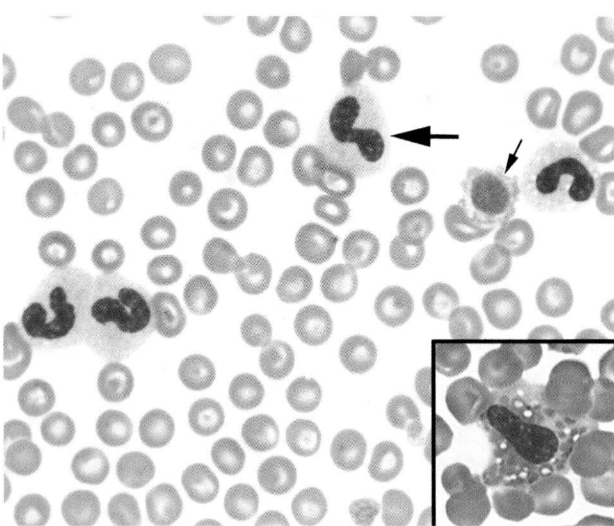

Figure 13.7 Granulocytes from a dog with Pelger-Huët anomaly. Four hyposegmented neutrophils (thick arrow) are present. The lower right inset shows a hyposegmented eosinophil. A macroplatelet, present by coincidence, is indicated by the thin arrow. Wright-Giemsa stain, high magnification.

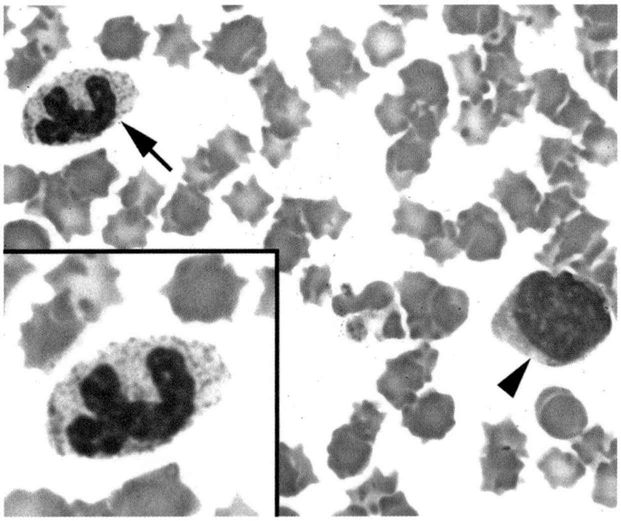

Figure 13.8 Granulated neutrophil from a cat with Birman cat neutrophil granulation anomaly (arrow). The lower left inset shows an enlarged view of the same cell. Note the fine granulation as compared with mucopolysaccharidosis (see Figure 13.9). Lymphocytes (arrowhead) are not affected. Wright-Giemsa stain, high magnification.

rare, and from that seen in neutrophils from cats with mucopolysaccharidosis (MPS), which usually is coarser.

Mucopolysaccharidoses

Neutrophils from animals with MPS typically contain numerous distinct, dark-purple or magenta-colored granules (Figure 13.9). Lymphocytes also usually contain granules and vacuoles.

MPS is a group of heritable, lysosomal storage disorders caused by a deficiency of lysosomal enzymes needed for the stepwise degradation of glycosaminoglycans (i.e., mucopolysaccharides). Common features include dwarfism (except feline MPS I), severe bone disease, degenerative joint disease including hip subluxation, facial dysmorphia, hepatomegaly (except feline MPS VI), corneal clouding, enlarged tongue (canine MPS), heart-valve thickening, excess urinary excretion of glycosaminoglycans, and metachromatic granules (i.e., Alder-Reilly bodies) in blood leukocytes. These granules are more distinct in MPS VI and VII than in MPS I. Granules usually are not apparent when stained with Diff-Quik. The disease is progressive, with clinical signs becoming apparent at 2–4 months of age. Affected animals may live several years, but locomotor difficulty is progressive.

Chédiak-Higashi syndrome

Neutrophils in cats affected by Chédiak-Higashi syndrome have large, fused, lysosomes that stain lightly pink or eosinophilic within the cytoplasm (Figure 13.10). Approximately one in three or four neutrophils contain one to four fused lysosomes. Eosinophilic granules appear slightly plump and large. These cats have a slight tendency to bleed, because platelet function is abnormal. Although neutrophil function is also abnormal, cats are generally healthy. The syndrome has been reported in cats of Persian ancestry and is inherited in an autosomal recessive manner.

Bovine leukocyte adhesion deficiency (BLAD)

Bovine leukocyte adhesion deficiency is a lethal, autosomal recessive disorder identified in Holstein cattle. The defect is

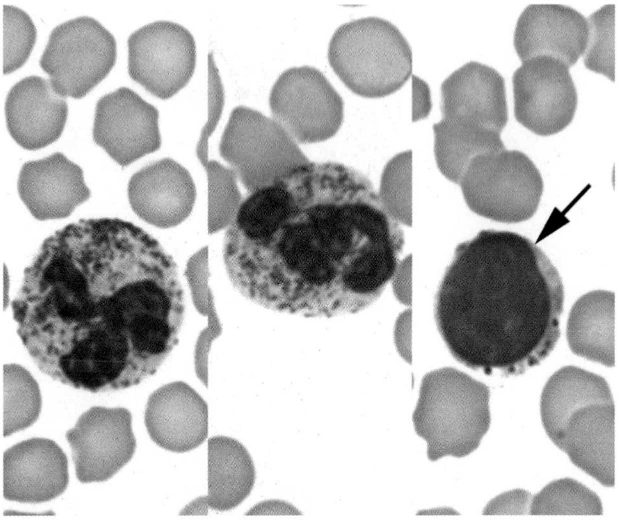

Figure 13.9 Granulated leukocytes from a cat with mucopolysaccharidosis VI. Note the prominently granulated neutrophils at the left and center. A lymphocyte with sparse granulation is typical of mucopolysaccharidosis (arrow). Wright-Giemsa stain, high magnification.

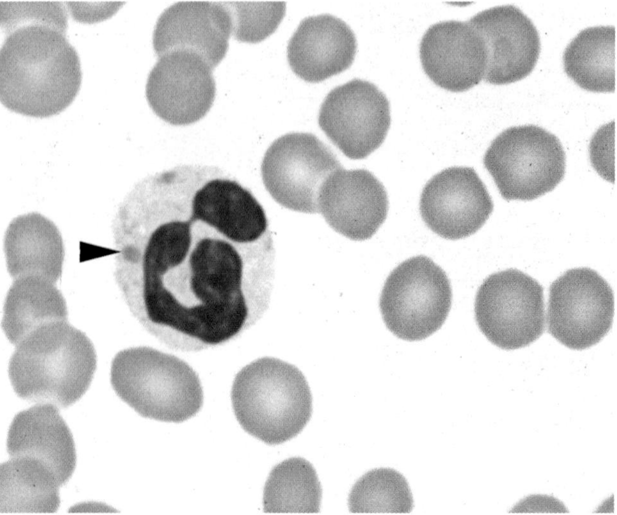

Figure 13.10 Neutrophil from a cat with Chédiak-Higashi syndrome. Note the large eosinophilic granule in the cytoplasm (arrowhead). Wright-Giemsa stain, high magnification.

a mutation in the CD 18 gene. This results in neutrophils with a deficiency of beta-2 integrin surface molecules that are essential for normal leukocyte adherence and emigration into tissues; hence there is a functional defect. Clinical signs of "poor doing" appear at 1–2 weeks of age. Affected calves may appear stunted and have signs related to respiratory and gastrointestinal tracts. They are predisposed to recurring bacterial infections and typically do not live beyond 2–8 months of age. A hematologic feature is marked, persistent neutrophilia (often >100,000/µL) with no left shift. On examination of tissues, there are few neutrophils, except within vessel lumens, because they persist in the circulation and have impaired entry into the tissues. Testing is available to detect carriers. Incidence of the defect is decreasing due to testing for the carrier state and removal of carriers from breeding stock.

Inherited abnormalities of lymphocyte morphology

Cytoplasmic vacuolization is the most significant inherited abnormality of lymphocytes and usually is associated with lysosomal storage disorders (Figure 13.11). Those lysosomal storage diseases described in domestic animals that result in vacuoles within the cytoplasm of lymphocytes include MPS (also have granules in neutrophils); G_{M1} and G_{M2} gangliosidosis (G_{M2} gangliosidosis also has granules in lymphocytes and neutrophils) (Figure 13.12); alpha-mannosidosis; Niemann-Pick types A, B, and C; acid-lipase deficiency; and fucosidosis. All these disorders, except for MPS and acid-lipase deficiency, result in severe, progressive neurologic disease that is ultimately fatal.

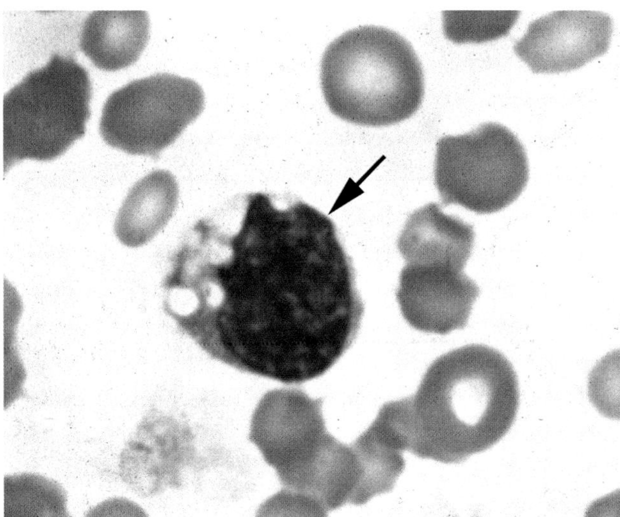

Figure 13.11 Cytoplasmic vacuolation of a lymphocyte (arrow) from a cat with a lysosomal storage disorder (alpha-mannosidosis). Wright-Giemsa stain, high magnification.

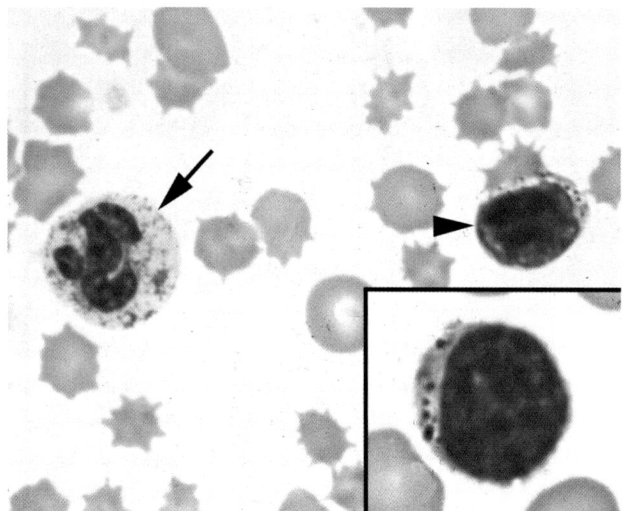

Figure 13.12 Leukocytes from a cat with G_{M2} gangliosidosis. Neutrophils (arrow) may have granulation similar to that seen with mucopolysaccharidosis. Lymphocytes (arrowhead) also have small numbers of granules with some degree of cytoplasmic vacuolation. The lower right inset shows an enlarged lymphocyte. Wright-Giemsa stain, high magnification.

Interpretation of leukocyte responses

Perspective

Most leukocyte response patterns are not interpreted into specific diagnoses, although leukemias may be an exception. Instead, responses are interpreted into basic processes occurring in the animal. These processes must then be coupled with other clinical information to work toward a clinical diagnosis.

Hematologic response to inflammation

Inflammation is the most important – and one of the most common – blood leukocyte responses. The nature of the response is best understood by considering a modified neutrophil trafficking model (Figure 13.13). It also may be helpful to review the steady-state neutrophil trafficking model in Chapter 12 (see Figure 12.3). When inflammation is established, an orchestra of chemical mediators modulates many events. Vasodilation and chemotactic substances work to increase the egress of neutrophils from the local marginated pool into the inflammatory lesion. Cytokines released from local mononuclear cells (see Figure 12.4) make their way to the bone marrow, where they increase the rate of release of maturing neutrophils and the rate of production by increasing stem cell entry, proliferative events, and maturation events. The net result is that the marrow response dramatically increases the delivery rate of neutrophils to blood. In summary, a complete cycle of consumption, production, and release is activated, with the goal

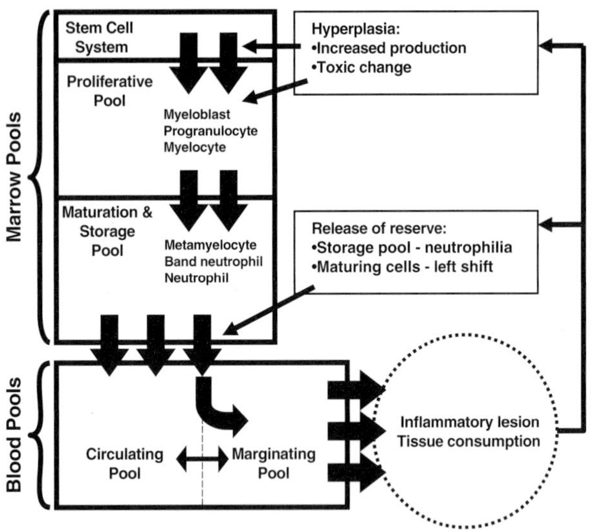

Figure 13.13 Modified neutrophil trafficking model illustrating effects of the inflammatory response on blood and bone marrow. Note the cycle of events leading to increased neutrophil delivery to blood and tissues at the inflammatory site: release of mediators from an inflammatory lesion, increased marrow hyperplasia, increased delivery from marrow to blood, and increased consumption at the site of inflammation.

of delivering a supply of neutrophils to the inflammatory lesion until it resolves.

The pattern of neutrophil concentrations seen in blood may vary from severely decreased to markedly increased. It is helpful to think of the pattern being dependent on a balance between consumption by the lesion and production and release by the marrow (Figure 13.14). This balance may

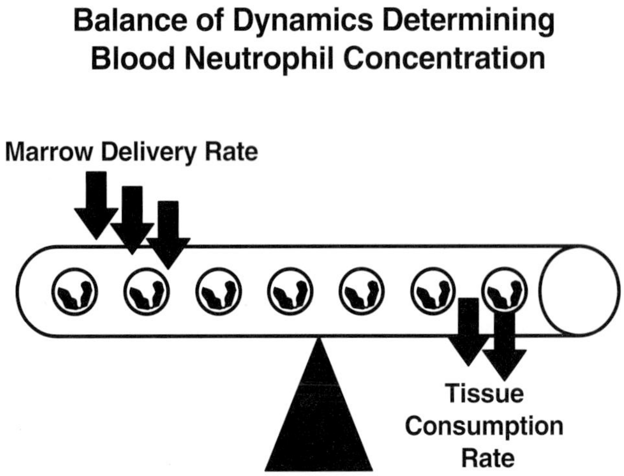

Balance of Dynamics Determining Blood Neutrophil Concentration

Marrow Delivery Rate

Tissue Consumption Rate

Figure 13.14 Balance between production and consumption. All inflammatory processes may be understood as a balance between marrow delivery and inflammatory-site consumption. When marrow delivery exceeds consumption, blood neutrophilia develops. When tissue consumption exceeds marrow delivery, neutropenia with a left shift develops.

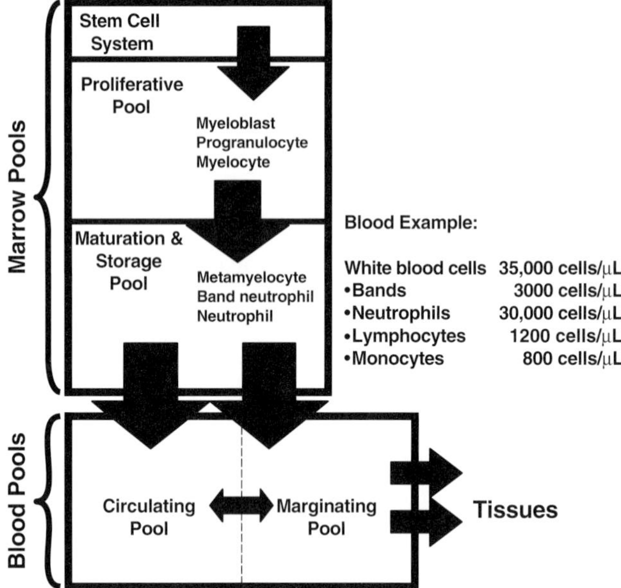

Figure 13.15 Modified neutrophil trafficking model used to illustrate a moderate inflammatory response. Also illustrated is an example of the balance between production and consumption. Note that in this case, marrow delivery exceeds tissue consumption. The example is described as leukocytosis caused by neutrophilia (30,000 cells/μL) and a left shift (3000 bands/μL). The neutrophil pattern is interpreted as inflammation.

explain all neutrophil concentration patterns encountered during inflammation. In small animals, most inflammatory processes result in some degree of neutrophilia, indicating that marrow releases more cells to blood than are consumed at the site of inflammation. This is illustrated using the neutrophil trafficking model in Figure 13.15. Inflammatory patterns manifesting in neutrophilia may be regarded as mild to severe responses that are managing the lesion. The severity of the process may be roughly predicted by the magnitude of the left shift and the presence of toxic change in neutrophils.

Very severe – and typically acute – inflammatory lesions, on the other hand, may consume neutrophils more rapidly than the neutrophils can be delivered to blood. When this occurs, neutropenia develops, as shown in the neutrophil trafficking model in Figure 13.16. In this case, a left shift is expected. At one or more time points, the concentration of bands and other left shift cells may be greater than that of segmented neutrophils.

The balance between neutrophil consumption and delivery by bone marrow is affected by species differences, as outlined in Table 13.1. Species may vary in the amount of neutrophil reserve and in the proliferative capacity of the marrow. Dogs have the largest reserve and the greatest ability to produce neutrophils; cows and other ruminants form the other extreme. Cats and horses are somewhat intermediate in their capacities to deliver cells to blood.

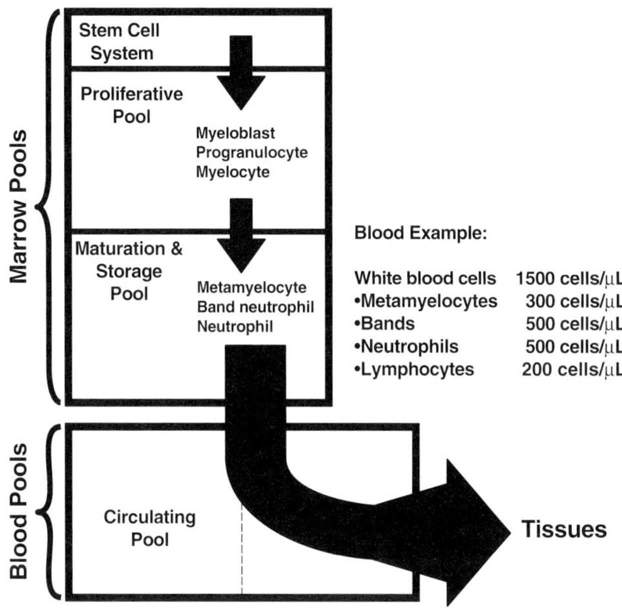

Figure 13.16 Modified neutrophil trafficking model used to illustrate a severe inflammatory response. Also illustrated is an example of the balance between production and consumption. Note that in this case, tissue consumption exceeds marrow delivery. The example is described as leukopenia caused by neutropenia (500 cells/μL) and a left shift (300 metamyelocytes/μL and 500 bands/μL). The neutrophil pattern is interpreted as severe, acute inflammation.

Table 13.1 Comparative bone marrow contribution to neutrophil trafficking and relationship to ranges of neutrophilia seen with the inflammatory response in various species.

Species	Marrow reserve	Regenerative capacity
Dog	Relatively high	Rapid
Cat	Intermediate	Intermediate
Horse	Intermediate	Intermediate
Cow	Relatively low	Slow
	Range of possible neutrophilia (neutrophils/μL)	
Dog	20,000–120,000	
Cat	20,000–60,000	
Horse	15,000–30,000	
Cow	10,000–25,000	
	Interpretation of neutropenia during acute inflammation	
Dog	Very severe lesion	
Cat	Very severe lesion	
Horse	Probable severe lesion	
Cow	Usual findings, regardless of severity	

These differences translate into magnitudes of neutrophilia that can occur with inflammatory disease in each species. They also influence how neutrophil concentrations are interpreted with respect to chronicity and severity of the process in various species. For example, in chronic, closed-cavity inflammatory processes, neutrophilia may go as high as 120,000 cells/μL in dogs, but a corresponding process in cows will result in a maximum of approximately 25,000 cells/μL. Cats and horses will be intermediate, as indicated in Table 13.1.

Similarly, bone marrow behavior influences how neutropenia is interpreted during acute inflammation. Because of the canine ability to deliver cells to blood, neutropenia only occurs with inflammatory states involving severe consumption. Neutropenia caused by inflammation may be regarded as a medical emergency in dogs; to some extent, this is also true in cats and horses. Neutropenia in cows is interpreted differently. Because of the minimal neutrophil reserve in this species, the expected response in the acute bovine inflammatory leukogram is neutropenia. Acute inflammatory lesions in cows consume neutrophils from the blood and marrow within a matter of hours. The result may be profound neutropenia that lasts for a few days. After that time, repopulation of blood with neutrophils, with a left shift, occurs as the marrow production increases.

Factors modulating the magnitude of neutrophilia in the inflammatory response

The type of inflammatory lesion may influence the balance between consumption and marrow release. Acute inflammation is a lesion with increased local blood flow and swelling. This results from inflammatory mediators that promote local vascular dilation. Chemotactic factors released within the lesion in conjunction with the vascular events have ample opportunity to promote consumption of neutrophils. An example is cellulitis associated with a bite wound, which results in a balance between consumption and production that is reasonably well matched. The blood inflammatory pattern then consists of mild to moderate neutrophilia with a variable left shift, depending on the severity of the lesion. Acute peritonitis due to gut rupture is an example of a major consumer of neutrophils that may exceed the marrow capacity for production; in this example, it is possible to see neutropenia with a prominent left shift.

Chronic, walled-off inflammatory lesions, on the other hand, may result in very high neutrophil concentrations. Examples include pyometra in dogs or a chronic, walled-off abscess that does not resolve. These are also known as closed-cavity inflammatory lesions (as opposed to diffuse inflammation; discussed above). These lesions continue to stimulate the marrow to achieve maximal production; however, the rate of consumption is curtailed by the nature of the lesion, thus tipping the balance toward production exceeding consumption. In these cases, neutrophil concentrations may approach 70,000–120,000 cells/μL in dogs.

Excitement response: epinephrine release

The excitement response is an immediate change associated with epinephrine release and is also known as the "fight-or-flight" response. Epinephrine release results in cardiovascular events that, in turn, result in increased blood flow through the microcirculation, particularly in muscle. Strenuous exercise just before bleeding may have the same effect. This results in a shift of leukocytes from the marginated pool to the circulating pool, as depicted in the neutrophil trafficking model (Figure 13.17). On the leukogram, this manifests as an approximate doubling of leukocytes and is noted in the neutrophils and/or lymphocytes. Within the neutrophil population, no left shift occurs, because mature cells in the microcirculation being flushed to the circulating pool cause the neutrophilia.

The excitement response is recognized most frequently in cats. Lymphocytosis up to a maximum of approximately 20,000 cells/μL is the prominent feature of the feline excitement response. Mature neutrophilia may occur if the resting neutrophil concentration was at the upper end of normal before initiation of the excitement response. In large animals, the excitement response is recognized in association with exercise before bleeding or events that may induce excitement, such as trucking or movement through chutes for blood collection. The excitement response is least common in dogs, because this species is usually accustomed to physical handling related to blood collection.

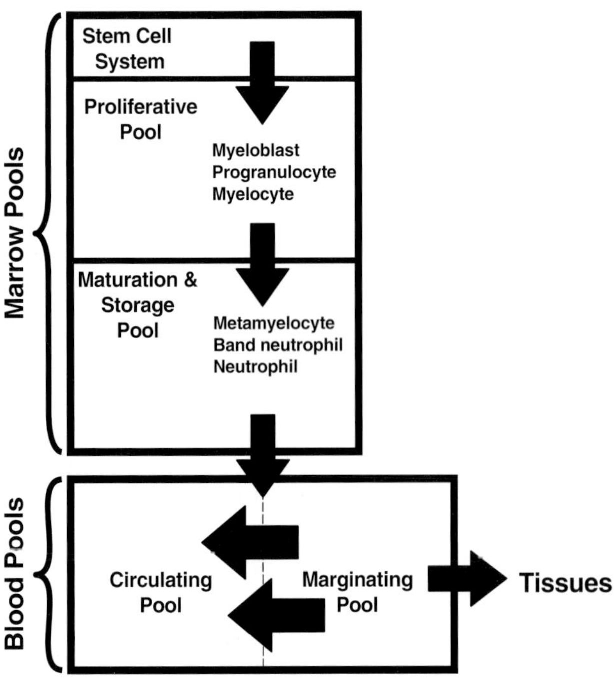

Figure 13.17 Modified neutrophil trafficking model used to illustrate the excitement response. Note that the change involves cell movement from the marginating pool to the circulating pool, resulting in an approximate doubling of resting leukocyte concentrations. Marrow delivery and tissue consumption are unchanged.

Stress response: corticosteroid release or administration

This is likely the most common leukocyte response. Physiologic stress is a body response mediated by release of adrenocorticotropic hormone by the pituitary gland and resultant release of cortisol by the adrenal gland. This occurs in response to major systemic illnesses, metabolic disturbances, and pain. Examples of conditions eliciting the stress response include renal failure, diabetic ketoacidosis, dehydration, inflammatory disease, and pain associated with trauma. The response may be detected in the leukogram by changes in multiple cell types.

The most consistent change is lymphopenia. Steroids may induce lymphocyte apoptosis and may alter patterns of recirculation. The second most consistent change is an approximate doubling of the circulating neutrophils. Steroids cause decreased stickiness and impaired margination, resulting in slightly longer than normal retention in the circulation. As a result, hypersegmentation may be observed. When the resting neutrophil concentration is in the upper 50th percentile of the normal range, neutrophilia is expected. A left shift will not occur unless inflammation is superimposed. Eosinopenia is the next most consistent change. Monocytosis is variable and occurs most consistently in dogs. The importance of interpreting the steroid leukogram is to look for an underlying physiologic disturbance (if it has not yet been recognized) and to avoid interpreting a simple steroid pattern as inflammation. An inflammatory condition may frequently cause a combined inflammatory and steroid response. The inflammatory component will take priority in determination of the magnitude of neutrophilia and any associated left shift. The steroid component may only be recognizable by the concurrent presence of lymphopenia.

Lastly, it is important to note that a steroid response not being present in a very sick animal should prompt the consideration of hypoadrenocorticism (i.e., Addison disease; see Chapter 33).

Summary: approach to neutrophilia

In summary, neutrophilia has three causes. Thus, it is useful to develop an orderly approach to looking at the leukogram to rapidly arrive at the proper interpretation of the neutrophilia. The flowchart in Figure 13.18 develops this approach. When neutrophilia is identified, one should next examine the leukogram for the presence of a left shift. If a left shift is present, the interpretation is inflammation. If a left shift is not present, the lymphocyte concentration should be examined. If lymphopenia is found with a neutrophilia and no left shift, the interpretation is steroid

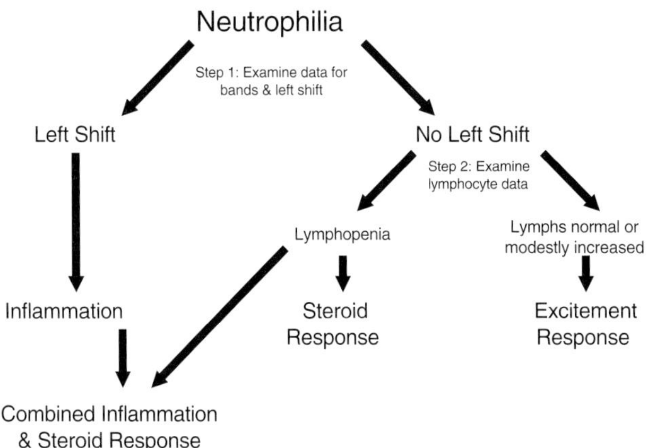

Figure 13.18 Summary flow chart for interpretation of neutrophilias. When neutrophilia is seen, the observer should examine the data for a left shift (step 1). If a left shift is present, then the interpretation is inflammation. If no left shift is present, then the observer should examine the lymphocyte data (step 2). Lymphopenia in conjunction with a mature neutrophilia indicates a steroid response. If the lymphocyte concentration is normal to increased, an excitement response should be considered. Also, note that an inflammatory pattern may have a superimposed steroid response that is recognized as lymphopenia occurring in conjunction with the inflammatory pattern.

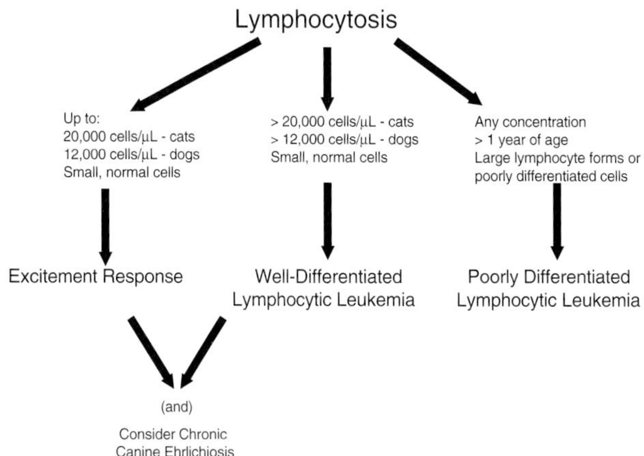

Figure 13.19 Summary approach to interpretation of lymphocytosis. This flow chart may be useful for distinguishing the excitement response from lymphocytic leukemias based on lymphocyte concentration and morphology guidelines. Inflammatory disease is rarely associated with lymphocytosis; however, chronic canine ehrlichiosis is an exception. See text for discussion.

response. If the lymphocyte concentration is upper normal or increased within certain limits, the interpretation of excitement response should be considered. Keep in mind that clear neutrophilia with a left-shift inflammatory pattern may have a superimposed steroid response; this is identified by the presence of lymphopenia in conjunction with the neutrophil inflammatory pattern.

Lymphocytosis

Lymphocytosis has two common causes. The first is the excitement response (discussed above), and the second is lymphocytic leukemia. The approach to interpreting lymphocytosis involves analysis of both cell concentration and cell morphology (Figure 13.19). The lymphocyte morphology should be critically examined when lymphocytosis is present. If the cell concentration is only modestly increased and the cells are morphologically small, normal-appearing lymphocytes, then an excitement response should be considered. As a guideline, this modest increase is suggested to be a lymphocyte concentration of up to approximately 12,000 and 20,000 cells/μL in dogs and cats, respectively. If the concentrations exceed this guideline or the animal was not excited, then a lymphocytic leukemia should be considered. Repeating the hemogram the next day while making note of the possibility of excitement during blood collection also may be helpful. When the lymphocyte concentration is of this magnitude with normal morphology, the confirmation of the diagnosis of leukemia is usually difficult. It involves exclusion and more extensive diagnostics; see Chapter 14. The higher the concentration, the greater the probability that the cause is a lymphoproliferative disorder with leukemia.

A common misconception is that lymphocytosis may occur with chronic inflammatory diseases. This concept likely is extrapolated from the knowledge that inflammatory disease results in an immune system response that includes lymphoid hyperplasia. This process does occur, but the expansion is confined to lymphoid tissues and rarely manifests as lymphocytosis in blood. An exception is the chronic form of canine ehrlichiosis, which has been documented to occasionally result in lymphocytosis and also a possible monoclonal gammopathy. The monoclonal gammopathy is expected to be superimposed on an underlying polyclonal gammopathy. When the lymphocytosis is examined, a high proportion of large granular lymphocytes (see Figure 11.4) may be observed. In dogs, chronic ehrlichiosis should be considered in an endemic region coupled with appropriate clinical signs when there is a lymphocyte concentration up to about 30,000 cells/μL.

Abnormal lymphocyte morphology in conjunction with lymphocytosis makes the diagnosis of leukemia less difficult. Abnormal morphology generally means lymphocyte forms that are normally not found in blood. These cells have one or more features of a cell undergoing proliferation, as opposed to the small, resting lymphocyte that is ordinarily seen in blood (Figure 13.20). These features may include a diameter larger than that of adjacent neutrophils, a fine chromatin pattern resulting in a lighter-staining nucleus, a visible nucleolus, and increased cytoplasm (Figures 13.20 and 13.21). If cells with abnormal features for blood, e.g., prolymphocytes and/or lymphoblasts, are present in the

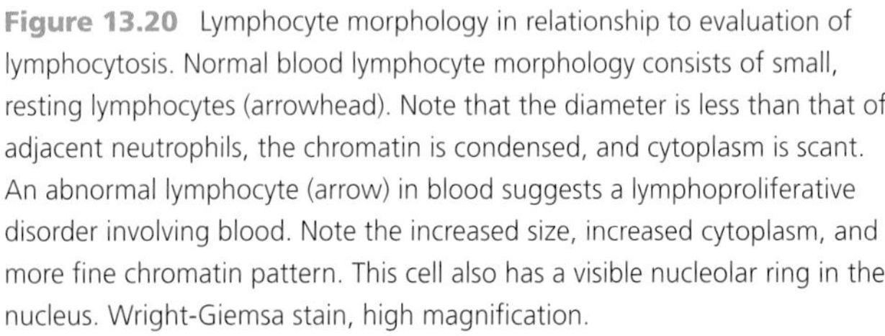

Figure 13.20 Lymphocyte morphology in relationship to evaluation of lymphocytosis. Normal blood lymphocyte morphology consists of small, resting lymphocytes (arrowhead). Note that the diameter is less than that of adjacent neutrophils, the chromatin is condensed, and cytoplasm is scant. An abnormal lymphocyte (arrow) in blood suggests a lymphoproliferative disorder involving blood. Note the increased size, increased cytoplasm, and more fine chromatin pattern. This cell also has a visible nucleolar ring in the nucleus. Wright-Giemsa stain, high magnification.

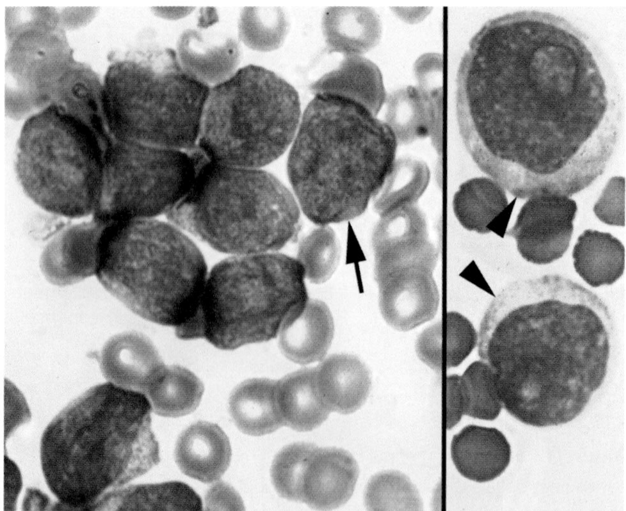

Figure 13.21 The left pane shows large, abnormal lymphocytes (arrow) from a dog with lymphoblastic leukemia (~70,000 lymphocytes/μL). Note the fine, granular chromatin pattern as well as the occasional, faint nucleoli and the large size. The right panel shows two lymphoblasts (arrowheads) from a cat with lymphoblastic leukemia. Note the large cell size, fine chromatin pattern, and prominent nucleolar rings. Wright-Giemsa stain, high magnification.

circulation, leukemia is a diagnostic consideration even with normal to mildly increased lymphocyte concentrations. Molecular diagnostics for lymphoproliferative disorders and lymphocytic leukemia are presented in Chapter 15.

Bovine persistent lymphocytosis may occur in cattle infected with bovine leukemia virus (BLV). Persistent lymphocytosis is defined as a lymphocyte concentration of greater than 7500 cells/μL on two or more hemograms. The morphology may be normal. Persistent lymphocytosis is part of a continuum in BLV-infected cows that eventually may progress to a diagnosis of lymphocytic leukemia or lymphosarcoma. Historically, hemograms, with an emphasis on the lymphocyte concentration, have been used as a screening test for BLV infection.

Neutropenia

Neutropenia resulting from acute inflammatory consumption

Neutropenia resulting from overwhelming consumption by an inflammatory lesion was discussed earlier (with the inflammatory response). Neutropenia resulting from consumption is associated with a left shift. Toxic changes are also expected within a few days of the onset of the process. An alternative form of consumptive neutropenia is immune-mediated neutropenia in which immunoglobulin that recognizes epitope(s) on the neutrophil surface or adsorbed onto the surface results in destruction of both circulating neutrophils and late stages of maturation within the marrow. This may result in profound neutropenia not associated with a demonstrable inflammatory lesion.

Neutropenia resulting from stem cell injuries

The various stem cell injuries may be considered modifications of the neutrophil trafficking model in Figure 13.22. Stem cell injuries have numerous causes, ranging from very acute, transient injury of variable duration to permanent, irreversible injuries. Stem cell injuries are nonspecific in that all cell lines of marrow are involved. Evidence of marrow failure manifested in blood is related to the duration of the injury in relationship to the circulating time or life span of various cell types. Because neutrophils are renewed in blood most rapidly, neutropenia develops first with a stem cell injury. Thrombocytopenia is seen second, because platelets last approximately 7 days in the circulation. Nonregenerative anemia occurs last because of the relatively long erythrocyte life span.

Neutropenia caused by reversible stem cell injuries

Several acute, transient stem cell injuries are caused by the tropism of viruses for rapidly dividing cells. Canine parvovirus and feline panleukopenia are notable examples; these result in injury to intestinal lining, lymphoid cells, and the bone marrow stem cell system. Profound neutropenia is attributable to two mechanisms. First, stem cell injury

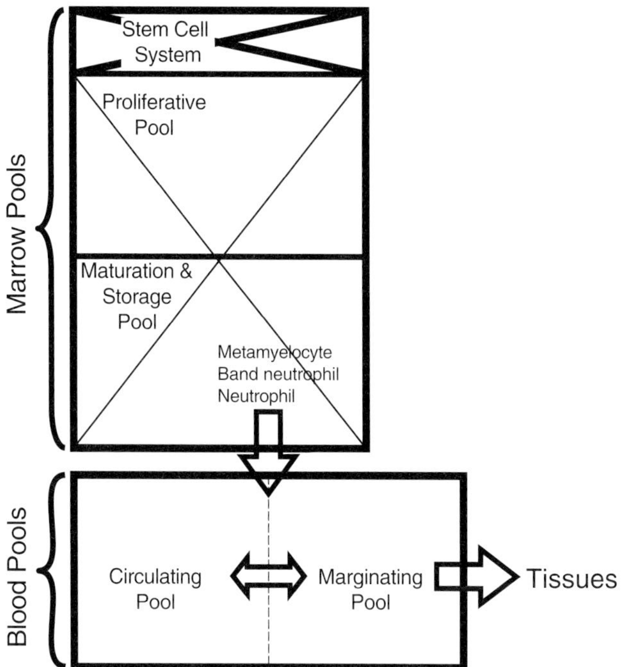

Figure 13.22 Modified neutrophil trafficking model used to illustrate neutropenias caused by stem cell injury. Injury occurs to the stem cell system, which results in a lack of recruited cells to proceed through the proliferative and maturation stages. The end result is interruption in the supply of neutrophils to blood. Because tissue consumption is not interrupted, profound neutropenia in the blood pools may occur within a few days or less.

results in transient failure of production. Second, neutrophil consumption increases at the site of gastrointestinal injury. The stem cell injury involves all marrow cell lines but is so transient that marrow repopulation occurs before thrombocytopenia and nonregenerative anemia can develop. If anemia is observed, it likely is caused by blood loss into the gastrointestinal tract. Acute neutropenia persists for only 24–48 hours. During the short period of neutropenia, a left shift is not observed. As the marrow repopulates, a left shift with progressively increasing neutrophil concentration is observed as recovery progresses. An inflammatory pattern, consisting of neutrophilia and left shift, is usually observed during recovery.

Reversible stem cell injury of varying duration also has numerous causes. These generally are present for days or longer; thus, varying degrees of thrombocytopenia and nonregenerative anemia accompany the neutropenia. One group of causes is chemicals or drugs that injure rapidly dividing cells. Most chemotherapeutic drugs are in this category. Estrogen overdosage and phenylbutazone administration are characterized toxicities in dogs. Very high, repeated doses of estradiol may cause stem cell injury in dogs, but not in cats. Historically, an alternate form of a long-acting, potent estrogen – estradiol cypionate – has been used to prevent unwanted pregnancies in dogs. This drug has been used safely in small doses to treat incontinence. Naturally occurring estrogen toxicity may occur in ferrets if ovulation is not stimulated. Phenylbutazone, a common medication for pain and lameness that is used safely in horses, may cause marked stem cell injury in dogs. An example of an infectious cause is ehrlichiosis in dogs; ehrlichiosis may induce cytopenias, possibly by an immune-mediated mechanism that appears to act on cells in the marrow.

Neutropenia caused by irreversible stem cell injuries

This category of stem cell injury may be regarded as a continuum of proliferative abnormalities of the bone marrow stem cell system. The underlying nature and mechanism of these injuries are poorly understood. Causes include feline leukemia virus, idiopathic hypoproliferative disorders, myelodysplasias, and myeloproliferative disorders. Because these are long-standing disorders, any combination of neutropenia, nonregenerative anemia, and thrombocytopenia may occur. These relatively irreversible stem cell injuries are considered in detail in Chapter 15.

Approach to neutropenia

The approach to interpretation of neutropenia is summarized in Figure 13.23. The observer should first determine if the neutropenia is associated with a left shift. If a prominent left

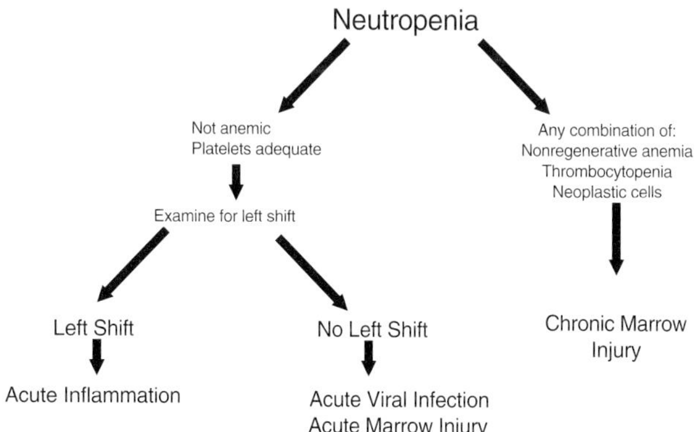

Figure 13.23 Summary approach to interpretation of neutropenia. This flow chart may be useful for distinguishing the various causes of neutropenia. When confronted with neutropenia, the observer should first examine the platelet and erythrocyte data for evidence of production problems. If these cell lines appear to have normal production, then a selective neutropenia is present. The observer should next examine the data for a left shift. If a left shift is found, then the interpretation is severe, acute inflammation (e.g., see Figure 13.16). If no left shift is found, then an acute failure to produce neutrophils should be considered (as in Figure 13.22). If the neutropenia is accompanied by evidence of failure to produce other cell lines (e.g., platelets and/or erythrocytes), then a more chronic marrow injury should be considered. The presence of neoplastic cells may indicate an underlying hematopoietic cell neoplasm and is also a possible cause of marrow failure. See text for discussion.

shift is observed with toxic change, then an inflammatory disease or recovery from viral marrow injury is the cause of the neutropenia. If no left shift is seen, then the other cell lines should be assessed. If any combination of thrombocytopenia, nonregenerative anemia, or evidence of hematopoietic cell neoplasia is found, then marrow injury should be considered.

Lymphopenia

Lymphopenia is usually attributable to a steroid response; other causes are uncommon to rare. Lympholytic acute viral infections induce lymphopenia that is accompanied by neutropenia; however, neutropenia is the more important finding. Combined immunodeficiency syndrome of Arabian foals is an inherited disorder with severe deficiency of both T- and B-cell lymphocyte functions. The lymphocyte concentration may be used as a screening test for this disorder in newborn Arabian foals. A lymphocyte concentration of greater than 1000 cells/μL is a finding that rules out the disease. If lymphopenia is found, more confirmatory tests may be performed.

Monocytosis

Monocytosis is a relatively unimportant change. It may accompany both acute and chronic inflammatory responses. Monocytosis that accompanies an inflammatory response is interpreted as a response to increased demand for mononuclear cells in tissues. Monocytes in blood are regarded as immature cells that become macrophages after migration to tissue sites. Monocytosis also may occur in the steroid response, particularly in dogs.

Eosinophilia

Eosinophilia is interpreted as a nonspecific response that requires consideration of parasitism, hypersensitivity, or an unusual lesion producing eosinophil chemoattractants such as mast cell tumor. Tissue-invading parasitisms are frequently associated with eosinophilia. Notable examples include heartworm disease and hookworm infestation in dogs. Inflammation at epithelial surfaces rich in mast cells (e.g., skin, respiratory tract, gastrointestinal tract) may be associated with eosinophilia, particularly if a component of hypersensitivity is present. Examples include fleabite allergic dermatitis, inhalant allergen disease or asthma-like syndromes, feline hypereosinophilic syndromes, and poorly characterized gastroenteritis that may have an allergic component.

Basophilia

Basophilia is uncommon. In fact, basophils are so rare in normal animals that they usually are not encountered in the 100-cell microscopy differential. The interpretation of basophilia is unknown or not clear. It most frequently accompanies eosinophilia. When this happens, it is described as eosinophilia and basophilia, but it is eosinophilia that is interpreted as indicated earlier.

14 Molecular Diagnostics of Hematologic Malignancies

Emily D. Rout and Anne C. Avery

Department of Microbiology, Immunology, and Pathology, Colorado State University, Fort Collins, CO, USA

Overview

Hematologic malignancies are a broad group of neoplasms arising from bone marrow derived cells. These include tumors derived from lymphocytes (lymphomas, lymphocytic leukemias, and plasma cell tumors) and from myeloid lineage cells (chronic myelogenous leukemia and other myeloproliferative disorders, acute myeloid leukemia, and mast cell tumors). This chapter will focus primarily on lymphoid tumors.

There are more than 15 subtypes of lymphoma and leukemia described in dogs, and they are highly variable in their presentation and outcome. This is because each different subtype of tumor is derived from a normal lymphocyte at a different stage in development with different function and oncogenic potential. For example, canine acute T-cell leukemia is a tumor of an immature T cell developing in the bone marrow or thymus. This disease has a dismal prognosis, even with aggressive chemotherapy. Canine T-zone lymphoma (TZL), on the other hand, is a tumor of mature, activated, or memory T cells and has a very good prognosis.

The goal of the testing described in this chapter is to (i) differentiate neoplastic from reactive lymphocytes and (ii) determine what subtype of lymphoma or leukemia is present to provide prognostic information for owners to help them make decisions about treatment.

Clonality testing

Lymphocytes have unique DNA sequences

The development of cancer is the result of a series of genetic mutations that render a cell resistant to growth controls. The cell divides unchecked, resulting in a tumor mass that is derived from that single original cell, and harboring the mutations – unique DNA sequences – of the original cell. Lymphocytes are further unique in the body in that even normal lymphocytes carry a genetic fingerprint specific to that individual cell. During lymphocyte development, the genes that encode antigen receptors (immunoglobulin for B cells and T-cell receptor for T cells) are assembled at random from a pool of genes. The random nature of this process means that each B and T cell will have a genetically unique antigen receptor. Additionally, nucleotides are trimmed or added at the junctions between genes, further increasing diversity. When these cells divide, as a result of antigenic stimulation or cancer, the daughter cells inherit the antigen receptor genes. The detection of oncogenes and unique lymphocyte genes gives us a very powerful diagnostic tool for detecting malignancy and for making predictions about prognosis and treatment.

Generation of antigen receptors in lymphocytes

To understand how the unique DNA sequences in lymphocytes can be used for diagnostic purposes, it is first important to understand how these sequences are generated. Lymphocytes develop in the bone marrow (B cells) with T cells finalizing their development in the thymus. The job of these cells is to identify the millions of different foreign antigens carried by potential pathogens. To accomplish this, lymphocytes have developed a system to generate enormous diversity in the antigen binding portion of their receptors. The B-cell immunoglobulin receptor for antigen is an antibody that consists of a heavy chain and a light chain, and the T-cell receptor for antigen is called the T-cell receptor, also consisting of two polypeptides (alpha and beta, or gamma and delta). Each of these proteins is a heterodimer with each protein chain encoded by a different gene. The genes encoding these two proteins use the same process for generating diversity, so only antibody heavy chain genes will be discussed.

The antigen binding region of an antibody (the variable region) is generated by bringing together three different genes – V (variable) genes, D (diversity) genes, and J (joining) genes. In the dog, there are 89 variable region genes

Veterinary Hematology, Clinical Chemistry, and Cytology, Third Edition. Edited by Mary Anna Thrall, Glade Weiser, Robin W. Allison and Terry W. Campbell.

Companion website: www.wiley.com/go/thrall/veterinary

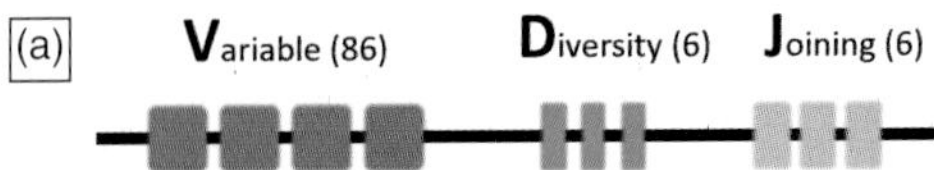

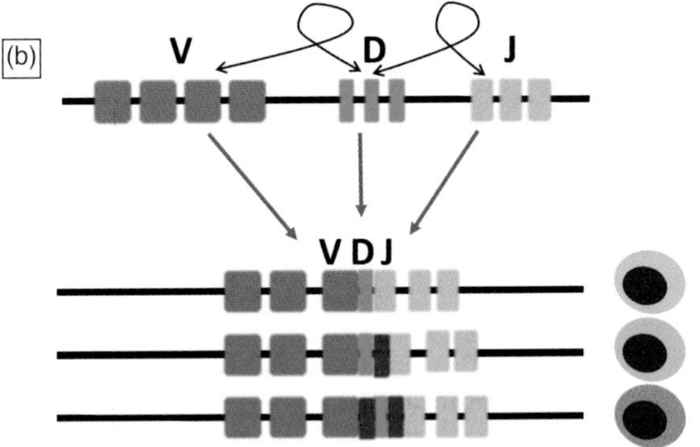

Figure 14.1 Arrangement of immunoglobulin gene segments on canine chromosome 8. (a) There are approximately 89 variable region genes (V, blue), 6 diversity genes (D, green), and 6 joining genes (J, orange). The black line between genes indicates noncoding DNA. This diagram is not to scale. (b) During B-cell development in the bone marrow, DNA between D and J and V and D genes is excised to bring together one V, one D, and one J gene. During this process, varying numbers of nucleotides are added between the genes (red). This process results in different B cells having immunoglobulin gene rearrangements of different lengths. The three VDJ gene rearrangements here would be found in three different B cells.

found on chromosome 8. Each gene is approximately 300 bases long, but the genes are separated by thousands of bases of noncoding DNA. Dogs have 6 D genes, ranging from 12 to 30 bases, and 6 J genes of approximately 50 bases (see http://www.imgt.org). The arrangement of the genes is shown schematically in Figure 14.1.

The arrangement of genes in Figure 14.1a is called the germline configuration. This is the arrangement of genes found in all cells of the body except fully developed B cells. During the development of a B cell, the V, D, and J genes of the antibody heavy chain are brought together so they form one contiguous gene in a process called recombination. Recombination is essentially random, so that any V can be combined with any D and any J. While V region genes have similar sequences, they are not identical. The same is true for D and J genes – they are similar to one another but not identical.

This random recombination alone creates a tremendous number of different genes, but in addition, nucleotides can be added between segments during the process, or trimmed from the ends of V, D, and J genes (Figure 14.1b). The process is again random. Thus, any given B cell will have not only a unique concatenation of V, D, and J genes, but within this new rearrangement will be further diversity as a result of nucleotides being added and trimmed. The result is that virtually every newly developed B cell will carry a unique DNA sequence. The length of the new VDJ gene rearrangement will also be different because of the addition and trimming of nucleotides. The same is true for T cells, because the T-cell receptor beta and delta gene loci are also composed of multiple V, D, and J genes. The antibody light chain genes and T-cell receptor alpha and gamma genes all undergo a similar process, with the exception that none of these gene rearrangements contain a D [1] gene.

Clonal versus polyclonal lymphocyte expansion

When mature lymphocytes with their unique antigen receptors encounter an antigen recognized by those receptors, they are stimulated to divide. The progeny cells contain the same antigen receptor gene rearrangement. Similarly, if a lymphocyte becomes neoplastic at some time during its development and divides unchecked, all of the progeny cells of this cancer will have the same antigen receptor gene rearrangement.

The response to a pathogen will involve hundreds to thousands of molecularly different B and T cells. This is because even the simplest pathogen is composed of multiple proteins, which can be recognized by the antigen receptors of many different lymphocytes. Even a single protein has many different antigenic structures and can stimulate the division of multiple lymphocytes. This response would be called polyclonal. Cancer, on the other hand, is characterized by the unrestricted division of a single cell, called clonal proliferation. Thus, a population of lymphocytes that are all the progeny of a single clone is most likely cancer, and a population of lymphocytes that have multiple different types of cells (called polyclonal) is most likely reactive.

The ability to distinguish a clonal from a polyclonal population of lymphocytes has many diagnostic applications. For example, a dog with dental disease presents to his veterinarian because his mandibular lymph nodes are enlarged. The enlarged lymph nodes can be due to antigenic stimulation by a heavy burden of oral pathogens. Other clinical factors, however, may raise concern for lymphoma – these can include age, breed, and cytologically suspicious cells. To distinguish a purely reactive process from a neoplastic one, it is possible to determine if the lymphocytes are mainly derived from a single clone (neoplastic) or multiple lymphocytes. The assay used to make this distinction is called a clonality assay and can also be called PARR (PCR for antigen receptor rearrangements) [2].

Molecular biology of the PARR assay

The PARR assay measures the size of all of the gene rearrangements in a collection of lymphocytes. If all of the lymphocytes have the same-sized gene rearrangement, the lymphocytes are considered clonal (Figure 14.2). If, however, there are multiple-sized gene rearrangements, then the population is polyclonal. To accomplish this, DNA is

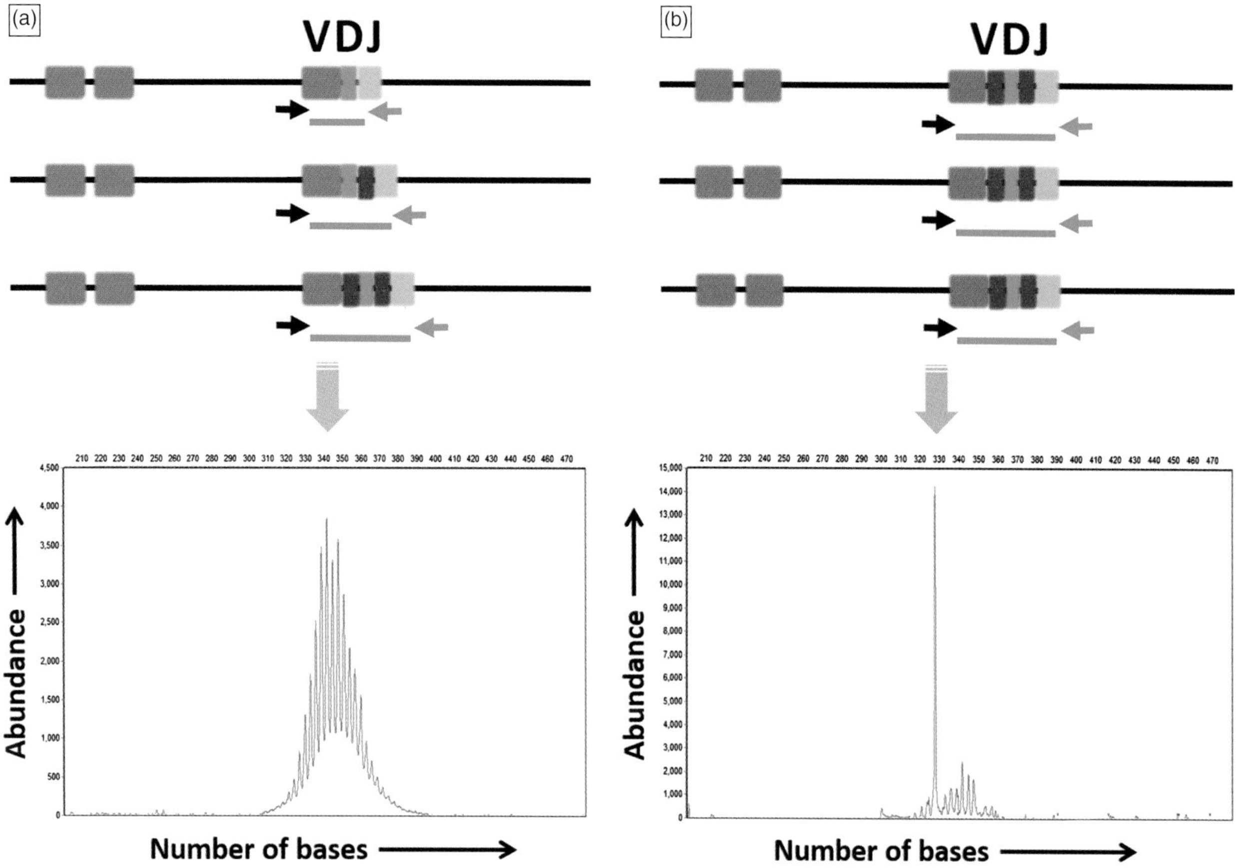

Figure 14.2 Placement of PCR primers and separation of PCR products by size. PCR primers (indicated by the arrows) placed as shown will amplify the VDJ gene rearrangement. One primer is conjugated to a fluorescent molecule (green). (a) Multiple-sized PCR products will be amplified when DNA is extracted from normal lymphocytes. The bottom histogram depicts separation of PCR products by size. (b) A single-sized PCR product is observed when the majority of DNA is derived from neoplastic lymphocytes, all of which are derived from the same original clone and carry the same-sized immunoglobulin gene rearrangement.

extracted from the lymphocytes in question – for example in the case above, a dog with enlarged mandibular nodes and dental disease, lymphocytes would be collected by aspiration from the mandibular node. Polymerase chain reaction (PCR) primers that will amplify the entire VDJ rearrangement will be added as shown in Figure 14.2.

The resultant DNA products are separated by size using any one of a variety of methods. A dominant single-sized product indicates that the population of cells was derived from a single clone. On the other hand, the presence of products of multiple sizes indicates that a heterogeneous population of lymphocytes is present, and the process is most likely reactive. Figure 14.2 shows the results of the PARR assay analyzed by capillary gel electrophoresis to demonstrate what each of these two results would look like. In practice, only 1–10% of the cells in any given sample need to be neoplastic for the result to be interpreted as clonal. This is because the remaining non-neoplastic cells are so heterogeneous that the PCR products from these varied cells are outcompeted by homogeneous product from the neoplastic cells. This idea is not necessarily intuitive but has been demonstrated experimentally.

Interpretation and uses of the PARR assay

The PARR assay is used when there is suspicion of lymphoma by cytology or histology but not a definitive diagnosis. Some common reasons for carrying out the assay are enlarged lymph nodes where the cytology or histology cannot definitively conclude that lymphoma is present, pleural or peritoneal fluid characterized by occasional suspicious-looking cells, and the presence of atypical-appearing lymphocytes on a peripheral blood film.

In most cases, the assay is performed by using multiple sets of PCR primers – some of which detect immunoglobulin gene rearrangements, and some of which detect T-cell receptor gene rearrangements. B-cell lymphomas will be characterized by single-sized PCR products when the immunoglobulin primers are used, but multiple products or no products at all when T-cell receptor primers are used. T-cell lymphomas, conversely, will be characterized by single-sized products when T-cell receptor primers are used and multiple or no products when immunoglobulin primers are used. Thus, the nature of the clonal PCR product is a clue to the lineage of the neoplasm. As with any assay, there are exceptions to this rule, but for most cases, the clonally rearranged gene reflects the lineage of the tumor. Plasma cell tumors and multiple myeloma are B-cell-origin tumors and will have clonally rearranged immunoglobulin genes.

Not all cases of lymphoma and leukemia can be detected by PARR. This is because there are likely to be V and J region genes whose sequences differ enough from the PCR primers that the primers will not bind. If the patient's tumor uses one of these V or J genes, then no amplification of tumor DNA will be seen. Therefore, as with many tests, the PARR assay cannot be used to rule out neoplasia, only to support a positive diagnosis.

Detection of genetic alterations in cancer cells

Principles

Almost all human cancers can be characterized by an array of genetic aberrations. These include chromosomal translocations, which bring two genes together that normally exist on different chromosomes, duplications or deletions of a part or a whole chromosome, and mutations within individual genes. Detection of such genetic changes is common practice in human oncology and is used for making an initial diagnosis as well as identifying clinically relevant subtypes of disease – subtypes that will be more or less aggressive or that will respond to specific targeted therapies.

Routine genetic testing in veterinary medicine is uncommon but likely to increase significantly in the next few years because of the enormous amount of genetic information available from high-throughput sequencing studies of veterinary cancers. Currently, there are commercially available tests for individual mutations in canine mast cell tumors and transitional cell carcinomas.

Testing for the *CKIT* mutation in mast cell tumors

Approximately 20% of canine mast cell tumors harbor a mutation in a gene called *CKIT* [3]. *CKIT* is the tyrosine kinase receptor for the growth factor called stem cell factor. The mutations result in the *CKIT* gene being permanently phosphorylated, resulting in a constitutive "on" signal. This means that the cells are continuously being stimulated to divide.

The most common mutations in this gene are called internal tandem duplications, in which a small segment of the gene is duplicated, such that a given sequence is repeated in tandem. One of these mutations is found in exon 11, where a variable-length segment is duplicated, creating a slightly larger version of the gene [4]. The mutation is readily detectable by PCR amplification of exon 11, since it will result in a larger product. Figure 14.3 shows the placement of PCR primers and what the product will look like.

Detection of an internal tandem duplication in mast cell tumors can provide objective prognostic information. High-grade mast cell tumors, a designation determined by the histologic appearance of the tumor, tend to be more aggressive and require more intensive therapy. Low-grade mast cell tumors may be cured by surgical excision alone. Many mast cell tumors, however, fall in the gray area

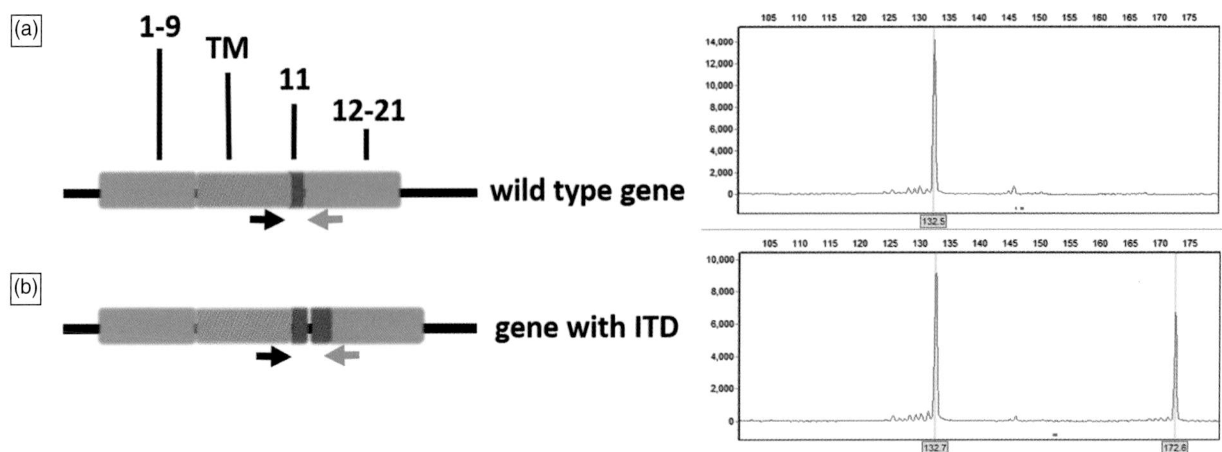

Figure 14.3 PCR amplification of c-kit exon 11. (a) The *CKIT* gene consists of 21 exons, which are indicated by numbers. Exons 11–21 are intracellular, TM = transmembrane (exon 10). PCR amplification with primers surrounding exon 11, indicated by the arrows, results in a single product shown in the histogram on the right. This is the wild-type form of the gene. (b) The *CKIT* gene with an internal tandem duplication (ITD) of exon 11 (red) is amplified with the same primer set. The ITD results in a larger-size PCR product shown in the histogram on the right. Both the smaller, wild-type product and the larger one are present because only one copy of the gene is mutated. In addition, there is invariably normal tissue in any mast cell tumor sample.

between low- and high-grade histologically, and the histologic assessment of the degree of aggressiveness of these tumors may differ between pathologists. Detection of *CKIT* mutation may help shift the designation of a tumor being more likely high grade, with a less positive prognosis. There is also conflicting data about the use of this mutation to guide the choice of chemotherapy [5].

CKIT mutations are relatively straightforward to detect because the mutation changes the size of the PCR product. Some cancers will have predictable, single-base mutations that do not change the size of the PCR product. Standard sequencing can detect such mutations, but sequencing is generally too labor-intensive and insensitive for clinical purposes. An example of this type of mutation is the *BRAF* mutation – this is found in 80% of cases of canine transitional cell carcinoma. The single nucleotide change found in the canine gene is equivalent to a *BRAF* mutation common in a variety of human cancers and causes constitutive activation of the BRAF protein. BRAF is a serine/threonine kinase that activates a series of downstream signaling pathways to drive cellular metabolism and proliferation. Detection of the *BRAF* mutation relies on a technique called droplet digital PCR [6], which is a sensitive method for detecting such changes. The *BRAF* mutation is unusual, however, in that it is the same in all tumors. Most mutations affecting oncogenes will not be found in exactly the same site but would be seen in a variety of locations within the gene. As noted below, these kinds of mutations will be best detected using high-throughput or next-gen sequencing methods.

High-throughput sequencing in diagnostics

The PCR methods described above for detection of clonally rearranged antigen receptor genes and mutation analysis will almost certainly be replaced by high-throughput or next-gen sequencing techniques in the coming years. These are techniques that will allow for sequencing of multiple genes (including entire genomes) simultaneously. Oncology research increasingly focuses on mutational "landscapes" in tumors, which involve cataloging an array (tens to hundreds) of individual mutations to characterize individual neoplasms. The technology is readily available, but a great deal of additional research on the effects of individual mutations in hematopoietic and other forms of cancer is necessary before such testing is appropriate.

Flow cytometry

In the context of hematologic malignancy, flow cytometry is used to identify proteins on the surface of lymphocytes, although the technology has a large variety of other uses. As discussed above, lymphoma and leukemia are the result of unchecked expansion of a single cell. The progeny cells resemble the original cancerous clone. Therefore, another way to determine if a population of lymphocytes is neoplastic would be to show they are all the same phenotype – all B cells, CD4 T cells, or CD8 T cells. This is not equivalent to showing that the cells are all derived from the same clone, but in practical terms, homogeneous expansion of a single lymphocyte subset is usually neoplastic, because reactive processes will result in the expansion of many different lymphocyte subtypes. Thus, if the lymphocytes in a mandibular lymph node aspirate consist of 98% B cells, the process in that node is almost certainly neoplastic. If the lymph node aspirate, however, consists of 30% B cells, 50% CD4 T cells, and 20% CD8 T cells, this finding is more consistent with a reactive process – response to infection or autoimmune disease or response to a metastatic tumor of nonlymphoid origin. In addition to evaluating the proportions of different lymphocyte subsets, flow cytometry can detect aberrancies of lymphocyte populations, including a lymphocyte population composed of atypically large-sized lymphocytes or a population that has aberrant protein expression on the cell surface.

Cell surface antigens

Most proteins found on the surface of hematopoietic cells are identified by a number, preceded by the letters "CD" (CD stands for "cluster of differentiation," a term that partly reflects the fact that different proteins are expressed at different points in the life of a cell). CD3, CD4, CD5, and CD8 are all proteins found on the surface of T cells and were among the earliest identified. CD21 and CD22 are proteins found on B cells but not on T cells. Monoclonal antibodies specific for virtually all CD antigens are available for both people and mice, and a significant repertoire is also available for dogs, horses, cattle, and sheep. There are fewer antibodies for cats. These antibodies are generally (but not always) species specific – an antibody to canine CD4 will not recognize feline CD4, and vice versa.

To determine how many CD4 T cells, CD8 T cells, and B cells there are in any given collection of lymphocytes, commercially available monoclonal antibodies are incubated with the cells in question (e.g., cells from a lymph node aspirate). The antibodies are conjugated to fluorescent molecules that come in a large array of different colors. Thus, if the antibody to CD4 is conjugated to a red molecule, cells that have red fluorescence are CD4+ T cells. If the antibody to CD8 is conjugated to a green molecule, cells that have green fluorescence are CD8+ T cells. A flow cytometer is used to count the number of cells bearing different fluorescent molecules, and the process of enumerating cells of different subtypes is called *immunophenotyping*.

Principles of flow cytometry

Flow cytometry is the analysis of cells and particles in liquid suspension. Flow cytometers are equipped with one or more lasers, which emit light of a single wavelength. The suspension to be analyzed is focused into a narrow stream that passes in front of the laser one particle or cell at a time. When a cell passes through the beam, several aspects of the interaction between the cell and the light are recorded by detectors. First, the cell scatters light in several ways. The *forward light scatter* is an estimate of the size of the cells – large cells produce greater forward light scatter. The complexity of a cell's cytoplasm is indicated by the *side scatter*. Cells such as eosinophils and neutrophils, with granules in their cytoplasm, have high side scatter, whereas lymphocytes, which have little cytoplasm, have low side scatter (Figure 14.4a).

The other important parameter detected by the flow cytometer is the amount and color of the fluorescent molecules bound to the cell. That characteristic is determined by which, if any, monoclonal antibodies specific for CD antigens have bound. The laser light is a single wavelength of light, which excites the fluorescent dye. That dye then emits light of a narrow spectrum – what our eyes would see as green, red, blue, etc. A detector records the amount of fluorescence for each cell that passes in front of the laser and stores it together with forward and side-scatter information. The amount of fluorescence is proportional to the number of antibody molecules on the cell, which is proportional to the number of CD proteins recognized by that antibody. This principle is illustrated in Figure 14.4b.

Clinical applications of flow cytometry

Flow cytometry is most useful for determining if an expanded population of lymphocytes is neoplastic (homogeneous) or reactive (heterogeneous). Flow cytometry can identify the lineage of a neoplasm, and it can also provide prognostic information in some cases. An example is shown in Figure 14.5. These are two cases of T-cell lymphoma. Figure 14.5a shows a flow cytometry study of a lymph node from a dog with a T-cell neoplasm called T-zone lymphoma (TZL). Figure 14.5b shows flow cytometry of a lymph node from a dog with a different form of T-cell lymphoma called peripheral T-cell lymphoma (PTCL). While both dogs have T-cell lymphoma, they are two entirely different forms of T-cell lymphoma with different antigenic characteristics. They also have vastly different outcomes.

TZL is an indolent disease, sometimes not requiring treatment. It is characterized by T cells that do not express the pan-leukocyte antigen CD45 and that express high levels of class II MHC. PTCL, on the other hand, is an aggressive disease with a poor outcome. Most dogs require multiagent chemotherapy and have a median survival of 5 months. PTCL is characterized by T cells that do express CD45 but do not express class II MHC. Flow cytometry is a noninvasive way of distinguishing these two types of T-cell lymphoma and providing prognostic information for veterinarians and owners [7].

Immunocytochemistry

There are some circumstances where flow cytometry is not possible, or where the antigens to be assessed are not on the surface of the cell. In these cases, immunocytochemistry (ICC) can be used to evaluate antigen expression. The equivalent technique in formalin-fixed biopsy tissue is called immunohistochemistry.

Like flow cytometry, ICC uses antibodies specific for different antigens to determine the nature of the cells of interest.

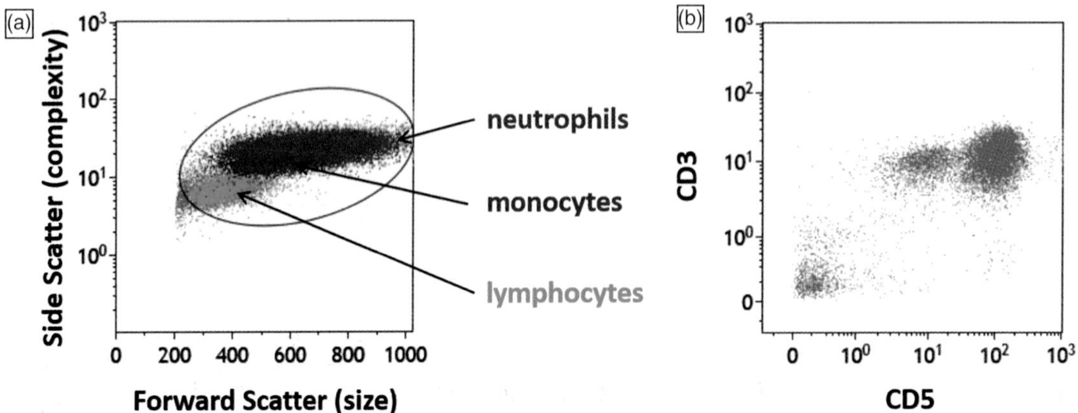

Figure 14.4 Flow cytometry of canine peripheral blood. (a) Light scatter properties of canine peripheral blood. Each dot represents a cell, and each cell is plotted along the *x* and *y* axes based on their forward and side light scatter properties. Light scatter values do not have units. In this example, forward scatter is a linear scale and side scatter a log scale. Side scatter is also often depicted on a linear scale. (b) Expression of two T-cell proteins on the surface of lymphocytes, CD3 and CD5. This histogram shows that the majority of cells express both proteins, but a subset of cells express lower levels of CD5. This illustrates how flow cytometry can be used to determine the relative abundance of proteins on the surface of cells.

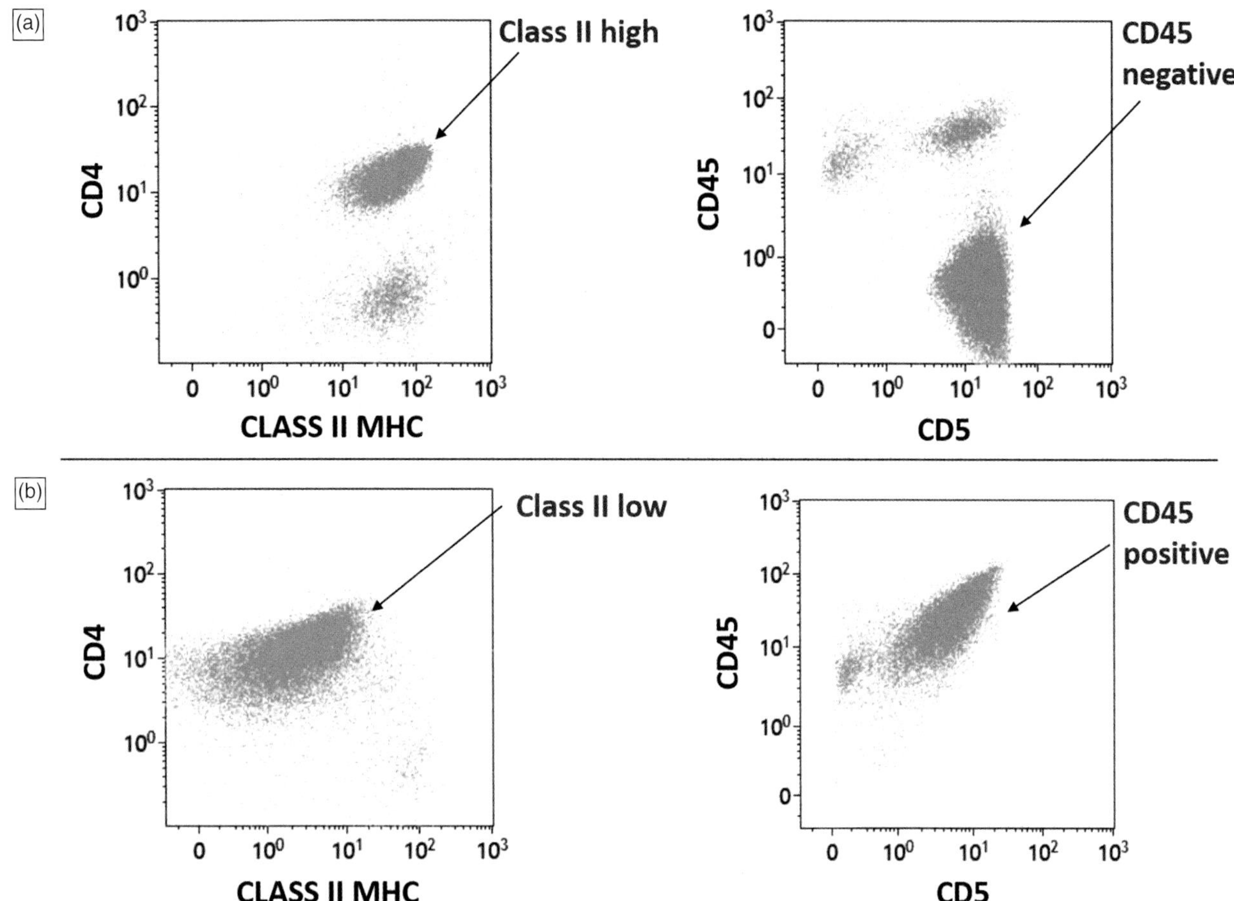

Figure 14.5 Two different types of T-cell lymphoma with different outcomes. This figure shows the expression of two proteins that are found on all normal peripheral canine lymphocytes (CD45 and class II MHC), and two proteins found on normal canine T cells (CD4 on a subset of T cells and CD5 on all T cells). (a) A T-zone lymphoma that expresses the T-cell antigen CD4 and high levels of class II MHC (left) but does not express CD45 (right). (b) A peripheral T-cell lymphoma that expresses the T-cell antigen CD4 and low levels of class II MHC (left) but expresses normal levels of CD45 (right).

However, ICC differs from flow cytometry in a number of ways: (i) the results are usually visualized with an enzymatic reaction that causes a color change that can be seen under the microscope when an antibody binds to a cell, rather than by fluorescence; (ii) ICC is performed on cytology slide preparations from bone marrow, blood, and tissues and does not require fresh, viable cells; (iii) the process of staining cells for ICC results in permeabilization of the cells so that antibodies can bind to antigens found in the cytoplasm or nucleus; and (iv) with typical methods, only one antigen can be detected at a time, which is a significant limitation of the technique, though methods have been developed that are capable of detecting multiple antigens at once.

An example illustrating the utility of ICC is shown in Figure 14.6. A dog with significant leukocytosis was examined by cytology and determined to have a lymphoid neoplasm with an uncertain lineage. A new sample was submitted for flow cytometry, but the flow cytometry assay found that the cells did not express proteins typically found on B cells or T cells, leaving a question as to their origin. They could be highly aberrant neoplastic B or T cells, which have lost expression of normal cell surface proteins, or a different cell type such as plasma cell. In this case, ICC of a blood smear revealed that the cells express the protein MUM1 (also called IRF4), which is most commonly seen in plasma cells or B cells differentiating toward plasma cells. Because this antigen is located in the nucleus, it cannot be detected by conventional flow cytometry techniques but is readily detectable by ICC.

Flow cytometry is by far preferable to ICC in most circumstances, because the ability to identify and quantify the expression of many antigens simultaneously means that a tumor can be subclassified into prognostically important groups. Typically, ICC only evaluates a small number of proteins, and while it can be used to determine if a tumor is T or B cell in origin, it cannot be used to subtype them. The two diseases shown in Figure 14.5, for example, cannot be distinguished by ICC.

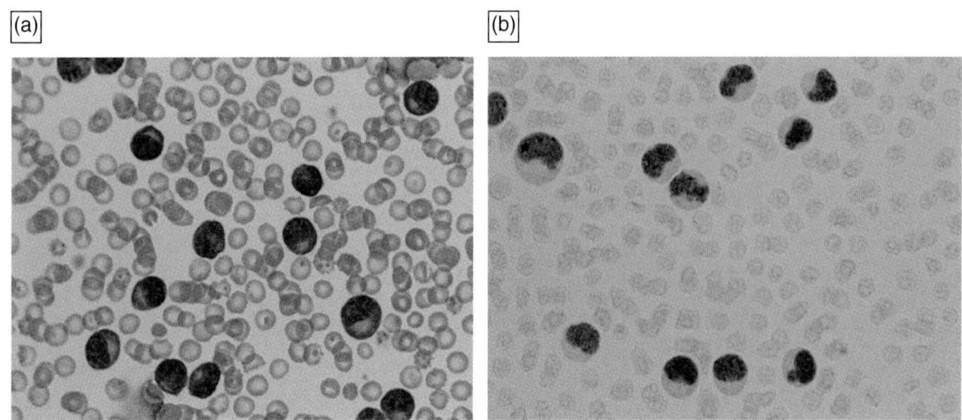

Figure 14.6 Peripheral blood from a dog with leukemia and circulating neoplastic cells of undetermined origin. Flow cytometry of the peripheral blood showed that the cells did not express any cell-surface, lineage-specific antigens (CD3, CD5, CD4, CD8, CD21). (a) Wright-Giemsa stain of the peripheral blood smear. (b) Immunocytochemistry showing MUM1/IRF4 staining with nuclear localization, indicating that these cells are most likely plasma cells.

Summary

Molecular diagnostic techniques such as clonality, detection of oncogenes, and flow cytometry can be used to diagnose lymphoma and leukemia. Many of these assays are widely available and now used routinely. They can provide objective confirmation of diagnoses made by cytology and histology and can help clarify an equivocal diagnosis made by more subjective methods. It is likely that a great many more molecular diagnostic assays will become available within a few years because rapid sequencing technologies allow for much more efficient identification of oncogenes and other genetic alterations in cancer.

Case Example 14.1. Homogeneous lymphocyte expansion

A 13-year-old female Chihuahua presents for a routine dentistry. Presurgical blood work showed that her lymphocyte count was 10,235 cells/μL, but all her other complete blood count (CBC) and biochemical data were normal. Her physical exam did not detect enlarged lymph nodes. No other imaging was performed. The lymphocytes were described as small and mature. Differentials for lymphocytosis of mature-appearing cells in dogs include lymphoproliferative disease, thymoma, Addison's disease, and chronic infection (particularly *Ehrlichia canis* infection).

Flow cytometry is a good diagnostic test in this case, because it will tell you the phenotype of the lymphocytes and may provide prognostic information. The results showed that 75% of the cells in the blood were B cells, resulting in a B-cell count of 7723 cells/μL (normal for this reference lab is <724 cells/μL) (Figure 14.7). T-cell counts were within normal range. This homogeneous expansion of small B cells is most consistent with B-cell chronic lymphocytic leukemia, which is common in older, small-breed dogs [8]. This disease often has an indolent clinical course.

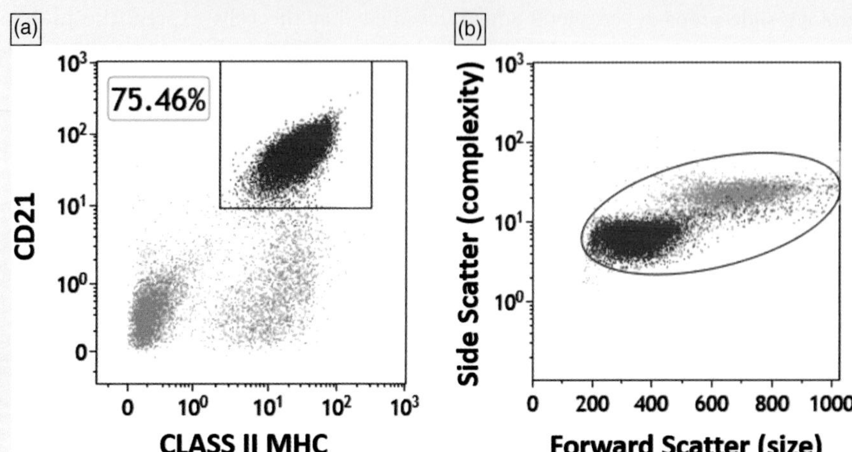

Figure 14.7 Flow cytometry of peripheral blood from a patient with B-cell chronic lymphocytic leukemia. (a) B cells are identified by expression of CD21 and class II MHC. The gate drawn around these cells indicates that 75.46% of all the cells in the blood are B cells. (b) In this plot, the B cells identified in (a) are colored red so that their light scatter properties can be visualized. The B cells are small lymphocytes, as can be seen by comparison with the neutrophils (gray cells).

Case Example 14.2. Heterogeneous lymphocyte expansion

A dog presents as above (same signalment and blood work). In this case, however, the results show that there are 2000 B cells/μL (normal high 724 cells/μL), 4000 CD4 T cells/μL (normal high 2063 cells/μL), and 4000 CD8 T cells/μL (normal high 968 cells/μL). In this case, there is a heterogeneous expansion of all lymphocyte subsets. Although this finding doesn't rule out leukemia, it is more consistent with a reactive or physiologic process. Given the normal biochemical data, atypical Addison's disease involving only glucocorticoid deficiency would be one possibility. Thymomas typically involve expansion of T-cell subsets but not B cells, so this would be lower on the differential list. Chronic infection, including chronic *E. canis*, would also be a consideration.

To further investigate the possibility that one of the three lymphocyte subsets was neoplastic, the PARR assay was performed (Figure 14.8). Amplification of the immunoglobulin and T-cell receptor gene rearrangements indicates that there are polyclonal, not monoclonal, B- and T-cell populations in this dog's blood. This finding indicates that this is most likely a reactive or physiologic process, consistent with the flow cytometry results.

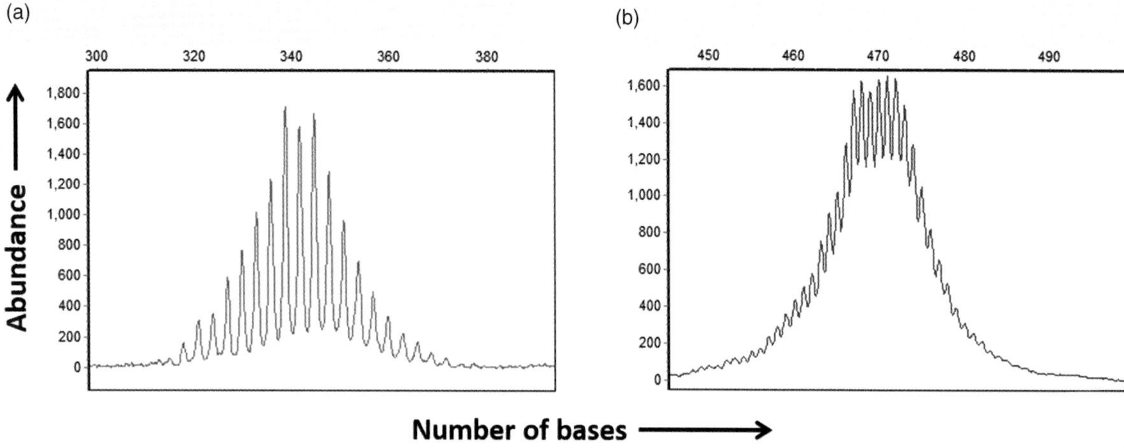

Figure 14.8 PCR for antigen receptor rearrangements showing that the B and T cells in the peripheral blood of a dog with a heterogeneous lymphocyte expansion are polyclonal, exhibiting multiple different-sized PCR products. (a) PCR products detected when DNA from the peripheral blood is amplified by primers specific for immunoglobulin heavy chain V and J genes. (b) PCR products detected when DNA from the peripheral blood is amplified by primers specific for the T-cell receptor gamma V and J genes.

Case Example 14.3. Cells with an abnormal phenotype

An 11-year-old golden retriever presents with adult-onset demodex and a lymphocyte count that is just outside the normal range (5500 lymphocytes/μL). The remainder of the blood work is normal. Mandibular lymph nodes palpate larger than normal and firm. Flow cytometry of a lymph node aspirate is shown in Figure 14.9.

The results indicate that there is a population of T cells with an aberrant phenotype – the cells do not express the pan-leukocyte antigen CD45, which is found on all normal cells in a lymph node. The presence of a marked expansion of aberrant lymphocytes is diagnostic for neoplasia. Furthermore, the specific type of neoplasm can be determined because loss of CD45 expression is the hallmark of TZL. This indolent disease is common in golden retrievers and in most cases progresses slowly [9].

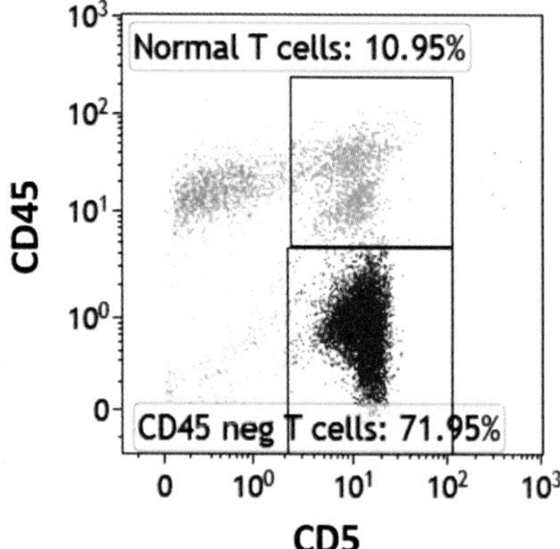

Figure 14.9 Flow cytometry of a lymph node from a dog with T-zone lymphoma. Normal T cells express CD45 but only comprise 11% of this lymph node. The majority of cells are T cells (CD5+) that do not express CD45. This abnormal phenotype can be considered diagnostic for T-zone lymphoma.

15 Laboratory Evaluation of Bone Marrow

Mary Anna Thrall[1] and Glade Weiser[2]

[1]Ross University School of Veterinary Medicine, Basseterre, Saint Kitts and Nevis
[2]Loveland, CO, USA

Cytologic evaluation of a bone marrow aspiration biopsy specimen is helpful in animals with unexplained hematologic abnormalities when a diagnosis cannot be established based on examination of the blood. Examples of such abnormalities include nonregenerative anemia, neutropenia, thrombocytopenia, gammopathy, and suspicion of neoplastic marrow disease (e.g., lymphoma). In horses, bone marrow aspirates are useful to determine if anemias are regenerative, because equine species do not release immature erythrocytes into the blood. Contraindications to bone marrow aspiration are few, but marrow aspirates from the ribs or sternum of horses with clotting disorders have resulted in death because of hemothorax or cardiac tamponade. Hemorrhage usually can be prevented in thrombocytopenic animals by applying pressure to the aspiration site for several minutes. Bone marrow aspiration technique is discussed in Chapter 2.

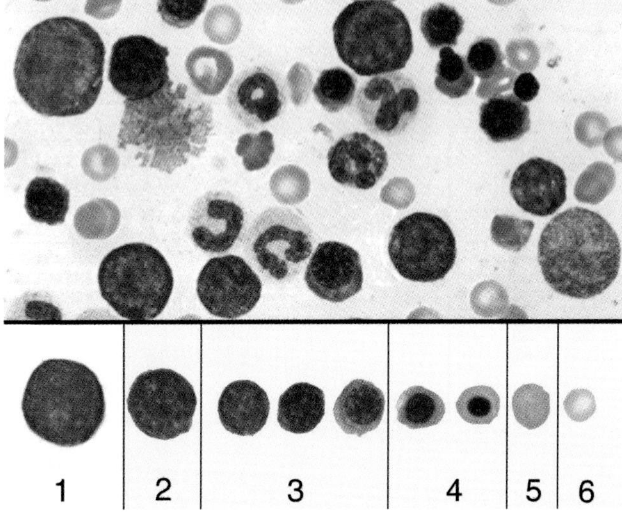

Figure 15.1 Top. Bone marrow aspirate from a dog showing numerous erythroid precursors with round nuclei, coarse chromatin, and blue- to hemoglobin-colored cytoplasm. Bottom. Maturation stages of erythroid precursors, from immature to mature. 1, rubriblast; 2, prorubricyte; 3, rubricytes; 4, metarubricytes; 5, polychromatophilic erythrocyte; 6, mature erythrocyte. Wright stain.

Cells encountered in bone marrow films

Erythroid series

Erythroid precursors tend to have round nuclei, coarse chromatin, and moderate to deep blue cytoplasm that becomes more pink in color as hemoglobin is produced by more-differentiated cells. The developmental stages of the erythroid series, from immature to mature, are the rubriblast, prorubricyte, rubricyte, metarubricyte, polychromatophilic erythrocyte, and mature erythrocyte (Figure 15.1).

Rubriblasts are the most immature cells that are recognizable in the erythroid series. These cells are relatively large, have round nuclei, slightly coarse chromatin, and nucleoli. The nucleus : cytoplasm ratio is high, with a scant amount of deeply basophilic cytoplasm. A clear Golgi zone may be present as well.

Prorubricytes, which are the next stage in erythrocyte maturation, have a round nucleus, slightly more coarse chromatin, and no visible nucleolus. The cytoplasm is slightly less blue, and it is also more abundant than that of the rubriblast.

Rubricytes are the most mature stage of maturation in which mitosis can still occur. These cells have smaller nuclei, very coarse chromatin, and blue to blue-pink (i.e., polychromatophilic) cytoplasm.

Metarubricytes are the most mature cells of the erythroid series that still contain a nucleus. The nucleus is very small, dark, and dense, and the cytoplasm is either polychromatophilic or the red-orange color of mature erythrocytes. Nuclei are extruded from metarubricytes, thereby resulting in polychromatophilic erythrocytes.

Polychromatophilic erythrocytes are anucleate, blue-pink in color, and larger than mature erythrocytes. They also may contain nuclear remnants (i.e., Howell-Jolly bodies). When stained with supravital stains (e.g., new methylene or brilliant cresyl blue), their mRNA and organelles clump,

Veterinary Hematology, Clinical Chemistry, and Cytology, Third Edition. Edited by Mary Anna Thrall, Glade Weiser, Robin W. Allison and Terry W. Campbell.

Companion website: www.wiley.com/go/thrall/veterinary

thereby resulting in blue-staining dots and fibrils (i.e., reticulum) throughout the cells. When stained in this manner, polychromatophilic erythrocytes are termed reticulocytes.

Mature erythrocytes are red-orange in color. Evaluation of mature erythrocyte morphology in bone marrow preparations usually is not indicated, but it can be diagnostically useful in that abnormalities such as red cell parasites, spherocytes, or hypochromasia occasionally may be observed. Such abnormalities are typically confirmed by blood film review.

Granulocyte (myeloid) series

Granulocytic precursors tend to have irregularly shaped and, sometimes, eccentric nuclei, with fine to stippled chromatin patterns and abundant, lavender-colored cytoplasm. At certain stages of maturation, they contain azurophilic (i.e., red-purple) to pink granules within the cytoplasm. As the cells mature, the nuclei elongate, from amoeboid or round in shape to kidney-bean- or horseshoe-shaped to segmented. The developmental stages of the myeloid series, from immature to mature, are the myeloblast, progranulocyte (promyelocyte), myelocyte, metamyelocyte, band granulocyte, and segmented granulocyte (Figure 15.2). When the maturation process is hastened, whether resulting from inflammation or other causes, the cytoplasm of the myeloid precursors at all stages of maturation is more basophilic and sometimes vacuolated.

Myeloblasts are subclassified into type I and type II. Type I myeloblasts, which are the most immature cells that are still recognizable in the granulocytic series, are large cells with round to oval nuclei, finely stippled or smooth nuclear chromatin, one or more nucleoli, a small amount of moderately blue cytoplasm, and no azurophilic granules. The nucleus usually is centrally located, and the nuclear outline may be slightly irregular. The nucleus : cytoplasm ratio is high (>1.5), and the cell size is approximately 1.5–3.0 times greater than the red cell diameter. The cytoplasm has a "ground-glass" appearance and, rarely, contains small vacuoles. Type II myeloblasts are very similar to type I, except that some small, azurophilic granules (primary granules) are scattered in the cytoplasm and the nucleus may be central or eccentric.

Promyelocytes are cells with smooth or slightly stippled nuclear chromatin, with or without a nucleolus, and many distinct azurophilic granules dispersed in slightly to moderately blue cytoplasm. The nucleus is central or eccentric. Prominent nucleoli may be present, even in cells with a high concentration of granules. A clear Golgi zone may be present as well.

Myelocytes, which are the last maturation stage in which mitosis can occur, are smaller than progranulocytes, have round to oval nuclei, light blue cytoplasm, and no primary granules within the cytoplasm. In these cells, the primary granules have been replaced by secondary (i.e., specific) granules, which are difficult to see in neutrophil precursors but are very distinct in eosinophil and basophil precursors. Eosinophil precursors contain pink (i.e., eosinophilic) granules, and basophil precursors contain azurophilic to dark purple granules (Figure 15.3).

Metamyelocytes have kidney bean–shaped nuclei. The cytoplasm is similar in appearance to that of myelocytes.

Band granulocytes have nuclei that are curved and elongated, with parallel sides. Some chromatin clumping is present, and the cytoplasm is similar to that of myelocytes and metamyelocytes.

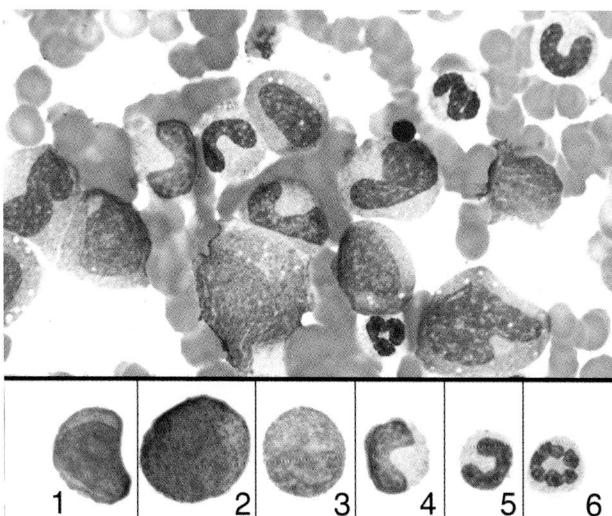

Figure 15.2 Top. Bone marrow aspirate from a dog showing numerous granulocytic (myeloid) precursors. Note the irregularly shaped nuclei, fine chromatin patterns, and lavender-colored cytoplasm. Bottom. Maturation stages of myeloid precursors, from immature to mature. 1, myeloblast; 2, promyelocyte; 3, myelocyte; 4, metamyelocyte; 5, band neutrophil; 6, segmented neutrophil. Wright stain.

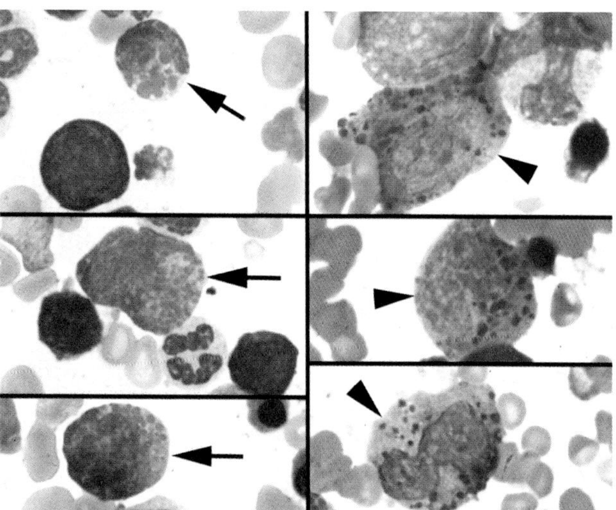

Figure 15.3 Left. Various maturation stages of eosinophil precursors (arrows). Right. Various maturation stages of basophil precursors (arrowheads). Granules may obscure the nucleus, thus making identification of specific maturation stage difficult. Wright stain.

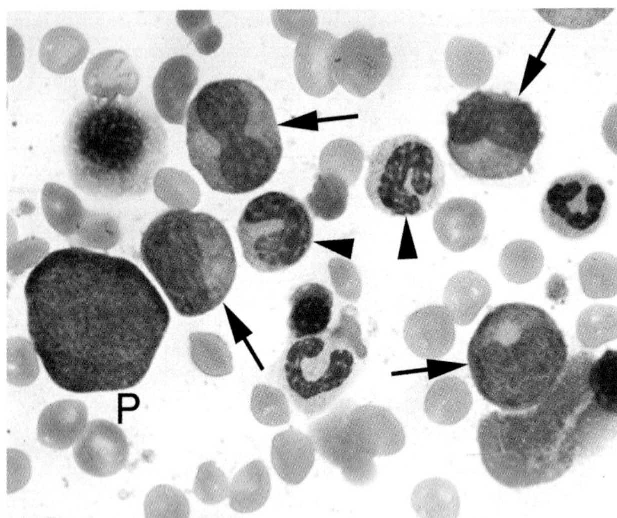

Figure 15.4 Bone marrow aspirate from dog with granulocytic and monocytic hyperplasia. Monocyte precursors (arrows) are difficult to distinguish from granulocytic precursors (arrowheads). Chromatin pattern is more coarse in granulocytic precursors. P, progranulocyte. Wright stain.

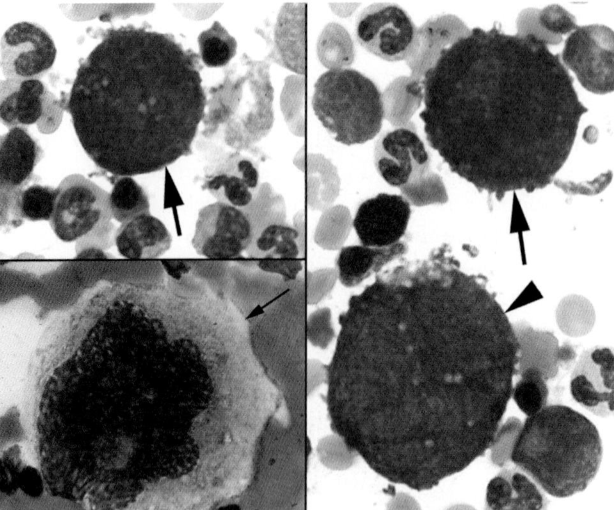

Figure 15.5 Various maturation stages of megakaryocyte series. Large arrows, megakaryoblasts; arrowhead, promegakaryocyte; small arrow, mature megakaryocyte. Wright stain.

Segmented granulocytes have lobulated or markedly constricted nuclei, with large and dense chromatin clumps. The cytoplasmic characteristics are generally similar to those of myelocytes, metamyelocytes, and bands.

Monocyte series

Cells of the monocyte series are relatively few in concentration, and they are very difficult to distinguish from those of the myeloid series in normal marrow. A distinctive feature is their irregular nuclear outlines. Monoblasts appear similar to myeloblasts, and promonocytes appear similar to myelocytes and metamyelocytes. Mature monocytes have the same appearance as monocytes in blood (Figure 15.4). Monocyte precursors usually are recognizable only in animals with monocytic leukemia.

Monoblasts are large cells with round, irregular or folded nuclei and finely reticular nuclear chromatin, one or more prominent nucleoli, and a moderate amount of basophilic, agranular cytoplasm. A Golgi zone often is prominent at the site of nuclear indentation. The nucleus : cytoplasm ratio usually is less than that of myeloblasts.

Promonocytes are large cells with cerebriform nuclei and prominent nuclear folds, stippled or lacy chromatin, and no distinct nucleolus. They also have more abundant and less basophilic "ground-glass" cytoplasm than that of monoblasts.

Megakaryocyte series

Megakaryocytes are very large cells, and their cytoplasmic fragments become platelets, which are important in the clotting process. Although these cells undergo mitosis, they do not divide, thus becoming very large and multinucleated, with as many as 16 or more nuclei. The nuclei are not separate entities, however, and they appear as a large, multilobulated structure in the center of the cell. The developmental stages of the megakaryocyte series, from immature to mature, are the megakaryoblast, promegakaryocyte, and megakaryocyte (Figure 15.5).

Megakaryoblasts are first recognizable when their size exceeds that of other types of precursors. The nuclei usually appear to be more dense than those of other types of blast cells, and the cytoplasm usually is deeply basophilic.

Promegakaryocytes have from two to four nuclei, which usually are connected by thin strands of nuclear material and deep blue agranular cytoplasm. They also usually are several-fold larger than rubriblasts or myeloblasts.

Megakaryocytes are very large (diameter, 50–200 μm), with numerous nuclei that form a lobulated mass of nuclear material. The cytoplasm stains more lightly than that of promegakaryocytes. As megakaryocytes mature, they become larger, gain more nuclei, and contain cytoplasm that becomes granular and, sometimes, light pink in color. Naked nuclei of megakaryocytes commonly are observed in bone marrow films.

Other cells

Small lymphocytes in bone marrow appear as they do in blood, with a round and usually indented nucleus, a diffuse chromatin pattern without visible nucleoli, and scant, light blue cytoplasm. They are slightly smaller than neutrophils (Figure 15.6). Plasma cells are differentiated lymphocytes that produce immunoglobulin, and they are similar in size to neutrophils. The appearance of plasma cells is very similar to that of rubricytes, except that the cytoplasm of plasma cells is light blue and more abundant, with a clear Golgi zone adjacent to the often-eccentric nucleus sometimes being apparent (Figure 15.6). The nuclei are round, with very coarse and dense chromatin, and nucleoli are inapparent. The cytoplasm of plasma cells occasionally may contain either very eosinophilic material (i.e., "flame cells") or round, clear to light blue structures that represent immunoglobulin (i.e., Russell bodies). Plasma cells that contain Russell bodies are called Mott cells (Figure 15.7).

Lymphoblasts rarely are seen in the bone marrow aspirates from normal animals, and their presence often is indicative of a lymphoproliferative disorder. Lymphoblasts are small to large cells with a round to oval nucleus, finely stippled to slightly course nuclear chromatin, one or more nucleoli, and a small to moderate amount of pale blue cytoplasm without azurophilic granules. The nuclear outline may appear to be slightly indented or irregular. The nucleus : cytoplasm ratio usually is greater than that of myeloblasts. Lymphoblasts are distinguished from myeloblasts by the slightly more coarse chromatin, less cytoplasm, and the absence of azurophilic granules. Lymphoblasts may appear similar to rubriblasts, but the nuclei of lymphoblasts are less perfectly round.

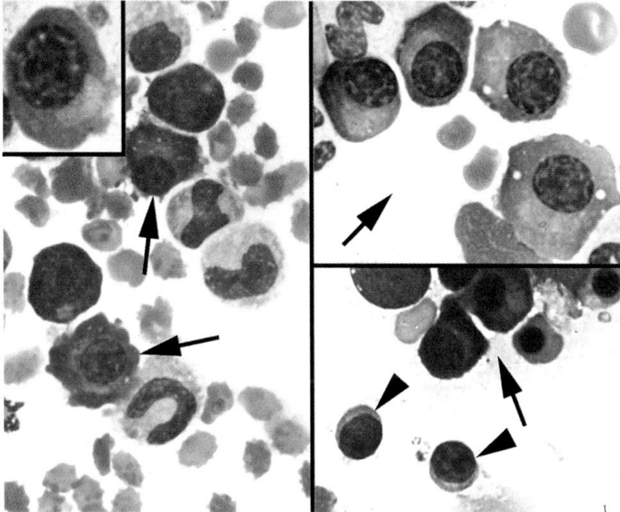

Figure 15.6 Plasma cells (arrows) have a variable appearance, depending on thickness of preparation and degree of flattening of the cells. Flattened plasma cells usually appear to have abundant cytoplasm and obvious, clear Golgi areas. Inset. Higher magnification of a plasma cell. Note the coarse chromatin and clear Golgi area. Lymphocytes (arrowheads) have a small amount of cytoplasm. Wright stain.

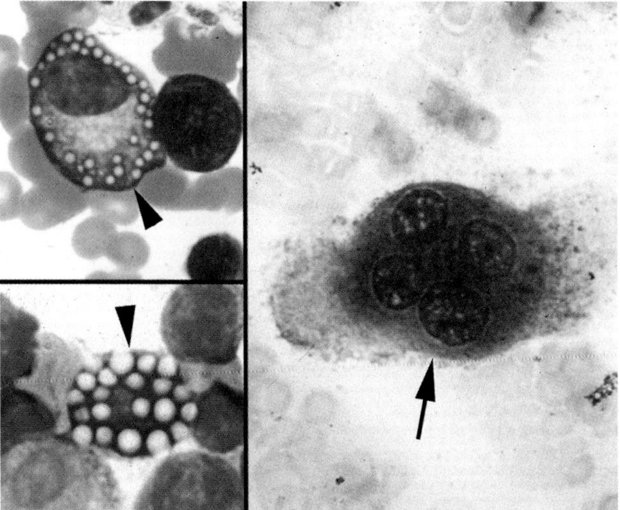

Figure 15.7 Left. Vacuolated plasma cells (Mott cells) containing packets of immunoglobulin (Russell bodies). Right. Osteoclast, which can be differentiated from a megakaryocyte because the osteoclast nuclei are separate rather than lobulated. Wright stain.

Macrophages derive from monocytes and are present at a low concentration in normal bone marrow. The appearance of macrophages is highly variable. The nuclei usually are round to slightly kidney bean in shape, and the nucleoli usually are small and inconspicuous. The cytoplasm is gray-blue and usually vacuolated; small, pink granules may be present in the cytoplasm as well. Macrophage nuclei may contain several small nucleoli. Macrophages commonly phagocytize cellular debris, including nuclei that have been extruded from metarubricytes, and they often contain hemosiderin, which is a red cell breakdown product containing iron.

Osteoblasts and osteoclasts may be seen in the bone marrow aspirates from young animals and from those in which bone remodeling is occurring. Osteoclasts are very large, multinucleated cells that may appear similar to megakaryocytes, but their nuclei are individual and not connected to each other (unlike those of megakaryocytes). The cytoplasm is basophilic, and may contain a few pink to azurophilic granules. Osteoclasts are specialized macrophages that derive from monocytes, and they function in the lysis of bone (Figure 15.7). Osteoblasts are similar in appearance to plasma cells but are larger (Figure 15.8). They have eccentric, round to oval nuclei that appear to be falling out of one end of the cell; they also have abundant basophilic cytoplasm and a clear Golgi area. Small pink or azurophilic granules may be present in the cytoplasm as well.

Mast cells are easily recognized in the bone marrow, and although rarely observed, they normally are present at very low concentrations. Mast cells are large, round, and discrete cells with abundant small metachromatic granules in the cytoplasm (Figure 15.8). They usually can be distinguished from basophil myelocytes, because mast cell granules are smaller and more numerous. Mast cells are more apparent and, possibly, increased in concentration in bone marrow that is hypocellular, such as that which may be seen with ehrlichiosis. When mast cells are abundant, infiltration by mast cell neoplasia is likely.

Fibrocytes and fibroblasts are seen only infrequently, even in aspirates from animals with myelofibrosis, because they do not exfoliate easily. The nuclei are round to oval, and the cytoplasm is lightly basophilic and spindle-shaped.

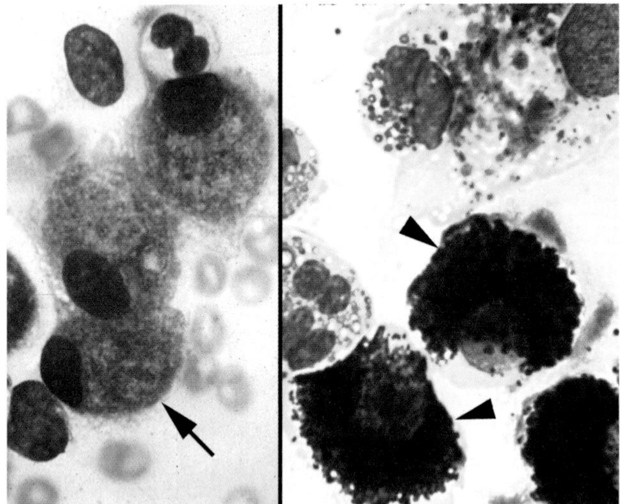

Figure 15.8 Left. Osteoblasts, which have a similar appearance to plasma cells but are larger, with a less condensed chromatin pattern and less distinct cytoplasmic margins (arrow). Right. Mast cells with abundant cytoplasmic granules that tend to obscure the round nucleus (arrowheads). Wright stain.

Cytochemistry and immunophenotyping

Cytochemical reactions sometimes are useful in the process of cell identification. These stain reactions are based on various cell types having different amounts, distribution, and types of enzyme activities. The stains most commonly used include peroxidase, Sudan black B, chloroacetate esterase, α-naphthyl acetate esterase, α-naphthyl butyrate esterase, and alkaline phosphatase (ALP). Peroxidase, Sudan black B, and chloroacetate esterase are myeloid (i.e., granulocytic) markers. The nonspecific esterases α-naphthyl acetate esterase and α-naphthyl butyrate esterase, which can be inhibited by sodium fluoride, and are monocyte markers, but their staining patterns vary. Monocytes may have a few small, round granules that stain positive for Sudan black B. Reactivity for ALP is somewhat confusing, however, because ALP positivity is rare in the immature neutrophils of normal animals but ALP-positive myeloid cells are common in animals with acute myelogenous leukemia. Moreover, ALP activity is present in some types of lymphoid cells as well as in cells with monocytic differentiation in animals with acute myelomonocytic leukemia. Cytochemical staining of blood and bone marrow films can facilitate the classification of neoplastic cells, but in many cases, negative staining occurs, perhaps because of abnormalities in hematopoietic differentiation that are associated with the neoplastic process.

Immunophenotypic analysis is based on using monoclonal antibodies that are directed against antigens on the surface of hematopoietic cells to determine the phenotypic profile of those cells, thus identifying the cell type. Very little sample quantity usually is necessary, and flow cytometric analysis using the antibodies makes the technique relatively simple to perform. Briefly, monoclonal anti bodies directed against cell surface proteins are conjugated to fluorescent molecules and then mixed with the cells, after which the cells are analyzed by flow cytometry. Flow cytometry provides information regarding the size of the cells, expression of any particular surface protein, and concentration of the surface protein. Phenotypes of both normal and neoplastic cells are continuously being classified as more monoclonal antibodies become available. Immunophenotyping likely will eventually replace cytochemistry for use in the classification of hematopoietic cells. See Chapter 14 for more discussion.

Evaluation and interpretation of bone marrow films

Bone marrow films must be evaluated and interpreted in conjunction with the analysis of concurrent complete blood count (CBC) data. For example, if an animal has a decreased platelet concentration (i.e., thrombocytopenia), the megakaryocyte concentration is particularly important to evaluate.

Cellularity

The low-power (×10) objective should be used to scan the slide at ×100 magnification to assess the degree of cellularity and amount of fat that is present (Figure 15.9). Hemodiluted marrow samples are difficult to evaluate for cellularity. Normal marrow cellularity varies, but in general, approximately 50% of the marrow consists of fat and 50%

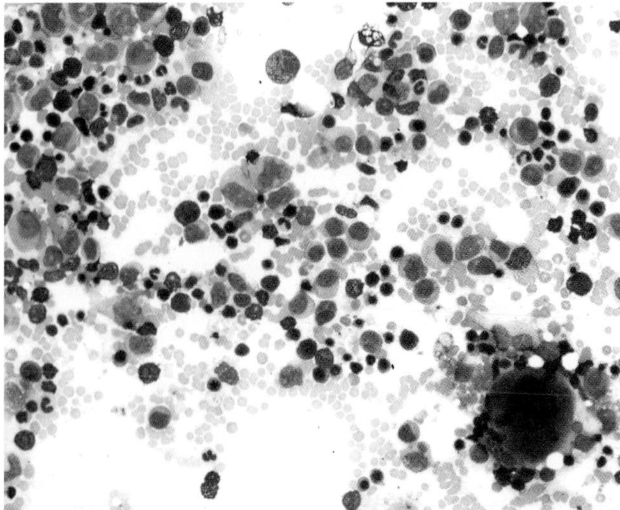

Figure 15.9 Bone marrow aspirate from a dog, low magnification. The degree of cellularity is adequate to increased. Cellularity is judged by the density of sheets of cells, as exemplified in this figure, or by estimating the ratio of fat to cells in particles. Wright stain, low power.

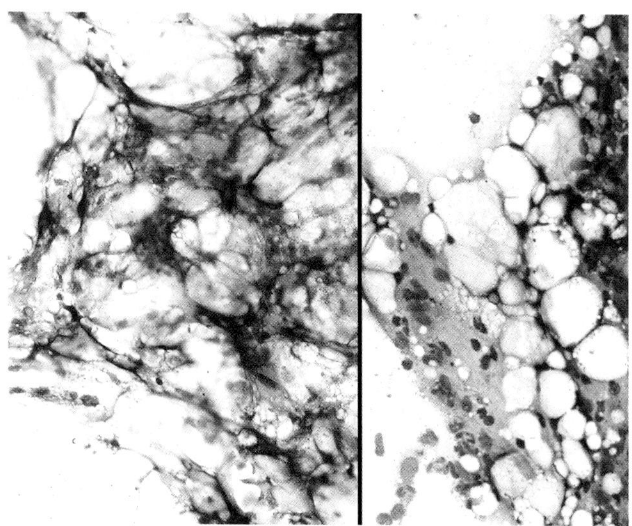

Figure 15.10 Bone marrow aspirate from a cat with generalized marrow hypoplasia, low magnification. Right. Numerous adipocytes are present, with very little hematopoietic cellularity. Left. Broken adipocytes and stroma are present, with few hematopoietic cells. Wright stain, low power.

of cells. Cellularity is increased when production in either the myeloid or the erythroid cell line is increased in response to cell loss, destruction, or consumption. Abnormal causes of increased cellularity include lymphoproliferative and myeloproliferative disorders as well as other neoplastic disorders. Overall cellularity may be decreased with disorders such as myelofibrosis, certain infectious agents (including *Ehrlichia* sp. in dogs and feline leukemia virus [FeLV]), estrogen toxicity (in dogs and ferrets), drug toxicities (including some commonly used chemotherapeutic agents), chemicals that are toxic to the marrow, radiation, and immune-mediated disorders in which stem cells are destroyed (Figure 15.10). A decrease in cellularity is termed hypoplasia, and a complete absence of cells is termed aplasia. Hypoplasia of only one cell line is relatively common, whereas aplasia usually involves all cell lines. Erythroid or myeloid aplasia is rare. Histopathologic evaluation of a core biopsy specimen is indicated when the cellularity is very low or cannot be determined by examination of the marrow aspirate.

Megakaryocytes

Using the low-power (10×) objective, the megakaryocyte concentration should be estimated as either increased (i.e., hyperplasia), decreased (i.e., hypoplasia), or adequate. Interpretation of this estimate depends on the platelet concentration in the blood. Areas with high cellularity normally contain at least a few megakaryocytes, and unless the sample is markedly hemodiluted, at least 5–10 megakaryocytes should be present on the slide. In animals with increased platelet consumption (e.g., animals with disseminated intravascular coagulopathy) or destruction (e.g., animals with immune-mediated thrombocytopenia), the megakaryocyte concentration in the marrow should be increased. Animals with megakaryocytic hyperplasia may have as many as 50 or more megakaryocytes in cellular areas of the slide. Increased concentrations of megakaryoblasts, promegakaryocytes, and smaller, more immature megakaryocytes typically are seen with megakaryocytic hyperplasia. In thrombocytopenic patients with megakaryocytic hyperplasia, the platelet size usually is increased because of the early release of platelets; this increase in size is analogous to the increased size of immature erythrocytes. Animals that are thrombocytopenic because of the lack of platelet production have very few – or even no – megakaryocytes in the marrow film. Megakaryocytic hypoplasia without erythroid and myeloid hypoplasia is rare and may be caused by immune-mediated destruction of megakaryocytes.

Myeloid : erythroid ratio

Using the ×10 objective, appropriate areas that are not too thick and in which cells are not broken can be chosen for further examination of the bone marrow using the ×50 or ×100 oil objectives (to magnify 500- and 1000-fold, respectively). At these higher magnifications, erythroid and myeloid precursors can be identified, and the myeloid : erythroid (M : E) ratio can be estimated (Figure 15.11). Usually, estimation of this ratio is just as informative as actual quantification. To quantify the M : E ratio, 300–500 nucleated cells are classified as being either myeloid or erythroid. This classification should be performed while examining several different areas, because some fields may be predominantly granulocytic and other areas predominantly erythroid.

Normal M : E ratios differ with the species, but in general, they range from 0.5 : 1 to 3 : 1. Decreased or increased production of either cell line shifts the M : E ratio, and such shifts

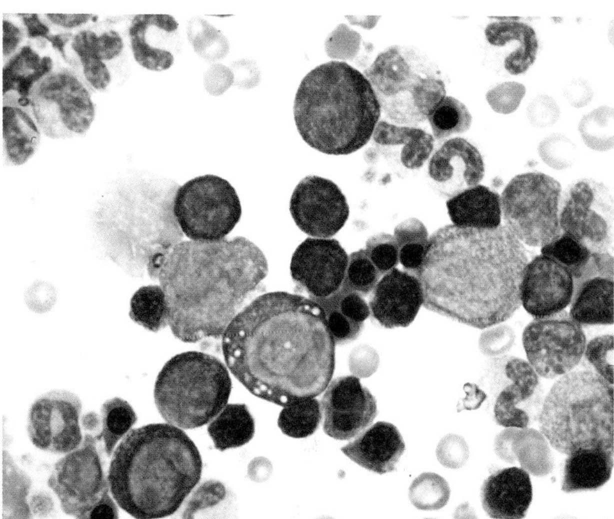

Figure 15.11 Bone marrow aspirate from a dog. Both myeloid and erythroid precursors are present, with a normal myeloid : erythroid ratio of approximately 1. Wright stain.

must be interpreted in light of the CBC results, particularly the packed cell volume and the neutrophil concentration. For example, if the M : E ratio is increased, the animal is anemic, and the blood neutrophil concentration is normal, then the ratio is increased because of a decrease in red cell production rather than an increase in neutrophil production. Conversely, if the animal is not anemic and the neutrophil concentration is increased, then the increased M : E ratio results from an increased neutrophil production rather than a decreased erythrocyte production.

Decreased M : E ratio

A decreased M : E ratio may be indicative of increased red cell production, such as that seen with a regenerative anemia (i.e., erythroid hyperplasia); a decreased neutrophil production (i.e., myeloid hypoplasia); or a combination of the two (Figure 15.12). Myeloid hypoplasia without erythroid hypoplasia is rare but, when present, usually is associated with myelodysplasia or myeloproliferative disorder.

Increased M : E ratio

An increased M : E ratio may be indicative of increased granulocyte production (i.e., myeloid hyperplasia), decreased in red cell production (i.e., erythroid hypoplasia), or both (Figure 15.13). Granulocytic hyperplasia usually results from inflammation, but it also may be seen in animals with immune-mediated destruction of neutrophils and in those recovering from viral-induced marrow damage, such as parvovirus infections in dogs (i.e., parvoviral enteritis) and cats (i.e., panleukopenia). Causes of erythroid hypoplasia are discussed in Chapter 8 and include renal failure, endocrinopathies, and anemia of inflammatory disease. Anemia of inflammatory disease (i.e., anemia of chronic disease) is one of the more common causes of mild erythroid hypoplasia in domestic animals. Granulocytic hyperplasia and increased iron stores (i.e., hemosiderin) also usually are seen in the marrow from these patients. Pure red cell aplasia is rare but, when present, usually is caused by immune-mediated destruction of very early erythroid precursors.

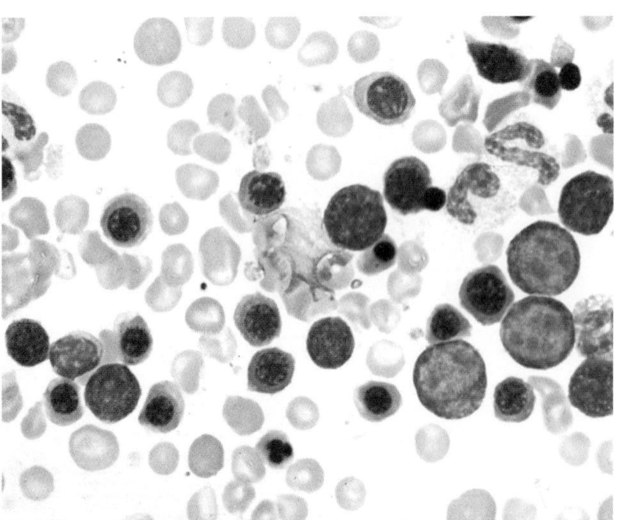

Figure 15.12 Bone marrow aspirate from a dog with regenerative anemia. The myeloid : erythroid ratio is decreased because of increased red cell production (erythroid hyperplasia). Wright stain.

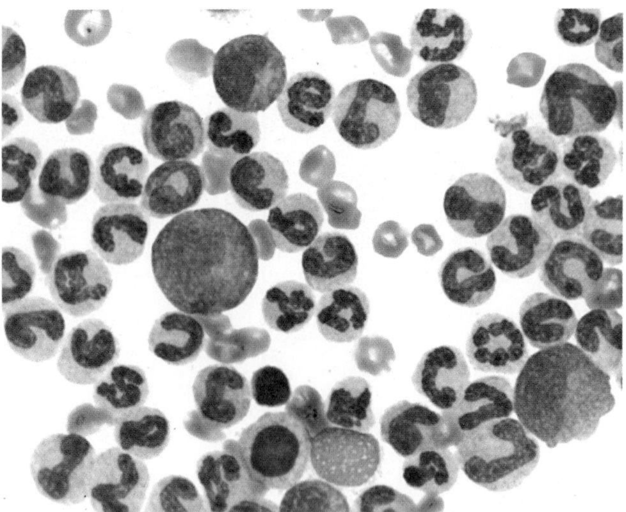

Figure 15.13 Bone marrow aspirate from a dog. The myeloid : erythroid ratio is markedly increased because of increased granulocyte production (myeloid hyperplasia). Wright stain.

Orderliness of maturation

The orderliness and completion of maturation in erythroid and myeloid cells should be determined. Blast cells divide to ultimately produce 16–32 mature cells. Thus, approximately 80–90% of the cells should be more mature forms (i.e., metamyelocytes, bands, and neutrophils in the myeloid series, and rubricytes and metarubricytes in the erythroid series), and polychromatophilic erythrocytes should be present. Orderly progression of maturation usually is referred to as a "pyramid," with the few immature forms comprising the top and the numerous more mature forms comprising the broad bottom (Figure 15.14).

Disorderly maturation of erythroid and myeloid precursors commonly is seen in animals with leukemia and myelodysplasia, but it also may be seen in animals with nonneoplastic conditions. An apparent arrest in maturation of the erythroid series, often at the rubricyte stage of maturity, may be seen in animals with immune-mediated destruction of immature erythroid cells. These animals do not have a typical regenerative response, such as that usually seen in animals with immune-mediated hemolytic anemia. Metarubricytes and polychromatophilic erythrocytes often are decreased to absent in the marrow from such patients.

A similar apparent arrest of maturation in the granulocytic series, which often occurs in conjunction with marked

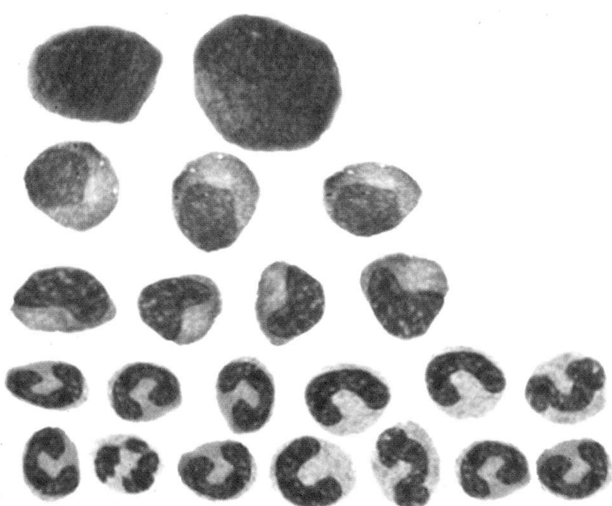

Figure 15.14 A normal "pyramid," illustrating an orderly maturation of myeloid precursors. A few very immature cells form the top of the pyramid, with numerous more mature cells forming the bottom.

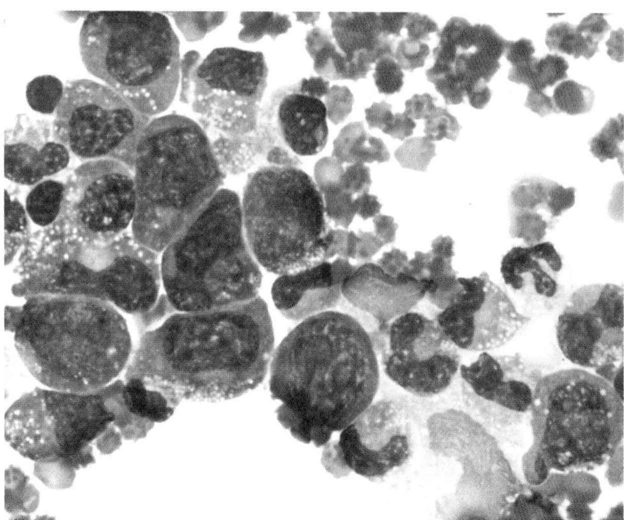

Figure 15.15 Bone marrow aspirate from a dog with immune-mediated neutropenia. Marked myeloid hyperplasia is evident, with an increased proportion of more immature granulocyte precursors and few mature granulocytes because of the immune-mediated destruction of more mature cells. Note that the cytoplasm is basophilic and vacuolated, likely because of the increased rate of cell production. Wright stain.

myeloid hyperplasia, commonly is seen in marrow aspirates from animals with immune-mediated neutropenia (Figure 15.15). This "arrest" may appear at any stage of granulocytic maturity, but it often occurs at the metamyelocyte stage. Marrow from animals with immune-mediated destruction can appear similar to that from patients with granulocytic leukemia, but the concentration of myeloblasts usually is lower in those with immune-mediated disease. Other conditions that cause disorderly maturation of granulocytes include marked inflammatory disease (with consumption of more mature forms) and recovery from viral-induced neutropenia.

Macrophages and iron stores

Macrophages (i.e., histiocytes) normally are present in small concentrations (<1% of nucleated cells), and phagocytosis of red cells and nuclear debris by macrophages occasionally may be seen in normal animals. The concentration of macrophages may be increased in animals with immune-mediated disorders, and macrophages that have phagocytized nucleated red cells, platelets, and neutrophils occasionally are observed (Figure 15.16). Other causes of increased cell destruction, such as marrow necrosis secondary to drugs, toxins, or radiation, may result in increased macrophage concentration. In these cases, other morphologic evidence of necrosis, such as pyknosis and increased cytoplasmic vacuolation, usually is observed.

A marked increase in the concentration of macrophages may be seen in animals with hemophagocytic syndrome, which also is called hemophagocytic histiocytosis and is a condition characterized by a benign, histiocytic proliferation secondary to infectious, neoplastic, or metabolic diseases. One retrospective study [1] found hemophagocytic syndrome in 3.9% of dogs that had bone marrow aspiration. This syndrome is associated with cytopenia of at least two cell lines and greater than 2% hemophagocytic macrophages in the marrow. It must be distinguished, on the basis of red cell morphology (i.e., lack of spherocytes and agglutination) and a negative Coombs test, from the much more commonly occurring immune-mediated diseases. Macrophages are a prominent cellular component in the marrow from animals with hemophagocytic syndrome, and they appear

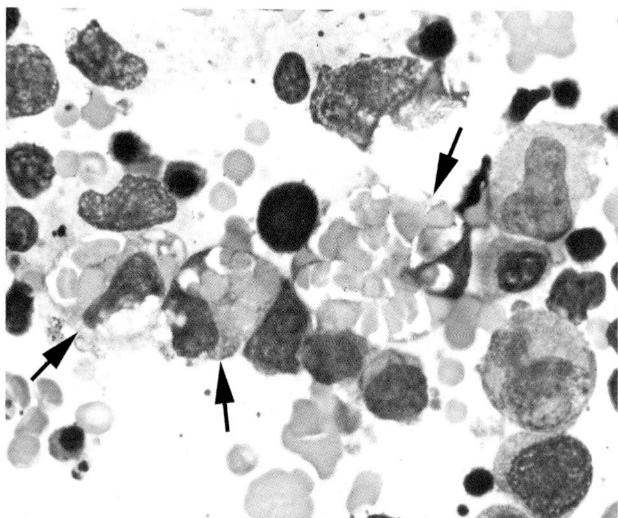

Figure 15.16 Bone marrow aspirate from a cat. Macrophages (arrows) are increased and have phagocytized many erythrocytes. This degree of phagocytic activity is abnormal and suggestive of either immune-mediated destruction of red cells or hemophagocytic syndrome. Wright stain.

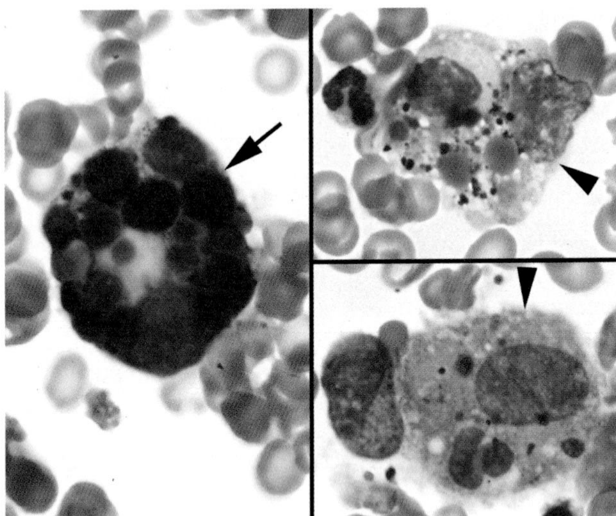

Figure 15.17 Bone marrow aspirate from a dog. Left. A macrophage (arrow) that has phagocytized erythrocytes as well as nucleated erythrocytes. Upper right. A macrophage (arrowhead) that has phagocytized erythrocytes, a large nucleated cell, platelets, and cellular debris. Lower right. A macrophage (arrowhead) that has phagocytized a neutrophil and contains hemosiderin. Phagocytosis of platelets and immature cells may be seen with immune-mediated disease and with hemophagocytic syndrome. Wright stain.

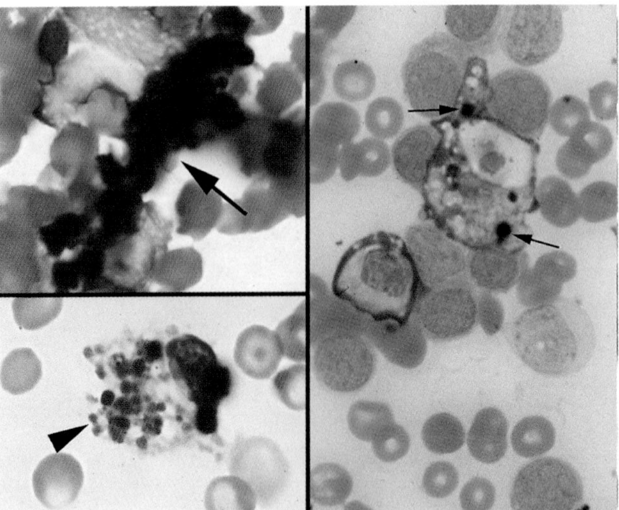

Figure 15.18 Bone marrow aspirate from a dog. Upper left. A clump of hemosiderin (storage iron; arrow) from a broken macrophage. Wright stain. Lower left. A macrophage (arrowhead) containing hemosiderin. Wright stain. Right. Prussian blue iron stain, showing the presence of blue-staining iron (small arrows).

to be normal and well differentiated, with amoeboid nuclei and abundant, light blue cytoplasm. Many macrophages are observed with phagocytized hematopoietic cells within their cytoplasm (Figure 15.17). Dogs with hemophagocytic syndrome often exhibit fever, icterus, splenomegaly, hepatomegaly, and diarrhea, and those with infection-associated hemophagocytic syndrome are thought to have a better survival rate than dogs with other causes of hemophagocytic syndrome. An increased concentration of macrophages also is seen in animals with malignant histiocytosis, which is a neoplastic proliferation of histiocytes (see below).

The presence or absence of hemosiderin (i.e., iron stores) in macrophages should be noted (Figure 15.18). Special stains for iron, such as a Prussian blue stain (Figure 15.18), usually are not necessary, because hemosiderin can be readily visualized with use of Romanowsky stains. Hemosiderin rarely is seen in the marrow aspirates from normal cats, but it usually is abundant in that from normal dogs and horses. Animals with iron deficiency anemia lack iron stores in the marrow, and animals with anemia of inflammatory disease may have increased iron stores.

Other cells

The presence and percentage of other types of cells, such as lymphocytes and plasma cells, should be noted as well. In animals that have been antigenically stimulated, the plasma cell concentration may be markedly increased, and the plasma cells may be present in small groups. Normally, approximately 2% or less of the marrow cells are plasma cells. Approximately 15% or less of the cells observed in a bone marrow film from healthy dogs may be lymphocytes, whereas as much as 20% of the cells may be lymphocytes in normal cats. The concentrations of plasma cells and lymphocytes in the bone marrow film usually vary from one area of the film to the next.

Microorganisms

Microorganisms occasionally may be found in bone marrow aspirates. Bacteria very rarely are seen, but *Histoplasma capsulatum* (Figure 15.19), *Toxoplasma gondii* (Figure 15.20),

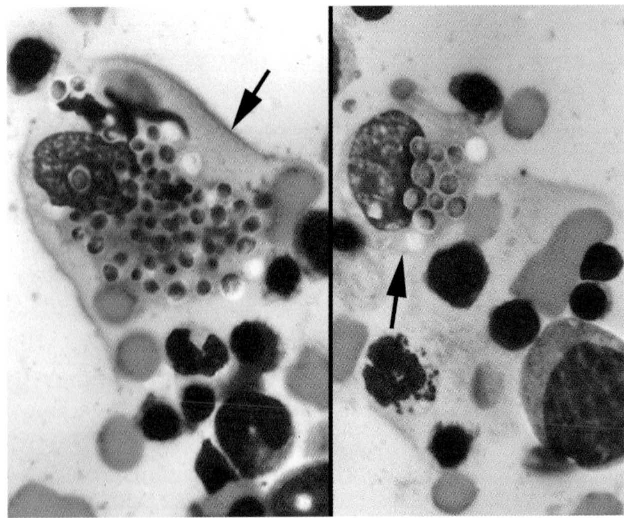

Figure 15.19 Bone marrow aspirate from a cat. Macrophages (arrows) contain numerous *Histoplasma capsulatum* organisms, which are round yeast cells with a well-defined, thin capsule. Wright stain. Source: Specimen courtesy of Antech Diagnostics.

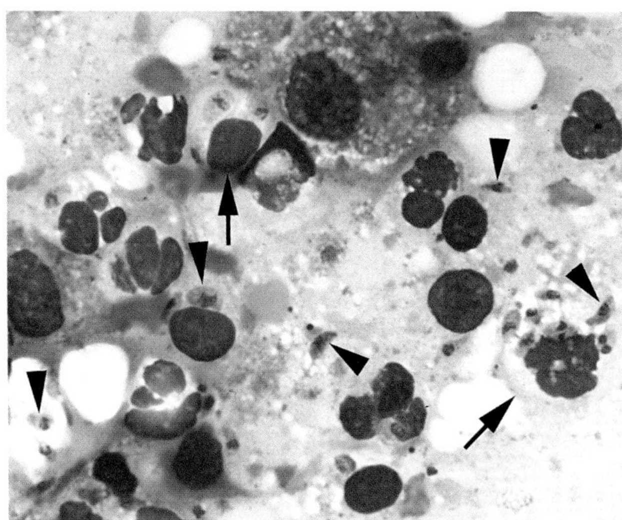

Figure 15.20 Bone marrow aspirate from a cat. Macrophages (arrows) contain trophozoites of *Toxoplasma gondii*. Individual trophozoites (arrowheads) have a characteristic crescent shape and a central nucleus. Wright stain.

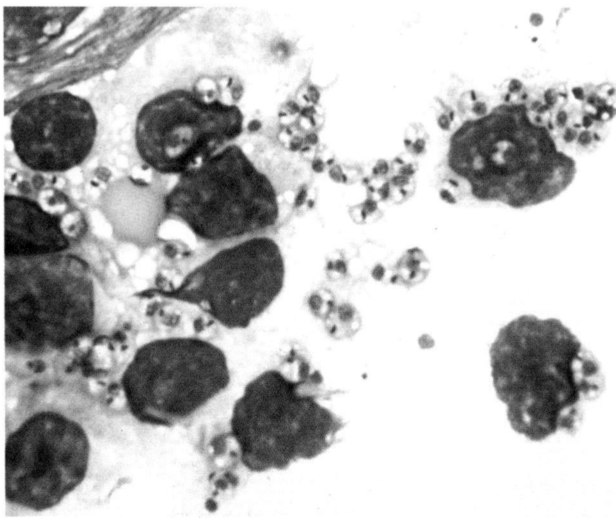

Figure 15.21 Bone marrow aspirate from a dog. Note the broken mononuclear cells with numerous *Leishmania donovani* organisms. These organisms are oval, with a typical, dark-staining, rod-shaped structure (kinetoplast). Wright stain.

Leishmania donovani (Figure 15.21), *Cytauxzoon felis*, and rarely, *Ehrlichia* sp. can be observed. Red cell parasites such as *Mycoplasma* sp. or *Babesia* sp. also may be observed in marrow aspirates.

Stem cell disorders of marrow

Reversible stem cell injuries

Reversible injury is transient in nature and, therefore, usually manifests as neutropenia because of the short half-life of neutrophils in blood (see Chapter 12). Causes include viral injury, drugs or chemicals, and chemotherapeutic drugs, such as doxorubricin, that injure rapidly dividing cells. Although neutropenia is recognized initially, thrombocytopenia and nonregenerative anemia may occur if the injury lasts for more than 1–2 weeks. In general, if the animal does not have complications associated with the cytopenias, the stem cell system can be expected to recover and repopulate the blood with normal concentrations of cells.

Some drugs and chemicals apparently are directly cytotoxic to stem cells. Drugs that have been associated with stem cell injury in animals include estrogen (in dogs and ferrets), phenylbutazone (in dogs), and albendazole, which is a broadspectrum anthelmintic (in dogs and cats). Estrogen toxicosis may occur in bitches given exogenous estrogen for mismating, termination of pseudopregnancy, or urinary incontinence. Myelosuppression may occur either from administration of excessive amounts of estrogen or from an idiosyncratic sensitivity to estrogen. Endogenous estrogen, either because of Sertoli cell tumors in male dogs or cystic ovaries in female dogs, also may result in bone marrow suppression. Because ferrets are induced ovulators, marrow suppression from endogenous estrogen is a common and potentially fatal disorder in this species. The mechanism of estrogen toxicosis is unclear but is thought to result from secretion, by thymic stromal cells, of an estrogen-induced substance that inhibits stem cells. Marrow suppression is paradoxically preceded by an initial thrombocytosis and neutrophilia.

Other drugs may induce cell destruction by immune-mediated mechanisms. In dogs, trimethoprim-sulfadiazine, cephalosporin, and phenobarbital have been associated with pancytopenia that may be immune-mediated. Methimazole, which is used for treating cats with hyperthyroidism, is associated with neutropenia and thrombocytopenia in approximately 20% of the cats given this drug. Stem cell injury that is drug related and immune-mediated usually responds to discontinuation of the drug. Idiopathic immune-mediated stem cell injury usually responds to immunosuppressive therapy; however, it may take several weeks to respond and, often, requires long-term treatment for resolution.

Myelofibrosis may develop in response to various types of marrow injury. Any agent that is directly toxic to hematopoietic cells presumably may damage the microvasculature of the marrow, thereby leading to necrosis and subsequent fibrosis. Myelofibrosis also has been associated with myeloproliferative and lymphoproliferative disorders, other types of neoplasia, chronic hemolytic anemia secondary to pyruvate kinase deficiency, radiation, and other unidentified causes.

Irreversible stem cell injuries

In contrast to reversible stem cell injuries, irreversible injuries result from an intrinsic defect in proliferative

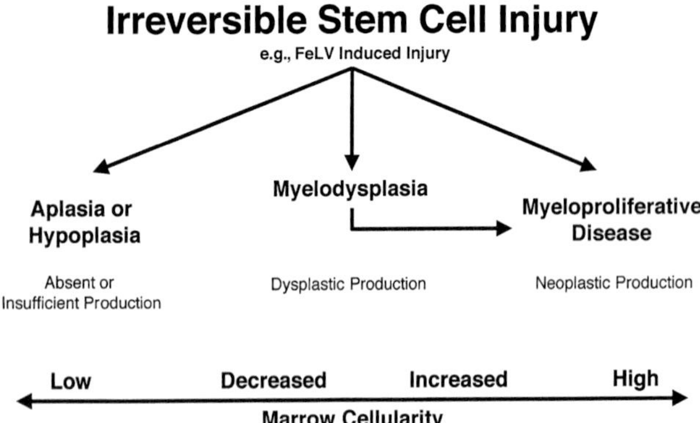

Figure 15.22 Organizational diagram of irreversible stem cell disorders. Myelodysplasia may progress to neoplasia over time. Expected cellularity of proliferative abnormalities is indicated at the bottom.

behavior or regulation of stem cell entry into differentiated hematopoiesis. These types of injuries generally are regarded as being irreversible, because they do not spontaneously correct themselves and therapeutic intervention almost never corrects the proliferative abnormality (with the exception of bone marrow transplantation, in which defective stem cells are replaced by normal donor stem cells). The causes of this form of stem cell injury are not well understood. The best-characterized causative association in domestic animals, however, is infection with FeLV in cats. In other domestic animals, the cause almost always is unknown. Chronic exposure to benzene-related chemical compounds is an employment hazard in humans and, rarely, may cause similar injury in animals. Radiation also may induce such an injury in a number of species. Manifestations of stem cell injury are highly variable (Figure 15.22). These manifestations are best regarded as being a continuum, from lack of cell production on one extreme to uncontrolled, neoplastic proliferation at the other. In the middle of this continuum is dysplastic cell production, which usually is associated with one or more cytopenias and with subtle morphologic abnormalities of the blood cells. Many cases likely begin as dysplasia and then, with time, progress to either hypoplasia or neoplasia. The stage observed at the initial examination is variable, depending on when during the course of the disease the animal is presented to the veterinarian. (More detailed descriptions of the points on this continuum are presented in Chapter 16.)

Aplasia or hypoplasia

Marrow aplasia is a relatively rare disorder in dogs and cats. Causes include chronic ehrlichiosis, Parvovirus, and FeLV infections; drug and toxin exposure; and idiopathic causes. Diagnosis is based on cytopenias in the blood and hypoplastic to aplastic bone marrow, with the marrow space replaced by adipose tissue. Treatment is dependent on determining the underlying cause of the bone marrow failure, and the outcome is variable. The hematologic result may be either somewhat selective, severe, and nonregenerative anemia (i.e., pure red cell aplasia or hypoplasia) or pancytopenia in which neutropenia and thrombocytopenia accompany the anemia (i.e., aplastic anemia). Establishing the morphologic diagnosis depends on the examination of marrow particles or histopathology to distinguish the hypocellularity from a hemodiluted marrow sample. Plasmacytosis of the marrow, in conjunction with the lack of hematopoietic cells, is often present with chronic ehrlichiosis, and is sometimes so marked that it must be distinguished from multiple myeloma (see Chapter 14). Most cases of pure red cell aplasia in dogs, as well as those that are not associated with FeLV in cats, likely are immune-mediated, and many respond to immunosuppressive therapy.

Dysmyelopoiesis

Dysmyelopoiesis is defined as a hematologic disorder characterized by the presence of cytopenias in the blood and dysplastic cells in one or more hematologic cell lines in the blood or bone marrow. The causes of dysmyelopoiesis include acquired mutations in hematopoietic stem cells (myelodysplastic syndromes) congenital defects in hematopoiesis, and secondary dysmyelopoietic conditions associated with various diseases, drugs, or toxins. Causes of secondary dysmyelopoiesis include immune-mediated hematologic diseases, lymphoid malignancies, and exposure to chemotherapeutic drugs. Secondary dysmyelopoiesis is also referred to as nonneoplastic syndromes of ineffective hematopoiesis in which dysmorphic maturation of cells occurs. Without methods to confirm clonality by cytogenetic analysis, the diagnosis of neoplastic myelodysplasia in dogs is based on light microscopic examination of bone marrow films (see Chapter 16). The characteristic morphologic and cytochemical features of neoplastic myelodysplasia and nonneoplastic ineffective hematopoiesis in dogs are discussed elsewhere in detail [2].

Neoplastic disorders involving bone marrow other than lymphoproliferative or myeloproliferative disorders

Mast cell leukemia may be seen in dogs and cats with systemic mastocytosis secondary to mast cell tumors (Figure 15.23). Although examinations of bone marrow aspirate commonly are performed to stage mast cell tumors, involvement of the marrow by mast cell tumors very rarely is observed. Buffy coat examination for mast cells also rarely is useful, because circulating mast cells occasionally may be seen in animals without mast cell tumors. The current recommendation is that bone marrow aspiration not be performed for routine staging but may be indicated for those dogs having either an abnormal CBC or presenting for tumor regrowth, progression, or new occurrence.

Malignant histiocytosis is a rapidly progressive – and ultimately fatal – proliferative disorder of the mononuclear

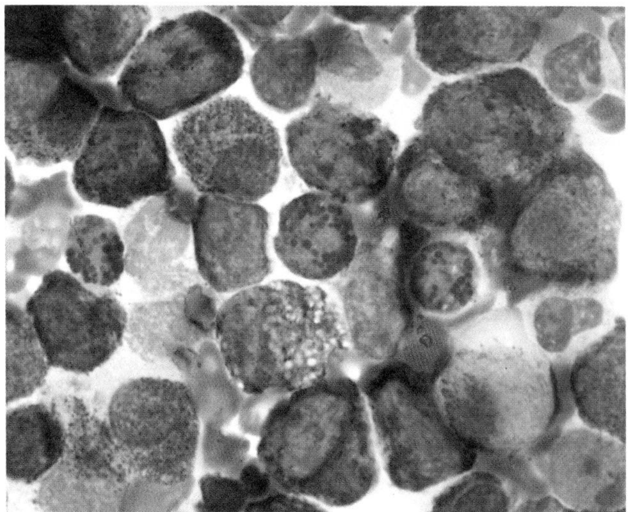

Figure 15.23 Bone marrow aspirate from a dog with poorly differentiated mast cell leukemia. Almost all of the cells present are mast cells with metachromatic cytoplasmic granules. This dog also had mast cells on the blood film. Wright stain.

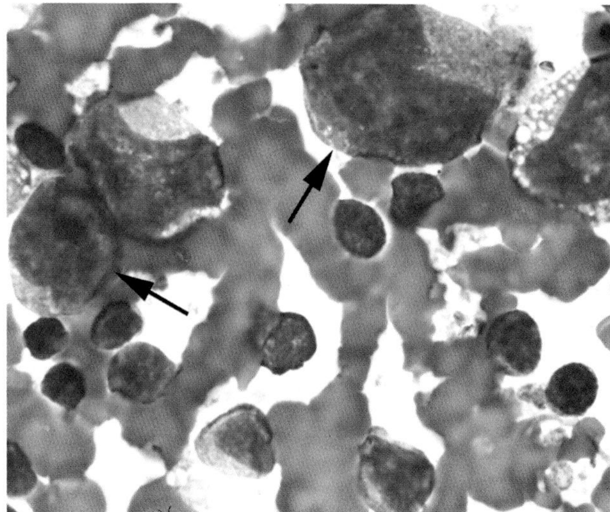

Figure 15.24 Bone marrow aspirate from a dog with malignant histiocytosis. Note the large, neoplastic histiocytic cells with prominent, irregularly shaped nucleoli (arrows). Most of the other nucleated cells in the field are small lymphocytes. Wright stain.

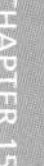

phagocyte system that has been described in adult dogs, including Bernese mountain dogs and other breeds. An increased incidence of the disorder has been suggested to occur in the golden retriever and flat-coated retriever breeds. The disorder often is characterized by the systemic proliferation of large, pleomorphic, single, and multinucleated histiocytes with marked cellular atypia and phagocytosis of erythrocytes and leukocytes. The bone marrow as well as lung, lymph nodes, liver, spleen, and central nervous system commonly are involved. Positive reactivity of neoplastic cells to histiocytic markers (e.g., lysozyme and α_1-antitrypsin) can be demonstrated by immunohistochemistry (IHC). This immunohistochemical reactivity aids in the differentiation of neoplastic histiocytic cells from lymphoid and epithelial neoplasms, and it is important for establishing a definitive diagnosis of the neoplasm. The cellularity of bone marrow aspirates containing neoplastic histiocytes is consistently very high. These histiocytes are pleomorphic, large, discrete, and markedly atypical mononuclear cells, and the nuclei are round to oval or reniform. Features of malignancy include marked anisocytosis and anisokaryosis, prominent nucleoli, bizarre mitotic figures, marked phagocytosis of erythrocytes, leukocytes, other tumor cells, and moderate amounts of lightly basophilic, vacuolated cytoplasm (Figure 15.24). The presence of multinucleated giant cells also is supportive of the diagnosis. Other findings vary and may include erythroid hypoplasia, with prominent cytophagia of marrow elements, or generalized marrow hypoplasia, with neoplastic infiltration of atypical histiocytes and marked phagocytosis. Hematologic abnormalities such as anemia and mild to marked thrombocytopenia also may be present, correlating with marrow changes.

Epithelial and mesenchymal tumors rarely metastasize to the bone marrow. Epithelial tumors (i.e., carcinomas) tend to form groups of cohesive cells that are easy to distinguish from normal hematopoietic cells (Figures 15.25 and 15.26). Metastatic sarcomas are more difficult to diagnose, however, and are characterized by large, discrete, spindle-shaped cells that meet multiple criteria for malignancy (Figure 15.27). These cells must be distinguished from fibroblasts that may be observed in myelofibrosis.

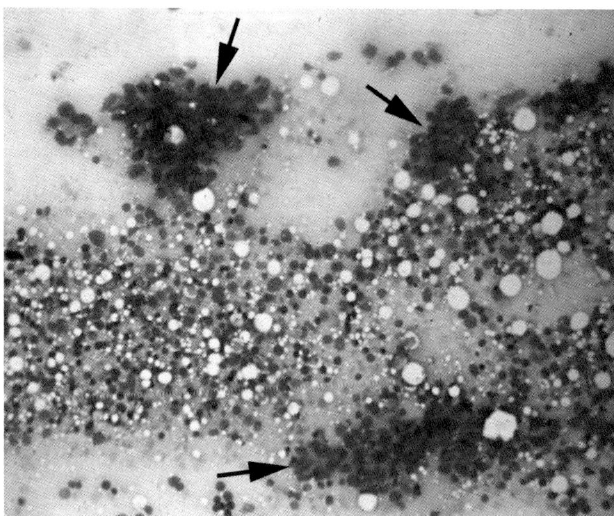

Figure 15.25 Bone marrow aspirate from a dog with metastatic mammary carcinoma, low magnification. The islands of cells (arrows) are neoplastic epithelial cells and can be differentiated from the normal hematopoietic cells by their tendency to adhere to each other. Wright stain. Low power.

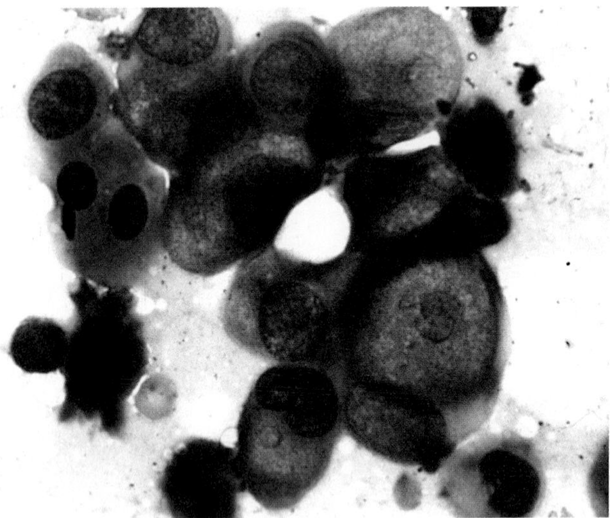

Figure 15.26 Bone marrow aspirate shown in Figure 15.25, high magnification. Note the large epithelial cells that exhibit numerous criteria of malignancy, including nuclear molding, binucelate cells, and prominent nucleoli. Wright stain.

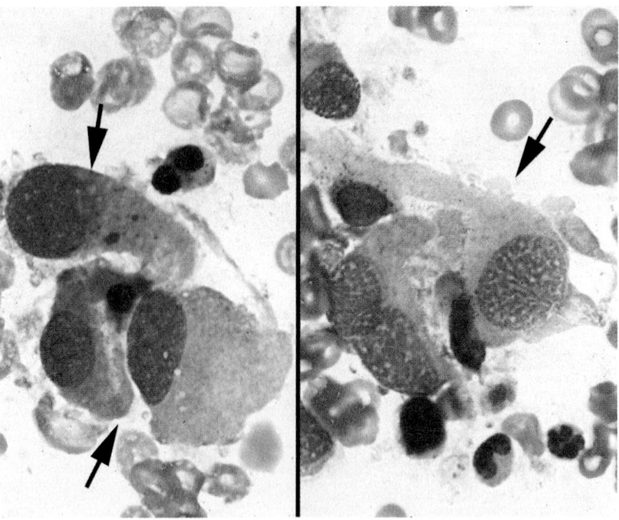

Figure 15.27 Bone marrow aspirate from a dog with metastatic hemangiosarcoma. Spindle-shaped neoplastic cells (arrows) exhibit numerous criteria of malignancy, including variability in nuclear size, variability in cell size, ropy chromatin, and prominent nucleoli. Note that some cells have fine, azurophilic granules in their cytoplasm. Wright stain. Source: Specimen courtesy of Dr. Kyra Somers, Idexx.

16 Lymphoproliferative Disorders and Myeloid Neoplasms

Mary Anna Thrall

Department of Biomedical Sciences, Ross University School of Veterinary Medicine, Basseterre, Saint Kitts and Nevis

Overview of myeloproliferative and lymphoproliferative disorders (leukemia)

Leukemia, a neoplastic proliferation of hematopoietic cells within the bone marrow, is defined by the presence of neoplastic blood cells in the peripheral blood, or bone marrow, and is classified broadly into myeloid neoplasms and lymphoproliferative disorders. The diagnosis of these disorders is established based on finding characteristic cells in the blood or bone marrow and associated hematologic abnormalities. Specific cell types are identified by their morphologic appearance in Wright-stained blood and bone marrow films, cytochemical staining properties, electron microscopic appearance, and monoclonal antibody binding to surface antigens. In some cases, cells may appear so morphologically undifferentiated that classifying the disorder into either the myeloproliferative or the lymphoproliferative category may be difficult (Figure 16.1). Myeloid neoplasms include neoplastic proliferation of erythrocytes, granulocytes, monocytes, and megakaryocytes. Multiple cell lines may be neoplastic if the affected stem cell is multipotential; an example is myelomonocytic leukemia, in which both neutrophils and monocytes have been neoplastically transformed. Lymphoproliferative disorders include acute lymphoblastic leukemia (ALL), chronic lymphocytic leukemia (CLL), and multiple myeloma.

Leukemias are also classified according to the concentration of neoplastic cells that are circulating in the blood. With leukemic leukemias, many neoplastic cells are circulating, thereby resulting in a markedly increased nucleated cell count. In patients with subleukemic leukemias, however, the nucleated cell count is near normal, with only a few neoplastic cells circulating. No circulating cells are observed on blood films from patients with aleukemic leukemia. Establishing the diagnosis of leukemia when few or no cells are circulating usually is based on examination of the marrow aspirate.

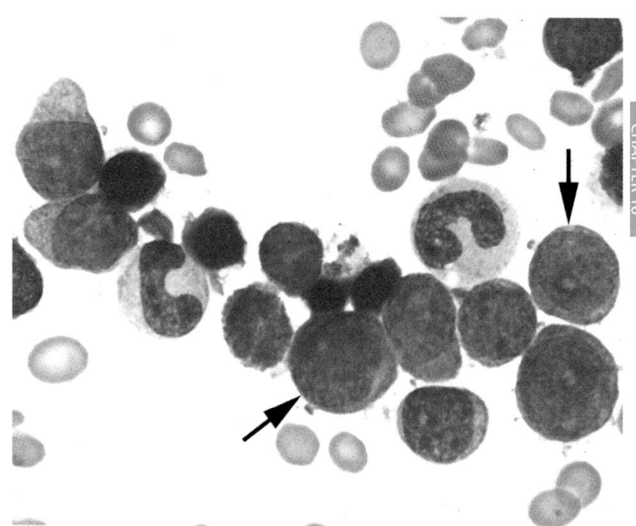

Figure 16.1 Bone marrow aspirate from a cat. Large undifferentiated cells (arrows) are difficult to classify based on their morphologic appearance. Cells may be lymphoblasts or type 1 myeloblasts. Wright stain.

Leukemias are also classified as either acute or chronic based primarily on the maturity or degree of neoplastic cell differentiation as well as by the clinical course. The neoplastic cells in acute leukemias are immature, often with an apparent nucleolus (blast), and the patient survival time usually is quite short. By definition, 20% or more blast cells in the marrow is diagnostic of acute myeloid leukemia (AML). The percentage of blast cells in the blood, however, is quite variable in these patients. Acute leukemias can be either myeloid (AML) or lymphoid (ALL), and neoplastic cells in most cases of acute leukemias express CD34, a marker for hematopoietic stem/precursor cells that also functions in cell migration. See Chapter 14 for discussion of CD (cluster of differentiation) protein expression on cell surfaces that identify various types of hematopoietic cells by using antibodies against those proteins. Both myeloid

Veterinary Hematology, Clinical Chemistry, and Cytology, Third Edition. Edited by Mary Anna Thrall, Glade Weiser, Robin W. Allison and Terry W. Campbell.

Companion website: www.wiley.com/go/thrall/veterinary

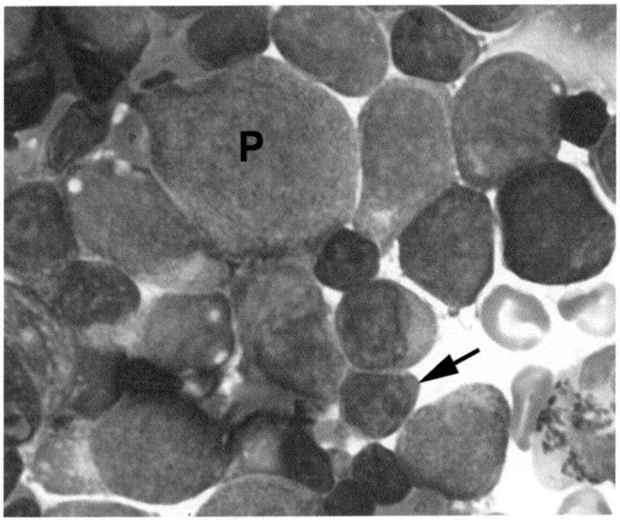

Figure 16.2 Lymph node aspirate from a dog with granulocytic leukemia (M2). Most of the large blast cells cannot be differentiated from lymphoblasts based on their morphology, but some are differentiating toward promyelocytes (P). Note the small lymphocyte (arrow). Wright stain.

and lymphoid acute leukemias occur most commonly in middle-aged dogs (median age is 7–8 years). Differentiating acute lymphoid from myeloid leukemia can be difficult and is based on morphology, expression of cell surface proteins, and cytochemistry. Some cells do not express cell-lineage proteins and remain unclassified. Chronic leukemias are characterized by the predominance of mature, more well-differentiated cells in the blood and marrow, and the patient survival time is longer. Neoplastic cells commonly can be found in organs other than the bone marrow in patients with leukemia. The spleen may be involved, and the liver and lymph nodes also may contain neoplastic cells (Figure 16.2).

Numerous genetic mutations have been identified in people with leukemia, and prognosis and therapy are often determined by the type of genetic mutation. Genetic mutations similar to those seen in people have been described in small numbers of dogs with lymphoid and myeloid leukemia, as well as in dogs with lymphoma. Several genes, including TRAF3 (tumor necrosis factor receptor associated factor 3), a negative and positive regulator of innate and adaptive immune responses, and POT1 (protection of telomeres protein 1), a telomere length regulator, are mutated in some cases of canine B cell lymphoma and may be involved in the pathogenesis. An excellent review of gene expression and mutational features of canine lymphoma and leukemia has been published [1]. The most recent version of the World Health Organization (WHO) classification system for human hematopoietic malignancies uses a combination of immunophenotyping, chromosomal aberrations, mutational analysis, and gene expression profiling to identify different types of leukemia.

In one study of 210 dogs with leukemia, 51 had ALL, 33 had AML, 61 had CLL, and 65 had grade V lymphoma with involvement of bone marrow [2]. Anemia, neutropenia, and thrombocytopenia were more common and severe in dogs with acute leukemias than in dogs with stage V lymphoma or chronic leukemias. Similar results were observed in a series of 64 dogs [3]. Twenty-five dogs had ALL, 22 had AML, and 17 had CLL. Golden retriever dogs in the study population were overrepresented in comparison with a control population of dogs. Various types of leukemias are discussed in more detail below.

Myeloid neoplasms

Myeloid neoplasms are cancers of hematopoietic cells, and are distinct from cancers of lymphoid cells. They manifest as either a lack of normal blood cells, or an increase in neoplastic cells in blood. While lymphoid leukemia may predominantly affect bone marrow, it is not referred to as a myeloid neoplasm. Myeloid neoplasms include cancers associated with both rapid and gradual disease progression. Percentage of blast cells in marrow is used to distinguish rapid (acute) from gradual (chronic). The rapidly progressing myeloid cancers are referred to as AMLs, and the myeloid cancers with more gradual progression are classified as either myelodysplastic syndromes (MDSs) or myeloproliferative neoplasms (MPN) (formerly termed "chronic leukemias").

Myelodysplastic syndromes

MDS is a variable manifestation with some subtle, morphologic changes in blood cells. The hematologic manifestations almost always involve some form of cytopenia, and this may include any single abnormality or combination of nonregenerative anemia, thrombocytopenia, and neutropenia. Cellularity of marrow is variable. The marrow may be hypocellular, of normal cellularity, or hypercellular, thereby making it difficult to distinguish this condition from a myeloproliferative disorder. Characteristic morphologic abnormalities include large, highly variable erythroid precursor size and dysynchrony of nuclear and cytoplasmic maturation events (Figure 16.3). The disturbed erythroid production in cats commonly leads to establishment of marked macrocytosis and increased erythrocyte volume heterogeneity (i.e., anisocytosis) seen as a widening of the erythrocyte histogram. Cats that are positive for feline leukemia virus (FeLV) infection may have mean red cell volumes of 70 fL or greater (reference interval, 40–55 fL) and macrocytic anemias have also been associated with feline immunodeficiency virus (FIV). Macrocytosis also has been reported in dogs with myelodysplasia. Other features in blood may include extreme platelet macrocytosis

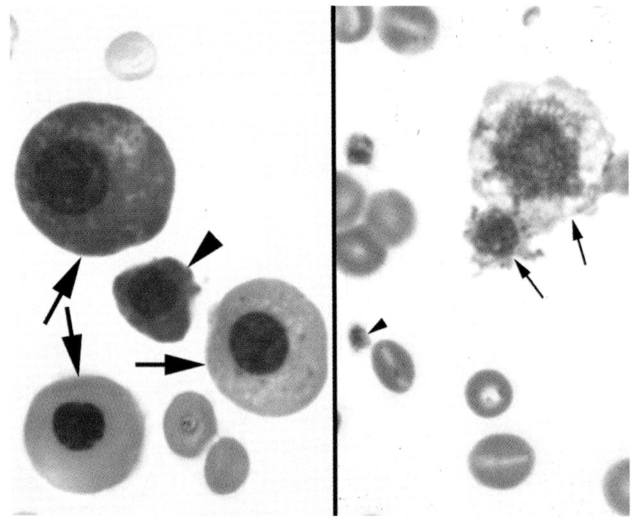

Figure 16.3 Left. Bone marrow aspirate from a cat with myelodysplasia. Note the three rubricytes with dysynchrony of nuclear and cytoplasmic maturation (arrows) and the more normal-appearing metarubricyte (arrowhead). Right. Blood film from a cat with myelodysplasia. Note the giant atypical platelets (small arrows) and the normal-appearing platelet (small arrowhead). Wright stain.

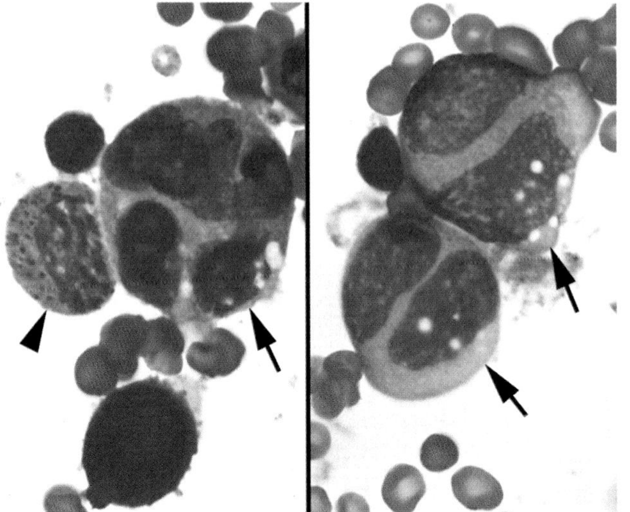

Figure 16.4 Left. Bone marrow aspirate from a cat with myelodysplasia. Note the dysplastic megakaryocyte (arrow) and the granulocytic precursor with retained primary granules (arrowhead). Right. Dysplastic megakaryocytes with hypolobulation of the nuclei (arrows). Wright stain.

(Figure 16.3). Megakaryocyte differentiation may be altered as well, with both hypo- and hyperlobulation of nuclei (Figure 16.4). Neutrophils of unusually large diameter may be observed, with nuclear changes that may include both hyper- and hyposegmentation (Figure 16.5). Very early precursors are not found in blood.

Several prognostic scoring systems based on number of bone marrow blast cells, cytogenetic findings, number of hematopoietic lines affected by cytopenia, and transfusion

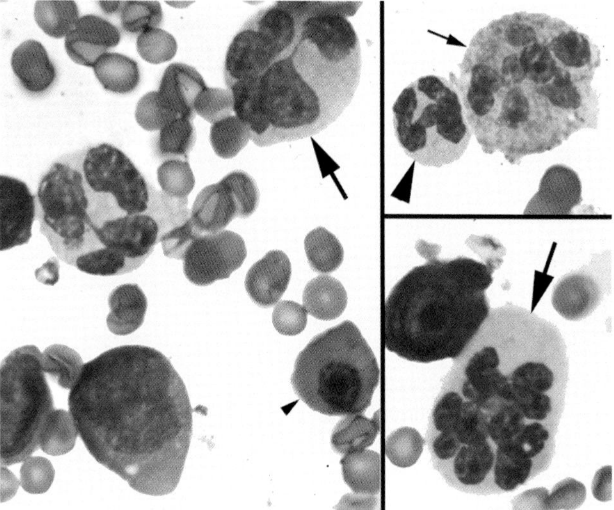

Figure 16.5 Bone marrow aspirate from a cat with myelodysplasia. Left and lower right. Note the giant hypersegmented neutrophils (arrows) and megaloblastic erythrocyte precursor (small arrow head). Upper right. Note the giant hypersegmented neutrophil (small arrow) and the neutrophil of normal size (large arrowhead). Wright stain.

dependence have been developed for use in humans with MDS. Classification schemes used for animals are quite simple in comparison. The Animal Leukemia Study Group in 1991 recommended two MDS categories: MDS (M : E >1.0) and MDS-erythroid (M : E <1.0). Since that time, recommendations for three subtypes have been made: (i) myelodysplastic syndrome with excess blasts (MDS-EB) has blast cell percentages in marrow that are equal to or greater than 5% but less than 20%; (ii) myelodysplastic syndrome with refractory cytopenia (MDS-RC), which has blast cell counts of less than 5%, can have an indolent course; (iii) MDS-ER (M : E ratio <1.0), which has a poor prognosis and short survival time. In general, high blast percentages (>5%) multiple cytopenias, and marked morphologic atypia are usually considered negative prognostic markers.

Other differential diagnoses for hypercellular marrow and cytopenias include the recovery stage of marrow damage, such as might be seen with parvovirus infection; immune-mediated disease, with destruction of more mature cells; and consumption of neutrophils due to an overwhelming inflammatory process.

MDSs have been reported in cats, dogs and one horse. Miniature dachshunds appear to have a higher incidence of myelodysplasia than do other breeds. Cats with myelodysplasia are commonly positive for FeLV. FIV has also been associated with myelodysplasia and is referred to as FIV-myelopathy. Clinical signs usually include lethargy, anorexia, and weight loss. Animals may die within weeks of diagnosis, without progression to leukemia, but overt leukemia is a common sequela. In a retrospective study of 152 bone marrow aspirates in cats that were performed for cytopenias or suspected leukemia, 15% were diagnosed with MDS.

Overview of acute myeloid leukemias and myeloproliferative neoplasms

AML is a neoplasm of hematopoietic cells resulting in rapid progression of disease. MPN comprise various types of clonal neoplastic conditions of hematopoietic tissue characterized by gradual disease progression. In general, these neoplasms are characterized by bone marrow hypercellularity, loss of orderliness in maturation, and a tendency for neoplastic cells to be released into the blood. Myeloid neoplasms are more common in cats than in other domestic animals and, as mentioned, usually are associated with FeLV infection. Hematopoietic precursors are infected by FeLV, and viral proteins are thought to interact with host cell products that are important in cell proliferation, resulting in recombination or rearrangement events involving host gene sequences that encode products involved in the normal regulation of cell growth. FIV also appears to be associated with stem cell disorders of cats, although FIV does not directly infect myeloid or erythroid precursors. The mechanism probably relates to infection of other cells in the bone marrow microenvironment or to the virus or viral antigen affecting hematopoiesis in some way. Cats with FIV are approximately five times more likely to develop leukemia.

Clinical signs usually relate to the crowding out of normal hematopoietic cells in the bone marrow, but they may also result from the infiltration of different organs by neoplastic cells. Lethargy, weakness, pallor, bleeding, shifting leg lameness, and bone pain frequently are seen, as are hepatomegaly and splenomegaly. Typical CBC findings include an increased nucleated cell count, neoplastic cells in the peripheral blood, nonregenerative anemia, and thrombocytopenia, although thrombocytosis may be present, particularly in cats. Other abnormal laboratory findings are variable, depending on the type and degree of organ dysfunction.

The response of these disorders in dogs and cats to therapy usually is disappointing, and the prognosis is poor, particularly in animals with AML. Chemotherapeutic drugs may produce remissions of very short duration (usually only a few weeks). Types of recommended chemotherapy differ with the type of leukemia and the species. A veterinary oncologist should be consulted for advice on new protocols for therapy. Bone marrow transplantation offers the potential for a complete cure but is expensive and requires intensive care. Cats that are negative for FeLV and FIV and have a sibling that can serve as a marrow donor are reasonably good candidates for bone marrow transplantation. Animals with MPN have a longer survival time after the diagnosis is established, but they almost always eventually develop a terminal blast crisis and die.

Classification of acute myeloid leukemias (AMLs)

AML is morphologically and biologically variable. Most cases of AML in humans are associated with genetic abnormalities that affect myeloid cellular proliferation and maturation. Thus, cytogenetic analysis is a routine component of the diagnosis in people, and plays a significant role in treatment modality and prognosis. Traditionally, AMLs in domestic animals have been characterized as being granulocytic (i.e., myeloid, neutrophilic), myelomonocytic (i.e., neutrophils and monocytes), monocytic, eosinophilic, basophilic, megakaryocytic, erythroid, or erythroleukemia (i.e., erythrocytes and granulocytes). Diagnostic criteria have varied considerably, however, and agreement on nomenclature and classification of hematopoietic neoplasms has been lacking. In the 1970s, a group of French, American, and British (FAB) leukemia experts in human medicine divided AML into subtypes, M0 through M7, based on the type of cell the leukemia develops from and how mature the cells appear, primarily based on morphology of the leukemia cells with routine blood staining. Because of potential differences in response to various treatment protocols and prognosis, in 1991 an animal leukemia study group standardized the definitions for AMLs by using a human classification scheme based primarily on the number and morphology of blast cells in Wright-stained blood and bone marrow films. To classify a myeloproliferative or myelodysplastic disorder, 200 cells are differentiated to calculate an M:E ratio and to determine the percentages of blast and other cell types. Blast cell percentages in the bone marrow are calculated in relation to all nucleated cells as well as to nonerythroid cells. Lymphocytes, macrophages, mast cells, and plasma cells are excluded for all-nucleated-cell counts, and erythrocyte precursors are excluded for nonerythroid cell counts. At the time of this study, 30% blasts in the marrow was considered the lowest percentage that could be present and still diagnose AML. Our physician counterparts, in collaboration with oncologists, have since constructed a new WHO standard, which lowered the blast threshold from 30% to 20% for diagnosing AML. The AML alphanumeric designations (M1, M2, etc.) described below have been largely discontinued in humans as numbers of subtypes have increased. The veterinary system established in 1991 has also been revised to lower the blast threshold to 20%.

The most recent modification by the WHO in 2016 classifies AML into the following categories: (i) AML with genetic (gene or chromosome) abnormalities (of which at least 11 have been identified), (ii) AML with myelodysplasia-related changes, (iii) AML related to previous chemotherapy or radiation, (iv) AML not otherwise specified (NOS), (v) myeloid sarcoma, (vi) myeloid proliferations related to

Down syndrome, and (vii) undifferentiated and biphenotypic acute leukemias that are not strictly AML and have both lymphocytic and myeloid features, sometimes called mixed phenotype acute leukemias (MPALs). Subgroups of "AML not otherwise specified" is similar to the previous FAB classification and include AML with minimal differentiation (FAB M0), AML without maturation (FAB M1), AML with maturation (FAB M2), acute myelomonocytic leukemia (FAB M4), acute monoblastic/monocytic leukemia (FAB M5), pure erythroid leukemia (FAB M6), acute megakaryoblastic leukemia (FAB M7), acute basophilic leukemia, and acute panmyelosis with fibrosis AML that develops in cats with FeLV and is most similar to the human "AML with myelodysplasia-related changes," but most of the cases in domestic animals are comparable to "AML not otherwise categorized." The alphanumeric designations and blast threshold should be formally reassessed by veterinary clinical pathologists and oncologists as to their accuracy and usefulness. Prognosis in humans with AML is primarily based on types of chromosomal translocations, types of gene mutations, cell marker expression, age, leukocyte concentration, presence of infection, prior diagnosis of myelodysplasia, and if leukemic cells have invaded the central nervous system.

Cytochemical stains that can identify myeloid-associated enzymes such as alkaline phosphatase and chloroacetate esterase, and immunophenotyping, as discussed earlier, may be useful adjuncts in the classification of leukemia (Figures 16.6 and 16.7). Flow cytometry can be used to identify surface antigens typical of myeloid origin such CD11b,

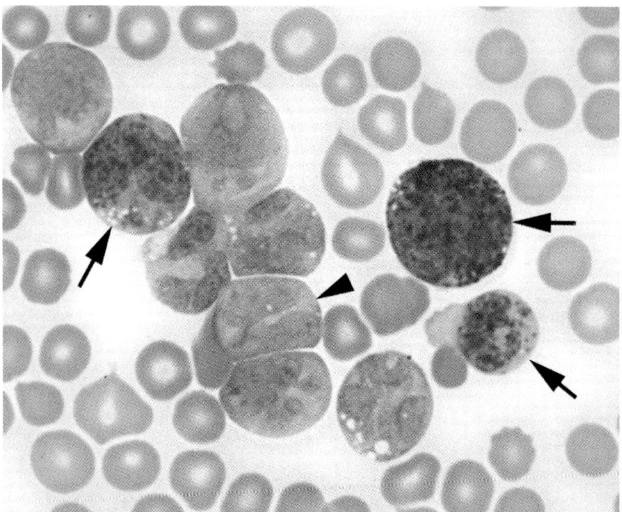

Figure 16.6 Blood film from a dog with myelomonocytic leukemia (M4) stained with chloracetate esterase (CAE), a granulocyte marker. Note the metamyelocyte and neutrophil with red-staining granules in the cytoplasm (arrows). Several monocytes (arrowhead) are present that do not stain positive with CAE. Source: Specimen courtesy of Dr. Wendy Sprague, Colorado State University.

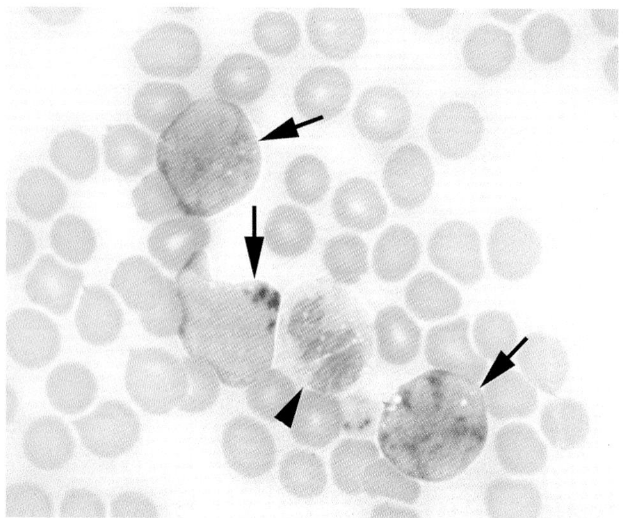

Figure 16.7 Blood film from dog with myelomonocytic leukemia (M4) stained with α-naphthyl butyrate esterase (ANBE), a monocyte marker. Note the brown-staining granules in the monocytes (arrows) and the neutrophil (arrowhead) that does not stain with ANBE. Source: Specimen courtesy of Dr. Wendy Sprague, Colorado State University.

CD11c, and CD14. Cells of myeloid origin do not express T or B cell markers. The clinical relevance of cytomorphologic, cytochemical, and immunophenotypic characterization of acute myeloproliferative diseases in animals remains to be determined, although given the importance of karyotyping in human AML, prognostically significant chromosomal abnormalities are likely present in animals with AML. Moreover, the classification of leukemia in a patient, especially cats with FeLV, may change as the disease progresses; for example, red cell leukemia may convert to erythroleukemia or acute myelogenous leukemia. A classification scheme showing historically used terminology, current terminology, and a summary of bone marrow findings is presented in Table 16.1.

Undifferentiated leukemia (M0)

The diagnosis of undifferentiated leukemia is established when approximately 100% of the cells in the bone marrow are blast cells that cannot be properly classified according to the usual morphologic and cytochemical criteria. The diagnosis can be based on electron microscopy, ultrastructural cytochemistry, or immunophenotyping. Included in this category are cases of what previously were termed reticuloendotheliosis in cats, in which a predominance of blast cells have pseudopodia, eccentric nuclei, and sometimes, features of both erythroblasts and myeloblasts (Figures 16.8 and 16.9). Some cells may contain azurophilic granules. If the neoplastic cells do not appear to be maturing toward erythroid or myeloid cells, they are categorized as being undifferentiated.

Table 16.1 Classification of leukemias.

Historical terminology	FAB	Description
Acute leukemias (≥20% blasts in marrow)		
Reticuloendotheliosis	AUL	Acute undifferentiated leukemia, myeloid and erythroid features
Granulocytic leukemia	M1	Myeloblastic leukemia with differentiation
Granulocytic leukemia	M2	Myeloblastic leukemia with neutrophilic differentiation
Myelomonocytic leukemia	M4	Combination of myeloblasts and monoblasts
Monocytic leukemia	M5a	Monocytic leukemia without differentiation
Monocytic leukemia	M5b	Monocytic leukemia with differentiation
Erythroleukemia	M6	Combination of myeloblasts and rubriblasts
Erythremic myelosis	M6Er	Erythroid leukemia
Megakaryoblastic leukemia	M7	Increased megakaryoblasts in blood and marrow
Chronic myeloid leukemias (<20% blasts in marrow)		
Chronic granulocytic leukemia		Mature neutrophilia, left shift, similar to granulocytic hyperplasia
Chronic myelomonocytic leukemia		Combination of mature neutrophilia, left shift, and monocytosis
Chronic monocytic leukemia		Mature monocytosis in blood and bone marrow
Chronic eosinophilic leukemia		Eosinophilia with left shift, basophilic predominance in marrow
Chronic basophilic leukemia		Basophilia with left shift, basophilic predominance in marrow
Essential thrombocythemia		Marked increase in platelets, megakaryocytic hyperplasia in marrow
Polycythemia vera (erythrocytosis)		Mature erythroid proliferative disorder, erythroid hyperplasia
Lymphoid leukemia		
Acute lymphoblastic leukemia		Lymphoblasts in blood or bone marrow
Chronic lymphocytic leukemia		Lymphocytosis, >30% lymphocytes in marrow

FAB, French-American-British.

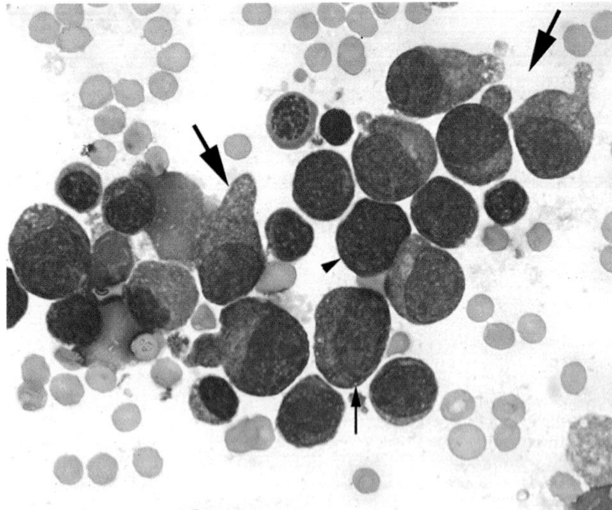

Figure 16.8 Bone marrow aspirate from a cat with undifferentiated leukemia. The cells have features of both erythroid and myeloid precursors. Cytoplasmic pseudopodia (large arrows) typically are present. Note the cell with obvious erythroid characteristics (arrowhead) and the cell with myeloid features and primary granules (small arrow). Wright stain.

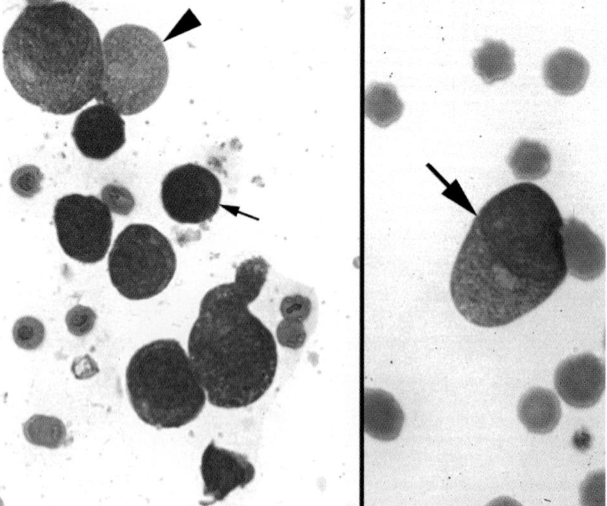

Figure 16.9 Left. Bone marrow aspirate from a cat with undifferentiated leukemia. Note the cytoplasmic pseudopodia that has detached from the cell (arrowhead). When present in blood, these cytoplasmic fragments may be mistaken for platelets. Note the rubricyte (small arrow) as well. Right. Blood film from a cat with undifferentiated leukemia. Note the typical undifferentiated cell with primary granules and an eccentric nucleus (large arrow). Wright stain.

Myeloblastic leukemia (M1)

The predominant cell in the bone marrow in animals with myeloblastic leukemia is the type I myeloblast; type II myeloblasts are only seen infrequently (Figure 16.10). Both types of blasts comprise more than 90% of all nucleated cells. Differentiated granulocytes (promyelocytes to neutrophils and eosinophils) comprise less than 10% of the nonerythroid cells.

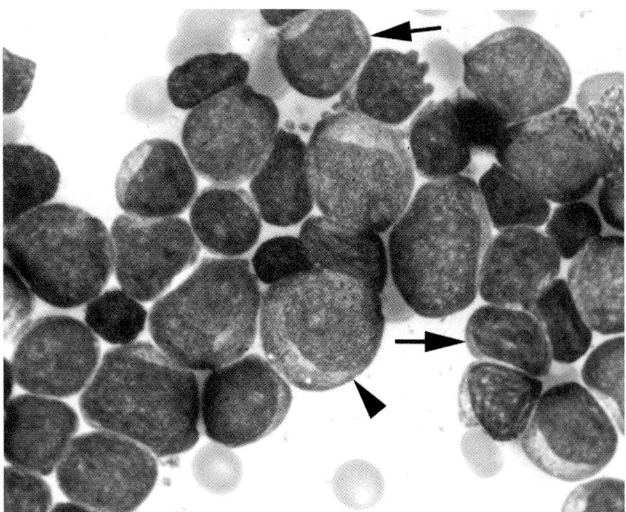

Figure 16.10 Bone marrow aspirate from a dog with granulocytic (myeloblastic) leukemia (M1). Almost all of the cells present are type 1 myeloblasts (arrows). A type II myeloblast with cytoplasmic primary granules (arrowhead) is present as well. Type I myeloblasts are morphologically similar to lymphoblasts, and without the presence of more differentiated cells, immunophenotyping may be necessary to correctly classify the leukemia. Wright stain.

Myeloblastic leukemia with maturation (M2)

Myeloblasts constitute from more than 20% to less than 90% of all nucleated cells, with a variable number of type II myeloblasts being present (Figures 16.11 and 16.12). Differentiated granulocytes comprise more than 10% of the nonerythroid cells, usually with a predominance of promyelocytes.

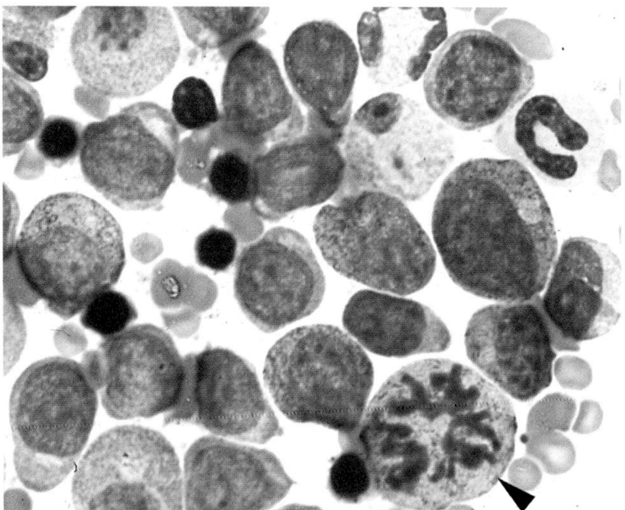

Figure 16.11 Bone marrow aspirate from a cat with granulocytic (myeloblastic) leukemia (M2). Numerous type II myeloblasts with cytoplasmic granules are present, as is a cell in mitosis (arrowhead). Note that cells are more differentiated than those seen in marrow aspirates of patients with M1. Wright stain.

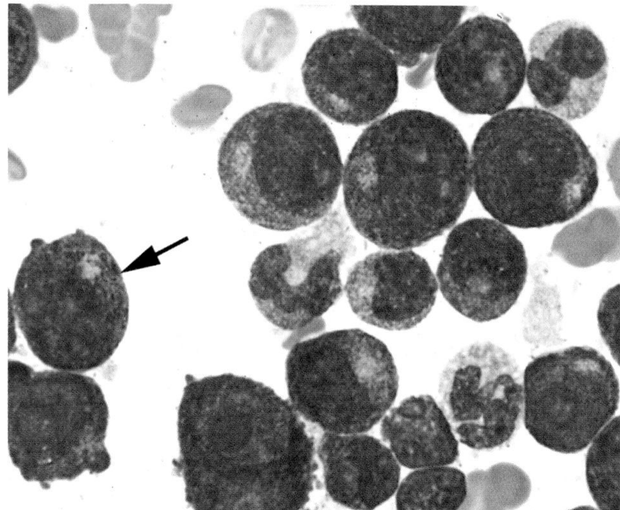

Figure 16.12 Bone marrow aspirate from a cat with granulocytic (myeloblastic) leukemia (M2). Note that most of the cells present are type II myeloblasts or progranulocytes (arrow). Most of these cells have clear Golgi areas. A few more differentiated myeloid precursors are present as well. Wright stain.

Myeloblastic leukemia with maturation and atypical granulation of promyelocytes (M3)

Although myeloblastic leukemia with maturation and atypical granulation of promyelocytes is one of the classifications for human leukemia, no such cases have been reported in domestic animals. This type of myeloblastic leukemia is characterized by either hypergranular, hypogranular, or microgranular promyelocytes with folded, reniform, or bilobed nuclei.

Myelomonocytic leukemia (M4)

Myeloblasts and monoblasts together constitute more than 20% of all nucleated cells, and differentiated granulocytes and monocytes comprise more than 20% nonerythroid cells (Figures 16.13 and 16.14).

Monocytic Leukemia (M5)

The predominant population is monocytic, as determined by the characteristic nuclear morphology and confirmed by cytochemical staining for nonspecific esterase. Monoblasts and promonocytes constitute more than 80% of nonerythroid cells in M5a (Figures 16.15 and 16.16), while M5b has more than 20% to less than 80% monoblasts and promonocytes with prominent differentiation to monocytes (Figures 16.17 and 16.18). The granulocytic component is less than 20%.

Erythroleukemia (M6)

The erythroid compartment in M6 is more than 50%, and the myeloblasts and monoblasts combined are less than 20% of all nucleated cells. The M6 classification is recognized

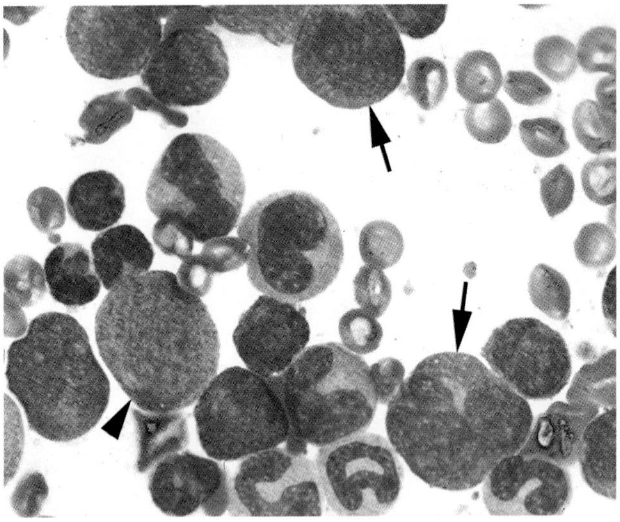

Figure 16.13 Bone marrow aspirate from a dog with myelomonocytic leukemia (M4). Both monocyte precursors (arrows) and myeloid precursors (arrowhead) are present. Wright stain.

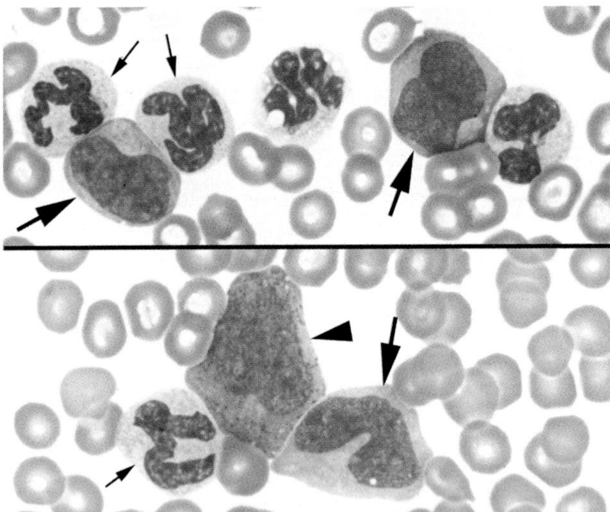

Figure 16.14 Blood film from a dog with myelomonocytic leukemia (M4). Top. Note the monoblasts (large arrows) and normal-appearing, segmented neutrophils (small arrows). Bottom. Note the segmented neutrophil (small arrow), monocyte (large arrow), and type II myeloblast (arrowhead). Wright stain.

when either of the following criteria are met: myeloblasts and monoblasts constitute more than 20% of nonerythroid cells, or blast cells (including rubriblasts) constitute more than 20% of all nucleated cells. An M6Er designation is used to define the latter situation when there is a predominance of rubriblasts in the erythroid component. Myeloproliferative disorders of erythroid precursors may fall under the designation of M6Er or MDS-Er, because the erythroid component constitutes more than 50% of all nucleated cells and the blast cell concentration, (including rubriblasts) may

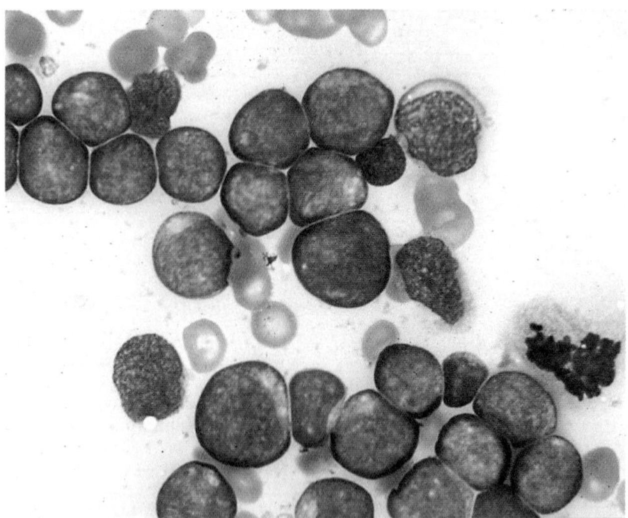

Figure 16.15 Bone marrow aspirate from a dog with monocytic leukemia (M5a). Almost all of the cells present are undifferentiated monoblasts. These cells appear to be morphologically similar to lymphoblasts and type I myeloblasts, but immunophenotyping and cytochemistry determined this was a very undifferentiated type of monocytic leukemia. Wright stain.

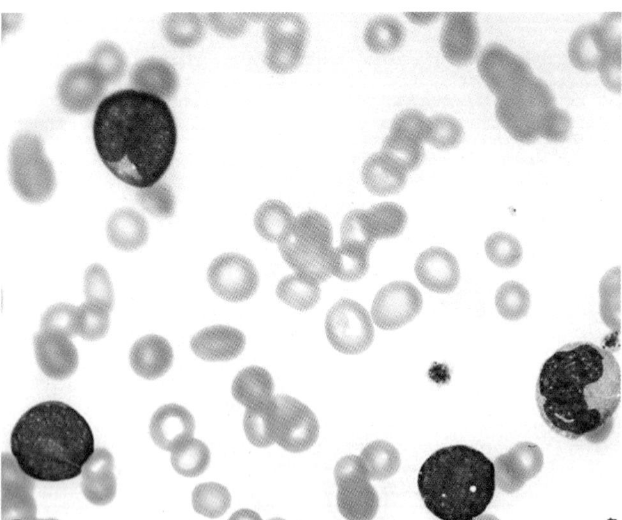

Figure 16.16 Blood film from a dog with monocytic leukemia (M5a). Cells were classified as monoblasts based on the presence of other cells that appeared to be differentiating to monocytes as well as on the results of cytochemical analysis and immunophenotyping. Wright stain.

constitute more than 20% (i.e., M6ER) or less than 20% (i.e., MDS-Er) (Figures 16.19 and 16.20).

Megakaryoblastic leukemia (M7)

More than 20% of all nucleated cells or nonerythroid cells is comprised of megakaryoblasts in the M7 stage. An increased concentration of megakaryocytes may be present as well, and megakaryoblasts usually are detected

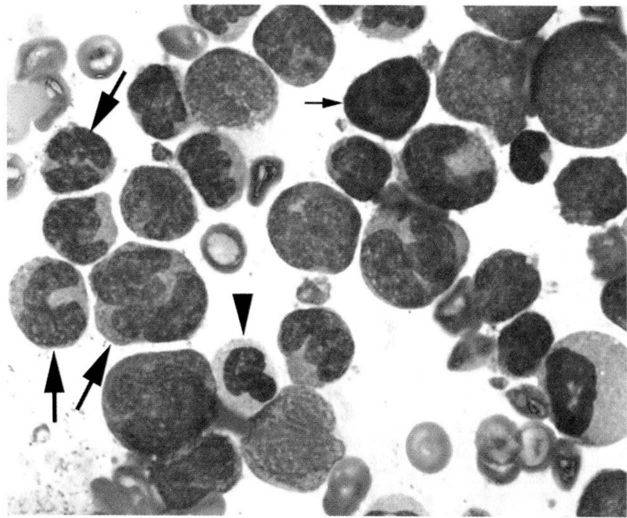

Figure 16.17 Bone marrow aspirate from a dog with monocytic leukemia (M5b). Note the numerous monocytes in various stages of maturation (large arrows), the segmented neutrophil (arrowhead), and the plasma cell (small arrow). Wright stain.

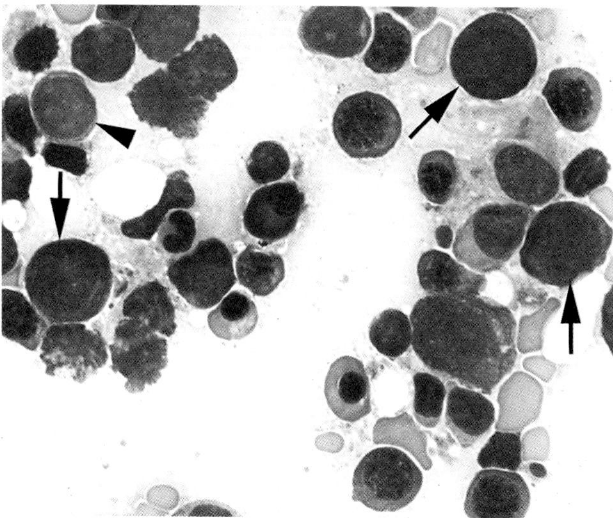

Figure 16.19 Bone marrow aspirate from a cat with erythremic myelosis (M6Er). Almost all of the cells present are erythroid precursors. Note the rubriblasts (large arrows) and the nonerythroid blast (arrowhead), which probably is a myeloblast. Wright stain.

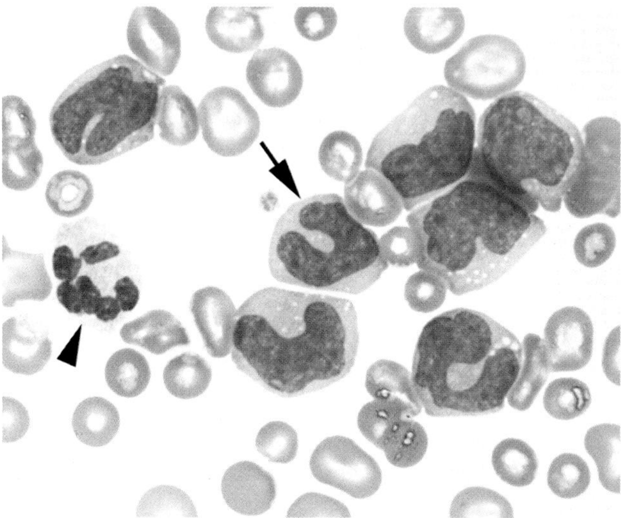

Figure 16.18 Blood film from a dog with monocytic leukemia (M5b). Note the numerous monocytes (large arrow), and compare the blue color of the cytoplasm and density of the nuclear chromatin with that of a segmented neutrophil, which has more dense nuclear chromatin and pink cytoplasm (arrowhead). Wright stain.

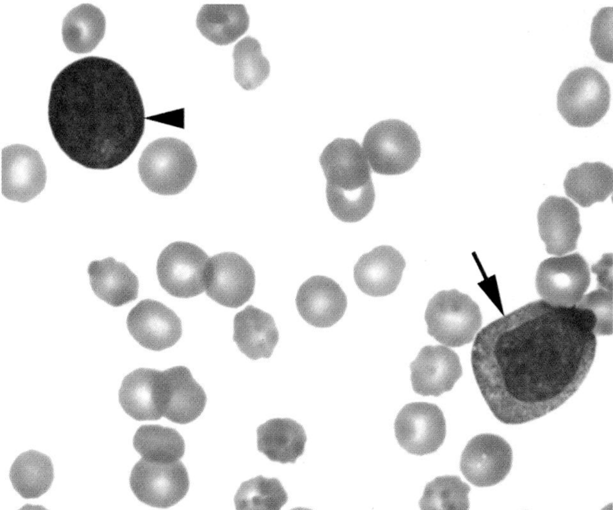

Figure 16.20 Blood film from a dog with erythroleukemia (M6). Note the rubriblast (arrowhead) and myeloblast (arrow). Also note the typical lack of polychromasia, because the erythroid precursors do not mature normally. Wright stain.

in the blood (Figure 16.21). Animals often are thrombocytopenic, although thrombocytosis has been reported. Immunohistochemical techniques to detect reactivity for factor VIII–related antigen and platelet glycoprotein IIIa sometimes are necessary to definitively identify megakaryoblasts. Primitive megakaryoblasts may also stain positive for acetylcholine esterase, a specific cytochemical marker for this cell line. This leukemia is rare in animals. While most cases of AML are rapidly fatal in domestic animals, one dog survived 2 years while being treated with chemotherapy for acute megakaryoblastic leukemia.

Dendritic cell leukemia

Dendritic cell leukemia has been reported in one dog with what appeared to be disseminated malignant histiocytosis. The cells appeared similar to histiocytes and flow cytometry of the abnormal circulating cells revealed CD1c, CD11c, and major histocompatibility complex (MHC) Class II expression without expression of CD11d or lymphoid markers, consistent with myeloid dendritic antigen-presenting cells.

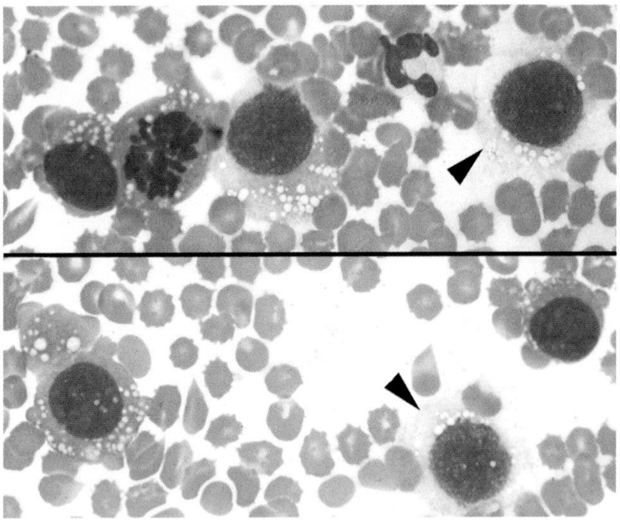

Figure 16.21 Blood film from a dog with megakaryoblastic leukemia (M7). Top. Note the numerous megakaryoblasts (arrowhead), one of which is in mitosis. Also note the abundant vacuolated cytoplasm with ruffled borders. Bottom. Note the broken megakaryoblast (arrowhead). Wright stain.

Chronic myeloproliferative neoplasms

Myelopoliferative neoplasms in people are classified as chronic myelogenous leukemia (CML), chronic neutrophilic leukemia (CNL), polycythemia vera (PV), essential thrombocythemia (ET), primary myelofibrosis (PMF), chronic eosinophilic leukemia (CEL) and CEL not otherwise specified (CEL, NOS), mastocytosis, and myeloproliferative neoplasm unclassifiable (MPN, U). The phenotypic diversity among these neoplasms is attributable to various chromosomal translocations and genetic mutations. Best characterized and first discovered among these mutations is a gene mutation that codes for a tyrosine kinase with increased enzymatic activity, resulting from a translocation between chromosomes 9 and 20 called the Philadelphia chromosome that is associated with CML, which is often treated successfully. Other mutations have been discovered for most of the other types of MPN. CML in people is a clonal stem cell disorder with proliferations involving several or all of the hematopoietic cell lineages, and is characterized by neutrophilia, basophilia, and eosinophilia. CNL in people is rare, and characterized by a marked leukocytosis composed of segmented neutrophils and band forms. Polycythemia and essential thrombocythemia have a relatively indolent course that results in a slight decrease in lifespan. Polycythemia in people may transform to AML. PMF is characterized by proliferation of megakaryocytes and granulocytic precursors, with progressive myelofibrosis. CEL and CEL, NOS result in persistent blood, bone marrow and tissue eosinophilia and must be distinguished from hypereosinophilia. Mastocytosis in people results from clonal expansion of mast cells, and is divided into localized or diffuse cutaneous mastocytosis, and systemic mastocytosis with variable involvement of bone marrow. Systemic mastocytosis has three possible manifestations: accumulations of mast cells in lymph nodes, spleen, liver, and GI tract with an indolent course; mast cell leukemia with a rapid course, and mast cell sarcoma with development of mast cell leukemia. Most of the unclassifiable MPN are early stages of other types of MPN that have not developed diagnostic features. This section presents a brief discussion of these relatively rare disorders in animals. Polycythemia vera, a chronic myeloproliferative disorder of erythrocytes, is discussed in Chapter 10.

In animals, the diagnosis is usually based on clinical and morphologic features. Cells are usually relatively normal to mildly dysplastic. CMLs can be difficult to distinguish from hyperplasia as a result of inflammation, and in the case of polycythemia vera, must be distinguished from other causes of erythrocytosis.

Chronic granulocytic (myelogenous) leukemia

The disorder that has been historically described in dogs and cats as CML more closely resembles human CNL, as neutrophilia predominates, and there is usually an absence of eosinophilia and basophilia. The morphologic equivalent of human CML has not been described in detail in animals. These chronic leukemias are rare in domestic animals and are characterized by marked neutrophilia, a left shift that often is disorderly, and anemia. A monocytosis may be present as well. CML has been reported more frequently in dogs than in cats. Dysgranulopoiesis may be present and include hypersegmented nuclei and giant metamyelocytes

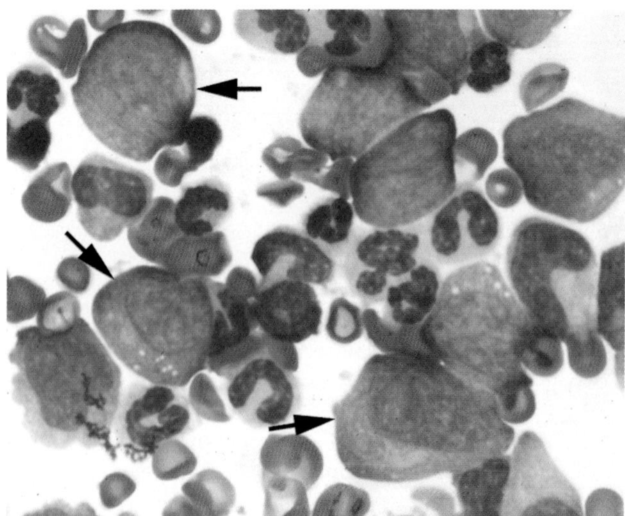

Figure 16.22 Bone marrow aspirate from a dog with chronic myelogenous leukemia. Note the increased concentration of myeloblasts (arrows). Although some degree of maturation to segmented neutrophils is occurring, the maturation appears to be disorderly. Very few erythroid precursors were present in the marrow, and none are present in this field. Wright stain.

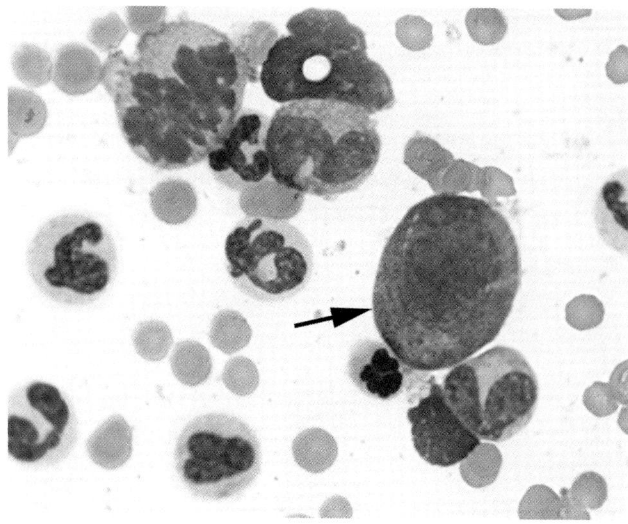

Figure 16.23 Blood film from a dog with chronic myelogenous leukemia in blast crisis. Note the cell in mitosis (upper left corner) and the myeloblast (arrow). The nucleated cell concentration in this dog was 150,000 cells/μL^{-1}. Wright stain.

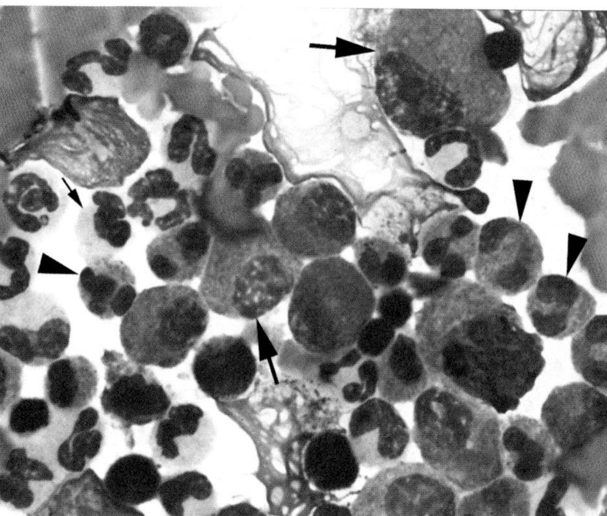

Figure 16.24 Bone marrow aspirate from a cat with eosinophilic leukemia or hypereosinophilic syndrome. Note the eosinophil precursors (large arrows) and the numerous, mature eosinophils (arrowheads). For comparison, note the neutrophil (small arrow). Wright stain. Source: Specimen courtesy of Antech Diagnostics.

and bands (Figure 16.22). These leukemias, however, can be differentiated from MDS by the marked leukocytosis in the blood. Inflammatory responses can mimic MPN, and such "leukemoid reactions" often are misdiagnosed as leukemias. Marrow examination may not be helpful in distinguishing the two, because marked inflammatory leukograms can be associated with marked granulocytic hyperplasia and a pronounced increase in the M : E ratio and the orderliness of maturation may be disrupted. Histopathologic evaluation of the spleen and liver is not always helpful, because these organs may exhibit marked granulopoiesis with some types of inflammatory disease. Animals with MPN usually eventually develop a disorderly left shift, and have a "blast crisis," during which myeloblasts appear in the blood (Figure 16.23). Animals with MPN also usually develop much more severe anemia than animals with inflammatory disease.

Differential diagnoses for a marked neutrophilia >50,000/μL and occasionally >100,000/μL include paraneoplastic responses, leukocyte adhesion deficiency (LAD), granulocyte-colony stimulating factor administration, infection with *Hepatozoon americanum*, and inflammation secondary to infections or immune mediated disease. LAD has been described in people, dogs, cats, and cattle. LAD is an autosomal recessive disorder caused by mutations in the integrin beta-2 subunit (ITGB2) gene resulting in a deficiency of the leukocyte integrin that is expressed on all leukocyte surface membranes, mediate strong neutrophil adhesion, and serve as co- receptors for activation of T-lymphocyte proliferation. The disorder results in chronic and overwhelming infections and poor wound healing. Affected animals are often young, since they may die before adulthood unless treated with antibiotics. They have a persistent marked mature neutrophilia; increased immature neutrophil concentration is not usually observed. Neutrophils may be hypersegmented due to aging within the circulation. Monocytosis and lymphocytosis may also be observed.

Eosinophilic leukemia

Eosinophilic leukemia is rare but has been reported primarily in FeLV-negative cats. It is characterized by eosinophilia, immature eosinophils in the blood, eosinophil predominance in the marrow (Figure 16.24), and infiltration of various organs with eosinophils. This disorder is difficult to differentiate from feline hypereosinophilic syndrome, in which the same characteristics can be seen, although the eosinophilic left shift may be more orderly with hypereosinophilic syndrome. Intestinal involvement is typical as well. Recent reports are suggestive that the separation between the two disorders may be artificial, and that they both may represent a neoplastic proliferation of eosinophils. Clinical signs are similar to those seen in animals with other myeloproliferative disorders. Typically, however, they also include thickened bowel loops, diarrhea, and vomiting, because the intestine usually is infiltrated. Most cats die within 6 months of the diagnosis being established, but hydroxyurea in combination with prednisone may prolong survival.

Chronic basophilic leukemia

Chronic basophilic leukemia is very rare but has been reported in dogs, cats, horses, and a calf. Abnormal blood findings include marked basophilia with an orderly left shift of the basophilic series, anemia, and occasionally thrombocytosis. Multiple organs usually are infiltrated. Chronic basophilic leukemia must be differentiated from mast cell leukemia. Basophils have segmented nuclei, whereas mast cells have round nuclei. Basophilic myelocytes, however, may be difficult to differentiate from mast cells, and animals with systemic mast cell neoplasia may have a mild basophilia.

Essential thrombocythemia

Essential thrombocythemia is a very rare chronic myeloproliferative disorder that is characterized by a marked increase in the platelet concentration (>1,000,000). Platelets may appear atypical, with hypo- or hypergranularity, and giant forms may be present. The concentrations of megakaryocytes and megakaryoblasts usually are increased in the bone marrow as well. The platelet concentration may be increased secondary to many other disorders, such as iron deficiency anemia, inflammation, antineoplastic drug therapy, corticosteroids, and neoplasia (particularly lymphoma).

Lymphoproliferative disorders

Although the term lymphoproliferative disorder can be used to describe any abnormal proliferation of lymphoid cells, it more commonly is used to describe neoplastic proliferations. Tumors that derive from lymphocytes or plasma cells are classified as lymphoproliferative, or lymphoid neoplasms. Lymphoproliferative disorders are more common than myeloproliferative disorders in domestic animals. As with myeloproliferative disorders, cats with certain types of lymphoproliferative disorders usually test positive for FeLV, FIV, or both. Lymphoproliferative disorders generally are categorized as primary lymphoid leukemia, lymphoma, or plasma cell tumors, including multiple myeloma and solitary plasma cell tumors. In turn, the leukemias can be classified as either acute or chronic, as discussed earlier, and are termed ALL or CLL. Clonality testing using polymerase chain reaction for rearrangements in the complementarity-determining region 3 of the immunoglobulin heavy chain of B lymphocytes (B cell receptor) and the T cell receptor of T lymphocytes helps distinguish between clonal and nonclonal expansions of lymphocytes. Another way to determine if a population of lymphocytes is neoplastic is to show that they are all of the same phenotype (all B cells or all T cells) using monoclonal antibodies to cell surface proteins and flow cytometry (see Chapter 14). Interestingly, clonally rearranged T and B cell receptors can be seen in a high percentage of dogs with AML, suggesting that clonality testing alone should not be used to distinguish AML from ALL.

Lymphoid leukemia differs from malignant lymphoma primarily in the anatomic distribution. Solid neoplastic masses are present in lymphoma but are less common in patients with primary lymphoid leukemia. At least 10–25% of dogs and cats with lymphoma develop leukemia, however, and some investigators report that approximately 65% of dogs with multicentric lymphoma are leukemic at the time of presentation (if the determination of leukemia is based on the evaluation of blood, bone marrow aspirates, and marrow core biopsy specimens). Dogs with lymphoid leukemia also commonly have lymph node and spleen involvement. While lymphoid leukemia is usually defined as proliferation of neoplastic lymphoid cells in the bone marrow, they may originate in the spleen, and may or may not be circulating in the peripheral blood.

Acute lymphoblastic leukemia (ALL)

ALL is characterized by the presence of lymphoblasts in the blood and bone marrow (Figures 16.25–16.28). In both ALL and the leukemic phase of multicentric lymphoma (stage V), however, lymphoblasts can be found in the blood and bone marrow, thereby making these two disorders difficult to differentiate. A general rule is that if lymphadenopathy is not present, the disorder most likely is ALL rather than lymphoma. Approximately half of the dogs with ALL, however, also have lymphadenopathy. As with the myeloproliferative disorders, clinical signs relate either to a lack of normal hematopoietic cells or to the infiltration of organs by neoplastic cells. Common findings include pale mucous membranes, splenomegaly, and hepatomegaly, lethargy, and weight loss. Common CBC abnormalities include anemia, thrombocytopenia, lymphocytosis, and lymphoblasts in the blood.

Lymphoblasts usually can be differentiated from other types of immature cells based on their characteristic morphology, as described earlier. Occasionally, however, certain types of lymphoblasts (e.g., large granular lymphoblasts) may contain a few fine to coarse azurophilic granules (Figure 16.29). These cells may be difficult to distinguish from myeloblasts, in which case immunophenotyping (using

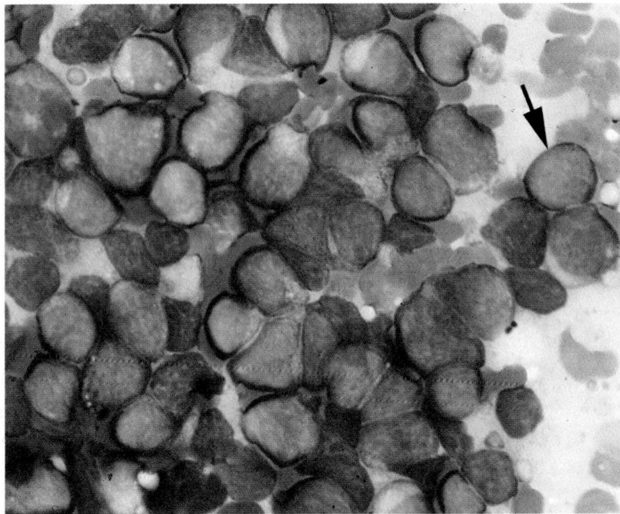

Figure 16.25 Bone marrow aspirate from a dog with acute lymphoblastic leukemia. Note that normal hematopoietic cells are absent, having been replaced by lymphoblasts (arrow). Wright stain.

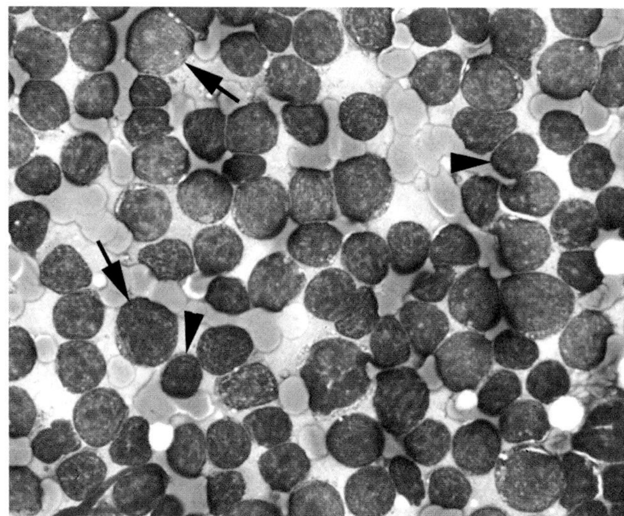

Figure 16.26 Bone marrow aspirate from a dog with acute lymphoblastic leukemia. Numerous intermediate-sized lymphoid cells are present and have completely replaced the normal marrow elements. Note the lymphoblasts (arrows) and lymphocytes (arrowheads). Wright stain.

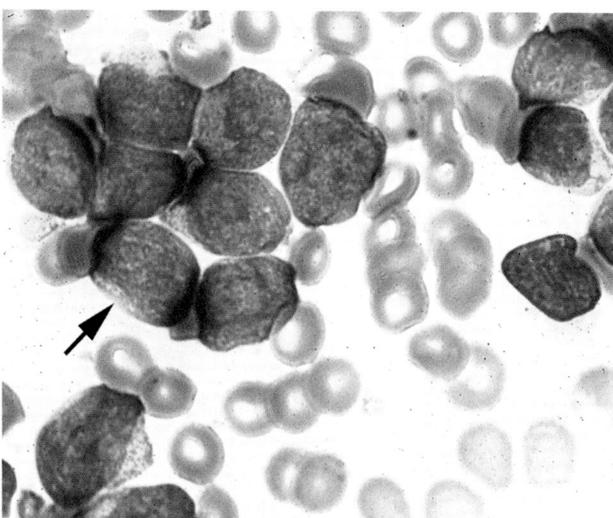

Figure 16.28 Blood film from a dog with acute lymphoblastic leukemia and a nucleated cell count of 300,000 cells/μL^{-1}. All of the cells present are lymphoblasts (arrow). Note the large size, high nucleus : cytoplasm ratio, and nucleoli with the nuclei. Wright stain.

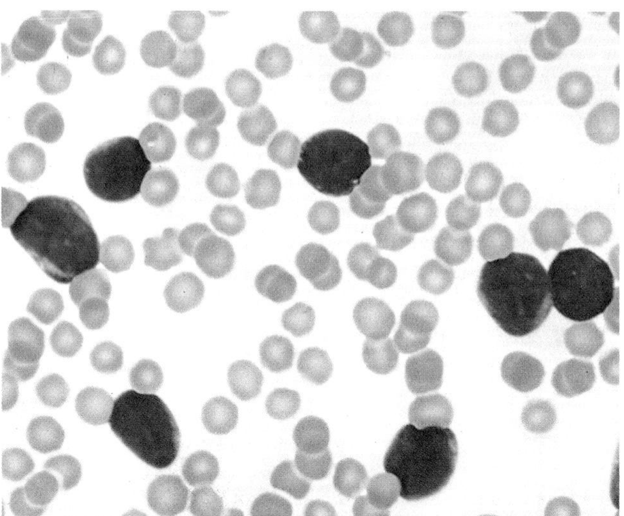

Figure 16.27 Blood film from a dog with acute lymphoblastic leukemia. Note the numerous large lymphoblasts. Wright stain.

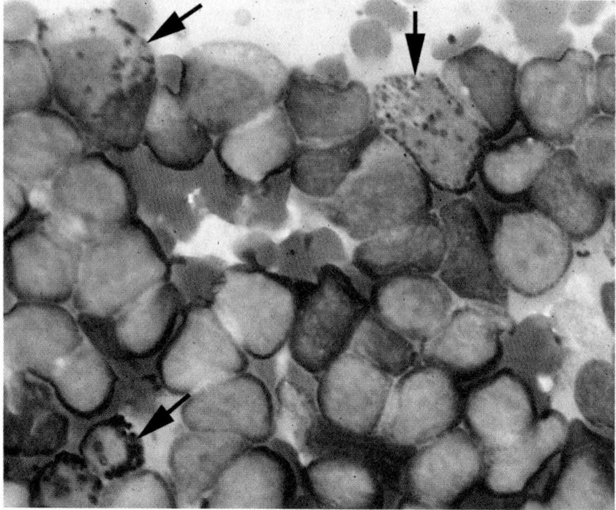

Figure 16.29 Bone marrow aspirate from a dog with lymphoblastic leukemia. Note the presence of a few cells with azurophilic granules within the cytoplasm (arrows), which are referred to as large granular lymphoblasts. These granules make this type of leukemia difficult to distinguish from M1 based on cell morphology alone. Wright stain.

monoclonal antibodies directed against proteins on the surface of leukocytes) may be very helpful. Large granular lymphocytes (LGL) leukemias of T cell origin are seen occasionally in cats with T cell lymphoma of the intestine (see Section VII, Case 13). Cytochemical reactions also may be helpful, because lymphoblasts typically are negative for most of the cytochemical stains except nonspecific esterase. Middle-aged to older dogs are usually affected. Cats are usually younger and FeLV positive. The majority of ALLs and leukemias associated with stage V lymphoma in dogs were thought to be of B cell origin, although one study found that the prevalence of B and T immunophenotypes in ALL and CLL was not statistically different [3]. Conversely, some authors are of the opinion that almost all cases of ALL are of T cell origin and that some cases were erroneously classified as B-ALL based on expression of CD79a, which does not have high lineage fidelity [1].

In a retrospective study of 50 dogs with ALL, the majority were of T cell lineage and approximately 1/3 had mediastinal lymphadenopathy. Age ranged from 2 to 14 years of age with a median of 7 years. Sixty-eight percent of dogs were anemic, 86% were thrombocytopenic, 22% were markedly neutropenic, and the median leukemic cell count was 73,500/μL. Hypercalcemia was seen in six dogs, all of which had T cell leukemia [4].

Chemotherapy, usually involving a combination of vincristine, cyclophosphamide, and prednisone, may result in remission in approximately 1/3 of patients with ALL, although usually of very short duration. The clinical course is typically rapid and progressive. Improvement in survival times will require substantial advances in chemotherapy protocols and the use of more targeted therapeutic agents. In people with ALL, cytogenetic discoveries have led to targeted therapy against oncogenes that have dramatically improved survival times, and analogous discoveries in dogs and cats will likely lead to better outcomes.

Chronic lymphocyte leukemia (CLL)

CLL is much more common than ALL, and T-CLL is more common than B-CLL. In animals with CLL, the lymphocytes are small and appear well-differentiated (Figure 16.30). CLL is more common in dogs than in other domestic animals. This type of leukemia, however, must be differentiated from physiologic lymphocytosis in excited cats (usually kittens and young adult cats), in which the absolute lymphocyte count may reach 20,000 cells/μL^{-1}. Other differential diagnoses include lymphocytosis induced by chronic antigenic stimulation, such as that seen in dogs with chronic ehrlichiosis. Lymphocytosis is rare and usually mild (<10,000 lymphocytes/μL^{-1}) with other types of antigenic stimulation, however. Lymphocytosis predominated by LGL may be seen in animals with ehrlichiosis or T-CLL.

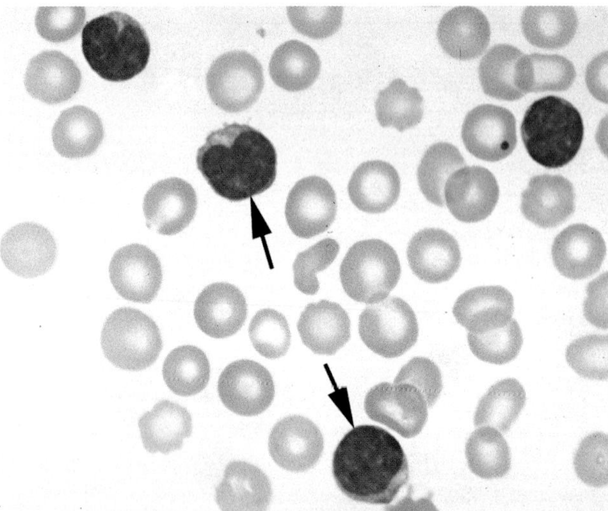

Figure 16.30 Blood film from a dog with chronic lymphocytic leukemia. Note the relatively small, normal-appearing lymphocytes (arrows). The diagnosis of leukemia was based on the high concentration of small lymphocytes in the blood (40,000 cells/μL^{-1}) and by polymerase chain reaction results. Wright stain.

Mild to moderate lymphocytosis has been reported as an infrequent finding in cats infected with *Bartonella henselae*. The list of major differentials for persistent nonneoplastic lymphocyte expansion in adult dogs and cats is short and includes tick-borne disease, especially canine monocytic ehrlichiosis, hypoadrenocorticism, and thymoma. Persistent lymphocytosis of small, mature, or reactive lymphocytes is most commonly the result of CLL or lymphoma. The first step in distinguishing nonneoplastic from neoplastic lymphocytosis is immunophenotyping by flow cytometry to determine the phenotypic diversity of the circulating cells. Clonality testing using the polymerase chain reaction for antigen receptor rearrangements assay is a useful second step in cases in which the phenotype data are equivocal. Once the diagnosis of malignancy has been established, the immunophenotype (see Chapter 14) also provides prognostic information in dogs.

Clinical signs and abnormalities found in ill animals are similar to those seen in animals with other types of leukemia, including lethargy, anorexia, pale mucous membranes, lymphadenopathy, splenomegaly, and hepatomegaly. However, some animals are asymptomatic, and the lymphocytosis is discovered during a wellness examination or presurgical screening. The most striking CBC abnormality is the lymphocytosis, which may range from increased slightly above the reference interval to greater than 300,000/μL^{-1}. Anemia and thrombocytopenia may be present, but the anemia usually is not as severe as that seen in animals with ALL. The concentration of small lymphocytes in the marrow is greater than normal, being reported to range from 25% to 93% of cells. Monoclonal gammopathies occasionally are seen in animals with CLL. A small percentage of dogs and people with CLL develop an aggressive diffuse large B cell lymphoma (Richter's syndrome) [5].

Three primary subtypes of CLL, based primarily on immunophenotyping, have been reported: (i) T-CLL, which is the most common form in dogs and cats, with cells in the many cases being CD3^{+}/CD8^{+} granular lymphocytes; (ii) B-CLL (CD21^{+}), which is the next most common subtype; and (iii) atypical CLL, which represents a combination of immunophenotypes. Patients that have CD34+ cells are typically classified as having ALL. Some of the dogs with T cell leukemia have LGL leukemia, and T cells sometimes proliferate in the spleen. Most dogs with T-zone lymphoma, an indolent disease with long survival times, have leukemia (see chapter 45). This T-cell leukemia is unique in that the cells express CD21, which is a B-cell marker. Immunophenotyping provides an objective method for determining prognosis in dogs with CLL. Expression of CD34 predicts poor outcome with much shorter survival compared with other phenotypes. Within the CD8+ phenotype, dogs presenting with a >30,000 lymphocytes/μL^{-1} have significantly shorter median survival than those presenting with <30,000 lymphocytes/μL^{-1}. Within the T cell leukemias, dogs with CD4-8-5+ leukemia and dogs with the CD8+ T cell phenotype have a similar survival time. A CD21+ B cell lymphocytosis composed of large cells was associated with shorter survival time than those with smaller circulating cells. In another study, old dogs with B-CLL survived longer than young dogs, and anemic dogs with T-CLL survived a shorter time than dogs without anemia.

B cell chronic lymphocytic leukemia (B-CLL) is the most common hematopoietic malignancy in people, and B cell leukemia in dogs may provide an animal model as the disease appears to be similar in dogs and people. Unlike the human disease, canine B-CLL cells do not express CD5. In people with B-CLL, analysis of the immunoglobulin genes has been crucial in understanding pathogenesis and prognosis, and preliminary studies show that these analyses may also be useful in dogs [6]. In a retrospective study of 491 dogs with B-CLL, the median age was 11 years and small breeds had significantly greater odds of having B-CLL [7]. Lymphadenopathy was present in 46%, splenomegaly in 51%, hepatomegaly in 29%, and visceral lymphadenopathy in 23%. Twenty-six percent of dogs were anemic, 26% were hyperglobulinemic, and only 5% were hypercalcemic. The median lymphocyte concentration was 24,600/μl with a range of 5000-812,544/μL, and the median percentage of lymphocytes that were B cells was 94%. Neutropenia and mild thrombocytopenia were rarely observed (1% and 7% respectively). English bulldogs had a unique presentation in that they were diagnosed at a median age of 6 years, and expressed lower class II MHC and CD25.

Therapeutic intervention is controversial, because untreated animals may live for months to years. Recommendations for chemotherapy in dogs and cats include a combination of chlorambucil and prednisone; long remissions and survival can be achieved. The median survival time for dogs is more than 1 year. Survival time has been reported to be significantly different in untreated dogs with CLL (~450 days), as compared to that of dogs with ALL (~65 days). CLL in cats is rarely associated with FeLV infection.

Enzootic bovine leukosis

Enzootic bovine leukosis, the most common neoplastic disease of cattle, is a B cell lymphoproliferative disorder of cattle that is caused by the bovine leukemia virus (BLV), an oncogenic retrovirus that infects lymphocytes and can result in a persistent lymphocytosis, and sometimes leukemia and lymphoma. The virus is transmitted through the blood, either iatrogenically or by biting flies. It is also spread vertically, either through the placenta or by colostrum. Virus specific antibodies are found in serum and milk. No vaccine is available, and therapy is not instituted. It occurs worldwide and is a significant problem for the beef and dairy cattle industries. Diagnosis is usually made by detecting the antibody to the virus or detecting the virus by quantitative PCR. Approximately 40% of cow-calf beef herds and 10% of individual beef cows in the US are BLV seropositive. Approximately 70% of BLV infected animals are asymptomatic carriers of the virus. Approximately one-third of infected cattle develop a benign form of nonmalignant persistent lymphocytosis of untransformed lymphocytes, characterized by increased concentration of $CD5^+$ IgM^+ B cells. Because absolute lymphocyte concentration is significantly increased by BLV infection, even in clinically healthy cattle, reference intervals should be derived from animals that are not infected with BLV and patient BLV status must be considered for meaningful interpretation of lymphocyte concentration.

Less than 5% of infected cattle develop malignant B cell lymphoma originating from mono- or oligo-clonal accumulation of B cells after a usually long period of latency. This malignant form of B cell lymphoma is predominantly detected in cattle over 4–5 years of age, although calves as young as 3 months of age have been reported. Lymph nodes, spleen, and other organs such as the heart, intestine, kidney lung, liver and uterus may be involved. BLV infection causes abnormal immune function, even in clinically healthy animals, affecting both the innate and adaptive immune system and altering proper functioning of uninfected cells.

Plasma cell myeloma (multiple myeloma, disseminated plasma cell neoplasia)

Plasma cell myeloma is a relatively rare lymphoproliferative neoplasm in which plasma cells or their precursors proliferate abnormally (Figures 16.31–16.33). As implied by the term multiple myeloma, plasma cells proliferate in the bone marrow at multiple sites. Plasma cell myeloma, also referred to as disseminated plasma cell neoplasia, accounts

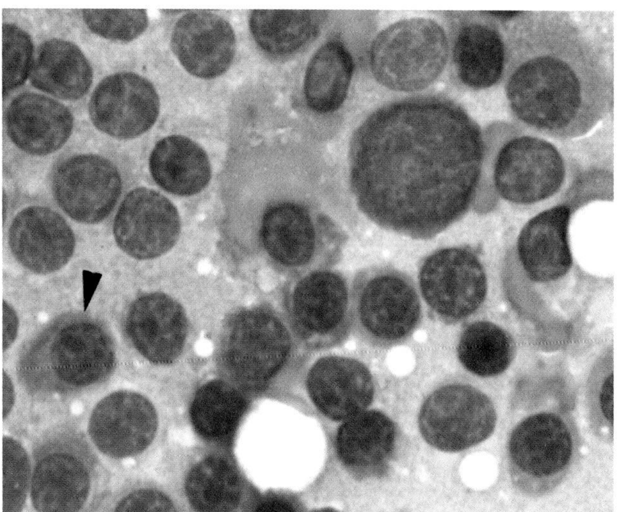

Figure 16.31 Bone marrow aspirate taken at autopsy from a dog with plasma cell myeloma. Almost all of the cells present are plasma cells. Note the more typical plasma cell with an eccentric nucleus and abundant cytoplasm (arrowhead). Wright stain.

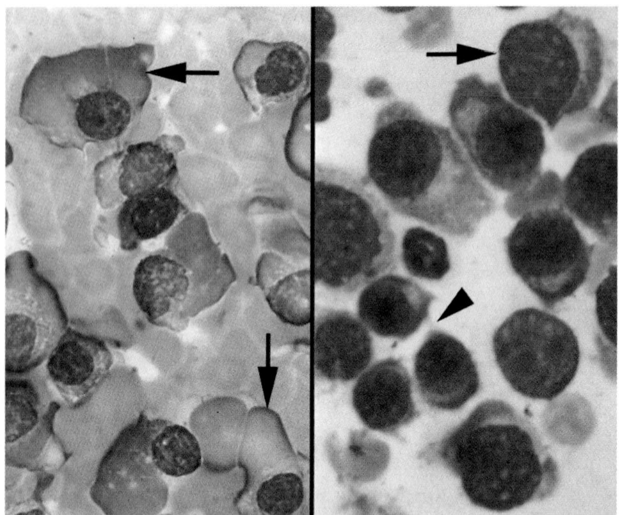

Figure 16.32 Left. Bone marrow aspirate from a dog with plasma cell myeloma. These plasma cells have eosinophilic-colored cytoplasm that is ruffled, and they sometimes are referred to as flame cells. The cytoplasm is filled with immunoglobulin. Right. Bone marrow aspirate from a dog with plasma cell myeloma. Note the variation in cell size, ranging from the large, immature plasma cell with loose chromatin (arrow) to the small cells with more condensed chromatin (arrowhead). Wright stain.

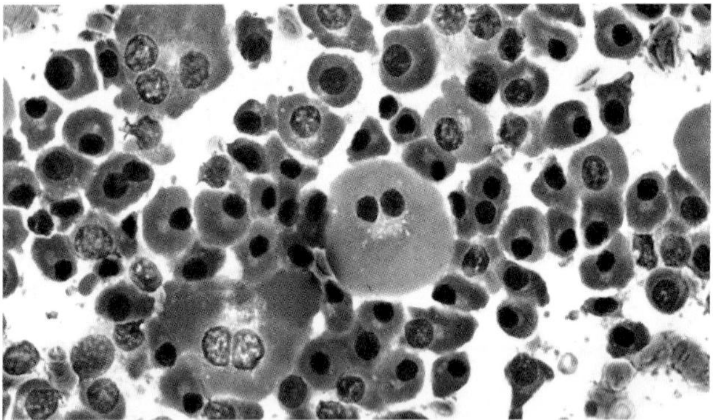

Figure 16.33 Bone marrow aspirate from a dog with plasma cell myeloma. Note the binucleate cells and abundant pink immunoglobulin in the cytoplasm. Wright stain. Source: Courtesy Dr. Clarissa Freemyer, North Carolina State University.

for approximately 10% of all hematopoietic malignancies in dogs and people. The incidence of multiple myeloma in cats is thought to be even less than that in dogs and usually is not associated with FeLV or FIV infections. Plasma cell myeloma has been reported infrequently in horses and twice in swine.

Neoplastic plasma cell proliferations are commonly detected on bone marrow films, but plasma cells only rarely are seen on blood films. When circulating neoplastic plasma cells are present, the survival time usually is less. Markedly increased plasma cell concentration in the bone marrow (>20% of all nucleated cells) often results from plasma cell neoplasia, but plasma cell proliferation also may occur secondary to chronic antigenic stimulation such as is seen with canine monocytic ehrlichiosis. Neoplastic plasma cells often are seen in large aggregates and sometimes appear slightly abnormal or immature, with occasional multinucleated plasma cells being present. Neoplastic cells may appear to be very well-differentiated, however, in which case they are difficult to distinguish from normal plasma cells. Plasma cells occasionally may have a ruffled eosinophilic cytoplasmic margin that appears similar to a flame; these are termed flaming plasma cells or flame cells (Figures 16.32 and 16.33). When plasma cells are poorly differentiated, they may be difficult to differentiate from other types of neoplastic cells, including lymphocytes, osteoblasts and malignant histiocytes. Immunocytochemistry using a monoclonal mouse anti-human MUM1 (multiple myeloma oncogene 1) antibody can be used to help identify plasma cells.

Plasma cells derive from B-lymphocytes and typically secrete immunoglobulins. A very common manifestation of plasma cell myeloma is a monoclonal or biclonal gammopathy, usually immunoglobulin G or A but, occasionally, immunoglobulin M (Figure 16.34). Patients with a monoclonal gammopathy may or may not be hyperglobulinemic. The immunoglobulins synthesized by malignant plasma cells also are known as paraproteins or monoclonal proteins (M-proteins). Serum protein electrophoresis (SPE) using a densitometer detects M-proteins, which are usually represented by a peak taller than albumin (see "Protein Electrophoresis" in Chapter 1). SPE can be performed using either agarose gel electrophoresis (AGE) or capillary zone electrophoresis (CZE) based techniques. Immunotyping is another electrophoretic-based technique that uses labeling antibodies to identify immunoglobulin fractions within a serum sample. Immunofixation using gel electrophoresis

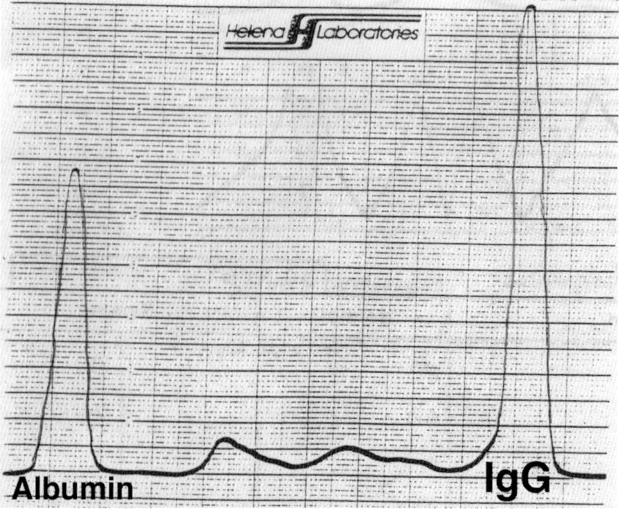

Figure 16.34 Protein electrophoretogram from a dog with plasma cell myeloma and monoclonal gammopathy. Note the monoclonal immunoglobulin (IgG) spike at the right. Albumin is represented by the smaller spike to the left. Wright stain.

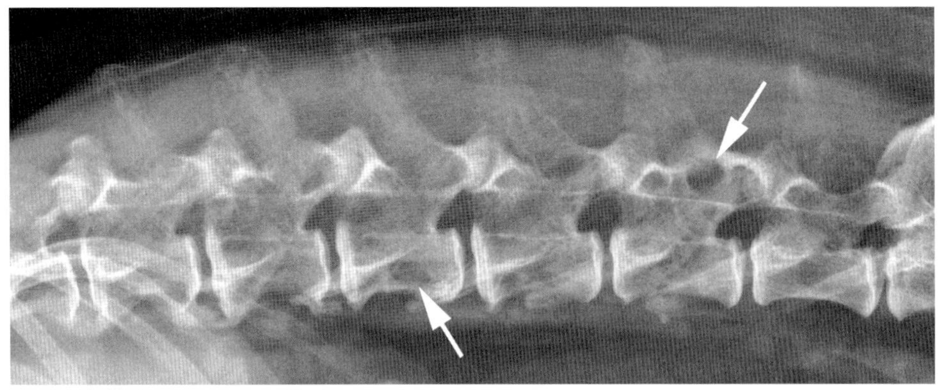

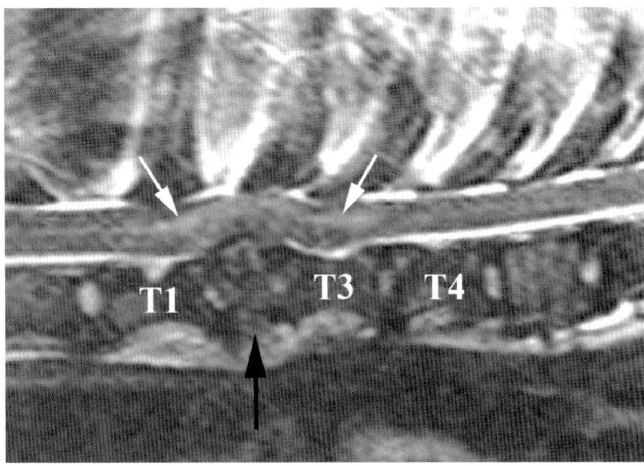

Figure 16.35 (a) Lateral lumbar radiograph of a dog with multiple myeloma. There are numerous small lucencies in the spinous processes and larger lucent lesions in the body of L3 and the lamina of L5 (white arrows) due to bone effacement from neoplastic cells. (b) Sagittal T2-weighted magnetic resonance image of the thoracic spine of a dog with multiple myeloma. Effacement of the second thoracic vertebral body by neoplastic cells has led to a pathologic fracture. Note the foreshortened irregular shape (black arrow) compared to the adjacent normal first, third, and fourth thoracic vertebrae (T1, T3, and T4, respectively). A portion of the fractured vertebra is protruding into the vertebral canal and causing spinal cord compression. The increased signal (whiteness) of the spinal cord (white arrows) is due to edema and inflammation. Vertebral fracture causing paralysis or paresis is a relatively common complication of multiple myeloma. Source: Courtesy Dr. Donald Thrall, North Carolina State University.

defines M-proteins typically composed of both heavy and light chains and evaluates IgG, IgA, and IgM heavy chain and light chain. In summary, AGE, CZE, and species-specific immunofixation can be used alone or in combination to detect M-protein.

Rarely, the neoplastic plasma cells produce only the light chain component of the immunoglobulin that readily passes through the glomerulus due to its small molecular size. Thus, a monoclonal gammopathy is not seen and these patients often go undiagnosed. The Bence-Jones proteins are not detected on dipsticks for urine protein, which are specific for detecting albumin. However, the light chain immunoglobulins can be detected by sulfosalicylic acid precipitation and confirmed by urine protein electrophoresis that will show a urine monoclonal gammopathy. Even more rarely, dogs with multiple myeloma will not have evidence of M-proteins in either their blood or urine. These nonsecretory myelomas (NSM) are further categorized as either "true" NSM, in which the neoplastic plasma cells are not synthesizing M-proteins, or "false" NSM, in which the plasma cells are not releasing M-proteins or the M-protein cannot be measured by conventional methods. Other diagnostic features of plasma cell myeloma include Bence-Jones protein (i.e., light chains of immunoglobulins) in the urine, and radiographic evidence of osteolysis (Figure 16.35). Two or three of these four features traditionally are considered to be essential for the diagnosis of plasma cell myeloma. However, diagnosis of multiple myeloma in humans no longer requires the documentation of complete M-proteins, since nonsecretory myelomas comprise up to 5% of all cases of multiple myeloma in people.

Differential diagnoses include canine monocytic ehrlichiosis, a disease with which a monoclonal gammopathy may very rarely be seen, usually within a polyclonal gammopathy. Dogs with ehrlichiosis commonly have a markedly increased concentration of plasma cells in the bone marrow. Other disorders in which monoclonal gammopathies have been reported include B cell chronic lymphocytic leukemia, B cell lymphoma, extramedullary plasmacytoma, and feline infectious peritonitis (rarely).

Plasma cells do not normally proliferate, but oncogenic mutations impart cell proliferation capability that results in progressive disease that eventually becomes symptomatic. Clinical signs associated with multiple myeloma are usually associated with plasma cell infiltration of the bone marrow and other organs or with increased concentration of circulating immunoglobulins, which may result in increased viscosity of the blood (i.e., hyperviscosity syndrome). Lethargy, anorexia, lameness, bleeding from the nares, paresis, polyuria, and polydipsia are relatively common. Fundoscopic changes such as retinal hemorrhages and engorged retinal blood vessels commonly are observed as well. Renal disease is relatively common and usually associated with the abnormal proteins interfering with tubular and glomerular function, but it sometimes occurs secondary to hypercalcemia with subsequent calcification of renal tissue. Central nervous system impairment may result from serum hyperviscosity and subsequent sludging of blood in small vessels. Bleeding diatheses, which are seen in approximately one-third of dogs with multiple myeloma, may result from thrombocytopenia, but it also can result from the abnormal immunoglobulins interfering with platelet function. Common findings in feline multiple myeloma include atypical plasma cell morphology, hypocholesterolemia, anemia, bone lesions, and multiorgan involvement. In one retrospective study, all of the affected cats examined had noncutaneous, extramedullary tumors of the spleen, liver, or lymph nodes.

Mephalan, an alkylating agent, is usually used to treat multiple myeloma in dogs, often in combination with prednisone. Response rate is usually good, with a mean survival time of approximately 18 months to 3 years. Mephalan or cyclophosphamide sometimes in combination with prednisone are preferred therapy for multiple myeloma in cats; cyclophosphamide is usually tolerated better than mephalan. Reported survival times in treated cats average approximately 1 year. Animals with multiple myeloma that are azotemic or have severe anemia, neutropenia, or thrombocytopenia usually have a shorter survival time. Hypercalcemia, Bence-Jones proteinuria, plasma cell leukemia, and extensive bony lesions also are associated with a poorer prognosis. In humans, stem cell transplantation offers significantly improved prognosis and survival rates.

17 Disorders of Hemostasis

James Meinkoth

Department of Veterinary Pathobiology, Oklahoma State University, Stillwater, OK, USA

Hemostasis is the physiologic cessation of bleeding. Patients demonstrating excessive or abnormal bleeding are fairly common in veterinary practice and are often presented as emergencies. A few simple laboratory tests are available that help to determine two things:

1. Whether the bleeding is the result of a defect in hemostasis versus local tissue disease (tissue trauma, neoplasia, infection, etc.).

2. In the event that a hemostatic defect *is* present, localize the problem to a particular segment of the hemostatic system and thus narrow the list of potential differentials that may be causing the presenting problem.

This chapter will (i) review the physiology of hemostasis to the level required to interpret common tests of hemostasis, (ii) discuss some clinical information that must be considered in a patient presenting for excessive bleeding, (iii) describe the routine tests used to evaluate hemostasis, and (iv) discuss some of the most common diseases in veterinary medicine that result in abnormal bleeding.

Review of physiology of hemostasis

The physiology of hemostasis is amazingly complex and can be quite intimidating. Fortunately, it is not necessary to know a tremendous amount of detail to appropriately interpret the common hemostatic tests. A quick overview of hemostasis will be presented followed by a bit more detail about each of the major steps. The process of hemostasis is reviewed here at a basic level with specific details added when they pertain to a relevant disease process. Far more detailed reviews are available for those who are interested (and slightly masochistic) and wish to pursue the topic in more depth [1–7].

The "big picture" overview

Blood is normally maintained in a fluid state within vessels, but if vascular injury occurs, then rapid hemostasis is necessary to prevent severe bleeding. The hemostatic system is amazingly efficient and able to (i) respond rapidly, thus limiting the amount of bleeding, and also to (ii) limit coagulation to the site of injury, which prevents pathologic coagulation or thrombosis. The essential components that are required for hemostasis to occur, *blood platelets* and certain proteins called *soluble coagulation factors*, are present preformed within circulation and available to act if vascular injury occurs.

Coagulation does not normally occur without vascular injury because the coagulation factors are mostly present in an inactive form and the endothelial cells that line all blood vessels function both *passively and actively* to inhibit clotting. The normal endothelial lining of blood vessels is a *nonthrombogenic surface* (meaning it does not activate platelets or coagulation factors) and also actively produces factors that inhibit the various components of hemostasis. In contrast to the endothelium, the connective tissues (e.g., collagen), which are just under the endothelial cells and thus termed the *subendothelium*, are extremely thrombogenic and start the hemostatic process when exposed by vessel injury. The endothelial cells surrounding a site of injury may actively switch from a nonthrombogenic state to a thrombogenic state, at least temporarily. They do this by reducing production or expression of inhibitors of hemostasis and expressing or secreting other components that promote the activation of platelets and coagulation factors.

> ***Major concept:*** There are always processes both favoring and opposing hemostasis occurring simultaneously. This leads to some confusion when first reading the details of hemostasis. Whether or not clotting occurs at any given time depends on the balance of these forces. Much of this balance is dependent on the function of the endothelial cells. Having both processes occurring at low levels all the time and opposing each other allows the process to be started and stopped faster than if they were dormant and needed to be "geared up."

Step 1: primary hemostasis

The initial event in hemostasis following vascular injury is a reflex constriction of local blood vessels. This limits blood flow in the affected area to reduce bleeding. It also slows the

Veterinary Hematology, Clinical Chemistry, and Cytology, Third Edition. Edited by Mary Anna Thrall, Glade Weiser, Robin W. Allison and Terry W. Campbell.

Companion website: www.wiley.com/go/thrall/veterinary

flow of platelets and coagulation factors, keeping them from being swept away from the area after they are activated. The first cellular event is that platelets bind to subendothelial collagen exposed at the area of the injury; this is called *platelet adhesion*. After adhesion, platelets become activated. Activated platelets quickly (i) change shape to spread out and cover more surface area, (ii) expose certain membrane receptors for adhesive proteins, and (iii) secrete substances called *platelet agonists*. These agonists recruit and activate additional platelets. Soon, newly arrived platelets bind to other platelets, a process called *platelet aggregation*. Platelet aggregation continues until a mass of platelets (*platelet plug*) completely fills the defect. The process of forming a platelet plug at the site of injury is referred to as *primary hemostasis*.

Step 2: secondary hemostasis

The initial platelet plug may transiently stop the bleeding but is not very stable. It is sufficient to stop bleeding only from very small wounds. With larger wounds, hydrostatic pressure within blood vessels would disrupt the platelet plug leading to *rebleeding*. This is where the soluble coagulation factors come in. The soluble coagulation factors are a group of proteins mainly produced by the liver. They are traditionally identified by roman numerals (i.e., Factor II) with the addition of an *"a"* (i.e., Factor IIa) to indicate the active form. They also have common names, some of which are used more frequently than the roman numerals (Table 17.1). These proteins are mostly proteases, secreted in an inactive proenzyme form, that cleave and thus activate each other in a sequential order termed the *coagulation cascade*.

The end result of the coagulation cascade is that fibrinogen (a.k.a., Factor I) is converted to fibrin at the site of the platelet plug. Fibrin is an adhesive protein that forms long strands and can bind to both other fibrin strands (called *cross-linking*) as well as platelets. This forms a fibrin mesh around the platelets within the platelet plug. Fibrin acts like a biological glue to stabilize the platelet plug and permanently stop bleeding. The process of coagulation factors working in sequence to produce fibrin to stabilize the platelet plug is called *secondary hemostasis*.

> ***Major concept:*** Why is it important to divide this process into primary and secondary hemostasis? First, the types of clinical signs seen with defects of primary hemostasis are often sufficiently different from those seen with defects of secondary hemostasis, so that you can predict which system is affected from the clinical signs. Second, most basic laboratory tests evaluate either primary or secondary hemostasis, so you must know what physiologic functions are being tested. Finally, the potential disease processes that must be considered for any given clinical problem (i.e., the differential diagnoses) are different depending on which portion of the hemostatic process is affected.

Step 3: fibrinolysis (clot breakdown)

Eventually, after the underlying damage is repaired, the formed clot is broken down so that blood flow through the vessel is restored. This process is called *fibrinolysis*, and it is the result of the enzyme *plasmin*, which cleaves the fibrin clot at various places. As this occurs, small fragments of cleaved fibrin termed *fibrin degradation products (FDPs)* are released into circulation. These can be measured in the blood and are an indicator of clot breakdown. One specific group of FDPs are called *D-dimers*. These can be measured by a test that is currently used to detect the formation and breakdown of clots at an accelerated rate within the vasculature.

Details about primary hemostasis (platelet plug formation)

von Willebrand factor and platelet adhesion

As mentioned earlier, the first cellular event in hemostasis is platelet adhesion to collagen in the subendothelium. This adhesion requires a serum protein called *von Willebrand factor (vWf)*. vWf is not one of the soluble coagulation factors and is not directly involved in secondary hemostasis. It is produced primarily by vascular endothelial cells and to some degree by megakaryocytes and ends up stored inside platelet granules. vWf is an adhesive protein that can form long strands. It binds both to exposed collagen at the site of vessel injury and also to receptors on platelet membranes. In doing this, it acts to link platelets to the vessel wall (Figure 17.1). While other proteins, such as fibrinogen, can also bind to both platelets and the vessel wall, vWf is the only protein that can adequately mediate platelet adhesion in the high sheer force created by flowing blood within areas of the vasculature.

As the endothelial cells make vWf, they secrete it both from their basal surface, where it binds to subendothelial collagen, and from their luminal surface, where it ends up in circulation (Figure 17.2). Circulating vWf does not bind platelets, or it would result in thrombosis. vWf must bind subendothelium first, which causes a conformational shift allowing it to bind platelets. In addition, the endothelial cells store vWf within intracellular granules. This stored vWf can be released following injury. Thus, when endothelial cells are removed as a result of injury, vWf is already present bound to the exposed collagen as well as in the blood flowing over this defect. In addition, it is released from the endothelial cells surrounding the injury and the platelets that are recruited to the site. All of these processes results in a high concentration of vWf at the site of injury, which is important for effective platelet adhesion. von Willebrand disease (vWd) is a genetic deficiency of vWf. It is common in both humans and dogs and results in defective primary hemostasis and bleeding tendencies.

Fibrinogen and platelet aggregation

Platelet aggregation, the process of platelets binding to other platelets in the growing platelet plug, is mediated primarily

Table 17.1 Coagulation factors: common names and their functions.

Factor number	Common name	Pathway involved	Comments/function
Factor I	Fibrinogen	Common	Converted by thrombin to the adhesive protein fibrin as the final step of coagulation cascade Also active in primary hemostasis (mediates platelet aggregation)
Factor II	Prothrombin	Common	Proenzyme Active form cleaves fibrinogen (also activates many other factors as amplification loop) Vitamin K dependent
Factor III	Tissue factor, tissue thromboplastin	Extrinsic[a]	Lipoprotein that can be expressed on cell membrane of various cells Serves a cofactor for FVII, initiating extrinsic coagulation cascade
Factor IV	Calcium	All	Required for surface dependent coagulation factors to bind to phospholipid surfaces of platelets and participate in coagulation reactions
Factor V	Proaccelerin	Common	When activated, serves as cofactor for Factor X
Factor VI	—	—	There is no Factor VI
Factor VII	Proconvertin	Extrinsic	Proenzyme Active form activates Factor X (and Factor IX) Vitamin K dependent
Factor VIII	Antihemophilic factor	Intrinsic[b]	When activated, serves as cofactor for Factor IX
Factor IX	Christmas factor	Intrinsic	Proenzyme Active form activates Factor X Vitamin K dependent
Factor X	Stuart-Prower factor	Common	Proenzyme Active form activates Factor II Vitamin K dependent
Factor XI	Plasma thromboplastin antecedent	Intrinsic	Proenzyme Active form activates Factor IX
Factor XII	Hageman factor	Intrinsic	Proenzyme Active form activates Factor XI (and other contact factors)
Factor XIII	Fibrin-stabilizing factor	Common	Cross-links fibrin strands, thus stabilizing them
Prekallikrein	Fletcher factor	Intrinsic	Proenzyme Active form activates Factor XII
HMWK[c]	Fitzgerald factor	Intrinsic	Cofactor Activates Factors XII, XI

[a]The extrinsic pathway is now typically referred to as the "tissue factor pathway."
[b]The intrinsic pathway is now typically referred to as the "contact pathway" or "surface dependent pathway."
[c]HMWK = high molecular weight kininogen.

by fibrinogen (Figure 17.1). vWf can act in platelet aggregation also, but fibrinogen is present in the blood in much higher concentrations than vWf. Fibrinogen is also stored in platelet granules and released during platelet plug formation to further increase the concentration of this protein at the site of the platelet plug. Remember that fibrinogen, which helps bind platelets to each other, is what will be converted to fibrin by the secondary hemostatic system to stabilize the platelet plug, so it makes sense to have it within the platelet plug.

While deficiencies in fibrinogen would obviously lead to defects in primary hemostasis, they also affect the secondary hemostatic system, so it is not usually considered in the differential of a patient with a defect in only primary hemostasis. Inherited deficiencies or abnormalities of fibrinogen are extremely rare in veterinary medicine. Acquired

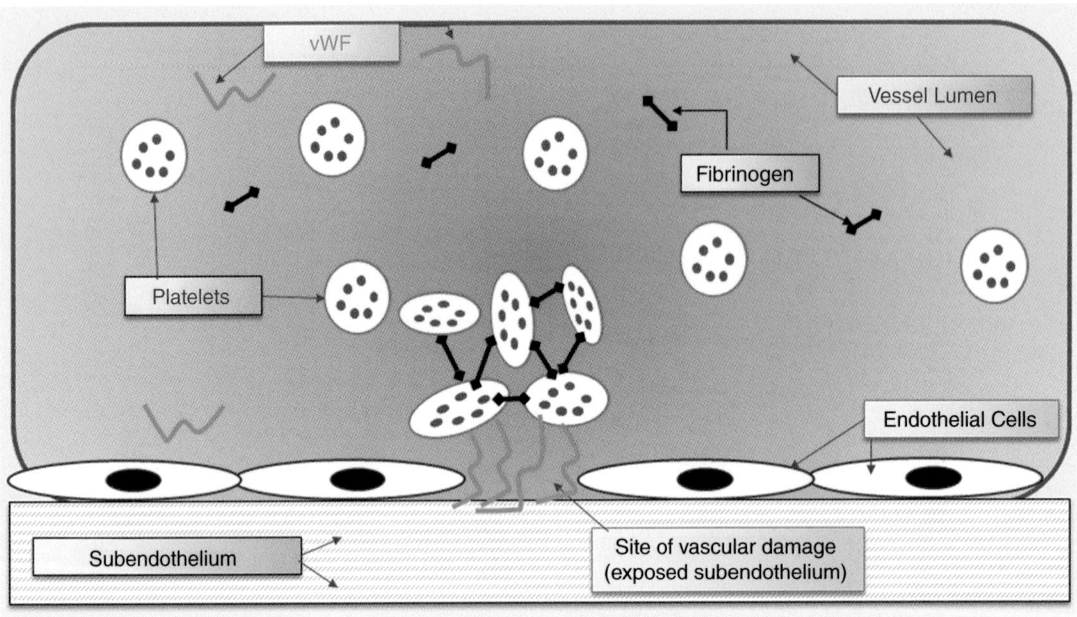

Figure 17.1 Schematic of components of primary hemostasis or production of the platelet plug. vWf (blue lines) mediates the adhesion of platelets to the exposed subendothelium following vascular damage. Fibrinogen (black arrows) mediates platelet aggregation to other platelets.

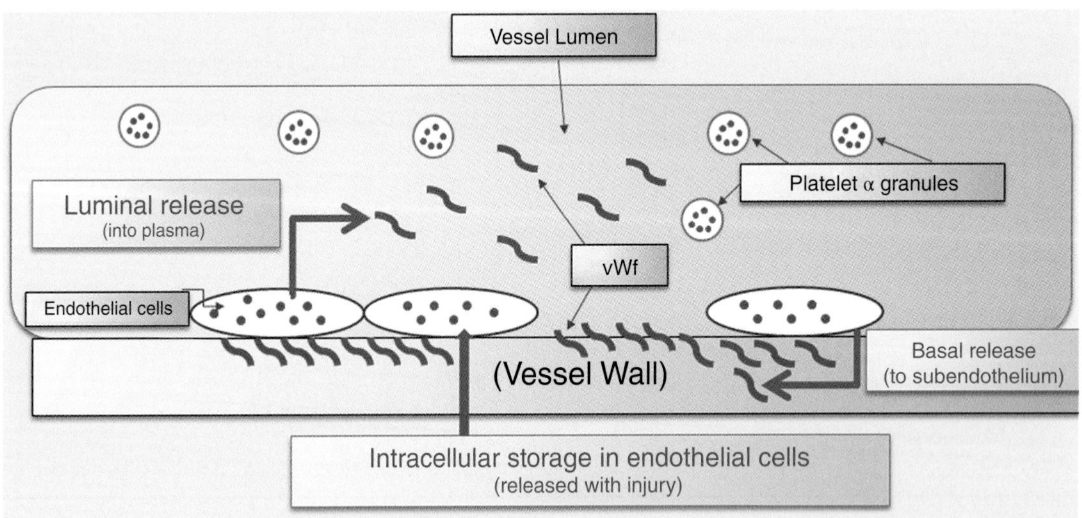

Figure 17.2 Schematic of vWf production. The production, storage, and release of vWf work together to create high concentrations of vWf at the site of platelet plug formation. vWf from endothelial cells is released both into the plasma and into the subendothelium. In addition, both platelets and endothelial cells contain vWf within intracellular granules. This stored vWf can be released during platelet plug formation to further increase the local concentrations.

deficiency of fibrinogen can occur due to excessive consumption in the disease *disseminated intravascular coagulation (DIC)*, which is discussed in more detail later.

Platelet numbers and function

The platelets themselves play an active part in hemostasis. First of all, adequate numbers of platelets are needed for the platelet plug to form. Thrombocytopenia, a decreased platelet concentration, is extremely common and is the most common cause of abnormal bleeding seen in veterinary medicine.

In addition to having sufficient platelets, they must be functional since they actively participate in both primary and secondary hemostasis. Platelet activation and normal platelet function are very complex, and much of the detail is beyond what is needed for interpretations of hemostatic tests. As a simplified overview, platelet functions involve (i) expression of surface membrane receptors, (ii) release

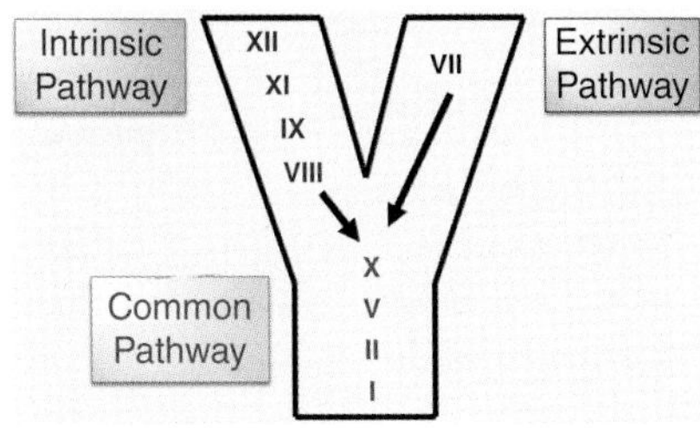

Figure 17.3 Schematic of the coagulation factor pathways, as they relate to coagulation testing results. Physiologically, the extrinsic pathway (a.k.a. tissue factor pathway) is of primary importance, and the intrinsic pathway serves primarily in amplification of the process. Also, there is cross-over between the two pathways as Factor VII (extrinsic pathway) may directly activate Factor IX (intrinsic pathway) in addition to its downstream activation of Factor X.

of granule contents, and (iii) initiation of a variety of intracellular signaling pathways.

Platelet function: surface receptors

Platelet receptors allow them to (i) bind to adhesive proteins and thus participate in adhesion and aggregation and (ii) respond to platelet agonists resulting in activation (Figures 17.3 and 17.4). The receptor for vWf is platelet *glycoprotein Ib* (GP Ib) and the receptor for fibrinogen is *glycoprotein IIb/IIIa* (GP IIb/IIIa). Inherited mutations of these receptors can lead to abnormal bleeding, with GP IIb/IIIa being most important in veterinary medicine. There are receptors for platelet agonists such as adenosine diphosphate (ADP) and thrombin. These receptors are the target of therapeutic interventions aimed at preventing thrombosis. An important example is the drug *clopidogrel* (Plavix®), which inhibits one of the ADP receptors.

Platelet function: granule contents

Platelets have dense granules and alpha granules, whose contents promote hemostasis and are released following platelet activation to increase their concentration in the microenvironment where the clot is forming. The *alpha granules* contain mainly a variety of adhesive proteins and coagulation factor proteins, while the *dense granules* contain nonprotein mediators of hemostasis (Table 17.2). Inherited defects of these granules and their release exist (e.g., Chédiak-Higashi syndrome), but these are extremely rare.

Platelet function: intracellular signaling pathways

Numerous intracellular biochemical pathways are initiated during platelet activation, which ultimately results in platelet shape change (allows the platelet to spread out and cover the defect), platelet cytoskeletal contraction (retracts and further strengthens the platelet plug), expression and activation of the previously mentioned membrane receptors (promotes aggregation), and release of the previously mentioned granules (further promotes adhesion, aggregation, and activation).

One important intracellular signaling pathway is arachadonic acid metabolism, which results in the production of thromboxane A2 (TXA2), a platelet agonist. This pathway is inhibited by aspirin and other NSAIDs, thus inhibiting platelet function. These drugs can be used therapeutically to prevent thrombosis but may also cause excessive bleeding.

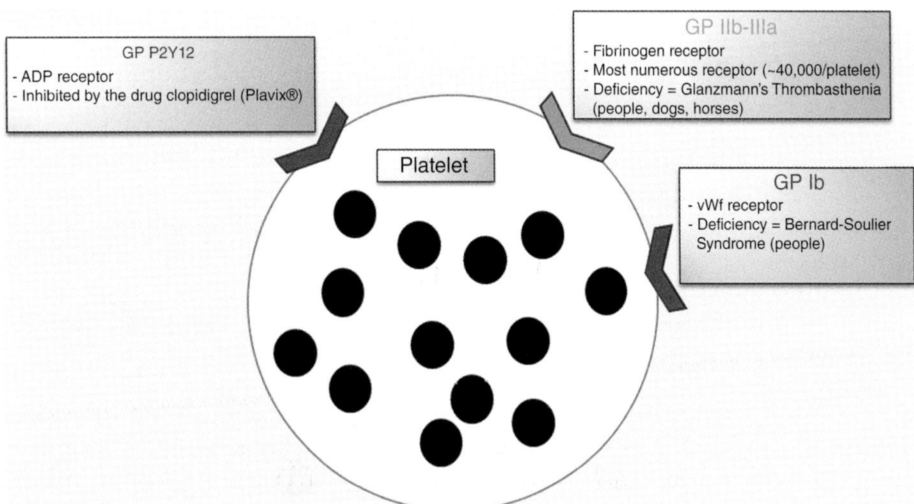

Figure 17.4 Selected platelet receptors and their ligands. There are many more receptors for both adhesive proteins (e.g., collagen receptors) as well as platelet agonists (e.g., additional ADP receptors, thrombin receptors), but these are the primary ones for which disease-causing mutations have been reported or pharmaceutical interventions have been directed. Platelet receptors are the targets of many new pharmacologic agents given the importance of thrombotic disease in people.

Table 17.2 Platelet granules and their contents.

Alpha granules contents	Dense granule contents
Adhesive proteins	ADP
– vWf	Adenosine triphosphate
– Fibrinogen	Calcium
– Vitronectin	Serotonin
– Fibronectin	
Coagulation factors	
– Factor V	
– Factor XI	
Growth factors	
– Platelet-derived growth factor	
– Endothelial cell growth factor	
– Epidermal growth factor	
Inhibitors of fibrinolysis	
– Plasminogen activator inhibitor	

> ***Major concept:*** Physiologically, the major things required for primary hemostasis to occur are (i) normal subendothelium, (ii) adequate numbers of platelets, (iii) normal platelet function, (iv) von Willebrand factor, and (v) fibrinogen (Figure 17.1). However, abnormalities of subendothelium are extremely rare, and fibrinogen deficiency affects secondary hemostasis as well as primary hemostasis. So, neither of these are commonly considered in patients with disorders limited to primary hemostasis. *Thus, the main differential diagnoses for such patients are (i) thrombocytopenia, (ii) von Willebrand disease, and (iii) abnormal platelet function.*

Details about secondary hemostasis (fibrin clot formation)

Coagulation vs. hemostasis

As discussed previously, secondary hemostasis involves the sequential activation of a group of serum proteins, most of them proteases, with the ultimate goal of converting fibrinogen to fibrin, which stabilizes the platelet plug. This process of fibrin formation from activation of these serum proteins is termed *coagulation*. Thus, the terms "coagulation" and "hemostasis" are not technically synonymous although they often get used as such.

Coagulation pathways

Traditionally, coagulation has been thought of as existing in two completely separate "arms" (the *intrinsic* and the *extrinsic* pathways) that converge into a single *common* pathway. The intrinsic system was so named because its activation occurred from within (or *intrinsic* to) the vascular system, usually by exposure to negatively charged surfaces such as collagen exposed by endothelial damage. The extrinsic system was so named because it was activated by the *tissue factor (Factor III)*, which comes from outside (or *extrinsic* to) the vasculature. Tissue factor is constitutively expressed by many extravascular cells that are exposed following vascular injury, such as smooth muscle cells and fibroblasts. It is not normally expressed by endothelial cells but potentially can be under pathologic conditions. Thus, this system is activated when there is damage to or inflammatory activation of a portion of the vasculature. This classic scheme is outlined in Figure 17.3.

Physiologic coagulation vs. coagulation testing

It is now known that activation of the extrinsic pathway is by far the most important physiologic initiator of hemostasis and the intrinsic pathway primarily acts as an amplification loop following the formation of small amounts of thrombin. There is a lot of cross-over between these two systems as well as many feedback loops, which amplify the process and help coagulation to occur quickly. In reality, this division into two systems is largely artificial and based on some *in vitro* coagulation tests. However, these tests are still commonly used to evaluate hemostasis and so the classic scheme is still a useful concept to memorize for interpreting these tests. Fibrinogen (Factor I), thrombin (Factor II), and tissue factor (Factor III) are often referred to by their common names, while the other factors are typically referred to only by their roman numeral designation.

Memorizing the coagulation pathways

It is helpful to memorize which factors are in the various pathways when interpreting the results of coagulation testing. The intrinsic system can be easily remembered as the "Walmart" cascade (thanks to Drs. Rick Cowell and Ron Tyler). To make an item sell better, rather than selling it for $12.00, it is put on "sale" for $11.98. *The intrinsic cascade comprises Factors 12, 11, 9, and 8, in that order*. The common pathway is where the two others meet, so it is the *crossroads* or *"X" roads*. They meet at Factor X. For the rest of the common pathway, simply cut the number in half each time, eliminating any fractions. *The common pathway comprises Factors 10, 5, 2, 1 in that order*. Factor 7 is all by itself in the extrinsic pathway.

Production and function of the coagulation factors

With the exception of Factor III (tissue factor) and Factor IV (calcium), coagulation factors are predominantly synthesized by the liver and circulate in the blood as inactive precursors. Most of these factors are enzymes, which act to cleave the next factor in the system, activating it. Some factors are not proteases. Tissue factor (Factor III) is a membrane receptor expressed on several cell types. It functions as a cofactor for Factor VII, resulting in initiation of the extrinsic pathway following vascular injury. Factors V and VIII are cofactors that act to increase the activity of some of the enzymatic factors (X and IX, respectively). Finally, fibrinogen, after conversion to fibrin, is an adhesive protein that stabilizes the clot and is the ultimate result of the cascade.

Factors II, VII, IX, and X are vitamin K–dependent factors, which is of tremendous clinical importance. When first produced by the liver, they are in an inactive form. They require the activity of vitamin K, which adds carboxyl groups to their glutamic acid residues (*"gamma carboxylation"*). This makes them fully functional by allowing them to interact with calcium and thus localize to phospholipid surfaces, typically the membranes of platelets and red cells incorporated into the platelet plug. Localizing the coagulation factors to phospholipid surfaces brings them into proximity, and thus the reactions occur far faster than if the factors were in solution.

Vitamin K antagonists, including some rat poisons, are a common cause of coagulopathy in veterinary medicine and one of the few easily treatable disorders of coagulation. Factor VII, one of the vitamin K–dependent factors, has a much shorter half-life than the other factors. In vitamin K antagonism, Factor VII becomes depleted first. This is important in interpreting the results of coagulation testing in cases of vitamin K antagonism.

Inhibitors of coagulation factors

There are naturally occurring inhibitors of the coagulation factors that serve to limit the action of these proteins to the site of vascular injury and prevent widespread activation of coagulation, which would lead to thrombotic disease.

Antithrombin

Antithrombin (previously referred to as Antithrombin III) is a protein that binds to and inactivates thrombin and also most of the other serine protease factors. The activity of antithrombin is enhanced by binding to heparin or heparan sulfates that are present on endothelial cells. This mechanism is the basis for use of heparin as an anitcoagulant, both therapeutically as well as in blood collection tubes.

Protein C

Protein C is a protease that cleaves and thus inactivates the coagulation factors that function as cofactors, Factor V and Factor VIII. Protein C is produced by the liver in an inactive form. Protein C is activated by thrombin but only when thrombin is bound to the protein *thrombomudulin*, which is expressed on endothelial cells. Thus, thrombin is a potent promoter of the coagulation cascade but can be switched to have an anticoagulant activity when bound to thrombomulin. Inherited Protein C deficiencies in humans result in thrombotic tendencies.

Tissue factor pathway inhibitor (TFPI)

The tissue factor pathway is the primary physiologic initiator of hemostasis, and TFPI is the primary regulator of this pathway. TFPI is a protein produced by endothelial cells but also many other cell types [2]. TFPI has separate binding sites for Factor Xa as well as Factor VIIa/tissue factor complex, thus inhibiting both the enzyme of the TF pathway as well as its substrate.

Details about fibrinolysis (fibrin clot breakdown)

Breakdown of the formed clot occurs concurrently with repair of the underlying defect in the vascular system. When this occurs completely, patency of the vessel and normal blood flow is restored. Similar to coagulation, this is a highly regulated process and one that should be limited to the site of clot formation and not occur systemically. Plasmin is formed as an inactive precursor called *plasminogen* by the liver. This precursor has affinity for fibrin and is incorporated into the clot as it forms. Plasminogen is converted to active plasmin by the enzyme *tissue plasminogen activator (TPA)*. TPA is produced by endothelial cells, but only when there are appropriate stimuli. So, TPA production is stimulated in close proximity to the clot. Furthermore, TPA only interacts with plasminogen that is bound to the fibrin clot, not free in plasma, so production of active enzyme is limited to its site of action rather than occurring systemically. As an added protection against systemic spread of fibrinolysis, there are circulating proteins (e.g., alpha-2-antiplasmin) that inhibit any active plasmin that escapes the fibrin clot. These circulating inhibitors cannot inactivate plasmin bound to fibrin, thus plasmin can perform its function at the appropriate site but is quickly inactivated should it break free from the clot.

"Orchestration" of hemostasis: role of endothelium

Much of the complexity of hemostasis and difficulty in understanding its processes are due to fact that each component has both activators and inhibitors, which often seem to be produced by the same cells, mainly endothelial cells. However, these seemingly contradictory responses actually make sense when you consider that they are occurring in cells in slightly different *locations* and they act in concert to simultaneously *promote rapid hemostasis* in the microenvironment where it is needed and also *prevent it from spreading* where it is not.

Under normal circumstances, endothelial cells actively produce many products that inhibit both primary and secondary hemostasis, which maintains blood in its normal fluid state (Table 17.3). When there is vascular damage, several things occur simultaneously: (i) anticoagulant functions are lost with removal of the endothelial cells, (ii) the strongly procoagulant subendothelial collagen is exposed, and (iii) the endothelial cells in the immediate site of the developing clot are stimulated to shift from having anticoagulant to procoagulant properties (Table 17.4). Endothelial cells farther away from the damage are not exposed to the associated stimuli and retain their anticoagulant nature, thus limiting the developing clots to the immediate site.

Table 17.3 Anticoagulant functions of resting endothelial cells.

Product	Function
Prostacyclin	Platelet inhibitor
Nitric oxide	Platelet inhibitor
ADPase	Degrades ADP, a platelet agonist
Heparan sulfate	Expressed on EC surface Activates antithrombin, an inhibitor of enzymatic coagulation factors
Thrombomodulin	Activates Protein C (via thrombin). Protein C inactivates Factors V, VIII
Protein S	Cofactor for Protein C
TPA	Activates fibrinolysis (plasminogen) breaking down any clot formed

Table 17.4 Procoagulant functions of activated endothelial cells.

Product	Function
vWf	Promotes platelet adhesion
Platelet activating factor	Platelet agonist
Thromboxane	Platelet agonist
Tissue factor	Stimulates extrinsic coagulation cascade
Plasminogen activator inhibitor	Inhibits TPA, inhibiting fibrinolysis
Reduced expression of heparin sulfate	Loss of anticoagulant activity
Reduced expression of thrombomodulin	Loss of anticoagulant activity

Clinical approach to the bleeding patient

Interpretation of laboratory test results always needs to be considered in terms of the clinical presentation of the patient and considering a differential diagnosis list of common potential underlying diseases. It is generally most productive if testing is done to answer a specific clinical question. Before discussing coagulation tests themselves, it is helpful to consider some of the clinical context.

Hemostatic defect vs. trauma-/disease-induced hemorrhage?

The first question when faced with a bleeding animal is whether the bleeding is due to (i) a generalized defect in hemostasis (these can be either congenital or acquired) or (ii) local tissue trauma/disease resulting in hemorrhage despite normal hemostatic function. For example, a dog with severe epistaxis may have a hemostatic defect such as thrombocytopenia or may have local nasal disease such as a nasal tumor, foreign body, trauma, or severe inflammatory disease. Physical exam findings, hemostasis testing and other tests such as imaging may help answer this question. However, some historical things and physical exam findings that should first be considered include

Has the animal had previous bleeding episodes? Numerous prior episodes of abnormal bleeding would make you consider a hemostatic defect, potentially congenital.

Has the animal had previous challenges, such as surgery, when it has not bled? This might make congenital defects less likely, although recently acquired hemostatic problems could not be ruled out.

Is the bleeding spontaneous or trauma induced? Spontaneous bleeding is more likely to be the result of a hemostatic defect than is bleeding induced by trauma. If the bleeding is trauma induced, consider if the severity/duration of bleeding is expected for the degree of trauma or if it seems exaggerated. Prolonged or more severe bleeding than expected following a minor insult would suggest a hemostatic defect.

Is the animal bleeding from multiple sites? This would also suggest the presence of a hemostatic defect, but it could possibly result from multifocal tissue damage, such as systemic vasculitis secondary to an infectious disease.

What is the color of the urine, feces? Bleeding can sometimes be occult. Bleeding into the gastrointestinal tract or urinary tract may not be easily recognized. Also, bleeding into body cavities can be occult and should be considered if there is evidence of pleural or peritoneal effusion.

Has the animal been exposed to drugs/diseases that affect hemostasis? For this, it is important to know the common causes of bleeding disorders. Certain drugs such as aspirin or NSAIDs may interfere with platelet function. Potential exposure to anticoagulant rodenticides is important to determine, especially in an animal housed outdoors or allowed to roam.

What species/breed is the patient? Certain breeds are predisposed to inherited hemostatic defects for which they are routinely screened, sometimes even if they are asymptomatic.

Primary vs. secondary hemostatic defects?

The clinical nature of bleeding is often different when there is a defect in primary hemostasis versus one of secondary hemostasis. Lab testing will help to confirm which portion of the hemostatic mechanisms are affected, but clinical findings are often highly suggestive.

Signs associated with defects in primary hemostasis

Petechiae are small, pinpoint hemorrhages in the skin or mucous membranes. Petechiae are strongly suggestive of a primary hemostatic defect; they do not generally occur in secondary defects. More specifically, they are more commonly associated with *thrombocytopenia* rather than other primary defects such as platelet function defects or vWd. Petechiae may also occur with any disease that causes vasculitis, such as certain infectious diseases and immune-mediated vasculitis. *Ecchymoses* are larger cutaneous hemorrhages that may occur in either primary or secondary defects.

Bleeding due to primary hemostatic defects is usually from mucosal surfaces. Common sites include bleeding from the nose (epistaxis), gums, genitourinary tract (e.g., hematuria, vaginal bleeding), or gastrointestinal tract (evidenced as either "melena" or "hematochezia"). Slow, prolonged oozing of blood spontaneously or from small, minor wounds is common. These are often "nuisance" bleeds. The most clinically concerning bleed would be cerebral hemorrhage, a site where even a relatively minor bleed could have significant clinical consequences.

Signs associated with defects of secondary hemostasis

Bleeding from secondary defects is often overt hemorrhage from a single site. Large hematoma formation is classic. Ecchymoses and hematomas may arise from minor insults. While hematoma formation is common with defects of secondary hemostasis, hematomas are not specific. They may also occur with tissue trauma in animals with primary hemostatic defects. For example, a hematoma may form at the site of blood collection in a thrombocytopenic animal.

Bleeding into body cavities is another classic finding with secondary hemostatic defects. This may manifest as bleeding into the abdominal cavity (*hemoabdomen*), thoracic cavity (*hemothorax*), or synovial spaces (*hemarthrosis*). Body cavity bleeds are the most common presenting signs of animals with vitamin K antagonism. Animals may present with dyspnea if there is a hemothorax.

Tests used to evaluate hemostasis

Tests of primary hemostasis

Buccal mucosal bleeding time (BMBT)

This test is often referred to as simply the "bleeding time" [8]. The bleeding time is an in-clinic screening test that evaluates all of the primary hemostatic system. The bleeding time measures the amount of time it takes for bleeding to stop from a small standardized stab incision. Following the creation of the incision, the blood is wicked away with absorbent paper without disturbing the wound until bleeding ceases. The normal bleeding time for dogs is less than ~3.5 minutes. This test is not commonly performed on dogs and is rarely done in any other species [9].

Abnormal bleeding times result from any problem in primary hemostasis: thrombocytopenia, platelet function defects, or von Willebrand factor deficiency (von Willebrand disease). Some important considerations are listed below.

Reliability: Results are very operator dependent, so published reference intervals are only a general estimate. The more experience a person has with performing the test, the more consistent the results will be. Even with a trained person running the test, it is *not very sensitive,* and some animals with primary hemostatic defects will have a normal BMBT [10].

Equipment: To be accurate, the incision must be small and have a standardized length and depth. The incision must be small enough that the bleeding can be stopped with only the formation of a platelet plug (i.e., secondary hemostasis is not involved). Template bleeding time devices (Simplate® or Surgicutt®) must be used, and there are differences in results depending on the device used [11]. It is not acceptable to just use a scalpel blade and make a small cut since it is not possible to standardize the length and depth of incision in this manner. Also, many people try to measure the duration of bleeding after clipping a toenail. While some authors recommend this, the length of bleeding in this case is going to vary according to the depth of the cut.

Location: In people, the bleeding time is done on the skin of the forearm. In dogs, the skin is too thick and variable in thickness for this to work. The test must be done on the inner surface of the lip. The patient must be cooperative for this to be done without sedation.

Indications: This test is NOT run very often in clinics because most veterinarians are not trained on it, it is not very sensitive, and alternative testing exists for most diseases. The causes of primary hemostatic disorders are thrombocytopenia, vWd, and platelet function defects. Of these, thrombocytopenia is most common, and a complete blood count (CBC) is used to assess platelet numbers. If an animal is suspected of having vWd, a vWf assay can be run and will be more precise than a bleeding time. However, it is very difficult to test for platelet function problems. Most labs do not offer this testing, and the testing must be performed within a few hours of sample collection, so mailing the sample to a specialized lab is not an option. *Thus, BMBT may be run in patients who have signs of primary hemostasis but have a normal platelet count and vWf concentration, to indirectly document a platelet function disorder.*

It can be used as a presurgical screen if there is clinical concern for a primary hemostatic defect. It is also performed in emergency clinics or referral practices in animals with nonspecific bleeding signs to quickly assess if there is a hemostatic defect vs. bleeding from tissue trauma of some kind while awaiting the results of other tests. If an animal is markedly thrombocytopenic (<20,000/μL), then there is also no point in running the test since a low platelet count by itself can prolong the BMBT.

Platelet concentration (platelet "count")

A platelet count can be done using an automated hematology analyzer or can be estimated from a blood film (or BOTH!). *Thrombocytopenia is probably the most common cause of abnormal bleeding of any kind in veterinary medicine, particularly in dogs*. Therefore, a platelet count should be obtained in any bleeding animal. Platelet counts are typically run from blood submitted in ethylenediaminetetraacetic acid (EDTA) tubes for a CBC.

Platelet numbers must be extremely low for animals to show spontaneous hemorrhage. Normal platelet counts for most domestic species range from ~200,000–500,000/μL (horses typically have fewer with the lower end of reference interval being about 100,000/μL). In general, platelet concentration must drop to *below* 20,000/μL to induce spontaneous bleeding. Platelet counts *below* 50,000/μL can result in hemorrhage secondary to trauma.

Platelets easily clump in the tube. This is especially a problem in cats and in any species when there is difficulty with blood collection. *However, clumping can happen in any sample and should always be considered*. Furthermore, clumping can occur if the blood sample sits for hours before running the test. It is best if the platelet count is run within ~5 hours of blood collection. When platelets clump, the platelet count will be artificially low because the clumped platelets are not counted by the analyzer. Platelet clumps can be seen on the feathered edge of a blood film and should be noted in the comments section of a CBC if the sample is sent to a commercial lab. If significant platelet clumping is present, a new sample is needed to get an accurate platelet count. The count from the clumped sample can be considered a minimum number of platelets. If a CBC is performed and a blood film is not examined for clumping, any low platelet count is suspect.

Artifact due to platelet clumping is the most common cause of a low platelet count in cats and is common in all others species as well. More than half of all feline blood samples submitted for CBC can have low platelet counts due to clumping [12].

Automated platelet counts can also be inaccurate (depending on the specific analyzer methodology) when a high percentage of large platelets are present. This occurs when the analyzer cannot distinguish large platelets from erythrocytes. This is also common in cats, whose platelets tend to be large and whose red cells tend to be small. It also occurs in goats, which have very small red cells. Cavalier King Charles spaniels may have an inherited abnormality called *macrothrombocytopenia* in which many of their platelets are abnormally large [13–15]. The reported platelet counts in this breed are often artifactually very low. The true platelet count can be normal or may be low, but the total platelet mass (*"platelet-crit,"* measured by some automated analyzers) is usually normal because the platelets present are larger than normal [16]. The condition is asymptomatic and animals do not have clinical bleeding episodes even if their true platelet count is somewhat decreased.

For the purpose of ruling out thrombocytopenia as a potential cause of bleeding in a patient when a platelet count is not available or when a low platelet count may be an artifact, platelet numbers can be estimated from a blood film. When viewing a slide using the 100×, oil immersion lens in the monolayer of a film, normal animals should have at least seven platelets per field on average. As an estimate, every platelet seen in a 100× field represents about 15,000/μL [17]. So, if an animal has an average of four platelets/hpf, its platelet count is probably ~60,000/μL. Since spontaneous hemorrhage does not occur until platelets decrease to <20,000/μL, an animal bleeding as the result of a thrombocytopenia will typically consistently have only ~0–2 platelets/hpf.

> ***Major concept:*** Automated platelet counts are the most commonly inaccurate result from a CBC. *Every* low platelet count should be confirmed by a review of a blood film – both looking at the feathered edge for clumps and looking at the number of platelets in the body of the film. *It is not acceptable to simply run the sample through an in-house hematology analyzer and trust that value.*

vWf assays

Assays for vWf concentration are performed in a few specialized labs. Most large diagnostic labs will either run it or relay it to the appropriate lab, but results often take a couple of days. Samples for vWf assay are typically submitted in citrate tubes (blue top) but may also be run from EDTA plasma. Ideally, samples should be centrifuged and the plasma removed and frozen until shipped, then shipped overnight with cold packs. vWf concentration has been shown to be stable through repeated freeze/thaw cycles and stable for at least 8 hours at room temperature when stored either as citrated plasma before freezing or whole blood before centrifugation [18–20].

Values are reported as "%," which refers to percent of "normal," rather than getting a specific quantity such as mg/dL. Labs running the assay collect plasma from a group of dogs and combine it into a *plasma pool*, which is arbitrarily designated as 100%. Because of this, results from a patient may be >100%. Reference intervals for vWf will vary from lab to lab, but typically >70% is normal. Most animals bleeding from vWd have values less than 30% [21].

Since vWd is an inherited condition, detecting carriers is often a concern of breeders. Asymptomatic carriers cannot be accurately identified by vWf concentration in the blood [22]. DNA tests are now available for many breeds of dogs (www.vetgen.com). DNA tests can determine if the animal is carrying one or two genes for the vWd defect. DNA testing generally evaluates for a single specific mutation. There are literally hundreds of different mutations identified in humans, and many exist in animals. Fortunately, a single mutation accounts for most cases in any given breed. So, the DNA testing must be specific for the breed of patient.

Platelet function testing

Various tests of platelet function are run in certain specialized hemostasis labs. The standard test is called *aggregometry*, which tests the ability of the platelets to aggregate in response to the addition of various agonists known to activate platelets. Unfortunately, aggregometry is only run in a few research labs. Also, it is generally recommended that samples are run within 4 hours of collection, thus mailing samples, even by overnight courier, is not suitable [23]. Because of this, platelet function testing is difficult in the vast majority of practices. Platelet function defects often are presumed based on a diagnosis of exclusion. An animal that has an abnormal BMBT but normal platelet count and normal vWf levels probably has a platelet function defect.

There are newer automated analyzers available that test either (i) all of primary hemostasis similar to BMBT (e.g., PFA-100®),or (ii) all aspects of both primary and secondary hemostasis in whole blood (e.g. Sonoclot®) [24, 25]. These could be used in place of BMBT to test for platelet function defects, again by exclusion after combining results with a normal platelet count and BMBT. These are not yet widely available but are being used in some specialty practices. Over time, it is likely that more analyzers that screen for all aspects of hemostasis will become more common.

Tests of secondary hemostasis

Activated clotting time (ACT)

Performing the test

The ACT is an in-clinic test used as a screening test of secondary hemostasis. It is usually followed by definitive coagulation testing if a coagulopathy is indicated. The original ACT tubes made by Becton Dickinson (BD, Franklin Lakes, NJ) contained diatomaceous earth, but production of these tubes has been discontinued [26]. Currently available tubes may alternatively contain kaolin, glass beads, or multiple activators [26]. The premise is to activate Factor XII and initiate the intrinsic coagulation pathways. Performing the test is relatively simple. A sample of whole blood is collected into the ACT tube, which is kept at 37 °C. Ideally, this is done in a heat block but can be done by holding the tube in the operator's axilla [27]. The tube is checked every 10 seconds for evidence of clot formation. At the first sign of clot formation, the test is ended and the time recorded.

ACT tube manufacturers typically recommend a two-tube method using a Vacutainer needle. The first 2 mL of blood is collected in one tube that is discarded to remove blood potentially contaminated with tissue factor during venipuncture. A second tube is then filled from the Vacutainer needle and used for the test. However, studies to date have not shown a difference in results whether or not the initial blood is discarded, at least in healthy animals [26, 28]. It makes sense that the sample should be collected with minimal time and trauma.

Interpretation

Published studies using the original Becton Dickinson ACT tubes suggested times of <95–125 seconds for healthy dogs and <165 seconds for healthy cats [28–30]. A more recent study using currently available tubes suggested a reference interval of <80 seconds for dogs and less than <85 seconds for cats [26]. However, this is an operator-dependent test and depends not only on the brand of tube used but also on the ability of the operator to detect the first signs of a clot. Therefore, it is essential for reference intervals to be determined by each operator by performing the test on clinically healthy patients in their particular setting [29].

Because the ACT tube activates the intrinsic system, any deficiency of a coagulation factor in either the intrinsic or common pathways will prolong the ACT. Essentially the only factor that does not affect the ACT is Factor VII. This makes the ACT a good general screening test of secondary hemostasis.

The test is fairly insensitive, so any given coagulation factor must be reduced to less than ~5% of normal to prolong results. With vitamin K antagonism, one of the more common conditions for which the ACT test is used, the factor activities are dramatically inhibited, and ACT results are usually prolonged despite this insensitivity. In the ACT test, the phospholipid surface needed for the coagulation factor reactions to occur is provided by platelets. So, even though the test is not designed to evaluate platelet numbers, a severe thrombocytopenia (<10,000/μL) may potentially cause a mild prolongation of the ACT, although this is not well documented, and any effect is likely minor.

Activated partial thromboplastin time ("APTT" or commonly just "PTT")

This test evaluates the intrinsic and common pathways of coagulation. It tests the same pathways as the ACT but is a more precise and sensitive test. It is typically run along with a PT, which is discussed next.

Blood is collected in a citrate tube (blue top), spun down, and the plasma is used for testing. In this test and the PT, a reagent is added to provide a phospholipid surface, which eliminates the need for platelets. So, these tests will not be affected at all by a low platelet count.

For the partial thromboplastin time (PTT), a reagent is added to initiate the intrinsic coagulation cascade. Because the blood is collected in citrate, which is a calcium chelator, the reaction does not proceed since most of the enzymatic coagulation factors are calcium dependent. After the reagent has been added to the plasma sample and allowed to incubate, sufficient calcium is added to overcome the action of the citrate, and the number of seconds that it takes for a clot to form is recorded. Because this test initiates the intrinsic coagulation cascade at Factor XII and ends with the formation of a fibrin clot (Factor I), the PTT will be prolonged with a deficiency of any one or more factors in either the intrinsic or the common coagulation pathway. Interpretation of both the PT and PTT is further discussed in the next sections.

One-stage prothrombin time ("OSPT" or commonly just "PT")

This concept of this test is similar to the PTT; however, the reagents activate the extrinsic system rather than the intrinsic system. So, this test evaluates the extrinsic and common pathways. Typically, the PT and PTT are both run on the same sample.

Some specific points about interpreting both the PT and PTT

Units reported

Both tests are reported in seconds. This is the number of seconds that it takes for a clot to form following addition of the final reagent, calcium. Increased values indicate that it took longer for a clot to form and suggest reduced concentrations of one or more factors in the affected pathway.

Relative sensitivity

For either the PT or PTT to be prolonged, the concentration of one or more of the coagulation factors tested must be below about 30% of normal. While this may seem to lack sensitivity, animals generally do not show evidence of bleeding unless coagulation factors are reduced to these same levels. Individual assays offered by various labs may vary in the methodology, reagents, and protocols used. Therefore, reference intervals from the individual labs may vary significantly and cannot be generalized.

Artifacts related to sample handling

Citrate tubes come in 3.2% and 3.8% concentrations. Historically, 3.8% was used in the United States, while 3.2% was standard in Europe, but now both tubes are commonly available in the United States. Studies in a limited number of dogs, both clinically healthy ones and those with hemostatic disorders, have not shown significant differences in results of PT or PTT tests between samples collected in 3.2 vs 3.8% citrate and run on various instruments [31, 32].

Underfilling the citrate tube with blood will result in a *relative excess* of anticoagulant (i.e., the same amount of citrate is in the tube but it is being diluted in less blood, so the concentration is higher). This can result in artificial prolongation of the PT/PTT. It is important to fill tubes to their intended volume. This effect may be more pronounced if using 3.8% citrate tubes [33].

A similar phenomenon occurs in animals with polycythemia. If a patient has a markedly increased hematocrit, there is less plasma for a given volume of whole blood. Less plasma volume again results in a relative excess of anticoagulant. Mild prolongations in PT and PTT are observed in animals with an increased hematocrit. Typically, however, coagulation testing is not being run on polycythemic patients.

Coagulation factors are labile. Ideally, the blood should be separated and plasma removed within 1 hour and the sample run within 4 hours. If the sample is to be mailed to an outside lab, the citrated plasma can be removed from the red cells and frozen. Although these recommendations make intuitive sense and are probably safest to ensure sample quality of all specimens, several studies of human samples suggest that most samples for PT and PTT may be stable for much longer periods, and plasma may be separated from the cells at 8–24 hours after collection with no clinically significant effect [34, 35]. Studies on canine samples suggest that valid PT and PTT results can be obtained from citrated plasma removed from red blood cells and stored for up to 48 hours when refrigerated or even at room temperature, at least in healthy animals [36].

Localizing a defect

By comparing the results of the PT and PTT, it is sometimes possible to localize which factors might be deficient. With a prolonged PTT (which tests intrinsic and common pathways) but a normal PT (which tests extrinsic and common), then one of the factors in the intrinsic pathway is deficient. The normal PT indicates that the common pathway is functioning normally. Conversely, if you have a prolonged PT but normal PTT, the problem is in the extrinsic pathway (Factor VII). If both are prolonged (which is the typical case), then the results do not localize the problem to a specific arm of the coagulation cascade, but the presence of a coagulopathy is confirmed. Either there is a deficiency in the common pathway or there are multiple factors being affected that involve both the intrinsic and extrinsic systems.

Specific factor analysis

If the results of the PT and/or PTT are abnormal, it is sometimes helpful to know the concentration of a specific coagulation factor. Some of the larger hemostasis labs offer these assays. Quantitative fibrinogen concentration (Factor I) is often included in a basic coagulation profile to test for reduced concentrations of fibrinogen resulting from increased consumption in disseminated intravascular coagulation. Specific factor analysis is also run on citrated plasma, so the same sample used to test PT/PTT can be used, if needed. Results for most factors are reported as % of a pool of plasma from normal animals, similar to vWf.

Tests of fibrinolysis (fibrin clot breakdown)

Fibrin(ogen) degradation products (FDPs) and D-dimers

Pathophysiology of D-dimer formation

FDPs refer to any of the various protein fragments produced when fibrin is cleaved by plasmin in the process of fibrinolysis. They can also be formed when fibrinogen (i.e., that which has not yet converted into fibrin and incorporated into a clot) is cleaved by plasmin.

D-dimers are a specific subset of FDPs. The fibrinogen molecule has three protein domains. There are two identical "D" domains on either end and an "E" domain in the middle. D-dimers are fragments that contain two "D" domains that have been cross-linked together. These can be formed only by the breakdown of cross-linked fibrin and not fibrinogen itself. Thus D-dimers are more specific to breakdown of clots and suggest that there is increased activity of concurrent coagulation and fibrinolysis. The D-dimer assay has essentially replaced the FDP test in clinical diagnostics. Citrated plasma is used for the D-dimer assay as with most other tests of coagulation.

Interpretation

In the normal animal, low levels of FDPs are constantly generated due to low levels of coagulation and fibrinolysis that occur normally to maintain vascular integrity as endothelial cells die and are replaced. These FDPs are quickly removed by macrophages in the liver and spleen. Thus, they are generally present in the blood in concentrations below detectable limits in healthy animals.

Increased concentrations of D-dimers indicate that coagulation and fibrinolysis are occurring at an accelerated rate. This usually occurs following formation of a large thrombus or multiple thrombi, which are subsequently degraded. *Thus, increased concentrations of FDPs or D-dimers is a marker of thrombotic disease.*

In addition to thrombotic disease, mild increases in FDP concentrations may be seen in animals with significant hemorrhage into body cavities (e.g., hemoabdomen) or tissues (e.g., trauma, postsurgery), as these conditions will result in subsequent coagulation and lysis of the clots. Increases can also occur with widespread inflammatory diseases, such as sepsis, which can also activate the coagulation system with subsequent fibrinolysis. Finally, since FDPs are cleared by the liver, animals with reduced hepatic function may have increased FDP concentrations as a result of reduced clearance [37, 38]. Thus, increased concentrations are not specific for thrombotic disease [37, 39].

The higher the concentration of D-dimers, the greater the likelihood of thromboembolic disease. Results up to 500–1000 ng/mL are often seen with trauma, postsurgery, liver disease, etc. If other findings suggest thromboembolism, mild to moderate increases up to this concentration may still be significant. Concentrations of 1000–2000 ng/mL or >2000 ng/mL are more specific for thromboembolism because other conditions do not usually result in increases of this magnitude [37, 39].

Hemostasis profiles (or "coagulation profiles")

Clinics may run ACT tubes and potentially BMBT in-house as rapid screens to evaluate secondary and primary hemostasis, respectively. More comprehensive testing may be done through private laboratories or in-house analyzers. Laboratories will typically offer different coagulation profiles, with variable numbers of tests included, depending on the specific condition suspected. *A general screen might include a platelet count (as part of a CBC), PT, PTT, D-dimers, and quantitative fibrinogen.* This would provide a good general screen for the most common defects of primary hemostasis (i.e., thrombocytopenia), secondary hemostasis, and evidence of thrombotic disease including DIC. Specific tests such as vWf concentration are added based on clinical suspicion. A smaller profile including platelet count, PT, and PTT might be used as a presurgical screen in an apparently healthy patient.

Common hemostatic disease in veterinary medicine

Once hemostasis testing has (i) confirmed that a hemostatic defect is present and (ii) localized it to a condition affecting primary hemostasis, secondary hemostasis, or both, then the presenting findings of the patient can be compared with a differential list of common diseases to attempt a specific diagnosis. There are a few common conditions that will account for the majority of hemostatic defects seen in practice.

Diseases affecting primary hemostasis

Thrombocytopenia

Thrombocytopenia is a common cause of abnormal bleeding, particularly in dogs. Since it is easy to obtain a platelet count, this should always be part of the workup of a bleeding animal. There are many specific causes of thrombocytopenia, which results in a huge differential list for this specific finding. Mild to moderate thrombocytopenia (platelet counts not lower than 50,000/μL) can be seen with numerous bacterial and viral infections, neoplasia, following hemorrhage (where it results from both loss of platelets and also use of platelets in attempts to clot), secondary to vasculitis (where the platelets are used for repairing endothelium), following vaccination, and many other causes [40–44]. Often, the thrombocytopenia is not the major/only finding in a very ill animal with systemic disease. These conditions are generally recognized by their more prominent findings.

There are fewer conditions in which (i) the thrombocytopenia is severe enough to result in spontaneous bleeding (i.e., less than 20,000/μL) and (ii) the thrombocytopenia and associated bleeding manifestations are the main or only abnormal finding in the patient. The major conditions that should be considered in these cases are:

a. *Rickettsial disease:* Many species of *Ehrlichia (E. canis, E. ewingii)* and *Anaplasma (A. phagocytophilum, A. platys)* can infect dogs [45]. These are regionally common diseases. Infection with these organisms can result in a marked thrombocytopenia in the acute stages of infection. Animals may present with petechiae or mucosal bleeding such as epistaxis. Thrombocytopenia may be severe (<10,000/μL) in the acute stages of infection. In chronic *E. canis* infection, there is sometimes a generalized hypoplasia of the bone marrow, and a pancytopenia may result. Rocky Mountain spotted fever also causes a thrombocytopenia, but it is usually not as severe as that seen with ehrlichiosis, although the clinical disease may be quite severe [46].

   Ehrlichia canis organisms are not typically present in numbers great enough to identify in peripheral blood films, although they may rarely be seen. Organisms are present in relatively greater numbers in acute *E. ewingii* and *A. phagocytophilum* infections [47, 48]. In endemic areas, these conditions may be identified by finding morulae in neutrophils on a peripheral blood smear. Even in these diseases, however, the parasitemia is short lived.

   Diagnosis is typically confirmed by running in-clinic tests (i.e. SNAP tests), antibody titers, or polymerase chain reaction (PCR) for detecting the DNA of the organism. It is important to consider that a positive antibody test means past exposure but not necessarily active disease.

b. *Immune-mediated thrombocytopenia (ITP):* Similar to immune-mediated hemolytic anemia, antibodies may be directed against platelet antigens and result in their removal. This is common in dogs but much less common in other species [40, 42, 43]. Like hemolytic anemia, ITP can be primary, in which there is no underlying cause detectable, or it can be secondary to other conditions such as administration of drugs, infections, or as a paraneoplastic response.

   Affected animals often have no other signs of systemic illness and are apparently healthy other than having a markedly decreased platelet count. ITP is often a diagnosis made by excluding other causes and then supported by response to treatment. It is possible to test for platelet surface-associated immunoglobulin by flow cytometry [49–51]. In addition to confirming an immune mechanism as the cause of the thrombocytopenia, patients are usually screened for possible underlying infectious (serology, PCR) or neoplastic (diagnostic imaging) causes.

c. *DIC:* In DIC, there first is widespread, uncontrolled activation of the hemostatic system throughout the body [52]. This is in contrast to normal hemostasis, which is limited to a site of vascular injury. If severe enough and prolonged enough, this widespread hemostatic response ends up consuming both platelets and coagulation factors, resulting in thrombocytopenia and reduced concentration of coagulation factors. DIC is thus initially *hypercoagulable* with thrombosis occurring throughout the body, but eventually the animal becomes *hypocoagulable* and may show hemorrhagic tendencies because of the depletion of platelets and coagulation factors. Because of this, DIC is sometimes called a *consumptive coagulopathy*.

   DIC is not a specific disease but is a common result of a variety of underlying disorders that share common properties of either inducing vascular damage, exposing massive amounts of tissue factor, or directly activating the intrinsic coagulation cascade. Common triggers for DIC include sepsis, widespread tissue trauma, heatstroke, neoplasia, and severe systemic inflammatory diseases such as pancreatitis or peritonitis [52, 53]. These diseases can cause widespread activation of hemostasis and overwhelm the normal regulatory processes that limit it in health.

   Animals with DIC are usually overtly clinically ill from their underlying disease. Along with the thrombocytopenia, there can be prolongations in the coagulation tests (PT, PTT) and increased concentrations of D-dimers. Not all tests are abnormal simultaneously in every case of DIC. This makes laboratory confirmation of DIC subjective, and there is no accepted consensus regarding a laboratory diagnosis of DIC in veterinary medicine [52, 53].

   In dogs with DIC, thrombocytopenia is reported in a greater percentage of cases than prolongations in PT or PTT. Evidence of excessive fibrinolysis from increased D-dimers is usually present. Other tests that are sometimes run to evaluate suspect cases of DIC are quantitative fibrinogen and antithrombin concentrations, both of which may be decreased if consumption is great enough to exceed production. Schistocytes may be noted in the peripheral blood of animals in overt DIC. In two reviews of cats with DIC, prolongations in PT, PTT were more frequent than thrombocytopenia [54, 55]. PTT was prolonged in 100% of the cats in both studies, while thrombocytopenia was detected in 50% or less of the cases. It is important to realize that the percentage of abnormal tests in all studies may depend significantly on the criteria used to define DIC and include or exclude cases. Given the lack of a "gold standard" to diagnose DIC, and considering the fact that it is a complication of underlying disease processes rather than a distinct entity unto itself, it may be more practical to think of DIC as a spectrum of activation (or loss of control of the activation) of the hemostatic system rather than something that is a dichotomous entity that is either "present" or "absent" [55]. DIC may be present with subclinical (compensated) or overt manifestations.

d. *Bone marrow disease:* The diseases listed previously each result in thrombocytopenia primarily as a result of increased consumption or destruction of platelets. Thrombocytopenia may also occur from decreased bone marrow production of platelets.

One of the most common causes of this type of thrombocytopenia is hematopoietic neoplasia of the bone marrow. With infiltration of the bone marrow by either lymphoma or acute leukemia, neoplastic cells can crowd out the normal hematopoietic tissue. This crowding out of normal bone marrow tissue by an abnormal cell type is termed *myelophthisis* or *myelophthisic disease*. Another less common cause of myelophthisis is myelofibrosis, in which the marrow is replaced by fibrous connective tissue. This is usually the result of prior bone marrow injury that has resulted in repair by fibrosis.

Apart from myelophthisic disease, toxic injury to marrow stem cells can result in lack of production of hematopoietic precursors and result in marrow hypoplasia or aplasia. A variety of drugs, including estrogen and chemotherapeutic agents, and even certain infectious diseases can be injurious to marrow stem cells. Depending on the specific drug or infectious agent, there may be a selective decrease of any one of the hematopoietic cell line (erythrocytes, leukocytes, or platelets), or there may be a reduction in multiple cell lines.

Because bone marrow disease often affects multiple cells lines, the index of suspicion for it should be increased in thrombocytopenic animals who also have a severe, nonregenerative anemia, neutropenia, or both. However, sometimes animals that appear to have widespread myelophthisic disease have only a single peripheral cytopenia. A bone marrow aspirate +/− core biopsy can allow evaluation of the number of megakaryocytes present and their maturation and help differentiate lack of production from either increased consumption or destruction of platelets as a cause of thrombocytopenia.

von Willebrand disease

vWd is predominantly an inherited deficiency of vWf [56]. Acquired deficiencies of vWf have been reported but are not common [56]. vWd is the most common of the *inherited* bleeding disorders in both humans and in dogs, having a far higher incidence than the more widely known hemophilia [56]. It has been reported in numerous breeds of dogs and is extremely common in certain breeds. At one point in time, it was estimated that up to 70% of Doberman pinschers had low vWf concentrations [57]. Other commonly affected breeds include Shetland sheepdogs, German shorthaired pointers, German wirehaired pointers, and Scottish terriers [58–61]. There are three forms of vWd (type I, type II, type III) described depending on whether there is strictly a quantitative decrease (type I), also a qualitative defect of the multimeric structure (type II), or complete absence (type III) of vWF [56, 57]. In dogs, the type of vWd present often depends on the breed affected, and the bleeding manifestations observed with type II and type III may be more severe.

Patients with vWd may present with mild to severe bleeding that is typical of primary hemostatic defect bleeds. Some patients will not show any bleeding tendencies unless stressed in some way, such as a surgical challenge or trauma. Diagnosis usually starts with an index of suspicion because of the breed or because the patient presents with mucosal-type hemorrhages and has a normal platelet count. The diagnosis is confirmed by assaying levels of vWf in plasma. Animals with vWd generally bleed only if the vWf concentration is below ~30% of normal [21]. Platelet counts will be normal unless the animal has lost significant amounts of blood, and even then, they will only be mildly decreased at most. The bleeding manifestations can be mild. Thus, despite being an inherited condition, many patients are not diagnosed until middle age or older. In people, diagnosis often is not made until the third or fourth decade of life.

Platelet function defects

Platelet function defects are termed either *thrombopathia* or *thrombopathy*. They are less common that thrombocytopenia. Platelet function defects can be acquired or inherited.

Inherited platelet function defects have been reported in several breeds of dogs (basset hound, otterhound, cocker spaniel, spitz, Great Pyrenees), cats (Persian), horses, and in Simmental cattle [62]. The defect in otterhounds, Great Pyrenees, and horses are all related to a lack of GPIIb/IIIa, the fibrinogen receptor. The defect in basset hounds, spitz dogs, and Simmental cattle results from an intracellular signaling defect that prevents normal platelet activation. Genetic testing is available for some of the breed-specific disorders.

Acquired platelet function defects can be seen with administration of certain drugs and with several disease states. Aspirin and other NSAIDs inhibit cyclooxygenase (COX), the enzyme involved in production of thromboxane, which is a platelet agonist. Most NSAIDs only reversibly inhibit COX. Thus, once the drug is cleared, platelet function returns to normal. Aspirin irreversibly inhibits COX, and since platelets are anucleate and cannot synthesize new enzyme, aspirin's effect on platelets is irreversible for the lifespan of the platelet. Common disease states in which there are acquired defects of platelet function include uremia, hepatic failure, and marked hyperproteinemia.

Animals with platelet function defects have normal platelet counts and normal vWf levels but may have a prolonged BMBT. As stated before, it is difficult to definitively diagnose because there are very few labs that do platelet function testing. Diagnosis is usually made by excluding other primary hemostatic defects in a bleeding animal and identifying an underlying disease known to affect platelet function.

Diseases affecting secondary hemostasis

Vitamin K antagonism

Pathogenesis

Vitamin K antagonism is a common problem in veterinary medicine and is probably the most commonly encountered disease affecting the coagulation proteins [63–66]. Factors II, VII, IX, and X are *vitamin K–dependent* coagulation factors. When these factors are first produced by the liver, they are inactive and need enzymatic action (carboxylation of glutamic acid residues) by vitamin K to become functional [67]. When vitamin K activates a single coagulation factor molecule, the vitamin K molecule itself becomes oxidized, and it is no longer functional. This oxidized vitamin K must be reduced back to its active form by an enzyme called *vitamin K epoxide reductase* to act on additional coagulation factor molecules (see Figure 17.5) [67]. Normally, one molecule of vitamin K is recycled many times by this enzyme and activates numerous coagulation factor molecules. Therefore, the body needs fewer molecules of vitamin K than if it was just used once. Vitamin K antagonists *do not inhibit the action of reduced vitamin K directly; instead, they inactivate the vitamin K epoxide reductase enzyme,* which regenerates the active form of vitamin K. Thus, when a molecule of vitamin K activates a single coagulation factor molecule, it becomes oxidized (nonfunctional) and is not reactivated. In this situation, all vitamin K molecules are quickly converted to their oxidized form, and no further activation of the vitamin K–dependent factors can occur.

An animal ingesting vitamin K antagonists initially has normal concentrations of fully activated factors, but no *new* factors can be activated. The concentration of active factors then starts to decline at a rate depending on their individual half-life, and bleeding manifestations begin once concentrations of any one or more factors drop below critical levels. Intoxication with vitamin K antagonists thus results in deficiencies of the active forms of Factors II, VII, IX, and X. However, the inactive forms continue to be produced and build up in the blood. These inactive coagulation factors are referred to as "PIVKAs" [proteins induced by vitamin k antagonism (absence)].

Diagnostic findings

Since the vitamin K–dependent factors are in the intrinsic, extrinsic, and common pathways, both PT and PTT are classically prolonged [63]. Because multiple factors in all pathways are affected, and because the concentration of active factors is markedly reduced, the prolongations in the tests are often dramatic. In many cases, an end point (clot) is not reached, and results are simply reported out as "greater than 100 seconds" or however long the lab establishes before stopping the test. Since Factor VII has the shortest half-life, it decreases most quickly. Therefore, testing very early after ingestion (within the first 24–48 hours) may show a prolongation of the PT before the PTT. Both tests will typically be markedly prolonged by the time clinical signs have developed. Platelet counts may be normal or may be mildly reduced if there is significant hemorrhage [63].

Other than signs related to their coagulopathy, these patients are not systemically ill. Animals typically present with body cavity hemorrhages. Dyspnea due to hemothorax is a common presenting finding [63, 64]. Hematoma formation may be noted at sites of venipuncture.

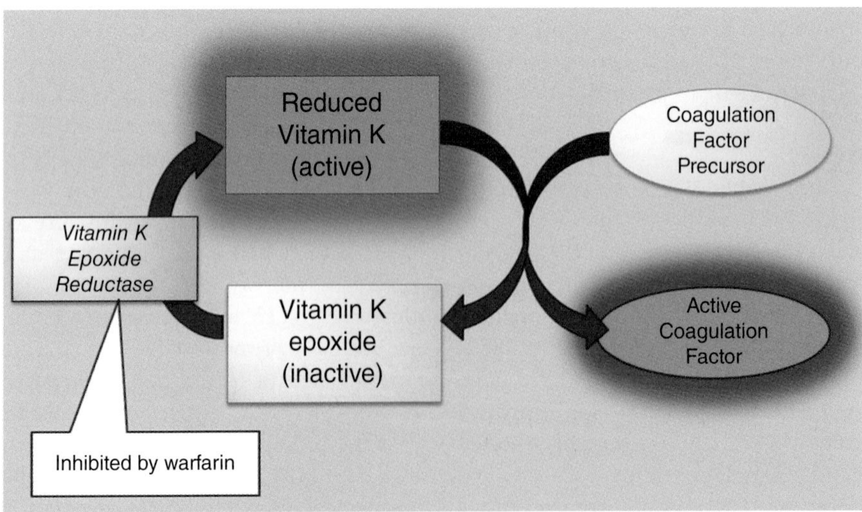

Figure 17.5 The vitamin K cycle. Vitamin K is needed for activation of precursors of Factors II, VII, IX, and X. When vitamin K activates a coagulation factor precursor, it becomes oxidized itself and is no longer functional until it is reduced back to its active form by the enzyme *vitamin K epoxide reductase*. Warfarin and warfarin-like molecules (including rodenticides) inhibit vitamin K epoxide reductase, resulting in reduced concentrations of the vitamin K–dependent factors.

Causes

Dietary deficiency of vitamin K is not generally a problem. Anticoagulant rodenticides are the most common source of vitamin K antagonism. These products are usually warfarin-like molecules, although some rodenticides have a completely different mechanism of action that does not affect hemostasis. The newer-generation anticoagulant rodenticides have a very long half-life that necessitates prolonged treatment with vitamin K. Ingestion of moldy sweet clover also causes a vitamin K antagonism in cattle. Since vitamin K is a fat-soluble vitamin and requires bile acids for absorption from the gut, vitamin K deficiency due to poor intestinal absorption can be seen in animals with severe cholestatic liver disease [66]. Sulfaquinoxaline, a coccidiostat, also has inhibitory effects on vitamin K.

Treatment

Since the inhibition is not direct, affected animals can be treated by administering active vitamin K. Response to administration of vitamin K is very rapid, usually within 24 hours [63, 65]. This rapid response occurs because the inactive PIVKAs are already produced and in circulation, simply requiring enzymatic activation. If faster response is needed in an acutely ill animal with life-threatening bleeding, administration of fresh or fresh-frozen plasma can provide active coagulation factors until the body has time to respond to vitamin K administration. Because even the newly administered vitamin K cannot be recycled as long as the antagonist is present, the animal must be treated for an extended time until the toxin is cleared from the body. The newer rodenticides have very long half-lives. Once treatment is discontinued, it is wise to screen the patient's PT at 48 and 96 hours after treatment is stopped to make sure there is no residual toxin remaining in the body [63].

Liver failure

Pathogenesis

Liver diseases of various types can result in reduced concentrations of coagulation factors by two different mechanisms. First, since all of the soluble coagulation factors are produced in the liver, liver failure can result directly in decreased production of these proteins. This generally requires a marked reduction in hepatic function, given the normal excess of functional capacity of most major organs in the body. Secondly, liver diseases that are cholestatic lead to a reduction in normal bile flow. Bile secreted by the liver into the intestines aids in fat absorption, so animals with cholestasis can have reduced fat absorption. Vitamin K is a fat-soluble vitamin, and cholestasis can result in decreased vitamin K absorption and deficiency.

Diagnostic findings

This is not usually a diagnostic challenge from the standpoint of trying to figure out why an animal is bleeding. Animals with liver disease severe enough to cause coagulation defects will usually have clinical signs (e.g., icterus) or lab findings (e.g., increased liver enzymes, increased bilirubin or abnormal liver function tests) that suggest liver disease.

More often, liver disease has already been recognized, and the concern is that the patient may have excessive bleeding from invasive procedures such as a liver biopsy. So, patients may be screened for coagulation abnormalities before a liver biopsy or other invasive procedure. Patients with severe cholestatic disease may be pretreated with vitamin K prophylactically before such a procedure. PT and PTT may both be prolonged since any or all of the factors may be deficient. Whether both are prolonged or just one depends on the severity of the hepatic dysfunction and relative reduction in the concentrations of the individual factors. Interestingly, many animals with chronic liver failure that have abnormal coagulation test results do not show significant bleeding manifestations following surgery or biopsy. Since the liver is involved in production and/or metabolism of both procoagulant factors as well as anticoagulant factors, evaluating only one arm, as is done with the PT and PTT, does not always reflects the true physiologic condition. Unfortunately, the results of the PT and PTT are not reliable in predicting which animals might bleed and which will not.

DIC

DIC was previously discussed under causes of thrombocytopenia. DIC is the one disease that commonly affects both primary and secondary hemostasis and should be considered in a clinically ill patient with both thrombocytopenia and evidence of a coagulopathy.

Inherited defects

Inherited defects of most of the coagulation factors have been reported, although none are common (Table 17.5) [68]. The most frequently encountered inherited defect is of Factor VIII. Given the intentional inbreeding associated with purebred animals, inherited defects may be propagated within a specific breed. However, once a condition is recognized, screening and selective breeding efforts often reduce the incidence, so the relative incidence of these diseases in a specific breed can change over time. Depending on the specific mutation involved, the magnitude of the decrease of the affected coagulation factor can be variable and thus so can the severity of clinical signs.

Diagnostic findings

Inherited coagulopathies usually have strong breed associations and may be associated with specific lines within a breed. An exception is Factor VIII deficiency, which has been reported in many different breeds of dogs as well as mixed-breed animals [68]. If dealing with a pure-breed dog, it is always worth researching to see if a certain inherited disorder has been reported in that breed.

Table 17.5 Inherited coagulopathies reported in animals.

Factor affected	Species/breed reported	Comments
Prekallikrein	Dogs: poodle Horses: Belgian, miniature horses	Not typically associated with clinical bleeding tendencies
Factor XII	Dogs: miniature poodle, Shar Pei Cats: DSH, DLH, Siamese, Himalayan	Not typically associated with clinical bleeding tendencies Relatively common in cats as an incidental finding of markedly prolonged aPTT
Factor XI	Dogs: springer spaniel, Weimaraner, Great Pyrenees, Kerry blue terrier Cats: DSH Cattle: Holstein	Clinical bleeding tendencies are generally mild
Factor X	Dogs: Jack Russell terrier, cocker spaniel Cats: DSH	Rare Severe clinical bleeding tendencies
Factor IX	Dogs: any breed, mixed breed Cats: any breed, mixed breed	Sex-linked, primarily seen in males De novo mutations relatively common resulting in cases with no prior familial history Second-most-common symptomatic, inherited coagulopathy (termed "*Hemophilia B*") Severity of clinical bleeding tendencies relates to residual factor activity, which is variable depending on specific mutation (hundreds identified in humans)
Factor VIII	Dogs: any breed (German shepherd common), mixed breed Cats: any breed, mixed breed Horses: any breed Sheep: White Alpine	Sex-linked, primarily seen in males De novo mutations relatively common resulting in cases with no prior familial history Most common symptomatic, inherited coagulopathy (termed "*Hemophilia A*") Severity of clinical bleeding tendencies relates to residual factor activity, which is variable depending on specific mutation (hundreds identified in humans)
Factor VII	Dogs: Alaskan Klee Kai, beagle, boxer, bulldog, dachshund, malamute, schnauzer Cats: DSH	Clinical bleeding tendencies are variable, even among related patients
Factor V	Not yet reported in animals	
Factor II	Dogs: boxer, English cocker spaniel	Rare In boxer, defect was functional (normal concentrations of an abnormal protein)
Factor I	Dogs: bichon frise, Borzoi, collie, Russian wolfhound Cats: DSH Goats: Saanen Sheep: Leicester	Acquired deficiencies (e.g., DIC, hepatic failure) are more common than inherited Both quantitative and function inherited defects are reported but uncommon Clinical bleeding tendencies range from mild to severe
Multiple: vitamin K–dependent factors	Dogs: Labrador retriever Cats: Devon rex Sheep: Rambouillet	Defect involves enzymes involved in vitamin K recycling leading to function deficiencies of vitamin K–dependent factors Clinical bleeding tendencies are moderate to severe Some cases respond to vitamin K administration

Sources: Based on Brooks M. Hereditary Coagulopathies In: Weiss DJ Wardrop KJ, ed. Schalm's Veterinary Hematology. 6th ed. Ames, IA: Blackwell, 2010; and Boudreaux, M. Hemostasis Lecture Notes 2011. Deer Park, NY: Linus Publications, Inc. 2011.

Animals with inherited coagulopathies usually do not have signs of systemic illness other than their bleeding manifestations, unless there is a concurrent illness. Bleeding manifestations common to most coagulation factor deficiencies include hemarthrosis, hematoma formation, and prolonged bleeding in response to minor injuries [68].

Animals with inherited coagulopathies should have normal platelet counts and other tests related to primary hemostasis. The coagulation testing results will depend upon in which system the deficient factor is located. Deficiencies of factors in the intrinsic cascade typically have a prolonged PTT and normal PT, while Factor VII deficiency would be expected to have the opposite results. Common pathway factor deficiencies would be expected to have prolongations of both PT and PTT. Typically, the magnitude of the prolongation in these tests is not nearly as dramatic as that seen with rodenticide toxicity.

Of particularly note, Factor XII deficiency is well characterized in cats and fairly common compared to other inherited coagulopathies. Interestingly, these cats *do not* show abnormal bleeding episodes, and they are usually clinically asymptomatic despite having markedly prolonged PTT results. These cases are usually picked up on presurgical hemostasis testing.

18 Principles of Blood Transfusion and Crossmatching

Linda M. Vap[1] and Karl E. Jandrey[2]

[1]Department of Microbiology, Immunology, and Pathology, Colorado State University, Fort Collins, CO, USA
[2]Clinical Small Animal Emergency and Critical Care, University of California- Davis, Davis, CA, USA

The treatment advancements with blood products for veterinary patients are due not only to the improved access to blood products by the growth of commercial and in-house donor programs but also advances in point-of-care assessment to increase safety in storage and administration to the recipient. Many regional blood banks and improved or expanded local programs within hospitals deliver a safe product beyond fresh whole blood (FWB). Hospitals without ready access to a safe and steady supply of blood products should consider referring their patients to one of these centers. Emergency or specialty hospitals in most metropolitan and suburban areas likely host a small animal or equine blood donor program and blood bank, some even selling their blood commercially while complying with local laws. These centers house the people, materials, and equipment that host a functional and profitable blood bank. The increased access and development of patient-side blood type and crossmatch technology has also added to the feasibility and improved delivery of quality transfusion therapy for some species. This chapter discusses crossmatching and blood typing products commercially available.

Blood groups

Blood groups or types are classifications made based on species-specific antigens on the surface of erythrocytes and are important in inducing immune-mediated reactions in host animals during transfusion therapies. Antigens associated with platelets, leukocytes, and plasma proteins may be important as well. Naturally occurring alloantibodies against another blood type can be present in an animal's plasma despite lack of prior exposure to those erythrocyte antigens. More commonly, antibodies against erythrocyte antigens are induced in response to exposure, either via blood transfusion, transplacental exposure, or, in the case of neonatal isoerythrolysis (NI), through colostrum. Blood groups in the common domestic and pet exotic species are described here and presented in Table 18.1.

Dogs

The dog erythrocyte antigen or blood type system is known as the DEA system and has historically included DEA 1 (1 neg, 1.1, 1.2, 1.3) and DEAs 3–8. Recent reports indicate DEA 1.1 and 1.2 are the same antigen with varying strengths of expression [7, 8]. Furthermore, it has been shown that dogs with weak red-cell DEA 1 expression do not develop antibodies when transfused with those of strong DEA 1 expression [9]. Henceforth, DEA 1.1 and DEA 1.2 will be referred to as DEA 1. DEA 1.3 has been described in German shepherd dogs in Australia [10]. However, to the authors' knowledge, no further evidence has been published confirming its continued existence. The most important canine blood type is DEA 1, which is present in approximately 60% of the canine population [11]. While naturally occurring DEA 1 alloantibodies have not been described, this antigen will induce severe transfusion reactions in previously sensitized dogs. Other DEA alloantibodies are reportedly of limited clinical significance in dogs, unlike the situation in cats, but may exist in some dogs [11–13]. DEA 4 is a high-frequency antigen that can result in hemolytic transfusion reactions in DEA 4-negative dogs previously sensitized by DEA 4-positive blood transfusions [14]. In addition, DEA 7 may elicit an antibody response in dogs that lack it, and DEAs 3 and 5 are low-incidence antigens in which naturally occurring alloantibodies can occur; anti-DEA 3, 5, and 7 can result in delayed transfusion reactions [15–19]. The high-frequency *Dal* erythrocyte antigen was so named as it was originally identified after accidental sensitization of a Dalmatian dog by transfusion of *Dal*-positive blood. It has since been demonstrated as lacking in up to 12% of Dalmatians, 42% of Doberman pinschers, and 57% of Shih Tzus within North

Veterinary Hematology, Clinical Chemistry, and Cytology, Third Edition. Edited by Mary Anna Thrall, Glade Weiser, Robin W. Allison and Terry W. Campbell.

Companion website: www.wiley.com/go/thrall/veterinary

Table 18.1 Antigens and pertinent factors in veterinary transfusion medicine.

Species	Major immunogenic antigens	Naturally occurring alloantibodies	Recommended donor type	First transfusion risks and recommendations	Matched transfused RBC half-life (d)
Dog	DEA 1	Rare; DEA 3, 5, 7; cold reacting	DEA 1 type-matched or DEA 1 negative for first transfusion. Crossmatch-compatible for repeat transfusions. *No* prior transfusion.	Low. Use of universal donor minimizes sensitization risk. Crossmatch if ≥4 d since prior transfusion.	24 [1]
Cat	A most common	Common. Anti-B, usually mild in type A cats.	Type A	Low if A/B type-matched. High if A/B type mismatched. Crossmatching always recommended.	29–39 [2]
	B rare except select breeds.	Common. Anti-A, strong in type B cats.	Type B		
	AB very rare – in breeds that also have B.	No anti-A or anti-B	Type AB if available (rare); Type A		
	Mik	Anti-*Mik* reported in DSH	A/B type-specific crossmatch compatible	6% in type A/B-matched blood. Crossmatch recommended.	
Horse	Complex system of 30+ antigens in seven blood groups. Donkey RBC antigen.	Occur. Anti-Aa, -Qa most important. Probably none.	None. Aa/Qa negative or same breed class is best starting choice.	Considerable; use least incompatible. High neonatal isoerythrolysis risk for mule foals.	9 [3], 24–43 [4]
Cattle	Eleven blood groups: B and J most important. B very complex in ruminants.	Occasionally anti-J.	J-negative.	Low for first transfusion. Close match difficult. Hemolytic crossmatch recommended.	12–20 [5]
Sheep Goat	Seven blood groups in sheep: sheep R similar to cattle J; sheep B similar to cattle and goat B. Five blood groups in goat: similar to sheep.	Weak. Goat anti-R.	Not defined	Low for first transfusion. Hemolytic crossmatch recommended. Hemolytic crisis rare in sheep.	16 [6]
Ferret	None identified	None identified	Not applicable	No risk identified	Unknown

America, varying with geographical regions [20]. There is a relatively high potential for clinically important transfusion reactions in those breeds [21]. Since less than 3% of mixed and other breeds are type *Dal* -, extended blood typing to include Dal antigen is recommended when there is suspicion for a transfusion reaction in any breed [20].

Cats

Three blood types are routinely recognized in the feline AB blood group system. Type A is the most common and occurs in more than 95% of domestic shorthair (DSH) and domestic longhair (DLH) cats in the United States [12, 22]. Type B occurs with varied frequency (<5–25%) in the Abyssinian, Birman, Himalayan, Scottish fold, Somali, Sphinx, Maine coon, Norwegian forest, and Persian cat breeds, whereas the highest frequency (25–50%) has been reported in the British shorthair, Cornish rex, Devon rex, and Turkish angora/van breeds [12, 22]. A higher percentage of DSH/DLH cats in the west coast region of the United States, Europe, Japan, India, Turkey, and Australia are reportedly type B [12, 23, 24]; one report found up to 30% of DSH/DLH cats were type B in the United Kingdom [25]. To date, type B has not been found in the Siamese, Burmese, Oriental shorthair, Tonkinese, American shorthair, or Russian blue breeds. Type AB is extremely rare but has been reported in DSH/DLH cats and in certain families of breeds in which type B blood also occurs, including the Abyssinian, Birman, British shorthair, Norwegian forest, Somali, Scottish fold, and Persian [26]. A novel erythrocyte antigen, *Mik*, has been described in DSH cats [27]. It is important to consider that geographical variation of feline blood types is significant, even in mixed-breed cats, and the risk of administering a potentially fatal type A or AB blood transfusion to a type B cat, at least in some populations, may be as high as one in five [25, 28].

Cats have naturally occurring anti-A, anti-B, and Anti-*Mik* alloantibodies [27, 29]. All type B cats have high serum concentrations of alloantibodies that are strong hemagglutinins and hemolysins against type A erythrocytes. Type A cats generally have weak hemagglutinins and hemolysins against type B erythrocytes. Newborn kittens have no alloantibodies because of their endotheliochorial placenta, but colostral transfer of immunoglobulin (primarily IgG) occurs. NI occurs in type A or AB suckling kittens born to type B queens with transfer of the anti-A alloantibodies via the colostrum [23, 29, 30]. Because DSH/DLH cats have a low frequency of type B blood, less than 2% of random matings produce litters at risk for NI, whereas Birman and Devon rex matings carry a risk of 15% and 25%, respectively, for producing NI [30]. The *Mik* antigen is clinically relevant in that approximately 6% of AB-matched blood transfusions can result in acute post-transfusion hemolysis if the patient blood is negative and the donor blood is positive for this antigen [27].

Horses and donkeys

The seven internationally recognized blood groups in the horse, A, C, D, K, P, Q, U, include more than 30 antigens [31, 32]. Because of various antigenic combinations, no universal donor exists. To minimize transfusion reactions, blood typing of the donor and recipient is ideal but often impractical. An earlier report indicating short transfused cell life span and limited utility of compatibility testing in horses has recently been refuted [4, 33]. At the very least, crossmatching prior to transfusion is recommended [34]. Aa and Qa alloantigens are extremely immunogenic; both are hemolysins, and most cases of NI are associated with anti-Aa or -Qa antibodies. In addition, anti-Aa and -Ca are agglutinating antibodies. It is important to note that Qa will not be detected with an agglutination test. Blood types vary among horse breeds, with Thoroughbreds and Arabians having a high prevalence of antigens Aa or Qa compared to other breeds, and Standardbreds lacking the Qa antigen [31, 35]. A unique donkey and mule erythrocyte antigen (donkey factor), not found in the horse, puts all mule pregnancies at risk for NI [36, 37]. Although erythrocyte antigens Aa or Qa have been associated with approximately 90% of equine NI cases [38], other antigens including Ab, Dc, Db, De, Dg, Pa, Qc, and Ua have rarely been associated with NI in foals [31, 35, 38, 39]. Reportedly, the anti-Ca antibody does not cause NI and, in fact, may actually prevent NI by removal of potentially sensitizing cells from the circulation [40].

Cattle, sheep, and goats

The 11 recognized blood groups in cattle are A, B, C, F, J, L, M, R, S, T, and Z with groups B and J being the most clinically relevant. The B group itself has more than 60 antigens, thereby making closely matched blood transfusions difficult. The J antigen is a lipid found in plasma that is not a true erythrocyte antigen; it is usually acquired to varying degrees early in life. Cattle with anti-J antibodies, despite having erythrocytes with a small amount of adsorbed J antigen that apparently type negative, can develop transfusion reactions when receiving J-positive blood [31, 41]. Vaccinations of blood origin (some anaplasmosis and babesiosis vaccines) may sensitize cattle to erythrocyte antigens that could result in NI in subsequent calves [31].

Seven blood groups have been identified in sheep (A, B, C, D, M, R, X). The B system has more than 52 factors [31]. The R system is similar to the J system in cattle (i.e., antigens are soluble and passively adsorbed to erythrocytes). The M-L blood group in sheep is related to active potassium transport in reticulocytes [42, 43]. The blood groups of the goat (A, B, C, M, J) are very similar to those of sheep, with the B system equally complex [44]. Many of the reagents used for blood typing of sheep also have been used to type goats.

Exotic pets

No blood groups have been identified to date in ferrets [45]. Blood transfusions can be administered safely without the need for crossmatching even when multiple transfusions are indicated, such as for severe estrus-induced aplastic anemia [46].

Little to no information is available on blood groups in rabbits and exotic pet species of birds or reptiles. In these cases, crossmatching prior to transfusion is recommended, and homologous transfusions using species-specific blood are advised. A low-volume simplified crossmatch procedure (see "Procedures for Crossmatching") can be used in these species, particularly for cases in which a prior transfusion has been administered [47, 48].

Donor selection

Blood typing should be performed to select permanent dog, cat, and horse blood donors. All donors should be healthy young adults that have never received a blood transfusion. In addition, donors must undergo routine physical examinations as well as hematology and clinical chemistry evaluations, receive vaccinations, and be tested free of blood parasites and other infectious diseases. There are consensus statements in both the United States and Europe that have recommendations for prevention and monitoring of infectious disease potentially transmitted through blood donations from dogs and cats [49, 50]. Donors should have normal baseline packed cell volume (PCV) and total protein concentrations prior to any donation. Blood should be collected aseptically, usually via jugular venipuncture. To avoid interference with platelet function, donors should not be sedated with acepromazine. Blood collection methods for different species have been reviewed in detail elsewhere [17, 47, 48, 51–53].

Dogs

Dogs can donate approximately 15 mL of blood per kilogram (kg) of body weight every 6 weeks [17]. A history of prior transfusion precludes a dog from being a prospective donor [12], whereas a history of prior pregnancy does not [54]. For first-time transfusion recipients, donors negative for DEA 1 can be considered universal donors and, for this situation, routine typing for other blood types is not clinically warranted [12]. A dog is considered a universal donor when negative for DEA 1, 3, 5, 7, and positive for DEA 4 [11, 17]. To minimize potential sensitization of the recipient and improve the odds of identifying compatible donors, the use of universal donors is recommended when periodic transfusions are anticipated. Since about half of dogs are DEA 1-positive and testing for DEA 1 is a practical procedure, having DEA 1-positive donor blood available for DEA 1-positive recipients is prudent [11, 12]. A practical summary is that DEA 1-negative dogs are ideal for first-time transfusions regardless of recipient blood type, and DEA 1-positive donors should be limited to DEA 1-positive recipients.

Dog donors should be greater than 25–30 kg, bled less than once per month to prevent iron deficiency, and well nourished, including supplementation with oral iron if collected frequently. To ensure general good health, donors should have negative fecal and heartworm disease examinations. According to the American College of Veterinary Internal Medicine's (ACVIM) Consensus Statement, donors should test negative for transmissible infectious diseases including babesiosis, leishmaniasis (especially foxhounds) [55], brucellosis, ehrlichiosis, anaplasmosis, and neorickettsiosis. The Consensus Statement should be consulted for specific recommendations on diseases relevant to particular geographical regions, such as trypanosomiasis, bartonellosis, and hemoplasmosis [16].

Cats

Donor cats can donate between 10 and 12 mL of blood/kg body weight. Healthy adult cats can donate 45–60 mL every 6 weeks and usually require sedation for blood collection [52, 56]. Like dogs, donor cats should have negative fecal and heartworm disease examinations as part of a general health screening. Since the majority of cats in the United States are type A, donors should also be type A, but type B and AB donors may also be required depending on geography and breed prevalence. Because of the cat's naturally occurring alloantibodies, there is no universal cat donor. Donor cats should be negative for feline leukemia virus (FeLV), feline immunodeficiency virus (FIV), cytauxzoonosis, and hemoplasmosis.

Horses

Adult horses can safely donate approximately 6–8 L of blood. Whole blood (WB) can be collected every 2–4 weeks and plasma collected every week if the erythrocytes are returned to the donor [57]. Donors should be in good health, and male donors may be preferred as they are less likely to have been previously sensitized [53]. Additionally, screening for equine infectious anemia and ensuring PCV and plasma protein concentrations are within normal limits are recommended. Mares that have been pregnant or foaled and horses that have received blood or erythrocyte-contaminated plasma transfusions should be excluded as potential donors. A totally compatible blood transfusion is unlikely to be achieved in the horse. Crossmatching to identify the least incompatible donor is recommended to minimize adverse transfusion reactions but will not identify all donor/recipient incompatibilities [34]. Because Aa and Qa erythrocyte antigens are extremely immunogenic, Aa- and Qa-negative donors are the best choice as donors to recipients of unknown blood type. In cases of NI, the dam's washed erythrocytes may be used for transfusion to severely anemic foals, whereas a transfusion from the sire to foal would be contraindicated [31, 58]. While blood transfusion can be life-saving to foals with NI, number and volume of transfusions must be limited; one study demonstrated that each administration of a blood product to a foal with NI increased its likelihood of *nonsurvival* by greater than eightfold, and administration of 4 or more liters (total volume) of blood products significantly increased the risk for liver failure in foals [59]. Mule foals with NI could receive a transfusion from a horse not previously sensitized by pregnancy against donkey factor, since horses are known to be free of naturally occurring antibodies against donkey factor, the implicated antigen in cases of NI in mules.

Cattle, sheep, and goats

Ruminants can donate 10–15 mL/kg of body weight. Closely matched transfusions are very difficult in cattle; first transfusions are generally low risk, but ideally a donor would be negative for the J antigen [41, 51]. Similarly, typing and matching blood for sheep or goat transfusions is impractical [60]. Prion diseases have been shown to be transmitted by blood transfusion in sheep [61] and should, therefore, be a consideration for disease screening prior to blood transfusion in ruminants.

Exotics

Large, vaccinated adult male ferrets are the best choice as blood donors and should have a normal PCV and total protein, be negative for Aleutian mink disease virus, and be screened for heartworm microfilaria [47, 62]. These ferrets can donate a total of 6–10 mL of blood depending on body weight [62]. When collected in anticoagulant solution containing citrate, phosphate, dextrose, and adenine (CPDA-1), stored blood should be used within 7 days of collection [63].

For pet birds and reptiles, since blood typing is not generally available, using a healthy donor of the same species as the recipient may minimize the likelihood or severity of transfusion reaction and will reportedly result in longer survival of transfused erythrocytes [48, 64]. Ideally a bird donor would be negative for chlamydiosis, psittacine beak and feather disease, and polyoma virus [47].

Indications for and general principles of transfusion therapy in dogs and cats

The prescription of blood products should be considered just like any other drug and requires a clear indication. Critical knowledge about the pros and cons of transfusion therapy is also necessary. The dose, administration, monitoring, and side effects must be clearly known to select the right product for the right patient at the right time. Commonly used products include WB, packed erythrocytes (packed red blood cells [PRBCs]), and a variety of plasma products including fresh frozen plasma (FFP), frozen plasma (FP), and plasma. The two most common reasons to use blood products are for the treatment of anemia (by increasing red blood cell [RBC] mass) or a secondary coagulopathy. RBC transfusions are commonly used to treat a patient's clinical signs of poor oxygen-carrying capacity determined by physical examination and clinicopathologic data such as hemoglobin concentration, PCV, or hematocrit. Other objective measures that may help in the decision-making process to trigger a transfusion include venous oxygen tension and lactate concentration. As oxygen delivery to the tissues falls but the tissue extraction remains the same, less venous oxygen is found in the measurement of PvO_2. However, this may also reflect increased oxygen demand by the tissues. Alternatively, an increase in lactate concentration is a readily available marker of poor perfusion.

Shock identified in a patient must first be resolved using isotonic crystalloids to improve perfusion while the best blood product is obtained. The transfusion should be considered as soon as the patient's cardiovascular status is jeopardized by the blood loss. Clinical signs include:

- Abnormal perfusion parameters: tachycardia, pale mucous membranes, prolonged capillary refill time, weak pulses, cold extremities, altered mentation.
- Signs of anemia: pale mucous membrane color and poor pulse quality, which may be difficult to differentiate from hypoperfusion/shock and need to be reassessed after initial isotonic fluid resuscitation.
- Downstream perfusion markers: increased lactate, decreased blood pressure, and urine output.
- Respiratory function: increased respiratory rate and effort, blood gas analysis.

Recent evidence from the human medical literature and adapted to clinical veterinary medicine (dogs and cats) considers treatment with PRBCs when the hemoglobin drops below 7 g/dL (or a PCV ≤ 20%) [65]. However, the acuity or chronicity of that anemia also plays a role in the decision making. Most patients with a Hgb below 4 g/dL (or a PCV ≤ 12%) require RBC transfusions due to life-threatening cellular energy depletion from inadequate oxygen-carrying capacity. A quick rule of thumb is to calculate the amount of RBCs needed to restore the PCV to 20–25%. This is a reasonable clinical goal to balance the costs and risks of a transfusion with the physiologic need for oxygen-carrying capacity to tissues. Most transfusions using 1 mL/kg PRBCs will raise the patient's PCV 1%. Alternatively, it takes 2 mL/kg to raise a patient's PCV 1% when using FWB. There are formulae in both dogs and cats that are more accurate [66, 67].

Patients with disorders of secondary hemostasis (e.g., hereditary factor deficiency, vitamin K antagonism) are unable to make sufficient fibrin to stabilize the platelet plug. Treatment with plasma for these patients attempts to normalize the timed coagulation tests that confirmed the presence of hemostatic dysfunction. The reader is referred to Chapter 17 for a review of hemostasis. The goal of therapy is to restore coagulation factors to levels that reduce the chance for hemorrhage to persist. In general, 10–20 mL/kg of FFP will restore coagulation factors to a level to normalize the coagulation tests. The improvement in clinical bleeding and the coagulation test results seem to parallel one another. FFP should be administered within 4 hours of thawing at a rate such that the patient is not at risk for fluid overload or acute hemolytic transfusion reaction.

Primary hemostasis is the formation of a platelet plug at the site of endothelial damage. Defects in primary hemostasis are most often caused by thrombocytopenia, von Willebrand disease, or thrombocytopathy (abnormal platelet function). Thrombocytopenia is much more common than thrombocytopathy (see Chapter 17 for details of hemostasis). The treatment of a defect in primary hemostasis involves the removal of the underlying cause if possible. Transfusion of platelets is challenging due to their reactive nature and special handling requirements. The donation of blood and placement into collection bags can activate platelets to form clumps. Platelets also activate at cold temperatures; therefore, all platelet transfusion must be completed using fresh blood products, either FWB, platelet-rich plasma, or a platelet concentrate. The access to platelet products is very limited, which makes complete resolution of a primary hemostatic defect often best addressed in hospitals with specialized blood banks and hemostasis centers.

Blood products

Blood collected from donors is often processed into components, each with unique qualities that make them ideal in certain situations in transfusion therapy (see Figure 18.1).

Blood should be refrigerated in plastic blood collection bags containing 1 mL of anticoagulant for every 7 mL of blood. CPDA-1 is the anticoagulant of choice because it maintains higher levels of 2,3-disphosphoglycerate (2,3-DPG) and adenosine triphosphate (ATP), allowing for approximately 35 days of refrigerated shelf life [68]. Heparin activates platelets and is not recommended for blood collection, but if heparin is used as the anticoagulant (5 U per mL of blood) [17], blood must be used immediately. Blood collected for transfusion in pet birds must be administered immediately because use of available storage media will result in a blood product that contains dangerously high potassium concentrations [64].

The most common product used in practices without developed blood banks or high volume of purchased products is likely FWB (drawn and used within 6 hours). FWB contains RBCs, platelets, and plasma (and white blood cells unless leukoreduced) and is often used for patients that not only have anemia but also coagulation defects and need volume. Care must be taken if the patient does not need all three of these components. Monitor for and address volume overload while the patient is at an increased risk of immunologic transfusion reactions. WB may be stored for up to 1 month at 4 °C. Stored whole blood (SWB) has viable RBCs only, as platelets quickly activate with cold and coagulation factors degrade during storage. More details on the preparation of blood components are available elsewhere [51, 52, 58, 69].

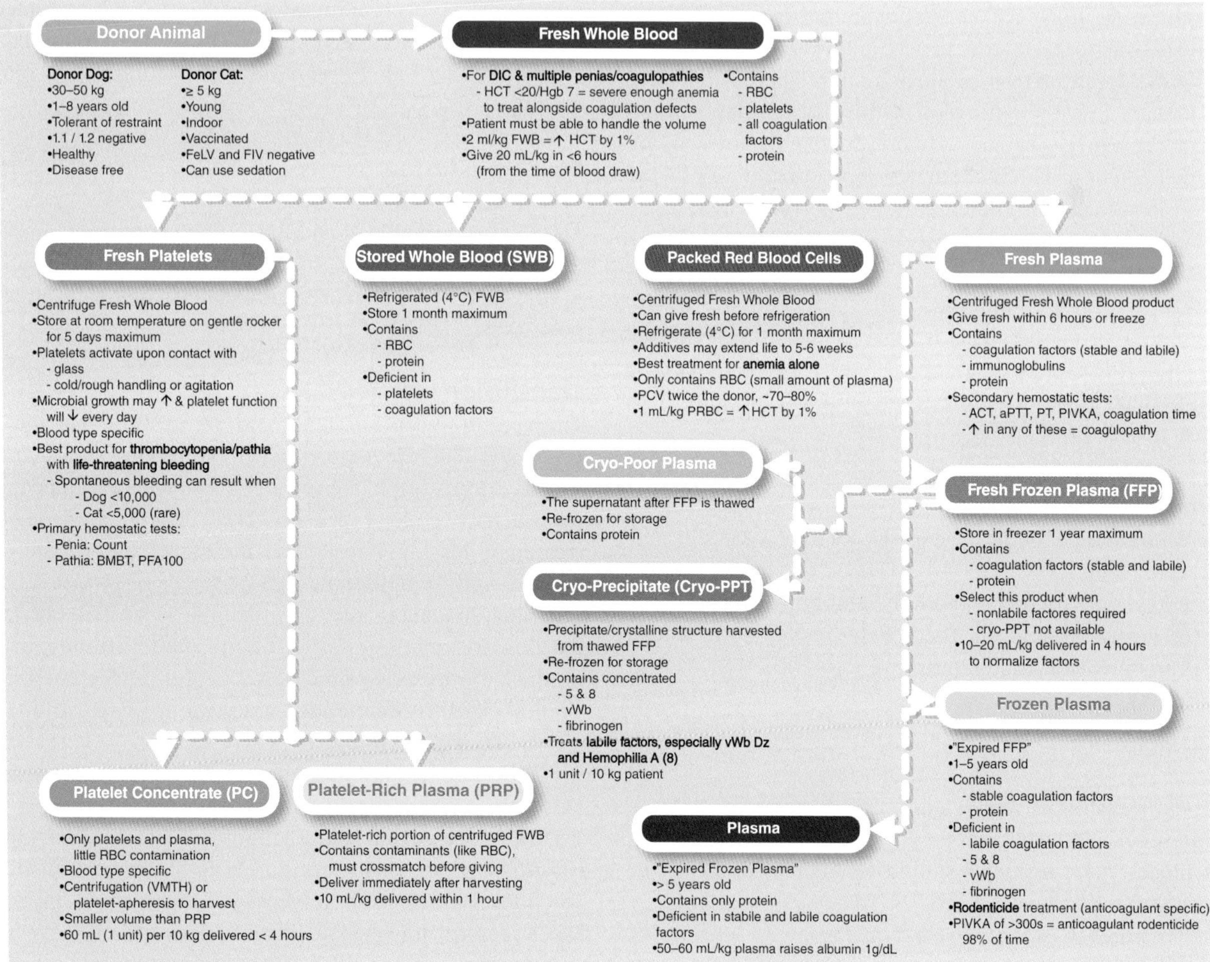

Figure 18.1 Blood component preparations.

When FWB is centrifuged and processed within 6 hours of collection, many products can be made. PRBCs, fresh plasma, and platelet products, each with unique processing and storage conditions, can be stored for later use. PRBCs are viable for about 1 month when stored at 4 °C. This product generally has a PCV twice that of the donor; thus, 1 mL/kg can raise the recipient's PCV 1%. Fresh plasma is more commonly frozen shortly after processing for thaw and use at the time it is needed. Fresh plasma or FFP has high concentrations of all coagulation factors. Calves, foals, puppies, and kittens with failure of passive transfer may benefit from FFP [51, 70, 71]. The concentration of labile factors (e.g., V, VIII, and von Willebrand factor) declines within the first year of storage. Therefore, after 1 year of FFP storage, the product is relabeled as FP. FP still has adequate concentrations of the stabile coagulation factors (II, VII, IX, X) for the treatment of vitamin K antagonist intoxication. FP maintains strong concentrations of these factors for up to 5 years [17]. After 5 years, FP products will not contain robust concentrations of coagulation factors for treatment of coagulopathies. Relabeled as plasma, it maintains adequate concentrations of plasma proteins and is a good source of albumin. To raise the patient albumin concentration, however, one generally needs to administer 50–60 mL/kg to raise the patient albumin concentration by 1 g/dL. Fresh platelet products require special handling and rapidly lose their function within their 5-day storage time [72]. Novel platelet ("freeze-dried," lyophilized, or bioengineered) products are in development and may be on the horizon for clinical practice in the near future [73].

Cryoprecipitate (Cryo-PPT) is a specialized product that requires a controlled freeze–thaw cycle. Cryo-PPT has the highest concentrations of the labile factors in the smallest amount of plasma. This is ideal for patients with von Willebrand disease or hemophilia A as a pretreatment or used perioperatively to prevent uncontrolled bleeding. The typical dose is 1 unit/10 kg.

Administration

The assumption for blood products is that they were collected and stored aseptically.

The following protocol for administration is adapted from the University of California, Davis, Veterinary Medical Teaching Hospital, Small Animal Intensive Care Unit.

Pretransfusion

- Blood transfusion can be administered intravenously or intraosseously in small patients (i.e., pediatrics or exotics).
- A blood type/crossmatch should be completed; ideally in dogs and horses, always in cats.
- FFP requires thawing at room temperature for 20 minutes before defrosting in warm water. (Note: FFP can be defrosted without thawing first in emergent situations.) Alternatively, use a commercial plasma thawer according to manufacturer directions.
- Set up a Y-type administration set with a filter for the blood. Attach blood bag with one of the two ports; the second one will be used for the 0.9% NaCl flush if indicated.
- If administering the blood product via syringe, insert an injection port into the bag. Draw the blood product into a syringe; attach a filter between the syringe and extension set.
- Place indwelling rectal temperature probe into the patient. Get a baseline TPR and vitals.

Transfusion

- Transfuse the blood product at 2.5–10 mL/kg/h. Usually, the transfusion is given in 4 hours to decrease the risk of bacterial contamination (rate of 2.5–10 mL/kg/h) using the lower rate at the beginning and increasing it if the patient tolerates the transfusion. In emergent situations, the blood product can be bolused more rapidly.
- Monitor temperature continuously and monitor respiratory rate, effort, and mentation every hour.
- Monitor vital parameters every 15–30 minutes for the first hour, and then every hour until the transfusion is completed.
- When transfusion is completed, flush the administration with 0.9% NaCl at the same rate until fluid line is mostly clear.

Post-transfusion

- Disconnect the blood administration set or fluid line from catheter and flush the catheter with heparinized saline.
- Draw blood for PCV/TP immediately, or up to an hour post-transfusion.

Transfusion reactions

The common clinical signs of a transfusion reaction are (in descending frequency) fever, vomiting, and hemolysis. The transfusion should be immediately stopped and investigated if these are observed. There is no specific treatment for these reactions; therefore, appropriate supportive and symptomatic treatments are recommended. True anaphylaxis is rare. Treat similar to any anaphylactic reaction including cessation of the administration of the product, intravenous fluid resuscitation, and epinephrine. Clinical signs, recommended investigatory steps, and treatments for hypersensitivity-related reactions are presented in Table 18.2. Additional details may be found elsewhere [11, 70].

Other causes of adverse reactions to blood product administration include many non-immune-mediated transfusion reactions. Hemolysis may occur by destruction of the donor RBCs before transfusion from inappropriate collection, storage, or administration [74]. Hemolysis will decrease the efficiency and efficacy of the transfusion. Intracellular

Table 18.2 Hypersensitivity-related reactions to blood products.

Hypersensitivity reaction	Clinical signs	Investigation	Discontinue the transfusion and then provide treatment(s) below
Type I: allergic	Urticaria, pruritus, angioedema	Transfusion history typically includes plasma products	Administer antihistamines or low dose of steroids.
Type I: anaphylactic shock	Cardiovascular collapse, dyspnea, seizures		Treat shock with IV fluid bolus, epinephrine.
Type II: hemolytic	Vomiting, hypotension, tachycardia, tachypnea, pyrexia	Examine patient samples for hemoglobinemia and/or hemoglobinuria; coagulation studies for evidence of DIC; repeat type and crossmatch of patient and donor; Coombs test	Treat symptomatically, IV fluids
Febrile: leukocyte and platelet sensitivity	Body temperature increase >1 °C	Rule out other causes of fever	Reassess patient, transfusion may be restarted at a slower rate

potassium is released into the product after RBC hemolysis and may contribute to hyperkalemia in the recipient. Hypothermia may occur if rapid transfusion occurs with an inappropriately warmed product. Because citrate binds calcium, massive transfusions of blood collected into CPDA-1 have the potential to cause hypocalcemia. The clinical signs of muscle tremors or weakness associated with hypocalcemia are treated with calcium gluconate infusion. Bacterial contamination of blood products is uncommon with proper handling but has been reported in the veterinary literature [74]. As mentioned previously, volume overload may occur, so close monitoring of the patient and use of appropriate component therapy will decrease the incidence.

How to type and crossmatch

In-house blood typing has become more common thanks to commercially available blood-typing products. Ethylenediaminetetraacetic acid (EDTA)-anticoagulated whole blood is generally required as other anticoagulants, such as heparin or citrate, have not been validated. Two popular typing methods amenable for in-clinic use include immunochromatography housed within a cartridge and agglutination performed on a card. These test for the DEA 1 antigen in dogs and A, B, or AB in cats and take just minutes to complete.

Cartridge methods are based on the migration of RBCs on a treated membrane under the capillary action of a buffer after undergoing lateral (RapidVet-H®, DMS Laboratories, Inc.) or vertical (Alvedia Quick Test®, Alice Veterinary Diagnostic) flow (Figure 18.2). These methods require a simple dilution of blood in provided diluent and application of sample to the test membrane. When the blood suspension has reached the control line, the reaction can be read.

Autoagglutination does not appear to interfere with typing results in dogs when using the cartridge system [75]. There is a similar system available for Ca typing in horses (Alvedia Quick Test, Alice Veterinary Diagnostic).

The card agglutination system (RapidVet-H) tests blood against antigens via a murine monoclonal antibody specific to DEA 1, which is lyophilized on the test card (Figure 18.3). Diluent is applied to the test card to reconstitute the lyophilized antibody and then one drop (or 10 μL) of the patient's blood is stirred into the mixture and the card is rocked, then evaluated for agglutination. Autoagglutination may interfere with interpretation of results. Alternatively, blood can be typed by sending a sample to an outside veterinary reference laboratory, and select locations offer a more complete typing service than available to the clinic setting.

Once the patient's blood type is determined, the next step is to crossmatch. Crossmatching is performed to help determine compatible red-cell products so as to reduce adverse transfusion reactions. A "major" crossmatch is performed to detect antibodies in the recipient's serum that may agglutinate or lyse the donor's erythrocytes. A "minor" crossmatch is performed to detect antibodies in the donor plasma directed against the recipient's erythrocytes. The antibodies detected may be naturally occurring or induced. The agglutination technique is adequate for the dog and cat [76], whereas testing for both agglutinating and hemolytic antibodies in the horse is necessary [32]. Cattle, sheep, and goats have minimal agglutinating antibodies, thus the use of a hemolytic test is warranted [41, 51, 76].

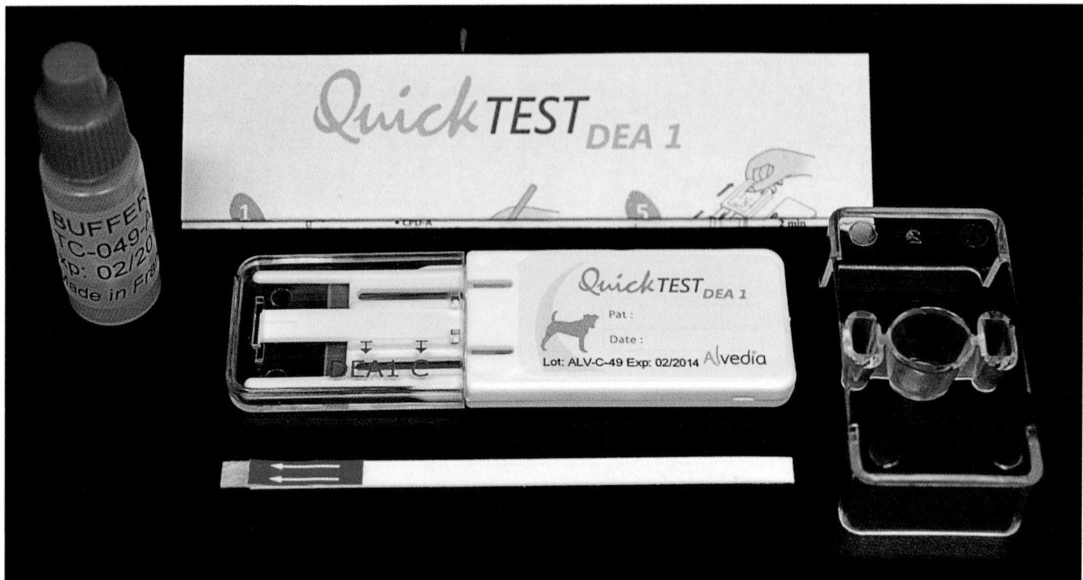

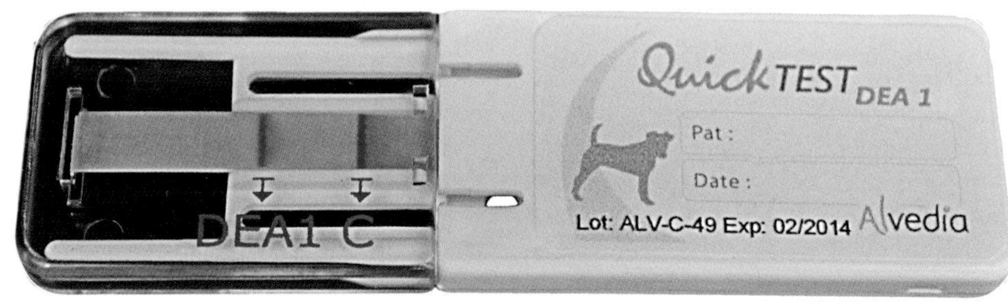

Figure 18.2 Immunochromatographic typing kit supplies (top) and column indicating type DEA 1 in a dog (bottom). Source: Courtesy of Alvedia.

A major crossmatch should always be performed in animals that have strong naturally occurring antibodies, as in cats, or in those that may have induced antibodies from prior transfusions. The latter is true even if the same donor blood is intended for repeated transfusion beyond a span of several days. The time required to mount an antibody response to transfused cells appears to vary slightly between species and author opinions. Erring on the side of caution, repeat crossmatching is recommended when there is a span of greater than 2 days in horses and cattle [51, 77] and 4 or more days in dogs and cats [78, 79] since a prior transfusion.

The minor crossmatch is considered less important, purportedly because the plasma volume is small in the donated product compared to the recipient, and is ultimately diluted, particularly when packed erythrocytes are transfused [80]. Exceptions have been documented when transfusing dogs [81] and horses [34]. Administration of packed erythrocytes may contain sufficient antibodies against recipient erythrocytes to induce adverse reactions in these species.

For exotic and feline species in which test volumes are limited, one can perform a simplified crossmatch procedure, as follows. For the major crossmatch, mix two drops of recipient plasma with one drop of blood from the donor on a clean glass slide at room temperature. Observe for macroscopic agglutination within 1 minute (Figure 18.4). Repeat the previous steps for the minor crossmatch using two drops of donor plasma and one drop of recipient blood. Grossly visible agglutination indicates incompatibility. Note that this method will not detect potentially fatal hemolytic antibodies [47, 78, 82].

Serum is preferred over EDTA plasma because plasma contributes to increased rouleaux formation and difficult interpretation of agglutination, particularly in the horse. Ideally, samples should be free of autoagglutination, hemolysis, and lipemia to aid in the interpretation of the reactions. When autoagglutination is present, or when no compatible units are available, transfusing the least incompatible unit may be a necessity, albeit not without significant risk. Test transfusing even a small volume of unmatched blood is an unsafe practice and never recommended [78].

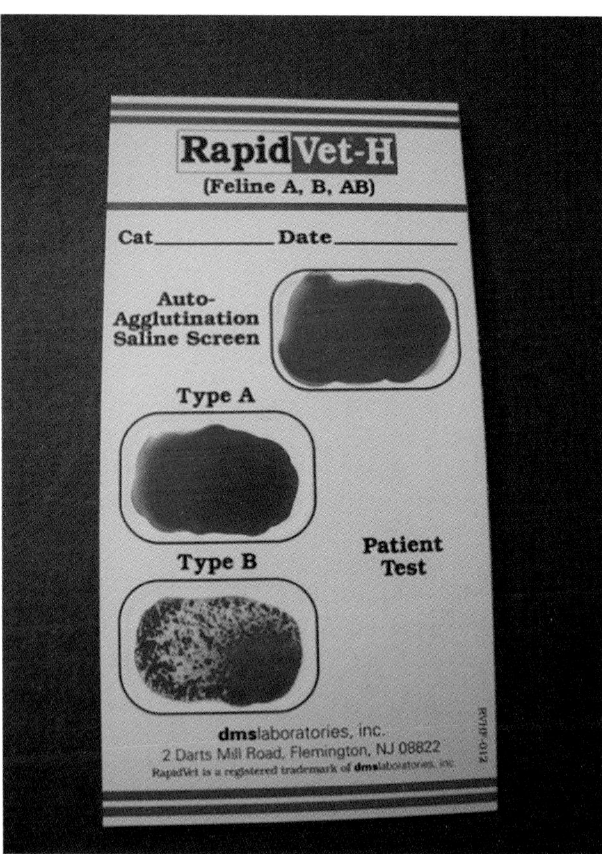

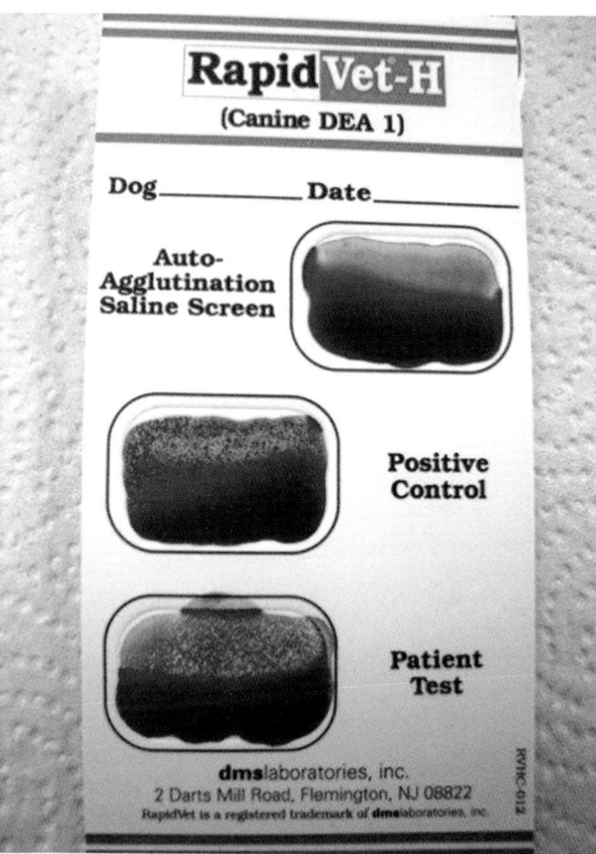

Figure 18.3 RapidVet-H typing cards demonstrating type B in a cat (left) and type DEA 1 in a dog (right), both with negative autoagglutination reactions. Source: Courtesy of DMS Laboratories, Inc.

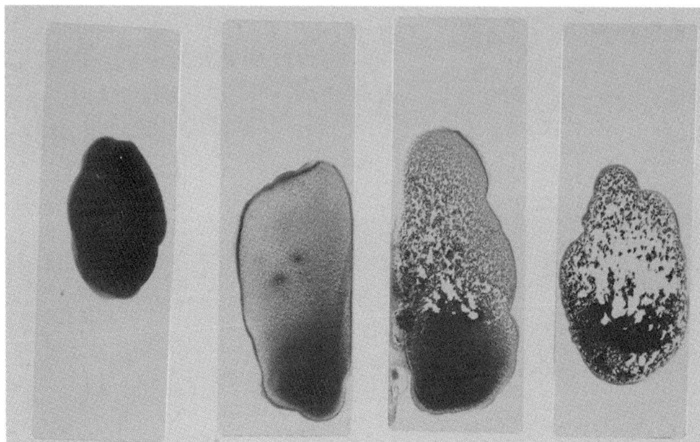

Figure 18.4 Slide crossmatch. Results demonstrate (from left to right) compatible (no agglutination), and 1+ to 3+ incompatible (agglutination) reactions.

Sample requirements and preparation for sending samples to reference laboratories

Large-animal blood typing requires ACD-anticoagulated blood for longer cell preservation. Usually, EDTA-anticoagulated whole blood is adequate for small-animal blood typing. Gently mix, not shake, samples collected with an anticoagulant immediately after collection. The EDTA-anticoagulated whole blood should be shipped cool (with, but not touching, a cold pack). Harvested patient serum is required for crossmatching; however, use of serum obtained from SST is not acceptable. Protect all samples from temperature extremes and ship by overnight delivery. Contact the reference laboratory to obtain specific requirements regarding sample type, handling, and shipping. Most laboratories performing parental exclusion typing supply blood collection kits or mailers. Harvested serum is required for antibody screening; handling is as for whole blood.

Appendix 18.1 Procedures for Crossmatching

Procedures

The procedure described here is modified from tube crossmatch standard operating procedures (SOPs) utilized by Colorado State University Veterinary Teaching Hospital, originally modified from that described by Jain [76], and the University of California, Davis School of Veterinary Medicine.

Tube agglutination crossmatch

Application

The tube agglutination crossmatch is appropriate for dogs and cats and is used in conjunction with the lytic test for horses. In dogs previously transfused with nonuniversal donor blood, an extra autocontrol and major crossmatch tube can be set up and incubated at 4 °C to detect cold reacting antibodies (i.e., anti-DEA 3, 4, 5, and 7) [15, 83]. Minor crossmatches are recommended for cats. Have a means of logging typing and crossmatching results available. A recipient autocontrol tube is included because some recipients may have autoagglutination interfering with the crossmatch. Donor autocontrols are optional, as currently healthy qualified donors should lack autoagglutination.

Procedure

1. Collect 0.5–2 mL whole blood in a clearly labeled EDTA and clot tube (not SST) from both the recipient and donor. If using a donor unit, a tubing segment (a.k.a. "pigtail") may be used for the source of erythrocytes and plasma.

2. Allow sufficient time for the nonadditive tube to clot. Centrifuge the tubes (~1000–1500 g for 3–5 minutes) to ensure the RBCs separate from the plasma and serum. If a centrifuge is not available, allow the RBCs to sediment in the EDTA tubes at room temperature for 1 or more hours.

3. Pipette off the serum/plasma into separate prelabeled glass test tubes.

4. Pipette 0.1–0.2 mL packed RBCs into saline-filled (phosphate buffered saline is recommended) 10 × 75 prelabeled disposable glass tubes (creating a 2–4% RBC suspension) for both the donor and recipient.

5. Centrifuge (45 seconds to 1 minute) to obtain a cell pellet, decant saline, and resuspend the pellet by gently flicking the bottom of the tube. A serofuge (e.g., Becton Dickinson or Clay Adams) with a fixed angle rotor is commonly used in blood bank facilities.

6. Wash the cells twice more (thrice for horses) by forcefully adding saline until the tubes are nearly full, and repeat step 5. After the last wash, resuspend the cells in saline to achieve a 2–4% erythrocyte solution.

7. Label clear glass tubes (typically 10 × 75 mm glass tubes are used) with "Donor Control," "Major," "Minor" (if performing), and "Recipient Control." To each of the following labeled tubes, add samples as described.

- Donor Control: two drops of the donor RBC solution and two drops of donor serum or plasma.
- Major: two drops of the donor RBC solution and two drops of the recipient's serum.
- Minor: two drops of the recipient RBC solution and two drops of donor plasma.
- Recipient Control: two drops of recipient RBC solution and two drops of recipient plasma.

8. Mix by flicking the bottom of each tube or gently shake the rack of tubes, and incubate at 37 °C for 30 minutes.

9. Centrifuge at a low speed for 15–30 seconds.

10. Examine the supernatant for hemolysis and record if present.

11. Gently rock the tubes to resuspend the cells and observe how the cells disperse.

12. Hold the tubes up to an agglutination viewer (or light) to observe for macroscopic agglutination or complete hemolysis (Figure 18.5).

13. Log macroscopic agglutination reactions as negative, 1+, 2+, 3+, or 4+.

14. If there is no agglutination observed grossly, or strong rouleaux is suspected, transfer a small amount to a glass slide and then examine under low power of the microscope. Lower the condenser to increase the contrast.

18.1 Erythrocytes are evenly dispersed if no agglutination is present (Figure 18.6).

18.2 Microscopic agglutination appears as grape-like clusters of erythrocytes (Figure 18.7).

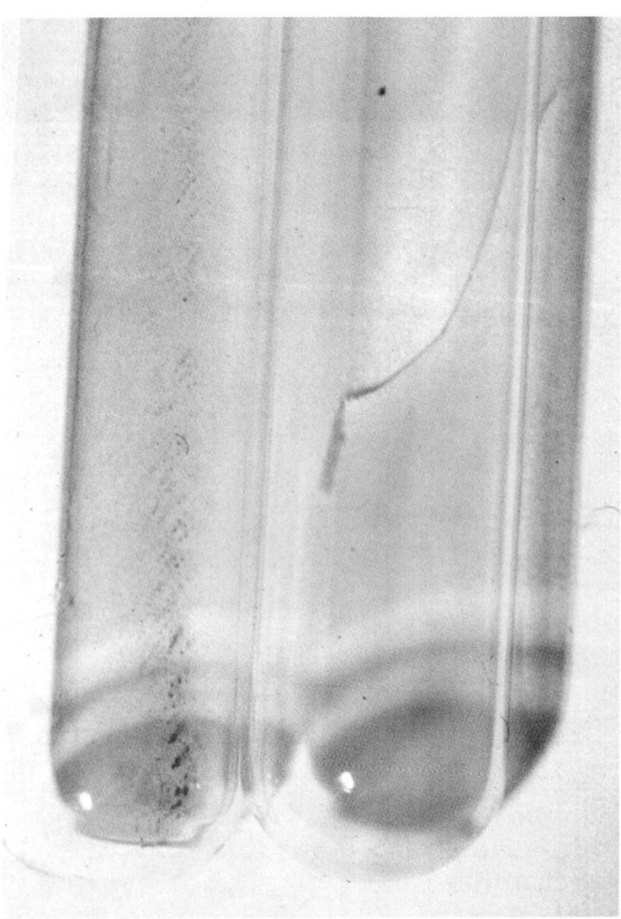

Figure 18.5 Tube crossmatch. Incompatible (2+ agglutination, left) and negative autocontrol (no agglutination, right).

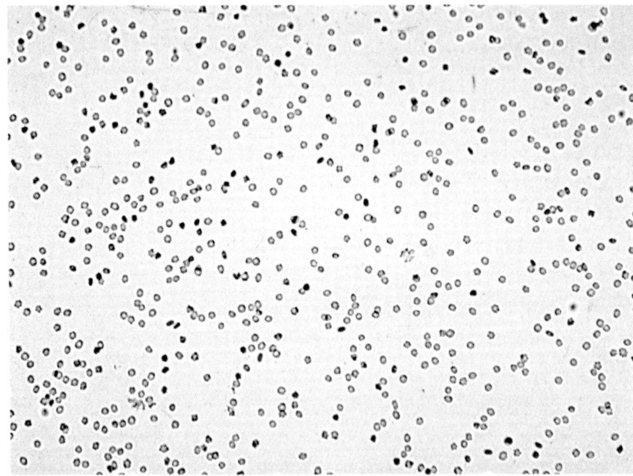

Figure 18.6 Negative microscopic agglutination. All the cells are evenly dispersed.

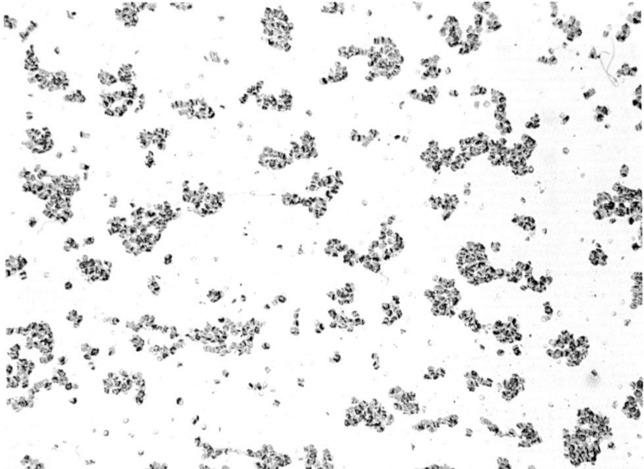

Figure 18.7 Microscopic 4+ agglutination. Note the irregular grape-like clusters. A microscopic reaction of this strength may also be detectable macroscopically as fine agglutination.

18.3 Rouleaux can be confused with agglutination. Rouleaux formation (Figure 18.8) is common in blood from horses and animals with high protein or globulin concentration, and it appears as stacks of coins. When strong, the stack may topple over on itself, mimicking agglutination.

Differentiate rouleaux from true agglutination with the following saline replacement procedure:

18.3.1 Centrifuge the tube for 15 seconds, remove the serum by pipette, and replace with two drops of PBS.

18.3.2 Mix and then centrifuge at 3400 rpm for 15 seconds.

18.3.3 Read for microscopic agglutination.

18.4 Saline replacement interpretation:

18.4.1 Erythrocytes should dissipate with rouleaux, whereas erythrocytes should remain in clusters with agglutination.

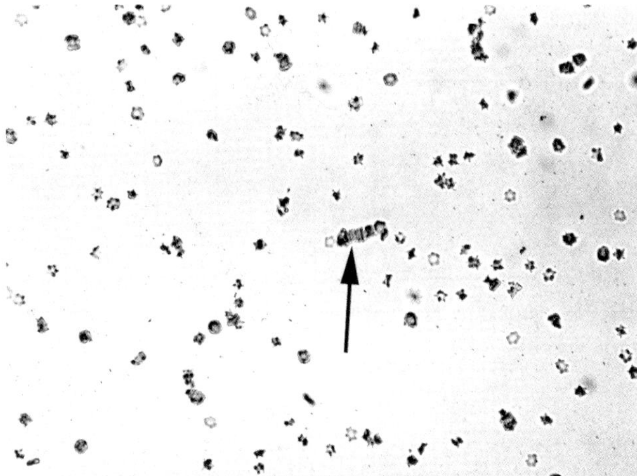

Figure 18.8 Rouleaux (con-stacking phenomenon). This must not be confused with agglutination, may indicate insufficient cell washing, and is common with equine samples.

15. Crossmatch interpretation:

19.1 Any macroscopic agglutination, significant hemolysis, or microscopic agglutination in the major or minor crossmatch (but not the control) indicates an incompatibility and the need to choose a new donor.

19.2 Slight hemolysis in canine crossmatches is nonspecific [76].

19.3 A negative result suggests the recipient is not likely to be at risk for an immediate transfusion reaction from the donor; however, it does not guarantee prevention of a delayed reaction.

19.4 Strong incompatibility in the minor crossmatch, as might be observed in mismatched cats, indicates the need to select a new donor; otherwise, packed or washed erythrocytes minimize transfusion of donor antibodies.

19.5 Agglutination in control tubes indicates autoagglutination or contaminated reagents, thereby rendering positive crossmatch tubes uninterpretable. Further patient workup such as Coombs testing may be warranted.

19.6 In horses, hemolysis in the agglutination test most likely indicates fragile or old cells rather than incompatibility. Therefore, hemolysis at this stage of testing in horses should be ignored; however, if all cells are hemolyzed, then agglutination is impossible to detect.

Hemolytic crossmatch test

Application

The hemolytic crossmatch test is required in crossmatching blood from goats, sheep, and cattle, because erythrocytes from these species tend not to agglutinate [51]. Most equine isoantibodies act as hemolysins; thus, performing both the agglutination and hemolytic test in horses is prudent. In this test, fresh rabbit serum is the source of complement. Because all rabbits possess naturally occurring anti-erythrocyte antibodies, the antibodies must be removed before using the serum as a complement source.

The following procedure is modified from that described by Jain [76].

Procedure

1. Follow steps 1–4 of the agglutination crossmatch adding serum and cell suspensions to appropriately labeled tubes; if performing the agglutination and hemolytic crossmatches concurrently (as for horses), set up four additional tubes labeled to identify them as major hemolytic and minor hemolytic tubes and recipient and donor hemolytic control tubes.
2. Add one drop of rabbit complement (absorbed for horses, sheep, and goats; refer to the complement absorption procedure that follows) to the hemolytic phase crossmatch and control tubes.
3. Shake the rack to mix, and then incubate at 37 °C for 30 minutes.
4. Centrifuge the tubes at 3400 rpm (1000 g) for 15 seconds. Observe the supernatant in each "hemolytic" tube for hemolysis; there is no need to check these tubes for agglutination.

Interpretation

A positive autocontrol indicates the presence of an autoantibody and may cause uninterpretable results in the crossmatch tubes. The major crossmatch is "incompatible" if the recipient's serum reacts with the donor's erythrocytes, and in this case, the donor blood should not be transfused. The minor crossmatch is incompatible if the donor serum reacts with the recipient's erythrocytes. In this case, only packed or washed erythrocytes are generally safe for transfusion.

Absorbed complement preparation; for use in the hemolytic crossmatch in horses, sheep, and goats [84]

Reagents

1. Lyophilized rabbit complement, unadsorbed (Pel-Freez Biologicals, Rogers, AR), store frozen.
2. $CaCL_2$-$MgCl_2$ solution, store refrigerated.
  a. $CaCL_2$, 14.7 g.
  b. $MgCl_2$, 20.35 g.
  c. Distilled H_2O, approximately 2 L.
3. Na2-EDTA solution.
  a. 74.4 g per 2 L of distilled H_2O.
    or
  b. Sequester-Sol® (Cambridge Diagnostic Products, Inc.).
4. PBS (Sigma Diagnostics, catalog no. 1000-3), store refrigerated.
5. Normal erythrocytes from the species to be tested, i.e., horse, sheep, or goat. (Two lavender-top [EDTA], 10 mL tubes from one donor are adequate.)

Procedure of the University of California, Davis Veterinary Genetics Laboratory

1. Dilute each of three vials of thawed rabbit complement with 1 mL of distilled water.
2. Add 1 part EDTA (0.3 mL) to 10 parts (3 mL) complement.
3. Centrifuge the EDTA-anticoagulated whole blood, and remove the plasma. Wash two aliquots of erythrocytes three times with PBS; make enough for two absorptions.
4. Add 1.1 mL of packed, washed erythrocytes to the complement solution. Incubate at room temperature for 30 minutes.
5. Harvest the complement solution, and repeat the absorption using fresh erythrocytes and incubating on ice instead of at room temperature for 30 minutes.
6. Centrifuge, collect absorbed rabbit complement (C′) into a flask on ice, and add 0.3 mL of $CaCL_2$-$MgCl_2$.
7. Aliquot the C′ in volumes of 0.5 mL in bullet tubes, and freeze at once. Label with the date and contents. Do not refreeze complement once thawed; use immediately or discard. (Do not store in a self-defrosting freezer, because the C′ thaws with each defrost cycle.)

Jaundiced foal agglutination test (colostrum crossmatch) [85]

The jaundiced foal agglutination test correlates highly with hemolytic blood group tests at 1 : 16 dilutions. Lower dilutions have poorer correlations because of the viscosity of colostrum [85].

Materials

1. Centrifuge (300–600 g).
2. Test tube rack.
3. Disposable glass test tubes (12 × 75 mm).
4. Saline.
5. Colostrum (or serum) and EDTA whole blood from mare (erythrocytes teased from clotted blood may be used).
6. EDTA whole blood from foal (erythrocytes teased from clotted blood may be used).

Method

1. Label tubes for 1 : 2, 1 : 4, 1 : 8, 1 : 16, and 1 : 32 dilutions for the foal.
2. Add 1 mL of saline to all tubes.
3. Add 1 mL of colostrum to the tubes labeled as foal 1 : 2. Mix and remove 1 mL of the dilution and then add to the next consecutive tube. Repeat the procedure, discarding 1 mL from the 1 : 32 tube. Discard tube labeled "1 : 8."
4. Add one drop of foal's whole blood to each tube and mix.
5. Centrifuge the tubes for 2–3 minutes at medium speed (300–600 g).
6. Invert all four tubes simultaneously (to make comparing reactions easier) and hold upside down, pouring out the liquid contents, and observe the status of the button of erythrocytes at the bottom of each tube. Grade for macroscopic

agglutination by observing how the cells flow down the side of the tube as follows:

0 No agglutination; cells flow easily.

1 Weak agglutination; cells in small clumps.

2 Strong agglutination; cells in large clumps.

3 Complete agglutination; cells remain packed in a button.

7. If no agglutination is present, report the test as being negative at all dilutions.

8. If agglutination is present, grade the reactions and continue with controls. (Controls may be set up along with the patient tubes during step 1 to save time.)

Controls

1. Foal autocontrol with 1 mL of saline and one drop of foal whole blood.

2. Mare colostrum/autocontrol, prepared by repeating steps 1 through 7 described earlier using colostrum and mare erythrocytes.

Interpretation

If all controls are negative, report the reactions of colostrum versus foal erythrocytes at all dilutions. A reaction at a dilution of 1 : 16 or greater is considered to be a high titer, and the colostrum should not be used. A positive foal autocontrol indicates autoagglutination and the possibility that the foal has already nursed. A positive mare colostrum/autocontrol indicates interference from the viscosity of the colostrum or a technical problem. Compare reaction grades for the same dilution between the mare autocontrol and the foal crossmatch tubes.

III

Hematology of Common Nondomestic Mammals, Birds, Reptiles, Fish, and Amphibians

19 Mammalian Hematology: Laboratory Animals and Miscellaneous Species

Terry W. Campbell

Department of Clinical Sciences, College of Veterinary Medicine and Biomedical Sciences, Colorado State University, Fort Collins, Colorado, USA

Blood collection and handling

Blood collection from small mammals can be challenging due to the small blood volume available for sampling. The manual or chemical restraint necessary to obtain a sample may alter the results of some laboratory tests. Blood collection studies in rats (*Rattus norvegicus*) used as laboratory animals have demonstrated that removal of 7.5% of the total blood volume over a 24-hour period did not have a biological effect, with complete recovery within 48 hours. The total blood volume of a rat has been determined to be 7.2 ± 1.19 mL/100 g body weight. Removal of blood volumes that exceed 7.5% will have a biological effect, the degree of which and time of complete recovery depend upon the amount removed. Blood collected up to 20% of the total blood volume of healthy rats does not affect the health of the rat.

In the clinical setting and for the ease of calculation, the maximum amount of blood that can be safely withdrawn from a single draw is presumed to be 1% of the animal's body weight or up to 10% of the total blood volume. This practice, however, may overestimate the safe amount that should be withdrawn during blood sampling. For example, on the average, a healthy 300 g rat has a total blood volume (based upon 7.2 mL/100 g body weight) of 21.6 mL. Removal of 7.5% of the total blood volume (considered to be a safe amount) represents 1.62 mL. If the same rat was sampled based upon 1% of the body weight, then the blood volume collected would be 3.0 mL or nearly twice the recommended safe amount. If up to 20% of the total blood volume can be safely removed from healthy rats, then a 4.32 mL blood sample could be obtained in the example above without causing ill effects. With this consideration, the 1% of the body weight rule for blood sample collection would indeed be within safe limits. This assumes the animal is healthy, and smaller blood volumes should be sampled when dealing with an unhealthy animal.

Total blood volumes reported for the mouse (*Mus musculus*) vary, with some reporting a range of 5–12 mL/100 g body weight and others a range of 7–8 mL/100 g body weight. The same guidelines recommended for laboratory rats likely apply to the laboratory mouse. Therefore, a 20 g mouse is likely to have a blood volume of 1.44 mL with a safe blood withdrawal volume of 0.1 mL. Using the 1% of the body weight guideline, the sample volume would be twice as much.

Although the blood volume will be restored within 48 hours of blood collection in most healthy mammals, it may take 2 weeks or longer for all of the blood constituents to return to normal and likely much longer in unhealthy animals. If blood collection is required more frequently than every 2 weeks, a smaller sample size such as 0.5% of the body weight (if using the 1% body weight rule) each week should be drawn. It is important to adhere to these recommended limits to prevent hypovolemic shock and anemia.

Blood collected from small mammals is typically placed in lithium heparin because the blood sample volume is small. The heparinized blood can then be used for hematologic studies and clinical chemistries.

The choice of blood collection method to be used is dependent upon the amount of blood required, frequency of sampling, technical skill of the one obtaining the sample, and parameters measured. A number of collection sites are used to obtain blood from small animals. Blood samples are often difficult to obtain from small mammals; they lack superficial vessels, and the deeper vessels may be covered with fat. In some cases, chemical restraint may be necessary to safely handle mammals for blood collection.

Most rodents will tolerate manual restraint alone for venipuncture; however, it is important to remember that the handling and restraint, as well as transport to the veterinary hospital and the hospital environment itself, are very stressful to these prey species. It is vital to approach these animals

Veterinary Hematology, Clinical Chemistry, and Cytology, Third Edition. Edited by Mary Anna Thrall, Glade Weiser, Robin W. Allison and Terry W. Campbell.

Companion website: www.wiley.com/go/thrall/veterinary

calmly and confidently and to minimize visual, olfactory, and auditory stimuli.

Small rodents, such as mice and rats, that are accustomed to being handled can be grasped gently at the base of the tail and lifted with the opposite hand placed underneath the body for support. Aggressive rodents can be picked up by the base of the tail or scruff of the neck using rubber-tipped forceps or coaxed, head first, into an appropriately sized disposable plastic syringe cover or commercially available restraint device, leaving the tail exposed for blood collection.

Rats, mice, gerbils (*Meriones unguiculatus*), and other small rodents with tails can be restrained by grasping the base of the tail and placing it on the cage lid or similar rough surface, allowing the animal to attempt to move forward while grasping the surface with its forepaws. These animals, especially gerbils, should not be picked up by the tip of the tail due to the risk of degloving injury. The handler can quickly tuck the base of the tail between the third and fourth finger while firmly grasping the rodent by the scruff with the same hand holding onto the tail. A proper scruff-hold prevents the rodent from twisting or turning to bite the handler. The scruff-hold should be brief because it can impede respiratory movements and lead to asphyxiation as indicated by cyanosis of the pinna, nose, and paws.

Manual restraint of hamsters (*Mesocricetus auratus*) can be performed by gathering the loose skin over the scruff of the neck in one hand using the scruff-hold method for rats, mice, and gerbils. Because these rodents have an abundant amount of loose skin, caution should be taken as to gather enough skin to prevent the animal from turning and biting the handler. Therefore, care should be taken to gather enough of the hamster's loose skin into the scruff-hold such that the corners of the mouth are drawn back into a smile.

Large rats can be restrained by the thoracic encirclement method, using a commercially available restraint device, or in a towel. The thoracic encirclement method can be performed by grasping the rat by the base of the tail with the dominant hand followed by placement of the nondominant hand over the back of the rat and grasping the rat around the thorax with the head of the rat between the index and middle fingers. The body of the rat can be stabilized by the handler's other hand, arm, or body. Alternatively, the rat can be grasped around the thorax, immediately under the shoulder blades, while pushing the rat's forearms cranially with the thumb and index finger so they cross under the chin, preventing the animal from biting the handler. Commercially available plastic restraint devices allow for easier blood collection from rats.

Guinea pigs become distressed when a restraint attempt is made with the scruff-hold method used on other rodents. When picking up the guinea pig for examination or to move it from one area to another, a hand should be placed over the dorsum, behind the shoulders, while grasping the animal gently with the thumb and fingers around the rib cage. The hindquarters should be supported when lifting a guinea pig to prevent spinal injury. Because guinea pigs may become distressed if restrained in lateral or dorsal recumbency, chemical restraint is frequently used when obtaining blood samples.

A rabbit's hindquarters should be supported whenever it is restrained to avoid injury to its spine. Although manual restraint can be used when obtaining blood samples from a rabbit, the use of additional restraint devices helps to reduce the risk of injury to the patient and to the technician or veterinarian. A cloth cat restraint bag can be used to restrain a rabbit, or it can be wrapped in a bath towel with its head exposed.

The restraint method used for blood collection in a ferret depends upon the collection site and preference of the phlebotomist. Most restraint methods are comparable to those used to restrain a domestic cat during blood collection. For example, a ferret may be placed in dorsal or lateral recumbency with the head extended and the front legs pulled caudally when performing a jugular venipuncture, or the animal could be placed in sternal recumbency with the front legs pulled downward over the edge of the exam table with the head flexed in a caudal direction.

A number of published chemical protocols are available that can be used for the sedation, tranquilization, and anesthesia of small mammals. Inhalant anesthetics, such as isoflurane, are commonly used to provide rapid induction and anesthesia of small mammals for blood collection. Although anesthesia is often needed for adequate restraint to obtain samples from small mammals, the anesthesia alone may produce changes, such as decreased hematocrit (HCT), hemoglobin level, and red blood cell count (RBC), in the hemogram. For example, it has been demonstrated that 5 minutes of 4% isoflurane anesthesia results in a slight decrease in the erythrocyte parameters and potassium and increase in glucose. Similar results have been reported in the ferret. Coagulation times may also be affected by anesthesia. As a result, a limit of 3 minutes of 4% isoflurane anesthesia is recommended to avoid these changes.

In the clinical setting, the tail vein is the site of choice for blood collection from small mammalian patients with tails (e.g., mice and rats). The lateral tail veins run the length of the tail and are more readily visualized in nonpigmented animals. These veins can be dilated by placing the tail in warm water or under a heat lamp prior to blood collection. Vasodilation can also be accomplished by placing the animal in an isolator at 104 °F for a few minutes or applying a warm water compress. "Milking" the vein by applying slight compression and stroking from base to tip in an attempt to push blood from the vein should be avoided, as this causes artifactual leukocytosis of the sample. A tourniquet can be placed at the base of the tail if necessary. After swabbing the venipuncture site with an appropriate disinfectant, a sterile hypodermic needle (25-gauge needle) or a sterile lancet is used to prick the vein, allowing blood to be collected into a microcollection device, such as a microhematocrit or Microtainer (Becton Dickinson, Rutherford, NJ) tube as it drips from the needle hub or skin. Gentle pressure should be applied over the venipuncture site to stop the bleeding. Blood for hematology is collected into tubes containing an anticoagulant, such as ethylenediaminetetraacetic acid (EDTA) or heparin. Blood collected for clinical biochemistry analysis is collected into tubes containing heparin or no anticoagulant.

A blood sample can also be obtained from the ventral caudal (tail) artery of a rodent with a tail (e.g., mouse or rat) placed in dorsal recumbency and under a general anesthetic. The artery runs the length of the tail but is not readily visualized. The collection site is disinfected before inserting a 23–25-gauge needle (depending on the size of the animal) into the ventral midline of the tail, approximately one-third the distance from the body to the tip. The needle is inserted at a 30° angle, in a cranial direction, until blood begins to flow from its lumen. If bone of the ventral surface of the caudal vertebra is contacted, then the needle is withdrawn and redirected slightly until blood begins to flow through the needle. Blood can be collected in a microhematocrit tube as it flows from the needle hub. In larger rodents, such as rats, a 22-gauge or smaller needle attached to a 1 or 3 mL syringe with plunger removed is used to collect the sample. Blood fills the syringe from the pressure of the artery once the vessel has been penetrated. Although rarely needed, puncture of the tail artery can also be attempted for blood collection in ferrets. The artery is approached along the ventral midline of the tail with a 22- or 21-gauge needle directed toward the caudal vertebrae. The artery is usually located 2–3 mm under the skin. After blood collection, gentle pressure should be applied to the arterial puncture site for several minutes to prevent continued blood flow.

Blood may be collected from the lateral saphenous vein in small animals by applying digital pressure or a tourniquet above the stifle after clipping the hair. Shaving the hair from the lateral aspect of the tibia exposes the vein. The lateral saphenous vein is typically small and will easily collapse, making the collection of large sample volumes difficult. Blood can be collected from the lateral saphenous veins and dorsal metatarsal veins of small rodents, such as mice, rats, hamsters, gerbils, and guinea pigs. To induce vasodilation and facilitate blood collection, small rodents can be placed in an incubator set at 104 °F for several minutes, or a warm water compress (e.g., an exam glove filled with warm water and tied off) can be applied to the venipuncture site for about a minute. After clipping the hair, the venipuncture site is swabbed with an appropriate disinfectant solution. The lateral saphenous vein runs dorsoventrally down the leg and courses laterally over the tarsal joint. With the leg extended in traction, the handler generally applies digital pressure by gently squeezing the leg between the thumb and forefinger just proximal to the venipuncture site. Blood collection may be accomplished using a needle and syringe in larger animals, such as the rabbit, or the vessel may be pricked/punctured using a sterile needle or sterile lancet in smaller animals. With the needle and syringe method, a 23–25-gauge needle with attached syringe (1.0–3.0 mL) is inserted into the vein in a distal to proximal direction, and blood is collected by slow aspiration to avoid collapse of the vein. For the "free-flow" method, digital pressure is applied to dilate the vein before the vein is pricked using a sterile 20–23-gauge needle or sterile lancet. The free-flowing blood is collected in a microcollection device, such as a microhematocrit, Microtainer tube, Pasteur pipette, or a snap-cap microcentrifuge tube that contains an appropriate volume of anticoagulant solution. Following the collection method, gentle pressure should be applied to the venipuncture site to stop the flow of blood and to prevent hematoma formation. The dorsal metatarsal vein may also be used for blood collection, using the same techniques described for lateral saphenous venipuncture. The lateral saphenous may be used for collecting small amounts of blood for packed cell volume (PCV) or complete blood count in the ferret.

Blood collection from the retro-orbital venous plexus is often performed in rodents in research laboratories and requires technical skill and general anesthesia. A heparinized microhematocrit tube is placed in the medial canthus of the eye and directed under the globe to the orbital venous plexus. With the rodent in lateral recumbency, the microhematocrit tube is rotated along its long axis as it is advanced toward the venous plexus along the caudal one-half to two-thirds of the orbit. Following blood collection, pressure on the area is required for hemostasis.

Blood is often collected from blood vessels in the ear of rabbits because of the ease of blood collection and the use of a safer manual restraint method. The two primary vessels used for blood collection from a rabbit are the marginal ear vein, yielding small to moderate quantities of blood (depending on the experience and expertise of the phlebotomist), and the central auricular artery, from which a larger volume of blood can be collected. A 22–25-gauge needle can be used to puncture the vessel, and blood collection is performed by a simple drip method, vacuum ear bleeder, Vacutainer (Becton Dickinson) method, or with a syringe. Blood collected as it drips (drip method) from the needle hub into a microcollection device minimizes hematoma formation during sampling. Aspiration into a syringe or Vacutainer tube often results in collapse of the vessel in small rabbits. Blood is slowly aspirated into a syringe when using that method, and if blood flow stops, the procedure is briefly paused until the flow starts again or the needle is slowly rotated if the bevel has been closed off by the vessel wall. A vacuum ear bleeder method is performed by lacerating an ear vessel and placing the ear inside a flask with a side arm that is attached to a vacuum line and held firmly against the rabbit's head. This method is generally used for research rabbits where large sample volumes are needed. The central auricular artery and the marginal ear vein(s) are located on the outer, haired surface of the ear. After the fur is plucked over the intended venipuncture site, the skin is cleansed with a disinfectant solution or alcohol (this may result in vasoconstriction). Ear vessels can be dilated prior to blood collection by applying a warm-water compress (e.g., a tied-off exam glove filled with warm water) over the ear for 1 minute; swabbing a small amount of oil of wintergreen to the vessel to be punctured and allowing 1–2 minutes prior to blood collection; administering acepromazine subcutaneously (0.5–1.0 mg/kg) about 15–20 minutes before venipuncture; or gently stroking ("milking") the vessel with the thumb and forefinger from the base of the ear toward the tip of the ear. Venipuncture of the marginal ear vein (typically the lateral one) is approached by directing the needle toward the base of the ear while the holder applies digital pressure to the base of the ear. Following the withdrawal of the needle from any of the venipuncture sites, gentle pressure should be applied with a cotton swab or sterile gauze pad for about 1–2 minutes to prevent hematoma formation.

Jugular venipuncture can be attempted in small mammals, although the jugular veins may be difficult to locate, and positioning the animals for the procedure can be stressful to them. Jugular venipuncture may require the use of sedation or general anesthesia is some mammals (e.g., ferrets, guinea pigs, hedgehogs, and rabbits). Blood collection in ferrets is commonly performed by jugular venipuncture, and simply allowing the ferret to lick food at the time of the procedure may be adequate to limit movement without the need of anesthesia. After the neck has been shaved and extended, blood is collected from the jugular vein using a 22–25- gauge needle and a 3 mL syringe. The jugular vein of ferrets is usually more lateral than those of dogs and cats and generally runs between the thoracic inlet and the angle of the mandible when the head and neck are extended. Often, the vein cannot be visualized, especially in large males. Blood collection from the jugular vein of hedgehogs usually requires sedation or anesthesia to prevent the animal from balling and to protect the handler from the animal's quills. Because the jugular vein is protected by thick skin in the ventral neck area, it can be difficult to sample blood from hedgehogs (*Atelerix albiventris*) using this technique.

Blood is frequently collected from the cranial vena cava in small mammals, especially the ferret, but may result in bleeding into the thoracic cavity. Chemical restraint is often used when performing venipuncture of the cranial vena cava to reduce movement during the procedure and the risk of laceration of the vessel by the needle resulting in significant internal hemorrhage. The animal, such as a ferret, is held in dorsal recumbency with the forelimbs held along its sides and the head and neck extended. A 25–27-gauge needle attached to a 3 mL syringe is inserted into the right sternal notch between the first rib and the manubrium, advanced caudally at a 30° angle to the body, and directed toward the left rear limb. The plunger is pulled back as the needle is slowly advanced or withdrawn, to allow blood to enter the syringe. Depending upon the depth of penetration of the needle, jugular venipuncture may actually occur using this technique in the ferret as the jugular vein lies just under the skin in the area of the sternal notch. The cranial vena cava is the most commonly used site for blood collection from hedgehogs and other small mammals using the same technique as described for the ferret. The heart in these animals, however, has a more cranial location compared to the ferret, and the phlebotomist must take this into consideration when using this approach.

General hematologic features of small mammals

The hematology of laboratory and other small mammals is similar to that of domestic mammals. However, obtaining meaningful reference values can be difficult because of variations associated with blood collection, environmental factors, and laboratory procedures. Blood collection often causes stress or requires chemical restraint. The hemogram can vary with age, environmental conditions, diet, gender, and reproductive status. Also, laboratory procedures and sample handling are not standardized, creating variability between data sets. Tables 19.1 and 19.2 provide suggested reference intervals for erythrocyte and leukocyte parameters, respectively, for small mammals.

The erythrocytes of mammals are small, compared to the nucleated erythrocytes of other vertebrates. The small, non-nucleated, biconcave shape minimizes the hemoglobin to surface distance during gas exchange and increases cell plasticity to improve movement through blood vessels, increasing oxygen delivery to tissues. The hemoglobin content and packed cell volume remain relatively constant among the mammals, but the total erythrocyte count and mean cell size varies. An inverse relationship between cell size and number exists. In general, only decreases greater than 10% in the erythrocyte parameters (RBC; hemoglobin concentration, Hb; and HCT) have biological significance.

The granulocytes of nondomestic mammals vary in appearance but can be classified as neutrophils or heterophils, eosinophils, and basophils. The heterophils of rabbits and some rodents were previously called pseudoeosinophils because their granules do not stain neutral with Romanowsky stains but are distinctly eosinophilic. Neutrophils of mice often have nonlobed nuclei, and those of normal primates appear hypersegmented. Cytochemical and ultrastructural features of cells differ between species. For example, lysozyme activity is lacking in the neutrophils of hamsters, and alkaline phosphatase activity is less in neutrophils of mice. Neutrophils of mammals are

Table 19.1 Erythrocyte parameters for laboratory animals and miscellaneous species (reference interval).

	RBC[a] (×10⁶/μL)	PCV (%)	Hb (g/dL)	MCV (fL)	MCH (pg)	MCHC (%)	Platelets (×10³/μL)
Rat ♂	8.2–9.8	44–50	13.4–15.8	50–58	14–18	26–35	150–450
Rat ♀	6.8–9.2	38–51	11.5–16.1	51–66	16–19	27–36	160–460
Mouse ♂	6.9–11.3	33–50	11.1–11.5	48–51	12–13	23–31	157–412
Mouse ♀	6.9–11.3	40–45	10.7–11.1	47–52	11–13	22–30	170–410
Hamster ♂	4.7–10.3	48–57	14.4–19.2	65–78	20–25	28–37	367–573
Hamster ♀	4.0–10.0	39–59	13.1–18.9	64–76	20–26	28–37	300–490
Gerbil ♂	7.1–8.6	42–49	12.1–13.8	47–60	16–19	31–33	432–710
Gerbil ♀	8.0–9.4	43–50	13.1–16.9	47–60	16–19	31–33	540–632
Guinea pig ♂	4.4–6.8	37–47	11.6–17.2	71–83	24–27	30–39	260–740
Guinea pig ♀	3.4–6.2	41–50	11.4–17.0	86–96	23–26	28–34	266–634
Guinea pig juvenile	4.1–6.0	34–49	10.1–15.1	78–89	–	28–32	–
Rabbit ♂	5.5–8.0	33–50	10.4–17.4	58–67	19–23	33–50	304–656
Rabbit ♀	5.1–6.5	31–49	9.8–15.8	58–65	17–24	29–36	270–630
Rabbit juvenile	5.2–6.5	38–44	10.7–13.9	66–80	20–23	24–33	–
Ferret ♂	6.5–13.2	34–50	12.0–18.2	44–53	17–20	34–42	297–730
Ferret ♀	6.7–9.3	36–55	12.9–17.4	44–54	16–19	33–35	310–910
Ferret juvenile	4.8–7.8	27–39	9.6–13.8	48–58	18–23	35–37	–

[a]Modified from Campbell TW (ed.). Hematology. *Vet. Clin. North Am. Exot. Anim. Pract.* vol. 18 (2015).

Table 19.2 Leukocyte parameters of laboratory animals and miscellaneous species (reference intervals).

	WBC[a] (x10³/μL)	Neutrophils (%)	Lymphocytes (%)	Eosinophils (%)	Basophils (%)	Monocytes (%)
Rat ♂	8.0–11.8	6–43	58–83	0–1	0–1	0–1
Rat ♀	6.6–12.6	4–49	50–85	0–2	0–0.4	0–2
Mouse ♂	12.5–15.9	13–22	62–83	1–3	0–1	2–2.5
Mouse ♀	12.1–13.7	16–19	66–78	2–3	0–1	0–1
Hamster ♂	5.0–10.2	17–27	55–92	0–2	0–5	1–4
Hamster ♀	6.5–10.6	23–35	51–85	0–1	0–2	0–4
Gerbil ♂	4.3–12.3	9–24	68–77	0–2	0–2	0–7
Gerbil ♀	5.6–12.8	11–26	59–78	0–2	0–1	2–6
Guinea pig ♂	5.5–17.5	28–56	40–63	1–7	0–2	3–5
Guinea pig ♀	5–16	20–42	46–80	0–7	0–1	1–3
Guinea pig juvenile	2.7–10.1	15–43	53–83	0–4	0–1	0–4
Rabbit ♂	5.5–12.5	38–54	28–50	1–4	3–8	4–12
Rabbit ♀	5.2–10.6	36–50	32–52	1–3	2–6	7–13
Rabbit juvenile	4.1–9.8	19–46	45–78	0–2	0–5	0–13
Ferret ♂	4.4–15.4	24–76	12–67	0–9	0–3	0–8
Ferret ♀	2.5–18.2	43–78	12–67	0–9	0–3	1–6
Ferret juvenile	5.3–12.6	46–77	42–68	2–7	0–1	1–5

[a]Modified from Campbell TW (ed.). Hematology. Vet. Clin. North Am. Exot. Anim. Pract. vol. 18 (2015).

phagocytic; one of their primary functions is to destroy microorganisms. Circulating neutrophil concentration increases with inflammation, especially that associated with invading microorganisms such as bacteria. Toxic changes in neutrophils and heterophils represent accelerated marrow production and shortened maturation time and are represented by the presence of small basophilic Döhle bodies, increased cytoplasmic basophilia, and occasionally increased cytoplasmic vacuolation. Typically reduced nuclear segmentation (bands, left shift) accompanies these toxic changes and can in most cases be viewed as a marker for presence of inflammation.

The granules of eosinophils become intensely eosinophilic with maturation as a result of the basic protein content. The ultrastructure of the granules in mammalian eosinophils reveals a distinct crystalline shape that varies with species; for instance, a trapezoidal pattern is found in the eosinophils of guinea pigs and true rodents, and a needle-shaped pattern is found in rabbit eosinophils. Mammalian eosinophils have phagocytic activity similar to that of neutrophils but are less effective. Mammalian eosinophils respond to metazoan infections (especially those involving helminth larvae), allergic inflammation (especially those associated with mast cell and basophil degranulation), and antigen–antibody complexes. Therefore, eosinophilia suggests one of these processes.

Mammalian basophils have characteristic cytoplasmic granules that are strongly basophilic in Romanowsky stained blood films. Unlike basophils of lower vertebrates, those of mammals tend to have lobed nuclei. The ultrastructural appearance of the granules varies with species; for instance, a coiled threaded pattern is observed in basophil granules from primates and rabbits and a homogenous pattern is observed in rodents. Basophils participate in allergic and delayed hypersensitivity reactions.

Mammalian monocytes generally are the largest leukocytes in peripheral blood films and do not vary grossly in appearance between species. The monocyte nucleus varies in shape, and the moderately abundant cytoplasm is typically light blue-gray. The granules, when present, are very fine and appear azurophilic in Romanowsky stained preparations. Monocytes engulf and degrade microorganisms, abnormal cells, and cell debris. Monocytes also regulate immune responses and myelopoiesis.

The appearance of mammalian lymphocytes varies depending upon the species, lymphocyte type, and degree of activation. Mammalian lymphocytes vary in size, color of cytoplasm (light to dark blue), and degree of nuclear chromatin condensation. Variability depends on the degree of antigenic stimulation and type of lymphocyte.

A variety of factors can influence the total leukocyte and differential counts of small mammals. These include circadian rhythm (time of day the sample is collected), time of last feeding, breed, and gender. In general, the leukocyte morphology of nondomestic mammals is a reliable indication of disease. The presence of immature cells, toxic neutrophils, and Döhle bodies is more reliable criteria for infectious diseases than are total leukocyte and differential counts, given the amount of information known regarding various strains and breeds.

The blood films of small mammals contain high numbers of platelets that appear as irregular oval (2–3 µm diameter) cytoplasmic fragments with inner more darkly and concentric outer lighter staining regions.

Hematologic features of rodents

Mice (*Mus musculus*) and Rats (*Rattus norvegicus*)

Hematologic parameters of mice and rats are influenced by a variety of factors, including site of sample collection, age, gender, strain, anesthesia, method of restraint, temperature, and stress. In rats, collection of blood from the heart results in a significant decrease in the erythrocyte and leukocyte counts, hemoglobin concentration, and HCT compared to samples taken from the retro-orbital venous sinus and tail. A distinct circadian rhythm affects peripheral leukocyte concentrations with an increase in circulating leukocyte concentration occurring during the light phase and a decrease during the dark phase. A distinct decrease in the total leukocyte count associated with a decrease in lymphocytes occurs in mice following the stress, such as occurs during transportation. Thus, it is difficult to establish reference hematologic values for mice and rats because of the large number of strains and variations in blood collection methods, handling techniques, and environmental conditions.

Published reference intervals for several strains of rats and mice are available, and the reader should refer to the "Suggested Reading" section at the end of this chapter. Erythrocytes of healthy rats and mice vary in size with a range between 5 and 7 µm in diameter; therefore, a marked anisocytosis is common (Table 19.1). Polychromasia is also common, with polychromatic cells representing 1–18% of the erythrocyte population (Figures 19.1 and 19.2). This is likely related to the relative short erythrocyte half-life of 56–69 days for rats, 41–52 days for mice, 50–78 days for hamsters, and 10 days for the gerbil. Hibernation (pseudohibernation) in hamsters prolongs the life span of their erythrocytes, and the end of hibernation generally reveals an increase in reticulocyte numbers. Adult rats and mice normally have a high degree of reticulocytosis with means that average between 2 and 5%; the young have even higher numbers ranging between 10 and 20%. Neonatal gerbils have erythrocyte counts that are approximately one-half adult values but increase to adult values by about 8 weeks of age. Gerbils up to 20 weeks old have a large number of circulating reticulocytes and erythrocytes with basophilic stippling and polychromasia, but these cells are also abundant in older gerbils and are likely associated with the short erythrocyte life span. Erythrocyte concentrations in females tend to be less than those of males. The normal PCV is 39–54% for rats and 35–45% for mice. The hemoglobin concentration generally ranges between 13.4 and 15.8 g/dL with a mean of 14.6 g/dL. Howell-Jolly bodies and nucleated erythrocytes are found in small numbers of erythrocytes in normal rats and mice (Figure 19.1). Rouleaux formation of erythrocytes is rarely seen, even with inflammatory disease.

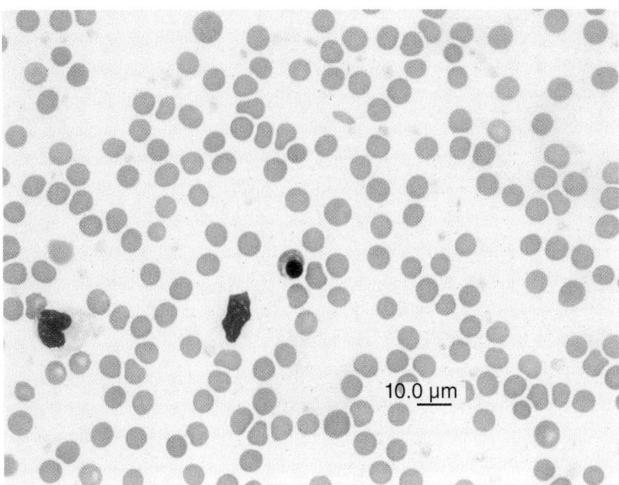

Figure 19.1 Polychromatic erythrocytes and a nucleated erythrocyte in the blood of a rat. Wright-Giemsa stain.

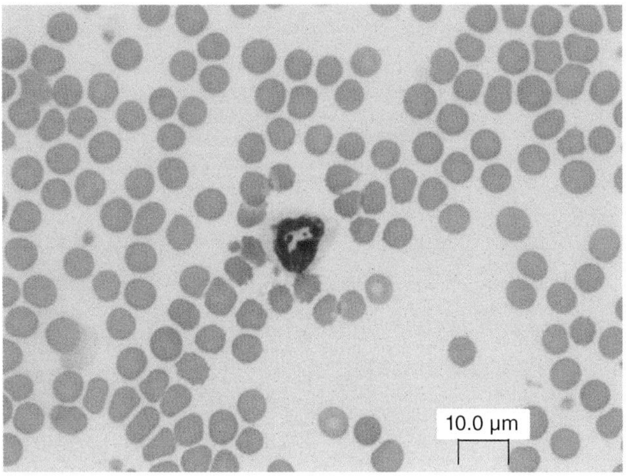

Figure 19.3 A neutrophil with a nucleus forming a ring in the blood of a mouse. Wright-Giemsa stain.

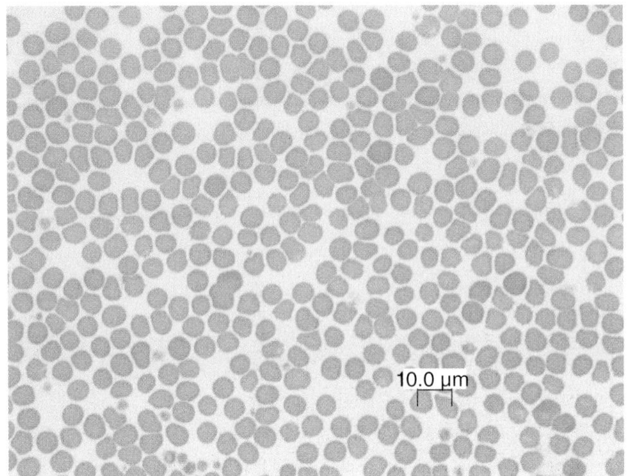

Figure 19.2 Polychromatic erythrocytes in the blood of a mouse. Wright-Giemsa stain.

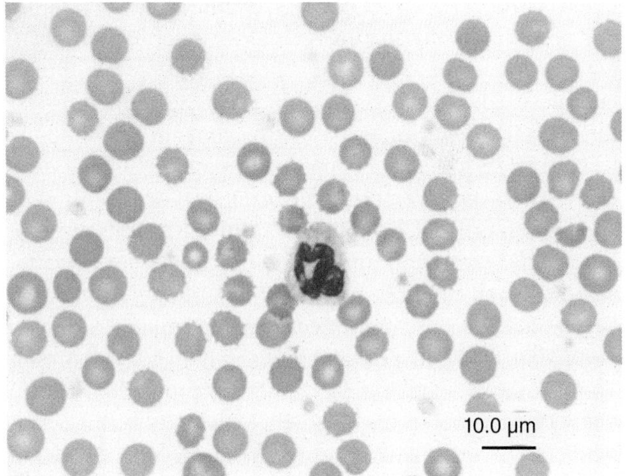

Figure 19.4 A neutrophil with fine, pink cytoplasmic granules in the blood of a rat. Wright-Giemsa stain.

Granulocytes of mice and rats often have nuclei without distinct lobes and typically have a horseshoe, sausage, or ring (doughnut) shape (Figures 19.3 and 19.5). The ring shape results from a gradually increasing hole that develops in the nucleus during maturation of the granulocyte. Nuclear segmentation occurs as the ring breaks during maturation and begins to form constrictions.

The nucleus of the neutrophil in rodents often has several indentations that result in a hypersegmentation. Band cells may be seen in normal animals, but this is usually seen in association with inflammation. Neutrophils with ring-shaped nuclei are considered to be associated with accelerated granulopoiesis. Neutrophils usually have a colorless cytoplasm but may contain a few dustlike red granules, thus appearing diffusely pink with Romanowsky stains (Figure 19.4). Hamster neutrophils (heterophils) have a lobed nucleus and dense pink cytoplasmic granules. Rat neutrophils measure 11 μm in diameter. In general, the neutrophil represents 12–38% of the leukocyte differential. Eosinophils have nuclei that are typically less segmented than those of neutrophils (often ring- or band-shaped), a basophilic cytoplasm, and numerous eosinophilic cytoplasmic granules that may be arranged in small clumps (Figure 19.5). In mice, eosinophils have large, round, nearly uniformly sized, reddish-brown to red granules with indistinct borders. In rats, eosinophils have small, round, reddish granules that fill the cytoplasm. In hamsters, the cytoplasm of eosinophils is tightly packed with rod-shaped azurophilic granules that create a narrow zone around the nucleus. Eosinophils generally compose 0–7% of the leukocyte differential. Basophils are present in small numbers (0–1%) and contain numerous basophilic granules. In rats, mice, and hamsters, basophils are rarely observed on peripheral

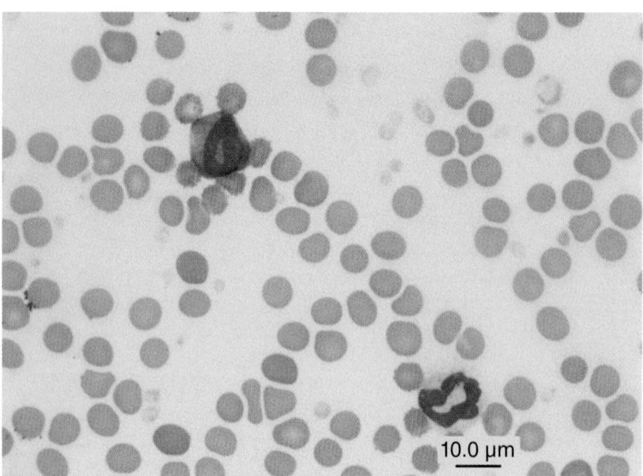

Figure 19.5 An eosinophil (cell on top) and a neutrophil each with a nucleus forming a ring in the blood of a rat. Wright-Giemsa stain.

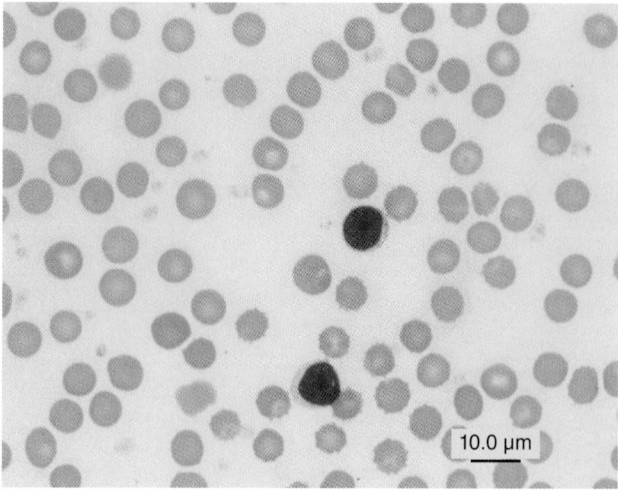

Figure 19.6 Lymphocytes in the blood of a rat. Wright-Giemsa stain.

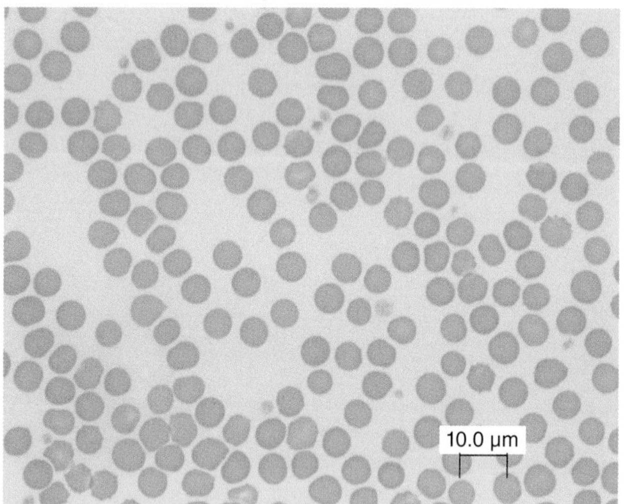

Figure 19.7 Numerous platelets in the blood film of a mouse. Wright-Giemsa stain.

blood smears. They lack tertiary granules but have larger and less numerous mature granules. Basophil nuclei are lobulated, and the cytoplasm contains large, round, purple granules that may be few in number or so numerous that they obscure the nucleus. Basophils should be differentiated from mast cells that may appear in peripheral blood, especially when cardiocentesis is performed. Basophil numbers appear higher in blood collected from the tail of mice and rats when excessive trauma is involved, such as laceration technique and compressing the tail to facilitate blood flow.

Lymphocytes are the predominant leukocyte in the peripheral blood of rats and mice, where they represent 60–75% and 70–80% of the leukocyte population, respectively (Figure 19.6). Likewise, lymphocytes comprise greater than 75% of the leukocyte population in the peripheral blood of hamsters and gerbils. The size of lymphocytes ranges from the size of erythrocytes to the size of neutrophils. The cytoplasm of lymphocytes stains light blue, and azurophilic cytoplasmic granules are occasionally found in large lymphocytes. The lymphocytes of hamsters are small round cells with a dark blue nucleus that fills most of the cell and is surrounded by a rim of lighter blue cytoplasm.

Monocytes (17 µm diameter) are the largest leukocyte found in the peripheral blood of rats and mice. They account for 1–6% of the leukocyte population in rats and 0–2% in mice. Monocytes have a variably shaped nucleus with the kidney-bean shape being the most common form. The abundant blue-gray cytoplasm often contains fine azurophilic granules and occasional vacuoles.

Leukocyte concentrations of mice and rats not only demonstrate a distinct diurnal variation but also vary markedly between strains; thus, lab results will vary by the time of day of blood sample collection and the strain. There is also an age-dependent variation in the neutrophil to lymphocyte ratio, with the lymphocyte concentration decreasing and neutrophil concentration increasing as a rodent ages. Acute stress in rats results in elevated serum corticosterone but with a normal neutrophil–lymphocyte ratio, whereas chronic stress (distress) yields the opposite – normal serum corticosterone concentrations with an elevated neutrophil–lymphocyte ratio.

Platelet concentrations in rodents tend to be high compared to those of larger domestic mammals (Figure 19.7). Platelet concentrations greater than 1×10^6 per µL are common.

Guinea pigs (*Cavia porcellus*)

Guinea pig erythrocytes are biconcave disks that, with a mean cell volume (MCV) of 84 fL, are larger in comparison to the erythrocytes of other common laboratory animal species. A moderate anisocytosis is common with cell widths ranging between 6.6 and 7.9 µm. The total erythrocyte

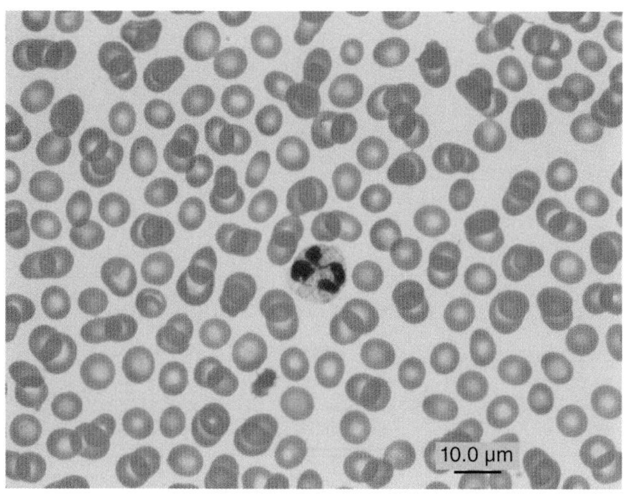

Figure 19.8 A neutrophil in the blood of a guinea pig. Wright-Giemsa stain.

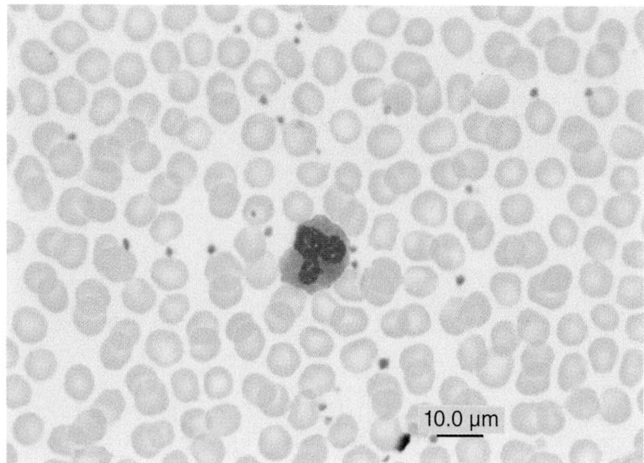

Figure 19.9 An eosinophil in the blood of a guinea pig. Wright-Giemsa stain.

count and the hemoglobin concentration of guinea pigs are generally lower than those of true rodents. Blood films from normal nonanemic guinea pigs exhibit polychromasia that varies with age: polychromatic erythrocytes may represent 25% of circulating erythrocytes in neonate, 4.5% in juvenile, and 1.5% in adult. Polychromasia and a macrocytosis characterize regenerative responses to anemia.

The neutrophils of guinea pigs measure 10–12 μm in diameter, have a pyknotic segmented nucleus, and contain pale cytoplasmic granules that stain eosinophilic that generally cause them to be referred to as heterophils or pseudoeosinophils (Figure 19.8). Although they stain differently than the neutrophils of domestic mammals with Romanowsky stains, the neutrophils of guinea pigs are equivalent in function. Guinea pig eosinophils (10–15 μm in diameter) are larger in size with less nuclear segmentation when compared to the neutrophils and have larger, rod-shaped (more pointed), bright red cytoplasmic granules, making eosinophils easy to differentiate from neutrophils (Figure 19.9). Basophils are slightly larger than heterophils, with a lobulated nucleus and many round variably sized reddish-purple to black cytoplasm granules (Figure 19.10).

Like those of rats and mice, lymphocytes are the predominant leukocyte in the differential of healthy guinea pigs, and small lymphocytes (approximately the size of erythrocytes) are the most common form. Large lymphocytes are almost twice as large as small lymphocytes, have a slightly smaller nucleus:cytoplasmic ratio, and often contain azurophilic granules. Approximately 3–4% of the lymphocytes or 1–2% of the total number of leukocytes in the peripheral blood of adult guinea pigs are large mononuclear cells that contain a single, large (1–8 μm wide) cytoplasmic inclusion referred to as a Kurloff body (Figure 19.11). These Foa-Kurloff cells are unique to cavies, such as guinea pigs, and are considered

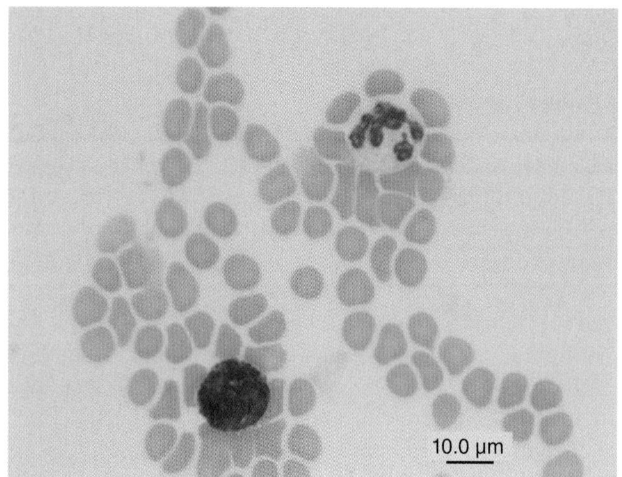

Figure 19.10 A basophil (cell on bottom) and neutrophil in the blood of a guinea pig. Wright-Giemsa stain.

to be of lymphoid cells. The finely granular and occasionally vacuolated Kurloff bodies stain homogeneously red with Romanowsky stains, and because they consist of a mucopolysaccharide, they stain positive with toluidine blue, periodic acid–Schiff, and Lendrum stains. Their numbers appear to be influenced by sex hormones and occur in low numbers in immature male guinea pigs. The exact origin and function of these cells is unknown, although it has been speculated that they may function as natural killer (NK) cells in the general circulation or as protectors of fetal antigen in the placenta because their numbers can increase under the influence of increased estrogens. Guinea pig monocytes are morphologically similar to those seen in common domestic mammals. They are large cells with an oval to amoeboid nucleus having loose lacy chromatin and an abundant gray-blue cytoplasm.

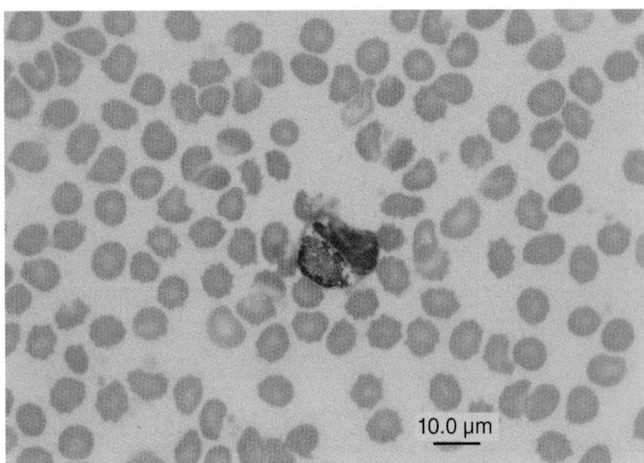

Figure 19.11 A lymphocyte containing a Kurloff body in the blood of a guinea pig. Wright-Giemsa stain.

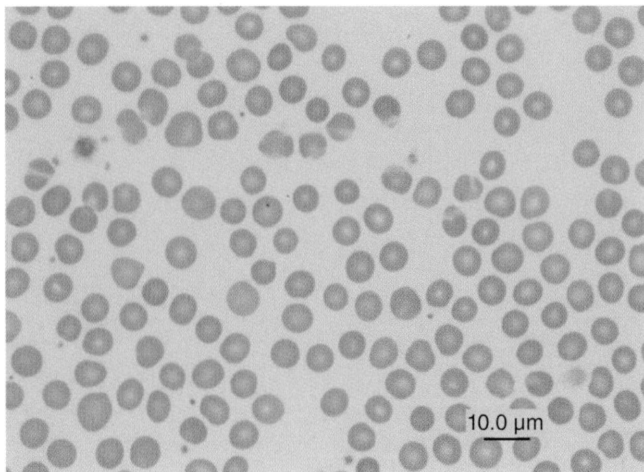

Figure 19.12 Erythrocytes in the blood of a rabbit. Wright-Giemsa stain.

Blood films of guinea pig contain large numbers of platelets. The normal platelet count ranges between 120 and 850/mm.

Other rodents

The hematologic features of hamsters (*M. auratus*), gerbils (*M. unguiculatus*), and chinchillas (*Chinchilla lanieger*) resemble those of mice and rats. As with rats and mice, polychromasia is a normal finding in blood film from hamsters and gerbils, and Howell-Jolly bodies are common. Nucleated red blood cells may account for up to 2% of the erythrocytes in blood films of normal hamsters. The neutrophils of chinchillas are typically hyposegmented and resemble neutrophils of dogs with the Pelger-Huet anomaly. Hamster neutrophils contain prominent round to rod-shaped eosinophilic cytoplasmic granules and are frequently referred to as heterophils. Lymphocytes are the predominate leukocyte in the differential of gerbils; however, a diurnal variation occurs in the numbers and types of leukocytes in the blood of hamsters. Leukocyte numbers of hamsters, a nocturnal animal, increase significantly at night when they are most active, with neutrophils rather than lymphocytes being responsible for the increase. Small and large lymphocytes are found in the blood of hamsters, but unlike other rodents, neutrophils tend to be the predominate leukocyte in the leukogram differential. Like the guinea pig, the chinchilla is normally lymphocytic; therefore, the hemic response in early inflammation often reveals an increase in heterophils and a decrease in lymphocytes with either a normal leukocyte count or a leukopenia.

Hematologic features of rabbits (*Oryctolagus cuniculus*)

The PCV of healthy rabbits generally ranges between 30 and 50%. The rabbit erythrocyte is a biconcave disk with an average diameter of 6.8 µm; however, the presence of erythrocytes with a range of 5.0–7.8 µm makes reporting of a significant anisocytosis a common finding in the hemogram of normal rabbits (Figure 19.12). Like rodents, polychromatic erythrocytes and reticulocytes are common in blood films of normal rabbits. Polychromasia is commonly observed in 2–4% of the erythrocyte population of normal rabbits. Nucleated erythrocytes and Howell-Jolly bodies are occasionally observed. The estimated half-life of rabbit erythrocytes is between 57 and 67 days. Male rabbits tend to have higher erythrocyte counts and hemoglobin concentrations than females. The total erythrocyte count, hemoglobin concentration, and HCT values can be significantly lower in pregnant rabbits in the third trimester compared to non-pregnant rabbits; however, the MCV value increases. Use of a general anesthetic does not appear to have an effect on the hematologic test results in rabbits. Erythrocyte fragility studies in rabbits based upon the sodium chloride concentrations indicate the first detectable hemolysis at 0.5–0.3% NaCl. As with most other species of mammals, a regenerative response to an anemia is characterized by increased anisocytosis, polychromasia, nucleated erythrocytes, and presence of Howell-Jolly bodies. Anemia is commonly associated with a variety of diseases in rabbits. Infectious diseases often result in increases in the number of nucleated erythrocytes.

Because the rabbit neutrophil contains small acidophilic granules and varying numbers of large red granules, it is generally referred to as a heterophil (or pseudoeosinophils in older literature). The smaller granules outnumber the larger granules by 80–90%. The rabbit neutrophil is between 10 and 15 µm in diameter. The polymorphic nucleus stains light blue to purple with Romanowsky stains. The cytoplasm of rabbit neutrophil typically stains diffusely pink with Romanowsky stains due to the fusion of the many small acidophilic granules (primary granules) (Figures 19.13 and 19.16). Rabbit neutrophils (heterophils) are ultrastructurally, functionally, and biochemically equivalent to neutrophils

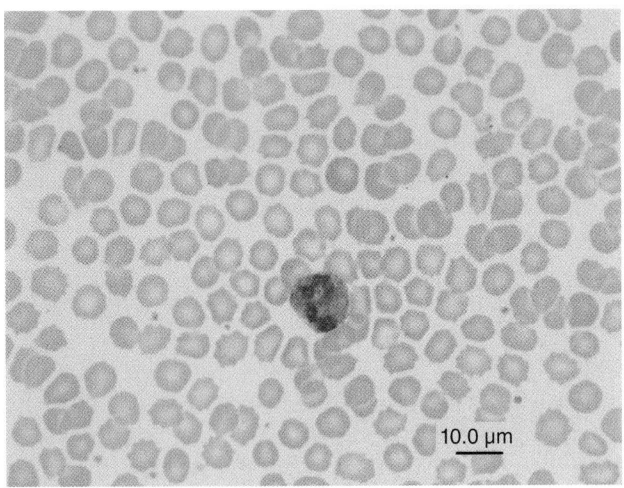

Figure 19.13 A neutrophil (heterophil) in the blood of a rabbit. Wright-Giemsa stain.

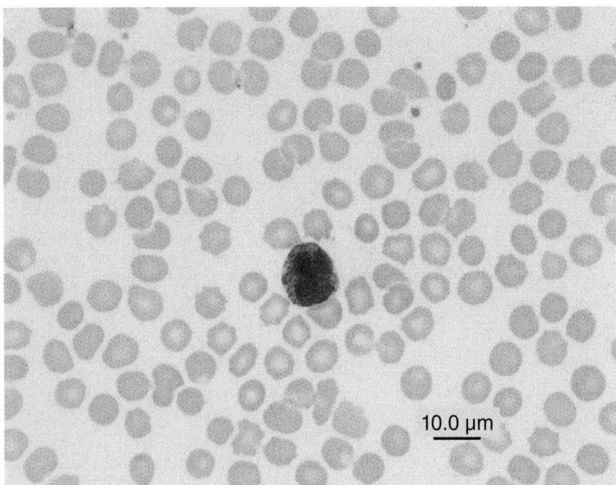

Figure 19.15 A basophil in the blood of a rabbit. Wright-Giemsa stain.

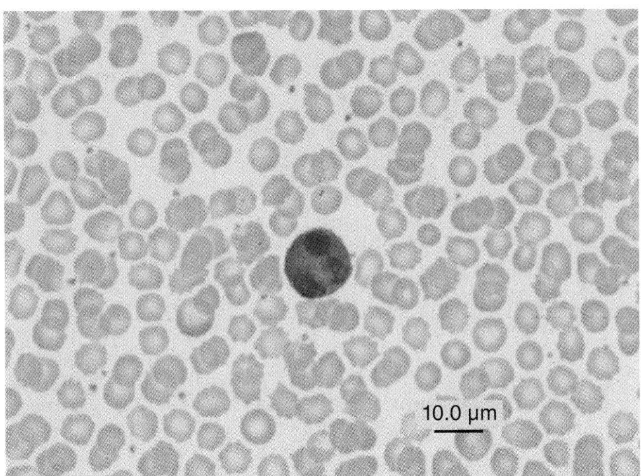

Figure 19.14 An eosinophil in the blood of a rabbit. Wright-Giemsa stain.

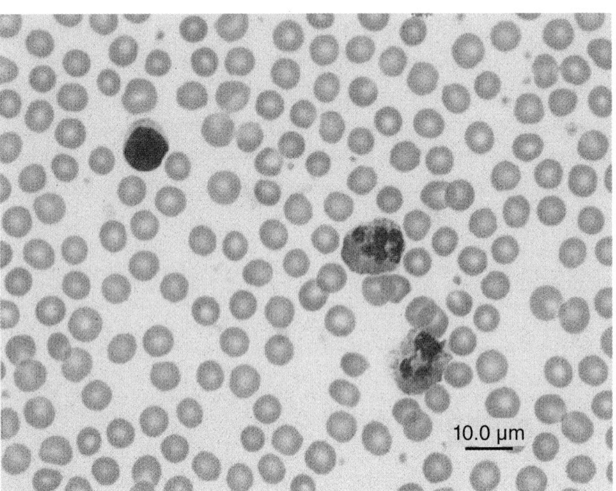

Figure 19.16 A lymphocyte and two neutrophils (heterophils) in the blood of a rabbit. Wright-Giemsa stain.

from other domestic mammals and humans. Occasional neutrophils with characteristics of the Pelger-Huet anomaly may be observed in blood films from normal rabbits. Rabbit neutrophils are easily distinguished from the eosinophils, which have large eosinophilic granules.

The eosinophils of rabbits are larger than the neutrophils and are between 12 and 16 μm in diameter (Figure 19.14). The large acidophilic cytoplasmic granules of the eosinophil are three to four times larger than those in the neutrophil and are more numerous in comparison, occupying much of the cytoplasm. Eosinophil granules are poorly defined and stain intensely pink to a dull pink-orange with Romanowsky stains, creating a tinctorial quality that differs from the neutrophil granules. The nucleus of the eosinophil is often bilobed to U-shaped. A low or absent eosinophil count is commonly observed in healthy rabbits.

Rabbits typically have more basophils than do other species; commonly 5% of the leukocytes are basophils, but they can be as high as 30% in rabbits with no apparent abnormalities. The rabbit basophil is about the same size as the rabbit neutrophil, and the purple to black metachromic cytoplasmic granules resemble those of basophils from other domestic mammals (Figure 19.15).

Rabbit lymphocytes are morphologically similar to those of other domestic mammals and humans. The majority of lymphocytes are small, between 7 and 10 μm in diameter; however, large lymphocytes between 10 and 15 μm in diameter may also be present (Figure 19.16). Azurophilic granules are often commonly present in the cytoplasm of the large lymphocytes.

Rabbit monocytes are similar to those found in other domestic mammals. The nucleus varies from lobulated to

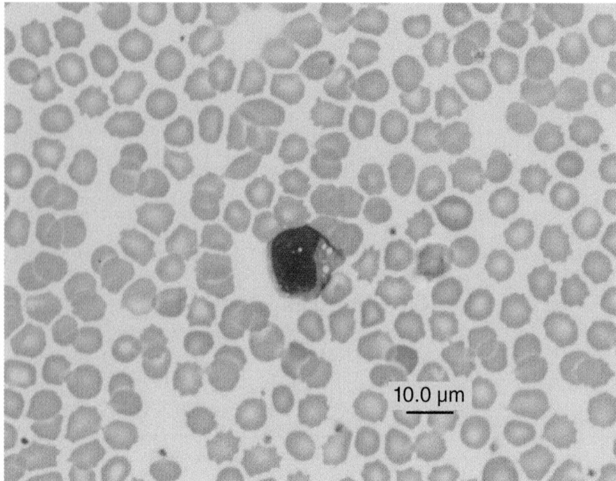

Figure 19.17 Monocytes in the blood of a rabbit. Wright-Giemsa stain.

bean-shaped, and the cytoplasm stains blue and may contain a few vacuoles (Figure 19.17).

The normal leukocyte concentration of rabbits is typically reported to range between 7000 and 9000/µL. Variations occur with age, restraint methods, methods of blood collection that may alter the neutrophil:lymphocyte (N:L) ratio, pregnancy, circadian rhythms (diurnal fluctuations and variation within a month), nutritional status and dietary differences, and differences in gender and breed. The number of circulating neutrophils is lower in the early morning and highest in the late afternoon and evening, and the opposite occurs with lymphocyte numbers. A bimodal increase in the leukocyte concentration is seen with increasing age, with highest lymphocyte concentration occurring at 3 months of age, then slowly declining, and highest neutrophil concentrations occurring in older animals. The normal neutrophil:lymphocyte ratio of 33 : 60 at 2 months of age changes to 45 : 45 by 12 months of age. Therefore, rabbits younger than 12 months of age are expected to have lower N:L ratios than do older rabbits, which typically have equal numbers of neutrophils and lymphocytes. A stress response associated with restraint during blood collection procedures can result in as much as a 15–30% decrease in the total leukocyte concentration. A mature neutrophilia and lymphopenia characterize glucocorticoid-mediated changes in the leukogram. Pregnant rabbits demonstrate a slight increase in total leukocyte counts during the first half of gestation, owing to an increase in lymphocyte numbers; however, a significant decrease can occur in the second half, owing to a decrease in lymphocytes and/or neutrophil numbers. Rabbits exposed to 28 °C (82.4 °F) for 1–3 hours are found to have an elevated PCV, lymphocytopenia, and leukocytosis.

Rabbits generally do not develop a leukocytosis with bacterial infections but will have a reversal of the N:L ratio; N:L ratio reversal is also associated with increases in serum cortisol concentrations. Therefore, evaluation of the N:L ratio appears to be the more reliable indicator of inflammatory disorders than are total leukocyte concentrations. Rabbits with acute infections may demonstrate a leukopenia with a normal leukocyte differential. Rabbits with septicemia and overwhelming bacterial infections often demonstrate a leukopenia with a degenerative left shift.

Rabbits presenting with an infectious disease do not typically have a higher white blood cell (WBC) count but rather have a shift from lymphocyte-predominant to neutrophil-predominant differential counts. Sometimes rabbits with acute infections may have a normal differential count but a decrease in total WBC count. Leukemias are infrequently reported in rabbits, usually presented as lymphoblastic leukemia. In cases of septicemia and in overwhelming bacterial infections, leucopenia with a degenerative left shift will be observed.

Rabbits with acute infectious processes commonly reveal a decrease in thrombocytes and an increase in nucleated erythrocytes.

Hematologic features of ferrets (*Mustela putorius*)

The hematology of ferrets resembles that of domestic carnivores. Ferrets are commonly anesthetized to restrain them for blood collection. The use of inhalant anesthetics such as isoflurane, enflurane, and halothane results in significant and rapid decreases in the RBC, HCT, and hemoglobin concentration. As much as a 33% decrease in the hemoglobin concentration occurs with the use of these inhalant anesthetics. Splenic sequestration and anesthetic-induced hypotension are possible causes for this response in ferrets. The erythron returns to normal within 45 minutes of recovery from the anesthetic. Either the use of manual restraint or injectable anesthesia such as ketamine or rapid blood collection following anesthetic induction (less than 3 minutes) is required to avoid this effect in the erythron.

Hematologic values of ferrets are similar to those of other domestic carnivores; however, the HCT, hemoglobin, and total erythrocyte and reticulocyte counts in ferrets are generally higher than those of domestic dogs or cats. The mean red blood cell diameter for ferrets is reported to range between 4.6 and 7.7 µm. The hemogram of domestic ferrets is influenced by gender and age. Young hobs (males) have lower RBCs, HCTs, and hemoglobin concentrations than adult hobs and young jills (females). Jills have a decrease in the HCT with age. The HCT of ferrets ranges between 30 and 61%, but usually averages between 40 and 50% for adult ferrets and between 32 and 39% for juvenile ferrets. The mean percentage of reticulocytes is reported to be 4%

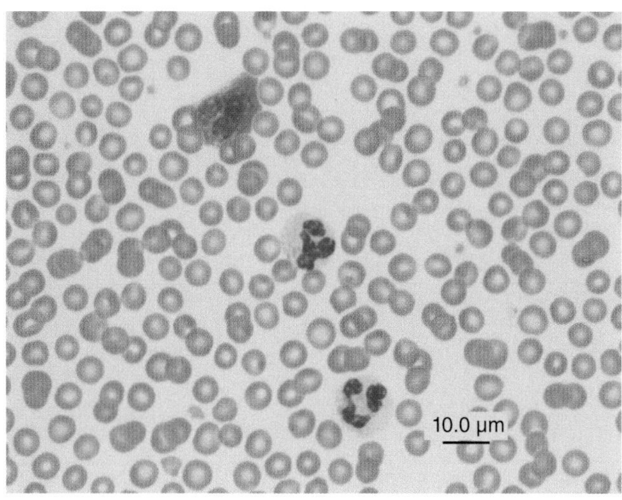

Figure 19.18 Two neutrophils and an eosinophil (cell on top) in the blood of a ferret. Wright-Giemsa stain.

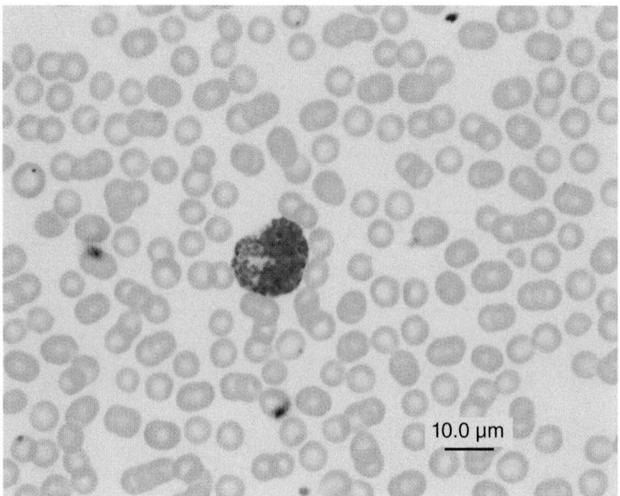

Figure 19.19 A basophil in the blood of a ferret. Wright-Giemsa stain.

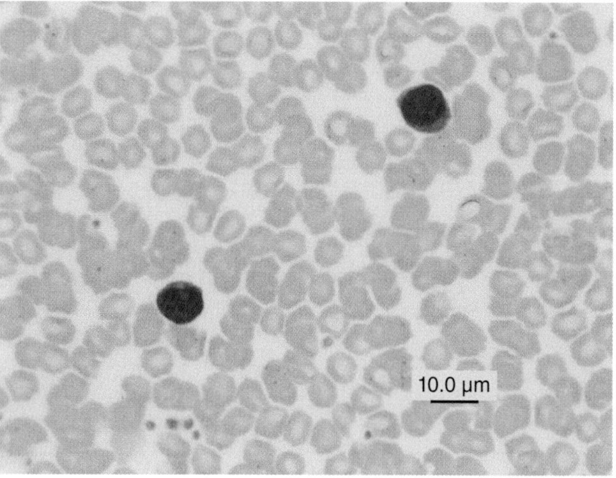

Figure 19.20 Lymphocytes in the blood of a ferret. Wright-Giemsa stain.

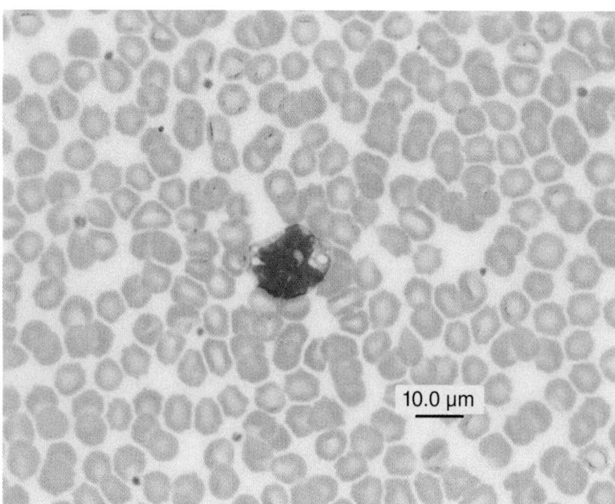

Figure 19.21 A monocyte in the blood of a ferret. Wright-Giemsa stain.

(range of 1–12%) in male ferrets and 5.3% (range of 2–14%) in female ferrets.

The morphology of ferret leukocytes is similar to that of dogs (Figures 19.18–19.21). The neutrophil is the predominant leukocyte in the peripheral blood of ferrets. The ranges in size for the various ferret granulocytes are 10–13 μm for neutrophils in males and 9–10 μm in females; and 12 and 14 μm for eosinophils and basophils, respectively, regardless of gender. The size of small lymphocytes ranges between 6 and 9 μm in male ferrets and 8 and 10 μm in females. Large lymphocytes and monocytes measure 11–12 μm and 12–18 μm in both sexes, respectively. Neutrophil concentrations are higher than lymphocyte concentrations in normal ferrets. Ferrets have an increase in neutrophil concentration and decrease in lymphocyte concentration with increasing age. The total leukocyte count of healthy ferrets can be as low as 3000/μL. In general, ferrets are unable to develop a marked leukocytosis with inflammatory disease, and concentrations greater than 20,000/μL are unusual and a left shift is rare.

Results of coagulation studies in ferrets vary depending upon methodology. For example, a significant prothrombin time was obtained using a manual method (12.3 ± 0.3 seconds) compared to an automated method (10.9 ± 0.3 seconds). Activated partial thromboplastin time; however was not significantly different between the two methods (18.7 ± 0.9 for the manual method and 18.1 ± 1.1 seconds for the automated method). Fibrinogen concentration for ferrets is reported as 107.4 ± 19.8 mg/dL and antithrombin activity is 96 ± 12.7%.

Common causes of nonregenerative anemia in domestic ferrets include malignant neoplasia such as lymphoma, systemic infections, and hyperestrogenism in intact females

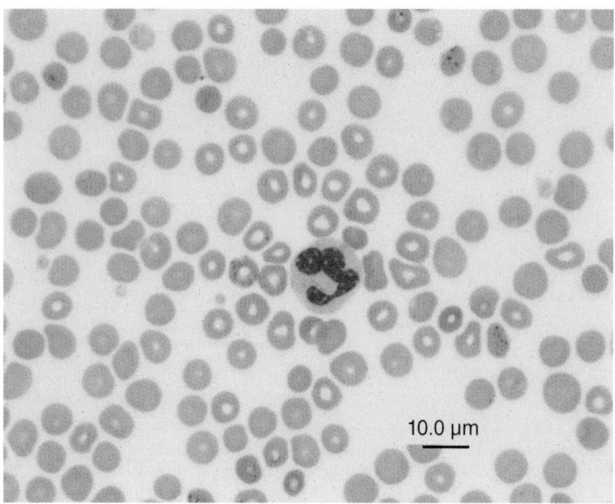

Figure 19.22 A neutrophil in the blood of a hedgehog. Wright-Giemsa stain.

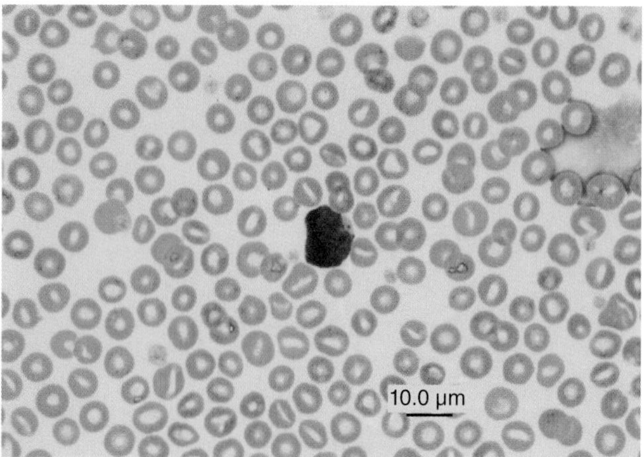

Figure 19.24 A basophil in the blood of a hedgehog. Wright-Giemsa stain.

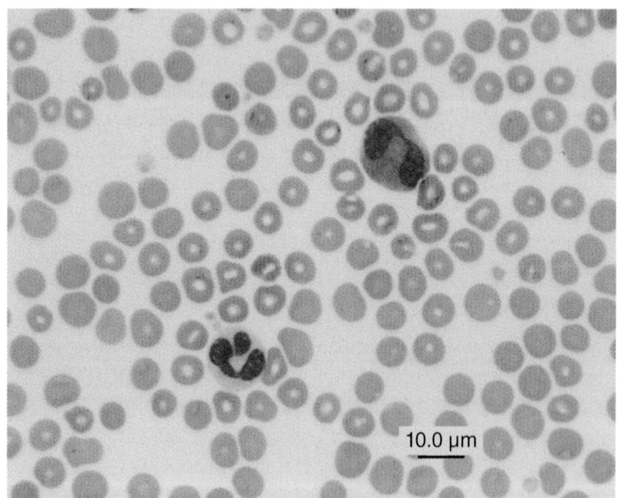

Figure 19.23 A neutrophil and eosinophil (cell on top) in the blood of a hedgehog. Wright-Giemsa stain.

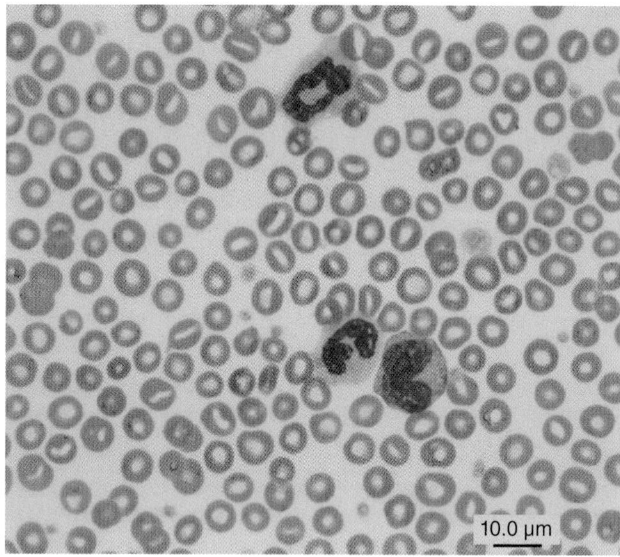

Figure 19.25 A neutrophil and monocyte (cell on the right) in the blood of a hedgehog. Wright-Giemsa stain.

(jills). Because jills are induced ovulators, an individual who does not breed during estrus may exhibit prolonged estrus throughout the breeding season. After a month of prolonged estrus, high levels of estrogen in the bloodstream may cause bone marrow suppression with leukopenia, thrombocytopenia, and aplastic anemia as indicated by a decrease in the PCV and total erythrocyte count. Jills in estrus with a PCV between 15 and 25% are given a guarded prognosis and those less than 15% a grave prognosis. Gastrointestinal ulcers are a common cause of blood loss anemia. Polychromasia is indicative of bone marrow erythroid hyperplasia in response to anemia.

Hematologic features of African hedgehogs (*Atelerix albiventris*)

The hematology of African hedgehogs resembles that of domestic carnivores (Figures 19.22–19.26). The morphology of erythrocytes and leukocytes is similar to that of other small mammals. Likewise, interpretation of changes in the hemogram is based upon those same changes in other small mammals.

Hematologic features of primates

The mature erythrocytes of primates are biconcave discs of approximately 7.5 μm in diameter. The red blood cell

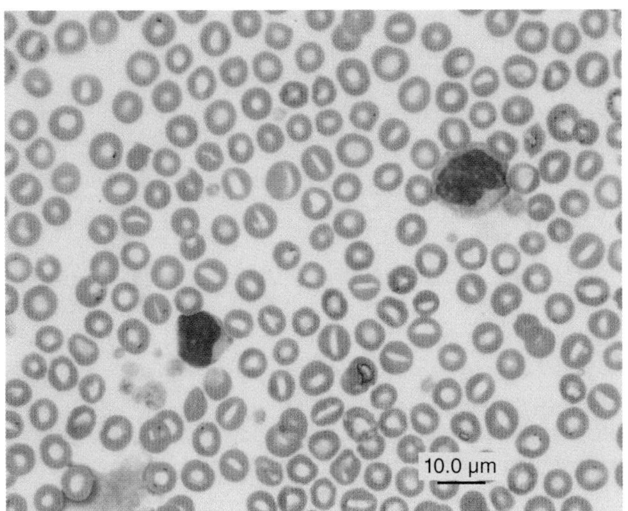

Figure 19.26 A lymphocyte (cell on the left) and monocyte in the blood of a hedgehog. Wright-Giemsa stain.

parameters of primates vary with age and gender. Neonates have higher total erythrocyte concentration, hemoglobin concentration, and PCV compared to adults. The erythron rapidly decreases as animals become subadults but then increases after puberty. Adult male primates have a higher erythrocyte concentration, hemoglobin concentration, and PCV compared with adult female primates. The reticulocyte concentration of most normal primates is less than 2.0%. Small numbers of Howell-Jolly bodies may be seen in the blood films from primates. Erythrocyte Rouleaux formation occurs with inflammatory disease.

Excitement and exertion associated with capture and restraint produce splenic contraction and a corresponding increase in the PCV. Use of an anesthetic (e.g., ketamine) reduces this effect.

Neutrophils of some primates, such as orangutans (*Pongo pygmaeus*), have very small eosinophilic granules, whereas those of others, such as chimpanzees (*Pan* sp.), have very small basophilic granules. Lymphocytosis, which is associated with restraint-related epinephrine release, can be prevented with use of ketamine anesthesia. Occasional binucleated lymphocytes are found in the blood of normal primates.

Leukocyte concentrations as great as 15,000 cells/μL are more typical of nonexcited primates; however, concentrations as great as 30,000 cells/μL can occur with excitement. An increased number of immature neutrophils (i.e., band cells) is indicative of inflammation. Most species demonstrate toxic neutrophils with inflammation associated with infections, and some species, such as rhesus monkeys (*Macaca mulatta*) and orangutans commonly exhibit neutrophil toxicity in the form of Döhle bodies. A marked, transient leukocytosis with lymphocytosis occurs in primates in response to antigenic challenges (e.g., adenovirus infection). Leukemia associated with high concentrations of large lymphocytes often has a viral etiology, such as *Herpesvirus saimiri* and RNA oncornavirus infection.

Blood parasites, including microfilaria and trypanosomes, commonly are present in wild-caught primates, especially New World monkeys. These parasites have a low virulence, however, and generally are considered to be an incidental finding. Plasmodium gametocytes and schizonts often appear as incidental findings in the erythrocytes of asymptomatic wild-caught primates. Gametocytes of *Hepatocystis*, which is a mildly pathogenic parasite, may be seen in the blood films of some African monkeys.

Hematologic features of minipigs

The hemograms of minipigs (e.g., pot-bellied pigs) do not vary significantly from those of domestic pigs. Therefore, hematologic studies of minipigs are interpreted in the same manner as those of domestic pigs. Erythrocyte spiculation, which is characterized by sharp, pointed projections from the cells, is common in the blood film of normal minipigs.

The neutrophils of pigs have irregularly stained nuclei with irregular margins, and they often are coiled and lack complete lobation. The cytoplasm of porcine neutrophils contains small, pink granules with Romanowsky stains. Porcine eosinophils have round to oval, orange cytoplasmic granules. The nucleus often appears to be a band. Normal minipigs have total leukocyte concentrations as great as 22,000 cells/μL because of the excitement leukocytosis associated with handling for blood collection. The lymphocyte concentration is greater than the neutrophil concentration in healthy pigs. Physiologic leukocytosis results from a transient neutrophilia and lymphocytosis. Minipigs, like other animals with low N:L ratios mount a lower leukocyte response than animals with high N:L ratios with inflammatory diseases; they may show only a reversal of the N:L ratio with mild inflammatory diseases. Marked neutrophilia is associated with more severe inflammatory diseases.

Hematologic features of camelids

The hematology of camelids, including camels, alpaca, and llamas, is similar to that of other mammals, except for the presence of numerous small, thin, flat, elliptical erythrocytes. Because the oval camelid erythrocytes are not biconcave discs as observed in most mammals, they lack central pallor. The flat contour lends them to a folding artifact. A few erythrocytes may contain rhomboid or hexagonal hemoglobin crystals, an intriguing but idiopathic and apparently nonpathogenic phenomenon. Camelids adapted to living at high altitudes, such as llamas, have erythrocytes that function at low atmospheric oxygen tension without the development of polycythemia and dissociated high blood viscosity. The elliptical shape may allow for easier passage through the capillaries, and the thin, flat contour allows for rapid gas exchange. Camelid erythrocytes are small in volume, and their numbers are significantly more numerous than those of most mammalian erythrocytes, with an upper limit of normal that approaches 18 million/μL. Although camelids have high erythrocyte concentrations, their small size results in relatively small PCVs. Healthy llamas have small MCV, ranging between 20 and 30 fL, and a relatively high mean cell hemoglobin concentration ranging between 40 and 45 g/dL. Camelid erythrocytes are more resistant to hemolysis in hypotonic saline than those of other mammals.

Because erythrocyte concentration of camelid blood is often two to three times that of common domestic species, blood samples from these animals must be properly diluted to avoid analytical error when using impedance – or flow cytometry – methods for cell counting. Counting errors in these hematologic analyzers occur when cells pass through the aperture or in front of the laser in pairs rather than singly, causing the two small cells passing through the measuring device to be counted as one large cell. In addition, sizing thresholds may not be set sufficiently low enough to capture the smallest cells of the erythrocyte population; therefore, the instrument may report erroneously low erythrocyte counts with an accurate hemoglobin concentration. When this occurs, a physiologically impossible high mean corpuscular hemoglobin concentration (MCHC) will be reported, indicating instrument error if hemolysis and lipemia are not the cause. Published quality control guidelines are available to ensure the instrument is providing accurate results and the veterinarian is provided with reliable data.

The reticulocyte count in healthy camelid blood is low (less than 1 per 1000× field); however, when exposed to altitudes of 14,000 ft or higher, the number of reticulocytes may represent 1.5% of the erythrocyte population. They appear polychromatophilic with Romanowsky-type stains and are larger and plumper than the mature cells. The polychromatic nucleated erythrocytes (nRBCs), which are occasionally observed in healthy camelids, appear more rounded than more mature polychromatophilic erythrocytes and have a rounded nucleus.

Hypochromic, macrocytic anemia with or without evidence of regeneration may be associated with iron deficiency, chronic inflammation, endo- and ectoparasitism, and copper deficiency. An increase in the number of folded cells and microcytosis is suggestive of chronic iron deficiency. Morphologic erythrocyte irregularities such as dacryocytes (teardrop-shaped cells), spindloid cells, and irregular hemoglobin distribution may also be observed with iron deficiency but can also occur with anemia from other pathogeneses. Maple leaf toxicity resulting in Heinz body–related hemolytic anemia can occur with maple leaf toxicity in camelids. *Mycoplasma haemolamae* (previously known as *Eperythrozoon*) is identified under high-resolution light microscopy as a small rod or circular structure on the surface of the erythrocyte. Because this bacterium will fall off the cells within a few hours after collection, examination of freshly prepared films is crucial.

A reliable nucleated cell count (NCC), which includes neutrophils, lymphocytes, and nRBCs, can be obtained from most automated methods, which are preferred over manual methods for accuracy, precision, and reduced technical time. Eosinophil concentrations tend to run higher in camelids than many mammals, and when sufficiently high enough, they may also be accurately counted by automated methods. As a general rule of thumb, monocytes and basophils are present in proportions too low to be accurately measured, but this variability is rarely clinically significant. A quick scan of a blood film can assess whether automated differentials appear reasonable. Camelid neutrophils, lymphocytes, monocytes, eosinophils, and basophils resemble those of most other mammals on Romanowsky-stained blood films. Healthy camelids tend to have small, intermediate, and large lymphocytes that are represented by a relatively high proportion with granulated cytoplasm (most noticeable with the alcohol-based Romanowsky stains). Camelid eosinophils typically have hyposegmented nuclei.

Like many animals, young camelids tend to have higher lymphocyte counts as compared to adults. Also, a mature neutrophilia and lymphopenia is consistent with stress (an eosinopenia may also be present). A neutrophilia with a left shift is indicative of inflammation, often with the presence of toxic changes within neutrophils (indicating accelerated bone marrow production and shortened maturation time) and hyperfibrinogenemia.

Because camelid platelets tend to be smaller and more numerous than other mammalian species, some automated analyzers may not recognize them and report erroneously low results. Therefore, a semiquantitative (e.g., low or adequate) estimate from the blood film is often used in reporting platelet numbers.

Hematologic features of deer

Erythrocytes in most species of normal deer exhibit *in vitro* sickling. The erythrocytes circulate as round cells, but sickling occurs during preparation of blood films after blood collection. Sickling occurs when the cells are exposed to oxygen and also appears to be affected by pH. Nearly all erythrocytes sickle at a pH of 7.4. Sickling can be prevented, however, by acidifying the blood. Sickled cells appear as crescent, holly leaf, matchstick, and burr shapes depending on the hemoglobin variant. Deer blood contains several hemoglobin types that polymerize or crystallize in the oxygenated state, thereby leading to sickle cell formation.

Excitement and stress during restraint result in high erythrocyte and leukocyte counts. Male deer have higher PCVs and erythrocyte counts compared with female deer. Erythrocytes in deer exhibit a high degree of Rouleaux formation with inflammatory disease.

Lymphocytes are the predominant leukocyte in normal deer. During the rutting period, male deer have higher neutrophil concentration compared with female deer.

20 Hematology of Birds

Terry W. Campbell

Department of Clinical Sciences, College of Veterinary Medicine and Biomedical Sciences, Colorado State University, Fort Collins, CO, USA

The original hematology studies in birds were based on Galliformes, such as chickens and turkeys, as the animal model; however, since that time, the majority of information concerning the hematology parameters of birds are based primarily on psittacines and raptors, two groups of birds most commonly presented to veterinarians in clinical practice. The normal values for the hematologic parameters of each species of bird have a broad range because of the influences of various intrinsic and extrinsic factors. In general, avian hematological values are subject to extensive variability resulting from different environment and management practices, which can affect physiological responses. For example, heterophil numbers are altered by seasonal changes, diurnal rhythm, gender and age, and diet. Normal hematologic values vary between the species as well. The different avian species from which blood samples are submitted to veterinary laboratories creates a significant logistical challenge to the development of clinically relevant normal values. Thus, published references should only be used as guidelines.

Avian hematology is approached in a manner similar to that of human and mammalian hematology, but a few differences require modification of the hematologic procedures. Major differences include the presence of nucleated erythrocytes, thrombocytes, and heterophil granulocytes in the peripheral blood of birds.

Collection and handling of blood samples

Blood collection should be performed safely and quickly. The stress associated with the capture and restraint of the avian patient, especially those that are ill or those not accustomed to being handled, can further compromise the health of the patient and may affect the hematologic indices. Proper restraint of birds has been previously described in other texts and is not discussed in complete detail. Many birds can be physically restrained without anesthesia for venipuncture. Cloth towels may be used to restrain most of the common pet psittacine and passerine birds. Birds should be held in an upright position or parallel to the floor and should not be held upside down because this may compromise their respiration. Birds must be able to move the keel (sternum) in order to breathe; therefore, excessive restraint around the body should be avoided to prevent asphyxiation. The wings and legs should be supported during the process of blood collection to prevent injury to those limbs. Many birds become tractable when the head is covered to reduce vision using a snug-fitting lightweight cloth or hood (birds used for falconry or those in raptor rehabilitation facilities often have properly fitting leather hoods available). Proper restraint of the avian patient should be safe for both the bird and the handler. Some species of birds are capable of inflicting serious injury to the handler. The talons of raptors and the spurs of Galliformes can injure handlers, so care should be taken to properly and safely restrain the legs of these birds during venipuncture. The beak of many birds can also serve as a weapon; therefore, proper restraint of the head is required to protect the handlers. Large birds, such as ratites, are especially dangerous as their kicks are potentially lethal to the handlers.

The amount of blood that can be safely removed from a bird depends on its body size and health status. A blood volume representing 1% or less of body weight usually can be withdrawn from healthy birds without detrimental effects. For example; a healthy, 80 g cockatiel (*Nymphicus hollandicus*) can easily tolerate removal of a 0.8 mL blood sample. The sample size taken from severely ill birds, however, must be reduced. For routine hematologic evaluations in birds, a sample size of 0.2 mL usually is adequate. A variety of collection methods have been used to obtain blood from birds, and the method chosen depends on the size of the bird, peculiarities of the species, preference of the collector, volume of blood needed, and physical condition of the patient.

Venous blood provides the best sample for hematologic studies. Blood collected from capillary beds (i.e., clipping of a toenail) usually results in abnormal cell distributions and contains both cells and other substances not found in

Veterinary Hematology, Clinical Chemistry, and Cytology, Third Edition. Edited by Mary Anna Thrall, Glade Weiser, Robin W. Allison and Terry W. Campbell.

Companion website: www.wiley.com/go/thrall/veterinary

venous blood, such as tissue fluid, macrophages, and cellular debris. Veins commonly used for venipuncture include the jugular, basilic (cutaneous ulnar, wing, or brachial), and medial metatarsal (caudal tibial). Blood can be collected using a needle and syringe when performing venipuncture on the jugular or other large veins. A short (1 in. or smaller) 25–22-G needle attached to a 3–6 mL syringe commonly is used for jugular venipuncture. A needle with an extension tube, such as a butterfly catheter (Abbott Hospitals, North Chicago, IL), aids in stabilization of the needle during sample collection. Blood also can be collected after venipuncture by allowing it to flow through the needle and drip into a microcollection device. Collecting blood by allowing it to flow through the needle, rather than by aspirating it into a syringe, minimizes hematoma formation. A variety of these devices (Microtainer tubes, Becton-Dickinson, Rutherford, NJ) are available. Microcollection tubes containing ethylenediaminetetraacetic acid (EDTA) are available for hematologic studies, but they also are available as plain tubes, with or without a serum separator, and as tubes containing heparin (lithium heparin is preferred) for studies of blood chemistry.

Jugular venipuncture most commonly is used for collecting blood from birds, because most small birds do not have other veins that are large enough for venipuncture. The right jugular vein is the vein of choice for this procedure, because it either is the only jugular vein present or is the larger of the two jugular veins. The jugular vein tends to be highly movable and is surrounded by a large subcutaneous space that predisposes it to hematoma formation during venipuncture. Therefore, the jugular vein must be stabilized before attempting venipuncture. Following adequate restraint, extend the bird's head and neck to allow the jugular vein to fall into the jugular furrow along the lateral side of the neck (Figure 20.1). Lightly wet the feathers with alcohol to expose the featherless tract (apterium) that overlies the jugular furrow. With a few exceptions (pigeons and doves), the jugular vein is visible through the thin skin on the neck. Pressure should be applied to the jugular vein just cranial to the thoracic inlet to occlude and distend the vein, which will facilitate the blood-collection process. Jugular venipuncture should be performed using an appropriate-sized needle and syringe because the large flow rate and the volume of blood present make it difficult to collect blood as it flows from a needle alone. Introduce the needle into the vein and collect the blood sample by applying only enough negative pressure on the syringe to allow blood to enter the syringe. More vigorous aspiration will cause collapse of the vein, promote hematoma formation of the vessel, and may cause hemolysis of the sample. Collection of blood with vacuum tubes is not recommended because of the excessive negative pressure that occurs.

The basilic (cutaneous ulnar, wing, or brachial) vein is a blood collection site that may be used in medium to large birds. This method of blood collection will require

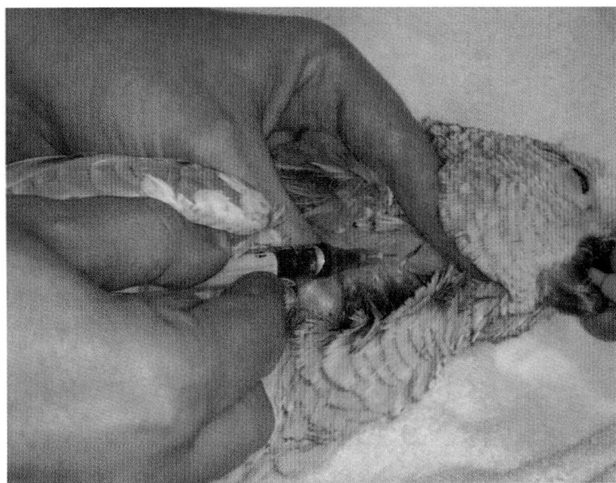

Figure 20.1 Jugular venipuncture in a parrot (*Amazona* sp.).

an assistant to restrain the bird and to apply pressure to the humeral area in order to occlude the vein, because proper restraint is crucial to prevent wing movement and hematoma formation. Typically, the bird is restrained in dorsal recumbency. One wing is then stretched away from the bird's body, with the elbow almost fully extended. Anesthesia may be required to facilitate restraint because many birds (i.e., psittacine birds) will struggle during this procedure. The basilic vein crosses the ventral surface of the humeral-radioulnar joint (elbow) directly beneath the skin and is easily visualized by wetting the area lightly with alcohol. Using an appropriate-sized needle, blood can be collected following cannulation of this vein either by aspiration into a syringe or by allowing the blood to drip from the needle hub into a microcollection tube (Figure 20.2). To prevent needle movement while aspirating blood into a syringe, the needle can be stabilized by the phlebotomist. This is accomplished by placing the index finger of the free hand alongside the ulna where the basilic vein crosses the elbow. The needle can then be supported as it rests on top of the index finger while it is guided into the vein. If necessary, additional support can be provided by placing the thumb of the free hand on top of the needle. A needle with an extension tube may also minimize needle movement when using a syringe. Hematoma formation is the most common complication associated with this procedure because of movement of the wing or the needle following venipuncture.

Venipuncture of the medial metatarsal (caudal tibial) vein is another common blood-collection method in medium to large birds. The medial metatarsal vein is located on the caudo-medial aspect of the tibiotarsus just above the tibiotarsus-tarsometatarsal joint and often hides beneath the calcaneal tendon. To access this vein, the bird should be restrained in dorsal or lateral recumbency, with the leg extended. Once the leg is extended and stabilized, a needle

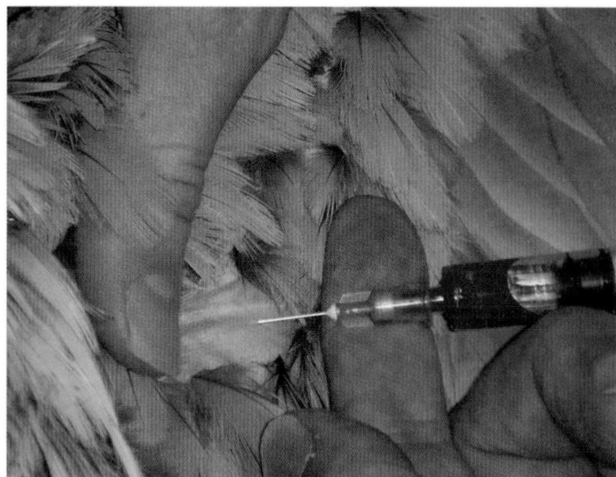

Figure 20.2 Blood collection from the basilic vein in a parrot (*Amazona* sp).

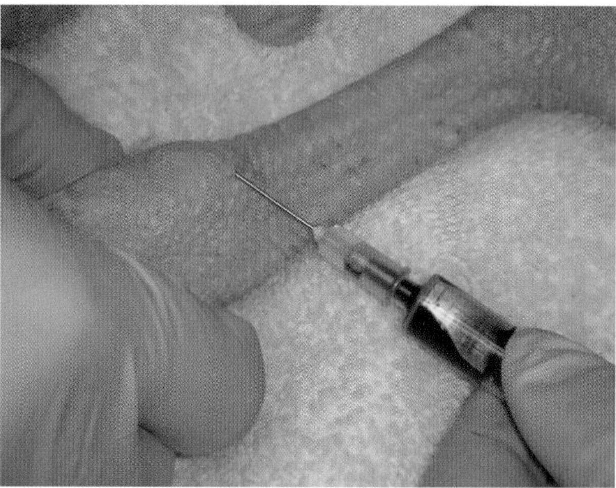

Figure 20.3 Blood collection from the medial metatarsal vein in a turkey poult (*Meleagris gallopavo*).

is introduced into the medial metatarsal vein at a shallow angle. Blood can be collected by aspiration into a syringe or by allowing blood to drip from the needle hub into a collection tube. Compared to venipuncture of the jugular and basilic veins, hematoma formation is typically minimal following venipuncture at this site because the leg is relatively easy to restrain, and the vein is protected by the surrounding muscles of the leg (Figure 20.3).

Clipping the toenail and lancet wounding are two other methods of blood collection, but these should be reserved for very small birds or for when attempts at venipuncture have failed. After alcohol cleansing, the toenail is clipped until blood flows freely for collection into a microcollection tube. After blood collection from the cut nail, hemostasis is accomplished by applying a hemostatic agent such as silver nitrate or ferrous subsulfate. Blood collection by this technique yields a poor sample for hematologic studies, however, because the blood is from the capillary bed and usually contains microclots, which interfere with cell counts. Capillary blood is also frequently contaminated with tissue fluid that affects hematologic data. Toenail clipping may result in temporary lameness because of nail damage. An alternative to nail clipping for blood collection from small birds is to collect blood after lancet wounding of vascular structures, such as the cutaneous ulnar vein, medial metatarsal vein, or external thoracic vein. After alcohol cleansing of the skin overlying the vein, the vessel is punctured through the skin using a lancet (i.e., needle), and the blood is allowed to drip into a microcollection tube.

Large volumes of blood can be collected from birds by cardiac puncture or occipital venous sinus puncture. These procedures are potentially dangerous, however, and should be reserved for birds that are used for research or are to be euthanized. Cardiac puncture can be performed using an anterior or a lateral approach. The heart is approached anteriorly by inserting a needle along the ventral floor of the thoracic inlet with the bird in dorsal recumbency. Care should be taken to avoid the ingluvies (crop) in some avian species. The needle is inserted near the "V" that is formed by the furcula, and it is directed toward the bird's dorsum and caudal toward the heart. Once the heart is penetrated, the vibration can be felt to ensure proper needle placement, and blood is then aspirated. In Galliforme birds, the heart can be approached laterally by inserting the needle in the fourth intercostal space near the sternum (keel) with the bird held in lateral recumbency. This approach, however, may vary with the species.

Blood collection from the occipital venous sinus requires use of evacuated glass tubes with appropriate needles and needle holders. The occipital venous sinus is located at the junction of the dorsal base of the skull and the first cervical vertebra, and it can be located by palpation while holding the bird's head firmly flexed and positioned in a straight line with the cervical vertebrae. A needle is inserted through the skin at a 30°–40° angle to the vertebrae. As soon as the needle penetrates the skin, the rubber stopper of the evacuated tube is perforated gently and the needle advanced until the sinus is reached. Penetration of the sinus results in a rapid flow of blood into the tube. Blood collection by puncture of either the heart or the occipital venous sinus requires proper restraint and technique to avoid permanent damage to the heart or brainstem – and even possible death of the patient.

The method of storage and handling of blood samples can have a significant influence on the hematological results. Blood samples collected without use of an anticoagulant require immediate processing. Dilutions for cell counting and preparation for blood films must be quickly performed with such samples. Because of the urgency for rapid processing of nonanticoagulated blood, most avian blood samples are collected into tubes containing an anticoagulant. EDTA, heparin, and sodium citrate are commonly used, and each has both advantages and disadvantages. The anticoagulant of choice for avian hematology is EDTA, because it allows for proper staining of cells and does not tend to clump leukocytes. Hematologic testing, however, should be performed soon after blood collection to avoid artifacts, such as increased cell smudging, which is created by prolonged exposure to any anticoagulant. Excessive liquid anticoagulants dilute the blood sample, thereby resulting in artifactually decreased hematocrit and total cell concentrations, and excessive dry anticoagulants may cause shrinkage of red blood cells, thus affecting the hematocrit. Blood from certain avian groups, such as crows and jays, may show incomplete anticoagulation or partial hemolysis when collected in EDTA. Heparin has the advantage of providing anticoagulated blood for hematology and plasma for evaluations of blood chemistry. Heparinized blood, however, may result in improper staining of cells, thereby resulting in erroneous leukocyte counts and poor cellular morphology in stained blood films. Heparin also causes clumping of leukocytes and thrombocytes and resultant inaccurate cell counts. A 3.8% sodium citrate solution, used in a ratio of one part citrate solution to nine parts blood, is the anticoagulant of choice for coagulation studies; however, it should not be used for other hematologic evaluations. Consistent use of the same anticoagulant is an important consideration with serial evaluation of the hemogram in the avian patient. For example, it has been demonstrated that although most hematologic parameters are in agreement between blood samples collected into heparin and EDTA, plasma protein and the packed cell volume (PCV) are significantly lower and lymphocyte counts are significantly higher in the heparinized samples.

Blood sampled during field studies often does not have the advantage of immediate processing following blood collection; therefore, artifactual changes may occur during storage. The period of stability of the sample is influenced by temperature, time, and species. In general, avian blood samples collected into EDTA can be stored at 4 °C for up to 72 hours and provide reliable results for PCV, hemoglobin (Hgb) concentration, total red blood cell count (RBC), mean corpuscular hemoglobin (MCH) values, and mean corpuscular hemoglobin concentration (MCHC), and up to 30 hours with reliable results for mean corpuscular volume (MCV) and the total white blood cell count (WBC).

A stained blood film is an essential part of the hematologic examination because it provides the opportunity to determine the differential leukocyte count and allows assessment of pathologic abnormalities of the various blood cells. A properly made blood film should have areas with a cellular monolayer that contains evenly distributed individually dispersed cells. Blood films are made using blood with or without an anticoagulant and using a variety of techniques. Avian blood cells are easily ruptured with improper blood film preparation techniques; therefore, it is advisable to use precleaned, bevel-edged microscope slides to minimize cell damage during blood film preparation. The standard or push-slide method commonly used for preparing human and mammalian blood films can be used to create blood films for avian hematology. This method involves placement of a drop of blood near one end of a microscope slide that is supported by a solid surface, such as a countertop. The second (pusher or spreader) slide is placed on top of the first slide to form a "wedge" at a 30°–45° angle in front of the drop of blood. The pusher slide is backed into the drop of blood and quickly advanced forward in one rapid motion to create the blood film. This method usually provides good cellular distribution and adequate monolayer fields for proper slide evaluation; however, cells are commonly damaged when too much pressure is applied to the pusher slide. To minimize cell damage, a drop of commercially available purified bovine albumin can be applied to a glass microscope slide, followed by an equal amount of blood placed on top of the albumin prior to making the blood film. The albumin should not be allowed to dry before making the blood film. Another method of blood film preparation using the two-slide wedge technique may aid in minimizing cell damage. Hold the slides rather than allowing one of the slides to rest on a firm surface. The slide intended to contain the blood film is held in one hand while the pusher slide is held in the other hand (Figures 20.4–20.6). A drop of blood is placed near the end of the slide farthest from the person making the blood film, and the pusher slide is immediately placed in front of the drop of blood. The pusher slide is then quickly backed completely through the drop of blood while being held at an angle of approximately 30°–45° to the blood film slide. The direction of the pusher slide is immediately reversed toward the opposite end of the blood film slide to make the blood film. The pusher slide, therefore, is brought toward the person making the blood film rather than being pushed away. Most people have better control of the spreader slide when it is being pushed toward them as opposed to being pushed away. This step should be performed in one rapid motion that involves a flip of the wrist holding the pusher slide. The advantage of holding the slides rather than allowing the blood film slide to rest on a solid surface is that less downward pressure can be applied to the pusher slide when making the blood film, which creates less cell damage. Alternately, blood films can be prepared by using a slide and coverslip, or two coverslips. With proper attention to technique, these methods minimize cellular disruption and maintain good cellular distribution with monolayered areas for examination. These methods utilize a coverslip that is pulled across a drop of blood that has been placed on a glass microscope slide or another coverslip. Primary disadvantages of this method include the inability to use an automatic stainer and the potential for cell rupture

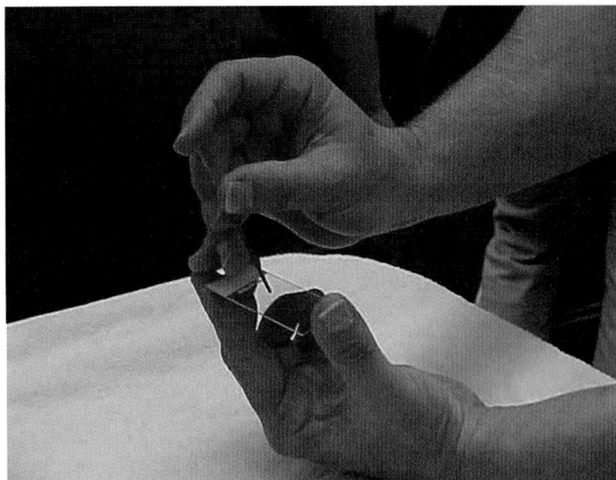

Figure 20.4 Making a blood film 1: The slide intended to contain the blood film is held in one hand.

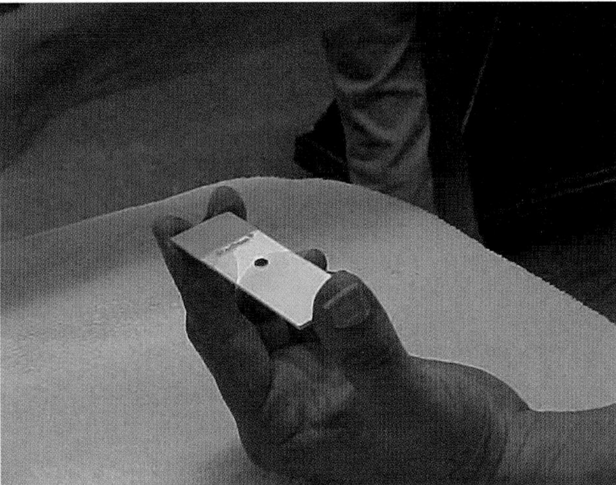

Figure 20.5 Making a blood film 2 : A drop of blood is placed near the end of the slide farthest from the person making the blood film.

(smudge cell formation) and improper cell distribution when improper technique is used.

Wright, Wright-Giemsa, Wright-Leishman, and May Grünwald-Giemsa stains have been used for staining air-dried, avian blood films for hematologic examination. Quick stains or modified Wright stains (Diff-Quik, American Scientific Products, Division of American Hospital Supply Corporation, McGraw Park, IL; Hemacolor, Miles Laboratories, Elkhart, IN) also can be used to stain avian blood films. Use of automatic slide stainers (Hema-Tek, Ames Division of Miles Laboratories, Elkhart, IN; Harleco Midas II, EM Diagnostic Systems, Gibbstown, NJ) simplifies the staining procedure and provides a means for consistency and high-quality staining of blood films. Automatic stainers remove much of the staining variation that occurs with hand-staining methods.

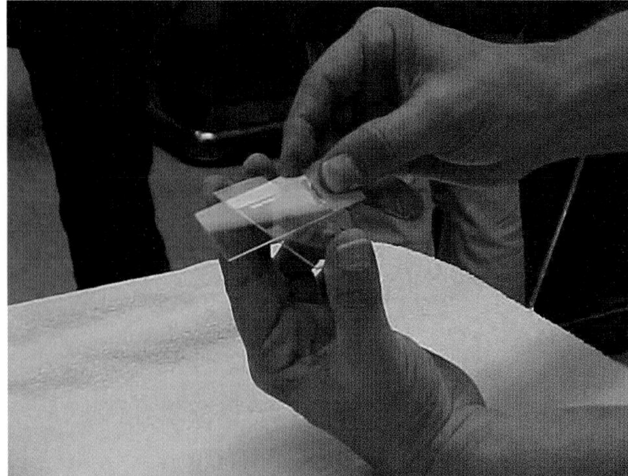

Figure 20.6 Making a blood film 3: The pusher slide is immediately placed in front of the drop of blood. The pusher slide is then quickly backed completely through the drop of blood while being held at an angle of approximately 30°–45° to the blood film slide. The direction of the pusher slide is immediately reversed toward the opposite end of the blood film slide to make the blood film. The pusher slide, therefore, is brought toward the person making the blood film rather than being pushed away.

Erythrocytes

Morphology

Evaluation of avian erythrocyte morphology involves observation of the cells in a monolayer ×1000 field in which approximately half the erythrocytes are touching one another. In general, such fields represent approximately 200 erythrocytes in most species of birds. Monolayer fields may be difficult to achieve, however, in severely anemic birds (i.e., films are too thin) or in poorly prepared blood films (i.e., films made too thick or thin). Avian erythrocytes should be evaluated on the basis of size, shape, color, nucleus, and presence of cellular inclusions. A semiquantitative scale can be used to estimate the number of abnormal erythrocytes based on the average number per monolayer ×1000 field (Table 20.1).

Mature avian erythrocytes generally are larger than mammalian erythrocytes but smaller than reptilian erythrocytes. Avian erythrocytes vary in size depending on the species, but they generally range between 10.7 × 6.1 μm to 15.8 × 10.2 μm. Erythrocytes of adult *Coturnix* quail, for example, measure 11.06 ± 0.70 μm in length and 6.80 ± 0.67 μm in width in males and 11.40 ± 0.63 μm in length and 6.73 ± 0.45 μm in width in females. Mature avian erythrocytes are elliptical and have an elliptical, centrally positioned nucleus. Nuclear chromatin is uniformly clumped and becomes increasingly condensed with age. In Wright-stained blood films, the nucleus stains purple, whereas the cytoplasm stains orange-pink with a uniform texture (Figure 20.7).

Table 20.1 Semiquantitative microscopic evaluation of avian erythrocyte morphology.

	1+	2+	3+	4+
Anisocytosis	5–10	11–20	21–30	>30
Polychromasia	2–10	11–14	15–30	>30
Hypochromasia	1–2	3–5	6–10	>10
Poikilocytosis	5–10	11–20	21–50	>50
Erythroplastids	1–2	3–5	6–10	>10

Based on the average number of abnormal cells per 1000x monolayer field.

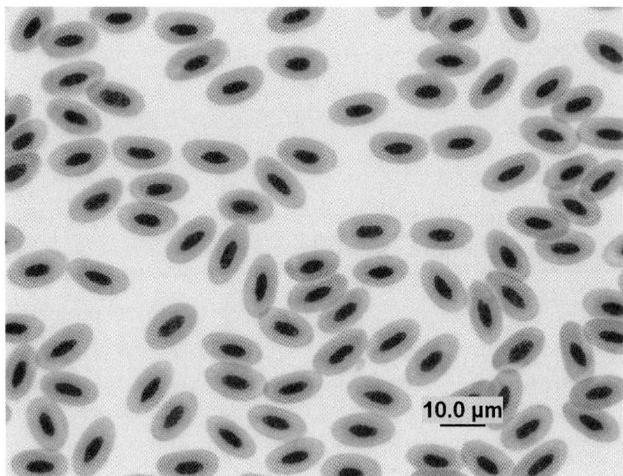

Figure 20.7 Normal erythrocytes in the blood film of a hawk (*Buteo jamaicensis*). Wright-Giemsa stain.

Variations from the normal erythrocyte morphology occur in blood films from normal healthy birds as well as those with medical disorders. Careful examination of erythrocyte morphology may reveal significant clues in the detection of disorders affecting avian erythrocytes. It is important to note, however, that the presence of atypical erythrocytes in a blood film may sometimes be associated with poor technique in blood film preparation. Disruption and/or smudging of avian erythrocytes are common artifacts of slide preparation. Severely ruptured cells result in the presence of purple, amorphous, nuclear material in the blood film. A semiquantitative scale can be used to estimate the number of abnormal erythrocytes based on the average number per monolayer ×1000 field (Table 20.1).

Changes in the size of avian erythrocytes include microcytosis, macrocytosis, and anisocytosis. A significant change in the mean size of the erythrocyte is reflected in the MCV. The presence of macrocytes or microcytes also should be noted during assessment of the blood film. The degree of variation in the size of erythrocytes (anisocytosis) can be scored from 1+ to 4+ based on the number of variable-sized erythrocytes in a monolayer field (Table 20.1). Erythrocyte subpopulations have been reported in ducks, in which larger erythrocytes (MCV 308 fL/cell) most likely represent those most recently released from the hematopoietic tissue and smaller cells (MCV 128 fL/cell) most likely represent the older, aging cells. Microcytic, hypochromic, nonregenerative anemia is often associated with chronic inflammatory diseases in birds, especially those with an infectious etiology.

Variations in erythrocyte color include polychromasia and hypochromasia. Polychromatophilic erythrocytes occur in low numbers (usually <5% of erythrocytes) in the peripheral blood of most normal birds. The degree of polychromasia can be graded according to the guideline presented in Table 20.1. The cytoplasm of polychromatophilic erythrocytes is weakly basophilic, and the nucleus is less condensed than in mature erythrocytes (Figure 20.8). Polychromatophilic erythrocytes are similar in size to mature erythrocytes, and they appear as reticulocytes when stained with vital stains such as new methylene blue.

Reticulocytes are the penultimate cell in the erythrocyte maturation series, and their presence in the peripheral blood of normal birds suggests that the final stages of red-cell maturation occur in circulating blood. Reticulocytes tend to be smaller in size and less elongated compared to the mature erythrocyte. For example reticulocytes of adult *Coturnix* quail measure 9.80 ± 0.77 µm in length and 8.23 ± 0.72 µm in width in males and 9.80 ± 0.77 µm in length and 7.73 ± 0.70 µm in width in females. Determination of the reticulocyte concentration can be made by staining erythrocytes with a vital stain such as new methylene blue. Reticulocytes have a distinct ring of aggregated reticular material that encircles the nucleus (Figure 20.9). As the cells mature, the amount of aggregated reticular material decreases and becomes more dispersed throughout the

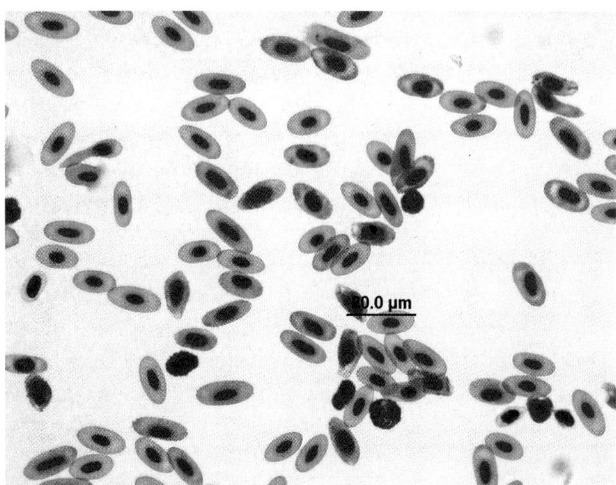

Figure 20.8 Polychromatic erythrocytes in the blood film of a hawk (*Buteo jamaicensis*). Wright-Giemsa stain.

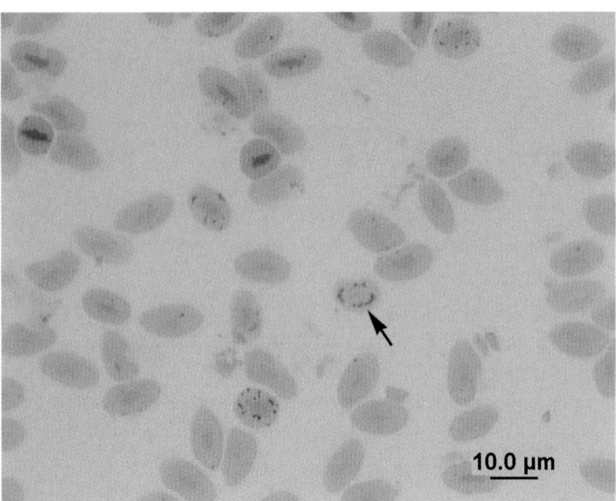

Figure 20.9 Reticulocyte (arrow) with a distinct ring of aggregated reticulum encircling the red-cell nucleus in the blood film of a parrot (*Psittacus erithacus*). Brilliant cresyl blue stain.

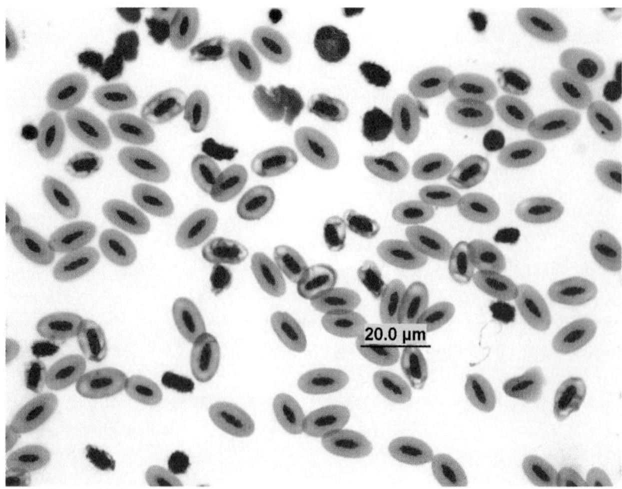

Figure 20.10 Hypochromatic erythrocytes in the blood film of a parrot (*Eclectus roratus*). Wright-Giemsa stain.

cytoplasm. With further maturation, the reticular material becomes nonaggregated, thereby resembling the "punctate" reticulocytes of felids. Most mature avian erythrocytes contain a varying amount of aggregate or punctate reticulum. Reticulocytes that reflect the current erythrocyte regenerative response, however, are those with a distinct ring of aggregated reticulum that encircles the red-cell nucleus. Significantly high numbers of these cells would represent a regenerative response to anemia.

Hypochromatic erythrocytes are abnormally pale in color compared with mature erythrocytes, and they have an area of cytoplasmic pallor that is greater than half the cytoplasmic volume (Figure 20.10). They also may have cytoplasmic vacuoles and round, pyknotic nuclei. A significant hypochromasia is reflected as a decrease in the MCHC and MCH values. The degree of hypochromasia can be estimated using the scale presented in Table 20.1.

In most species of birds, the shape of erythrocytes is relatively uniform. The degree of poikilocytosis can be estimated using the scale outlined in Table 20.1. Atypical erythrocytes occasionally are present in the peripheral blood of normal birds, and such erythrocytes may represent artifacts associated with preparation of the blood film. Careful examination of erythrocyte morphology may reveal significant clues in the detection of disorders affecting avian erythrocytes. As mentioned, the degree of polychromasia and reticulocytosis and the presence of immature erythrocytes in the peripheral blood aid in the assessment of red-blood-cell regeneration. The presence of many hypochromatic erythrocytes (i.e., 2+ hypochromasia or greater) indicates an erythrocyte disorder such as iron deficiency.

Atypical erythrocytes may vary in both size and shape. A slight variation in the size of erythrocytes (1+ anisocytosis) is considered to be normal for birds. A greater degree of anisocytosis, however, usually is observed in birds with a regenerative anemia and is associated with polychromasia. Likewise, minor deviations from the normal shape of avian erythrocytes (1+ poikilocytosis) are considered to be normal in the peripheral blood of birds, but marked poikilocytosis may indicate erythrocytic dysgenesis. Round erythrocytes with oval nuclei occasionally are found in the blood films of anemic birds and suggest a dysmaturation of the cell cytoplasm and nucleus, which may be a result of accelerated erythropoiesis. Automated methods of performing erythrocyte counts can calculate the degree of anisocytosis using the red cell distribution width (RDW), which measures variation in red blood cell size, or MCV. Normal psittacine RDW range between 10 and 11; whereas greater values indicate an increase in anisocytosis.

The nucleus may vary in its cellular location and contain indentions, protrusions, or constrictions. Anucleated erythrocytes (erythroplastids) or cytoplasmic fragments occasionally are found in normal avian blood films (Figure 20.11). The nucleus may contain chromophobic streaking, which suggests chromatolysis, or achromic bands, which indicate nuclear fracture with displacement of the fragments (Figure 20.12). Mitotic activity associated with erythrocytes in blood films suggests a marked regenerative response or erythrocytic dyscrasia. Perinuclear rings are common artifacts of improper slide preparation (e.g., exposure to solvent or formalin fumes, or allowing the slide to dry too slowly), and they represent nuclear shrinkage. Clear, irregular, refractile spaces in the cytoplasm occur when blood films are allowed to dry too slowly. This artifact, which is a form of erythrocyte crenation, should not be confused with avian blood parasites, such as gametocytes of *Hemoproteus* and *Plasmodium*. Disruption or smudging of avian erythrocytes is the most common artifact of slide

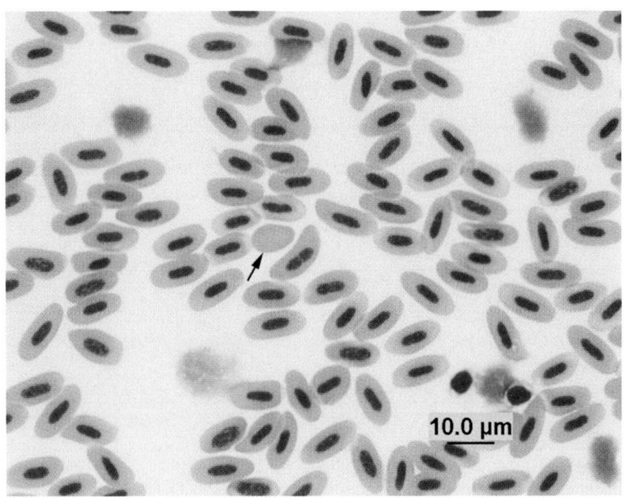

Figure 20.11 Erythroplastid (arrow) in a blood film of a budgerigar (*Melopsittacus undulatus*). Wright-Giemsa stain.

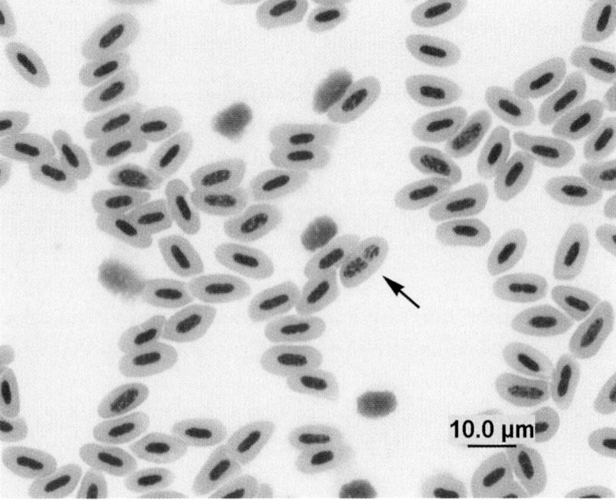

Figure 20.12 An erythrocyte nucleus exhibiting chromophobic streaking (arrow) in the blood film of a budgerigar (*Melopsittacus undulatus*). Wright-Giemsa stain.

preparation. Severely ruptured cells result in the presence of purple, amorphous nuclear material in the blood film.

Binucleate erythrocytes rarely occur in the blood films of normal birds. Large numbers of binucleated erythrocytes plus other features of red-blood-cell dyscrasia, however, suggest neoplastic, viral, or genetic disease.

Punctate basophilia is characterized by punctate aggregations of small, irregular, basophilic-staining granules throughout the cytoplasm of erythrocytes in Wright-stained smears. As in mammalian hematology, punctate basophilia is most likely associated with degenerative changes in ribosomal ribonucleic acid and is indicative of a response to anemia or, rarely, lead poisoning. Basophilic stippling can be affected by preparation and staining of the blood film. Using fresh blood without an anticoagulant or rapid drying of blood films made from EDTA-anticoagulated blood provides the best films for demonstrating basophilic stippling. Such stippling is less apparent when alcohol fixation of blood is used. Heinz bodies rarely are reported in birds and are the result of hemoglobin denaturation (oxidized hemoglobin). Heinz bodies appear as round to irregularly shaped, pale blue, cytoplasmic inclusions with new methylene blue stain; as round to irregular inclusions of densely stained hemoglobin with Wright stain; or as refractile inclusions in unstained erythrocytes. Agglutination of erythrocytes and erythrophagocytosis in blood films are rare abnormal findings that are suggestive of immune-mediated disease. Agglutination is represented by clumping of erythrocytes on the blood film. Red cell agglutination is best observed on low magnification. Erythrophagocytosis is identified by phagocytosis of whole red blood cells or iron pigment from hemoglobin degradation in the cytoplasm of leukocytes, typically monocytes.

Laboratory evaluation

Laboratory evaluation of avian erythrocytes involves the same routine procedures as that used in mammalian hematology, but with a few modifications. The standard manual technique for using microhematocrit capillary tubes and centrifugation (12,000 g for 5 minutes) can be used to obtain a PCV (hematocrit). Hemoglobin concentration is measured using the same methods for mammalian blood samples; however, removal of free erythrocyte nuclei by centrifugation is required.

The PCV is the quickest and most practical method for evaluating the red cell mass of birds. Much as in mammals, the PCV of birds is affected by the number and size of the erythrocytes, as well as changes in the plasma volume that do not affect total cell mass. These changes include increased plasma volume (hemodilution), decreased plasma volume (hemoconcentration), improper blood sampling (hemodilution), and epinephrine administration and hypothermia, which may result in hemoconcentration.

The total erythrocyte concentration in birds can be determined using the same automated or manual methods as those used for obtaining the total erythrocyte counts in mammalian blood. Automated cell counters provide a rapid, reliable method for obtaining total red-blood-cell concentrations. Two manual methods for obtaining total red-blood-cell count in birds are the erythrocyte Unopette (Becton-Dickinson) method used in mammalian hematology and the Natt-Herricks method, which involves preparation of Natt-Herricks solution to be used as a stain and diluent (Table 20.2). A 1 : 200 dilution of the blood is made using the Natt and Herricks solution and red-blood-cell diluting pipettes. After mixing, the diluted blood is discharged into a hemacytometer counting chamber, and the cells are allowed to settle for 5 minutes, to the ruled surface, before counting.

Table 20.2 Natt and Herricks solution and stain.

Sodium chloride (NaCl)	3.88 g
Sodium sulfate (Na SO_4)	2.50 g
Sodium phosphate (Na_2HPO_4)	1.74 g
Potassium phosphate (KH_2PO_4)	0.25 g
Formalin (37%)	7.50 mL
Methyl violet	0.10 g

Bring to 1000 mL with distilled water and filter through Whatman #10 medium filter paper.

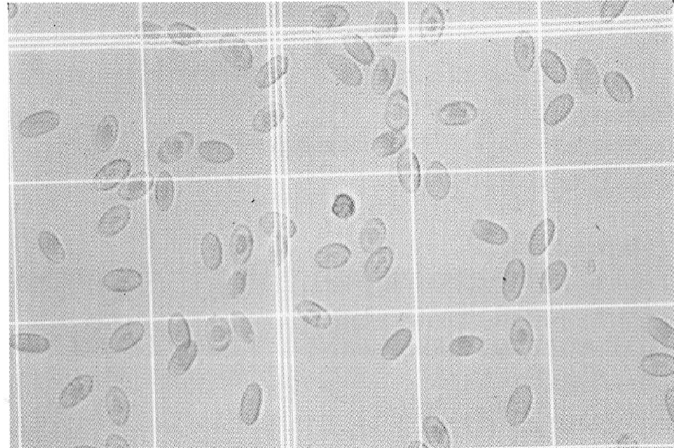

Figure 20.13 Appearance of avian erythrocytes and a leukocyte (center) in a hemocytometer using the erythrocyte Unopette method. Source: Image from Campbell TW. *Exotic Animal Hematology and Cytology*, 4th ed. Ames, IA: Wiley Blackwell, 2015, p. 200.

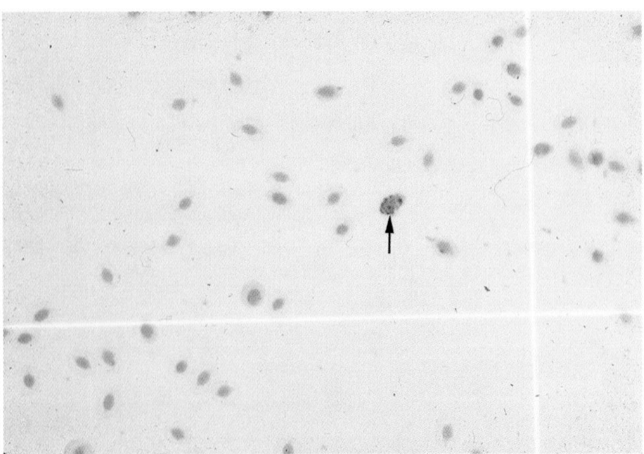

Figure 20.14 Appearance of avian erythrocytes and a granulocyte (arrow) in a hemocytometer using Natt and Herricks method. Source: Image from Campbell TW. *Exotic Animal Hematology and Cytology*, 4th ed. Ames, IA: Wiley Blackwell, 2015, p. 201.

Erythrocytes located in the four corner and the central squares of the hemacytometer chamber are counted when using either of the manual methods (Figures 20.13 and 20.14). The number obtained then is multiplied by 10,000 to calculate the total red-blood-cell count per microliter (μL) of blood. Commercially prepared Natt-Herricks solution kit (Natt-Pette) makes the procedure easier and more accurate. The kit contains prefilled Natt-Herricks stain reservoirs, a pipette calibrated for 5 μL (to make the 1 : 200 dilution), and tips for the pipette. The diluted blood is then discharged onto the hemocytometer counting chamber and is allowed to settle for a minimum of 5 minutes before counting. With these stains, the oval erythrocytes show a small, dark blue nucleus that is surrounded by a colorless to faint pink cytoplasm. The total number of erythrocytes in the four corner and central squares in the central, large square of a Neubauer-ruled hemocytometer chamber is obtained using ×40 (high dry) magnification. The TRBC is calculated by multiplying the numbers of erythrocytes by 10,000.

The red blood cell indices (i.e., mean erythrocyte volume [MCV], MCHC, and mean cell hemoglobin [MCH]) can be calculated using standard formulas. However, the direct, electronic measurement of MCV appears to be more sensitive for detecting changes in the erythrocyte size in birds.

Normal erythrocyte physiology

Normal reference values vary among species of birds; however, with a few exceptions, psittacine birds in captivity have similar erythrocyte parameters: PCV of 35–55%; RBC count of 2.4–5.0 × 10^6/μL; hemoglobin concentration of 11–16 mg/dL; MCV of 90–200 fL; and MCHC of 22–33% (Table 20.3).

It should be noted that a proportional relationship exists between Hgb concentration and PCV in avian blood samples. A simplified relationship of Hgb (g/dL) = 0.30 × PCV provides a reasonable estimate of Hgb concentration from the PCV of birds from the orders Anseriformes, Columbiformes, Falconiformes, Galliformes, Passeriformes, Psittaciformes, Sphenisciformes, and Strigiformes, but a separate relationship of Hgb = 0.217 × PCV + 6.69 might be warranted for the order Phoenicopteriformes.

The total erythrocyte concentration and PCV of birds are influenced by species, age, sex, hormonal influences, hypoxia, environmental factors, and disease. In general, the total erythrocyte count, PCV, and MCV increase with age. The Hgb does not appear to be affected by age; therefore, a decline in MCHC is a function of the increase in MCV.

Total erythrocyte counts and PCV tend to be higher in male compared to female birds. The reason for this may be a hormonal effect where estrogen depresses erythropoiesis, whereas androgens and thyroxin stimulate erythropoiesis. Variations in erythrocyte parameters associated with gender in birds are generally not statistically significant; however, reported differences between males and females have been reported and reflect a seasonal variation, where females tend to have higher PCV, Hgb, TRBC, and MCHC values compared to males in the prenesting period.

Table 20.3 Erythrocyte parameters for selected birds.

	PCV (%)	RBC ($\times 10^6/\mu L$)	Hgb (g/dL)	MCV (fL)	MCHC (%)
Psittacines					
African gray parrot	43–55	2.4–4.5	11.0–16.0	90–180	23–33
Amazon parrot	45–55	2.5–4.5	12.5–25	160–175	29.1–31.0
Blue-fronted Amazon	44–58	2.1–3.5	16.0–18.4	163–209	31.7–37.8
Cuban Amazon	44–54	3.1–3.5	15.2–17.7	142–162	31.4–37.2
Festive Amazon	47–53	3.1–3.8	16.1–17.4	135–164	31.5–34.5
Orange-wing Amazon	46–51	2.8–3.3	15.5–17.5	151–166	32.1–36.0
Vinaceous Amazon	46–52	3.0–3.3	15.0–17.5	145–174	31.7–35.6
Yellow Amazon	38–51	2.1–3.5	12.1–17.4	135–175	31.0–34.1
Budgerigar	44–58	2.3–3.9	13–18	90–190	22–32
Cockatiel	45–54	2.5–4.7	11–16	90–200	22–33
Cockatoos	42–54	2–4	12–16	120–175	28–33
Black cockatoo	40–46	2.4–2.7	12–17	154–184	32–37
Goffin's cockatoo	37–47	2.4–3.4	12–16	119–175	33–39
Palm cockatoo	36–47	2.0–3.6	13–17	131–235	31–36
White cockatoo	37–48	2.8–3.2	14–18	132–171	30–39
Conure	42–54	2.9–4.5	12–16	90–190	23–31
Golden conure	50–54	3.6–4.0	17.6–20.4	126–144	33.9–40.7
Patagonian conure	45–52	3.2–4.1	14.3–16.2	127–146	30.9–32.3
Eclectus parrot	45–55	2.7–3.8	13.5–16.0	125–175	29–32
Jardine's parrot	35–48	2.4–4.0	11–16	90–190	21–33
Lovebird	44–57	3.0–5.1	13–18	90–190	22–32
Macaw	47–55	2.7–4.5	15–17	125–170	29–35
Green-wing macaw	39–54	2.7–4.1	9.6–18.7	116–177	21.9–34.9
Military macaw	37–55	2.7–5.2	11.1–19.6	106–173	33.9–40.7
Scarlet macaw	40–54	2.3–3.7	13.1–19.9	135–169	29.7–37.3
Pionus parrot	35–54	2.4–4.0	11–16	85–210	24–31
Quaker	30–58	2.8–3.9	11–15	90–200	22–32
Senegal parrot	36–48	2.4–4.0	11–16	90–200	23–32
Others					
Canary	37–49	2.5–3.8	12–16	90–210	22–32
Pigeon	38–50	3.1–4.5	13–17.5	85–200	22–33
Chicken	23–55	1.3–4.5	7.0–18.6	100–139	20–34
Turkey	30.4–45.6	1.74–3.70	8.8–13.4	112–168	23.2–35.3
Quail	30.0–45.1	4.0–5.2	10.7–14.3	60–100	28.0–38.5
Canada goose	38–58	1.6–2.6	12.7–19.1	118–144	20–30
Mallard duck[a]	46–51	3.05–3.65	14.8–16.4	134–162	31.4–31.8
Mallard duck[b]	34–44	1.61–2.41	11–13	172–227	27–31
Peregrine falcon	37–53	3–4	11.8–18.8	118–146	31.9–35.2
Red tailed hawk	31–43	2.41–3.59	10.7–16.6	150–178	29.7–34.5
Tawny owl	29–47	1.5–2.4	8.0–13.3	154–221	33.1–62.1
White-back vulture	35–54	21–3.0	1632–1623.0	186–208	36.2–42.3

[a] January.
[b] June.
Sources: Based on Pollack et al. (2005); Tell and Citino (1992); Cray (2000); Campbell (2000); Polo et al. (1998); Spagnolo et al. (2008); and Naidoo et al. (2008).

Studies with free-ranging ducks and geese have shown that averages for PCV, Hgb, TRBC, and MCHC values tend to be higher in the winter and prenesting period in adults regardless of gender compared to the postnesting period and fall. During migration, ducks tend to have slightly lower erythrocyte counts compared to wintering ducks and postnesting MCV averages for these birds tend to be higher in the winter or prenesting periods. Interestingly, these changes also occur in captive ducks that are not able to migrate. Feather molting, a seasonal event, has an effect on the hemogram where the PCV, RBC, and Hgb have been shown to decrease in ducks during and after remige molt.

The normal erythrocyte parameters vary among avian species. For example, in Anseriformes, mallard ducks (*Anas platyrhynchos*), a dabbling duck, have higher average PCV and TRBC values in the winter and prenesting period compared to diving ducks (*Aythya* spp. and *Oxyura jamaicensis*); whereas, diving ducks have higher MCV values during the winter and prenesting period compared to mallards. In general, ducks tend to have higher TRBC values than geese, but geese have higher MCV and Hgb than ducks during the winter.

Birds, like mammals, respond to blood loss and blood destruction by increasing erythropoietin production, which stimulates erythropoiesis. Avian erythropoietin (a glycoprotein produced by the kidney) acts directly on the bone marrow to increase erythrocyte production. Avian erythropoietin does not stimulate mammalian erythropoiesis, however, and mammalian erythropoietin has no effect on avian hematopoiesis.

Avian hemoglobin has four iron-containing heme subunits, as with mammalian hemoglobin, but the protein moieties (i.e., globulins) are different. In avian erythrocytes, the phosphate compounds influencing the affinity of hemoglobin for oxygen also differ from those in mammals. The hemoglobin of mature birds contains myoinositol pentophosphate, not the 2,3-diphosglycerate as in mammals. Inositol pentophosphate causes hemoglobin to have a lower affinity for oxygen, and it shifts the oxygen dissociation curve to the right of the mammalian curve. Therefore, avian tissues can extract oxygen more readily from hemoglobin than mammalian tissues can.

Responses in disease

The normal PCV for many species of birds ranges between 35% and 55%. Therefore, a PCV of less than 35% suggests anemia, and a PCV of greater than 55% suggests dehydration or erythrocytosis (polycythemia). The latter condition can be differentiated by the total serum protein: increased total protein indicates dehydration, whereas normal or low total protein indicates erythrocytosis.

Typically, polychromatic erythrocytes make up 5% or less of the erythrocyte population in blood films from normal birds. The degree of erythrocyte polychromasia and reticulocytosis indicates the degree of erythrogenesis. Anemic birds with greater than 10% polychromasia (3+ and 4+ polychromasia) are exhibiting an appropriate regenerative response to their anemia. Those with a smaller response, however, are not. The number of reticulocytes also indicates a bird's current response to anemia. Therefore, the reticulocyte count can be used in conjunction with assessment of the degree of polychromasia to determine the bird's current erythropoietic response.

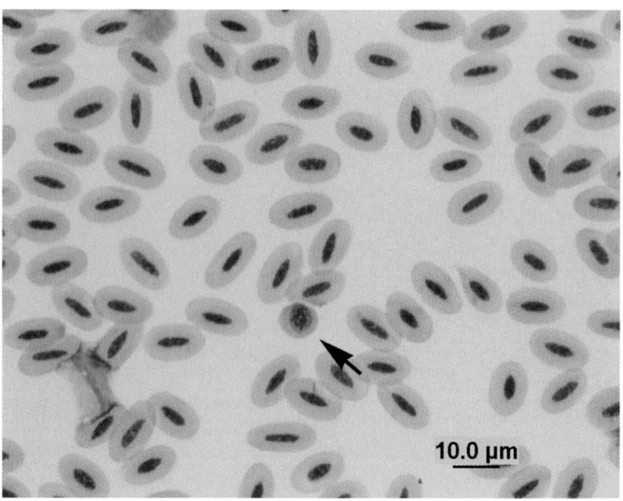

Figure 20.15 Immature erythrocyte (a mid-polychromatic rubricyte, arrow) in the blood film of an eagle (*Haliaeetus leucocephalus*). Wright-Giemsa stain.

Other evidence of active erythropoiesis is the presence of binucleate, immature erythrocytes and an increased number of normal, immature erythrocytes in the peripheral blood. Immature erythrocytes (i.e., rubricytes) in peripheral blood films in addition to increased polychromasia indicate a marked erythrocyte response (Figure 20.15). In cases of nonanemic birds, however, these cells indicate abnormal erythropoiesis. Immature erythrocytes also may suggest early release from the hematopoietic tissue after anoxic insult or toxicity (i.e., lead poisoning).

The causes of anemia in birds include blood loss (hemorrhagic anemia), increased red cell destruction (hemolytic anemia), and decreased red cell production (depression anemia). The most common causes of hemorrhagic anemia in birds include traumatic injury, bloodsucking parasites, coagulopathies, and hemorrhagic lesions of internal organs, such as ulcerated neoplasms, gastric ulcerations, and rupture of the liver or spleen. Heavy infestation with bloodsucking ectoparasites such as ticks or mites (i.e., *Dermanyssus* mites) or with gastrointestinal parasites such as coccidia can lead to severe blood loss anemia in birds. Coagulopathies that result in blood loss anemia usually are acquired and often are associated with toxicities such as aflatoxicosis or coumarin poisoning or severe liver disease such as papovavirus infections. Birds can tolerate acute blood loss better than mammals and diving and flying birds are more resistant to blood loss than nondiving birds such as Galliformes. The mobilization and restoration of fluid during the first 90 minutes after bleeding in chickens is approximately 13–17% of the initial blood volume per hour, which is twice that of dogs.

With hemolytic anemia, the destruction rate of erythrocytes is higher than normal resulting in an increase in erythrocyte production to compensate for the loss, which is indicated by an increase in the presence of immature erythrocyte stages in the circulating blood. Hemolytic anemia can result from systemic or hematogenous bacterial infection (septicemia), infectious disease, hemoparasites, and toxicities. Most avian blood parasites have the potential to cause anemia in the host; however, the two parasites that most frequently are associated with hemolytic anemia are *Plasmodium* and *Aegyptianella*. Salmonellosis or spirochetoses commonly cause bacterial septicemia that result in severe hemolytic anemia. Toxicoses that lead to increased erythrocyte destruction include aflatoxins, certain plant chemicals (i.e., mustards), drugs, and petroleum products. Ingestion of petroleum products may produce a Heinz body anemia. Hemolytic anemia occurs in marine birds associated with oil pollution and is characterized by low red-cell indices and numerous immature erythrocytes. Heavy metals such as lead and zinc are associated with hemolytic anemia in a variety of avian species, and are considered by some authors as the most common cause of this condition in companion birds. Although rare, immune-mediated anemia may result in hemolysis, with red-cell agglutination being present in the blood film. Hemolytic anemias typically are characterized by a marked regenerative response. Although hemochromatosis usually does not affect the hemogram, a report by Rupiper and Read of a psittacine with hemochromatosis described a severe anemia with a marked regenerative response (4+ polychromasia and immature erythrocytes as early as prorubricytes). The hemochromatosis may have altered the maturation of erythrocytes as a result of defective iron uptake.

A nonregenerative, normocytic, normochromic anemia indicates decreased erythropoiesis (depression anemia), which can develop rapidly in birds with inflammatory diseases, especially those involving infectious agents. Birds appear to develop anemias from a lack of erythropoiesis more quickly than mammals, perhaps because of the relatively short erythrocyte half-life in birds compared with that in mammals. Although the avian erythrocyte life span varies with the species, it is generally shorter than those in mammals. For example, the erythrocyte life span is 28–35 days in chickens, 42 days in pigs, 35–45 days in pigeons, and 33–35 days in quail. The degree of polychromasia or reticulocytosis is poor to absent in birds with depression anemias. Infectious diseases frequently associated with depression anemia in birds include tuberculosis, aspergillosis, and chlamydophilosis. Chronic hepatic and renal disease and hypothyroidism can also result in a depression anemia. Neoplasia resulting in infiltration of neoplastic cells into the bone marrow can also cause a depression anemia. Treatment with myelosuppressive medication for neoplastic lesions can also lead to depression anemia. Nonregenerative anemia can also be associated with parasites, such as *Baylisascaris procyonis* infections. Chronic inflammation in birds is often associated with a marked nonregenerative anemia, leukocytosis, and heterophilia.

Hypochromasia can be seen with iron deficiency, chronic inflammatory diseases, and lead toxicosis. Hypochromatic erythrocytes frequently appear in the blood films from birds with chronic inflammatory diseases, presumably related to iron sequestration as part of the bird's defense against infectious agents. In such cases, hypochromatic cells often are observed in blood films before the red-cell indices (MCHC and MCH) suggest hypochromasia (Figure 20.10).

Heavy metal poisoning, especially with lead and zinc intoxication, can result in the appearance of immature and abnormal erythrocytes in the peripheral blood. Chronic lead toxicosis also may be associated with an in appropriate release of normal-appearing, immature erythrocytes into the peripheral blood of nonanemic birds (Figure 20.16). In this condition, the blood film reveals small, senescent, mature erythrocytes with pyknotic nuclei and immature erythrocytes (usually rubricytes) without the presence of normal, mature erythrocytes. This hematologic response resembles the inappropriate release of nucleated erythrocytes in the blood of nonanemic dogs affected by chronic lead poisoning. Basophilic stippling in the cytoplasm of erythrocytes may be seen with lead poisoning in birds but can also be associated with erythrocyte regeneration and hypochromic anemia. Changes in PCV, Hb, and MCHC occur in a predictable manner with increasing blood lead concentrations in birds. Erythrocyte morphological changes tend to occur when blood lead concentrations are greater than 3 mg/L and therefore are associated with severe lead toxicosis. A decreased MCHC is a more sensitive indicator of lead poisoning in birds than is hypochromasia.

A macrocytic, normochromic anemia occurs in birds with food restriction or folic acid deficiency. Folic acid deficiency

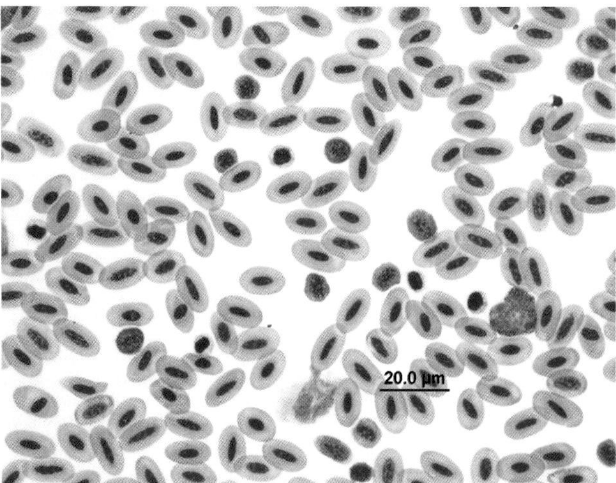

Figure 20.16 Marked numbers of immature erythrocytes and a heterophil in a blood film from a vulture (*Cathartes aura*) with a normal packed cell volume (46%). The vulture has lead poisoning. Wright-Giemsa stain.

causes defective DNA synthesis, thereby causing nuclear maturation to be out of step with hemoglobinization of the cytoplasm. Food restriction anemia also is associated with leukopenia, thrombocytopenia, abnormal erythrocyte shapes (marked poikilocytosis), and hypersegmentation of granulocytes.

Erythrocytosis (polycythemia) as indicated by an elevated PCV and erythrocyte count is rarely reported in birds. Relative polycythemia associated with redistribution of erythrocytes does not occur in birds because they do not store reserve erythrocytes in their spleens. The conditions associated with polycythemia in mammals most likely cause polycythemia in birds as well. A primary erythrocytosis (polycythemia vera) is a myeloproliferative disorder resulting in an absolute erythrocytosis and a rare condition in birds. Most reported cases of an absolute erythrocytosis (PCV usually >70%) in birds are secondary as a response to hypoxia that results in an increased production of erythropoietin. Disease conditions that lead to secondary polycythemia include chronic pulmonary diseases, cardiac disease, iron storage disease, rickets, renal disease or renal neoplasia, or a physiologic response to high altitude. A relative erythrocytosis associated with dehydration is responsible for most avian cases with an erythrocytosis.

The presence of numerous immature erythrocytes (especially rubriblasts) and abnormal-appearing immature erythrocytes in the peripheral blood of birds indicates erythrocytic neoplasia. Erythroblastosis in poultry with avian leukosis complex is an example of this condition.

The genotoxicity of cyclophosphamide and mitomycin-C cause a decrease in the PCV and the formation of erythrocytes with micronuclei and nuclear budding. The micronuclei are seen in erythrocytes at the rubriblasts and prorubricytes stages of development. These effects are seen up to day 8 following secession of cyclophosphamide therapy. Recovery is signaled by a large increase in immature erythrocytes with complete resolution by day 13. Thus, detection of nuclear budding and micronuclei in avian erythrocytes in blood films is an indication of exposure to a therapeutic or environmental genotoxin.

Leukocytes

Morphology

Leukopoiesis in normal birds appears to be similar to that in mammals, in that leukocytes are released into the peripheral circulation only when they are mature. Leukocytes in avian blood include lymphocytes, monocytes, and granulocytes. The granulocytes are classified as heterophils, eosinophils, and basophils. Heterophils are the most abundant granulocyte in most birds. The cytoplasm of normal, mature heterophils appears colorless and contains eosinophilic granules (dark orange to brown-red) with Romanowsky stains (Figures 20.16 and 20.17). The cytoplasmic granules typically are elongate (rod or spiculated shaped), but they may appear oval to round in some species. Heterophil granules frequently have a distinct central body that appears to be refractile. The granules may be affected by the staining process and appear atypical (i.e., poorly stained, partially dissolved, or fused). The nucleus of mature heterophils is lobed (usually two to three lobes) with coarse, clumped chromatin that stains purple. The nucleus often is partially hidden by the cytoplasmic granules.

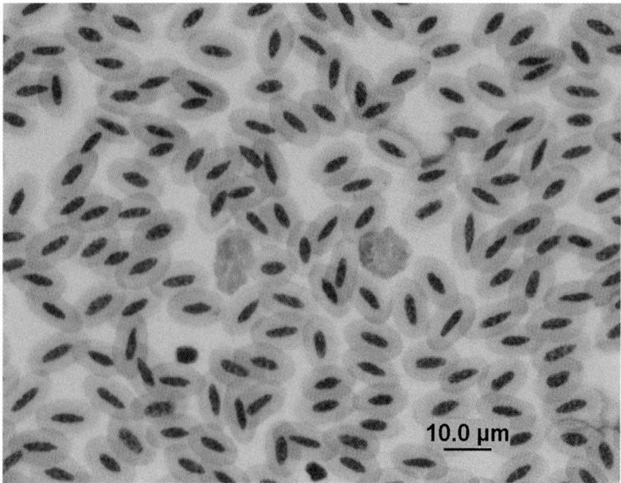

Figure 20.17 Normal heterophils in the blood film of an eagle (*Haliaeetus leucocephalus*). Wright-Giemsa stain.

Avian heterophils are considered to be functionally equivalent to mammalian neutrophils; however, there are differences. They actively participate in inflammatory lesions, and they are phagocytic. The cytoplasmic granules of heterophils contain lysozyme and proteins needed for bactericidal activity, although some avian species, such as chickens, have heterophils that lack peroxidase activity. Heterophils phagocytize microorganisms and destroy them by oxygen-dependent and -independent mechanisms. Although chicken heterophils lack the alkaline phosphatase, catalase, and myeloperoxidase needed for oxygen-dependent killing of microorganisms, they do consume oxygen and produce oxygen radicals and hydrogen peroxide, but to a lesser extent than in mammalian neutrophils. Therefore, avian heterophils rely more heavily on oxygen-independent mechanisms, lysozyme, and cationic proteins (i.e., acid hydrolases and cathepsin) to destroy microorganisms. Avian (chicken and turkey) heterophils do not respond to the chemoattractant formyl-methionyl-leucyl-phenylalanine (fMLP) as do mammalian neutrophils.

Ultrastructural studies of avian heterophils reveal primary, secondary, and tertiary granules. Primary granules are the most numerous, and they appear as electron-dense, fusiform rods (1.5 × 0.5 µm) with a circular central body.

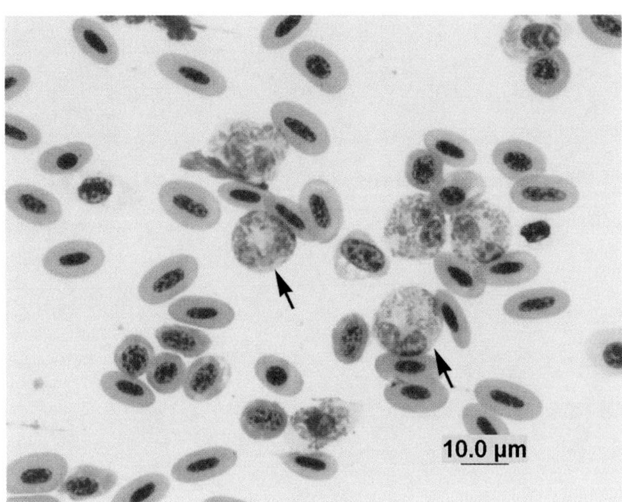

Figure 20.18 Heterophil metamyelocytes (arrows) in the blood film of a hawk (*Buteo regalis*). Wright-Giemsa stain.

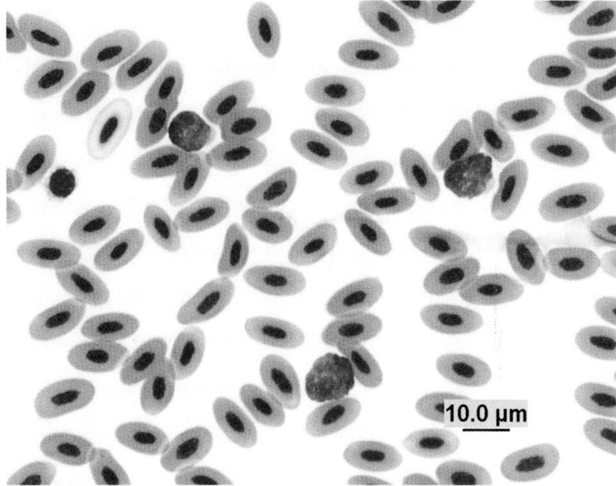

Figure 20.19 Mildly toxic (1+) heterophils (note the slight cytoplasmic basophilia) in the blood film of a macaw (*Ara chloropterus*). Wright-Giemsa stain.

Secondary granules (diameter, 0.5 μm) are less dense and contain eccentric inclusions composed of loose, filamentous material. Tertiary granules (0.1 μm) have a dense core that is separated from a membranous envelope of an electron-lucent area. Based on the results of biochemical evaluations of chicken heterophils, myeloperoxidase and alkaline phosphatase are absent. Chicken heterophil granules do not stain with alkaline phosphatase, peroxidase, Sudan black B, acid phosphatase, naphthol AS-D chloroacetate esterase methods, or periodic acid–Schiff. Small and medium granules may be seen ultrastructurally in avian heterophils, and these probably represent maturation stages of the cytoplasmic granules.

Abnormal appearing heterophils in blood films include both immature and toxic heterophils. Immature heterophils have increased cytoplasmic basophilia, nonsegmented nuclei, and immature cytoplasmic granules compared with normal, mature heterophils (Figure 20.18). Immature heterophils most frequently encountered in the blood are myelocytes and metamyelocytes. Heterophil myelocytes are larger than mature heterophils, and they have blue cytoplasm as well as secondary, rod-shaped granules, which occupy less than half the cytoplasmic volume, and a round to oval, nonsegmented nucleus. Heterophil metamyelocytes resemble myelocytes, except that the nucleus is indented and the rod-shaped granules occupy more than half the cytoplasmic volume. Band heterophils resemble mature heterophils, except that the nucleus is not lobed. It often is difficult to recognize a band cell because the nucleus is hidden by the cytoplasmic granules. Therefore, a true assessment regarding the concentration of band cells in avian blood films requires use of a nuclear stain, such as hematoxylin, which stains only the nucleus and not the cytoplasmic granules.

In response to severe systemic illness, avian heterophils exhibit toxic changes similar to those in mammalian neutrophils. Toxic changes in avian heterophils are subjectively quantified as to the number of toxic cells and the severity of toxicity, as in mammalian hematology. Toxic heterophils have increased cytoplasmic basophilia, vacuolization, abnormal granulation (degranulation, granules that appear deeply basophilic, and granules that appear to coalesce into large, round granules), and degeneration of the cell nucleus (Figures 20.19–20.22). The degree of heterophil toxicity can be rated subjectively on a scale of 1+ to 4+. A 1+ degree of toxicity or mild toxicity is assigned when heterophils exhibit increased cytoplasmic basophilia. A 2+ or mild to moderate degree of toxicity is assigned when heterophils have deeper cytoplasmic basophilia and partial degranulation. A 3+ degree of toxicity or moderate toxicity is assigned when heterophils exhibit deep cytoplasmic basophilia, moderate degranulation, abnormal granules, and cytoplasmic vacuolization, and a 4+ or marked degree of toxicity is assigned when heterophils exhibit deep cytoplasmic basophilia, moderate to marked degranulation with abnormal granules, cytoplasmic vacuolization, and karyorrhexis or karyolysis. The number of toxic heterophils are graded as few (5–10%), moderate (11–30%), and marked (>30%).

Most avian eosinophils are nearly the same size as heterophils in most blood films. For example, heterophils of adult *Coturnix* quail measure 10.22 ± 1.20 μm in diameter for males and 9.80 ± 1.14 μm in diameter in females compared to eosinophils that measured 9.76 ± 1.13 μm in diameter for males and 9.55 ± 1.23 μm in diameter in females. In contrast to mature heterophils, avian eosinophils in general have round, strongly eosinophilic cytoplasmic granules, although the granules in some species are oval to elongate. In general, eosinophil granules stain more intensely that

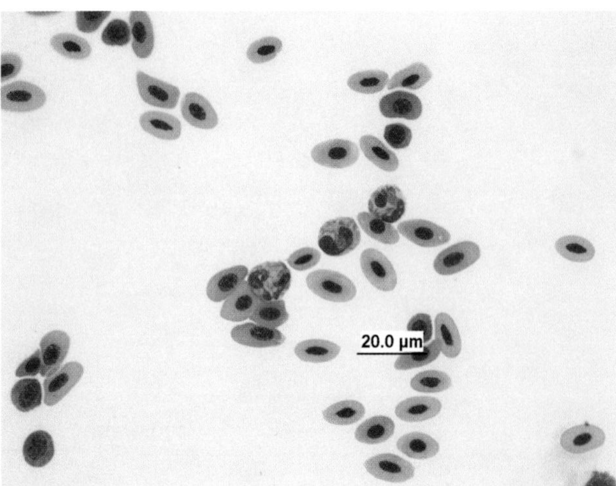

Figure 20.20 Moderately toxic (2+) heterophils (note the darker cytoplasmic basophilia and reduction of the number of rod-shaped cytoplasmic granules as indicated by increased visible cytoplasm) in the blood film of a hawk (*Buteo jamaicensis*). Wright-Giemsa stain.

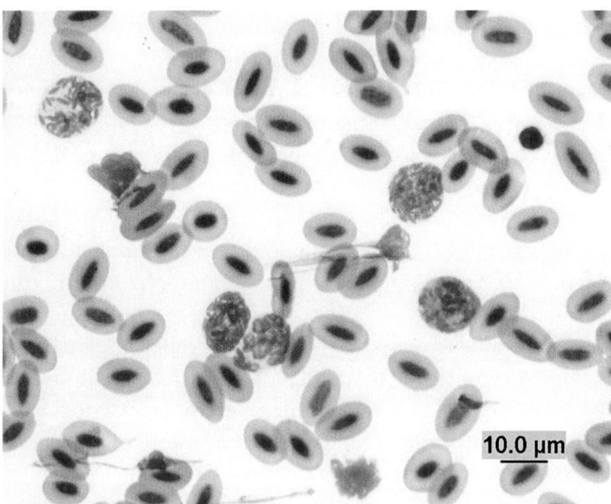

Figure 20.21 Moderately toxic (2+) heterophils (note the darker cytoplasmic basophilia and reduction of the number of rod-shaped cytoplasmic granules as indicated by increased visible cytoplasm) in two of the heterophils in the blood film of an eagle (*Haliaeetus leucocephalus*). Wright-Giemsa stain.

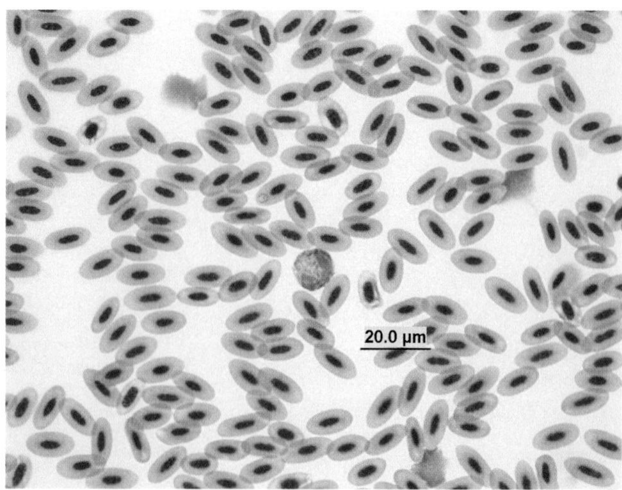

Figure 20.22 A heterophil (band cell) exhibiting marked (3+) toxicity (note the dark cytoplasmic basophilia, reduction of rod-shaped granules, and cytoplasmic vacuolization) in the blood film of a parrot (*Eclectus roratus*). Wright-Giemsa stain.

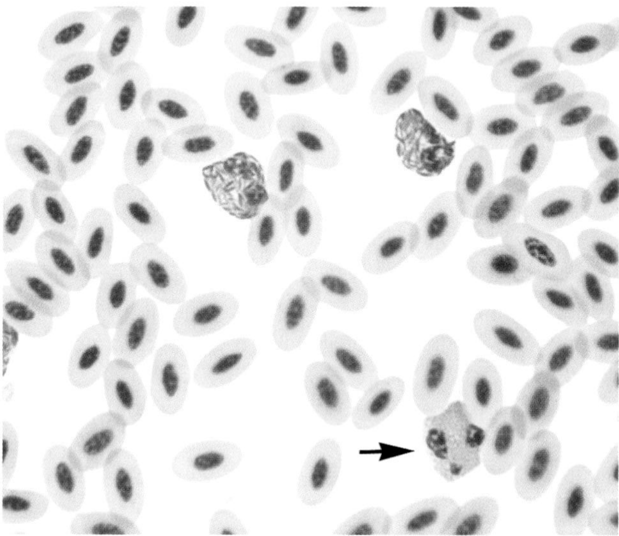

Figure 20.23 An eosinophil (arrow) and two heterophils in the blood film of a hawk (*Buteo jamaicensis*). Wright-Giemsa stain.

heterophil granules (Figures 20.23–20.25). The cytoplasmic granules of eosinophils lack the central, refractile body seen in many avian heterophils. The cytoplasm of eosinophils stains clear blue, in contrast to the colorless cytoplasm of normal, mature heterophils. The nuclei of eosinophils are lobed and usually stain darker than heterophil nuclei. The cytoplasmic granules of eosinophils frequently are affected by Romanowsky stains. The granules may appear to be large, swollen, and round, and they also may appear colorless or to stain pale blue (Figure 20.26). Eosinophils vary in appearance among species of birds.

Avian eosinophils have some features in common with mammalian eosinophils. The ultrastructure of avian eosinophils reveals large, spherical, primary granules and mature, rod-shaped, specific granules. In some birds, the specific granules possess a crystalline core, a prominent feature of mammalian eosinophils; however, this feature is missing in other species (e.g., chicken and duck). The larger primary granules most likely are precursors to the smaller, specific granules. Similar to mammalian eosinophils, specific granules possess a high concentration of arginine and enzymes, such as peroxidase, acid phosphatase, and arylsulfatase. Cytochemical staining of chicken eosinophils indicates a positive reactivity for peroxidase, acid phosphatase, and

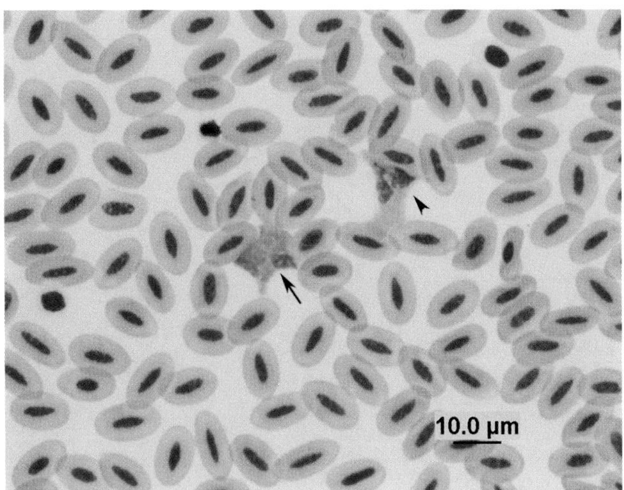

Figure 20.24 An eosinophil (arrowhead) and a heterophil (arrow) in the blood film of an eagle (*Haliaeetus leucocephalus*). Wright-Giemsa stain.

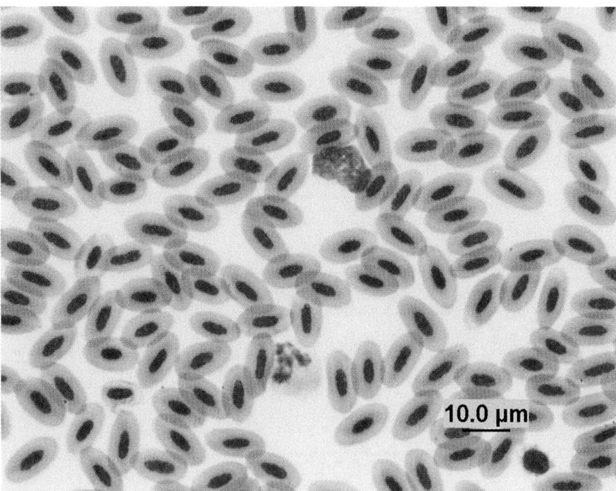

Figure 20.26 An eosinophil with blue-staining granules and a heterophil in the blood film of a parrot (*Psitticus erithacus*). Wright-Giemsa stain.

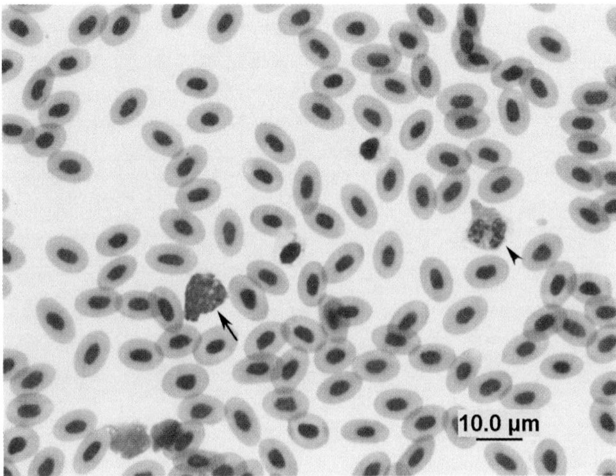

Figure 20.25 An eosinophil (arrowhead) and a heterophil (arrow) in the blood film of a chicken (*Gallus gallus domesticus*). Wright-Giemsa stain.

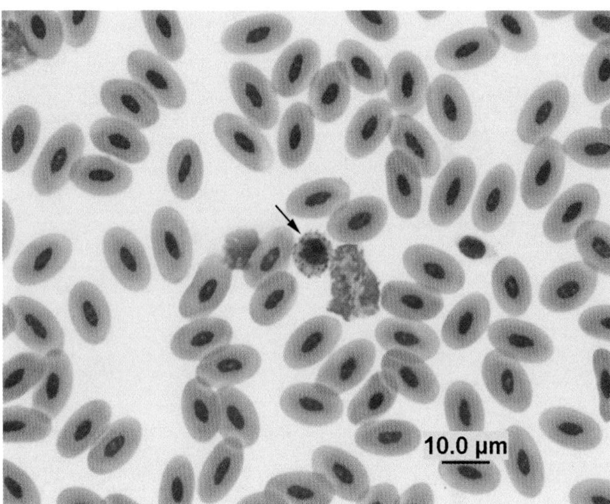

Figure 20.27 A basophil (arrow) and a heterophil in the blood film of a grebe (*Podiceps auritus*). Wright-Giemsa stain.

Sudan black B. Avian eosinophils (chicken and duck) contain major basic protein, a principal protein in mammalian eosinophils but not in mammalian neutrophils. Therefore, these reactions can be used to distinguish eosinophils from heterophils. Unlike heterophils, avian eosinophils, although they are immotile and nonphagocytic, do respond to fMLP by forming surface projections and clumping to form large aggregates. Avian eosinophils have been shown to participate in delayed hypersensitivity reactions, a feature not seen with mammalian eosinophils.

Avian basophils tend to be smaller than heterophils and eosinophils. For example, basophils of adult *Coturnix* quail measure 9.23 ± 1.35 μm in diameter for males and 9.55 ± 1.26 μm in diameter in females. Avian basophils contain deeply metachromic granules that often obscure the nucleus. The nucleus usually is nonlobed, thereby causing avian basophils to resemble mammalian mast cells (Figures 20.27 and 20.28). The cytoplasmic granules of basophils frequently are affected by alcohol-solubilized stains, and they may partially dissolve or coalesce and appear abnormal in blood films stained with Romanowsky stains. Avian basophils frequently are found in the peripheral blood, in contrast to mammalian basophils, which rarely are found in the blood films of normal animals. The function of avian basophils is not known. However, it is presumed to be similar to that of mammalian basophils and mast cells, because their cytoplasmic granules contain histamine. They also participate in acute inflammatory and type IV hypersensitivity reactions.

Avian lymphocytes resemble mammalian lymphocytes and generally come in two sizes, small and medium

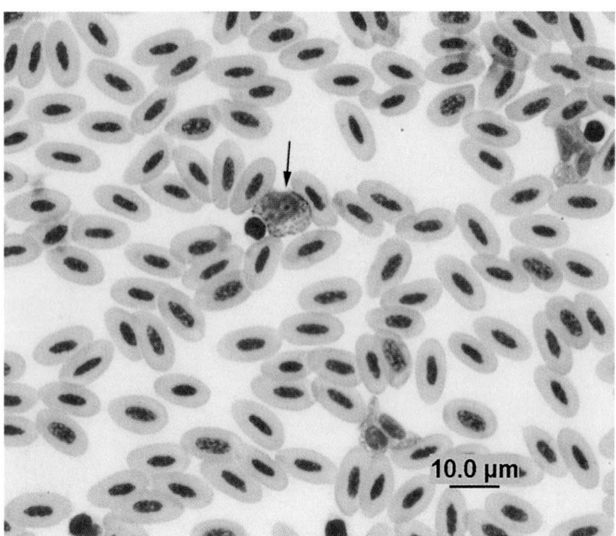

Figure 20.28 A basophil (arrow) in the blood film of a parrot (*Myiopsitta monachus*). Wright-Giemsa stain.

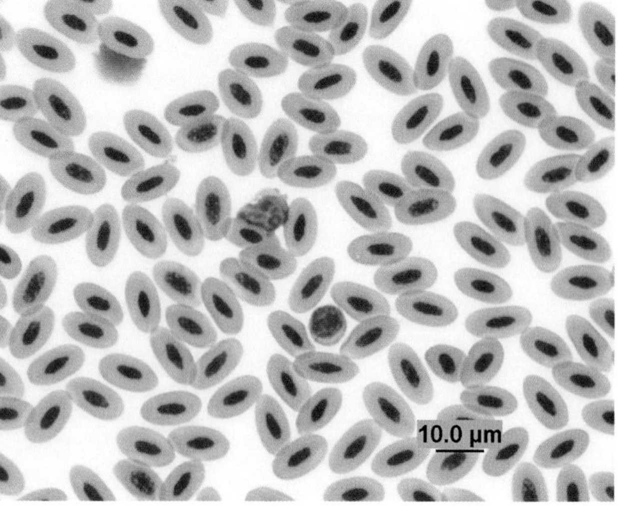

Figure 20.30 Medium lymphocytes in the blood film of a parrot (*Pionus menstruus*). Wright-Giemsa stain.

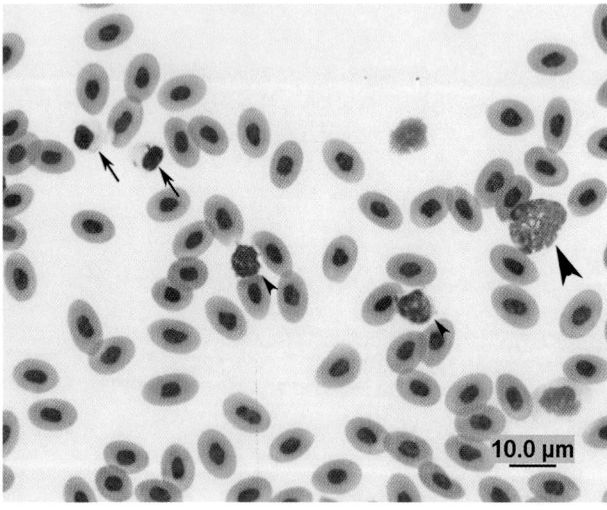

Figure 20.29 Small lymphocytes (small arrowheads), a heterophil (large arrowhead), and thrombocytes (arrows) in the blood film of a chicken (*Gallus gallus domesticus*). Wright-Giemsa stain.

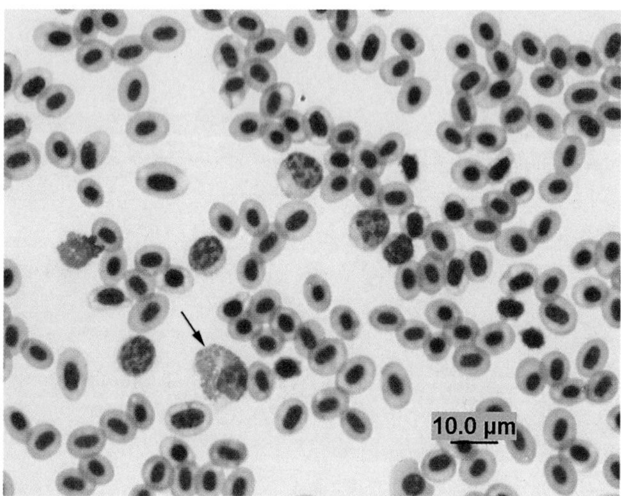

Figure 20.31 Large and medium lymphocytes and a heterophil (arrow) in the blood film of a macaw (*Ara glaucogularis*). Many of the erythrocytes are polychromatophils. Wright-Giemsa stain.

(Figures 20.29–20.33). Small lymphocytes of adult *Coturnix* quail measure 4.83 ± 0.24 μm in diameter for males and 4.86 ± 0.22 μm in diameter in females, whereas medium lymphocytes measure 7.73 ± 1.33 μm in diameter for males and 8.53 ± 1.40 μm in diameter in females. Typically, they are round cells that often show cytoplasmic irregularity when they mold around adjacent erythrocytes in the blood film. Lymphocytes have a round, occasionally slightly indented, centrally or slightly eccentrically positioned nucleus. The nuclear chromatin is heavily clumped or reticulated in mature lymphocytes, and the cytoplasm typically is scant, except in large lymphocytes, thereby giving lymphocytes their high nucleus:cytoplasm (N : C) ratio. Large lymphocytes that resemble those found in bovine blood films can also be found in the blood of normal birds. Large lymphocytes can be confused with monocytes, however, because of their size, cytoplasmic volume, and pale-staining nuclei. The lymphocyte cytoplasm usually appears to be homogenous and weakly basophilic (pale blue), and it lacks both vacuoles and granules. Cytoplasmic features are important when differentiating small lymphocytes from thrombocytes (Figures 20.29, 20.34–20.36). The latter have clear, colorless cytoplasm that often appears to be vacuolated, with a few distinct specific granules. Occasionally, cells in the blood films of birds have features of both thrombocytes and lymphocytes. These intermediate cells have small, round to oval

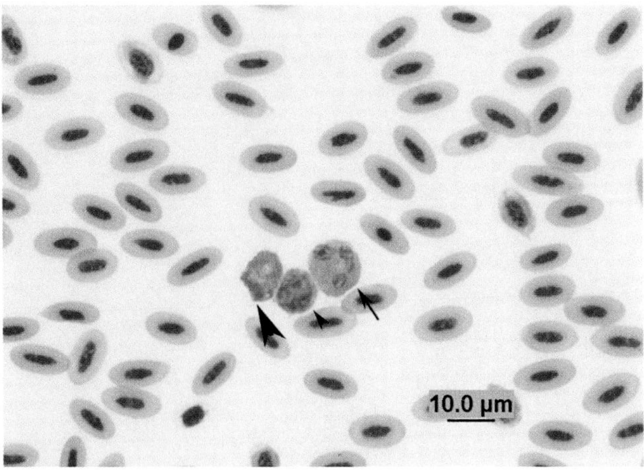

Figure 20.32 A large lymphocyte (small arrowhead), heterophil (large arrowhead), and eosinophil (arrow) in the blood film of a duck (*Anas platyrhynchos domesticus*). Wright-Giemsa stain.

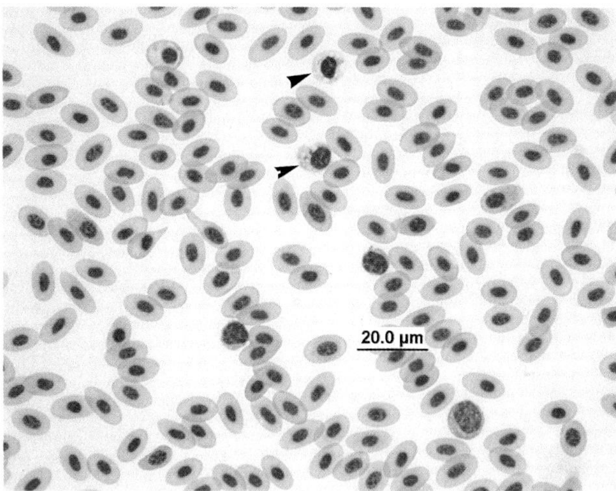

Figure 20.34 Lymphocytes and thrombocytes (arrowheads) in the blood film of a chicken (*Gallus gallus domesticus*). Wright-Giemsa stain.

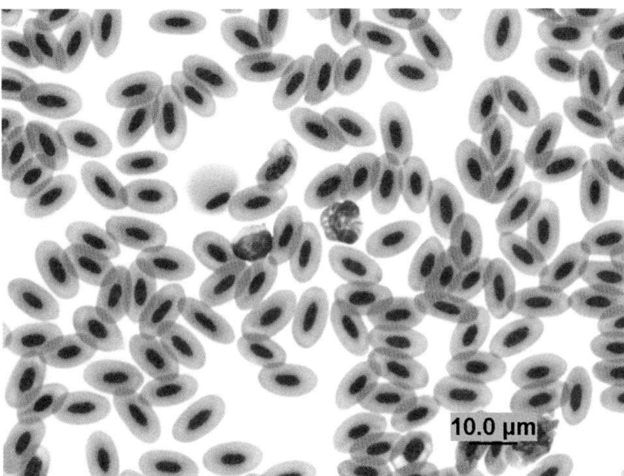

Figure 20.33 A large lymphocyte and a heterophil in the blood film of a parrot (*Psittacula krameri*). Wright-Giemsa stain.

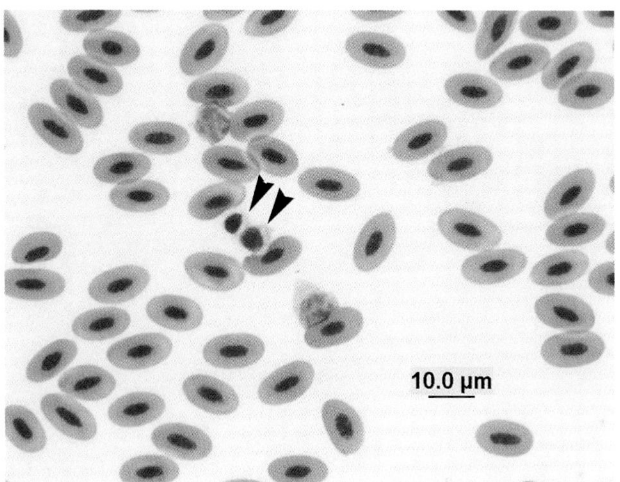

Figure 20.35 Lymphocytes and thrombocytes (arrowheads) in the blood film of a hawk (*Buteo jamaicensis*). Wright-Giemsa stain.

nuclei with coarsely clumped chromatin and moderately abundant, blue-tinged cytoplasm that lacks both vacuoles and granules. Cytochemical properties indicate these cells are lymphocytes.

Occasionally, lymphocytes may contain large distinct azurophilic granules or irregular cytoplasmic projections. Although sometimes considered to be natural killer cells, the significance of lymphocytes with azurophilic granules is not known. Irregular cytoplasmic projections are indicative of cellular degeneration, a significant finding if represented by the majority of lymphocytes.

Abnormal lymphocytes are classified as either reactive or blast-transformed lymphocytes. Reactive lymphocytes are small to medium lymphocytes with heavily clumped nuclear chromatin and deeply basophilic cytoplasm. Lymphocytes develop into reactive lymphocytes when antigenically stimulated. Blast-transformed lymphocytes are large lymphocytes with dispersed, smooth nuclear chromatin, which may contain nucleoli (Figure 20.37). They have basophilic cytoplasm that may exhibit a prominent, clear, perinuclear halo or Golgi zone. These lymphocytes have anaplastic features and may be neoplastic, but they also may result from immunologic stimulation. Plasma cells also can be found in the peripheral blood of birds. These are large B lymphocytes with eccentrically positioned mature nuclei, abundant, deeply basophilic cytoplasm and a distinct Golgi zone. Lymphocytes that contain prominent azurophilic granules are also considered to be reactive.

Avian monocytes typically are the largest leukocyte and they resemble their mammalian counterpart, varying in shape from round to ameboid. For example, monocytes of adult *Coturnix* quail measure 13.53 ± 0.74 μm in diameter

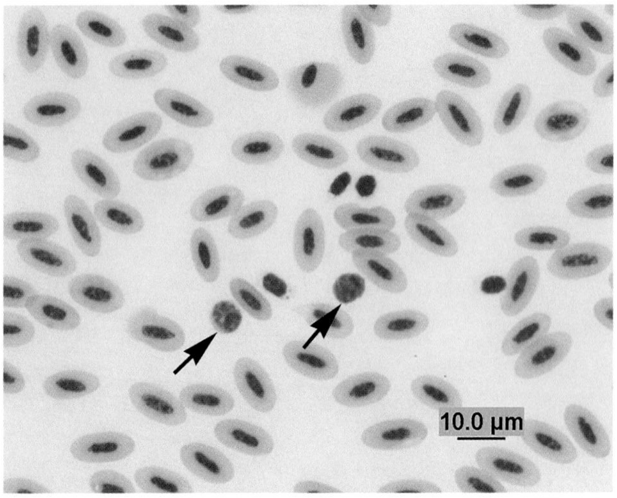

Figure 20.36 Lymphocytes (arrows) and thrombocytes in the blood film of a duck (*Anas platyrhynchos domesticus*). Wright-Giemsa stain.

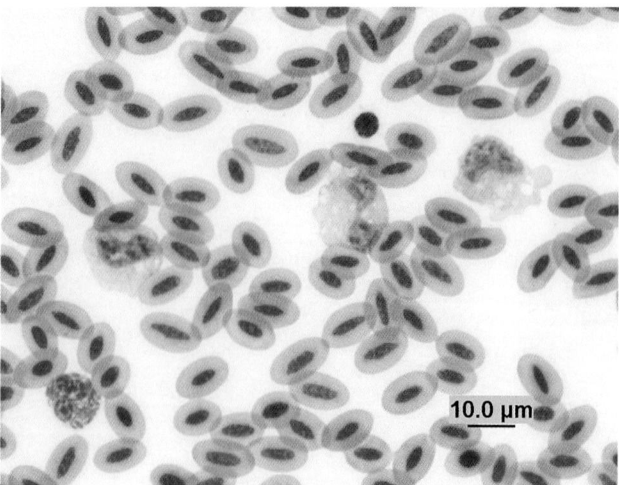

Figure 20.38 Three monocytes in the blood film of an eagle (*Haliaeetus leucocephalus*). A heterophil and a thrombocyte are also present in the image. Wright-Giemsa stain.

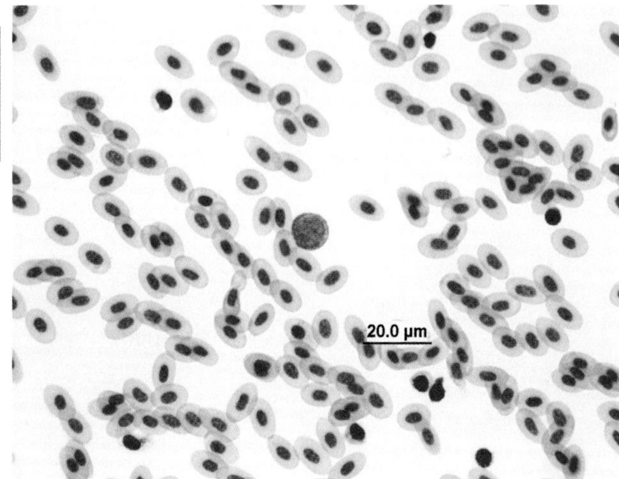

Figure 20.37 A reactive lymphocyte (center) in the blood film of a chicken (*Gallus gallus domesticus*). Wright-Giemsa stain.

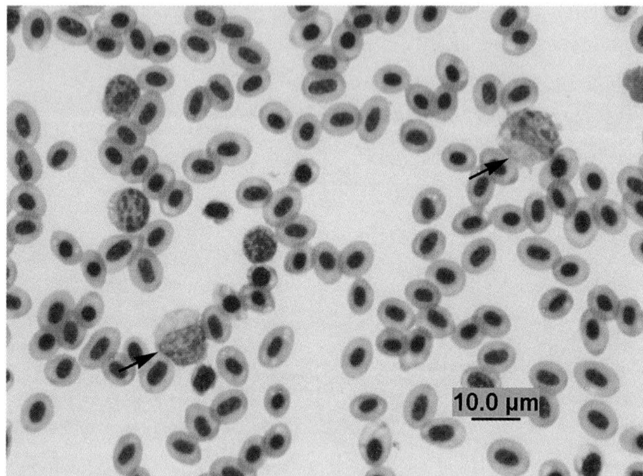

Figure 20.39 Monocytes (arrows) and large and medium lymphocytes in the blood film of a macaw (*Ara glaucogularis*). Wright-Giemsa stain.

for males and 13.26 ± 0.45 μm in diameter in females. Monocytes have abundant, blue-gray cytoplasm that may appear to be slightly opaque, and they contain vacuoles or fine, dust-like eosinophilic granules (Figures 20.38–20.40). Avian monocytes frequently exhibit two distinct zones in the cytoplasm: a light-staining perinuclear area, and a darker-staining area. The monocyte nucleus can vary in shape and is relatively pale, with less chromatin clumping compared with lymphocyte nuclei. The ultrastructure of avian monocytes and macrophages reveals a cytoplasmic membrane that is composed of blebs or filaments, a prominent Golgi apparatus, many ribosomes, and a variable number of pinocytic vesicles and lysosomes. Monocytes exhibit phagocytic activity and migrate into tissues to become macrophages. They possess biologically active chemicals that are involved in inflammation and oxidative destruction of invading organisms. Monocytes also have an important immunologic role in antigen processing.

Laboratory evaluation

Leukocyte counts may be obtained using manual and automated methods. However, significant differences may occur between the manual absolute and relative microscopic leukocyte differential count and the automated absolute and relative leukocyte count techniques. Manual methods for the determination of a leukocyte differential have a greater variability compared to automated methods. The presence of nucleated erythrocytes and thrombocytes in the blood of

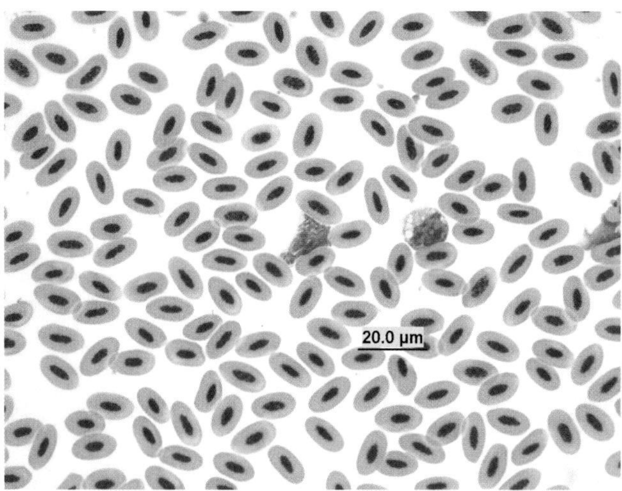

Figure 20.40 A monocyte and a heterophil in the blood film of a parrot (*Eclectus roratus*). Wright-Giemsa stain.

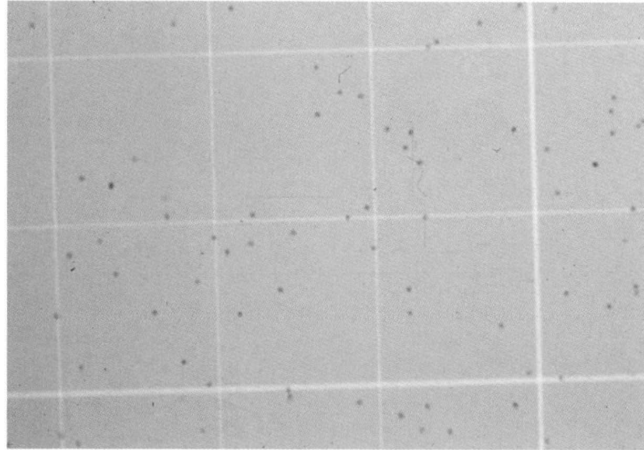

Figure 20.41 The appearance of acidophils stained with phloxine dye in a hemocytometer chamber, 100×. Source: Image from Campbell TW. *Exotic Animal Hematology and Cytology*, 4th ed. Ames, IA: Wiley Blackwell, 2015, p. 202.

lower vertebrates, such as birds, presents a challenge when attempting to apply the automated counting methods used for obtaining mammalian white blood cells counts. The fact that these animals have a nucleated erythrocyte that is similar in size to many of the leukocytes, small lymphocytes, and thrombocytes presents an additional challenge. Automated methods tend to yield a higher percentage of monocytes and lower percentage of basophils compared to manual methods when using avian blood; however, there appears to be no difference between the mean percentage of heterophils and lymphocytes. This makes automated methods suitable for determination of heterophil/lymphocyte (H/L) ratios in birds.

Direct and semidirect manual methods for obtaining total leukocyte concentrations in birds have been developed. A commonly used semidirect method involves the staining of avian heterophils and eosinophils with phloxine B as the diluent. Phloxine B commonly is used as a specific stain for eosinophils in mammalian blood. The procedure is simplified and made more accurate by using a commercially prepared Phloxine B solution kit (Eopette, Exotic Animal Solutions, Inc., Hueytown, AL). The kit contains prefilled Phloxine B stain reservoirs, a pipette calibrated for 25 μL to make the proper 1 : 32 dilution. The diluted blood is then discharged onto the hemocytometer counting chamber and is allowed to settle for a minimum of 5 minutes before counting. When properly prepared, only heterophils and eosinophils stain red with Phloxine B. The hemocytometer should be loaded immediately after proper mixing of the blood and phloxine diluent, because red blood cells also may stain after prolonged exposure. The red-stained cells are counted in both sides of the chamber (18 large squares) (Figure 20.41). Next, the total leukocyte concentration (TWBC/mm^3) is calculated after completing a leukocyte differential to obtain the percent heterophils and eosinophils on the stained blood film using the following equation:

$$\frac{(\text{Average count from } \textbf{both} \text{ sides of chamber} + 10\%) \times 32 \times 100}{\%\text{heterophils} + \%\text{eosinophils on differential}} = \text{WBC/mm}^3$$

For example: The total number of eosin-stained cells counted in the nine large squares on both sides of a Neubauer-ruled hemocytometer chamber (total of 18 squares) is 80 and the differential leukocyte count revealed 35% heterophils and 2% eosinophils, then using the above formulas, the TWBC/mm^3 is 7611/mm^3 when rounded to the nearest whole number.

A direct method for obtaining total leukocyte concentrations in avian blood is to make a 1 : 200 dilution with Natt-Herricks solution (Table 20.2) using a standard red blood cell–diluting pipette or by adding 20 μL of blood to 4 mL of the Natt-Herricks solution (Figure 20.14). The total leukocyte concentration is obtained by counting all of the leukocytes (dark blue cells) in the nine large squares in the ruled area of the hemocytometer chamber using the following formula:

$$\text{TWBC/mm}^3 = (\text{Total cells in nine large squares} + 10\%) \times 200$$

Commercially prepared Natt-Herricks solution kit (Natt-Pette) makes the procedure easier and more accurate. The kit contains prefilled Natt-Herricks stain reservoirs, a pipette calibrated for 5 μL (to make the 1 : 200 dilution), and tips for the pipette. The advantage to this method is that a total erythrocyte and thrombocyte count also can be obtained using the same charged hemocytometer. A disadvantage is that differentiating thrombocytes from small lymphocytes often is difficult, thus creating errors in the counts. Staining for 60 minutes in the Natt-Herricks solution, however, improves the differentiation between small lymphocytes and thrombocytes.

A second method for obtaining a direct total leukocyte count in birds is to dilute the anticoagulated blood 1 : 100 with 0.01% toluidine blue in phosphate-buffered saline before charging a Neubauer-ruled hemocytometer. Cells that are equal to or larger than the width of the erythrocytes are counted in the nine large squares of the hemocytometer. The total leukocyte count is calculated using the standard formula:

$$\text{TWBC/mm}^3 = \frac{\text{No. cells} \times 10 \times 100}{9}$$

Or, to simplify the math,

$$\text{TWBC/mm}^3 = (\text{Number of cells} + 10\%) \times 100$$

Toluidine blue stains leukocytes blue, erythrocytes pale orange, and thrombocytes pale blue. Counting cells that are equal to or larger than the width of erythrocytes should rule out thrombocytes, which tend to be smaller in width than erythrocytes. Small lymphocytes tend to be equal to or larger than the width of erythrocytes. Immature erythrocytes are distinguished from small lymphocytes by their round to irregular shape; their round, centrally positioned nucleus with dark, irregularly clumped chromatin; and their moderate volume of basophilic hyaline cytoplasm. A corrected total leukocyte concentration can be obtained when a large number of immature erythrocytes are present by using the following formula:

$$\text{Corrected TWBC/mm}^3 = \frac{\text{TWBC} \times 100}{\begin{array}{c}100 + \text{No. immature RBCs} \\ \text{per 100 leukocytes}\end{array}}$$

With counting methods requiring use of a hemocytometer, the difference between the counts obtained from each chamber should not exceed 10% to ensure accuracy between the two sides. If the difference does exceed 10%, the procedure should be repeated. The semidirect method using the phloxine stain is easier to perform and is more precise for hemocytometer counting than the Natt and Herricks method. To our knowledge, no comparisons have been made for the toluidine blue method; however, the results should be similar to those with the Natt and Herricks method. Because the semidirect method using phloxine B stain for determination of total leukocyte counts in birds depends on the leukocyte differential, especially the number of heterophils and eosinophils, it likely becomes less accurate as the level of mononuclear leukocytes exceeds that of the granulocytes.

Accurate interpretation of leukocyte counts, especially when determined by the semidirect method, depends on the accurate identification and differentiation of leukocytes in the blood film. The leukocyte differential is performed during the microscopic evaluation of Romanowsky-stained blood films. Blood samples collected into heparin make it necessary to prepare the blood films immediately following sample collection in order to decrease the incidence of cell clumping. Whenever possible, preparing blood films using blood containing no anticoagulant is preferred. The differential leukocyte count is performed by counting a minimum of 100 leukocytes in a monolayer area in the blood film. The cells counted are those consecutively encountered as one moves from one counting field to the next. The cells are classified as heterophils, eosinophils, basophils, lymphocytes, and monocytes. The number of each cell type becomes a fraction of the total or a percentage of the leukocyte population. Absolute numbers of each cell type are obtained by multiplying the total leukocyte concentration by the percentage of that type of leukocyte from the differential count.

Responses in disease

Avian leukograms often vary widely between normal birds of the same species (Table 20.4). Because birds often become excited when handled, the blood collection process usually results in a physiologic leukocytosis, and this physiologic response increases the concentration of heterophils and lymphocytes in the peripheral blood. Normal total leukocyte reference intervals obtained from birds generally are broader than those obtained from domestic mammals. Thus, avian leukogram values must differ greatly from the normal reference intervals to have diagnostic significance.

In general, gender differences in the normal leukogram of birds are not clinically significant; however, age differences can be. Generally, percentages of heterophils and lymphocytes and absolute lymphocyte counts vary significantly between adult and juvenile birds where younger birds tend to have higher lymphocyte counts. The leukogram may also be affected by seasonal influences, especially in free-ranging birds. For example, the absolute leukocyte, heterophil, and lymphocyte counts of ducks decrease during and after the remige molt, a seasonal event.

Leukocytosis and heterophilia

A leukocyte differential aids in the assessment of a leukocytosis. Because leukocytosis often is caused by inflammation, a heterophilia usually is present as well. The magnitude of the heterophilia depends on both the cause and the severity of the inflammation: the greater the degree of heterophilia, the greater the severity of the inflammation. A leukocytosis and heterophilia can be associated with inflammation in response to localized or systemic infections caused by a spectrum of infectious agents (i.e., bacteria, fungi,

Table 20.4 Leukocyte parameters for selected birds.

	WBC × $10^3/\mu L$	Heterophils %	Lymphocytes %	Monocytes %	Eosinophils %	Basophils %
Psittacines						
African gray parrot	5–15	45–75	20–50	0–3	0–2	0–22
Gray parrot	4.0–20.0	29–83	16–68	1–6	0–3	0
Amazon parrot	6–11	30–75	20–65	0–3	0–1	0–5
Blue-fronted Amazon	4.7–11.0	12–47	52–84	1–3	0–1	0–1
Cuban Amazon	1.9–24.7	19–28	71–75	0–5	0–5	0–1
Festive Amazon	2.2–7.0	22–32	66–76	0–4	0–2	0
Orange-wing Amazon	1.2–10.1	22–41	56–73	2–5	0–5	0–2
Yellow Amazon	2.2–7.2	12–52	48–80	0–8	0–1	0–1
Budgerigar	3–8	40–65	20–45	0–1	0–1	0–1
Caique	8–15	39–72	20–61	0–2	0–2	0–2
Cockatiel	5–13	40–70	25–55	0–2	0–2	0–6
Cockatoo	5–10	55–80	20–45	0–2	0–1	0–3
Black cockatoo	3.7–22.1	7–61	33–90	3–7	0	0–2
Palm cockatoo	1.4–17.6	24–75	24–69	1–7	0–1	0–1
White cockatoo	1.3–18.7	18–83	15–80	0–4	0–1	0–1
Conure	4–13	40–70	20–50	0–3	0–3	0–5
Golden conure	4.2–8.0	22–49	49–69	1–3	0–2	0
Patagonian conure	2.5–8.7	24–63	35–66	0–3	0–1	0
Eclectus parrot	9–20	35–50	45–65	0–2	0–1	0–3
Gray-cheek parakeet	4.5–12.0	40–75	20–60	0–3	0–1	0–5
Jardine's parrot	4–10	55–75	25–45	0–2	0–1	0–1
Lory	8–13	40–60	22–69	0–2	0–1	0–1
Red Lory	0.8–9.0	26–79	19–70	0–5	0–5	0–1
Lovebird	3–16	40–75	20–55	0–2	0–1	0–6
Macaw	7–22	40–60	35–60	0–3	0–1	0–1
Blue and gold macaw	1.7–36.0	13–60	36–84	0–2	0–2	0–2
Green-wing macaw	3.8–30.0	14–62	35–84	0–8	0–3	0–2
Hyacinthine macaw	1.5–19.2	52–89	10–77	0–2	0–4	0
Military macaw	13.7–18.0	12–63	43–80	0–8	0–2	0–1
Scarlet macaw	4.7–22.0	26–67	36–68	0–8	0–4	0–2
Pionus parrot	4.0–11.5	50–75	25–45	0–2	0–2	0–1
Quaker	4–10	55–80	20–45	0–4	0–2	0–6
Senegal parrot	4–14	55–75	25–45	0–2	0–1	0–1
Others						
Canary	4–9	50–80	20–45	0–1	0–2	0–1
Finch	3–8	20–65	20–65	0–1	0–1	0–5
Mynah	6–11	25–65	20–60	0–3	0–3	0–7
Toucan	4–10	35–65	25–50		0–4	0–5
Pigeon	1.3–2.3	50–60	20–40	0–3	0–3	0–3
Chicken	0.9–3.2	15–50	29–84	0–7	0–16	0–8
Ringneck pheasant	1.8–3.9	12–30	63–83	2–9	0–1	0–3
Turkey	1.6–2.5	29–52	35–48	3–10	0–5	0–9
Quail	1.3–2.5	25–50	50–70	0–4	0–15	0–2
Canada goose	1.3–1.9					
Mallard duck[a]	2.3–2.5	35–40	52–56	0–6	0–1	0–4
Mallard duck[b]	2.3–2.5	27–31	64–68	0–3	0–1	0–3
Golden eagle	1.2–1.5	81–86	14–22	0–1	2–5	0–1
Peregrine falcon	3.3–11.0	1–9	1–3	0–1	0–1	0–1
Tawny owl	4.0–59.0	1.6–9.6 × $10^3/\mu L$	2.1–7.2 × $10^3/\mu L$	0–0.5 × $10^3/\mu L$	0.2–3.0 × $10^3/\mu L$	0.1–0.4 × $10^3/\mu L$
White-back vulture	1.3–2.0	1.5–25.9 × $10^3/\mu L$	0–4.8 × $10^3/\mu L$	0–3.7 × $10^3/\mu L$	0–2.2 × $10^3/\mu L$	0–0 × $10^3/\mu L$

[a] January.

[b] June.

Sources: Based on Pollack et al. (2005); Tell and Citino (1992); Cray (2000); Campbell (2000); Polo et al. (1998); Spagnolo et al. (2008); and Naidoo et al. (2008).

Chlamydophila, viruses, and parasites) and noninfectious causes (i.e., traumatic injury, foreign bodies, or toxicities). A marked leukocytosis and heterophilia often are associated with diseases produced by common avian pathogens, such as *Chlamydophila*, *Mycobacterium*, and *Aspergillus*. Persistent inflammatory leukograms may occur with long standing inflammation, such as the presence of granulomas. Viral diseases can also result in a marked leukocytosis; however, they are not typically associated with a heterophilic leukocytosis. These include avian leukosis virus, reticuloendotheliosis virus, Marek's disease (herpesvirus), myeloblastosis (retrovirus), and lymphoid leukosis (reticuloendotheliosis virus and avian leukosis virus).

An absolute leukocytosis with a moderate mature heterophilia and lymphopenia are typically the hallmarks of a stress leukogram. The mechanisms mediating these cellular changes are poorly defined in birds but appear to be associated with changes in endogenous corticosteroid levels. Corticosteroid levels change rapidly during stress; however, absolute leukocyte numbers change more slowly (30 minutes to 20 hours) in response to stress and are less variable but more enduring. Blood samples ideally should be collected quickly with minimal stress to the patient to avoid leukogram changes associated with handling. When working with wild birds, blood collection should be performed immediately after capture. An absolute leukocytosis may also occur when exogenous glucocorticoids are administered to birds. The stimulus for heterophil recruitment or mobilization arises from bone marrow interactions with the hypothalamic-pituitary-adrenal cortical axis.

Stressors increase the number of heterophils and reduce the number of lymphocytes. Consequently, the heterophil/lymphocyte ratio (H/L ratio) has been used as an index of stress in birds since the early 1980s. The H/L ratio has been shown to be a reliable indicator of stress associated with injury, reproductive cycles, and seasonal changes in birds in both captive and field situations. The H/L ratio appears to be the most accurate indicator of stress because it is less variable than the number of heterophils or lymphocytes alone. In free-living birds, H/L ratios may be more useful than a single measure of plasma corticosterone in assessing response to chronic stressors like injury or crowded conditions in the breeding colony, and H/L ratios have been shown to be a valuable tool to measure stress in passerine birds and to evaluate management practices for critically endangered passerines. In the poultry industry, H/L reference values of 0.20, 0.50, and 0.80 are characteristic of low, optimal, and high degrees of stress, respectively. However, there are limitations to the accuracy of the H/L ratio as an indicator of stress in birds. Recent studies suggest that the H : L ratio appears to be an unreliable indicator of stress owing to the lack of correlation between that ratio and plasma corticosterone concentrations. The magnitude of leukocytosis and heterophilia during disease or corticosteroid excess varies with the H : L ratio, with greater responses being seen in species with normal H : L ratios of 3.0 : 1 versus those with ratios of 0.5 : 1. Initially, species that normally have high numbers of circulating lymphocytes (e.g., Anseriformes) may show a leukopenia but, later (i.e., up to 12 hours) demonstrate typical leukocytosis, heterophilia, and lymphopenia. Species that normally have greater numbers of circulating heterophils (e.g., Galliformes) show a less dramatic change in the stress leukogram. The H/L ratio may vary with conditions that affect heterophil and lymphocyte numbers, such as age and inflammatory disease. There may also be species variation in the hemic response to corticosteroids and stress, which would in turn affect the magnitude of the; in some extreme circumstances, a bird may even exhibit a heteropenia and basophilia.

Although the nature of the immune response to bacterial infections in birds has not yet been fully elucidated, nonlymphoid cells, such as macrophages and heterophils, play a crucial role in immunity to bacteria. Therefore, increases in the numbers of heterophils and monocytes in the peripheral blood would be expected with bacterial infections. The degree of the inflammatory response present in the blood may be associated with the location of the bacterial infection. For example, psittacine birds with varying degrees and causes of sinusitis often exhibit normal complete blood cell counts or have only a mild inflammatory leukogram, perhaps because the lesions remained a focal one.

Common hematologic abnormalities associated with avian mycobacteriosis include mild to moderate nonregenerative anemia, marked to severe leukocytosis, heterophilia, lymphopenia, monocytosis, eosinophilia, and immature heterophils. Thrombocytosis has also been reported in birds with mycobacteriosis. Laboratory findings can be variable and reflect the stage of the disease, presence of concurrent illness, and species differences. Initial hematological results may be normal in some individuals. In such cases, repeat and serial complete blood cell counts may be useful in the diagnosis of mycobacteriosis. A leukocytosis with a moderate to marked monocytosis, with or without heterophilia, is supportive of possible mycobacteriosis. High leukocyte counts are typically seen in birds with advanced mycobacteriosis. When present, immature heterophils indicate a poor prognosis.

An inflammatory leukogram characterized by heterophilia and/or monocytosis is often associated with infections with *Chlamydophila* or mycotic infections, such as aspergillosis. The presence of toxic or immature heterophils indicates severe inflammation and a poor prognosis for survival.

An inflammatory leukogram characterized by heterophilia, lymphopenia, and monocytosis may be associated with neoplastic diseases such as squamous cell carcinoma, papillomatosis, and other neoplasias in birds. Bacterial or fungal infections within the lesions may be responsible for this; however, tissue necrosis and granulocyte breakdown can also stimulate the inflammatory response. Some tumors may produce a hematopoietic factor capable of promoting a leukocytosis, which could cause an inflammatory leukogram.

Immature heterophils rarely are present in the peripheral blood of normal birds. When they do occur, however, their presence usually results from excessive peripheral utilization of mature heterophils with depletion of the mature storage pool in the hematopoietic tissue, which indicates a severe inflammatory response, especially when associated with a leukopenia. Marked increases in the concentration of immature heterophils also may result from granulocytic leukemia, which is a rare condition in birds.

Toxic heterophils are associated with severe, systemic illness such as septicemia, viremia, chlamydophilosis, mycotic infections, and severe tissue necrosis. The degree of heterophil toxicity usually indicates the severity of the bird's condition, and a marked number of 4+ toxic heterophils indicates a grave prognosis.

Hematological indicators of inflammation are species and etiology dependent; however, the presence of a mild to moderate anemia, heterophilia, monocytosis, and heterophil morphological atypia appears to be the most consistent hematologic changes associated with inflammation in birds. Interpretive guidelines have been developed for some species of birds. For example, in free-ranging black cockatoos (*Calyptorhynchus* spp.), anemia can be graded based upon a PCV of 30–35% as a mild anemia, 20–30% as moderate anemia, and less than 20% as severe anemia. A mild leukocytosis in black cockatoos is represented by a leukocyte count less than 25,000/μL, whereas a count between 25,000 and 40,000/μL and greater than 40,000/μL represent moderate and severe responses respectively. Significant heterophilias in black cockatoos are represented by counts less than 20,000/μL as mild, 21,000–30,000/μL as moderate, and greater than 30,000/μL as severe. Toxic heterophils were not a common finding in black cockatoos with inflammatory disorders.

In contrast to black cockatoos, the inflammatory response in falcons (*Falco* spp.) appears different. Normal falcons in general are reported to have a PCV between 37% and 53%, hemoglobin concentration between 12 and 21 g/dL, total leukocyte count between 3000 and 11,000 μL, and an absolute heterophil count greater than the absolute lymphocyte count. Falcons rarely exhibit a leukocytosis greater than 17,000/μL in response to inflammation regardless of the etiology. Aspergillosis, a common mycotic disease of birds, frequently causes a severe inflammatory disease in birds; however that response is variable between the species. For example, falcons (*Falco* spp.) with aspergillosis develop a relatively mild leukocytosis compared to *Buteo* hawks that demonstrate a severe leukocytosis.

Leukopenia

Leukopenia is associated with either consumption of peripheral leukocytes or decreased production. In many species of birds, an absolute heteropenia is the cause of a leukopenia. Heteropenia results from decreased survival of mature heterophils or from decreased or ineffective production. Leukopenias associated with heteropenias can occur with severe bacterial infections or certain viral diseases (e.g., Pacheco's parrot disease). Severe leukopenia is commonly associated with parrots infected with psittacine circovirus, where peracute infections can present with leukopenia, anemia, or pancytopenia. Leukopenia and heteropenia with the presence of immature heterophils suggest exhaustion of the mature heterophil storage pool because of excessive peripheral demand for heterophils, as seen with severe inflammation. A degenerative left shift is reflected by an absolute heteropenia in conjunction with immature heterophilia and toxicity that indicates either an overwhelming demand for heterophils in the periphery due to bacterial sepsis or viral disease, a reduced production of heterophils in the bone marrow, or an ineffective granulopoiesis due to maturation arrest. Degenerative left shifts and depletion are differentiated by the presence of toxic heterophils or by following the decreasing leukocyte count with serial leukograms. Bone marrow evaluation may be helpful in the rule-out of these conditions. In general, a degenerative left shift in the leukogram of a bird indicates a poor prognosis for survival. As discussed, leukopenia and lymphopenia can occur as an early, corticosteroid-induced leukogram response in some species of birds. Leukopenias and lymphopenia also may suggest a viral cause, although such causes have been poorly documented in birds. Leukopenia and lymphopenia has been associated with mycotoxins poisoning and other toxicities in birds. Leukopenia associated with a heteropenia, marked anemia, and thrombocytopenia (pancytopenia) suggests injury to the bone marrow, which can be associated with certain neoplastic conditions and other causes of bone marrow injury discussed below.

Heteropenia

Heteropenia is seen with acute inflammatory disease or in those with marked severity resulting from heterophils being consumed at a faster rate than being produced and released to peripheral circulation. A heteropenia with a left shift and toxic changes is indicative of an acute inflammatory response associated with excessive peripheral utilization of heterophils. Immune-mediated heteropenia, should it occur in birds, would result in a profound heteropenia in the peripheral blood and depletion of the maturation pool in the bone marrow. Injury to the stem cells in the bone marrow can occur with chemicals, drugs, or infectious agents, such as viral agents, that affect rapidly dividing cells resulting in a profound heteropenia. Stem cell injury would first appear as a profound heteropenia followed by a thrombocytopenia and eventually a nonregenerative anemia. A heteropenia with a left shift, no anemia, and adequate thrombocytes is indicative of an acute inflammatory response with exhaustion of the mature heterophil storage pool caused by excessive peripheral utilization of heterophils. A heteropenia with no left shift, no anemia, and adequate thrombocytes is indicative of an acute viral infection or acute marrow injury. This has been shown with psittacine birds experimentally infected with the herpesvirus that causes Pacheco's disease that developed severe heteropenia. A heteropenia associated with a nonregenerative anemia and possibly a thrombocytopenia is indicative of a chronic marrow injury. Fenbendazole toxicity in birds produces a bone marrow toxicosis that results in a transient leukopenia, severe heteropenia, and anemia as the result of a compromise to cellular division impacting rapidly dividing. Leukopenia associated with a heteropenia, marked anemia, and thrombocytopenia suggestive of stem cell injury to the bone marrow can be associated with certain neoplastic conditions. Absolute heteropenia in conjunction with immature heterophilia and heterophil toxicity indicates either an overwhelming demand for heterophils in the periphery due to bacterial sepsis or viral disease, a reduced production of heterophils in the bone marrow, or ineffective granulopoiesis. This type of leukogram carries a poor prognosis.

Lymphocytosis

Lymphocytosis may occur with antigenic stimulation. An occasional reactive lymphocyte may be found in blood films from normal birds; however, many reactive lymphocytes suggest antigenic stimulation associated with infectious disease (Figure 20.37). Lymphocytosis also can occur with lymphocytic leukemia (e.g., avian leukosis). In some cases of lymphocytic leukemia, immature lymphocytes may be present in the blood film. A marked lymphocytosis in which most lymphocytes appear as small, mature lymphocytes with scalloped cytoplasmic margins also has been associated with lymphoid neoplasia.

Lymphopenia

Lymphopenia can occur with glucocorticosteroid excess, which may be more pronounced in some avian species than others. Immunosuppressive drugs other than corticosteroids, such as chemotherapeutic agents, may also cause lymphopenia. Lymphopenia may also be associated with toxicities, such as zinc intoxication. A lymphopenia with numerous atypical large lymphocytes containing scalloped cytoplasmic margins has been documented in birds with lymphoma.

Monocytosis

A monocytosis can be seen with acute and chronic inflammation and occurs with an increased demand for monocytes. Monocytosis in avian patients is typically associated with infectious and inflammatory disease, especially those associated with granulomatous inflammation. Other causes of monocytosis may include hemic reaction to a foreign body and certain nutritional deficiencies, such as zinc. Anemia and leukocytosis with increases in monocyte, heterophil, and basophil numbers are a common hematologic feature of chronic inflammation in birds. Early in the inflammatory process an initial leukocytosis and heterophilia generally occurs; however, some infectious agents may elicit an acute monocytosis. For example, acute *Mycoplasma* infections can result in heterophilia, lymphopenia, monocytosis, and eosinophilia. Anemia and monocytosis then develop as the inflammation becomes chronic. Organisms such as *Mycobacterium*, *Chlamydophila*, and fungi such as *Aspergillus* typically cause granulomatous inflammation in birds and are often associated with monocytosis. A profound nonregenerative anemia and severe monocytosis can occur with chronic clostridial infections. Neoplasia may cause monocytosis in some birds; for example, quail exposed experimentally to Rous sarcoma virus developed a leukocytosis as tumor growth developed. The leukocyte counts returned to normal in birds that showed regression of the tumors; however, those with progression of tumor growth continued to exhibit a leukocytosis with heterophilia, monocytosis, and lymphopenia.

Eosinophilia

Because the exact functions of avian eosinophils are not known, interpreting the cause of peripheral eosinophilia is difficult in birds. Although this avian granulocyte was given the name "eosinophil," avian eosinophils may behave differently than mammalian eosinophils. Studies have shown that avian eosinophils may participate in delayed (type IV) hypersensitivity reactions, which does not occur with mammalian eosinophils. Experiments using parasite antigens have failed to induce peripheral eosinophilias, although eosinophilias associated with gastrointestinal nematode infestations have been reported. The responses of avian eosinophils to inflammation are variable and have not been reliably associated with a specific etiology. Despite limited knowledge regarding the function of avian eosinophils, peripheral eosinophilia in birds can be loosely interpreted as being a response to internal or external parasitism or exposure to foreign antigens (i.e., hypersensitivity response). It has been noted; however, that parasitic infections may not elicit a peripheral eosinophilia in birds.

Eosinopenia

Eosinopenia may be difficult to document in birds. If present, it is expected to be associated with a stress response or with administration of glucocorticosteroids.

Basophilia

Basophilia is rare in birds. Because avian basophils produce, store, and release histamine, they may have a function similar to that of mammalian basophils. Therefore, avian basophils may participate in immediate hypersensitivity reactions, release mediators for thrombocyte activation, cause smooth muscle contractions, initiate edema, and affect coagulation. Basophils appear to participate in the initial phase of acute inflammation in birds; however, this usually is not reflected as a basophilia on the leukogram. Peripheral basophilia may suggest early inflammation or an immediate hypersensitivity reaction in birds. A stress-related basophilia occurs in chickens subjected to food restriction, but this response may be age or duration dependent.

Thrombocytes and hemostasis

Morphology

Avian thrombocytes are nucleated cells that are the second most numerous cell (after erythrocytes) found in the blood. Thrombocytes are typically small, round to oval cells (smaller than erythrocytes) with a round to oval nucleus that contains densely clumped chromatin. The nucleus is more rounded than an erythrocyte nucleus and thrombocytes tend to have a high N : C ratio. They are generally the smallest cell in the peripheral blood but only slightly smaller than small mature lymphocytes. For example, thrombocyte measurements for adult *Coturnix* quail are 4.10 ± 0.30 μm in diameter for males and 4.06 ± 0.32 μm in diameter for females. Normal, mature thrombocytes have a colorless to pale gray cytoplasm, which often has a reticulated appearance. The appearance of the cytoplasm is an important feature in differentiating thrombocytes from small, mature lymphocytes (Figures 20.34–20.36 and 20.42). Cytoplasmic vacuolation can occur in activated or phagocytic thrombocytes. Thrombocytes frequently contain one or more distinct eosinophilic (dense) granules, which usually are located in one area of the cytoplasm. Thrombocytes participate in the hemostatic process and, like mammalian platelets; therefore, they secrete thromboplastin, which polymerizes fibrinogen in the formation of clots in blood coagulation. Activated thrombocytes occurring in aggregates may have indistinct cellular outlines or cytoplasmic pseudopodia, and may demonstrate degranulation of dense granules, cellular degeneration, and nuclear pyknosis. Ultrastructurally, the cytoplasm resembles that of mammalian platelets. The granules that frequently are seen in thrombocytes at light microscopy appear as aggregates of many small granules at electron microscopy. The dense granules contain primarily 5′-hydroxytryptamine, and they are an unlikely source of thromboplastin. Thrombocytes aggregated in clumps show degranulation of dense granules, cellular degeneration, and nuclear pyknosis. Avian thrombocytes contain a large amount of serotonin, and some studies suggest that they are capable of phagocytosis and may participate in removing foreign materials from the blood.

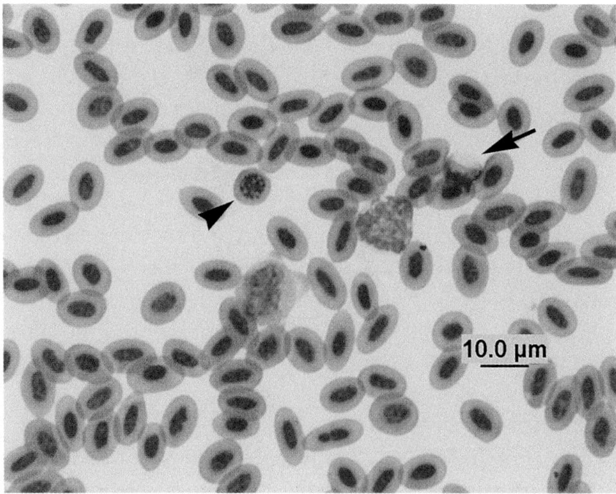

Figure 20.42 A monocyte, immature erythrocyte (mid-polychromatic rubricyte, arrowhead), medium lymphocyte (arrow), and heterophil in the blood film of a chicken (*Gallus gallus domesticus*). Wright-Giemsa stain.

Avian thrombocytes may play a role in innate immunity because they are capable of phagocytosis and may participate in removing foreign materials from the blood. Theoretically, even though thrombocytes are less phagocytic than heterophils, avian thrombocytes may act as a nonspecific "scavenging" phagocyte, capable of clearing a wide range of foreign objects, including bacteria. Therefore, thrombocytes may play a role in fighting bacterial infection, although the mechanisms, by which thrombocytes interact with, adhere to, or respond to bacteria are largely unknown. Light and electron microscopy has demonstrated that thrombocytes contain lysosomal vesicles and are actively phagocytic *in vitro* for vital dyes and Gram-positive bacteria. Oxidative burst activity has been demonstrated in avian thrombocytes after phagocytosis of bacteria. In some studies, oxygen radicals were detected in thrombocytes after activation by binding the monoclonal antibody 11C3 that targets the avian homolog of the platelet integrin GPIIb-IIIa. Further studies on how thrombocytes interact with other cells and the role of complement and Fc receptors in phagocytosis and antimicrobial activity are needed to determine specific roles of thrombocytes in avian immunity.

Laboratory evaluation

The thrombocyte concentration of most avian species studied ranges between 20,000 and 30,000 cells/μL, or 10–15 thrombocytes per 1000 erythrocytes. The actual thrombocyte concentration is difficult to determine, because thrombocytes tend to clump. Therefore, their concentration often is reported as either normal, increased, or decreased, based on estimates made from peripheral blood films. Approximately one to five thrombocytes can be seen in a monolayer ×1000 (oil-immersion) field in a blood film from a normal bird, unless the thrombocytes clump excessively during preparation. Thrombocytopenia is suggested by thrombocyte numbers less than one per monolayer ×1000 field, and thrombocytosis is suggested by numbers greater than five in an average monolayer ×1000 field. A thrombocyte concentration can be obtained with the same hemocytometer used for obtaining total leukocyte and erythrocyte counts with the Natt and Herricks method. The number of thrombocytes counted in the central large square on both sides of the Neubauer-ruled hemocytometer is multiplied by 1000 to obtain the number of thrombocytes per microliter of blood.

Responses in disease

Avian thrombocytes are derived from mononuclear precursors in the bone marrow. Immature thrombocytes occasionally are present in the peripheral blood of birds. They are round to oval cells with round to oval nuclei and basophilic cytoplasm compared with mature thrombocytes (Figure 20.43). The mid and late immature thrombocytes most commonly are seen when immature cells are present. The presence of immature thrombocytes usually indicates a regenerative response to excessive utilization of thrombocytes.

Young birds tend to have relatively higher numbers of circulating thrombocytes than adult birds. Thrombocytosis associated with large thrombocytes has been reported in birds with chronic inflammation, which may be related to the thrombocytes' phagocytic role in inflammatory disease.

Thrombocytopenia is usually the result of decreased bone marrow production or excessive peripheral utilization or destruction, and may be associated with severe septicemia and possibly disseminated intravascular coagulation (DIC). Thrombocytosis associated with large thrombocytes has been reported in birds with chronic inflammation, which may be related to the thrombocytes' phagocytic role in inflammatory disease.

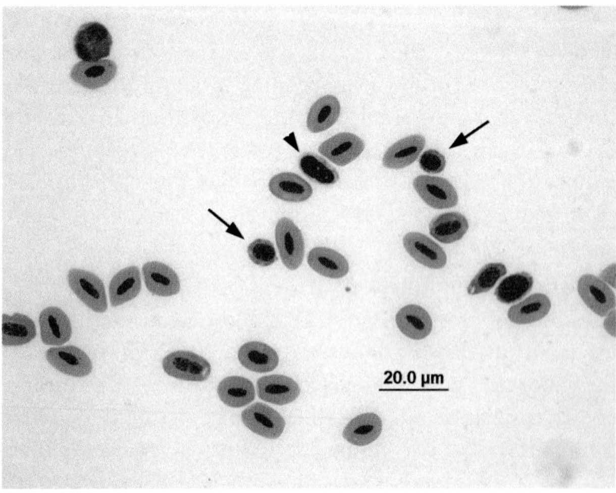

Figure 20.43 Immature thrombocytes (arrows) and a mature thrombocyte (arrowhead) in the blood film of a parrot (*Eclectus roratus*). Wright-Giemsa stain.

The initial hemostatic plug of birds is formed through the adhesion and aggregation of thrombocytes, and the secondary hemostatic plug develops through the coagulation cascade after injury to a blood vessel wall. Most clotting factors involved in avian blood coagulation are similar to those in mammals. Although evidence suggests an intrinsic clotting mechanism in some avian species, coagulation of avian blood appears to depend on the extrinsic clotting system, which involves the release of tissue thromboplastin (i.e., factor III). The extrinsic and common pathways can be evaluated using a one-step prothrombin time test. Avian brain thromboplastin is required for avian prothrombin time testing because commercially available mammalian sources of thromboplastin give unreliable results in birds. Studies suggest that the source of thromboplastin should be from the brain of the same species of bird as the patient for prothrombin time determinations. The normal prothrombin time for most birds is 13 seconds or less. Increased prothrombin time is produced by a defect in the intrinsic or common pathway of coagulation and is caused by a deficiency of factors V, VII, X, fibrinogen, and prothrombin (factor II). Increased prothrombin times in affected birds can be related to the presence and the severity of hepatic lesions. Whole blood (capillary) clotting times in birds usually are less than 5 minutes; however, normal values appear to range between 2 and 10 minutes. The whole-blood clotting time is more variable than the prothrombin time.

Blood parasites

The three genera of hemosporidian parasites most commonly found in the peripheral blood of birds are *Hemoproteus, Plasmodium*, and *Leukocytozoon*. Microfilaria of filarial nematodes are also commonly found in blood films of wild birds. Microfilaria are typically found between the cells, whereas the merozoites of *Hemoproteus, Plasmodium*, and *Leukocytozoon* invade erythrocytes and their gametocytes are found within the erythrocyte. In general, the presence of blood parasites in wild birds has no effect on the health of the bird, although combined infections with *Hemoproteus* and *Leukocytozoon* can produce a fatal anemia in young birds. Birds may be infected with a single blood parasite, or may have mixed infections based on examination of stained blood films. Populations of certain free-ranging species of birds in various parts of the world appear to be free of blood parasites, whereas birds in other areas often have multiple infections. Avian hemosporidian parasites can vary in their degree of host specificity and even have a broad host range likely relying on a key host species. Free-living birds may exhibit seasonal variation in the degree of parasitemia. The age and effects of captivity may affect the occurrence of blood parasites in birds. For example, Blanco et al. reported that *Hemoproteus* and *Leukocytozoon* were more commonly found in birds held in captivity for longer than 365 days and *Leukocytozoon* was found more commonly in adults and juveniles than nestlings. Identification of avian blood parasites can usually be made using stains commonly used for evaluation of blood cells. Films made from fresh blood, without the addition of an anticoagulant, provide samples with fewer artifacts affecting the parasite.

Haemoproteus

Protozoan blood parasites of the genus *Haemoproteus* are common in many species of wild birds. The only forms of the parasite in the peripheral blood of birds are gametocytes, which range in size from small, developing, ring forms to the elongate, crescent-shaped, mature gametocyte that partially encircles the erythrocyte nucleus to form the characteristic "halter shape" (Figures 20.44 and 20.45). The mature gametocyte typically occupies greater than half the cytoplasmic volume of the host erythrocyte and it causes minimal displacement of the host cell nucleus; the nucleus is never pushed to the cell margin. *Haemoproteus* gametocytes contain refractile, yellow to brown pigment granules (hemozoin) that represent iron pigment deposited as a result of hemoglobin utilization. Macrogametocytes stain dark blue with Romanowsky stains and have iron pigment dispersed throughout the cytoplasm of the parasite, whereas microgametocytes stain pale blue to pink and have iron pigment aggregated into a spherical mass. Erythrocytes parasitized by *Hemoproteus* are larger than normal erythrocytes, which likely causes the cells to become fragile. PCR (polymerase chain reaction) analysis for *Hemoproteus* can be used to detect low parasitemia.

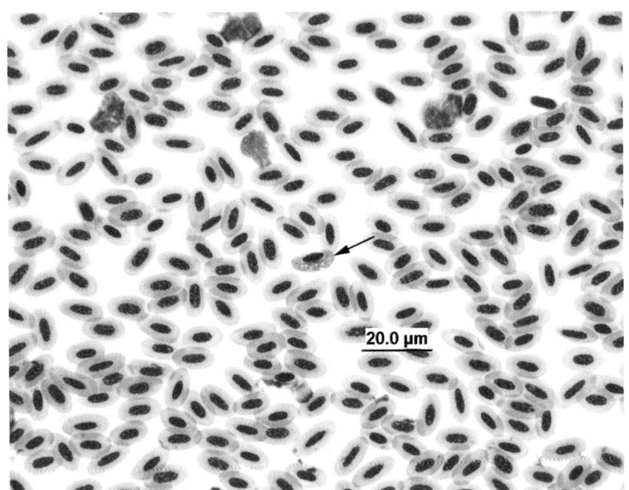

Figure 20.44 Haemoproteus gametocyte (arrow) in the blood film of a pigeon (*Columba livia domestica*). Wright-Giemsa stain.

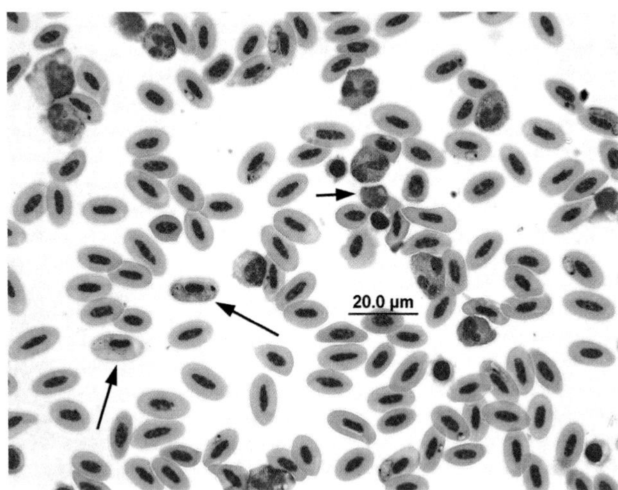

Figure 20.45 *Haemoproteus* gametocytes (long arrows) and an extracellular macrogametocyte (short arrow) in the blood film of an owl (*Bubo virginianus*). Wright-Giemsa stain.

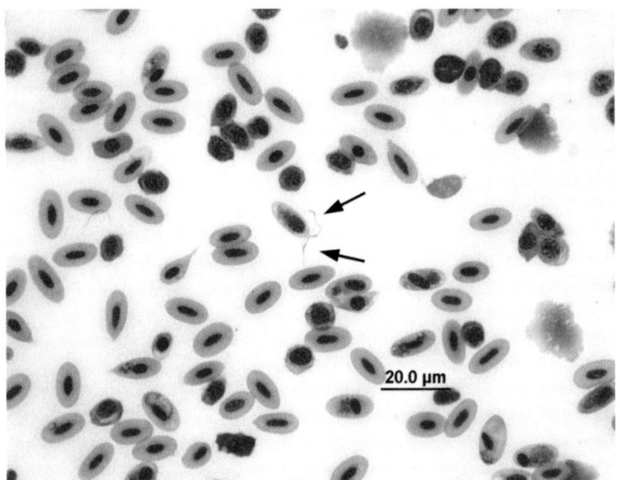

Figure 20.46 *Haemoproteus* gametocytes and an extracellular microgametocyte (arrows) in the blood film of a kestrel (*Falco sparverius*). Wright-Giemsa stain.

Occasionally, extraerythrocytic macrogametes and microgametes can be found in blood films, especially those made from blood collected several hours prior to preparing the film (Figures 20.45 and 20.46). Extraerythrocytic macrogametes are round and resemble the gametocytes normally seen within the erythrocyte. Microgametes are small spindle-shaped structures scattered throughout the blood film (Figure 20.46). Typically these forms are found in the midgut of the insect host following a blood meal but can appear in blood films when erythrocytes begin to deteriorate as the blood sample ages.

A banana-shaped ookinete, the zygote formed by the union of a macrogametocyte and a microgametocyte may

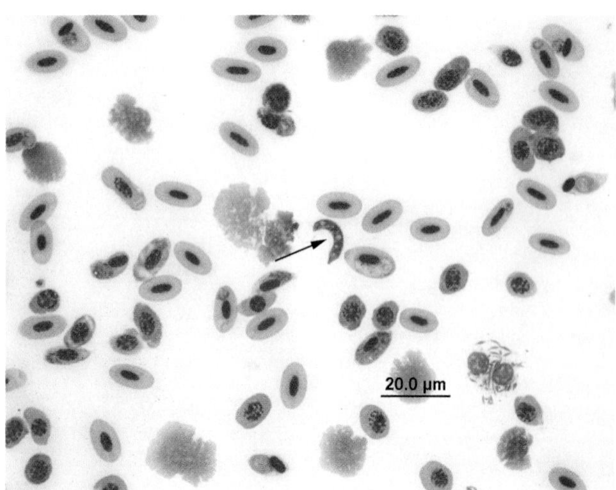

Figure 20.47 A banana-shaped ookinete (arrow) in the blood film of a kestrel (*Falco sparverius*). Wright-Giemsa stain.

also be found in the blood film (Figure 20.47). Macrogametocytes, microgametocytes, and ookinetes are rarely found in the peripheral blood films of animals and when this occurs, it is likely associated with a substantial delay between blood collection and preparation of the blood film. It is difficult to determine if the ookinete is from the *Hemoproteus* or another parasite, *Plasmodium*. A delay between blood collection and blood film preparation also creates an increased number of smudge cells on the blood film.

Bloodsucking insect vectors, such as hippoboscid flies (Hippoboscidae) and midges of the genus *Culicoides* (Ceratopogonidae), transmit *Haemoproteus*. The insect host ingests gametocytes when it feeds and the parasites then undergo a series of developmental stages to become sporozoites within the salivary gland. Sporozoites are injected into the new avian host when the insect feeds. The sporozoites enter the bird's vascular endothelial cells in various tissues (primarily the lung, liver, bone marrow, and spleen) and then undergo schizogony. *Haemoproteus* schizonts occasionally are found in cytologic or histologic samples of infected tissue, and they appear as large, round cysts containing numerous multinucleated bodies or cytomeres. Each cytomere produces numerous merozoites that escape into the bloodstream when the endothelial cell and cytomeres rupture. Merozoites enter erythrocytes to become gametocytes, which then are ingested by insect hosts to complete the cycle.

The pathogenicity of *Haemoproteus* generally is low, and parasitized birds rarely show evidence of disease. Clinical disease, however, can occur in certain avian species, such as pigeons, jays, and quail, nestlings, and in birds suffering from other diseases that, perhaps, result in immunodeficiencies. Mortalities associated with this parasite may also be the result of infections in aberrant hosts. The clinical signs include hemolytic anemia, anorexia, and depression. Hemolytic anemia is probably a sequela to lysis of the fragile parasitized erythrocyte as it passes through the fine trabecular network of the spleen. Other hematological changes that may occur during the erythrocytic phase of infection include leukocytosis, heterophilia, lymphocytosis, eosinophilia, and monocytosis. Death may be associated with severe anemia and hepatic necrosis resulting in hemorrhage related to megaloschizont-associated lesions (pre-erythrocytic stage) rather than the intraerythrocytic gametocytes. Hepatomegaly and splenomegaly may be observed at postmortem evaluation.

The degree of *Haemoproteus* parasitemia can be graded semiquantitatively based on the number of gametocytes per field when viewed under 400× magnification and used as an index to assess the recovery of birds, especially raptors, from traumatic injuries or diseases. A score of 0 is assigned if no parasites are observed, a 1 with less than 1 parasite, a 2 if 1–5 parasites, a 3 if 6–10 parasites, and a 4 if greater than 10 parasites. For example, an injured raptor that presents with *Haemoproteus* parasitemia score of 3 or 4 will dramatically drop to a score of 1 or 2 as it recovers from its injuries. Presumably, this represents an improved immune status of the bird. The intensity of the hematozoan infection can also be calculated from manual quantification of 2000 erythrocytes; however, the results from this method are significantly lower than the intensity calculated from digital quantification of 50,000 erythrocytes. The later allows for a precise method to quantify infections of low to moderate intensity.

Plasmodium

Parasites of the genus *Plasmodium* can be pathogenic and responsible for malaria, which affects certain species of birds (e.g., canaries, penguins, ducks, pigeons, raptors, and domestic poultry). Many avian species appear to be asymptomatic carriers of the parasite, however, and do not develop the clinical disease. Outbreaks of avian malaria occur sporadically in endemic areas, especially during seasons associated with increased mosquito populations. Clinical signs associated with avian malaria include anemia, anorexia, depression, and acute death. The hemogram often reveals hemolytic anemia, leukocytosis, and lymphocytosis. Hemoglobinuria or biliverdinuria also may occur. Splenomegaly and hepatomegaly often are seen on postmortem examination.

Blood smear examination is a definitive diagnostic method for detecting *Plasmodium* spp. because the intermediate forms (trophozoites, schizonts, and gametocytes) can be seen in the cells. In both *Plasmodium* spp. and *Hemoproteus* spp., refractile yellow-to-brown pigmented granules (hemozoin) are observed because schizonts ingest and metabolize hemoglobin resulting in refractile granule formation. Unlike *Haemoproteus*, stages other than the gametocyte, such as schizonts and trophozoites, can be found within erythrocytes, thrombocytes, and leukocytes (Figures 20.48–20.50). Certain *Plasmodium* sp. have round to irregular gametocytes that cause marked displacement of the host-cell nucleus,

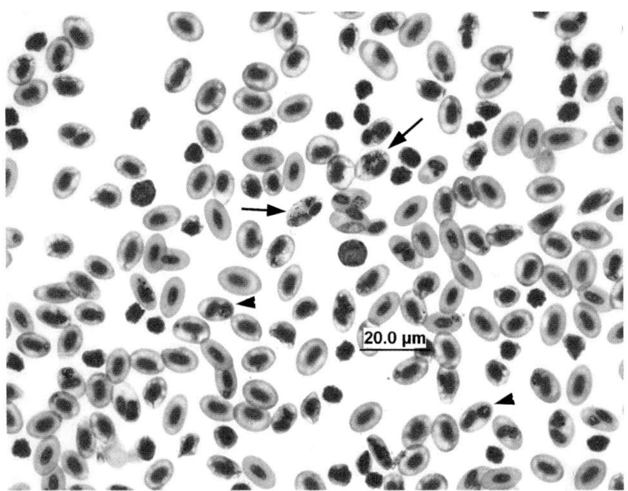

Figure 20.48 *Plasmodium* gametocytes (arrows) and schizogony (arrowhead) in the blood film of a skua (*Stercorarius skua*). Wright-Giemsa stain.

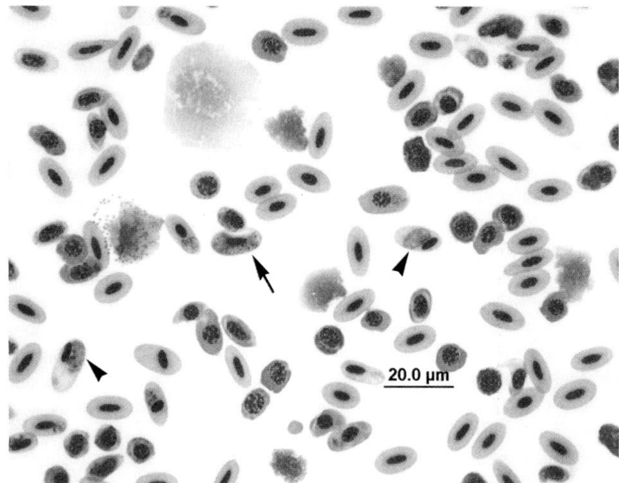

Figure 20.50 *Haemoproteus* gametocyte (arrow) and *Plasmodium* gametocytes (arrowheads) in the blood film of a kestrel (*Falco sparverius*) with marked polychromasia. Wright-Giemsa stain.

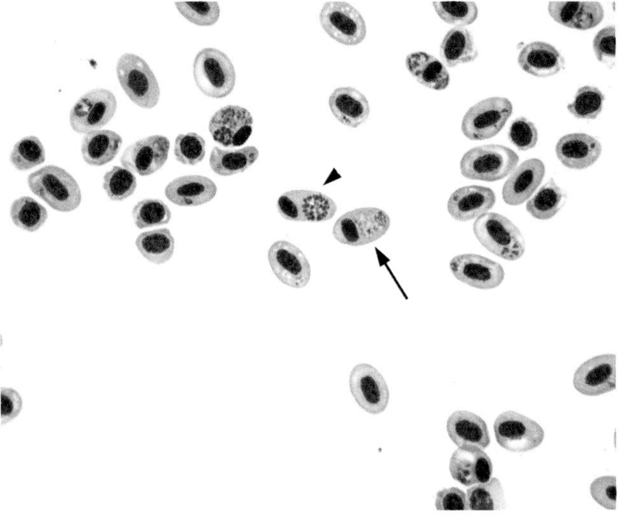

Figure 20.49 *Plasmodium* gametocytes (arrow) and schizogony (arrowhead) in the blood film of a skua (*Stercorarius skua*). Wright-Giemsa stain.

whereas other species have elongate gametocytes that do not displace the host-cell nucleus. Like those of *Haemoproteus*, *Plasmodium* gametocytes contain refractile, yellow to brown, iron pigment granules, which tend to be scattered, and macrogametocytes stain deeper blue than microgametocytes. *Plasmodium* trophozoites are small, round to oval, ameboid forms containing a large vacuole that pushes the parasite nucleus to one edge, thereby giving the trophozoite a "signet-ring" appearance. Schizonts are round to oval inclusions that contain several deeply staining merozoites; the number of merozoites is used to determine the *Plasmodium* species. Schizonts with developing merozoites exhibit clusters of merozoites that appear to be fused, which is in contrast to mature merozoites, which appear to be distinct bodies and separate from each other. Identification of the *Plasmodium* species depends on the location and appearance of the schizonts and gametocytes. The key features used to differentiate *Plasmodium* from *Haemoproteus* are the presence of schizogony in the peripheral blood, parasite stages within thrombocytes and leukocytes, and gametocytes causing marked displacement of the erythrocyte nucleus.

The organism is transmitted from infected to uninfected birds by mosquitoes (Culicidae) when, during feeding, sporozoites from the mosquito salivary glands invade host tissues and reproduce as schizonts to produce numerous merozoites. Unlike *Hemoproteus* spp., the merozoites of *Plasmodium* spp. penetrate erythrocytes, leukocytes, and thrombocytes and become ring-shaped trophozoites that mature into schizonts or infectious gametocytes. The schizonts rupture, killing the infected cells and releasing merozoites to infect more blood cells.

Leukocytozoon

Leukocytozoon, which is a protozoan parasite commonly found in the blood of wild birds, is identified by large, dark-staining macrogametocytes or light-staining microgametocytes on Romanowsky-stained blood films. The large gametocytes grossly distort the infected host cell, thereby elongating and distending the cell and making the identification of the cell difficult (Figure 20.51). The macrogametocyte appears as a parasite inclusion that occupies 77% of the area of the host cell-parasite complex. Microgametocytes are similar in morphology but are usually 5–10% smaller. Some parasitologists believe that immature erythrocytes rather than leukocytes, as suggested by the name of the parasite, serve as the host cell for *Leukocytozoon*. As with *Haemoproteus*, only the gametocytes of *Leukocytozoon* occur in the peripheral blood.

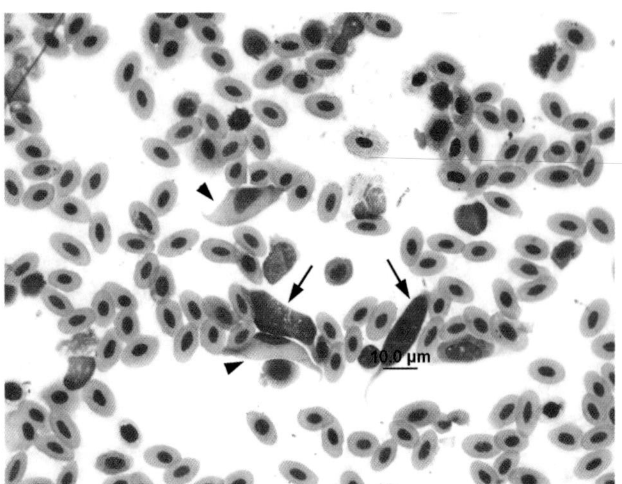

Figure 20.51 *Leukocytozoon* macrogametocytes (arrows) and microgametocytes (arrowheads) in the blood film of a hawk (*Buteo jamaicensis*). Wright-Giemsa stain.

Parasitized cells appear to have two nuclei: a dark-staining, host-cell nucleus that lies along the cell membrane, and a pale pink–staining, parasite nucleus that lies adjacent to the host-cell nucleus. *Leukocytozoon* gametocytes do not contain the refractile pigment granules seen in the gametocytes of *Haemoproteus* and *Plasmodium*. Appearance of the gametes in the peripheral blood can vary depending upon the species of *Leukocytozoon* present. For example, gametocytes *of Leukocytozoon sakharoffi*, the *Leukocytozoon* parasite of birds in the family Corvidae (crows, jays, and magpies), are round, and the host cell nucleus covers nearly 80% of the periphery of the parasite.

Leukocytozoon is transmitted by black flies (Simuliidae), which act as intermediate hosts and inject sporozoites into the blood of susceptible avian species. The sporozoites invade the endothelial and parenchymal cells of various tissues such as the liver, heart, and kidney, in which schizogony occurs. Primary schizogony typically occurs in the liver. When the schizonts mature they release thousands of merozoites, which then initiate a second generation of schizonts in the liver and in phagocytic cells throughout the body. The schizonts in phagocytic cells become very large and are called megaschizonts. The megaschizonts release millions of merozoites that can either initiate schizogony elsewhere or enter circulating erythrocytes (or perhaps leukocytes), where they develop into macrogametes or microgametes.

The pathogenicity of *Leukocytozoon* usually is low; however, certain species can be highly pathogenic for some birds, such as young waterfowl and turkeys. The clinical signs associated with this parasite include anemia, anorexia, and lelthargy. Clinical laboratory evaluation may reveal a hemolytic anemia, leukocytosis, and elevated serum enzymes such as aspartate aminotransferase or alanine aminotransferase, thereby suggesting hepatocellular necrosis. Postmortem findings may include splenomegaly and hepatomegaly with hepatic necrosis.

Microfilaria

Microfilaria are minute larvae of parasitic filarial nematodes measuring 5–7 µm in diameter and 200–300 µm in length that are commonly found in the peripheral blood of many species of birds. The adult filarial nematodes usually are not seen unless they occur in peripheral locations, such as in the fluid of distended joints. Adult filarial nematodes may occur anywhere within the body of birds, but they most frequently are seen in the air sacs, subcutaneously, or in the body cavities. Most of these parasites are considered to be nonpathogenic and cause little harm to their host.

Less common avian blood parasites

Other parasites that are seen less frequently in the peripheral blood of birds include *Atoxoplasma*, *Aegyptianella*, *Trypanosoma*, and *Borrelia*. *Atoxoplasma* is a coccidian parasite that often is found in passerine birds, which can be highly pathogenic, especially to canaries. It is transmitted directly via oocysts in the feces. Atoxoplasmosis is diagnosed on the basis of demonstrating characteristic sporozoites within the lymphocytes on peripheral blood films or cytologic imprints of the liver, spleen, or lung. The sporozoites appear as pale, eosinophilic, round to oval, intracytoplasmic inclusions within lymphocytes, monocytes, or macrophages in Romanowsky-stained preparations (Figure 20.52). The sporozoites indent the host lymphocyte nucleus, thereby resulting in a characteristic crescent shape. Sporozoites of *Atoxoplasma* lack pigment granules. Detection of *Atoxoplasma* in the peripheral blood can be improved by using a preparation of a buffy-coat film to concentrate the leukocytes for examination.

Aegyptianella is a minute parasite of avian erythrocytes that lacks pigment granules. It is a piroplasma that can affect

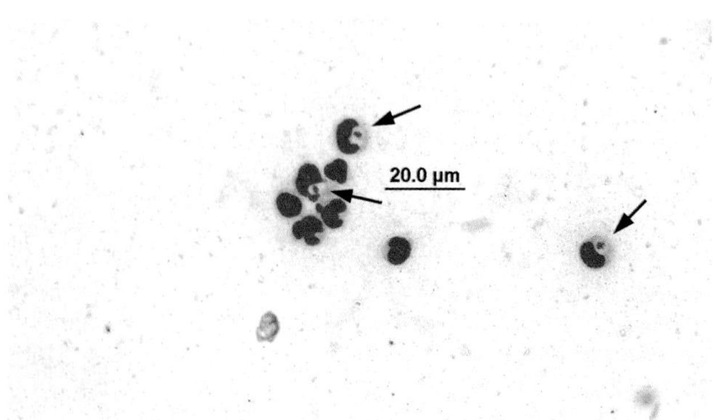

Figure 20.52 *Atoxoplasma* inclusions within lymphocytes from a buffy coat film of a thrush (*Garrulax chinensis*). Wright-Giemsa stain.

several avian species, usually those originating in tropical or subtropical climates. *Aegyptianella pullorum* occurs in chickens, geese, ducks, and turkeys. The organism is detected by demonstrating the developing forms within erythrocytes in blood films. Three forms can occur. One form, the initial body, is a small structure that is less than 1 mm in diameter and appears as a round, basophilic, intracytoplasmic inclusion similar to *Anaplasma marginale*. A second form is a round- to piriform-shaped inclusion with pale blue cytoplasm and a chromatin body at one pole resembling *Babesia*. The third form is a larger (2–4 μm), round to elliptical inclusion. *Aegyptianella* can be pathogenic, resulting in anemia, anorexia, and diarrhea. Postmortem findings include splenomegaly, hepatomegaly, and hepatic as well as renal degeneration.

Trypanosomes (*Trypanosoma*) occasionally are found in the peripheral blood of wild birds, especially passerines, Galliformes, waterfowl, and pigeons. They are transmitted by biting insects such as mosquitoes, hippoboscid flies, and blackflies or mites. Avian trypanosomes resemble those found in mammals. They have an undulating membrane, a slender, tapering posterior end, and a short, anteriorly directed flagellum. Trypanosomes usually are considered to be an incidental finding.

Borrelia anserina is the causative agent of avian spirochetosis, which can affect several species of birds, especially Galliformes and waterfowl. It is transmitted by arthropod vectors such as ticks and mites. *Borrelia* is a loosely spiraled spirochete that tapers into fine filaments and is found free in the plasma. During the acute stages of the disease, the organism is spiral shaped; however, as the disease progresses and the bird nears death, the organism may appear abnormal or clumped and often is difficult to find. In acute avian spirochetosis, affected birds are lethargic, anemic, and weak. Postmortem findings include splenomegaly and hepatomegaly. Birds recovering from the disease exhibit a regenerative anemia.

Hematopoiesis

Bone marrow

The bone marrow is the primary site for erythropoiesis, granulopoiesis, and thrombopoiesis during late embryonic development and hatched birds. In some adult birds, such as chickens, the hematopoietic activity of the bone marrow primarily is associated with erythropoiesis and, possibly, thrombopoiesis, with only a small reserve of granulopoiesis compared to that of mammalian bone marrow. Therefore, compared with mammals, granulopoiesis in mature birds is more diffuse and is found in a variety of tissues. During embryonic development, granulocyte stem cells colonize to create foci of granulopoiesis in the spleen, kidney, lungs, thymus, gonad, pancreas, and other tissues, including the bone marrow. The bone marrow also provides an environment for lymphocyte maturation. Because it is the most readily available source of hematopoietic tissue in birds, the bone marrow is used to evaluate disorders of blood cells. Cytologic evaluation of the bone marrow is indicated in avian patients with nonregenerative anemia, heteropenia, and other unexplained alterations involving the cellular elements in circulating blood.

Bone marrow collection

Marrow samples for cytologic evaluation can be successfully obtained in most avian species via bone marrow aspiration. The best source of bone marrow for most birds is the proximal tibiotarsus because the procedure at this location is relatively simple. Marrow may also be collected from the sternum (keel), however, and from most of the long bones, except the pneumatic bones. A general anesthetic usually is not required, but a local anesthetic can be used with caution in large birds. The type of biopsy needle used for aspiration depends on the size of the bird, location of the biopsy site, and preference of the cytologist. Biopsy needles commonly used for bone marrow collection in both domestic mammals and humans (Jamshidi bone marrow biopsy–aspiration needles and disposable Jamshidi Illinois-Sternal/Iliac aspiration needles, Kormed Corp., Minneapolis, MN) can be used for marrow collection in birds. The pediatric sizes are preferred, however, because of the relatively small bone size in most birds compared with mammals. Spinal needles containing a stylet can be used for marrow collection in very small birds.

The procedure for collecting bone marrow from the proximal tibiotarsus begins with application of a skin disinfectant, as for any surgical procedure. The medial or cranial aspect of the proximal tibiotarsus just below the femoral-tibiotarsal joint is a suitable location for aspiration because only a minimal amount of soft tissue overlies the bone in this area. After application of a local anesthetic, a small incision is made using a scalpel blade to facilitate passage of the needle through the skin. The needle with stylet is placed against the bone (Figure 20.53), and using gentle pressure and rotary movements, the needle then is advanced into the marrow cavity. A perpendicular approach to the bone should be used. The hand not being used to manipulate the needle is used to stabilize the tibiotarsus. Once the needle is positioned into the marrow cavity, the stylet is removed, and a 6–12 mL syringe is attached (Figure 20.54). Marrow is aspirated into the lumen of the needle by applying negative pressure to the syringe using the syringe plunger (Figure 20.55). Excessive or prolonged negative pressure should be avoided to minimize blood contamination of the marrow sample. Unlike collection of bone marrow from most mammals, avian marrow should not appear in the syringe (except in very large birds) because of the small marrow volume in

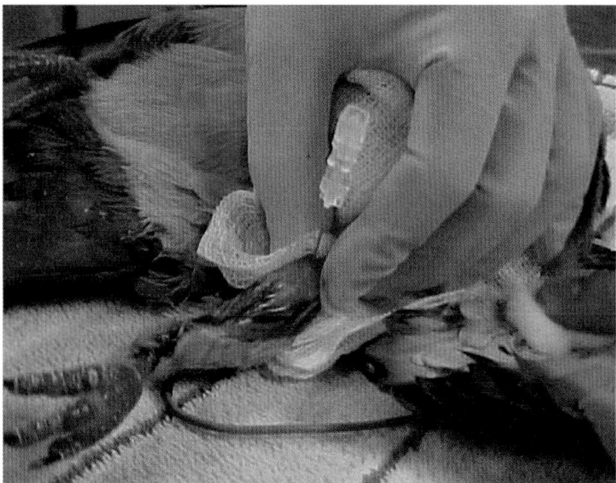

Figure 20.53 Placement of a spinal needle in the proximal tibiotarsus of a pigeon (*Columba livia*).

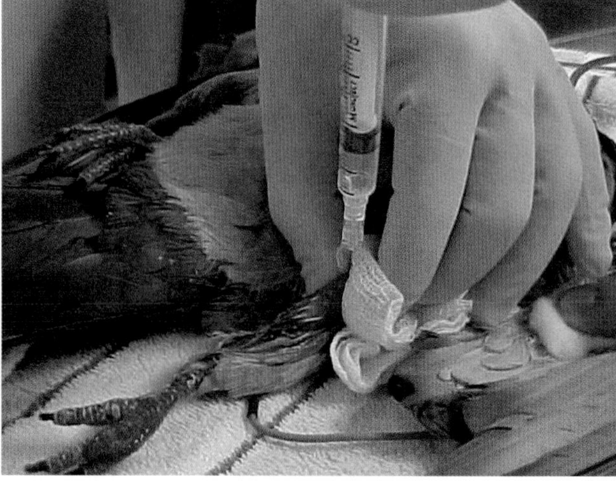

Figure 20.55 Aspiration of a bone marrow sample from a spinal needle placed in the proximal tibiotarsus of a pigeon (*Columba livia*).

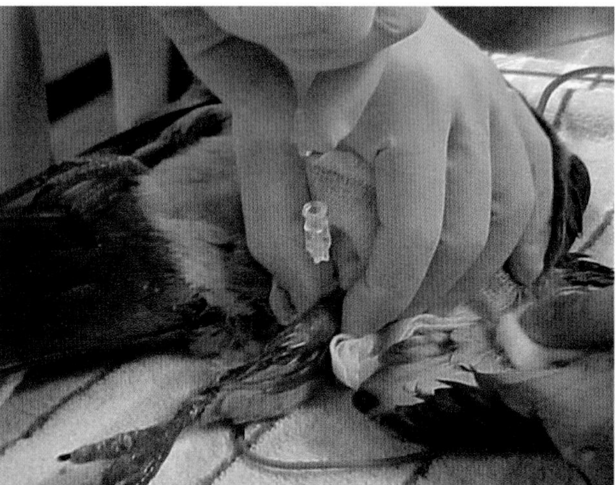

Figure 20.54 Removal of the stylet from a spinal needle placed in the proximal tibiotarsus of a pigeon (*Columba livia*).

most birds. Therefore, the marrow sample is found in the lumen of the biopsy needle.

When aspiration is completed, the needle and syringe are removed from the tibiotarsus while making sure that negative pressure is not being applied to the syringe. The needle is removed from the syringe, and the syringe is filled with air to force the marrow from the lumen onto a glass microscope slide. A second glass microscope slide is placed atop of the marrow sample, and the marrow is allowed to spread between the two slides as they are pulled apart. Bone marrow samples also can be obtained from the keel (sternum) of some birds, such as Galliformes; the biopsy needle is introduced into the widest part of the sternal ridge in the manner as described for the proximal tibiotarsus.

Marrow core biopsies for histologic evaluation can be obtained from birds using a technique similar to that of marrow aspiration. Once the biopsy needle is introduced into the bone marrow space, the stylet is removed, and the needle is advanced deeper into the marrow cavity, toward the opposite cortex. Once the opposite cortex has been reached, the needle is twisted and redirected slightly to detach the marrow plug within the lumen of the needle. Gentle vacuum may be applied to the syringe to aid in holding the marrow plug in the needle as the needle is withdrawn from the marrow cavity. The marrow core sample is removed by reinsertion of the stylet (usually beginning at the tip of the needle) to push the sample out of the needle. Imprint films can be made from the core sample for cytologic evaluation before the sample is placed in 10% neutral-buffered formalin. A sample holder often is required to maintain the marrow core while it is being fixed in the formalin solution.

Examination of avian bone marrow

Bone marrow slides are stained with the same Romanowsky stains used for blood films. Interpretation of avian bone marrow begins with scanning of the marrow film using the 10× microscope objective to evaluate both the number and the distribution of cells. Because an actual cell count of a bone marrow sample cannot be obtained, the cellularity is estimated by evaluating the ratio of fat and cells in marrow particles and is compared with the cellularity of normal bone marrow. The degree of cellularity is estimated as poor, normal, or high.

The distribution of cells can be estimated as well. Myeloid, erythroid, and thrombocytic elements may appear to be normal, hypoplastic (decreased), or hyperplastic (increased). A more objective approach is to perform an actual differential count based on 1000 cells or more, but this is more time-consuming and may not provide more information.

In addition to estimating the degree of cellularity and evaluating the distribution of cell types in the marrow sample, the cytologist also should estimate the myeloid: erythroid (M : E) ratio. Any changes involving the maturation sequence of each cell line should be noted as well. The cell lines include erythrocytes, granulocytes (heterophils, eosinophils, and basophils), monocytes, and thrombocytes. Other cells that occasionally are found include lymphocytes, plasma cells, osteoblasts, and osteoclasts. The presence of abnormal cells also should be noted.

The normal M : E ratio varies with species; however, the ratio in most species is approximately 1.0. For example, the M : E ratio is 1.23 ± 0.17 in. blackheaded gulls (*Larus ridibundus*) where the mean percentage of erythroid cells is 39.91 ± 3.26%; of myeloid cells is 49.37 ± 4.86%; of thrombocyte precursors is 5.95 ± 0.79%; and all other cells is 4.77 ± 0.53%.

An accurate interpretation of the bone marrow response can be made only in conjunction with knowledge regarding the current peripheral blood cellular response. Therefore, a hemogram from a blood sample collected at the same time as the bone marrow sample should be evaluated.

Erythropoiesis

Avian erythropoiesis occurs within the lumen of the vascular sinusoids in the bone marrow. These sinuses are lined by elongated endothelial cells that are associated with the most immature cells of the erythroid series. The more mature cells are located in the lumen of the sinuses. The vascular sinuses communicate with a central vein.

Avian erythropoietin, which is a glycoprotein that differs structurally from mammalian erythropoietin, is necessary for the multiplication and differentiation of precursor stem cells committed to the erythroid series. Erythropoietin can be collected from the blood of anemic birds, and the site of its production is considered to be the kidney.

The stages of maturation in normal avian erythropoiesis appear to be similar to those of mammals. The terminology used for the different stages of erythrocyte maturation, however, varies in the literature. In general, seven stages are recognizable in red blood cell development based on findings with Romanowsky stains. These include rubriblasts (proerythroblasts), prorubricytes (basophilic erythroblasts), basophilic rubricytes (early polychromatic erythroblasts), early polychromatic rubricytes (late polychromatic erythroblasts), late polychromatic rubricytes (orthochromic erythroblasts), polychromatic erythrocytes, and mature erythrocytes. As erythroid cells mature, the nuclear size decreases, the chromatin becomes increasingly condensed, the nuclear shape changes from round to ellipsoid, the amount of cytoplasm increases, the hemoglobin concentration increases (resulting in increasing eosinophilia), and the cell shape changes from round to ellipsoid. Unlike mammalian erythrocytes, avian erythrocytes normally retain their nucleus.

Rubriblasts

Rubriblasts are large, round, deeply basophilic cells with a large, round, central nucleus that results in a high N : C ratio (Figures 20.56–20.58 and 20.60). The nuclear chromatin typically is coarsely granular, and large, prominent nucleoli or nucleolar rings are present. The cytoplasm is deeply basophilic, with clear spaces most likely representing mitochondria.

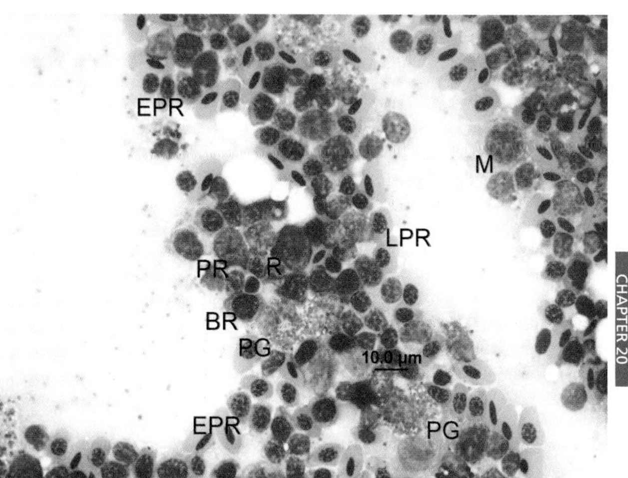

Figure 20.56 A rubriblast (R), prorubricyte (PR), basophilic rubricyte (BR), early polychromatic rubricytes (EPR), late polychromatic rubricyte (LPR), myeloblast (M), and progranulocyte (PG) in the bone marrow aspirate of a conure (*Aratinga solstitialis*). Wright-Giemsa stain.

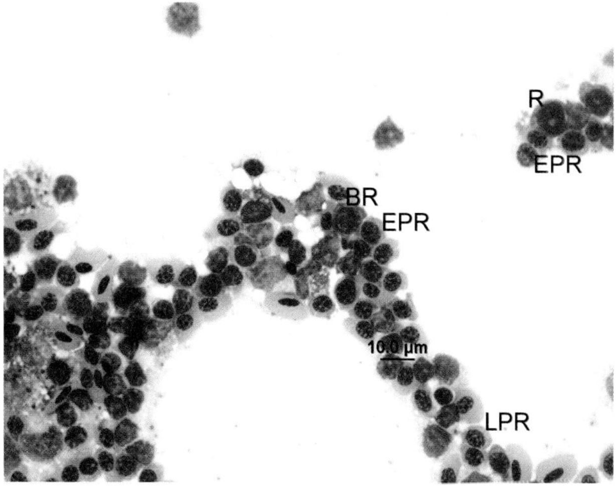

Figure 20.57 A rubriblast (R), basophilic rubricyte (BR), early polychromatic rubricyte (EPR), and late polychromatic rubricyte (LPR) in the bone marrow aspirate of a conure (*Aratinga solstitialis*). Wright-Giemsa stain.

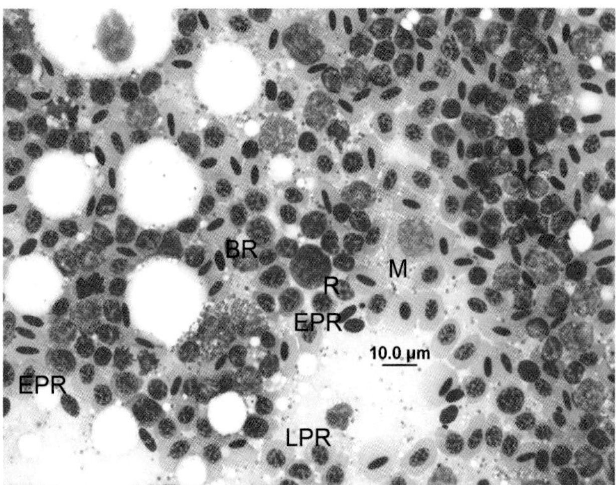

Figure 20.58 A rubriblast (R), basophilic rubricyte (BR), early polychromatic rubricytes (EPR), late polychromatic rubricyte (LPR), and myeloblast (M) in the bone marrow aspirate of a conure (*Aratinga solstitialis*). Wright-Giemsa stain.

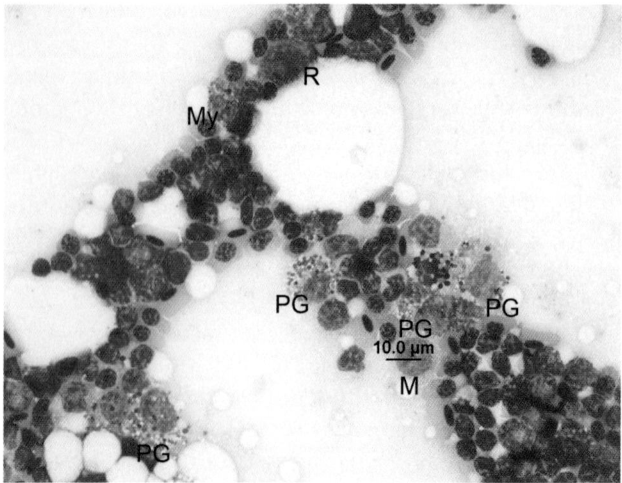

Figure 20.60 A rubriblast (R), myeloblast (M), progranulocytes (PG), and myelocyte (My) in the bone marrow aspirate of a conure (*Aratinga solstitialis*). Wright-Giemsa stain.

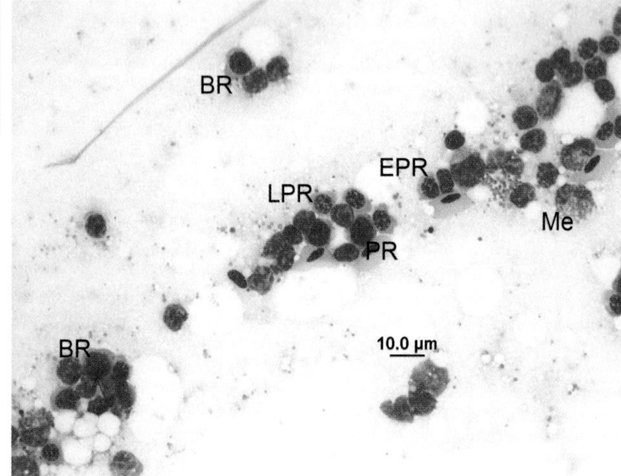

Figure 20.59 A prorubricyte (PR), basophilic rubricytes (BR), early polychromatic rubricyte (EPR), late polychromatic rubricyte (LPR), and metamyelocyte (Me) in the bone marrow aspirate of a conure (*Aratinga solstitialis*). Wright-Giemsa stain.

Prorubricyte

The prorubricyte resembles the rubriblast, but it lacks the prominent nucleoli (Figures 20.56 and 20.59). The N : C ratio is high, and the large nucleus usually is surrounded by a narrow rim of blue cytoplasm. The cytoplasm is predominantly basophilic but may contain spots of reddish material, suggesting the beginning of hemoglobin development. The cytoplasm lacks the mitochondrial spaces of the rubriblast.

Rubricyte

Rubricytes are round cells that are smaller than rubriblasts and prorubricytes. They can be divided into three stages, based primarily on the appearance of the cytoplasm. The basophilic rubricyte is the earliest rubricyte stage and is characterized by a homogenous, basophilic cytoplasm and a round nucleus with clumped chromatin (Figures 20.56–20.59). The next stage, the early polychromatophilic rubricyte, is smaller than the basophilic rubricyte and has a gray (basophilic to slightly eosinophilic) cytoplasm because of increased hemoglobin production (Figures 20.56–20.59). The nucleus of early polychromatophilic rubricytes contains clumped chromatin and is small in relation to the amount of cytoplasm. The final rubricyte stage, the late polychromatophilic rubricyte, is ellipsoid and has more eosinophilic (eosinophilic gray to weakly eosinophilic) cytoplasm than earlier stages (Figures 20.56–20.59). The nucleus of late polychromatophilic rubricytes varies from round to slightly ellipsoid, with irregularly clumped chromatin.

Polychromatophilic erythrocytes and mature erythrocytes

Cells in the final stages of erythropoiesis are the polychromatophilic erythrocyte and the mature erythrocyte. These cells are found in the peripheral blood of normal birds and were described earlier. The mature erythrocyte has a flattened, ellipsoid shape. The nuclear chromatin is condensed and transcriptionally inactive.

Granulopoiesis

Avian granulocytes appear to develop in a manner similar to those of mammals. The maturation stages have been described based on their morphologic appearance, primarily in chicken bone marrow. Thus, the study of avian hematopoiesis lags behind research in mammalian hematopoiesis, in which morphologic criteria are only part of the overall evaluation. Avian granulocytes show a progressive decrease in size and cytoplasmic basophilia as they mature, which is similar to the granulocytes of mammals. Specific cytoplasmic granules appear during the later stages of development and then progressively increase in number, until a full complement is reached in the cytoplasm of the mature granulocyte. The nuclei of granulocytes initially are round and progress toward segmentation, except for basophils, which do not segment, and the nuclear chromatin becomes increasingly condensed with maturity. The developmental stages of avian granulocytes include, in order of maturation, myeloblasts (granuloblasts), progranulocytes (promyelocytes), myelocytes, metamyelocytes, band cells, and mature granulocytes.

Myeloblasts

Avian myeloblasts are large, round cells with a high N : C ratio (Figures 20.56, 20.58, 20.60, and 20.61). The cytoplasm stains a lighter blue than that of rubriblasts. Myeloblast nuclei typically are round, with delicate reticular (fine) chromatin and prominent nucleoli. Myeloblasts do not contain specific cytoplasmic granules and, possibly, represent a stage that is common to all granulocytes. Myeloblasts frequently are associated with other developing granulocytes, especially on imprints of bone marrow core biopsy specimens.

Progranulocytes

Avian progranulocytes are large cells with light blue cytoplasm and slightly eccentric nuclei (Figures 20.56 and 20.60). The N : C ratio is lower than that of myeloblasts because of an increase in cytoplasm. The nuclear chromatin often has a delicate reticular pattern. Nucleoli are absent, and nuclear margins may be indistinct. Progranulocytes contain primary granules that vary in appearance among the types of granulocytes. Heterophil progranulocytes contain primary granules that vary in color and shape. They often appear as orange spheres and rings or as deeply basophilic spheres and rings. Eosinophil progranulocytes contain only brightly staining, orange, primary granules, and they appear to lack the dark magenta granules and rings found in heterophil progranulocytes. Basophil progranulocytes contain basophilic granules that appear to be smaller than the specific basophilic granules and the immature granules of the heterophil series. Fewer ring forms are seen in basophil progranulocytes.

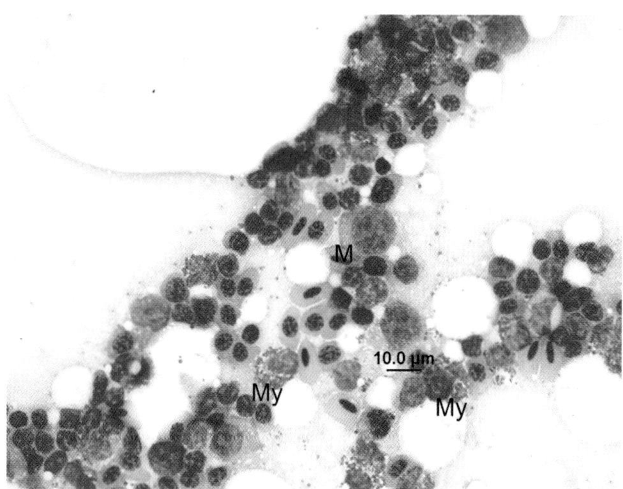

Figure 20.61 A myeloblast (M) and myelocytes (My) in the bone marrow aspirate of a conure (*Aratinga solstitialis*). Wright-Giemsa stain.

Myelocytes

Myelocytes are smaller than myeloblasts and progranulocytes, and they contain the secondary or specific granules of the mature granulocytes, thereby making identification of this cell somewhat simple (Figures 20.60 and 20.61). The round to oval nucleus of the myelocyte appears to be more condensed than the nuclei of myeloblasts and progranulocytes. Heterophil myelocytes typically are round cells, with a light blue cytoplasm that contains a mixture of rod-shaped specific granules and primary granules and rings. The eosinophilic, rod-shaped specific granules occupy less than half the cytoplasmic volume. Eosinophil myelocytes lack the deeply basophilic granules and rings that occasionally are found in early heterophil myelocytes. Basophil myelocytes contain basophilic specific granules that occupy less than half the cytoplasmic volume. The specific basophil granules have a slightly eosinophilic tinge, compared with the deep violet of the smaller primary granules that also may be present.

Metamyelocytes

Metamyelocytes are slightly smaller than myelocytes, have slightly indented nuclei, and possess specific cytoplasmic granules that occupy greater than half the cytoplasmic volume (Figure 20.59). Heterophil and basophil metamyelocytes have fewer primary granules than myelocytes and progranulocytes.

Band cells and mature granulocytes

Band cells resemble mature granulocytes, except that the nucleus appears as a curved or coiled band rather than segmented. Identifying band cells often is difficult, because the exact shape of the nucleus is obscured by specific cytoplasmic granules. A specific nuclear stain such as hematoxylin usually is required to determine the concentration of band cells. Because mature basophils lack a segmented nucleus, the band stage of basophils is not apparent. Mature granulocytes generally are the most abundant cell of each granulocytic cell line in the bone marrow of normal birds and were described earlier.

Thrombocytes

Avian thrombocytes appear to derive from a distinct line of mononuclear cells in the bone marrow, unlike mammalian platelets, which are cytoplasmic fragments of large, multinucleated megakaryocytes. The thrombocyte series consists of thromboblasts, immature thrombocytes, and mature thrombocytes. Thromboblasts resemble rubriblasts, but they tend to be smaller, with round nuclei having fine to punctate nuclear chromatin and one or more nucleoli. The cytoplasm is scant, stains deeply basophilic, and may contain clear spaces. They tend to be round to oval, with cytoplasmic blebs.

Immature thrombocytes are divided into three groups – early, mid, and late immature thrombocytes – based on their degree of maturity (Figure 20.43). Early immature thrombocytes are intermediate in size between thromboblasts and more mature stages. They tend to be round to oval and have more abundant cytoplasm than thromboblasts. The cytoplasm is basophilic and may contain vacuoles. The nuclear chromatin is aggregated into irregular clumps. Mid immature thrombocytes are slightly elongate or irregular, with pale blue cytoplasm. Cytoplasmic dense granules and vacuoles occasionally are seen at this stage of development. The nucleus contains heavy chromatin clumping. Late immature thrombocytes are oval and slightly smaller than the mid immature stage. The cytoplasm stains pale blue, with vaguely defined, clear areas. Dense granules frequently are seen at one pole of the cell. The nucleus is oval and has densely packed chromatin. The mature thrombocyte is the definitive cell in the thrombocyte series and was described earlier.

Other cells in avian bone marrow

Monocytes and macrophages

Monocytopoiesis is poorly defined in birds. Granulocytic precursor cells may be similar to, or even the same as, monocytic precursor cells. Monocytes originating in hematopoietic tissues become the monocytes and macrophages found in blood and body tissues, respectively. A variety of tissues, notably bone marrow, embryonic yolk sac, and spleen, can produce macrophage colonies. Mature monocytes are described in the discussion of leukocytes. Macrophages within the bone marrow are involved with iron metabolism during hemoglobin synthesis and catabolism and may contain red cell breakdown products such as hemosiderin or hematoidin in their cytoplasm. Hemosiderin contains iron and may appear as gray to black granulation; hematoidin lacks iron and is a golden, crystalline material.

Lymphocytes

Aggregates of lymphocytes are found within the bone marrow of birds, although major sites of lymphopoiesis in adult birds are located in the spleen, liver, intestines, and cecal tonsils. Avian lymphocytes can be classified as B lymphocytes (providing humoral immunity) or T lymphocytes (responsible for cell mediated immunity), but these two cell types usually cannot be differentiated based on morphology alone. B lymphocytes differentiate in the bursa of Fabricius, and T lymphocytes differentiate in the thymus.

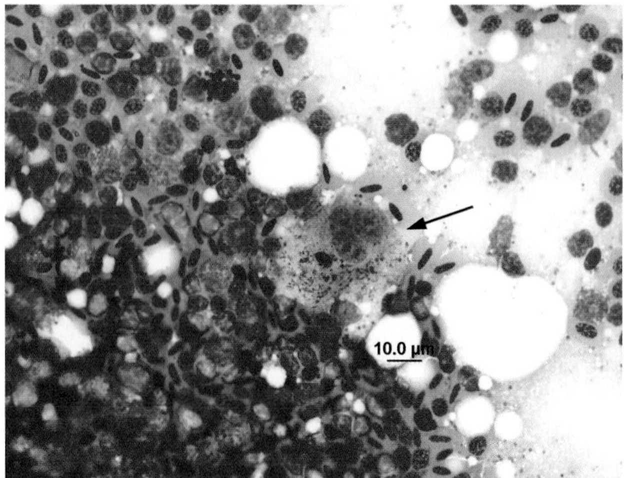

Figure 20.62 An osteoclast (arrow) in the bone marrow aspirate of a conure (*Aratinga solstitialis*). Wright-Giemsa stain.

Immature avian lymphocytes are larger than mature lymphocytes, and they are classified as either lymphoblasts or prolymphocytes based on morphology. Lymphoblasts have large nuclei with fine chromatin, and they contain one or more prominent nucleoli. The cytoplasm is relatively abundant and deeply basophilic. Prolymphocytes resemble lymphoblasts, but their nuclear chromatin is coarser and nucleoli are not present. Mature lymphocytes have coarse chromatin that typically is clumped. Cytoplasm is scant and stains light blue.

Osteoblasts

Avian osteoblasts are large cells found in the bone marrow that resemble those of mammals. They have abundant, lightly basophilic cytoplasm with a distinct, clear Golgi apparatus. The nucleus is round to oval and eccentrically located in the cell, contains reticular to coarsely granular chromatin, and possesses one or more distinct nucleoli. Osteoblasts are polygonal to fusiform, and they may have indistinct cytoplasmic margins.

Osteoclasts

Osteoclasts are large, multinucleated, giant cells with an ameboid shape (Figure 20.62). The cytoplasm is weakly basophilic and vacuolated, and red cytoplasmic granules may be present. Nuclei are round to oval and often contain prominent nucleoli.

Hematopoietic tissues other than bone marrow

Bursa of Fabricius

Based on research using domestic chicken and quail embryos, lymphoid cells first appear in the developing bursa of the

13–15-day embryo. Granulopoiesis also occurs in the developing bursa of the 12–13-day chicken embryo, but it disappears either at or just before hatching. The bursa reaches its maximum growth around 4 weeks after hatching then gradually undergoes involution during a 2–3-month period.

During development, the bursa contains numerous deeply basophilic, lymphoid precursor cells. Lymphoid precursors reach a maximum number in the 13–25-day embryo and then decline as lymphoid differentiation progresses. Lymphoid precursors may originate from an external source, such as the yolk sac or bone marrow. Seeding of the bursa with lymphoid precursor cells appears to occur in the 7–14-day embryo, depending on the species. Thus, the sole source of B lymphocytes in the adult bird are the self-regenerating aggregates of B lymphocytes that originated in the bursa and then spread to the spleen, liver, intestines, and cecal tonsils.

Thymus

The thymus is organized into a cortex consisting of densely packed lymphoid cells and a medulla. Lymphoid precursors originating from the yolk sac or bone marrow begin to colonize the thymus during the first 4–8 days of development, depending on the species. The influx of lymphoid precursors appears to last from 24 to 36 hours and then ends abruptly. The invasion of the thymus by precursors is followed by a 4–5-day refractory period before another influx occurs. This cyclic colonization of the thymus by lymphoid stem cells consists of two to three colonization periods, which may extend into the posthatchling period, depending on the species. This contrasts with colonization of the bursa, which occurs during a distinct, single episode in the embryo before hatching. T lymphocytes acquire their T antigen during a 24-hour period of development around the time of the second wave of colonization, between days 12–15 of embryonic life. T lymphocytes originating in the thymus spread to the spleen, liver, intestines, and cecal tonsils, and they are the predominant lymphoid cells of the spleen and peripheral blood of hatched birds.

Spleen

T and B lymphocytes appear at different locations in the white pulp of the spleen. The central arteries of the white pulp are surrounded by a periarteriolar lymphoid sheath, which is composed of densely packed T lymphocytes. Capillaries branching at right angles from the central arteries are surrounded by periellipsoid lymphoid tissue consisting of B lymphocytes. B lymphocytes also are found at the germinal centers located within the periarteriolar lymphoid sheath. During embryonic development, the spleen participates in erythropoiesis and granulopoiesis. Granulopoiesis becomes more predominant as the embryo matures. At hatching, however, the granulocytes begin to disappear, and by 3 days, they are replaced by lymphocytes.

21 Hematology of Reptiles

Terry W. Campbell

Department of Clinical Sciences, College of Veterinary Medicine and Biomedical Sciences, Colorado State University, Fort Collins, Colorado, USA

CHAPTER 21

Evaluation of the hemogram and blood film is part of the laboratory evaluation of reptilian patients. Hematology is used to detect conditions such as anemia, inflammatory diseases, parasitemias, hematopoietic disorders, and hemostatic alterations. Hematologic evaluation involves examination of the erythrocytes, leukocytes, and thrombocytes in the peripheral blood.

When evaluating the hematologic responses of reptiles, external factors such as environmental conditions that may enhance or inhibit the animal's response to disease should not be overlooked. The cellular responses in the blood of reptiles are less predictable than those in the blood of endothermic mammals and birds whose cellular microenvironments are more stable. A number of intrinsic factors, such as age and gender, also affect the hematologic data from reptiles. In addition, a number of sample-handling factors, such as the site of blood collection, type of anticoagulant used, method of cell counting, and type of stain used, add to the variability of reptilian hemogram values. All of these factors complicate the establishment of normal reference values in reptiles. Therefore, total and differential leukocyte counts must differ greatly (i.e., twofold or greater increase or decrease) from normal reference values to be considered significant.

Blood collection and handling

Blood samples for hematologic and blood biochemical studies can be collected from reptiles using a variety of methods, with the choice depending on the peculiarities of the species, volume of blood needed, size of the reptile, physical condition of the patient, and preference of the collector. The site of blood sample collection will influence the hematologic values because lymphatic vessels often accompany blood vessels in reptiles; frequently a mixture of blood and lymph occurs with venipuncture of peripheral vessels. Lymph often appears as transparent fluid entering the syringe immediately prior to the appearance of blood. If this occurs, discard the syringe and attempt sample collection again. The quantity of lymphatic fluid that mixes with the blood sample is variable and will dilute the cellular components of the blood, resulting in lower packed cell volume (PCV), hemoglobin concentration (Hb), erythrocyte count (TRBC), and leukocyte count (TWBC).

The use of a general anesthetic may be required as a method of restraint for blood collection in some reptiles, such as chelonians that can hide within their carapace and plastron. A number of published chemical protocols are available that can be used for the sedation and anesthesia of reptiles. Ketamine hydrochloride used alone or in combination with xylazine or midazolam are commonly used anesthetics for this purpose. It has been shown that anesthesia with ketamine does not affect the hemogram in some reptiles.

Jugular venipuncture can be used to collect blood from reptiles, especially chelonians (turtles and tortoises), and is the preferred site of blood collection by some authors (Figure 21.1). Jugular venipuncture is a useful method for obtaining blood samples from large lizards, such as green iguanas (*Iguana iguana*) and monitor lizards (*Varanus* spp.). Blood collection via jugular venipuncture is recommended in some species of reptiles, e.g., chameleons, to minimize unwanted effects, such as skin darkening, which occurs with blood collection from other sites. One advantage of jugular venipuncture is that the chances of sample hemodilution with lymphatic fluid are minimized owing to the size of the vessels.

The jugular vein of certain species of tortoises (e.g., desert tortoise, *Gopherus agassizii*) may be visible; however, this vein is rarely visible in most species. Some species of chelonians have dorsal and ventral jugular veins that lie on either side of a large cervical lymphatic vessel (superficial jugular trunk), and the right jugular vein may be larger than the left in some species of reptile. Chelonians may be restrained by an assistant with the head and neck extended to expose the lateral

Veterinary Hematology, Clinical Chemistry, and Cytology, Third Edition. Edited by Mary Anna Thrall, Glade Weiser, Robin W. Allison and Terry W. Campbell.

Companion website: www.wiley.com/go/thrall/veterinary

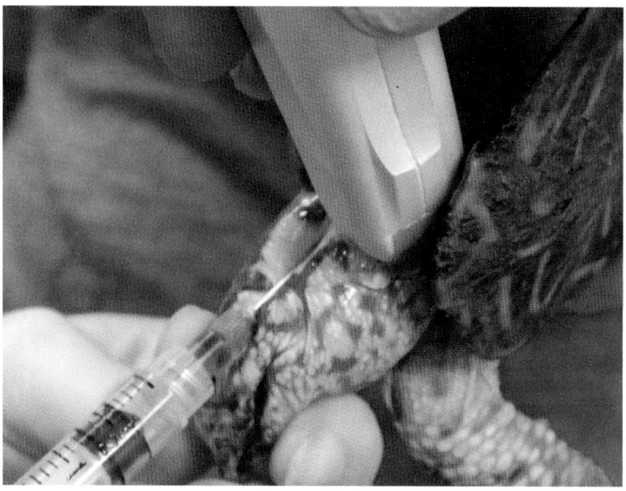

Figure 21.1 Blood collection by jugular venipuncture in a turtle (*Terrapene carolina*) using ultrasound to find the vein.

aspect of the neck. Chemical restraint may be required to aid in sample collection in some chelonians. The jugular vein (or veins) course caudally in a line extending from the angle of the mandible to the cranial carapacial inlet. The dorsal jugular vein extends from the dorsal edge of the tympanic membrane to the carapacial inlet when present. The jugular veins are relatively superficial; deep insertion of a needle may result in sample collection from the carotid artery.

The jugular vein of lizards lies deep along the lateral aspect of the neck. The vein is rarely visible and is approached blindly by directing the needle caudally along a line that runs behind the tympanum along the stretched neck of the lizard held in lateral recumbency. The right jugular vein is generally larger than the left, which is an aid to blood collection.

The supravertebral sinus (dorsal cervical venous, postoccipital, or occipital sinus) is a common location for obtaining blood samples in sea turtles. With the neck extended and the head held downward slightly, the sinus can be located just lateral to the cervical vertebrae. The sinus is approached by inserting the needle into the neck at a location one-third the distance from the base of the head to the carapace and one-third the distance from the dorsal midline to the lateral edge of the neck (Figure 21.2). This site can also be used for blood collection in freshwater turtles. A 20–22-gauge, 1–1 1/2 in. needle is inserted at a 30° angle, and the blood sample is collected with a syringe or evacuated tube. While the head is restrained, the needle is inserted just lateral to the dorsal midline on the right side of the neck.

The supravertebral vein is commonly used for blood collection in large crocodilians. The needle used for blood collection is inserted just behind the nuchal crest or occiput on the dorsal midline. Slight negative pressure is applied to the syringe as the needle is advanced until the sinus is entered. Spinal trauma is possible if the needle is inserted too deeply.

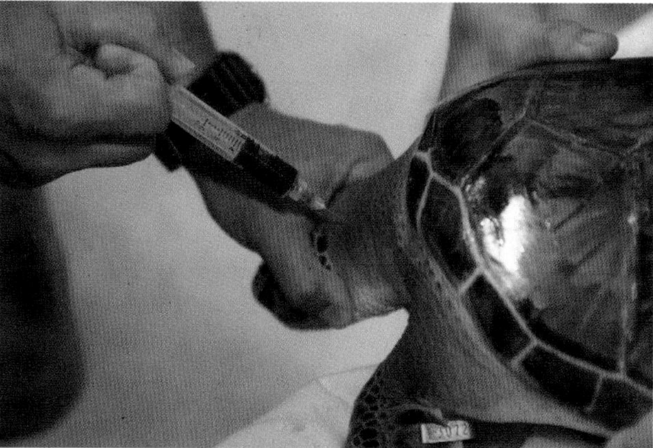

Figure 21.2 Blood collection from the supravertebral sinus (dorsal postoccipital vein) of a turtle (*Chelonia mydas*).

A dorsal vertebral blood vessel can be used to obtain a blood sample from large boid snakes (boas and pythons). With the back of the snake held in a tight flexed position, a needle is inserted between the vertebrae while negative pressure is applied to the syringe as the needle advances (Figure 21.3). Once blood enters the syringe, advancement of the needle is stopped and blood is collected into the syringe.

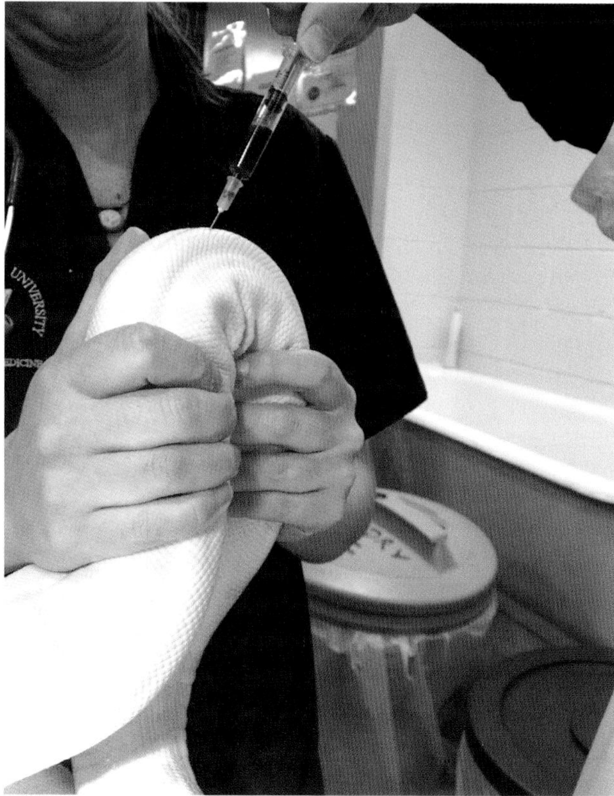

Figure 21.3 Blood collection from the dorsal vertebral vessels of a snake (*Boa constrictor*). Source: Image from Campbell TW. *Exotic Animal Hematology and Cytology*, 4th ed. Ames, IA: Wiley Blackwell, 2015, p. 174.

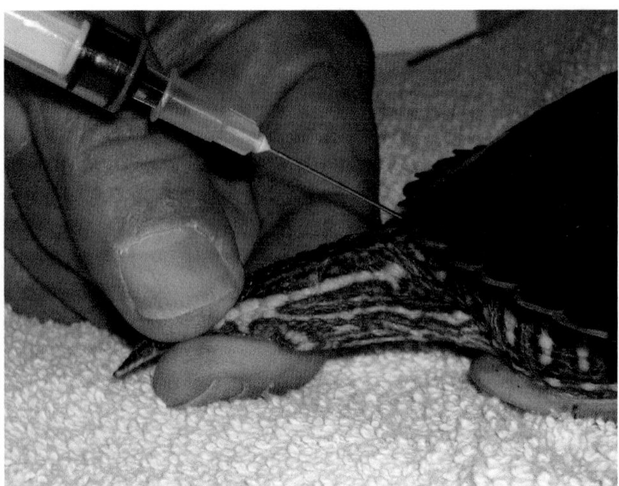

Figure 21.4 Blood collection from the dorsal coccygeal venous sinus (dorsal coccygeal vein) of a turtle (*Trachemys scripta elegans*). Source: Image from Campbell TW. *Exotic Animal Hematology and Cytology*, 4th ed. Ames, IA: Wiley Blackwell, 2015, p. 175.

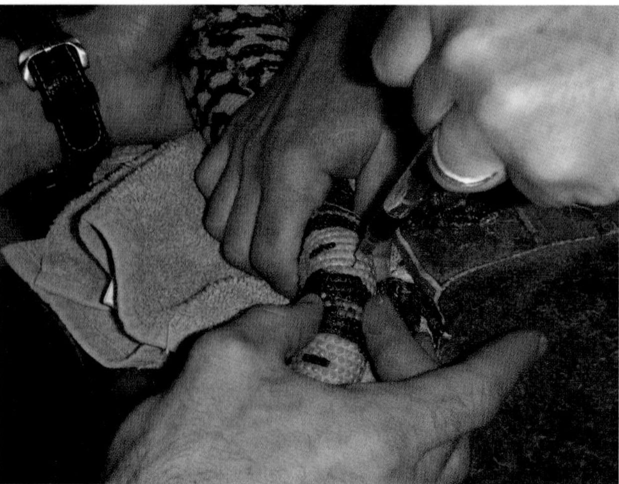

Figure 21.5 Blood collection by venipuncture of the ventral coccygeal vein in the tail of a lizard (*Heloderma suspectum*) using the ventral approach.

A dorsal coccygeal venous sinus (dorsal coccygeal vein) is present in many species of chelonians and is located on the dorsal midline of the tail. Blood collected from this site is often diluted with lymph. Venipuncture requires an assistant to restrain the chelonian. Insert a 22–25-gauge needle attached to a 1–3 mL syringe on the dorsal midline at the base of the tail at a 30°–60° angle (Figure 21.4).

The ventral coccygeal vein (ventral caudal or tail vein) lies just ventral to the caudal vertebrae and is a common site for blood collection in reptiles, especially lizards, large snakes, and crocodilians. Blood samples may be collected using a 22–23-gauge, 1 in. needle inserted under a ventral scale on the ventral midline and directed toward the vertebrae (Figure 21.5). The location of the needle insertion should be some distance caudal to the vent (e.g., 25–50% of the distance from the vent to the tip of the tail in snakes) to avoid the hemipenes of males or musk glands of snakes. Slight negative pressure should be applied to the syringe as the needle is advanced. If the needle contacts bone (a vertebra) before blood enters the needle, withdraw the needle slowly and change the direction of the needle (either cranially, caudally, left, or right) until blood flows into the syringe. Lizards can be restrained for this procedure by holding them vertically, by allowing them to cling to a cage door, or by allowing the lizard to sit on a table with the tail extending over the edge. These methods of restraint are better tolerated by the reptile compared to restraining them in dorsal recumbency. A lateral approach can also be used, especially in lizards and crocodilians, by inserting the needle along the middle of the lateral aspect of the tail in an area where a natural groove or line created by muscles in the tail occurs (Figure 21.6). The needle tip should be placed just beneath the caudal vertebra and into the vein. Crocodilians

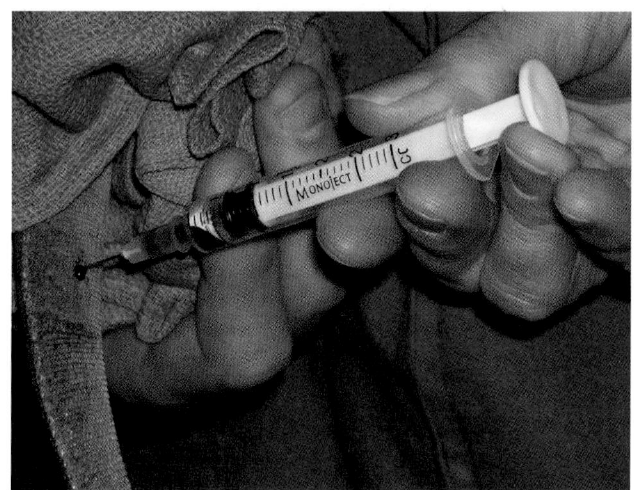

Figure 21.6 Blood collection by venipuncture of the ventral coccygeal vein in the tail of a lizard (*Iguana iguana*) using the lateral approach. Source: Image from Campbell TW. *Exotic Animal Hematology and Cytology*, 4th ed. Ames, IA: Wiley Blackwell, 2015, p. 175.

may be restrained on a tabletop, and either the ventral or lateral approach may be used. It should be noted that some lizards have tail autotomy (the ability to quickly shed the tail, usually as a defensive mechanism); therefore, part of the tail could be lost during the mishandling of these lizards for blood collection.

The subcarapacial (subvertebral) venous sinus may be used for blood collection in chelonians. The subcarapacial venous sinus is located caudal to the nuchal scute at the level of the eighth cervical vertebra and is made up of a collection of blood vessels (internal jugular vein, anterior pulmonic vein and artery, vertebral veins and arteries, and

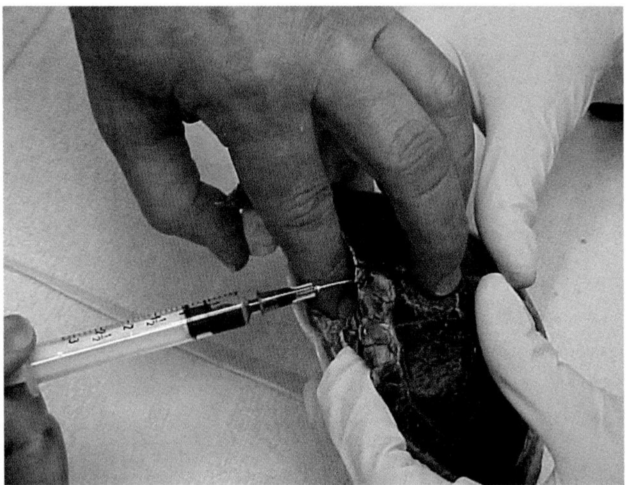

Figure 21.7 Blood collection from the subcarapacial (subvertebral) venous sinus in a turtle (*Trachemys scripta elegans*) with the head pushed into the shell.

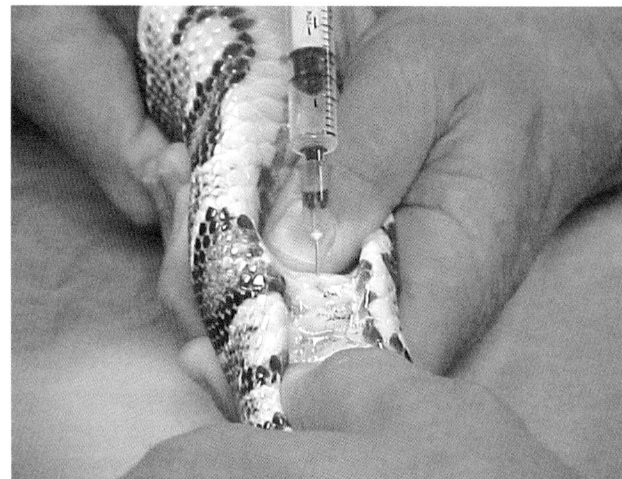

Figure 21.8 Blood collection by cardiocentesis of a snake (*Boa constrictor*).

subclavian veins and arteries) and lymphatic vessels. Blood collected from this site may not be adequate for hematologic evaluation because marked dilution with lymphatic fluid may occur. For sample collection, insert a needle dorsal to the neck at the carapacial inlet and angle it up toward the ventral aspect of the carapace (Figure 21.7). This can be performed with the head and neck extended or retracted. If the needle touches bone (either a vertebra or the carapace) before blood enters the syringe, withdraw the needle slightly and redirect it caudally. The major lymphatic vessels are located cranial to the venous sinus; therefore, subsequent attempts at sample collection should be made caudal to the site of the first attempt.

Blood may be collected from the ulnar (radiohumeral) venous sinus of reptiles. Blood is collected by extending the front leg of the reptile and inserting a needle at a perpendicular angle to the body behind the tendon that lies on the caudal aspect of the radiohumeral joint. Advance the needle toward the radiohumeral joint while applying gentle pressure to the attached syringe.

Cardiocentesis is commonly performed for blood collection from snakes. The exact location of the heart varies depending on the species but in general lies in the cranial one-third of the body. With the snake held in dorsal recumbency, the heart is located by palpation, by observing the movement of the ventral scutes for heartbeats, or by use of a Doppler. The heart can move cranially and caudally and should be stabilized at the apex and base during sample collection. A 22–23-gauge needle attached to a 3–6 cc syringe needle is inserted under (not through) the scute and advanced into the heart (Figure 21.8). The syringe typically fills slowly as the heart pulsates. Sedation of the snake prior to cardiocentesis is recommended to avoid excessive movement and possible cardiac trauma.

Cardiocentesis may be performed in other reptile species as well. Cardiocentesis of chelonians is performed by passing a needle through the plastron on the ventral midline at the junction of the humeral and pectoral scutes. A needle can be passed through the soft plastron of soft-shelled turtles (*Trionyx* spp.), neonates, or those affected by secondary nutritional hyperparathyroidism. Otherwise, an access hole may be drilled through the plastron with an 18–20-gauge needle in small chelonians; a sterile drill bit may be required for larger chelonians. Following sample collection, the hole should be sealed with an epoxy. If multiple samples are required, a larger hole can be drilled through the plastron and plugged with a rubber stopper from a blood collection tube. The rubber stopper must then be sealed in position with epoxy, and it serves as an access port to the heart for blood collection. Cardiocentesis is not recommended for routine blood collection from lizard species.

Other, less commonly used blood collection sites include the brachial vein or artery, the palatine-pterygoid vein, the ventral abdominal vein, and toenails. Blood collection from the brachial vein or artery is a blind approach and may be attempted in chelonians or lizards. Samples obtained by this method are often diluted with lymph, although blood collected from this site in tortoises may be more reliable for hematologic study than blood collected from the dorsal coccygeal. Blood can be collected from the palatine-pterygoid veins in the oral cavity of medium- to large-sized snakes but will require general anesthesia or an extremely cooperative patient. These veins are fragile and easily lacerated. Blood can be collected by syringe or by allowing the blood to flow from the needle hub into a microcollection tube. Lizards have a large ventral abdominal vein present on the ventral midline of the abdomen. This vein is easily located but can be easily lacerated, and hemostasis following venipuncture can be problematic. The needle is inserted through the ventral midline usually just cranial to the umbilicus in a cranial-dorsal direction to reach the vein just below the body wall. The vein can be cannulated with a needle and blood collected from the needle hub into a microcollection tube or aspirated into a syringe. Blood collected from capillary beds (toenails) do not provide optimal samples for hematologic studies but may be the only procedure available for blood collection in very small reptiles (<30 g). The humane aspects of toenail clipping should be considered as this method causes pain and trauma to the patient. The toenail should be thoroughly cleaned and is clipped using nail trimmers. Blood is then collected into a microcollection tube. A styptic powder or solution should be applied to the clipped nail to aid in hemostasis.

The total blood volume of reptiles is estimated to range between 5% and 8% of the body weight. For example, the total blood volume of desert tortoises (*Gopherus polyphemus*), freshwater turtles (*Chelydra serpentina*), and marine turtles is 4.9–7.2%, 3.8–5.6%, and 5.2–7.9% of the body weight, respectively. Most reptile species can tolerate withdrawal of up to 10% of the total blood volume (1% of the body weight) without detrimental effects. The maximum blood sample volume recommended for collection from chelonians is 3 mL/kg body weight, and a smaller volume representing 0.5% of the body weight has been recommended for sick animals. Typically, only 0.2–0.3 mL of blood is required for routine hematologic studies; most reptiles will tolerate this loss.

Blood should be collected into an anticoagulant for hematologic evaluation. Lithium heparin is the anticoagulant of choice for many reptilian blood samples intended for hematologic evaluation because ethylenediaminetetraacetic acid (EDTA) can cause hemolysis, especially in chelonian blood. Lithium heparin will cause clumping of leukocytes and thrombocytes, which can make it difficult to obtain accurate cell counts. Evaluation of cell morphology may be difficult as well due to the clumping and because lithium heparin creates a blue tinge to blood films. Blood samples collected in lithium heparin do not stain well if several hours pass prior to processing. In some species of reptiles, such as the green iguana (*I. iguana*), Chinese water dragon (*Physignathus concincinus*), and perhaps most species of lizards, EDTA can be used and is considered to be the anticoagulant of choice, allowing for better staining of the cells and, therefore, making cell identification easier than when cells are exposed to heparin. To minimize staining artifacts associated with an anticoagulant, the blood sample should be processed as soon as possible after collection. Blood films should be quickly prepared from a drop of blood containing no anticoagulant that is taken from the needle immediately following collection to avoid interference during staining.

Some authors feel that preparation of blood films using the two-microscope slide wedge method is more likely to cause cell lysis than use of a coverslip method. It has been the experience of this author (Campbell) that coverslip smears can also result in excessive cell lysis; therefore, the method chosen appears to be a matter of technical skill. Experienced medical technologists working with blood collected from lower vertebrates, such as reptiles, routinely prepare blood films using the conventional methods using two microscope slides without creating cell lysis.

Erythrocytes

Morphology

Mature erythrocytes of reptiles are typically larger than erythrocytes of birds, bony fish, and mammals but are smaller than the erythrocytes of most amphibians. Erythrocytes of reptiles are blunt-ended ellipsoidal cells with permanent, centrally positioned, oval to round nuclei containing dense purple chromatin (Figure 21.9). Unlike the smooth nuclear margins of avian erythrocytes, those of reptiles tend to be irregular. The cytoplasm stains uniformly orange-pink with Romanowsky stains such as Wright's stain. Polychromatophilic erythrocytes have nuclear chromatin

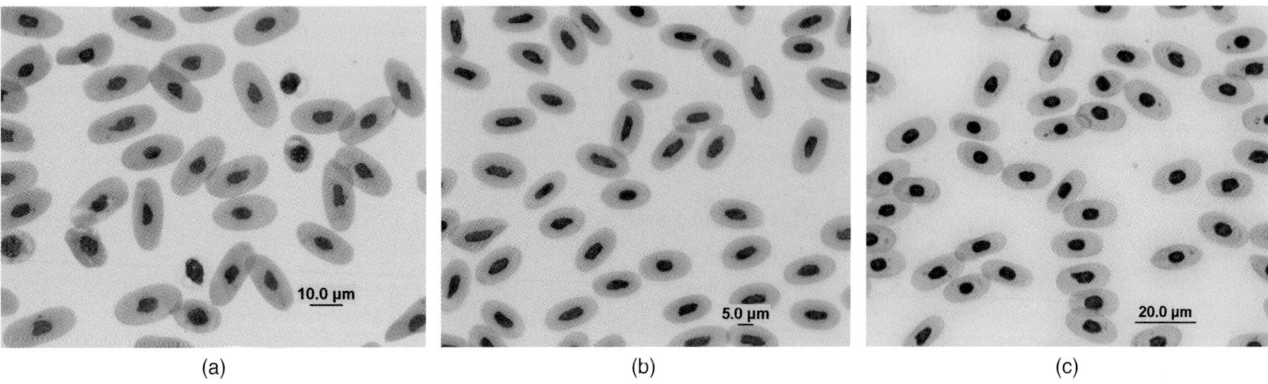

Figure 21.9 (a) Normal erythrocytes in the blood film of a snake (*Boa constrictor*). Wright-Giemsa stain. (b) Normal erythrocytes in the blood film of a lizard (*Chamaeleo calyptratus*). Wright-Giemsa stain. (c) Normal erythrocytes in the blood film of a chelonian (*Terrapene carolina*). Wright-Giemsa stain.

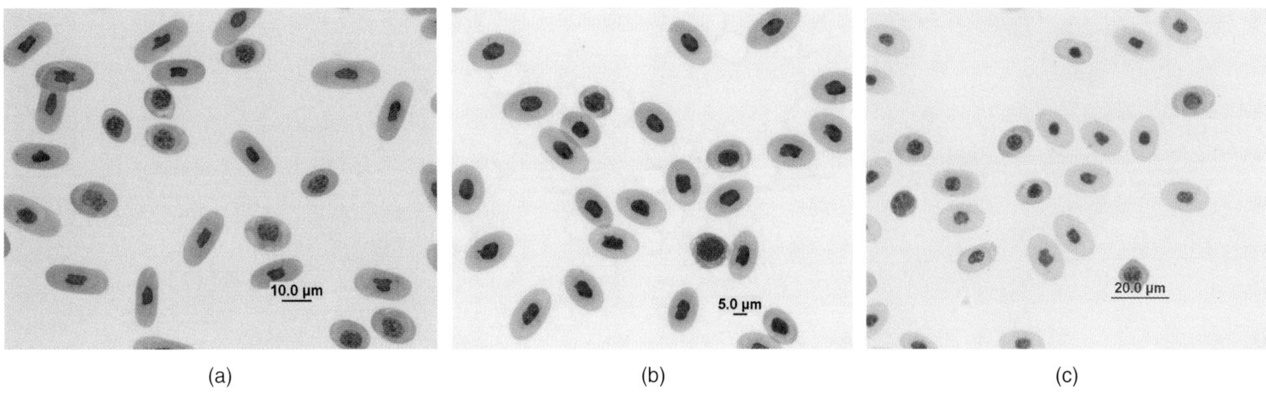

Figure 21.10 (a) Increased polychromasia in the blood film of a snake (*Boa constrictor*). Wright-Giemsa stain. (b) Increased polychromasia and an immature erythrocyte (basophilic rubricyte) in the blood film of a lizard (*Pogona vitticeps*). Wright-Giemsa stain. (c) Increased polychromasia in the blood film of a chelonian (*Mauremys reevesii*). Wright-Giemsa stain.

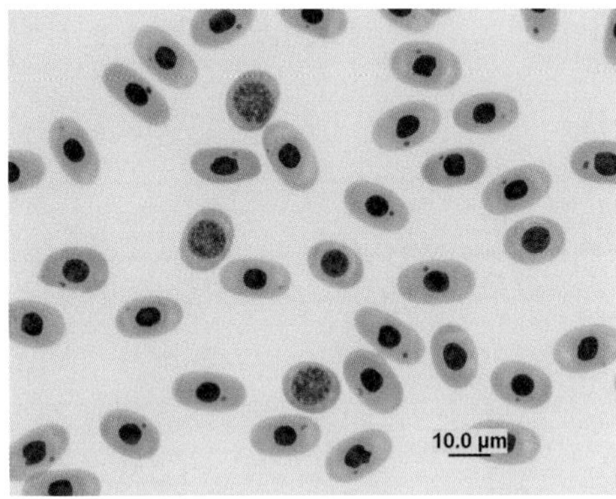

Figure 21.11 Immature erythrocytes (basophilic and midpolychromatic rubricytes) in the blood film of a chelonian (*Cuora amboinensis*). Wright-Giemsa stain.

that is less dense and cytoplasm that is more basophilic than mature erythrocytes (Figure 21.10). Immature erythrocytes are occasionally seen in the peripheral blood of reptiles, especially very young animals or those undergoing ecdysis. I'mmature erythrocytes are round to slightly irregular cells with large round nuclei and basophilic cytoplasm (Figures 21.10b and 21.11). The nucleus lacks the dense chromatin clumping of the mature cell. Immature erythrocytes often appear smaller than mature erythrocytes, probably because they are spherical in shape and have yet to become flattened ellipsoid cells. Mitotic activity associated with erythrocytes is common in the peripheral blood of reptiles (Figure 21.12).

Reticulocytes are detected by staining cells with a vital stain such as new methylene blue or brilliant cresyl blue. Reptilian reticulocytes, like avian reticulocytes, have a distinct ring of aggregated reticulum that encircles the red-cell nucleus (Figure 21.13). These cells best correspond to the polychromatophilic erythrocytes found in Romanowsky-stained blood films, and they probably are the cells that were recently released from erythropoietic tissues. Basophilic stippling commonly occurs in polychromatophilic erythrocytes stained with Romanowsky stains.

Round to irregular basophilic inclusions are frequently seen in the cytoplasm of erythrocytes in peripheral blood films from many species of reptiles (Figure 21.14). These inclusions most likely represent an artifact of slide preparation since blood films made repeatedly from the same blood sample often reveal varying degrees of these inclusions and are not considered to be clinically significant. Electron microscopy suggests these inclusions are degenerate organelles, such as clumping of the endoplasmic reticulum. Other artifacts found in the erythrocyte cytoplasm include vacuoles and refractile clear areas. These can be minimized with careful blood film preparation.

Laboratory evaluation

Laboratory evaluation of the reptilian erythron involves determination of the PCV, TRBC, and Hb of blood (see Table 21.1). The PCV is obtained by microhematocrit centrifugation. A PCV also can be calculated by electronic cell counters that are accurately adjusted for each species according to differences in erythrocyte sizes. Microhematocrit centrifugation, however, is the most practical method for obtaining PCVs of reptilian blood.

The total erythrocyte concentration of reptiles can be determined using the same automated or manual methods used for the determination of total erythrocyte counts in mammalian blood. Electronic impedance cell counters provide a rapid, reliable method for obtaining total red blood cell concentrations. Erythrocyte counts with electronic cell counters are slightly inflated by the inclusion of leukocytes and thrombocytes in the count; however, these additional cells are not significant in most samples as they make up approximately 0.1% of the peripheral blood cell population. Although rarely performed, manual methods for obtaining total red blood cell counts in reptiles can be obtained using the Natt and Herrick's method, which involves the

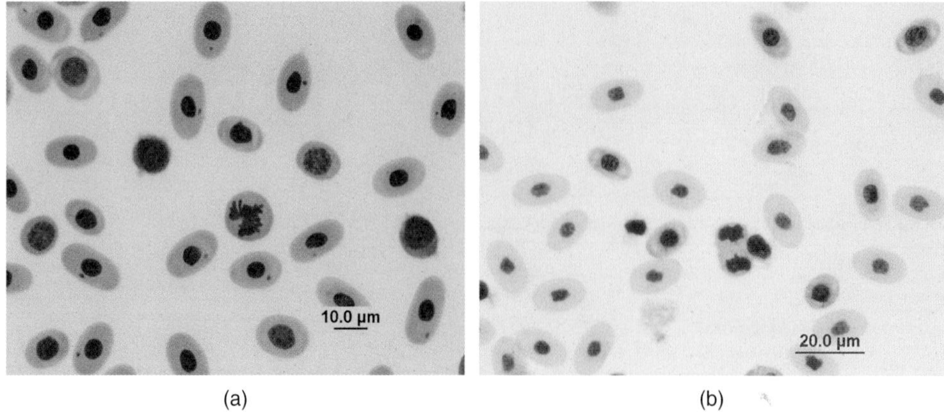

Figure 21.12 (a) An erythrocyte exhibiting mitotic activity in the peripheral blood of a chelonian (*Cuora amboinensis*). Wright-Giemsa stain. (b) Mitotic activity (either an erythrocyte or thrombocyte) in the peripheral blood of a chelonian (*Mauremys reevesii*). Wright-Giemsa stain.

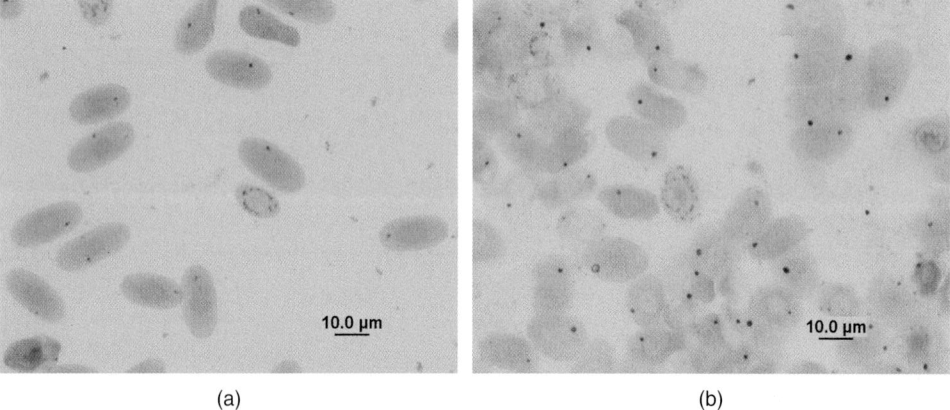

Figure 21.13 (a) Reticulocyte with a distinct ring of aggregated reticulum encircling the red-cell nucleus in the blood film of a snake (*Boa constrictor*). Brilliant cresyl blue stain. (b) Reticulocyte with a distinct ring of aggregated reticulum encircling the red-cell nucleus in the blood film of a chelonian (*Cuora amboinensis*). Brilliant cresyl blue stain.

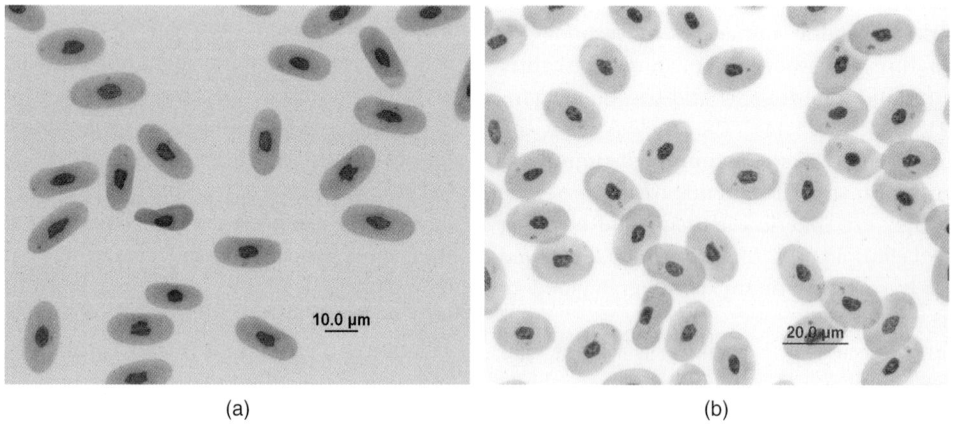

Figure 21.14 (a) Basophilic erythrocyte inclusions considered to be artifacts in the blood film of a snake (*Boa constrictor*). Wright-Giemsa stain. (b) Basophilic erythrocyte inclusions considered to be artifacts in the blood film of a chelonian (*Chelonia mydas*). Wright-Giemsa stain.

CHAPTER 21

Table 21.1 Erythrocyte parameters for selected reptiles.

	PCV [%]	RBC [×10⁶/μL]	Hb [g/dL]	MCV [fL]	MCHC [g/dL]
Lizards					
Argentine lizard[a] winter	24–28	0.8–1.1	10–14	252–300	36–48
Argentine lizard[a] summer	18–26	0.8–1.1	7–13	198–262	41–49
Adult male iguana[b]	29–39	1.0–1.7	6.7–10.2	228–303	22.7–28.0
Adult female iguana[b]	33–44	1.2–1.8	9.1–12.2	235–331	24.9–31.0
Juvenile iguana[b]	30–47	1.3–1.6	9.2–10.1	–	–
Prehensile-tailed skink[c]	24–60	0.8–1.4	7.4–11.6	152–600	17–56
Snakes					
Boa constrictor[d e]	24–40	1.0–2.5	3.3–15.3	159–625	21–42
Ball python[f]	16–21	0.3–1.3	5.5–7.9	211–540	25–40
Yellow rat snake[g]	9–46	0.2–1.6	2.8–15.2	179–961	26–54
Jungle carpet python[h]	23–37	0.5–1.3	4.0–15.5	178–414	23.5–53.2
Chelonians					
Aldabra tortoise[i]	11–17	0.3–0.7	3.2–8.0	375–537	28–40
Desert tortoise[j]	23–37	1.2–3.0	6.9–7.7	377–607	19–34

[a]Troiano JC, Gould EG, Gould I. Hematological reference intervals in argentine lizard *Tupinambis merianae* [Sauria-Teiidae]. *Comp Clin Pathol* 17: 93–7. 2008.

[b]Harr KE, Alleman AR, Dennis PM, et al. Morphologic and cytochemical characteristics of blood cells and hematologic and plasma biochemical reference intervals in green iguanas. *JAVMA* 218: 915–21. 2001.

[c]Wright KM, Skeba S. Hematology and plasma chemistries of captive prehensile-tailed skinks [*Corcucia zebrata*]. *J Zoo Wildl Med* 23: 429–32. 1992.

[d]Chiodini RJ, Sundberg JP. Blood chemical values of the common boa constrictor [*Constrictor constrictor*]. *Am J Vet Res* 43: 1701–2. 1982.

[e]Rosskopf WJ, Woerpel RW, Yanoff SR. Normal hemogram and blood chemistry values for boa constrictors and pythons. *Vet Med Small Anim Clin* May: 822–3. 1982.

[f]Johnson JH, Benson PA. Laboratory reference values for a group of captive ball pythons [*Python regius*]. *Am J Vet Res* 57: 1304–7. 1996.

[g]Ramsey EC, Dotson TK. Tissue and serum enzyme activities in the yellow rat snake [*Elaphe obsolete quadrivitatta*]. *Am J Vet Res* 56: 423–8. 1995.

[h]Centini R, Klaphake E. Hematologic values and cytology in a population of captive jungle carpet pythons, *Morelia spilota cheynei*. *Proc Assoc Rept Amph Vet*, pp. 107–11. 2002.

[i]Carpenter JW. *Exotic Animal Formulary*, 3rd ed. St. Louis: Elsevier Saunders, p. 107. 2001.

[j]Gottdenker NL, Jacobson ER. Effect of venipuncture sites on hematologic and clinical biochemical values in desert tortoises [*Gopherus agassizii*]. *Am J Vet Res* 56: 19–21. 1995.

preparation of Natt and Herrick's solution to be used as a stain and diluent (see Chapter 20 on avian hematology).

Total hemoglobin concentration for reptiles is typically determined using the standard cyanmethemoglobin method with one modification: the cyanmethemoglobin reagent-blood mixture should be centrifuged prior to analysis. The free nuclei from lysed erythrocytes are removed before obtaining the optical density value, in order to avoid an overestimation of the hemoglobin concentration. Published hemoglobin concentration values for reptiles are usually low; often less than 10 g/dL.

After the primary hematologic indices (PCV, erythrocyte count, and hemoglobin concentration) have been determined, the secondary hematologic indices can be determined. These include the mean cell volume (MCV) or mean erythrocyte volume (MEV), mean cell hemoglobin (MCH), or mean erythrocyte hemoglobin (MEH), and mean cell hemoglobin concentration (MCHC) or mean erythrocyte hemoglobin concentration (MECH). The mean corpuscular volume (MCV) is an index of red cell volume. The mean corpuscular hemoglobin concentration (MCHC) is an index denoting the proportion of hemoglobin present in an average erythrocyte. Published MCV values for reptiles generally range between 160 and 950 fL (femtoliters, mm^3) and MCHC values typically range between 20 and 40 g/dL.

Reference intervals for the TRBC, Hb, and PCV are difficult to establish for reptiles and other ectotherms, as mentioned above. Intrinsic factors include species, gender, age, and the physiologic status of the reptile. Extrinsic factors include season, temperature, habitat, diet, disease, stress associated with captivity, and the venipuncture site. When establishing reference intervals, the intrinsic and extrinsic factors affecting the reference population must be documented in order to ensure that the physiologic data are collected under consistent circumstances. It has been recommended that a minimum of 97 samples is required from a reference population to provide statistically meaningful intervals.

Disparity in erythrocytic values may be related to gender in some reptile species. Male reptiles typically have higher erythrocytic values than females; however, this is not always the case. Seasonal changes in environment, physical condition, and age can affect the hematologic parameters of reptiles. For example, adult crocodiles have higher red blood cell counts compared to juveniles, and the hemogram of free-ranging tortoises is influenced by physical condition, availability of forage, and the rainfall patterns of the environment. Significant seasonal variations in hematologic values have also been reported in snakes. The normal PCVs of green iguanas (*I. iguana*) housed outdoors with significant exposure to direct sunlight and a slightly higher environmental temperatures (80–100 °F) exhibit a slightly wider range (28–46%) compared to the PCV (25–38%) of the same species housed indoors exposed to artificial lighting and lower environmental temperature (74–95 °F). Hibernation will affect erythrocytic values in some reptile species. In general, erythrocyte values are highest prior to and lowest immediately after hibernation, although some reptile species do not appear to be affected by hibernation.

Chronic stressors such as captivity and inappropriate habitat or diet will affect the hemogram. The effects of acute stressors, such as capture, handling, and restraint for venipuncture, are unknown but are likely to affect erythrocyte values as well. In one study, captive-bred snakes had higher red blood mass compared to wild-caught snakes of the same species.

The site and method of blood collection can affect the hemogram. As previously mentioned, lymphatic vessels often accompany blood vessels in reptiles, commonly resulting in a mixture of blood and lymph during venipuncture. The subsequent lymphodilution of the blood sample will affect the hemogram by decreasing the PCV, Hb concentration, TRBC, and TWBC.

Responses in disease

Published normal PCVs of most reptile ranges between 15 and 55%. Values greater than 55% suggest either hemoconcentration or erythrocytosis (polycythemia), while a PCV less than 15% is suggestive of anemia if hemodilution of lymph is not a factor.

The causes of anemia in reptiles are similar to those described for birds and mammals. Anemia can be classified as hemorrhagic (i.e., blood loss), hemolytic (i.e,. increased red-cell destruction), or depression anemia (i.e., decreased red-cell production). Hemorrhagic anemias usually result from traumatic injuries or bloodsucking parasites; however, other causes, such as a coagulopathy or an ulcerative lesion, should be considered as well. Hemolytic anemia can result from septicemia, parasitemia, or toxemia. Bone marrow depression anemia (nonregenerative anemia) usually is associated with chronic inflammatory diseases, especially those associated with an infectious agent. Other causes that should be considered for nonregenerative anemia in reptiles include chronic renal or hepatic disease, neoplasia, chemicals, and possibly, hypothyroidism.

The degree of polychromasia or reticulocytosis in the blood films of normal reptiles generally is low, and it represents less than 1% of the erythrocyte population. This may be associated with the long erythrocyte life span (600–800 days in some species) and, therefore, with the slow turnover rate of reptilian erythrocytes compared with those of birds and mammals. The relatively low metabolic rate of reptiles also may be a factor. Young reptiles tend to have a greater degree of polychromasia than adults.

Slight anisocytosis and poikilocytosis are considered to be normal for most reptilian erythrocytes. Moderate to marked anisocytosis and poikilocytosis are associated with erythrocytic regenerative responses and, less commonly, with erythrocyte disorders. An increased polychromasia and number of immature erythrocytes is seen in reptiles responding to anemic conditions. Young reptiles or those undergoing ecdysis also may exhibit increased polychromasia and immature erythrocyte concentration. Erythrocytes exhibiting binucleation, abnormal nuclear shapes (anisokaryosis), or mitotic activity can be associated with marked regenerative responses (Figures 21.12b and 21.15). These nuclear findings, however, also may occur in reptiles awakening from hibernation or in association with severe inflammatory disease, malnutrition, and starvation. Basophilic stippling usually suggests a regenerative response, but it may also be seen in patients with lead toxicosis. Hypochromatic erythrocytes are associated with iron deficiency or chronic inflammatory disease, presumably in association with iron sequestration.

Erythrocytic intracytoplasmic inclusions in reptilian blood films can be caused by viruses or blood parasites (see section on blood parasites). Viral inclusions caused by an iridovirus

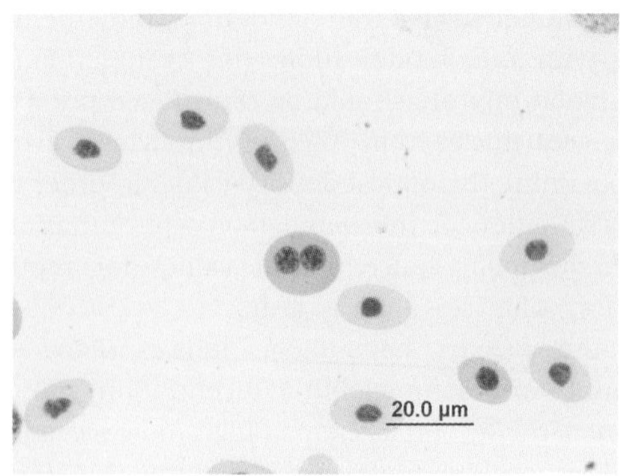

Figure 21.15 A binucleated erythrocyte in the peripheral blood of a chelonian (*Mauremys reevesii*). Wright-Giemsa stain.

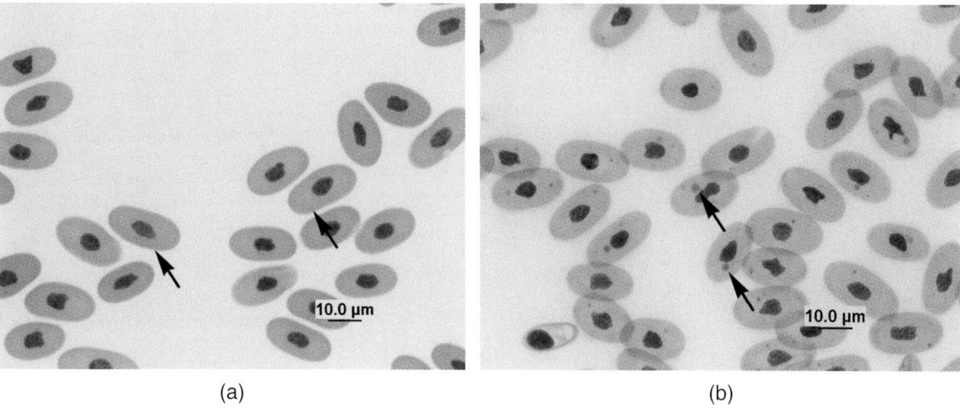

Figure 21.16 (a) Intracytoplasmic inclusions (arrows) in the erythrocytes in the peripheral blood of a snake (*Boa constrictor*) with inclusion body disease. Wright-Giemsa stain. (b) Intracytoplasmic inclusions (arrows) in the erythrocytes in the peripheral blood of a snake (*Boa constrictor*) with inclusion body disease. Diff-Quik stain.

are represented by snake and lizard erythrocyte viruses (formerly known as *Pirhemocyton*) and are identified as small round (punctate to oval) red-staining (Giemsa stain) inclusions that may be associated with rectangular or hexagonal translucent, crystalline, or albuminoid vacuoles. The iridovirus inclusion of box turtles appears as round to oval pink granular inclusions in the cytoplasm of leukocytes.

Inclusion body disease (IBD), suspected to be caused by an arenavirus, is a common and highly contagious disease seen worldwide in snakes of the families Boidae and Pythonida. Blood films from boid snakes affected with IBD may reveal inclusions within the cytoplasm of erythrocytes, lymphocytes, or heterophils. IBD inclusions stained with Wright–Giemsa appear as lightly basophilic homogenous intracytoplasmic inclusions of varying size and shape (Figure 21.16). The inclusions may stain darker with Diff-Quik stain. A lymphocytosis may also be present, presumably due to chronic antigenic stimulation from the infectious agent.

Leukocytes

Morphology

Classification of reptilian leukocytes can be problematic in part due the presence of morphologic variation among the different reptilian species. Classification can be further complicated by the presence of differing descriptive nomenclature in the literature. For example, some sources differentiate the reptilian granulocytes into three cell groups – eosinophils, azurophils, and neutrophils – while other sources only differentiate two – eosinophils and heterophils, or eosinophils and neutrophils. In general, the leukocytes of reptiles can be divided into two groups: the granulocytes and the mononuclear leukocytes. The granulocytes of reptiles can be further classified into two groups – acidophils and basophils – based upon their appearance in blood films stained with Romanowsky stains. The acidophils are further divided into heterophils and eosinophils. Heterophils and eosinophils may then be distinguished from each other by the shape and color of their granules. The basophils, lymphocytes, and monocytes found in reptilian blood closely resemble those of mammals and birds and are classified accordingly. A sixth cell type, the azurophil, is often described in the literature and could be considered to be a monocyte with azurophilic granules. Attempts using cytochemical staining reactions for normal leukocytes and thrombocytes in various reptiles have been made to help in the classification of reptilian leukocytes.

Reptilian heterophils generally are large (10–23 µm), round cells with a colorless cytoplasm containing eosinophilic (bright orange), refractile, rod- to spindle-shaped cytoplasmic granules (Figure 21.17). Occasionally degranulated heterophils can be found in the blood film of normal reptiles. The cell margins may appear irregular, and pseudopodia may be present under certain circumstances. The nucleus of the mature heterophil is typically eccentrically positioned in the cell and is round to oval with densely clumped nuclear chromatin. Some species of lizards (i.e., green iguanas, *I. iguana*) have heterophils with lobed nuclei. When toxic changes are present, the cytoplasm appears blue in color and contains abnormal purple-colored granules and vacuoles. Reptilian heterophils are functionally equivalent to mammalian neutrophils but probably behave like avian heterophils in that they rely primarily on oxygen-independent mechanisms to destroy phagocytized microorganisms. Except for a few species of snakes and lizards, reptilian heterophils do not stain for alkaline phosphatase, and are usually peroxidase negative.

Eosinophils in most reptilian blood films are large (11–17 µm) round cells with light blue cytoplasm, a round to oval to possibly lobed, slightly eccentric nucleus, and large numbers of spherical eosinophilic cytoplasmic granules

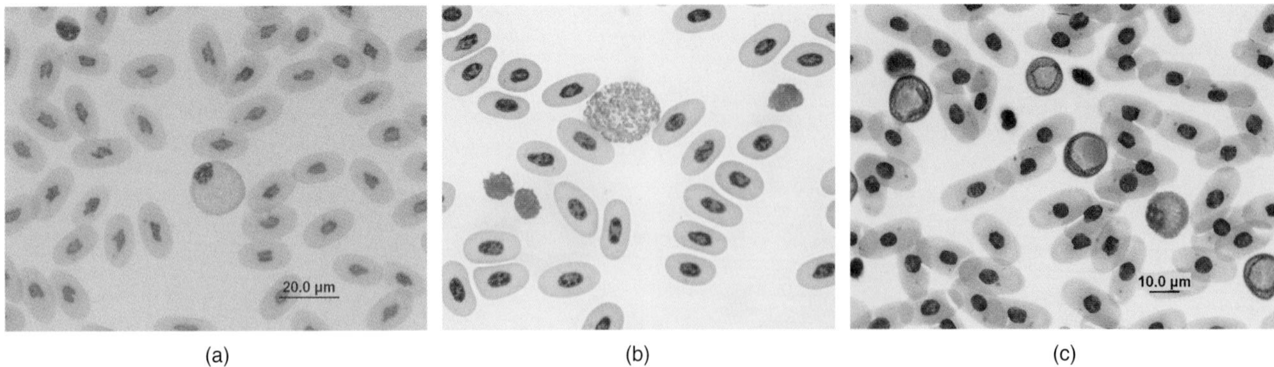

Figure 21.17 (a) A heterophil in the blood film of a snake (*Boa constrictor*). Wright-Giemsa stain. (b) A heterophil in the blood film of a lizard (*Salvator merianae*). Wright-Giemsa stain. (c) Heterophils in the blood film of a chelonian (*Mauremys mutica*). Wright-Giemsa stain.

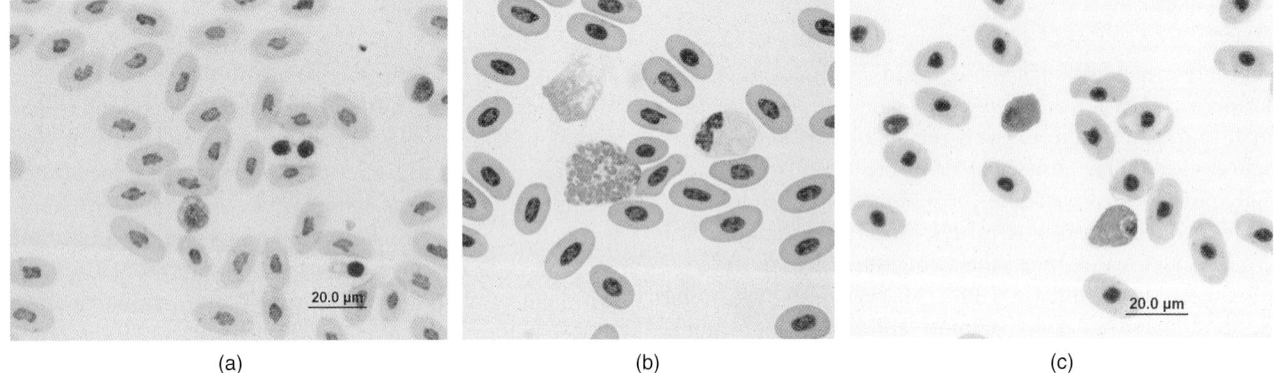

Figure 21.18 (a) An eosinophil in the blood film of a snake (*Boa constrictor*). Wright-Giemsa stain. (b) An eosinophil with pale blue granules (granulocyte on the right) and a heterophil in the blood film of a lizard (*Salvator merianae*). Wright-Giemsa stain. (c) An eosinophil (granulocyte on top) and a heterophil in the blood film of a chelonian (*Batagur borneoensis*). Wright-Giemsa stain.

(Figure. 21.18). The cytoplasmic granules of some reptilian species, such as iguanas, stain blue with Romanowsky stains, and will stain positive for peroxidase in some species of reptiles, allowing differentiation between eosinophils and heterophils (Figures 21.18b and 21.19). The nucleus is typically centrally located but may be eccentrically located in some cases. The size of the eosinophil is species variable. For example, snakes have the largest eosinophils and lizards have the smallest. Reptilian eosinophils contain glycogen, myeloperoxidase, and basic proteins. The latter are known potent toxins for parasites, especially helminthes, inactivating leukotrienes, and causing histamine release from mast cells.

Basophils are small (8–15 µm) round cells, typically smaller than heterophils and eosinophils, that contain variable numbers of round basophilic (i.e., dark blue to purple) metachromatic cytoplasmic granules (Figure 21.20). The nucleus is often obscured by the granules but when visible is nonlobed and slightly eccentric in position. Alcohol fixation and use of Romanowsky stains provide the best staining for reptilian basophils because basophil granules are frequently affected by water-based stains and will partially dissolve.

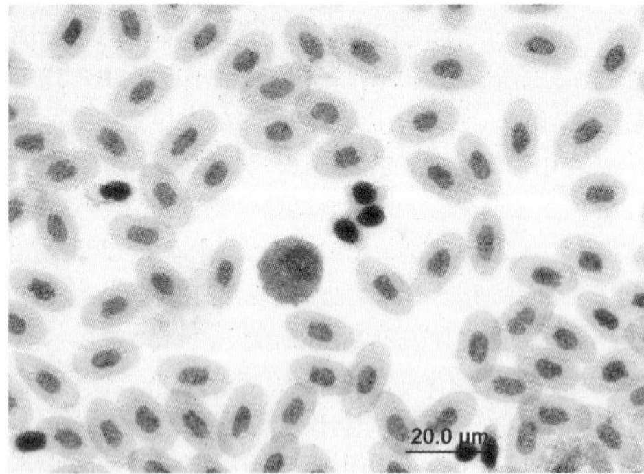

Figure 21.19 An eosinophil with blue cytoplasmic granules in the blood film of a lizard (*Iguana iguana*). Wright-Giemsa stain. Source: Image from Campbell TW. *Exotic Animal Hematology and Cytology*, 4th ed. Ames, IA: Wiley Blackwell, 2015, p. 74.

Species differences in basophil sizes do occur; lizards tend to have smaller basophils than those observed in turtles and crocodiles.

Reptilian lymphocytes resemble those of birds and mammals. They vary in size from small (5–10 µm) to large

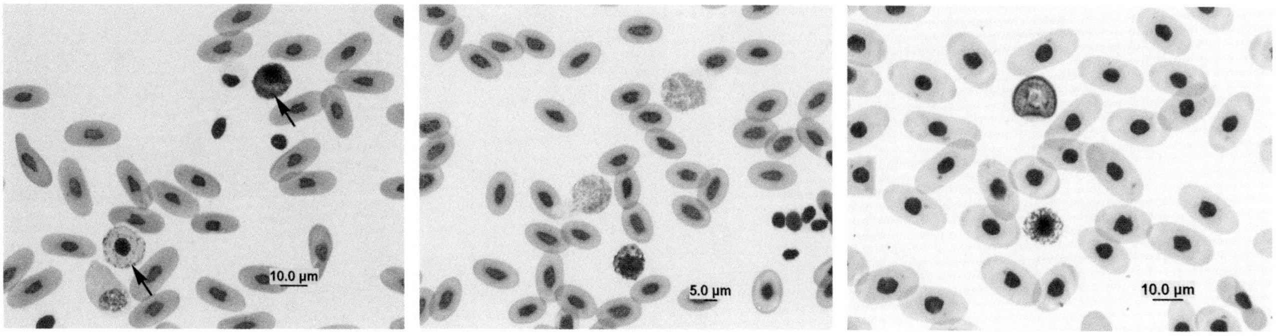

(a) (b) (c)

Figure 21.20 (a) Basophils (arrows), a monocyte, and thrombocyte in the blood film of a snake (*Boa constrictor*). Wright-Giemsa stain. (b) Basophil (granulocyte on the bottom) and heterophils in the blood film of a lizard (*Pogona vitticeps*). Wright-Giemsa stain. (c) Basophil (granulocyte on the bottom) and heterophil in the blood film of a chelonian (*Mauremys mutica*). Wright-Giemsa stain.

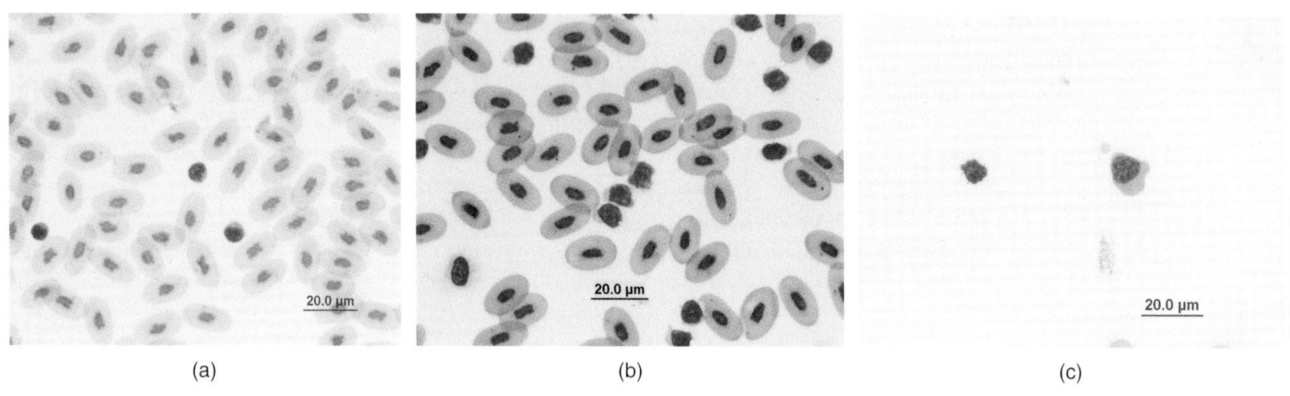

(a) (b) (c)

Figure 21.21 (a) Lymphocytes in the blood film of a snake (*Boa constrictor*). Wright-Giemsa stain. (b) Lymphocytes in the blood film of a lizard (*Pogona vitticeps*) with lymphocytosis. Wright-Giemsa stain. (c) A small and a large lymphocyte in the blood film of a chelonian (*Glyptemys insculpta*). Wright-Giemsa stain.

(15 µm). Lymphocytes are round cells that exhibit irregularity when they mold around adjacent cells in the blood film or fold at their cytoplasmic margin (Figure 21.21). They have a round or slightly indented nucleus that is centrally or slightly eccentrically positioned in the cell; nuclear chromatin is heavily clumped in mature lymphocytes. Typically, lymphocytes have a large nucleus: cytoplasm (N : C) ratio. The typical small, mature lymphocyte has scant slightly basophilic (pale blue) cytoplasm. Large lymphocytes have more cytoplasmic volume compared with small lymphocytes, and the nucleus often is pale staining. The cytoplasm of a normal lymphocyte appears to be homogenous and lacks both vacuoles and granules. Plasma cells may be observed in the blood film of reptiles, and are slightly larger than normal lymphocytes. The nucleus is eccentrically placed, is round to oval, and contains clumped chromatin. The cytoplasm of plasma cells stains deep blue, and a perinuclear halo representative of the Golgi is present (Figure 21.22).

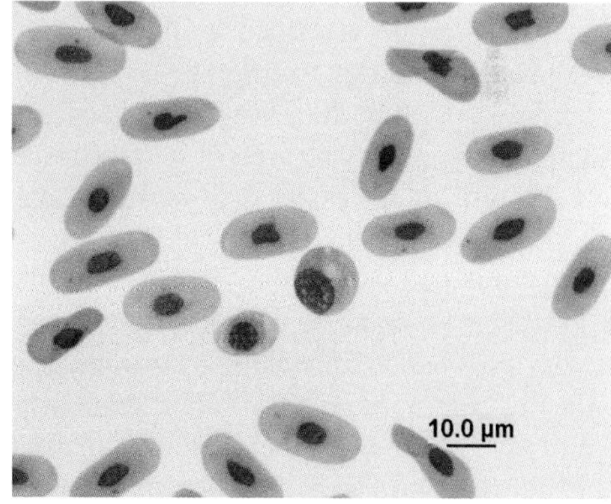

Figure 21.22 A plasma cell in the blood film of a snake (*Boa constrictor*). Wright-Giemsa stain.

Reptilian monocytes resemble those of birds and mammals and are generally the largest leukocytes in peripheral blood (often one-half to two times the size of erythrocytes in the same blood film) (Figure 21.23). Monocytes vary in shape from round to amoeboid, and contain a variably shaped nucleus that ranges in shape from round to oval to lobed or bean-shaped. The nuclear chromatin of the monocyte is less condensed and paler staining compared

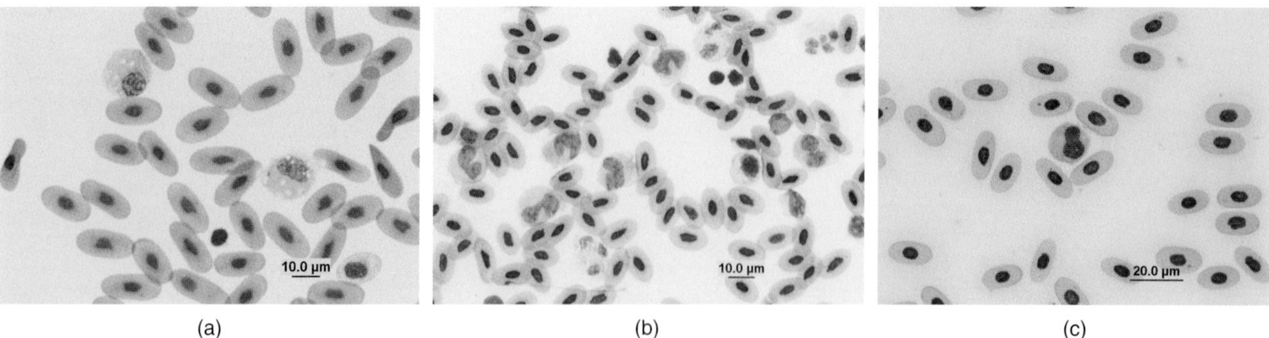

Figure 21.23 (a) Monocytes with azurophilic granules (azurophils) in the blood film of a snake (*Boa constrictor*). Wright-Giemsa stain. (b) Numerous monocytes in the blood film of a lizard (*Pogona vitticeps*) with monocytosis. Three heterophils, a basophil, two lymphocytes, and three thrombocytes are also present. Wright-Giemsa stain. (c) A monocyte in the blood film of a chelonian (*Terrapene carolina*). Wright-Giemsa stain.

to the nuclear chromatin of lymphocytes. The cytoplasm is abundant, stains pale blue-gray, and may be slightly opaque or foamy in appearance. Phagocytized material, vacuoles, or fine eosinophilic or azurophilic granules may be present in the cytoplasm of some monocytes. Monocytic cells of reptiles have been referred to as monocytes, monocytoid azurophils, azurophilic monocytes, or azurophils (Figure 21.23a). Azurophilic leukocytes are often noted in the blood film of reptiles, and historically there has been much confusion surrounding the classification and identification of these cells. Some consider azurophils to be unique to reptiles because they are often found in low numbers in the blood of lizards, chelonians, and crocodilians but in high numbers in snakes. The azurophil is described as an irregularly shaped cell that is slightly smaller in size than the monocyte. The nucleus is nonsegmented and is irregularly round to oval to bilobed. The nuclear chromatin is coarse in appearance. The cytoplasm is basophilic and darker than that of the monocyte, and may be described as blue to lavender in color. Small numbers of dull azurophilic granules of various sizes are present within the cytoplasm. Vacuolation and phagocytosed material may be present within the cytoplasm of these cells, and pseudopodia may be noted on the cell margins. The granulopoietic origin of the azurophil has not been documented. At various times in the literature, this cell has been classified as a granulocyte, a neutrophil, or a monocyte. By light microscopy, azurophils resemble the monocytes that contain azurophilic granules that are occasionally noted in the peripheral blood of mammals and birds, and ultrastructurally and cytochemically, these cells are similar to monocytes. There may be species differences in the characteristics of the cells. For example, the cytochemical properties of all monocytic cells (monocytes and azurophils) of green iguanas (*I. iguana*) are characteristic of monocytes but differ from those of snakes. The azurophils of snakes stain positive for peroxidase, Sudan black B, and PAS, whereas those of the green iguanas do not. Monocytic cells of other reptiles, even those from snakes, have cytochemical properties similar to those of green iguanas (*I. iguana*); however, there is some variability. For example, monocytic cells in some lizards stain positive for peroxidase, but those from alligators do not. Most, if not all, stain PAS and acid phosphatase positive. These facts support the hypothesis that azurophils should be considered monocytes and not a separate distinct cell type. There is little clinical advantage in separating azurophils from monocytes in the leukocyte differential of reptiles, and these cells should be counted as monocytes just as they are in mammals and birds. Azurophils could represent an immature form of the monocyte.

Laboratory evaluation

Evaluation of the reptilian leukogram involves determination of a total and a differential leukocyte count and examination of the leukocyte morphology on a stained blood film. Manual counting methods are used to obtain total leukocyte concentrations in reptiles for the same reasons they are used in avian hematology: the presence of nucleated erythrocytes and thrombocytes in the blood of reptiles precludes the use of electronic cell-counting procedures. Two manual methods commonly used to obtain a total leukocyte count in reptilian blood are the Natt and Herrick method and the phloxine B method (see Chapter 20 on avian hematology). In species of reptiles that normally have higher numbers of circulating lymphocytes than of heterophils, the Natt and Herrick method is preferred, because the accuracy of the phloxine B method relies on large numbers of heterophils and eosinophils.

Responses in disease

Establishment of reference values for the total leukocyte count and leukocyte differential is difficult in reptiles and other ectotherms for the same reasons described in the erythrocytes section. Physiologic adaptations to the intrinsic and extrinsic factors previously described may affect the leukogram of the individual reptile. The same guidelines used for establishing erythrocyte intervals should be considered when developing meaningful statistically accurate leukocyte intervals. Intrinsic factors such as species, gender, age, and the physiologic status of the reptile will affect the leukogram. Differences in the leukogram may occur broadly across the reptile species but can occur within the same genus as well. For example, significant differences in heterophil, monocyte, and lymphocyte counts have been documented among different species of *Gallotia* lizards. Gender and age differences may affect the leukocyte parameters. For example, male crocodiles have higher total leukocyte and heterophil counts compared to females and adult crocodiles have lower total leukocyte counts compared to juveniles. The reproductive status of a reptile may also influence the hemogram. For example, female chameleons may demonstrate a heterophilia after egg-laying; however, being gravid in turtles appears to have no physiological effects on blood parameters or morphometrics. Extrinsic factors include season, temperature, habitat, diet, disease, stress associated with captivity, and even the venipuncture site. For example, factors including season, location, surgical radiotransmitter placement, and anesthetic state can influence blood parameters in snakes. The leukogram of free-ranging tortoises is related to seasonal and annual differences in rainfall patterns, forage availability, and physiological condition. Young crocodiles housed in low temperature (28 °C) environments for 10 days had lower total leukocyte and lymphocyte counts compared to young crocodiles housed in high temperature (38 °C) environments and both sets of these crocodiles had leukocyte counts that were abnormal compared to crocodiles housed at normal temperature (32 °C). Some species of reptile may not be affected by season or temperature; no differences in the pre- and posthibernation hematologic parameters were noted in temperate species of snakes. Stress associated with captivity may affect the leukogram of some reptile species. For example, captive-bred cobras have higher red blood cell parameters and lymphocyte numbers but lower monocyte (azurophil) and heterophil numbers compared to wild-caught cobras. Although the results of the hemogram may vary with the site of venipuncture in some species, it may have no effect in others.

The primary function of the heterophil is phagocytosis. In general, heterophils of most reptiles, like those of birds, do not stain positive with benzidine peroxidase and Sudan black B; therefore, they appear to produce less oxidative responses in their bactericidal function compared to mammalian neutrophils. There is evidence, however, that heterophils from some lizards may have oxidative properties similar to mammalian neutrophils based on their benzidine peroxidase activity. The percentage of heterophils in the leukocyte differential of normal reptiles varies with the species (Tables 21.2 and 21.3). Heterophils can represent as much as 40% of the leukocytes in some normal reptilian species. The heterophil concentration in reptiles also is influenced by seasonal factors. For example, the heterophil concentration is highest during the summer months and is lowest during hibernation.

Because the primary function of heterophils is phagocytosis, significant increases in the heterophil count of reptiles usually are associated with inflammatory disease, especially microbial and parasitic infections or tissue injury. Noninflammatory conditions that may result in heterophilia include stress (i.e., glucocorticosteroid excess), neoplasia, and heterophilic leukemia. The high initial leukocyte counts that commonly occur in cold-stunned turtles are likely a reflection of inflammation, immune response, physiologic stress, or systemic pathologic conditions.

Heterophils may appear to be abnormal in reptiles suffering from a variety of diseases. For example, heterophils may exhibit varying degrees of toxicity with inflammatory diseases, especially those involving infectious agents such as bacteria. Toxic heterophils exhibit increased cytoplasmic basophilia, abnormal granulation (i.e., dark blue to purple granules or granules with abnormal shapes and staining),

Table 21.2 Leukocyte parameters for selected reptiles.

	WBC × $10^3/\mu L$	Heterophils × $10^3/\mu L$	Lymphocytes × $10^3/\mu L$	Monocytes × $10^3/\mu L$	Eosinophils × $10^3/\mu L$	Basophils × $10^3/\mu L$
Lizards						
Argentine lizard[a] winter	13.1–18.1	1.5–2.2	6.7–7.7	1.8–3.0	3.4–4.4	0.2–0.4
Argentine lizard[a] summer	16.0–20.8	1.9–2.9	7.8–8.5	1.6–2.6	3.8–5.0	0.3–0.5
Adult male iguana[b]	11.1–24.6	1.0–5.4	5.0–16.5	0.2–2.7	0.0–0.3	0.1–1.0
Adult female iguana[b]	8.2–25.2	0.6–6.4	5.2–14.4	0.4–2.3	0.0–0.4	0.2–1.2
Juvenile iguana[b]	8.0–22.0	1.0–3.8	6.2–17.2	0.3–0.6	0.0–0.4	0.1–0.7

[a]Troiano JC, Gould EG, Gould I. Hematological reference intervals in argentine lizard *Tupinambis merianae* [Sauria-Teiidae]. *Comp Clin Pathol* 17: 93–7. 2008.

[b]Harr KE, Alleman AR, Dennis PM, Maxwell LK, Lock BA, Bennett RA, Jacobson ER. Morphologic and cytochemical characteristics of blood cells and hematologic and plasma biochemical reference intervals in green iguanas. *JAVMA* 218: 915–21. 2001.

Table 21.3 Leukocyte parameters for selected reptiles.

	WBC × $10^3/\mu L$	Heterophils %	Lymphocytes %	Monocytes %	Eosinophils %	Basophils %
Lizards						
Prehensile-tailed skink[a]	3.9–22.4	16–58	2–40	0–6	0–18	4–26
Snakes						
Boa constrictor[b c]	4–10	20–65	10–60	0–6	0–3	0–20
Ball pythons[d]	7.9–16.4	56–67	7–21	12–22	–	0–2
Yellow rat snake[e]	0.4–32.0	–	–	–	–	–
Jungle carpet python[f]						
Chelonians						
Aldabra tortoise[g]	1.0–8.3	32–79	2–40	0–8	0–7	0–4
Desert tortoise[h]	6.6–8.9	35–60	25–50	0–4	0–4	2–15

[a]Wright KM, Skeba S. Hematology and plasma chemistries of captive prehensile-tailed skinks [*Corcucia zebrata*]. *J Zoo Wildl Med* 23: 429–32. 1992.
[b]Chiodini RJ, Sundberg JP. Blood chemical values of the common boa constrictor [*Constrictor constrictor*]. *Am J Vet Res* 43: 1701–2. 1982.
[c]Rosskopf WJ, Woerpel RW, Yanoff SR. Normal hemogram and blood chemistry values for boa constrictors and pythons. *Vet Med Small Anim Clin* May:822–3. 1982.
[d]Johnson JH, Benson PA. Laboratory reference values for a group of captive ball pythons [*Python regius*]. *Am J Vet Res* 57: 1304–7. 1996.
[e]Ramsey EC, Dotson TK. Tissue and serum enzyme activities in the yellow rat snake [*Elaphe obsolete quadrivitatta*]. *Am J Vet Res* 56: 423–8. 1995.
[f]Centini R, Klaphake E. Hematologic values and cytology in a population of captive jungle carpet pythons, *Morelia spilota cheynei*. *Proc Assoc Rept Amph Vet* 107–11. 2002.
[g]Carpenter JW. *Exotic Animal Formulary*, 3rd ed. St. Louis: Elsevier Saunders, p. 107. 2001.
[h]Gottdenker NL, Jacobson ER. Effect of venipuncture sites on hematologic and clinical biochemical values in desert tortoises [*Gopherus agassizii*]. *Am J Vet Res* 56: 19–21. 1995.

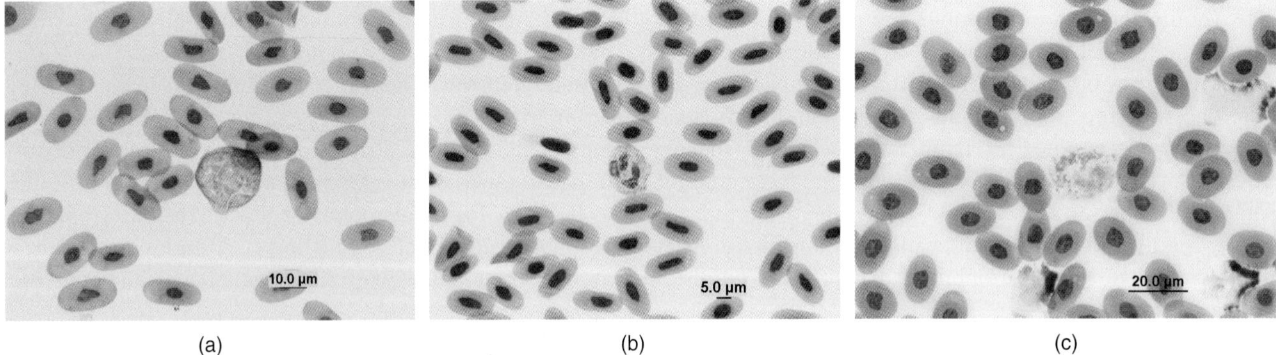

Figure 21.24 (a) A toxic heterophil (1+) in the blood film of a snake (*Boa constrictor*). Wright-Giemsa stain. (b) A toxic heterophil (2+) in the blood film of a lizard (*Chamaeleo calyptratus*). Wright-Giemsa stain. (c) A toxic heterophil (3+) in the blood film of a chelonian (*Centrochelys sulcata*). Wright-Giemsa stain.

and cytoplasmic vacuolation (Figure 21.24). Degranulated heterophils may be associated with artifacts of blood-film preparation or represent toxic changes. Nuclear lobation in species that normally do not lobate their heterophil nuclei also is an abnormal finding and suggests severe inflammation.

The presence of immature heterophils (left shift) in the blood film of reptiles exhibiting a heterophilia is indicative of an inflammatory disease. A left shift in the presence of a heteropenia is indicative of an overwhelming inflammatory response that is likely associated with an infectious etiology. Reptiles often develop a marked leukocytosis and heterophilia with the presence of many immature heterophils, often as early as progranulocytes or myeloblasts, with severe inflammatory diseases, especially those with a bacterial etiology.

Disease and exposure to environmental or chemical toxins can affect the leukogram of reptiles. Tortoises affected with herpesvirus infection often demonstrate heteropenia and lymphocytosis, toxic heterophils, and lymphocytes with pale blue, eccentric intracytoplasmic inclusions. Abnormal heterophil: lymphocyte ratios appear to be related to the circulating blood concentration of organochlorine exposure in sea turtles.

The number of circulating eosinophils in normal reptiles is variable. In general, lizards tend to have low numbers of eosinophils compared with some species of turtles, which can have as much as 20% eosinophils. Like heterophils, the number of eosinophils present in the peripheral blood is influenced by environmental factors, such as seasonal changes. The number of eosinophils generally is lower during the summer months and highest during hibernation in some species. Eosinophilia may be associated with parasitic infections and stimulation of the immune system.

The percentage of basophils in the differential leukocyte count of normal reptiles can range from 0 to 40%. Seasonal variation in basophil concentration is minimal compared to the heterophil and eosinophil concentrations. Some species of reptiles normally have high numbers of circulating basophils. For example, some species of turtles typically have circulating basophil numbers that represent as much as 40% of the leukocyte differential, although the reason for this is unknown. Based on the results of cytochemical and ultrastructural studies, reptilian basophils most likely function in a manner similar to that of mammalian basophils. They appear to process surface immunoglobulins and to release histamine on degranulation. Basophilia has been associated with parasitic and viral infections.

The lymphocyte concentration in reptilian blood also varies. Many healthy reptiles have a higher lymphocyte count than heterophil count and they can represent more than 80% of the normal leukocyte differential in some species. Lymphocyte numbers are influenced by several intrinsic and extrinsic factors. Like heterophils and eosinophils, lymphocytes also are influenced by seasonal change; lymphocyte counts tend to be lowest during the winter months and highest during the summer months. Temperate reptiles have a decreased concentration of lymphocytes during hibernation, after which the lymphocyte concentration increases. Tropical reptiles also demonstrate decreased numbers of circulating lymphocytes during the winter months despite their lack of hibernation. Lymphocyte concentrations also are affected by gender, with the female members of some species having significantly higher lymphocyte concentrations than males of the same species. Reptilian lymphocytes function in a manner similar to those of birds and mammals. They have the same major classes of lymphocytes, B and T lymphocytes that are involved with a variety of immunologic functions. Unlike those in birds and mammals, however, the immunologic responses of ectothermic reptiles are influenced greatly by the environment. For example, low temperatures may suppress or even inhibit the immune response in reptiles.

Lymphopenia often is associated with malnutrition or is secondary to a number of diseases because of stress and immunosuppression. Lymphocytosis occurs during wound healing, inflammatory disease, parasitic infection (e.g., anasakiasis and spirorchidiasis), and viral infections. Lymphocytosis also occurs during ecdysis. The presence of reactive lymphocytes and, less commonly, of plasma cells suggests stimulation of the immune system (Figure 21.22). These cells resemble those of birds and mammals. Reactive lymphocytes have more abundant, deeply basophilic cytoplasm compared with normal lymphocytes, and their nuclear chromatin may appear to be less condensed. Plasma cells have abundant, intensely basophilic cytoplasm that contains a distinct Golgi zone and an eccentrically positioned nucleus.

Monocytes generally occur in low numbers in the blood films of normal reptiles, ranging between 0 and 10% of the leukocyte differential. Snakes typically have monocytes with an azurophilic appearance to the cytoplasm, which frequently is referred to as azurophils in the literature (Figure 21.23a). The monocyte concentration changes little with seasonal variation. Monocytosis suggests inflammatory diseases, especially granulomatous inflammation. For example, chameleons with dystocia often demonstrate a monocytosis in the absence of peritonitis and a progressive increase in monocyte numbers along with the total leukocyte count and heterophil numbers have been associated with an increase in the tumor score of green turtles (*Chelonia mydas*) with fibropapillomastosis. Significant increases in monocytes (azurophils) have been noted in lizards with *Karyolysus* and snakes with *Hepatozoon* parasitemia. The cause of this was not determined but could be related to an inflammatory response to the parasites.

Monocytes in the peripheral blood of reptiles often reveal phagocytic activity. Erythrophagocytosis and leukophagocytosis by can be associated with anemia and infectious diseases. Circulating siderophagocytes and erythrophagocytes can be transiently found to be part of the postsurgical removal of extravasated blood in reptiles recovering from intracoelomic surgery, during which time the PCV remains relatively stable. Circulating siderophagocytes in the blood may reflect differences in the circulation of macrophages in snakes compared with mammals. In mammals, intraperitoneal macrophages are drained via lymphatics to lymph nodes, where they accumulate in the sinuses resulting in posthemorrhagic lymph nodes that contain large numbers of hemosiderin-laden macrophages. Because reptiles have no lymph nodes to filter out these cells, it is likely the coelomic macrophages reenter circulating blood from the lymphatic system to be transported either directly to bone marrow or to the spleen. Therefore, circulating siderophagocytes in postoperative blood films in reptiles can be interpreted as recirculating macrophages involved in the removal of blood from the coelomic cavity following mild postsurgical hemorrhage. Macrophages containing melanin (melanomacrophages) are common in lower vertebrates. These cells can be found in peripheral blood films of reptiles with inflammatory diseases.

Leukemia has been reported rarely in reptiles. Myeloproliferative diseases of reptiles are classified in the same manner as in mammals. Special cytochemical studies may be required to identify the abnormal cells. Lymphoid leukemia and other hematopoietic neoplasia have been reported in reptiles. Affected animals frequently present with a marked to severe leukocytosis due to high numbers of atypical cells, usually blasts. Lymphoid leukemia is indicated by the presence of large number of immature and abnormal lymphocytes. The lymphocytes can be medium-sized cells with round to pleomorphic nuclei, slightly clumped chromatin, indistinct nucleoli, and scant moderate-to-dark blue cytoplasm with occasional red-to-purple cytoplasmic granulation. Advanced diagnostic tools, such as cytochemical and immunochemical staining and transmission electron microscopy, are needed to further evaluate and differentiate the neoplastic hemic cell population of hematopoietic neoplasms of reptiles. For example, the diagnosis of T-cell lymphoid leukemia can be based on positive cytochemical staining with α-naphthyl butyrate esterase using mammalian controls.

Considerations in the interpretation of the reptilian hemogram

Hematology is a valuable diagnostic tool that can be used to assess the response of a reptilian patient to disease or therapy. An example of a favorable response in the leukogram would be a shift from a leukocytosis or leukopenia to a normal leukocyte concentration. A normal heterophil, eosinophil, or monocyte count following a heterophilia, eosinophilia, or monocytosis, respectively, would usually indicate improvement as well. The disappearance of toxic heterophils, reactive lymphocytes, and plasma cells from a blood film during or after therapy indicates improvement and a favorable response to therapy. Anemic reptiles that exhibit an erythrocytic regenerative response have a better prognosis compared to those with little or no response. Similarly, a normal thrombocyte concentration following thrombocytopenia indicates a favorable response.

When evaluating the hematologic responses of reptiles, the effects that intrinsic and extrinsic factors may have on the animal's response to disease cannot be overlooked. The cellular responses in reptilian blood are less predictable than those of endothermic mammals and birds whose cellular microenvironments are more stable. Reptilian hemogram values may be affected by a number of sample-handling factors as well. The blood collection site, type of anticoagulant used, method of cell counting, type of stain used, and experience of the technician add to the variability of reptilian hemogram values. All of these factors can complicate the establishment and validation of normal reference intervals in reptiles. Because of this variability, total and differential leukocyte concentrations must be increased or decreased at least twofold from normal reference intervals in order to be considered significant.

Thrombocytes and hemostasis

Morphology

Thrombocytes of reptiles appear as small (generally smaller than erythrocytes), elliptical to fusiform, nucleated cells (Figure 21.25). The round to oval centrally positioned nucleus has dense nuclear chromatin that stains purple, whereas the cytoplasm typically is colorless to pale blue and may contain a few azurophilic granules. Some nuclei may contain a pale line that extends across the width of the nucleus. Activated thrombocytes are common and appear as clusters of cells with irregular cytoplasmic margins and vacuoles. Thrombocytes appear to be devoid of cytoplasm when aggregated. Indistinct cytoplasmic margins may be noted on some individual thrombocytes, and are probably a product of age, artifact, or function.

Laboratory evaluation

The actual thrombocyte concentration may be difficult to determine, because thrombocytes tend to clump especially when exposed to heparin, which is a commonly used anticoagulant in reptilian hematology. The thrombocyte concentration can be measured using the Natt and Herrick

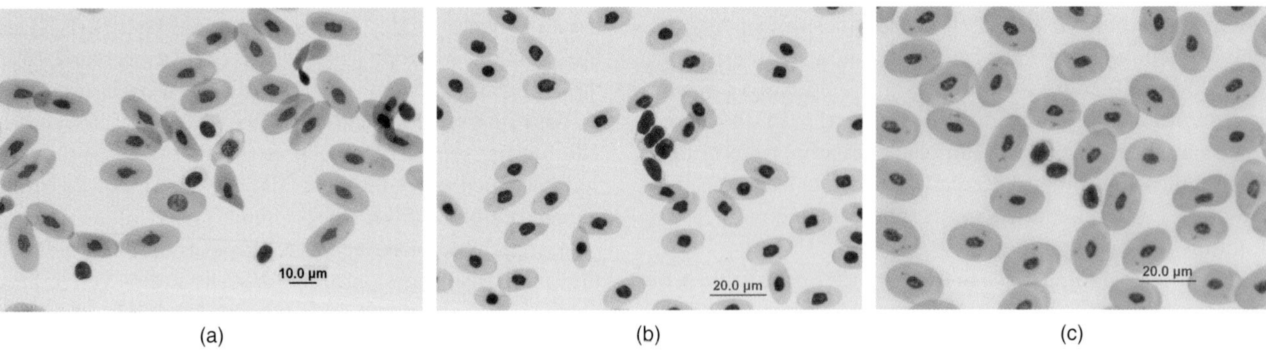

Figure 21.25 (a) Thrombocytes in the blood film of a snake (*Boa constrictor*). Wright-Giemsa stain. (b) Thrombocytes in the blood film of a lizard (*Iguana iguana*). Wright-Giemsa stain. (c) Thrombocytes in the blood film of a chelonian (*Chelonia mydas*). Wright-Giemsa stain.

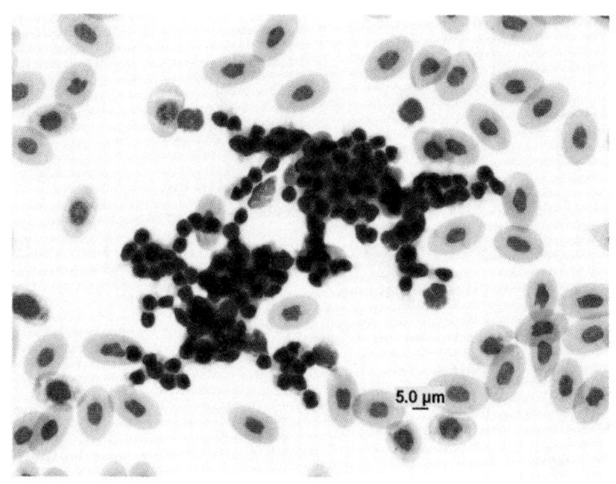

Figure 21.26 Clusters of activated thrombocytes in the blood film of a lizard (*Pogona vitticeps*). Wright-Giemsa stain.

method for obtained erythrocyte and leukocyte counts. After preparing the 1 : 200 dilution of the blood with Natt-Herrick solution and charging a Neubauer-ruled hemocytometer, the number of thrombocytes in the entire central ruled area (i.e., the central, large square) are counted on both sides of the hemocytometer. The number of thrombocytes per microliter of blood is obtained by multiplying that number by 1000. A subjective thrombocyte concentration can be determined based on the number of thrombocytes that appear in a stained blood film and it can be reported as either reduced, normal, or increased. Thrombocyte concentration typically ranges between 25 and 35 thrombocytes per 100 leukocytes in the blood film of normal reptiles (Figure 21.26).

Responses to disease

Reptilian thrombocyte numbers vary with species and seasons. For example, the mean absolute thrombocyte count of the argentine lizard (*Tupinambis merianae*) is $7.2 \times 10^3/\mu L$ during the winter months but $9.1 \times 10^3/\mu L$ during the summer. Reptilian thrombocytes have a significant role in thrombus formation, and they function similarly to avian thrombocytes and mammalian platelets. The ultrastructural features of activated reptilian thrombocytes include pseudopodia with fine, granular material and many fibrin-like filaments radiating both between and around the cells. Immature thrombocytes of reptiles resemble the immature thrombocytes of birds and, when present in blood films, represent a regenerative response. Thrombocytopenias of reptiles most likely result from excessive peripheral utilization of thrombocytes or decreased thrombocyte production. Thrombocytes with polymorphic nuclei are considered to be abnormal, and may be associated with severe inflammatory disease.

Blood parasites

Blood parasites are common in reptiles. Their presence usually is considered to be an incidental finding; however, some have the potential of causing disease, such as hemolytic anemia.

Common hemoprotozoa include the hemogregarines, trypanosomes, and *Plasmodium*. Less commonly encountered hemoprotozoans include *Leishmania*, *Saurocytozoon*, *Haemoproteus*, and *Schellackia*, and the piroplasmids. Microfilaria are commonly found in the peripheral blood films of some reptiles.

Hemogregarines

Hemogregarines are the most common group of sporozoan hemoparasites affecting reptiles, especially snakes. The three genera of hemogregarines that are common in reptiles are *Hemogregarina*, *Hepatozoon*, and *Karyolysus*. Accurate classification of the hemogregarines into their appropriate genus cannot be accomplished based on their appearance in the blood film alone. Therefore, the general term "hemogregarine" is used when reporting their presence in blood films during hematologic examinations.

Hemogregarines are identified by the presence of intracytoplasmic gametocytes in erythrocytes (Figure 21.27). The sausage-shaped gametocytes have a colorless to pale purple cytoplasm that lacks the refractile pigment granules found in the gametocytes of *Plasmodium* and *Haemoproteus*, and they distort the host cell by creating a bulge in the cytoplasm. Typically, only one gametocyte is found per erythrocyte; however, in heavy infections, two gametocytes may be found in one cell.

Hemogregarines have a lifecycle that involves sexual reproduction (sporogony) in an invertebrate host and asexual multiplication (merogony) in a reptilian host. The parasite infects the reptilian host when the sporozoites are transmitted from the invertebrate host as it feeds on the blood of the reptile or is ingested by the reptile. Several biting, invertebrate hosts (i.e., mites, ticks, mosquitoes, flies, and true bugs) can transmit the parasite to terrestrial reptiles, whereas leeches appear to be the primary intermediate host for the hemogregarines of aquatic reptiles. Reptilian

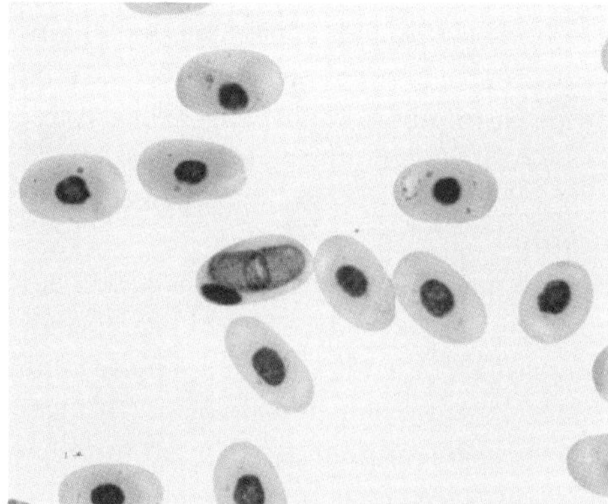

Figure 21.27 A hemogregarine gametocyte within an erythrocyte in the blood film of a chelonian (*Trachemys scripta elegans*). Wright-Giemsa stain. Source: Image from Campbell TW. *Exotic Animal Hematology and Cytology*, 4th ed. Ames, IA: Wiley Blackwell, 2015, p. 123.

hemogregarines are well adapted to their natural host and do not cause clinical disease; however, because they are relatively not host-specific, they can cause significant clinical disease in unnatural or aberrant host species. Such infections result in severe inflammatory lesions associated with schizonts in a variety of organs.

Intraleukocytic (i.e., heterophils) forms of hemogregarines appear to be parasites phagocytized by leukocytes as part of an immune response in the vertebrate host. A high level of intraleukocytic hemogregarines may represent a stage in the infection cycle where the reptilian host is clearing the parasite infection from its blood cells. The increased number of intraleukocytic forms has a seasonal appearance that may represent a more efficient immune response during warmer months. Infection intensity varies with fluctuations in vector abundance; both seasonally and spatially, whereas patterns of infection within exposed populations can vary with host body size and perhaps reproductive status. For example, the hemogregarine parasitemia has been shown to decline with increasing host body size.

Snakes are more commonly infected with hemogregarine parasites compared to other reptile species. The hemogregarines found in snakes are typically of the genus *Hepatozoon*. Hemogregarines may be found in semiaquatic freshwater turtles and are usually of the genus *Hemogregarina*. *Karyolysus* typically occurs in old world lizards and possibly tree snakes. There are no reported cases of hemogregariniasis in sea turtles, and the parasites are rare in tortoises. Hemogregarine parasites have been noted in the peripheral blood films of American alligators (*Alligator mississippiensis*) and are considered to be an incidental finding.

Trypanosomes

The trypanosomes found in reptiles resemble those found in mammals and birds. They are large, extracellular, flagellate protozoa with a bladelike shape, a single flagellum, and a prominent, undulating membrane. For transmission, they require a bloodsucking invertebrate host, such as biting flies for terrestrial reptiles or leeches for aquatic reptiles. Trypanosomes have been found in all orders of reptiles, have a worldwide distribution, rarely cause clinical disease, and often are associated with lifelong infections.

Plasmodium

More than 60 species of *Plasmodium* have been described in reptiles; most have been identified in lizards and a few in snakes. *Plasmodium* in reptiles resembles those found in birds (see Chapter 20 on avian hematology). The gametocytes have refractile pigment granules that aid in differentiation between *Plasmodium* and hemogregarines. Also, unlike hemogregarines, *Plasmodium* schizogony (packets of merozoites) can occur in blood cells. The trophozoites are small, signet-ring structures in the cytoplasm of erythrocytes. The lifecycle of *Plasmodium* involves a sporogony stage in an insect host (e.g., mosquito) and schizogony and gametogony in a reptile host. Infections with *Plasmodium* can result in a severe hemolytic anemia.

Leishmania or *Sauroleishmania*

Leishmania or *Sauroleishmania* rarely are seen in blood films of reptiles. The organism is related to trypanosomes, and it primarily infects lizards. When present, the organism (i.e., amastigote or leishmanial stage) appears as a round to oval inclusion of 2–4 μm with blue cytoplasm and an oval, red nucleus in the cytoplasm of thrombocytes or mononuclear leukocytes.

Saurocytozoon

Saurocytozoon produce large, round gametocytes that lack pigment granules in the cytoplasm of leukocytes in peripheral blood films. Only the gametocyte stage is found in the peripheral blood, and schizogony occurs in the tissues. The organism resembles *Leukocytozoon* of birds, because it grossly distorts the host cell that it parasitizes (see Chapter 20). As indicated by its name, this is a parasite of lizards and, most likely, is transmitted by mosquitoes.

Lainsonia and *Schellackia*

Lainsonia and *Schellackia* are coccidian parasites of lizards and snakes. They produce schizonts that can be found in the intestinal epithelium and sporozoites that can be found in the peripheral blood. The sporozoites are intracytoplasmic inclusions that are seen in erythrocytes and mononuclear leukocytes, primarily lymphocytes; they resemble *Atoxoplasma* in birds (see Chapter 20). The parasite is identified by the round to oval, pale-staining, nonpigmented inclusions that deform the host-cell nucleus into a crescent shape. *Schellackia* and *Lainsonia* are transmitted by mites or, possibly, by ingestion of oocysts from feces. *Lainsonia iguanae* is frequently found in the blood of normal green iguanas (*I. iguana*) housed outdoors and is not associated with health problems.

Piroplasmids

The piroplasmids of reptiles include *Babesia*, *Aegyptianella* (*Tunetella*), and *Sauroplasma* or *Serpentoplasma*. They have been reported in chelonians, lizards, and snakes and appear as small, nonpigmented inclusions in the cytoplasm of erythrocytes. The inclusions are small, round to piriform, nonpigmented, and signet ring–like vacuoles measuring from 1 to 2 μm in diameter. Piroplasmids commonly found in the peripheral blood erythrocytes of lizards are referred to as *Sauroplasma*, whereas the same organisms in the blood of snakes are called *Serpentoplasma*. The piroplasmids are transmitted by biting insects or arthropods. They reproduce by either schizogony or binary fission.

Pirohemocyton

Pirhemocytonosis is characterized as the presence of red, punctate to oval, erythrocytic inclusions that increase in size (0.5–1.5 µm) as infection develops. Pirhemocytonosis is typically reported in lizards, although similar inclusions have been reported in snakes and turtles as well. Inclusions may be associated with vacuoles or irregular pale-staining areas in the cytoplasm of erythrocytes in Giemsa-stained blood films. A single inclusion per erythrocyte is typical; however, two inclusions per cell may occur on occasion. These intraerythrocytic inclusions were previously considered to be piroplasmids and were referred to as *Pirhemocyton*, until ultrastructural studies revealed the presence of a virus consistent with members of the Iridoviridae family. Natural infections with this erythrocytic virus appear to be nonfatal, even when high viremia is present (i.e., greater than 85% of the erythrocytes are infected). Erythrocytes may appear spindle-shaped or thin and elongated. One report of pirhemocytonosis in snakes was suggestive of an oncornavirus based upon ultrastructural studies. Square to rectangular, pale, crystalline-like cytoplasmic inclusions are commonly found in the erythrocyte cytoplasm of green iguanas (*I. iguana*) (Figure 21.28). One report determined that 20% of iguanas examined had these inclusions in 1–5% of their erythrocytes. Although some consider these to be viral or *Pirhemocyton* inclusions, the exact cause for these is unknown and they do not appear to be associated with hematologic abnormalities or disease.

Hemoproteus

Hemoproteus (*Haemocystidium*) has been reported in lizards, turtles, and snakes. They resemble the *Hemoproteus* found in birds; only the gametocytes with refractile pigment granules are found in the peripheral blood films (see Chapter 20).

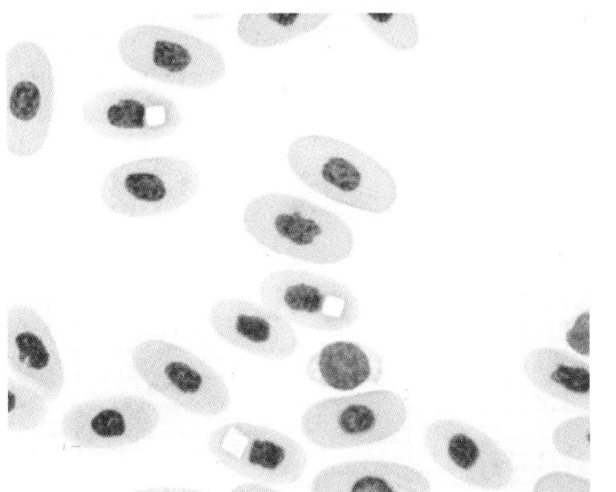

Figure 21.28 Clear, square, vacuole-like cytoplasmic inclusion in the erythrocyte in the blood film of a lizard (*Iguana iguana*). Wright-Giemsa stain. Source: Image from Campbell TW. *Exotic Animal Hematology and Cytology*, 4th ed. Ames, IA: Wiley Blackwell, 2015, p. 125.

Microfilaria

Microfilaremia in reptiles typically is not associated with clinical signs of illness or changes in the hemogram or blood biochemical profile. The reptile typically survives for years with these parasites, and microfilaria are detected as an incidental finding on examination of routine Romanowsky-stained blood films. Microfilarias are produced by adult female filarid nematodes, which can live in various locations in the body of a reptile. Microfilarias are ingested by a suitable bloodsucking arthropod (i.e., tick or mite) or insect (i.e., mosquito), in which they develop into the infective, third-stage larval form. The lifecycle is complete when the infective form enters a new reptilian host during intermediate-host feeding.

Hematopoiesis

The bone marrow appears to be the primary site for erythropoiesis, granulopoiesis, and thrombopoiesis in adult reptiles. The bone marrow of some reptiles, especially turtles and tortoises, is not gelatinous, and hematopoietic cells may be difficult to sample for study. A saline-soak technique can be used for turtles in which a 2 mm thickness of bone is allowed to soak for 18–24 hours at 4 °C and then agitated for 30 minutes, and the solution centrifuged to obtain the hematopoietic cells.

Erythropoiesis in the bone marrow occurs within the vascular space of the reticular stroma. Foci of extramedullary erythropoiesis, in the liver and spleen, are common. The stages of reptilian erythrocyte maturation appear to be similar to those of birds and mammals; however, during the final stages of maturation, the mature reptilian erythrocytes are often larger than the immature erythrocytes – a distinctive difference compared to mammals. In general, seven recognizable stages are involved in erythrocyte development: rubriblasts, prorubricytes, basophilic rubricytes, early polychromatic rubricytes, late polychromatic rubricytes, polychromatic erythrocytes, and mature erythrocytes. The morphologic features of these cells are similar to those described in birds (see Chapter 20).

The rubriblast (proerythroblast, pronormoblast) is the first progenitor cell that can be visually identified and appears as a round cell with a large round nucleus, delicate uncondensed chromatin, and one or two nucleoli. The cytoplasm is basophilic and agranular and typically appears as a narrow band surrounding the nucleus. Pinocytotic vesicles may be found along the cell margin and are a characteristic feature of early reptilian erythroid cells. These vesicles make up the process for ferritin incorporation used in hemoglobin synthesis.

The prorubricyte (basophilic erythroblast) is similar to the rubriblast. The cell is round, and the nucleus lacks nucleoli and contains a slightly more condensed chromatin network. The cytoplasm of the prorubricyte stains basophilic.

The rubricyte (polychromatic erythroblasts) is the third stage in erythrocyte maturation. During this stage of development, the cell is smaller in size and is still spherical or just beginning to develop an oval shape. The size of the nucleus is reduced, and the chromatin appears more condensed and clumped. The cytoplasm of the rubricyte is scant and lighter in color due to hemoglobin synthesis and may be classified as basophilic, early polychromatic, or late polychromatic. Reptilian erythrocytes are typically released into the peripheral circulation in the rubricyte stage.

Reticulocytes (polychromatic erythrocyte, acidophilic or orthochromatic erythroblast, proerythrocyte) make up the next stage of erythrocyte maturation and resemble mature erythrocytes. The cell is larger in size, and the shape resembles a flattened ellipsoid. Reticulocytes may be differentiated from the mature erythrocyte based on the presence of abundant slightly basophilic cytoplasm and nuclear chromatin that is not fully condensed. The presence of reticulocytes in peripheral blood may vary with species. Some authors describe them as a common finding, and others describe them as rare.

Mature erythrocytes (normocytes) are morphologically similar among most reptiles. The mature erythrocyte is a flattened oval and has a centrally positioned nucleus with condensed nuclear chromatin. The nuclear margins may be irregular. The nucleus is ellipsoid in many species of reptile; however, in some species (turtles, tortoises), the nucleus may appear round. The cytoplasm stains light red to yellowish in color. As erythrocytes age, the nucleus becomes more condensed and darker staining. In summary, as the reptilian erythrocyte matures, the cell becomes larger and the cytoplasm increasingly eosinophilic because of increased hemoglobin synthesis. A clear, size-related progression in erythrocyte development may not be evident in some species, but the shape of the cell changes from spherical to a flattened ellipsoid with maturation. The erythrocyte nucleus also decreases in size, with its shape changing from round to ellipsoid, and the nuclear chromatin becomes increasingly condensed as the cell matures. Sudan black B stain can be used as an erythrocyte marker that stains the cytoplasm of erythrocyte precursors and mature erythrocytes dark gray to black.

Developing granulocytes are morphologically similar to mammalian granulocytes and are associated with the extravascular spaces of the bone marrow reticular stroma. The maturing granulocytes migrate through the endothelial cells of the sinusoids to enter the bloodstream. The maturation stages of the granulocytes of reptiles also resemble those of birds (see Chapter 20 on avian hematology). As the granulocyte matures, the cell decreases in size, and the cytoplasm becomes less basophilic. Specific, characteristic granules appear in the myelocyte and metamyelocyte stages of development, and these increase in number with maturation. The nuclear chromatin becomes increasingly condensed with maturity, and in those species that lobate their nuclei, the nucleus changes from round to segmented. Mature and immature heterophils from some species stain positive with chloroacetate esterase, α-naphthyl butyrate esterase, α-naphthyl acetate esterase, and leukocyte alkaline phosphatase chemical stains. The cytoplasmic granules of the eosinophils of some reptiles typically are large, round, and pink with Romanowsky stains and golden brown with benzedrine peroxidase, which helps in the differentiation of eosinophil precursors from heterophil precursors.

Granulopoiesis begins with the myeloblast. Myeloblasts have a moderate amount of agranular, slightly basophilic cytoplasm and a large, central to slightly eccentric ovoid, vesicular nucleus with a large nucleolus or prominent nucleoli. As maturation takes place, the cells decrease in size, the cytoplasm becomes less basophilic, the nuclear chromatin becomes increasingly condensed, and the nucleus changes shape from round to segmented in those reptile species that lobate their nuclei. The acidophils (heterophils and eosinophils) are derived from separate cell lines, and their specific characteristic cytoplasmic granules appear in the myelocyte and metamyelocyte stages of development. These granules increase in number as maturation continues.

The cytoplasmic granules of the eosinophils of some reptiles are typically large, round, and pink with Romanowsky stains and golden brown with benzidine peroxidase to help in the differentiation of eosinophil precursors from those of heterophils. Mature and immature heterophils from some reptile species stain positive with chloroacetate esterase, a-naphthyl butyrate esterase, a-naphthyl acetate esterase, and leukocyte alkaline phosphatase chemical stains.

Thrombopoiesis in reptiles is similar to that in birds (see Chapter 20 on avian hematology). The elliptical, mature thrombocytes are derived from round precursor cells. The thrombocyte series consists of thromboblasts, immature thrombocytes, and mature thrombocytes. Reptilian thrombocytes are derived from a distinct line of mononuclear cells found in the bone marrow or other hematopoietic tissue. Thromboblasts appear as small, round to oval cells that resemble rubriblasts and contain round nuclei with fine to punctate nuclear chromatin and one or more nucleoli. Immature thrombocytes may be divided into three groups: early, mid-, and late-immature thrombocytes, based upon their degree of maturity. As thrombocytes develop, they decrease in size, the cytoplasm becomes less basophilic, and the shape of the cell changes from round to elliptical. The nucleus changes from round to oval in shape as well. In later stages of maturation, the nuclear chromatin becomes densely packed, and specific cytoplasmic granules may appear. It often is difficult to differentiate thrombocytes from lymphocytes in hematopoietic specimens. Special chemical stains may be used to differentiate the two in some species, in which thrombocytes stain positive with periodic acid–Schiff, acid phosphatase, and α-naphthyl butyrate esterase and lymphocytes do not.

Lymphopoiesis of reptiles resembles that of mammals and birds. Reptilian lymphoblasts, prolymphocytes, and mature lymphocytes appear identical to those found in birds and mammals and can be found in lymphopoietic tissues such as the spleen and liver. The lymphocytes are derived from blood-borne stem cells, which most likely originated from the embryonic yolk sac. Lymphoid precursors originating from the yolk sac or bone marrow colonize the thymus during embryonic development. The thymus is the first lymphoid organ to develop in reptiles, and it is likely that T lymphocytes are the predominant lymphoid cells of the spleen and peripheral blood of posthatched reptiles. T cells that originate in the thymus spread to spleen, liver, intestines, and other tissues containing lymphoid aggregates. The origin of the immunoglobulin-producing cells (B lymphocytes) is unknown since a reptilian equivalent to the avian bursa of Fabricius has not been found. The spleen functions as an organ of leukopoiesis in reptiles. During early stages of splenic development, large numbers of granulocytes are found, indicating that the organ is involved in granulopoiesis. During later development, the spleen becomes primarily involved with lymphopoiesis.

22 Hematology of Fish

Terry W. Campbell

Department of Clinical Sciences, College of Veterinary Medicine and Biomedical Sciences, Colorado State University, Fort Collins, Colorado, USA

Published hematologic reference intervals for fish and the interpretation of piscine blood test results are limited when compared to what is available for mammals and birds. This is expected given the diversity of fish, a group of animals represented by approximately 27,300 species; a number that exceeds that of all other vertebrates combined. Regardless of these limitations, hematologic evaluation of the piscine patient can be useful in the detection of diseases affecting the cellular components of blood. Certain diseases of fish result in anemia, leukopenia, leukocytosis, thrombocytopenia, and other abnormal changes of the blood cells. Evaluation of the hemogram also may be useful in following the progress of the disease or the response to therapy.

Blood collection and handling

Blood for diagnostic sampling can be collected safely from fish that are greater than 3 in. (8 cm) in length. The collection procedure itself should be accomplished in less than 30 seconds, however, because fish that are held out of water for longer periods suffer from respiratory distress and electrolyte imbalance. Blood collection from fish may be accomplished with either physical or chemical restraint. Physical restraint is used if the patient is cooperative or severely debilitated and when the procedure can be performed without causing added stress to the animal. Because their integument has many important metabolic functions, fish should be handled cautiously, and every attempt should be made to protect the skin and mucous coating. Therefore, examination or surgical gloves that contain no powder should be worn to protect the skin and mucous layer of the fish as well as the hands of the handler from zoonotic disease and the physical and chemical defense mechanisms of the fish. In general, small fish can be restrained by using one hand to grasp near the base of the tail while supporting the body with the other hand. Larger fish may require the use of ancillary equipment, such as nets or stretchers, for restraint and handling. Some elasmobranchs may enter a hypnotic state referred to as tonic immobility when placed in dorsal recumbency. Tonic immobility has been noted in several species and offers a short duration of decreased activity allowing for minor procedures such as physical or ultrasonographic examination, venipuncture, or administration of medications. When physical restraint cannot be safely accomplished, then chemical restraint is commonly used. A number of chemical agents can be used to provide sedation or anesthesia in fish; however, the most commonly used Food and Drug Administration–approved agent is tricaine methanesulfonate (Tricaine-S, previously Finquel; also referred to as tricaine or MS-222). Tricaine methanesulfonate requires buffering with two parts sodium bicarbonate and is used as an immersion bath to create sedation and anesthesia. Factors such as physical characteristics of the fish and environmental conditions may affect the outcome of a chemical agent used for sedation or anesthesia. Suggested sedation and anesthetic doses for tricaine methanesulfonate range from 50 to 400 mg/L; however, the commonly used induction dose for most fish ranges between 50 and 150 mg/L – it is recommended to begin conservatively.

The amount of blood that can be safely obtained from a healthy fish has been reported at 30–50% of total blood volume; however, a sample representing 1% of the body weight is typically collected in most clinical situations. Blood for hematologic evaluation should be collected in either heparin or ethylenediaminetetraacetic acid (EDTA) as an anticoagulant. Disadvantages of heparin include the tendency for leukocytes and thrombocytes to clump and the creation of a blue tinge to blood films with Romanowsky stains. In addition, if the blood sample contains a small clot, heparin may not prevent coagulation once it has started. Disadvantages of EDTA include the hemolysis of erythrocytes in some fish species, such as elasmobranchs. For elasmobranch blood, although heparin can be used, a combination of heparin and EDTA or use of another modified anticoagulant solution is ideal to match the osmolarity of the blood. Hemolysis also

Veterinary Hematology, Clinical Chemistry, and Cytology, Third Edition. Edited by Mary Anna Thrall, Glade Weiser, Robin W. Allison and Terry W. Campbell.

Companion website: www.wiley.com/go/thrall/veterinary

can occur with the use of tricaine sedation or anesthesia, but cooling the blood sample to 25 °C and rapidly preparing the film can minimize the hemolysis associated with tricaine. To avoid staining artifacts caused by an anticoagulant, a freshly prepared blood film should be made at the time of blood collection.

Blood can be collected from fish via the caudal vertebral vein or artery. Venipuncture of these vessels can be accomplished with or without sedation or anesthesia, and the caudal vertebral vein or artery can be approached either ventrally or laterally. The ventral approach used for teleosts (bony fish) and small elasmobranchs begins with the fish in dorsal recumbency followed by the insertion of the needle under a scale (teleost fish) along the ventral midline near the base of the caudal peduncle (Figure 22.1). The needle is then directed toward the vertebral bodies. Slight aspiration of the plunger is applied once the needle has penetrated the skin, and advanced deeper into the tissue until blood enters the syringe. After reaching the vertebral bodies and no blood has been obtained, the needle is withdrawn slightly; both ventrally and laterally, with continued negative pressure applied to the syringe. Once the vessels have been entered, blood will begin to enter the syringe. The needle may need to be rotated slightly to properly position the needle hub in the vessel to facilitate collection of the blood.

The lateral approach in teleosts begins with the fish in lateral recumbency and identification of the lateral line. The needle is inserted into the skin between the scales, if applicable, a few millimeters below the lateral line near the base of the caudal peduncle. As the needle penetrates through the skin, mild negative pressure can be applied to the syringe as the needle is advanced deeper into the tissue toward the midline and under the vertebral bodies until blood enters the syringe (Figure 22.2). If bone is detected with the needle, the needle should be repositioned ventrally (below the spine).

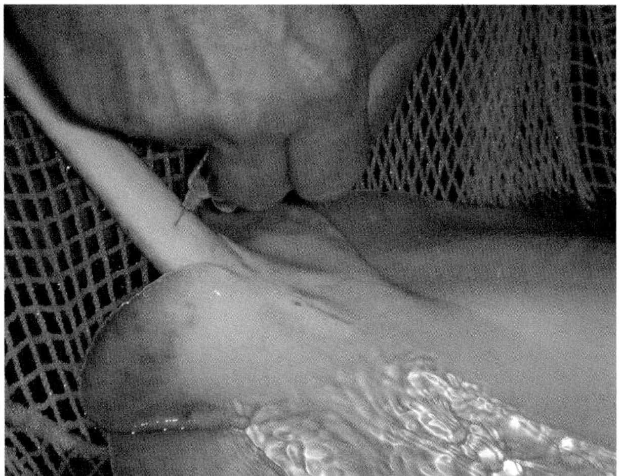

Figure 22.1 Venipuncture of the caudal vein using the ventral approach in an elasmobranch fish (*Dasyatis americana*) using the ventral approach.

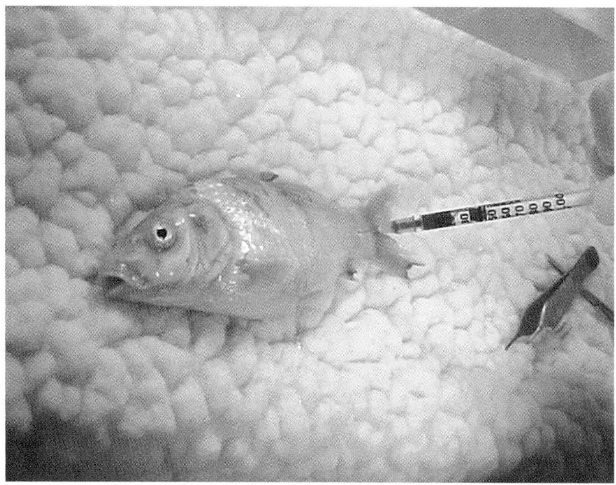

Figure 22.2 Venipuncture of the caudal vein using the lateral approach in a teleost fish (*Carassius auratus*) using the lateral approach.

Blood can be collected from the heart or bulbous arteriosus using a ventral approach. The needle is inserted slightly caudal to the apex of the V-shaped notch formed by the gill covers (opercula) and isthmus, and it is then advanced toward the heart while a slight vacuum is applied to the syringe. Blood will enter the syringe once the heart is penetrated. An anterolateral approach through an opened gill opercular cover also can be used to reach the heart. In this approach, the needle is directed caudally, from a point one-third of the distance between the ventral limit of the cavity (gill chamber) and medial to the bony support of the caudal wall of the opercular cavity. The needle is then advanced toward the heart using a slight vacuum. Cardiocentesis carries a greater risk of damage to the fish than use of the caudal vertebral vessels for blood collection.

Blood can be collected from large sharks using the dorsal venous sinus that courses caudal and slightly ventral to the dorsal fins. With the shark restrained in ventral recumbency or in a sling with its back exposed, a needle is inserted through the soft skin just under the caudal aspect of a dorsal fin (caudal flap) as it is lifted dorsally (Figure 22.3). The needle is then directed under the dorsal fin but is kept to the back and slightly off the midline. Use of a needle with an extension tube is often helpful for keeping the needle in position should the shark move during the procedure. Advantages of this method compared with venipuncture of the caudal vertebral vessels in large sharks include ease of access to the vessel and restraint of large sharks when using the dorsal fin approach.

Erythrocytes

Morphology

The transportation of oxygen is the primary function of fish erythrocytes, the extent of which depends on the

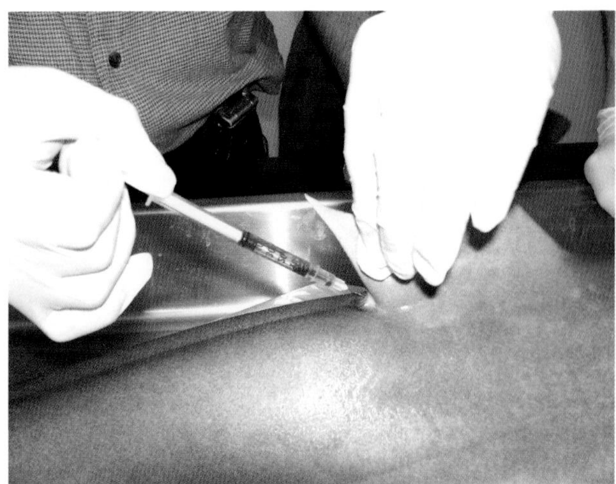

Figure 22.3 Blood collection from a shark (*Carcharhinus plumbeus*) using the blood vessel under the dorsal fin. Source: Image from Campbell TW. *Exotic Animal Hematology and Cytology*, 4th ed. Ames, IA: Wiley Blackwell, 2015, p. 185.

amount of hemoglobin concentration within the cell and the gas-exchange mechanism. Normal, mature erythrocytes of the majority of fish species are oval to ellipsoidal, have abundant pale eosinophilic cytoplasm, and include a centrally positioned, oval to ellipsoidal basophilic nucleus in Romanowsky-stained blood films (Figure 22.4). The long axis of the nucleus is parallel to that of the cell, except in a few species with round erythrocyte nuclei. The nuclei of fish erythrocytes can be large, occupying as much as one-fourth (or more) of the cell volume. The nuclear chromatin is densely clumped and stains dark purple. A few species of fish (e.g., certain species in the Gonostomidae family) have anucleated erythrocytes. The cytoplasm of fish erythrocytes when viewed on the stained blood film is typically homogeneous, but it may contain variable amounts of rarefied or pale-staining areas or vacuoles associated with the degeneration of organelles.

Both the size and number of erythrocytes vary between species of fish and, depending on the physiologic conditions, even within a single species. For example, the erythrocytes of fish belonging to the class Chondrichthyes (sharks and rays) generally are larger and more rounded than those of the class Osteichthyes (bony fish). Mature erythrocytes of some fish are biconvex, with a central swelling that corresponds to the position of the nucleus, whereas those of other species are flattened and biconcave.

Slight to moderate anisocytosis and polychromasia are normal in many species of fish. Polychromatic erythrocytes have a pale blue cytoplasm compared with that of mature erythrocytes (Figure 22.5). They also may appear to be more rounded and to have a less condensed nuclear chromatin.

Because erythropoiesis occurs in the peripheral blood of normal fish, immature erythrocytes may be found in blood films. An estimated 1% of the erythrocytes in peripheral blood are derived from circulatory erythropoiesis. Immature erythrocytes contribute to the degree of polychromasia and anisocytosis. As in the blood films of birds and reptiles, immature erythrocytes of fish have larger, less condensed nuclei and less cytoplasm than mature erythrocytes. Immature erythrocytes (i.e., rubriblasts, prorubricytes, and rubricytes) are round cells with centrally positioned, round nuclei. Depending on the stage of development, the cytoplasmic volume varies in both the amount and intensity of basophilic staining with Romanowsky stains. Erythroid cells in mitosis also may be present in the peripheral blood films from normal fish. Although erythropoiesis occurs in peripheral blood, the primary site of hematopoiesis in general is the

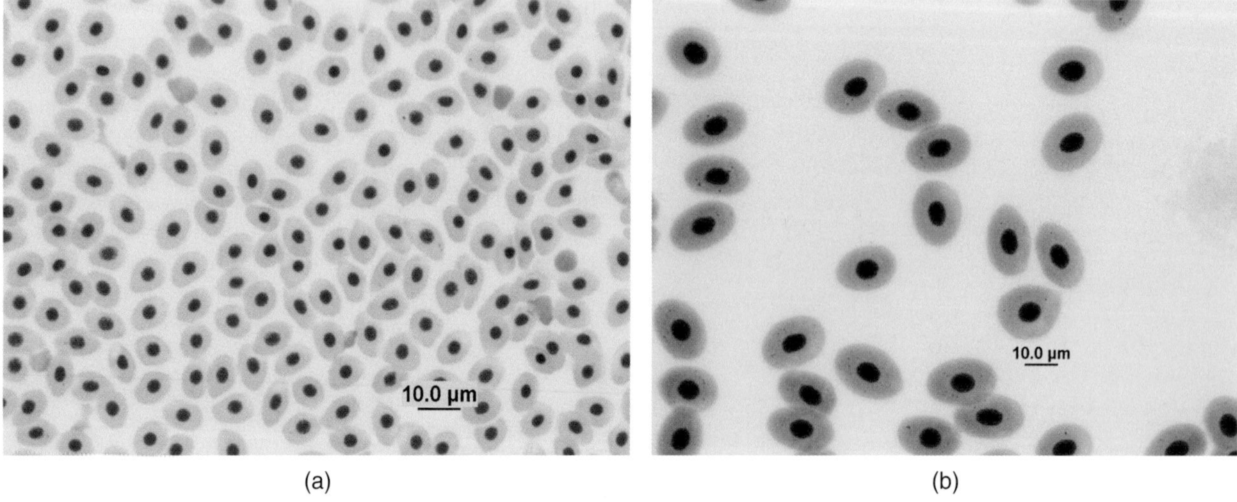

Figure 22.4 (a) Normal mature erythrocytes in the blood film of a bony fish (*Roncador stearnsii*). Wright-Giemsa stain. (b) Normal mature erythrocytes in the blood film of a cartilaginous fish (*Rhinoptera bonasus*). Wright-Giemsa stain.

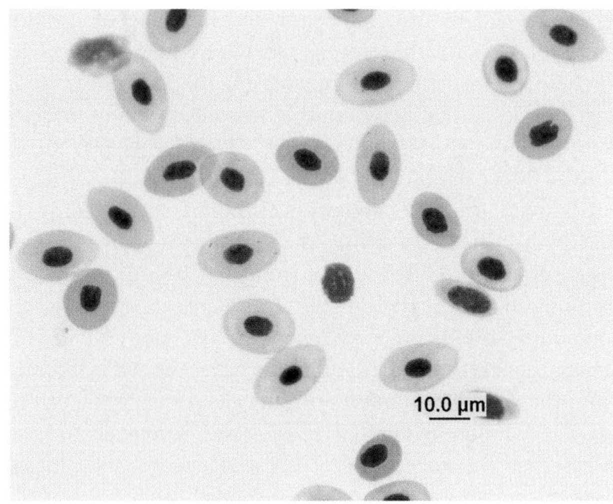

Figure 22.5 Increased polychromasia in the blood film of a bony fish (*Opsanus tau*). Wright-Giemsa stain.

kidney in teleosts and the Leydig organ, epigonal organ, thymus, and spleen in the elasmobranch.

Ultrastructurally, mature fish erythrocytes have a finely granular cytoplasm with no inclusions, whereas immature erythrocytes have a cytoplasm with mitochondria, Golgi complex, and small vacuoles.

Laboratory evaluation

Determination of packed cell volume (PCV) is the most commonly used method for evaluating the red cell mass of fish. The microhematocrit method is used for obtaining a PCV of fish blood. The normal range in bony fish is between 20 and 45%. The normal range in elasmobranchs may be similar; however, results vary based on venipuncture site. The PCV tends to be lower in samples collected from the venous sinus near the dorsal fin than from those collected from the caudal vein of the tail. Other factors that may contribute to PCV variation in healthy animals include stress (handling, anesthesia, water intake), physical characteristics (size, species), sex, environmental factors (water temperature, dissolved oxygen, population density, photoperiod), activity level (thermodynamics), reproductive status, life stage, and diet.

Although a variety of methods have been used to determine the hemoglobin concentration in fish blood, the cyanmethemoglobin method provides the most consistent results. As with avian and reptilian hemoglobin determinations, this procedure requires centrifugation of the blood–cyanmethemoglobin reagent mixture to remove the free erythrocyte nuclei before measurement of optical density. Most teleost hemoglobin concentrations range from 5 to 10 g/dL.

A total erythrocyte count (TRBC) in fish can be determined by a manual counting method using a hemocytometer or by an electronic cell counter. Three manual methods that can be used to obtain TRBCs in fish blood use the Erythro-pette™ system (Exotic Animal Solutions, Inc. Hueytown, AL, USA), Natt-Herricks solution (see Chapter 20 on avian hematology), or modified Dacie's solution (Table 22.1). The Erythro-pette™ method is the easiest of the three, because the 1 : 200 dilution of whole anticoagulated blood is made

Table 22.1 Erythrocyte parameters for selected teleost fish.

	PCV [%]	RBC [$\times 10^6/\mu L$]	Hb [g/dL]	MCV [fL]	MCHC [g/dL]
Bass, hybrid[a]	23–47	3.66–4.96	8–12	81–106	22–30
Channel catfish[b]	40	2.44	–	–	–
Flounder[c]	17–26	1.7–2.6	4.2–6.0	90–126	–
Goldfish[d]	38–40	1.6–1.8	9.7–10.6	241–245	26
Red pacu[e]	25	1.68	–	–	–
Tilapia[f]	27–37	1.91–2.83	7.0–9.8	115–183	22–29
Trout[g]	21–44	0.77–1.67	1.5–7.7	192–420	14.4–70.0

[a]Hrubec TC, Smith SA, Robertson JL, et al. Comparison of hematologic reference intervals between cultured system and type of hybrid striped bass. *Am J Vet Res* 57: 618–23. 1996.

[b]Grizzle JM, Rogers WA. *Anatomy and Histology of the Channel Catfish*. Opelika, AL: Craftmaster Printers, p. 18. 1976.

[c]Bridges DW, Cech JJ Jr., Pedro DN. Seasonal hematological changes in winter flounder *Pseudopleuronectes americanus*. *Trans Am Fish Soc* 105: 596–600. 1976.

[d]Burton CB, Murray SA. Effects of density on goldfish blood: I, hematology. *Comp Biochem Physiol* 62A: 555–8. 1979.

[e]Tocidlowski ME, Lewbart GA, Stoskopf MK. Hematologic study of the red pacu [*Colossoma brachypornum*]. *Vet Clin Pathol* 26: 119–25. 1997.

[f]Hrubec TC, Cardinale JL, Smith SA. Hematology and plasma chemistry reference intervals for cultured tilapia [*Oreochromis hybrid*]. *Vet Clin Pathol* 29: 7–12. 2000.

[g]Miller WR, Hendricks AC, Cairns J. Normal ranges for diagnostically important hematological and blood chemistry characteristics of rainbow trout [*Salmo gairdneri*]. *Can J Fish Aquat Sci* 40: 420–5. 1983.

using the diluent, pipette, and mixing vial provided with the kit. The Natt-Herricks method is also easy and practical as total leukocyte and thrombocyte counts can also be obtained on the same charged hemocytometer. The modified Dacie's staining methods require preparation of the diluent/stain solution and use of the red blood cell–diluting pipette. Blood is drawn to the 0.5 mark on the pipette, and either Natt-Herricks or modified Dacie's stain is drawn to the 101 mark to prepare the 1 : 200 dilution. Commercially prepared Natt-Herricks solution kit (Natt-Pette) makes the procedure easier and more accurate. The kit contains prefilled Natt-Herricks stain reservoirs, a pipette calibrated for 5 μL (to make the 1 : 200 dilution), and tips for the pipette. The diluted blood is then discharged onto the hemocytometer counting chamber and is allowed to settle for a minimum of 5 minutes before counting. With these stains, the oval erythrocytes show a small, dark blue nucleus that is surrounded by a colorless to faint pink cytoplasm. The total number of erythrocytes in the four corner and central squares in the central, large square of a Neubauer-ruled hemocytometer chamber is obtained using ×40 (high dry) magnification. The TRBC is calculated by multiplying the numbers of erythrocytes by 10,000.

The red blood cell indices (i.e., mean erythrocyte volume [MCV], mean corpuscular hemoglobin concentration [MCHC], and mean cell hemoglobin [MCH]) can be calculated using standard formulas. However, the direct, electronic measurement of MCV appears to be more sensitive for detecting changes in the erythrocyte size in fish and is more reproducible than the calculated MCV. Table 22.1 offers erythrocyte reference values for selected teleost fish. The intervals shown are merely an estimate, as many factors may contribute to slight variation. For example, active fish will have a higher demand for oxygen and, therefore, a smaller red cell concentration (RBC) count and a lower MCV. Elasmobranchs, in general, have larger and fewer erythrocytes that contain more hemoglobin in comparison with bony fish, which translates into increased MCV, MCHC, and MCH but decreased PCV, hemoglobin concentration, and total RBCs. Similar to PCV, other factors that may contribute to changes in these values are cell maturity (the more mature, the larger the cell, thereby increasing values), species, season, and diet.

Responses in disease

In general, a PCV less than 20% indicates anemia in fish. Anemia may be due to blood loss (hemorrhagic anemia), cell destruction (hemolytic anemia), or decreased production (hypoplastic anemia). Polycythemia is classified as hematocrit greater than 45% and may due to dehydration, sexually mature males, hypoxia, stress, splenic contraction, or erythrocyte swelling.

The standard practices for collecting, handling, and analyzing blood from mammals and birds can be misleading when applied to fish. Emersion and handling of fish for venipuncture or cardiocentesis can have a marked effect on the hemogram, significantly increasing the hematocrit by as much as 25%. The magnitude of this effect relates directly to the handling and analytic time. Handling of fish for as little as 20 seconds results in the release of catecholamines, which tend to cause hemoconcentration and swelling of the erythrocytes. Therefore, the hematocrit increases, but the hemoglobin concentration remains the same, thereby resulting in a decreased MCHC. The increase in blood catecholamines causes ion exchanges (Na^+/H^+ and Cl^-/HCO^-) across the erythrocyte membrane; thus, as Na^+ and Cl^- enter the cell, water follows osmotically, causing the cell to swell. Cannulation methods have been developed for use in research fish to minimize these effects; however, these methods are impractical for use in clinical studies.

In general, the PCV of fish is lower than that of mammals and birds. Hematocrits vary both between and within fish species, and they appear to correlate with the normal activity of the fish, with less active fish having lower hematocrits than active, fast-swimming fish. Hematocrits also vary during the life cycle of fish. For example, during prespawning conditions, Atlantic salmon (*Salmo salar*) have high hematocrits compared with those during spawning. Age, sex, water temperature, photoperiod, and seasonal variation also may influence the PCV of fish. In fact, the PCV in some species of male fish are large enough to require two reference intervals.

Cartilaginous fish (sharks and rays) and bony fish appear to have different gas transport systems, which affect their erythrocyte parameters. Bony fish exhibit a high cardiac workload and blood pressure, which are associated with a higher PCV and smaller erythrocytes. Sharks and rays, however, exhibit relatively modest cardiac work load, higher cardiac output, higher blood volumes, and increased flow rates, which are associated with lower concentrations of larger cells.

In general, fish with PCVs less than 20% are considered to be anemic and associated with blood loss (hemorrhagic anemia), cell destruction (hemolytic anemia), or decreased production (hypoplastic anemia). However, for some species, such as the Port Jackson shark (*Heterodontus portusjacksoni*), a normal PCVs may be as low as 20%.

Polycythemia is classified as hematocrit greater than 45% and may due to dehydration, sexually mature males, hypoxia, stress, splenic contraction, or erythrocyte swelling. A high PCV associated with dehydration is supported by increased serum osmolality or total protein.

Fish with regenerative anemia often have an increased concentration of polychromatic and immature erythrocytes in their blood films. Anemic fish that exhibit little or no polychromasia have nonresponsive anemia. A microcytic normochromic anemia has been associated with environmental stresses, such as increased population densities. A microcytic hypochromic anemia with marked poikilocytosis has been reported in trout (*Salmo gairdneri*) that were fed diets containing yeast, thereby resulting in oxidative damage to erythrocytes. Anemias associated with erythrocytes having pyknotic nuclei, erythroplastids (i.e., erythrocytes without nuclei), and red-blood-cell fragmentation have been associated with conditions that interfere with the splenic removal of senescent red blood cells from the peripheral circulation. Abnormal erythrocyte nuclei (i.e., amitosis, segmentation, and fragmentation) as well as formation of erythroplastids may relate to nutritional disorders, such as deficiency of folic acid or vitamin E and toxicosis from rancid oils and environmental pollutants.

Because the immature erythrocytes of fish are smaller than the mature erythrocytes, microcytosis often is associated with marked hemorrhagic or hemolytic anemias, in which the regenerating, immature erythrocytes represent the majority of the peripheral blood erythrocytes. Hemorrhagic anemias of fish are associated with trauma, bloodsucking parasites, vitamin K deficiency, and septicemia (bacteria or viral). For example, enteric red mouth disease (yersiniosis) of fish produces a hemorrhagic septicemia and a hemogram that is characterized by leukocytosis, low PCV, and reticulocytosis. Hemolytic anemias of fish may be associated with toxins (bacterial or environmental), viral infections (erythrocytic necrosis virus), certain nutritional deficiencies, and hemoparasites. Cadmium is a calcium channel blocker that impedes normal membrane function in erythrocytes resulting in hemolytic anemia in freshwater teleost fish exposed to toxic levels of cadmium in the water. Nitrite poisoning (brown blood disease or new tank syndrome) of fish also results in severe hemolytic anemia. Nitrite is readily absorbed from the gills and enters into the blood, where it then oxidizes hemoglobin to methemoglobin, which in turn gradually changes the blood from red to brown in color. A hemolytic anemia results as splenic macrophages remove the affected erythrocytes from the circulation.

Several nutritional deficiencies have been produced experimentally in fish. For example, folic acid deficiencies result in normochromic macrocytic anemias, and vitamin B_{12} deficiencies result in hypochromic anemias. Folate deficiency has been suggested as being a cause of the chronic hemolytic anemia that occurs in channel catfish (*Ictalurus punctatus*).

Leukocytes

Fish have granulocytic and agranulocytic leukocytes, with the latter represented by lymphocytes and monocytes. Leukocytes (especially the granulocytes) exhibit a wide variation in appearance among fish species. This has led to controversy and confusion when applying the nomenclature and classification of piscine leukocytes on the basis of such descriptions from avian and mammalian Romanowsky-stained blood films. Some fish granulocytes have an appearance similar to that of the avian heterophil, while others to the mammalian neutrophil, hence the adoption of those terms in some cases. Evaluation of the cellular ultrastructure, differential cytochemical staining, immunofluorescence, and function testing of fish leukocytes, however, has helped to alleviate some of this controversy in some species.

Leukocytes of commonly studied bony fish

Channel catfish (*Ictalurus punctatus*)

One study identified these fish as having neutrophils, basophils, lymphocytes, and monocytes using both electron microscopy and cytochemical staining while another declared heterophils as the primary granulocyte, using electron microscopy only. Ultrastructural and cytochemical studies have identified heterophils, basophils, lymphocytes, and monocytes in the peripheral blood of channel catfish. These results support the general classification of these cells in Romanowsky-stained blood films of this species.

Goldfish (*Carassius auratus*) and koi (*Carassius carpio*)

On the basis of electron microscopy, leukocytes found in the peripheral blood of goldfish can be classified as lymphocytes, monocytes, heterophils, eosinophils, and rarely, basophils. On the basis of cytochemical reaction, goldfish leukocytes can be classified as lymphocytes, heterophils, monocytes, and an atypical, segmented granulocyte. Electron microscopy and cytochemical staining indicate that koi, *Cyprinus carpio*, possess neutrophils, eosinophils, basophils, lymphocytes, and monocytes. It has been suggested that cell identification might be more effectively accomplished by using more than one evaluation method.

Red pacu (*Colossoma brachypomum*)

Six types of cells are classified as leukocytes in blood films from red pacu (*Colossoma brachypomum*). The four common types are classified as heterophils, eosinophils, lymphocytes, and monocytes. Nonstaining granulocytes are reported to occur in a frequency similar to that of eosinophils and are considered to be heterophils that failed to stain properly. The sixth cell type is referred to as a "granular-lymphocytoid cell" because it resembles a medium-sized lymphocyte containing one or more dull, fusiform eosinophilic granules. This cell type represents a significant population of the blood leukocytes of red pacu.

Salmonids (trout and salmon, *Salmo* spp.)

On the basis of cytochemical staining, salmonids appear to have three types of leukocytes: lymphocytes, neutrophils, and monocytes.

Striped bass (*Morone saxatulis*)

Striped bass leukocytes are classified as lymphocytes, neutrophils, and monocytes.

Tilapia (*Oreochromis spp.*)

The leukocytes of tilapia (*Oreochromis spp.*) are classified as neutrophils, eosinophils, lymphocytes, and monocytes.

White sturgeon (*Acipenser transmontanus*)

Four types of leukocytes – lymphocytes, monocytes, neutrophils, and eosinophils – have been described in white sturgeon.

Summary

Cytochemical studies of piscine leukocytes appear to support the use of mammalian leukocyte terminology as a classification scheme because they are considered to be analogous to mammalian leukocytes based upon cytochemical and ultrastructural studies. In general, neutrophils or heterophils, lymphocytes, and monocytes commonly are reported in the peripheral blood films of fish belonging to the class Osteichthyes (teleost or bony fish). Myeloperoxidase stain is used to differentiate neutrophils from true heterophils, because neutrophils stain positive and heterophils stain negative. In general, fish heterophils are neutrophils, based on myeloperoxidase staining, but are called heterophils because of the presence of prominent eosinophilic cytoplasmic granules with Romanowsky stains. Eosinophils and basophils are rare in the peripheral blood of bony fish.

Leukocytes of sharks and rays

The peripheral blood of fish belonging to the class Chondrichthyes (cartilaginous fish, such as sharks and rays) contain leukocytes that can be classified as granulocytes, lymphocytes, or monocytes. The granulocytes exhibit marked variation in both numbers and types between species, and the granulocyte classification scheme is based on the results of ultrastructural and cytochemical studies performed in blood samples from the lesser spotted dogfish (*Scliorrhinus canicula*), which has been used as a model for cartilaginous fish. The granulocytes are classified as either G_1 (type I), G_2 (type II), or G_3 (type III). To simplify the identification of these cells using familiar terminology, the G_1 granulocytes resemble the avian or reptilian heterophil, the G_2 granulocyte resembles the mammalian neutrophil, and the G_3 granulocyte resembles the eosinophil based upon the cell's appearance on Romanowsky-stained blood films. Basophils also can be found in the peripheral blood of cartilaginous fish.

Morphology

Neutrophils of bony fish

The neutrophils of bony fish tend to be round to slightly oval cells with eccentric nuclei (Figure 22.6). The nucleus of mature neutrophils vary in shape, being round, oval, indented (metamyelocyte type), elongated (band cell type), or segmented, and usually with two to three lobes. Nonsegmented nuclei are the most common in the granulocytes of bony fish. The nuclear chromatin is coarsely clumped, and it stains deeply basophilic in Romanowsky-stained blood films. The neutrophils of bony fish have abundant colorless, grayish, or slightly acidophilic-staining (light pink) cytoplasm; small cytoplasmic granules and vacuoles also may be present. The staining of the granules varies, however, and depends on the species or the maturity of the cell. The small, cytoplasmic granules of the neutrophils vary from gray to pale blue or red. Interspecies differences in the cytochemical reactions of bony fish neutrophils are observed; however, in general, they resemble the neutrophils of mammals.

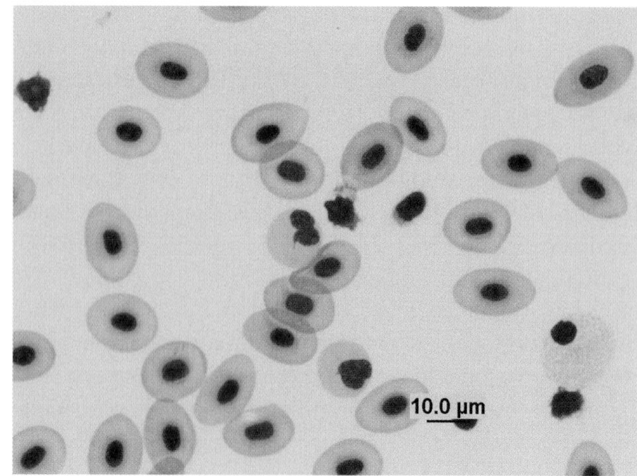

Figure 22.6 Neutrophils in the blood film of a bony fish (*Opsanus tau*). Wright-Giemsa stain.

Piscine neutrophils that exhibit distinct, rod-shaped cytoplasmic granules on Romanowsky stains often are classified in the literature as heterophils. Some species, such as goldfish and carp (*C. carpio*), have granulocytes with distinct and slightly acidophilic cytoplasmic granules, colorless cytoplasm, and eccentric, partially lobed nuclei on Romanowsky stains. These cells often are classified as heterophils rather than neutrophils, although they do have cytochemical properties similar to those of neutrophils in other fish. They measure approximately 9–10 in. diameter (some as large as 20 µm). These heterophils are peroxidase and Sudan black B positive when the granules are immature, but they are peroxidase negative in mature granules. Neutrophils from channel catfish and certain species of eel also contain prominent eosinophilic, rod-shaped cytoplasmic granules resembling those of avian heterophils on the basis of Romanowsky stains. The granules of these cells are strongly peroxidase positive. Similar cells have been found in a number of other bony fish as well. In salmonids, such as rainbow trout (*Onchorhynchus mykiss*) and coho salmon (*Onchorhynchus kisutch*), these neutrophils are the predominant granulocyte, as in most bony fish. Piscine neutrophils often reveal artifacts of blood film preparation, causing the cells to appear large and with swollen, pale nuclear chromatin (karyolysis).

Eosinophils of bony fish

Eosinophils rarely are reported in the blood films from bony fish, and some investigators doubt whether they exist at all in some species. When present, however, they appear as intermediate to large granulocytes, with distinct eosinophilic granules and pale blue cytoplasm. The nucleus varies from round (more common) to segmented. They can be distinguished from heterophils on the basis of cytochemistry and ultrastructural findings, although the absence of crystalloids (used as a fingerprint for mammalian eosinophils) often is the rule with piscine eosinophils. Eosinophils have been reported in goldfish, white sturgeon, and channel catfish. Piscine eosinophils tend to be round, with round to rod-shaped eosinophilic-stained cytoplasmic granules with Romanowsky stain (Figures 22.7 and 22.11b). The granules of piscine eosinophils often are less distinct compared with those of birds and mammals. These granules also have a tinctorial quality that differs from those of heterophils with distinct eosinophilic granules.

Fish eosinophils generally measure 9–14 μm in diameter, for example eosinophils of carp are approximately 7.5 in. diameter and have an eccentric nucleus that is indented, sausage-shaped, or bilobate as well as eosinophilic, cytoplasmic granules that are larger than those of the heterophils (neutrophils).

Basophils of bony fish

Basophils are rare in the peripheral blood of bony fish and have been reported only in a few species. Basophils are identified as round cells that have round, basophilic cytoplasmic granules that often obscure the cell nucleus. The nucleus is large, eccentric, and round. The nuclear chromatin is homogeneous. The basophils of carp measure between 10 and 20 μm. When present, basophils occur in low numbers.

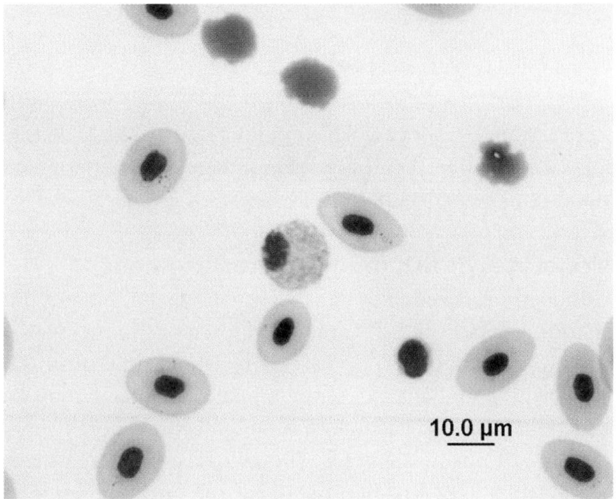

Figure 22.7 An eosinophil in the blood film of a bony fish (*Opsanus tau*). Wright-Giemsa stain.

Granulocytes of elasmobranchs (sharks and rays)

The elasmobranchs (or cartilaginous fish) appear to have the same types of leukocytes as described for other vertebrates; however, there is often disagreement associated with terms used for their granulocytes. The granulocytic leukocytes of elasmobranchs have been determined to be G_1 (also referred to as type I, heterophil, and fine eosinophilic granulocyte or FEG), G_2 (also referred to as type II and neutrophil), and G_3 (also referred to as type III, eosinophil, and coarse eosinophilic granulocyte or CEG). These cells tend to be similar in size. Some species of elasmobranchs may contain G_1, G_2, and G_3 granulocytes in their blood film. The G_1 granulocytes are typically round cells with an eccentric, irregular, nonlobed nucleus; colorless cytoplasm; and fine round to oval, eosinophilic cytoplasmic granules (Figures 22.8–22.10, 22.11a, and 22.16). The nucleus may be lobed in some species. These cells resemble avian heterophils, and they often are the most common form of the granulocytes. The G_2 granulocytes are typically round cells with a lobed nucleus and a colorless cytoplasm that lacks distinct granules (Figure 22.9). The granules and margin of the cell are often difficult to view and can be easily overlooked. These cells resemble mammalian neutrophils. The G_3 granulocytes are round cells characterized by a round to lobed nucleus (in some species), pale blue cytoplasm, and strongly eosinophilic, round to rod-shaped cytoplasmic granules (Figures 22.10 and 22.14). The cytoplasmic granules in the G_3 granulocytes have tinctorial qualities that differ from those of the G_1 granulocytes in the same blood film. The G_3 granulocytes of cartilaginous fish resemble avian eosinophils.

The granulocytes of sharks and rays tend to stain negatively for peroxidase, β-glucuronidase, and Sudan black B but positive for acid phosphatase, arylsulfatase, and acid naphthyl AS-D chloroacetate esterase. The eosinophilic granulocytes (G_1 and G_3) of the elasmobranchs share few morphologic and cytochemical characteristics with mammalian eosinophils. The function and interrelationships of the granulocytes in cartilaginous fish are not known; however, they appear to be separate cell types rather than intermediate stages of one cell type. Not all species of cartilaginous fish exhibit all of the granulocytes described for the lesser spotted dogfish (*S. canicula*). For example, only G_1 and G_3 granulocytes have been found in the rays *Raja clavata* and *Raja microcellata*. Basophils occasionally are found in peripheral blood films of some species of cartilaginous fish.

Basophils may occasionally be found in the peripheral blood of elasmobranchs, appearing as round cells with dark purple–stained granules. The amount of granules varies from sparse to obliterating the nucleus.

Lymphocytes of fish (bony and cartilaginous)

Lymphocytes frequently are the most abundant leukocyte in peripheral blood films of fish, and they resemble

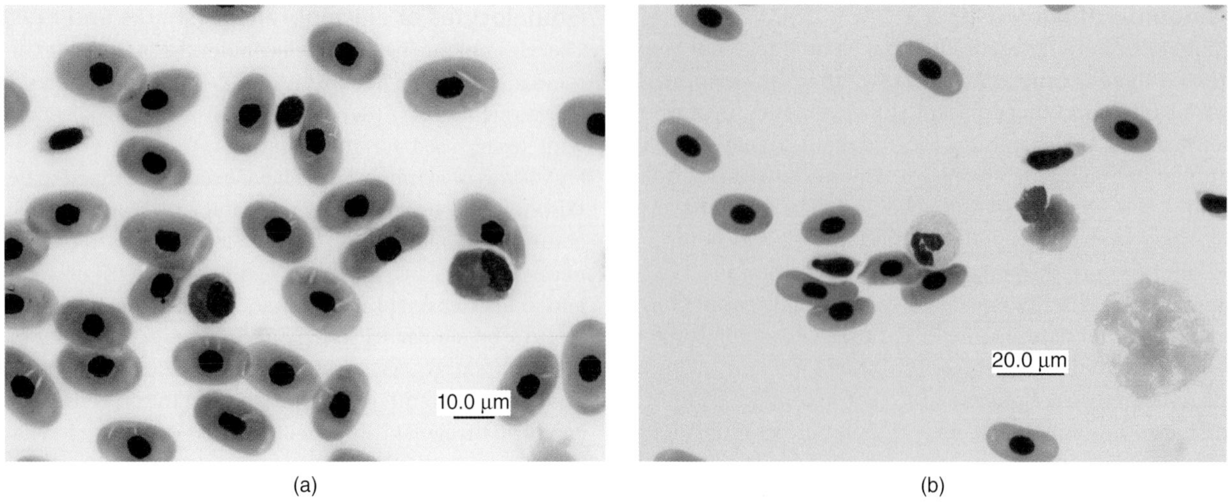

Figure 22.8 (a) G_1 granulocytes (heterophils) in the blood film of a cartilaginous fish (*Ginglymostoma cirratum*). Wright-Giemsa stain. (b) A G_1 granulocyte (heterophil) in the blood film of a cartilaginous fish (*Chiloscyllium plagiosum*). Wright-Giemsa stain.

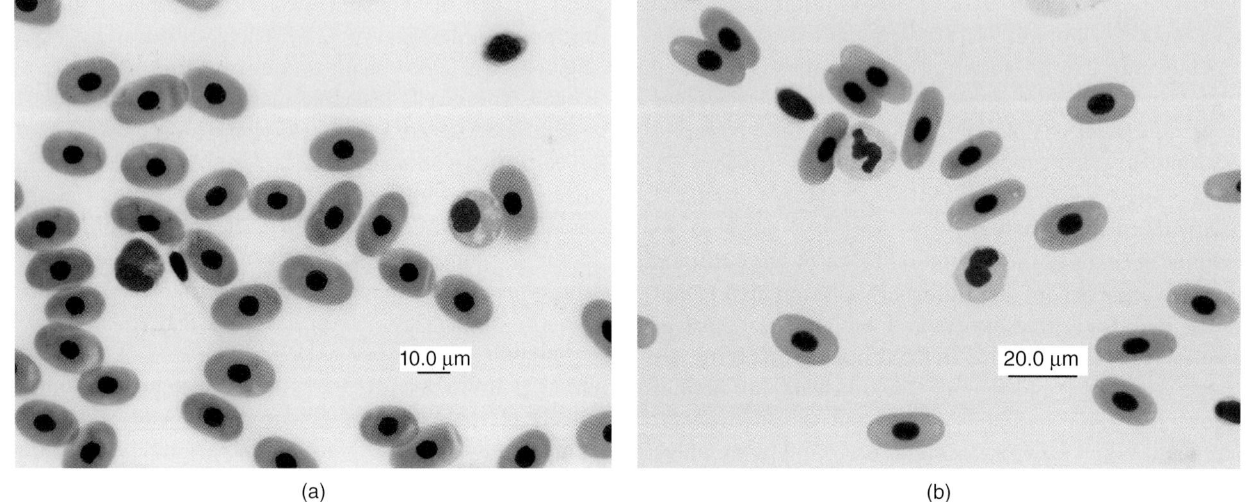

Figure 22.9 (a) A G_2 granulocyte or neutrophil (granulocyte on the right) and a G_1 granulocyte (heterophil) in the blood film of a cartilaginous fish (*Ginglymostoma cirratum)*. Wright-Giemsa stain. (b) A G_2 granulocyte or neutrophil (granulocyte near the center) and a G_1 granulocyte or heterophil (granulocyte nearest the top) in the blood film of a cartilaginous fish (*Chiloscyllium plagiosum*). Wright-Giemsa stain.

their counterparts in avian and mammalian blood films (Figures 22.11). Lymphocytes are often described by size – small, medium, and large. The small lymphocytes are considered to be more mature. Combinations of different sizes may appear in one sample. Fish lymphocytes typically measure between 5 and 10 μm in diameter. Lymphocytes tend to be round, but they may mold around adjacent cells in the blood film. They have a high nucleus:cytoplasm (N:C) ratio, with coarsely clumped, deeply basophilic nuclear chromatin. The scant cytoplasm of small mature lymphocytes stains a homogenous pale blue. An occasional lymphocyte possesses azurophilic cytoplasmic granules. Reactive lymphocytes in blood films from fish resemble those of birds and mammals, with abundant, deeply basophilic cytoplasm and an occasional, distinct Golgi complex (Figure 22.12). Plasma cells also may be seen in small numbers on the peripheral blood films of many species of fish.

Monocytes of fish (bony and cartilaginous)

Monocytes occasionally are reported in the blood films of most species of fish, and they resemble monocytes of birds and mammals. They are large, mononuclear leukocytes, with abundant blue-gray to blue agranular cytoplasm, which may contain vacuoles. Fish monocytes generally measure 10–20 μm in diameter. The cytoplasmic margins may be indistinct or ragged because of the presence of pseudopodia. The nucleus varies in shape (round to kidney-shaped to bilobate) and generally occupies less than 50% of the

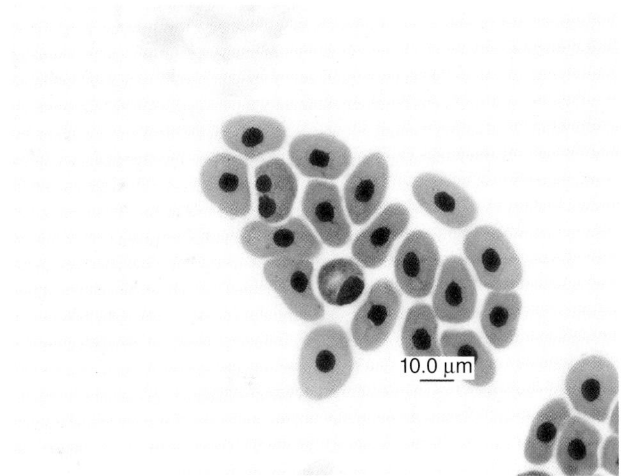

Figure 22.10 A G_3 granulocyte or eosinophil (granulocyte nearest the top) and a G_1 granulocyte or heterophil (granulocyte near the middle) in the blood film of a cartilaginous fish (*Ginglymostoma cirratum*). Wright-Giemsa stain.

cytoplasmic volume. The nuclear chromatin of monocytes generally is more granular and less clumped compared with that of lymphocyte nuclei. Results of ultrastructural studies indicate that monocytes in all species of fish are similar to those in other vertebrates. The term monocyte/macrophage frequently is used to classify piscine monocytes, because cells resembling transformational forms between monocytes and macrophages often are found in peripheral blood films (Figure 22.13). The term monocyte, however, is reserved for those found in peripheral blood, and the term macrophage is reserved for those found elsewhere. Fish monocytes can be differentiated from immature granulocytes and lymphocytes by the positive, nonspecific esterase reaction in monocytes.

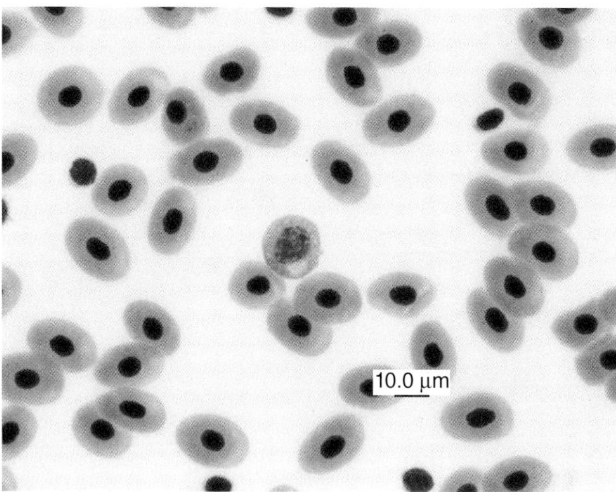

Figure 22.12 A reactive lymphocyte in the blood of a cartilaginous fish (*Rhinoptera bonasus*). Wright-Giemsa stain.

Laboratory evaluation

The same problems associated with obtaining total leukocyte counts in birds and reptiles also apply in fish. Because fish have nucleated erythrocytes and thrombocytes, manual counting methods are used. Direct leukocyte counting methods using a Neubauer-ruled hemocytometer and a variety of staining and diluting solutions have been used. Natt and Herricks method commonly is used, and the procedure is the same as that described for obtaining total leukocyte counts in avian and reptilian blood (see Chapters 20, on avian hematology, and 21, on reptilian hematology). The leukocytes appear blue and stain darker than erythrocytes stained with Natt-Herricks. It may be difficult to distinguish small, mature lymphocytes from thrombocytes if the counts are made using a ×10 objective; cells are more accurately

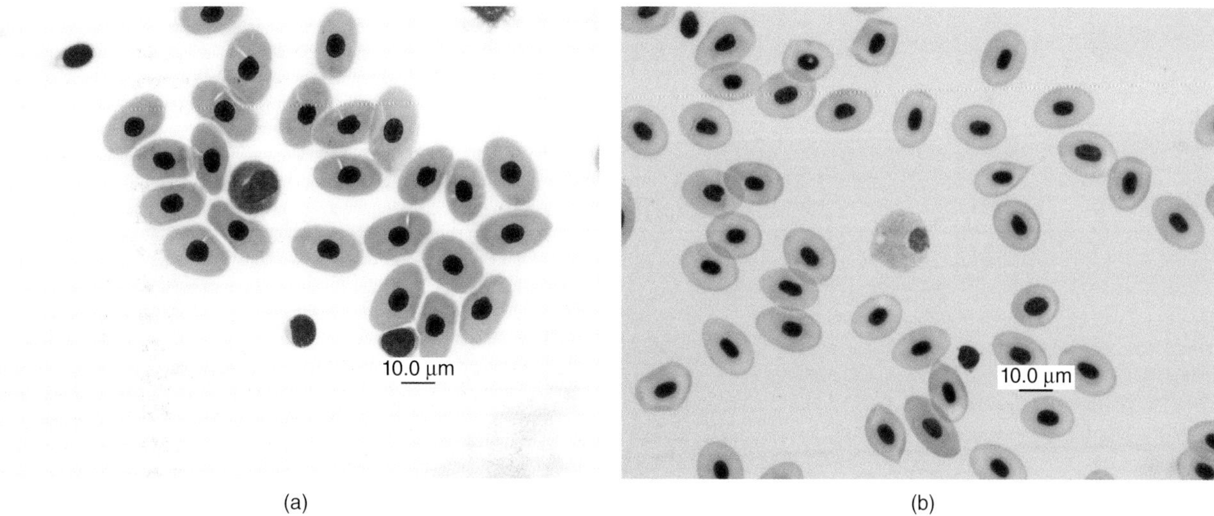

Figure 22.11 (a) A G_1 granulocyte (heterophil) and two lymphocytes in the blood of a cartilaginous fish (*Ginglymostoma cirratum*). Wright-Giemsa stain. (b) An eosinophil and small lymphocyte in the blood of a bony fish (*Opsanus tau*). Wright-Giemsa stain.

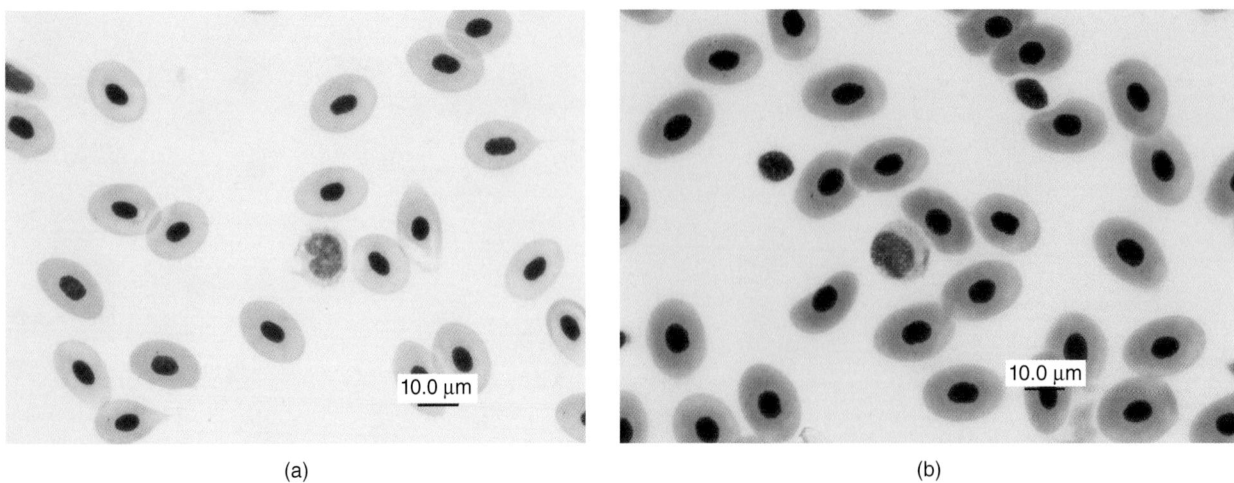

Figure 22.13 (a) A monocyte in the blood of a bony fish (*Opsanus tau*). Wright-Giemsa stain. (b) A monocyte in the blood of a cartilaginous fish (*Rhinoptera bonasus*). Wright-Giemsa stain.

identified at higher magnifications. Staining for 60 minutes in Natt-Herricks solution also may improve the differentiation between small lymphocytes and thrombocytes. Alternatively, thrombocytes can be included in the hemocytometer count and the differential count from the blood film. The total thrombocyte count can then be subtracted from the total cell count to obtain the WBC. Advantages of the Natt and Herricks procedure include the ability to obtain a total erythrocyte, leukocyte, and thrombocyte count using the same charged hemocytometer. In addition, the technique can be applied to blood samples obtained from all lower vertebrates.

A leukocyte differential is obtained from a Romanowsky-stained blood film. Applying a drop of albumin to the slide during preparation of the blood film often is advantageous to minimize smudging of the cells. Quickly drying the blood film using a hair dryer also may help to alleviate cellular artifacts associated with blood film preparation.

Table 22.2 offers leukocyte reference values for selected teleost fish.

Table 22.2 Leukocyte parameters for selected teleost fish.

	WBC × $10^3/\mu L$	Neut/Heterophils × $10^3/\mu L$	Lymphocytes × $10^3/\mu L$	Monocytes × $10^3/\mu L$	Eosinophils × $10^3/\mu L$	Basophils × $10^3/\mu L$
Bass, hybrid[a]	32.6–115.1	0.4–3.5	22.5–115.1	1.5–7.5	0–0.4	0
Channel catfish[b]	8.9–124.0	4.5–86.8	1.4–23.6	0.7–14.7	0	0–7.1
Flounder[c]	88.0–282.0	2.5–26.6	38.7–154.5	–	–	–
Goldfish[d]	10.1–14.7	–	9.5–13.7	–	–	–
Red pacu[e]	33.5	3.2	21.0	1.2	0.2	0
Tilapia[f]	21.6–154.7	0.6–9.9	6.8–136.4	0.4–4.3	0–1.6	0
Trout[g]	21.0	1.6	18.8	0.6	0	0

[a]Hrubec TC, Smith SA, Robertson JL, et al. Comparison of hematologic reference intervals between cultured system and type of hybrid striped bass. *Am J Vet Res* 57: 618–23. 1996.
[b]Tavares-Dias M, de Moraes FR. Leukocyte and thrombocyte reference values for channel catfish [*Ictalurus punctatus* Raf], with an assessment of morphologic, cytochemical, and ultrastructural features. *Vet Clin Pathol* 36: 49–54. 2007.
[c]Bridges DW, Cech JJ Jr., Pedro DN. Seasonal hematological changes in winter flounder *Pseudopleuronectes americanus*. *Trans Am Fish Soc* 105: 596–600. 1976.
[d]Murray SA, Burton CB. Effects of density on goldfish blood: II, cell morphology. *Comp Biochem Physiol* 62A: 559–62. 1979.
[e]Iocidlowski ME, Lewbart GA, Stoskopf MK. Hematologic study of the red pacu [*Colossoma brachypornum*]. *Vet Clin Pathol* 26: 119–25. 1997.
[f]Hrubec TC, Cardinale JL, Smith SA. Hematology and plasma chemistry reference intervals for cultured tilapia [*Oreochromis hybrid*]. *Vet Clin Pathol* 29: 7–12. 2000.
[g]Hunn JB, Wiedmeyer RH, Greer IE, Grady AW. Blood chemistry of laboratory-reared golden trout. *J Aquat Anim Health* 4: 218–21. 1992.

Responses in disease

The leukocyte response of fish is affected by stress, inflammatory and infectious diseases, and nutritional disorders as well as other intrinsic and extrinsic factors. Total leukocyte counts vary with species, physiologic age, sex, season, and methods of rearing and nutrition. Normal physiological factors and various other stressors such as environmental factors and handling can cause leukocyte concentrations to range into or slightly above the upper limits of normal. Normal physiological factors include age, population densities, water quality, and other factors. For example, age-related changes in the total leukocyte and lymphocyte counts of fish are similar to those described in mammals. Juvenile fish have notably higher total leukocyte counts and lymphocyte concentrations compared to adults. High Total leukocyte counts and lymphocyte concentrations are also associated with fish kept in high-density production systems where there is constant exposure to high concentrations of bacteria in the water and poor water quality parameters.

Stress factors can cause a response similar to that of higher vertebrates in which a rapid increase in the release of catecholamines occurs followed by the release of corticosteroids. In general, the effect of stress on the leukogram of fish is manifested as a leukopenia with a lymphopenia and a relative granulocytosis (heterophilia or neutrophilia) because lymphocytes are the predominate leukocyte in the peripheral blood of most fish. Hematologic changes associated with stress may persist for several days after the removal of the stressor.

Interpretation of changes in granulocyte concentrations in the peripheral blood of fish can be, at times, challenging. Piscine neutrophils and heterophils participate in inflammatory responses; however, it would be inappropriate to view them as homologous to the granulocytes of higher vertebrates because the exact function of fish granulocytes is not known. Fish granulocytes are not always phagocytic, and little is known about their methods of intracellular killing, digestion of phagocytized organisms, and other functions. Until further studies are performed that determine the function and responses of piscine granulocytes to disease, only broad generalizations about changes in the leukocyte counts of fish can be made.

In general, increases in the concentration of fish neutrophils or heterophils are often associated with inflammatory diseases, especially those associated with infectious agents. They are known to phagocytize bacteria and yeast and their methods of intracellular killing and digestion of phagocytized organisms appear to be similar to mammals in some species. Fish neutrophils migrate to inflammatory sites to kill bacteria by producing a series of reactive oxygen species where the respiratory burst and the peroxidase contained in the neutrophils contribute to microbial killing activity during phagocytosis. A granulocytosis (neutrophilia) can also occur with inflammation associated with

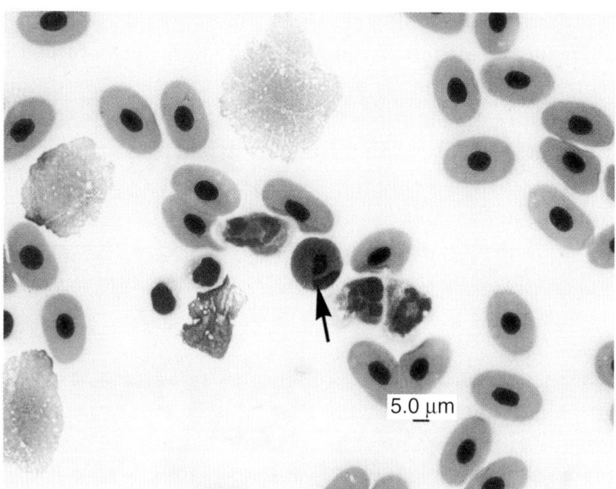

Figure 22.14 Toxic G_1 granulocytes (heterophils), a G_3 granulocyte or eosinophil (arrow), and two thrombocytes in the blood film of an elasmobranch fish (*Dasyatis americana*). Wright-Giemsa stain.

parasitic and viral diseases. A relative neutrophilia or heterophilia often is associated with lymphopenias, which can be interpreted as a stress response in fish.

In response to severe systemic illness, piscine neutrophils and heterophils exhibit toxic changes similar to those in mammalian neutrophils and avian and reptilian heterophils. Toxic neutrophils and heterophils of fish have increased cytoplasmic basophilia, vacuolization, abnormal granulation (degranulation of heterophils, granules that appear deeply basophilic, and heterophils granules that appear to coalesce into large, round granules), and degeneration of the cell nucleus (Figure 22.14). Toxic neutrophils and heterophils in fish are associated with severe, systemic illness such as septicemia, mycotic infections, and severe tissue necrosis. The degree of toxicity usually indicates the severity of the fish's condition, and a marked number of neutrophils or heterophils exhibiting marked (4+) toxicity indicates a grave prognosis.

Eosinophils are found in low concentrations (0–3% of the leukocyte differential) in the peripheral blood of normal fish. Piscine eosinophils participate in inflammatory responses along with neutrophils (heterophils) and macrophages, and they appear to have a limited phagocytic capability. Piscine eosinophils apparently are involved in the control of infections with metazoan parasites, and they participate in the immune responses to antigenic stimulation. Therefore, an increased eosinophil concentration in the peripheral blood of fish suggests an inflammatory response associated with parasitic infections or antigenic stimulation.

The granulocytes of cartilaginous fish do appear to participate in inflammatory responses. It is important to note that because the granulocytes make up 20%–30% of the total leukocyte population in sharks and rays, the normal granulocyte to lymphocyte (G:L) ratio is typically low (i.e., less than 0.5). An increase in granulocyte concentration is indicative of an inflammatory response. A decrease in the lymphocyte concentration typically results from conditions that reduce the number of circulating lymphocytes, such as stress responses, for example. In sharks, increases in granulocyte concentrations and decreases in lymphocyte concentrations can be associated with bacterial septicemias. The presence of toxicity in the granulocytes as indicated by increased cytoplasmic basophilia and vacuolation is indicative of a severe inflammatory leukogram regardless of the cell count.

The functions of the granulocytes of cartilaginous fish are not known; however, they appear to participate in inflammatory responses. Because the granulocytes account for 20–30% of the leukocytes in sharks and rays, the normal granulocyte: lymphocyte ratio typically is low (<0.5). An increase in the granulocyte concentration is indicative of an inflammatory response. A decrease in the lymphocyte concentration results from conditions that reduce the number of circulating lymphocytes, such as stress responses. Both increases in the granulocyte concentrations and decreases in the lymphocyte concentrations of sharks can be associated with bacterial septicemias. The presence of toxicity in the granulocytes as indicated by increased cytoplasmic basophilia and vacuolation is indicative of a severe inflammatory leukogram regardless of the cell count. The leukogram of cartilaginous fish can be used to follow the progress of these fish during the course of the disease or in response to therapy. For example, an initial increase in the granulocyte concentration or decrease in the lymphocyte concentration that has returned to normal indicates a favorable response to therapy and prognosis.

In one study, male White-spotted bamboo sharks (*Chiloscyllium plagiosum*) with traumatic clasper wounds developed a marked anemia, leukocytosis, and heterophilia (increase in G_1 granulocytes). Surgical removal of the affected claspers as a treatment option resulted in a return of the abnormal hemogram results to normal values indicating that the hematologic differences present in males with clasper wounds were capable of mounting a significant inflammatory hemic response.

Monocytes occur in low numbers (i.e., less than 5%) in the leukocyte differential of normal bony and cartilaginous fish. Piscine monocytes are actively phagocytic cells, and they participate in acute inflammatory responses in fish. Morphologic, cytochemical, and functional studies indicate that teleost monocytes resemble those of mammals. Monocytes and macrophages appear to be the primary phagocytic cells of fish. Fish monocytes can also phagocytize melanosomes when released, suggesting a relationship to melanomacrophages. A monocytosis is suggestive of an inflammatory response in fish, perhaps associated with an infectious agent, although monocyte numbers will also increase following injections of foreign material.

Lymphocytes are the most commonly observed leukocytes in the peripheral blood of most normal fish, in which they typically represent greater than 60% (and as much as 85% in some species) of the leukocyte differential. Lymphocytes play a major role in the humoral and cell-mediated immunity of fish. Monocyte or lymphocyte have been shown to have cytotoxic reactions similar to those described as mediated by mammalian cytotoxic cells. B lymphocytes in teleost fish function in the same manner as mammalian B-1 cells and produce immunoglobulin M (IgM). Therefore, lymphocytosis is suggestive of immunogenic stimulation, whereas lymphopenia is suggestive of immunosuppressive conditions, such as stress or excess exogenous glucocorticosteroids. Interestingly, B lymphocytes from teleost fish also demonstrate phagocytic and microbicidal activity. Bacterial septicemias commonly affect fish and result in marked leukopenias and lymphopenias. Environmental conditions, such as prolonged photoperiod and elevated water temperature that cause a stress response in fish will also result in a leukopenia associated with a lymphopenia.

Thrombocytes and hemostasis

The blood of fish clots in response to injury, as it does in other vertebrates. The speed and effectiveness in fish, however, are variable. Clotting is much more rapid in bony fish compared with sharks and rays. Sharks and rays appear to rely primarily on the extrinsic pathways of coagulation; the addition of skin, high calcium solutions, sea water, or other extrinsic factors enhances clotting. Clot formation in bony fish usually occurs within 5 minutes, whereas clotting in samples taken from sharks and rays can take 20 minutes or longer.

Morphology

Fish thrombocytes are smaller than erythrocytes, vary in shape, and can be round, elongate, or spindle-shaped. In addition, the shape may vary with the stage of maturity or the degree of reactivity. The oval and elongated forms tend to be nonreactive, mature thrombocytes (Figure 22.15) (Thrombocytes can also be found in Figures 22.5, 22.8, 22.9, 22.11a, and 22.13). Immature thrombocytes are round in some species, whereas spindle-shaped thrombocytes appear to be reactive forms and often are found in clumps. The cytoplasm of the piscine thrombocyte is colorless to faint blue; the nucleus is condensed and follows the shape of the cell. Fish thrombocytes also may contain a variable amount of eosinophilic cytoplasmic granules (Figure 22.16).

Like those in birds and reptiles, thrombocytes in fish often are confused with small, mature lymphocytes. Lymphocytes, however, have slightly more abundant, mildly basophilic cytoplasm compared with thrombocytes (Figure 22.17). The nucleus of the lymphocyte also usually is larger and less

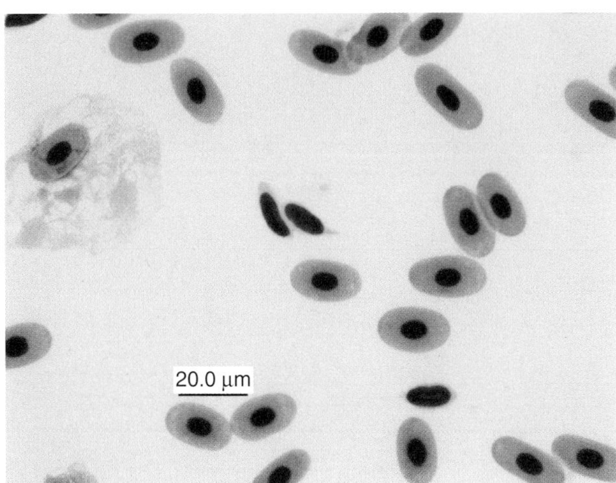

Figure 22.15 Thrombocytes in the blood film of a cartilaginous fish (*Chiloscyllium plagiosum*). Wright-Giemsa stain.

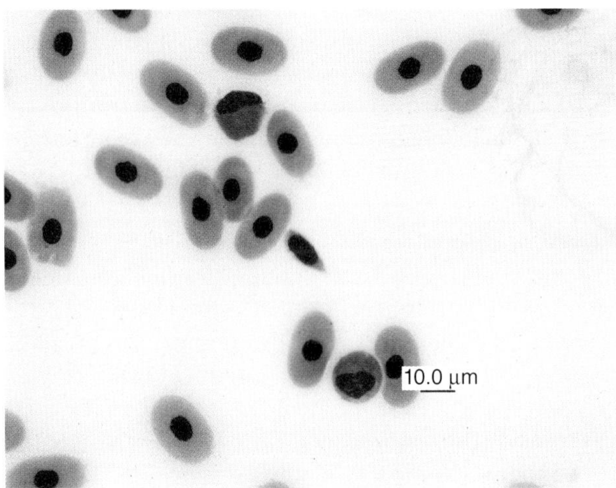

Figure 22.16 G_1 granulocytes (heterophils) and a thrombocyte with eosinophilic cytoplasmic granules (cell in the center) in the blood of a cartilaginous fish (*Ginglymostoma cirratum*). Wright-Giemsa stain.

condensed compared with that of the thrombocyte. Fish thrombocytes usually stain weakly positive with periodic acid–Schiff and positive for acid phosphatase.

Laboratory evaluation

The total thrombocyte count can be obtained via the same hemocytometer charged with diluting solutions (i.e., Natt-Herricks solution) used to obtain a total erythrocyte and leukocyte count. The thrombocytes resemble erythrocytes in the hemocytometer, but they are much smaller and appear to be round to oval, with a greater nucleus:cytoplasm (N:C) ratio compared to erythrocytes. All squares in the central, large square of a Neubauer hemocytometer are counted on both sides. The average number of thrombocytes in one large hemocytometer square is calculated and then multiplied by 2000 to obtain the total thrombocyte count per microliter. Because thrombocytes tend to clump, however, accurate counts may be difficult to achieve.

Responses in disease

During the clotting process in fish, fibrinopeptides are formed after the cleavage of fibrinogen, which is under the control of thrombin. These fibrinopeptides differ from those produced by mammals; however, the basic structure of fibrin in fish, though much larger than its mammalian counterpart, is the same as that in mammals. Fish thrombocyte aggregation differs from mammalian platelet aggregation. For example, fish thrombocytes convert arachidonic acid to prostaglandins with little, if any, thromboxane formation, whereas thromboxane is a potent inducer of platelet aggregation in mammals. Thrombocyte aggregation in sharks is temperature reversible, which is a feature not seen with mammalian platelet aggregation. Shark thrombocyte aggregation also is independent of thrombin and adenosine diphosphate. Therefore, both the control and the outcome of thrombocyte aggregation in fish may not be the same as mammals.

Glucocorticoid excess in fish tends to decrease the thrombocyte concentration and increase the clotting time. Environmental stressors, such as a prolonged photoperiod and elevated water temperature will result in a thrombopenia. Prolonged clotting times also occur with vitamin K deficiency; dietary requirements for vitamin K have been determined for salmonids and channel catfish.

Thrombocytosis and hypercoagulability of whole blood has been associated with exposure to toxic levels of cadmium (126 mg/L) in freshwater teleosts.

Blood parasites

Hemogregarina

Hemogregarina sp. affecting fish resemble those described in the blood films of reptiles, and they are identified by characteristic gametocytes in the cytoplasm of erythrocytes (see Chapter 21 on reptilian hematology). The gametocytes lack refractile pigment granules and may create a bulge in the cytoplasmic membrane. Little is known regarding the life cycle of fish hemogregarines, but they most likely require a blood-feeding, intermediate host, such as leeches, copepods, and isopods. Therefore, they more frequently are found in wild-caught fish. Often, the *Hemogregarina* sp. gametocytes in the peripheral blood of fish are considered to be an incidental finding; however, some species can cause anemia, leukocytosis with a marked left shift, and large granulomas in internal organs.

Trypanosomes

Trypanosomes occasionally may be found in blood films of fish, especially wild-caught, cold-water species. They can

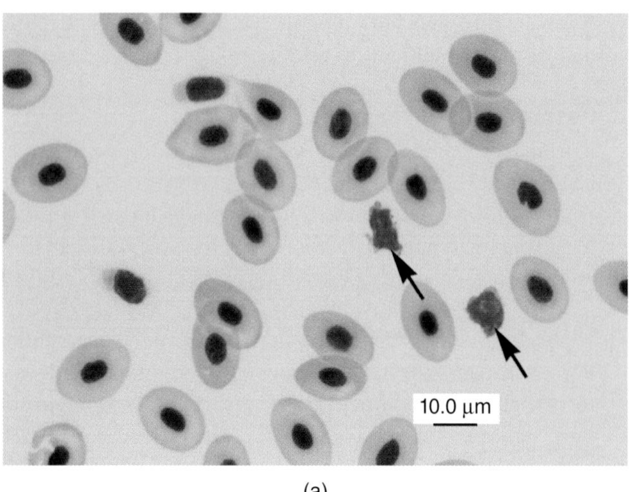

(a)

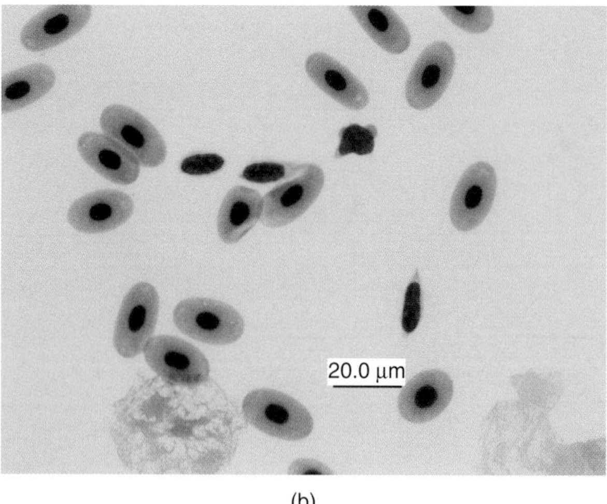

(b)

Figure 22.17 (a) Thrombocytes and lymphocytes in the blood film of a bony fish (*Opsanus tau*). Wright-Giemsa stain. (b) Thrombocytes and a lymphocyte in the blood film of a cartilaginous fish (*Chiloscyllium plagiosum*). Wright-Giemsa stain.

occur in high concentration (1,000,000 organisms/mL) and are especially prevalent in the imprints of kidney tissue. Infections with trypanosomes can result in fatal anemias. Leeches act as the intermediate host for the trypanosomes, and the infective trypomastigotes develop and then enter the fish host when the leech takes a blood meal. Trypanosomes are identified by their slender and serpentine shape, single anterior flagellum, prominent and undulating membrane, nucleus, and kinetoplast. On wet-mount preparations, the trypanosomes exhibit rapid, wriggling movements but have no forward motion.

Trypanoplasms

Trypanoplasms are hemoparasites that resemble trypanosomes morphologically, except that they are more pleomorphic (a slender, serpentine shape is most common), have two flagella (one directed anteriorly and one posteriorly), and kinetosomes. Their life cycle is similar to that of the trypanosomes. A prepatent period occurs after infection followed by a parasitemia (i.e., cryptobiasis) resulting in either death of the fish or disappearance of the trypanoplasms from the blood. *Trypanoplasma borreli* causes a severe anemia in cyprinids (i.e., koi, goldfish, and carp), and the disease is referred to as sleeping sickness. Anemia, exophthalmia, ascites, and splenomegaly occur in freshwater salmonids (i.e., trout) with *T. salmositica*; *T. bullocki* infects marine fish, especially flatfish species along the western Atlantic and Gulf of Mexico. On wet-mount preparations, trypanoplasms exhibit flowing, ameboid motility, which aids in their identification.

Piroplasmids

Babesiosoma, *Haemohormidium*, *Haematractidium*, and *Mesnilium* are genera of piroplasmids that have been described in fish. As with the hemogregarines, little is known regarding their life cycle, which most likely requires a blood-feeding, intermediate host. Piroplasmids are identified by their intracytoplasmic inclusions in circulating erythrocytes, which can vary from small, ringlike forms to anaplasma-like inclusions. Piroplasmids may cause hemolytic anemia in fish.

Microsporidians

Enterocytozoon salmonis is an intranuclear microsporidium that primarily infects hematopoietic cells of salmonids. The infected cells exhibit intranuclear inclusions. This organism was once considered to be the causative agent of plasmacytoid leukemia of Chinook salmon (*Onchorhynchus tshawytscha*). The presence of high reverse-transcriptase activity in the affected tissues from these fish, however, suggests that an oncogenic retrovirus may be the causative agent for that disease.

Viral inclusions

Intracytoplasmic inclusions occur in the erythrocytes of fish with viral erythrocytic necrosis (i.e., piscine erythrocytic necrosis), erythrocytic inclusion body syndrome, and coho anemia. Viral erythrocytic necrosis occurs in a variety of marine fish, including salmon, cod, and herring. The disease is characterized by marked poikilocytosis, a single intracytoplasmic inclusion (0.3–4.0 μm) within the erythrocytes, and karyolysis of the red-blood-cell nuclei. Erythrocytic inclusion body syndrome of young salmonids is characterized by progressive, severe anemia, which is caused by a viral agent that creates 0.8–3.0 μm intracytoplasmic inclusions within the erythrocytes. A Leishman-Giemsa stain provides the best results for demonstrating the inclusions. An anemia that occurs in seawater-reared coho salmon (*O. kisutch*) results from 0.1 to 2.0 μm intracytoplasmic inclusions, which often are rod-shaped within the erythrocytes.

Hematopoiesis

Cartilaginous fish (Chondrichthyes) lack bone marrow and lymph nodes, but they do have a lymphoid thymus, spleen, and other lymphomyeloid tissues. Significant hematopoietic activity occurs in the sinusoids of the red pulp area of the spleen, where erythrocytes, thrombocytes, and lymphocytes develop. Little evidence, however, suggests that granulopoiesis occurs in the spleen of these fish. Development of erythrocytes in these fish appears to occur in the same manner as that in mammals. The peripheral blood may be an important component of erythropoiesis, because several stages of erythrocyte development can be found in the routine blood films from cartilaginous fish. The epigonal organ, which is associated with the gonad, and Leydig's organ, which is situated in the submucosa of the alimentary tract, are the major sites for granulopoiesis in cartilaginous fish. Myeloblasts, progranulocytes, myelocytes, metamyelocytes, and mature granulocytes have been described in these unique lymphomyeloid tissues.

The principal lymphomyeloid tissues of bony fish (Osteichthyes) are the thymus, spleen, and kidney. The thymus, which is the first lymphoid organ to develop, seeds the spleen and kidney with lymphocytes. The kidney is a major blood-forming organ in bony fish; the pronephric (anterior or head) and opisthonephric (main or trunk) kidneys are the sites of hematopoiesis in these fish. The opisthonephric kidney also functions as an excretory organ. Therefore, the kidney (primarily the pronephros) is the principal site for the differentiation and development of erythrocytes, granulocytes, lymphocytes, monocytes, and, possibly, thrombocytes in most bony fish. The typical stages of granulocyte development have been identified for each type of granulocyte in the kidney of bony fish. The spleen of teleost fish is similar to that of elasmobranchs, but it typically has a secondary role in hematopoiesis, except in some species in which it is the only hematopoietic organ.

23 Hematology of Amphibians

Terry W. Campbell

Department of Clinical Sciences, College of Veterinary Medicine and Biomedical Sciences, Colorado State University, Fort Collins, CO, USA

Compared with other vertebrates seen in veterinary practices, amphibians are unique because their normal life cycle includes a metamorphosis from a larval to an adult form. Amphibians have adapted to aquatic, terrestrial, fossorial, and alpine environments, and their normal hematologic parameters vary accordingly. Amphibians are grouped into three orders: Caudata (Urodela), which includes salamanders and newts; Anura (Salientia), which includes frogs and toads; and Apoda (Gymnophiona), which includes the caecilians. Amphibians, especially frogs of the Ranidae family, are often used in research, but hematologic evaluation of amphibians is not routinely used in establishing the diagnosis of amphibian diseases. Hematologic evaluation may be used to monitor the health status of an amphibian as long as the reported reference intervals and interpretations account for the intrinsic and extrinsic factors that affect the hemic response. Extrinsic factors, such as environmental temperature, photoperiod, season, water-quality parameters, diet, and population density, should be noted whenever reference values are reported. Adaptation to a specific environment also influences the hematologic parameters. Important intrinsic factors include gender and age; larval and adult stages should be considered as separate entities, each with their own reference interval. Hematology can be useful in the detection of diseases that affect the cellular components of blood, such as anemia, leukopenia, leukocytosis, thrombocytopenia, and other abnormal changes of blood cells, and may also be useful in following the progression of a disease or a response to therapy.

Collection and handling of blood

The approximate blood volume of many species of aquatic amphibians ranges between 13% and 25% of the body weight and between 7% and 10% of the body weight for most terrestrial amphibians. In general, it is considered "safe" to draw a blood sample equaling 1% of the total body weight of an individual amphibian at one time. Sites for blood collection include the heart, ventral abdominal vein, ventral caudal vein, and lingual vein. Some amphibians may be manually restrained for blood collection, and others may require sedation or anesthesia. Submersion of the amphibian in a 0.05% solution of tricaine methanesulfonate is one method of restraint that may be considered for use in blood sample collection of amphibian patients. Moistened powder-free latex gloves should be worn when handling amphibians for examination, restraint, or blood collection in order to protect their skin. Small-gauge needles and small syringes are typically used to collect blood samples from amphibians. Consequently, blood flow into the syringe is usually slow. Many amphibian patients are small, making it necessary to use microhematocrit tubes with inner diameters that are smaller than regular hematocrit tubes in order to obtain a packed cell volume (PCV). Use of these small microhematocrit tubes will also help maximize the amount of hematologic testing that can be performed on small blood samples.

Blood can be collected from frogs, toads, salamanders and newts by venipuncture of the ventral abdominal or lingual vein. This vein lies under the linea alba along the ventral midline of the coelomic cavity. Venipuncture is performed by inserting a 25-gauge needle in a craniodorsal direction midway along a line of sight extending from the sternum and pelvis (Figure 23.1). Use of a Doppler probe to locate this vein may be required in species where the vein is not clearly visible. Blood may then be collected by the drip method or by aspiration of blood into a small syringe. Because lymphatic vessels accompany blood vessels in amphibians, a mixture of blood and lymph frequently occurs with venipuncture of the ventral abdominal vein. This mixing of lymphatic fluid with the blood sample is variable, but it will dilute the cellular components of the blood, thereby resulting in lower PCV, hemoglobin concentration, and erythrocyte and leukocyte concentrations.

Blood can be collected from frogs and toads by venipuncture of the lingual vein. Venipuncture of the lingual vein may be performed after gently opening the patient's mouth and

Veterinary Hematology, Clinical Chemistry, and Cytology, Third Edition. Edited by Mary Anna Thrall, Glade Weiser, Robin W. Allison and Terry W. Campbell.

Companion website: www.wiley.com/go/thrall/veterinary

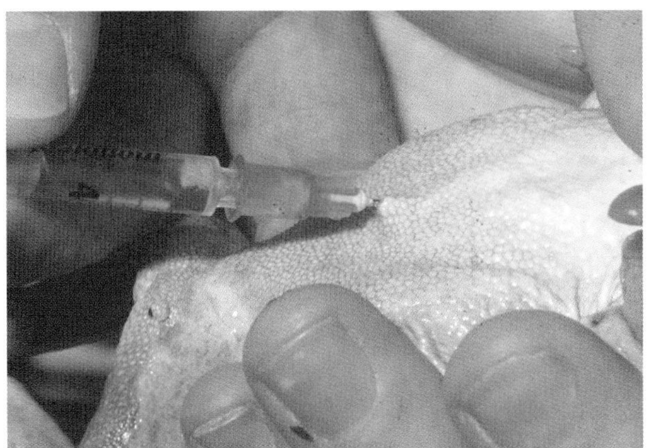

Figure 23.1 Blood collection from a tree frog (*Litoria caterulea*) using the ventral abdominal vein. Source: Image from Campbell TW. *Exotic Animal Hematology and Cytology*, 4th ed. Ames, IA: Wiley Blackwell, 2015, p. 182.

moving the tongue forward and upward using a cotton tip applicator to expose the lingual venous plexus that lies on the ventral aspect of the tongue on the floor of the mouth. Care must be taken to avoid breaking the fragile mandibular bones while holding the mouth open to collect blood from the lingual vein. Excess saliva is swabbed from below the tongue, after which a large vein of the lingual venous plexus on the ventral aspect of the tongue is punctured with a 25-G needle or smaller. Blood should be collected by the drip method into a microcollection tube or microhematocrit tube instead of by aspiration into a syringe in order to minimize the potential for hematoma formation.

Cardiocentesis is performed by placing the frog, toad, salamander, or newt in dorsal recumbency and locating the heart either by visualizing the pulsing heart, by use of a Doppler scan, or by transillumination. Cardiocentesis in amphibians often requires sedation or general anesthesia using tricaine methanesulfonate to prevent movement and potential damage to the heart and great vessels. Visualization of the heart can also be accomplished in some species via transillumination by use of the cool light from a rigid arthroscope inserted into the stomach. Once the heart is located, a 25-G needle is inserted into the ventricle, and blood is aspirated into a syringe.

Venipuncture of the ventral caudal vein (ventral coccygeal vein, tail vein) may be used for blood collection from some species of salamanders and newts and is performed in the same manner described for venipuncture of the ventral caudal vein in reptiles. This technique should not be performed in salamanders and newts that have tail autotomy (a natural ability to lose their tails) because their tails may break off during the procedure. The salamander or newt is held in dorsal recumbency to perform a venipuncture of the ventral coccygeal vein. A 25-gauge needle is inserted into the ventral midline of the tail and directed to a point just below the coccygeal vertebrae. The needle is then advanced while applying negative pressure to the syringe until blood can be aspirated into the syringe barrel.

Blood for hematologic studies in amphibians should be collected using lithium heparin as an anticoagulant. In general, ethylenediaminetetraacetic acid (EDTA) usually causes lysis of erythrocytes in the blood of amphibians and should be avoided; however, a 3% EDTA solution with distilled water may be used as an anticoagulant in some species to avoid the erythrocyte lysis effect. Syringes may be pretreated with lithium heparin or blood can be allowed to drip from the needle hub into a microcollection tube containing lithium heparin.

Erythrocytes

Morphology

Erythrocytes of amphibians are large nucleated, elliptic discs (Figure 23.2). The cells usually have a distinct nuclear bulge, and the nuclear margins often are irregular. Some amphibians, such as the slender salamander (*Batrachoceps attenuatus*), do not have nucleated red blood cells. Amphibian erythrocytes are large compared with those of other vertebrates with sizes that vary from 10 to 70 μm in diameter and typically have mean cell volume (MCV) values ranging from 390 and 14,000. The cytoplasm of frog and toad erythrocytes is homogenous and packed with hemoglobin. Ultrastructural analysis reveals rare organelles. Because the erythrocytes of salamanders and newts complete their maturation in the peripheral circulation, the cytoplasm is not homogenous, and ultrastructural examination demonstrates clusters of granular and vacuolar bodies.

There is considerable interspecies variation in the erythrocyte parameters of amphibians and they can be dramatically different from other vertebrates, especially mammals (Table 23.1). Normal amphibian erythrocytes do exhibit slight anisocytosis; however, increased anisocytosis suggests an increased concentration of large red cells due to erythroid regeneration or erythroid dyscrasia. This may be seen in association with a regenerative response to a hemolytic or hemorrhagic anemia. Conditions that result in erythroid dyscrasia may indicate a nutritional deficiency or toxicity; however, these have not been documented in the literature.

Two forms of erythrocytes differentiated by size and morphology appear to occur in amphibians. One form, a larger elongated form is considered to be the larval form, whereas a smaller, rounded form is considered to be the adult form. The transition from the larval form to the adult form begins at the onset of metamorphosis, and by day 12 a complete transformation to all adult forms occurs. There is a positive relationship between body size and erythrocyte width in salamanders. As salamanders grow, their erythrocytes become more rounded. This morphological change does not affect the overall area, however.

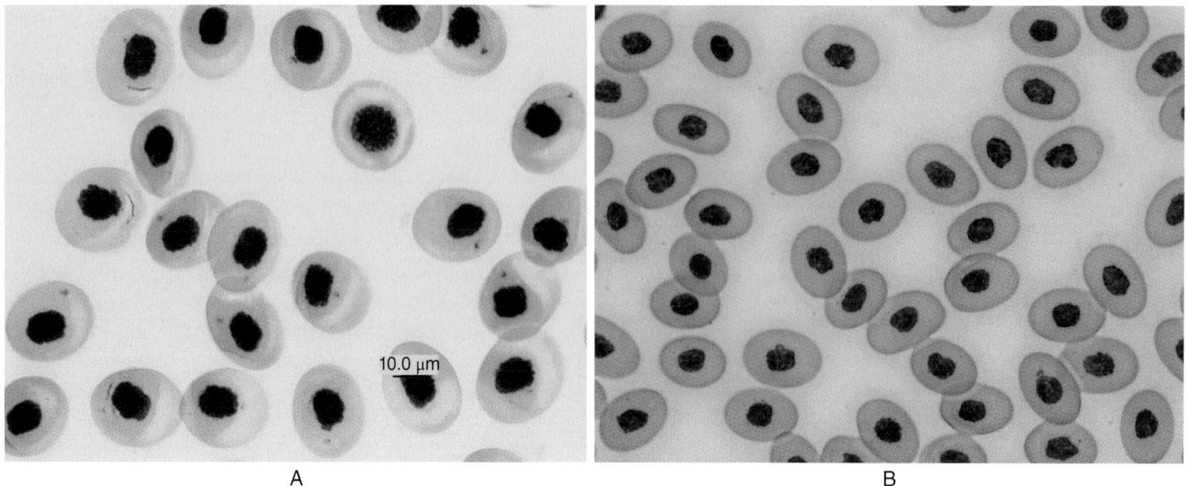

Figure 23.2 (a) Erythrocytes in the blood film of a salamander (*Ambystoma tigrunum*). Wright-Giemsa stain. (b) Erythrocytes in the blood film of a toad (*Incillius alvarius*). Wright-Giemsa stain, ×1000.

Table 23.1 Erythrocyte parameters for selected amphibians.

	PCV (%)	RBC ($\times 10^6/\mu L$)	Hb (g/dL)	MCV (fL)	MCHC (g/dL)
American bullfrog[a, b]	39–42	0.450	9.3–9.7	—	21.1–25.9
Cuban tree frog[a]	20–24	—	5.6–6.8	—	25–31
Fire-bellied toad (male)[c]	14–26	0.190–0.465	5.0–12.2	412–758	29–55
Fire-bellied toad (female)[c]	12–23	0.240–0.355	3.4–8.3	363–917	19–60
Leopard frog (male)[a]	19–52	0.227–0.767	3.8–14.6	722–916	23–27
Leopard frog (female)[a]	16–51	0.174–0.701	2.7–14.0	730–916	20–28
Mudpuppy[a]	21	0.020	4.6	10070	22
Tiger salamander[a]	40	1.657	9.4		

[a]Wright KM. Amphibians. In: *Exotic Animal* Formulary, 3rd ed., J. Carpenter (ed.). St. Louis, MO: Elsevier Saunders, p. 46. 2005.
[b]Cathers T, Lewbart GA, Correa M, Stevens JB. Serum chemistry and hematology values for anesthetized American bull frogs [*Rana catesbeiana*]. *J Zoo and Wildlife Medicine* 28: 171–4. 1997.
[c]Wojtaszek J, Adamowicz A. Haematology of the fire-bellied toad, *Bombina bombina*. *L. Comp Clin Path* 12: 129–34. 2003.

The appearance of the nucleus of the amphibian erythrocyte also changes as the cell matures. The nuclear chromatin of immature erythrocytes lacks the dense chromatin clumping of the mature cell (Figure 23.3). Older senescent cells have pyknotic nuclei.

The cytoplasm of the immature cells also stains more basophilic compared to mature cells with Wright's stain (Figure 23.4). The blue staining of the amphibian erythrocyte cytoplasm may also be associated, in part, with the effects of heparin on Wright's-stained blood films as heparin is a commonly used anticoagulant during blood collection in amphibians. The staining effects caused by heparin can be prevented if a blood film is made from a drop of blood remaining in the needle that does not contain heparin after blood collection.

Increased numbers of immature erythrocytes may be indicative of a disease such as iridovirus infection, or may indicate the presence of a regenerative response. Iridovirus infections have been associated with disease outbreaks associated with high mortalities in wild frogs and salamanders. Intranuclear inclusions of the iridovirus are found in the erythrocytes on histologic specimens. Irregular immature erythrocytes with characteristics reminiscent of cells in mammalian erythroid leukemia or exuberant responses can be found in blood films of clinically healthy frogs and may be indicative of rapid cell turnover or a result of environmental stressors.

Laboratory evaluation

The microhematocrit method is used for obtaining a PCV, which is the most common method for evaluating the red

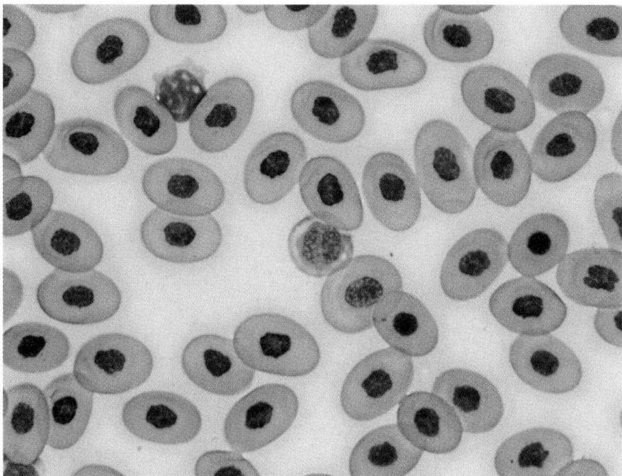

Figure 23.3 A polychromatic erythrocyte and lymphocyte in the blood film of a toad (*Incillius alvarius*). Wright-Giemsa stain.

cell mass of amphibians. The cyanmethemoglobin method commonly is used to determine the hemoglobin concentration in amphibian blood. As with blood hemoglobin determinations in birds, reptiles, and fish, this procedure requires centrifugation of the blood–cyanmethemoglobin mixture to remove the free erythrocyte nuclei before the optical density is measured. The total erythrocyte count in amphibians can be determined either by manual counting with a hemocytometer or by an electronic cell counter. Manual counting methods to obtain red cell concentrations in amphibian blood use of the Erythro-pette™ system (Exotic Animal Solutions, Inc. Hueytown, AL, USA) and Natt and Herricks method. These methods are the same as those described for use in avian blood (see Chapter 20).

Responses in disease

The average amphibian erythrocyte life span is considered to be greater than 100 days, which may have an impact on the erythrocytic response. Because newts and salamanders generally are more fishlike than toads and frogs, interpretation of their hemograms may be more like those of fish, whereas hematologic changes in toads and frogs may be more like those of reptiles. In general, amphibian PCVs are lower than those of mammals and birds, and these values vary with species, age, gender, environmental temperature, photoperiod, and husbandry of the amphibian (Table 23.1). The peripheral erythrocyte count of amphibians is affected by seasonal activity. An increase in bone marrow erythropoiesis occurs during the spring and following hibernation; therefore, the highest number of circulating erythrocytes occurs at this time. In some studies, males have higher erythrocyte counts than females. Also, numbers of immature erythrocytes (as early as rubriblasts) in the peripheral blood tend to be greater in males where they can represent as high as 2% of the erythrocyte population (Figure 23.4). Captive amphibians may have more stable erythrocyte parameters than their wild counterparts due to the stability of the environment in which most captive amphibians reside. Because amphibians are ectothermic, the rapidity of their hematologic responses can be manipulated by changes in the environment, such as temperature fluctuation.

Leukocytes

Morphology

In general, amphibian leukocytes resemble those of mammals but are larger (10 and 25 μm in diameter for most

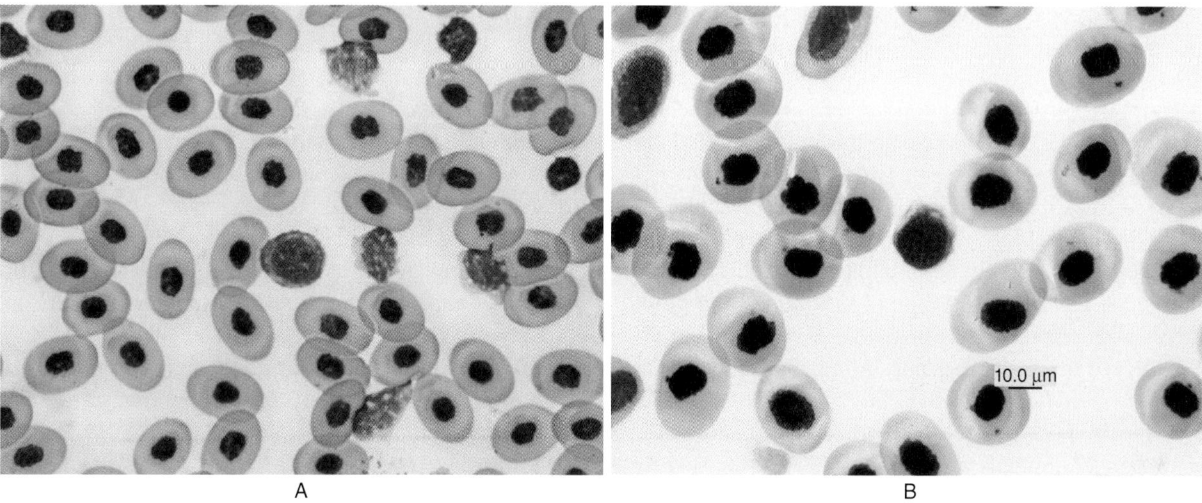

Figure 23.4 (a) An immature erythrocyte (basophilic rubricyte) and lymphocytes in the blood film of a toad (*Incillius alvarius*). Wright-Giemsa stain. (b) An immature erythrocyte (early basophilic rubricyte) in the blood film of a salamander (*Ambystoma tigrunum*). Wright-Giemsa stain.

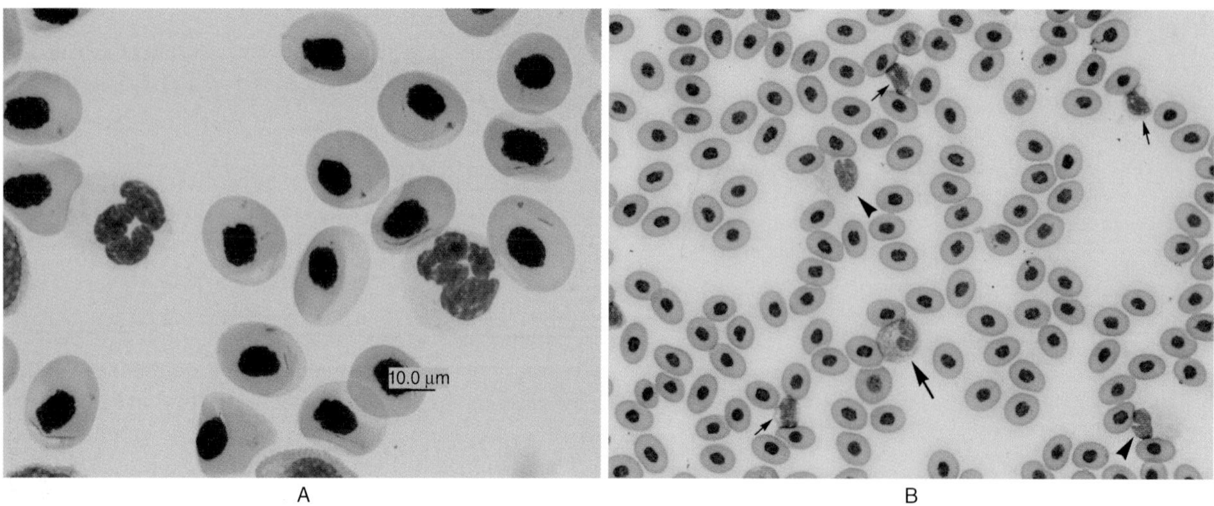

Figure 23.5 (a) Neutrophils in the blood film of a salamander (*Ambystoma tigrunum*). Wright-Giemsa stain. (b) Two neutrophils (arrowheads), an eosinophil (large arrow), and three lymphocytes (small arrows) in the blood film of a toad (*Incillius alvarius*). Wright-Giemsa stain, ×500.

species) comparatively. Amphibian leukocytes are typically classified based upon their appearance in blood smears stained with Wright-Giemsa stain and their resemblance to mammalian leukocytes; therefore, they have been classified as neutrophils, eosinophils, basophils, lymphocytes, and monocytes. Other classification schemes present in the literature use heterophils instead of neutrophils and identify some cells as azurophils instead of or in addition to monocytes. Some references also include different combinations of heterophil, azurophil, and neutrophil to describe the granulocytic cells present. Amphibian granulocytes (neutrophils or heterophils, eosinophils, and basophils) have multilobed nuclei with small cytoplasmic granules that are variable in size, shape, and ultrastructure depending on the species.

Amphibian neutrophils resemble those of mammals, and they range from 10 to 25 μm in diameter for most species (Figure 23.5). When stained with Romanowsky stains, they are generally round cells with a lobed nucleus and neutral (colorless) staining cytoplasm. The small cytoplasmic granules vary in size, shape, and ultrastructure between species. Cells with small eosinophilic cytoplasmic granules often are referred to as heterophils, whereas those cells that do not are referred to as neutrophils. Some species of amphibians may exhibit neutrophils with large irregular cytoplasmic granules that stain slightly eosinophilic (light pink). These cells resemble the neutrophils found in humans and other mammals with Chediak-Higashi syndrome but are considered to be normal in amphibians. Amphibian neutrophils typically are peroxidase positive, but phosphatase activity varies with the species.

Amphibian eosinophils are similar in size to or slightly larger than the neutrophils found in the same blood film. Eosinophils have a slightly basophilic cytoplasm compared to neutrophils and have small to moderate-sized round to oval eosinophilic cytoplasmic granules (Figures 23.5b and 23.6). The nuclei of eosinophils are often less lobed than those of neutrophils; however, this may not be true of all species. Eosinophils are peroxidase negative, and the phosphatase activity varies with species. The eosinophils of some species are negative for aryl sulfatase and β-glucuronidase activity. Some amphibian eosinophil granules have a crystalloid ultrastructure, but others lack the crystalloid structures that are typical of the ultrastructural morphology of eosinophils from higher vertebrates.

The size of amphibian basophils varies between species. Typically, these basophils have nonsegmented nuclei and large, metachromatic granules (Figure 23.7). The nucleus is often obscured by the granules but when visible is nonlobed and slightly eccentric in position. Alcohol fixation and use of Romanowsky stains provide the best staining for amphibian basophils because basophil granules are frequently affected by water-based stains and will partially dissolve. The granules contain acid mucopolysaccharides (i.e., glycosaminoglycans) that are less sulfated than those of mammals, and the histamine content is lower than that of mammals. Ultrastructural analysis demonstrates large numbers of membrane-bound cytoplasmic granules with small numbers of organelles.

The lymphocytes of amphibians resemble those of other vertebrates morphologically. Small lymphocytes are more abundant than larger forms in the blood films of normal amphibians. The lymphocytes are round with round nuclei containing densely clumped chromatin and a scant amount of pale-blue cytoplasm (Figures 23.3, 23.4a, 23.5b, 23.7b, 23.8, and 23.9). Many of the lymphocytes from frogs of the family Ranidae have distinct azurophilic granules. Amphibian lymphocytes, like mammalian lymphocytes, are nonspecific esterase positive and peroxidase negative

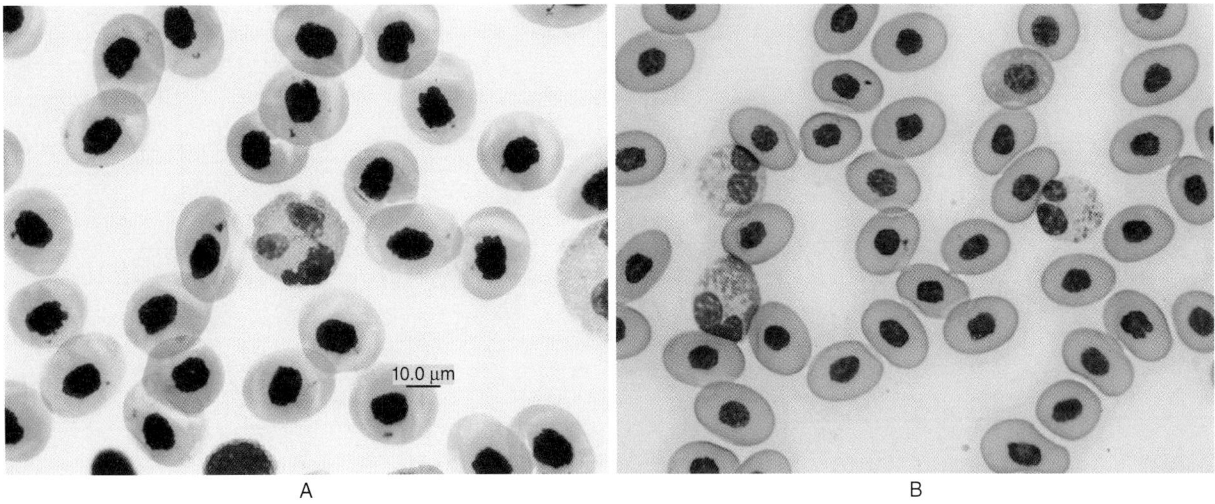

Figure 23.6 (a) An eosinophil in the blood film of a salamander (*Ambystoma tigrunum*). Wright-Giemsa stain. (b) Eosinophils in the blood film of a toad (*Incillius alvarius*). Wright-Giemsa stain.

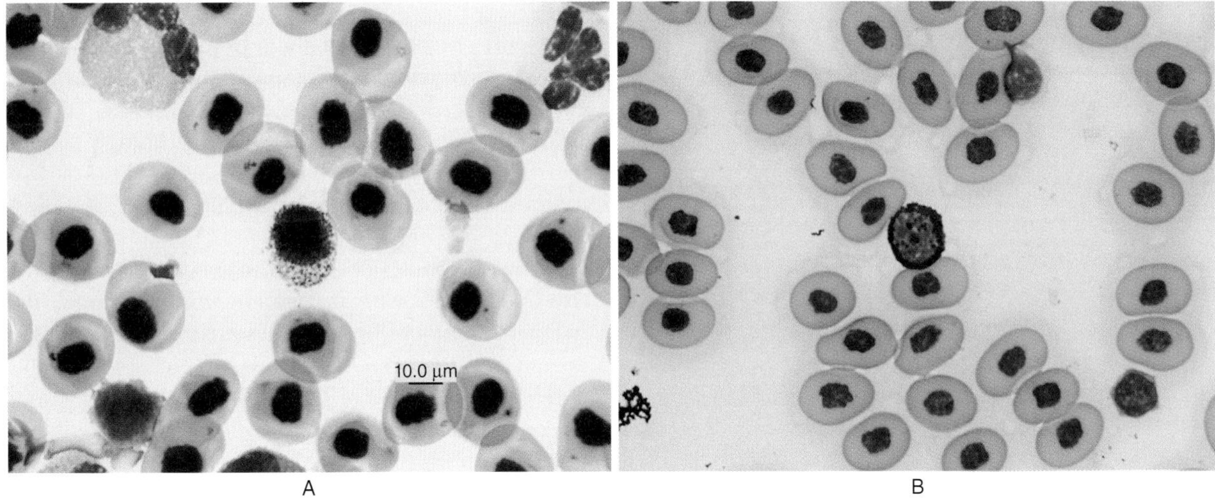

Figure 23.7 (a) A basophil in the blood film of a salamander (*Ambystoma tigrunum*). Wright-Giemsa stain. (b) A basophil and lymphocyte in the blood film of a toad (*Incillius alvarius*). Wright-Giemsa stain.

but, unlike mammalian lymphocytes, are negative for β-glucuronidase and aryl sulfatase.

Monocytes in amphibian blood films are similar to those of other vertebrates. They are characterized by their large size, abundant, blue-gray cytoplasm that may be foamy or vacuolated, and a variably shaped nucleus with less chromatin clumping than seen in lymphocyte nuclei (Figure 23.9). The cytoplasm of amphibian monocytes may contain fine, azurophilic granulation and pseudopodia. Amphibian monocytes are peroxidase positive and contain some of the same hydrolytic enzymes found in mammalian monocytes.

Some amphibian leukocytes have been classified as azurophils. These cells have features commonly associated with monocytes and are considered to be monocytes by some authors. Other authors hypothesize that the amphibian azurophil is either an immature or senescent granulocyte or monocyte. There is little advantage in classifying these cells as separate cells from the monocyte population in the blood when interpreting the hemogram of amphibians. Therefore, they should be classified as monocytes until further evidence justifies classifying them as a different cell type.

Cytochemical characteristics have been applied to amphibian blood cells in an effort to characterize the cells as an aid for interpretation of cellular responses. Frog leukocytes have been described using a number of Romanowsky–type stains and cytochemical stains, including peroxidase, acid phosphatase, alkaline phosphatase, nonspecific esterase, basic protein, periodic acid–Schiff (PAS), Alcian blue, and toluidine blue, and evaluating serotonin fluorescence. For example, in the bullfrog (*Rana* (Aquarana) *catesbeiana*) and

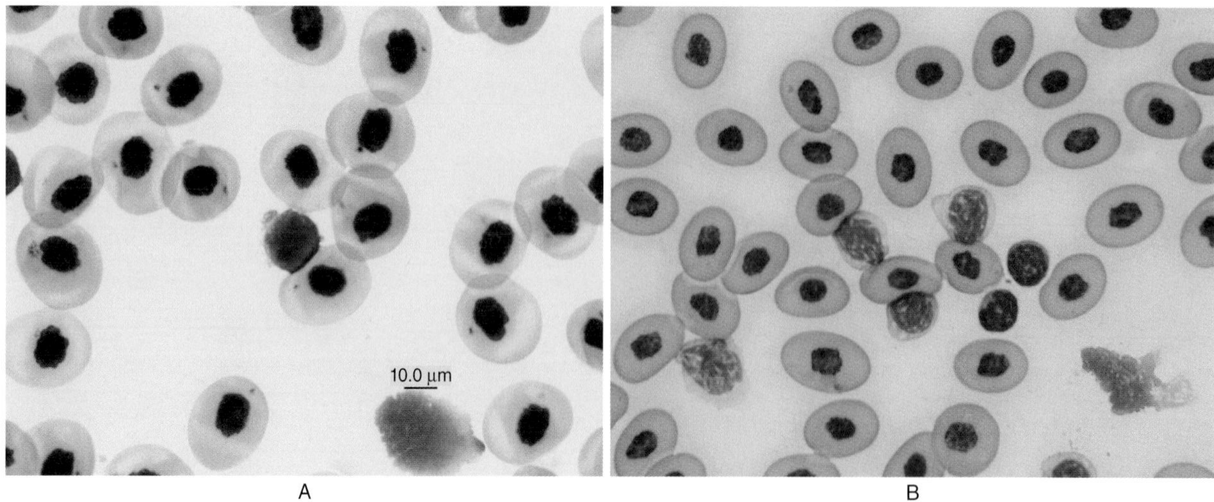

Figure 23.8 (a) A lymphocyte in the blood film of a salamander (*Ambystoma tigrunum*). Wright-Giemsa stain. (b) Lymphocytes (small, medium, and large) in the blood film of a toad (*Incillius alvarius*). Wright-Giemsa stain.

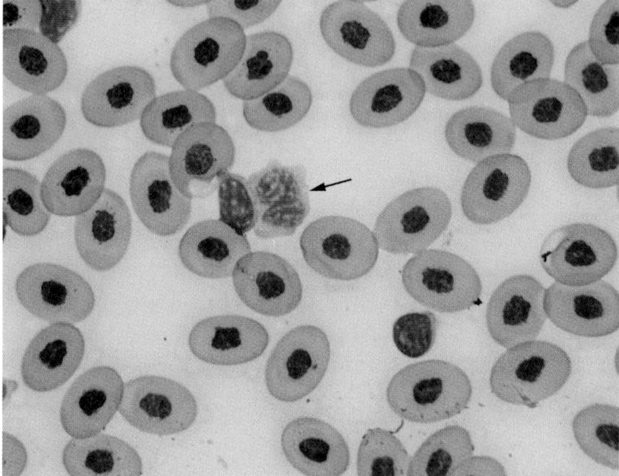

Figure 23.9 A monocyte (arrow) and lymphocytes in the blood film of a toad (*Incillius alvarius*). Wright-Giemsa stain, ×1000.

clawed frog (*Xenopus laevis*), neutrophils, eosinophils, and monocytes were positive for some or all of the following: α-naphthyl butyrate esterase (NBE), chloroacetate esterase (CAE), myeloperoxidase (PER), and Sudan black B (SBB). Lymphocytes occasionally were positive for CAE. Lymphocytes in these species were negative for all cytochemical stains and leukocyte alkaline phosphatase (LAP) was not a useful marker for any leukocyte type. Peripheral blood lymphocytes in these frogs were strongly immunoreactive for CD3ε, CD79a, and BLA.36. Also, basophils from the African clawed frog had different enzymatic activity than basophils of the bullfrog, which may suggest different functions for the basophils of these two species. Some cytochemical reactions, including PER and SBB in neutrophils, CAE in monocytes, and PER in eosinophils, were consistent across the species, suggesting they may be helpful in characterizing leukocytes from a variety of frog species. Some leukocytes were only noted occasionally in frogs, including azurophils, large granular lymphocytes, and, in the case of clawed frogs, eosinophils.

Granulopoiesis occurs in the liver, kidney, and bone marrow of amphibians; however, some species lack bone marrow. Myeloblasts and progranulocytes have not been positively described in amphibians. Immature neutrophils have small granules of various shapes that increase in both size and density with maturation until the larger, definitive peroxidase-positive granules are formed. Some species do not develop primary granules; rather, they produce a different population of granules. Evidence suggests that in some species, eosinophils begin as round cells with a round nucleus and scant cytoplasm that contains large, dense, and round primary granules. Further development of eosinophils results in a mixture of the larger primary granules and the smaller secondary granules. The monocyte is the first leukocyte to appear in the peripheral blood of bullfrog (*Rana catesbeiana*) larvae, in which immature monocytes with linear nuclear chromatin appear 15 days after hatching and mature monocytes with round nuclei, which develop into kidney-shaped or lobed nuclei, appear 22 days after hatching. Definitive neutrophils, eosinophils, and basophils in larval bullfrogs appear in the peripheral blood at the same time, late during development of the frog. Lymphopoiesis in amphibians resembles that in other vertebrates. Small lymphocytes are the most common, but larger lymphocytes also may be seen.

Laboratory evaluation

As in other nonmammalian vertebrates, amphibians have nucleated erythrocytes and thrombocytes that interfere with automated methods for counting leukocytes; therefore,

Table 23.2 Leukocyte parameters for selected amphibians.

	WBC ($\times10^3/\mu L$)	Neut/Heterophils ($\times10^3/\mu L$)	Lymphocytes ($\times10^3/\mu L$)	Monocytes ($\times10^3/\mu L$)	Eosinophils ($\times10^3/\mu L$)	Basophils ($\times10^3/\mu L$)
Fire-bellied toad (male)[a]	2.21–18.48	0.20–5.70	2.30–10.80	0.20–1.80	0–0.90	0.10–4.20
Fire-bellied toad (female)[a]	1.04–14.25	0.10–4.40	0.70–7.10	0.10–1.60	0–0.80	0.10–2.30

[a]Wojtaszek J, Adamowicz A. Haematology of the fire-bellied toad, *Bombina bombina*. *L. Comp Clin Path* 12: 129–34. 2003.

Table 23.3 Leukocyte parameters for selected amphibians.

	WBC ($\times10^3/\mu L$)	Neut/Heterophils (%)	Lymphocytes (%)	Monocytes (%)	Eosinophils (%)	Basophils (%)
African clawed frog[a]	8.2	6.9–9.1	62.6–68.0	0–1	0	7.1–9.9
American bullfrog[a, b]	2.3–8.1	6.8–37.2	47.9–77.9	0–2	2.8–15.0	0–6
Edible frog[a]	6.1	6.7–10.9	48.7–55.3	0–2	18.1–20.7	15.3–17.9
Grass frog[a]	14.4	5.5–7.51.5	65.6–71.4	0–1	11.6–17.4	22–26.4
Japanese newt[c]	1.51–2.09	25.4–30.6	2.6–3.4	5–7	3.3–4.7	53.8–60.2

[a]Wright KM. Amphibians. In: *Exotic Animal* Formulary, 3rd ed., J. Carpenter (ed.). St. Louis, MO: Elsevier Saunders, p. 46. 2005.
[b]Cathers T, Lewbart GA, Correa M, Stevens JB. Serum chemistry and hematology values for anesthetized American bull frogs [*Rana catesbeiana*]. *J Zoo and Wildlife Medicine* 28: 171–4. 1997.
[c]Pfeiffer CJ, Pyle H, Asashima M. Blood cell morphology and counts in the Japanese newt [*Cynops pyrrhogaster*]. *J Zoo and Wildlife Medicine* 21: 56–64. 1990.

manual counting methods are used. The Natt and Herricks or phloxine B method, as described for birds in Chapter 20, can be used to obtain a total leukocyte concentration in amphibian blood.

The leukocyte differential is performed manually using Romanowsky-stained blood films (Tables 23.2 and 23.3). Because most blood samples from amphibians are collected into heparin, making blood films either with blood containing no anticoagulant or immediately after mixing of the blood with the heparin (to decrease cell clumping and improve staining) is best.

Responses in disease

Hematologic evaluation is not used routinely in veterinary medicine as a means of evaluating the health or diseased state of amphibian patients. Reasons for this include the difficulty in obtaining amphibian blood samples without affecting the hemogram results, the challenges involved in obtaining cell counts, and the lack of meaningful reference intervals. Absolute numbers of each cell type are expected to vary considerably with season, temperature, species, habitat, and a number of other extrinsic considerations. Many published reference intervals fail to include information involving intrinsic (i.e., gender and age) and extrinsic (i.e., environmental temperature, photoperiod, water quality parameters, diet, population density, and season) factors, which may influence the hematology values. Some publications do include some of this information, and whenever possible these sources should be used when interpreting amphibian hematological results. Normal total leukocyte counts exhibit inter- and intraspecies variation. The lymphocyte is generally the most numerous leukocyte and the neutrophil is the most numerous granulocyte in the peripheral blood of most amphibian species studied.

Little is known regarding the function of the various amphibian leukocytes. The process of interpreting the amphibian leukogram is extrapolated from that used with other vertebrates. Amphibian neutrophils have both migratory and phagocytic activity, and they participate in inflammation. Likewise, amphibian monocytes are phagocytic and, most likely, function in a manner similar to those of other vertebrates. Therefore, increases in the neutrophil and monocyte counts likely suggest an inflammatory response. More studies that evaluate the types of blood cells that increase or decrease during different disease states are needed to better determine the function of each cell type and their clinical importance.

The presence of a peripheral eosinophilia may be suggestive of parasitic infections. Amphibian eosinophils appear to have an inferior ability to phagocytize particles or microorganisms compared to neutrophils but do respond to metazoan parasitic infections. Increased frequency of eosinophils has also been documented in frogs from polluted areas, perhaps a reflection of stimulation of the immune system.

Amphibian basophils may function in a manner similar to those of mammals. They rarely are found in the peripheral blood of some species but are abundant in others. For example, they occur in high numbers in the blood of the African clawed frog (*X. laevis*), an aquatic species, compared to their absence or low numbers in the semiaquatic bullfrog (*Rana* [*Aquarana*]) and Colorado River toad (*Incilius alvarus*). The difference may be reflective of their environment, as has been suggested for aquatic reptiles, such as aquatic turtles that are noted for their high numbers of circulating basophils. Another example is the aquatic Japanese newt (*Cynops pyrrhogaster*), which normally has a differential leukocyte count that includes up to 60% basophils. Basophils of this species are considered to play a significant role in immunosurveillance.

Lymphocytes of frogs and toads demonstrate an immunologic sophistication similar to those of higher vertebrates. The lymphocytes can be classified as B cells that produce immunoglobulins or as T cells with populations of functional diversity, such as helpers and different effectors. Contrast, the lymphocytes of newts and salamanders appear to lack such refinement. A lymphocytosis is suggestive of an excitement response, stimulation of the immune system, or possibly lymphoid leukemia. A transitory lymphocytosis following tail amputation for blood collection has been demonstrated in the Japanese newt (*C. pyrrhogaster*), suggesting either an excitement response or recruitment of lymphocytes.

Thrombocytes

Morphology

Amphibian thrombocytes are nucleated cells that resemble those described for birds, reptiles, and fish, although anucleated thrombocytes that resemble mammalian platelets have been described in certain species. Amphibian thrombocytes typically vary in shape from oval to spindle-shaped (Figure 23.8). When the cells are in a nonreactive state, they tend to be oval in shape. Once activated, the cells become spindle-shaped. The nucleus is dense and round to oval. Thrombocyte cytoplasm is abundant and colorless; however, when they become reactive the cytoplasm may contain numerous eosinophilic granules. Amphibian thrombocytes are often confused with small lymphocytes but may be differentiated based on the appearance of the cytoplasm. The cytoplasmic volume of small lymphocytes tends to be small and the cytoplasm stains blue. Ultrastructurally, the thrombocytes of some amphibian species, such as *Xenops* and *Rana*, are alkaline phosphatase positive, whereas the lymphocytes are negative.

Laboratory evaluation

The total thrombocyte count can be obtained from the same charged hemocytometer used to obtain the total erythrocyte and leukocyte count. The thrombocytes resemble the erythrocytes in the hemocytometer, but they are smaller and appear to be round to oval with a greater nucleus:cytoplasm (N:C) ratio compared to the erythrocytes. All squares in the central large square of a Neubauer-ruled hemocytometer are counted on both sides, and the average number of thrombocytes in one large square is calculated and multiplied by 2000 to obtain the total thrombocyte count per microliter. Accurate counts may be difficult to achieve, however, because thrombocytes tend to clump (Table 23.4).

Responses in disease

Functionally, thrombocytes are equivalent to mammalian platelets and they participate in coagulation. Immature forms of thrombocytes (round cells with round nuclei) are not normally found in the peripheral blood of amphibians; therefore, their presence suggests either a regenerative response or dyscrasia. Developing thrombocytes include thromboblasts, prothrombocytes, and immature thrombocytes. Thromboblasts are round to oval with weakly basophilic cytoplasm and a round to oval nucleus that contains fine nuclear chromatin and a large, irregular, eccentric nucleolus. Prothrombocytes have elongate nuclei and vacuolated cytoplasm with pale blue granules. Immature thrombocytes resemble those described in avian hematology. They are intermediate in size between thromboblasts and mature thrombocytes and appear as round to oval cells containing more abundant cytoplasm than the thromboblasts. The color of the cytoplasm of immature thrombocytes varies with cell development, and changes from a basophilic color in the early developing cells to a pale blue or colorless cytoplasm in the later stages. These cells may contain cytoplasmic vacuoles. The nuclear chromatin of the earlier immature thrombocytes is aggregated into irregular clumps that become more densely packed as the cell matures. Low and high thrombocyte counts are interpreted in the same manner as those described for other nonmammalian vertebrates, such as birds (see Chapter 20).

Blood parasites

Wet-mount evaluation of a whole blood sample may be utilized as a means to detect the movement of common extracellular blood parasites such as trypanosomes and microfilaria in amphibian blood. Common differentials for amphibian intraerythrocytic inclusions found on Romanowsky-stained blood films include hemogregarines, such as those described in reptiles (see Chapter 21on hematology of reptiles), *Aegyptianella* spp., and a *Pirohemocyton*-like

Table 23.4 Thrombocyte counts for selected amphibians.

	African clawed frog[a]	Edible frog[a]	Fire-bellied toad (male)[b]	Fire-bellied toad (female)[b]	Grass frog[a]
Thrombocytes $\times 10^3/\mu L$	17.7	16.3	2.76–10.69	1.43–19.47	20.8

[a]Wright KM. Amphibians. In: *Exotic Animal* Formulary, 3rd ed., J. Carpenter (ed.). St. Louis, MO: Elsevier Saunders, p. 46. 2005.
[b]Wojtaszek J, Adamowicz A. Haematology of the fire-bellied toad, *Bombina bombina. L. Comp Clin Path* 12: 129–34. 2003.

virus. *Lankesterella* spp. may also be found within the cytoplasm of lymphocytes. *Toxoplasma, Isospora,* and *Leptotheca* are also found on occasion. In general, these organisms are considered to be an incidental finding; however, they may be pathogenic when they are found in the blood of anemic patients, suggesting a possible etiology for the anemia.

Hematopoiesis

Development of the amphibian erythrocyte is similar to that described for other vertebrates with nucleated erythrocytes. Maturation of the rubriblast to the mature erythrocyte involves a progressive change of cytoplasmic basophilia to eosinophilia, a change from round to an elongated shape, a decrease in the nuclear and nucleolar size, and an increased chromatin density.

The liver is the predominant erythropoietic tissue of both larval and adult frogs. Larval amphibians may have two populations of morphologically different erythrocytes, which have different origins. One population, originating in the liver, has a centrally positioned nucleus; the other, originating in the kidney, has a peripherally located nucleus. The different erythrocyte populations also have different larval hemoglobins. During metamorphosis, a third population of erythrocytes appears, and this population persists in adults. Dark-field illumination can be used to differentiate larval erythrocytes, which have a white to gray, granular luminescence, from adult erythrocytes, which lack luminescence.

The metamorphosis from larval to adult amphibians is accompanied by the synthesis of hemoglobins with different oxygen affinities and various intracellular modulators of hemoglobin–oxygen affinity. Gilled larval amphibians have blood with a higher affinity for oxygen than that of air-breathing adults. The tetrameric hemoglobin of amphibians consists of two α-like and two β-like globin chains, thereby creating four larval-type and four adult-type hemoglobins. No globin chains are shared between larval and adult amphibians. Adult hemoglobin begins to appear in frogs during tail regression, and it is the only hemoglobin found 3 weeks after metamorphosis. Adult amphibians have higher hemoglobin concentrations and PCVs compared with the larval forms. Metamorphosis results in decreases in adenosine triphosphate (ATP) and guanosine triphosphate concentrations in the erythrocytes, thus suggesting a change in the phosphate regulation of hemoglobin in adults compared with larval forms.

Metamorphosis in newts and salamanders is not always associated with a transition in hemoglobin such as that occurring in frogs and toads. When newts and salamanders change from aquatic to aerobic respiration at metamorphosis, the larval and adult hemoglobins have the same affinity for oxygen. The reduced oxygen affinity of the blood in adults, however, frequently is achieved by an increased erythrocyte concentration of ATP. Even so, some species, such as the tiger salamander (*Ambystoma tigrinum*), experience no decrease in the oxygen affinity of blood at metamorphosis, and the hemoglobin and total erythrocytic organic phosphate concentrations remain unchanged.

Toads, which primarily rely on aerobic respiration, tend to have higher hemoglobin and erythrocyte phosphate concentrations and a lower blood oxygen affinity compared with frogs, which primarily rely on anaerobic respiration. Aquatic amphibians do not have the same association between high erythrocyte phosphate concentrations and dependence on aerobic production of energy for activity as terrestrial amphibians do. The exchange of gases from the blood to the surrounding water occurs through the skin of aquatic amphibians.

IV

Clinical Chemistry of Common Domestic Species

24 Laboratory Evaluation and Interpretation of the Urinary System

Donald Meuten[1] and Saundra Sample[2]

[1]North Carolina State University, Raleigh, NC, USA
[2]University of Missouri College of Veterinary Medicine, Columbia, MO, USA

Introduction

Diseases of the urinary system are common in all animal species, and clinical pathology is an essential tool for evaluation of the urinary system. The primary reasons for assessing the urinary system are to recognize renal failure or diseases in the urinary bladder, or as part of an annual health check. Laboratory abnormalities that indicate renal failure will not appear until so many nephrons are damaged that the remaining nephrons can no longer compensate for the damaged ones. Once identified, renal failure is then categorized as acute or chronic. This identification is further narrowed down to the renal structure that is diseased, and sometimes a specific diagnosis. For example, the disease may be centered on the glomeruli (glomerulonephritis or amyloidosis), tubules (nephrosis), interstitium (interstitial nephritis), renal pelvis (pyelonephritis), or excretory system (cystitis, obstruction, or rupture). Chronic kidney disease (CKD) is further classified into stages defined by the International Renal Interest Society (IRIS) that are based on severity of disease. There are multiple causes of CKD, and it is difficult to identify the initiating insult. Identification of a cause is not needed for patient management. A relatively common and somewhat confusing term is "acute on chronic kidney disease." This implies a disease process where underlying CKD has acutely exacerbated. Often this is due to acute dehydration. Occasionally acute on CKD occurs when the chronic disease has progressed or a second disease process is superimposed on the first (e.g., an ascending infection from the lower urinary tract damages an already diseased kidney).

The most accurate way to identify or monitor renal failure is to directly measure glomerular filtration rate (GFR); however, in veterinary medicine this is rarely done. Instead, we use indirect evidence to estimate reductions in GFR, and from this to imply that renal failure is present. Laboratory analyses of the serum biochemical profile, complete blood count (CBC), and complete urinalysis (UA) are more practical means to assess renal function and are performed daily in veterinary hospitals. If a more precise assessment of renal function is desired, then GFR can be measured by clearance studies.

There are many ways to recognize failure of the urinary system based on the history, biochemical profile, and evaluation of urine. These include identification of anuria, polyuria, azotemia, uremia, electrolyte abnormalities, hypoalbuminemia, inappropriate urine specific gravity (USG), casts, cystitis, and hematuria, to list a few (see definitions). When renal failure is severe, the clinical recognition is easy. When failure is mild and/or the disease is in the earliest stages, then recognition can be difficult and may require ancillary diagnostic tests such as creatinine clearance, fractional excretion of sodium, assessment of proteinuria, or ultrasonography. These ancillary tests are also useful to monitor the patient's response to treatments.

Understanding the physiology of the kidney makes the understanding of clinical pathology simple. If structures are damaged, then functions are lost, and if the remaining nephrons cannot compensate a clinical laboratory or physical examination finding will generally be obvious. For example, glomeruli exclude albumin from the ultrafiltrate; if glomerulonephrhitis is present, then this exclusionary function is lost. If the disease is severe enough and the remaining nephrons cannot compensate, there will be proteinuria, hypoalbuminemia, and, potentially, ascites and dependent edema (nephrotic syndrome; Table 24.1).

Laboratory abnormalities may be nonexistent, mild, moderate, or marked depending on severity and chronicity of disease as well as any treatments that have been undertaken to slow disease progression. Guidelines for the staging and management of chronic renal disease have been developed by IRIS and are based on severity of clinical signs, physical examination findings, and laboratory

Veterinary Hematology, Clinical Chemistry, and Cytology, Third Edition. Edited by Mary Anna Thrall, Glade Weiser, Robin W. Allison and Terry W. Campbell.

Companion website: www.wiley.com/go/thrall/veterinary

Table 24.1 The concentration of certain substances measured in serum or plasma is affected by renal function.

Substance	Function lost	Abnormality
UN Ct	Excretion	Azotemia
Water	Balance	Polyuria, anuria, oliguria
P	Excrete	Hyperphosphatemia
Na Cl	Conserve	Normo- to hyponatremia, hypochloremia
K	Excrete	Hyperkalemia
Ca	Conserve	Hypocalcemia
Acid base	Balance	Acidosis metabolic; alkalosis cow
Albumin	Conserve	Proteinuria, hypoalbuminemia, ascites
Erythropoietin	Produce	Anemia, nonregenerative
Vitamin D	Produce	Hypocalcemia, osteodystrophy
Lipase, amylase	Excrete	Increased one- to threefold
Antithrombin III	Conserve	Decreased AT III, thrombi

Damage to specific renal structures results in damage to renal function. The abnormalities listed are generalizations and not constants. Their presence will depend on the severity of the lesion, chronicity, treatments, and compensatory ability of surviving nephrons.

abnormalities. The stage of the renal disease correlates with the severity of the renal lesions and reflects prognosis. As the stage of the renal disease progresses, so does the severity of the laboratory abnormalities. Laboratory abnormalities will not appear until enough nephrons are impaired and the remaining nephrons cannot compensate. Two classic examples are isosthenuria and azotemia. Isosthenuria occurs when approximately 66% of nephrons are not functioning properly. Azotemia is not seen until approximately 75% of nephrons are compromised. Bear in mind that analytes are not meant to be interpreted in isolation but rather must be carefully considered with the patient's clinical signs, physical exam findings, and complete laboratory data.

This chapter will follow the functions of the urinary system, predict clinical pathology results and diagnoses, and provide case examples. The emphasis is on interpretation of laboratory data with less focus on methodology, which is covered exhaustively in other excellent resources. The chapter is organized by evaluation of renal function, urinalysis, diseases of the urinary system, definitions, and glossary of terms. Students learning this body of information for the first time should consider reading the definitions and glossary first. A glossary of terms is at the end of chapter.

Laboratory evaluation of renal function: bloodwork

GFR is the volume of plasma filtered at the glomerular capillaries into Bowman's space per unit of time. It is the best predictor of renal function because it is directly related to total functional renal mass or, in other words, to the number of functioning nephrons. It is dependent on adequate blood flow to the kidneys, blood pressure, interstitial, and intratubular pressures, as well as number of functioning nephrons. A GFR of 3–6 mL/min/kg is normal for a dog and 2–4 mL/min/kg is normal for a cat. A decrease in GFR indicates decreased renal function. GFR can be used to stage renal disease and monitor the progression of renal disease. It is not easy to measure GFR directly, but it can be measured by studies that use substances that are freely filtered by the glomerulus and that are neither secreted nor reabsorbed, such as inulin, iohexol, mannitol, *p*-amminohippuric acid, and exogenous creatinine. GFR can also be estimated by endogenous creatinine clearance studies. The methodologies of these and other tests can be found in many other resources.

Because of the complexity of direct GFR measurement studies, it is seldom measured in veterinary medicine. Instead, indirect evidence of decreased GFR is derived from serum urea nitrogen concentration (UN), creatinine concentration (Ct), symmetric dimethylarginine concentration (SDMA), and phosphorus concentration (P). Additional data are derived from serum calcium concentration (Ca), electrolytes (sodium, potassium, chloride), the complete urinalysis, and/or urinary protein and creatinine clearance, as well as the fractional excretion of sodium.

A decreasing GFR is the best indicator of renal insufficiency, and because UN and Ct are freely filtered by the glomerulus, they are the analytes traditionally used to estimate GFR (Figure 24.1). As the GFR decreases, plasma UN and Ct concentrations increase; however, renal mass must be reduced 75% before UN and Ct concentrations increase in blood plasma. Because azotemia is not evident until 75% of nephrons are no longer functioning adequately, and because the ability to concentrate urine is lost after 66% of nephrons are compromised, azotemia and dilute urine or polyuria caused by renal failure are not detected until a large portion of the total renal mass is compromised. Therefore, they are not early indicators of renal failure. These percentages indicate the tremendous reserve of renal function, because only 25% of total renal mass is needed to excrete sufficient nitrogenous waste to prevent azotemia, and only 33% is needed to concentrate urine and preserve the body's fluid volume.

It should be noted that no serum biochemical abnormalities indicate irreversibility of renal damage, for, while glomeruli have no regenerative capabilities, tubules have tremendous regenerative capacity if basement membranes are preserved. If glomeruli and tubules sustain severe damage, the remaining nephrons compensate by hypertrophy, especially in CKD. Therefore, when azotemia is detected, the total nephron mass not functioning adequately may actually be greater than 75%. The remaining nephrons compensate and maintain the overall GFR such that serum UN and Ct stay within the reference interval (WRI), delaying azotemia until more nephrons are lost. For example, if a dog with normal serum Ct of 0.5 mg/dL developed renal disease such that serum Ct increased to 1.0 mg/dL, then theoretically 50% of its nephrons are now not functioning properly. However, because that value of serum Ct concentration is still WRI, that 50% loss of function would not be detected by measuring Ct or UN concentrations because the renal reserve, or compensation via hypertrophy of remaining nephrons, would work to maintain serum Ct WRI of a "normal" dog. However, and very importantly, once Ct is increased above the upper reference interval, then every doubling of serum Ct indicates a loss of function of 50% of the remaining renal mass. Conversely, the recovery of nephrons from an insult can be monitored, for every 50% reduction in serum Ct or UN indicates that 50% of the nephrons have returned to function. This is because there is a logarithmic relationship of serum Ct to GFR (Figure 24.1). It is this principle that allows us to monitor progression of renal disease through measurement of serum Ct, once the upper limit of the reference interval has been surpassed. The great amount of renal functional reserve sometimes requires more sophisticated methods to determine if renal disease is present when serum Ct is not increased, e.g., the tests of endogenous or exogenous creatinine clearance, inulin clearance, clearance of radioisotopes, SDMA, and assessment of fractional excretion of electrolytes, etc.

It should be noted that serum Ct is a better indicator of GFR than serum UN because its rates of production and excretion are fairly constant, and extrarenal or renal processes do not metabolize it. In contrast, serum UN is influenced by more nonrenal factors than is Ct, and a significant proportion of UN excreted into the glomerular filtrate is reabsorbed (approximately 66%). Furthermore, the rate of reabsorption of UN varies with the hydration status of the animal as well as the speed of flow of the glomerular filtrate within the tubules.

Serum Ct WRI does not mean the kidneys are normal, it means that 25% of the renal mass is functioning adequately enough to excrete creatinine and keep it WRI. An endogenous creatinine clearance study is a better indicator of renal function than serum Ct or UN. Endogenous Ct clearance can be used to estimate GFR because the production of Ct is relatively constant, and essentially 100% is excreted via the kidneys (the small amount that is secreted by proximal tubules is negligible for this estimation). Creatinine clearance is useful when renal disease is suspected but the serum concentrations of Ct and UN are not increased. Creatinine clearance can be calculated from the Ct, urine Ct, the volume of urine produced in a defined period, and the weight of the patient.

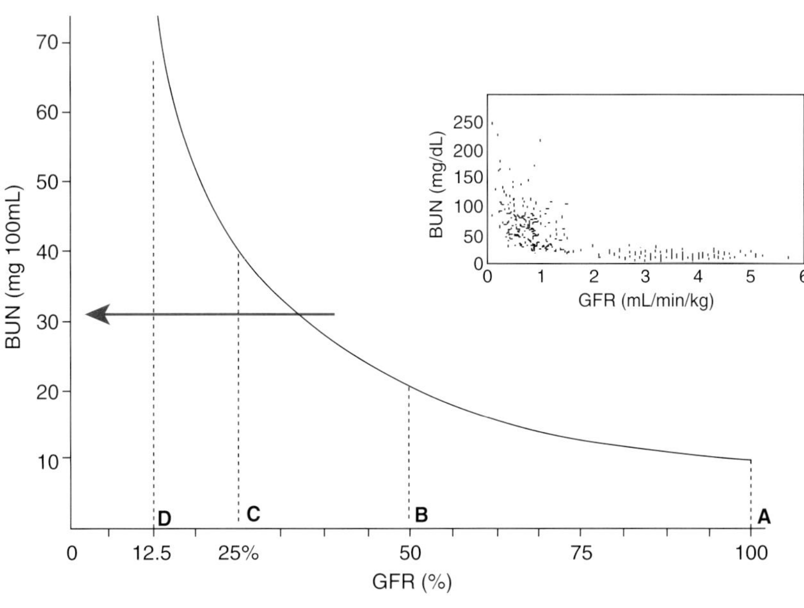

Figure 24.1 Glomerular filtration rate (GFR) as mL/min/kg body weight (inset) and as % functioning nephron units. A GFR of 3–6 mL/min/kg is normal for dogs and the BUN is less than 30 mg/dL, and as GFR decreases the BUN increases (inset). In the example provided, (A) correlates with 100% functional nephron units and a BUN of approximately 12 mg/dL. When 50% of the nephron units are compromised (GFR decreased 50%) the BUN has doubled to approximately 24 mg/dL, but it is still in reference interval (occult renal issues). Not until approximately 75% of the nephron units are compromised (GFR is now 25% of normal) is the dog azotemic (C). Therefore, BUN and serum creatinine (Ct) are poor indicators of early renal insufficiency. If the GFR is decreased by half again (D) by advancing renal disease, then a rule of thumb is the BUN and Ct will double. Likewise, a decrease in BUN and Ct by half indicates the GFR has doubled, meaning there is improvement in renal function, e.g., more nephrons are functioning. Monitoring BUN or Ct to assess deterioration or improvement of renal function can be done only after they are increased, but GFR can be used to monitor patients with renal insufficiency at any time.

Case Example 24.1. 40 kg dog with normal serum Ct and reduced Ct clearance

Canine creatinine clearance reference interval is 3–6 mL/min/kg. Serum Ct 1.0 mg/dL; over 1 hour, patient produces 30 mLs of urine with a urine Ct of 200 mg/dL.

The dog has reduced Ct clearance not reflected by the serum Ct, which is WRI. This may be seen in post-treatment of renal failure when serum Ct has returned to the reference interval. The patient feels better but there is still compromised renal function (e.g., some renal lesions may persist, such as interstitial fibrosis). These patients will benefit from dietary changes and ad libitum access to water. This might be predicted from clinical experience, but it would not be known without assessment of urinary creatinine clearance. In a 24-hour study of endogenous creatinine clearance, the urinary bladder is emptied of urine at the start of the study, the volume of urine produced in 24 hours is measured, and a serum sample is collected usually in the middle or at the end of the study.

The urinary bladder is completely emptied of urine at the start of the study, and the volume of urine produced in the duration of the study is measured.

Endogenous creatinine clearance can also be used in the diagnostic evaluation of a patient in which occult renal disease is suspected. This patient is not azotemic but has polyuria, polydipsia, and dilute urine. This situation may be observed when functional renal mass is reduced to between 66% and 75%. If more accurate assessment of renal function is desired, then clearance of exogenous creatinine, inulin, or iohexol can be performed as well as injected radioisotopes or renal scintigraphy. These studies are usually only performed in specialty hospitals and when the clinician and owner want the patient monitored closely.

Biological markers of the glomerular filtration rate

Urea nitrogen (UN)

The serum urea nitrogen and creatinine concentrations should always be correlated with the urine specific gravity and clinical findings; calculate the UN/Ct ratio.

The term "blood urea nitrogen" (BUN) is no longer a relevant term because of changes in measurement methodology. Originally, a urease method released nitrogen from urea and the amount of nitrogen was measured, i.e., BUN. Now urea is measured from the release of ammonium ions via urease. "Urea" is not a substance defined by the International Clinical Chemistry Federation, rather they use the term "carbamide." It has been difficult to switch clinicians from BUN to UN, and impossible to force the acceptance of carbamide, so throughout this chapter, the term UN will be used.

Urea is a 60 Da molecule produced in the liver. It is derived from proteins (amino acids) absorbed through the intestines and catabolized by the liver into ammonium. Likewise, the rate of urea production is dependent upon two factors, liver function and the amount of protein in the diet. Urea is the main method of nitrogen excretion in animals. UN is freely filtered by glomeruli, and approximately 50% is reabsorbed passively by the proximal tubules, with ~10% being actively reabsorbed by the collecting tubules. The amount of urea reabsorbed varies with the rate of flow through the tubules. For example, during dehydration, the tubular flow rate slows, and more UN is reabsorbed through the tubules, increasing serum UN. A portion of urea is also excreted via salivary glands into the gastrointestinal (GI) tract, where it is degraded by bacteria into ammonium. Ammonium is then absorbed and converted back into urea by the liver. Thus, there is no net excretion of UN via the gastrointestinal system in most species.

All species can excrete UN through their salivary glands. However, only ruminants and horses have unique microflora that convert the UN into amino acids. The amino acids are then reabsorbed, leading to a net excretion of UN. This is the logic of feeding cattle liquid urea as a source of protein. Cattle are so efficient with this mechanism that it may take up to 1 week post–bilateral nephrectomy before serum UN increases. Cattle on a nitrogen-deficient diet or those that are severely anorectic will excrete the majority of their UN via the GI tract. This makes it is especially critical in ruminants to rely on Ct and USG to predict renal disease. Horses are not as efficient at converting UN into amino acids with the microflora in their cecum and colon but can accomplish some net excretion of UN (case examples are found later in this chapter). Thus, in horses, serum UN is used in the assessment of renal function along with Ct and USG.

Because serum UN is dependent upon both production and excretion of UN, there are multiple factors that may contribute to changes in serum UN besides renal disease. Increases in serum UN may be due to increased dietary protein; intestinal hemorrhage (hemoglobin in blood is a very high concentration of protein); sepsis and fasting, which increase protein catabolism; decreased renal perfusion (favors increased tubular reabsorption); and most importantly, renal disease. For example, normal dogs fed a high-protein meal may have a slight increase in their serum UN peaking at 6 hours and lasting up to 18 hours. The protein is broken down in the GI tract and the ammonium produced is reabsorbed and converted into UN by the liver. This is the principle of feeding reduced-protein diets to patients in renal failure. These patients may benefit from a low-protein diet that results in less UN production and therefore reduces some of the work performed by the kidneys. All nonrenal causes of increased serum UN cause only a mild increase, usually less than 30–35 mg/dL.

Decreased serum UN is uncommon. A decreased serum UN implies decreased production of urea. Conditions that may decrease UN production are intra- or extrahepatic shunts, chronic liver failure, malnutrition, hyperthyroidism (increased catabolism and increased GFR; hyperthyroidism may also decrease Ct due to cachexia), and diuresis. Hepatic shunts are probably the most common cause of decreased serum UN. If a shunt or chronic liver failure causes a decrease in serum UN, there will be other clinical and laboratory abnormalities suggestive of these problems, e.g., decreased mean cell volume, albumin, glucose, cholesterol, ammonium biurate crystals in the urine, to name a few.

Serum reagent strips that use urease to estimate serum UN are less accurate than strips that assay the release of ammonia, which is a semiquantitative determination. These methods are somewhat useful for broadly estimating "normal" or "increased" serum UN in after-hours situations but are not reliable for patient monitoring over time. They are good at identifying low or normal values and are not adequate to quantify abnormally high values. If the strip indicates that a patient is azotemic, then it would be preferable to determine serum UN via quantitative chemical methodology prior to fluid therapy. If serum strips are used to assess uroabdomen, then the measurement difference between abdominal fluid and serum should be definitive, and it is recommended that results be confirmed with quantitation of UN or Ct in fluid and serum (refer to the "Uroabdomen" section). As in any case, all of the pieces of data should be integrated. Reagent strips are a benefit for after-hours estimations but should not replace chemical measurement of urea, UN.

Creatinine (Ct)

Creatinine (from the Greek word for flesh *kreas*) is a waste product of creatine and creatine phosphate found in muscle. It is a ring structure with a molecular weight of 113 Da. Creatine is produced in the liver with a minor role from the pancreas, transported to skeletal muscle, where 95% of the total body creatine is located. In skeletal muscle, creatine is converted into creatine phosphate via the enzyme creatine kinase. Creatine phosphate serves as an energy store for production of adenosine triphophate (ATP) and, along with creatine, is spontaneously degraded in muscles to creatinine. Creatinine production is relatively constant (1–2%/d) and is roughly proportional to muscle mass. Creatinine has no charge and freely passes out of muscle cells. The majority of circulating Ct is filtered freely through the glomeruli and not resorbed by the tubules. It is generally considered a reliable marker of GFR. As an aside, a small amount of Ct is secreted by the proximal tubules of male dogs, but this is clinically inconsequential; cats and ponies do not secrete or reabsorb Ct in their kidneys.

Increases in serum Ct may be due to either physiologic or pathologic etiologies, and the most important is renal disease. Physiologic minimal increases are frequently associated with heavily muscled animals. For example, greyhounds have a higher serum Ct than the average dog. Factors that increase endogenous muscle catabolism such as sepsis, developing cachexia, can increase the release of creatine and, hence, the quantity of creatinine that is produced. However, these increases are mild and rarely interfere with clinical interpretation. Increases in serum Ct may also be observed in neonatal foals born to dams with dysfunctional placentas. The excess Ct typically resolves the first few days after birth. Pathologic causes of increased serum Ct are almost exclusively associated with decreased GFR. These differentials are discussed in detail below (see "Azotemia").

Decreased serum Ct or at least decreased synthesis of Ct is seen with conditions that decrease muscle mass such as chronic cachexia. It is occasionally observed in feline hyperthyroidism as patients with this condition develop an increased GFR. Hyperthyroidism may mask the development of azotemia in geriatric cats with concurrent chronic renal disease [1]. A decrease is observed rarely with chronic liver failure. Otherwise, decreased serum Ct is not considered clinically significant and has no meaningful interpretation.

Creatinine is measured spectrophotometrically, and any chromogenic substance (or noncreatinine chromogen) will also be measured, resulting in a false increase in the measured serum Ct. The most common noncreatinine chromogens are ketones, glucose, carotenes, and vitamin A (substances that tend to be higher in herbivores) as well as pyruvate, ascorbic acid, and uric acid (Table 24.2). The Jaffé reagent is used most frequently in veterinary laboratories to measure creatinine, and it reacts with many noncreatinine chromogens. At normal concentrations of serum Ct, noncreatinine chromogens can contribute up to 50% of the measured serum Ct. There are several situations where these noncreatinine chromogens contribute to the measured Ct such that they will interfere with clinical interpretation. Cattle and horses occasionally have disproportionate increases in serum Ct as compared to UN, and this may be due to an increase in noncreatinine chromogens that falsely increase serum Ct.

Table 24.2 Nonrenal factors that increase serum UN and Ct.

Both	UN	Ct
Dehydration	GI hemorrhage	Noncreatinine chromogens
Hypovolemia		Oxyglobin
Shock		Glucose
		Ketones
		Carotenes
		Uric acid
		Vitamins A and C

Protein-rich meals, fever, sepsis, and anorexia are listed as factors that will increase serum UN. While sepsis and developing cachexia can lead to increased release of creatine and increased creatinine production, these increases tend to be mild and do not interfere with clinical interpretation.

This is seen with some regularity in horses with colic. In horses, when Ct is disproportionately higher than UN, such that the serum UN:Ct ratio is 5 or less, then noncreatinine chromogens are a likely cause. This is particularly likely if UN is within or only mildly increased, above the RI, but Ct is clearly increased (3–6 mg/dL). The easiest way to determine if the increase in Ct is due to renal or nonrenal causes is to compare the USG and the serum UN. If the USG and the serum Ct are increased but UN is within the RI, then the horse has noncreatinine chromogens artifactually increasing the serum Ct. If the USG is increased and UN is increased, but Ct is disproportionately higher than the increase in UN, then the horse has prerenal azotemia and noncreatinine chromogens are contributing to the Ct measurement. If USG is isosthenuric and there is azotemia, then the animal has renal azotemia. This presents a clinical dilemma, which is compounded when the UN is not increased as much as the Ct due to the enteric excretion of UN in horses and cattle.

In small animals, false-high Ct is seen almost exclusively with artificial transfusates such as oxyglobin products. The serum Ct can be increased as high as 20 mg/dL, but serum UN will remain WRI. In addition to other analytes, these animals will have falsely increased serum hepatic enzymes, and the serum may be yellow-orange, depending on the dose of artificial transfusate administered as well as the cause of the anemia.

Azotemia

A major function of the urinary system is to excrete UN and Ct. When this function is lost, serum concentrations of UN and Ct increase – a condition termed azotemia. Traditionally, azotemia is the single best laboratory abnormality that indicates problems in the urinary system. When UN and Ct are not excreted in adequate amounts, their concentration increases in serum (azotemia), and this may lead to the clinical signs of urinary toxin accumulation in the patient, known as uremia. Both UN and Ct are reported in the biochemical profile, and an increased concentration of either implies a decreased GFR. Neither substance increases until approximately 75% of nephrons are nonfunctional. In fact, this percentage is probably closer to 80–90%. The remaining nephrons compensate by hypertrophy, especially in CKD. Therefore, when azotemia is detected, the total nephron mass not functioning adequately may actually be greater than 75%. The remaining nephrons compensate and maintain the overall GFR such that serum UN and Ct stay WRI, delaying azotemia until more nephrons are lost. Because serum UN and Ct do not increase until 75% of the nephrons are compromised, they are not useful in the detection of early renal failure, i.e., they are insensitive indicators of lower levels of renal dysfunction. However, they are fairly specific as relatively few nonrenal factors cause their increase. Table 24.2 lists nonrenal factors that increase these substances. The most common causes are dehydration (hypovolemia) and GI hemorrhage.

Once azotemia is identified, the next step is to determine if the cause is prerenal, renal, or postrenal. It is important to remember that categorizing the azotemia should not be done in isolation. Rather, findings from the urinalysis (USG, urine volume) and clinical presentation (dehydrated?) are important considerations in obtaining an accurate diagnosis. The magnitude of azotemia also factors in to the clinical assessment. Mild azotemia is characterized by a serum Ct (in mg/dL) of 1.5–2.0 in the dog, 1.6–3.0 in the cat; moderate azotemia, 2.1–5.0 dogs, 3.0–5.0 cats; and severe azotemia is >5.0 in both the dog and cat. Extreme values >10.0 may be observed when hypovolemia (e.g., dehydration) is superimposed on renal or postrenal causes of azotemia. The magnitude of serum UN or Ct does not predict a prerenal, renal, or postrenal cause of azotemia. In general, if serum Ct is your shoe size or greater, your patient has marked azotemia, but it could be reversible.

The UN:Ct Ratio

Urine Ct:serum Ct ratios can be used to distinguish renal and prerenal azotemias. The ratio of serum UN:Ct in small animals is approximately 20 : 1 and in large animals 10 : 1. An increased ratio is associated with dehydration or intestinal bleeding. A decreased ratio is associated with fluid diuresis, the presence of noncreatinine chromogens, or the unique ability of cows and horses to metabolize and excrete UN through their gastrointestinal tracts. Ratios >50 : 1 indicate prerenal azotemia and ratios <37 : 1 indicate renal azotemia.

Prerenal Azotemia

Prerenal azotemia describes etiologies that contribute to a decreased GFR that occurs outside of the urinary tract. The primary mechanism of prerenal azotemia is failure to deliver blood to the kidneys. This is most commonly associated with dehydration, shock, and cardiac insufficiency of which dehydration is the most common cause. Azotemia occurs because there is continual basal production of UN and Ct in the face of a decreased GFR. The decreased GFR results from the decreased blood volume causing inadequate blood flow to glomeruli. Characteristic findings in bloodwork and urinalysis include an increased serum UN and Ct, concentrated USG, decreased urine volume, increased packed cell volume (PCV) and serum albumin, and clinical signs of dehydration (Figure 24.2).

In cases of prerenal azotemia (e.g., dehydration) urine production should decrease as the body attempts to conserve serum volume (water), thereby increasing the USG. Increases in the PCV and albumin further support a diagnosis of prerenal azotemia. The increases in UN and Ct observed with dehydration are usually mild to moderate (e.g., serum UN 35–120 mg/dL and Ct 2–5 mg/dL). UN to creatinine ratios of >50 : 1 usually indicate a prerenal azotemia. In cases of

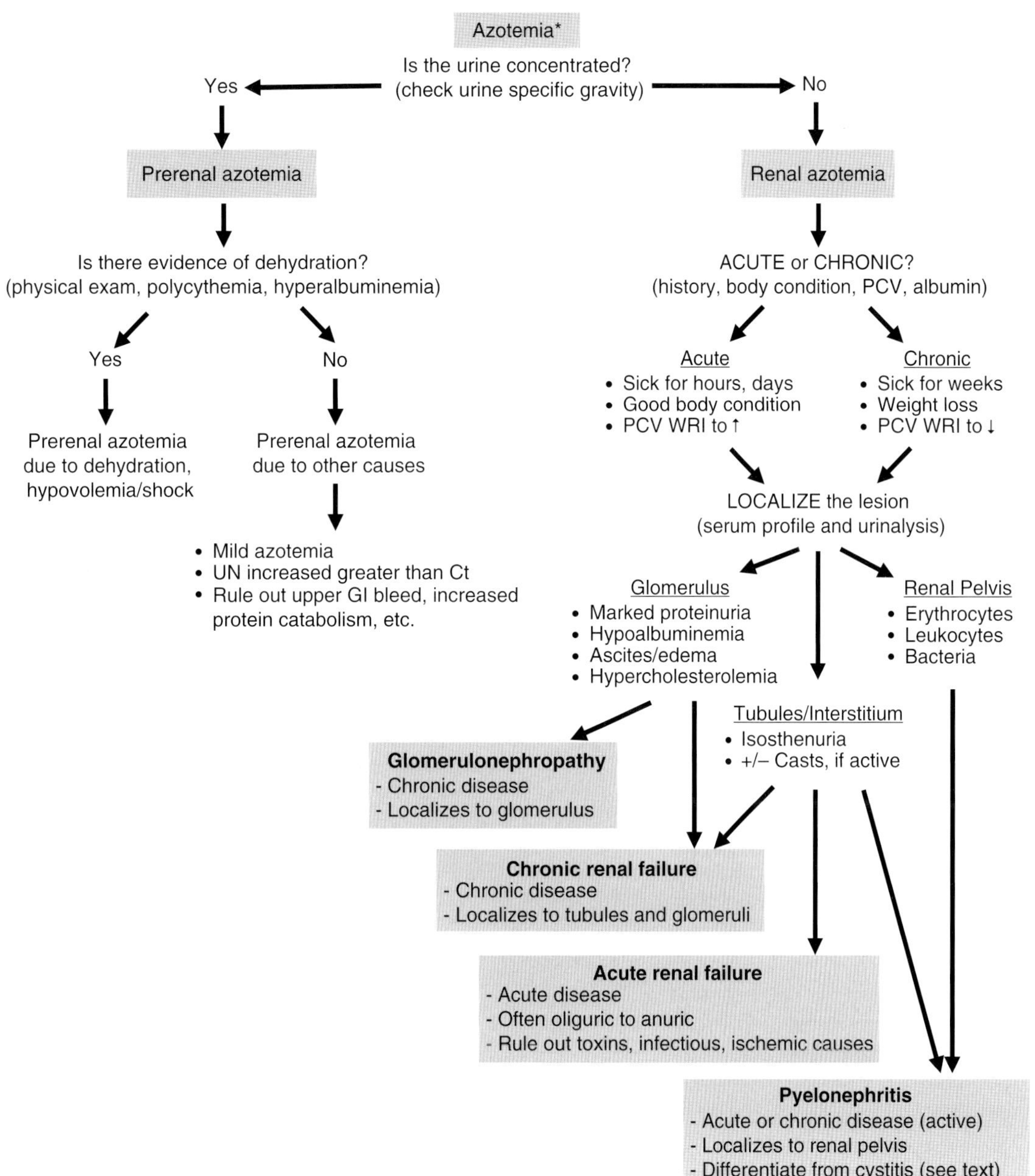

* Remember patients can have poorly concentrated urine and be dehydrated. Examples include: decreased ADH (e.g., diabetes insipidus), hypercalcemia, medullary washout (e.g., hypoadrenocorticism, hepatic shunt), excessive glucocorticoids (e.g., hyperadrenocorticism, exogenous), pyometra, osmotic diuresis (e.g., diabetes mellitus).

Figure 24.2 General approaches to azotemia in kidney disease. Correlate azotemia with USG, PCV, albumin, and hydration status to determine if azotemia is prerenal, renal, or a combination. Azotemia with concentrated urine is indicative of a prerenal azotemia. Urine is considered concentrated when the USG is >1.030 for a dog and >1.040 for a cat. As the USG increases, confidence in the kidney's ability to concentrate urine increases. Postrenal azotemia is due to obstruction of outflow (calculi) or rupture of the urinary bladder and is not part of this algorithm. Azotemia with urine that is not adequately concentrated (≤1.030 for a dog, ≤1.040 for a cat) suggests renal disease. It should be noted that azotemia is often exacerbated in clinically dehydrated patients, leading to a prerenal azotemia superimposed on a renal azotemia. Sometimes this is referred to as acute on chronic renal disease. In these cases, kidney disease is the primary differential. Once azotemia is identified to be caused by kidney disease, a patient's history, body condition, urine volume, PCV, and albumin are used to determine chronicity (acute injury vs. chronic disease). The lesion is then localized within the kidney (glomeruli, tubules, interstitium, pelvis) using the urinalysis and serum chemistry. There are other differentials for a patient with azotemia and unconcentrated urine. Differentials include decreased ADH (diabetes insipidus), substances that interfere with renal ADH receptors (hypercalcemia, glucocorticoids, bacterial endotoxin, etc.), medullary washout (hyponatremia secondary to hypoadrenocorticism, decreased UN in liver insufficiency, prolonged IV fluids therapy), or osmotic diuresis due to substances excreted in the urine with strong osmotic pull (glucose, ketones, mannitol, etc.). In these cases, the classical presentation is a mild azotemia with a USG <1.013. If there is no concurrent renal disease the azotemia is prerenal in origin, as patients are unable to keep up with water losses. Each of these differentials may also present with USG <1.013 and no azotemia (they are not dehydrated).

prerenal azotemia, the fractional excretion of sodium is <1% as the kidney attempts to retain sodium and thereby water.

Diagnosing a prerenal azotemia may be complicated as the classic pattern of a mild to moderate azotemia with decreased urine production and concentrated urine can vary with underlying disease. For example, the severity of the azotemia may be exaggerated if the dehydration is superimposed on a case of true renal failure. In these cases, the azotemia can be severe (e.g., UN >200 mg/dL, Ct >10 mg/dL). Fluid therapy may remove the prerenal contribution and decrease serum UN and Ct. The point at which these values plateau is the degree of azotemia that is due to the true renal insufficiency.

Additionally, a prerenal azotemia may be present in a disease process that prevents the concentration of urine. These include primary and secondary diabetes insipidus, hypercalcemia, steroids, pyometra, and medullary washout. Despite clinical dehydration, the kidneys cannot concentrate urine adequately because there is inadequate antidiuretic hormone (ADH), or a substance is interfering with ADH, or the renal medullary interstitium is no longer saturated with sodium and urea. Calcium interferes with the action of ADH and when hypercalcemia is present urine is often dilute, even if the animal is dehydrated and azotemic. Azotemia is present in 90% of dogs with hypoadrenocorticism (Addison's disease) due to dehydration, and a small percentage of these may have dilute urine because of chronic hyponatremia and resultant medullary washout. Because the constellation of laboratory and clinical signs associated with hypoadrenocorticism are similar to those caused by renal failure (namely, azotemia, inadequately concentrated urine [e.g., USG <1.020], anorexia, and vomiting), Addisonian dogs may be initially misdiagnosed. Fluid therapy will rapidly correct the azotemia in these dogs, and when fluid therapy reverses azotemia overnight or in hours, then true renal failure was not present.

Utilizing physical exam findings consistent with dehydration (tacky mucus membranes, skin tents, etc.) as well as other hematology and chemistry analytes (PCV, albumin) can assist in diagnosing prerenal azotemia in complicated cases. Bear in mind that if the PCV was decreased prior to onset of dehydration then the PCV may shift upward to WRI during dehydration, which may mask an underlying anemia.

GI hemorrhage will increase UN without increasing Ct. Blood in the GI tract is broken down, reabsorbed as amino acids and ammonia, delivered to the liver, and converted into UN for excretion by the kidneys. Hemorrhage does not have to be so severe as to cause anemia, and in fact, hemorrhage may be mild enough that it requires an occult blood test on feces to be certain it is present. Other "high-protein meals" may increase UN production postprandially, but they do not cause azotemia in healthy patients. The increase in UN is offset by a concurrent increase in GFR stimulated by the meal. The increase in Ct from the meat is so mild that the postprandial increase in GFR actually decreases the serum concentration of Ct within 2 hours of the meal. Excess muscle catabolism (e.g., starvation or fever) could increase the production of UN, but it rarely produces azotemia. If there is an increase it will be mild and will not interfere with clinical interpretation.

Case Example 24.2. 1-year-old small breed dog, poor growth, thin, and bizarre behavior (snapping at objects, not playful)

UN 5 mg/dL (RI 10–30), Ct 1.1 mg/dL (RI <1.5), UN:Ct ratio 45 : 1, USG 1.012, Serum albumin 1.8 g/dL (RI 2.6–3.9); liver enzymes are WRI (RI = reference interval, WRI = within reference interval)

Interpretation: Decreased UN and albumin in a young dog with possible central nervous system (CNS) disturbances (snapping at objects) and dilute urine is likely caused by congenital hepatic shunt and decreased synthesis of UN and albumin by the liver. Inability to concentrate urine is due to a renal medullary interstitium that never developed a high UN, resulting in an inability to produce concentrated urine (medullary washout). It would be a classical sign of congenital hepatic shunt if ammonium biurate crystals were observed in the urine. These crystals and ammonium biurate uroliths (green, green-brown [Figures 24.A.18 and 24.A.19]) are caused by the markedly elevated ammonia concentration in plasma, which, because it is freely filtered at the glomerulus, contributes to an ultrafiltrate that is both supersaturated with ammonia and alkaline in pH and leads to ammonia crystallization. Most cases of congenital liver shunts have no to only mild increases in serum liver enzymes and are not bilirubinemic. This is in contrast to most cases of acquired liver shunts, which have moderate to marked increases in liver enzymes and bilirubinemia because the severe liver lesion precedes the development of the shunt.

Renal azotemia

Renal azotemia describes failure within the kidneys and is caused by lesions in one of five locations: glomeruli, tubules, interstitium, renal pelvis, or blood vessels. Any renal disease that causes damage to greater than 75% of the nephrons and reduces GFR below 25% will decrease the excretion of UN and Ct. Azotemia with unconcentrated urine is of renal origin (Figure 24.2). The azotemia may be mild, moderate, or severe azotemia depending on the severity and distribution of the underlying pathology. Urine volume may also be variable (polyuria, oliguria, anuria). For example, in cases of acute severe renal failure, urine volume will be decreased (oliguria or anuria). In cases of CKD, urine production will be increased (polyuria). Patients with renal azotemia will have isosthenuric or possibly hyposthenuric urine.

Case Example 24.3. 11-year-old Labrador Retriever treated with NSAIDs for chronic arthritis

UN 78 mg/dL (RI 10–30), Ct 1.2 mg/dL (RI <1.5), UN:Ct ratio 65 : 1, USG 1.034

First interpretation: A disproportionate increase in UN relative to Ct coupled with a concentrated urine is most likely due to GI hemorrhage secondary to gastric erosions and ulcerations, related to NSAID use.

Further tests: Occult blood test on feces and/or suspension of NSAIDs and evaluation of hydration status.

Second interpretation: Dehydration resulting in increased renal retention of UN. However, because UN is increased and Ct is WRI, GI hemorrhage is more likely than dehydration. Evaluate hydration status.

Dehydration can increase UN without a commensurate increase in Ct, and the UN:Ct ratio may be high, i.e., >20 : 1. One hundred percent of creatinine excreted in the glomerular filtrate passes out in the urine. However, approximately 50% of UN excreted in glomerular filtrate is reabsorbed via the tubules. The amount reabsorbed is a function of health of the tubules and the flow rate of filtrate through the tubules. The slower the flow rate (dehydration), the greater the reabsorption of UN; up to 70% of urea may be reabsorbed versus the expected 50%. The faster the flow rate (diuresis), the lower the amount of UN reabsorption; perhaps only 40% or less is reabsorbed. Therefore, with dehydration UN increases more than Ct, and with diuresis UN decreases faster than Ct, and both of these situations may be seen clinically. The faster decrease in UN during fluid therapy is due to increased production of glomerular filtrate, leading to a faster transit time of fluid in tubules, and therefore reduced time to reabsorb UN.

Case Example 24.4. 9-year-old dog, 6% clinically dehydrated

UN 88 mg/dL (RI 10–30), Ct 2.8 mg/dL (RI <1.5), UN:Ct ratio 31 : 1, USG 1.058

Interpretation: Prerenal azotemia, as evidenced by a disproportionate increase of UN compared to Ct, with a highly concentrated urine and clinical signs of dehydration. Urea reabsorption is increased secondary to decreased flow of glomerular filtrate caused by the hypovolemia of dehydration. The PCV and albumin may also be increased if dehydration is severe enough and if neither PCV nor albumin were decreased below the lower reference interval prior to the onset of dehydration. If the dog was not anemic, then PCV may be increased; however, if the dog was anemic prior to the onset of dehydration, then the decrease in plasma volume may cause an increase in the PCV to WRI, thus masking the anemia.

Once renal failure is recognized, the next steps are to determine which region of the kidney is diseased and to determine whether the renal failure is acute or chronic (Table 24.3). This distinction is critical, because acute kidney injury (AKI) may be reversible whereas CKD is not.

Table 24.3 Expected results in acute versus chronic kidney disease.

	Acute	Chronic
PCV	WRI	Decreased
Albumin	WRI	Decreased
K	Increased, variable	Decreased
Urine volume	Anuria, oliguria	Polyuria, polydipsia
Body condition	Good	Poor
History	Sudden onset	Gradual deterioration
Size of kidneys	Normal to enlarged	Small, irregular contours

These are generalizations and there is a range of actual results and species variations. WRI, within the reference interval.

Characteristic features of AKI are variable but generally include a good body condition, sudden onset (the animal often being reported as "fine yesterday"), depression, lethargy, and decreased to absent urine output. Laboratory data will include PCV and albumin concentration WRI (or increased if dehydration is present) and increased potassium concentration.

The most common cause of AKI is nephrosis, meaning tubular degeneration and necrosis, which is most commonly caused by a nephrotoxin. Acute nephrosis will be reflected in the urinalysis by isosthenuria, numerous casts, mild proteinuria, mild glucosuria in the face of normal blood glucose concentration, and variable cellular abnormalities in the sediment. If the kidneys can be imaged or palpated, they will be normal sized or enlarged and have regular contours.

CKD can be the result of glomerular diseases as well as chronic interstitial nephritis, pyelonephritis, progressive familial nephropathy, and even bilateral staghorn calculi. In short, anything that can cause enough tissue damage may result in end-stage renal failure. Characteristic features of CKD are steady weight loss, mediocre to poor body

Case Example 24.5. Mixed-breed dog, 6% clinically dehydrated

Initial results: UN 120 mg/dL (RI 10–30), Ct 4.5 mg/dL (RI < 1.5), UN:Ct ratio 26 : 1, USG 1.062

Post-IV fluids: UN 34 mg/dL (RI 10–30), Ct 4.5 mg/dL (RI < 1.5), UN:Ct ratio 12 : 1, USG 1.008

Interpretation: Prerenal azotemia; disproportionate increase of UN to Ct with concentrated urine and clinical dehydration. Dog is still mildly azotemic post–fluid therapy and the decrease in UN is of greater magnitude (70% less) than the decrease in Ct (33%). Serum UN is almost WRI, and Ct is nearly twice the upper reference interval value. This is due to the increased flow of filtrate through the tubules caused by the fluid therapy, which allowed less time for UN and water to be reabsorbed, and, therefore, more UN and fluid remained in the plasma ultrafiltrate, allowing more to be excreted (polyuria). This led to a faster decrease in UN than Ct. During fluid diuresis the increased flow of fluid through the kidneys decreases the reabsorption of UN to <40%, and therefore BUN decreases faster than creatinine during fluid therapy.

Approximately 40–60% of the UN excreted in the glomerular filtrate is reabsorbed via the tubules by passive (proximal tubules) and active mechanisms (via ADH in collecting ducts). There are urea transporters (UT1, UT2, UT3) that are active in different regions of the tubules to accomplish urea reabsorption. The amount reabsorbed is a function of the health of tubules and the rate of flow in the glomerular filtrate. A portion of the UN remains in the interstitium, along with sodium and chloride, and contributes to the hypertonicity of medulla that is part of the countercurrent multiplier system. The degree of saturation in the interstitium is proportional to the concentration of UN, sodium, and chloride in the medulla, which makes it hypertonic compared to the fluid in the tubules, and this gradient is needed to help concentrate the glomerular filtrate as it is processed into urine. Urea and sodium are the two substances primarily responsible for the passive reabsorption of water from tubules in the descending limb of the loop of Henle. If a patient has prolonged decreases in plasma sodium or UN, it may result in decreased concentrations of either substance in the interstitium, leading to a decreased ability to reabsorb water passively and, therefore, to a decreased ability to concentrate urine. Hence, a dilute urine results that is noted clinically as polyuria. This combination of events that leads to decreased medullary tonicity is referred to as medullary washout. It is seen with hypoadrenocorticism (prolonged hyponatremia) and with prolonged decreased production of UN due to hepatic shunts (congenital or acquired) as well as severe chronic liver failure. Urea is synthesized in the liver, and chronic liver failure can result in decreased production and therefore decreased plasma UN. Single-digit UN combined with hypoalbuminemia and microcytosis may be subtle clues that indicate hepatic shunts.

Psychogenic polydipsia will wash out the medullary interstitium of UN and sodium via marked diuresis. resulting in hyposthenuria and polyuria/polydipsia (PU/PD).

condition, lethargy, polyuria, polydipsia, and laboratory data that include nonregenerative anemia, hypoalbuminemia, and hypocalcemia (the latter is uncommon in horses). Hypokalemia is often seen in cattle and cats. If the kidneys can be imaged, they will be small and have irregular contours, especially when the disease is fully developed.

To monitor these patients over time, practical parameters would include patient weight, water intake, urine volume, USG, and serum UN and Ct. If closer monitoring was desired, or if you wanted to more accurately determine the functional renal mass, then specialized studies such as exogenous or endogenous creatinine clearance, fractional excretion of sodium, microproteinuria, or ultrasonography could be offered or performed.

Postrenal azotemia

Postrenal azotemia is due to either obstruction of outflow occurring after the nephron or a rupture in the urinary outflow tract. Azotemia is present due to the continued production of UN and Ct and an inability to excrete UN and Ct from the body. In cases of urinary bladder or urethral rupture, there is additional reabsorption of UN and Ct from the abdomen or the subcutis. Postrenal azotemia is generally considered to produce the greatest and most rapid increases in serum creatinine but is not diagnostic. Urine production is decreased (oliguria) or absent (anuria), and the USG may be variable. The diagnosis of postrenal azotemia is made more from historical and physical examination findings than through laboratory evaluation and is dependent on determining that urine is not being excreted.

Most cases of postrenal azotemia are associated with urolithiasis in males due to their narrow urethra. On physical examination, the bladder will be enlarged on palpation if the obstruction is distal to the bladder. Urine obtained via cystocentesis in an obstructed animal is often red, and examination of the sediment reveals many red blood cells (RBCs) and inflammatory cells. Hyperkalemia can be severe (>8 mEq/L) and life-threatening, especially in male cats with a complete urethral obstruction. Blocked intact male cats can have rapid and marked increases of UN and Ct with Ct > 15 mg/dL. The azotemia decreases rapidly following relief of the obstruction.

In cats, sheep, goats, and cattle, uroabdomen is classically a disease of males due to their narrow urethra that is more easily obstructed than wider female urethra. As urine accumulates in the bladder, it distends and eventually ruptures. In horses, uroabdomen occurs in male foals <7 days old when the urinary bladder is ruptured during birth. In dogs, uroabdomen is frequently associated with trauma (e.g., hit by car), especially in males. On physical examination, the bladder is small and/or difficult to palpate, and a palpable abdominal fluid wave may be present. Azotemia is variable and is often associated with electrolyte derangements. Uroabdomen is confirmed by an abdominal fluid Ct > serum Ct and is discussed under diseases in this chapter.

In large animals, a disproportionate increase in serum Ct is seen most frequently in cases of equine colic and is attributed to an increase in chromogens other than creatinine. When Ct is disproportionately higher than UN, such that the serum UN:Ct ratio is 5 or less, then noncreatinine chromogens are a likely cause, especially in horses. This is particularly likely if UN is within or only mildly increased, above the RI, but Ct is clearly increased (3–6 mg/dL). The easiest way to determine if the increase in Ct is due to renal or nonrenal causes is to compare the USG and the serum UN. If the USG and the serum Ct are increased but UN is within the RI, then the horse has noncreatinine chromogens artifactually increasing the serum Ct. If the USG is increased and UN is increased but Ct is disproportionately higher than the increase in UN, then the horse has prerenal azotemia and noncreatinine chromogens are contributing to the Ct measurement. If USG is isosthenuric and there is azotemia, then the animal has renal azotemia. This presents a clinical dilemma, which is compounded when the UN is not increased as much as the Ct due to the enteric excretion of UN in horses and cattle.

Case Example 24.6. 10-year-old horse with colic, clinical signs of dehydration are equivocal

UN 35 mg/dL, Ct 5.1 mg/dL, UN:Ct ratio 7 : 1, urine not obtained

Interpretation: Disproportionate increase of Ct to UN due to noncreatinine chromogens and/or possible excretion of UN in gastrointestinal tract. A UN of 35 mg/dL is mild to insignificant; however, a Ct of 5.1 mg/dL is a moderate increase and is of concern. This is especially true if banamine and/or phenylbutazone are to be administered to alleviate pain and aid in the prevention of laminitis. NSAIDs are contraindicated if the horse is dehydrated, not drinking, or azotemic as the propensity for NSAIDs to cause medullary crest necrosis in the kidneys is enhanced in these situations. This is a practical clinical dilemma. If the increase in Ct is due to noncreatinine chromogens, then the horse would benefit from NSAIDs. However, prerenal azotemia may be present in this horse, so obtaining the USG *before* fluid therapy is the best means to determine if there is a renal contribution to the azotemia. Fractional excretion of sodium <1% would be definitive evidence of no renal involvement, whereas fractional excretion of sodium >1% indicates renal disease. In the latter case NSAIDs are contraindicated. If they occur, the renal lesions induced by NSAIDs in horses are usually mild. From a practical view, colic is much more common than renal failure in horses, and therefore odds are that the increase in Ct is due to noncreatinine chromogens.

Symmetric dimethylarginine (SDMA)

SDMA is a natural byproduct of intranuclear protein metabolism that is continually produced in the nucleus of cells and excreted in urine via GFR. Its small molecular weight (202 g/mmol) and positive electrical charge allow the molecule to be freely filtered by the glomerulus (net negative charge). SDMA is a strong marker of kidney function in humans [2] and is a component of a chemistry panel offered by IDEXX Laboratories. Approximately 90% of SDMA is eliminated by the kidneys [3]. SDMA serum concentration is inversely proportional to GFR [4–6] and is positively correlated to serum creatinine concentration [4–7]. SDMA has been shown to increase earlier in kidney disease than creatinine in both cats [4] and dogs [6], increasing as early as 40% reduction in GFR. It is considered a more specific indicator of renal disease because it is not affected by extrarenal factors such as lean body mass or GI bleeding [3, 8]. Thus, it is a useful marker for identifying renal disease in patients with muscle loss (e.g., hyperthyroid cats). SDMA is measured by liquid chromatography-mass spectroscopy [4] and has been validated as a clinically relevant and reliable indicator of kidney disease in dogs and cats using propriety technology [6].

As with all renal analytes, SDMA is not a standalone test. It needs to be interpreted with clinical findings, PCV, UN, Ct, and USG. If UN and Ct are increased in a patient with isosthenuria, there is no need to request SDMA. Serial Ct and USG can be monitored to follow the progression of renal disease or GFR clearance studies can be offered. If the concentration of SDMA (reported in μg/dL) is increased in the absence of definitive clinical signs or other laboratory evidence of kidney disease, rechecking SDMA and other clinical chemistry results in 2–4 weeks is suggested. At that time, if values are still increased, pursuing a full renal workup including urinalysis and culture, diagnostic imaging, etc. is warranted (Figure 24.3). Consider SDMA as a screening test for annual wellness checks, especially in geriatric patients or breeds that have familial renal diseases. Measurement of SDMA can be helpful in the evaluation of patients with PU/PD and concentrations of UN and Ct WRI. An increased SDMA at this time suggests that occult renal disease is likely. However, if SDMA is not increased, then other causes of inadequately concentrated urine are more likely (Table 24.4).

SDMA is still in the early stages of evaluation as a renal marker in veterinary medicine. It has been shown to successfully diagnose CKD in dogs and cats; however, it is

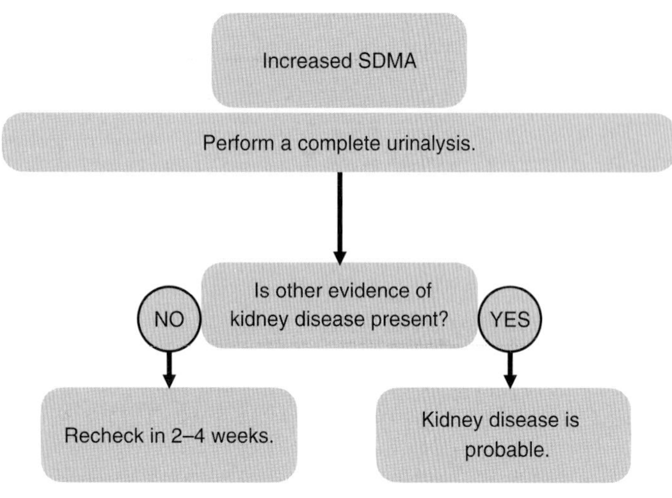

Figure 24.3 Algorithm for increased SDMA. SDMA is a relatively new test for the detection of occult renal disease; it increases in serum concentration earlier than traditional renal markers (isosthenuria, increased serum UN, Ct). SDMA is used as a screening test in animals at risk for renal disease (e.g., geriatric patients) or if early renal disease is suspected. It is a redundant test in azotemic patients.

Table 24.4 Causes of polyuria (polydipsia) and dilute urine.

Decreased ADH – central diabetes insipidus (DI)
Pituitary (hypothalamic rare) tumor, abscess, idiopathic, congenital
Inadequate response of tubular cells to adequate ADH – nephrogenic DI
Hypercalcemia, steroids, hypokalemia, pyometra, *E. coli* endotoxin, congenital lack of response of tubular cells to ADH
Decreased renal mass = lesions in kidneys, loss of tubular cells
With azotemia = >75% involvement; especially if lesions in medulla and pelvis
Without azotemia = 66–75% involvement of total renal mass
Excess fluid intake
Psychogenic polydipsia
Fluid overload diuresis
Medullary washout – medullary interstitium not saturated with sodium and urea
Addison's – prolonged hyponatremia
Liver failure – decreased urea nitrogen (other laboratory data will also support); congenital and acquired shunts; end-stage liver disease
Psychogenic polydipsia
Fluid overload diuresis
Solute overload
Diabetes mellitus, acromegaly, Fanconi syndrome, salt toxicity
Diuretics – many with actions at different regions of the tubules
Others/incompletely understood mechanisms
Hypoparathyroidism, hyperthyroidism, polycythemia, myeloma without hypercalcemia

unable to differentiate between CKD and AKI [9]. Similar to serum UN and Ct concentrations, SDMA will increase with a reduction of GFR caused by prerenal, renal (acute or chronic), and postrenal etiologies. Increases in SDMA do not help differentiate between these mechanisms. Identification of renal disease using SDMA requires the same steps as used for distinguishing causes of increased serum UN and Ct. Likewise, an increase in SDMA does not imply permanent loss of renal function. SDMA has not been correlated with specific diseases other than chronic and acute kidney disease. Nevertheless, it appears to be a promising analyte and will gain value as it continues to be evaluated by independent investigators.

Electrolyte abnormalities

There is a tremendous amount of information on how and where in the tubules electrolytes, ions, and other substances are reabsorbed and excreted. This section focuses on the abnormalities seen with renal failure and related diseases more than the physiology. Electrolyte abnormalities are common in renal failure and generalizations are predictable; however, the severity of the renal failure and the stage of compensation make accurate predictions difficult and therefore serum electrolytes must be measured. Hyperphosphatemia is expected anytime GFR is reduced. If CKD is in a compensatory state then sodium, potassium, and chloride will likely be within reference intervals. If chronic or AKI

Case Example 24.7. Categorize the azotemia: normal, prerenal, renal

Patient	A	B	C	D	E	F
Serum UN (10–30)	28	85	190	110	60	63
Serum Ct (<1.5)	1.1	4	9.2	3.2	3	3.1
Serum UN: Ct ratio	28 : 1	21 : 1	21 : 1	34 : 1	20 : 1	21 : 1
USG	1.034	1.006	1.010	1.058	1.014	1.044

(reference intervals are provided in parentheses; serum UN, Ct mg/dL)

A. "Normal": all results are within reference intervals, and USG indicates adequate concentrating capacity.
B. Renal azotemia: serum UN and Ct increased, and USG dilute.
C. Renal azotemia: UN and Ct increased and USG indicates isosthenuria; repeat USG to see if concentration increases out of the 1.007–1.013 range.
D. Prerenal azotemia: UN and Ct increased and USG elevated (concentrated); UN/Ct ratio increased to 34, which also suggests prerenal; dehydration likely, evaluate hydration status.
E. Renal azotemia: UN and Ct increased and USG close to isosthenuric range, need repeat USG to see if patient can concentrate its urine.
F. Prerenal azotemia: UN and Ct increased and USG concentrated; nearly identical values to example "E" but different causes based on results of USG; there are no values for UN and Ct that are too high for prerenal azotemia; however, often the greatest increases are seen when there is a combination of prerenal and renal azotemia.

Case Example 24.8. Match the patient to the diagnosis

Patient	A	B	C	D	E
Serum UN (10–30)	22	5	180	90	55
Serum Ct (<1.5)	1.5	1	9	2	10.2
Serum UN: Ct ratio	16:1	5 : 1	20 : 1	45 : 1	5.5 : 1
USG	1.024	1.005	1.010	1.055	Not performed

(reference intervals are provided in parentheses; serum UN, Ct mg/dL)
Possible diagnoses: normal, prerenal azotemia, renal azotemia, azotemia in a horse, hepatic shunt
Interpretation:

A. "Normal": at least all results are within reference intervals, and USG indicates some concentrating capacity. Recall that any USG is possible on a random urine sample.
B. Hepatic shunt: UN is decreased and urine is hyposthenuric, implying renal ability to dilute urine, but it may not be able to concentrate, need more USG to identify a pattern. The decreased UN is attributable to decreased hepatic production; recommend evaluation of liver function.
C. Renal azotemia: UN and Ct are increased and USG indicates isosthenuria. The USG should be repeated to determine whether it will rise out of the 1.007–1.013 range. Dilute urine suggests tubular lesions, but we need to know the rapidity of onset, body condition of the animal, serum albumin, and PCV to differentiate acute from chronic renal disease.
D. Prerenal azotemia: UN and Ct increased and high UN/Ct ratio suggestive of prerenal cause (e.g., dehydration leading to decreased GFR) with high USG (concentrated urine). One could observe similar values with GI hemorrhage, increased substrate delivery to liver for increased UN production (e.g., bleeding ulcer, hookworm infection, NSAIDs, etc.).
E. Horse: disproportionate increase in Ct relative to UN resulting in low UN/Ct ratio. Differential diagnoses include an increase in noncreatinine chromogens combined with dehydration (e.g., noted with colic). Similar results are expected in cattle with renal failure coupled with GI excretion of UN, a urinalysis and especially USG would help differentiate these possibilities. If isosthenuric urine is observed, then the results are consistent with renal failure. If urine is adequately concentrated, then the results are consistent with prerenal azotemia and the presence of noncreatinine chromogens.

is not compensated then there will be disturbances of these electrolytes that run the gamut of increased to decreased.

Phosphorus and calcium

Evaluate these two electrolytes together. Most dogs and cats with renal failure will have normocalcemia and hyperphosphatemia, next most frequent is hypocalcemia and hyperphosphatemia. Hyperphosphatemia is a nearly constant association with CKD in all species except the horse. Horses tend to have hypercalcemia and hypophosphatemia. As renal failure progresses from stage 1 to stage 4, the serum concentrations of UN, creatinine, and phosphorus

Case Example 24.9. Categorize the azotemia (normal, prerenal, renal) and list differentials

1. Categorize the Azotemia: normal, prerenal, renal
2. What are your differentials?

Patient	A	B	C	D	E-1	E-2 with fluid therapy
Serum UN (10–30)	20	98	121	220	225	68
Serum Ct (<1.5)	1.0	2	6	11	12	6.2
Serum UN:Ct ratio	20 : 1	50 : 1	20 : 1	20 : 1	20 : 1	10 : 1
PCV (30–50)	42	59	48	21	62	41
Albumin (2.8–4.0)	3.0	4.8	5.1	1.9	4.9	3.0
USG	1.022	1.044	1.059	1.009	1.006	1.010

(reference intervals are provided in parentheses; serum UN, Ct mg/dL, PCV %, albumin g/dL)

Interpretations:

A. Normal.

B. Azotemia with concentrated USG, increased UN/Ct ratio, polycythemia, and increased serum albumin all attributable to dehydration causing a prerenal azotemia. GI hemorrhage could produce similar results, the PCV does not need to be decreased for GI hemorrhage to cause an increase in UN but an increased PCV fits better with dehydration, and an increase in albumin confirms dehydration.

C. Prerenal azotemia, there is not an increase in the UN/Ct ratio in this example; the *only* cause of increased serum albumin is dehydration (bisalbuminemia or a hepatocellular carcinoma causing increased albumin either through increased production by neoplastic hepatocytes or due to reduced negative feedback on production; both conditions are incredibly rare).

D. Azotemia with isosthenuric urine indicates renal failure. The low PCV and low albumin indicate CKD. Correlate laboratory results with body condition of patient, physical exam results, and history. Ultrasonography of kidneys may reveal small, fibrotic kidneys.

E-1. Azotemia with unconcentrated urine indicates there is renal disease but that the kidneys are functional to some degree because they are able to produce urine more dilute than plasma. The increases in albumin concentration and PCV indicate a prerenal component and indicate the renal failure is probably acute and therefore tubular lesions are likely, possibly a nephrosis; this is an example of renal and prerenal azotemia, but it cannot be determined what portion of the azotemia is due to each of these factors. These data warrant performing serial urinalyses to monitor USG.

E-2. IV fluid therapy resulted in decreased azotemia supporting the interpretation that part of the azotemia was of prerenal azotemia. There is a greater decrease in UN relative to Ct, which is typical of fluid diuresis and is caused by the increased rate of flow of filtrate leading to decreased reabsorption of UN in tubules. The decrease in PCV and albumin is due to fluid therapy; the second USG is isosthenuric and is expected following fluid therapy (i.e., it cannot be interpreted). A large portion of the azotemia before fluid therapy was due to dehydration. Fluid therapy should continue to determine if fluids and other treatments can lower the azotemia further. The point at which fluid therapy cannot decrease the azotemia further is the UN and Ct concentrations that are due to the true renal lesions. The patient can be further treated and monitored. Azotemia is not a death sentence. Many dogs and especially cats can be maintained with a low degree of azotemia and inability to concentrate urine for months or years with periodic treatments and monitoring the progression or improvement of their renal disease.

increase accordingly as well as the Ca × P product. At stage 1 (mild renal disease), hyperphosphatemia is observed in approximately 20% of dogs and the magnitude is mild, e.g., 6–8 mg/dL. Hyperphosphatemia progresses to 100% of dogs in stage 4 (severe end stage) and increases are severe, 17–25 mg/dL. Similarly, parathyroid hormone (PTH) increases over time. About 33% of dogs will have increased values at stage 1 and 100% at stage 4.

Phosphorus

Approximately 80% of phosphorus entering the glomerular filtrate is reabsorbed in the proximal tubules and 20% is excreted. The most common cause of hyperphosphatemia in veterinary medicine is decreased GFR. Pre-, renal, and postrenal causes, acute, and CKD all do this. In dogs with CKD increases in serum phosphorus (P) are roughly parallel to increases in UN. In a ruptured urinary bladder, phosphorus increases in the serum because it is reabsorbed along its concentration gradient from a high concentration in the urine/abdominal fluid across the peritoneum and into the blood. Serum phosphorus may increase before azotemia in some patients with ethylene glycol toxicity if the antifreeze product ingested also contains a phosphate rust inhibitor.

Case Example 24.10. What is your diagnosis? Acute vs. chronic kidney disease

Patient	A	B	C
History	Fine yesterday	Week's weight loss	Week's weight loss
Body condition	Good	Poor	Poor, dehydrated 5%
Serum UN (10–30)	200	221	120
Serum Ct (<1.5)	10	11	5
Serum UN:Ct ratio	20 : 1	20 : 1	22 : 1
PCV (30–50)	42	19	32
Albumin (2.8–4.0)	3.0	2.2	2.8
USG	1.012	1.009	1.006
Urine volume	Small amount	Increased	Increased

(reference intervals are provided in parentheses; serum UN, Ct mg/dL, PCV %, albumin g/dL)

Interpretation:

A. Azotemia, isosthenuric urine, history, and all other data point to acute tubular disease; therefore, suspect toxic or infectious nephrosis.

B. Azotemia, isosthenuric urine, history, and all other data point to chronic renal disease/failure.

C. Azotemia, lack of concentrated urine, history, urine volume, and body condition all point to chronic renal disease/failure but PCV and albumin do not support this interpretation; suspect concurrent dehydration detected on physical exam has raised these analytes into reference interval and after fluid therapy both will be decreased; seems likely given they are at low end of reference interval and dehydration is 5%.

Hyperphosphatemia greater than 10 mg/dL is common; it can be as severe as >15 mg/dL. At these concentrations, phosphorus may amplify renal failure via mineralization of tubular cells and cellular organelles, direct nephrotoxicity, and vasoconstriction. When the serum Ca × P product is >70, soft-tissue mineralization is possible, and if it is >100, soft-tissue mineralization is occurring. Soft-tissue mineralization is enhanced in renal failure due to underlying vasculitis that damages tissues. Phosphorus is more important in mineralization than is Ca; therefore, mineralization of soft tissues will be occurring even if there is hypocalcemia as long as there is hyperphosphatemia. For example, a patient with a serum total Ca of 7.8 mg/dL and serum P of 16 mg/dL has a Ca × P product of 125. Soft-tissue mineralization is occurring even though there is hypocalcemia. Mineralization occurs outside the kidneys as well and predisposed sites are blood vessels throughout the body, mid-zonal gastric mucosa, lungs, and heart. On rare occasions, the mineralization in blood vessels is severe enough to be seen in radiographs. This metastatic calcification is very harmful and contributes to mortality in animals with renal failure. Treatment of renal failure includes dietary changes and medicinal products to bind phosphorus and decrease GI absorption in an attempt to lower serum phosphorus.

A normal serum P concentration in an azotemic patient is unusual and should prompt consideration that there is another disease lowering the serum P such as primary hyperparathyroidism or, more likely, hypercalcemia of malignancy.

Hypophosphatemia occurs in some horses with renal failure but does not occur in small animals unless it is caused by treatment. It is estimated that approximately 66% of horses in renal failure will be hypercalcemic and 50% will have hypophosphatemia. The mechanism is not clear. It is relatively easy to hypothesize on the hypercalcemia, but hypophosphatemia is problematic; there may be increased P excretion in the intestines. Some horses may adapt to the high calcium diet in alfalfa by excreting calcium and reabsorbing phosphorus in their kidneys. These horses may then retain calcium and excrete phosphorus during renal failure. This is the opposite of normal renal physiology. Hypercalcemia and hypophosphatemia in a horse is most likely due to renal failure, but in a dog hypercalcemia of malignancy is the most likely diagnosis.

PTH inhibits P reabsorption in the proximal tubules and therefore promotes phosphaturia. Increased concentrations of PTH help prevent hyperphosphatemia in renal failure for some time, but when the GFR is decreased below 20% of normal, this compensatory adaptation is overwhelmed and hyperphosphatemia develops. Hyperphosphatemia and hypocalcemia are the major stimulatory factors for renal secondary hyperparathyroidism.

Calcium

Normocalcemia is seen most frequently in animals with renal failure (50–75%); hypocalcemia is relatively common (up to 40%). Hypercalcemia is sometimes seen and is dependent upon species, stage of compensation of the renal failure, and methodology for calcium measurement.

Hypocalcemia can be explained via six mechanisms: decreased tubular cells to reabsorb the Ca, decreased concentrations of vitamin D, decreased albumin, soft-tissue mineralization, reciprocal decrease in serum due to increased P, and if renal failure is due to ethylene glycol toxicity, the chelating effect of oxalate on calcium. The hypocalcemia seen with AKI caused by ethylene glycol can be severe, <6 mg/dL. Hypocalcemia is more common with chronic than AKI and usually is mild to moderate, 7–8 mg/dL, and asymptomatic. The rate-limiting step in the synthesis of vitamin D is in the kidney, hence CKD is associated with decreased production of vitamin D. Prolonged hypocalcemia stimulates parathyroid hyperplasia, which may lead to metabolic bone demineralization disease, osteopenia, or renal fibrous osteodystrophy, or "rubber jaw." Although the bone lesions are generalized, they are best seen radiographically in the mandible and maxillae.

The changes seen in total serum calcium are usually the same for ionized calcium, but some cases of renal failure in dogs may have decreased ionized calcium while total serum calcium is normal or increased. Rarely are there clinical signs in these patients referable to this change in calcium. If measurement of ionized calcium is available, it is the best fraction to measure to predict biologic action of calcium. If fluid therapy corrects the metabolic acidosis rapidly, then these patients may develop tremors, tetany, and neuromuscular signs that could be due to the shift of calcium from ionized (acidosis) to protein or complexed compartments (alkalosis). Use of calcium products to correct this possible effect is probably contraindicated as the administered calcium would combine with the existing hyperphosphatemia to speed soft-tissue mineralization. Hypocalcemia is expected in cows with renal failure due to the mechanisms listed above as well as the tendency for cattle to develop alkalosis with renal failure and the observations that many sick cattle with a variety of diseases will have mild hypocalcemia.

Hypercalcemia is seen in cases of canine and feline renal failure (10–20%) and equine renal failure (66%). The mechanism is not clear. It is hypothesized that there is an acquired defect in the calcium-sensing protein receptor. This protein is critical for the parathyroid gland to recognize the concentration of calcium and adjust synthesis and secretion of PTH appropriately to normalize serum calcium. If the molecule is abnormal, as in congenital and acquired disorders in humans, the parathyroid cells do not decrease their secretion of PTH. Continued secretion of PTH stimulates calcium reabsorption in the proximal convoluted tubules and osteoclastic osteolysis, further contributing to the hypercalcemia. Hypercalcemia with canine renal failure is seen most frequently in young dogs with progressive familial renal nephropathy. It is seen with other types of renal failure as well. Dogs and cats with renal failure–associated hypercalcemia will have hyperphosphatemia, and the threat of soft-tissue mineralization is high.

Renal failure is the second to third most common cause of hypercalcemia in dogs regardless of whether total serum calcium or ionized calcium is used to assess the calcium status. Several studies have highlighted that total serum calcium does not correlate with the ionized calcium in up to one-third of the cases of CKD in dogs. Approximately 4–10% of dogs with renal failure will have increased ionized calcium, and 5–15% will have increased total serum calcium.

Total serum calcium also may not reflect the ionized calcium in cats with CKD. Ionized calcium increased in 6% vs. 20% via total calcium and ionized calcium decreased in 25% vs. 8% with total calcium. The measurement of ionized calcium is preferred to accurately assess calcium biologic status. However, it is recommended to use the total serum calcium for calculating the Ca × P product.

Hypercalcemia is associated with dilute urine and PU/PD. There are multiple mechanisms for this including interference with the action of ADH, decreasing the movement of AQP2 to the apical membrane and effectively preventing water reabsorption, blocking receptors on renal epithelial cells, and mineralization of cells. Biochemical steps may be reversed, but structural lesions induced by mineralization may not. Basement membranes and cellular organelles will become mineralized and lead to death of cells, further contributing to both concentrating defects and renal azotemia.

Hypercalcemia, steroids (hyperadrenocorticism), and pyometra (*Escherichia coli* endotoxin) are examples of diseases or substances that interfere with the action of ADH and frequently result in dilute urine and PU/PD. If these patients are also azotemic, it can be difficult to differentiate prerenal from renal azotemia. This is because they will have dilute urine due to the inhibitory substance, but the azotemia may actually be due to concurrent dehydration and the kidneys are fine.

Calcium-oxalate urolithiasis or crystalluria are clues to look for hypercalcemia in small animals. Usually they are dihydrate oxalate crystals, but both dihydrate and monohydrate forms have been seen in dogs and cats with hypercalcemia, e.g., primary hyperparathyroidism and idiopathic hypercalcemia of cats. Hyperparathyroidism is often asymptomatic, and it is the presence of hypercalcemia found on a routine chemistry panel or calcium crystalluria that is the first clue that this disease is present. Calcium-oxalate monohydrate and dihydrate crystals can also be normal findings. They are also highly associated with ethylene glycol toxicity in dogs and cats, therefore their presence must be correlated with all of the clinical and lab data. Calcium-oxalate monohydrate and dihydrate crystals are seen in normal horses, rabbits, and guinea pigs. Horses and rabbits have cloudy urine and excessive mucus in their urine and have reference interval serum calcium values greater than other species, up to 13 mg/dL depending on the lab and methodology.

Calcium in complicated renal failure cases

Deciding if renal failure is the cause or the result of the hypercalcemia is problematic. The easiest way to decide is to look at all of the data and see if a primary diagnosis is evident. For example, if CKD can be established based on laboratory data, breed disposition, biopsy, etc., then that is the most likely cause of hypercalcemia. However, if a dog has lymphoma, azotemia, and hypercalcemia then hypercalcemia is probably due to lymphoma. The marked hypercalcemia can cause renal impairment. In lymphoma, hypercalcemia is a paraneoplastic syndrome associated with parathyroid hormone related protein (PTH-rp) that stimulates urinary phosphorus excretion and calcium reabsorption. The ionized calcium may be markedly increased. The azotemia is secondary to possible dehydration, soft-tissue mineralization, and/or lymphoma in the kidneys. The serum P in these dogs will not be markedly increased despite azotemia due to the phosphaturic effect of PTH-rp. Inability to concentrate urine can be due to hypercalcemia or renal failure so USG is not a distinguishing feature.

If a primary diagnosis is not evident, then the greater the serum Ca the more likely there is a primary calcium disease, and the greater the serum P the more likely it is primary renal failure. The lower the serum P, the more likely there is a primary disease causing the hypercalcemia such as primary hyperparathyroidism or hypercalcemia of malignancy, both of which stimulate phosphaturia and a decrease in serum phosphorus. However, only 5% of dogs with primary hyperparathyroidism have azotemia so it is much more likely they have hypercalcemia of malignancy as azotemia is fairly common in these dogs. If serum phosphorus is WRI in an azotemic patient with hypercalcemia, then there is a primary calcium disease and a hormone that is stimulating phosphaturia. If the total serum calcium is increased but the ionized calcium is normal or decreased, then renal failure is the more likely cause of the hypercalcemia.

Sodium and chloride

Essentially 100% of sodium in the glomerular filtrate is reabsorbed: 65% in proximal convoluted tubules, 25% in the ascending loop of Henle, 5% in each distal tubule and collecting ducts. Most cases of renal failure have normal concentrations of serum sodium and chloride; however, CKD is associated with hyponatremia and hypochloremia, especially in horses and cattle. Hyponatremia and hypochloremia can be seen in dogs and cats with CKD. If the fractional excretion of sodium exceeds 1%, it indicates renal tubular failure. Additionally, hyponatremia and hypochloremia are characteristic electrolyte abnormalities of uroabdomen in all species.

Potassium and magnesium

Most potassium entering the filtrate is reabsorbed in the proximal tubules, and potassium is excreted in collecting tubules via aldosterone stimulation of cellular channels. Potassium increases in the serum with postrenal azotemia and in some cases of AKI, especially if oliguria/anuria are present because of inability to excrete potassium. This is often exacerbated by a concurrent inorganic acidosis that shifts intracellular potassium to the extracellular space, in an exchange for hydrogen ions to maintain intracellular electroneutrality. Potassium may increase to life-threatening concentrations (>8 mEq/L) in obstructed male cats.

Potassium decreases with CKD especially if polyuria is present (increased tubular flow). It may also decrease during the diuretic phase of AKI if dietary intake does not match renal loss. Cattle with renal failure have hypokalemia from renal loss, salivary loss, anorexia, and metabolic alkalosis. Alkalosis shifts potassium into cells in exchange for a hydrogen ion to buffer excess serum bicarbonate. Alkalosis is due to ileus and forestomach atony secondary to uremia.

Historically, approximately 30% of cats with CKD developed hypokalemia with an increased fractional excretion of potassium. When severe, the hypokalemia caused myopathy, generalized muscle weakness, and cervical ventroflexion. The mechanisms are not clear and likely multifactorial. Treatment of this syndrome has been somewhat addressed with current feline renal foods that are supplemented with potassium. Hypokalemia may also contribute to renal failure by causing degeneration of tubular cells, and it also interferes with ability to concentrate urine by decreasing the responsiveness of tubular epithelial cells to ADH. The condition is known as feline kaliopenic polymyopathy-nephropathy syndrome.

Magnesium entering the glomerular filtrate is reabsorbed via active and passive routes in the proximal tubule and in the thick ascending loop of Henle. The primary route of magnesium excretion is via the kidney and therefore serum magnesium concentrations increase with renal failure in most species, although it is seldom measured. Horses with blister beetle intoxication tend to have severe hypocalcemia and hypomagnesemia. These horses have hemorrhages in numerous tissues including the urinary bladder that result in hematuria.

Blood gas

Metabolic acidosis is expected with renal failure in all species. It is dependent upon the severity of the renal failure, the presence of concurrent diseases, and compensatory mechanisms. Compensated renal failure patients have normal blood gas values and uncompensated renal failure patients may have severe acidosis. Acidosis is usually associated with hyperkalemia. In renal failure, hydrogen ion excretion is decreased in the tubules, leading to acidemia. Hydrogen ions will shift into cells in exchange for potassium ions, a mechanism used to maintain intracellular electroneutrality. This will increase the serum potassium. Total CO_2 concentration <15 mEq/L and an increased anion gap indicated a titrational metabolic acidosis due to retention of uremic acids; these patients will have acidic urine as well.

Vomiting uremic dogs and cats will develop a hypochloremic metabolic alkalosis. This results from the loss of hydrogen and chloride ions in the vomitus, and the retention of their counterparts, bicarbonate and sodium ions, respectively, within the body. This is often a subtle finding in the chemistry panel identified by a disproportionate hypochloremia (with respect to hyponatremia), as the alkalosis is frequently masked by the acidosis developed from renal failure. Some cattle develop metabolic alkalosis due to ileus and forestomach atony secondary to uremia. The result is sequestration of acid-rich secretions in the abomasum and rumen. These cows will also have hypochloremia, hyponatremia, hypokalemia, and an increased anion gap due to retained uremic acids.

If patients with hypochloremic metabolic alkalosis are also severely dehydrated, they may develop paradoxical aciduria. Paradoxical aciduria is an uncommon event that happens most commonly in dairy cattle with displaced abomasum, especially right-sided. These cows have severe metabolic alkalosis and severe hypochloremia due to trapping of chloride-rich fluid in the displaced abomasum. They are also dehydrated, hypokalemic, and hyponatremic, and this combination leads to paradoxical aciduria. Dehydration drives the process through activation of the renin-angiotensin-aldosterone system. Aldosterone stimulates sodium and water resorption in the renal tubules. In health, the kidney resorbs chloride with the sodium to maintain electroneutrality. However, in the face of hypochloremia, the kidney uses a back-up plan of excreting a cation. As potassium is depleted, the kidney excretes hydrogen ions, leading to the acidification of urine. The excretion of hydrogen ions potentiates tubular formation of bicarbonate, which is reabsorbed. The reabsorption of bicarbonate ion further exacerbates the alkalosis, and the hydrogen ion excretion results in acidic urine. Until the displaced abomasum is replaced and the severe hypochloremia is corrected, the paradoxical aciduria with metabolic alkalosis will persist.

Protein abnormalities

Albumin

An increased concentration of serum albumin is seen only with dehydration. There is no specific correlation of hyperalbuminemia with renal diseases, but dehydration is often present in patients with renal failure. These patients will have multiple mechanisms characterizing their azotemia including both prerenal and renal etiologies. The distinction of prerenal and renal azotemia is made by measuring the USG while assessing skin turgidity, PCV, and serum albumin to assess hydration. Decreased serum albumin is seen with glomerular diseases and end-stage renal disease. It may also be seen with diseases in the gastrointestinal, liver, and cardiovascular systems. Hypoalbuminemia due to glomerular disease is discussed in detail in the "Glomerular Proteinuria" section later in this chapter.

Antithrombin

Antithrombin (AT) (also known as antithrombin III) is a small alpha globulin synthesized in the liver and lost in the urine of patients with glomerular diseases. AT has a molecular weight just lower than albumin; hence both proteins are lost in the filtrate of patients with glomerular diseases. Antithrombin is the most potent inhibitor of the coagulation cascade. When AT is decreased, a prothrombotic state exists. The most common location of thrombi is in the pulmonary artery, but thrombi are also located in the aortic quadrification and in many other vessels if they are examined. The hypoalbuminemia also stimulates platelet hypersensitivity that further contributes to the formation of thrombi. In contrast, many cases of severe renal failure tend to bleed due to several mechanisms: concurrent disseminated intravascular coagulation (DIC), as uremia alters platelet function leading to prolonged bleeding times, and increased clotting associated with uremia-induced vasculitis.

Fibrinogen

Small animals tend to have increased fibrinogen associated with chronic renal disease. Cattle in renal failure tend to have marked increases in fibrinogen, 1000–2000 mg/dL.

Other abnormalities

Generally, as the renal disease progresses from stage 1 to stage 4 (mild to severe), the laboratory abnormalities worsen in their magnitude and/or the percentage of patients with each abnormality increases.

Packed cell volume; erythroid

CKD is characterized by nonregenerative anemia in all species. Horses will have an anemia due to CKD, but distinction of regenerative versus nonregenerative is not practical in horses. Decreased production of erythropoietin in the kidneys is the main cause; however, other factors that contribute to anemia are decreased life span of erythrocytes, blood loss due to tendency of uremic patients to bleed, anemia of chronic inflammatory disease, bone marrow suppression, hyperphosphatemia, and increased serum PTH concentration. The anemia of CKD is usually mild to moderate; a PCV in high teens to twenties is typical. If the anemia is severe, such as low teens or single digits, then search for an additional cause and/or gastrointestinal bleeding.

Rarely a renal tumor produces erythropoietin and increases the PCV. Any tumor in the kidney can produce this paraneoplastic syndrome. The result is an absolute polycythemia, and it has been reported with non-neoplastic renal masses as well.

Cholesterol

Increased cholesterol is seen with the nephrotic syndrome. The mechanism is not known, but there are numerous publications that make the association and attempt to explain hypercholesterolemia: increased hepatic production of lipoproteins, defective lipolysis of lipoproteins, and decreased conversion of cholesterol into bile acids are some of the hypotheses.

Parathyroid hormone

CKD patients will have parathyroid hyperplasia and hypertrophy secondary to hypocalcemia and hyperphosphatemia. This may result in clinically detectable fibrous osteodystrophy and osteopenia due to increased bone resorption triggered by increased serum concentrations of PTH. PTH will be increased due to decreased renal clearance and concurrent production and release in the hyperplastic parathyroid glands. These mechanisms result in increased PTH no matter what assay is used. As renal failure progresses from stage 1 to stage 4, PTH concentrations increase (along with increases in serum UN, creatinine, and phosphorus). About 33% of dogs will have increased serum PTH at stage 1 and 100% at stage 4. There is ample evidence that increased serum PTH concentrations are one of the uremic toxins that contribute to the vasculitis and suppress bone marrow function.

Vitamin D

Vitamin D concentrations will eventually decrease in patients with renal failure as the rate-limiting step in the synthesis of vitamin D is in the kidneys. The decreased serum concentration of vitamin D contributes to hypocalcemia and hyperparathyroidism. It is not necessary to measure serum vitamin D concentration in patients with renal failure, but knowledge of the possible consequences of reduced vitamin D may be useful.

Lipase and amylase in serum

These enzymes are inactivated or excreted through the urinary system, and any cause of azotemia (decreased GFR) may result in increased serum concentrations of one or both. The magnitude of increase is usually one to threefold. If the increase in lipase is greater than threefold, then a purely renal contribution is unlikely and pancreatitis should be considered. An increase of fivefold or greater is usually indicative of pancreatitis. Prerenal azotemia can produce as great an increase in lipase or amylase as renal azotemia. Expect amylase or lipase or both to increase in 70% of patients with spontaneous renal failure. Approximately 33% of azotemic patients will have an increase in both; 33% will have increased lipase only and 33% increased amylase only.

Urinalysis

No other body system has an excretory product that is produced regularly, is easy to obtain, and that informs us so vividly on the health of the parent organ. A UA is an essential component of the evaluation of the urinary system. Urinalyses have an excellent benefit-cost ratio as a screening test in all species. It is an absolute requirement for the diagnosis or to rule out urinary diseases. It is excellent as a follow-up test to determine the progression or improvement of urinary diseases. It is very useful in the diagnosis of some nonurinary diseases. It should be part of all geriatric exams, is performed in-practice, and costs almost nothing. Some of the nonurinary diseases a UA helps diagnose are hyperadrenocorticism (Cushing's disease), diabetes mellitus, hepatic diseases, hemolytic diseases, rhabdomyolysis, psychogenic polydipsia, and central diabetes insipidus. It is essential in distinguishing prerenal from renal azotemia.

Early detection of disease

In renal disease, changes in the urinalysis frequently precede changes in the serum biochemistry profile. For example, in glomerular disease proteinuria is the first abnormality and precedes hypoalbuminemia, nephrotic syndrome, and azotemia. Persistent proteinuria found in a symptomatic or asymptomatic patient should prompt evaluation for glomerulonephritis, amyloidosis, and multiple myeloma. Renal disease, especially in geriatric patients, is typified by the inability to concentrate urine adequately, often before there is azotemia (exception: some cats). Hematuria is a common clinical pathology abnormality and is detected with uroliths, transitional cell carcinoma (TCC), and several other diseases.

Monitoring of renal patients

Urinalysis and especially USG are excellent inexpensive tests for following patients post-treatment to assess the progression or improvement of disease, especially if the patient is no longer azotemic. Persistent inability to concentrate urine in a previously azotemic patient suggests that the disease is still present or that over 66% of the nephrons are still not functioning adequately. It is likely that the disease process has destroyed nephrons and fibrosis has replaced much of the renal mass. Return of concentrating ability indicates that the disease has improved and at least less than 66% of the nephrons are still damaged. The presence of waxy casts in the urine sediment suggests persistence and chronicity of the disease.

Gross, microscopic, and chemical determinations are the key components of a UA. Table 24.5 summarizes expected results in normal animals. Table 24.6 provides guidelines for urinalysis findings to predict renal site of pathology that may be present. Urine composition is determined by the serum constituents and the quantity of serum presented to the kidneys, renal function, and material added to the glomerular filtrate as it passes through the kidneys, bladder, urethra, and lower urinary tract. Urine examination should be done in-practice; there is no reason to send it out. Urinalyses should be performed on fresh urine (<½-hour old), and if the macroscopic and reagent strip evaluations have no abnormalities, then performing the microscopic examination is optional because the sediment is rarely abnormal if the macroscopic exam and reagent strips are normal. This is especially true if the UA is being used to screen an apparently healthy patient.

Table 24.5 "Normal"/expected findings in UA.

Urinalysis parameter	Dog	Cat	Horse	Cow
Color	Yellow	Yellow	Yellow	Yellow
Clarity	Clear	Clear	Cloudy	Clear
SG	1.020–1.045	1.020–1.050	1.020–1.045	1.020–1.045
pH	5–7	5–7	7–8	7–8
Protein	Neg to trace	Neg	Neg	Neg
Bilirubin	Trace	Neg	Neg	Neg
Blood[a]	Neg	Neg	Neg	Neg
Glucose	Neg	Neg	Neg	Neg
Ketones	Neg	Neg	Neg	Neg
Urobilinogen	Do not use	Do not use	Do not use	Do not use
WBCs	0–5	0–5	0–5	0–5
RBCs	0–5	0–5	0–5	0–5
Epithelial	0–5/few	0–5	0–5	0–5
Casts	Neg/none	Neg	Neg	Neg
Crystals	None	None	Ca carbonate/oxalate	None
Other	None	None	Mucus	None

[a]Small to trace amount with cystocentesis or catheterization collections.

Summary

- Excellent benefit-cost ratio, low costs.
- Essential to distinguish prerenal from renal-origin azotemia.
- Detects diseases in early stages.
- Detects nonrenal diseases.
- Useful for monitoring patients.
- If the macroscopic and reagent strips have no abnormalities, then performing the microscopic examination is optional; UA should be performed in-house.

Collection

- *Voided, free catch* – morning sample preferred when urine is usually at maximal concentration; may add contamination of cells and bacteria from lower urogenital tract. Lower urethra has resident bacterial population, but upper urethra and bladder are sterile. Bacteria and leukocytes are common in the prepuce. Epithelial cells are added from genital tract and distal urethra.
- *Catheterization* – may induce a small amount of hemorrhage and introduces epithelial cells from urethra.
- *Cystocentesis* – preferred for culture, commonly introduces small amount of hemorrhage especially in cats.

Urinalyses are often not performed in large animals simply due to difficulty in collecting a sample. Horses often require catheterization, but placing a horse in a stall and whistling is a commonly used technique for racehorses. Gentle rubbing below the ventral commissure of the vulva causes micturition in dairy cattle. Manually occluding the nares will cause sheep to urinate.

Timing

Perform on fresh urine, ideally less than ½ hour after collection, otherwise refrigerate (do not freeze) in an opaque airtight container to avoid deterioration of cellular components and metabolism or escape of analytes. If left at room temperature, cells and casts will lyse; glucose is metabolized; ketones and bilirubin decrease; pH increases as urea is converted into ammonia; CO_2 escapes; bacteria proliferate. Refrigeration can encourage crystal formation, so samples must be rewarmed for 20 minutes on the benchtop and mixed gently to resuspend any settled particles. Rewarm refrigerated urine to room temperature before performing a urinalysis – cold temperatures will lower USG and may influence dipstick results.

Expected volume in healthy dogs and cats

Dogs = 20–40 mL/kg/d; Cats = 10–20 mL/kg/d

Physical examination of urine

Color and clarity

Normal urine is yellow and clear, concentrated urine is deep amber, and dilute urine is clear to pale yellow. Red, brown, and various shades in between are seen commonly with hematuria, hemoglobinuria, and myoglobinuria. Uncommon differential diagnoses for red or brown urine include porphyria and administration of phenothiazine anthelmintics or aminopyrine (uncommon, given as urinary analgesic). See Table 24.7 for the differentiation of hematuria, hemoglobinuria, and myoglobinuria, and the specific diseases that cause them. Horse and rabbit urine may be cloudy in normal animals due to normal urinary

Table 24.6 Renal azotemia and predicting location of lesion.[a]

	Glomerular	Tubular (interstitial)	Tubular (interstitial)	Pelvis
Disease progression	Chronic	Acute	Chronic[a]	Chronic, acute exacerbations
Clinical presentation	• Thin body condition • Weight loss • Polyuria • Ascites	• Good body condition • Anuria/oliguria	• Thin body condition; weight loss • Polyuria • Hypertension	
Kidney size, shape	• Normal to small	• Normal to enlarged	• Small • Normal to irregular contours	• Normal to irregular contours • Dilated irregularly shaped pelvis
Hematology and serum chemistry	• Hypoalbuminemia • Increased cholesterol • +/− azotemia • NRA	• Azotemia • Hyperphosphatemia	• Nonregenerative anemia • Azotemia • Hyperphosphatemia • Hypokalemia (cats)	• Azotemia
USG	• Variable	• Isosthenuria	• Isosthenuria	• Variable
Urine chemistry	• Proteinuria	• Glucosuria • Proteinuria	• Proteinuria	
Urine sediment		• Casts • RBCs, WBCs • Bacteria		• WBCs • WBC casts, cellular casts • Bacteria
Biopsy?	• Biopsy	• Do not biopsy	• Do not biopsy	• Avoid biopsy
Potential etiologies	• Amyloidosis • Glomerulonephritis	• Toxins • Infectious • Lepto	• Lepto	• Ascending infection

[a]This is assuming the diseases are behaving in a characteristic manner. Glomerular diseases usually present when chronic; tubular diseases are commonly acute, but if they survive they can end up as chronic PU/PD patients. Pyelonephritis is in an active phase when the infection is present. All of these diseases will change over time and depending on severity (mild, moderate, severe) and treatments. All of these diseases may have acute kidney injury superimposed on a chronic disease, e.g., patient becomes dehydrated, a second renal disease develops, the primary chronic problem progresses, and the patient goes into what appears to be acute kidney injury.

tract mucus production and numerous calcium carbonate crystals. Guinea pigs may also have abundant calcium carbonate crystalluria. Cloudiness is caused by suspended solids (crystals, mucus, casts, cells, etc.) that do not change the specific gravity (SG) but may interfere with reading of the refractometric SG line. Cloudy urine in species other than those listed here is abnormal and should be assessed microscopically for the presence of cells, bacteria, casts, crystals, sperm, powder, contaminants, etc. If urine is so turbid that it is difficult to see the calibrations in an optical refractometer, then use the supernatant from a centrifuged sample to determine USG.

Hematuria, hemoglobinuria, myoglobinuria – red, red-brown urine

The main differential diagnoses for urine discolored red to red-brown are hematuria, hemoglobinuria, and myoglobinuria. Uncommon causes are aminopyrine (urinary

Table 24.7 Differentiating hematuria, hemoglobinuria, and myoglobinuria.

	Hematuria	Hemoglobinuria	Myoglobinuria
Signalment	Any	Any	Horse, exotics
History	Dysuria/obstructed	Variable	Exercise
PCV	Normal (RI)	Decreased	Normal to increased
Plasma	Clear	Pink to icteric	Clear
CPK	Normal (RI)	Normal, mild inc.	Markedly inc. 5+
AST	Normal (RI)	Normal, mild inc.	Markedly inc. 5+
Azotemia	No If obstructed yes	Possible Can be high	Likely May be lethal
Urine	Red	Red-brown	Red-brown-black
Blood	4+	4+	4+
RBCs	TNTC	None, few	None few
WBCs	+++	None, few	None few
Casts	None	Variable, many	Variable, many
Urine color postcentrifugation	Yellow, pink	Red	Red-brown
Ammonium sulfate ppt.	Not performed	Red pellet Supernatant clearer	No pellet Supernatant red-brown
Etiologies	Obstruction urolithiasis, trauma neoplasia, biopsy	Red maple, copper, zinc, IHA, postparturient hemoglobinuria water intoxication, *Babesia*	Exertional rhabdomyolysis capture myopathy, aortic thrombus

RI, reference interval.

analgesic), porphyria, and phenothiazine anthelmintics. When all of the data are considered, distinguishing the common causes of red urine is straightforward (Table 24.7). One of the easiest procedures is to simply look at the urine before and after centrifugation. If the color is cleared or greatly reduced by centrifugation, then the diagnosis is hematuria; if the color persists after centrifugation, then hemoglobinuria or myoglobinuria is present. If the color remains postcentrifugation, look at all of the data to distinguish these two differentials and if it is still not obvious, then ask a lab to perform an ammonium sulfate precipitation test on the supernatant. This will precipitate hemoglobin such that after centrifugation a red pellet forms and all or the majority of the supernatant is cleared and is now yellow or semiclear to light pink. An 80% saturated solution of ammonium sulfate will not precipitate myoglobin and the supernatant remains red-brown. If there is still doubt there are additional tests that can be requested: electrophoresis, spectroscopic, immunoprecipitation, and ultrafiltration. Hematuria, hemoglobinuria, and myoglobinuria will all produce positive reactions to blood and protein on urine strips.

Hematuria will have numerous RBCs in the urine (too numerous to count [TNTC]) and will likely have numerous white blood cells (WBCs) due to inflammation triggered by the cause of the hematuria: infection, cystitis, urolithiasis, trauma, neoplasia, etc. Depending on the amount of hemorrhage, the PCV will be normal or decreased; a normal or reference interval PCV is most likely. If the urine has a pink hue postcentrifugation, it is due to hemolysis *in vitro*, which can be due to alkaline urine, USG <1.008, prolonged storage, and/or rough handling.

Hemoglobinuria is due to intravascular hemolysis (not extravascular) of such magnitude that the buffering mechanisms are overloaded and free hemoglobin spills into the glomerular filtrate. Plasma during the hemolytic event will be pink to red, the mean corpuscular hemoglobin concentration (MCHC) will be increased (artifact of free hemoglobin), and gradually the plasma and the patient will become icteric. Heinz bodies should be searched for in all species with this problem. The PCV is decreased to variable degrees depending on the severity of the hemolysis. Etiologies to consider are those that cause intravascular hemolysis: most cases of immune-mediated hemolytic anemia (IHA) are actually extravascular, but intravascular hemolysis can occur; parasites that are in the RBCs (*Babesia*) as opposed to on the surface (*Mycoplasma*); metals such as zinc or copper; water intoxication in cattle (osmotic lysis); *Clostridium hemolyticum*; postparturient hemoglobinuria in cattle; Heinz body anemias; and acetaminophen, onions, garlic, baby food, and red maple toxicity in horses.

Myoglobinuria is rarely seen in dogs (racing, crush injuries), cats (aortic thrombus, crush injury), or cattle. It is relatively common in horses and captured wild animals.

Of the many types of equine myopathies, the most common form associated with myoglobinuria is exertional rhabdomyolysis, which has various common names: azoturia, Monday morning disease, tying up syndrome, and capture myopathy. In these situations, there is massive muscle necrosis and release of myoglobin. Myoglobin is of a small molecular weight compared to hemoglobin (18,000 vs. 68,000 Da) such that it readily passes into the glomerular filtrate, discoloring the urine. The plasma may remain clear. In horses the plasma and the patient may turn icteric due to concurrent anorexia. The PCV will be in reference interval or increased due to concurrent dehydration and/or splenic contraction secondary to pain. Muscle enzymes will be markedly increased. The serum CPK can be as high as 1,000,000 IU/mL in horses with this disease. An increased CPK means the muscle necrosis is still active. CPK increases first; it is cleared rapidly once the muscle necrosis stops and is followed by increases in AST within hours to days of the onset of the disease. This disease can be lethal and requires immediate treatment. It is typically seen in horses that are over-exercised following periods of rest and full feed ("couch potatoes"), large-breed horses undergoing prolonged anesthetic procedures (pressure necrosis and ischemia of muscles), and wild animals that are chased for prolonged periods, equidae, ruminants, etc. It is rarely seen in domestic ruminants even with severe vitamin E Se responsive disease but can be seen in young ruminants chased excessively, similar to capture myopathy of exotics.

Hematuria is not associated with azotemia unless the cause of the hematuria is obstruction of urine outflow. Azotemia is expected with myoglobinuria and often occurs with severe cases of hemoglobinuria. Neither hemoglobin nor myoglobin is the nephrotoxin; apparently small molecular weight substances released concurrently are the toxic substances. Regardless, azotemia is possible and intravenous fluid therapy to help prevent "hemoglobinuric and myoglobinuric nephrosis" is warranted. Interestingly, some cases of severe myoglobinuria do not develop azotemia even when the muscle enzymes are markedly increased (>500,000 IU/mL) and the urine is brown-black. These cases have a better prognosis, and the absence of azotemia may be due to the absence of the nephrotoxic substance in the muscles of these horses. Casts are anticipated with hemoglobinuria and myoglobinuria and should not be present with hematuria. The casts may be of any type due to concurrent nephrosis or they may be characteristic for the diseases: myoglobin or hemoglobin casts.

Urine concentration and urine specific gravity

Correlate the urine specific gravity with serum UN and Ct, as well as all of the other case data. Measuring USG is a simple and effective test to assess renal function. Generalizations: azotemia and concentrated urine = prerenal cause; azotemia and unconcentrated urine = renal tubular disease/involvement.

See "Urine Concentration" and Tables 24.7 and 24.8 for the range of possible values.

Urine concentration

Kidneys reabsorb more than 99% of the water that enters the tubules. Water is reabsorbed in the proximal tubules passively, in the descending loop of Henle passively due to the osmotic pull of the saturated medullary interstitium (countercurrent multiplier system), passively in the distal tubules, and actively in the collecting ducts through the actions of ADH. Failure in one or more of these locations may result in polyuria. Interference with of one or more of these mechanisms is used by different diuretics to stimulate water excretion.

The ability to produce concentrated urine is dependent on several factors. At least one-third of the renal mass must be functional, adequate amounts of ADH must be produced, the medullary interstitium must be saturated, the hydration status must be conducive, and there must be an absence of concurrent diseases. Therefore, animals with impaired urine concentration will have one or more of the following: lesions in two-thirds of the renal mass (tubules or interstitium), decreased ADH production (central diabetes insipidus), refractoriness to ADH (nephrogenic diabetes insipidus, hypercalcemia, excess glucocorticoids, pyometra, or hypokalemia), decreased medullary hypertonicity

Table 24.8 USG – expected, maximal, adequate, isosthenuric, and hyposthenuric concentration ranges.

	Dog	Cat[a]	Horse	Cow
Expected	1.020–1.045	1.020–1.050	1.020–1.045	1.020–1.045
Max. conc.	1.060>	1.080>	1.050>	1.050>
Adequate	1.030>	1.035>	1.025>	1.025>
Isosthenuria	1.007–1.013	1.007–1.013	1.007–1.013	1.007–1.013
Hyposthenuria	<1.007	<1.007	<1.007	<1.007
With 5% dehydration	1.040–1.075	1.045–1.088		

[a]Some cats with renal azotemia can concentrate urine.

(medullary washout), over-hydration, or solute overload (diabetes mellitus, diuretic administration).

Kidneys concentrate and dilute the glomerular filtrate as it passes through tubules by removing solutes and water in different segments of the nephron. Glomerular filtrate is plasma minus albumin, and it starts with an SG approximately 1.010 (300 mOsm/kg), and in an animal with normal hydration, it finishes with a concentrated SG.

Urine specific gravity

Measuring osmolality via freezing point depression is the gold standard for evaluating urine concentration. This methodology is generally confined to reference laboratories, as the equipment is either too expensive, or used too infrequently to make it practical for use in private practice. Instead, urine concentration is determined by measuring USG with a refractometer.

Measurement of specific gravity

SG is a ratio of the density of urine to the density of pure water (1.000) at a given temperature [10, 11]. This differs from urine osmolality for, in addition to the number of particles, SG is also affected by the size (molecular mass) of the particles. As a result, the presence of heavy molecules like glucose, proteins, and radiocontrast may cause a disproportionate increase in USG compared with urine osmolality [10]. Nonetheless, there is a linear relationship between USG and urine osmolality [10], which makes clinical decisions based on SG generally acceptable.

Refractometry measures the SG indirectly by using the urine's refractive index to estimate USG. The refractive index is the ratio of the velocity of light in air to the velocity of light in a solution [10] and is proportional to the number and type of particles in solution. Particles not in solution will not alter USG, even when the urine is turbid (cloudy). Substances in solution are dependent on temperature and pressure, therefore SG is determined at constant temperature (room temperature) and pressure (atmospheric).

There are two types of refractometers commonly used, an optical refractometer ("Goldberg-type") and digital refractometers. The scales in refractometers are calibrated to estimate SG and/or proteins. There is a maximum reading, e.g., 1.060. Urine can be diluted to determine the exact reading if clinically required. The scales are different for dogs, cats, and horses (and humans). The differences are minor and, ideally, the scale for one species should not be used for another; however, this is not always practical in the clinical setting. In a recent study, dog and cat urine were measured on five different currently available refractometers and compared to the weight of the dry matter in the urine samples. The findings showed a single sample of urine will have a small range of USG results, and thus refractometers are imprecise tools [11]. This lack of precision reduces the usefulness of strict cutoff values (e.g., 1.008, 1.012, 1.035, etc.) when classifying the concentrating ability of the kidneys [11]. Additionally, the study showed that refractometers designed specifically for cats underestimate the USG [11]. Nonetheless, refractometers are useful in all species to measure USG and estimate concentrating ability. However, their precision is such that strict cutoffs of USG should not be used to classify a disease state. Integrate the hydration status of the patient with several values of USG to determine if the urine is appropriately or inappropriately concentrated.

Refractometers require only a drop of urine, results can predict clinical problems, and it is a low-cost test that should be used in sick patients and annual wellness checks. USG is usually determined from a well-mixed sample of urine that has not been centrifuged. If the urine is too cloudy to see lines in the refractometer, then use the supernatant to determine USG. Usually, the USG values of the uncentrifuged urine and supernatant will be similar; any differences are typically minor and do not interfere with clinical interpretation.

Reagent strip tests estimate the SG indirectly based on pKa that uses a shift in the pH to produce a color change. Maximum concentration detected is 1.030, and this is inadequate to detect the concentration ranges in cats and dogs. Additionally, reagent strips do not correlate well with refractometer results; false positives and negatives are common. For these reasons, reagent strips are considered unreliable.

Interpretation of urine specific gravity

There is a wide range of reference values for USG (1.001–1.070), and depending on the patient's hydration status, any of these values can be considered "normal." The most important task is to determine the pattern of concentrating ability by correlating USG with hydration status, serum UN and Ct, urine volume, and the clinical data. In a healthy, euhydrated animal, there is an "expected range" of USG that varies slightly by species (Table 24.8). Knowing the "expected range" is important when attempting to determine if the kidneys are functioning and concentrating urine appropriately. Concentrated urine indicates good renal tubular function, as it implies removal of more water than solutes. The savvy clinical practitioner will interpret USG with respect to the patient's hydration status. For example, in a dehydrated dog with healthy kidneys, the USG is expected to be hypersthenuric (well-concentrated).

As a generality, only dilute urine is considered "abnormal"; however, dilute urine can be expected in an over-hydrated individual as the kidneys attempt to excrete the excess body water. For instance, dilute urine is expected in psychogenic polydipsia, during fluid therapy, and while patients are receiving diuretics. In contrast, isosthenuria in a dehydrated or azotemic patient is abnormal and suggests the renal lesion involves the tubules.

If a USG is dilute, the measurement should be repeated/confirmed at different times of the day to determine if urine can be concentrated and if there is a pattern. The first urine excreted in the morning is typically the urine with the highest USG. Additionally, if findings are nebulous or unclear, repeating USG on a fresh sample is an easy and inexpensive option. Persistently dilute urine in a nonazotemic patient is abnormal and could involve renal or nonrenal causes (Table 24.8).

When serial urinalyses reveal urine with an SG of 1.007–1.013, it indicates that the kidney neither concentrated nor diluted the glomerular filtrate. In other words, urine is isosthenuric with respect to blood plasma, which has an SG of approximately 1.007–1.013 and an osmolality of 295–300 mOsmo. This is the least favorable range of urine specific gravities to detect over time as it is strong evidence of renal disease that involves >66% functional loss of both kidneys. Urine specific gravities that are <1.007 or >1.013 imply some renal function. However, cutoffs should be used cautiously as refractometers are not precise measurements [11]. USGs 1.014–1.020 are "gray zone," meaning that USG could be abnormal, and repeating USG may be warranted based on the rest of the data. A USG of 1.014 is so close to the isosthenuric range that several additional USGs should be obtained to help determine if concentrating ability is present. Likewise, a single USG in the range of 1.006–1.008 is not clear evidence of a disease process. Repeating USG at different times of the day to determine the range for that patient usually clarifies these gray-zone cases. Repeated USGs on urine samples supplied by the owner can be done for no or minimal cost. Correlate USG with the other data in cases like this to help determine a course of action.

When dilute urine is attributed to renal disease, it implies that the lesion involves the tubules. Glomerular diseases may be associated with dilute urine because 90% of the vascular supply to tubules passes through glomerular capillaries. Therefore, if the glomerular lesion is severe enough it may eventually compromise tubular function. Interstitial diseases are often associated with dilute urine because tubules and interstitium are anatomically adjacent to each other, and eventually lesions in one area involve the other. These examples illustrate the nephron concept. That is, injury to one part of the nephron may eventually lead to injury of the rest of the nephron. When renal injury is suspected, following a patient's USG over time is a practical, affordable laboratory test to monitor the progression or improvement of renal function. Fractional excretion studies or creatinine clearance studies are other more discerning methods for evaluating renal injury.

Consistently hyposthenuric USG measurements (e.g., <1.007) are probably not due to renal lesions, especially if the animal is not azotemic. Dilute urine indicates that the kidney has enough function to remove more solutes than water, because dilution is an active process. Mechanisms for the production of hyposthenuric urine include excess fluid intake (IV fluids, psychogenic polydipsia), decreased ADH production (diabetes insipidus), tubules refractory to ADH (steroids, calcium, caffeine), decreased medullary hypertonicity, plasma solute overload, combinations of the foregoing, and other unknown mechanisms (Table 24.4).

Additionally, substances in solution influence SG measurements. For example, in cases of marked proteinuria or glucosuria, every 1 g/dL of protein or glucose that is added to urine will increase the USG approximately 0.004, yet these solutes have little effect on the osmolality. The increased USG caused by proteinuria or glucosuria could lead to an overestimation of the USG and, therefore, an overestimation of the concentrating ability of the kidneys. Additionally, adding the following substances to 1 mL of water will increase the SG by 0.001 units: NaCl 1.5 mg; urea 3.6 mg; glucose 2.7 mg; albumin 4.0 mg. Each time the urine glucose increases by 1 g/dL (1+ on the dipstick) the USG increases by 0.004. A 4+ urine glucose would increase USG by approximately 0.010 units. These estimates and the principles are nice to know, but they are not used to calculate or estimate a USG. It is best to simply measure USG and realize the magnitude of change that may occur with organic solutes such as protein and glucose.

An example of a potential clinical problem would be in a dog treated intravenously with an artificial colloid substance such as hetastarch (HES). This artificial volume-expanding solution contains molecules of various sizes, some of which can pass through the glomerulus. In normal dogs 20 mL/kg of HES will increase the USG without a concurrent increase in the urine osmolality. This is because the number of molecules per kg of water determines urine osmolality. In contrast, the USG is dependent upon the density of the urine, and density is dependent upon both the size and number of particles. If USG were increased by HES therapy, it could lead to an overestimation of renal concentrating ability and mask an inadequate renal concentrating ability [12].

Suspended particles, such as hemoglobin, mucus, crystals, and cells, do not affect USG because they are not dissolved; however, they can make the urine cloudy and may make reading the line on the refractometer difficult.

Urine specific gravity in puppies

Approximately 4 weeks of age is when pups are able to concentrate urine comparable to other canine age groups. USG is significantly lower in pups younger than 4 weeks of age as compared to pups 4–24 weeks of age, but there are no differences in protein, blood, glucose, ketones, or bilirubin.

Chemical examination of urine

There are numerous products to help analyze urine, but it is beyond the scope of this writing to list them all and their associated false-negative and false-positive results. This chapter will focus on semiquantitative reagent strips that are

Case Example 24.11. 12-year-old FS Boston terrier cross named "Poppy"

The patient presents for "urinating and drinking a lot." The physical exam is unremarkable. Owners approved CBC, chemistry panel, and complete urinalysis; only abnormality detected was a USG of 1.006. What are the next steps in working up this case?

1. "Urinating a lot" is a common owner concern and may suggest either pollakiuria or polyuria. Owners should be questioned carefully regarding the frequency and quantity of urine produced. Additionally, absence of abnormalities in cellular and sediment examination of urine makes cystitis unlikely (more common in female than male dogs).
2. The USG is at the cutoff between isosthenuria and hyposthenuria. Differentiating between this is important because the differential diagnoses for isosthenuria are quite different from hyposthenuria (Table 24.4). To determine which is more likely, ask the owners to collect a clean sample of urine when the dog first wakes in the morning. Measure USG in that sample and preferably in a sample from another time of the day and determine if Poppy can concentrate urine and if not, is there a pattern. A second complete UA is a good idea, and a urine culture should also be considered. There is no need to repeat CBC or chemistry panel.
3. Consider offering the owners SDMA. The prior results of UN, Ct, and P were WRI, if SDMA is WRI then renal disease is less likely and consider differentials for low USG (Table 24.8). If SDMA is increased then offer full "renal workup" and monitor dog periodically for progression of possible renal disease.

Cushing's is unlikely as alkaline phosphatase (ALP) was WRI (no chemistry abnormalities detected) and there were no PE abnormalities suggestive of hyperadrenocorticism (HAC). Ninety-five percent of HAC dogs will have an increase in ALP. Diabetes mellitus is unlikely because of absence of glucose in urine or hyperglycemia. Hypercalcemia was not detected. Pyometra is ruled out, FS. The results of basic laboratory tests and PE are practical means to distinguish the more common causes of PU/PD.

commonly used in veterinary practice. These provide a semi-quantitative analysis of the concentration of most substances of interest in urine. The strips contain pads impregnated with various chemicals that, rather than detecting a specific compound, detect the product of a chemical reaction involving the specific analyte. Formation of the product leads to a color change, and the degree of color change is proportional to the concentration of the analyte (Figure 24.4).

Product expiration dates should be adhered to because outdated strips can give false-negative results. During storage, containers must be kept tightly closed, as the reagent pads are sensitive to air and humidity. Additionally, reagent strips are designed for human urine and some of the reactions are not valid in animal urine. For example, these strips should not be used to determine WBCs, SG, urobilinogen, or nitrite concentration in animals.

After the urine sample is examined grossly for color and clarity, the reagent strip is immersed in a well-mixed sample of urine for the prescribed period (no longer or false increases will occur) and then removed with excess urine being drained while holding the stick laterally on a paper towel. Depending on the solute evaluated, the instructions will state how long after immersion that pad should be graded. Hold the reagent strip horizontally to prevent intermixing of reagents. The next step is to determine if a solute is present – a qualitative assessment. Proceeding by the time indicated on the container with the color grading scheme, the pads are read and graded, usually 1+ to 4+.

Results should be interpreted with USG because the concentration of the urine will affect the quantity of solutes. To illustrate this point, a 2+ protein in urine with an SG of 1.020 would be 1+ protein if that urine sample were diluted to 1.010 (i.e., diluted by half). A dog with a urine protein of 50 mg/dL and a USG of 1.010 is losing as much protein per day as a dog with a urine protein of 100 mg/dL and a USG of 1.020. In dogs, a 1+ proteinuria in urine with an inactive sediment and a USG of 1.060 is less significant than trace or 1+ proteinuria in urine with an SG of 1.008 and an inactive sediment. These reagent strips should be interpreted cautiously, as the various reagents are prone to false-negative and false-positive results (e.g., see "Glucose" below). If results on a strip are equivocal, there are chemical tablets available that are generally more sensitive for each substance on the strip and that can be used to clarify results.

pH

Dogs and cats have urine that is neutral to acidic, and herbivores, neutral to alkaline. The pH reagent pads contain dyes that change color based on the pH: red in acidic, yellow in neutral, and blue-green in alkaline urine. The range detected is approximately 5.0–9.0. Because urine is produced from filtration of blood plasma, urine pH reflects plasma pH. Additionally, it is a crude index of blood gas status. Urine pH may be compared with TCO_2 (bicarbonate) to determine if they correlate, and usually they do. Paradoxical aciduria is a unique situation seen most frequently in dairy cattle with a left or right displaced abomasum (described earlier). Alkaline urine in a dog with acidosis may be an indicator of "renal tubular acidosis," which indicates the inability to acidy urine in the face of metabolic acidosis. Urease splitting bacteria can cause alkalinization of urine, as will prolonged storage at room temperature and the presence of certain disinfectants (contamination of urine collection container).

Normal dog and cat urine has a pH of approximately 5–7. If urine pH is below 5 or above 7.5, the cause should be investigated. Alkaline urine with a pH >8 may result in lysis of RBCs, WBCs, and dissolution of casts. It has been reported

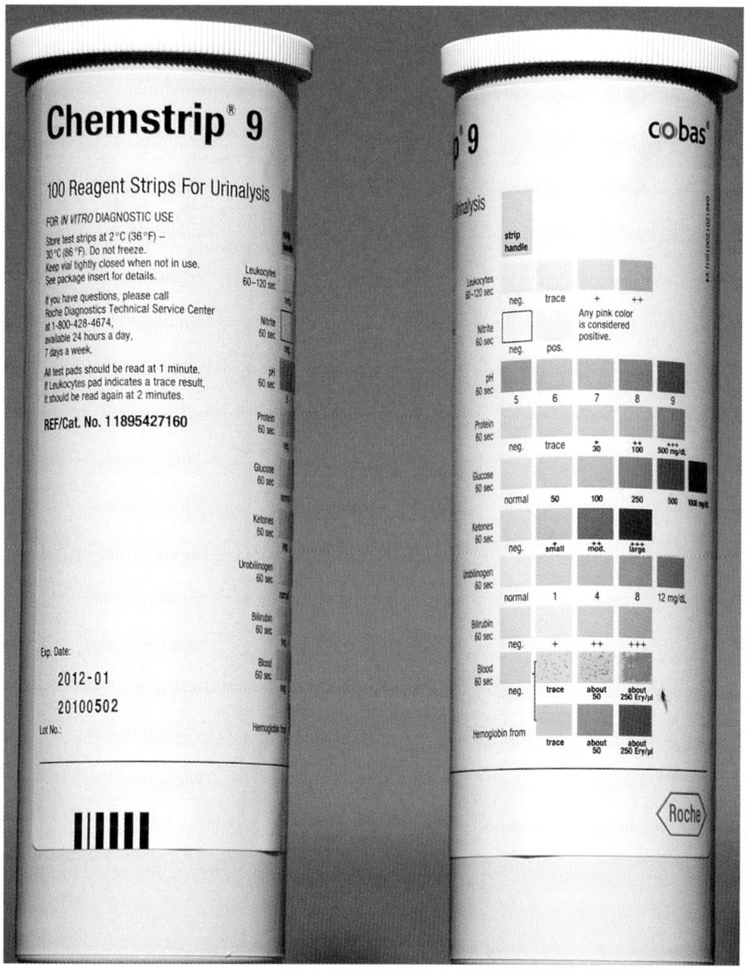

Figure 24.4 Two containers of representative urinalysis reagent strips. Container on left is oriented to show text labeling with storage and use directions and expiration date. Container on right is oriented to show a chart of reagent test pad color reactions. The patient urinalysis test strip must be read within the stated times for each reagent and is then compared to the color chart for recording results. Alternatively, an optical color reflectance reader device is used to determine the urinalysis test strip results.

that a pH >8 will falsely result in a 1+ protein on the reagent pad; however, recent studies suggest that this is no longer the case.

Protein

Proteinuria is a term used to describe the presence of any protein in urine, such as albumin, globulins, and Bence Jones proteins. Proteinuria has preglomerular, glomerular, and postglomerular causes (Table 24.9). However, it is used clinically to recognize renal disease, especially diseases affecting glomeruli. Quantification of renal proteinuria is a practical means to identify renal disease, predict glomerular disease, monitor renal disease, and formulate treatment plans. Colorimetric dipsticks, sulfosalicylic acid (SSA) turbidity testing, or other chemical assays detect excess protein in the urine.

Reagent pads

Most proteins produce a positive color change on the reagent strip pad, and the concentration of protein is assigned a trace to 4+. Chemical methods for protein determination are best at detecting albumin. Reagent pads on strips detect albumin up to 50 times better than globulins but are able to detect other globulins, Bence Jones proteins (if present in sufficient concentration), hemoglobin, and myoglobin relatively well. Bence Jones proteins are associated with multiple myeloma. Reagent strips do not easily recognize Bence Jones protein because light chain immunoglobulins have fewer free amino groups available to react with reagents. In general, approximately 25–50 mg/dL of Bence Jones proteins are required for a trace to 1+ reaction on the reagent pad. If concentrations are insufficient, a false-negative result will ensue.

Sulfosalicylic acid turbidity test

Protein is also determined and scored via SSA turbidity (1+ to 4+). SSA also detects albumin the best but does detect all proteins provided they are present in sufficient concentrations and is considered better than the reagent pad on the dipstick. If urine is cloudy, it should be centrifuged prior to performing the SSA turbidity test, because suspended solids can cause a false-positive result. False-positive results are also possible with certain drugs (penicillin and sulfonamides) and radiology contrast media. False-negative protein results are associated with the inability to read through very turbid

Table 24.9 Differentiating proteinuria.

Preglomerular	Glomerular	Postglomerular
• Physiologic • Fever • Exercise • Seizures • Hypertension • Pigments • Hemoglobinemia/-uria • Myoglobinemia/-uria • Neoplasia (Bence Jones proteins) • Multiple myeloma • Lymphoma	• Glomerulonephritis • Amyloidosis	• Hematuria • Cystitis (e.g., inflammation) • Tubular disease • Fanconi syndrome

Hyperadrenocorticism and exogenous steroids cause proteinuria with and without cystitis. The mechanisms when the urine sediment is inactive are not as clear; however, glucocorticoid therapy given to healthy dogs resulted in a mild increase in UPC (slightly greater than 1) and glomerular lesions. Others have shown that hydrocortisone will increase the blood pressure of dogs and cause proteinuria, both of which are reversible within 1 month of stopping the steroid.
Microproteinuria, microalbuminuria**:** <30 mg/dL, and albuminuria is >30 mg/dL.

urine and in markedly alkaline urine. If Bence Jones proteinuria and/or multiple myeloma are suspected, then consider sending urine to a reference laboratory to request SSA, and possibly urine and serum electrophoresis to determine if immunoglobulin light chains or a monoclonal gammopathy are present.

Spectrophotometry

Protein can be quantified by a spectrophotometer in a spot urine sample or in a 24-hour collection. The latter is not recommended as it is too labor-intensive, and there is good correlation between 24-hour collections and urine protein:Ct ratios from spot urine samples. For further information, see the section on "Protein Abnormalities" in this chapter.

Interpreting a positive protein

A positive protein reaction should always be correlated with USG, presence of blood in the urine, results of the serum biochemical profile, and results of the microscopic examination of urine sediment. Hemorrhage causes a positive pad result due to hemoglobin (a protein) being released from lysed RBCs, as well as any plasma proteins that may be exuded along with RBCs. If blood is positive on the strip and RBCs are seen microscopically, then it complicates interpretation of a proteinuria. If glomerular disease is suspected, the proteinuria will need to be assessed when the hemorrhage has resolved. In general, reagent pads are generally considered poorly reactive with proteins from WBCs and epithelial cells. In dogs, a trace protein reading is ≤0.1 g/dL (10 mg/dL; 0.1 g/L) and a 1+ result indicates the renal loss of 0.03 g/dL (30 mg/dL; 0.3 g/L). Both are considered normal if urine is concentrated but abnormal if urine is dilute and/or if there is a positive blood reaction or urine sediment abnormalities. False-positive dipstick protein results have been associated with excessive urine contact time, specific antibiotics, contamination of sample with disinfectants, and historically with highly alkaline urine.

Preglomerular proteinuria

Preglomerular diseases that result in marked hyperproteinemia may damage the filtration barrier, overload the proximal tubular capacity for reabsorption, and result in persistent proteinuria, referred to as "overload proteinuria." This is most commonly associated with hemoglobinemia, myoglobinemia, and paraproteins of small molecular weight (<45,000 Da) as seen in multiple myeloma, and recognition of one of these three problems is critical to the diagnosis of preglomerular proteinuria. Serum proteins in patients with multiple myeloma may exceed 9 g/dL, and this may induce preglomerular, overload proteinuria that is persistent. If hemoglobinemia is so severe it overwhelms carrying proteins such as haptoglobin, then excess hemoglobin will enter the glomerular filtrate. Myoglobin does not have carrier proteins, and it readily passes into the glomerular filtrate producing dipstick results that are positive for protein and blood. Mild, clinically insignificant preglomerular proteinuria is also associated with excess exercise, seizures, fever, stress, etc., and is referred to as functional proteinuria. This type of proteinuria is transient and is not significant. Historical and physical exam data and UA will identify these causes. One study demonstrated that exercise did not increase the urinary excretion of albumin in dogs.

Glomerular proteinuria

Glomeruli retain proteins larger than approximately 68,000 Da and that are negatively charged, thereby conserving albumin at the level of the glomerulus. In health, the small amounts of albumin that leak through are reabsorbed by tubular epithelium and degraded by cellular lysosomes. Although albuminuria may be due to tubular lesions, the amount of protein in the urine is small and this mechanism never results in hypoalbuminemia. In glomerular disease, glomeruli lose their negative charge because immunoglobulins (positively charged) are deposited in glomerular basement membranes as part of the pathogenesis of glomerulonephritis and amyloidosis. Albumin, with its small molecular size (66,000) and negative charge, leaks through the glomerular membrane. This occurs to such an extent that a patient will develop hypoalbuminemia, and the correlation of hypoalbuminemia with proteinuria is a cornerstone toward developing a diagnosis of glomerular disease. Furthermore, if glomerulonephritis and amyloidosis are severe enough, nephrotic syndrome may develop. Nephrotic syndrome is characterized by proteinuria, hypoalbuminemia, edema, ascites, thrombi, and hypercholesterolemia. Diagnosis of glomerular proteinuria requires persistent proteinuria with inactive urine sediment (free of RBCs, WBCs, etc.).

The distinction of glomerulonephritis and amyloidosis could have different treatment and prognostic implications, and therefore the differentiation of these two diseases is sometimes desired. The correlation of renal biopsy results with histologic sections taken at necropsy is 98%. This is because the lesions of glomerulonephritis and amyloidosis are diffuse. Essentially 100% of glomeruli have lesions to some degree, so biopsy, even if only one to three small pieces are obtained, will adequately sample the disease process as long as the cortex is sampled. The most common complication is minor hemorrhage, resulting in hematuria; but rarely, the complications are severe and life-threatening. Results of biopsy that indicate severe end-stage renal disease may influence the decision to treat.

The majority of dogs 9 years of age and older will have some form of microscopic glomerulonephritis. The majority of these cases are subclinical. The recognition of these animals with newer screening tests that detect microproteinuria (urine albumin <30 mg/dL, correlating to 1+ on the urine dipstick) may prove beneficial for long-term care. It is reported that 2% of clinically healthy dogs have proteinuria and 20% have microalbuminuria. Proteins that are leaking through diseased glomeruli may cause damage to tubules via cytokines, direct toxicity, and overload of lysosomal degradation mechanisms. Therefore, recognizing persistent proteinuria and preventing its progression may have beneficial effects for the health of the kidney and therefore the animal.

Postglomerular proteinuria

Postglomerular proteinuria is due to inflammation in the urogenital tract and is the most common cause of proteinuria. Postglomerular proteinuria should be considered when the urine sediment reveals evidence of inflammation, such as erythrocytes and/or leukocytes (i.e., "active sediment"). When an active sediment is seen, investigation into the underlying inflammatory cause should be sought. If the cause of the proteinuria is due to postglomerular inflammation, when the underlying cause has been managed, the proteinuria should also resolve. For example, cystitis is a common cause of postglomerular proteinuria. Attention is focused on the diagnosis and treatment of cystitis, not proteinuria. In most cases, the proteinuria is gone once the cystitis and associated inflammation is resolved. If proteinuria persists, then consideration is given to causes of persistent proteinuria. In rare occasions, postglomerular proteinuria may be due to in-tubular resorptive defects as seen in familial or acquired Fanconi syndrome.

Quantifying proteinuria

Once proteinuria has been diagnosed, and causes of prerenal and postrenal proteinuria have been ruled out, the next critical step is to determine if the proteinuria is persistent. A persistent proteinuria should be quantified, as this helps determine the severity of renal lesions and serves as a means of monitoring disease progression or response to treatment. This is most commonly done via urine protein to creatinine ratio (UPC). Determination of UPC is accomplished by collecting urine and serum simultaneously and chemically measuring the protein and creatinine in both samples. The amount of protein in the urine is divided by the amount of creatinine in the urine and a ratio is derived, Prot:Ct. Determining UPC ratios on several samples taken 24 hours or more apart is recommended for even more reliable results because there can be random variation in the amounts of albumin loss in any one sample. However, measuring serial UPC may be cost-prohibitive. In these situations, pooling one mL aliquots taken from three urine samples collected 24–48 hours apart yields results that are clinically useful and more cost-effective. The IRIS has proposed reference values for dogs and cats. A UPC <0.2 is considered normal in both species. In dogs a borderline proteinuria is 0.2–0.5 and is 0.2–0.4 in cats. A UPC of >0.5 in dogs and >0.4 in cats is indicative of glomerular disease or CKD, and UPCs of >2.0 are strongly suggestive of glomerular disease. To determine if the disease is progressing or improving, a change of at least 35% in UPC should be observed in high values, and 80% at low UPC values (near 0.5) is required.

Microproteinuria

Microproteinuria, microalbuminuria is an extension of proteinuria and refers to situations where the amount of protein in the urine is small or below the limit of detectability of most qualitative and some routine quantitative assays. A trace or 1+ protein in concentrated urine is considered insignificant; however, it can imply early or occult renal disease (minimal change nephropathy). The primary protein in the urine of these patients is albumin, and assays are now available to measure microalbuminuria. Microalbuminuria is albumin <30 mg/dL and albuminuria ("overt albuminuria") is urine albumin >30 mg/dL in urine normalized to SG of 1.010. The limit of detectability of dipstick colorimetric pads is approximately 6–10 mg/dL and SSA 5 mg/dL. If these trace amounts are detected in urine with an SG of 1.020, then the concentrations would double if the USG was 1.040. Similarly, trace amounts in urine with an SG of 1.020 would be undetectable with these qualitative methods in urine with an SG of 1.010

or less, yet this may be significant. The detection of microproteinuria may be of value in geriatric patients, patients with suspected occult renal disease, monitoring chronic renal patients, breeds with known familial nephropathies, or sick patients with an unknown diagnosis. Recognizing occult renal disease opens avenues for patient management such as restricted diets and angiotensin-converting enzyme (ACE) inhibitors. It is not known if these treatments can change the progress of the disease or are beneficial to these patients but it may prove helpful, and the first step is to recognize the problem exists. Although its use is implied to recognize occult glomerular or chronic renal disease, any cause of proteinuria, pre-, glomerular, and postglomerular, will be positive with these microalbumin assays. Therefore, these other causes must be ruled out before steps are taken to recognize occult renal disease. There are qualitative (reagent pad) and semiquantitative immunologic test strips (ELISA) available to estimate Prot:Ct ratios, but their clinical utility has not been proven.

The other methodologies, protein electrophoresis and immunoturbidimetric tests, are quantitative and are performed in reference labs. Semiquantitative immunologic test strips and protein electrophoresis are less accurate than automated immunoturbidimetric assays. Semiquantitative immunologic test strips are easy to use. Urine is diluted to an SG of 1.010 by adding distilled water, and the strip is immersed for 3 minutes and the color intensity compared to various categories. The sensitivity and specificity of the test strips are 91% and 92%, respectively. They have a false-positive rate of 8%, false-negative rate of 9%, and at the high and very high positive categories are detecting overt proteinuria that can be assessed with routine dipsticks.

Blood (occult blood, heme)

The reagent pad has a chromogen that changes to various shades of blue-green after oxidation of the enzyme. Anything that causes oxidation of the enzyme is detected and it implies blood is present only because that is how the pad is labeled and because iron in RBCs is the most common substance that will stimulate this oxidation reaction. However, a positive blue color change is also seen with iron in free hemoglobin, iron in myoglobin, peroxidase in plants and bacteria, and cleaning agents. The reaction is sensitive and the color intensity varies with the amount of "heme" detected; it is more sensitive to free hemoglobin than intact RBCs.

Method

Immerse the stick in well-mixed, noncentrifuged urine. A "speckled" pattern of green dots is due to individual RBCs that contact the pad and then lyse; this pattern is associated with microscopic hematuria. A uniform color change is due to a greater amount of hemorrhage, free hemoglobin, myoglobin, or contaminants. False negatives are uncommon but are associated with bacteria that produce nitrites and treatments with vitamin C. Ascorbic acid is a reducing substance that counteracts the oxidation reaction.

Correlate the results with microscopic enumeration of RBCs in urine, PCV, muscle enzymes, USG, and urine pH. Very dilute urine, less than 1.007, and alkaline urine may lyse RBCs and mask hematuria. Distinction of hematuria, hemoglobinuria, and myoglobinuria is clinically important and is described in the section on diseases.

Degrees of sensitivity of various tests to detect blood

Method	Positive	RBC/hpf
Hemastix, Labstix; hemolytic reagents in the stick lyse RBCs	1/8000	200 RBC/hpf
Occult test tablet	1/32,000	20 RBC/hpf
Microscope		<10 RBC/hpf

Glucose

There should be no glucose in the urine of healthy animals. Reagent strips are sensitive, and detect glucose via an oxidation reaction that produces a color change. False negatives are due to vitamin C and outdated strips. False negatives can occur if the glucose in urine is in low concentrations and one of these substances is present: vitamin C, formaldehyde, ketones, bilirubin (large amount), salicylates, or tetracyclines. False-positive results are observed when samples are contaminated with oxidizing cleaning agents and hydrogen peroxide. Cats with urethral obstruction reportedly have an unknown substance that reacts with the color indicator to produce false-positive results. In an animal (most commonly cat) with a positive urine glucose, it is important to correlate the dipstick result with serum glucose as stress can cause a transient hyperglycemia that results in a transient glucosuria.

Urine dipsticks are accurate to rule in glucosuria (high specificity) but not rule it out (low sensitivity). Therefore, if glucosuria is suspected but the dipstick is negative consider assessing for glucosuria with a different method. For example, submit a urine sample for analysis on a clinical chemical analyzer or request urine glucose to creatinine ratio (UGCR). Visual readings of urine dipsticks were more accurate than automated readings in this study that included more than 500 dog and cat urine samples. Automated reading of glucosuria was more accurate for cat than dog urine. This same study sought to establish a UCGR measurement as an additional clinical diagnostic test. Although the UCGR correlated well with the absolute measurement of urine glucose, it did not add any clinically useful information in these patients [13].

Tablets are available to detect glucose and do so through copper reduction. False negatives are due to outdated product and low glucose concentration in urine. False positives are fairly common as any reducing substance can cause the color change.

Always correlate results of urine glucose with serum glucose. The main clinical differential is transient (epinephrine, corticosteroids) versus persistent hyperglycemic disorders (diabetes mellitus, hyperadrenocorticism). When plasma glucose exceeds certain concentrations, the ability of the proximal tubules to reabsorb glucose is surpassed and glucose escapes into the urine. The renal threshold for glucose in dogs is approximately 200 mg/dL (range: 180–220 mg/dL), cats 300 mg/dL (range: 250–350 mg/dL), horses 150 mg/dL (range: 120–200 mg/dL), and cattle 100 mg/dL (range: 80–120 mg/dL). Positive urine glucose results coupled with serum glucose concentrations below the renal thresholds suggest a defect in tubular reabsorption mechanisms, and may be seen with nephrosis (toxic insults), tubular injury, primary or familial glucosuria, and Fanconi syndrome. Fanconi syndrome is a heritable or acquired disease characterized by defects in proximal tubular reabsorption of various substrates that include one or more of glucose, sodium, calcium, bicarbonate, amino acids, and phosphate. Primary glucosuria is seen in Scottish terriers, Norwegian elkhounds, and dogs of mixed breeding and is marked by glucosuria in the absence of hyperglycemia. Glucosuria without hyperglycemia may also be seen due to a time delay of urine collection relative to serum collection. The urine in the bladder may be several hours old relative to the serum and therefore a transient hyperglycemia may have occurred, while the serum glucose has meanwhile normalized. This can be seen with stress, postprandially, and after fluid therapy with glucose-enriched fluids. Glucosuria is common in cattle due to their low renal threshold for glucose and the ease of which cattle develop stress hyperglycemia. Cattle with CNS disease may have serum glucose values of 300 mg/dL or greater; pyloric obstruction can produce serum glucose values up to 500 mg/dL or greater.

Serum fructosamine is formed when sugar moieties become attached to plasma proteins, and its concentration can be used to distinguish transient from persistent hyperglycemia. The longer blood sugar has been elevated, the higher the serum fructosamine concentration. Serum fructosamine concentration reflects the average serum glucose concentration over the past 1–3 weeks (roughly the half-life of albumin and globulins), and will not be increased by transient hyperglycemia.

Postprandial glucosuria lasts for approximately 1.5 hours; glucosuria beyond 2 hours is abnormal and should prompt examination of serum glucose. Persistent hyperglycemia and glucosuria is seen commonly with diabetes mellitus and hyperadrenocorticism (Cushing's disease), and less frequently with pheochromocytoma, pancreatitis, acromegaly, progesterone administration, and some cases of sepsis. A urinalysis used to screen for glucosuria is an acceptable screening test for diabetes mellitus and in monitoring the effect of treatment for diabetes. Marked hyperglycemia, glucosuria, and ketonuria are diagnostic for diabetes mellitus.

Glucose increases the USG by approximately 0.004 units for each 1 g/dL of glucose in the urine. A 4+ urine glucose would increase USG by approximately 0.010 units. Glucosuria promotes bacterial and fungal growth.

Ketones

There should be no ketones in the urine of healthy animals. Reagent strips detect ketones via a reaction with nitroprusside that produces a purple color change proportional to the concentration of ketones present. Ketones enter the circulation first and then spill into the glomerular filtrate. Ketonuria can be detected in the absence of ketonemia. Ketogenesis produces three kinds of ketone bodies, but only two have the form of a true ketone and are detected by the nitroprusside reaction. The proportions of ketones excreted in the urine are approximately 78% beta-hydroxybutyrate, 20% acetoacetic acid and 2% acetone. The reaction mainly detects acetoacetic acid (approximately 90%), and reacts less efficiently with acetone (volatile). Beta-hydroxybutyrate, the most abundant product of ketogenesis, does not have the structure of a ketone and therefore is not detected. The most sensitive test for ketones in cattle is Ketostix™. Tablets are available but are less sensitive than Ketostix. Tablets rely on the same nitroprusside reaction as the urine reagent pads. Place one drop of urine (or blood, serum, plasma, or milk) on the tablet and read the color change in thirty seconds. Lavender to deep purple is positive and the intensity is proportional to the concentration of ketones present in the urine or blood. Tablets are more sensitive than strips and can detect ketones in the urine at 5 mg/dL, as opposed to 10 mg/dL for strips, and 10 mg/dL in blood.

If there is a trace ketone reaction on the dipstick consider confirming their presence with Ketostix, or the tablet method. A positive test result can be due to: excessive fat catabolism, as with negative energy balance, inadequate carbohydrate content in the diet, cachexia, starvation, anorexia, hyperthyroidism, pregnancy toxemia, and diabetes mellitus. Ketonuria occurs most commonly in high production dairy cattle, which enter a state of negative energy balance that promotes formation of ketones. Diabetes mellitus is the most common cause of ketonuria in dogs and cats. Ketones are negatively charged and force the excretion of a cation (sodium or potassium) when the kidney filters them. This may lead to hyponatremia and hypokalemia.

The chemicals used in the pads to detect ketones are light, humidity, heat, and date sensitive; therefore, do not use expired strips and keep the lid secured tightly.

Blood glucose	Urine glucose	Urine ketones	Diagnosis
High	Positive	Positive	Diabetes mellitus
High	Positive	Negative	Diabetes mellitus, hyperadrenocorticism; uncommon causes
High	Negative	Negative	Epinephrine or corticosteroids
Low	Negative	Positive	Starvation, pregnancy toxemia, etc.
Normal	Positive	Negative	Transient hyperglycemia, time delay, nephrosis, other tubular diseases, Fanconi

Bilirubin

Use fresh noncentrifuged urine for analysis. Reagent strips detect only conjugated bilirubin using a diazo methodology similar to Ictotest tablets. Since the color reaction is beige to pink to red, any substance that imparts a red color to urine may interfere with interpretation. Large quantities of vitamin C may cause false-negative results. As with all substances, correlate results with the USG. The sensitivity of strips is approximately 0.2–0.4 mg/dL, and tablets approximately 0.05–0.1 mg/dL. Tablet testing is recommended if interference is suspected (e.g., hemoglobinuria or myoglobinuria).

The reaction does not detect biliverdin, and conjugated bilirubin will hydrolyze to biliverdin in urine exposed to light, so analyze fresh urine. Conjugated bilirubin is water soluble and readily enters the glomerular filtrate in most species (cats have a higher threshold). Unconjugated bilirubin is bound to albumin and therefore should not pass through glomeruli.

Bilirubinuria indicates possible liver disease or hemolysis rather than disease in the kidneys. It is most commonly associated with cholestasis. Any positive reaction in a cat is considered abnormal and warrants further investigation. Dogs have a low renal threshold for bilirubin, and additionally, it can be conjugated in small quantities in tubular epithelial cells of normal dogs. In dogs, up to 1+ bilirubin in concentrated urine is considered normal and is common, especially in male dogs but the finding must correlate with other clinical abnormalities. Approximately 20–25% of normal dogs will have positive reaction for bilirubin in urine via reagent strips, and up to 60% with tablets. Bilirubinuria precedes bilirubinemia and icterus, and may therefore be an early indicator of hepatic disease.

Urobilinogen

Urobilinogen is present on reagent strips used for human patients but it is not present on reagent strips designed for animals as it has no value. The detection of urobilinogen indicates a patent bile duct and a fresh urine sample, and is ignored.

Nitrites

Detection of nitrites is indirect evidence of bacteriuria as some bacteria produce nitrite, however, the results are unreliable so do not use in animals. Determination of bacteriuria should be done by microscopic examination and culture of the urine.

Leukocytes

Reagent strips for WBCs recognize a specific leukocyte esterase that is found in human neutrophils, eosinophils, basophils, and monocytes but is not reliable for dogs and cats. Determination of leukocytes in the urine of animals should be done by microscopic examination.

Urine specific gravity

The reagent strip tests are considered unreliable in veterinary medicine. The strips indirectly estimate the SG based on pKa, the shift in the pH produces a color change. Maximum concentration detected is 1.030, and is inadequate for determination of concentration ranges in dogs and cats. Furthermore, results do not correlate well with refractometry measurements, and false positives and negatives are common. (See earlier discussion in the "Urine Specific Gravity" portion of this chapter.)

Microscopic sediment examination

It is standard to centrifuge 5–10 ml of well mixed fresh urine at 1500–2500 rpm for 5 minutes; however, the exact volume is not critical. It is recommended to use a consistent amount or whatever is available when collection volume is small. Pour off or aspirate and save the supernatant (for possible chemistry analysis) and resuspend the sediment in the urine that remains (0.5 ml is ideal and the amount left should be consistent) by flicking the tube several times with your finger until the pellet and its contents are well mixed. Place one unstained drop on a slide, add a coverslip and examine at low-power field (10× objective) for casts and crystals and at a high-power field (40× objective) for cells and bacteria. Reduce the light in the field by closing the iris diaphragm (preferable to lowering the condenser) until the material in the field is refractory. Scan the slide with the 10× objective and then record the results as number seen per low- or high-power field (#/lpf; #/hpf) by counting 10 fields and averaging the results. There also are manufactured systems that aid in these steps and results will be based on number seen per microliter. Change the focus during examination to better see the materials present as not all material is in the same plane of focus in wet-mount preparations. If the sample of urine is excessively turbid dilute it with additional supernatant or physiologic saline (but results per magnification are now reduced) and if RBCs are so numerous that it is difficult to see other structures then lyse the RBCs with 2% acetic acid (vinegar). All abnormalities can be seen in unstained preparations however if unusual structures are seen consider a wet-mount stain (follow directions) and/or prepare an air-dried film and stain it with a Diff-Quik type stain just like a cytology specimen; the latter is preferable. If neoplasia is suspected you may want a fresh sample of urine obtained with a wash as urine is harsh on cellular features and cells sitting in urine for several hours in the bladder will be visibly altered. Better yet is an ultrasound-guided aspirate from the mass. These slides should be air dried and stained with Diff-Quik type stains or Wright stains. Do not diagnose neoplasia on wet-mount preparations, use air-dried, monolayer preparations.

Always correlate results with mode of collection, USG, chemical results, and clinical findings. Examples: 2 casts/lpf in urine with a USG of 1.004 in an azotemic animal is very significant, whereas 2 casts/lpf in urine with a USG of 1.044 in a wellness check is probably normal. Leukocytes in a voided sample may be from the genital tract. Normal findings or results expected in normal patients are in Table 24.5.

Casts and heavier structures tend to aggregate along the edges of the coverslip so be sure to examine all regions of the cover slipped area. Count in a low-power field but proceed to high-power fields to better see their morphology and for more accurate identification.

Sources of technical error

Inexperience, open iris diaphragm, dirty objectives, old urine, poorly mixed urine, contamination, variable amounts of urine centrifuged, too much stain added, organisms growing in contaminated stain jars, random rather than systematic examination of 10 fields, and confusion of Brownian movement of small material with bacteria are all contributors to error.

Refer to Appendix 24.A for color imagery related to microscopic examination of urine; Figures 24.A.1–24.A.37.

Red blood cells

Hematuria occurs when there is greater than 5 RBCs per high-power field (/hpf). As with all cellular events in urine, correlate results with collection technique, SG, pH, reagent pad findings, and mode of collection. For example, cystocentesis and catheterization may induce minor hemorrhage; and RBCs lyse in urine with a USG of <1.008 and in alkaline urine. At USG >1.025 they tend to crenate (shrink and have irregular contours). At a USG in mid-ranges, erythrocytes are uniform, discoid, smoothly contoured, clear to light-yellow or rust-red, refractile, and have no internal detail. Results are recorded as number seen/hpf. Normal is considered <5/hpf, and the phrase "too numerous to count" (TNTC) is used when the field is crowded with RBCs.

There are too many causes of hematuria to produce a practical list. However, the common denominator is trauma: cystocentesis, catheterization, calculi, hit by car, obstruction, cancer, biopsy of kidney or bladder; and nonphysical traumatic events such as infection, estrus, nephrosis, feline lower urinary tract disease (formerly known as feline urologic syndrome), parasites, and bleeding disorders. RBC casts are rare but localize the hemorrhage to the renal tubules. RBC casts are very fragile and often disintegrate with handling of urine. RBCs may be confused with fat droplets, but fat droplets are not uniform in size, are more refractile, and some will be out of the plane of focus.

Leukocytes

Greater than five WBCs per high-power field (#/hpf) is abnormal and is termed pyuria. The magnitude of WBCs/hpf is the key and as always, the results should be correlated with USG, the rest of the data in the UA, other data in the case (steroids will decrease the number of WBCs in urine), mode of collection, urine pH, etc. WBCs lyse easily in alkaline urine and hypotonic urine (as do RBCs). Voided urine could have inflammation anywhere in the urogenital tract. Cystocentesis localizes the source of the inflammation to the kidneys or more likely the urinary bladder; however, reflux is possible, e.g., prostatitis.

WBCs are slightly larger than RBCs (1.5–2× larger), are spherical, granular, have internal structures, a nucleus, and appear singular, in clumps, or in casts. WBC casts localize their source to renal tubules and indicate pyelonephritis. Although any WBC could be seen they are almost always neutrophils and differentiation of the types of WBCs is not necessary but if desired will require examination of a stained film. Neutrophils indicate inflammation in the urogenital tract. They are usually accompanied by RBCs and bacteria should be searched for microscopically and via culture. Inflammation is also seen with cancer, calculi, cystitis, prostatitis, and pyelonephritis. Eosinophils are rarely seen, can be associated with parasitic diseases and in dogs consider eosinophilic polypoid cystitis. The latter is a common histologic diagnosis that causes persistent hematuria and produces a mass in the urinary bladder that resembles a tumor. The mass is infiltrated with eosinophils and there is eosinophilpoiesis within the mass. It requires surgical removal.

Epithelial cells

These cells may be squamous (urethra, genital, or skin), transitional (bladder), renal (tubules), or neoplastic (usually TCC). Squamous cells are huge (5× larger than WBCs, 10× larger than RBCs), have lined or sharp edges, with nuclei often not visible, and usually are in low numbers. If numerous squamous epithelial cells are seen in a free catch sample from a female dog in estrus. They are genital in origin and if numerous squamous epithelial cells are seen in a male dog consider a Sertoli cell neoplasm that is secreting estrogen and inducing squamous metaplasia of the prostate.

Transitional epithelial cells are from the bladder, ureter, or renal pelvis and most are from the bladder. Supposedly the depth of location in the urothelium changes their morphology enough to recognize the different sources, but this is difficult to discern and does not aid a diagnosis. In normal urine there are only a few epithelial cells: <5/hpf. When in large numbers they are usually accompanied by RBCs and WBCs and are associated with cystitis. If numerous and in rafts they may be due to catheterization. Their appearance has a wide range; they are approximately 2× larger than WBCs, round to polygonal, have a round nucleus, and are granular to homogenous appearing. These are the most common epithelial cell seen in urine.

Renal tubular epithelial cells are the least common or the least commonly recognized. They are approximately the size of WBCs and look like WBCs. They are round, granular, and have a central round nucleus. Different shapes and sizes may be localized to different regions of the kidneys but too little is known in veterinary medicine for this to be clinically useful.

Neoplastic transitional epithelial cells may be found in this chapter, under "Diagnoses."

Bacteria

The kidneys, ureters, bladder, and proximal urethra are sterile therefore urine should be sterile, at least until it passes through the distal urethra where normal flora can be added as a contaminant. Centrifugation at speeds used for urinalysis will not take bacteria out of suspension so the supernatant or the pellet is equally satisfactory for microscopic detection. Use the pellet as that is what is used for everything else in the microscopic examination and it will permit visualization of cells and therefore the possibility of seeing bacteria inside neutrophils. This will be seen best if a film is prepared and stained, rather than a wet mount. The key to seeing bacteria is the number present, the type of bacteria, and the observer's ability to see them. *Reduce the light considerably* to help outline them (decrease the iris diaphragm or lower the condenser to increase wet-mount contrast). The greater the numbers the more likely they will be seen. They are usually reported as few, moderate or many. Counting the number/field is impractical.

A bacterial infection should be confirmed with culture and preferably sensitivity. Bacteria can be seen in wet mounts with the 40× objective; however, Brownian movement of particulate matter is easily confused with bacteria and single cocci are easy to confuse with debris. If bacteria are seen but culture results are negative consider misinterpretation of particulate material and Brownian movement as a possible explanation. These "false-positive" observations are relatively common in clinical practice. Additional explanations for visualization of bacteria but culture negative include inhibition of growth by cold or frozen storage, or the patient has received antibiotics. It is not due to decreased sensitivity of culture technique, as culture is better to identify bacteria than is visualization. It takes about 10,000 rods/mL urine to see them and up to 100,000 cocci/mL to see them as opposed to only 1–10 bacteria/mL to produce a positive culture.

Localization of the infection is critical as they could be from kidney, bladder, urethra, prostate, uterus, prepuce, external genitalia, or the environment. If bacteria are detected in urine that was collected aseptically via cystocentesis an infection in the kidneys or bladder is the diagnosis. Correlate results with the rest of the urinalysis and if WBC casts are present (tubules involved), especially with concurrent azotemia, then pyelonephritis is the source. These patients may also have concurrent cystitis as an ascending infection from the bladder is the most common cause of pyelonephritis. Catheterized and voided samples that are positive for bacteria because of contamination will be culture positive, but bacteria are usually in too low a number to visualize. If cystocentesis is not possible then use a sterile catheter and take as many precautions as possible to reduce contamination from the catheter. If a voided sample is used for culture, clean the genitalia and catch a midstream sample. Voided samples are to be avoided to rule in an infection, but they can be used to rule out an infection. Most contaminants and normal flora are Gram positive. Bacteria can replicate in urine readily therefore examine and culture soon after collection. Refrigeration, and especially freezing, will inhibit growth and/or kill bacteria and therefore may result in false negatives. If samples are to be shipped to a lab, refrigerate and strive to have cultures prepared in <24 hours from collection; do not store at room temperature or freeze. Storage of canine urine at four degrees centigrade for 24 hours will not affect results of culture and susceptibility tests.

Bacterial infections should be accompanied by pyuria, hematuria, proteinuria and various clinical signs including dysuria, stranguria, etc., so correlate all of the data available. The presence of intracellular bacteria in neutrophils is good evidence for *in vivo* infection but can happen *in vitro* if samples are allowed to sit at room temperature. Results of urinalysis may look similar for cystitis and pyelonephritis. Cystitis will not have azotemia or casts in the urine. Pyelonephritis may be associated with azotemia and casts, especially if the disease is active and widely disseminated (>75% involvement of kidneys). Infectious cystitis is more common in females due to their wider urethra and predisposition to ascending infection. It should be treated aggressively as it may lead to an ascending pyelonephritis. Sterile cystitis can occur with uroliths and neoplasia but all cases of cystitis/pyuria should be cultured before they are determined to have a nonbacterial etiology. Bacterial infection may also be a secondary event. Regardless of cause, bactiuria requires therapy. Bacteriuria without neutrophils is a paradox but is associated with contamination,

Cushing's disease or exogenous steroids that inhibit the influx of neutrophils, dilute or alkaline urine that may lyse the neutrophils, and antibiotic therapy that inhibits growth but bacteria are still seen. Cushing's disease is associated with increased prevalence of urinary tract infection due to dilute urine and decreased urinary bladder immunity.

Microscopic absence of bacteria does not rule out an infection. Rule out requires negative cultures to be certain. Aerobic Gram-negative rods account for most infections in the urinary tract, and *E. coli* is the most common pathogen cultured. Commercial products are available to culture urine and/or enumerate colonies in practice but they will require an incubator. Results obtained can be correlated with results of UA and this is a rapid way to identify a urinary tract infection and/or differentiate the discrepancy of Brownian movement versus true bacteria. If bacteria are seen in practice and culture results from a commercial laboratory are negative, the likely explanations are (i) the purported "bacteria" were actually Brownian movement of small particles; or (ii) the patient is receiving antibiotics. Urine should be placed in the culture system as soon after collection as possible for best results. Some systems use select media that turn different colors around different bacterial colonies. If numerous different colors are identified consider contamination. In these systems, the colonies are enumerated or the entire Culturette can be sent to a referral lab for enumeration, culture, and identification. Positive results determined in practice should be confirmed, bacteria classified, and an antibiotic sensitivity recommended. In samples obtained by cystocentesis and enumerated with these products >1000 cfu/mL is significant, 100–1000 is suspect and <100 is probably contamination or unimportant. For samples obtained by catheterization these guidelines are increased by 10-fold. Point-of-care commercial systems are an alternative to sending out urine to a commercial laboratory [14]. A positive culture result is reliable; a negative result should be interpreted with caution, as the bacteria may not have been identified. Susceptibility results are part of these systems; however, they may be limited to five antimicrobials and results may not correlate with those from the commercial laboratory.

Quantitative bacterial culture results from a commercial laboratory are still the best means of determining if a bacterial infection is present. The number of colonies is reported as "colony forming units per milliliter of urine" (cfu/mL). The gold standard for documenting urinary tract infection is ≥10 [5] cfus/mL. Susceptibility testing is provided if requested. Most commercial laboratories provide interpretation and consultation of their results. Generally, bacterial growth from urine collected via sterile cystocentesis technique is interpreted as clinically significant. Approximately 20% of normal female dogs will have >100,000 cfu/mL urine via catheterization but normal male dogs rarely have >1000 cfu/mL via catheterization. The following numbers can be used as guidelines to diagnose true infection via collection technique when correlated with all of the other data:

- Catheterization female dog >100,000 cfu/mL.
- Catheterization male dog >1000 cfu/mL.
- Catheterization female and male cat >1000 cfu/mL.
- Cystocentesis cat or dog either sex >100 cfu/mL.

Voided urine is not reliable to rule in but can be used to rule out an infection.

Yeast and fungi

Fungal hyphae and yeast forms in urine sediment are most commonly due to overgrowth of contaminants in old samples, or from the skin, litter box, etc.; however, if they are seen in a fresh sample/cystocentesis collected, then a fungal infection of the kidneys and/or bladder should be suspected. They are colorless, often plentiful when present; appear as long hyphae or budding ovals and spheres when in yeast forms. They tend to occur in immune-suppressed patients or patients on long-term antibiotic therapy. If noted in a feline, the feline immunodeficiency virus and feline leukemia virus status should be determined.

Parasites

Capillaria plica or *felis, Dioctophyma renale*, and *D. immitis* are seen rarely in urine of dogs and cats. *Klosiella* spp. in horse urine has been seen but is exceedingly rare. Capillaria ova look like whipworm ova, with oval shape, bipolar plugs, rough surface, and colorless to light yellow-tan. Check a fecal float for *Trichuris* and differentiate fecal contamination from dual infection. Microfilaria of heartworm may be seen due to hematuria, and a heartworm check should be performed if the status is not already known. Adult *D. renale*, or the kidney worm, is sometimes seen during a laparotomy and the ova are rarely seen in urine as large oval-shaped structures with an internal structure and a pitted tan to light brown surface.

Debris

Spermatozoa, talc crystals from gloves, pollen, fibers, and hair are some of the more common large "debris" seen with the 10 or 20× objectives. Brownian movement that can be confused with bacteria is seen with 40, 50, or 100× objectives.

Lipid

Lipid droplets are clear, variable in size, refractile, round, in different planes of focus, and common in cat urine. They may appear gray to black at low magnification and rarely can be seen grossly in urine from cats. Cat kidneys have considerable amounts of lipid in tubular epithelium and presumably this is the source of the lipid. There is no correlation between lipiduria and lipemia in these individuals.

Casts

Casts are molds of tubular lumens. Their primary component is the Tamm-Horsfall mucoprotein that is secreted by tubular epithelial cells. Casts may contain variable amounts of cells, lipid, and debris. When present in significant numbers they reflect active disease in renal tubules, nephrosis, which usually has an acute toxic etiology. Casts are not a reliable marker of onset, severity, or reversibility of the tubular disease, but they do imply that the disease is still active and is in the kidneys. Tubules have excellent regenerative capabilities if the basement membrane remains intact. Casts form in the loops of Henle, distal tubules and the collecting ducts. Absence of casts does not rule out tubular involvement. If they are not reported but tubular disease is suspected then repeat the UA as they may be shed intermittently or in showers. If casts continue to be shed post-treatment, they indicate the disease is still active. Waxy casts are often seen in chronic progressive tubulointerstitial renal disease.

Casts are classified based on their microscopic appearance and an attempt is made to correlate their appearance with a pathologic process, which has variable success. They are reported as the number seen/lpf (10× objective) and they are seen more easily if contrast is increased by closing the iris diaphragm. Normal urine should have no casts or only a few casts, and 1–2 hyaline or fine granular casts/lpf in concentrated urine is considered acceptable. Correlate number of casts with the USG as 1–2 casts in dilute urine, especially if other abnormalities are present, is abnormal. Increased number of casts is termed cylindruria.

Hyaline casts

These are the most difficult to see, are clear, have rounded or blunt ends, tend to dissolve in dilute or alkaline urine, and are composed almost entirely of mucoprotein and albumin with no cells or granularity. In elevated numbers, they imply glomerular disease or, less likely, a preglomerular proteinuria. The albumin that leaks through glomeruli apparently stimulates excess secretion and precipitation of tubular Tamm-Horsfall mucoprotein leading to formation of these casts. A few hyaline casts in concentrated urine are normal, a few in dilute urine and many in urine of any SG are abnormal. When they are observed, the possibility of glomerular disease or, less likely, multiple myeloma (Bence Jones proteinuria) should be pursued.

Granular casts

These are clear to tan-brown, easy to see, and consist of cells and mucoprotein. They are from epithelial cells that recently sloughed, became entrapped in the mucoprotein, and formed a cast. They indicate possible nephrosis, pyelonephritis, or infarction. The longer the casts are in the tubules before they are released, the more their granular appearance changes from rough and coarse to fine and then waxy, which is the final stage of degeneration of granular casts. Differentiation of coarse and fine granular casts is not necessary. One to two fine granular casts per lpf in concentrated urine are considered normal, but the presence of coarse granular and elevated numbers of fine granular casts is abnormal.

Waxy casts

Waxy casts are clear, with no internal structure, and they have sharply defined margins and squared-off ends as they are brittle and break. To the novice, they may resemble hyaline casts that are smoother and the ends are more rounded. Waxy casts imply chronicity and indicate a pathologic process when found in large numbers.

Cellular casts

These can be composed of epithelial, red, or WBCs, and all can have a granular appearance (granular casts). If RBCs are recognized in the cast it indicates hemorrhage in the tubules and if WBCs are recognized in the cast it indicates pyelonephritis. It can be difficult to recognize the type of cells in casts as the cells are degenerating and they are not stained well; RBC casts tend to be fragile.

Lipid casts

These are composed of lipid and are seen in cats; one may see refractile droplets in the casts. These casts are associated with tubular disease (degeneration) and diabetes mellitus. Confirmation of lipid content may require use of fat stains such as Sudan black B or Oil-red-O.

Hemoglobin and myoglobin casts

These are seen rarely and indicate intravascular hemolysis or myoglobinuria, respectively. They are yellow to pink-red to brown, homogeneous and smooth or may be granular if tubular cells are dying and sloughing into the lumens of the tubules. Correlate their presence with the rest of the case data.

Crystalluria (see Appendix 24.A for visual examples)

Crystalluria is the term used to describe the presence of crystals in the urine. Crystals may be found in normal patients (incidental finding, no treatment needed) or sick patients wherein the crystals may correlate with a known disease or they may indicate a primary disease that was formerly unidentified. For example, calcium oxalate dihydrate may indicate a hypercalcemic disorder; calcium oxalate monohydrate may indicate ethylene glycol toxicity; and ammonium biurate may indicate liver failure. Crystals in urine are often incidental and of no diagnostic significance; struvite, carbonate, and oxalate crystals can be present in urine from normal patients. The observation of crystalluria should be correlated with clinical and other clinical pathology data. Crystals are only one of several risk factors for urolithiasis. For crystals to form, the urine must be supersaturated and therefore the potential for nephrolith or urolith formation is present but not guaranteed. Stones must be analyzed to identify them properly as urinary crystals may or may not be the same as the urolith. Analyses of uroliths always require a send out test. Urethral obstruction in most species is due to a urolith and is almost exclusive to males. However, obstructions in male cats are usually due to a plug of mucoid material and phosphate crystals rather than a stone.

Crystals should be identified in fresh urine, as storage, refrigeration, and preservatives may influence their formation or dissolution. Delaying examination for 6–24 hours can induce crystal formation especially in refrigerated samples. The formation of crystals depends on multiple factors including, species, breed, pH, hydration, diet, and underlying diseases. Urine pH influences precipitation of some crystals and changing urinary pH through diet modification can lead to crystal dissolution.

There are general guidelines for expected pH ranges for different crystals. However, urinary pH does not establish identification of the crystal. Identification is done visually by matching photos with what is seen in the urine; shape, color, and size of crystal are all used. Rarely, chemical analyses or X-ray diffraction are used for crystal identification.

Ammonium biurate

These are brown, tan, yellow, or greenish spiky spheres. They often have protrusions giving a "mite-like" or "thorn-apple" appearance. These can be seen in normal animals, especially in Dalmatians and English bulldogs. They may also be suggestive of liver failure, congenital or acquired shunts, in which there is decreased conversion of ammonia to urea. In these cases the serum UN may be decreased while serum ammonia is increased and excreted in urine where it forms urate crystals, and may lead to nephrolith or urolith formation (tan to green in color). Their formation is generally favored in lower pH urine, but they can form in any pH. Patients in liver failure may have concurrent hypoalbuminemia, microcytosis, decreased serum cholesterol, and variable liver-derived serum enzyme activity.

Bilirubin

These are yellow, yellow-red, or red and usually needle-shaped or granules. They are associated with bilirubinemia and bilirubinuria but these abnormalities do not have to be present to form bilirubin crystals. They are common in canine urine, especially in concentrated specimens. They are abnormal in urine of other species. They typically are associated with a pH <7 and may resemble tyrosine crystals.

Calcium carbonate

These are colorless, tan, or brown. They are large and may have radial striations. Shape may include spheres and dumbbell-shapes. They are commonly seen in herbivores, such as horses, rabbits, and guinea pigs. They are not seen in the dog or cat. Dumbbell-shaped crystals in a dog or cat are more likely to be calcium oxalate monohydrate.

Calcium oxalate dihydrate

These are colorless with an "x" pattern through the crystal that imparts a "Maltese cross" or "envelope" pattern in square to rectangular shape. These are common in horses and cows and associated with ingestion of oxalate-rich plants. They may be seen in normal dogs and cats but also suggest hypercalcemia and hypercalciuria. If numerous, their presence should prompt investigation of a potential hypercalcemic disorder, such as hyperparathyroidism or idiopathic hypercalcemia. These crystals are seen in conjunction with calcium oxalate monohydrate crystals in ethylene glycol toxicity.

Calcium oxalate monohydrate

These are colorless with shapes including "Washington monument," "double-ended picket fence" (may look like double-ended hippuric acid crystals), dumbbell (may look like calcium carbonate), spindle, sheaths, and hemp seed-like. They can be normal in herbivores, dogs, and cats. However, their presence in prominent numbers suggests ethylene glycol toxicity (correlate with signs and laboratory data). When observed in dilute urine in any number from a dog or cat with AKI they indicate the possibility of ethylene glycol toxicity. One should also consider hypercalcemic diseases in dogs and cats, especially if dihydrate forms are also present.

Calcium phosphate

These are colorless to tan with shapes including amorphous aggregates, spheres, elongated prisms, and needles that may aggregate into sheaths or rosettes. They can be normal in dogs but may form uroliths. They are typically associated with alkaline urine.

Cholesterol

These are colorless and transparent large flat plates occurring in rectangles, often with a notch in one corner. They may stack on top of each other. They are birefringent and colorful with polarized light. They may be present in normal dogs but also may suggest hypercholesterolemic syndromes and protein losing nephropathy.

Cystine

These are colorless with hexagonal shape with a tendency to stack on top of each other. They are rare and not always abnormal. They may be seen with the rare inherited metabolic disorder cystinuria. This may occur in both male and female dogs, but clinical signs are observed almost exclusively in male dogs. This has occurred in Newfoundland, Australian cattle dogs, Mastiffs, Scottish deerhounds, English bulldogs, and Dachshunds.

Drug-associated

These are dark to light brown in color and typically form needles arranged in sheaves, bundles, fans, and radiating spokes. They are occasionally seen with sulfa family drugs, ampicillin, allopurinol, xanthine crystals, radiographic contrast media, and others. Correlate this finding with history of drug administration.

Hippuric acid

These are distinguished from calcium oxalate monohydrate by noting single-ended points, but distinction is difficult.

Leucine

These are yellow or brown spheres with concentrically radiating circles. They are rarely identified in animals but are suggestive of liver disease.

Magnesium ammonium phosphate – struvite – triple phosphate (a misnomer)

These are colorless with variable shapes including a "coffin-shaped" pattern, prisms, and plates. They are variably three-dimensional with have to six sides and oblique ends. They are a very common crystal in dogs and cats and tend to occur in alkaline urine. Urease splitting bacteria that produce free ammonia and alkaline urine enhance their formation. They can be numerous in normal dogs and cats, especially in concentrated urine. They commonly form uroliths.

Struvite

See "Magnesium Ammonium Phosphate" (above).

Tyrosine

These are colorless or yellow with needle-like shape and can resemble bilirubin crystals. They are rare and suggest liver disease.

Urate ammonium

See "Ammonium Biurate" (above).

Uric acid

These are yellow, yellow-brown; diamonds, rhomboid, rosettes; imply the same as urates. Uric acid is produced during purine degradation. Dalmatian dogs have a genetic defect in the gene for a uric acid transporter resulting in failure to metabolize uric acid and leads to increased plasma and urine concentrations of uric acid. These dogs have adequate uricase in hepatocytes as compared to an absence of this enzyme in people but Dalmatians cannot transport uric acid into hepatocytes for uricase to convert uric acid to allantoin. Increased uric acid is excreted in the urine. Their importance should be correlated with clinical signs. These crystals may also be seen in dogs with primary hepatic disease in which there is failure to convert uric acid to allantoin and ammonia to urea.

Xanthine

These are brown or tan. They appear similar to ammonium biurate crystals, but xanthine crystals usually form after treatment with allopurinol, a xanthine oxidase inhibitor to prevent formation of uric acid in dogs with urate calculi. They may be familial in Cavalier King Charles spaniels and dachshunds.

Fractional excretion of electrolytes

Fractional excretion of all of the electrolytes can be calculated, but sodium, potassium, and phosphorus are most clinically useful. Fractional excretion of electrolytes is performed to determine whether there is renal tubular failure in an animal that is hyponatremic or hypokalemic. They are used to determine the contribution of the kidney to the respective electrolyte decrease. Fractional excretion of phosphorus is examined to determine the likelihood of increased PTH in a nonazotemic animal. Single-spot urine and serum samples are adequate and are preferred over 24-hour urine collections for clinical assessment. Collect a serum sample close to the time of the urine sample and submit both for measurement of the electrolyte(s) desired and creatinine in serum and urine. The reference laboratory should calculate the result or use this formula:

$$\text{Fx exc of electrolyte} = \frac{\text{Serum Ct}}{\text{Urine Ct}} \times \frac{\text{Urine electrolyte}}{\text{Serum electrolyte}} \times 100$$

About 99% of the sodium entering the filtrate is normally reabsorbed. Increased FE_{Na} >1% is consistent with tubular failure or decreased aldosterone activity. The result should correlated with all other data. FE_{Na} in an azotemic patient <1% is consistent with prerenal azotemia, and if hyponatremia is observed, is consistent with sodium loss via the GI.

FE_P > reference interval indicates increased serum PTH or PTH-rp.

Reference intervals

Fx excretion, %	Dog	Cat
Sodium	<1	<1
Potassium	<6–20	<6–20
Chloride	<1	<1.5
Phosphorus	<20	<73

Fractional excretion of sodium in normal horses is 0.01–0.70; 0.80–10.10 in horses with renal failure, and 0.02–0.50 in horses with prerenal azotemia. It can also be used to determine if renal failure is present in nonazotemic patients and to follow recovery post-treatment of an azotemic patient.

PTH and PTH-rp stimulate phosphorus excretion. Animals with hypercalcemia and primary hyperparathyroidism or humoral hypercalcemia of malignancy (if mediated by PTH-rp) will both have increased fractional excretion of phosphorus and, therefore, measuring the fractional excretion of phosphorus does not help distinguish these two diseases. Physical examination to locate the cancer is the best means to distinguish these differential diagnoses. If that is inconclusive then concurrent measurement of PTH, PTH-rp and serum calcium usually is definitive with or without imaging techniques of the parathyroid-thyroid region of the neck.

Enzymes in urine

Gamma glutamyltransferase (GGT) and N-acetyl-glucosaminidase (NAG).

Enzymes found in urine have two sources, filtered at glomeruli or released from tubular epithelium. Enzymes that are too large to be filtered at glomeruli but that are released from damaged tubular epithelial cells can be a useful adjunct to determine if there is an acute tubular lesion before azotemia develops. Two such enzymes are GGT and NAG. GGT is a membrane-bound enzyme and NAG is a lysosomal enzyme. Although both enzymes are produced in other tissues neither is filtered at the glomerulus, and therefore, any amount in the urine reflects a tubular source. Proximal tubular epithelium contains more of these enzymes than other tubular cells, and most toxins affect the proximal convoluted tubules preferentially due to their high metabolic rate. These enzymes are measured in a random urine sample along with urine Ct, and the ratio of enzyme to Ct is reported. Samples should be refrigerated but not frozen as freeze thawing destroys the activity of enzymes. Enzymes cannot accumulate in the urine because they are voided from the bladder on urination. Therefore, the amount measured indicates the amount released since the last urination, and an increased amount implies that the lesion is active or ongoing. These enzymes are not absorbed into the circulation. GGT and NAG have proven useful in dogs, cats, horses, sheep, and cattle, particularly in cases of drug-induced tubular injury (e.g., gentamicin, neomycin, NSAIDs). Urinary NAG varies with sex, being twofold greater in male dogs.

Reference values should be obtained from the laboratory and not the literature due to analytical variation in how the enzymes are measured. Despite the early detection of renal tubular disease afforded by urinary enzymes, they are seldom measured. This may be because the by the time animals with spontaneous renal diseases present the diagnosis of AKI is easily made and use of urinary enzymes is unnecessary. A potential use would be to monitor an animal placed on a nephrotoxic drug such as an NSAID or gentamicin, where an increase in these enzymes would warrant discontinuing drug therapy. In experimental gentamicin nephrotoxicity, increased tubular enzymes occurs before increased fractional excretion of electrolytes, and precedes azotemia by 7–8 days and decreased creatinine clearance by 4–6 days (Figure 24.5). Increases in C-reactive protein and retinol binding protein also occur with tubular disease and may be future useful disease markers.

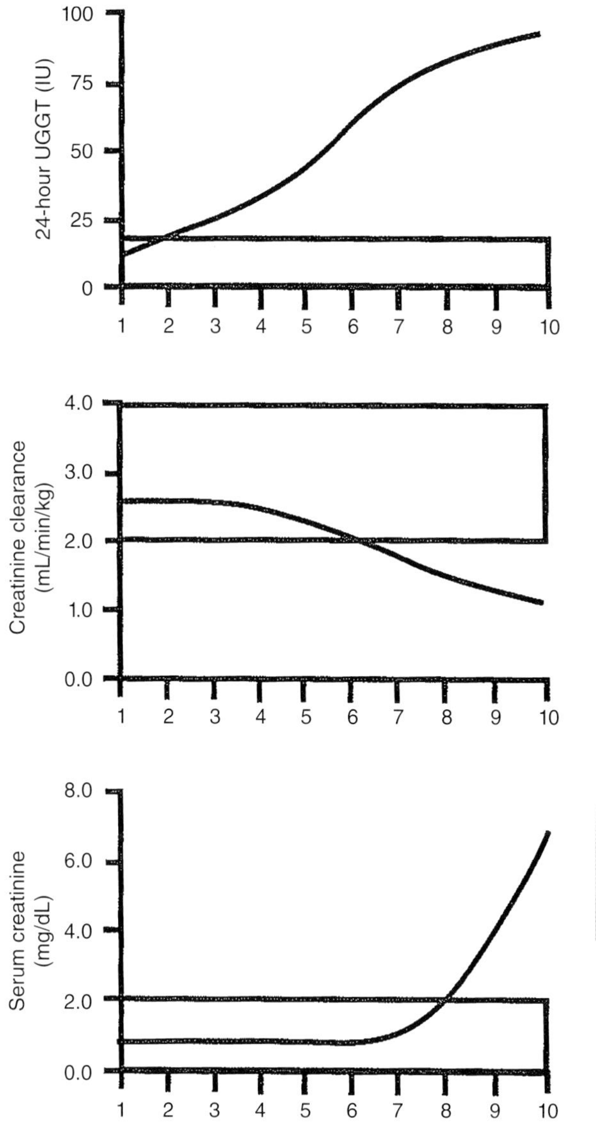

Figure 24.5 Serum creatinine, 24-hour endogenous creatinine clearance, and 24-hour urine GGT activity in experimental gentamicin nephrotoxicosis.

Diseases/syndromes

Chronic kidney disease

CKD is a common problem in older cats and dogs, and is the most common cause of renal failure in cats [15]. In cats, this disease most commonly manifests in the adult to geriatric patient [16]. It is a clinical term for animals with the following chronic renal diseases: chronic glomerulonephritis, amyloidosis, chronic interstitial nephritis, chronic pyelonephritis, progressive familial renal nephropathy, and even staghorn calculi. If none of these are confirmed then generic terms applied are CKD, chronic nephrosclerosis, or, if severe, end-stage kidney disease. If the kidney is biopsied or an autopsy is performed one of those diseases may be recognized. However, the lesions may be so chronic that the primary disease process can no longer be recognized. At the late stage, it may not matter as the kidneys contain fibrous connective tissue and chronic inflammation with an overall irreversible reduction in tubules and glomeruli (loss of renal mass). The underlying etiology is seldom known. A large number of potential etiologies have been proposed ranging from toxic insults, tissue hypoxia, infectious etiologies, neoplasms, polycystic kidney disease, and some congenital disorders have been implicated [17]. Dogs progress more rapidly, and once clinical signs and lab data worsen they will only live months or less, but the lives of cats may be extended for years. The diagnosis is usually easy. Patients present with weight loss, inappetence, and poor body condition score, PU/PD, dehydration, and hypertension. Clinicopathologic findings include a nonregenerative anemia, increased Ct and UN concentrations, and inappropriately low USG measurements (isosthenuric) [17, 18]. Kidneys are small with irregular renal contours. All of these signs range from mild to marked depending on the severity of the disease and when the patient is seen. Once baseline clinical signs and laboratory data are documented they can be used to monitor the progression of the disease.

The IRIS has published guidelines for the staging of CKD in both cats and dogs (Table 24.10). The stages presently used range from asymptomatic but at risk for development of CKD through degrees of severity based on increasing serum Ct concentration and increased clinical abnormalities. Staging of CKD is done following diagnosis to facilitate appropriate treatment and monitoring of the patient. It is based on fasting serum Ct evaluated at least twice in the stable patient (see Table 24.10). Once a stage is determined, the patient may be sub-staged based on proteinuria and blood pressure. Early data derived from the use of SDMA in veterinary patients is being considered for IRIS staging. Currently, if patients are diagnosed with CKD using SDMA before azotemia develops, patients are considered to be IRIS stage 1.

The International Society of Feline Medicine (ISFM) recently published consensus guidelines for the diagnosis and management of feline CKD in the *Journal of Feline Medicine and Surgery* [17]. In patients with suspected CKD, recommendations include a minimum routine database starting with a complete history and physical examination. A routine urinalysis, serum biochemistry, and hematology, along with a systolic blood pressure, and renal diagnostic imaging are considered ideal in the workup process. Monitoring of CKD should include clinical signs, patient's condition, and regular monitoring of blood pressure, azotemia, proteinuria, hypokalemia, hyperphosphatemia, anemia, and urinary tract infections. Following diagnosis, initial reevaluations should be done every 1–4 weeks based on clinical needs. Patient's undergoing long-term management should be reevaluated at least every 3–6 months. Management of CKD is centered around supportive care and increasing the patient's quality of life. Many think some aspects of management slows disease progression, aside from diet modification. However, the veterinary literature lacks data to support this assumption. Therapy predominately involves maintaining hydration and diet modification. Additional therapeutics targeted at various other disease manifestations (nausea, electrolyte and mineral imbalances, hypertension, proteinuria, anemia, etc.) are commonly utilized. Therapeutic plans are developed around each individual patient's needs and are frequently correlated with the IRIS stage [17].

Table 24.10 IRIS staging of chronic kidney disease.

Stage	Blood creatinine (mg/dL)		Comments
	Dogs	Cats	
At risk	<1.4	<1.6	History suggests the animal is at increased risk of developing CKD in the future because of a number of factors (e.g., exposure to nephrotoxic drugs, breed, high prevalence of infectious diseases in the area, old age).
1	<1.4	<1.6	Nonazotemic. Some other renal abnormality present (e.g., lower than anticipated USG).
2	1.4–2.0	1.6–2.8	Mild renal azotemia. Clinical signs usually mild or absent.
3	2.1–5.0	2.9–5.0	Moderate renal azotemia. Many extrarenal clinical signs may be present.
4	>5.0	>5.0	Increasing risk of systemic clinical signs and uremic crises.

Ethylene glycol intoxication

Ethylene glycol (EG) is sweet tasting and is one of the most common lethal toxins in veterinary medicine. First it causes vomiting, ataxia, and CNS depression such that owners might think their pet is "drunk." At this stage, a UV light may reveal fluorescence in the oral cavity, in vomitus, and in urine. Fluorescent dye is commonly present in commercial antifreeze preparations (the dye helps detect radiator leaks). Negative fluorescence does not rule out EG ingestion as not all antifreeze products add this dye. EG itself is not nephrotoxic, but alcohol dehydrogenase converts EG to toxic metabolites, principally oxalic acid. Competitive inhibition of alcohol dehydrogenase by ethanol is the treatment of choice for cats as 4-methylpyrazole (fomepizole) does not work well in cats. 4-Methylpyrazole directly inhibits alcohol dehydrogenase in dogs and is therefore recommended to treat dogs exposed to antifreeze.

Key to successful treatment is to confirm the diagnosis before the patient becomes azotemic. Azotemia is usually not present until about 24 hours postexposure, and therefore the goal is to diagnose AKI in a patient that is not azotemic. Five ways to accomplish this are: UV fluorescence, visualize calcium oxalate monohydrate crystals in urine (present in 3 hours postexposure in cats and 6 hours postexposure in dogs), increased serum osmolality and increased serum osmole gap (both occur in first hour postingestion), increased anion gap (3–6 hours postingestion), and perhaps the easiest way is a test kit that can be used in-house. Additionally, the FE_{Na} will be increased in the first 3 hours postexposure prior to the onset of azotemia.

The commercial diagnostic kit detects serum EG via a color change. The test takes 15 minutes to perform. The test is designed for serum and packet directions state it is useful only in the first 12 hours postexposure as it recognizes the parent compound, but not metabolites. We have used the kit on aqueous humor, serum, and urine up to 2 days postexposure with positive results achieved along with the diagnosis confirmed by histology. However, this is too late for effective therapy to be implemented. Commercial kits: Ethylene glycol test kits (Allelic Biosystems, Kearneysville, WV, and PRN Pharmacal, Pensacola, FL).

Serum phosphorus may increase before azotemia if the antifreeze product ingested also contains a phosphate rust inhibitor. Calcium oxalate monohydrate crystals are more plentiful in EG toxicity than are dihydrate crystals. Both types can be seen in urinalyses but they require careful searching with increased contrast as there may only be low numbers.

Osmole gap

Markedly increased osmole gap is diagnostic for EG. The increased osmolality and the gap are due to the parent compound ethylene glycol. Both are increased within one hour of ingestion. Osmolality is measured in serum by freezing-point depression. Serum osmolarity is calculated using the following formula, and osmole gap is calculated by subtracting the calculated osmolarity from the measured osmolality:

$$\text{Calculated osmolarity} = 1.86\,(\text{Na} + \text{K} + \text{Glucose}/18 + \text{UN}/2.8)$$

$$\text{Osmole gap} = \text{measured osmolality} - \text{calculated osmolarity}$$

Osmole gap interpretive guideline is: > 20 suggestive, > 30 diagnostic

Serum osmolality is rarely measured in private practices and the blood sample must be kept cool in transit to the referral laboratory. The technique to measure serum osmolality is based on the freezing point depression of a fluid. Ethylene glycol (antifreeze) is a small molecular weight molecule that lowers the freezing point of serum and therefore increases the measured osmolality and does so within an hour of ingestion.

The increased anion gap (AG) is due to the metabolites of EG and therefore an increased AG is seen after the increased osmole gap, usually around 3–6 hours postingestion. Most laboratories now report the AG in a chemistry panel, but it can be calculated via the following equation:

$$\text{Anion gap} = \text{Na} + \text{K} - \text{CL} - \text{HCO}_3$$

An AG >35 is suggestive of EG toxicity and >45 is highly suggestive. However, it is important to correlate the results with all of the other data in the case. Diagnosis of ethylene glycol toxicity should not be diagnosed by an increased anion gap alone.

Hypocalcemia often develops because the toxic metabolite, oxalate, will chelate calcium in the serum. This may produce marked hypocalcemia, in the range of 4–5 mg/dL total serum calcium. Many of the other laboratory and clinical abnormalities present in patients with antifreeze toxicity are not unique to this toxicity but are part of AKI. These include oliguria to anuria, dilute urine, casts in UA, and hyperphosphatemia. Azotemia does not develop for almost 24 hours postingestion of EG.

Diethylene glycol

This compound is related to ethylene glycol; however, it is less nephrotoxic. It is found in a variety of industrial products such as brake fluid, dyes, oils, ink, glue, lubricants, and heating/cooking fuel, as well as personal care products such as skin creams, deodorants, and toothpastes, and as an adulterant to create sweet wine or sweeten cough syrups. It is metabolized in the liver into various aldehydes and the acid 2-hydroxyethoxyacetic acid (HEAA) that is believed to be the nephrotoxic metabolite. Much like EG toxicity, the first phases of diethylene glycol (DEG) toxicity affect the GI and central nervous systems, producing an inebriation-like state that is followed by renal failure. Similar to EG toxicity both ethanol and fomepizole are used in the treatment (to prevent the formation of HEAA), but unlike EG there are no calcium oxalate crystals in the kidneys. Scattered cases in pets have been observed. The LD 50 for small mammals is between 2 and 25 g/kg.

Uroabdomen

Abdominal fluid Ct > serum Ct in concurrent samples; hyponatremia, hyperkalemia, hypochloremia, hyperphosphatemia; hole is usually located dorsally in the bladder; some animals can urinate and retain contrast dye; more common in males.

The best method to confirm uroabdomen is to measure creatinine in the abdominal fluid and serum concurrently. Abdominal fluid creatinine greater than serum creatinine is diagnostic. The slower diffusion of creatinine as opposed to UN (4 hours vs. 90 minutes) is why creatinine is measured preferential to UN in the diagnosis of uroabdomen, but either can be used. This difference in diffusion rates may be due to the difference in sizes of these molecules (UN is 60 Da and creatinine 113 Da) or their shape (urea is a simple chain and creatinine a ring structure). If the serum creatinine is increased in a patient with uroabdomen then the abdominal fluid creatinine will always be greater than the serum Ct concentration. The greater the difference between the serum and abdominal Ct values the greater the level of confidence of the diagnosis. The abdominal fluid creatinine does not have to be twice as high as the serum creatinine to confirm the diagnosis. Do not wait for a threefold or greater difference as the patient will benefit from surgical correction as early as possible. Because the hole in the bladder is almost always located dorsally the patient may still be able to urinate and retain radiopaque dye in the bladder. Cytologic examination of the abdominal fluid is not useful to establish the diagnosis. On rare occasions, urinary crystals and/or sperm may be seen in the abdominal fluid. These findings also confirm the diagnosis of uroabdomen. Classically uroabdomen is a disease of males due to their narrow urethra that is more easily obstructed than the wider urethra of females. In horses uroabdomen occurs most frequently in male foals less than 7 days old that were fine for several days postbirth and now are lethargic and anorectic. The urinary bladder ruptured during birth and there are no calculi. Uroabdomen in sheep, goats, cattle, and cats occur in males that have a calculus or mucus plug (cats) lodged in the most narrow portion of the urethra. The narrow portion in sheep and goats is the urethral appendage; in cattle it is the sigmoid flexure. In steers the rupture may also occur in the urethra. The bladder is intact and these individuals tend to have less severe clinical pathology abnormalities and a better surgical prognosis. In dogs uroabdomen is most typically seen post-trauma, e.g., hit by car. The characteristic serum electrolyte abnormalities include hyponatremia, hyperkalemia, and hypochloremia, along with hyperphosphatemia. In the experimental induction of uroabdomen in dogs these electrolyte abnormalities develop slowly over a 48-hour period.

Substances that are excreted into the urine in high concentration are now greater in the abdominal fluid than the blood and diffuse from the abdominal fluid into the blood, following their concentration gradient and gradually increase the serum concentration of UN, Ct, K, and P. Substances such as Na and Cl that are excreted into the urine in low concentration are lower in the abdominal fluid than the blood and therefore diffuse from the blood into the abdominal fluid gradually decreasing their serum concentrations. This is most notable for Na and Cl. Additionally fluid will flow into the abdominal cavity due to the irritation and increased osmolality from the urine mixing with the peritoneal fluid producing a third space and dilution effect on multiple analytes.

Differential diagnoses for hyponatremia, hyperkalemia, and hypochloremia are uroabdomen, Addison's disease, renal failure, GI disease (whipworms, salmonella, colibacillosis), Akita and other dog and sheep breeds with potassium-rich RBCs, chylothorax with repetitive drainage, and others (see Addison's disease in this book).

Patients in renal failure and with an intact urinary bladder will have increased concentrations of Ct and UN in all body fluids due to diffusion of Ct and UN from the blood. Therefore, Ct is increased in comparable amounts in abdominal fluid, thoracic fluid, cerebrospinal fluid, aqueous, and blood; however, the increase in these fluids will be less or nearly the same as the increased serum Ct concentration. The diffusion of Ct into other fluids is the basis of peritoneal dialysis in patients with renal failure.

Examples:

	Uroabdomen			Renal failure		Healthy
	Case 1	Case 2	Case 3	Case 4	Case 5	Case 6
Serum Ct mg/dL	8.1	4.5	5	6.3	11	1.2
Abdominal Ct mg/dL	13.4	6.2	15	6.1	10	0.9

The first three examples are all characteristic of uroabdomen. The next two examples are azotemia with an intact bladder and the last example is a "normal" or at least nonazotemic patient. The patients with an intact bladder and azotemia may benefit from peritoneal dialysis. The procedure involves abdominal fluid removal, injection of warm saline into the abdomen, allow time for Ct to diffuse from the blood into the saline and remove the fluid. This cycle is repeated until serum creatinine is reduced to an acceptable concentration. In AKI, peritoneal dialysis may, along with other treatments, permit the patient to survive long enough for tubules to regenerate.

Azostick determination of abdominal versus blood UN has been used to diagnose uroabdomen and may be beneficial if after-hour chemical measurements are not available. However, the color differences should be obvious and the qualitative results confirmed with chemical measurements and/or all of the data should correlate superbly. This includes a male animal that cannot urinate or does so in small volumes, a bladder that is small or collapsed, excess fluid in abdomen, azotemia, and characteristic electrolyte abnormalities.

Medullary washout

Primary diseases: Psychogenic polydipsia, liver failure, and hypoadrenocorticism.

Urea and sodium chloride are the main solutes that saturate the renal medullary interstitium. This hypertonic medullary intersitium combined with the vasa recta form the *counter current multiplier system*. This system is responsible for the passive absorption of water from the proximal convoluted tubules and is the first step in the process of concentrating the glomerular filtrate. If either urea or sodium, or both, are decreased in the interstitium of the medulla then passive absorption of water from the tubules is compromised and the filtrate concentration is impaired. Two syndromes that do this are chronic liver failure, such as acquired and congenital shunts (decreased urea) and hypoadrenocorticism (chronic hyponatremia). Liver failure caused by congenital shunts will have decreased serum concentrations of other substances produced by the liver such as albumin and cholesterol, and may have microcytosis as clues that this disease is present. Addison's patients will have azotemia, a Na: K ratio <23, and basal cortisol <2 µg/dL.

Psychogenic polydipsia will "wash out" the medullary interstitium via marked diuresis that provides insufficient time for urea and sodium reabsorption.

Fanconi syndrome

This is a heritable or acquired disease characterized by defects in proximal tubular reabsorption of various solutes that include one or more of glucose, sodium, calcium, bicarbonate, amino acids, and phosphate. Abnormal lab data includes dilute urine, inappropriate glucosuria, and proteinuria, increased fractional excretion of electrolytes, cystinuria, and aminoaciduria. Clinical signs range from asymptomatic to marked clinical alterations and death from renal failure. The disease is heritable and is present in 10–33% of Basenjis and is seen in Norwegian elkhounds, Shetland sheepdogs, and Schnauzers. It is recognized by breed susceptibility, clinical signs, and UA.

Nephrotic syndrome

Proteinuria, hypoproteinemia, hypoalbuminemia, ascites, and hypercholesterolemia, with or without azotemia, define this syndrome.

The combination of proteinuria, hypoalbuminemia, edema, ascites, and hypercholesterolemia are the classical features of the nephrotic syndrome but not all are present in every case, or are not detected. Ascites and edema may not always be present, but if the rest of the features are present, that is adequate to use this term (see section on "Protein Abnormalities" and tables and figures in this chapter). The nephrotic syndrome implies a lesion is present in glomeruli, either amyloidosis or glomerulonephritis. End-stage kidneys from any cause could present with similar features. Dogs with severe and chronic lesion pathology usually have peripheral edema and some develop thrombi due to a decrease in antithrombin III (AT III). This is a common syndrome in veterinary medicine because glomerulonephritis is so common in older dogs.

Proteinuria will precede azotemia in most cases. The more severe the lesions the more likely azotemia will be present. Approximately half of the dogs with glomerulonephritis will be azotemic and 75% of the dogs with amyloidosis will be azotemic. Dogs that are azotemic at initial diagnosis have the shortest survivals. Dilute urine will be seen in 50–60% of the cases. Casts are often present and they can be hyaline (protein-rich) or of other types. Amyloidosis may account for more cases simply because the glomerular lesions are more severe and therefore there is greater proteinuria. There is no effective treatment for amyloidosis. Glomeruli cannot regenerate, but if the lesions are mild and the underlying cause of inflammation predisposing to glomerulonephritis can be removed it is possible glomerulonephritis patients can survive for several years.

Progressive familial renal nephropathy/dysplasia

Chronic progressive familial nephropathy (renal dysplasia) is one of the most common causes of renal failure in young dogs, with some presenting as early as eight weeks of age. This is not hypoplasia as the kidneys start with a normal number of nephrons and then progressively lose nephrons over time. In severe cases the kidneys are shrunken and fibrotic, but there often are regions of embryonic glomeruli, tubules, and interstitium. There also are other familial glomerulopathies that look similar clinically and histologically. Regardless of nomenclature there are several diseases of high prevalence in many purebred animals that present at a young age. Amyolidosis has breed predilections as well. The lesions vary in severity, as do the laboratory findings. Clinical pathology results look like CKD. The kidneys appear shrunken on imaging, but the patient is a young or middle-aged purebred dog. Of all of the causes of renal failure, these diseases probably have the highest incidence of concurrent hypercalcemia. Hyperphosphatemia will accompany the azotemia, and therefore soft-tissue mineralization is prominent. Some breed-specific anomalies include the following:

- Progressive familial renal nephropathy is observed in the Lhasa Apso, Shih Tzu, soft-coated Wheaten terrier, standard poodle, miniature schnauzer, Alaskan malamute, golden retriever, Norwegian elkhound, and Doberman breeds.
- Inherited glomerulopathies have been documented in the Samoyed, Bernese mountain dog, bull terrier, chow chow, English cocker spaniel, and Rottweiler breeds.

- Amyloidosis is noted in Abyssinian, Siamese, and Oriental shorthair cats and in Shar Pei, beagle, and English foxhound dogs.
- Polycystic kidney disease is observed in the Persian cat, West Highland white and Cairn terrier, and bull terrier.

Neoplasms

Lymphoma is the most common tumor in the kidneys of animals but is a secondary tumor, metastatic to this site. Primary tumors are uncommon and split approximately equally between mesenchymal and epithelial. Primary renal tumors are tubular adenomas and carcinomas, nephroblastomas in young animals, fibromas, and hemangiosarcomas. Other neoplasms of the kidneys are infrequent and detailed descriptions can be found in other resources [19].

Bladder tumors account for approximately 1.0% of all canine neoplasms. Approximately 90% of urinary bladder neoplasms in dogs, cats, and horses are epithelial and malignant. Urothelial carcinoma (UC) or transitional cell carcinoma (TCC) is the most common tumor of the bladder in all species. Tumors in the kidney and bladder are difficult to diagnose clinically. Clinical signs and laboratory data are not specific. Urinalysis abnormalities are seen in 90% of dogs with tumors of the urinary bladder, but these abnormalities are also nonspecific. The most common UA abnormalities are hematuria (>75%), pyuria (50%), proteinuria (30%), and bacteriuria (30%). Cystitis or uroliths are much more likely to cause these abnormalities than is neoplasia. Hypertrophic osteopathy occurs with several different bladder tumors. There are numerous reports of hypertrophic osteopathy with bladder rhabdomyosarcomas in young dogs, but this is an uncommon tumor.

Renal lymphoma

Rarely is a renal tumor diagnosed from examination of cells in the urine; most cases will be diagnosed from ultrasound-guided fine needle aspiration into the focal renal mass. Lymphoma, however, can cause marked bilateral renomegaly and aspirational cytology of an enlarged kidney without ultrasound guidance can be performed to diagnose lymphoma in these cases. Neoplastic lymphoid cells appear as they do in lymph nodes and other organs infiltrated with lymphoma. Sometimes renal tubules are aspirated concurrently (Figure 24.A.7). If lymphoma is in the kidneys it will also be located elsewhere. An unusual feature of lymphoma in the kidneys is the occasional tumor that stimulates erythropoietin production resulting in polycythemia. This is not unique to lymphoma and has been seen with other neoplasms and non-neoplastic renal masses. A nonregenerative anemia due to decreased erythropoietin production combined with anemia of chronic inflammatory disease is much more likely than polycythemia.

Transitional cell carcinoma

TCC of the urinary tract is synonymous with UC. It is the most common tumor in the urinary system from the renal pelvis to the distal urethra. Clinical signs are similar across species. In dogs they include weight loss, weakness, dysuria (85%), pollakiuria (40%), and incontinence (10%). The Scottish terrier has 20-fold greater likelihood of developing UC than mixed breeds. Etiology is multifactorial and likely involves interactions of susceptible genes and environmental factors. Interestingly, consumption of cruciferous vegetables may help reduce the risk of bladder cancer in humans and dogs [20].

Activation of BRAF mutation is present in canine UC tissue and was detectable in the urine of dogs with UC [21]. The mutation was found on chromosome 16 in canine UC cell lines and in >80% of 62 naturally occurring canine UC cases [21]. BRAF mutation is rare (<1%) in human UC, which also tends to be much less invasive than canine UC. A genomic test is available for early and noninvasive diagnosis of canine UC in patients with this mutation. The test requires a urine sample with a low number of neoplastic cells [22]. Approximately 80% of dogs with TCC have a single point mutation in the BRAF gene; likewise, the test has a high specificity and moderate sensitivity. The test is not affected by the presence of blood or bacteria in the urine sample [22]. Fluorescence in situ hybridization (FISH) is used to detect chromosomal aneuploidy in cells present in the urine of humans with suspected bladder cancer and has been developed for use in dogs [23]. If molecular changes precede morphologic changes, then these tests could be used to screen or detect bladder cancer early and monitor recurrence. Molecular tests do not replace traditional diagnostic methods but can be used in tandem to help establish a diagnosis or to determine if further testing is warranted. Other molecular based tests include a PCR based assay, *BRAF* mutation, calgranulins, microRNAs, and peptide cancer-binding ligands. If tests can be developed that use urine samples to differentiate dogs with TCC/UC from dogs with diseases that have similar clinical problems such as cystitis or urolithiasis than we may be able to recognize the tumor early in its course when treatments are more effective. Presently, by the time we recognize TCC/UC the tumor has already invaded the bladder wall or has metastasized. Screening tests are useful in annual wellness exams, especially for breeds with high a prevalence of TCC/UC such as the Scottish terrier.

We need tests that can recognize UC earlier because 20% of dogs have clinically detectable metastases at the time of clinical diagnosis. Of these, 50% actually have metastases and 90% are expected to develop metastases if the tumor is allowed to progress. This is likely due to the combination of a highly malignant tumor, which remains occult and for which early diagnostic tests are not performed. Most cases of bladder cancer are recognized when the tumor is advanced, and therefore the prognosis is uniformly poor.

TCC can be diagnosed by finding neoplastic cells in the urine (Figures 24.A.4–24.A.6). Approximately 30% of UC/TCC can be diagnosed via urine cytology, 75% via urethral or prostatic washes, and 90% via aspiration cytology of the mass. Cytological diagnosis of neoplastic cells in the urine seems a logical diagnostic aid but must be interpreted cautiously as inflammation of the urinary tract stimulates hyperplasia and dysplasia of transitional epithelium, making the distinction of hyperplasia from dysplasia or neoplasia difficult. Furthermore, urine is caustic to cells and will cause cellular deterioration if preparations are not made promptly.

The best method to diagnose TCC in urine is to collect a fresh sample, centrifuge the urine to prepare a concentrated preparation, pour off the supernatant, make a film of the sediment, and stain with a Romanowsky stain (do not diagnose from a wet-mount, sedi-stain preparation). Additionally, a diagnostic laboratory can prepare a cellblock of the sediment and prepare a histologic section. Tumor cells will be in clusters or individual, neoplastic cells will be extremely large (>40 μm diameter), and will have marked cytologic and nuclear atypia (various sizes and shapes of cells, nuclei, and nucleoli). Some cells will contain Melamed-Wolinska bodies, which are large cytoplasmic vacuoles diagnostic for UC (Figures 24.A.5 and 24.A.6). The more numerous these abnormalities and the less inflammation present, the more likely the cells are neoplastic. If only a few of these cytologic abnormalities are identified and there is inflammation, then the cellular atypia is more likely due to dysplasia or hyperplasia than to neoplasia. Correlate results with other data, such as a mass in the trigone region of the bladder, unresponsive hematuria, and age of patient. TCC can seed and grow in the abdominal incision site used for surgical removal of the tumor. This occurs in approximately 10% of cystotomies performed on dogs with UC [24]. A few reports exist of seeding from fine needle aspiration cytology, but this should not prevent attempts to diagnose the tumor via this means. Other means of confirming the diagnosis (catheterization, wash) can be tried first. Seeding of TCC/UC in the abdominal wall from FNA is unlikely but owners should be made aware of this possibility and that it could complicate treatments. There are also reported cases of abdominal wall TCC/UC in dogs in which a contributing cause could not be found [24].

Basic fibroblast growth factor (bFGF) is a pro-angiogenic peptide used as a marker for urologic and nonurologic tumors in humans and has been detected in high concentrations in the urine of dogs with bladder cancer. Although the numbers of dogs were small, one study demonstrated significantly higher concentrations of bFGF in dogs with bladder cancer than in normal dogs or dogs with urinary tract infection (UTI). Results are expressed as ng/g creatinine, and the median concentration of bFGF was 2.23 in normal dogs, 2.45 in dogs with UTI, and 9.86 in dogs with bladder cancer. Of dogs with cancer 86% could be correctly identified by increased concentrations of bFGF, and 90% of dogs with UTI did not have increased concentrations. The commercially available ELISA test kit uses a monoclonal antibody to recognize natural and recombinant human bFGF.

Another commercially available test is the bladder tumor-associated antigen (BTA). The assay detects a glycoprotein antigen complex that is of host basement membrane origin and partly of tumor origin. The dipstick test was used on 65 dogs, 20 with TCC, 19 healthy controls, and 26 controls. Test sensitivity (dogs with cancer have positive results) was reported to be 78% and the specificity (dogs without cancer have negative results) 90%. Results are not quantified, they are either positive or negative. False-positive results can be seen with pyuria, hematuria, proteinuria, and glucosuria. When these abnormalities are present the utility of the dipstick test is greatly limited, and if used, the test should be performed in conjunction with cytology and other ancillary tests. The dipstick test may be more appropriately applied as a screening test in older dogs for bladder cancer; however, cost and index of suspicion may limit utility.

Second-generation BTA statistical tests use a monoclonal antibody to recognize a human complement complex that is secreted into the urine of humans with bladder cancer. When applied to dogs with TCC the results have been negative, and they were attributed to the lack of cross-reactivity of the monoclonal antibody to canine TCC generated antigens.

Definitions, glossary, and principles

Definitions

Urea nitrogen (UN)

This is produced in the liver from ammonium and bicarbonate, and is excreted from the body via glomerular filtration through the kidneys. The most common cause for an increase in serum UN is decreased GFR, less common causes, and to lesser magnitudes include high-protein diet, hemorrhage into the GI tract, increased catabolism, and fever. An increase in UN due to a decrease in GFR will not be detected until approximately 75% of both kidneys are not filtering adequately. A decrease in UN is usually due to chronic liver disease. The units of serum or plasma UN are reported in mg/dL, and as μmol/L, internationally. The conversion factor between these units is: 1 mg/dL × 0.7140 = μmol/L (e.g., 10 mg/dL UN is 7.1 μmol/L). The atomic weight of urea is 60 Da. Approximately half of the UN excreted into the tubules is reabsorbed passively in the proximal tubule and actively by the cells of the collecting ducts. Urea is held in the medullary interstitium and in combination with Na make the necessary concentration gradient for the "counter current multiplier" system (CCM). If UN and/or Na are not in sufficient concentration in the interstitium the CCM is compromised and dilute urine is produced. Renal, prerenal and postrenal diseases can increase serum UN and the increase is comparable for all three causes.

Creatinine (Ct)

Creatinine is a breakdown product of muscle creatine and creatine phosphate. It is excreted via glomerular filtration in the kidneys. It is produced at a fairly constant rate dependent on muscle mass; 1–2% of muscle creatine is converted to creatinine/day (human). The most common cause for an increase in serum Ct is decreased GFR. Less common minimal causes include increase breakdown of muscle, increased catabolism, and fever. An increase in Ct due to a decrease in GFR will not be detected until approximately 75% of both kidneys are not filtering adequately. Creatinine concentration is reported in mg/dL and as μmol/L internationally. The conversion factor between these units is: 1 mg/dL × 88.4 = μmol/L (e.g., 1 mg/dL Ct is 88.4 μmol/L). Minimal to no creatinine is reabsorbed in tubules and therefore endogenous Ct clearance can be measured to indicate GFR. Noncreatinine chromogens, such as glucose, ketones, vitamins A and C, carotenes, oxyglobin, pyruvate, and uric acid, may falsely increase measured creatinine. This occurs most frequently in cows and horses. Approximately 50% of measured serum creatinine consists of noncreatinine chromogens. If creatinine is increased due to renal failure then the majority of the increased serum Ct is from decreased GFR and not noncreatinine chromogens. Renal, prerenal and postrenal diseases can increase serum Ct and the increase is comparable for all three causes.

Azotemia

This is the most commonly used laboratory indicator of decreased GFR (renal dysfunction) and occurs when the serum concentration of UN and/or Ct concentrations are increased, to any degree. An increase in UN or Ct due to a decrease in GFR will not be detected until approximately 75% of both kidneys are not filtering adequately. Azotemia indicates the kidneys are not functioning adequately. However, this may be due to diseases that are in front of kidneys (prerenal), in the kidneys (renal: glomerular, tubular, interstitial, pelvis), or after the kidneys (postrenal), or due to combinations of each. The greater the concentration of UN/Ct the more likely the disease is severe, but there are no concentrations that indicate irreversibility or that distinguish prerenal, renal, postrenal, or combinations. Patients may be azotemic but are not yet necessarily uremic (see below). Although azotemia means UN/Ct are increased in the blood both substances are also increased in "all" bodily fluids (CSF, aqueous, peritoneum, joint, etc.). This occurs because both UN and Ct have small molecular weights and they diffuse freely across membranes.

Uremia

This is the term used when clinical signs are attributed to azotemia. Uremia results in anorexia, weight loss, depression, stupor, vomiting, oral ulcers, anemia, mineralization, electrolyte and fluid imbalances, and hormone deficits and/or increases. This is caused by accumulation of nitrogenous waste products and uremic toxins in blood. Uremic toxins is an umbrella term for the retention of all solutes, many of which are unmeasured, normally excreted by a healthy kidney that contribute to "uremia."

Prerenal azotemia

This is recognized when azotemia is present and USG is concentrated. To be considered concentrated, USG should be greater than 1.030 in dogs, 1.035 in cats, and 1.025 in horses and cattle. The urine s.g. is often >1.050 when the azotemia is due to dehydration. Causes of prerenal azotemia include any state that results in a decreased renal blood flow, including hypovolemia due to dehydration, shock, and cardiac insufficiency. Prerenal conditions are the most common cause of azotemia. If these conditions persist, they can lead to kidney damage and renal azotemia. Prerenal azotemia is often superimposed on either renal or postrenal, usually due to concurrent dehydration. If the azotemia is only due to prerenal causes it is usually mild e.g., <100 mg/dL. However, there are no concentrations of UN/Ct that rule out prerenal as the cause. Dehydration will cause a more rapid increase in serum UN than Ct and a disproportionate increase in UN to Ct (increased UN/Ct ratio). Ratio of UN/Ct is now reported by some clinical laboratories to help identify prerenal azotemia.

Renal azotemia

This is recognized when azotemia is coupled with inability to concentrate urine, especially isosthenuric urine, as indicated by a USG between 1.007 and 1.013 (do not use strict cutoffs of a single USG to define isosthenuria). Isosthenuria implies that the kidneys are damaged to such an extent that they are no longer able to concentrate or dilute the plasma ultra-filtrate (urine). An SG of 1.007–1.013 is approximately the SG of plasma (295–300 mOsm/L). Renal azotemia can be due to acute or CKD. The defect in renal function may arise from many different diseases of the glomeruli, tubules, interstitium, renal pelvis, and, least likely, from renal blood vessels. Renal azotemia identifies the lesion is in the kidneys, but it does not localize the disease to a structure, type of disease, or etiology.

Postrenal azotemia

This is associated with any obstruction to the outflow of urine or rupture of urinary bladder or urethra. Oliguria or anuria will be observed, and any USG is possible. In theory, the nephrons (kidneys) are excreting UN and Ct adequately into the ultra-filtrate, but UN and Ct are not excreted from the body. If the cause is obstruction then some UN/Ct can be reabsorbed through the bladder wall but more importantly backpressure from the obstruction causes structural lesions (hydronephrosis) and/or functional lesions in all renal structures. A ruptured bladder or urethra cause azotemia when UN and Ct are reabsorbed through the peritoneum (ruptured bladder) or subcutaneous tissues (ruptured urethra). Both molecules are small (low atomic weight) and are passively reabsorbed easily from regions of high concentration gradient (peritoneum) to lower concentration gradient (blood).

Nephrons

These are the smallest individual anatomic units in the kidney, and are composed of a glomerulus, tubule, and collecting tubule. There are approximately one million glomeruli per kidney.

Renal disease

This is classified as a structural or biochemical lesion in kidney. If the lesion is focal, it may never produce clinical problems (such as with the interstitial nephritis caused by ascarid migration). Renal disease is a continuum that begins with renal insufficiency and finishes with end-stage renal disease.

Renal insufficiency

This is a state in which nephrons are functionally impaired but not yet sufficiently damaged as to result in clinically apparent disease. Unaffected individual nephrons compensate for these losses by hypertrophy, but with progression of disease, enough nephrons become impaired so that they are unable to maintain the health of the animal.

Renal failure

This exists when roughly at least two-thirds of functional renal mass is impaired. Urine cannot be concentrated adequately and polyuria, oliguria, or anuria results. When three-quarters of nephrons are dysfunctional, remaining nephrons cannot compensate and azotemia is detected.

Clinical signs associated with renal failure are attributable to a loss of functional renal tissue, and accumulation of nitrogenous and other waste products in blood. Signs may include anemia, vomiting, lethargy, anorexia, weight loss, vasculitis, glossal, and/oral ulcers, gastric erosions or ulcers, bleeding diatheses, petechiae, thrombosis, gastrointestinal tract bleeding, parathyroid hyperplasia, mineralization of soft tissues, and fibrous osteodystrophy.

Glossary

Anuria: Refers to a state wherein there is no urine output.

Dysuria: Describes painful or difficult urination.

Glomerular filtration rate (GFR): The volume of plasma filtered by the glomerular capillaries into Bowman's space per unit of time. A GFR of 3–6 mL/min/kg is normal for dogs and 2–4 mL/min/kg is considered normal in cats. A decrease in GFR can occur due to prerenal, renal or postrenal causes.

Microalbuminuria: Describes a state in which small quantities of protein are lost in urine but are below the limit of detection of reagent sticks. Microalbuminuria is urinary albumin 1–30 mg/dL and albuminuria ("overt albuminuria") is urine albumin >30 mg/dL in urine normalized to a USG of 1.010. Persistent microalbuminuria may indicate early or mild renal disease.

Oliguria: Indicates reduced urine output.

Pollakiuria: A term indicating an increased frequency of urination. However, the total volume of urine produced may not be increased. Pollakiuria is associated with diseases of the urinary bladder, urethra, and vaginal canal.

Polydipsia (PD): A term denoting an increased volume of water is consumed within a 24-hour period. It is associated with renal failure and multiple other causes. This usually occurs secondary to polyuria caused by the loss of urinary concentrating ability. In dogs, polydipsia is considered as drinking >90 mL/kg/d, and in cats >45 mL/kg/d.

Polyuria (PU): A term denoting an increased total volume of urine produced within 24 hours. The normal range in dogs is 20–40 mL/kg/d (1 mL/kg/hr), and in cats, 10–20 mL/kg/d.

Proteinuria: Refers to protein in the urine as detected by reagent sticks or SSA protein precipitation methods. It is caused by preglomerular, glomerular, or postglomerular causes. Persistent proteinuria coupled with a quiescent urine analysis suggests a glomerular lesion, such as amyloidosis or glomerulonephritis.

Stranguria: Refers to straining to urinate.

Principles

The ability of the kidneys to concentrate urine is a good indicator of renal function. Loss of this capability is one of the earliest signs of renal failure, preceding azotemia in all species except cats.

Expected urine specific gravity: The expected USG of a random urine sample from a healthy domestic animals 1.020–1.045 for dog, horse, cattle, and 1.025–1.050 for cat. The USG must always be considered in conjunction with the hydration status. On any random urine sample, an adequate USG is considered to be >1.030 in the dog; >1.035 in cat; and >1.025 in horse and bovine. Dogs are not born with an adult's level of concentrating capacity, and dilute urine is expected up to four weeks of age. There are no differences in protein, blood, glucose, ketones, or bilirubin based on age.

Dilute urine specific gravity: For the purposes of this chapter, dilute urine refers to urine that is inappropriately concentrated for the patient's hydration status. In many instances this will match with hyposthenuria. However, there are clinical situations in which the USG is >1.020, and yet this is inappropriately concentrated. For example, in the clinical setting adequate renal function in a healthy cat is generally associated with a USG of >1.035. If a dehydrated cat presents, the USG is expected to be >1.035 (and often >1.060). However, if this same patient presents with a USG 1.025, the urine is considered inappropriately concentrated (i.e., dilute for this cat). The next step is to verify this clinical finding (as described above) and begin an investigation to determine the underlying cause (e.g., osmotic diuresis/glucosuria, pyelonephritis, CKD, etc.) by evaluating clinical signs, complete bloodwork, diagnostic imaging, urine culture and sensitivity.

Hyposthenuria occurs when the kidneys actively produce urine with a USG <1.007, or with an osmolality less than that of plasma, e.g., <300 mOsm/kg. Hyposthenuria has several renal and nonrenal causes, and indicates that the kidneys are healthy enough to actively dilute the plasma ultrafiltrate.

Isosthenuria indicates a USG similar to the SG of plasma, i.e., 1.008–1.012 and 1.007–1.013 are reported in different sources. This USG implies that the nephrons were unable to either concentrate or dilute the plasma ultrafiltrate. Isosthenuric urine with concurrent azotemia indicate renal failure and the lesion involves the tubules or the medulla. If the disease was confined to the glomeruli then tubules should be able to concentrate urine, in principle. However, 90% of blood supply to the tubules passes through glomeruli therefore glomerular diseases will secondarily affect tubules and ability to concentrate urine is compromised.

Hypersthenuria, or baruria, are two rarely used terms that describe urine with an SG greater than 1.013. These terms imply that urine has been concentrated to greater than the isosthenuric range.

Differential diagnoses for polyuria and polydipsia (PU/PD) include renal failure (with or without azotemia), diabetes mellitus, primary or secondary diabetes insipidus, hyperadrenocorticism, hypercalcemia, pyometra, psychogenic polydipsia, and medullary washout (associated with hypoadrenocorticism or liver failure). A complete list is in Table 24.4.

Water reabsorption occurs passively/osmotically in the proximal convoluted tubules and descending loop of Henle. It is actively reabsorbed in the collecting tubules through the actions of antidiuretic hormone (ADH).

Medullary washout occurs when the solutes urea and sodium chloride, located in the interstitium of the renal medulla, are decreased. This loss of hypertonicity in the medulla results in production of a dilute urine, and the clinical signs of PU/PD. Decreased urea happens with hepatic shunts and severe chronic liver disease. Decreased sodium happens with hypoadrenocorticism.

Creatinine clearance is the volume of plasma that is cleared of creatinine per unit time and can be used to estimate GFR. In dogs essentially 100% of creatinine entering the filtrate is excreted (male dogs also secrete a small amount of Ct via the proximal tubules). However, 40–60% of UN is reabsorbed from the filtrate and the amount reabsorbed varies with hydration status. Therefore, creatinine clearance is an acceptable means to estimate GFR and UN clearance is not acceptable.

Acute kidney injury (AKI): The onset of AKI is swift. It is commonly due to a nephrotoxin that causes necrosis of tubules (nephrosis), and less commonly due to an infectious etiology (e.g., leptospirosis), or ischemic injury. AKI is typified by azotemia and inability to concentrate urine coupled with hyperphosphatemia, variable changes in potassium, a normal to increased PCV, and good body condition. Potassium >8 mEq/L can be life-threatening. It is generally accompanied by anuria or oliguria. This term is used interchangeably with acute renal injury, acute renal failure, acute kidney failure, acute renal insufficiency, acute kidney insufficiency.

Chronic kidney disease (CKD) can be due to chronic glomerulonephritis, amyloidosis, chronic interstitial nephritis, chronic pyelonephritis, progressive familial renal dysplasia, etc. Lab data include azotemia, inability to concentrate urine, and mild nonregenerative anemia. If the disease process involves the glomeruli, there may be hypoalbuminemia. The onset of CKD is chronic, progressing over months to years. As a result, the patient has poor to thin body condition. The etiology is often unknown as the primary event was months to years previous to diagnosis. This term is used interchangeably with chronic renal disease, renal failure, and chronic kidney failure.

Acute on chronic renal failure implies there is underlying CKD and now something else has acutely made the renal failure "worse." There are multiple potential etiologies for the acute exacerbation, including dehydration, progression of the chronic primary disease and/or a second disease process superimposed on the first (e.g., pylenonephritis occurring in a cat with CKD).

Formed elements in urine: Casts may be observed during microscopic examination of urine, and suggest tubular disease. They are formed in the loop of Henle and in the distal and convoluted tubules. Rare hyaline and fine granular casts (1–2/low-power field) may be observed in concentrated urine and are considered normal; however, casts found in dilute urine are considered abnormal.

Crystalluria refers to crystals in urine. *Nephroliths* are stones found in the kidney, while the term *urolith* indicates the presence of stones in the bladder or urethra.

Staging renal disease: The severity of renal disease is graded as 1, 2, 3, or 4 based on severity of clinical signs, physical examination results, and laboratory abnormalities. As the stage of renal disease progresses so do the severity of the laboratory abnormalities and the percentage of animals that have an abnormality. For example, 20% of azotemic dogs also have mild hyperphosphatemia (~6 mg/dL) in stage 1. This percentage increases to 100% of dogs in stage 4 renal failure, where the serum phosphorus will be markedly increased (>20 mg/dL).

The *nephrotic syndrome* is due to chronic glomerular disease. It is characterized by proteinuria, hypoproteinemia, hypercholesterolemia, ascites, and edema. There may or may not be an azotemia. With nephrotic syndrome, the lesion is in glomeruli, e.g., amyloidosis or glomerulonephritis.

Other terms, disease conditions, and methods of analyzing renal function

Chronic progressive familial nephropathy (renal dysplasia) is one of the most common causes of renal failure in young dogs, and it has a high prevalence in many purebred breeds. In severe cases, kidneys are shrunken and fibrotic and look like any end-stage kidney disease. They retain regions of embryonic glomeruli, tubules, and interstitium.

Uroabdomen or uroperitoneum is typified by hyponatremia, hypochloremia, and hyperkalemia. Serum Ct and UN are variable, but abdominal fluid Ct:serum Ct is ≥ 1.5–2 : 1. This commonly occurs in males due to their narrow urethra that becomes obstructed, or in male foals in which the dorsal bladder wall ruptures during birth or from being stepped on.

Paradoxical aciduria is a unique situation seen in dairy cattle with displaced abomasums, or other animals with proximal duodenal blockage, and is typified by profound hypochloremia, severe metabolic alkalosis, and acidic urine.

Transitional cell carcinoma (TCC) is a highly malignant tumor of transitional epithelium and is the most common tumor of the urinary bladder and the urinary excretory system.

Monitoring renal disease patients over time is advisable for purposes of prognostication and for monitoring response to therapy. Practical methods include accurate weight of the patient, water intake and urine volume measurement, USG, and periodic serum UN and Ct. If closer monitoring is desired, then specialized studies such as ultrasonography, endogenous or exogenous creatinine clearance, fractional excretion of sodium, monitoring of microproteinuria, clearance studies of inulin, iohexol, radioisotopes, and renal scintigraphy can be undertaken.

Essentially 100% of sodium is reabsorbed from the glomerular ultrafiltrate and therefore less than 1% is excreted in the urine of animals with normal renal function. If there is increased renal loss of sodium as measured by an increase in the urinary fractional excretion of sodium (>1%) it indicates renal insufficiency or failure. A fractional excretion of sodium is <1% indicates prerenal azotemia.

Urinary protein:Ct ratio (UPC): The concentration of protein and creatinine are measured in a random urine sample, and urine protein concentration is divided by urine Ct concentration. This is used to quantify the degree of proteinuria, and to identify what the most likely disease process affecting the kidneys is.

In dogs, a UPC <0.5 is considered normal, 0.5–1 is inconclusive, and >1 is considered abnormal.

Urine cortisol:Ct ratio (UCCR): Urinary cortisol concentration is a good estimate of cortisol production over the preceding 24 hours, and the UCCR is used to rule out hyperadrenocorticism (Cushing's disease). Of dogs with normal UCCR 90% do not have hyperadrenocorticism. About 95% of dogs with hyperadrenocorticism have increased UCCR, but 80% of dogs with nonadrenal disease have increased UCCR. The latter animals are generally sick and stressed, and the finding of an increased UCCR in these individuals is considered a false-positive result. Creatinine and cortisol are measured in a sample of urine collected at home first thing in the morning.

Urine bile acid:Ct ratio: With increased production, bile acids are excreted in the urine. Increased urine bile acid:Ct ratios have the same diagnostic value as measuring serum bile acid. Creatinine and total bile acids, or bile acid components, are measured in a random urine sample from a nonfasted dog or cat, a ratio is calculated and compared to published data or the reference laboratory's reference interval.

Appendix 24.1

A Urinalysis and Urinary System Imagery

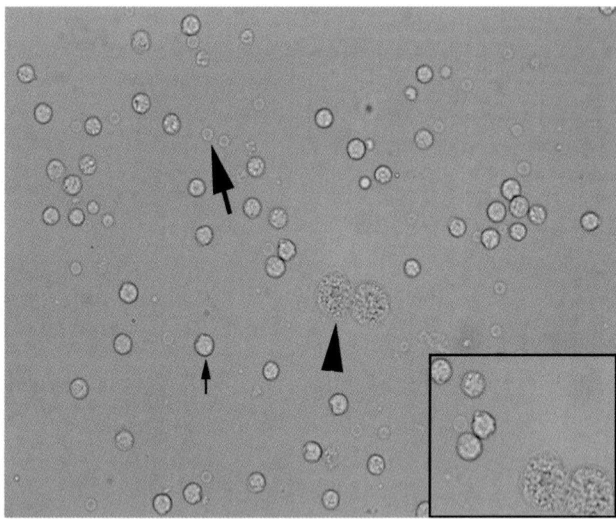

Figure 24.A.1 Urine sediment, unstained. There are numerous leukocytes (small arrow), fewer erythrocytes (large arrow), and two epithelial cells (arrowhead). Despite the number of white cells, there are no bacteria visible. A culture of the urine is required to verify there are no bacteria. ×400.

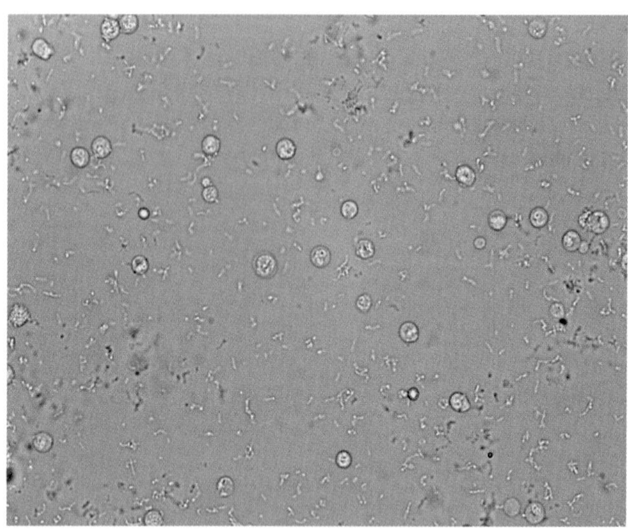

Figure 24.A.3 Urine sediment, unstained. There are numerous leukocytes and rod-shaped bacteria present, indicating bacterial urinary tract infection. ×400.

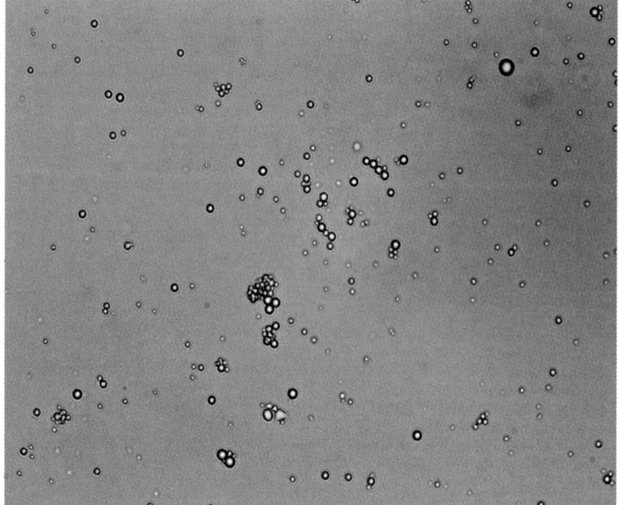

Figure 24.A.2 The numerous lipid droplets present are frequently noted in feline urine and are suspected to come from renal tubular epithelium but have unknown significance. They may be mistaken for red blood cells, but lipid droplets are variably sized and are in a different plane of focus from cellular elements in the urine due to their lower density. ×100.

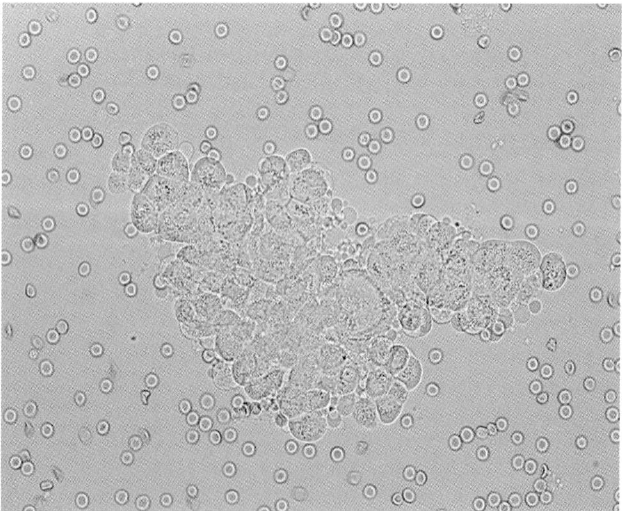

Figure 24.A.4 Urine sediment, unstained. Note the large cluster of many pleomorphic epithelial cells on a background of erythrocytes. This dog had a lesion in the trigone of the urinary bladder confirmed as transitional cell carcinoma. ×400.

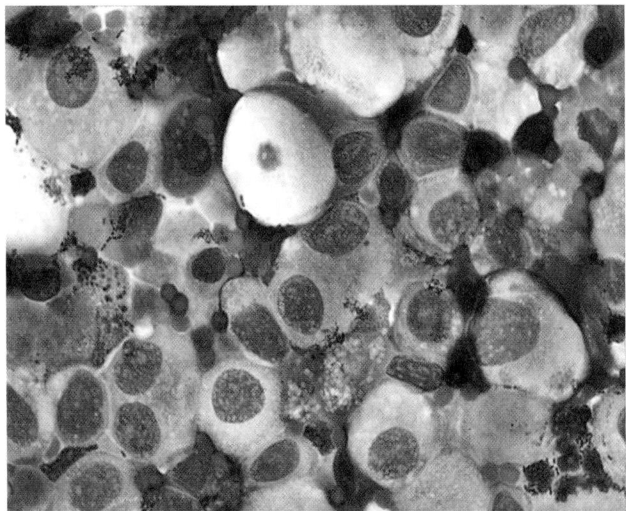

Figure 24.A.5 Urine sediment, Wright-Giemsa stain. There are many pleomorphic epithelial cells without any inflammation consistent with transitional cell carcinoma. Key to the diagnosis is the overall number of epithelial cells, the variability in sizes and shapes of these cells, and the absence of inflammation. ×1000.

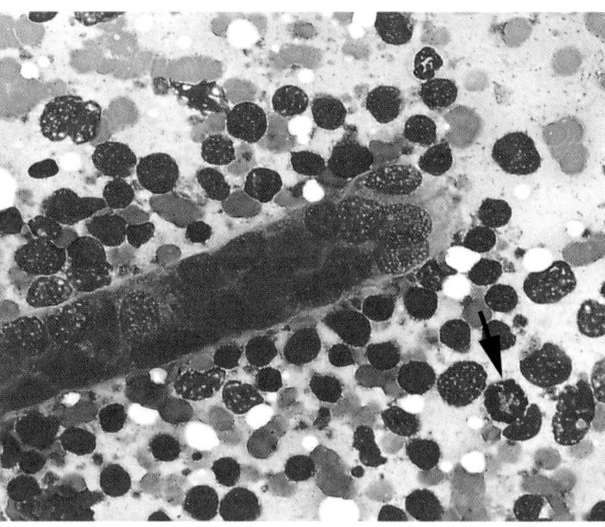

Figure 24.A.7 Kidney aspirate, Wright-Giemsa stain. A renal tubule is surrounded by numerous intermediate to large lymphoid cells with one mitotic figure (arrow); diagnosis is renal lymphoma. ×500.

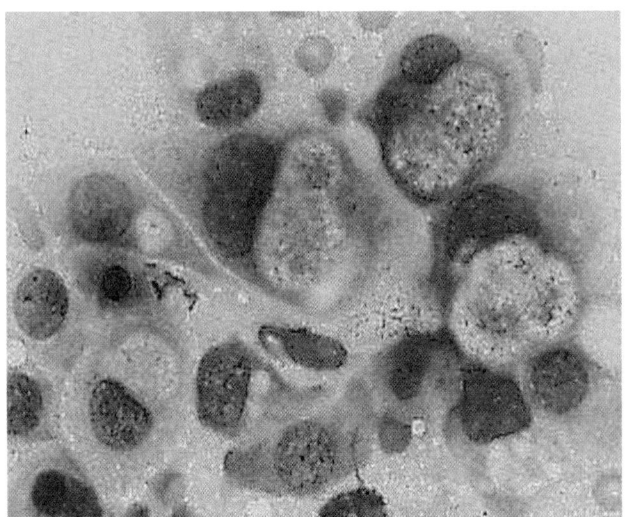

Figure 24.A.6 Urine sediment, Wright-Giemsa stain. These pleomorphic epithelial cells, seen in the absence of inflammation, occasionally have large cytoplasmic vacuoles containing pink material characteristic of transitional cell carcinomas. ×1000.

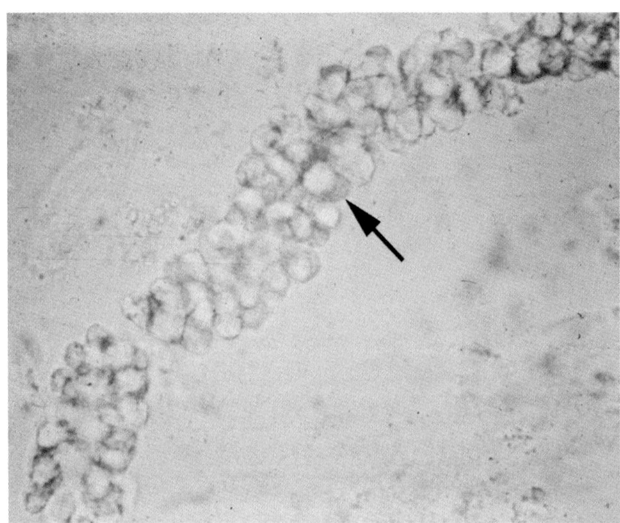

Figure 24.A.8 Urine sediment, unstained. Leukocyte casts (arrow) are quite fragile, seen infrequently, indicate inflammation is in renal tubules and therefore suggests pyelonephritis. ×400.

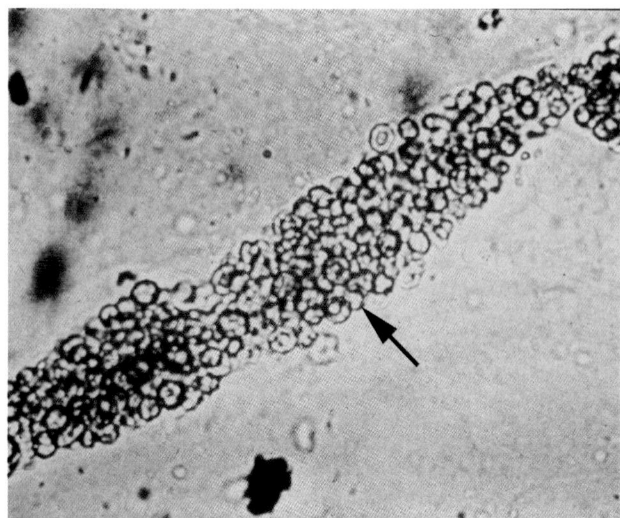

Figure 24.A.9 Urine sediment, unstained. Erythrocyte casts (arrow) are fragile and infrequently seen. When present, they indicate hemorrhage within the renal tubules. ×400.

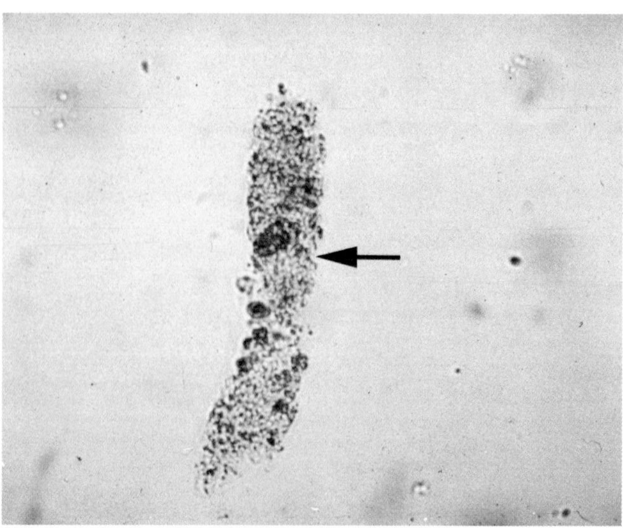

Figure 24.A.11 Urine sediment, unstained. The coarse granular cast (arrow) shown here is seen most frequently with a toxic insult (nephrosis) and can be caused by renal ischemia. ×400.

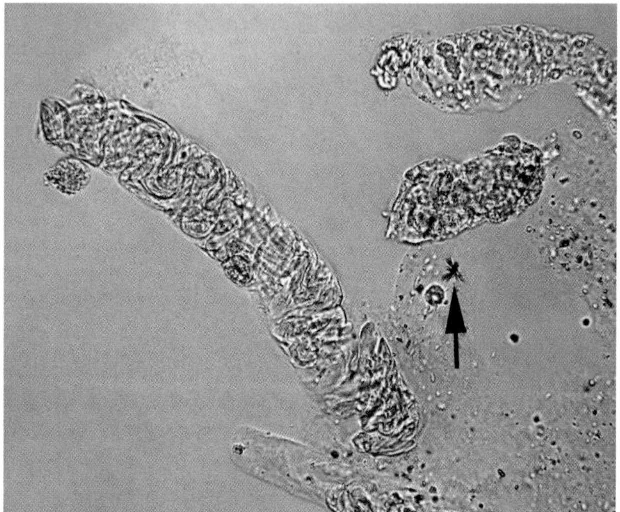

Figure 24.A.10 Urine sediment, unstained. Note the cellular casts and bilirubin crystal (arrow) present. ×400.

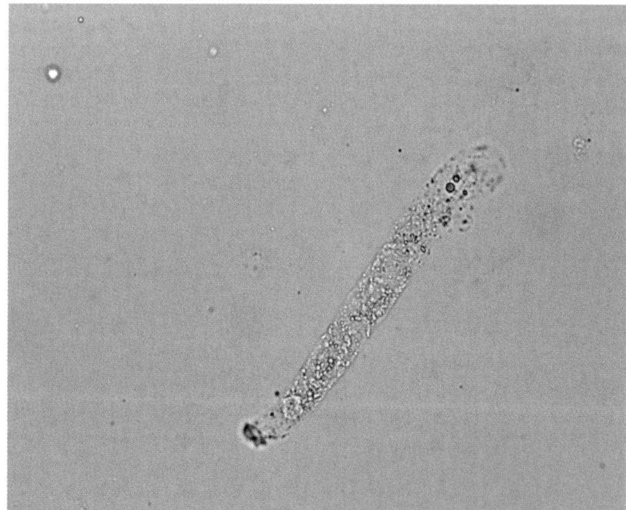

Figure 24.A.12 Urine sediment, unstained. The granular cast is progressing from coarse to finely granular; the distinction is not important, the critical factor is that these type of casts indicate an active tubular lesion when they are numerous and if urine is not concentrated. ×400.

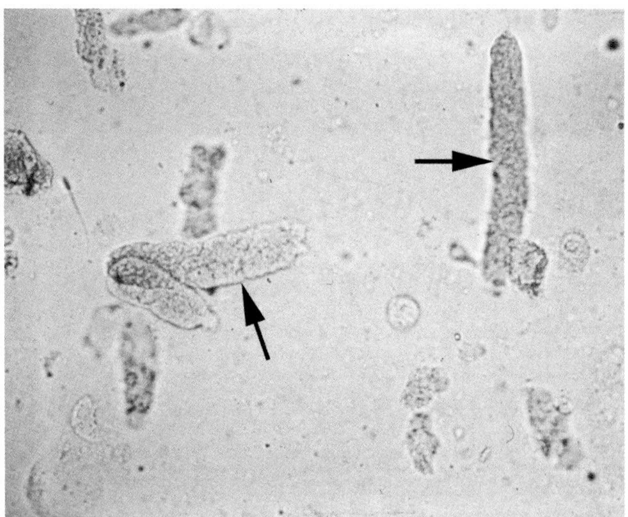

Figure 24.A.13 Urine sediment, unstained. These fine granular casts (arrows) occur under the same circumstances as coarse granular casts. ×100.

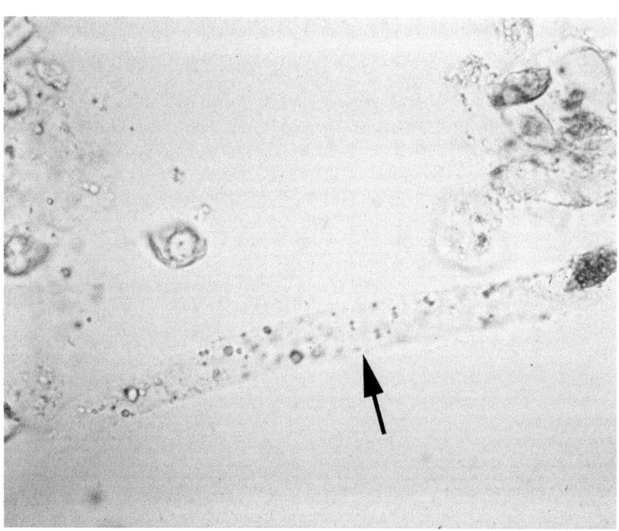

Figure 24.A.15 Unstained urine sediment with a hyaline cast (arrow). These casts can be seen in low numbers in healthy patients that have concentrated urine; they also are associated with proteinuria (particularly the nephrotic syndrome). ×400.

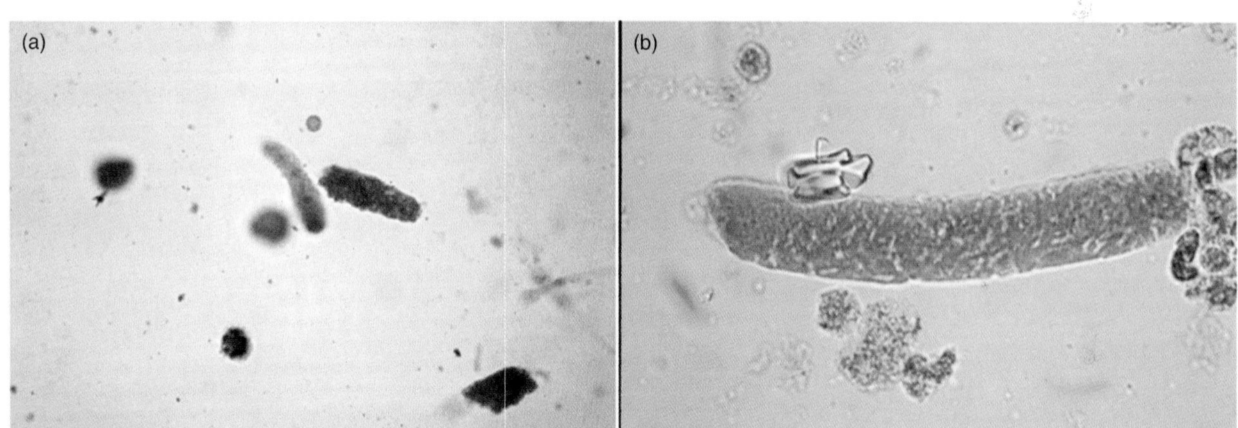

Figure 24.A.14 Urine sediment, sedi-stain. The multiple granular casts present at (a) low power (×100) and (b) at high power (×400) were found in urine with an SG of 1.008, indicating hyposthenuria and active tubular disease (nephrosis).

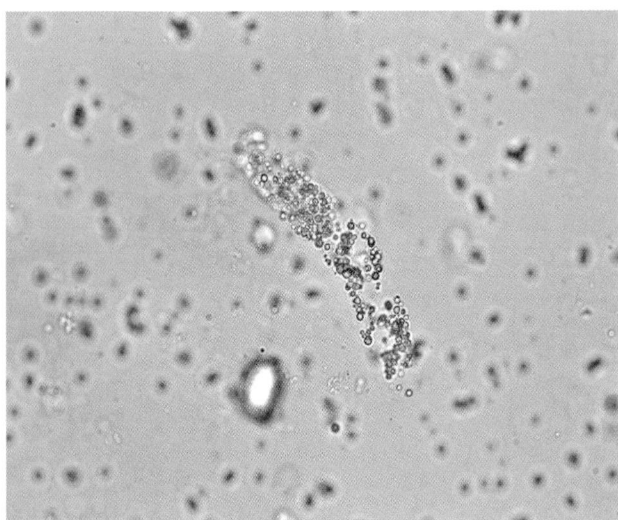

Figure 24.A.16 Urine sediment, unstained. Note the lipid (fatty) cast. ×400.

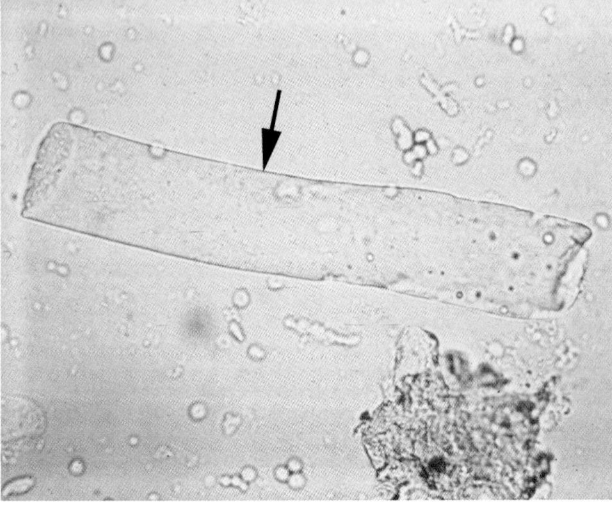

Figure 24.A.17 Urine sediment, unstained. The waxy cast (arrow) depicted here has sharp, linear edges with blunt ends and has a brittle appearance. When seen, waxy casts indicate prolonged periods of decreased tubular flow, most likely due to chronic renal lesions. ×400.

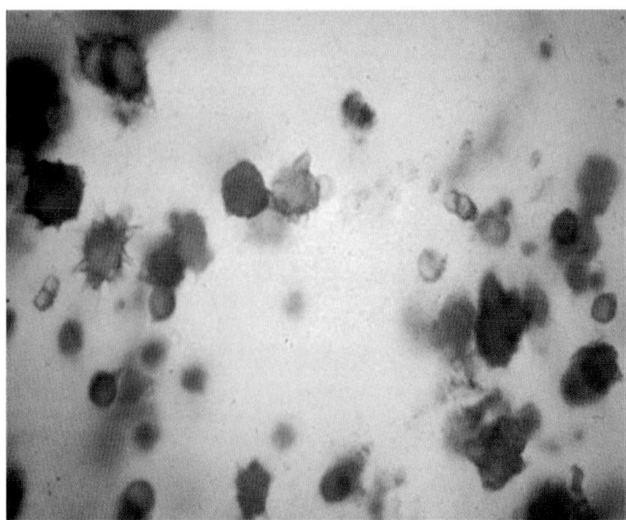

Figure 24.A.18 Note the many crystals with a thorn-apple appearance typical of ammonium biurate, which can be seen in health in English bulldogs and Dalmatians and are also associated with portosystemic shunts and severe liver failure. Clinical chemistry should be performed to identify low BUN, glucose, cholesterol, and albumin confirming decreased synthesis of these substances by the liver.

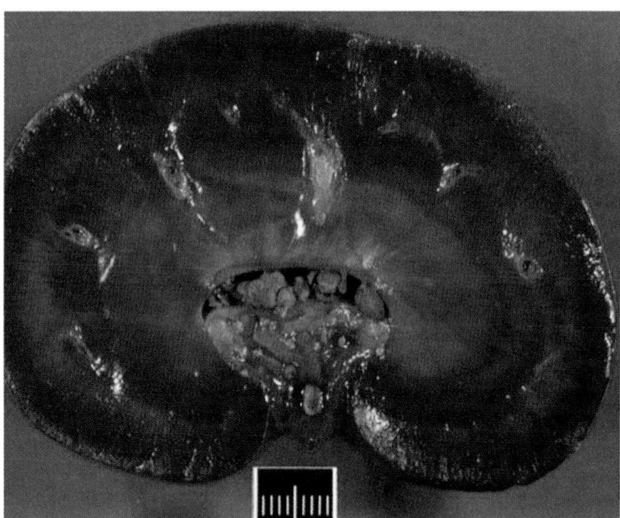

Figure 24.A.19 These variably sized green calculi located in the renal pelvis are nephroliths. This dog had a portosystemic shunt as well as the ammonium biurate crystals seen on sediment analysis in Figure 24.A.18.

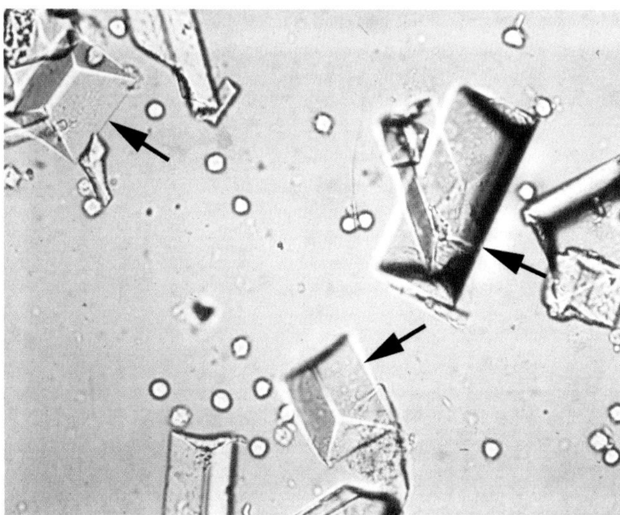

Figure 24.A.20 Urine sediment, unstained. Note the magnesium ammonium phosphate crystals (arrows) and the prism-like appearance. These are the most common crystals seen in cats and dogs. In dogs, they are associated with bacterial urinary tract infection. ×400.

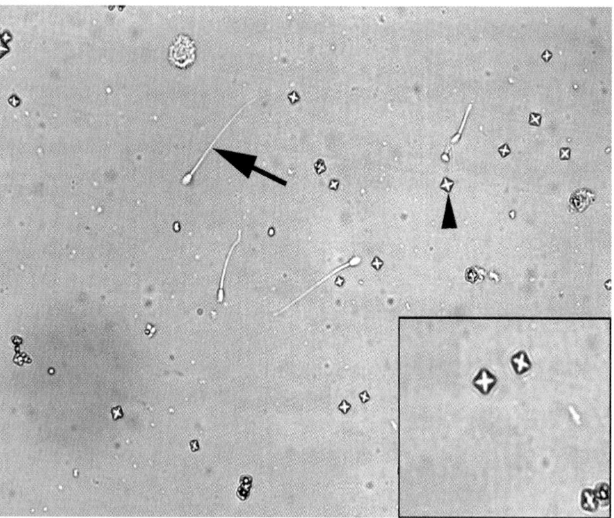

Figure 24.A.22 Urine sediment, unstained. The many crystals (arrowhead) depicted here have a Maltese cross appearance typical of calcium oxalate dihydrate. These crystals are seen in neutral to acidic urine. They can occasionally be seen in normal urine although when seen persistently are a clue to investigate hypercalcemic disorders. These crystals can be seen alone or with calcium oxalate monohydrate in ethylene glycol toxicity. There are also occasional sperm (arrow) present. ×100.

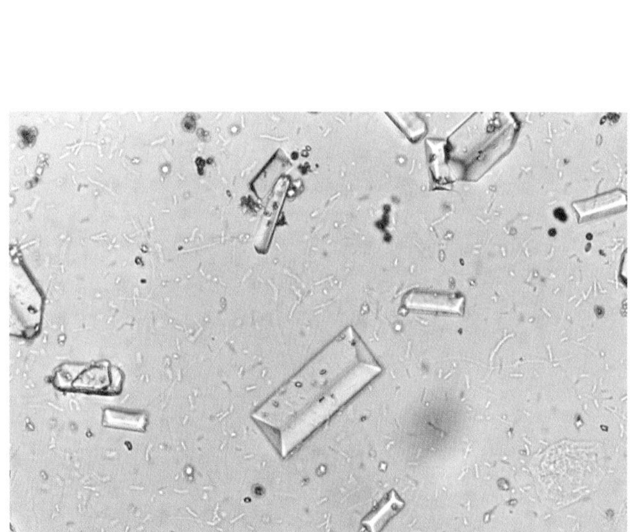

Figure 24.A.21 These multiple struvite crystals present on a background of many rod bacteria indicate bacterial overgrowth, as evidenced by the lack of leukocytes. ×400.

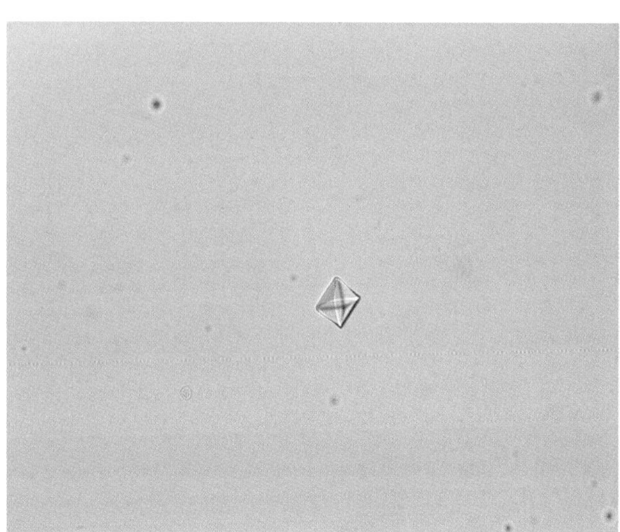

Figure 24.A.23 Urine sediment, unstained. Note the calcium oxalate dihydrate crystal at high power. ×400.

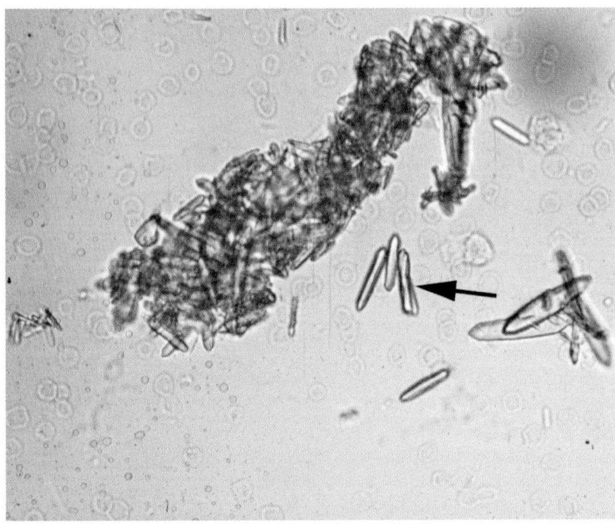

Figure 24.A.24 Urine sediment, unstained. These calcium oxalate monohydrate crystals shown here are present individually and in aggregate. If these crystals are found in a patient with acute kidney injury, they are diagnostic for ethylene glycol intoxication. Intoxication can be confirmed with the ethylene glycol test kit, or a marked osmolar and anion gap. ×400.

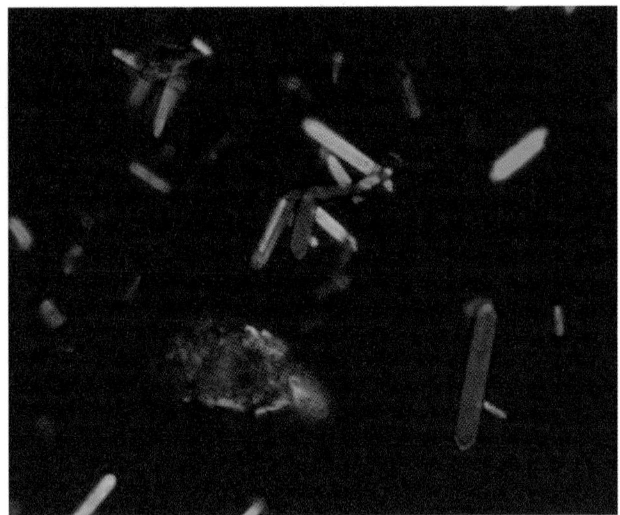

Figure 24.A.25 Urine sediment, unstained under polarized light. Note the many "picket-fence" calcium oxalate monohydrate crystals seen with ethylene glycol toxicity.

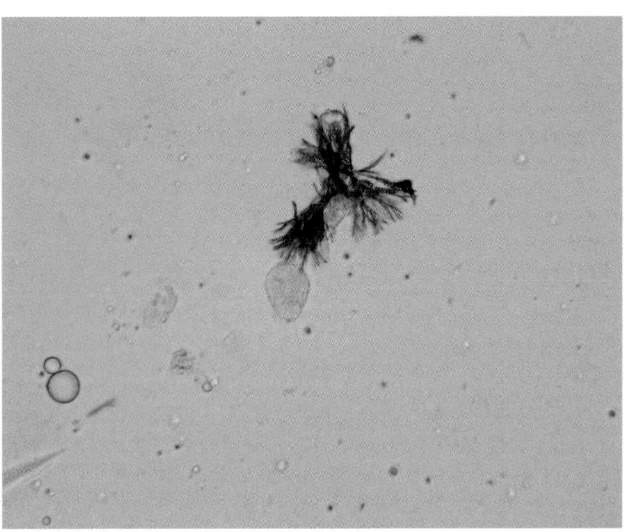

Figure 24.A.26 Urine sediment, unstained. This cluster of crystals is bilirubin, which can be seen with hemolysis, hepatocellular disease, or intra or extrahepatic cholestasis. The cellular elements present are also stained with bilirubin. ×400.

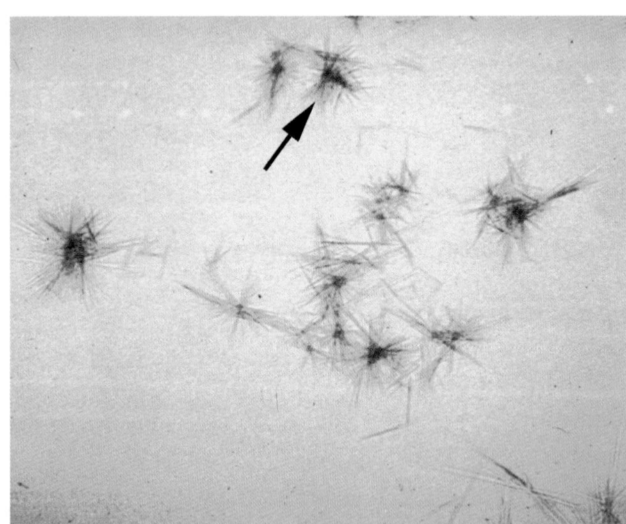

Figure 24.A.27 Urine sediment, unstained. Numerous tyrosine crystals (arrow) are present. These crystals are associated with hepatic disease, resemble bilirubin crystals, and occur under similar circumstances. ×400.

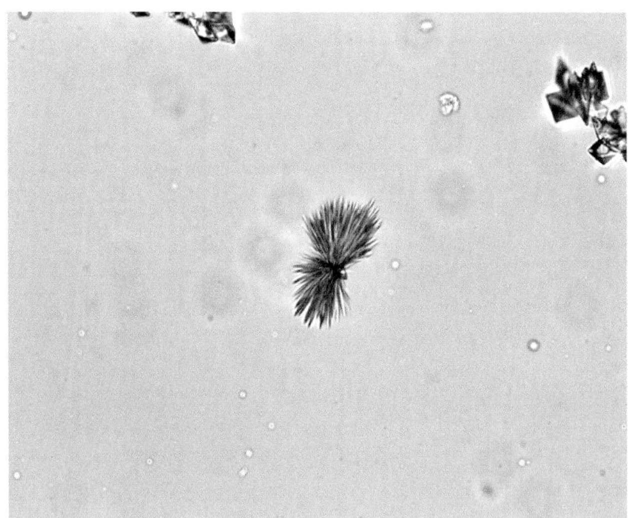

Figure 24.A.28 Urine sediment, unstained. Note the radiographic contrast crystal. These can be seen after intravenous contrast studies are performed. ×400.

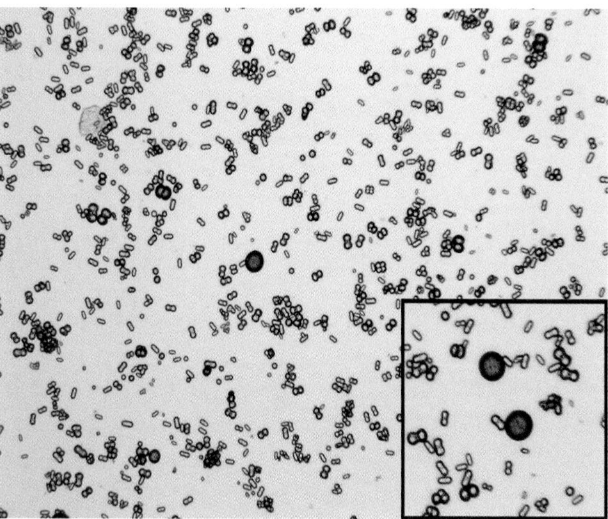

Figure 24.A.30 Urine sediment, unstained. Note the calcium carbonate crystals seen commonly in horses, rabbits, and guinea pigs, predominantly in the spherical forms. ×400.

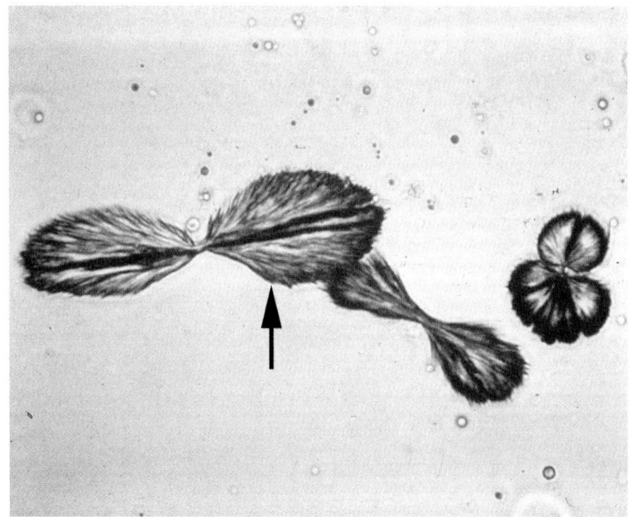

Figure 24.A.29 Urine sediment, unstained. Note the sulfonamide crystals (arrow). Nephrotoxic drugs may lead to the appearance of bizarre crystals in urine. ×400.

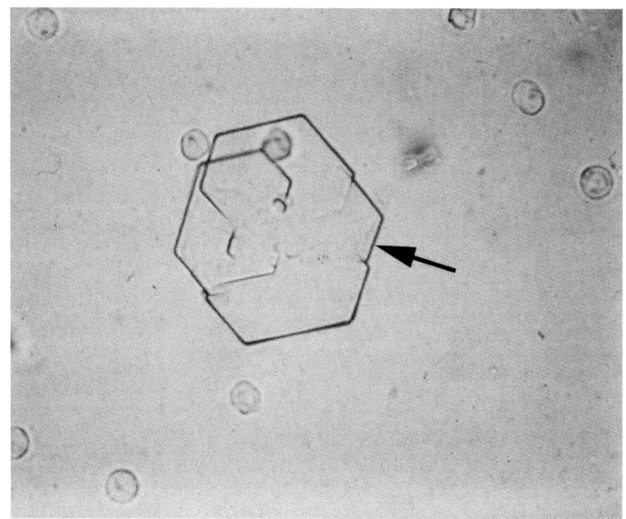

Figure 24.A.31 Urine sediment, unstained. The cystine crystals (arrow) seen here are always an abnormal finding and indicate cystinuria, which is due to a tubular defect heritable in English bulldogs, mastiffs, Chihuahuas, dachshunds, Newfoundlands, Australian cattle dogs, and American Staffordshire terriers. ×400.

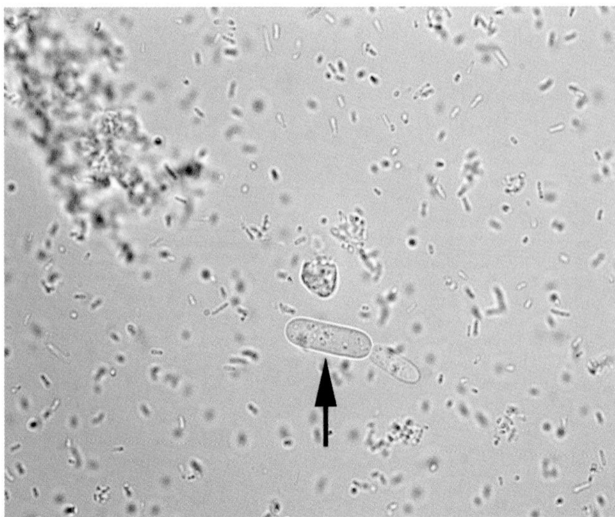

Figure 24.A.32 Urine sediment, unstained. The large, cylindrical-shaped budding yeast structure here is typical of *Cyniclomyces guttulatus*. The *Cyniclomyces* yeast can be seen in urine due to fecal contamination. This yeast is seen uncommonly, is regarded as nonpathogenic, and can be seen due to ingestion of rabbit feces. Many rod bacteria are also present within the background. ×1000.

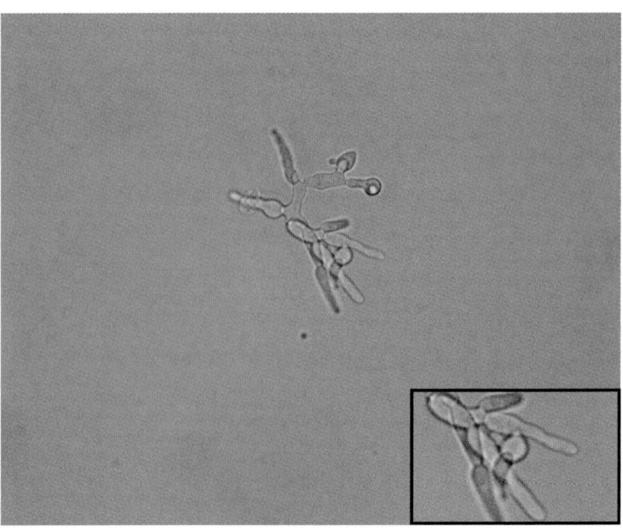

Figure 24.A.34 Urine sediment, unstained. Note the pseudohyphae and budding yeast forms in a young golden retriever with an incompetent urethral sphincter treated chronically with antibiotics and subsequently diagnosed with *Candida albicans* cystitis. ×500.

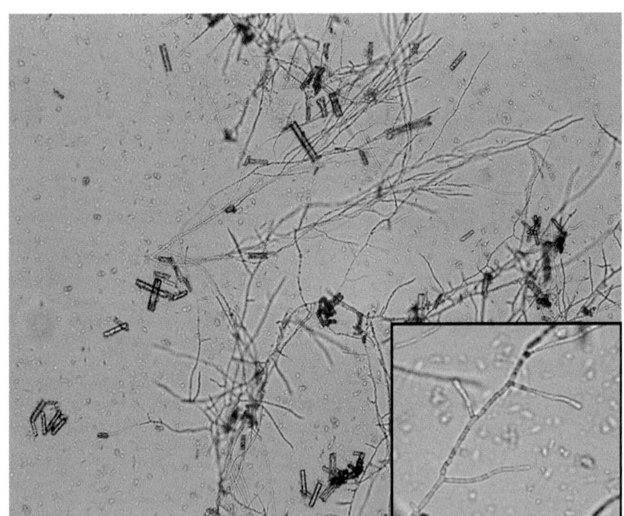

Figure 24.A.33 Urine sediment, unstained. Note the pseudohyphae and budding yeast forms in a pet with confirmed *Candida albicans* cystitis. These can also be contaminants; therefore, correlate presence of organisms with presence or absence of inflammation and clinical findings. ×500.

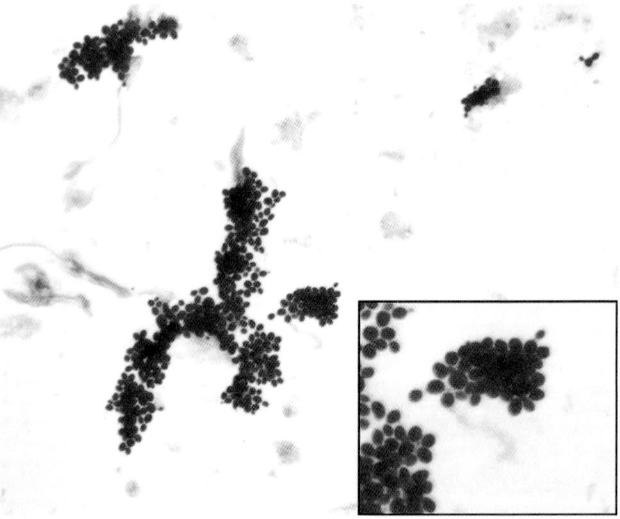

Figure 24.A.35 Urine sediment, Wright-Giemsa stain. There are numerous budding yeast present confirmed on culture as *Candida albicans*. These organisms are larger than bacteria and smaller than red blood cells, despite the lack of cells in this field for size comparison. This feline patient was a newly diagnosed diabetic with a history of multiple urinary tract infections and was chronically treated with antibiotics. ×500.

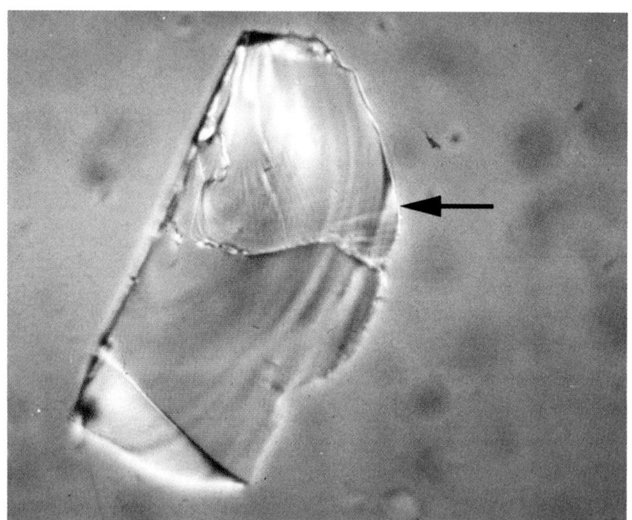

Figure 24.A.36 Urine sediment, unstained. The glass fragment (arrow) seen here may be from urine specimen containers or environmental contamination. It is important that this and other debris not be mistaken for crystals of pathologic significance. ×400.

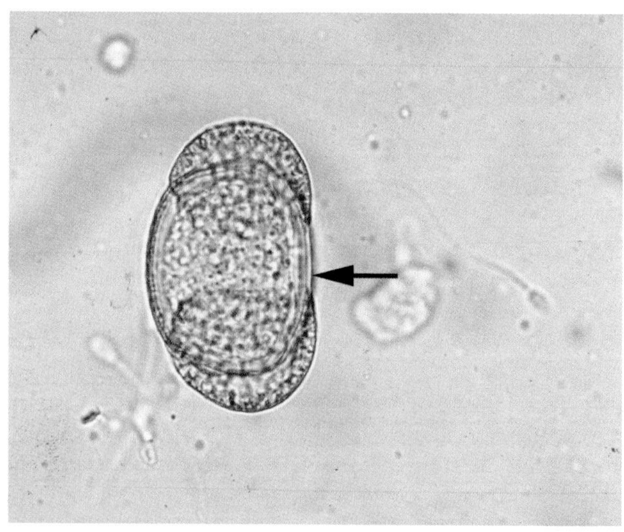

Figure 24.A.37 Urine sediment, unstained. The pine pollen (arrow) shown here can be commonly seen in free-catch urine specimens. ×400.

25 Laboratory Evaluation of Electrolytes

Andrea A. Bohn

Department of Microbiology, Immunology and Pathology, College of Veterinary Medicine and Biomedical Sciences, Colorado State University, Fort Collins, CO, USA

Evaluation of electrolyte concentrations is often used to assess severity of disease and guide treatment but can also aid in the diagnosis of disorders. Electrolytes are present in all intracellular and extracellular body fluids, but we typically measure their concentration in blood, plasma, or serum. The serum electrolyte concentration may not accurately reflect the balance of that particular electrolyte within the whole body, especially for electrolytes that are predominantly intracellular. Sodium and chloride are the electrolytes whose concentrations are greatest in extracellular fluid (ECF). The concentration of potassium, calcium, phosphorus, and magnesium are highest in intracellular fluid (ICF). Maintaining the intra- and extracellular concentration of each electrolyte within narrow limits is essential to life.

Intake of all of the electrolytes is via the oral route. The common organs that are important in maintaining all serum electrolyte levels are the gastrointestinal (GI) system and the kidneys. Additional regulatory mechanisms as well as the consequences and causes of imbalances for each individual electrolyte will be covered when each electrolyte is discussed in more detail.

Sodium

Sodium has many important functions, including maintaining normal blood pressure and volume and maintaining normal function of muscles and nerves. These functions are dependent on keeping plasma sodium concentrations within a narrow range. The concentration of sodium in the blood is predominantly a balance between what is consumed in food and drink and what is excreted in urine. Only a small amount is normally lost through stool and sweat, but these routes can become more important in certain disease or physiological states, depending on species.

The regulation of sodium cannot be discussed without also discussing water balance since these substances are intricately tied together. Water comprises approximately 60% of body weight, with about two-thirds in ICF and one-third in ECF. Approximately one quarter of ECF is within the vasculature while three quarters is present in the interstitium. Water balance between different compartments is dependent on osmotic pressures. As the most abundant cation of plasma, sodium, along with its associated anions, is the major determinant of extracellular osmolality. (For further information on osmolality, see Box 25.1) Sodium pumps maintain concentration differences across cell membranes, but sodium can freely cross vascular walls, equilibrating between interstitial and vascular spaces. Serum concentration of sodium reflects its ratio with water and does not necessarily reflect whole body sodium content. Abnormalities in serum sodium concentration are more likely due to abnormalities in water than sodium content.

Water and sodium regulation is associated with maintaining normal blood volume and osmolality. Sensors of osmolality and vascular pressure, including hypothalamic osmoreceptors, arterial, and atrial baroreceptors, and the juxtaglomerular apparatus, result in changes of sodium and/or water handling by the kidney. As little as a 1–2% increase in plasma osmolality will be detected by osmoreceptors in the hypothalamus, resulting in vasopressin (antidiuretic hormone or ADH) secretion from the posterior pituitary. By contrast, baroreceptors must perceive rather large deficits of blood volume (≥10%) to result in vasopressin release; in these instances maintaining blood volume is prioritized over maintaining osmolality. Vasopressin enhances water reabsorption in the renal collecting duct to replenish vascular water. Osmoreceptor cells are also involved in the sensation of thirst as an additional mechanism to replenish body water. Atrial baroreceptors that sense elevated blood pressure or blood volume signal the hypothalamus to inhibit

Veterinary Hematology, Clinical Chemistry, and Cytology, Third Edition. Edited by Mary Anna Thrall, Glade Weiser, Robin W. Allison and Terry W. Campbell.

Companion website: www.wiley.com/go/thrall/veterinary

Box 25.1 Osmolality

Solutes = Substances that are dissolved in plasma (electrolytes, proteins, etc).
Osmolality = The concentration of solutes in plasma (only the number matters, not size or weight).
In plasma, osmolality and osmolarity are nearly equal and can be used interchangeably.
Definitions are: the concentration of osmotically active particles *per kilogram solvent* (osmolality) vs. *in one liter of solution* (osmolarity).
Effect = Water will flow from low to high osmolar solutions.
Measurement = Osmolality is measured by determining either the freezing point depression or vapor-point elevation of a solution compared to water.
Calculated estimate =
2[Na] + [glucose (mg/dL)]/18 + [urea (mg/dL)]/2.8
Calculated osmolality is typically about 300–310 mOsm/L.
Osmolar gap = Measured mOsm - Calculated mOsm
In a healthy state, calculated mOsm is ~10 mOsm/L less than the measured value.
Increased osmolar gap indicates an increase in or presence of osmolar substances not included in the calculation (mannitol, ethylene glycol, etc.)

vasopressin release and decrease sodium reabsorption in the distal nephron.

While osmolality is regulated by water intake and excretion, sodium balance is regulated by sodium excretion, largely by the renal system. The juxtaglomerular cells of the kidney act as baroreceptors that detect low blood pressure. These cells activate the renin-angiotensin-aldosterone system (RAAS) by secreting renin. Renin cleaves angiotensinogen to angiotensin I, which is then converted to angiotensin II by angiotensin-converting enzyme. Angiotensin II causes the release of aldosterone from the adrenal glands, increases secretion of vasopressin, and stimulates thirst centers. Aldosterone acts on the renal cortical collecting tubules to reabsorb sodium. The reabsorption of sodium is coupled with either the secretion of potassium (another very important function of aldosterone) or the absorption of chloride to maintain electroneutrality.

When evaluating serum sodium concentration, the animal's total body water must be taken into consideration. Is there clinical or biochemical evidence of low body water (dehydration; Boxes 25.2 and 25.3) or does it appear normal or, possibly, increased? An increase in serum sodium concentration can be due to more sodium, less water, or a combination of causes. A decrease in serum sodium concentration can be due to less sodium, more water, or a combination of causes.

Box 25.2 Physical and biochemical parameters used in the assessment of hydration status

Assessment of body water content:
Physical exam
Skin turgor = interstitial tissue consistency
Capillary refill time = peripheral vascular blood flow
Change in body weight
Biochemical analysis
PCV and plasma protein concentration
Serum urea concentration
Serum sodium concentration

Hypernatremia

Hypernatremia (Figure 25.1) is most commonly associated with an imbalance in body water; it is usually easy to prevent with normal vasopressin and thirst responses, but there are conditions in which it occurs. Hypernatremia can happen with either decreased water intake or loss of water that exceeds the loss of electrolytes. Decreased intake can be due to water deprivation, defective thirst response, or a physical inability to drink. Loss of water can occur through insensible losses (respiratory or skin losses) or loss from the kidney or gastrointestinal systems.

For hypernatremia to develop, more water needs to be lost than electrolytes. Pure water loss occurs when there is an increase in insensible fluid losses, fever, and heat stroke are examples, or when the kidney cannot conserve water, as with diabetes insipidus. Whether vasopressin is deficient, as with central diabetes insipidus, or ineffective, as with congenital or acquired nephrogenic diabetes insipidus, a concurrent decrease in water intake is typically required for hypernatremia to occur. In many instances of water loss, electrolytes are also lost, as with vomiting, diarrhea (osmotic diarrhea, ruminal acidosis), osmotic diuresis, chronic or acute nonoliguric renal disease, or burns. Animals that lose electrolytes with water will become hypovolemic. With pure water loss or inadequate intake of water, the total body sodium content is normal, and intracellular water is drawn into the extracellular spaces, maintaining plasma volume (isovolemic hypernatremia).

Sodium excess is an uncommon cause of hypernatremia; either concurrent fresh water restriction or lack of urine concentration is usually necessary for hypernatremia to occur. Hypernatremia can occur either by ingesting excess salt (salt licks, sea water) or iatrogenically with the administration of hypertonic fluids. Decreased excretion of sodium can also lead to sodium excess; this can occur with the rare condition of hyperaldosteronism. These animals will become hypervolemic. If excess sodium is present in ECF, intracellular water will shift to the ECF and cells will become dehydrated.

Box 25.3 Manifestations and underlying processes of the various states of dehydration

Isotonic dehydration: proportional loss of NaCl and water
Some diarrheas and renal diseases
[Na] and [Cl] do not change.
PCV and [plasma protein] increase.
No change in osmolality; water does not shift between ICF and ECF, therefore ECF volume decreases.

Hypertonic dehydration: (ECF becomes hypertonic)
Water loss > NaCl loss.
- Diabetes insipidus
- Water deprivation/hypodipsia
- Respiratory loss with high temperature/panting
- Osmotic diuresis
- Diarrhea

[Na] and [Cl] increase.
PCV and [plasma protein] increase.
Osmolality increases; water shifts from ICF to ECF to maintain ECF volume.

Hypotonic dehydration: (ECF is hypotonic)
NaCl loss > water loss.
- Secretory diarrhea
- Vomiting
- Third-space loss
- Equine sweat

[Na] and [Cl] decrease.
PCV and [plasma protein] increase.
Osmolality decreases; water shifts from ECF to ICF, leading to volume depletion.

Protein and/or PCV may not appear increased if there is concurrent protein loss and/or anemia.

In a retrospective study that looked at hypernatremia in dogs and cats, disease processes and pathophysiologic factors were described for animals with moderate to severe hypernatremia (>10 mEq/L above reference interval) [1]. Over half of the cats had urological disease processes. Neurological disease was common in both dogs and cats and dogs had a higher incidence of neoplasia. Some of the other disease processes associated with cases of hypernatremia involved the respiratory, hepatobiliary, and gastrointestinal systems. Underlying pathophysiologic factors were commonly related to the renal system in cats. Gastrointestinal loss was common in both dogs and cats; in many instances, vomiting and diarrhea were likely secondary to another disease process rather than a primary gastrointestinal disorder. Central diabetes insipidus and fever/hyperthermia were also common factors in dogs. Osmotic diuresis and nephrogenic diabetes insipidus were among other causes. Common clinical signs in animals with hypernatremia were obtundation, vomiting, lethargy, weakness, and ataxia; it is not clear whether these signs were more likely due to the underlying disease process or the electrolyte imbalance.

When considering differentials for hypernatremia, along with other biochemical data, urinalysis and history are also important to consider [2, 3]. Concentrated urine indicates that extrarenal water loss is present and very dilute urine (hyposthenuric) is an indication of free water loss from the kidney. It is also important to know if the animal is polyuric and polydipsic, has had adequate access to water, has demonstrated any changes in mentation or shown neurological signs, or has had any recent significant events (burns, urinary obstruction, etc.) or therapies (fluid administration, etc.).

Hyponatremia

Hyponatremia (Figure 25.2) may be either due to sodium loss that exceeds water loss or an increase in body water. Hyponatremia is associated with hypo-osmolality except in cases of pseudohyponatremia or in translocational hyponatremia, in which large numbers of alternative osmoles are present.

Pseudohyponatremia can occur when sodium concentration is measured in whole plasma and not just plasma water because sodium is only dissolved in the water component of plasma. Marked hyperlipidemia or hyperproteinemia cause volume displacement and decrease the percent of serum or plasma that is water (known as the electrolyte exclusion effect). If the method used to measure sodium dilutes the sample (as with the majority of large chemistry analyzers), an artifactually low sodium concentration may be obtained, although measured plasma osmolality is normal. Direct ion-specific electrode potentiometry (the method used by most point of care and blood gas analyzers) uses undiluted samples and measures sodium concentration in just the water component of plasma so that pseudohyponatremia will not occur.

Translocational hyponatremia is due to the presence of other substances in the plasma causing hyperosmolality. Substances that readily cross cell membranes, like urea, will not cause translocational hyponatremia. Tonic substances,

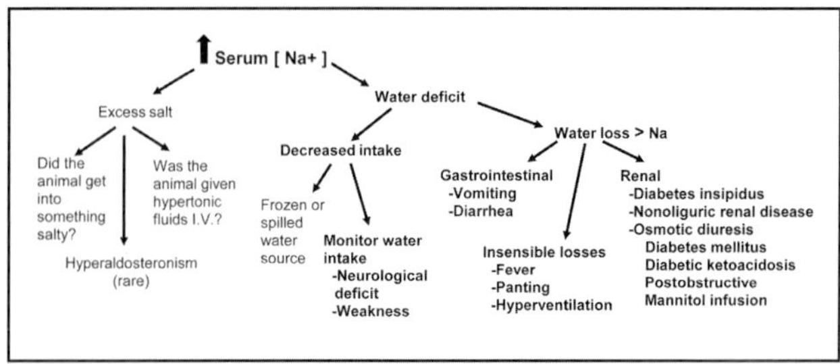

Figure 25.1 Algorithm for causes of hypernatremia (the more common causes are bolded).

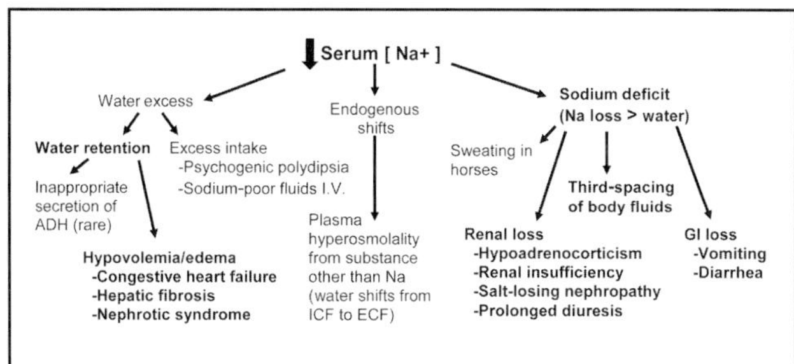

Figure 25.2 Algorithm for causes of hyponatremia (the more common causes are bolded).

osmolar substances that cannot easily cross cell membranes, will draw water from the ICF to the higher osmolality of the ECF, diluting out the sodium that is present. If glucose cannot enter cells due to the lack of insulin or its actions, hyperglycemia can result in translocational hyponatremia. In this case, measured and calculated osmolality will be similar. Exogenous substances (mannitol, ethylene glycol) that cause translocational hyponatremia will result in an increase in osmolar gap.

Hypo-osmolar hyponatremia occurs because of either increased water content or decreased sodium content. Increased water content occurs if there is impaired renal excretion of either dilute urine or free water or if water intake exceeds the maximal renal excretory capacity. Excess water intake is rare but can occur with psychogenic polydipsia. With excess intake, urine osmolality as well as plasma osmolality will be low.

Decreased renal excretion of free water in response to perceived hypovolemia can lead to an increase in total body water. This occurs due to third-spacing of fluid (accumulation within body cavities) associated with congestive heart failure, cirrhosis of the liver, or nephrotic syndrome. Vasopressin is released in response to perceived hypovolemia, resulting in increased reabsorption of water. Impaired renal excretion of water due to renal failure can also lead to hyponatremia with hypervolemia.

Hypovolemia typically accompanies loss of sodium from the body. Sodium is rarely lost from the body without some water, but to become hyponatremic there either has to be loss of hypertonic fluid (more sodium lost than water) or isotonic or hypotonic fluid loss resulting in volume depletion, which stimulates drinking and renal water retention, diluting the remaining body fluids. Hypovolemic, hypo-osmolar hyponatremia can result from gastrointestinal loss (vomiting, diarrhea), renal loss (hypoadrenocorticism, prolonged diuresis), third-space loss (body cavity effusions), or sweating in horses. Primary hypoadrenocorticism (Addison's disease) is associated with aldosterone deficiency, resulting in decreased renal reabsorption of sodium, increased retention of potassium in cortical collecting tubules, and a decreased sodium potassium ratio (Box 25.4).

It is important to keep in mind that an animal may be normonatremic in many of the conditions listed above despite being dehydrated or hypervolemic if there is a net loss or gain of isotonic fluids or if an equilibrium has been reached. Hypovolemia not only stimulates vasopressin release but triggers the RAAS, which leads to sodium retention.

Hyponatremia is more common than hypernatremia and was present in 49.4% of hospitalized cats and 25.5% of hospitalized dogs in a recent study [4]. In that study, disease processes and pathophysiologic factors were described for animals with moderate to severe hyponatremia (>10 mEq/L below reference interval), which comprised 4% of dogs and 8% of cats. The most common disease processes in this subset of cats were urological and cardiovascular and, in dogs, gastrointestinal and urological. Some of the other disease processes associated with hyponatremia were neoplasia, diabetes mellitus, hypoadrenocorticism, and respiratory, hepatobiliary, and pancreatic disorders. The most common pathophysiologic factors were gastrointestinal loss from vomiting and diarrhea, third space loss ± decreased effective circulating blood volume, and factors associated with urological diseases. Common clinical signs in animals with hyponatremia, were obtundation, vomiting, lethargy, and weakness; it is not clear whether these signs were more likely due to the underlying disease process or the electrolyte imbalance.

Determining the cause of hyponatremia is often achieved after considering history, physical exam findings (ECF volume status, presence of body cavity effusions, jaundice, heart murmur, etc.), the rest of the serum biochemical panel and urinalysis. For challenging cases, one may wish to measure urine fractional excretion (see the "Fractional Excretion of Electrolytes" section in Chapter 24) to differentiate appropriate from inappropriate vasopressin secretion or to determine if there is an inappropriate amount of sodium getting excreted by the kidneys. Syndrome of inappropriate antidiuretic hormone secretion (SIADH) is a syndrome where urine is inappropriately being concentrated without the kidneys being in a state of sodium retention (which would be an appropriate response if the animal was hypovolemic). Urine electrolyte and osmolality measurements are necessary for the diagnosis of SIADH [5].

Chloride

Chloride is the major anion in the ECF and, similar to sodium, chloride is important in the regulation of body fluids. Chloride also plays an important role in digestion and muscular activity and serves as a conjugate anion in acid base metabolism. To maintain electroneutrality, chloride either moves in the same direction of the positively charged sodium or exchanges with the negatively charged bicarbonate ions. When evaluating an abnormality in serum

Box 25.4 Sodium potassium ratio

Reference interval ~ 27 : 1 to 40 : 1

Ratios <27 : 1 can be due to either an absolute or relative increase in potassium, decrease in sodium, or a combination of these changes; increased potassium is the most common reason.

Low ratios are commonly associated with hypoadrenocorticism.

Hypoadrenocorticism should always be a differential with a decreased Na:K ratio BUT not the only one.

Other diseases/conditions commonly associated with low Na:K ratios include

- Renal/urinary tract disease.
- Gastrointestinal disease; parasitism in dogs.
- Body cavity effusions.

Low Na:K ratios have also been reported with:

- Diabetes mellitus, pancreatitis, cardiorespiratory disease, pyometra, disseminated neoplasia, grade III patellar luxation, mushroom poisoning, behavior problem, ocular disease, skin disease.

Na:K ratios <15 are more commonly associated with hypoadrenocorticism in dogs.

A small percent of dogs with primary hypoadrenocorticism have a normal ratio.

The ratio is often normal in dogs with secondary hypoadrenocorticism (low ACTH).

Sources: Bell et al. [6], Feldman and Nelson [7], Lifton et al. [8], Nielsen et al. [9], Pak [10], Peterson et al. [11], and Roth and Tyler [12].

Box 25.5 Using sodium to correct chloride concentration in the analysis of chloride abnormalities

Correction of chloride for water imbalance

Can the abnormality in chloride be attributed to the water imbalance that is affecting sodium concentration?

This can be estimated by proportionally correcting chloride using the sodium concentration. The middle of the reference interval (RI) can be used as the "normal" sodium value. Divide this value by the measured sodium concentration to arrive at the factor with which to multiply the measured chloride concentration. The corrected chloride concentration can then be compared to the RI for chloride.

Normal sodium/Measured sodium × Measured chloride = Corrected chloride

Example 1: Na = 164 mEq/L (RI 134–144 mEq/L; middle = 139)
Cl = 136 mEq/L (RI 105–125 mEq/L)
Corrected chloride = 139/164 × 136 = 115
Therefore, Cl shifts are due to same process as Na shifts.

Example 2: Na = 124 mEq/L (RI 134–144 mEq/L; middle = 139)
Cl = 75 mEq/L (RI 105–125 mEq/L)
Corrected chloride = 139/124 × 75 = 84
The corrected chloride concentration is still markedly outside of the RI. Bicarbonate is expected to be increased.

chloride concentration, it is important to compare chloride levels with sodium levels and to the animal's acid base status. If abnormalities in chloride concentration appear to be in proportion to abnormalities in sodium concentration (Box 25.5), differentials to consider are similar to those given for hyponatremia or hypernatremia above. If the change in chloride concentration appears greater than a change in sodium concentration, bicarbonate concentration should be evaluated and a blood gas analysis may be indicated (Chapter 26).

Hyperchloremia

If the degree of hyperchloremia is proportional to concurrent hypernatremia (Box 25.5), consider the same differentials as hypernatremia. Hyperchloremia is usually associated with a water deficit.

Alternatively, hyperchloremia can be related to hypobicarbonatemia (Figure 25.3). Loss of bicarbonate can occur from the gastrointestinal tract with diarrhea, loss of saliva in cattle that contains a high bicarbonate concentration, or vomiting intestinal contents as can occur with intestinal obstruction. Biliary, pancreatic, and duodenal secretions contain high concentrations of bicarbonate, the addition of which requires exchange with chloride at the luminal cell membrane. The secreted bicarbonate is normally resorbed in the jejunum, but when resorption does not occur, hyperchloremia will result. Additional regulation of bicarbonate occurs in enterocytes of the ileum and distal colon, where secretion of bicarbonate is, again, dependent on exchange with chloride; hypersecretory states result in hypobicarbonatemia and hyperchloremia, most commonly seen with secretory diarrhea in calves.

Renal loss of bicarbonate (and therefore chloride retention) occurs with proximal or distal renal tubular acidosis (RTA), which can be primary or acquired. Proximal RTA is due to a lack of bicarbonate absorption in the proximal tubules and subsequent loss. Distal RTA is due to decreased ability to secrete an acid load in the distal tubules, which would otherwise be accompanied by bicarbonate absorption and concurrent chloride excretion. Some of the diverse disease processes that result in RTA are congenital tubular defects, hypoadrenocorticism, and renal tubular disease.

In a physiologic compensatory response to chronic respiratory alkalosis, the kidneys decrease acid secretion and bicarbonate resorption, resulting in retention of chloride. Mild alkalosis associated with hypoalbuminemia may also lead to mild hyperchloremia [13].

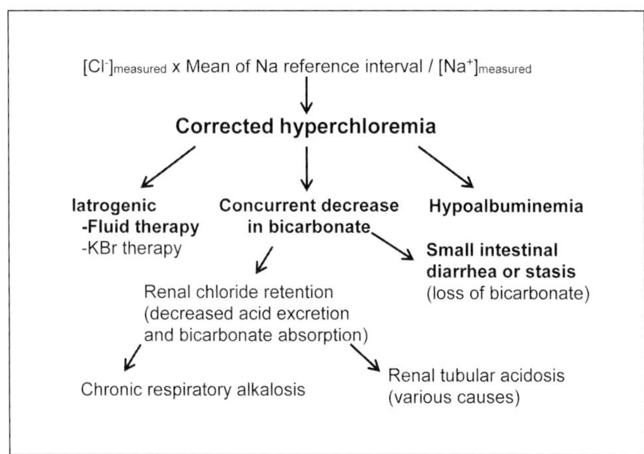

Figure 25.3 Algorithm for causes of corrected hyperchloremia (the more common causes are bolded).

Hyperchloremia can occur iatrogenically if administered solutions contain proportionally greater amounts of chloride than sodium: 0.9% sodium chloride (chloride is proportionally higher in saline than ECF), hypertonic saline, ammonium chloride, potassium chloride, and cationic amino acids (e.g., total parenteral nutrition). Administration of halides (e.g., bromide, iodide, fluoride) can result in artifactual hyperchloremia because ion selective electrodes are not specific and these substances are measured as chloride. A false elevation in chloride is often seen in animals receiving potassium bromide as an anticonvulsant.

Hypochloremia

If the degree of hypochloremia is proportional to the degree of hyponatremia (Box 25.5), the same differentials listed for hyponatremia apply.

If chloride is decreased to a greater degree than sodium, differentials related to metabolic alkalosis must be considered (Figure 25.4). In the process of secreting HCl into the stomach, serum chloride is decreased and serum bicarbonate is increased. These changes are normally reversed when hydrogen and chloride ions and water are reabsorbed in the intestines. If gastric fluid is lost due to vomiting or sequestered due to a displaced abomasum, pyloric obstruction, or functional obstruction, serum chloride will remain low and bicarbonate will remain elevated.

In a physiologic compensatory response to chronic respiratory acidosis, the kidneys increase acid secretion and bicarbonate resorption, resulting in chloride secretion and hypochloremia.

The chloride concentration in equine sweat is up to twice as much as in plasma and it is higher than sodium concentration. After sweat loss, hypochloremia can be present even after correcting for hyponatremia. Bicarbonate will be elevated.

Iatrogenic hypochloremia is fairly common. Loop diuretics (furosemide) and thiazides cause a proportionally greater

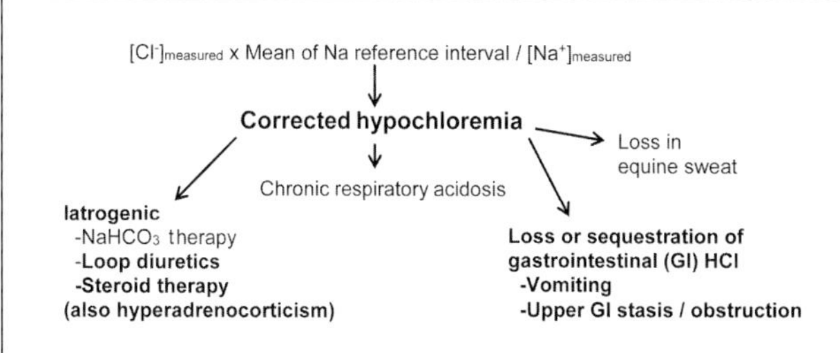

Figure 25.4 Algorithm for causes of corrected hypochloremia (the more common causes are bolded).

loss of chloride than sodium. Glucocorticoids have been associated with mild hypochloremia, likely an effect on cortical collecting ducts. Administration of solutions containing sodium and without chloride (e.g., sodium bicarbonate) may also result in corrected hypochloremia.

Potassium

Potassium is a major intracellular cation that plays an important role in resting cell membrane potential. Clinical signs associated with abnormal serum potassium concentrations manifest as cardiac and skeletal muscle dysfunction, and hyperkalemia can have life-threatening effects on cardiac conduction. Therefore, it is important to maintain serum potassium concentrations within narrow limits. Total body potassium is a balance between what is ingested (100%) and what is excreted from the kidneys (normally ~90–95%) and colon (normally ~5–10%). The concentration of ECF (serum) potassium is also reliant on the translocation of potassium between the ECF and ICF. Less than 5% of total body potassium is present in the ECF; therefore serum potassium concentration is an unpredictable representation of total body potassium content.

Hyperkalemia

Hyperkalemia (Figure 25.5) occurs if there is an increased potassium load, a decrease in potassium excretion, or a shift of potassium from ICF to ECF. Increased ingestion of potassium is unlikely to result in hyperkalemia unless there is a concurrent decrease in renal excretion. An increase in potassium load can occur iatrogenically and may result in death when fluids containing high concentrations of potassium are mistakenly given.

Decreased renal excretion of potassium is a common cause of hyperkalemia and can result from renal or postrenal diseases of the urinary tract. In anuric or oliguric renal failure the kidney itself does not have the capacity to remove excess potassium from the body. Postrenal processes that result in decreased removal of urine from the body, such as urethral obstruction or ruptured urinary bladder, can also result in hyperkalemia.

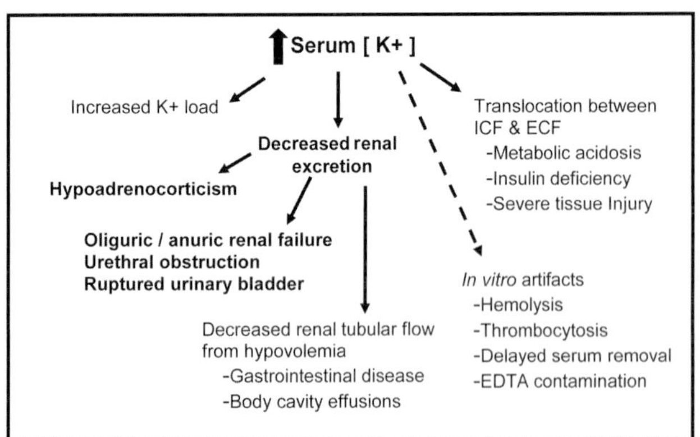

Figure 25.5 Algorithm for causes of hyperkalemia (the more common causes are bolded).

Aldosterone acts to increase serum sodium and decrease serum potassium concentrations by reabsorbing sodium and excreting potassium in the renal cortical collecting tubules and, to a lesser extent, in the colon. Aldosterone deficiency results in decreased excretion of potassium, thus hypoadrenocorticism is commonly associated with hyperkalemia, hyponatremia, and decreased sodium potassium ratio (Box 25.4).

Potassium renal excretion is decreased with a decrease in tubular flow rate, which can occur with hypovolemia. This is thought to be the reason for increased serum potassium concentrations associated with body cavity effusions and gastrointestinal disease. Hypovolemia and hyponatremia become more severe with repeated drainage of body cavity effusions, and hyperkalemia is more commonly seen with effusions that have been repeatedly drained. The gastrointestinal disease that is most commonly associated with hyperkalemia in dogs is severe whipworm infestation. The hyperkalemia seen with neonatal calf diarrhea is predominantly attributed to the degree of dehydration and prerenal azotemia in the calves [14].

Translocation between ECF and ICF plays a large role in maintaining serum potassium concentrations. A condition that moves potassium from the ICF to ECF causing hyperkalemia is the movement of acid (H^+) into cells with metabolic acidosis. Experimentally, this has been reproduced only with non–anion gap metabolic acidosis. Since insulin is important in normal movement of potassium from the ECF to ICF, insulin deficiency can result in hyperkalemia. Given the high concentration of intracellular potassium, potassium released from injured cells can increase its concentration in the ECF, especially if there is also decreased renal excretion. A large degree of tissue injury is typically necessary to result in hyperkalemia, which can occur with tumor lysis syndrome, rhabdomyolysis, or severe trauma. Potassium can also be released from muscle during exercise and transient hyperkalemia may be seen during and shortly after exercise in horses [15].

Pseudohyperkalemia occurs if large amounts of potassium leak out of cells during or after blood is drawn. Platelets contain abundant intracellular potassium that is released upon activation. Blood clotting, therefore, can result in an elevation in serum potassium concentration, especially if a thrombocytosis is present. Reference intervals for serum potassium are typically about 0.5 mEq/L higher than for plasma. Hemolysis causes potassium to leak from erythrocytes. The amount of potassium in erythrocytes varies with species and even breed. Horses, pigs, and cattle have high erythrocyte potassium concentrations. Cats and dogs typically have lower erythrocyte potassium except for the Akita and other Japanese dog breeds.

False increases in potassium also occur if a sample has been contamination with potassium ethylenediaminetetraacetic acid (EDTA). In this case, calcium and magnesium should be very low.

Hypokalemia

Hypokalemia (Figure 25.6) is one of the more common electrolyte disturbances in critically ill veterinary patients, although a definitive cause cannot always be identified. Hypokalemia may be due to decreased intake, increased excretion or loss, shifts between the ECF and ICF, or (often) a combination of these. Decreased intake from diet can contribute to hypokalemia. This is usually not a cause on its own, although it may play a larger role in ruminants where potassium absorption is reliant on ruminal potassium concentration. A significant decrease in plasma potassium concentration was shown in as little as 18 hours of food withholding from steers [16]. Hypokalemia can also be caused iatrogenically with potassium-poor fluids.

Loss of potassium occurs from the gastrointestinal or renal systems. Vomiting and small intestinal diarrhea can result in hypokalemia. Renal losses can occur for a variety of reasons. Hypokalemia associated with chronic renal failure occurs more commonly in cats. Distal RTA, postobstructive diuresis, diabetic ketoacidosis, acquired or congenital Fanconi syndrome, and diuretic administration all can lead to increased

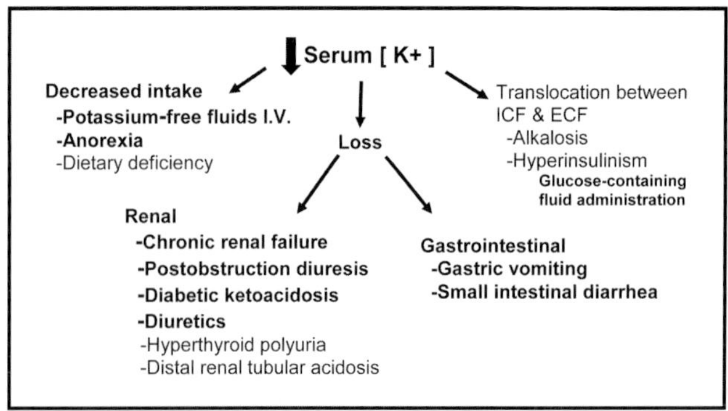

Figure 25.6 Algorithm for causes of hypokalemia (the more common causes are bolded).

Box 25.6 Calculation of the anion gap

Na^+ and K^+ are the major cations; all other cations are classified as unmeasured cations (UC^+).
Cl^- and HCO_3^- are the major anions; all other anions are classified as unmeasured anions (UA^-).
Given the law of electoneutrality:

$$Na^+ + K^+ + UC^+ = Cl^- + HCO_3^- + UA^-$$

Subtracting UC^+ and Cl^- and HCO_3^- from both sides:

$$\mathbf{Na^+ + K^+ - Cl^- - HCO_3^-} = UA^- - UC^+ = \textbf{Anion gap}$$

potassium excretion and hypokalemia. Hyperaldosteronism is a rare cause of hypokalemia, but repeated administration of isoflupredone acetate is a potential cause of hypokalemia syndrome in cattle [17].

Increased movement of potassium from the ECF to ICF can cause hypokalemia. This can be due to an excess of insulin, a glucose infusion, or alkalosis. Hypokalemia due to xylitol toxicity in dogs is because of insulin release and its effect of moving potassium into cells along with glucose. Alkalosis is thought to play a large role in the frequent occurrence of hypokalemia in cattle with displaced abomasums [16]. Catecholamines can also cause a shift of potassium from ECF to ICF secondary to pain, sepsis, or trauma.

Anion gap

We measure several anions and cations in the blood, but there are many others that are not routinely measured. The predominant cations of ECF are sodium, potassium, calcium, and magnesium, and the predominant anions are chloride, bicarbonate, plasma proteins, organic acid ions, phosphate, and sulfate. The number of unmeasured anions is greater than the number of unmeasured cations, and the difference between these is called the anion gap. The greatest change in the anion gap is when an increase occurs owing to an increase of organic acids in the circulation. The anion gap, therefore, is important in determination of the acid-base status of an animal (Chapter 26). The anion gap is essentially used to determine the cause of decreased blood bicarbonate concentrations (metabolic acidosis) or to detect metabolic acidosis during a mixed acid-base disorder in which bicarbonate may be normal or increased.

An indirect method is used to calculate the anion gap (Box 25.6). The calculation is based on the law of electroneutrality (i.e., the number of positive charges need to equal the number of negative charges in the body). The cations and anions that are considered "measured" are sodium & potassium and chloride & bicarbonate, respectively. The anion gap is the difference between these anions and cations as illustrated in Figure 25.7.

Because cations rarely change enough to affect the anion gap, a decrease in bicarbonate has to be accompanied by either an increase in unmeasured anions or a decrease in chloride to keep the equation equal and to maintain electroneutrality. (Figure 25.7) Unmeasured anions that have the most effect on anion gap are the endogenous products lactate, ketones, and uremic acids, as well as the exogenous substances salicylate and the metabolites of ethylene glycol toxicity. Lactic acidosis is produced during hypoxia and anaerobic metabolism. Keto acids are produced when there is a negative energy balance and metabolism switches from primarily glycolysis to lipolysis. Uremic acids are phosphates, sulfates, and organic acids that are no longer adequately filtered because of decreased glomerular filtration rate (GFR). Decreases in anion gap are typically due to hypoalbuminemia, as the predominant unmeasured anion in health is albumin. For further utilization of the anion gap, see Chapter 26.

Calcium, phosphorus, and magnesium

Calcium, phosphate, and magnesium are required for vital extra- and intracellular functions. Like potassium and in contrast to sodium and chloride, intracellular concentrations of calcium, phosphate, and magnesium are higher than extracellular concentrations. As with the other electrolytes, their intake is by ingestion and the regulation of their blood concentration involves the kidneys and gastrointestinal tract. Bone is another essential player in regulation, as the majority of total body calcium, phosphate, and magnesium are stored in bone. Maintaining appropriate circulating concentrations of these electrolytes is largely dependent on hormonal control. Regulatory hormones are shared by these electrolytes, with magnesium regulation being less well understood. The main hormones that function to maintain normal calcium and phosphate levels are calcitonin, parathyroid hormone (PTH), and 1,25-dihydroxyvitamin D (calcitriol or vitamin D).

Calcitonin is produced by thyroid parafollicular cells (C- cells). It is released in response to hypercalcemia and its release is inhibited by hypocalcemia. The main function of calcitonin is to limit postprandial hypercalcemia by inhibiting osteoclastic bone resorption and decreasing reabsorption of calcium and phosphate by the kidney tubules. Its overall effect is to decrease serum calcium and phosphate concentrations (Figure 25.8).

PTH is produced by chief cells in the parathyroid gland and is the principle hormone in fine, minute-to-minute blood calcium regulation. It is released in response to hypocalcemia and its release is inhibited by elevated calcium levels and vitamin D. PTH acts to increase the activity of vitamin D, increase calcium and phosphate reabsorption from bone, and increase

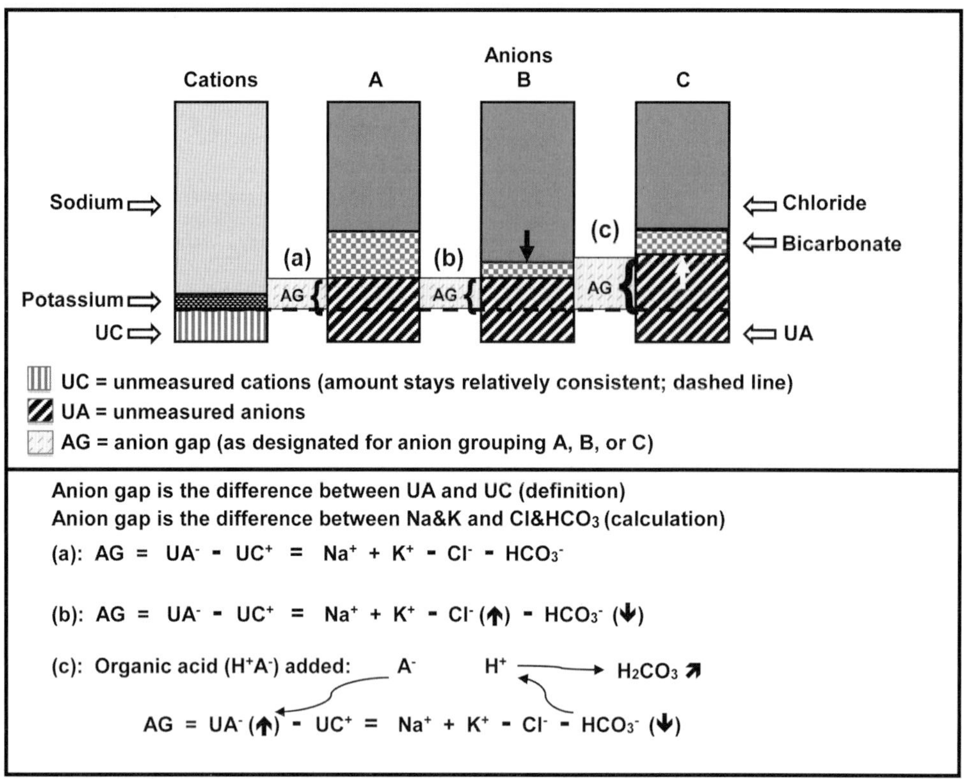

Figure 25.7 Demonstration of how anion gap is affected in different situations resulting in metabolic acidosis. Anions A: normal acid base status; normal anion gap (a). Anions B: Nonanion gap (secretional) metabolic acidosis. Bicarbonate is exchanged for chloride (solid black arrow); anion gap is not affected (b). Anions C: Anion gap (titrational) metabolic acidosis. As organic acids are introduced, bicarbonate is utilized to buffer the hydrogen ion while the leftover anion adds to the unmeasured anion pool (solid white arrow); anion gap is increased (c).

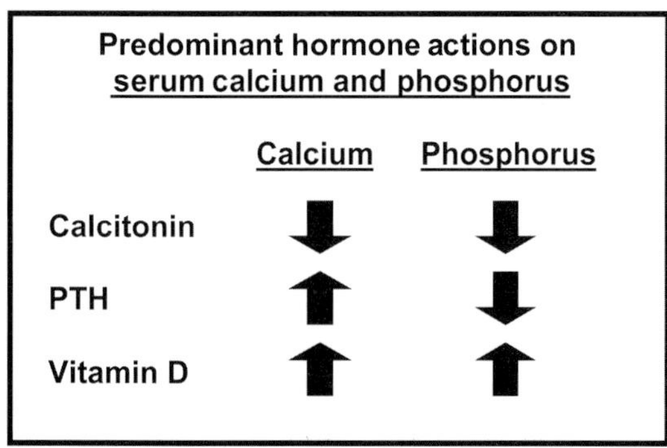

Figure 25.8 The effect of hormones on blood calcium and phosphorus concentrations.

calcium while decreasing phosphate reabsorption by the kidneys. Because of its potent phosphaturic action, the overall effect of PTH is to increase serum calcium and decrease serum phosphate concentrations (Figure 25.8).

Vitamin D comes from diet or is synthesized in the skin from sunlight exposure. In dogs and cats, diet is the only significant source. The dietary or synthesized form of vitamin D is inactive and must be metabolized in the liver and kidney for activation. Cholecalciferol is metabolized to calcidiol in the liver under fairly loose regulation. Renal metabolism of calcidiol is more tightly regulated and generates active calcitriol under the influence of PTH. The activation of calcitriol is influenced by serum calcium, phosphate, PTH, and calcitriol concentrations and the effects of calcium and calcitriol concentrations on PTH release. Vitamin D predominantly acts to increase the absorption of calcium and phosphate from the gastrointestinal tract. Its overall action is to increase both serum calcium and phosphate concentrations (Figure 25.8).

Calcium

Why is calcium measured? One reason is that alterations in blood calcium concentrations can result in severe clinical problems, including death. Another reason is that recognizing and pursuing the cause of calcium abnormalities often aids in diagnosing the underlying disease process.

When measuring serum concentrations of calcium, it is important to understand the difference between the measurement of total calcium (tCa) and free, ionized calcium (iCa). Free (unbound) iCa is the biologically active, hormonally regulated fraction that comprises approximately 50% of tCa. Measuring the concentration of iCa is necessary to confirm if abnormalities in tCa concentrations are significant or if calcitonin, PTH, and vitamin D concentrations are appropriate. Ionized calcium is not routinely included in serum chemistry panels because it is measured by an ion-selective electrode methodology that is not typically used in the large chemistry analyzers. Total calcium is what is routinely reported on a serum biochemical panel; it is measured via a colorimetric technique. The tCa measurement includes all calcium, whether bound or unbound. The bound fractions of tCa are those that are bound to protein (~40–45% of tCa) and complexed with nonprotein ions such as phosphates, citrate, lactate, etc. (5–10% of tCa). Changes in the amount of calcium bound to proteins or other ions will affect tCa but will not affect the concentration of iCa. Bound calcium is essentially removed from the biologically active pool of calcium. Therefore, as long as regulatory mechanisms are functioning properly, the iCa concentration typically remains within a narrow range, even if tCa concentrations decrease or increase because of changes in the amount of substances that bind calcium in the blood (Figure 25.9).

Ionized calcium is required for vital intracellular and extracellular functions, including muscle tone and contraction, nerve conduction, hormone secretion, enzymatic reactions, blood coagulation, and cell growth, division, and function. It is also required for skeletal support. Some of the more common sequelae to marked hypercalcemia include polyuria, constipation, acute renal failure, and cardiac arrhythmias. The majority of signs related to hypocalcemia are due to the importance of calcium in muscle function. Signs may include muscle fasciculations, tetany, seizures, paresis, tachycardia, hypotension, and respiratory arrest.

Box 25.7 An acronym to help remember the differentials for hypercalcemia

Acronym for most hypercalcemia differentials (tCa):

- **G** ranulomatous inflammation
- **O** steolytic lesions
- **S** purious results
- **H** yperparathyroidism (primary)
- **D** vitamin toxicity
- **A** ddison's disease
- **R** enal disease (chronic)
- **N** eoplasia
- **I** diopathic
- **T** ransient

Abnormalities in blood calcium concentration result from an imbalance in hormonal regulation, altered absorption from the gastrointestinal tract, pathologic excretion from the kidneys, or altered distribution involving bone or other tissues. This chapter will briefly cover differentials for calcium and phosphate abnormalities. For more in-depth discussion of regulation and pathophysiologic mechanisms, see Chapter 34.

Hypercalcemia

Hypercalcemia (Box 25.7), if ignored, can lead to serious consequences such as acute renal injury and failure. Therefore,

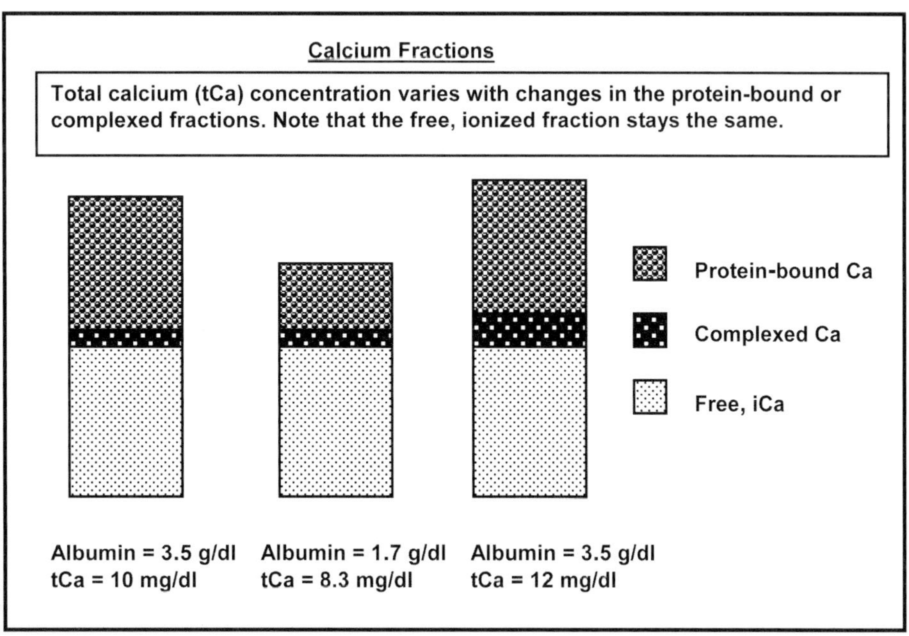

Figure 25.9 Ionized calcium, the biologically active fraction, normally stays within a very narrow range while total calcium concentration is affected by calcium that is bound or complexed and, therefore, inactive.

depending on the situation, if hypercalcemia is not immediately investigated, it is a good idea to at least determine persistence by rechecking or, ideally, to measure the iCa concentration when tCa is elevated. More routine measurement of iCa may be indicated when potential for a calcium disorder exists because concordance of tCa and iCa concentrations is poor; >60% of cats with elevated iCa had tCa concentration within reference intervals [18]. If the iCa concentration is normal, this suggests that abnormalities in tCa are due to changes in the amount of bound calcium and, therefore, an increase in the concentration of complexing or binding substances. If the iCa concentration is increased there is a problem with calcium regulation.

Hypercalcemia can occur due to an increase in PTH or PTH-like substances. High concentrations of calcium normally feed back to decrease PTH secretion. If PTH concentrations are higher than they should be in the face of hypercalcemia, the cells producing PTH are not responding to feedback signals, as occurs with parathyroid tumors. Primary hyperparathyroidism is most commonly associated with parathyroid adenomas; in this disease, the thyroid gland itself is inappropriately over-producing PTH. Along with increased iCa and PTH levels, hypophosphatemia is typically present, unless there is a concurrent decrease in GFR, with which normal or increased phosphate concentrations may be seen.

A substance that has similar actions to PTH is PTH-related protein (PTHrP). While this substance has normal functions, it becomes a problem when produced by neoplastic cells. One of the most common causes of hypercalcemia is neoplasia, and PTHrP is associated with many of these cases of humoral hypercalcemia of malignancy (also called pseudohyperparathyroidism). The more common neoplasms associated with humoral hypercalcemia of malignancy are lymphoid neoplasms (e.g., lymphoma) and apocrine gland adenocarcinoma of the anal sac, although many different tumors have been associated with hypercalcemia, including thymoma and various carcinomas. An assay to measure the concentration of PTHrP is available for dogs and cats. In cases of humoral hypercalcemia of malignancy, PTHrP is often increased, iCa concentrations are increased, and PTH is appropriately low. Phosphate levels are typically decreased, unless there is a concurrent decrease in GFR.

Vitamin D toxicity results in increased absorption of calcium from the gastrointestinal tract. Toxicity can occur with cholecalciferol rodenticide poisoning, ingestion of plants containing vitamin D glycosides (*Cestrum diurnum*, *Solanum malacoxylon*, and *Trisetum flavescens*), ingestion of calcipotriene, an analog of calcitriol found in a topical preparation used to treat psoriasis in people, or over-supplementation. Some granulomatous diseases as well as some neoplasms activate vitamin D precursors in an unregulated manner, resulting in hypercalcemia. Hypervitaminosis D results in increased iCa and phosphate and low PTH concentrations.

Renal disease can be associated with hypercalcemia but should only be attributed as the cause after other differentials are ruled out because hypercalcemia can induce renal failure.

Hypercalcemia is a common finding in chronic renal failure in horses, as the horse kidney plays a more important role in excreting excess calcium than in other species. In equine chronic renal failure, iCa is often high, phosphate low, and PTH appropriately low. Only approximately 10% of dogs with chronic renal failure are hypercalcemic; within this population, dogs with hereditary disease are more common. Hypercalcemia is also a common finding in dogs with grape or raisin-induced renal failure [19]. Hypercalcemia is more common in cats with chronic renal failure than in dogs. In cats and dogs, although tCa may be increased in chronic renal failure, iCa is usually normal or low, consistent with increased complexing of calcium, and PTH may be increased.

Hypoadrenocorticism (Addison's disease) is a common cause of hypercalcemia in dogs. Approximately 1/3 of dogs with hypoadrenocorticism are hypercalcemic. The mechanism of hypercalcemia is unclear and the concentration of iCa is variable [20, 21].

Because bone contains high amounts of calcium, osteolytic lesions occurring from inflammatory conditions or from metastatic neoplasia can result in hypercalcemia.

Idiopathic hypercalcemia is diagnosed if all other potential causes have been ruled out. This has become one of the most common causes of hypercalcemia in cats [18]. As the name implies, the underlying mechanism is unknown. Hypercalcemia is typically mild to moderate, with increased iCa, low to normal PTH, and normal vitamin D concentrations [22].

There can be nonpathological reasons for hypercalcemia. Mild, transient increases may occur postprandially. Dehydration concentrates proteins within the blood, which can result in mild increases in tCa concentration. Acidosis decreases calcium binding of serum proteins, which can result in increased iCa concentrations. Young, growing animals normally have higher calcium concentrations; consequently, if adult reference intervals are used, they will appear hypercalcemic when, in fact, their calcium concentrations are normal for their age. Depending on method of analysis, lipemia or marked hemolysis may interfere with the colorimetric measurement of tCa. If there is significant lipemia or hemolysis present in the sample, a new sample should be collected and measured or iCa determined.

Diagnostic tools for further working up the cause of a persistent hypercalcemia include laboratory techniques as well as other diagnostic modalities. If hypercalcemia was detected by measuring tCa, determining the iCa concentration is important in order to interpret the importance of the abnormality as well as helping differentiate between causes. A complete blood count (CBC), serum chemistry panel, and urinalysis are critical for the assessment of underlying disease processes. A thorough physical exam, including careful palpation of lymph nodes and the perianal area as well as radiographs and/or ultrasonography are valuable in the detection of masses or osteolyic lesions. Cytologic or histologic examination of mass lesions provides additional diagnostic information. It is possible to measure PTH and vitamin D concentrations as well as, in dogs and cats, PTHrP for assessment of hormonal status.

Hypocalcemia

It is uncommon for hypocalcemia (Box 25.8) to be severe enough to cause clinical signs, but mild hypocalcemia is often detected on a serum biochemistry panel when tCa is measured. The most common reason for hypocalcemia is a decrease in the protein-bound fraction when hypoalbuminemia is present. When this is the cause, the iCa concentration is normal. A simple correction factor is frequently used to correct for the decreased protein-bound fraction of calcium (3.5 − patient albumin + patient calcium = corrected calcium), but it must be kept in mind that this equation was determined only for dogs and is only a rough estimate that tends to underestimate the incidence of deficient iCa concentrations. While it serves as a reminder of the importance of albumin in tCa content, the use of the equation is no longer recommended since it does not accurately predict iCa concentrations [18]. It is more important to measure iCa in order to determine the significance of decreased tCa concentrations and if iCa is also low, especially in critically ill animals.

Primary hypoparathyroidism is an uncommon cause of hypocalcemia. It should be considered after other causes are ruled out. Iatrogenic hypoparathyroidism is more common and occurs if the parathyroid glands are mistakenly removed during thyroidectomy. With hypoparathyroidism, PTH is inappropriately low in the face of a low iCa concentration. Phosphate concentration is typically increased.

Dietary deficiency of calcium seldom leads to hypocalcemia because of the regulatory mechanisms in place to maintain normal blood calcium, but a severe decrease in absorption from the gastrointestinal tract caused by a malabsorption or maldigestion disease process or by cantharidiasis (blister beetle toxicity in horses) can result in hypocalcemia. Decreased absorption associated with vitamin D deficiency can also result in hypocalcemia along with hypophosphatemia.

Imbalances of other electrolytes can lead to hypocalcemia. Hypomagnesemia decreases PTH secretion and action, resulting in hypocalcemia. This is a common occurrence in bovine grass tetany but also occurs in other species. Hyperphosphatemia can also lead to hypocalcemia because high levels of phosphate decrease the activation of vitamin D and decrease the action of PTH on bone. This pattern of events is most commonly associated with renal disease (increased phosphate with decreased GFR) or nutritional imbalances (excess phosphate or low calcium:phosphate ratio) and is termed secondary hyperparathyroidism because PTH levels become increased secondarily to the persistent hypocalcemia.

During late pregnancy or lactation, the demand for calcium may be greater than the bearer's body can maintain. Puerperal hypocalcemia most commonly occurs a few weeks post-whelping in dogs and is rare in cats. Parturient paresis most commonly occurs within 3 days on either side of calving in cattle but can occur several weeks before or after parturition in sheep and goats. In horses, hypocalcemic tetany usually occurs 1–2 weeks after foaling (lactation tetany). Hypocalcemic tetany can also occur with increased calcium loss caused by excessive sweating in horses.

Transport tetany has occurred in cattle, small ruminants, and horses. Pregnancy or lactation can be a contributing factor, but the primary cause of the hypocalcemia is thought to be due to stress and decreased intake.

Altered distribution of calcium results in hypocalcemia when there is deposition of calcium in tissues as can occur with saponification of fat with pancreatitis or in massive tissue injury, including acute tumor lysis. Precipitation of calcium with oxalates occurs with ethylene glycol toxicity.

Although the mechanism is not completely understood, inflammatory mediators appear to influence calcium regulation. Hypocalcemia associated with sepsis and critical illness is well recognized in human medicine and has been reported in dogs with sepsis, [23–25] in cats with septic peritonitis [26], and with equine colic [27–30]. Total calcium concentrations and calcium concentrations corrected for albumin are not reliable indicators of iCa in these cases. Free, iCa

Box 25.8 An acronym to help remember the differentials for hypocalcemia

Acronym for most hypocalcemia differentials (tCa):

- **M** agnesium deficiency
- **I** njury to tissues (severe)
- **L** actation/pregnancy
- **D** vitamin deficiency
- **P** ancreatitis
- **R** enal disease
- **A** lbumin deficiency
- **I** ntake decreased (gastrointestinal)
- **S** epsis
- **E** thylene glycol toxicity

CHAPTER 25

should be measured in critically ill patients, especially if signs of hypocalcemia are evident.

Alkalosis promotes calcium binding to serum proteins and can cause a decrease in iCa concentrations.

Calcium chelators can result in decreased calcium measurements. Contamination of a sample with EDTA will result in a falsely low calcium value; magnesium is also low and potassium is typically increased.

Phosphorus

Phosphorus is required for energy metabolism, nucleic acid synthesis, and cell signaling. In the body, phosphorus is in the form of phosphate, a molecular anion that is in higher concentrations in ICF than ECF. It is an important buffer in blood and urine and an important component of bone and structural plasma membrane phospholipids and phosphoproteins. Abnormalities in serum phosphate concentrations can be due to abnormalities in hormonal balance, intestinal absorption, renal excretion, or tissue or cell distribution. Serum concentrations of phosphate may not reflect total body levels.

If there is a concurrent abnormality in serum calcium, pursuing and determining the cause of the calcium abnormality will often provide explanation for an abnormality in phosphate. Examining the pattern of change between calcium and phosphate can provide important clues.

Hyperphosphatemia

Hyperphosphatemia (Box 25.9) typically occurs when the phosphate load (from GI absorption, cellular release, or exogenous administration) exceeds excretion and tissue uptake. In most species, the primary route of phosphate excretion is via the kidneys, but in ruminants, it is via the gastrointestinal tract. The most common cause of hyperphosphatemia is decreased renal excretion associated with a decrease in GFR. Chronic renal failure is the most common cause of hyperphosphatemia in adult dogs and cats. In ruminants, upper GI obstruction can lead to hyperphosphatemia because of decreased gastrointestinal excretion.

Phosphate enters the body via the gastrointestinal tract, dependent on diet and hormonal regulation. The amount of phosphate absorbed in the small intestine is linearly related to its concentration in the intestinal lumen. Therefore, an excess phosphate load from high phosphate diets or ingestion of nondietary substances containing high concentrations of phosphate, such as ethylene glycol that contains phosphate rust inhibitors, will increase intestinal absorption. Hypervitaminosis D increases the amount of phosphate absorbed from the gastrointestinal tract, leading to hyperphosphatemia and hypercalcemia. Phosphate enemas can also lead to severe hyperphosphatemia.

Given that the majority of total body phosphate is stored in bone and that the concentration of intracellular phosphate is more than 10 times that of ECF, the redistribution of phosphate from bone or from the intracellular space can

Box 25.9 An outline for working through the differentials for hypophosphatemia and hyperphosphatemia

Working through phosphorus abnormalities

1. What is the serum calcium concentration?

- Is there a pattern consistent with hormonal imbalance?

Hypophosphatemia	Hyperphosphatemia
Hypercalcemia • Primary hyperparathyroidism? • Hypercalcemia of malignancy? Hypocalcemia • Vitamin D deficiency?	Hypercalcemia • Vitamin D toxicosis? Hypocalcemia • Hypoparathyroidism?

2. What do renal parameters look like?

- Is there evidence for decreased excretion or resorption?

Hypophosphatemia	Hyperphosphatemia
Prolonged diuresis? • Treatments? • Hyperglycemia? • Polyuria? • Dilute urine? Possible tubular defects? • Glucosuria? Horse with hypercalcemia and azotemia?	Is there evidence for decreased GFR?? • Elevated serum BUN and creatinine? **Most common cause of hyperphosphatemia.**

3. Is there any evidence of dietary or gastrointestinal problems?

Hypophosphatemia	Hyperphosphatemia
Prolonged anorexia? Diarrhea? Vomiting? Low phosphorus diet?	High phosphorous diet? Phosphate enema use? Ingestion of ethylene glycol with phosphate rust inhibitors? Ruminant with upper GI obstruction?

4. Could there be redistribution; a shift between the ICF and ECF?

Hypophosphatemia	Hyperphosphatemia
Insulin therapy? Carbohydrate loading? Alkalosis?	Evidence of extensive tissue damage? Presence of osteolytic bone lesion? Acidosis?

result in hyperphosphatemia. Release from bone can occur with osteolytic lesions. Release from cells occurs with injury, which must be extensive in order to significantly affect the serum concentration of phosphate; this can occur with acute tumor lysis or acute myopathies. Acidosis decreases the cellular uptake of phosphate and can contribute to hyperphosphatemia.

Improper sample handling may cause falsely increased serum phosphate concentrations. This includes hemolysis of the sample or a delay in the removal of serum from erythrocytes after collection. Mild, transient increases in serum phosphate concentration may occur postprandially. Young, growing animals have higher concentrations of serum phosphate; consequently, if adult reference intervals are used, they will appear hyperphosphatemic when, in fact, their phosphate concentrations are normal for their age.

Hypophosphatemia

Hypophosphatemia (Box 25.9) occurs from hormonal imbalances, decreased renal reabsorption, decreased intestinal absorption, or redistribution from ECF to ICF. Hormonal imbalances typically include concurrent calcium abnormalities, the pattern of which can aid diagnosis. A low phosphate with increased calcium concentration is the pattern seen with pseudo- or primary hyperparathyroidism. A decrease in both phosphate and calcium is the pattern seen with hypovitaminosis D. Hypophosphatemia can also occur due to elevated PTH in response to periparturient hypocalcemia (physiologic hyperparathyroidism).

Decreased renal phosphate reabsorption (increased phosphate excretion) leads to hypophosphatemia. This can occur because of congenital or acquired defects in the proximal tubules where the majority of reabsorption normally occurs, often called Fanconi's syndrome. Diuresis results in decreased renal phosphate reabsorption, which, when prolonged, can lead to hypophosphatemia. Diabetic ketoacidosis leads to hypophosphatemia because of osmotic diuresis, as well as phosphate's role as a buffer for excreted acid. Although the mechanism is poorly understood, hypophosphatemia is often seen with the hypercalcemia associated with chronic renal failure in horses. Increased phosphate excretion is also the mechanism of hypophosphatemia associated with hyperparathyroidism as PTH decreases reabsorption of phosphate in proximal renal tubules.

Decreased intestinal absorption of phosphate is an uncommon cause of hypophosphatemia as the body typically can maintain normal blood levels even with decreased intake, although anorexia or a low phosphate diet, if prolonged, may lead to hypophosphatemia. Impaired absorption because of vomiting, diarrhea, or an intestinal malabsorption disease can also lead to hypophosphatemia. Decreased intestinal absorption is the mechanism of hypophosphatemia with hypovitaminosis D.

Redistribution of phosphate from ECF to ICF can result in hypophosphatemia. Insulin causes phosphate to move into cells. Hypophosphatemia can occur with administration of insulin or with insulin-producing tumors. It can also occur with carbohydrate loading or intravenously administered glucose, which induces the secretion of insulin. Respiratory alkalosis has been associated with hypophosphatemia because phosphate shifts to the intracellular space when CO_2 moves out of the cell. Because phosphate is required for energy metabolism, accelerated metabolism, in general, will result in intracellular shifts of phosphate, decreasing extracellular concentrations.

Magnesium

Magnesium is primarily an intracellular ion and is a cofactor of many enzymatic reactions, including all reactions involving the formation and utilization of ATP and many mitochondrial reactions. It is also required for protein and nucleic acid synthesis. Vitamin D and PTH influence, but do not regulate, magnesium metabolism [31]. Homeostasis is primarily a balance between intestinal absorption and renal excretion. Magnesium has a similar charge as calcium and, as does calcium, exists in free ionized, protein-bound (approximately 30%), and complexed forms in serum. Serum magnesium contains only approximately 1% of total body magnesium and therefore is not necessarily an accurate representation of total body magnesium.

Hypomagnesemia

Hypomagnesemia is more commonly associated with morbidity than hypermagnesemia. Neuromuscular signs occur with hypomagnesemia, including hyperexcitability, muscle tremors, spasms, and fasciculations, and ataxia. Other complications associated with hypomagnesemia include the development of hypokalemia or hypocalcemia. These deficiencies may not be able to be corrected unless hypomagnesemia is corrected first.

Hypomagnesemia is typically associated with either increased loss or decreased intake. Losses, the most common cause of hypomagnesemia in small animals, are through the renal or gastrointestinal systems. Renal loss occurs due to lack of renal conservation of magnesium, typically associated with diuresis or tubular dysfunction. Causes of urinary magnesium loss include: diuretics, osmotic diuresis, diabetic ketoacidosis, postobstructive diuresis, polyuric renal failure, RTA, hyperthyroidism, hypercalcemia, and nephrotoxic drugs [32]. Malabsorption and diarrhea are causes of gastrointestinal magnesium loss.

Decreased intake is a common cause of hypomagnesemia in ruminants. Grass tetany is a disease that is associated with ruminants eating lush green pastures that are high in potassium and low in magnesium content. Increased potassium ingestion blocks normal magnesium absorption in the rumen. Milk tetany is a disease that is associated with older calves being fed milk-only diets. Prolonged anorexia or poor diet can lead to hypomagnesemia, especially if an animal is lactating. Prolonged intravenous fluids or parenteral nutrition can also lead to hypomagnesemia if magnesium supplementation is not included.

Other causes of hypomagnesemia include redistribution and hypoalbuminemia (if total magnesium is measured instead of free, ionized magnesium). Redistribution of magnesium is not well understood but may be influenced by administration of insulin or glucose, sepsis, trauma, or pancreatitis.

Hypermagnesemia

Hypermagnesemia is typically a less significant clinical problem, unless it develops acutely. It can result in cardiac or neurological problems and cause nausea and vomiting.

Hypermagnesemia can occur iatrogenically or due to decreased renal excretion, primarily associated with acute renal failure or urethral obstruction.

26 Laboratory Evaluation of Acid-Base Disorders

Glade Weiser
Loveland, CO, USA

Introduction

Acid-base analysis, also known as blood-gas analysis, has been a growing point-of-care diagnostic application established for complicated medical cases and in critical care settings. Assessment of acid-base status is typically done in conjunction with electrolyte evaluation to determine the presence and severity of fluid and electrolyte derangement attributable to the animal's underlying disease process. Advances in technology have made acid-base evaluation possible and even routine within the in-clinic laboratory. These determinations allow for correction of such clinical abnormalities, which in turn aids recovery time and may improve mortality outcome.

Blood-gas analysis has historically been regarded as complex and intimidating for many clinicians. This is likely because measurement and interpretation of partial pressures of gases in blood solution are less conceptually intuitive than concentration measurements dealt with in hematology and conventional clinical chemistry. The subject also is complicated by many derivative specialty calculations that may appear on laboratory reports. Sample transportation to a central laboratory, perceived complex sample handling, and a perception that blood-gas analysis necessitates arterial blood collection are factors that have contributed to adoption reluctance. However, the clinician is encouraged to embrace this capability made possible by the availability of simplified point-of-care analysis systems that eliminate most of these barriers.

Recommendations to facilitate use include the following. It may help to think of blood-gas analysis more simply as analysis of acid-base balance. This approach may be more intuitive. Today's point-of-care electrochemical analyzers make capability to evaluate acid-base status routine. Incorporation of this capability into the practice routine provides the use frequency needed to build and maintain interpretive skills. Users should focus on a few key values and not be overwhelmed by the various possible derivative calculations that may appear on laboratory reports. Most of the calculations may be ignored while initial interpretive skill is acquired. Users may then adopt a few selected calculations as skill is accumulated.

The purposes of this chapter are to present a background of the technical aspects of acid-base analysis and an introductory approach to interpretation of basic acid-base laboratory data. The introductory approach is designed to help the reader recognize and interpret basic, common acid-base abnormalities; there is no intention to discuss advanced concepts used by various specialties. The latter is left to literature and advanced training that exists for specialty applications.

Technical considerations

Measurement of acid-base parameters

Acid-base laboratory data are generated on electrochemical analyzers (Chapter 1). These typically use the same sample to simultaneously determine both electrolyte and acid-base determinations. Venous blood collection is adequate for evaluation of the metabolic complications of disease that result in acid-base and electrolyte disturbances. Arterial blood is typically only required when it is necessary to critically evaluate blood oxygenation.

While a number of parameters may appear on an acid-base report, there are very few direct measurements and calculations that are important for interpretation of acid-base balance. A systematic focus on this small number of parameters will simplify interpretation. These include the following.

pH

The primary measurement of blood acidity is pH. It is directly measured by an ion specific electrode (see Chapter 1). pH is the negative log of hydrogen ion concentration. Therefore, a decrease in pH value indicates an increase in free hydrogen ion concentration (relatively acidic) and an increase in

Veterinary Hematology, Clinical Chemistry, and Cytology, Third Edition. Edited by Mary Anna Thrall, Glade Weiser, Robin W. Allison and Terry W. Campbell.

Companion website: www.wiley.com/go/thrall/veterinary

pH indicates a decrease in free hydrogen ion concentration (relatively alkaline). pH is very tightly regulated in the body by a number of buffering systems.

PCO_2

The partial pressure of carbon dioxide (CO_2) gas dissolved in blood, measured in mm of mercury (mmHg). This may be measured in either venous or arterial blood.

HCO_3 or bicarbonate concentration

Using the pH and pCO_2 values, bicarbonate concentration is calculated by the instrumentation software. It is expressed in mmol/L. The pH and bicarbonate values are the most useful for interpretation of acid-base disturbances when venous blood is the sample.

PO_2

The partial pressure of oxygen (O_2) gas dissolved in blood, measured in mm of mercury (mmHg). This measurement is typically only useful for analysis of blood oxygenation and therefore is only of interpretive value when arterial blood is sampled specifically to evaluate the patient for oxygenation pathology.

Other calculated values

There are a number of possible calculated indices. The presentation of these on reports varies by the manufacturer. Their use is somewhat optional, and most are typically adopted by critical care specialists. Some relate to arterial human applications that are rarely used in animals.

Sample handling requirements

Proper sample handling instructions are available and are simplified by the capability provided by point-of-care analysis. pH may be affected by changes in pCO_2. Both CO_2 and O_2 may move toward ambient equilibrium in blood removed from the body if not properly handled. The following are proper sample handling guidelines for electrochemical analyses that should be supplemented by instructions accompanying point-of-care analyzers:

- Avoid manual heparinization of syringes. This can cause gross over-heparinization of the sample, leading to errors in any of the acid-base and electrolyte results.
- It is recommended to use a balanced heparin-containing syringe produced specifically for electrochemical analysis samples (see Chapter 2).
- Any gas bubbles in the collection syringe should be expelled.
- Unless the sample is introduced for analysis immediately after collection, the syringe should be capped to prevent sample contact with air. Recommended collection devices have a cap for this purpose.

Physiologic considerations

Regulation of blood pH

It is critical for most physiologic functions that acid-base balance be maintained within a narrow range of pH, typically 7.35–7.45, with some minor species variations indicated in reference interval tables. A number of pathologic conditions may add or subtract acid in blood and body fluids. The blood contains considerable buffering capacity to aid regulation of blood pH. Major buffers include hemoglobin and the bicarbonate buffer systems. Minor contributory buffers include inorganic phosphate and plasma proteins. Through equilibrium reactions, these molecules may incorporate or release hydrogen ions in the effort to maintain pH. The bicarbonate buffer system is important because of its rapid buffering capacity and because its components are readily measured for assessment blood pH and associated therapeutic monitoring. In addition, the bicarbonate system interacts with the mass quantity of hemoglobin in both pH regulation and gas exchange between tissues and respiration. The equilibria within the bicarbonate buffer system are shown in Figure 26.1.

The relationship of the bicarbonate buffer system to pH is described as:

$$pH = pK + \log \frac{[HCO_3^-]}{[H_2CO_3]}$$

where pK is the pH at which 50% of an acid is dissociated; this is ~6.1 for carbonic acid.

Because pCO_2 can be measured and the dissolved CO_2 in blood is proportional to the carbonic acid concentration, this relationship may be simplified to:

$$\text{Blood pH} = 6.1 + \log \frac{[HCO_3^-]}{\alpha pCO_2}$$

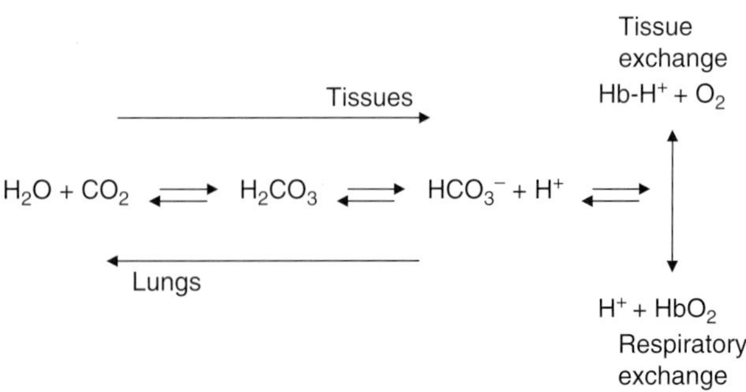

Figure 26.1 Bicarbonate buffer system interactions. At the lung level, hemoglobin binds oxygen; this creates a molecular change that favors dissociation of H^+ from hemoglobin. This will push the equilibrium to the left, yielding CO_2 and water that is expired. At the tissue level, metabolism yields CO_2 and considerable acid. Hemoglobin releases O_2 to tissues and deoxygenated hemoglobin then binds H^+. Thus, equilibrium is driven to the right.

where α pCO_2 is pCO_2 multiplied by its solubility constant to yield the amount of CO_2 gas dissolved in blood. Using the solubility constant, the above formula may be rearranged to:

$$\text{Blood pH} = 6.1 + \log \frac{[HCO_3^-]}{0.03 \times pCO_2}$$

Normally, the ratio of bicarbonate to CO_2 is 20 : 1. At this ratio, the log of 20 plus 6.1 yields the desired blood pH of 7.4. For interpretation purposes it is helpful to think of bicarbonate as being the metabolic component of blood pH regulation and pCO_2 as being the respiratory component of blood pH regulation. For example, if bicarbonate is utilized to buffer an increase in metabolic acid (H^+), a decrease in bicarbonate in the above equation results in a decrease in pH, or acidosis. In response, respiration may increase CO_2 expiration to partially normalize the ratio and is known as compensation. The compensation response attempts to normalize the ratio, which in turn helps normalize or regulate pH. This framework of metabolic and respiratory components in the above equation will be very helpful for identifying and interpreting acid-base abnormalities.

Acid-base balance pathology

General processes that may result in life-threatening abnormalities in acid-base balance are classified in the following four primary categories. Common disease entities that may result in these categories are outlined in Table 26.1. Metabolic acid-base disturbances develop relatively slowly, usually over a period of days, whereas respiratory acid-base disturbances may develop very acutely.

Bicarbonate (HCO_3^-) depletion – metabolic acidosis

This is due to pathologic metabolic production of acid in the form of hydrogen ions. The increased hydrogen ions are buffered by combining with bicarbonate to form carbonic acid that then dissociates to CO_2 gas and water. The CO_2 is then rapidly eliminated from the system via respiration. Common examples of pathologic metabolism resulting in metabolic acidosis include lactic acidosis, ketoacidosis, renal failure, and acid toxicities (e.g., ethylene glycol toxicity). Alternatively, bicarbonate may be lost from the system such as may occur with severe diarrhea. By any of these mechanisms, depletion of bicarbonate establishes metabolic acidosis.

Metabolic acidosis is the most common acid-base disturbance. This is attributed to the fact that dehydration and poor tissue perfusion leading to lactic acid production is a process common to many primary internal medical disorders. Renal failure and diabetes mellitus, relatively common disorders in veterinary patients, also contribute to the incidence of metabolic acidosis.

CO_2 retention due to hypoventilation – respiratory acidosis

This is due to acute respiratory failure with accumulation of CO_2. Causes include hypoventilation during anesthesia or any pathologic cause of acute spontaneous hypoventilation or severe impairment of gas exchange at the blood – lung interface.

Bicarbonate excess – metabolic alkalosis

This is due to metabolic production and accumulation of excess bicarbonate. Gastric parietal cells produce hydrogen

CHAPTER 26

Table 26.1 Acid-base disturbances resulting in abnormal blood pH.

Acid-base disturbance	Metabolic acidosis decreased pH	Metabolic alkalosis increased pH	Respiratory acidosis decreased pH	Respiratory alkalosis increased pH
Primary bicarbonate buffer alteration	Decreased bicarbonate	Increased bicarbonate	Increased CO_2	Decreased CO_2
Causes	Any cause of generalized poor perfusion leading to lactate production	Loss of acid due to vomiting or functional upper gastrointestinal obstruction	Any cause of respiratory failure, e.g.:	Pulmonary pathology resulting in impaired O_2 alveolar diffusion
	Diabetic ketoacidosis Lactic acidosis	Excess bicarbonate therapy	Severe pneumonia Pneumothorax Severe pleural fluid	Excess positive pressure ventilation during anesthesia
	Renal failure Ethylene glycol toxicity	Excess diuretic therapy	Airway obstruction Hypoventilation due to anesthetic overdose	
	Diarrhea			

For each disturbance category, the major abnormality in the bicarbonate buffer system is indicated. Also, common causes or processes that may cause a given disturbance are listed.

ions by combining CO_2 and water to form carbonic acid, which then dissociates to H^+ and bicarbonate. Bicarbonate is exchanged to the plasma for chloride ions. H^+ and Cl^- are then excreted into the gastric lumen as part of the gastric acid (H^+Cl^-) digestive response. The most common cause of metabolic alkalosis is upper gastrointestinal obstruction. The hydrogen ions are secreted into the stomach and are lost in the obstructive process, while bicarbonate is retained.

CO_2 loss due to hyperventilation – respiratory alkalosis

This may occur when there is hypoxemia that stimulates hyperventilation, as seen with some forms of pneumonia. With inflammatory or fluid pneumonia, the gas diffusion barrier is increased. Oxygen diffuses more slowly than CO_2 across such barriers. Increased ventilation due to poor oxygenation can result in loss of CO_2 since it diffuses more freely across the barrier. More severe pneumonia that impairs even CO_2 diffusion is more likely to lead to respiratory acidosis as a result of CO_2 retention. Excess positive pressure ventilation during anesthesia may also cause respiratory alkalosis.

Relationship of acid-base pathology to anion gap

The anion gap is discussed in Chapter 25. The anion gap is useful in classifying metabolic acidosis into one of two categories, which may help determine the cause of the acid-base disturbance. The most common pathway to metabolic acidosis is accumulation of acid due to either production of organic acid or the presence of an acid toxicity. The accumulation of a dissociable acid yields H^+ and the respective anion. As the H^+ is buffered by bicarbonate, the bicarbonate concentration decreases. The anion is unmeasured in calculation of anion gap and its accumulation results in the increased anion gap. Representative unmeasured anions associated with metabolic acidosis disorders are listed in Table 26.2.

The alternative cause of metabolic acidosis is due to a primary process of bicarbonate loss. This may be due to severe diarrhea or, less commonly, renal tubular acidosis in which there is pathologic renal loss of bicarbonate. In this situation, the anion gap will be normal because there is no accumulation of unmeasured anions. Increased serum chloride may develop with this type of acidosis. The kidneys will continue to reabsorb the vast majority of filtered sodium. Because active renal sodium reabsorption requires either bicarbonate or chloride as a counterion, more chloride may be retrieved when there is relatively severe deficit of bicarbonate. As a result, hyperchloremia may develop.

Table 26.2 Causes of metabolic acidosis with increased anion gap, with associated pathologic acids.

Disease with unmeasured anions	Pathologic acid(s)
Diabetes, unregulated	Ketoacids: acetoacetate, beta-hydroxybuterate
Renal failure	Sulfates, phosphates, and lactate when dehydrated
Hypoxemia and/or poor perfusion	Lactic acid
Acid toxicity, e.g., ethylene glycol toxicity	Metabolism to form oxalic and glycolic acids

Approach to interpretation of acid-base data

Evaluation of acid-base status begins with analysis of blood pH, bicarbonate concentration, and the partial pressure of carbon dioxide. It is desirable to develop a stepwise approach to interpretation of the acid-base data. A recommended stepwise approach is described below and diagrammed in Figure 26.2.

Step 1 – Evaluate pH. The pH is abnormal if either decreased or increased beyond the reference interval limits. If the pH is decreased, the animal by definition has acidemia. This is due to some process that is causing acidosis or accumulation of acid in the system. If the pH is increased, the animal by definition has alkalemia. This is due to some process that is causing alkalosis or accumulation of base in the system.

If the pH is within the reference interval, a major acid-base disturbance is unlikely. However, there is still merit in checking the bicarbonate buffer pair for abnormality. If the pH is near the lower or upper limit it should still be evaluated as a possible indicator of acidosis or alkalosis. Borderline pH values may be an indication that a process causing acidosis or alkalosis is present, but there has been compensation in an attempt to normalize the pH. Alternatively, a mixed acid-base disturbance may be due to severe disease but result in a relatively normal pH value. A mixed acid-base disturbance is due to two or more processes affecting acid and/or base addition to the system.

Because of the relationship between pH and HCO_3^- and pCO_2 described above, the bicarbonate buffer system should next be evaluated to determine the cause of the acid-base disturbance defined by the pH. This involves a determination of whether the metabolic component (HCO_3^-) or respiratory component (pCO_2) of the buffer system is responsible for the primary acid-base disturbance.

Step 2 – Evaluate bicarbonate (HCO_3^-) concentration. Interpret if the HCO_3^- value is below the reference interval limit, indicating increased metabolic acid (acidosis), or above the reference interval limit, indicating increased metabolic base (alkalosis).

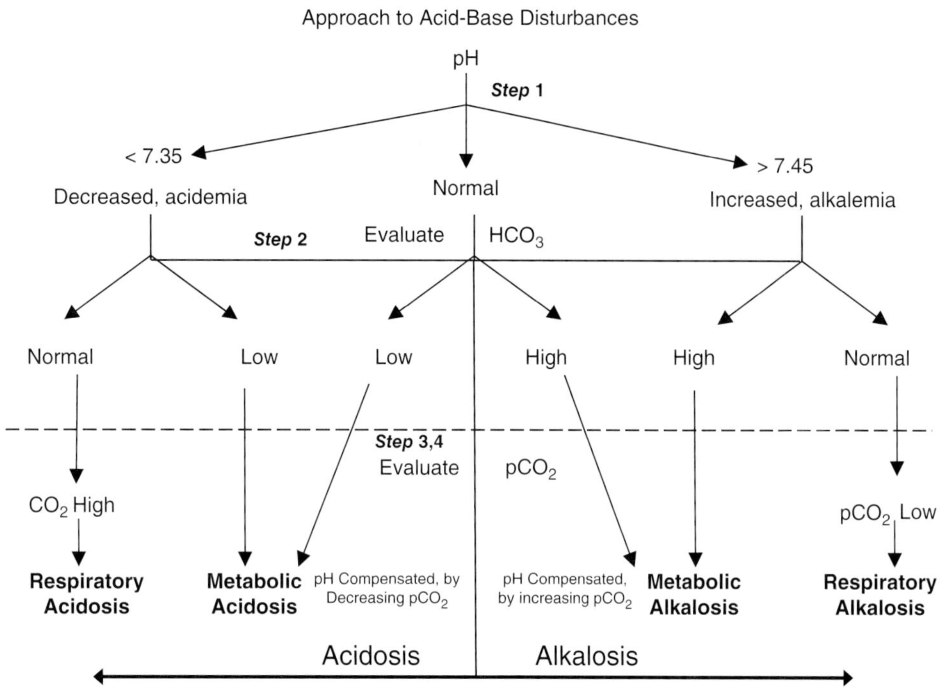

Approach to Acid-Base Disturbances

pH
Step 1
< 7.35 Decreased, acidemia | Normal | > 7.45 Increased, alkalemia
Step 2 Evaluate HCO_3
Normal | Low | Low | High | High | Normal
Step 3,4 Evaluate pCO_2
CO_2 High → Respiratory Acidosis
Low → Metabolic Acidosis
Low → pH Compensated, by Decreasing pCO_2 → Metabolic Acidosis
High → pH Compensated, by increasing pCO_2 → Metabolic Alkalosis
High → Metabolic Alkalosis
Normal → pCO_2 Low → Respiratory Alkalosis
Acidosis ← → Alkalosis

Figure 26.2 Stepwise approach to interpretation of acid-base disturbances. See text for narrative discussion.

Note that some references may suggest evaluation of pCO_2 first. However, because most acid-base disturbances identified in animals are due to metabolic disorders, evaluation of HCO_3^- first usually will readily define the acid-base disturbance.

Step 3 – Evaluate the pCO_2. If the pCO_2 value is normal, the acid-base disturbance is defined by the bicarbonate concentration abnormality. Interpret if the pCO_2 value is above the reference interval limit, indicating increased respiratory acid (acidosis), or below the reference interval limit, indicating increased respiratory base (alkalosis).

Step 4 – If needed, evaluate any combined abnormalities between HCO_3^- and pCO_2. If both the HCO_3^- and pCO_2 values are abnormal, the primary acid-base base disturbance is almost always due to the most abnormal value in the pair. The change in the least abnormal value is almost always due to a compensation response in an attempt to normalize the pH. In addition, the compensating value is either abnormal or moving toward abnormal in a direction *opposite* what would be required to cause the pH abnormality. This step may also aid in identification of acid-base disturbances due to more than one process, known as a mixed acid-base disturbance.

This approach may be illustrated in the following example of a common patient acid-base data, with comparison reference intervals (RI):

pH 7.21 RI = 7.35–7.45

decreased—indicates a primary acid disorder (acidemia)

HCO_3^- 12 mmol/L RI = 15–23 mmol/L

decreased—indicates acid response,

metabolic component of buffer system

pCO_2 30 mmHg RI = 35–40 mm Hg

decreased—indicates base response,

respiratory component of buffer system

Both determinants of the bicarbonate buffer system are abnormally decreased. The determinant abnormality that adds acid or base consistent with the pH change is the primary cause of the acid base disturbance. In this example, a decrease in HCO_3^- is interpreted as an addition of acid. The decrease in pCO_2 cannot explain the pH because this change would add base to the system, increasing the pH. Therefore, the concluding interpretation is metabolic acidosis with some respiratory compensation. The decrease in pCO_2 is a compensation response. Increased respiratory elimination of CO_2 tends to compensate to normalize the pH to some degree. Some will find it useful to utilize the formula of this relationship when making these interpretations:

$$\text{Blood pH} = 6.1 + \log \frac{[HCO_3^-]}{0.03 \times pCO_2}$$

Looking at this equation, it is apparent that either a decrease in HCO_3^- or an increase in pCO_2 would be required to decrease blood pH.

Table 26.3 Expected values for pH, HCO_3, and pCO_2 in various acid-base disturbances, including expected compensation responses.

Disturbance	pH	HCO_3	pCO_2
Metabolic acidosis	Dec	Dec	N
Metabolic acidosis, compensating	Dec or low N	Dec	Dec or low N
Metabolic alkalosis	Inc	Inc	N
Metabolic alkalosis, compensating	Inc or high N	Inc	Inc or high N
Respiratory acidosis	Dec	N	Inc
Respiratory acidosis, compensating	Dec	Inc or high N	Inc
Respiratory alkalosis	Inc	N	Dec
Respiratory alkalosis, compensating	Inc or high N	Dec or high N	Dec

N, normal value, within reference interval; Dec, decreased; Inc, increased.
Note that acute respiratory acidosis may not effectively compensate.

Compensation is a normal, active physiologic action to attempt pH correction in response to the primary acid-base disturbance. Unless the acid-base disturbance is very acute, a compensation response is expected. Typically, respiratory compensation for metabolic disorders occurs faster than metabolic compensation for respiratory disorders. Table 26.3 shows abnormalities in the bicarbonate buffer system for various acid-base disturbances and the expected respective compensation responses. It is important to note that compensation will move the pH toward normal but may at best only partially normalize the pH. For certain, mechanisms involved in compensation will not overcompensate pH normalization. This perspective is helpful for recognizing the presence of mixed acid-base disturbances.

More advanced considerations

Mixed acid-base disturbances

As mentioned above, a mixed acid-base disturbance is composed of two or more pathologic processes that affect pH. The pH value will reflect a balance of the contributing processes. An example of a mixed acid-base disturbance might be recognized in a dog with severe pancreatitis. In this situation, there may be dehydration with poor tissue perfusion and prerenal azotemia. These processes lead to metabolic acidosis. If there is also protracted or disproportionate vomiting, there is a superimposed process of metabolic alkalosis as a result of loss of gastric H^+Cl^-. The latter process may be suspected if there is a disproportionately decreased serum chloride concentration.

Recognition of a mixed acid-base disturbance should start with suspecting it based on diagnosis of the existing clinical problem or problems. Some example clinical scenarios that may result in mixed acid-base disorders include

- Hypoadrenocorticism with disproportionate vomiting – metabolic acidosis and alkalosis.
- Protracted vomiting and aspiration pneumonia – metabolic alkalosis and respiratory acidosis.
- Heart failure with severe pulmonary edema – metabolic and respiratory acidosis.
- Renal failure with disproportionate vomiting – metabolic acidosis and alkalosis.
- Gastric dilatation/volvulus – variable, depending on manifestations.
- Anesthesia in excess, with preexisting disorder – variable, depending on disorder.

The acid-base data may aid in confirming the presence of a mixed disturbance. Using the clinical findings and the most likely primary acid-base data abnormality, identify the primary acid-base disturbance. Then, predict the expected compensation response to the primary disturbance. Guidelines for magnitude of compensation changes in Table 26.4 may aid this determination. If the expected compensation response is either not present, excessive, or in the opposite direction of what is expected, then a second primary disturbance should be suspected, indicating a mixed acid-base disturbance. These guidelines should be used with considerable latitude and only large deviation from the expectation should be interpreted as inappropriate. By way of example, consider the following case data.

pH 6.99 RI = 7.35 – 7.45

severely decreased—indicates a primary acid disorder (acidemia)

HCO_3^- 12 mmol/L RI = 15 – 23 mmol/L

decreased—indicates acid response, metabolic component of buffer system

pCO_2 50 mm Hg RI = 35 – 40 mm Hg

increased—indicates acid response, respiratory component of buffer system

At first glance, this may appear confusing if one is suspecting a single primary disturbance. If it is initially assumed that metabolic acidosis is the primary abnormality, one would expect a compensatory decrease in pCO_2 of about 2 mmHg below the lower RI limit, or ~33 mmHg (Table 26.4). However, the pCO_2 result is grossly different from the

Table 26.4 Guidelines for expected magnitude of compensation of primary acid-base disturbances.

Acid-base disturbance	Metabolic acidosis decreased pH	Metabolic alkalosis increased pH	Respiratory acidosis decreased pH	Respiratory alkalosis increased pH
Primary bicarbonate buffer alteration	Decreased bicarbonate	Increased bicarbonate	Increased CO_2	Decreased CO_2
Expected compensation	Decrease pCO_2 by respiration change	Increase pCO_2 by respiration change	Increase HCO_3^- by metabolism	Decrease HCO_3^- by metabolism
Expected magnitude of compensation	0.7 mmHg per 1.0 $mmol/L^{-1}$ decrease in HCO_3^-	0.7 mmHg per 1.0 $mmol/L^{-1}$ increase in HCO_3^-	Acute: 1.5 mmol/L HCO_3^- per 10 mmHg increase in pCO_2 Chronic: may approximately double	Acute: 2.5 mmol/L HCO_3^- per 10 mmHg decrease in pCO_2 Chronic: may approximately double

For each acid-base disturbance, the table shows the associated primary alteration, action for compensation, and expected magnitude of change in the compensation response.

compensation expectation. If it is initially assumed that respiratory acidosis is the primary abnormality, one would expect an increase in HCO_3^- of about 1.5–3.0 mmol/L, or ~ 25 mmol/L. Again, the result is grossly different than the compensation expectation. This should prompt consideration of a mixed acid-base disturbance. In this case there are two acid responses consisting of both respiratory acidosis and metabolic acidosis. The two primary acid-base disturbances are recognized as a mixed disturbance. Therefore, both the pulmonary function and potential causes of metabolic acidosis should be investigated (Table 26.1).

Arterial blood oxygenation

A conventional blood-gas analyzer measures pO_2 along with other values discussed above. It then calculates or predicts the percent hemoglobin saturation with oxygen (SO_2) based on the expected behavior of hemoglobin affinity at a given pH, body temperature, and pO_2. The relationship between percentage saturation and these variables is characterized by the hemoglobin-oxygen dissociation curve. These values are present on all blood-gas analyzer reports but are typically only useful for arterial samples performed specifically to evaluate oxygenation. As an initial alternative to arterial sampling, a simpler approach is to use a pulse oximeter to measure hemoglobin percentage saturation as a screening measurement to rule out oxygenation defects.

When breathing ambient air and blood oxygenation is normal, the animal will have an arterial pO_2 in the range of 85–100 mmHg. At this level, the SO_2 is typically 95% or higher. Generally, a large pathologic change in pO_2, e.g., <60–70 mmHg, is required to result in clinically important changes in SO_2. The calculation of percentage saturation is reasonably accurate when hemoglobin is normal. However, it is not accurate in the presence of the toxicities such as methemoglobinemia and carboxyhemoglobinemia (below) and in some hemoglobin abnormalities present only in humans.

Base excess calculation

The base excess (BE) value is typically included on the acid-base data report. This value is calculated to account for the combined bicarbonate and hemoglobin buffering capacity of blood. This is a complex calculation that utilizes information from a nomogram built on the relationship between pH, pCO_2, and HCO_3^- in blood. This relationship is similar for human and dog but may vary with other species. Instrument software typically uses the human calculation to derive BE. The normal range of BE is slight positive and negative deviation around zero. A positive abnormal value indicates an excess of base, or alkalosis. A negative value indicates the magnitude of HCO_3^- deficit in mmol/L in metabolic acidosis. The amount of deficit may be useful in planning fluid and bicarbonate therapy in treatment of metabolic acidosis in conjunction with hydration.

The BE utility is for calculation of the amount of bicarbonate replacement in fluid therapy formulae. These calculations result in the target amount of bicarbonate that would be administered with fluids to normalize the bicarbonate concentration and pH. The calculation is based on body weight and the goal to deliver bicarbonate to the extracellular fluid space, which is approximately 30% of body weight. A representative formula using the absolute value of BE is:

$$\begin{array}{l}\text{Bicarbonate}\\ \text{dosage (mmol)}\end{array} = 0.3 \times \text{Body weight (kg)} \times \text{BE (mmol/L)}$$

One may encounter variations of the above formula, but the general principle is unchanged. The user must realize that bicarbonate replacement in acidosis is a moving target. The administration of bicarbonate is initially distributed to the extracellular fluid space, but there is movement intracellularly over time. Furthermore, the process(es) causing acid-base disturbance may change or continue to affect bicarbonate balance. As a result, the acid-base status should be monitored during replacement therapy and ongoing bicarbonate administration should be adjusted accordingly.

Co-oximetry

In contrast to measurement of pO_2, co-oximetry is the measurement of hemoglobin (HGB) spectrophotometrically using multiple wavelengths of light. HGB will absorb light maximally at different wavelengths depending on its configuration. The four common absorption maximum wavelengths used in these devices are to provide measurement of:

- Oxygenated hemoglobin (oxy-HGB or O_2-HGB), which is expressed as true, measured oxygen saturation percent.
- Unoxygenated hemoglobin (deoxy-HGB).
- Carboxyhemoglobin (CO-HGB) – used to detect the presence and severity of carbon monoxide poisoning.
- Methemoglobin (Met-HGB) – used to detect the presence and severity of methemoglobinemia.

Because co-oximetry is used to characterize HGB oxygenation, it is typically useful only for arterial blood analysis.

27 Laboratory Evaluation of the Liver

Robin W. Allison

Department of Veterinary Pathobiology, Oklahoma State University College of Veterinary Medicine, Stillwater, OK, USA

The liver functions in an amazing variety of biologic processes that are essential to life. These functions include metabolism of carbohydrates, lipids, proteins, hormones, and vitamins; detoxification and excretion of waste products and other toxic substances; digestion (especially of fats); and production of most clotting factors. The liver is highly vascular and uniquely situated to receive not only arterial blood via the hepatic artery but also venous blood via the portal vein. In fact, the majority (70–75%) of blood flow to the liver arrives from the portal circulation, and the liver's capacity to remove various solutes from portal blood is central to many of its functions [1]. Because of the liver's remarkable diversity, liver dysfunction may result in a variety of laboratory abnormalities.

Liver disease versus liver failure

Liver disease includes any process that results in hepatocyte injury, cholestasis, or both. These include hypoxia, metabolic diseases, toxicoses, inflammation, neoplasia, mechanical trauma, and intra-hepatic or extrahepatic bile duct blockage. It is important to realize that the liver is frequently secondarily affected by primary disease processes occurring in other tissues, such as inflammatory bowel disease and pancreatitis. Liver failure may result from liver disease, and is recognized both by failure to clear the blood of those substances normally eliminated by the liver and by failure to synthesize those substances normally produced by the liver. Liver disease, however, does not always result in liver failure. The liver has a marked reserve capacity, and 70–80% of the functional hepatic mass must be lost before liver failure occurs. Tests for liver disease or failure fall into three main categories:

- Serum enzyme assays that detect hepatocyte injury.
- Serum enzyme assays that detect cholestasis.
- Tests that evaluate liver function.

Introduction to enzymology

A basic understanding of diagnostic enzymology is necessary to interpret the results of serum enzyme assays used to detect liver disease. Principles of diagnostic enzymology include:

- Different organs, tissues, or cells contain different enzymes. In some cases, only a few organs or tissues contain a given enzyme; these "tissue-specific" enzymes tend to be the most diagnostically useful.
- Increased serum enzyme activity results when an increased quantity of the enzyme passes into the blood, either because of leakage from injured cells or because of increased production.
- Detection of increased serum enzyme activity, therefore, suggests either injury to the cells of origin or stimulation of the cells to produce increased quantities of the enzyme.
- Diagnostic enzymology is a means of locating where tissue injury or stimulation of increased enzyme production has occurred.
- Results of diagnostic enzymology, in combination with other clinical and laboratory data, are helpful in understanding the disease process and in making a diagnosis.
- Diagnostic enzymology does **NOT** provide information about tissue *function*.

In the body, enzymes catalyze biochemical reactions by converting a substrate into a product. For example,

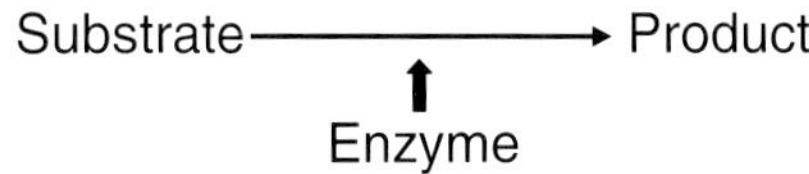

To measure enzyme activity, a standard quantity of serum containing the enzyme to be measured is mixed with a solution containing the substrate for that enzyme. The reaction is then allowed to occur, and the enzyme's activity is measured by the rate of either substrate disappearance or product formation. The more rapidly that either one occurs, the greater

Veterinary Hematology, Clinical Chemistry, and Cytology, Third Edition. Edited by Mary Anna Thrall, Glade Weiser, Robin W. Allison and Terry W. Campbell.

Companion website: www.wiley.com/go/thrall/veterinary

the patient's serum enzyme activity. Frequently, the product is not measured directly; rather, it is incorporated into a second reaction, which often involves the conversion of NAD^+ (or $NADP^+$) to NADH (or NADPH), or vice versa. This second reaction results in a change in the sample's light absorbance, which can be measured using a spectrophotometer [2].

Enzyme concentrations are not measured directly, but the serum activity of an enzyme is considered to be directly proportional to its concentration. Currently, enzyme activities are reported in terms of units per liter (U/L), with a unit defined as the quantity of enzyme that catalyzes the reaction of 1 μmol of substrate per minute [2]. Although this unit was historically referred to as an international unit (IU), the actual SI unit (Système International, for international uniformity) is the katal, which describes enzyme activity in moles per second. The SI system enzyme activity is reported in terms of katals per liter (kat/L) [2]. For conversion of units, IU/L × 0.01667 = μkat/L [3].

Basic concepts and information that must be considered to properly interpret the results of serum enzyme assays include:

- The difference between leakage enzymes and induced enzymes.
- The duration of enzyme activity after passage into the blood (i.e., the enzyme's biologic half-life in the blood).
- The tissue specificity of enzymes.
- The proper handling and storage of serum for enzyme assays.

CHAPTER 27

Leakage versus induced enzymes

Increased serum enzyme activities can result from either leakage or induction. Enzymes can be released when cell injury alters cell membranes; enzymes that pass into the extracellular space and then into the serum by this mechanism are termed *leakage enzymes* (Figure 27.1). The term is somewhat misleading, however. Although membranes of fatally injured cells can certainly leak enzymes as they degrade, sublethally injured cells may release membrane blebs that later rupture, resulting in increased serum enzyme activity [4]. Nevertheless, it is useful to think of the process in terms of leakage. By contrast, induction involves the increased production of an enzyme by cells that normally produce the enzyme in smaller quantities. This increased production is induced by some type of stimulus, and it results in increased release of the enzyme from the cells and subsequent increased activity of the enzyme in serum. Enzymes that pass into the serum by this mechanism are termed *induced enzymes* (Figure 27.2).

Leakage enzymes are present in the cytosol, organelles, or both, and escape following sub-lethal or lethal (i.e., necrosis) cell injury. Increased serum enzyme activities can be detected within hours of the injury [5]. By contrast, induced enzymes are attached to cell membranes. Increased serum activity of these enzymes depends primarily on increased production and develops more slowly (i.e., days rather than hours) [5].

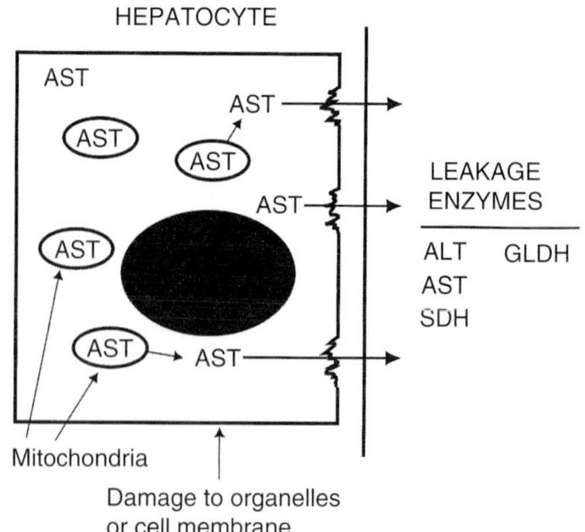

Figure 27.1 Leakage enzymes escape from the cell because of altered plasma membranes. Some leakage enzymes, such as AST, are also present in the organelles. More severe damage is required to cause leakage from these organelles.

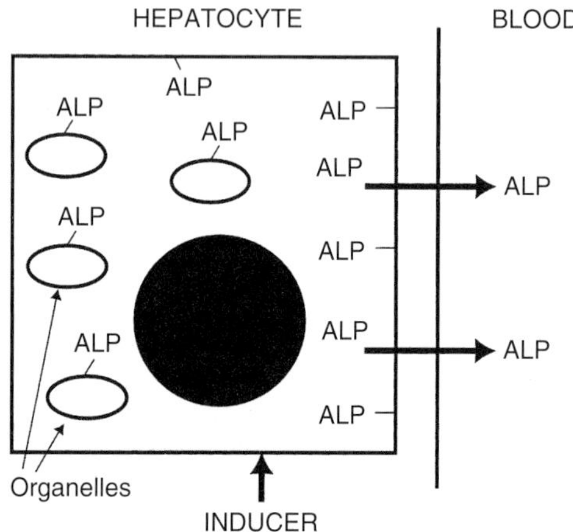

Figure 27.2 Increased serum activities of induced enzymes result, in part, from increased production of these enzymes, with a subsequent increase in secretion. This increased production is caused by some type of inducer.

The concept of leakage versus induced enzymes is important, but the difference is not entirely clear-cut in clinical situations. For example, acute hepatocyte injury can result in loss of leakage enzymes, but enzyme production may be upregulated in the subsequent reparative process of hepatic regeneration, resulting in a slower decline of serum enzyme activity than expected based on the enzyme half-life [6]. In addition, the release of membrane blebs containing membrane-bound enzymes may cause rapid but generally mild increases in serum activity of those "inducible" enzymes [5]. Release of induced enzymes can also occur secondary to less acute membrane alterations. The increased serum activities of alkaline phosphatase (ALP) and gamma glutamyltransferase (GGT) that occur as a result of cholestasis are examples. A portion of the increase in the serum activities of these enzymes probably results from increased enzyme production, but the bile acids sequestered in bile canaliculi and ducts can solubilize membranes of hepatocytes and bile duct epithelial cells, resulting in increased release of these enzymes [7, 8].

Although activities of both leakage and induced enzymes often increase during most types of liver disease, the relative magnitudes of the increases can provide a hint about the underlying liver lesions. In diseases characterized primarily by hepatocyte injury, the activities of leakage enzymes tend to be increased to a greater degree than are the activities of induced enzymes. Similarly, in diseases characterized primarily by cholestasis, the activities of induced enzymes tend to be increased to a greater degree than are the activities of leakage enzymes. However, many liver diseases (particularly chronic diseases) result in both hepatocyte injury and cholestasis, so these distinctions are not always useful.

Enzyme half-life

After leakage or secretion from cells, the enzymes eventually are degraded and/or excreted from the body. Some enzyme molecules also lose their activity in the serum over time. The rate at which the loss of activity, degradation, or excretion occurs determines the length of time during which the enzyme activity is detectable in the serum after leakage or secretion. The disappearance rate of enzyme activity typically is measured as the biologic half-life of the enzyme, which is the time required for one-half of that enzyme's activity to disappear from the serum. Knowledge of the average biologic half-life of an enzyme is helpful when assessing how recently leakage or increased production has occurred and whether these processes are continuing. The biologic half-lives of various diagnostic enzymes and the use of enzyme half-lives in assessing tissue injury are discussed later.

Tissue specificity

It is important to know from which tissue the enzyme most likely originated. Knowledge of tissue specificity allows the diagnostician to narrow the list of possible tissues that are involved in a disease process. Tissue specificity is a function of:

- The presence or absence of the enzyme in the tissue. When increased serum activity of an enzyme is detected, only the tissues in which that enzyme is normally present are considered potential sites of injury.
- The concentration of the enzyme in tissues. An enzyme can be present in many tissues but have high concentrations in only one or a few. When increased serum activity of an enzyme is detected, the tissues in which that enzyme is found at the highest concentrations are the most likely sites of injury.
- Where the enzyme goes after leakage or secretion. Enzymes that are detected in serum have either leaked or been secreted into the extracellular spaces and then passed into the serum. Some tissues may have high enzyme concentrations, but leaked or secreted enzymes are not readily accessible to blood. For example, injury to renal epithelial cells results in leakage of the enzyme GGT [9]. This enzyme leaks from the brush border of the cell into the lumens of the renal tubules, rather than into the extracellular space. Thus, increased GGT activity can be detected in the urine, but the serum activity does not increase.
- The half-life of different isoenzymes. Enzymes with the same catalytic activity might be produced in several different tissues, but these enzymes can vary regarding other properties. These different forms of enzymes are termed isoenzymes or isoforms (see later discussion of ALP isoenzymes versus isoforms), and they may have different half-lives in serum. If an isoenzyme has a very short half-life (e.g., minutes to a few hours), it is less likely to accumulate in the serum after leakage or secretion and, therefore, is less likely to be detected. If an enzyme originates from two different tissues but the half-life of the isoenzyme from one tissue is minutes and that of the isoenzyme from the second tissue is days, then the increased serum enzyme activity is more likely to have originated from the second tissue. For example, the placenta of dogs contains large quantities of the enzyme ALP, but the half-life of the placental isoenzyme is minutes. Therefore, the placenta is not considered to be a likely source when an increased serum ALP activity is detected [5].

The ideal diagnostic enzyme would be specific for only one tissue. Increased serum activities of such an enzyme would direct the diagnostician to that tissue as the site of a disease process. Almost no diagnostic enzymes are found in only one tissue; however, some are found in only a few tissues.

Diagnosticians sometimes attempt to relate the magnitude of increased serum enzyme activities with the type or degree of injury in a tissue. It is tempting to assume that higher enzyme activities are indicative of more severe tissue injury (especially in the case of leakage enzymes), but this assumption is not always true (Figure 27.3). Dead cells release all of their enzymes, and they produce no additional enzymes. Sublethally injured cells, however, lose only a portion of their enzyme content and continue to produce enzymes (possibly at an increased rate). Such cells can ultimately release more enzyme than can dead cells. In other words, necrosis can result in increased enzyme activity, but diffuse, sublethal injury to the same tissue can result in even greater serum enzyme activity. Thus, the magnitude of the serum enzyme activity is not a reliable indicator of the type or degree of tissue injury. The relative magnitude of increased serum enzyme activity is often referred to in terms of the fold increase above the upper reference limit (URL); for example, 3× URL signifies a threefold increase above the upper reference limit.

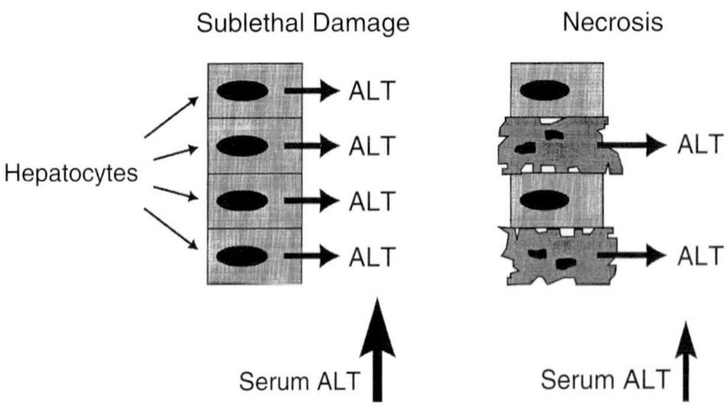

Figure 27.3 The magnitude of serum enzyme activity is not necessarily related to the severity of tissue injury. Serum ALT leaks from hepatocytes when their plasma membranes are injured. The resultant serum ALT activity can be greater after sublethal injury to many hepatocytes than after necrosis of a few hepatocytes.

Sample handling

Unlike substances in serum that are directly measured (e.g., urea, creatinine, electrolytes), serum enzyme concentrations are determined by measuring serum activity and assuming that the activity is proportional to the serum concentrations. If serum samples are not properly handled the enzyme activity can be altered leading to erroneous results. It is important to realize that serum enzymes are proteins that are subject to degradation or denaturation by heat, changes in pH, and exposure to various chemicals, any of which can result in loss of enzyme activity [2].

Regardless of whether serum enzyme activities are assayed in an in-clinic laboratory or a reference laboratory, some delay usually occurs between sample acquisition and testing, making proper sample handling essential. While serum to be used in these assays should be harvested and assayed as soon as possible, most enzymes are stable in refrigerated, separated serum for 24 hours. The degree of degradation that occurs after 24 hours varies considerably depending upon the particular enzyme [10]. Lipemia and *in vitro* hemolysis should be avoided because of the potential to interfere with spectrophotometric assays (increased serum bilirubin may also interfere but is not preventable). Some enzymes are present in erythrocytes, and hemolysis can also directly contribute to the increased enzyme activity (see Chapter 3).

Hepatocyte injury

Hepatocyte injury is detected by measuring the serum activities of hepatocellular leakage enzymes. The three serum enzymes that are commonly measured to provide information about hepatocyte injury include alanine aminotransferase (ALT), aspartate aminotransferase (AST), and sorbitol dehydrogenase (SDH). An additional enzyme, glutamate dehydrogenase (GLDH), is available but is primarily utilized in countries other than the United States. However, numerous other enzymes are utilized in laboratory animals as biomarkers of hepatic toxicity [11].

Alanine aminotransferase

ALT, previously referred to as serum glutamic pyruvic transaminase (SGPT), is a leakage enzyme that is free in the cytoplasm. In dogs and cats, the highest concentrations of ALT occur in hepatocytes (especially those in periportal regions), and the ALT assay is commonly included in the serum biochemical profiles of these species [12]. ALT activity is sometimes the only test used to detect hepatocyte injury in dogs and cats because ALT is much more liver specific than AST (discussed below). However, ALT is not totally liver specific; severe muscle damage or disease can cause increases in serum ALT activity [13]. ALT activity of muscle is less than that of the liver (in dogs, activities in skeletal and cardiac muscle are approximately 5% and 25% that of liver activity, respectively) [12]. Because the total mass of muscle is much greater than that of the liver, muscle can be a significant source of ALT leakage. While increased serum ALT activity in dogs and cats is usually indicative of either hepatocyte death or sublethal hepatocyte injury, necrosis or sublethal damage to muscle cells must be considered as well. When ALT activity is increased, measurement of a serum enzyme activity that is more muscle specific (e.g., creatine kinase [CK]) is helpful in order to determine if muscle damage is a possible source of the increased ALT.

Horses and ruminants have low ALT concentration in hepatocytes; consequently, serum ALT activity is not useful for detecting liver disease in these species [12]. Moderate amounts of ALT are present in the muscle of horses and ruminants, and moderate increases in the serum ALT activity occur with muscle injury in these species [12]; however, ALT is not usually included in large animal biochemical profiles. Other muscle-specific enzymes (e.g., CK) are more commonly used for detecting muscle injury in these species.

In dogs and cats, a wide variety of liver diseases can produce increased serum ALT activity. Hypoxia, metabolic alterations resulting in hepatocyte lipid accumulation, bacterial toxins, inflammation, hepatic neoplasia, and a multitude of toxic chemicals and drugs can cause hepatocyte injury, thereby resulting in ALT leakage. Acutely, the serum activity of ALT is proportional to the number of cells that are injured, but as illustrated in Figure 27.3, the magnitude of ALT activity is not indicative of the *cause* of the injury or of the *type* of damage to the hepatocytes (sublethal damage versus necrosis). After acute severe injury, such as from a toxin, serum ALT activity can increase markedly within a day or two [5]. If the injury is not ongoing, ALT activity slowly decreases over several weeks. Serum ALT activity can also be increased during recovery from liver injury when active hepatocyte regeneration is occurring; this may explain why ALT activity does not always return to normal as quickly as expected based on its serum half-life, which has been estimated at

17–60 hours in dogs and 3.5 hours in cats [12]. More chronic inflammatory liver diseases can result in periodic "flares" of increased ALT activity. Thus, repeated measurement of serum enzyme activity may give insight about the underlying disease process. However, it is important to recognize that in certain situations significant liver disease can occur with normal or only slightly increased serum ALT activity. For example, if liver disease is severe and the hepatic mass is markedly decreased there may be too few remaining hepatocytes to result in markedly increased serum activity, even if the remaining cells are injured and leaking ALT. Some chronic diseases may have little active hepatocyte injury taking place, resulting in little enzyme leakage. Also, a few toxins (aflatoxin, microcystin) seem to interfere with transaminase production; massive acute hepatic necrosis may occur with minimal increases in ALT (or AST) [5, 14].

Increases in serum ALT activity can also be observed in dogs with hyperadrenocorticism or that have been administered corticosteroids [15]. These increases are generally mild (two- to fivefold), but ALT activity increases can vary widely among dogs receiving corticosteroid therapy, depending on the dose and duration of treatment [16–18]. It is not entirely clear whether these increases in ALT activity are due to induction of enzyme production by steroids (as is well-documented for the induction enzymes ALP and GGT) or due to actual hepatocyte membrane injury; morphologic changes in hepatocytes develop within days after steroid therapy begins and resolve slowly after therapy ceases [16, 17, 19].

Anticonvulsant drugs (e.g., phenobarbital, primidone, phenytoin) also cause mildly increased serum ALT activity in dogs [20, 21]. Because most dogs remain clinically healthy and liver biopsies have not shown morphologic evidence of liver damage these increases have been attributed to induction (up-regulation of enzyme production); however, *in vitro* studies have not supported that hypothesis [22, 23]. In addition, some dogs receiving anticonvulsants will develop a toxic hepatopathy, in which case ALT activity may be markedly increased due to hepatocyte injury [24].

Aspartate aminotransferase

AST, previously termed serum glutamic oxaloacetic transaminase (SGOT), is present at highest concentrations in hepatocytes and muscle cells (both skeletal and cardiac) of all species [12]. Therefore, AST is not a liver-specific enzyme. AST is a leakage enzyme that is found predominantly in the cytoplasm with about 20% located within mitochondria [25]. In contrast to ALT, hepatocyte AST is in highest concentration in cells of the periacinar region, surrounding central veins (zone 3) [5]. Increased serum AST activity can result from lethal or sublethal injury to either hepatocytes or muscle cells.

In dogs and cats, serum AST activity will increase as a result of the same liver diseases previously listed for ALT and generally parallels ALT activity, but the magnitude of the increase may be less than that of ALT [5]. The serum AST activity may return to baseline faster than ALT following acute liver injury in some animals, making repeated measurements useful for monitoring disease resolution. Although AST is less liver specific than ALT, it may be more sensitive than ALT for detecting some liver diseases in dogs and cats [5]. For example, one study reported 89% of cats with hepatic lipidosis had increased AST activity compared to 72% for increased ALT activity [26].

Similar to ALT, mild increases in AST activity may be seen in dogs as a result of enzyme induction due to corticosteroids and possibly phenobarbital, although there is some controversy in the literature [21, 23, 27]. Because muscle is a possible source of serum AST activity, measurement of an enzyme specific for muscle injury (i.e., CK) is useful to determine if the increase in AST activity is due to muscle injury.

In horses and ruminants, AST is often used for the routine detection of hepatocyte injury since it is included in most large animal biochemical profiles and because of low hepatocyte ALT concentrations. In these species, an increased serum AST activity can result from the same spectrum of liver diseases (both sublethal and necrotic) as listed for ALT. The major problem with AST in detecting hepatocyte injury is its lack of liver specificity. As in dogs and cats, increased serum AST activity in horses and ruminants can result not only from hepatocyte injury but also from muscle injury. This problem can be mitigated to a certain extent by assaying a muscle-specific enzyme such as CK along with AST. Increased AST activity with normal CK activity may be seen if the source of the AST is the liver, suggesting hepatocyte injury has occurred. Uncertainty remains in such a case, however, because the half-life of CK is shorter than that of AST (Figure 27.4). Serum activities of both enzymes may increase as a result of muscle injury, but the CK activity may return to normal earlier than the AST activity [28]. These problems with use of AST in detecting hepatocyte injury in horses and ruminants have led to use of more liver-specific enzymes (such as SDH) in these species.

As discussed for ALT, the serum activity of AST may be normal or only slightly increased with significant liver diseases that are chronic and low-grade, that have resulted in markedly decreased hepatic mass, or that are due to toxins that inhibit transaminase activity. In dogs and cats, the half-life of AST is shorter than that of ALT and has been estimated between 4 and 12 hours in dogs and 77 minutes in cats [12, 29]. In horses, the half-life of AST has been estimated at 7–8 days [28].

Sorbitol dehydrogenase (iditol dehydrogenase)

SDH, also called iditol dehydrogenase (ID), is a leakage enzyme that is free in the cytoplasm. It is present at high concentrations in the hepatocytes of dogs, cats, horses, and ruminants, but its concentration in other tissues in

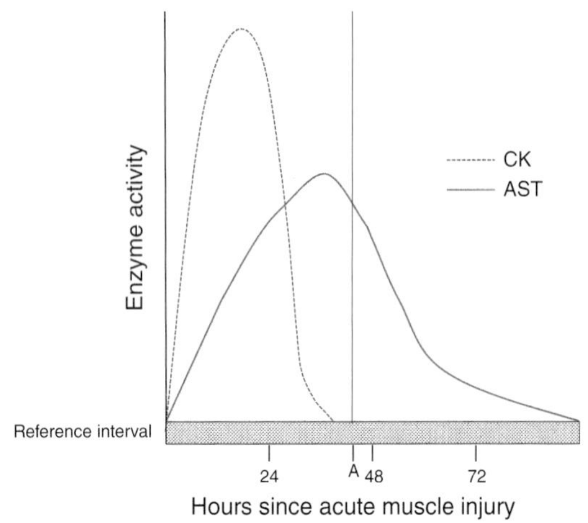

Figure 27.4 Serum activities of both AST and CK increase because of muscle injury. As illustrated here, these activities increase and decrease at different rates. Depending on when a blood sample is analyzed after muscle injury, it is possible to detect increased serum AST activity and normal serum CK activity (note time A) and to erroneously interpret this as being an indication of hepatic injury.

these species is low [12]. Therefore, SDH is a liver-specific enzyme. Increased serum SDH activity is suggestive of either hepatocyte death or sublethal hepatocyte injury. SDH is not superior to ALT for detecting hepatocyte injury in dogs and cats, and it is not commonly used in these species. In horses and ruminants, however, SDH is much more specific than AST for detecting hepatocyte injury. The half-life of SDH is very short (<2 days); serum activities may return to normal within 4–5 days after acute hepatocyte injury [30]. The main disadvantage to SDH is that it is less stable *in vitro* than most other diagnostic enzymes, and the stability varies by species. In both horses and cattle, however, SDH is stable in room temperature or refrigerated serum for as long as 5 hours (24 hours refrigerated in cattle), and for as long as 48 hours (72 hours in cattle) when frozen [31]. In llamas, SDH is stable in serum for 8 hours, and in refrigerated or frozen serum for up to 1 week [32]. In dogs, SDH is stable in serum for 4 hours at room temperature, 48 hours refrigerated, 1 week frozen at −20 °C, and one month frozen at −70 °C [33]. In most cases, these time periods should be sufficient to allow the delivery of serum to a laboratory for an SDH assay. Because SDH is preferable to AST for detecting hepatocyte injury in horses and ruminants, one should identify a laboratory that can perform this assay within the appropriate time frame.

Glutamate dehydrogenase

GLDH is a leakage enzyme present in highest concentrations within mitochondria of hepatocytes, predominantly in periportal regions [12]. The same types of reversible and nonreversible hepatocyte injury that cause increased serum activity of ALT will cause increased serum activity of GLDH. Increased serum concentration of this enzyme is reported to have excellent sensitivity for the detection of canine hepatic disease [10, 34]. The sensitivity for equine hepatic disease is reported to be good but slightly less than that of GGT [35]. GLDH activity is stable in canine serum for 2 days at room temperature, 7 days refrigerated at 4 °C, and 6 months frozen at −20 °C [34]. Serum activity of GLDH increased in dogs with hyperadrenocorticism; increases have also been documented in dogs receiving anticonvulsants [36]. Assays for this enzyme have not been routinely available in the United States but are used more commonly in other countries.

Cholestasis

Cholestasis (impaired bile flow) can be detected by measuring the serum activities of enzymes whose increased production is induced by cholestasis or by measuring the serum concentrations of substances (either endogenous or exogenous) that normally are considered tests of liver function and are discussed later. The two serum enzymes used to detect cholestasis are ALP and GGT.

Alkaline phosphatase

ALP is an induced enzyme that is attached to cell membranes and synthesized by many tissues such as liver, bone, kidney, intestine, pancreas, and placenta [12, 25, 37]. In domestic animals two ALP isoenzymes are produced from two different genes; these are referred to as the intestinal isoenzyme and the tissue-nonspecific isoenzyme [37]. The tissue-nonspecific isoenzyme undergoes further post-translational modification in different tissues resulting in different isoforms from liver (LALP), bone (BALP), kidney, and placenta. The intestinal isoenzyme can also undergo further modification to produce the unique corticosteroid induced isoform (CALP) in dogs. These different isoforms are often mistakenly referred to as different isoenzymes, but isoenzymes must be produced from different genes. Most of the normal serum ALP activity originates from the liver. The half-life of intestinal, renal, and placental ALP in dogs is approximately 6 minutes, and the half-life of intestinal ALP in cats is approximately 2 minutes, thus they are unlikely to cause increased serum ALP activity [37]. Increased ALP production and increased serum ALP activity commonly occur with cholestasis, increased osteoblastic activity, induction by certain drugs (primarily in dogs), and a variety of chronic diseases.

Increased serum alkaline phosphatase activity

Hepatobiliary disease

ALP in the liver is associated with biliary epithelial cells and canalicular membranes of hepatocytes [5]. A variety of hepatobiliary diseases can result in increased serum ALP activity due to increased enzyme production, solubilization of membranes by the action of bile salts, and release of membrane blebs after cell injury [4, 7, 8, 37]. Cholestatic diseases can result in marked increases in serum ALP activity in dogs (greater than 10-fold URL) but increases are more variable in other species [5, 37–39]. Disorders that impair bile flow in focal areas of the liver may result in variable increases in ALP activity. For example, dogs with hepatic nodular hyperplasia, which is a relatively common benign condition in older dogs, were reported to have ALP activities that were 2.5–14× URL [40]. Impaired bile flow induces increased ALP production, and sequestration of bile salts in the biliary system causes solubilization of ALP molecules attached to cell membranes, which are then released into the blood [7, 8, 41, 42]. The half-life of the cholestasis-induced LALP is approximately 3 days in dogs but only 6 hours in cats [5]. In cats, this short half-life, in addition to lower liver ALP concentration per gram of tissue, contribute to the relatively smaller magnitude of serum ALP activity increases seen with liver disease in cats compared to dogs [5]. However, ALP is still a useful enzyme to evaluate feline cholestatic liver disease if one keeps in mind that even mild increases (2–3× URL) can be significant [5]. The utility of ALP for detection of cholestasis in horses and ruminants is generally considered inferior to that of GGT (discussed later) [37, 39]. Wide reference intervals for ALP in horses and ruminants contribute to the reduced sensitivity of the serum ALP assay for the detection of liver disease in these species.

When cholestasis is the cause of increased serum ALP activity, serum total bilirubin and bile acid concentrations may be increased concurrently. In dogs with cholestasis, serum ALP activity often increases prior to increases in serum bilirubin concentration; thus ALP is a more sensitive indicator of cholestasis in dogs [10, 43]. However, even if the serum bilirubin concentration is normal, bilirubinuria may accompany cholestasis-induced increases in ALP. Whereas lesions primarily involving the intra- or extrahepatic biliary system are common causes of cholestasis, hepatic diseases resulting in significant hepatocyte swelling (e.g., lipidosis or inflammation of the hepatic parenchyma) can obstruct small bile canaliculi and also induce increased ALP production and release [44]. It is also important to realize that pancreatic and intestinal lesions can sometimes be the primary cause of cholestasis due to extrahepatic bile duct obstruction.

Osteoblastic activity

Increased serum ALP activity associated with increased osteoblastic activity occurs in all species. These increases are most often are detected in young, growing animals when the results of ALP assays are compared with adult reference intervals for ALP. For instance, the mean serum activity of alkaline phosphatase of bone origin (BALP) in immature cats in one study was more than 10 times that of adult cats, resulting in a mean total ALP activity more than twice that of the adults [45]. Another study found reference intervals for total ALP activity in 4-week old kittens was 97–274 U/L compared to 10–80 U/L for adult cats [46]. Puppies up to 8 weeks of age have been found to have total ALP activities greater than the adult reference interval [47, 48]. Since age-specific reference intervals are seldom provided, one must remember that young animals commonly have serum ALP activities greater than adult reference intervals. In puppies, kittens, and calves, ALP activity increases attributed to bone growth are generally mild (<4–5× URL), but foals may have increases up to 20× URL in the first 3 weeks of life [37, 49].

A few causes of increased osteoblastic activity in mature animals may result in mildly increased serum ALP activity due to production of BALP. Osteosarcoma and other bone neoplasms (both primary and secondary) inconsistently result in increased serum ALP activity because of osteoblast proliferation in these processes, and dogs with osteosarcoma and increased serum ALP activity appear to have a worse prognosis than those with normal ALP activity [37, 50, 51]. Fracture healing usually results in localized increases in osteoblastic activity and mild increases in serum ALP that may be useful for monitoring the progression of healing. In one study dogs with uncomplicated fracture healing had mild increases in serum ALP activity that returned to normal with bone union, while dogs with failure of bone union had no changes in serum ALP activity [52]. Canine hyperparathyroidism (primary or secondary) and feline hyperthyroidism may result in increased bone turnover and increased osteoblastic activity; mild increases in serum ALP may be detected in patients with these diseases [37].

Induction by drugs (dogs)

Serum ALP activity can be markedly increased when enzyme production is induced by certain drugs. Drug-induced ALP production is well documented in dogs but not in other species, thus the following discussion pertains to dogs only. Corticosteroids (exogenous or endogenous) and anticonvulsants (e.g., phenobarbitol, phenytoin, primidone) induce increased ALP production by canine hepatocytes. Exogenous corticosteroids in any form (oral, parenteral, topical, ophthalmic, and otic) have been implicated [53, 54]. Serum ALP activity increases induced by corticosteroids vary depending on dose and duration of exposure but can be marked (>20× URL) [5, 16]. Anticonvulsants generally cause somewhat milder increases (<10× URL) [5, 24, 55].

Corticosteroids induce production of a unique isoform (CALP) that is distinct from that produced by hepatocytes in response to cholestasis (LALP). Although it is possible to distinguish LALP from CALP with special laboratory tests, the clinical utility of such distinction is uncertain. In dogs given corticosteroids the initial rise in serum ALP activity is due to LALP, while CALP increases after a 10-day lag period, and there appears to be considerable individual variation in the degree of ALP induction caused by corticosteroids [17, 18, 56–58]. Although not specific, increased CALP activity is common in dogs with naturally occurring hyperadrenocorticism, and a *lack* of increased CALP argues against hyperadrenocorticism in suspect cases [57, 59]. Although many dogs with increased blood corticosteroid concentrations will have increased serum ALP activity due to induction, some will develop a steroid hepatopathy with swelling of hepatocytes due to glycogen deposition. Evidence of decreased hepatic function (increased total bilirubin or bile acids) is uncommon in these dogs but can occur, depending on severity of disease [5]. Chronic stress resulting in increased blood concentrations of endogenous steroids may also cause increases in CALP activity [5, 37].

To help distinguish cholestasis-induced from corticosteroid-induced increases in serum ALP in dogs, other tests can be performed. These tests include serum and urinary bilirubin concentrations, serum bile acid concentration, and tests to detect hyperadrenocorticism. A suggested approach is presented in Figure 27.5. The concurrent presence of increased ALP activity and hyperbilirubinemia is strongly suggestive of cholestasis, but the serum bilirubin concentration may be normal in some cases of cholestatic disease (e.g., early in the disease process or if only a portion of the biliary tree is obstructed). In the latter situation, the unobstructed portion of the biliary system excretes enough bilirubin that serum concentrations remain within the reference interval.

Dogs receiving anticonvulsant drugs (e.g., phenobarbitol, phenytoin, primidone) often have increased serum ALP activity, which may be due to LALP, CALP, or both [5, 55]. Most of these dogs remain clinically healthy, but anticonvulsants are also known to cause a toxic hepatopathy in some dogs. In healthy dogs the serum ALP increases have been attributed to induction, but this has not been confirmed by *in vitro* studies and remains controversial [22, 23]. Animals that develop a toxic hepatopathy will usually have other indications of decreased hepatic function (increased total bilirubin or serum bile acids), as well as histologic abnormalities [24].

Miscellaneous other causes

Neonates of several species have high serum ALP activity following ingestion of colostrum. During the first few days of life puppies, kittens, and lambs have transient marked increases in serum ALP activity (up to or >30× URL for adult animals) [46, 60, 61]. Foals and calves do not have such marked increases following colostrum ingestion, although serum ALP activity is increased compared to adults due to BALP, as discussed earlier [49, 62, 63].

A variety of endocrine diseases have been associated with increased serum ALP activity. Hyperadrenocorticism has already been discussed as a cause of often marked corticosteroid-induced ALP activity increases in dogs. The precise mechanisms for the generally mild increases seen with other endocrine diseases are not clearly defined but are likely multifactorial; remember that stress associated with any chronic disease may increase endogenous corticosteroids

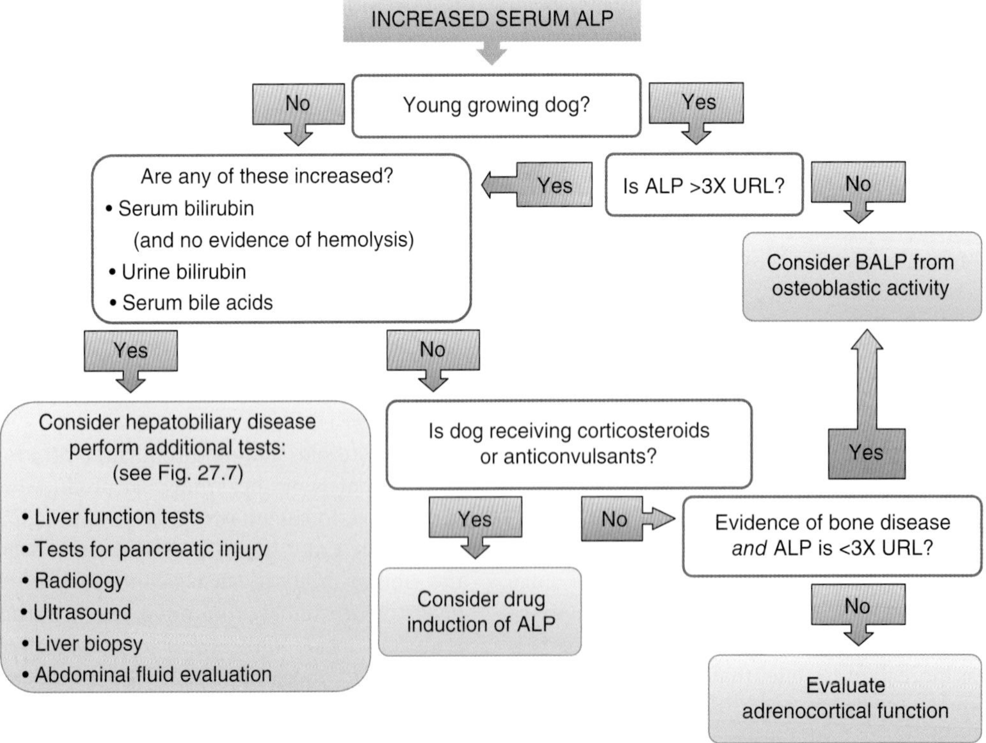

Figure 27.5 Flow chart for evaluating the possible causes of increased serum ALP activities in dogs.

and result in induction of CALP (at least in dogs). Such diseases include diabetes mellitus, canine hypothyroidism and hyperparathyroidism, and feline hyperthyroidism; as many as 80% of hyperthyroid cats are reported to have increased serum ALP activity (generally <4× URL, due to both BALP and LALP) [37, 64–67].

Neoplasia may be associated with increased serum ALP activity; hepatic neoplasia may directly cause cholestasis, and bone neoplasia may be associated with increased osteoblastic activity (both discussed earlier). In addition, mammary gland neoplasia, without metastases to bone or liver, has been identified as a cause of increased serum ALP activity in dogs. Serum ALP activity increases may be seen with benign or malignant mammary gland tumors, are generally mild (<8× URL), and do not appear to have prognostic value [68, 69].

In cattle, there are mild increases in ALP activity associated with pregnancy (mid to late gestation) and early lactation [70, 71]. In dogs, serum ALP activity increases slightly during pregnancy but remains within reference intervals [37].

Breed-related increases in serum ALP activity have been identified in Siberian husky and Scottish terrier dogs. ALP activity (characterized as BALP) in some Siberian huskies was >5× that of siblings in eight related litters; no underlying cause was identified and the condition was described as benign familial hyperphosphatasemia [72]. Increased serum ALP activity in comparison to other breeds has been reported in Scottish terriers, with ALP activity as high as 15× URL [73]. A study of 34 apparently healthy Scottish terriers found that CALP activity was significantly increased in 14 dogs with hyperphosphatasemia compared to 14 dogs with normal ALP activities [74]. The authors attributed these findings to hyperadrenocorticism based on exaggerated cortisol responses to ACTH administration. Histologic changes consistent with hyperadrenocorticism were observed in liver biopsies from both groups of dogs, but no dogs had clinical signs suggestive of hyperadrenocorticism.

γ-Glutamyltransferase

GGT is considered an induced enzyme. Acute hepatic injury, however, can produce rapid increases in serum GGT activity, likely due to release of membrane fragments to which GGT is attached [4]. Most body tissues synthesize GGT, with the highest concentrations occurring in the pancreas and kidney [12, 25, 75, 76]. It also is present at lower concentrations in the hepatocytes, bile duct epithelium, and intestinal mucosa and at high concentrations in the mammary glands of cattle, sheep, and dogs. Most of the serum GGT activity originates in the liver (except for neonates of some species, discussed later). Release from renal epithelial cells results in increased urinary GGT activity but not increased serum GGT activity (see Chapter 24). Similarly, GGT is released into pancreatic ducts by pancreatic cells, rather than into the blood.

Increased GGT production, release, and subsequent increased serum GGT activity occur with cholestasis and biliary hyperplasia [77, 78]. The increased serum GGT activity that occurs with cholestasis may result from both increased production and solubilization of GGT attached to cell membranes [5]. In dogs, increased GGT activity also occurs as a result of drug induction, similar to that described for ALP [5].

Experimentally, extrahepatic bile duct obstruction in dogs results in increases in GGT activity up to 50-fold within 2 weeks; similar studies in cats found increases up to 16-fold [5, 79, 80]. For the detection of liver disease in dogs, GGT is more specific, but less sensitive, than ALP [38]. For the detection of liver disease in cats, GGT is more sensitive, but less specific, than ALP (the exception is hepatic lipidosis, discussed below) [81]. In both dogs and cats, results of serum ALP and GGT assays performed in combination to detect hepatobiliary disease are more diagnostically valid than those of either enzyme assay used alone [38, 81]. Cats with hepatic lipidosis usually have greater relative increases in serum ALP activity compared to GGT, which may be within the reference interval or only minimally increased [5, 82]. However, if there is an underlying necroinflammatory disease present that is the primary cause of the hepatic lipidosis, GGT activity may be increased to a greater degree than is ALP activity [26, 81].

Similar to ALP, increases in serum GGT activity are seen in dogs receiving corticosteroids, but it is not clear whether these increases are due to increased GGT production or are secondary to steroid hepatopathy [19, 56]. When the increase in GGT activity is induced by corticosteroids, GGT activity increases more slowly and to a lesser degree than does ALP activity [16]. Drug induction of GGT activity has also been reported in dogs receiving anticonvulsant medication, but resulting increases are minimal (2–3× URL) and may not even exceed reference intervals [5, 23, 83]. If increases of greater magnitude are seen in dogs receiving such medications, they are more likely the result of cholestasis. Marked increases in the serum GGT activity of a dog being treated with anticonvulsant medication may be indicative of a drug-associated toxic hepatopathy with life-threatening implications [5, 84].

In horses and cattle, GGT is generally considered more sensitive than ALP for detection of cholestasis. In horses with experimental cholestasis induced by bile duct ligation, serum GGT activity increased to a greater degree than did ALP activity [39]. Cattle and horses with pyrrolizidine alkaloid toxicity, which causes marked biliary hyperplasia and eventual liver failure, consistently have early increases in serum GGT activity [85, 86]. However, ALP activity may be increased to a greater degree than GGT activity in more chronic cases [86]. Cattle with moderate to severe hepatic lipidosis have only mild increases in serum GGT activity (2–3× URL) [87].

High serum GGT activity in the colostrum of dogs, cattle and sheep can result in extremely high activities in the serum of young puppies, calves and lambs that have consumed colostrum [61, 88, 89]. In calves, the GGT activity can be >50× URL for adult animals during the first few days after birth [62, 63, 89]. Typically, the GGT activity declines over a period of weeks to reach normal adult levels by about 5 weeks of age. Lambs also have markedly increased serum GGT activity after colostrum consumption, with this activity falling to within the adult reference intervals by approximately 30 days of age [88]. In puppies, marked increases in GGT activity (up to 100× URL for adults) following colostrum ingestion return to normal adult levels more quickly, by about 10 days of age [61]. Increased serum GGT activity also occurs in foals and is typically 1.5–3× URL during the first month of life, but this enzyme activity is apparently not of colostral origin [90, 91].

Liver function

Tests of liver function include measurement of the serum concentrations of substances that normally are removed from the blood by the liver and then metabolized or excreted via the biliary system (e.g., bilirubin, bile acids, ammonia, cholesterol), and substances that normally are synthesized by the liver (e.g., albumin, globulins, urea, cholesterol, coagulation factors). Although abnormal blood concentrations of these substances can result from nonhepatic factors, the detection of abnormal concentrations *in addition to evidence of liver injury* (as detected by changes in leakage or induced enzyme activities) can supply further evidence of significant liver disease or liver failure. Often, however, liver biopsy is required for a definitive diagnosis.

Bilirubin

Normal bilirubin metabolism

Bilirubin is formed primarily from the degradation of hemoglobin (Figure 27.6), with a small contribution from other hemoproteins (e.g., myoglobin, cytochromes, peroxidase, catalase) [92]. Erythrocytes normally are destroyed at a constant rate because of aging, but they also can be destroyed at an increased rate because of hemolytic processes (discussed later). Senescent erythrocytes, which have reached the end of their normal life span, are phagocytized by mononuclear phagocytes primarily in the spleen but also in the liver and the bone marrow. These phagocytized erythrocytes are broken down, and their hemoglobin is dismantled. The globin portion is converted to amino acids, and the heme portion is split into iron and protoporphyrin. The iron is recycled, but the protoporphyrin is converted first to biliverdin and then to bilirubin. The newly formed unconjugated bilirubin (U-bilirubin, also called indirect bilirubin) is released from macrophages, noncovalently bound to albumin, and transported in blood to the liver sinusoids, where it is released from albumin and enters

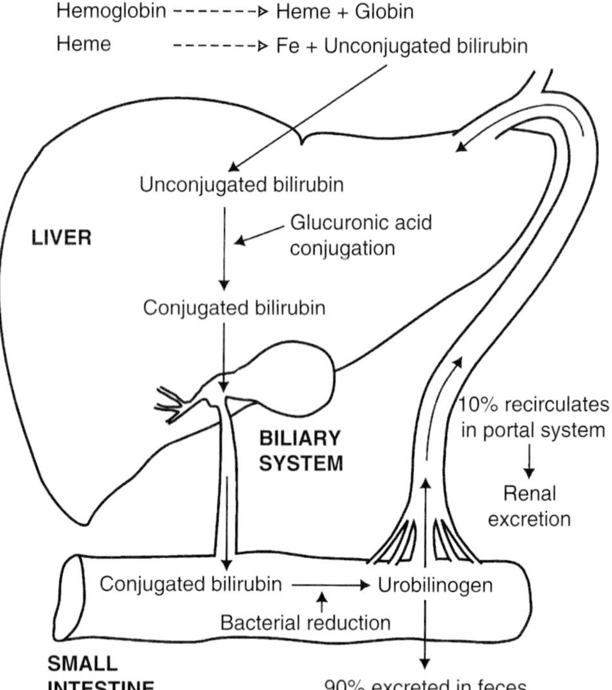

Figure 27.6 Normal bilirubin metabolism.

hepatocytes. Passage through the hepatocyte membrane is facilitated by a carrier, the capacity of which can be saturated if too much bilirubin is presented to the liver (as occurs with increased erythrocyte destruction).

Once inside the hepatocyte, U-bilirubin is bound by proteins (Y protein or ligandin, and Z protein), which limit efflux of U-bilirubin back into the plasma [93]. In the hepatocyte, U-bilirubin is conjugated to sugar groups forming conjugated bilirubin (C-bilirubin, also called direct bilirubin). In many mammals, the major sugar group to which bilirubin is conjugated is glucuronic acid, resulting in the formation of bilirubin glucuronide. This reaction is catalyzed by membrane-associated enzymes of the UDP-glucuronosyltransferase superfamily [94]. Both monoglucuronides and diglucuronides are formed in mammals, with the latter being the predominant form of conjugated bilirubin in bile. In addition to glucuronides, alternate conjugates (e.g., glucosides, glucoside-glucuronide mixed conjugates, xylosides) are produced in some species, with glucosides predominating in horses [95, 96]. Conjugated bilirubin is not tightly protein bound, and is more water soluble than the protein-bound, unconjugated bilirubin. Most C-bilirubin is actively transported against the concentration gradient into bile canaliculi and then excreted in the bile. A small amount of C-bilirubin normally passes through the sinusoidal side of the hepatocyte membrane and back into the blood. If this C-bilirubin remains unbound to protein, it is quickly excreted by the kidney via glomerular filtration. A portion of the C-bilirubin in the blood may become covalently bound to albumin and is termed biliprotein or delta bilirubin [97]. This form of C-bilirubin does not pass through the glomerulus and remains in the blood for a longer period of time. (The implications of delta bilirubin in the assessment of cholestatic disease are discussed later.)

Conjugated bilirubin that is secreted into bile canaliculi passes with the bile into the small intestine where it is converted to urobilinogen by bacterial reduction. Approximately 90% of the urobilinogen is excreted with the feces as stercobilinogen. The remaining 10% of urobilinogen is reabsorbed and enters the blood. A portion of this urobilinogen then is removed from the blood by the hepatocytes and is re-excreted. Another portion of the urobilinogen circulates to the kidneys, where it passes through the glomerulus and is excreted in the urine.

Abnormalities of bilirubin metabolism

Increased serum bilirubin concentrations (hyperbilirubinemia) can be caused by three main pathologic processes: increased bilirubin production (due to increased erythrocyte destruction), decreased bilirubin uptake or conjugation by hepatocytes, and decreased bilirubin excretion (cholestasis).

Increased production of bilirubin most often occurs due to hemolytic disease (extra- or intravascular hemolysis) but can also result from massive internal hemorrhage and subsequent breakdown of erythrocytes in the area of that hemorrhage. During the process of extravascular hemolysis, macrophages remove and destroy erythrocytes just as they do senescent erythrocytes but at an accelerated rate. Hemoglobin breakdown and bilirubin delivery to the liver then occurs in the normal way. During the process of intravascular hemolysis, the free hemoglobin that is released into the blood forms complexes with haptoglobin. These complexes are removed from the circulation by mononuclear phagocytes with subsequent breakdown of hemoglobin and U-bilirubin production. Whatever the specific underlying cause, increased erythrocyte destruction and production of increased amounts of U-bilirubin may overwhelm the liver's capacity for U-bilirubin uptake or C-bilirubin excretion, resulting in an increased serum bilirubin concentration. This is often referred to as prehepatic hyperbilirubinemia.

By contrast, hepatic hyperbilirubinemia may result from decreased uptake or conjugation of bilirubin by hepatocytes. (Intrahepatic cholestasis, discussed later, is also a cause of hepatic hyperbilirubinemia.) Decreased functional hepatic mass due to acute or chronic hepatic disease can cause both decreased bilirubin uptake and decreased bilirubin conjugation. Hereditary defects in conjugation due to enzyme deficiencies occur in people but have not been confirmed in domestic animals. There has been one report of persistent hyperbilirubinemia in a horse that appeared to have a congenital defect in an enzyme required for bilirubin conjugation, similar to Crigler-Najjar Syndrome in people; the exact enzymatic defect was not characterized [98]. Two forms of inherited hyperbilirubinemias have been identified in sheep. Mutant Southdown sheep can have hyperbilirubinemia associated with defective hepatocyte up take of bilirubin from the serum producing increased serum U-bilirubin concentrations; this is similar to Gilbert syndrome in humans [99]. Mutant Corriedale sheep can have hyperbilirubinemia associated with defective hepatic excretion of conjugated bilirubin producing increased serum C-bilirubin concentrations; this is similar to Dubin-Johnson syndrome in humans [100].

Decreased uptake of bilirubin occurs in some species secondary to fasting. This type of hyperbilirubinemia is most marked in horses and can result in serum bilirubin concentrations that plateau at 5–6 mg/dL by 64–136 hours after initial food deprivation; bilirubin concentrations up to 8.5 mg/dL have been reported due to fasting alone [101, 102]. Fasted cattle develop milder hyperbilirubinemia (<1.4 mg/dL) [103]. Small increases in the serum bilirubin concentration occur in other species when deprived of food. These increases result from an increased serum concentration of U-bilirubin, but they do not appear to relate to increased bilirubin production. The mechanisms responsible for fasting hyperbilirubinemia have not been determined, but increased blood fatty acid concentrations correlate with hyperbilirubinemia. Increased fatty acids in the blood may compete for binding to Y and Z proteins in hepatocytes, or may compete with membrane protein transport proteins [101, 102, 104].

Decreased bilirubin excretion (cholestasis) can be either hepatic or posthepatic in origin, and usually results from a blockage (partial or complete) in the biliary system that causes accumulation of bile. Blockage of bile flow results in regurgitation of C-bilirubin into the blood. Blockages are often caused by processes directly affecting the biliary tree, such as infections or neoplasms that compress or damage bile ducts, or biliary calculi. However, diseases that primarily affect the hepatic parenchyma can also result in cholestasis by causing hepatocyte swelling that blocks small bile canaliculi and prevents the normal flow of bile. Extrahepatic bile duct obstruction can also occur secondary to small intestinal or pancreatic lesions, which may cause severe cholestasis and hyperbilirubinemia. Leakage of bile into the abdominal cavity resulting from rupture of the gall bladder or bile duct can also result in hyperbilirubinemia.

Another type of intrahepatic cholestasis results not from obstruction but from impaired excretion of C-bilirubin secondary to extrahepatic bacterial infection, and has been termed functional or sepsis-associated cholestasis. Functional cholestasis has been well described in people but is likely under-recognized in animals. The pathogenesis involves the production of inflammatory cytokines (TNF, IL-6, IL-1β) that reduce bile flow by inhibiting hepatocellular transport mechanisms [105].

Whenever there is increased serum C-bilirubin concentration, a portion of the C-bilirubin may become tightly (covalently) bound to serum protein (biliprotein or delta bilirubin). Delta bilirubin is removed from circulation relatively slowly; it is eliminated at a rate approximately equal to the half-life of albumin (8–20 days) [106]. Delta bilirubin is included in the serum total bilirubin as measured by routine wet chemistry methods. Therefore, total bilirubin concentrations can occasionally be misleading since delta bilirubin may persist for a period of weeks in the serum of animals with resolved cholestatic disease. Such animals may have increased serum total bilirubin concentrations but normal urinary bilirubin concentrations, since tightly protein-bound delta bilirubin does not easily cross the glomerulus. Practical laboratory methods for the measurement of delta bilirubin concentration exist; dry chemical methods allow calculation of delta bilirubin concentrations. However, delta bilirubin is not currently routinely measured.

Historically, the measurement of serum bilirubin involved not only the measurement of total bilirubin but also the determination of the concentrations of both conjugated and unconjugated bilirubin. In theory, hyperbilirubinemia associated with hemolysis or reduced hepatic uptake of bilirubin should produce marked increases in U-bilirubin and smaller, if any, increases in C-bilirubin. Similarly, cholestasis or leakage of bile should produce marked increases in C-bilirubin and smaller, if any, increases in U-bilirubin. Such determinations, however, have proved unreliable in differentiating between causes of hyperbilirubinemia [97, 107]. If hyperbilirubinemia is detected, the patient history, physical findings, and results of other laboratory tests can be helpful in differentiating the potential causes. A flow chart for the evaluation of hyperbilirubinemic animals is presented in Figure 27.7.

Species differences should be considered when evaluating serum bilirubin concentrations. If cholestasis is the cause of hyperbilirubinemia, the serum ALP and GGT activities will likely also be increased and are considered more sensitive than serum bilirubin concentrations for cholestasis in dogs and cattle, but not cats and horses [10, 43]. Most species have a relatively low renal threshold for bilirubin, and because C-bilirubin is efficiently excreted by the kidney, bilirubinuria often precedes hyperbilirubinemia [108]. Healthy dogs, however, frequently exhibit mild bilirubinuria, likely due to the ability of the canine renal tubules to form and conjugate bilirubin [109]. Bilirubinuria in dogs should be interpreted in conjunction with the urine specific gravity; concentrated urine (specific gravity >1.025) may normally contain a small amount of bilirubin [108].

Serum total bilirubin concentrations in healthy horses tend to be greater than in other domestic species, so it is important to use species-specific reference intervals when

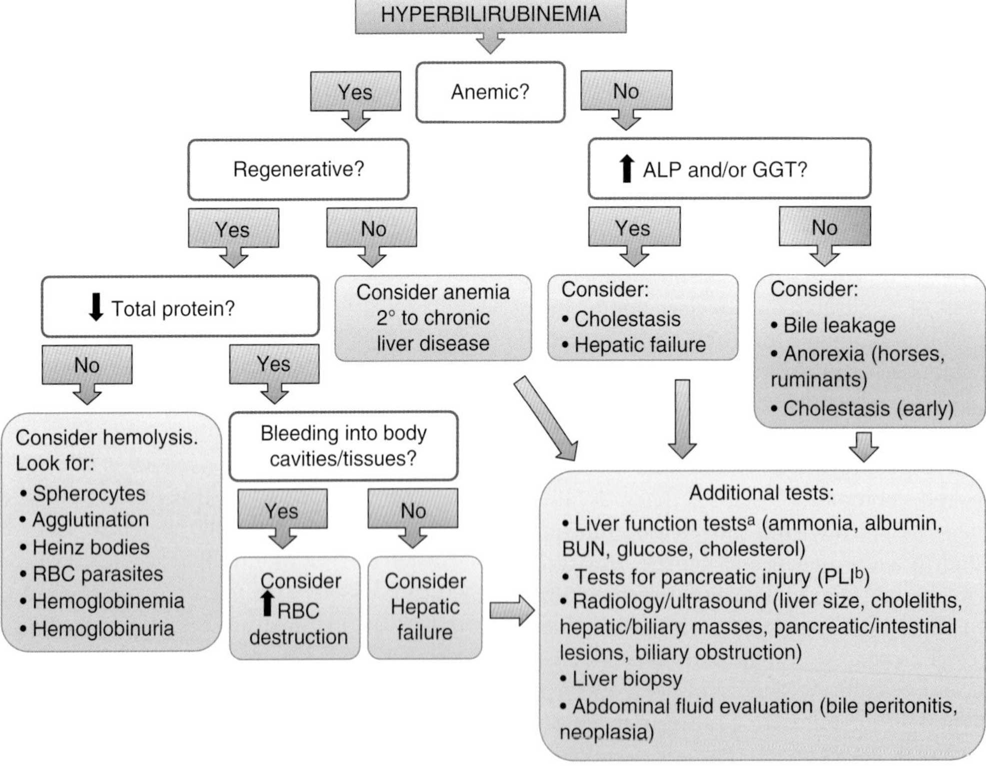

Figure 27.7 Flow chart for the evaluation of hyperbilirubinemic animals. [a]Serum bile acids are not usually useful in hyperbilirubinemic animals but may be helpful in anorexic horses or anemic animals (see text for details). [b]PLI, pancreatic lipase immunoreactivity.

interpreting test results. Hepatic necrosis, neoplasia, cirrhosis, lipidosis, fasting, and hemolysis are reported to cause hyperbilirubinemia in horses; biliary obstruction is a relatively uncommon cause [110]. Hyperbilirubinemia in horses with hemolysis can be marked; serum bilirubin concentrations approaching 50 mg/dL have been reported in foals with neonatal isoerythrolysis [111]. As noted earlier, anorexia or starvation can result in increased serum bilirubin concentrations in horses. Regardless of the cause of hyperbilirubinemia in horses, most of the bilirubin in the blood is unconjugated [112].

Hyperbilirubinemia is not consistent in ruminants with liver disease. Diffuse hepatic diseases such as hepatic lipidosis or chronic liver failure are most likely to cause hyberbilirubinemia [87, 113]. Primary diseases of the biliary tract and gallbladder are uncommon in ruminants. Significant hyperbilirubinemia most often results from hemolysis. Cattle that are ill with a variety of nonhemolytic, nonhepatic diseases may have hyperbilirubinemia associated with rumen stasis and anorexia [114].

Bile acids

Serum bile acids

Measurement of serum bile acid (SBA) concentrations is a routine diagnostic test for hepatic function, cholestasis, and abnormalities of portal circulation, and has replaced the more difficult to perform dye excretion tests (BSP, ICG). Bile acids are synthesized in hepatocytes from cholesterol (Figure 27.8). Cholic acid and chenodeoxycholic acid are the primary bile acids in most animals. After their synthesis, bile acids are conjugated to amino acids (primarily taurine in most animals) before secretion into bile. Bile acids are stored and concentrated in the gallbladder (in those species that have one). At the time of a meal, hormonal and neurohormonal factors stimulate gallbladder contraction and passage of bile acids into the small intestine, where dehydroxylation by anaerobic microorganisms results in the conversion of the primary bile acids to secondary bile acids. Thus, cholic acid is converted to deoxycholic acid, and chenodeoxycholic acid is converted to lithocholic acid. Bile acids emulsify fat and, therefore, promote both the digestion and absorption of fat as well as of fat-soluble vitamins. Most of the bile acids are reabsorbed from the ileum into the portal circulation (<5% of the bile acid pool is lost in the feces each day) [115]. Normally, bile acids are efficiently cleared from the portal circulation on their first pass through the liver; as a result, only a slight postprandial increase in SBA concentrations is seen in healthy animals. Bile acids that are cleared by hepatocytes are secreted into the biliary system and recirculate; a bile acid molecule recirculates several times after a meal.

There are three main pathologic processes involving the liver that result in increased SBA concentrations. Decreased SBA concentrations do not occur with hepatic disease but may occur with some intestinal disorders [115].

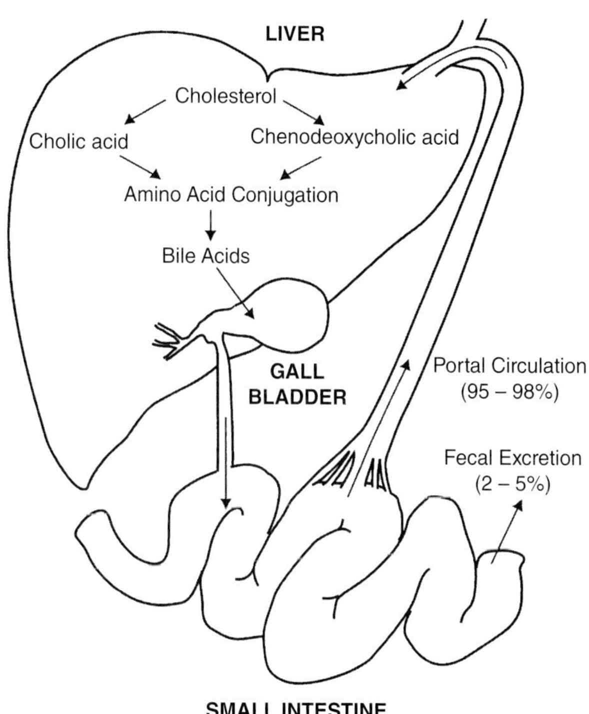

Figure 27.8 Normal production and circulation of bile acid.

1. Abnormalities of portal circulation (e.g., congenital portosystemic shunts, hepatoportal microvascular dysplasia, acquired shunts due to severe cirrhosis). In these situations, blood is shunted away from hepatocytes impairing first-pass clearing of bile acids from portal circulation; bile acids then enter the systemic circulation.

2. Decreased functional hepatic mass. This is a major factor in many diffuse liver diseases (e.g., hepatitis, necrosis, glucocorticoid hepatopathy) that result in sufficient hepatocyte damage that uptake of bile acids from portal blood is impaired.

3. Decreased bile acid excretion in bile. This can result from hepatic or posthepatic cholestasis from any cause (obstruction, hepatocyte swelling, neoplasia, inflammation), functional or sepsis-associated cholestasis, or leakage from the bile duct or gallbladder.

Bile acid assays are most useful for animals in which liver disease is suspected but not unequivocally proven on the basis of routine biochemical profile tests; for example, when serum liver enzyme activities are increased but serum total bilirubin concentrations are normal. SBA concentrations are a sensitive indicator of cholestasis, and it is important to recognize that patients already icteric due to cholestasis will always have increased SBA concentrations as well. However, measuring SBA concentrations may be helpful in differentiating hemolytic hyperbilirubinemia from hepatic or cholestatic hyperbilirubinemia in anemic patients for which a hemolytic cause is not obvious and liver enzyme activities are equivocal. Bile acids do not compete with bilirubin for uptake or metabolism by hepatocytes; therefore, a hemolytic hyperbilirubinemia can occur without a concurrent increase in SBA concentrations [115]. However, severe anemia can cause hepatocellular hypoxia leading to hepatic dysfunction, with subsequent increases in SBA concentrations [115]. In horses, SBA concentrations may also be helpful in discriminating fasting hyperbilirubinemia from hepatic or cholestatic hyperbilirubinemia. Bile acid concentrations do increase twofold to threefold after 3 days of fasting but generally stays below 25 μmol/L, and so may be only slightly outside of laboratory reference intervals [39, 116]. By contrast, horses with experimental bile duct obstruction or diffuse hepatic necrosis have SBA concentration increases exceeding 8- to 10-fold (50–100 μmol/L) after 3 days [39].

Bile acid assays are readily available. Bile acids are stable in serum at room temperature for several days, and serum for bile acid assays can be frozen. Depending upon the test method, hemolysis may cause false decreases and lipemia false increases in SBA concentrations [115]. Administration of ursodeoxycholic acid to dogs for the treatment of hepatobiliary disease has been shown to minimally increase SBA concentrations, usually still within the reference interval [117].

In dogs and cats, both fasting (preprandial) and postprandial samples are recommended for bile acid assays in order to provide the most reliable information. A standard procedure is the following:

1. The patient is fasted for 12 hours before collection of the first (fasting) serum sample.

2. A fat-containing diet of adequate volume and containing adequate fat to stimulate cholecystokinin secretion by the small intestine and subsequent gallbladder contraction is fed. Growth diets with higher fat content are recommended. In animals with potential hepatic encephalopathy, a restricted-protein diet can be used but should be supplemented with corn oil to increase the fat content to approximately 5%.

3. A serum sample is collected at 2 hours after feeding (postprandial sample).

4. Both fasting and postprandial bile acid concentrations are measured.

Fasting bile acid concentrations of >20 μmol/L and postprandial bile acid concentrations of >25 μmol/L are very specific for liver disease in dogs and cats [115]. A fasting bile acid concentration of <5 μmol/L is normal in dogs and cats, and concentrations between 5 and 20 μmol/L are suggestive of hepatic disease. However, fasting bile acid concentrations as great as 20 μmol/L occasionally occur in normal dogs and cats. Fasting bile acid concentrations between 5 and 20 μmol/L in dogs and cats should be interpreted in light of the patient history, clinical signs, and results of diagnostic imaging as well as other laboratory tests for hepatic disease or function.

In dogs, increased SBA concentrations can occur with a variety of liver diseases, including portosystemic shunts, hepatic microvascular dysplasia, cholestasis, cirrhosis, necrosis, hepatitis, hepatic lipidosis, glucocorticoid hepatopathy, and neoplasia [118, 119]. Exaggerated increases in postprandial bile acid concentrations are most consistent and marked in animals with portosystemic shunts [115]. However, defining the type of liver disease on the basis of the bile acid concentrations alone is not possible. Abnormal bile acid concentrations are an indication for further testing (e.g., liver biopsy, radiologic studies, ultrasound) aimed at identifying the specific type of liver disease that is present. Dogs with hepatic microvascular dysplasia may have subtle clinical signs and normal portograms but do have increases in SBAs; liver biopsy and histopathology is required for diagnosis [120]. Slight increases in SBA concentrations with an increased percentage of unconjugated bile acids have been reported in some dogs with small intestinal bacterial overgrowth [121]. Additionally, there is one report of increased SBA concentrations in healthy Maltese dogs [122]. The sometimes-marked increases were found with the routine enzymatic assay but not by an HPLC assay, suggesting presence of a cross-reacting substance or unusual bile acid.

In cats, increased SBA occurs with portosystemic shunts, cholestasis, cirrhosis, necrosis, hepatitis, hepatic lipidosis, and neoplasia [123, 124]. Fasting bile acid concentrations in cats with these diseases are less consistently increased than are postprandial concentrations, and measuring both is desirable.

Postprandial bile acid concentrations are occasionally lower than fasting bile acid concentrations in dogs and cats. This may result from spontaneous emptying of the gallbladder during the fasting period or to differences in gastrointestinal variables (gastric emptying time, intestinal transit time, intestinal flora) or the release of/response to cholecystokinin [115].

In horses, ruminants, and llamas, a single sample is usually collected for a bile acid assay. Reference intervals in these species tend to be wider than those in dogs and cats. Interpretation of SBA concentrations in cattle is hampered by the periodically interrupted flow of ingesta into the duodenum, which results in considerable hourly variation (differences up to 60 μmol/L) in SBA concentrations [125]. Differences also occur between dairy and beef breeds, and among age groups and stages of lactation [126]. However, despite relatively wide reference intervals SBA concentrations are still the most sensitive test for hepatobiliary diseases in cattle [113]. Fluctuations in SBA concentrations are less in llamas than in cattle, and increased SBA concentrations have been reported in llamas with hepatic lipidosis and portosystemic shunt [127–129]. Reported reference intervals for llamas ≤1 year of age are 2–50 μmol/L, and those for llamas >1 year of age are 1–23 μmol/L [127].

In horses, the SBA reference interval has varied in different studies, but the upper limit of this interval is <20 µmol/L [39, 130]. Horses continuously secrete bile into the intestinal tract because of their lack of a gallbladder and apparent weakness of the sphincter of the common bile duct. Increased SBA concentrations are sensitive indicators of hepatobiliary disease in horses with a variety of disorders including hepatic necrosis, hepatic lipidosis, neoplasia, and cirrhosis [110, 130]. The increases in SBA concentrations observed with these diseases are often marked (40 to >100 µmol/L).

Urine bile acids

Because the liver efficiently removes bile acids from portal circulation, in health only small amounts of bile acids enter systemic circulation to be eliminated in the urine. However, when SBA concentrations are increased there are increased amounts of bile acids excreted in urine. In theory, a one-time measurement of urine bile acid (UBA) concentration compared to urine creatinine concentration (UBA:creatinine ratio) might provide information similar to assays measuring SBA without the need for fasting and postprandial blood samples. Preliminary investigations of urine sulfated and nonsulfated bile acid:creatinine ratios have been performed in dogs and cats [131, 132]. In dogs, the ratio of unsulfated UBA:creatinine had excellent specificity (100%) but relatively poor sensitivity (63%) for liver disease [131]. In cats, the ratio of unsulfated UBA:creatinine had good specificity (88%) and sensitivity (87%) for liver disease [132]. The clinical utility of these ratios for diagnosis of various hepatic disorders awaits further study.

Plasma ammonia

Ammonia (predominantly ammonium, NH_4^+) is produced largely by bacteria in the GI tract during normal digestion and absorbed from the intestinal tract into the blood. It is removed from portal circulation by the liver, where it is used for urea and protein synthesis. Alterations in blood flow to the liver or markedly decreased numbers of functional hepatocytes can result in increased blood ammonia concentrations. Blood ammonia measurement or the ammonia tolerance test may be used to assess liver function. One advantage of measuring ammonia concentrations over SBA concentrations is that blood ammonia levels are not altered by cholestasis. Additionally, increased blood ammonia concentration is considered evidence for hepatic encephalopathy, although this is not a consistent finding. Increased blood ammonia concentrations are considered fairly specific but relatively insensitive for serious hepatic disease. Increased plasma ammonia concentrations are most common in animals with portosystemic shunting of blood (either congenital shunts or shunting secondary to severe cirrhosis). Increased blood ammonia concentrations also can occur with the loss of 60% or more of the hepatic functional mass [44].

In addition to decreased clearance of ammonia from portal circulation, as occurs with portosystemic shunting or decreased functional hepatic mass, there are additional situations in which blood ammonia concentrations may be increased. Increased ammonia intake and/or production have been documented in cattle with urea toxicosis or ingestion of contaminated feed [133, 134]. Strenuous exercise has been shown to increase ammonia levels in dogs and horses [135–137]. Intestinal disease in horses has occasionally been associated with increased ammonia concentrations and signs of hepatic encephalopathy [138–140]. Irish wolfhound puppies may have transient hyperammonemia that disappears in adulthood; however, Irish wolfhounds also have an increased incidence of inherited portosystemic shunts [141]. Finally, there are rare instances of inherited or acquired urea cycle defects that may cause hyperammonemia [108].

Ammonia concentrations are typically measured in plasma using an enzymatic method available in commercial laboratories. Ammonia concentrations in blood are very unstable after collection, however, which has been a deterrent to routine use of this test [142]. A procedure for the collection and storage of plasma for an ammonia assay is as follows [108]:

1. Simple-stomached animals are fasted for at least 8 hours before sampling.

2. Blood is collected and placed into EDTA or ammonia-free heparin anticoagulant, placed in an ice bath, and the plasma separated immediately (within 10 minutes). There should be minimal exposure to air. Delayed separation of plasma or storage at room temperature will cause falsely increased ammonia concentrations.

3. Plasma is refrigerated (4 °C) and assayed within 30–60 minutes.

Point-of-care analyzers that utilize whole blood samples have increased the usefulness of blood ammonia assays in clinical situations by eliminating the issues related to proper sample handling for timely delivery of plasma to a commercial laboratory [143, 144]. However, reference intervals for these point-of-care methods may need to be adjusted in order to minimize false-negative test results [143].

Assaying blood ammonia concentrations following administration of ammonium chloride (ammonia tolerance test) increases the diagnostic accuracy of the test [44, 145]. The ammonia tolerance test is usually performed on animals in which portosystemic shunt or decreased hepatic function are suspected but other tests are equivocal and fasting ammonia concentrations are normal. Ammonia tolerance tests should never be performed on animals with fasting hyperammonemia, as dangerously high blood ammonia concentrations may result causing acute ammonia toxicity. Ammonia tolerance tests involving both oral and rectal administration of ammonium chloride have been described.

A suggested procedure for the oral ammonia tolerance tests is as follows [44]:

1. A fasting (preadministration) heparinized (ammonia-free heparin) blood sample is obtained and processed as previously described.

2. Ammonium chloride solution (20 mg/mL) at a dosage of 100 mg/kg body weight is administered via a stomach tube.
3. A total dose of 3 g should not be exceeded.
4. A 30-minute postadministration heparinized blood sample is collected and processed.

The preadministration to postadministration increase of blood ammonia in normal dogs is from 2.0- to 2.5-fold. Most dogs with portosystemic shunts or severe hepatic insufficiency have postadministration increases of 3- to 10-fold.

A postprandial ammonia tolerance test has also been described for dogs, in which food instead of ammonium chloride is used as the challenge material [146]. This test had a sensitivity of 91% for detection of portosystemic shunts in dogs when the postadministration sample was collected 6 hours after feeding. However, it was not useful for detecting other liver diseases.

Albumin

Liver is the site of all albumin synthesis. Hypoalbuminemia usually is not noted until 60–80% of hepatic function is lost. There appear to be some species differences, however, in the incidence of hypoalbuminemia accompanying liver disease. Hypoalbuminemia is quite common in dogs with chronic liver diseases (>60% have hypoalbuminemia), but it does not appear to be as common in horses with chronic liver diseases (~20% have hypoalbuminemia) [35, 147, 148]. Many nonhepatic factors can influence blood albumin concentrations (see Chapter 30).

Globulins

Liver is the site of synthesis for the majority of globulins, with the exception of immunoglobulins synthesized in lymphoid tissue. Hepatic failure can result in decreased synthesis and, therefore, decreased serum concentrations of these globulins. However, globulin concentration usually does not decrease as much as the albumin concentration, and so the albumin: globulin ratio commonly decreases in hepatic failure. In many cases, globulin concentrations may increase with chronic liver disease, either as a result of increased acute phase protein production or immunoglobulin production [149]. This has been especially well documented for horses, in which more than 50% of those with chronic hepatic disease also have increased globulin concentrations [147]. In animals with severe liver disease, the clearance of foreign proteins by the Kupffer cells of the liver is theorized to be decreased. Such foreign proteins are thought to be absorbed from the intestine and carried to the liver by the portal circulation. Thus, when Kupffer cells fail to efficiently clear these proteins on their first passage through the liver, they come in contact with the immune system in other parts of the body resulting in an immune response and hyperglobulinemia.

Glucose

The liver plays a key role in glucose metabolism. Glucose that has been absorbed by the small intestine is transported to the liver via the portal circulation and then enters hepatocytes. The hepatocytes convert glucose to glycogen, which helps to regulate the blood glucose concentration. Hepatocytes also synthesize glucose via gluconeogenesis and release stored glucose via glycogenolysis. In animals with hepatic failure, glucose concentrations can vary from decreased to increased. Increased glucose concentrations may occur because of decreased hepatic glucose uptake, resulting in prolonged postprandial hyperglycemia. Conversely, decreased glucose concentrations may occur because of reduced hepatocytic gluconeogenesis or glycogenolysis. The liver has tremendous reserve capacity for maintaining normal blood glucose levels; 70% hepatectomy does not result in hypoglycemia [149].

Urea

Urea is synthesized by hepatocytes from ammonia. In animals with liver failure, the decrease in functional hepatic mass results in decreased conversion of ammonia to urea. Consequently, the blood ammonia concentration increases, and the blood urea (also known as BUN) concentration decreases. However, blood urea concentrations also may decrease because of numerous other disorders (see Chapter 24).

Cholesterol

Bile is a major route of cholesterol excretion from the body. Therefore, interference with bile flow (cholestasis) can result in increased serum cholesterol concentrations (hypercholesterolemia). Many other nonhepatic disorders, however, also can result in hypercholesterolemia (see Chapter 32).

The liver is also a major site of cholesterol synthesis. In some forms of hepatic failure, decreased cholesterol synthesis can lead to decreased blood cholesterol concentrations (hypocholesterolemia). The balance between decreased cholesterol synthesis and decreased cholesterol excretion varies with different types of liver disease. If decreased synthesis of cholesterol is the major alteration in hepatic failure, hypocholesterolemia can result; if cholestasis is the major alteration, hypercholesterolemia may occur. Many dogs and cats with portosystemic shunts (60–70%) have hypocholesterolemia [150]. However, many animals with liver failure have normal serum cholesterol concentrations.

Coagulation factors

The liver plays a central role in the regulation of coagulation as the sole source of synthesis for the majority of coagulation factors; it also produces anticoagulants such as antithrombin, protein C and protein S [33]. In addition, the blockage of bile flow can result in decreased absorption of vitamin K leading to decreased function of the vitamin K–dependent coagulation factors (factors II, VII, IX, and X) and anticoagulants (proteins C and S). Therefore, defects in both hemostasis and finbrinolysis may occur in animals with liver disease [149]. Accordingly, animals with liver disease may have abnormalities in a variety of coagulation tests including prothrombin time, activated partial thromboplastin time, antithrombin activity, protein C activity, and fibrinogen concentrations [151–156]. Although coagulation test abnormalities are frequent, clinical bleeding tendencies are recognized less often [153, 155, 157]. Platelet abnormalities including thrombocytopenia and decreased platelet function may also be associated with liver disease [33, 149]. Animals with evidence of liver disease and coagulation abnormalities have the potential for serious complications such as disseminated intravascular coagulation (DIC), and should be fully evaluated using the tests discussed in Chapter 17.

Patterns of laboratory abnormalities for specific diseases

The spectrum and potential magnitude of changes in laboratory test results for selected liver diseases are summarized in Table 27.1. The most common changes in different types of liver diseases are listed but one should be aware that there is a great deal of overlap.

Portosystemic shunt

Portosystemic shunting of blood can be acquired because of severe cirrhosis, and if this is the case, test results similar to those described for end-stage liver disease are expected. Early congenital portosystemic shunts usually do not produce much active hepatocyte damage. Consequently, leakage enzyme activities often are normal or only slightly increased. Cholestasis is not a feature of congenital portosystemic shunts; consequently increased production of ALP and GGT does not occur. However, because congenital shunts most commonly occur in young animals with growing bones, mildly increased serum ALP activity (due to BALP) is common. Because portal circulation to the liver is impaired, increased fasting or postprandial bile acid concentrations and increased blood ammonia concentrations are common. While fasting SBA increases may be marginal, postprandial SBA increases are often marked. The decreased hepatic blood flow can cause hepatic atrophy and decreased functional hepatic mass. Therefore, other tests of hepatic function may become abnormal in more chronic cases. Microcytosis, with or without mild anemia, is a relatively common hematologic finding in dogs with portosystemic shunts. The pathogenesis is uncertain, but abnormal iron metabolism associated with altered iron transport has been implicated [158–160].

Hepatic necrosis

Hepatic necrosis can vary from focal to multifocal to diffuse. Focal to multifocal hepatic necrosis can result in increased activities of leakage enzymes, but these increases are less frequent and of lesser magnitude than those resulting from diffuse necrosis. Focal necrosis usually does not cause significant cholestasis, and induced enzyme activities usually remain normal. Diffuse necrosis is more likely to compromise the flow of bile and cause cholestasis, resulting in induced enzyme activity increases. Bile acid concentrations usually are not affected by focal necrosis, but diffuse necrosis can produce increases in SBA concentrations because of decreased hepatocyte removal of bile acids from the portal circulation as well as cholestasis. Similarly, other tests of hepatic function are not affected by focal necrosis, but if more than 60–80% of the hepatic mass is lost because of diffuse necrosis, results of liver function tests (i.e., albumin, BUN, glucose, cholesterol, coagulation) may be abnormal.

Infiltrative disease, such as lymphoma or other hematopoietic cell neoplasia, can cause laboratory changes similar to those seen with diffuse necrosis. Modest increases in leakage enzyme activities may occur, with variable increases in induced enzyme activities depending on the degree of cholestasis. Liver function may eventually become impaired in advanced cases of infiltrative disease.

Hypoxia or mild toxic damage

Hypoxia (due to conditions such as anemia, hepatic congestion, heart or lung disease, and chronic tracheal collapse [161]) or mild toxic damage (possibly secondary to endotoxins, mycotoxins, or other toxicants) can result in mild injury to many hepatocytes. As a result, leakage enzyme activities can be mildly to moderately increased. Generally cholestasis does not occur, and the activities of induced enzymes usually are normal. However, cell swelling may occur and if it is severe enough, swollen hepatocytes can impinge on bile canaliculi and cause cholestasis as well as increased activities of induced enzymes. This cholestasis usually is not severe enough to result in increased serum bilirubin concentrations but may cause mild increases of SBA concentrations.

Focal lesions

Focal lesions such as abscesses, infarcts, or localized neoplasms may only cause local hepatocyte damage, in which case the activities of leakage enzymes are normal or mildly increased. The activities of these enzymes depend on the time and the extent of hepatocyte damage. Expansion of abscesses or neoplasms into the surrounding tissue may be slow and result in only a few hepatocytes being damaged during any given period of time. Activities of induced enzymes usually are normal but may be increased if the focal lesion causes significant cholestasis. Serum bilirubin or SBA concentrations occasionally are increased, however, the pathogenesis is not clear; focal lesions seldom occlude bile ducts that are large enough to interfere significantly with bile flow. Other tests of hepatic function usually are normal, because 60–80% of the hepatic mass is not lost with focal lesions.

Table 27.1 Common laboratory findings for various hepatic diseases.

Disorder	Leakage enzymes (ALT, AST)	Induced enzymes (ALP, GGT)	Bilirubin	Serum bile acids	Other function tests	Miscellaneous
Congenital portosystemic shunt	N to ↑	ALP = N to ↑ (due to BALP in young animals)	N	Fasting = N to ↑↑ Postprandial = ↑↑ to ↑↑↑	Ammonia = N to ↑ Albumin = N to ↓ BUN = N to ↓ Glucose = N to ↓ Cholesterol = N to ↓ Protein C = ↓ PT = N to prolonged	RBC microcytosis (60–70% of dogs) Ammonium biurate crystalluria
Necrosis – focal to multifocal	N to ↑↑	N	N	N	N	
Necrosis – diffuse, or infiltrative disease	↑↑ to ↑↑↑	N to ↑↑	N to ↑↑	Fasting = N to ↑↑ Postprandial = N to ↑↑	Variable	
Hypoxia or mild toxic insult	↑ to ↑↑	N to ↑	N	Fasting = N to ↑ Postprandial = N to ↑	N	
Focal abscesses, infarcts, neoplasms	N to ↑	N to ↑↑	N to ↑	Fasting = N to ↑ Postprandial = N to ↑	N	
Hepatic lipidosis (diffuse, cats)	N to ↑↑↑	ALP = N to ↑↑↑ GGT = N to ↑	N to ↑↑↑	Fasting = N to ↑↑↑ Postprandial = ↑ to ↑↑↑	PT, APTT = N to prolonged BUN = N to ↓	RBC poikilocytosis
Steroid hepatopathy (dogs)	N to ↑↑	↑ to ↑↑↑	N to ↑	Fasting = N to ↑ Postprandial = N to ↑	N	
Bile duct obstruction, cholangiohepatitis, cholangitis	↑ to ↑↑	ALP = ↑ to ↑↑↑ GGT = N to ↑↑↑	N to ↑↑↑	Fasting = N to ↑↑↑ Postprandial = ↑ to ↑↑↑	Variable PT, APTT prolonged if vit. K deficient	
Chronic liver disease or diffuse neoplasia	N to ↑↑	N to ↑↑↑	N to ↑↑	Fasting = N to ↑↑↑ Postprandial = N to ↑↑↑	Variable	
End-stage liver (liver failure)	N to ↑↑	N to ↑↑↑	↑↑ to ↑↑↑	Fasting = N to ↑↑↑ Postprandial = N to ↑↑↑	Ammonia = N to ↑ Albumin = N to ↓ BUN = N to ↓ Glucose = N to ↓ Cholesterol = N to ↓ Protein C = ↓ PT, APTT prolonged	

N, Normal; PT, prothrombin time; APTT, activated partial thromboplastin time.

CHAPTER 27

Hepatic lipidosis

Hepatic lipidosis occurs in many species, but the syndrome has been documented best in cats [26]. Serum activities of leakage enzymes (ALT, AST) are mildly to markedly increased in 70–90% of cats with hepatic lipidosis, likely from marked lipid accumulation in hepatocytes. More than 80% of cats with hepatic lipidosis have increased serum ALP activity, varying from mild to marked, whereas only approximately 16% have increased serum GGT activity [82]. However, cats with underlying necroinflammatory disorders may have relatively greater GGT activity compared to ALP activity [26]. Serum activities of these induced enzymes are most likely increased because lipid-laden hepatocytes impinge on bile canaliculi, with resultant cholestasis. The serum bilirubin concentrations are increased to some degree in the majority of cats (75–95%), probably because of cholestasis, and most cats have increased SBA concentrations. Other tests of hepatic function are inconsistently abnormal. If diabetes mellitus is the underlying problem in cats with hepatic lipidosis, blood glucose concentrations may be very high. Coagulation abnormalities (prolonged prothrombin time or activated partial thromboplastin time) occur in 25–40% of cats with hepatic lipidosis.

Steroid hepatopathy

Steroid hepatopathy is most common in dogs and can produce moderate damage to hepatocytes, largely due to distention of hepatocytes from glycogen accumulation. The serum activities of leakage enzymes usually are mildly increased in dogs with steroid hepatopathy, while serum activities of induced enzymes may be markedly increased because of corticosteroid-mediated induction of their synthesis. Serum bile acids may be modestly increased but total bilirubin concentration is rarely increased, and other tests of hepatic function are usually normal.

Biliary abnormalities

Cholangitis, cholangiohepatitis, and extrahepatic bile duct obstruction can occur in many different species. Because lesions usually are centered in the portal areas of the liver or outside of the liver, increased serum activities of leakage enzymes usually are mild and result from secondary damage to hepatocytes caused by increased intrabiliary pressure. The serum activities of induced enzymes are markedly increased and become progressively higher as the disease becomes more severe. Increased intrabiliary pressure induces hepatocytes and biliary epithelial cells to produce increased amounts of these enzymes. Serum bilirubin concentrations are moderately to markedly increased because of the blockage of bile flow. Both fasting and postprandial serum bile acid concentrations are usually increased and sometimes markedly so, resulting from the blockage of bile flow. Other tests of hepatic function are usually normal, unless these diseases progress to end-stage liver disease.

Chronic progressive liver diseases

Chronic progressive liver diseases can occur in many species but are most common in dogs. Moderate to severe inflammation is a common feature, and variable degrees of hepatocyte necrosis, fibrosis, and cirrhosis may also occur. Some cases of chronic hepatitis are associated with abnormal copper accumulation in the liver. Bedlington terriers have a well-described hereditary disorder resulting in hepatic copper accumulation and chronic hepatitis; the molecular defect in this disorder has been characterized [162]. A variety of other dog breeds have been identified that seem to have a predisposition to hepatic copper storage and chronic hepatitis, including West Highland white terriers, Skye terriers, Doberman pinschers, Dalmatians, and Labrador retrievers [163, 164]. Certain drugs (e.g., anticonvulsants) and infectious agents also may cause chronic hepatitis in dogs. Serum activities of leakage enzymes often are mildly or moderately increased because of progressive hepatocyte damage. If progression of the disease is slow, the release of these enzymes within a given period of time may be minimal, and serum activity may not increase. Many of these diseases ultimately result in varying degrees of hepatic fibrosis that may compromise bile flow. Therefore, serum activities of induced enzymes are often mildly or moderately increased. Serum bilirubin concentrations are normal in animals with the early, less severe forms but can be increased in those with later, more advanced disease. Fasting and postprandial SBA concentrations are inconsistently increased, depending on how far the disease has advanced. These increases probably relate to impaired blood flow to the liver, impaired clearance of bile acids by hepatocytes, and cholestasis. Other tests of hepatic function are normal, unless the disease has resulted in the loss of 60–80% of functional capacity. The coagulation status of dogs with chronic liver disease can be variable, with laboratory abnormalities suggestive of both hypo- and hypercoagulability. When evaluated with thromboelastography, which measures the dynamics of clot formation, 7 of 21 and 5 of 21 dogs with chronic hepatopathy were found to be hypercoagulable and hypocoagulable, respectively [165].

End-stage liver disease

End-stage liver disease occurs when more than 60–80% of the hepatic functional mass has been lost. The serum activities of leakage enzymes are normal to moderately increased. Normal serum activities of these enzymes may result from markedly decreased numbers of hepatocytes or minimal active hepatocyte damage. Serum activities of induced enzymes are moderately to markedly increased because of cholestasis. Serum bilirubin concentrations are usually moderately to markedly increased. Fasting or postprandial SBA concentrations are increased, and sometimes markedly so, resulting from decreased hepatic blood flow, impaired hepatocyte uptake of bile acids from portal blood, and cholestasis. Many other hepatic function tests are often abnormal, including increased blood ammonia concentrations, decreased blood glucose concentrations, decreased blood urea (BUN) concentrations, and decreased serum albumin concentrations. Serum globulin concentrations vary from mildly decreased to increased. Coagulation tests are also often abnormal in animals with end-stage liver disease.

Summary

Biochemical testing can suggest three basic categories of liver disease depending upon the pattern of abnormalities observed: hepatocellular injury, cholestasis, and decreased function. However, characterization of the specific type of liver disease usually requires additional tests (e.g., radiographic studies, ultrasound, liver fine needle aspirate, liver biopsy). If serum enzyme activity greater than 2× URL is persistently increased for more than 4–8 weeks, serum bile acids should be determined. If bile acids are increased, additional testing as previously described should be performed. Additionally, careful attention must be paid to the patient's clinical history, current medications, and physical examination findings in order to rule-out underlying conditions that could affect test results. Repeated biochemical testing is often useful for evaluating disease progression or response to therapy.

28 Laboratory Evaluation of the Pancreas and Glucose Metabolism

Robin W. Allison
Department of Veterinary Pathobiology, Oklahoma State University College of Veterinary Medicine, Stillwater, OK, USA

The pancreas is a compound organ with both exocrine and endocrine functions. The exocrine pancreas is composed of glandular epithelium that forms acinar lobules comprising about 80% of the pancreas [1], and the endocrine cells are concentrated in the islets of Langerhans.

The exocrine pancreas

The primary function of the exocrine pancreas is the synthesis and secretion of digestive enzymes. These enzymes include proteases that are stored in acinar cell zymogen granules and secreted as inactive proenzymes (e.g. trypsinogen, chymotrypsinogen, proelastase, and procarboxypeptidases), lipase, which hydrolyzes lipids; and amylase, which hydrolyzes starches [2]. The inactive proenzymes become activated by enzymatic cleavage of a small peptide (activation peptide). Normally, trypsinogen is cleaved by enterokinase in the intestine to form trypsin and trypsinogen activation peptide (TAP); trypsin then activates other proenzymes [3]. Unlike the proteases, amylase and lipase are secreted in active form [2].

Two major disorders of the exocrine pancreas can be detected by laboratory evaluation:

- Injury to the pancreatic parenchyma, usually due to pancreatitis. Inflammation may result in the premature activation and leakage of pancreatic enzymes into the pancreatic interstitium, peritoneal cavity, and vasculature. Pancreatitis is recognized most commonly in dogs and cats and may be acute or chronic. Intraperitoneal release of pancreatic enzymes causes tissue damage in the area of the pancreas, thereby increasing both the severity and the extent of the inflammation. Subsequent release of inflammatory mediators can result in a systemic inflammatory response [4].
- Exocrine pancreatic insufficiency (EPI), a disorder resulting in insufficient production and secretion of pancreatic enzymes. EPI is due to loss of pancreatic acinar cells and results in inadequate digestive function (maldigestion). The clinical signs are similar to intestinal disorders that result in inadequate absorption of adequately digested nutrients (malabsorption). Laboratory testing to differentiate maldigestion and malabsorption is discussed in Chapter 29.

Detection of pancreatic injury

The diagnosis of pancreatitis can be extremely difficult to establish, especially in cases of chronic or mild disease. Dogs with acute pancreatitis frequently exhibit vomiting and abdominal pain, but these clinical signs are less common in cats [4]. Cats seem to develop chronic pancreatitis more frequently than acute disease [5]. Necropsy studies indicate subclinical chronic pancreatitis occurs more often in both dogs and cats than previously appreciated [6–8]. Although most cases of pancreatitis are considered idiopathic, various risk factors have been identified. Some dog breeds (miniature schnauzers, Yorkshire terriers) seem to be at increased risk [8]. Idiopathic hyperlipidemia is also common in miniature schnauzers, and hyperlipidemia frequently occurs with acute canine pancreatitis; whether hyperlipidemia is a cause or effect of the pancreatitis is not clear [3]. Other risk factors in dogs include obesity, high fat diets, a wide variety of drugs, zinc toxicosis, hypercalcemia, trauma, ischemia, biliary tract obstruction, neoplasia, and infectious agents [3]. In cats, many cases of pancreatitis have been associated with inflammatory diseases of the bowel and biliary tract (often referred to as triaditis) [5, 9, 10]. Trematode infections of the liver or pancreas can cause pancreatitis [11–13]. Other risk factors in cats are similar to those in dogs [8, 14].

Because clinical signs are nonspecific and highly variable depending upon disease severity, laboratory testing, imaging studies, and sometimes pancreatic fine-needle aspiration (FNA) cytology or biopsy are employed to confirm the diagnosis. Many laboratory tests for pancreatitis have been developed, but most have significant limitations.

Veterinary Hematology, Clinical Chemistry, and Cytology, Third Edition. Edited by Mary Anna Thrall, Glade Weiser, Robin W. Allison and Terry W. Campbell.

Companion website: www.wiley.com/go/thrall/veterinary

Historically, serum activities of enzymes such as amylase and lipase were measured, but such tests have poor sensitivity and specificity for pancreatitis (discussed later). However, immunodiagnostic methods have greater utility, as detailed below.

Pancreatic lipase immunoreactivity

Pancreatic lipase immunoreactivity (PLI) tests are species-specific immunoassays that use antibodies to measure serum concentrations of lipase originating specifically from the pancreas [15, 16]. By contrast, older tests (discussed later) used enzymatic methods to measure serum enzyme activity of lipase, which includes lipase originating from many tissue sources (i.e., not pancreas-specific lipase) [17]. Radioimmunoassays have been developed to detect canine (cPLI) and feline (fPLI) pancreatic lipase immunoreactivity, and newer versions of these assays are available commercially (Spec cPL™ and Spec fPL™, IDEXX Laboratories, Westbrook, ME) [15, 16]. There are also rapid in-clinic tests available for cPLI (SNAP® cPL, IDEXX Laboratories) and fPLI (SNAP fPL, IDEXX Laboratories). In dogs, the sensitivity of the Spec cPL assay for the detection of pancreatitis has been estimated at 72–94% with a specificity of 66–96%, depending upon the cutoff value used and disease severity [18, 19]. False-negative results are considered more likely in cases of chronic pancreatitis [19]. Using that assay, a cPL concentration >400 μg/L is considered consistent with pancreatitis and concentrations between 200 and 400 μg/L are considered a gray zone, with retesting recommended [19]. The rapid SNAP test uses a reference spot that corresponds to the upper reference limit (URL) (200 μg/L for dogs and 3.5 μg/L for cats); if the sample test spot is darker than the reference spot the result is considered abnormal and could be either in the gray zone or consistent with pancreatitis [19]. Sensitivity in dogs has ranged between 92% and 94% and specificity between 71% and 78%, thus confidence in a negative test result is reasonably high [18]. Limited studies suggest that cPLI concentrations are minimally increased with renal failure and not affected by prednisone administration, in contrast to enzymatic serum lipase assays; however further studies in this area are needed [20, 21]. In cats, the sensitivity of fPLI for the detection of pancreatitis is 54–100%, depending upon disease severity, with a specificity of 91% [22]. Sensitivity and specificity of the feline SNAP test have not been published to date. Similar to the situation in dogs, a negative (normal) test result makes pancreatitis unlikely [19, 23]. These assays are most reliable for detection of moderate to severe pancreatitis, and currently are the most useful laboratory tests for diagnosis of pancreatitis in dogs and cats [4, 19, 23].

Serum trypsin-like immunoreactivity

Trypsinogen is synthesized only by the pancreas, and it is converted to the active proteolytic enzyme, trypsin, in the small intestine. The trypsin-like immunoreactivity (TLI) assay uses species-specific antibodies to detect both trypsinogen and trypsin in serum (hence, trypsin-like immunoreactivity). Currently, TLI assays are readily available for dogs and cats, and have been used experimentally in horses [24–26]. In healthy animals, a small amount of trypsinogen leaks into the extracellular space and then diffuses via the lymphatics into the blood. Thus, a normal serum TLI concentration is a good indicator of adequate pancreatic trypsinogen production [26].

Increased serum TLI is expected with pancreatitis due to leakage from damaged acinar cells; however, trypsinogen is cleared by glomerular filtration [27]; thus any disorder causing a decreased glomerular filtration rate (GFR) can increase serum TLI concentration. Activated trypsin, on the other hand, is quickly complexed with protease inhibitors in the blood, and these complexes are removed by the mononuclear phagocyte system [3]. The sensitivity of increased serum TLI concentration for diagnosis of pancreatitis in dogs and cats is 33–36%, less than that of PLI [4, 5]. Specificity has been reported between 65% and 90%, also less than that of PLI [4]. As a result, the serum TLI concentration is now principally applied to diagnosis of pancreatic exocrine insufficiency (see Chapter 29).

Acute and chronic pancreatitis have been recognized in horses, albeit infrequently, and an assay for equine TLI has been described [24, 28]. Information on the utility of this assay for diagnosis of equine pancreatitis awaits clinical trials. In one study, five of seven horses with strangulating intestinal obstructions had increased serum TLI, with the highest values in two horses that did not survive [24]. Serum TLI was not increased in three of three horses with nonstrangulating obstructions. Pancreatic histopathology was not performed. Plasma enzymatically active trypsin (EAT) activity has also been investigated in horses. In one study, 10 horses with acute abdominal disease and histologic evidence of pancreatic injury had increased plasma trypsin activity (mean 196 ng/mL) compared to that of three control horses (mean 28.5 mg/mL) [29].

Serum lipase activity

Enzymatic assays that measure serum lipase activity detect lipase from pancreas as well as other tissues [17]. Thus, increases in serum lipase activity are not specific for pancreatic injury. The utility of measuring serum lipase activity to detect pancreatitis varies between species. Serum lipase activity is frequently normal in cats with spontaneous pancreatitis, and therefore is not considered useful for the diagnosis of pancreatitis in this species [4, 5, 30]. Similarly, it is not considered helpful in the diagnosis of pancreatitis in horses or cattle, although there are rare reports of increased serum lipase activity with acute pancreatitis in these species [31–33]. Serum lipase activity has some utility as a screening test for detection of pancreatitis in dogs, and is frequently included on standard biochemical profiles. However, it is neither sensitive nor specific for canine pancreatitis [4, 34]. Generally, increases of serum lipase activity of greater than 3–5× the URL are interpreted as suggestive of pancreatitis in dogs, and should prompt further evaluation (cPLI, imaging, biopsy) [4]. However, in one study of dogs with fatal acute pancreatitis, serum lipase activity was increased in only 16 of 41 cases [35]. In dogs, increased serum lipase activity can result from a variety of conditions other than pancreatitis, including:

- Decreased GFR. Dogs with prerenal, renal, or postrenal azotemia can have increased serum lipase activity due to decreased renal excretion and/or inactivation of lipase [36–38]. Usually the increase is <4× URL, but increases up to 10× URL have been reported.
- Corticosteroid administration. Dexamethasone and, to a lesser extent, prednisone can cause increased serum lipase activity in dogs without pancreatitis [39, 40]. Increases are typically <2× URL but may be as much as 5× URL.
- Neoplasia. A variety of neoplasms involving the pancreas (carcinoma, adenocarcinoma), liver (hepatocellular carcinoma, bile duct carcinoma, lymphoma), gastrointestinal tract (lymphoma, adenocarcinoma), and heart (hemangiosarcoma) have been associated with increased serum lipase activity in dogs [38, 41].
- Hepatic disease. In addition to neoplasia, hepatic necrosis and fatty degeneration have been associated with increased serum lipase activity in dogs [38].
- Other. Gastrointestinal and hepatic tissues can be a source for serum lipase activity [42]. Increased serum lipase activity up to 5× URL has been reported in dogs with acute enteritis; however, pancreatitis was not ruled out in those dogs [43]. Mild transient increases in serum lipase activity (threefold baseline values) were reported in dogs following exploratory laparotomy that included manipulation of viscera; no histologic evidence of pancreatitis was present [44].

Serum amylase activity

Assays that measure serum amylase activity, similar to those for serum lipase activity, detect amylase from a variety of tissue sources in addition to the pancreas [17, 45]. Thus, increased serum amylase activity is not specific for pancreatic injury. In dogs, four amylase isoenzymes have been identified including amylase complexes bound to proteins (macroamylases), which have a longer serum half-life than uncomplexed amylase [45, 46].

Although serum amylase activity is readily available on standard biochemical profiles, its utility for the diagnosis of pancreatitis is limited. Cats with spontaneous or experimental pancreatitis typically have normal to minimally increased serum amylase activity, although decreased activity has also been reported [30, 47]. Therefore, serum amylase activity is not useful for diagnosis of pancreatitis in cats [5]. Increased serum amylase activity has rarely been reported with pancreatitis in cattle or horses [31–33], and may also occur with intestinal mucosal injury [48]. In dogs, increased serum amylase activity is neither sensitive nor specific for pancreatitis, and generally considered inferior to serum lipase activity as a screening test [4, 38, 49–51]. Increases of 3–5× URL may be interpreted as suggestive of pancreatitis, prompting further evaluation (cPLI, imaging, biopsy). However, in dogs without pancreatitis many of the same conditions that cause increased serum lipase activity (discussed earlier) can also cause increased canine serum amylase activity [4, 8, 36, 38, 44, 50]. The main exception is corticosteroid administration, which does not increase serum amylase activity and may actually decrease it [39, 40].

Peritoneal fluid amylase and lipase activities

If peritoneal fluid can be obtained from animals suspected of having pancreatic injury, measurement of amylase and lipase activities in this fluid may be diagnostically useful. With active pancreatic damage, these enzymes leak into the cavity resulting in increased fluid enzyme activity. Peritoneal fluid amylase or lipase activity that is higher than serum amylase or lipase activity is suggestive of pancreatic injury [31, 48, 52]. However, duodenal perforation can also result in increased peritoneal fluid amylase and lipase activities. The sensitivity and specificity of peritoneal fluid amylase and lipase activities for detecting pancreatic injury have not been determined.

Cytologic evaluation

Ultrasound-guided FNA of the pancreas for cytologic evaluation is becoming an accepted diagnostic tool, and a few recent studies have evaluated its usefulness in dogs and cats. In healthy dogs, pancreatic FNA did not cause significant increases in serum cPLI or TLI [53]. A study of 92 dogs that had pancreatic FNA for clinical evaluation estimated diagnostic yield of the procedure at 74% with few clinical complications; cytologic interpretations agreed with confirmatory test results in 10 of 11 cases [54]. In 73 cats with clinical evidence of pancreatic disease, pancreatic FNA was considered safe with a diagnostic yield of 67%; cytologic interpretations agreed with histopathologic diagnoses in seven of nine cases [55]. Results of these preliminary evaluations are promising, but additional studies are needed to further assess the safety and efficacy of pancreatic FNA.

Other laboratory abnormalities associated with pancreatic injury

None of the routine laboratory tests typically performed as part of the minimum database (complete blood count [CBC] and biochemical profile) are diagnostic for pancreatic injury, but the presence of several of these abnormalities in addition to physical findings suggestive of pancreatitis should prompt further evaluation using more sensitive and specific tests (cPLI, imaging, etc.). Laboratory abnormalities that can accompany pancreatic injury are discussed here. It is important to realize that some cases of pancreatitis, particularly chronic pancreatitis in cats, may have normal CBC and biochemical profile results [5, 8].

- Leukocytosis and neutrophilia with or without a left shift may be present. Hematologic evidence of inflammation occurs more often with severe pancreatitis in dogs (~55% of cases) and less often with pancreatitis in cats [4, 5]. Because pancreatitis can be very painful, neutrophilia induced both by epinephrine (excitement) and corticosteroids (stress) may also occur. Lymphopenia may also be present, due to either inflammation or stress.
- Increased hematocrit, hemoglobin concentration, and red blood cell count may be present if the animal is significantly dehydrated, which may occur secondary to vomiting and reduced fluid intake. Mild anemia, regenerative or nonregenerative, occurs occasionally in dogs and cats with pancreatitis.
- Azotemia, usually prerenal, is common in severe cases of pancreatitis and is caused by a combination of factors, including dehydration and hypovolemia that result in decreased GFR [4, 5]. Tubular concentrating ability is usually normal, and urine specific gravity is usually high. Urine specific gravity helps to differentiate prerenal azotemia accompanying pancreatitis from renal azotemia associated with renal failure. This is an important distinction, because pancreatitis and renal failure can cause increases in serum amylase and lipase activities of similar magnitude. In addition, the clinical signs of pancreatitis and renal failure can be similar. Analysis of urine collected at the time of blood sampling is important for animals in which pancreatitis or renal failure (or both) are possibilities; keep in mind that acute renal failure can occur in severe cases of pancreatitis. Details of differentiating prerenal from renal azotemia, including other potential causes of dilute urine in azotemic animals, are discussed in Chapter 24.
- Hyperglycemia is common in animals with acute pancreatic injury and, acutely, is the result of increased serum concentrations of corticosteroids, epinephrine, and glucagon [3]. In patients with chronic or recurring pancreatitis, hyperglycemia may be caused by diabetes mellitus resulting from islet cell injury.
- Mild to moderate hypocalcemia is inconsistently present in animals with pancreatic injury and seems more common in cats than in dogs [35, 56]. The exact pathogenesis of this hypocalcemia is not known but is likely multifactorial. Proposed mechanisms include calcium binding with fatty acids in plasma or those freed from peripancreatic fat by the action of pancreatic lipase (fat saponification), hormonal imbalances involving parathyroid hormone, glucagon, or calcitonin, and intracellular translocation of calcium [57]. In dogs with marked hypoproteinemia, hypoalbuminemia resulting in decreased protein-bound calcium also may contribute to the hypocalcemia. In one study of cats with acute pancreatitis, 19 of 46 cats had low total serum calcium, but 28 of 46 had low ionized calcium, and low ionized was associated with a poorer clinical outcome [56].
- Hypercalcemia has been reported in people with pancreatitis and has been suggested as a cause of pancreatitis in people with diseases such as hyperparathyroidism and lymphoid tumors, although the pathogenesis is unclear [58–60]. Hypercalcemia has been reported occasionally in dogs with pancreatitis [35]. One study in cats demonstrated that acute hypercalcemia increases the pancreatic duct permeability to large molecules, suggesting that pancreatic enzymes could leak and contribute to pancreatitis [61].
- Increased serum activity of leakage (alanine aminotransferase, aspartate aminotransferase) or induced (alkaline phosphatase, γ-glutamyltransferase) liver enzymes occurs frequently [3, 5]. Increased serum activity of leakage enzymes results from ischemic or toxic damage to hepatocytes secondary to pancreatic damage and release of pancreatic enzymes. Increased serum activity of induced enzymes may result from blockage of the common bile duct secondary to inflammation of tissue near both the pancreas and the bile duct. Hepatic lipidosis can occur with pancreatitis in anorexic cats and contribute to hepatic enzyme activity increases. Serum bilirubin concentration may be increased in dogs and cats with pancreatitis, particularly those with acute disease; potential causes include cholestasis (intra- or extrahepatic) and secondary hepatocyte injury [30, 35].
- Hypercholesterolemia and hypertriglyceridemia, often with gross plasma lipemia, are common in dogs with pancreatitis. Although the pathogenesis is not clear, altered lipoprotein processing is suspected, and cholestasis may contribute [62]. Hypertriglyceridemia may be either a cause or an effect of pancreatitis [63]. Hypercholesterolemia and, less commonly, lipemia have been reported in cats [5].
- Serum and plasma protein concentrations are variable in patients with pancreatitis. Exudation of protein-rich fluid into the peritoneal cavity, as a component of peritonitis, can decrease the serum protein concentration, but dehydration tends to increase the serum protein concentration. In some cases, these changes counterbalance each other.
- Disseminated intravascular coagulation can be a sequela to acute pancreatitis. Alterations in hemostatic function tests that occur with disseminated intravascular coagulation are discussed in Chapter 17. Because bile flow is essential for absorption of fat-soluble vitamins in the intestine, bile duct obstruction caused by pancreatic disease occasionally leads to vitamin K deficiency, causing altered hemostasis and abnormal coagulation test results.

The endocrine pancreas

The islets of Langerhans contain the cells of the endocrine pancreas (Figure 28.1). There are a variety of specialized

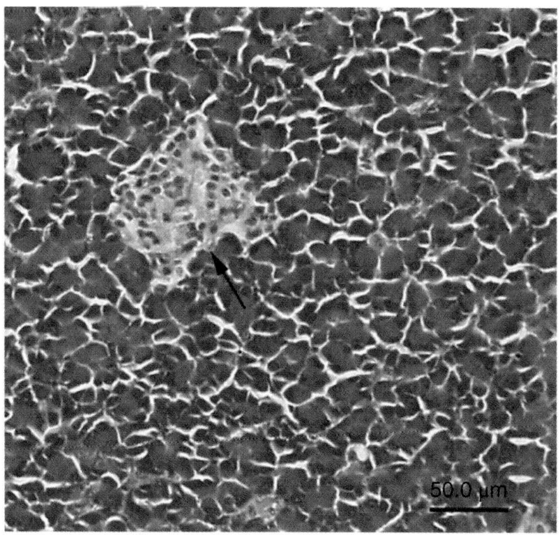

Figure 28.1 The islets of Langerhans (arrow) are the endocrine portion of the pancreas. Both deficient and excessive production of insulin by islet β cells result in abnormalities of glucose metabolism.

endocrine cells present in the islets, including α cells, which secrete glucagon, δ cells, which secrete somatostatin, and PP cells, which secrete pancreatic polypeptide. However, the most common functional abnormalities of the endocrine pancreas involve the β cells, which comprise 60–80% of all islet cells and secrete insulin [64]. Both deficient and excessive insulin production may result in serious abnormalities of glucose metabolism. Many factors in addition to the endocrine pancreas play key roles in glucose metabolism. This section reviews the major factors affecting glucose metabolism, discusses the causes of decreased blood glucose concentration (hypoglycemia) and increased blood glucose concentration (hyperglycemia), and describes tests for evaluating the status of glucose metabolism.

Glucose metabolism

Sources of blood glucose

Glucose in blood is derived from three sources:

• Intestinal absorption. Dietary carbohydrates are broken down and absorbed in the intestine. Intestinal absorption of glucose can increase blood glucose concentrations in monogastric animals for 2–4 hours after a meal.

• Hepatic production. Hepatic production of glucose results from gluconeogenesis and glycogenolysis. Gluconeogenesis is the formation of glucose from noncarbohydrate sources, primarily amino acids (from protein) and glycerol (from fat) in monogastric animals. Ruminants absorb volatile fatty acids rather than carbohydrates, and gluconeogenesis from propionic acid is a major source of blood glucose in ruminants. Glycogenolysis is the hydrolysis of glycogen to glucose.

• Kidney production. Although the liver is considered the primary source of glucose production, gluconeogenesis has also been documented in renal epithelial cells. One study in dogs demonstrated the kidney is responsible for about 30% of glucose turnover during fasting [65]. Renal gluconeogenesis occurs in the proximal tubule and is now understood to have a significant effect on glucose metabolism in both normal and abnormal physiological states [66].

Regulation of blood glucose concentration

Blood glucose concentrations are dependent on multiple interacting factors, including time since last meal, hormonal influences, and use of glucose by peripheral tissues such as skeletal muscle. Time since the last meal is important only in monogastric animals, in which food ingestion is followed by an increase in the blood glucose concentration.

Hormones affect the blood glucose concentration by regulating hepatic production and peripheral use of glucose (Table 28.1). Insulin is secreted by pancreatic islet β cells. Insulin lowers blood glucose concentrations by promoting glucose uptake by liver, skeletal muscle, and fat; by inhibiting gluconeogenesis in the liver; and by promoting the formation and storage of liver glycogen. Glucose uptake into myocytes and adipocytes is facilitated by a glucose transport protein called GLUT-4, which is translocated to plasma membranes after insulin binds to cell surface insulin receptors [64]. After a meal, approximately 1/3 of absorbed glucose is stored as glycogen within the liver, and approximately 2/3 is used as energy by other tissues [67]. Insulin also accelerates the conversion of glucose to fat, accelerates glucose oxidation, and promotes protein and glycogen synthesis in muscle. The net effect of these actions is increased hepatic and peripheral

Table 28.1 Effects of various hormones on glucose metabolism and blood glucose concentrations.

Hormone	Actions	Effect on blood [glucose]
Insulin	Promotes tissue glucose uptake Inhibits gluconeogenesis Promotes glycogen synthesis	Decrease
Glucagon	Promotes gluconeogenesis Promotes glycogenolysis Inhibits glycogen synthesis	Increase
Glucocorticoids	Promotes gluconeogenesis Promotes glucagon release Inhibits tissue glucose uptake	Increase
Catecholamines	Promotes glycogenolysis Inhibits insulin secretion Stimulates growth hormone release	Increase
Growth hormone	Inhibits tissue glucose uptake Inhibits insulin action Promotes glucose production	Increase

uptake and use of glucose, with decreased hepatic synthesis of glucose.

Glucagon is secreted by α cells of the pancreatic islets in response to insulin-induced hypoglycemia. In direct contrast to insulin, glucagon increases blood glucose concentrations by stimulating hepatic gluconeogenesis and hepatic glycogenolysis, and inhibiting hepatic glycogen synthesis [68].

Glucocorticoids increase blood glucose concentrations by promoting glucagon release, hepatic gluconeogenesis, and inducing a state of insulin resistance by affecting the ability of membrane proteins (such as GLUT-4) to transport glucose into cells [69]. The net effect of these actions is decreased peripheral use of glucose and increased hepatic synthesis of glucose.

Catecholamines (i.e., epinephrine and norepinephrine) increase blood glucose concentrations by increasing hepatic glycogenolysis, inhibiting insulin secretion, and stimulating growth hormone release [69]. The net effect of these actions is decreased peripheral use of glucose and increased hepatic synthesis and release of glucose.

Growth hormone increases blood glucose concentrations by inhibiting insulin-mediated uptake of glucose by hepatocytes, muscle cells, and adipose cells; by increasing hepatic production of glucose; and by exerting a post receptor influence within cells that inhibits the action of insulin on glucose metabolism [70, 71]. The net effect of these actions is decreased peripheral use of glucose and increased hepatic synthesis of glucose.

Extreme physical activity might result in a decreased blood glucose concentration because of increased use of glucose by tissues such as skeletal muscle. In normal animals, hormonal influences keep the blood glucose concentrations stable during most types of physical activity.

Causes of hypoglycemia

Conditions that can cause hypoglycemia are listed in Table 28.2. Additionally, delayed separation of serum from erythrocytes will result in artifactually decreased glucose concentrations (see later discussion in section on "Laboratory Evaluation of Glucose Metabolism").

- Drugs. Therapeutic insulin overdose may occur when treating an animal that has diabetes mellitus. Similarly, sulfonylurea medications such as glipizide and glyburide, which act by stimulating insulin secretion, may cause hypoglycemia. An increased insulin concentration decreases gluconeogenesis and glycogenolysis and increases cellular uptake and use of glucose.
- Extreme exertion. Hypoglycemia may occur in hunting dogs and endurance horses, if glycolysis demands more glucose than gluconeogenesis or glycogenolysis can produce [69].
- Glycogen storage diseases. These rare diseases are congenital deficiencies of the enzymes required for glycogenolysis, causing intracellular glycogen accumulation and possibly hypoglycemia. A variety of specific enzyme deficiencies have been reported in cattle, dogs, cats, and horses [72–76].
- Hepatic insufficiency/failure. Severe hepatic insufficiency or hepatic failure resulting from the loss of >70% of functional hepatic mass may cause hypoglycemia due to decreased gluconeogenesis and glycogenolysis. Other laboratory evidence of decreased hepatic function is expected to be present, such as hypoalbuminemia, decreased blood urea nitrogen (BUN) concentration, and increased serum bile acid concentration (see Chapter 27).
- Hypoadrenocorticism. Hypoglycemia occurs inconsistently in dogs with hypoadrenocorticism, likely caused by a lack of cortisol. Hypoglycemia is usually mild and probably results from decreased gluconeogenesis and increased insulin-mediated uptake of glucose by muscle tissue [77, 78].
- Hypopituitarism. Lack of adrenocorticotropic hormone (ACTH) secretion from the pituitary results in hypocortisolemia, which may cause mild hypoglycemia. Lack of growth hormone secretion may also contribute to hypoglycemia.
- Juvenile and neonatal hypoglycemia. Neonatal hypoglycemia is especially common in pigs, but it can occur in other species. It is usually associated with poor nursing secondary to diarrhea, dehydration, or hypothermia in the piglets or agalactia in the sow [79, 80]. Hypoglycemia during periods of decreased food intake in neonates results from inadequate storage pools of glycogen and protein, which could be used for glucose production. Juvenile hypoglycemia is a syndrome that usually is seen in toy breed puppies younger than 6 months [81, 82]. Clinical signs often are triggered by stressors such as diarrhea, fasting, or

Table 28.2 Causes of hypoglycemia.

Drugs
Insulin overdose
Sulfonylurea medications
Extreme exertion
Glycogen storage diseases
Hepatic insufficiency or failure [a]
Hypoadrenocorticism [a]
Hypopituitarism
Juvenile and neonatal hypoglycemia
Lactational hypoglycemia [a]
Neoplasia
β cell tumor (insulinoma) [a]
Non-β cell tumors
Pregnancy hypoglycemia
Sepsis [a]
Starvation or malabsorption
Xylitol toxicosis
Unripe ackee fruit poisoning

[a] Relatively common.

parasitism. As in neonatal hypoglycemia, inadequate storage pools of glycogen and protein probably play an important role in this syndrome. Inadequate levels of hepatic enzymes for gluconeogenesis also may contribute.

- Lactational hypoglycemia. This syndrome, also known as spontaneous bovine ketosis, occurs in cattle during periods of marked milk production [83]. Hepatic gluconeogenesis is unable to meet the demand for glucose production, and ketosis develops due to increased fat mobilization.
- Neoplasia. Neoplasms of the β cells of the pancreatic islets (insulinomas) are the most common tumors associated with hypoglycemia. Insulinomas have been reported in dogs, cats, and ferrets [84, 85]. Excess insulin production by the neoplastic β cells causes increased glucose utilization by tissues and decreased hepatic gluconeogenesis and glycogenolysis. Hypoglycemia may be sporadic but is often of sufficient magnitude to cause clinical signs of weakness and seizures. Non-β cell tumors of several types have also been associated with a paraneoplastic hypoglycemia. In dogs, many of these tumors have been mesenchymal (leiomyoma, leiomyosarcoma), but epithelial tumors (hepatic carcinoma, renal carcinoma, and others) and round cell tumors (lymphoma, plasma cell tumor) have also been reported [85]. Proposed mechanisms for the hypoglycemia include liver dysfunction, glucose utilization by neoplastic cells, and neoplastic cell production of insulin-like growth factor [86]. In horses, hypoglycemia has been reported in association with hepatic and renal neoplasia, peritoneal mesothelioma, and gastrointestinal stromal tumor [87–91].
- Pregnancy hypoglycemia. A syndrome of hypoglycemia and ketonemia may occur during late pregnancy in dogs and sheep [92, 93]. There is a decreased ability to produce glucose via gluconeogenesis, glycogenolysis, and lipolysis due to blunting of the normal responses to hypoglycemia. In sheep, this is referred to as pregnancy toxemia, which may be related to the number of fetuses and quality/quantity of feed. Pregnancy hypoglycemia appears to be uncommon in dogs.
- Sepsis. Hypoglycemia occurs inconsistently with sepsis, most often associated with endotoxemia. Experimentally, hyperglycemia occurs early, followed by hypoglycemia [94]. The causes of hypoglycemia that occurs in association with sepsis are not completely understood. Possible causes include impaired gluconeogenesis and glycogenolysis and increased use of glucose by tissues, including leukocytes. Hypoglycemia secondary to glucose consumption by large numbers of hemotropic mycoplasmas, bacteria that parasitize erythrocytes, has been reported in pigs, sheep, llamas, and calves. However, rapid bacterial glycolysis *in vitro* may also cause artifactually decreased blood glucose concentrations [95].
- Starvation or malabsorption. Decreased glucose absorption from the intestine is a rare cause of hypoglycemia. Hypoglycemia only occurs after long-term starvation or malabsorption, because gluconeogenesis helps to maintain a normal blood glucose concentration at the expense of other substances, principally protein.
- Xylitol toxicosis. Xylitol is used as a sugar substitute in various products and is a strong promoter of insulin release in dogs. Severe hypoglycemia has been reported in dogs following ingestion of xylitol-containing sugar-free products [96, 97]. Xylitol also causes marked changes in liver leakage enzymes, as described for diffuse hepatic necrosis (Chapter 27).
- Unripe ackee fruit poisoning. The ackee apple fruit is commonly found in West Africa and some islands of the Caribbean. The unripe fruit and seeds are toxic, containing hypoglycin A and B, respectively, so named for their ability to cause hypoglycemia [98, 99]. In people, consumption of the unripe fruit causes severe vomiting, marked hypoglycemia, and seizures, and may progress to coma and death. Although published reports in animals are lacking, unripe ackee fruit poisoning has been associated with hypoglycemia in dogs in the Caribbean islands (Mary Anna Thrall, personal communication).

Causes of hyperglycemia

Conditions that can cause hyperglycemia are listed in Table 28.3.

- Drugs or toxins. A variety of drugs are associated with transient mild hyperglycemia. The mechanisms of action differ. Detomidine, xylazine, propanolol, and thyroxine inhibit insulin release. Progestins and morphine stimulate growth hormone release; ketamine stimulates epinephrine release. Megestrol acetate acts as a steroid and also stimulates growth hormone release. The Somogyi effect is a paradoxical hyperglycemia that may occur in a diabetic animal in response to excess insulin administration. The actions of glucagon and glucocorticoids were described earlier (see "Regulation of Blood Glucose Concentration").
- Physiologic. Mild hyperglycemia can occur secondary to several physiologic responses. During diestrus, progesterone stimulates release of growth hormone, which decreases tissue glucose utilization. Catecholamine release (epinephrine and norepinephrine) associated with excitement, pain, or strenuous exertion stimulates growth hormone release, inhibits insulin secretion, and stimulates glycogenolyis. Cats frequently exhibit transient hyperglycemia related to struggling during blood collection; the magnitude of the hyperglycemia may reach 300 mg/dL or greater, and it may persist for 1.5–2 hours [100, 101]. A stress response, caused by endogenous corticosteroid release, stimulates gluconeogensis, glucagon release, and causes a state of insulin resistance. Corticosteroid and/or catecholamine release likely play a role in many different disease processes in which hyperglycemia occurs secondarily. Monogastric animals experience a normal postprandial increase in blood glucose concentrations that typically subsides within 4 hours.

Table 28.3 Causes of hyperglycemia.

Drugs or toxins
Detomidine
Ethylene glycol
Glucocorticoids
Glucagon
Insulin (Somogyi effect)
Intravenous glucose
Ketamine
Megestrol acetate
Morphine
Progestins
Propanolol
Thyroxine
Xylazine
Physiologic
Diestrus (progestins)
Exertion/excitement/pain (catecholamines)
Postprandial (monogastrics)
Stress (corticosteroids)
Pathologic
Diabetes mellitus
Hepatocutaneous syndrome (dogs)
Hyperammonemia (horses and cattle)
Metabolic syndrome (horses)
Milk fever (cattle)
Moribund animals
Neoplasia — acromegaly, glucagonoma, hyperadrenocorticism, pheochromocytoma, hyperthyroidism, hyperpituitarism
Pancreatitis
Proximal duodenal obstruction (cattle)

The magnitude of increase may be either constrained within the reference interval or result in an interpreted mild hyperglycemia.

• Diabetes mellitus. Diabetes mellitus is caused by a deficiency of insulin production or an interference with the action of insulin in target tissues, thereby resulting in abnormal glucose metabolism. Altered protein and lipid metabolism also occurs in diabetes mellitus. Diabetes is typically associated with the greatest degrees of hyperglycemia. Therefore, animals with diabetes mellitus usually have blood glucose concentrations greater than the renal threshold resulting in glucosuria. Glucosuria occurs less commonly with other causes of glucose intolerance. Diabetes mellitus has been classified according to the underlying cause as either type 1 or type 2, and by the dependence of the affected animal on insulin therapy as either insulin dependent (IDDM) or noninsulin dependent (NIDDM). These two classification schemes overlap, causing confusion regarding the types of diabetes mellitus occurring in animals. Type 1 diabetes mellitus results from immune-mediated destruction of pancreatic β cells, and animals with type 1 diabetes mellitus are insulin dependent. Type 1 diabetes is the most frequent cause of diabetes in dogs, but it has not been well documented in cats [102]. Insulin dependent diabetes mellitus can also occur secondary to other disease processes that destroy β cells (such as pancreatitis [102]) or cause β cell hypoplasia (genetic diabetes mellitus in keeshond dogs [103], and juvenile pancreatic atrophy in greyhounds [104].) Type 2 diabetes mellitus is characterized by a sluggish insulin response to hyperglycemia (i.e., decreased capacity to produce insulin) and a poor tissue response to insulin (i.e., insulin resistance). Animals with type 2 diabetes mellitus may be either insulin or noninsulin dependent. This is the most common type of diabetes mellitus in cats, but it can occur in dogs as well [102]. Approximately 70% of cats with type 2 diabetes mellitus are insulin dependent [105]. The pathogenesis of type 2 diabetes mellitus in cats is complex and incompletely understood. A consistent finding in more than 90% of diabetic cats is deposition of islet amyloid, derived from islet amyloid polypeptide (IAPP, or amylin) [106] (Figure 28.2). Pancreatic amyloidosis is toxic to β cells, causing cell death and decreased insulin secretion [106]. IAPP is secreted by β cells along with insulin, and states of insulin resistance (obesity, e.g.) cause increased secretion of both insulin and IAPP. In turn, circulating IAPP may contribute to peripheral insulin resistance. Obesity causes insulin resistance in several ways (downregulates insulin receptors, impairs receptor affinity for insulin, causes postreceptor defects in insulin action) and is considered a major risk factor for diabetes mellitus in cats [105, 107].

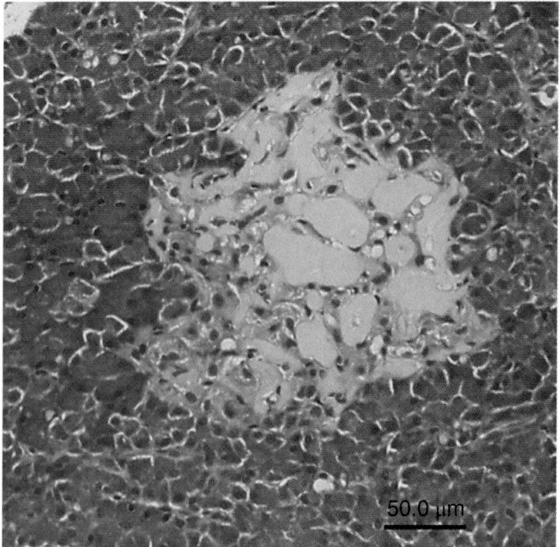

Figure 28.2 Pancreatic amyloidosis. Amyloid deposition surrounds β cells and has enlarged this islet of Langerhans. Amyloid deposition is toxic to β cells and hampers insulin secretion.

• Hepatocutaneous syndrome. This uncommon syndrome in dogs is characterized by liver disease in combination with superficial necrolytic dermatitis. Hyperglycemia is common, but the pathogenesis is not clear [108].

• Hyperammonemia. Hyperglycemia may occur in horses and cattle with hyperammonemia that is unrelated to liver disease (for example, excess ammonia production in the intestine, urea toxicosis, ammonia toxicosis). Proposed mechanisms include stimulation of gluconeogenesis and reduced tissue uptake of glucose [109, 110].

• Metabolic syndrome. Serum glucose concentrations may be increased or normal in horses with metabolic syndrome, which is a complex disorder that mimics Cushing's disease [111]. Affected horses are typically obese and insulin resistant and are prone to develop laminitis.

• Milk fever. Hyperglycemia, along with hypocalcemia and hypophosphatemia, is often present in cattle with milk fever (parturient paresis) [112]. Hypocalcemia suppresses insulin release [113]; catecholamine and/or corticosteroid release in "down" cows may also contribute to the hyperglycemia.

• Moribund animals. Hyperglycemia may occur in moribund animals, usually ruminants. Likely causes include catecholamine and/or corticosteroid release and decreased peripheral use of glucose.

• Neoplasia. A variety of neoplastic diseases can predispose to development of diabetes mellitus. Acromegaly is typically caused by a pituitary adenoma that secretes growth hormone and occurs most commonly in cats. Excess growth hormone promotes insulin resistance. Glucagonoma is a pancreatic α cell tumor that secretes glucagon, which increases hepatic glucose production. Hyperadrenocorticism, whether due to pituitary or adrenal neoplasia, results in excess cortisol production that increases hepatic gluconeogenesis and causes insulin resistance. Hyperadrenocorticism is a fairly common concurrent disorder in dogs diagnosed with diabetes mellitus [114]. Pheochromocytomas secrete catecholamines, which inhibit insulin secretion and stimulate glycogenolyis. A small percentage of cats with hyperthyroidism are persistently hyperglycemic, theorized to be due to insulin resistance; the mechanism is unknown [115]. Hyperpituitarism may be due to pituitary hyperplasia or neoplasia, with excess secretion of growth hormone or ACTH that causes insulin resistance and increased cortisol concentrations. Pituitary pars intermedia dysfunction in horses causes increased ACTH secretion and hyperglycemia [116].

• Pancreatitis. Destruction of β cells due to pancreatitis can lead to development of insulin dependent diabetes mellitus. This may be the underlying cause in up to 30% of canine IDDM cases [102].

• Proximal duodenal obstruction. Cattle with proximal duodenal obstruction may have marked hyperglycemia, up to 1000 mg/dL [117]. The proposed pathogenesis is a combination of stress and decreased peripheral glucose utilization. By contrast, cattle with abomasal volvulus have a much milder hyperglycemia, usually attributed to stress.

Laboratory evaluation of glucose metabolism

Blood glucose

Measurement of the blood glucose concentration is the initial step in evaluating glucose metabolism. After detection of either hyperglycemia or hypoglycemia, tests for more specific evaluation of glucose metabolism may be required. Analysis of blood glucose concentration can be performed by a reference laboratory and is usually part of the standard biochemical profile. Serum or plasma is the sample required by reference laboratories, and it must be separated from erythrocytes within 30 minutes of blood collection. Glycolysis in erythrocytes results in loss of 10% of glucose per hour if the serum or plasma remains in contact with erythrocytes. Sodium fluoride anticoagulant inhibits glycolysis and should be used if serum or plasma cannot be separated from cells promptly. All in-clinic clinical chemistry analyzers also have glucose methods, either as single tests or included in panels. Portable blood glucose meters (PBGMs) are also available that allow rapid and repeated measurements of whole blood glucose concentrations in clinic situations; some pet owners utilize these instruments to monitor diabetic pets at home [118–120]. Several of these instruments have been evaluated for use in animals; most of them provide results that differ to some degree from reference methods [121, 122]. In most cases (but not all), glucose concentrations determined by PBGMs are lower than those determined by reference methods. Therefore, it is important to consider test methodology when comparing results from any individual patient.

Because blood glucose concentrations in monogastric animals are increased for 2–4 hours postprandially, glucose concentrations should be measured after fasting. Dogs and cats should be fasted for 12 hours before sampling to avoid postprandial influences. Potentially hypoglycemic animals should not be fasted before sampling, however, because severe hypoglycemia may result. Horses usually are not fasted before collecting blood samples for glucose analysis; however, blood glucose concentrations might increase during a period of 2–4 hours after eating high-energy supplements. It is not necessary to fast ruminants before blood glucose analysis, because they primarily absorb volatile fatty acids rather than glucose from the gastrointestinal tract.

Artifactual hypoglycemia may occur due to *in vitro* consumption of glucose in cases of extreme leukocytosis and marked erythrocyte parasitemia with hemotropic mycoplasmas [95].

Urine glucose

Urine glucose measurement is discussed in Chapter 24. Glucosuria occurs when the blood glucose concentration exceeds the renal threshold, which varies by species. Renal thresholds are between 180 and 220 mg/dL in dogs [123],

200–300 mg/dL in cats [105], 180–200 mg/dL in horses [124], and 100 mg/dL in cattle [124]. Concurrent measurement of blood glucose is important when interpreting glucosuria; diabetic animals typically have both persistent hyperglycemia and glucosuria. Glucosuria can occur in the absence of hyperglycemia if the renal glucose threshold is decreased. Decreased renal thresholds usually result from proximal tubular abnormalities, which may be acquired or congenital. Acquired abnormalities include those caused by ischemia, nephrotoxins, and amyloidosis [125]; congenital disorders include primary renal glcosuria and Fanconi syndrome [126].

Serum insulin

Insulin concentrations can be determined in serum or heparinized plasma. These are usually immunoassays using antibodies developed to detect porcine or human insulin, but there is good cross-reactivity with canine insulin; assays should be validated for the species of interest. Serum insulin is stable for a week if kept refrigerated, and for several months if frozen [69].

Insulin concentrations are most frequently measured in hypoglycemic animals when insulinoma is suspected. Because animals with insulinoma may be euglycemic on a random blood sample, it is important to document inappropriate insulin levels at the same time that hypoglycemia is present. Normally, insulin concentrations should be very low when glucose concentrations are low. In dogs with a blood glucose <60 mg/dL, detection of insulin concentrations that are above the reference interval (usually >20 μU/mL) is strong evidence for insulinoma [85]. Insulinoma is possible in hypoglycemic dogs with insulin concentrations in the mid to upper reference interval (10–20 μU/mL). Fasting, with hourly evaluation of blood glucose concentrations, may be required to achieve the desired hypoglycemic state for accurate results. Dogs must be carefully monitored during this process to avoid life-threatening hypoglycemia. Following the test, the dog should be fed several small meals over several hours. Calculated ratios (insulin: glucose or amended insulin: glucose) are not reliable for diagnosis of insulinoma and are not recommended.

In theory, measurement of insulin levels in diabetic animals could help to classify their disease as IDDM or NIDDM. Practically, however, this has not proved to be very useful. The vast majority of dogs have IDDM with low serum insulin concentrations. Most cats with type 2 diabetes mellitus (insulin resistant) also have low serum insulin and require insulin therapy, although some only transiently. Prolonged hyperglycemia and glucose toxicity, which impairs β cell function, is thought to be responsible for this finding [105].

Fructosamine

Fructosamine is a general term that refers to any glycated protein (i.e., a protein with attached carbohydrate). Fructosamine is formed when glucose is linked irreversibly to amine groups of albumin and other proteins in the blood [127]. The serum fructosamine concentration is an indicator of blood glucose concentrations during the previous 2–3 weeks (based on the average life span of the proteins involved in this complex) [128]. Fructosamine provides more reliable information regarding the long-term state of glucose metabolism than the blood glucose concentration, which may be transiently increased in some situations. Fructosamine, therefore, has potential in establishing the diagnosis of diabetes mellitus and in monitoring therapy for diabetics.

Serum fructosamine assays are available at reference laboratories. Fructosamine appears to be quite stable in serum kept refrigerated (~10 days) or frozen (~30 days) [129, 130]. Hemolyzed samples may give erroneous results, and should be avoided. Hyperproteinemia and hyperbilirubinemia do not appear to affect test results [131].

Increased fructosamine concentrations

Increased fructosamine concentrations are indicative of persistently increased blood glucose concentrations and, in diabetic animals receiving insulin treatment, of a lack of therapeutic control of blood glucose concentrations during the previous 2–3 weeks. Because hyperglycemia is relatively common even in well-controlled diabetics, the cutoff value used for a determination of poor glycemic control is greater (typically >500 μmol/L) than the URL for nondiabetic animals (typically 365 μmol/L) [105, 123].

Fructosamine also is useful in distinguishing excitement-induced hyperglycemia from diabetic hyperglycemia in cats. Fructosamine concentrations are usually within the reference interval in cats with hyperglycemia caused by excitement, since hyperglycemia must be present for approximately 4 days before increased fructosamine concentrations are detected. The reported sensitivity of increased fructosamine concentration for detection of diabetes mellitus in cats is 93%, with a specificity of 86% [132]. The reported sensitivity and specificity of increased fructosamine concentration for detection of diabetes mellitus in dogs is 88% and 99%, respectively [133].

Mildly increased fructosamine concentrations have been reported in some dogs with hypothyroidism; however, those dogs were not hyperglycemic [134]. Prolonged albumin half-life due to decreased protein turnover is the proposed mechanism.

Decreased fructosamine concentrations

Decreased fructosamine concentrations are expected with persistent hypoglycemia, as occurs with insulinoma. However, because fructosamine is a measure of glycated proteins, hypoproteinemia may be a cause of decreased fructosamine concentrations. In one study, normoglycemic dogs had decreased fructosamine concentrations that correlated best with the degree of hypoalbuminemia, while normoglycemic cats had decreased fructosamine concentrations that correlated best with the degree of hypoproteinemia [131]. Based on these correlations, formulae have been suggested to correct fructosamine concentrations for protein abnormalities in dogs and cats. In these formulae, the reference interval median value is used for the "normal" albumin and total protein concentrations:

- Dogs: Corrected fructosamine = fructosamine × (normal albumin ÷ patient albumin).
- Cats: Corrected fructosamine = fructosamine × (normal total protein ÷ patient total protein).

Decreased fructosamine concentrations have been reported in normoglycemic cats with hyperthyroidism, likely due to increased protein turnover [135]. Decreased fructosamine concentrations in the absence of hypoglycemia or hypoproteinemia have also been reported in some animals with parasitic infections, including dogs with *Angiostrongylus vasorum* [136] and sheep with *Teladorsagia circumcincta* [137] infections. Increased protein turnover is suspected in these cases. Decreased fructosamine concentrations were reported in normoglycemic, normoproteinemic dogs (but not cats) that were hyperlipidemic or azotemic [131].

Glycated hemoglobin

Glycated hemoglobin (GHb) is formed in erythrocytes by an irreversible reaction between carbohydrates (especially glucose) and hemoglobin. GHb forms continuously during the life span of an erythrocyte; therefore, older erythrocytes usually contain more GHb compared with younger erythrocytes. The amount of GHb that is formed is proportional to the blood glucose concentration during the life span of the erythrocyte. The blood GHb concentration reflects glucose status during a longer period of time than does the serum fructosamine concentration, because of relatively long erythrocyte life spans (approximately 110 days in dogs, 70 days in cats, 150 days in cattle and horses) [138]. Increased GHb concentrations do not immediately return to normal after reestablishing more normal blood glucose concentrations, because this requires the removal of senescent erythrocytes with high GHb concentrations. Such decreases in GHb concentrations might be delayed for several weeks. GHb can be used in the same situations as fructosamine [139, 140]. However, fructosamine concentrations change faster with changes in blood glucose concentrations, which may be an advantage in many situations.

GHb is measured in EDTA-anticoagulated whole blood, and is stable for 7 days when refrigerated [123]. GHb will be decreased in anemic animals, due to decreased hemoglobin concentrations and/or increased numbers of reticulocytes present as part of a regenerative response [140]. Conversely, GHb will be increased in polycythemic animals.

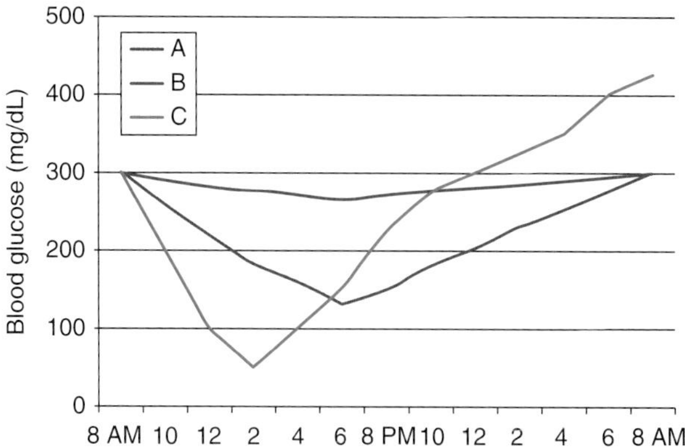

Figure 28.3 Hypothetical serial glucose curves in three diabetic cats receiving insulin at 8 AM. Cat A appears well controlled, with blood glucose concentrations reaching a nadir of about 125 mg/dL and staying between 125 and 300 mg/dL over a 24-hour period. Cat B exhibits a poor response to insulin, which may be related to insulin underdosage. Cat C becomes rapidly hypoglycemic, with rebound hyperglycemia. This is known as the Somogyi effect, which is due to hormonal responses following excess insulin administration.

Serial glucose curve

In diabetic animals receiving initial insulin therapy, measurement of blood glucose concentrations at one- to two-hour intervals throughout the day helps to assess the efficacy and appropriateness of the insulin dosage. These results, which are known as the serial glucose curve, are analyzed to ensure that the insulin therapy has lowered the blood glucose concentrations, that the lowest glucose concentration after insulin treatment (nadir) is in an appropriate range, and that the duration of the insulin effect is appropriate (Figure 28.3). Serial glucose curves are also useful when animals with previously well-controlled IDDM show clinical signs of hyperglycemia or hypoglycemia.

In diabetic dogs, the goal is to keep glucose concentrations between 100 and 250 mg/dL [123]. In diabetic cats, the goal range is 100–300 mg/dL [105]. Ideally, the blood glucose nadir should be 100–125 mg/dL for both dogs and cats. Many factors must be taken into account when interpreting serial glucose curves, including the type and duration of insulin being administered, time of feeding, and stress and/or excitement induced by hospitalization during the procedure. PBGMs are sometimes used by owners of diabetic pets to generate serial glucose curves at home, under the supervision of their veterinarian, to avoid the effects of stress or excitement [120].

Continuous glucose monitoring

New technological developments are providing advances in glucose monitoring of diabetic animals. A continuous glucose monitoring system (CGMS) utilizes a subcutaneous sensor that measures interstitial fluid glucose concentrations and stores up to 288 measurements in a 24-hour period [141]. Interstitial fluid glucose concentrations correlate well with blood glucose concentrations. Commercially available CGMS have been tested on dogs, cats, cattle and horses [142–145]. Use of these systems avoids limitations associated with traditional serial glucose curves such as repeated blood collection, patient restraint and hospitalization, and provides more detailed information about glucose metabolism since measurements are taken every 5 minutes. Brief periods of hypoglycemia and Somogyi phenomena can be easily identified using CGMS [142, 143].

Glucose tolerance tests

Oral or intravenous glucose tolerance tests can be performed to provide more information about glucose metabolism in animals suspected of having insulin resistance. These tests are labor and time intensive and rarely used in clinical small animal practice but are occasionally performed in horses that are suspected to have metabolic syndrome [146] and are used in research settings [147]. As discussed previously (see "Serum Insulin"), it is rarely clinically useful to document insulin resistance in animals that have been diagnosed with diabetes mellitus.

Basically, these tests involve administration of a glucose solution followed by blood collection at predetermined intervals; blood samples are analyzed for glucose concentrations and sometimes insulin levels. Intravenous tests are considered superior to oral tests because gastrointestinal factors are eliminated. Decreased glucose tolerance is suggested if glucose concentrations fail to return to baseline within the expected time period or if the calculated fractional glucose turnover rate is low. Insulin response tests can also be performed [148], and a test combining glucose tolerance with insulin response (combined glucose-insulin test) has been developed for horses [149].

Other laboratory abnormalities associated with diabetes mellitus:

- CBC findings may include increased packed cell volume/hematocrit and increased plasma protein concentrations due to dehydration. The leukogram may indicate stress or inflammation.
- Azotemia and dilute urine. Glomerular lesions have been reported in diabetic dogs and cats, but the occurrence of clinical renal disease in such animals is not well documented. Urine specific gravity usually is low in animals with glucosuria, generally because of the osmotic effect of glucose rather than from a defect in the ability of the tubules to concentrate urine. If dehydration is present, there may be a prerenal azotemia in addition to dilute urine, mimicking renal failure. The serum phosphorus concentration also may be increased in azotemic animals because of the decreased glomerular clearance of phosphorus. Some diabetic animals have hyperphosphatemia, but hypophosphatemia may occur in others (discussed later).
- Pyuria, hematuria, and proteinuria. Urinary tract infection is common in diabetic animals. Such infection can result in increased numbers of leukocytes, erythrocytes, and bacteria in the urine as well as in an increased concentration of protein. Increased urine protein concentration without evidence of inflammation could result from glomerular damage, which commonly occurs in humans with diabetes but is not well documented in animals with diabetes mellitus.
- Ketonemia and ketonuria. Ketones include acetoacetate, β-hydroxybutyrate (βHB), and acetone. Deficient insulin production in diabetes mellitus results in decreased incorporation of fatty acids into triglycerides (i.e., decreased lipogenesis). Fatty acids then are converted to acetyl–coenzyme A (acetyl-CoA). Almost all acetyl-CoA is converted to acetoacetate in animals with severe diabetes mellitus. Some of this acetoacetate then is converted to βHB and acetone. Increased blood ketone concentration (i.e., ketonemia) and increased urine ketone concentration (i.e., ketonuria) can result. Ketones are acids that dissociate into hydrogen ions and respective unmeasured anions. Their metabolic production therefore results in development of acidosis and increased anion gap. Impaired peripheral use of ketones because of insulin deficiency also contributes to ketonemia and ketonuria in diabetes mellitus. The renal threshold for ketones is low, and ketonuria often precedes ketonemia. The common method of detecting ketones used by urine dipsticks (nitroprusside reaction) detects acetoacetate and acetone, but it does not detect βHB. In some ketoacidotic patients, production of βHB can predominate, thereby resulting in failure to detect ketouria. Point-of-care (POC) methods for measuring concentrations in blood have proven useful in people and have recently been investigated for use in veterinary species [150–153]. In one study of 72 diabetic dogs, blood βHB concentration measured with a POC analyzer (MediSense Optium®, Abbott Laboratories) was superior to urine dipstick tests for identification of ketoacidosis [151]. Sensitivity and specificity varied with the cutoff value used for ketonemia; a cutoff value of 2.3 mmol/L had 100% sensitivity and 70% specificity, while a cutoff value of 4.3 mmol/L had 64% sensitivity and 100% specificity. The authors concluded that if the ketone concentration is <2.8 mmol/L the risk of ketoacidosis is very low [151]. A study in 62 cats using a different POC analyzer (Precision Xceed®, Abbott Laboratories) demonstrated that the analyzer was easy to use and results were in good agreement with the reference method when values were <4.0 mmol/L; concentrations >4.0 mmol/L were underestimated with the POC method [153]. In 138 diabetic cats, a cutoff value of 2.55 mmol/L had a sensitivity of 94% and specificity of 68% for diagnosing ketoacidosis using the POC analyzer Precision Xtra® (Abbott Laboratories) [154]. Causes of ketonemia and ketonuria, in addition to diabetes mellitus, include starvation, bovine ketosis, pregnancy toxemia in sheep, and hepatic lipidosis syndrome of cattle. In cattle, a meta-analysis

of 18 different studies concluded that a POC analyzer (Precision Xtra, Abbott Laboratories) had good sensitivity (95%) and specificity (98%) for detection of hyperketonemia at a cutoff value of 1.2 mmol/L [152].

• Electrolyte abnormalities. Osmotic diuresis and ketonuria cause the loss of sodium, chloride, potassium, and phosphorus in the urine. Hyponatremia, hypochloremia, and, less commonly, hypokalemia and hypophosphatemia may result. The serum potassium concentration may be normal or increased in diabetic animals, especially if the animals are acidotic, but the whole-body potassium concentration is often depleted. Potassium depletion results from hypoinsulinemia, which allows intracellular potassium to shift out of cells and into blood; this potassium then is lost via the urine. This has an important therapeutic implication because administration of insulin in treatment of the acute stage of diabetes will drive potassium back inside cells, which may cause severe hypokalemia. Phosphorus depletion results from multiple factors, including increased renal excretion, increased tissue catabolism, and in animals treated with insulin, shifting of phosphorus from the serum into cells. Serum phosphorus concentrations of less than 1.5 mg/dL may occur in diabetic dogs and cats, especially after the initiation of insulin therapy. Severe hypophosphatemia may potentially result in hemolysis, leukocyte or platelet dysfunction, neurologic disorders, and abnormal muscle function.

• Metabolic acidosis (ketoacidosis). Ketones are acidic, and increased concentrations lead to metabolic acidosis, which can be life-threatening.

• Increased anion gap. An increased anion gap usually results from increased ketoacid concentrations in the blood. Increased blood lactate concentration also can contribute to this gap.

• Hyperosmolarity. Hyperosmolarity usually occurs in animals with extremely high blood glucose concentrations (>600 mg/dL). A serum osmolarity of >350 mOsm/L can cause neurologic and gastrointestinal abnormalities.

• Increased hepatic and pancreatic enzyme activities. Metabolic alterations in hepatocytes can lead to the leakage of enzymes. Fatty change in hepatocytes results from the increased liberation of fatty acids from adipose tissue, influx of these fatty acids into hepatocytes, and incorporation of fatty acids into triglycerides. Activities of induced enzymes also increase if these alterations result in hepatocyte swelling and cholestasis. Pancreatitis can cause diabetes mellitus as a result of islet damage, and if active pancreatitis is present, serum activities of PLI, amylase, or lipase may be increased.

• Increased serum bilirubin concentration. Cholestasis secondary to the hepatocyte swelling that is associated with fatty change may lead to hyperbilirubinemia. Moreover, hemolysis resulting from Heinz-body formation can occur in diabetic cats and result in increased serum bilirubin concentrations.

• Hyperlipidemia. Increased blood concentrations of several lipids, including triglycerides, cholesterol, and free fatty acids, result from decreased incorporation of triglycerides into fat deposits, decreased hepatic degradation of cholesterol, and increased hepatic production of very low-density lipoproteins. Increased concentrations of these proteins often result in visible lipemia.

Other laboratory abnormalities associated with hyperinsulinism

In addition to hypoglycemia, the only laboratory abnormality that is frequently associated with hyperinsulinism is hypokalemia, which may result from insulin-mediated shifting of extracellular potassium into cells.

29 Laboratory Evaluation of Gastrointestinal Disease, Digestion, and Intestinal Absorption

Dawn Seddon
St. George's University, Grenada

CHAPTER 29

Introduction

Diarrhea, vomiting, and weight loss are clinical signs that are frequently seen with disease of the digestive system. These signs are not, however, indicative of a specific disease or cause. Laboratory tests that are specific for gastrointestinal (GI) disease are also limited, but tests that specifically evaluate the digestive system can provide important diagnostic information in these cases. Because many underlying disease processes can secondarily affect the gastrointestinal tract, basic laboratory tests such as a complete blood count (CBC), biochemical profile, urinalysis, and routine fecal examination are usually performed in animals with evidence of gastrointestinal disease prior to more specialized tests. Minimum data evaluating proteins, electrolytes, and packed cell volume (PCV) can provide significant information. Examples of some more specific laboratory tests used in small animals include trypsin-like immunoreactivity (TLI), pancreatic lipase immunoreactivity (PLI) [1], cobalamin (vitamin B_{12}) and folate, α1-proteinase inhibitor, canine microbiota dysbiosis index [2], etc.

Other modalities such as ultrasound, endoscopy, and/or biopsy of the affected area of the GI tract may be required to obtain a definitive diagnosis, but it must be borne in mind that there are a number of functions of the bowel such as motility, absorption, secretion, permeability, visceral sensitivity, and oral tolerance that may be compromised without evidence of structural or morphological anomalies [3]. The choice of laboratory tests to evaluate the digestive system depends on whether clinical signs are suggestive of acute or chronic disease. Vomition or diarrhea that persists for more than 3 weeks is regarded as chronic.

There are a number of breed-specific predispositions to various GI tract disturbances. In dogs, more than 400 inherited defects have been identified by molecular methods [4], using cheek swabs or whole blood. Only a few disorders are recognized in cats [5]. Knowledge of these diseases may help in the compilation of a differential list but should not be used in isolation to make a definitive diagnosis. Some of these are listed in Table 29.1.

Two important syndromes that cause signs of chronic gastrointestinal disease are maldigestion and malabsorption. Maldigestion is a failure to adequately digest food and usually results from extensive atrophy of exocrine pancreatic acinar cells, causing inadequate secretion of digestive enzymes. This is known as exocrine pancreatic insufficiency (EPI), which results secondarily in the inadequate absorption of nutrients. By contrast, malabsorption is failure of the intestinal tract to absorb adequately digested nutrients and results from a variety of small intestinal lesions. Clinical signs of these two syndromes can be similar, including increased fecal volume and poorly formed feces; however, the treatment for these conditions differs. This chapter describes the use of laboratory tests to differentiate maldigestion from malabsorption in animals showing signs of weight loss and to differentiate between EPI and other small intestinal disorders. In addition, several other laboratory tests to evaluate the digestive system are discussed.

Maldigestion and malabsorption in dogs and cats

The treatment and prognoses differ in maldigestion and malabsorption, thus distinguishing these two syndromes is important in small animals. Since malabsorption may result secondary to maldigestion, the clinical signs are similar regardless of which syndrome is the primary disease process.

Exocrine pancreatic insufficiency or maldigestion

Although EPI can occur at any age, it is usually recognized in young dogs (1 to 5 years of age). Dogs are thin, have a

Veterinary Hematology, Clinical Chemistry, and Cytology, Third Edition. Edited by Mary Anna Thrall, Glade Weiser, Robin W. Allison and Terry W. Campbell.

Companion website: www.wiley.com/go/thrall/veterinary

Table 29.1 Common breed-specific predispositions to various gastrointestinal disorders found in dogs and cats.

Gastrointestinal disorder	Breed	Notes
Antibiotic-responsive diarrhea/enteropathy [6, 7] (small intestinal bacterial overgrowth [SIBO])	Young, large-breed dogs, especially German shepherds [8, 9]	Genetic inheritance unknown Secretory dysregulation or deficiency of IgA [8, 10]
Cobalamin (vitamin B_{12}) deficiency (selective) [11]	Beagles [12]	
	Border collies [13, 14]	Puppies fail to thrive, have magaloblastic anemia and methylmalonic aciduria [13]
	Giant schnauzer [11, 17]	Autosomal recessive, with proteinuria
	Chinese Shar Peis [15, 16]	
Eosinophilic enteritis [18–21]	Boxers Chinese Shar Peis Doberman pinschers [22] German shepherds Rottweilers [19, 20]	
Exocrine pancreatic insufficiency [23]		Autosomal recessive [26]
	German shepherds	Age of onset 36 mo
	Rough collies [24]	Age of onset 36 mo
	Cavalier King Charles spaniels	Age of onset 72 mo
	Chow chows	Age of onset 16 mo
	English setters [25]	Age of onset 5 mo
Gastric carcinoma [26, 27]	Belgian shepherds Rough collies Norwegian Lundehunds	
Gastric dilatation volvulus [26]	Great Danes Irish setters	
Gluten-sensitive enteropathy [28]	Irish setters [28, 29]	Autosomal recessive clinical onset between 4 and 7 mo of age [28, 30] Weight loss with/without diarrhea [30]
Histiocytic ulcerative (granulomatous) colitis (HUC) [31]	Boxers [31–33]	Common in boxer dogs <2 yr of age [35] Genetic inheritance unknown Associated with mucosally invasive *E. coli* [31, 32, 35, 36]
	French bulldogs Mastiffs Alaskan malamutes Doberman pinschers [34]	
Hypertrophic pyloric gastropathy [26]	Lhasa Apsos Maltese Pekingese Shi Tzus Yorkshire terriers	
Inflammatory bowel disease (IBD) [36, 37]	German shepherds Shar Peis Siamese cats Soft-coated Wheaten terriers [37]	Interaction between genetic predisposition, dysbiosis [39], and dietary antigens Includes: antibiotic-responsive diarrhea [6, 7]/enteropathy, cobalamin deficiency [11, 40], gastric carcinoma [26], gluten sensitive enteropathy, granulomatous colitis [26], lymphangiectasia [41, 42], and PLEs [29, 41, 43]
	Basenjis [38]	Genetic inheritance unknown Including immunoproliferative small intestinal disease
Lymphangiectasia [41, 42]	Basenjis [38] Norwegian Lundehunds [42] Rottweilers Soft-coated Wheaten terriers Yorkshire terriers	Most common causes of PLE in dogs [41, 43] Genetic inheritance unknown
Lymphoplasmacytic enteritis [43, 44] and hypergammaglobulinemia	Basenjis [38] Boxers Chinese Shar Peis	

Table 29.1 *(continued)*

Gastrointestinal disorder	Breed	Notes
Megaesophagus [43]	German shepherds Irish setters [29] Labrador retrievers	
Protein losing enteropathies (PLEs) [29, 41, 43]	Basenjis [38] Chinese Shar Peis German shepherds Norwegian Lundehunds Rottweilers Soft-coated Wheaten terriers	Genetic inheritance unknown (the latter breed has also been documented with protein losing nephropathy [45])
Pyloric stenosis	Brachycephalic breeds [26]	

ravenous appetite, and typically have voluminous greasy, rancid, gray stools (steatorrhea), often with diarrhea. Signs of EPI generally do not occur until >90% of the functional capacity of the exocrine pancreas is lost [24]. Steiner [46] reports that lesions suggesting feline EPI have been found in 0.2% of the feline pancreata that he has examined. The most frequently reported clinical signs of EPI in cats include loss of weight, copious amounts of loose stools and oily soiling of the hair coat [46].

The serum TLI assay (discussed later) is the most common test used to diagnose EPI. There are no consistent hematological or biochemical changes with maldigestion and amylase and lipase values are usually normal in cases of EPI. Undigested fats may be found in the feces, but this is an inconsistent finding.

CHAPTER 29

A number of specific conditions are recognized:

1. **Idiopathic pancreatic acinar atrophy** is the most common cause of EPI in dogs but has not been reported in cats [47].
2. **Juvenile pancreatic acinar atrophy** is thought to be caused by hereditary immune-mediated lymphocytic pancreatitis and has been reported in German shepherd dogs and rough-coated collies [48, 49].
3. **EPI** may be acquired in dogs and cats secondary to chronic pancreatitis due to atrophy and/or fibrosis of the pancreas. There may be subsequent development of diabetes mellitus if there is concurrent islet cell destruction [50]. Chronic pancreatitis occurs more commonly in cats than dogs [51], and chronic pancreatitis is thought to be the most common cause of EPI in cats [47].
4. **Pancreatic duct obstruction** can occur in dogs and cats and may impair secretion of pancreatic enzymes into the intestine. This is usually associated with acute inflammation, but animals do not necessarily develop maldigestion. However, some cases of pancreatic neoplasia that cause obstruction of the pancreatic duct may lead to pancreatic atrophy [46, 47].

Infection with the fluke *Eurytrema procyonis* has also been reported to cause EPI in cats without previous evidence of pancreatitis, although this is extremely rare [52].

Malabsorption

There are many possible underlying causes of malabsorption, including inflammatory, infectious, and neoplastic processes. Chronic disease usually results in protein losing enteropathy (PLE). A list of possible causes of malabsorption syndromes in dogs (PLE) can be seen in Table 29.2. In young dogs with chronic intermittent diarrhea and protein loss, where hookworm has been ruled out, intussusception should be a consideration [26].

Specific function testing for intestinal absorption is not always necessary as syndromes such as osmotic diarrhea can usually be recognized clinically and signs generally tend to cease when the animal is fasted. Osmotic diarrhea is associated with water retention in the GIT, which results from the presence of osmotically active solutes in the intestine that are not absorbed. TLI testing can be used to differentiate osmotic diarrhea due to malabsorption from that due to maldigestion [3] (see later). Examples of osmotic and secretory diarrheas can be found in Table 29.3.

A variety of specialized tests, discussed later in this chapter, may be useful in cases of suspected malabsorption. Diagnostic tests such as endoscopy and intestinal biopsy rather than tests for intestinal absorption are usually recommended. Intestinal absorption tests that may be useful in the diagnosis of malabsorption include the breath hydrogen test (dogs) [76–78] or vitamin B_{12}/folate levels (dogs and cats). Orocecal transit time can be measured by means of the H_2 breath test, which has been validated in cats and dogs [79]. There are no consistent hematological or biochemical changes in cases of malabsorption, but more chronic cases may have decreased serum protein concentrations (often panhypoproteinemia) due to PLE, and lowered cholesterol.

Table 29.2 Causes of malabsorption syndromes in dogs (associated with PLE).

Disease syndrome	Breeds associated with disease syndrome and comments
Antibiotic responsive diarrhea (ARD)/bacterial overgrowth [7, 9]	German shepherds [8, 9]
Chronic inflammatory small intestinal enteropathies [26, 37, 53]	Basenjis [38], Norwegian Lundehunds, Chinese Shar Peis, German shepherds, Rottweilers, soft-coated Wheaten terriers
Defective brush-border enzymes [30]	Basenjis [38], Irish setters [28–30]
Eosinophilic enteritis [18–21]	Rottweilers, soft-coated Wheaten terriers [37, 53], Yorkshire terriers
Giardiasis [54]	See Table 29.5
Granulomatous enteritis [26, 45]	Norwegian Lundehunds, Rottweilers, and Yorkshire terriers
Histoplasmosis [45, 55]	
Intestinal lymphoma [16]/adenocarcinoma [26, 27]	Occult blood may be useful to evaluate gut bleeding in these cases
Lymphangiectasia [41, 42]	Basenjis [38], Lundehunds, soft-coated Wheaten terriers, and Yorkshire terriers
Lymphocytic-plasmacytic enteritis	Soft-coated Wheaten terriers [37, 53], Yorkshire terriers
Pythiosis [16, 45]	Pythium occurs in large-breed dogs. Can be cultured, ELISA, serology
Protothecosis [45]	
Villous atrophy [26]	German shepherds
Wheat-sensitive enteropathy [29]	Hereditary in Irish setters [28, 30]

Table 29.3 Examples of osmotic and secretory diarrheas.

Osmotic diarrheas	Secretory diarrheas
Intestinal malignant lymphoma	Endotoxemia
Johne's disease (*Mycobacterium avium* subspecies *paratuberculosis*) – cattle >18 mo of age	Enterotoxic colibacillosis
Lymphangiectasis	Salmonellosis – most commonly associated with increased sodium chloride loss induced by the enterotoxin that promotes active secretion into the gut lumen. Increased water loss follows this osmotic gradient
Magnesium cathartics	
Other maldigestion/malabsorption syndromes	
Protein losing enteropathies	
Proximal enteritis (horses)	

A failure of oral tolerance may result from food allergy that can cause acute or chronic gastrointestinal disease, which is difficult to differentiate from inflammatory bowel disease (IBD) without dietary elimination-challenge tests. Dietary trials should be a routine part of all gastrointestinal workups [3], but details are beyond the scope of this text.

Maldigestion and malabsorption in horses

Maldigestion alone is a rare cause of malassimilation in horses and maldigestion syndromes are uncommon in horses as compared with other domestic species. EPI is not recognized in cattle and horses [51], but Carlson [80] reported a few cases in ponies and draft horses where horses showed chronic weight loss and intermittent colic. Definitive diagnosis of chronic pancreatic necrosis was made on necropsy.

Malabsorption is more common in horses, and many horses with malabsorptive disease develop PLE and subsequent hypoproteinemia. A list of causes of PLEs in horses can be found in Table 29.4.

Maldigestion and malabsorption in ruminants

In ruminants, maldigestion syndromes are poorly understood and are generally uncommon. Main causes of maldigestion may be associated with changes in the rumen microflora or gastric function, overgrowth of small intestinal bacteria, or lactase deficiencies [85]. Variations in bile salt concentrations may exacerbate diarrhea in milk-fed neonates, but this does not interfere with digestion in the adult ruminant.

Malabsorption syndromes in cattle are poorly documented, but villous atrophy in calves secondary to viral infection (rotavirus, coronavirus), or cryptosporidia leads to maldigestion and malabsorption. Maldigestion results from villous destruction with subsequent hydrolytic enzyme deficiency (such as lactase) [85]. Other causes of malabsorption include congestive heart failure, which may result in localized or generalized ischemia, lymphatic obstruction, parasitism (trichostrongylosis of sheep and cattle), protein malnutrition, tuberculosis, and Johne's disease (*Mycobacterium avium* subspecies *paratuberculosis*, which can be found

Table 29.4 Causes of malabsorption and PLE in horses.

Syndrome	Examples
Biochemical or genetic abnormalities	Congenital or acquired lactase deficiency (lactose intolerance) [81, 82] Monosaccharide transport defects
Cellular infiltrates	Granulomatous enteritis [83] Eosinophilic gastroenteritis enterocolitis [21, 84] Lymphocytic, plasmacytic, or monocytic
Fungal (may be secondary to antibiotic [61] or corticosteroid therapy [85])	*Aspergillus fumigatus* [85] *Histoplasma capsulatum* [61]
Immune mediated	Amyloid A-associated gastroenteropathy [86]
Metabolic	Congestive heart failure, intestinal ischemia
Microbiological Bacterial	Chronic infectious granulomatous enterocolitis due to tuberculosis [86] Paratuberculosis Salmonellosis *Rhodococcus hoagie* *Lawsonia intracellularis* [86–89] Multiple abscessation *Clostridium* [88]
Neoplastic	Intestinal mural lymphoma [16, 90] Leiomyoma, leiomyosarcoma [84] Squamous cell carcinoma [91] Adenocarcinoma [92]
Nutritional	Dietary-induced enteropathy Zinc deficiency
Pancreatitis	
Parasitic	*Strongylus vulgaris* larvae, [93] and small strongyles – *Strongyloides westeri* (foals) causing ischemia and damage due to migration Cryptosporidia [93]
Toxic	Heavy metal toxicity
Viral (rotavirus, coronavirus) [94]	Villous damage or atrophy [71]

in cattle more than 18 months of age and can also be seen in sheep, goats, llamas and alpacas, deer and wildlife).

Screening tests in veterinary medicine

Several tests can be performed in a veterinary practice on animals with clinical signs and histories that are suggestive of digestive system disease. The results of these tests can be supportive of but are not always definitive for a specific diagnosis or etiology. Further confirmatory tests may need to be performed at a reference laboratory (discussed later).

Fecal assessment

Optimal fecal assessment involves systematic formulation of a differential list based on signalment, history, and clinical signs. The options for fecal testing surpass simple flotation for parasite ova, and it is essential to select appropriate tests for specific etiologies and to interpret them based on their relative sensitivity and specificity for the specific disease process [71]. Basic methods for the detection of parasitic ova, larvae, oocysts, cysts, and trophozoites are discussed here, but a parasitology textbook should be consulted for more detailed descriptions and interpretations of these techniques.

In small animals with vomition, fecal sedimentation or smears help in the detection of the stomach worm *Physaloptera rara,* and in cats examination of vomitus is useful for detection of feline stomach worm *Ollulanus tricuspis* [26]. In dogs and cats with diarrhea, fecal examination should include assessment for intestinal parasites (including coccidia, *Cryptosporidium, Giardia, Tritrichomonas,* hookworms [*Ancylostoma* and *Uncinaria*] and whipworms [*Trichuris vulpis, Trichuris campanula* in dogs and *Trichuris serrate* – rare in cats]) and culture for potentially pathogenic bacteria (including *Salmonella* and *Campylobacter*) [55]. In dogs, *Trichuris vulpis* is the most common cause of acute and chronic large intestinal diarrhea [34, 62, 95, 96]. Other infectious causes of diarrhea in cats include *Anerobiospirillum, Candida, Histoplasma, Pythium,* and viral (corona, feline leukemia virus [FeLV] or feline immunodeficiency virus [FIV]) associated diarrhea [62]. In young ruminants, *Yersinia* should also be considered in addition to the previously mentioned bacterial pathogens. There are numerous other nematodes and pathogens that are more species and age specific but these are beyond the scope of this text.

Feces starts deteriorating from the time a stool is passed and cells undergo degenerative changes, which makes identification difficult. Organisms such as *Giardia* and trichomonads are fragile and undergo rapid deterioration with time, refrigeration, or processing, and fecal samples that are more than 5 minutes old are inadequate for the detection of these organisms [67, 71, 97, 98]. Marks [67] suggests that feces should be less than 2 hours old, and if there is a delay in examination, the sample should be refrigerated at 4 °C [67, 68]. Nematode eggs undergo development or hatch, which makes identification difficult. Hookworm eggs tend to hatch within 24 hours in warm humid weather, giving rise to motile larvae. *Toxascaris* eggs embryonate within a few days in older fecal samples [98]. Variations in bacterial flora lead to overgrowth and sporulation of some species [71].

Fecal collection methods

The preferred collection method for fecal cytology is by means of digital rectal examination, but fecal loops are more practical for smaller animals where digital collection is inappropriate [71]. Rectal lavage may be useful for cytology, but the technique results in less fecal material with relatively more mucous secretion from the mucosal surface, and thus the amount of fecal material may be insufficient for some techniques. Flush samples have high yields of motile protozoa and bacteria as these organisms are usually more ubiquitous at the mucosal surface, whereas eggs and cysts are more common in fecal material [68].

Rectal wall scrapes [16] may be useful in cases with suspected infectious diseases of the gastrointestinal tract (e.g., *Aspergillus, Balantidium, Candida, Cryptococcus, Entamoeba, Histoplasma, Leishmania, Pentatrichomonas, Prototheca,* and *Pythium* [16]) or infiltrative disease such as inflammation or neoplasia [45]. Cell harvest from the rectal wall can be obtained by means of moistened cotton swabs, a gloved fingernail, or spatula (similar to those used for conjunctival scrapes). Slides are made by gently rolling the harvested material onto glass slides [16], which are subsequently stained with Diff-Quik® or Wright-Giemsa stains.

Voided fecal samples provide larger samples, which are required for fecal flotation, sedimentation and Baermann techniques [71]. Defecation should occur in uncontaminated areas, followed by timely collection and appropriate storage.

Adequate amounts of feces are required for various tests: 1–2 g feces is required for fecal flotation or sedimentation, 2–3 g feces are necessary for fecal culture [71], and up to 10 g of feces should be used for the evaluation of lungworm (Baermann technique) [68, 96]. Feces can be refrigerated for up to 24 hours for flotation or sedimentation techniques [71], and can be preserved in formalin for longer periods. Fecal antigen (mainly for polymerase chain reaction [PCR]) can be preserved by freezing feces [71] but culture requires transport medium [68].

Wet preparations

Wet mounts can be used to detect motile parasites (trophozoites of *Giardia* and *Tritrichomonas*). Direct smears should be carried out on fresh feces, which is ideally less than 5 minutes old [97] but not more than 2 hours old [67, 71, 97, 98].

A small sample (not larger than match head size) should be mixed with a drop of warm saline (0.9%) on a warmed glass slide with a wooden applicator stick, which is then covered with a coverslip. The smear preparation can then be examined on low power (×10) for eggs, cysts, and larvae. Other organisms may be found using higher magnification (×40). Motile organisms seen on wet mounts can also be assessed on dry mount and stained slides, but it is important not to make dry smears too thick [71], as trophozoites can be overlooked in thick smears. It should be possible to read print through the preparation. Prolonged survival of *Tritrichomonas* is facilitated by adding 3 mL of warmed 0.9% saline to 2–5 g feces. *Tritrichomonas* can be confused with *Giardia* and this misdiagnosis may often explain the lack of response to treatment. Direct smear examination for *Tritrichomonas* has low sensitivity (14%) [26].

Giardia cysts can also be mistaken for pollen grains or yeasts. Cysts are shed intermittently and numbers can vary significantly (from 1 or 2 to thousands) even in samples taken over 4 consecutive days, although the recommendations suggest higher sensitivity for examination of feces from three [16] non-consecutive stools over a period of 6–10 days [65–67]. The sensitivity for fecal flotation and examination for cysts has been quoted in a study as 85.3% in cats [72].

A list of potential fecal pathogens identifiable on wet and dry fecal mounts, including additional selected tests available for diagnosis, as well as the brief clinical implication, is presented in Table 29.5.

Fecal flotation and sedimentation

In many cases, low concentrations of parasites preclude their detection in direct fecal smears, and fecal flotation is required for examination of parasitic ova and oocysts. Samples for these tests should be refrigerated within an hour of collection, and should be sent chilled to the laboratory. The integrity of the sample for fecal flotation and sedimentation is maintained for up to 7 days in the fridge. Fecal flotation with zinc sulfate and centrifugation [99] is the most sensitive for the detection of whipworm eggs (*Trichuris vulpis*) [96]. Centrifugal flotation techniques show an 8× higher yield of organisms than gravitational flotation techniques. In dogs with large intestinal disease, presence of *Trichuris* can only be ruled out by testing at least three fecal samples, as whipworms produce eggs sporadically and in low numbers [69], and eggs are shed intermittently [95].

Other nematodes that may be found in the gut of young pups and kittens include *Toxocara canis* and *cati, Toxascaris leonina* and *Ancylostoma*.

Parasites from other organ systems may also be detected by fecal flotation, such as ova of Eucoleus aerophilus (formerly known as Capillaria aerophila) (lungworm of cats), *Oslerus osleri* (tracheal worm of dogs), and *Filaroides hirthi* (lungworm of dogs).

The typical fecal flotation technique involves mixing feces with water, removing large pieces of debris by straining the mixture, centrifuging the strained feces, followed by mixing the resulting sediment with flotation solutions composed of varying concentrations of sugar or salts, including sodium chloride [68, 98], magnesium sulfate (35%) [71], zinc sulfate (33%) [71, 96], or sodium nitrate [68, 100]. Flotation solutions are commercially available. The fecal sediment/flotation solution mixture is then centrifuged for 5–10 minutes or is allowed to stand for 30 minutes. The correct specific gravity (SG) should be maintained for flotation solutions to be effective [68]. Zinc sulfate (with an SG of 1.18–1.20) is a superior flotation solution for maintenance of the morphology of *Giardia* cysts as compared with other flotation solutions [67]. Sheather's solution [71, 96] is a sugar solution with a specific gravity high enough to float any ova. It is considered superior for isolation of most eggs and oocysts as it generally causes little distortion and it does

Table 29.5 Potential fecal pathogens identifiable on wet and dry stained mounts with other selected tests available for diagnosis.

Wet and dry preparations	Parasites	Microscopic characteristics, clinical implications, location and other tests available for diagnosis
Algae	*Prototheca* spp. [45, 55] *P. wickerhamii* and *P. zopfii*	**Microscopy:** Achlorophyllous algae – oval hyaline cells 1.2–16.1 μm long, 1.3–13.4 μm wide [55] Granular basophilic to magenta internal structure containing 2–20 or more small sporangiospores (endospores or autospores) Have a thick cell wall surrounded by a clear highly refractile capsule **Location:** Large intestine **Testing:** Feces, culture
	Pythium insidiosum [16, 45] Water mold (oomycete)	**Microscopy:** Wide, poorly staining occasionally branching pseudohyphae with parallel cell walls and occasional septae [45] Cannot be differentiated cytologically from *Lagenidium* **Location:** In stomach, small intestine, ileocolic junction **Testing:** Culture, serology, PCR
Bacteria	*Campylobacter* [56]	**Microscopy:** Spiral to rod or curved shape. Gram negative **Location:** Feces **Testing:** Culture, PCR (http://www.cvm.tamu.edu/gilab)
	Clostridium perfringens [45]	**Microscopy:** Large rectangular straight or curved Gram-positive bacilli with rounded or truncated ends, 3-8 μm × 0.4-1.2 μm, encapsulated **Testing:** Fecal enterotoxin ELISA, PCR
	Helicobacter [45, 57]	**Microscopy:** Commonly curved or spiral but some can be short, tapered rod shape, Gram negative, flagellated **Location:** Stomach (gastric mucosa) **Testing:** Culture Helicobacter may be implicated as a cause of vomition in some patients.
	Sarcina ventriculi [58]	**Microscopy:** Large Gram-positive cocci in bundles Abomasal bloat in small ruminants, gastric dilitation dogs [58]
Fungi [55]	*Blastomyces dermatitidis*	**Microscopy:** Yeast 7–15 μm, refractile, basophilic yeast with thick cell wall, with single broad-based bud **Location:** Stomach, intestine or colon **Testing:** Culture and cytopathology, antigen testing, antibody immunodiffusion, antigen enzyme immunoassays and PCR [60]
	Candida spp. [45, 56]	**Microscopy:** Yeast 3–6 μm, basophilic round to oval, clear cell wall, pseudohyphae and hyphae **Location:** Stomach intestine. Opportunistic pathogen **Testing:** Fungal culture, PCR
	Cryptococcus neoformans	**Microscopy:** Yeast 3.5–7 μm, with clear nonstaining capsule, narrow based budding **Testing:** Microscopic examination and/or culture of tissue or body fluids such as blood, cerebrospinal fluid and sputum. The cryptococcal latex antigen test is a rapid test that can be performed on blood and/or on cerebrospinal fluid
	Histoplasma capsulatum	**Microscopy:** Yeast, ovoid 2-4 μm, non-refractile walls, narrow based budding **Location:** Located in macrophages, intestine **Testing:** Fungal culture, PCR, latex agglutination
	Cyniclomyces guttulatus [45, 59] *(Saccharomycopsis guttulata)*	**Microscopy:** Oval to cylindrical yeast, 5–7 × 20 μm with a clear wall [45]. Nonpathogenic in canines that have ingested rabbit feces, but large numbers may be clinically significant in chronic diarrheas [61, 62] **Location:** Large intestine, feces **Testing:** Fungal culture, PCR

CHAPTER 29

Table 29.5 *(continued)*

Wet and dry preparations	Parasites	Microscopic characteristics, clinical implications, location and other tests available for diagnosis
Protozoa	*Balantidium* [63]	**Microscopy:** Trophozoite Oval pointed anterior end, 50–130 mm long by 20–70 mm wide Two nuclei – the macronucleus is long and kidney-shaped, with an adjacent spherical micronucleus A peristome is located at the pointed anterior end Covered in cilia – rotary motility Cyst stage is the infective stage – spherical 40–60 mm diam, thick, hard cyst wall with cilia Nonmotile **Testing:** IFA, PCR Infects dogs ingesting pig feces [55]
Protozoa	Coccidial oocysts [45, 63] Puppies: *Isospora canis, I. ohioensis* Kittens: *I. rivolta, I. felis*	**Microscopy:** Oocysts ovoid to ellipsoid in shape 10–40 μm long, 10–30 μm wide **Fecal flotation:** Sheather's sugar solution or wet preparations
Protozoa	*Cryptosporidium* [63] *C. parvum, C. canis & C. felis*	**Microscopy:** Spherical, red staining oocysts, 2–6 μm against a green or blue background – depends on counterstain. Difficult to see on smears Modified Ziehl-Neelsen (acid fast) stain **Testing:** **Concentration techniques:** Sheather sucrose or zinc sulfate flotation, saturated sodium [45] Sensitivity fecal flotation is as low as 21.4% in cats **Immunofluorescent antibody staining:** MeriFluor *Cryptosporidium* Direct immunofluorescence test kit: [56, 64, 65]. IFA (Texas A&M - fresh chilled feces, shipped on ice) Sensitivity of 77–91% and specificity of 94–95% in cats ProSpecT® *Cryptosporidium* Microplate Assay [66, 67] 71.4% sensitivity, 96.7% specificity in cats Coproantigen ELISA kit [63, 68] (PCR) [61, 69] **Polymerase chain reaction**: This is the most sensitive assay, detecting 100–1000 *Cryptosporidium* oocysts per gram of feces [69]. Occurs in young or immune-compromised adults. Can be asymptomatic or cause severe diarrhea and protein losing enteropathy. Shed intermittently *Cryptosporidium* can have up to a 6-month prepatent period [5]
Protozoa	*Entamoeba* sp. [54]	**Microscopy:** *Entamoeba histolytica* trophozoites 12–50 μm Large nucleus and central karyosome Cysts 10–20 μm, one to four nuclei Trichrome or methylene blue stains **Location:** In large intestine, feces **Testing:** Specific culture media [16] Antigen ELISA [67]
	Giardia [54, 70]	**Microscopy:** **Trophozoites** pear-shaped 15–10 μm long [45, 55] (four pairs flagella: one cranial, two posterior, one caudal) Appearance of a "smiling alien face" with two anterior nuclei, divided by a longitudinal axioneme and a posterior transverse median body **Giardia cysts** oval, 8–19 μm (average 11–14 μm) [45, 55] Immature cysts – two nuclei Mature cysts – four nuclei

Table 29.5 *(continued)*

Wet and dry preparations	Parasites	Microscopic characteristics, clinical implications, location and other tests available for diagnosis
Protozoa	*Giardia* [54, 70]	**Testing: Zinc sulfate centrifugation** of feces Sensitivity 85.3% cats [70] Specificity greater than 99.4% [70] Higher sensitivity if three nonconsecutive samples evaluated over 6–10 d [65, 67] Coproantigen ELISA kit [70, 71] **SNAP *Giardia* Antigen** ELISA from IDEXX (IDEXX Laboratories, Westbrook, ME) 85.3% [72], 92% [71] Sensitivity >99.4% [65, 66, 70]/100% [73] Increased sensitivity of 97.8% for *Giardia* when tested in parallel with fecal flotation This test detects cyst wall protein 1 The ELISA tests should not be used to monitor effectiveness of treatment, as any residual antigen present in the cyst wall will give a positive result ProSpecT Giardia Microplate Antigen ELISA (Remel Microbiology Products, Lenexa, KS) [56, 66, 72] Human immunoassays utilize different genotypes of *Giardia* to those found in dogs and cats. 91.2% sensitivity, 99.4% specificity in cats [66, 72] Direct IFA, PCR [45] Cysts shed intermittently – vary in number [54] Young kittens and puppies or immune-compromised adults Acute diarrhea may be intermittent and can become chronic (>3 wk duration) May be subclinical in adult animals, usually self-limiting [72] Feces may be transiently soft Infection usually from contaminated water May occur concurrently with *Cryptosporidium* Vomition is uncommon [73]
	Pentatrichomonas hominis [45]	**Microscopy:** Spindle to pear-shaped, five anterior flagella, one posterior flagellum, undulating membrane **Testing:** Motile in feces PCR
	Tritrichomonas foetus [54, 56]	**Microscopy:** Oval to pear-shaped, 5–20 x 3–14 μm [55] Highly motile – three anterior flagella, an undulating membrane, a longitudinal axostyle, an anterior nucleus, and a single posterior flagellum **Location:** Large intestine, feces **Testing:** Wet preparations – sensitivity 14% [26]. No cyst stage InPouch™ TF culture systems [63] (Biomed Diagnostics, San Jose, CA) Sensitivity 70–80% 0.05 g fresh feces is inoculated directly into the pouch Pouches are incubated for 24 h at 37 °C, followed by room temperature (25 °C) incubation for up to 10 d, with examination of pouches every 48 h PCR for *T. fetus* antigen in feces [55] sensitivity >90% [74] Affects young cats 3–9 months but can occur in aged cats Bengals and Abyssinian cats predisposed Foul-smelling large bowel diarrhea (colitis) but can cause diarrhea in puppies [72] May/may not cause bleeding Self-limiting but can take 2 years to resolve Some animals asymptomatic
Nematodes	*Nanophyetus salmincola* ova [75]	**Testing:** Fecal flotation
	Strongyloides larvae [63, 71]	**Testing:** Fecal flotation Can cause diarrhea in animals of all ages with anemia, colitis, weight loss, or poor weight gain

A brief clinical implication for each organism is also mentioned.

CHAPTER 29

not crystallize, but it does tend to distort *Giardia* and some lungworm larvae [67, 71].

A modified Sheather's solution (sugar) with a higher specific gravity (SG of 1.270) gives increased recovery of species with heavier eggs such as *Taenia* spp. [67]. Most parasitic ova and oocysts float to the surface of the mixture as they have a lower density than the flotation solution. They can be harvested by touching a coverslip to the surface. Microscopic observation of the material collected (×10 objective) reveals the presence of parasitic ova or oocysts, but the technique can be modified for counting ova and oocysts to assess their concentrations in feces.

The double centrifugation flotation technique [72, 101] (below) is regarded as the gold standard and is reported to have fewer false-negative results and allows higher recovery of more parasite eggs, cysts, and oocysts than passive (gravitational) flotation techniques (e.g., Ovassay®, Fecalyzer®, Ovatector®) [71, 101].

Double centrifugation/flotation technique [72, 101]:

1. Make a suspension of feces sample by mixing 1–5 g of feces, with 10–12 mL water in a beaker.

2. Pour the mixture through a fine sieve or tea strainer into another beaker, pressing feces in the strainer with a spatula, and discard the excess material in the strainer.

3. Pour strained solution into a 15 mL centrifuge tube and fill to the top with water.

4. The centrifuge should be balanced every time before use.

5. Centrifuge at 1200–1500 rpm for 5–10 minutes.

6. Decant the supernatant.

7. Resuspend the fecal pellet with flotation solution, stir, and fill tube with flotation solution to form a slight positive meniscus.

8. Place the tube in the centrifuge and position a coverslip on the meniscus. The coverslip will not fall off if using a free swing centrifuge. (If a fixed angle centrifuge is used, fill the tube to within 3 cm from the top of the tube, and spin without a coverslip (as it will fall off). Gently fill the tube with the flotation solution to form a positive meniscus, coverslip, and leave for 10 minutes before examination.)

9. Centrifuge at 1200–1500 rpm for 5–10 minutes.

10. Remove the tube and allow to stand for 10 minutes.

11. Remove the coverslip by lifting upwards and place on a clean slide.

12. Examine the entire coverslip at 100× magnification (10× objective).

13. A 40× objective can be used to confirm identification and measurement of parasites/eggs.

Fecal sedimentation is superior for the detection of fluke ova, even though they float in flotation solutions such as zinc sulfate. Sedimentation can also be used for detection of embryonated nematode eggs, such as *Physaloptera* spp. and *Spirocerca lupi* [71]. This method involves mixing feces with water or another appropriate flotation solution, straining off large pieces of debris, and centrifuging the strained feces at 1200 rpm (280 ×g) for 5 minutes [67]. Centrifugation of the mixture sediments the fluke ova, and the presence or absence of the parasite ova can then be demonstrated by microscopic examination of a few drops of the sediment. Saline is superior for sedimentation of fluke eggs, as they hatch in water [68].

Some GI parasites (e.g., *Strongyloides* sp.) produce larvae rather than ova. These larvae are not easily detected using flotation methods, but they may be detected using sedimentation techniques. The Baermann technique is the most sensitive for the detection of fecal larvae. Samples should ideally be less than 1 hour old and should not be refrigerated [29]. The technique involves placing warm water in a glass funnel that is plugged by a stopcock or rubber hose clamped at its end. A small amount of feces is wrapped in a double layer of gauze and placed in the water for 8 hours. During this time, larvae that are present in the feces pass into the water, and descend to the bottom of the funnel. After 8 hours, a small aliquot of fluid is collected from the base of the funnel and centrifuged. The resulting sediment is then examined microscopically for the presence of larvae. This method can be used for detection of various larvae such as lungworm (i.e. *Aelurostrongylus* and *Filaroides*) and small intestinal threadworms (i.e., *Strongyloides*). Hookworm eggs (i.e., *Ancylostoma* and *Uncinaria*) can hatch in fresh feces, producing active larvae [68].

Samples for enzyme-linked immunosorbent assay (ELISA), direct fluorescent antibodies (DFAs), or PCR

Fresh feces should be refrigerated within 1 hour of collection, and sent chilled to the lab.

Dry mount fecal cytology

Fecal cytology has the potential to provide a diagnosis for some animals with signs of GI disease, although there are mixed opinions on the usefulness of fecal cytology. Thin fecal smears are preferable over thick smears and a small sample not larger than match head size should be used [71]. Thin fecal smears may be stained with routine hematology stains (e.g., Wright-Giemsa or Diff-Quik stain [Dade Diagnostics of P.R., Inc., Aquada, Puerto Rico]). Bacteria and cell morphology are best assessed with oil immersion at 500 to 1000× magnification. Single smears may not be entirely representative and there may be variation of cells or organisms seen depending on how dilute/watery the stool sample is at the time of sampling.

Bacterial flora

The initial step in fecal cytology is assessment of the bacterial flora, which should be mixed in normal small domestic animals (Figure 29.1) with bacilli predominating [45]. Cocci should be in the minority (with only low numbers detected). Occasional extracellular yeasts may be observed

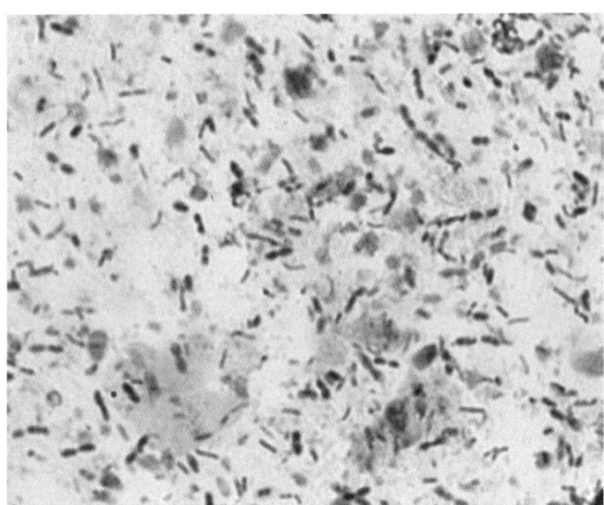

Figure 29.1 Wright-Giemsa-stained fecal smear from a dog showing a mixture of bacteria representing the mixed bacterial flora typical of normal animals. ×1000.

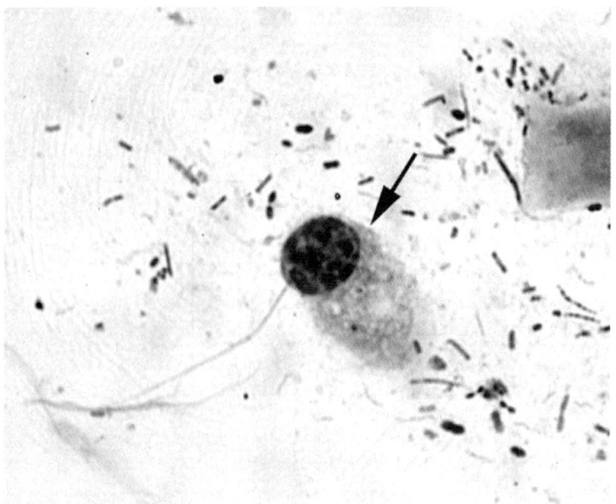

Figure 29.2 Wright-Giemsa-stained fecal smear from a dog. Epithelial cells (arrow) are interspersed with a variety of bacteria and amorphous material. Small numbers of epithelial cells are a normal finding in fecal smears. ×1000.

but it is unknown whether these are clinically significant [22]. If there is an obvious predominance of a single type of bacterium, this organism may be pathogenic, and bacterial culture is indicated. In animals with maldigestion or malabsorption, mixed flora is usually observed.

The small intestine contains primarily aerobic bacteria whereas anerobic and facultative anerobes are predominant in the large intestine and colon. *Helicobacter* colonizes the canine stomach and mucosa of the large intestine (amongst others), but very few are found in the mucosa of the small intestine.

Historically, culture of specific pathogens (such as *Campylobacter* or *Salmonella*) has been used for detection of organisms in the small animal GI tract, but more recently it has been shown to have low sensitivity [102]. Sequencing of bacterial DNA following PCR amplification of 16S rRNA can be used to identify bacteria present in the sample. At least 10^{12}–10^{14} bacteria in the GI tract constitute the intestinal microbiome [102]. Abnormal changes of the intestinal microbiome can manifest as acute hemorrhagic diarrhea, IBD and stress diarrhea. Using PCR sequencing, mucosally invasive *Escherichia coli* can be identified. This organism has been described in causing granulomatous colitis in French Bulldogs and Boxer dogs [32].

Epithelial cells

Small numbers of epithelial cells (Figure 29.2) can be found in fecal films from normal animals.

Neutrophils

The presence of neutrophils (Figure 29.3) in fecal smears is abnormal and suggestive of inflammation of the colon [71]. Neutrophils often appear degenerate as they undergo degenerative changes during their migration into the lumen of the small intestine in transit to the terminal colon. Invasive bacterial pathogens (e.g., *Salmonella*, *Campylobacter* sp., *Clostridium* and enterotoxigenic *E. coli*) should be considered as possible etiologic agents when neutrophils are present in feces, although the presence of clostridial spores is not specific for toxin-associated diarrhea [95]. Counts of clostridial endospores on smears are unreliable.

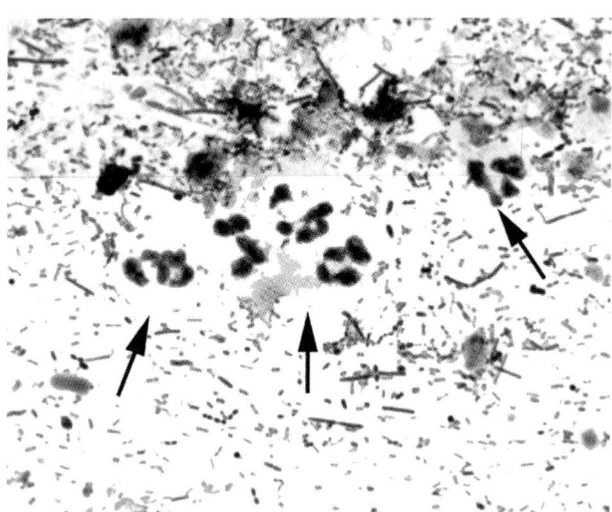

Figure 29.3 Wright-Giemsa-stained fecal smear from a dog. Large numbers of degenerate neutrophils are present (arrows). Neutrophils are abnormal in fecal smears from all species. ×1000.

Presence of fecal neutrophils can also be associated with whipworm and IBD in small animals. Viral disease is a consideration in puppies with hemorrhagic diarrhea if fecal neutrophils are absent [71].

Eosinophils

Eosinophils are also abnormal in fecal films and, when present, are suggestive of eosinophilic colitis, chronic endoparasitism or IBD. They may also be associated with GI lymphoma and mast cell tumor (the latter more commonly in small animals). Occasionally neoplastic lymphocytes can be seen in cases of gastrointestinal tract lymphoma [16]. Refer to Table 29.1 and 29.2 for breeds associated with eosinophilic inflammation. Eosinophilic infiltrates are occasionally seen in horses and can manifest as IBD (the main clinical sign is colic), which is characterized by a number of different syndromes (see section on IBD).

Macrophages

Granulomatous inflammation (predominantly macrophages) is associated with causes of chronic inflammation such as fungal or algal disease [22].

Granulomatous enteritis in horses has been associated with mycobacteria, and PCR is used for identification.

Infectious organisms

Clostridia are bacilli, which, in the sporulated form, have a "tennis racquet" or "safety pin" appearance (Figure 29.4) and can be identified microscopically. The spore causes distension of the bacillus, which then appears swollen and clear. However, recent studies have documented a poor correlation between fecal endospore numbers and the presence of enterotoxin [103]. Only certain strains of *Clostridium perfringens* produce toxins in the gut that can be associated with acute or chronic intermittent (every 4–6 weeks) hemorrhagic diarrhea. The latter can reoccur over months or years. It is thought that up to 20% of diarrhea cases in dogs are associated with *Cl. perfringens*, but it is less commonly seen in cats [27, 104].

Healthy cats can have large numbers of *Cl. perfringens* endospores in their stools, and thus one should be aware of the possibility of over-interpreting the presence of *Cl. perfringens* endospores in fecal smears obtained from cats with diarrhea [105]. *Cl. piliforme* also causes colitis and *Anaerobiospirillum* causes ileocolitis in cats [44]. *C. difficile* also produces specific enterotoxins and is a less common cause of colitis in dogs and horses (including foals). It is most commonly seen in animals treated inappropriately with antibiotics, which causes disturbances in the microbiota (normal flora)

Campylobacter sp. are recognized by their "seagull" or "W" shape (Figure 29.5), and spiriliform bacteria are commonly *Serpulina* spp., which are associated with mucoid diarrhea [22].

Examination of stained fecal smears can be useful for the detection of numerous pathogenic protozoa such as trophozoites of *Balantidium coli* (rectum), *Entamoeba histolytica*, *Giardia* and *Leishmania* [56] (Figure 29.6). Fecal films or scrapings from the colon may also reveal other infectious agents (e.g., fungal organisms such as *Aspergillus, Candida* [56], *Cryptococcus* (intestine), *Histoplasma* (intestine, rectum), *Pythium* and *Prototheca* (rectum) [55]) (Figure 29.7). Special stains may be required for different organisms, e.g., *Cryptosporidium* stains red with a modified acid fast stain. Various stains such as iodine (for *Giardia*), methylene blue (for *E. histolytica*), or acid methyl green (for *B. coli*) help to optimize recognition of some organisms.

Birds

In birds, Gram-positive cocci and bacilli predominate in cloacal films from noncarnivorous birds, and thus stains may be useful in these species. In avian feces, occasional *Candida*-like yeasts or Gram-negative bacterial rods (or even

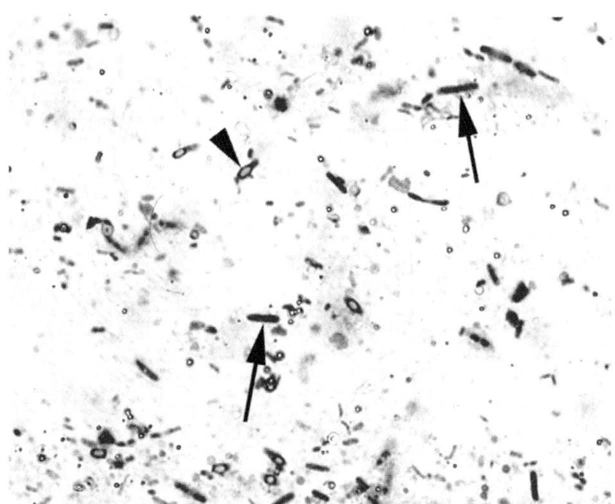

Figure 29.4 Wright-Giemsa-stained fecal smear from a dog showing an overgrowth of *Clostridium* sp. (arrows) that are recognized in the sporulated form ("safety pin" form, arrowhead). ×1000.

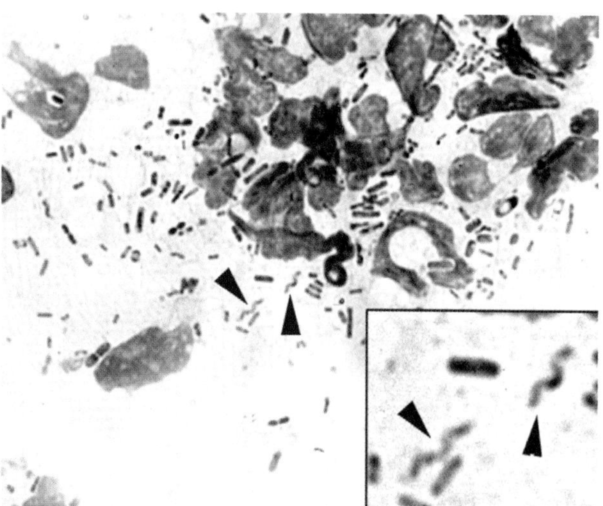

Figure 29.5 Wright-Giemsa-stained fecal smear from a dog showing an overgrowth of *Campylobacter* sp., which are recognized by a distinctive "sea gull" morphology (arrowheads). ×1000.

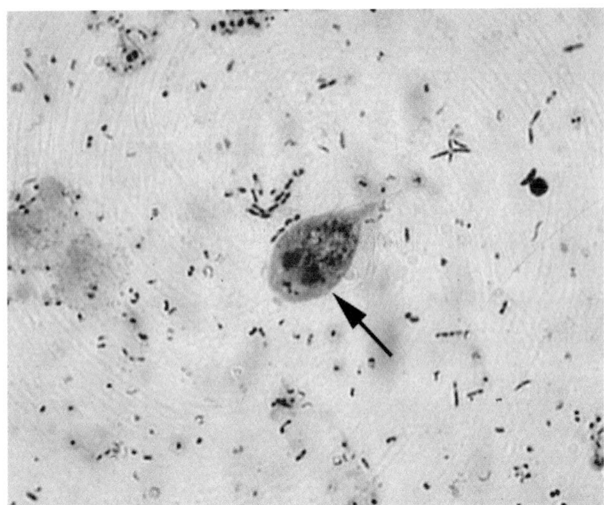

Figure 29.6 Wright-Giemsa-stained fecal smear from a dog showing a *Giardia* organism (arrow). ×1000.

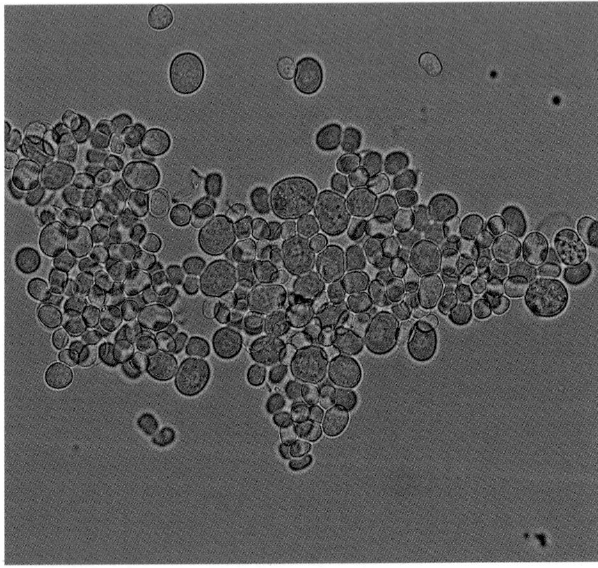

Figure 29.7 *Prototheca* organisms in a fecal wet preparation. ×500.

partial Gram-positive rods) per 1000× oil are regarded as normal. Gram-negative bacteria (bacilli) that are present in large numbers, increased numbers of filamentous Gram-positive bacteria or increased numbers of *Candida*-like yeasts, protozoa, or parasite ova are regarded as abnormal. Staining cloacal smears with carbol fuchsin or iodine may facilitate detection of *Giardia* on cytology [106].

Horses

Grindem et al. [61] suggest that fecal cytology may be of use in horses for the evaluation of variations to the GI flora or for the identification of precise etiologic agents, which may cause gastrointestinal disease. These authors prefer Romanowsky stains over Gram stains for detection of the presence of inflammatory cells or infectious agents during the initial evaluation of smears, as Romanowsky stains give better differentiation than Gram stains. With Gram stains, most cellular structures (including neutrophils) tend to stain Gram negative (red).

Fecal cytology may also be used to make a tentative diagnosis of chronic IBD in horses. These infiltrative bowel diseases include eosinophilic lymphoproliferative disorders and granulomatous gastroenteritis (the latter may be associated with mycobacteriosis, histoplasmosis, or parasitic larvae) [26]. Eosinophilic gastroenteritis may be part of a complex multisystemic epitheliotropic syndrome that may be associated with eosinophilic dermatitis and eosinophilic granulomatous pancreatitis [90, 107] (see later section on IBD).

Rectal biopsies in healthy horses may often contain eosinophils, thus making a definitive diagnosis of eosinophilic infiltrative disease difficult [92]. Ciliated protozoa such as *Tritrichomonas* and nonciliated protozoa such as *Eimeria* have been associated with chronic diarrhea in horses, but their pathogenicity is uncertain [93]. *Eimeria leuckarti* has been reported in North American horses and a study demonstrated a prevalence in foals from Kentucky, but the organism appears to be relatively harmless and clinical significance is questionable [63].

Cytology of biopsy samples

Intestinal biopsies [16] can be used to make scrape or impression smears for cytologic preparations. Ultrasound guided FNAs can be used to make rapid or tentative diagnoses of various disease syndromes such as malignant lymphoma, adenocarcinoma, mast cell tumors (cats) and adenocarcinoma and leiomyomas in dogs. Inflammatory infiltrates such as lymphoplasmacytic or eosinophilic enteritis can also be diagnosed in this manner. Impression smears of gastric mucosa or biopsies can be stained with routine methods for the evaluation of *Helicobacter* spp. [57], although this cannot be differentiated from *Gastrospirillum*-like bacteria on light microscopy [55]. Further clarification of the clinical significance of these organisms is required as they can also be seen in healthy animals [108].

Brush cytology

Brush cytology tends to exfoliate more cells as it represents deeper layers as compared with impression smears but can induce hemorrhage and inflammation [55]. Inflammation causes dysplastic change of epithelial and spindle cells, and over-interpretation of cytological changes must be avoided. Negative results do not rule out any differentials and full thickness gut biopsies for histopathology are the preferred sample in most cases for definitive diagnosis and confirmation of the cytological findings [109].

Fecal occult blood

A large amount of blood (life-threatening amounts) can be lost into the gut without evidence of external blood loss. Microcytic hypochromic, nonregenerative anemia (characteristic of iron deficiency) usually results from chronic gastrointestinal blood loss. Melena (black tarry feces) is usually due to digestion of blood when passing through the GI tract, and is most commonly due to bleeding of the proximal GI tract, but this is also dependent on the transit time. There are a number of drugs and foods (metronidazole, spinach and liver [26]) that can cause dark colored feces, which can be confused with melena. Fresh blood in feces (hematochezia) is usually associated with coagulopathies (rodenticides), colitis, foreign bodies and neoplasia.

Testing for fecal occult blood is a simple test, and is available for in-practice use. The test detects the pseudoperoxidase activity of fecal hemoglobin and picks up minute amounts of fecal blood at concentrations as low as 20× to 50× times less than those where blood is visible grossly [110]. A loss of 30–50% of the blood volume into the GI tract can occur without gross blood being visible in the feces. The test procedure involves application of the feces to the test paper, and when blood is present, the peroxidase activity results in the formation of a blue color (Figure 29.8).

There are two types of fecal occult blood tests available. The modified guaiac slide test is based on the detection of a conjugate product called quinone by chemical oxidation of guaiaconic acid, and the orthotolidine tablet test is based on the oxidation of tetramethylbenzidine. In both tests, a positive fecal blood is evidenced by the development of a blue color. In dogs, some authors report a higher threshold for peroxidase detection in the orthotolidine (o-tolidine) test [111, 112]. In a study by Rice et al. [112], the o-tolidine test was shown to be more specific as compared to the guaiac test, but these tests appear to have similar sensitivities. The clinical applications of the fecal occult blood test include testing animals with unexplained acute or chronic diarrhea, those with loose stools, or in cases of microcytic anemias, where the cause of chronic blood loss is not obvious. The test can also be used to monitor animals that are at risk of developing GI hemorrhage due of treatment with ulcerogenic drugs (e.g., nonsteroidal anti-inflammatory compounds [NSAIDs]) or those with a history of GI neoplasia [110].

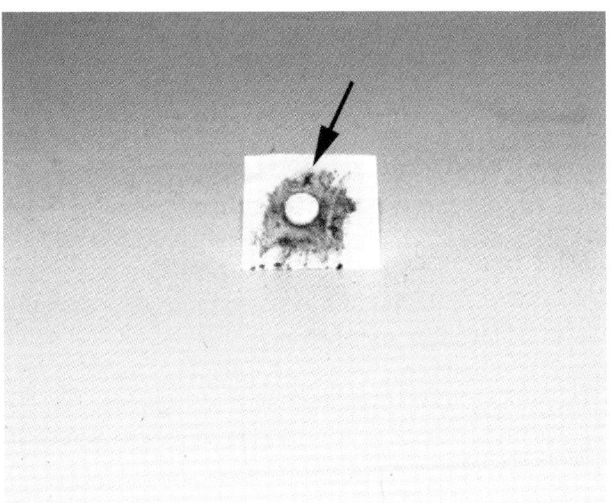

Figure 29.8 The occult blood test. This test is positive for occult blood, as indicated by the blue color on the filter pad.

The fecal occult blood test is extremely sensitive, and thus false positive results may be seen with meat or fish diets that contain myoglobin and hemoglobin, and some vegetable diets including plants such as brassicas [112] and citrus. The guaiac slide test is reported to be more likely to give false positive results than the orthotolodine tablet test, but this difference also depends on the composition of different diets [112].

It is important to observe strict dietary restriction for at least 3–5 days prior to performing the occult blood test as this decreases the number of false-positive results [16, 71]. Recommended feed restrictions include meat-free, low-peroxidase diets (e.g., rice or pasta with cottage cheese or egg as a protein source).

Cimetidine is reported to cause a false-positive hemoccult reaction in gastric juice but has not been shown to be associated with false-positive hemoccult reactions in feces [113].

Fecal immunochemical tests used for human testing detect globin in feces (rather than heme) and are human specific and do not work in veterinary species.

Positive results on the fecal occult blood test in the absence of grossly visible blood in the feces suggests the possibility of upper or lower (colon) [114] GI tract inflammation, ulceration, or neoplasia. Blood from the upper GI tract is usually digested and is not always grossly visible in the feces, but blood from the lower GI tract is undigested, and is normally evident grossly. Loss of large amounts of blood in the upper GI tract can cause rapid transit times, and occasionally, results in grossly visible blood in the feces. At least three consecutive tests for fecal occult blood should be carried out [71] to make a definitive diagnosis, as the sensitivity of the test increases when three tests are done as compared with a single test result. In a study by Smith [115], the fecal occult blood test in ruminants (Hematest, Miles Laboratories, Inc., Elkhart, IN) was reported to have a sensitivity of 77% and a specificity of 97% for abomasal ulceration, which was confirmed at surgery or necropsy [115, 116]. Serum pepsinogen is an indirect test for the detection of abomasal ulceration in young ruminants (usually <2 years of age).

Gastric ulceration in horses can result in constriction of mesenteric arteries, which can lead to necrosis of tissue supplied by these vessels, such as the pelvic flexure and distal ileum, which in turn can cause intermittent colic. Mild decreases in serum albumin can suggest GI ulceration. An Equine Fecal Blood Test™ marketed as SUCCEED® is a lateral flow species (antibody) specific colorimetric test that measures the presence of increased levels of albumin and hemoglobin in feces. This test can be used in the field and is suggested as a marker for hind gut lesions, as enzymatic activity in the area of the common bile duct causes digestion of albumin. Grade 2 ulcerative lesions are required before hemoglobin is found in feces [117].

Digestion/absorption screening tests

Historically there have been numerous screening tests performed on feces to try to evaluate maldigestion and/or malabsorption, which included microscopic examination for fecal starch, fat, and muscle protein, and tests for fecal proteolytic activity. These tests have become obsolete as they are subjective, imprecise, and interpretation is complicated by numerous factors including the variation associated with different diets and intestinal transit times. They have low sensitivity and specificity for diagnosis of GI disease, and are regarded by current leading experts and researchers as diagnostically useless and are not recommended for clinical use [16, 26, 29, 118]. The tests for fecal proteolytic activity are fraught with numerous false positive and negative results because of the daily fluctuations in fecal protease activity and the presence of protease inhibitors in the feces, and are not recommended even as a crude screening test [119, 120].

The plasma turbidity test for fat absorption has poor sensitivity (i.e., 80% or more of ingested fat is still absorbed in dogs with EPI). There can also be marked variation in the degree of lipemia that develops and in the length of time required for lipemia to develop in normal animals.

Tests in a reference laboratory

Serum trypsin-like immunoreactivity

Serum TLI (canine and feline specific cTLI and fTLI respectively) [121] is regarded as the most sensitive and specific laboratory test available for diagnosing EPI [121]. It should be part of any standard workup for canine small intestinal diarrhea [3]. TLI assay (GI Lab, Texas A&M University) utilizes species-specific antibody that detects cationic trypsin and trypsinogen, which are bound to protease inhibitors [51]. Immunoassays are currently available for dogs and cats. In healthy animals, trypsinogen is constantly produced by pancreatic acinar cells and small amounts leak continually into the peripheral circulation, thus most of the serum TLI measured is trypsinogen. Trypsinogen is converted in the small intestine to trypsin, which is the active form of the proteolytic enzyme, but this is not reabsorbed into circulation. In animals with EPI, TLI levels are severely decreased due to the marked depletion of functional exocrine pancreatic tissue. EPI can be treated successfully, which results in the resolution of the changes that usually occur in the small intestine, thus EPI should be ruled out as a differential before considering a diagnosis of primary intestinal disease. Commercially available Immulite® TLI testing (Siemens Medical Solutions Diagnostics) for dogs is a solid phase enzyme-labeled chemiluminescent immunometric assay but is not suitable for other species such as felines.

EPI can also cause cobalamin (vitamin B_{12}) malabsorption, which in turn, can hinder interpretation of serum cobalamin levels and thus the diagnosis of intestinal disease [122].

The following information should be considered when performing TLI:

- Animals should be fasted for a minimum of 12 hours prior to collection of a blood sample, as recent feeding may falsely increase TLI levels.
- 1 mL of nonhemolyzed serum is preferred, but EDTA or heparinized plasma may be used [51]. Severe lipemia will interfere with the radioimmunoassays commonly used for the measurement of TLI [118, 121].
- Serum TLI is stable for several days at room temperature and for several years when frozen. High temperatures will destroy TLI. Samples should be stored at 4 or −20 °C [51].
- Oral supplementation with pancreatic extracts (generally extracted from porcine pancreatic tissue) do not interfere with TLI assays or affect results [118].

Normal dogs have serum cTLI concentrations >5 μg/L (5–35 μg/L [123], 5.7–45.2 μg/L [124]). Serum TLI concentrations are dramatically decreased in dogs with EPI (<2.5 μg/L) [77]. In dogs with clinical signs of maldigestion due to EPI, the diagnostic sensitivity, specificity and accuracy of fasting serum cTLI is high (approaching 100%) [121]. Values between 2.5 and 5.0 μg/L are seldom associated with signs of EPI but may reflect subclinical pancreatic acinar cell destruction secondary to ongoing immune-mediated lymphocytic pancreatitis [125]. Dogs with reproducible subnormal results of between 2.5 and 5.0 μg/L may have subclinical disease (EPI) with partial pancreatic acinar atrophy and concurrent chronic diarrhea and weight loss.

The cTLI can decrease from the "gray" zone to a confirmatory level within a few weeks. In these cases the TLI assay should be repeated after 1 month, ensuring that food is withheld for 12–15 hours prior to blood sample collection. Other possible causes for results in this "gray" zone (2.5–5.0 μg/L) include:

- The dog is in the process of recovering pancreatic function after an episode of pancreatitis, and the results may be normal at retesting.
- The sample had a normal TLI when collected but was exposed to excessive heat during transit. Results may be normal at retesting.
- Food was not withdrawn for an adequate length of time prior to testing. Retesting may indicate that the dog has EPI.

In cats, values ≤8.0 µg/L are diagnostic for EPI [77, 121]. Values between 8.0 and 12.0 µg/L are equivocal and retesting in a month (as for dogs) is recommended [40, 126].

TLI concentrations are reported to be normal in cases where EPI is due either to obstructive pancreatic duct tumors or to congenital deficiencies of the enzymes other than trypsinogen [64]. Diseases causing decreased GFR are reported to increase TLI [124], and could potentially mask an abnormally low serum TLI concentration.

Assays for serum cobalamin (vitamin B_{12}) and folate are strongly recommended whenever serum TLI is assayed as serum vitamin abnormalities are common in dogs and especially cats with EPI.

High TLI values (>50 µg/L (dogs) and 100.0 µg/L (cats)) can be associated with pancreatitis but PLI testing is preferred for the diagnosis of pancreatitis (see Chapter 28).

Fecal elastase 1

The fecal elastase 1 (E1) is a canine monoclonal (species specific) immunoassay ELISA test (ScheBo®, BiotechUS) which claims a sensitivity of 97% and a specificity of 98% for the detection of canine pancreatic insufficiency [127]. Spillman et al. have demonstrated that fecal elastase has a lower specificity than cTLI [127]. In a recent study, Steiner quotes false positive rates up to 23.1% [26]. This test measures undegraded pancreatic elastase in feces, which reflects EPI.

The single advantage of this test over cTLI testing is that it does not require a 12-hour fast, but the disadvantages are that feces are required, it is a more cumbersome assay and may also be more expensive than TLI. Fecal elastase values <10 µg/g in dogs with appropriate clinical signs suggest severe dysfunction [123]. There are also marked daily variations in fecal elastase results, with no clear cut differentiation in results between subclinical and control dogs [125].

Fecal α_1-proteinase inhibitor concentration (α_1-PI)

Many gastrointestinal disorders can be associated with protein loss. In small animals the most common causes of GI protein loss include IBD, intestinal lymphoma, and lymphangiectasia [29].

α1-Proteinase inhibitor (PI) is a protein in feces that has a similar molecular mass to albumin but is not degraded by digestive or bacterial proteinases (as is albumin). It is lost at approximately the same rate as albumin and other plasma proteins into the GI lumen [128]. α1-Proteinase inhibitor is normally found in plasma, lymph, and interstitial fluid but is not normally present in the intestinal lumen [129]. In dogs with gastrointestinal protein loss, increases in fecal α_1PI concentrations may be seen before the protein loss becomes severe enough to observe hypoalbuminemia [130].

Confirmation of gastrointestinal protein loss in dogs, i.e., PLE, can be made by measurement of fecal α1-proteinase inhibitor by means of a validated ELISA assay [128]. The test is only valid in dogs more than one year of age. This assay is available through the Gastrointestinal Laboratory at Texas A&M University (College Station) [128, 131], and this test is no longer available for cats (http://www.cvm.tmu.edu/gilab).

There are daily fluctuations in fecal α_1-PI levels and excretion should preferably be measured over 24 hours, but a more realistic approach involves collection and evaluation of three individually voided fecal samples [71]. Fecal blood is reported to falsely increase α_1-PI [132]. Three different fecal samples (1 g) should be frozen immediately and shipped to the reference laboratory frozen [71], on dry ice for testing. They must be received in a frozen state by the testing laboratory.

Time and increased temperature decrease concentrations [128]. Samples kept at room temperature for 72 hours were shown to have only 66% of the prestorage concentrations [128].

Abnormal results in dogs are reported as a three day average of α_1-PI ≥13.9 µg/g feces or a α_1-PI in one individual sample of ≥21.0 µg/g feces [131]. When serum albumin decreases to a level of 1–2 g/dL, ascites and peripheral edema may result.

Serum vitamin B_{12} (cobalamin) and folate [40]

In dogs and cats that have unexplained weight loss or chronic small intestinal diarrhea, serum vitamin B_{12} and folate concentrations may be useful to evaluate intestinal function [16], but it must be remembered that a precise etiologic diagnosis based on these tests results is unlikely [16]. Results will be abnormal in animals with EPI, and thus animals should be evaluated for EPI prior to vitamin B_{12} or folate testing [40]. These tests are the most useful to diagnose small intestinal bacterial overgrowth (SIBO)/antibiotic responsive diarrhea, although sensitivity for B_{12} is reported as 25–55% and that of folate as 50–66% [11].

Serum is the preferred sample for both vitamin B_{12} and folate assays, but EDTA plasma may be used for folate only with some methodologies [51]. Assays should be validated for the species of interest. Vitamin B_{12} is stable in serum for 12 hours at 8 °C, and for up to 8 weeks at −20 °C. Folate is stable for 24 hours at 4 °C and for up to 8 weeks at −20 °C [51]. Exposure to light may cause false decreases in vitamin B_{12} values [16, 51, 133], whereas hemolysis falsely increases folate concentrations [16, 51, 118, 133]. Samples should preferably be frozen [40].

Texas A&M reference intervals for vitamin B_{12} (cobalamin) in dogs range from 251 to 908 ng/L and folate 7.7–24.4 µg/L. In cats the vitamin B_{12} range is from 290 to 1500 ng/L and folate 9.7–21.6 µg/L.

Deficiency of tissue cobalamin is also associated with increases of serum and urine methylmalonic acid (MMA) (produced by mitochondria) as an alternative pathway of cobalamin production [40].

Serum vitamin B_{12} (cobalamin)

Cobalamin is a large molecule that cannot pass through the intestinal epithelial barrier either by diffusion or by carrier-mediated transport, and thus vitamin B_{12} (cyanocobalamin/cobalamin) has a highly complex homeostasis, which primarily involves sequential metabolism by means of enterohepatic recirculation [29].

Secretions of pepsin and gastric acid (HCl) in the stomach mediate the release from dietary proteins. Free cobalamin then binds to specialized proteins (known as R proteins), which in turn renders cobalamin unavailable for absorption. This complex passes into the small intestine, where it subsequently becomes digested by pancreatic proteases, which in turn releases the vitamin B_{12} [77]. Intrinsic factor is produced primarily by the pancreas in dogs and cats [134], and also by the gastric mucosa in dogs [51], then binds to the free vitamin $B_{12.}$ This vitamin B_{12}-intrinsic factor complex is later absorbed in the distal small intestine, especially the ileum [18, 29].

The three main causes for decreased serum B_{12} (cobalamin) concentrations are:

- **Exocrine pancreatic insufficiency:** Either cobalamin is not released from R proteins because of insufficient secretion of bicarbonate-rich fluid into the duodenum, or there is decreased intrinsic factor production, especially in cats because they lack gastric intrinsic factor [135]. Low serum cobalamin levels are an indication for checking serum TLI.
- **Antibiotic responsive diarrhea/enteropathy – formerly known as small intestinal bacterial overgrowth (SIBO):** SIBO was defined as a specific number of colony-forming units/mL of duodenal juice [136], but further studies have shown that there is no correlation between bacterial counts and disease status [11, 16]. Bacteria involved are predominantly anerobes (*Clostridium* and *Bacteroides*). The amount of cobalamin bound to intestinal bacteria is increased, decreasing free cobalamin for absorption.

Increases in bile acids can also be seen in cases of intestinal overgrowth and EPI (without evidence of liver disease) [137]. This is due to the increased production of unconjugated bile acids by intestinal bacteria that are freely absorbed into portal circulation but fail to be cleared sufficiently [26].

- **Decreased absorption of cobalamin:** In the ileum of dogs and cats, decreased cobalamin absorption may be due to diseases damaging the ileum, such as IBD and neoplasia.

Additionally, congenital selective cobalamin malabsorption and cobalamin deficiency has been documented in cats [138], border collies [14], giant schnauzers [11, 17], Australian shepherd dogs, and beagles with defective ileal cobalamin–intrinsic factor receptor.

In a study at the GI Lab at Texas A&M, they report that approximately 70% of the serum samples tested from Shar Peis with GI disease have serum cobalamin B_{12} levels below the reference interval [15, 16], but these dogs do not appear to have abnormal pancreatic function. They also report that in nearly half of these dogs tested, the serum cobalamin could not be detected by normal methods [16].

Increased levels of serum cobalamin concentrations are relatively uncommon in dogs, but they may occur with supplementation of cobalamin, or they can also arise from hepatic parenchymal damage, as hepatocytes store cobalamin.

Low levels of cobalamin may reflect chronic malabsorption (often associated with chronic diarrheas), and should be treated appropriately. This can commonly be seen in young cats with chronic diarrhea. Cobalamin deficiency is also associated with mucosal inflammation, villous atrophy, immunodeficiency, and neuropathies [26].

Increased levels of serum cobalamin

Occasionally increased serum cobalamin concentrations are found and are generally attributed to either parenteral supplementation or dietary factors or are usually ignored. In man, hypercobalaminemia has, however, been associated with a number of diseases such as neoplasia and hepatic disease. Trehy et al. suggest that hypercobalaminemia in cats should not be ignored and that investigation to rule out hepatic disease or neoplasia should be undertaken [139].

Serum folate

Folate is ingested in the diet (green leafy plants) in the form of folate polyglutamate. It is conjugated with glutamic acid residues but is poorly absorbed. In the proximal small intestine, folate polyglutamate is deconjugated by folate deconjugase enzyme to folate monoglutamate [77], which is then absorbed by specific folate carriers in the proximal small intestine, especially the jejunum. Enteric bacteria also produce folate.

The main cause of decreased serum folate concentrations is the decrease of intestinal folate absorption due to proximal small intestinal disease. Many potential underlying causes are possible, such as IBD or infiltrative neoplasia such as lymphoma. Ingested antigens are in increased concentrations in the lumen of the proximal small intestine and this area is thus vulnerable to damage by specific diets, e.g., gluten enteropathy in Irish setters [28, 29]. Overuse of antibiotics with subsequent sterilization of the intestine can also lead to decreased serum folate levels. A functional folate deficiency may also occur in cases of cobalamin deficiency, and serum folate concentrations may be normal or be potentially increased in those animals due to the decreased utilization of folate [51].

There are several potential causes for increased serum folate concentrations, including excess supplementation or high dietary intake. Many different bacterial species synthesize folate and thus SIBO can lead to significant increases in serum folate concentrations [9]. Bacterial overgrowth may result secondary to EPI or a variety of underlying intestinal diseases that cause defects in the mucus barrier or decreased peristalsis. IgA deficiency in German shepherds has also been associated with intestinal bacterial overgrowth [8]. Greater folate absorption occurs at lower pH, which could be caused either by excess gastric acid secretion or decreased bicarbonate secretion. The latter can be seen in cases of EPI.

Interpretation of vitamin B_{12} and folate concentrations

Results are only meaningful if pancreatic function is normal and if the condition is sufficiently chronic for body reserves of vitamin B_{12} and folate to have been depleted. Dietary intake is a consideration as prolonged anorexia can affect serum concentrations. Misleading results can occur in cats or dogs with EPI and in patients who have bacterial overgrowth or are receiving vitamin supplements. In a survey by Hall et al. [140], the authors reported that 74% of dogs with EPI had decreased vitamin B_{12} and 32% had increased folate [140].

The combination of decreased vitamin B_{12} and increased folate concentrations with normal pancreatic exocrine function suggests SIBO [16], also known as antibiotic responsive diarrhea or bacterial dysbiosis [141]. In dogs, decreased B_{12} and increased folate concentrations have a low sensitivity (5%) for detecting bacterial overgrowth but have high specificity (almost 100%) [7].

Bacterial dysbiosis [2] is not a clinical condition that is commonly seen in cats, but serum cobalamin concentrations can be decreased due to binding by intestinal bacteria. In cats, low concentrations of serum cobalamin are most frequently associated with small intestinal disease, that is, if pancreatic insufficiency (EPI) has been excluded [29].

A decrease in serum concentrations of both vitamin B_{12} and folate suggests severe, chronic diffuse disease involving the entire small intestine (generalized malabsorption).

Decreased vitamin B_{12} and folate concentrations have been reported in cats with EPI. In a study by Simpson [32], in more than 50% of the cats tested at the time they were presented with GI disease, the cobalamin concentration was below normal, and some cats with GI lymphoma were also found to have concurrently low folate levels [32]. It is hypothesized that the reduced serum vitamin B_{12} concentration results from decreased secretion of pancreatic intrinsic factor, which is necessary for vitamin B_{12} absorption in cats. Decreased folate concentrations are thought to result from concurrent intestinal disease with EPI and the resultant decrease in folate absorption. Detection of decreased vitamin B_{12} and folate concentration in cats warrants consideration of EPI in addition to intestinal disease.

A decrease in vitamin B_{12} with normal folate concentration but normal pancreatic function suggests distal small intestinal disease, whereas decreased folate with normal B_{12} concentrations suggests proximal small intestinal disease. A decrease in vitamin B_{12} with or without increased folate in dogs (due to bacterial overgrowth) suggests EPI, and TLI testing is indicated. If both vitamin B_{12} and folate concentrations are increased, vitamin supplementation prior to sampling is the most likely explanation, because there is no disease process that should give rise to this change.

A summary of the interpretation of vitamin B_{12} and folate levels is presented in Table 29.6.

Table 29.6 Summary of the interpretation of vitamin B_{12} and folate levels.

SIBO – normal or ↓ vitamin B_{12}, folate ↑ (TLI measurement indicated)
EPI – slight ↓ vitamin B_{12} folate normal/↑ (ileal mucosal disease – TLI low)
Cats EPI – most ↓ vitamin B_{12}, >50% folate ↓
Vitamin supplementation – ↑ vitamin B_{12}, folate ↑
Severe, diffuse long-standing SI disease – usually ↓ vitamin $B_{12,}$ folate ↓ (IBD, lymphoma, or fungal disease)
Upper SI disease – usually normal or ↑ B_{12}, folate low (IBD, lymphoma or fungal disease)
Malabsorption – low folate
Hepatic disease or neoplasia - ↑Vitamin $B_{12,}$ folate within reference interval [139]

Methylmalonic acid [142]

MMA is most often used in conjunction with vitamin B_{12}, especially in cases where equivocal results are obtained for cobalamin. It is used to detect cobalamin (vitamin B_{12}) deficiency on a cellular level, which is more physiologically important as cobalamin co-reactions are intracellular. Fasted serum samples, shipped to the lab frozen are the preferred samples. Reported reference intervals (Texas A&M) for dogs are 414–1193 nmol/L and 139–897 nmol/L for cats [142].

Cobalamin in large animals

Cobalt is required for synthesis of cobalamin by ruminal bacteria, and thus cobalt deficiencies in ruminants can result in decreased serum cobalamin (vitamin B_{12}) [143]. Cobalamin deficiencies are shown to have repercussions on production in large animals, with manifestations of diarrhea, weight loss, ill thrift, pica, etc. [144].

Other tests that may be useful in assessing gastrointestinal disease

Canine microbiota dysbiosis index [145]

The GI Lab at Texas A&M offers a PCR test that is carried out on canine feces that quantifies eight fecal groups of bacteria and is expressed as a summary of these as a single number.

The secondary interpretation uses the microbial profile to predict conversion of primary to secondary fecal bile acids. Fecal dysbiosis is indicated by a dysbiosis index >0, which can be seen in cases of chronic enteropathies such as antibiotic responsive diarrhea, IBD, food responsive diarrhea, EPI, and dysbiosis [2] induced by antibiotic therapy.

Specificity is approximately 75% with 15% of normal dogs having false positive results within an equivocal range of 0–2. Feces is best shipped frozen.

Markers for gastric disease

Gastrin is a peptide hormone produced by the parietal cells of the stomach, G cells of the duodenum, and pancreas whose main function is to elicit the release of hydrochloric acid, and that plays a role in gastric motility.

Excessive amounts of gastrin can be associated with gastrin producing tumors (gastrinoma) of the duodenum or pancreas (Zollinger-Ellison syndrome) [146], immune mediated gastritis leading to low stomach acidity and compensatory over-secretion of gastrin, and chronic gastritis associated with *Helicobacter* infection.

Gastrin concentration in serum can be measured in dogs and cats. Gastrin is labile and serum should be separated immediately, frozen and shipped on ice. The diagnosis of gastrinoma is made on the basis of a 10× increase in gastrin levels as compared with fasting samples [26]. Chronic inflammation of the gastric lining causes damage to the gastric glands leading to atrophic gastritis and decreased secretion of gastrin, which is reported in Norwegian Lundehunds [147].

Damage and inflammation of the gastric mucosa elicits an increase in serum C-reactive protein concentrations in dogs that is highly sensitive but nonspecific [148].

Gastroscopy (beyond the scope of this text) is regarded as the gold standard for evaluation of gastric disease [77].

There are no specific markers for general gastric disease but anecdotally, gastric carcinoma is often associated with increases of ALP (usually accompanied by evidence of anemia on CBC).

Evaluation of ruminal fluid

When sampling the ruminal contents, it is important to avoid contamination with saliva, which has an alkaline pH.

Ruminal pH varies according to the type of feed, and time interval between feeding and sampling. The maximal decrease in pH occurs 5–6 hours postprandially due to production of volatile fatty acids. pH increases on exposure to air and thus should be measured immediately after sampling [149].

Normal rumen pH is reported to be between 5.5 and 7.2, with an average of 6.5–6.8 (on roughage) [149, 150]. Acidosis is evidenced by a pH less than 5.5–6.0 (usually due to grain overload or high concentrate diets) [151], although an animal with lactic acidosis with protracted anorexia may have a normal rumen fluid pH if there is persistent saliva production [144]. Alkalosis is associated with pH above 7 (8–10) and is due to high protein diets, saliva contamination of rumen content, or rumen putrefaction due to rumen stasis [149].

Microscopic examination of rumen fluid includes evaluation of the types of bacteria and types and motility of the protozoa present. It is important to mix the sample adequately prior to examination. Protozoal motility can be evaluated on wet preparations at low power that should be kept warm [152]. Numbers and morphology can be examined on wet mounts without stains (or by adding a drop of Lugol's iodine to the rumen contents) on a slide and covered with a coverslip. Normally a minimum of five to seven active protozoa should be seen per low-power field [149].

Ruminal bacteria are predominantly Gram negative but these may be replaced by Gram-positive organisms in cases of ruminal acidosis [149].

Normal rumen chloride is <30 mmol/L (10–25 mmol/L) in cattle and (<15 mmol/L) in sheep [149], and chloride concentration of the abomasum is (>90 mmol/L) [152]. Increases in rumen chloride are associated with abomasal reflux of HCl, ileus, or high salt intake [144, 149].

A list of additional tests that may be used for the evaluation of gastrointestinal disease is presented in Table 29.7.

Absorption tests

The functional assessment of small intestinal disease in small animals by measuring absorption of various substrates such as glucose, lactose, and starch are obsolete [16]. This is because concentrations of plasma glucose after dosing of these compounds depends on more than mucosal hydrolysis of starch and lactose, and absorption of glucose, making these tests unreliable [16]. Other insensitive tests that have also become outdated include vitamin A testing (previously used to assess malabsorption), D-xylose testing in small animals, and triglyceride absorption tests [16].

Some of these absorption tests however, are still used in large animals, such as xylose absorption, and are occasionally used in horses when malabsorption is suspected [162, 163]. This has largely been replaced by glucose absorption tests, which are used to assess chronic weight loss in horses [164]. An abnormal test result does not, unfortunately, provide a specific etiology for the weight loss. Both tests are influenced by the rate of gastric emptying, small intestinal transit time, diet and fasting period. Both tests require adequate fasting prior to testing, but this may be contraindicated in debilitated animals.

Xylose absorption tests depend largely on absorption of xylose whereas glucose absorption tests depend on intestinal absorption and utilization of glucose by hepatocytes and other tissues. Theoretically the xylose absorption test is preferred because xylose is not a normal metabolite, although the test has a number of disadvantages. The test is more expensive, xylose assays are less accessible, and results may be difficult to interpret [149]. Results are also affected by diet (horses on high energy diets show lower absorption curves). The glucose absorption test is more practical because glucose is readily available, less expensive, and assays are

Table 29.7 Additional tests that may be useful for the evaluation of gastrointestinal disease.

Test type	Purpose of test
Fecal antigen detection methods	Evaluation of microorganisms associated with diarrhea and/or vomition, e.g., ELISA for viruses (parvo [153], rota) Parvo ELISA is only positive during viral shedding (10–12 d postinfection) False positives seen if vaccinated with live attenuated vaccine within 10 d of testing [153] Also useful for panleukopenia in cats, along with severe leukopenia on leukogram PCR required to differentiate field from vaccinal strains
Fecal ELISA for bacterial enterotoxins	*Clostridium perfringens* [29] and *Clostridium difficile* [29, 154]
Fecal PCR or bacterial or fungal culture	Evaluation of microorganisms, associated diarrhea, and or vomition such as *Campylobacter* spp. [97, 155, 156], *Clostridium difficile* [45, 154], *Clostridium perfringens* [97, 103, 154], pathogenic strains of *Escherichia coli* [9, 32, 45, 97, 157] and *Salmonella* spp. [66, 71, 97], *Helicobacter* [57, 158], *Heterobilharzia americana* [159], *Histoplasma capsulatum* [45], *Tritrichomonas* [55, 74]
Hydrogen breath test [76–78]	Investigation of bacterial overgrowth and carbohydrate malabsorption secondary to EPI in dogs and cats [43, 160]
Intestinal biopsy	Evaluation of etiology of GI tract disease [16]/causes of malabsorption/ maldigestion [55]
Serum gastrin	Evaluation for gastrinoma (Zollinger-Ellison syndrome) [146]
Serum pepsinogen	Screening for abomasal ulceration/damage [151] in ruminants and screening test for *Teladorsagia* (ostertagiasis) [161] in young calves <2 yr of age

more accessible. Glucose absorption tests can be used in monogastrics and preruminant calves to assess intestinal absorption but cannot be used in adult ruminants as sugars are degraded in the rumen.

Oral D-xylose absorption tests in horses

Protocol:

• The animal is fasted for 12–18 hours [165].
• D-xylose is administered orally via nasogastric tube at a dosage of 0.5–1.0 g/kg (10% solution) in horses [149].
• Blood samples are collected into heparinized tubes for D-xylose determinations and are collected before D-xylose administration and at 30-minute intervals for up to 5 hours (30, 60, 90, 120, 180, 240, and 300 minutes) after administration. For routine diagnostic purposes, the 60- through 180-minute samples are the most important.

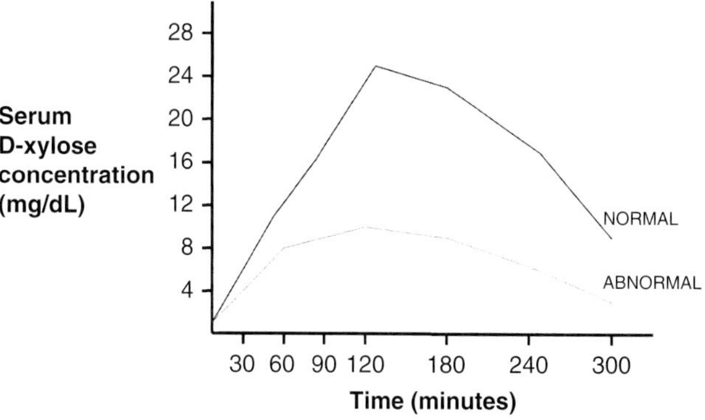

Figure 29.9 The D-xylose absorption curves from normal and abnormal horses. A normal D-xylose absorption curve in a horse peaks at greater than 20–30 mg/dL at 90–180 minutes after D-xylose administration.

D-xylose concentrations should represent a bell-shaped curve but should peak at greater than 20–30 mg/dL (1.34–2.01 mmol/L) at 90–180 minutes (Figure 29.9) [149]. In normal horses, peak values should be greater than 15 mg/dL (1.00 mmol/L) above baseline values. In normal foals the xylose peak is reached at 30–60 minutes, but peak concentrations are reported to vary with age [149]. A flattened D-xylose absorption curve is suggestive of malabsorption [149].

The D-xylose absorption test is insensitive, and thus a normal D-xylose absorption test does not rule out malabsorption. D-xylose absorption curves can be affected by many factors not directly related to malabsorption such as diet, anorexia, age, decreased renal clearance, infections, anemia, hypoxia, and in foals, the IgG concentration. D-xylose absorption can be falsely decreased (i.e., a falsely flattened curve or delay in reaching peak value) with delayed gastric emptying, bacterial overgrowth causing intraluminal bacterial breakdown of xylose, and sequestration of xylose in patients with abnormal extravascular fluid accumulation (e.g., edema, hydrothorax, or ascites).

Oral glucose absorption/tolerance test (OGTT) in horses

Protocol [164, 166–168]:

• The animal is fasted overnight (18–24 hours), and a baseline (0-hour) blood sample for glucose is drawn into a sodium fluoride oxalate tube.
• Glucose (20% solution) is administered at 1 g/kg body weight via nasogastric tube.
• Blood samples for glucose determination are collected into sodium fluoride tubes at 30, 60, 90, 120, and 180 minutes after glucose administration.

Normal horses should show increases in blood glucose concentrations of greater than 85–100% above the baseline concentration at 120 minutes [51, 83]. Results may be affected by a number of factors such as age and diet [166, 169], bacterial overgrowth, delayed gastric emptying (excitement) [164, 167, 168], small intestinal obstruction, reduced intestinal circulation, and sequestration in ascitic fluid. Anorexia or prolonged fasting may delay or decrease peak glucose concentrations, causing flatter curves due to decreased peristalsis.

The specificity of the oral glucose tolerance test was assessed in 42 cases of horses with chronic weight loss [167]. Specificity was found to be very good; normal OGTT results correlated well with normal histopathological findings of the small bowel, but severe infiltrative disease of the small intestine (such as lymphoma or granulomatous enteritis) was associated with a complete malabsorptive response [167]. Histopathological findings correlated poorly with a partial malabsorption response.

Tests for maldigestion in horses

Oral lactose tolerance test in horses

Maldigestion syndromes are infrequently observed in horses as compared with other species. In foals and young adults less than 3 years of age, lactase enzyme (found in the brush border of the small-intestinal enterocytes) hydrolyzes lactose into its two component sugars d-glucose and galactose before absorption occurs. Acquired lactase deficiency can be seen in foals and preruminant calves secondary to a number of causes of intestinal mucosal damage. These include viral (rotavirus), protozoal, or bacterial enteritis (*C. difficile* enterocolitis in foals) [82, 83] or other less specific causes of small intestinal disease [51]. Preruminant calves and lactose-deficient foals may develop osmotic diarrhea due to the presence of osmotically active particles (lactose) and subsequent retention of water and electrolytes in the small intestine. These two types of diarrhea may be difficult to differentiate clinially [88].

The lactose tolerance test does not distinguish maldigestion from malabsorption but is used principally in foals to identify lactase deficiency and for young foals and calves with diarrhea or poor growth. The test is inappropriate for adult ruminants and horses (the latter greater than 3 years of age as they are lactose-intolerant).

Protocol [51, 81, 164, 167]:

- Grain and hay should be withdrawn from the dam and foal for 18 hours and water removed 2 hours prior to testing. Muzzling of the foal is recommended 4 hours prior to testing, and the foal should remain muzzled for the duration of the test. A baseline (0-hour) blood sample for glucose is taken.
- Lactose monohydrate (20% solution) is dosed at 1 g/kg body weight via nasogastic tube [149].
- Blood samples for glucose assay are collected into sodium fluoride tubes at 30-, 60-, and 90-minute (120 minutes optional) intervals after lactose administration.

In healthy foals, the glucose concentration is reported to be 150–250% of baseline concentration at 60 or 90 minutes [81, 83] or should peak at least 35 mg/dL (1.94 mmol/L) greater than the baseline concentration [81]. Maldigestion or malabsorption will usually result in an inappropriate increase in the blood glucose concentrations after the administration of lactose. If the lactose tolerance test is abnormal, then either a glucose or D-xylose absorption test is recommended to evaluate for possible malabsorption. Casein hypersensitivity and lactose intolerance can be differentiated by evaluation of the foal's response to enzymatically treated and untreated milk. A definitive diagnosis of lactase deficiency can be confirmed by direct measurement of mucosal lactase activity in the intestinal tissue, but this is rarely performed in practice, as surgical biopsy of the mucosa is required.

Starch digestion test in horses

This is a test of small intestinal and pancreatic function.

Protocol [149]:

- The horse is fasted for 18 hours, after which a baseline sample for blood glucose is taken into a sodium fluoride tube.
- Cornstarch is dosed at 1 kg in 4 L of water or 2 g/kg body weight via nasogastric tube.
- Samples for blood glucose determinations are collected in sodium fluoride tubes at 15-, 30-, 60-, 90-, 120-minute intervals and then hourly for 6 hours.

Normal horses are reported to should show increases in blood glucose concentrations of approximately 30 mg/dL (1.67 mmol/L) with a peak at 60 minutes, and the curve should return to pretreatment levels within 3 hours. This pattern of response closely approximates results obtained by oral glucose absorption tests [170].

Other laboratory abnormalities associated with disease of the digestive system

Laboratory test abnormalities associated with gastrointestinal disease vary with the area of the system affected, the disease etiology, and the speed of onset and duration of the disease. Common abnormalities associated with acute or chronic diarrhea or vomiting are discussed here.

Other laboratory abnormalities associated with acute or chronic diarrhea (more than 3 weeks' duration) or vomiting

Dehydration and hemoconcentration

Dehydration and hemoconcentration are characterized by increased hematocrit, hemoglobin concentration, and erythrocyte count, as well as increased plasma and serum protein concentrations. These changes can occur with acute diarrhea or vomiting, and are due to the loss of fluid via the GI tract. Increases in blood urea nitrogen or (serum urea) and creatinine can occur secondary to dehydration (i.e., prerenal azotemia).

Leukogram

Variable abnormalities in the leukocyte concentration can occur with acute diarrhea. If the diarrhea results from an infectious agent that produces toxins, (such as *Salmonella*), then sequestration of neutrophils as well as strong tissue demand can result in marked neutropenia and leukopenia with or without a left shift and toxic change. Less severe endotoxemia or tissue demand can result in neutrophilia with a left shift.

- Eosinophilia may or may not be seen with hypersensitivity – allergy or intestinal parasitism, intestinal mast cell tumor, GI lymphoma, hypoadrenocorticism, eosinophillic enteritis, or hypereosinophilic syndrome.
- Lymphopenia may be seen with immunodeficiency, stress, or lymphangiectasia [16, 29, 34]. Severe lymphopenia in cats can also be associated with lymphoma [171] and FeLV/FIV infection.
- Thrombocytopenia, coagulopathies, and disseminated intravascular coagulation may be features of endotoxemia secondary to sepsis.

Acid-base and electrolyte abnormalities

Acid-base and electrolyte abnormalities can occur in animals with diarrhea or vomiting. These abnormalities, however, are variable and unpredictable. Assessment of acid-base and serum electrolyte status is important in such animals. In patients with secretory diarrheas, loss of Na, Cl, and occasionally K can result in decreased serum concentrations of these electrolytes. Hypokalemia is common in horses with long-standing colic with impaction of the large colon, or in horses that have been anorexic for a few days [149].

Increases in potassium with pseudohypoadrenocorticism (pseudoaddisons) is noted in some dogs with secretory diarrhea, especially with whipworm (*Trichuris*) infection [71, 172]. Bicarbonate is also lost in diarrhea, which can cause a metabolic acidosis. This in turn can result in a shift of K from intracellular to extracellular spaces as well as retention of K by the kidneys. Potassium shifts can lead to a normal or increased serum K concentration despite a loss of K in the feces. Vomiting animals may lose significant amounts of HCl in the vomitus, which often leads to hypochloremia and metabolic alkalosis. If the vomitus includes alkaline small intestinal contents, however, such animals may have normal acid-base results or metabolic acidosis.

Metabolic alkalosis in vomiting animals is associated with obstructive GI disease, and is caused by loss of HCl without loss of alkaline intestinal contents. No significant association was found by Boag et al. [173] between electrolyte or acid-base abnormalities and the site of foreign body; metabolic alkalosis with hypochloremia (disproportionate to sodium) and hypokalemia can be seen with both proximal and distal gastrointestinal foreign bodies. Linear as compared with discrete foreign bodies were more likely to be associated with lowered sodium concentrations [173].

A marked disproportionate decrease in chloride as compared to sodium may also be associated with left displacement of the abomasum (LDA) in ruminants with alkalosis and hypokalemia. This may be accompanied by paradoxic aciduria [149]. A less severely (but disproportionately) lowered chloride with low or low normal potassium and alkalosis has also been observed in cattle with ileus, vagal indigestion, or oversupplemented with magnesium.

Increased activities of hepatic leakage enzymes

Increased activities of hepatic leakage enzymes (mainly ALT [alanine aminotransferase] in dogs and cats or ALP [alkaline phosphatase] in dogs [16] and GLDH [glutamate dehydrogenase] in large animals) can occur with acute diarrhea, possibly because of hepatocyte damage resulting from toxins absorbed from the injured GI tract or seeding of the liver by bacteria from the gut or circulating inflammatory mediators and cytokines. The liver's dual blood supply and large blood flow make it sensitive to injury due to systemic disorders and diseases in organ systems drained by the portal circulation, especially the GI and pancreas.

Serum amylase and lipase

Serum amylase and lipase may be variably increased with gastrointestinal disease in dogs, including gastrointestinal space occupying lesions such as foreign body or neoplasia.

Hypocholesterolemia

Hypocholesterolemia although nonspecific, may be present in some cases of intestinal disease. Many dogs with PLE have hypocholesterolemia, which may be secondary to lymphangiectasia [16], and presumably results from fat malabsorption associated with failure of chylomicron transport.

Panhypoproteinemia

Panhypoproteinemia can be seen with PLEs [16, 34] including neoplasia. This should be differentiated from hypoalbuminemia secondary to protein losing nephropathies and liver failure [16]. Checking for urine protein with a dipstick is a simple means of looking for proteinuria (see Chapter 30). Chronic intussesception should be a consideration in young dogs with chronic diarrhea [174] and PLE that are negative for hookworm [26].

Coagulation defects

Coagulation defects can be seen in horses with severe colic and is characterized by low levels of antithrombin III and prolonged PT and APTT [175].

Other laboratory abnormalities associated with exocrine pancreatic insufficiency or malabsorption syndrome

Hematologic and serum biochemical tests usually are not helpful in establishing the diagnosis of EPI. Routine hematologic tests and biochemical profiles, however, may help to differentiate EPI from other disorders. Serum amylase and lipase activities may or may not decrease slightly with EPI, but these decreases usually are not recognized as being significant. Increased alanine aminotransferase (ALT) activities and decreased cholesterol concentrations occasionally are seen in dogs with EPI.

Other laboratory abnormalities that can occur with malabsorption syndrome include:

1. **Microcytic anemia** associated with iron deficiency, which commonly results from chronic blood loss via the GI tract [34]. Chronic GI blood loss can be associated with a variety of underlying conditions, including neoplasia and parasites.
2. **An inflammatory leukogram**, may be suggestive of significant inflammation or deep ulceration in the intestinal wall.
3. **Neutropenia** with or without a left shift. If neutrophils are toxic, then endotoxin absorption from the GI tract secondary to Gram-negative enteritis, intestinal stasis, septicemia, severe bacterial peritonitis secondary to intestinal perforation, or viral enteritis are possible.
4. **Eosinophilia**, may be associated with eosinophilic gastroenteritis or parasitism, is an inconsistent marker of eosinophilic gastroenteritis [16, 34]. Lack of eosinophilia does not rule out these differentials. Hall [16] states that in his experience, fewer than 50% of cases of biopsy-proven eosinophilic enteritis have peripheral eosinophilia and that mild eosinophilia can also be seen with other forms of IBD [16].
5. **Abnormal serum protein,** albumin, or globulin concentrations. Serum albumin and globulin concentrations are important in screening for protein losing enteropathies [34]. In these cases, both albumin and globulin concentrations are usually decreased. In other types of malabsorption or maldigestion, the only decrease, if any, occurs in the albumin concentration. An exception is immunoproliferative enteropathy of basenjis [16], in which globulin concentrations increase as part of an immune response. Similar immunoproliferative enteropathies with hyperglobulinemia may occur in other breeds of dogs, especially German shepherds.
6. **Prolonged coagulation times –** prothrombin time (PT), prolonged activated partial thromboplastin time (APTT), and prolonged activated clotting time (ACT) caused by vitamin K deficiency may be seen in animals with malabsorption syndrome. A suspected vitamin K–deficient bleeding syndrome has been reported in cats with malabsorption syndrome. Malabsorption of vitamin K, which is a fat-soluble vitamin, probably plays an important role in this syndrome, but the vitamin K deficiency in such animals also is potentiated by secondary hepatic diseases, thereby resulting in decreased production of vitamin K–dependent clotting factors; possible antibiotic therapy, thereby altering small intestinal bacterial flora and reducing bacterially derived vitamin K_2 production; and in some cases, severe dietary fat restriction, thereby reducing vitamin K uptake still further, because it is dependent on fat absorption. Before these changes are seen, the activity of vitamin K–dependent clotting factors decrease to less than 35% of the reference interval by which time these animals are markedly deficient and should receive parenteral vitamin K supplementation [176].

Specific gastrointestinal disease syndromes

Antibiotic responsive diarrhea (ARD)/enteropathy – formerly known as small intestinal bacterial overgrowth (SIBO) [6, 7]

SIBO was a syndrome that described animals with chronic GI disease that responded to antibiotic therapy [177]. These dogs were shown to have similar numbers of bacteria in their GI tracts to dogs with EPI, response to steroids or food trials, and normal dogs [6]. These animals may show histologic evidence of lymphocytic-plasmacytic IBD, and German shepherd dogs appear to be predisposed [9]. Patients with chronic or intermittent diarrhea are retrospectively diagnosed with this syndrome if they respond to a specific antibiotic such as Tylosin [178] (dogs usually respond within 3 days), doxycycline, oxytetracycline, or metronidazole [26, 178].

Gastrointestinal disease in working dogs

The most common manifestations seen in working dogs are vomition, diarrhea, and gastric ulceration. These can be associated with metabolic disease or can be psychological. Protracted physical exertion is associated with hyperthermia and oxidative stress [179] with production of reactive oxygen species, which increases intestinal permeability [180]. The energy requirement in these dogs is high and diets are usually high in fat, which is associated with maldigestion and malabsorption. As a consequence, bacterial flora is disturbed and there is inflammation of the mucosa and liquefaction of feces [181].

Chronic diarrhea in cats

The most common causes for chronic diarrhea in cats are parasites (especially protozoal infections), lymphoma, IBD, food hypersensitivity and hyperthyroidism. Intestinal lymphoma is the most common neoplastic condition in cats [182]. FNA of thickened intestines and or histopathology with immunocytochemistry or immunohistochemistry is required for diagnosis of lymphoma. Small intestinal lymphoma is most commonly small cell, T phenotype. Progression of the tumor can result in thickening of the gut wall, intestinal perforation and peritonitis. In the early stages of disease differentiation from IBD is necessary, but chronic IBD can progress to lymphoma in later stages of the disease. PCR for clonality is required [183].

Inflammatory bowel disease [36, 37]

IBD is defined as chronic persistent to intermittent inflammation of the GI tract, manifesting as chronic small intestinal diarrhea, and /or vomition (small animals), and/or weight loss, with accompanying alterations in the gut flora and changes in the mucosa associated bacteria (dysbiosis) [39], along with immune dysregulation and irregularities of pro- and anti-inflammatory cytokines and chemokines [39, 184, 185]. Dogs may show abnormal behavior [26].

There are canine breed predispositions to a number of IBD phenotypes [22], including antibiotic-responsive diarrhea [6, 7]/enteropathy, cobalamin deficiency [11, 40], gastric carcinoma [26], gluten sensitive enteropathy [28, 30], granulomatous colitis [26], lymphangiectasia [41, 42] and PLEs [29, 41, 43]. These are referred to in Tables 29.1 and 29.2. In cats the inflammation can extend to the liver and pancreas causing triaditis. Malabsorption may also be involved with a ravenous appetite and significant weight loss [186].

Because of the variety of potential etiologies (including idiopathic), the histopathological diagnoses should not be regarded as the diagnostic endpoint. There are a number of different breed predilections and phenotypes of IBD, and diagnosis is multifactorial (including histopathological findings that may represent the culmination of many different diseases) [36].

Infectious disease

Infectious disease should be considered in cases of a histopathological description of granulomatous or pyogranulomatous inflammation. Organisms involved include bacteria (*E. coli* [187], *Campylobacter, Streptococcus, Yersinia,* and *Mycobacteria*) [56], algae (*Prototheca*) [45, 55], or fungal infections (*Histopaslma*). Culture, PCR (16S rRNA amplification), or canine microbiota dysbiosis index may aid in further evaluation in these cases. *Campylobacter jejuni, C. coli,* and *C. upsaliensis* can be seen in large and small animals with diarrhea and healthy animals [155]. Shedding of *Campylobacter* is 2× higher in young dogs with diarrhea than healthy dogs [156]. Treatment with antibiotics usually prolongs shedding, as these infections are usually self- limiting.

In cats other differentials that need to be ruled out include hyperthyroidism, EPI, liver disease, lymphoma, giardiasis and other parasites, viral disease (FeLV, FIV, FIP), adenocarcinoma [26, 27] and lymphoma [16].

Eosinophilic infiltrates

Eosinophilic infiltrates are generally associated with hypersensitivity – allergic (dietary) or parasitic disease, but environmental triggers and genetics may also play a role [86]. GI tract thickening with small intestinal diarrhea, vomition, and weight loss are common manifestations, although large intestinal signs may also be seen. Animals may or may not have peripheral eosinophilia. Other disease processes with similar findings on CBC include Addison's disease (dogs), intestinal mast cell tumors (dogs and cats), lymphoma, and endoparasites.

Eosinophilic infiltrates in horses are part of the IBD syndrome [21, 84] and are characterized by several specific conditions. Eosinophilic enteritis (EE) is associated with eosinophilic and lymphocytic infiltrates. Idiopathic focal eosinophilic enteritis (IFEE), which involves the small intestine mainly in young horses <5 years of age, is associated with an eosinophilic-macrophage infiltrate with fibrous focal lesions causing obstruction. Eosinophilic colitis is also a disease of young horses with eosinophilic infiltrates into left dorsal colon, also with fibrous bands causing impaction. Carbohydrate tests may be abnormal. Multisystemic eosinophilic epitheliotropic disease (MEED) [21] is seen in horses >5 years of age, and is characterized by eosinophilic infiltrates of skin, liver, pancreas, lungs, and large intestine. Blood work and carbohydrate tests may be normal, but rectal biopsies may be diagnostic. Prognosis is poor.

Lymphoplasmacytic enteropathies

Lymphoplasmacytic enteropathies are the most commonly described PLEs (IBDs – see Tables 29.1 and 29.2) even though this diagnosis is controversial as healthy dogs [188] and cats [189] have similar numbers of lymphocytes and plasma cells as compared with affected animals. The World Small Animal Veterinary Association has made significant headway in defining this in the Gastrointestinal Standardization Group 2008 publication [109]. Dogs with chronic enteropathy that have low albumin [37] or cobalamin [190] have been shown to have a guarded prognosis, and hypokalemia in cats is also associated with a poor outcome. In horses, PLE, anemia, and abnormal carbohydrate absorption tests are inconsistent findings, and as for small animals, lymphoplasmacytic infiltrates from rectal mucosa are nonspecific and can be seen in normal or disease states of any age but are regarded as possible precursors to gastrointestinal malignant lymphoma. If biopsies are suggestive of lymphoma, PCR should be undertaken to determine clonality.

Granulomatous enteropathies [83]

Granulomatous enteropathies are seen in young horses (<4 years of age) and may be associated with mycobacteria, with accompanying skin and coronary band lesions, anemia, and PLE. Carbohydrate absorption tests are abnormal, and rectal biopsies may be diagnostic.

Lymphangiectasia [41, 42]

The majority of these animals have significant PLE, which is usually associated with chronic diarrhea and vomition, weight loss, ascites, and chylothorax. The Norwegian Lundehund [42] and Yorkshire terrier are overrepresented, and soft-coated Wheaten terriers appear to be predisposed. Associated serum biochemical changes include hypoproteinemia (albumin and globulins), with associated hypocalcaemia (40% total calcium is albumin bound), hypocholesterolemia, hypomagnesemia (vitamin D deficiency) [191], hypokalemia and hypochloremia, (vitamin D deficiency) [191], and the leukogram may show lymphopenia.

Chronic vomition

There are numerous potential underlying causes including obstruction, inflammation, drugs, metabolic and endocrine disease, toxins, neurological and numerous miscellaneous causes. Clinical pathology workup should include a full CBC, chemistry (with electrolytes), urinalysis, fecal examination, PLI (feline or canine), paired bile acids, serum B_{12} and folate, FeLV, FIV in cats, and T4 in cats older than 4 years of age (approximately 40% of hyperthyroid cats vomit chronically) [192]. A coagulation profile is indicated if there is hematemesis.

Chronic weight loss

More than 10% loss of body mass is clinically significant and >20% constitutes emaciation [75]. The most common causes of weight loss include decreased food intake or poor quality food, and systemic disease such as the various causes of PLE, PLN, and infiltrative intestinal disease including IBD and neoplasia. Other metabolic causes include renal, liver, pancreatic disease, and some endocrine disorders such as diabetes mellitus and hypoadrenocorticism (Addison's disease). Cardiovascular disease can result in cardiac cachexia (myo-, endo-, or pericarditis), and infectious causes include *Borrelia, Dirofilaria*, or *Trypanosoma*. Maldigestion and malabsorption is associated with IBD, antibiotic responsive diarrhea (SIBO), EPI and endoparasitism to name a few.

Pyrexia concurrent to weight loss occurs with a number of inflammatory, infectious (viral, bacterial, ehrlichial or rickettsial, systemic fungal), immune mediated (SLE, polyarthropathy) and intestinal neoplastic diseases (adenocarcinoma, lymphoma and leiomyosarcoma) [26]. Other SI tumors reported in dogs include fibrosarcoma, mast cell tumors (Maltese predisposed) [169] extramedullary plasmacytomas, and in cats, MCT, hemangiosarcoma [193], extraskeletal osteosarcomas [194].

Acute gastritis and enteritis

These are commonly caused by dietary indiscretion or hypersensitivity [195] but can also be associated with IBD, eosinophilic (idiopathic eosinophilic gastrointestinal masses, Rottweilers predisposed [19, 20], scirrhous eosinophilic gastritis/feline GI eosinophilic sclerosing fibroplasia), [196] lymphoplasmacytic (hyperplasia, atrophy, [41] parasites) or granulomatous [45] IBD or infectious agents including *Cryptococcus, Entamoeba, Histoplasma, Heterobilharzia americana* (causes hypercalcemia) [197], *Prototheca*, pythiosis, and *Neorickettsia*. Histiocytic ulcerative colitis (granulomatous colitis) in boxers is associated with *E. coli* [35, 187]. Feline infectious peritonitis (FIP) can cause granulomatous colitis and lymphadenitis.

Gastritis in horses is associated with a number of syndromes including equine gastric ulcer, glandular, and squamous ulcer syndrome. There are no specific diagnostic clinical pathology tests for these syndromes and gastroscopy is used for diagnosis. *Gasterophilus* can also cause gastritis, and diagnosis is difficult – larvae may been seen in feces or bot eggs on the hair.

Acute enteritis in horses (including duodenitis-proximal jejunitis [198] seen in horses >1.5 years of age) can be associated with infectious causes such as bacteria (*C. difficile* and *perfringens, E. coli* [187], *Salmonella*). *C. difficile* produces toxins A and B, which can be detected in feces. Viral enteritis is associated with rotavirus (foals) and coronavirus (adults) [94]. Acute bacterial enteritis can be associated with gastric reflux, and culture and PCR may be useful to diagnose a specific etiological agent.

Chronic enteritis is associated with equine proliferative enteropathy (*Lawsonia intracellularis* [87] (foals 4–7 months of age, affecting ileum and jejunum, with significant PLE) [89], *Rhodococcus hoagii* (young horses)), granulomatous (mycobacteria), and eosinophilic infiltrates. Abdominal effusion with a predominance of neutrophils with high protein and lactate content can be seen with strangulating lesions (higher than seen with infectious causes). Neutrophilic inflammation is usually associated with gastric ulceration that can be seen with irritation (foreign material), hormone secretions, or ulcerogenic drugs (including NSAIDs and steroids) [44].

Gastric neoplasia is relatively uncommon in small animals. Gastric lymphoma in cats and gastric carcinoma is the most common in dogs [43, 199].

Chronic gastritis

Chronic gastritis is a vague syndrome that may be associated with parasitism, metabolic or immune mediated disease or can be idiopathic, and is considered to be part of the IBD syndrome.

Colitis

In dogs and cats colitis is associated with large intestinal diarrhea, often with mucus and hematochezia [26]. Various causes of acute colitis include toxins (including drugs), foreign bodies, diet, and *Trichuris* infection (dogs). Chronic colitis is associated with IBD. *Cl. perfringens* infection with enterotoxin type A [200] is associated with both acute and chronic colitis. Diagnosis can be made using a Tox A/B II ELISA Kit (TECHLAB, Blacksburg, Virginia, USA). Diagnostic usefulness of culture and PCR are limited due to high prevalence in normal dogs [201]. Other infectious causes of chronic colitis are less common [26].

In horses, colitis involves colon and/or cecum (typhlitis), and is seen in horses average age 2–10 years. It can be acute or chronic, infectious or noninfectious. Infectious causes include various bacteria such as *Clostridium difficile* and *perfringens* [201], *E. coli, L. intracellularis, Neorickettsia risticii* (Potomac horse fever), *Salmonella,* rotavirus (foals) and coronaviruses, and small stronglyes [202]. Noninfectious causes include antibiotic responsive diarrhea, dietary, IBD, neoplasia, plant and drug toxicity (including NSAIDs), and sand impaction. NSAIDs can cause ulceration throughout the gut, but a right dorsal colitis [203] has been described using appropriate doses for less than a week [204] Clinicopathological findings of anemia with hypoproteinemia and hypocalcemia are typical although nonspecific. Occult blood testing is useful if there is no overt hematochezia or melena. Diagnostic workup should include routine CBC and chemistry, serum amyloid A, fecal testing for occult blood, specific bacterial culture, fecal examination for parasites, and PCR/ELISA testing.

Intestinal neoplasia

Gastrointestinal lymphoma is the most commonly diagnosed tumor in dogs and cats [171, 182]. Neoplasia of the intestines includes lymphoma, leiomyomas and sarcomas (now known as GI stromal tumors), mast cell tumors, plasmacytomas, rectal ganglioneuromas, neurilemomas, and carcinoids [26, 205]. Large intestinal tumors in dogs include carcinoma in situ and adenomatous polyps. Adenocarcinomas predominate in cats.

CHAPTER 29

30 Laboratory Evaluation of Plasma and Serum Proteins

Robin W. Allison

Department of Veterinary Pathobiology, Oklahoma State University College of Veterinary Medicine, Stillwater, OK, USA

Laboratory evaluation of plasma and serum protein concentrations is a part of both basic hematology and biochemistry testing in animals. Protein alterations occur commonly as secondary changes in a large number of diseases and may be the major abnormal finding in a few disease processes. Measurement of plasma or serum protein concentrations often yields important information that can be helpful in narrowing the list of diseases to be considered and, in some cases, in revealing the presence of a specific disease. This chapter discusses the types of proteins that are normally present in plasma and serum, the methods for analyzing these proteins, and the significance of abnormal protein concentrations.

Classification of plasma proteins

The two major types of proteins in plasma are albumin and the globulins. Albumin is one of the smallest of these proteins and the single most abundant, accounting for approximately 75% of the oncotic pressure (colloidal osmotic pressure) of plasma within the vasculature, which prevents water from diffusing from the blood into the tissues [1]. Albumin is an important carrier protein and plays a role in the transport of free fatty acids, bile acids, bilirubin, calcium, hormones, and drugs [2]. Albumin is synthesized by the liver, enters the blood, and is catabolized by most tissues. The half-life of a circulating albumin molecule varies in different species, ranging from approximately 8 days in dogs to approximately 20 days in horses [3, 4].

Globulins are a heterogeneous group of proteins that are variable in size but usually larger than albumin. Hundreds of different types of globulins are present in plasma, including the immunoglobulins (e.g., IgG, IgM, IgA), complement proteins, clotting factors, many different enzymes, and a variety of proteins that carry lipids, vitamins, hormones, extracellular hemoglobin, and metal ions (e.g., iron, copper) [1]. The majority of the globulins are produced in the liver, with the exception of immunoglobulins (antibodies) that are produced in lymphoid tissues. Globulins typically are classified as alpha, beta, or gamma on the basis of their electrophoretic mobility. (The separation and measurement of these globulins are discussed later.) A relatively small number of globulins are present in sufficient quantities to affect the electrophoretic pattern. Some of the major contributors to each fraction are listed below.

The alpha globulin fraction includes α_1-fetoprotein, α_1-acid glycoprotein (seromucoid), α_1-antitrypsin (protease inhibitor), α_1-antichymotrypsin (protease inhibitor), α_1-lipoprotein (HDL; transports lipid), ceruloplasmin (transports copper), haptoglobin (binds hemoglobin), α_2-macroglobulin (protease inhibitor), and serum amyloid-A [5, 6]. The beta globulin fraction includes β_2-lipoprotein (LDL; transport lipids), transferrin (transports iron), ferritin (iron storage), complement components (C3 and C4), and fibrinogen (in plasma but not serum) [5, 6]. Immunoglobulin molecules of the IgM and IgA type occasionally migrate in the beta fraction. The gamma globulin fraction is composed primarily of immunoglobulins (all types). These proteins are produced by plasma cells in the lymphoid tissues in response to antigenic stimulation. C-reactive protein migrates in this fraction in dogs but migrates between the beta and gamma fractions in horses [7, 8].

Acute phase proteins

Concentrations of a number of plasma proteins change significantly during the acute systemic response to inflammation; collectively these proteins are referred to as acute-phase proteins (APP). The acute-phase response occurs due to release of a variety of cytokines (e.g., IL-1, IL-6, and TNF-α) from the site of inflammation [9]. These cytokines affect the production of APP by the liver. The plasma concentrations of most APP increase; these proteins are called positive APP, and they generally reach maximal

Veterinary Hematology, Clinical Chemistry, and Cytology, Third Edition. Edited by Mary Anna Thrall, Glade Weiser, Robin W. Allison and Terry W. Campbell.

Companion website: www.wiley.com/go/thrall/veterinary

serum concentrations within a day or two after initiation of the response. Concentrations of some APP actually decrease; these are called negative APP. The specific pattern and magnitude of protein alterations during the acute-phase response is species-specific; however, the concentration of serum albumin (a negative APP) is consistently decreased by 10–30% [10]. Transferrin, measured in serum as the total iron-binding capacity (TIBC), is another negative APP. The positive APP are globulins; important ones in veterinary species include haptoglobin, fibrinogen, C-reactive protein, serum amyloid-A, and α_1-acid glycoprotein [9, 10]. Serum amyloid-A is a major APP of dogs, cats, pigs, and horses; haptoglobin is a major APP of cattle, sheep, and pigs; C-reactive protein is a major APP of dogs, horses, and pigs.

Measurement of plasma and serum proteins

Plasma versus serum

The two types of samples commonly used for clinical biochemistry analyses are plasma and serum. Plasma is the liquid portion of blood that has not clotted, thus the blood must be collected in an anticoagulant. Plasma contains all of the proteins described earlier. Serum is the liquid portion of the blood that remains after clotting. When a blood sample is collected without use of an anticoagulant, the subsequent clotting in that sample results in the conversion of all fibrinogen to fibrin. Therefore, serum is devoid of fibrinogen but contains albumin and the remaining globulins.

Total protein concentration

The total plasma or serum protein concentration can be estimated using a refractometer. Protein molecules in plasma or serum increase the refractive index of that fluid in proportion to their concentration. However, there are other molecules potentially present in plasma or serum that can increase the refractive index and artifactually increase the estimated protein concentration. Substances most likely to cause significant interference include lipoproteins (such as in lipemic serum), cholesterol, urea, and glucose [11]. Note that marked elevations in cholesterol concentrations will not result in visible lipemia but can artifactually increase the protein estimate. Plasma protein may be falsely increased by 0.6 g/dL by serum urea concentrations of 300 mg/dL or glucose concentrations of 700 mg/dL [5]. Synthetic colloid solutions, sometimes given as volume expanders, will artifactually increase the refractometer estimate of total protein. Hyperbilirubinemia and hemolyzed serum typically do not interfere with the total protein estimate, although hemolysis may obscure the line of demarcation on the refractometer [11].

The total protein concentration of serum is measured routinely in reference laboratories by spectrophotometry, most commonly the biuret method, which detects peptide bonds and is considered very specific. The serum total protein concentration obtained by this method will be less than the plasma protein estimation from a refractometer, due in part to the absence of fibrinogen from serum. Differences in protein measurements performed by different methods (refractometry versus spectrophotometry) should be expected, even for the same type of sample. In avian species, marked differences in total protein concentrations have been found depending upon the methodology used, with lower values determined with the biuret method versus refractometry [12, 13]. Use of method and species-specific reference intervals are necessary for accurate interpretation [14].

Albumin concentration

The albumin concentration is routinely measured spectrophotometrically using dye-binding methods, usually with bromcresol green (BCG). However, BCG is not specific for albumin and may bind to some globulins. As a result, the BCG method may overestimate the albumin concentration when it is very low (<1 g/dL). Other dye-binding methods sometimes used in human laboratories (BCP, HABA methods) are unreliable for accurate measurement of albumin concentrations in animals due to species variations. Albumin concentrations measured by the BCG method may be overestimated as much as 1.2 g/dL in canine heparinized plasma samples compared to serum samples, especially when fibrinogen concentrations are increased; this interference may be eliminated by changes in the specific method protocol [15]. In avian species, albumin concentrations measured by the BCG method often correlate poorly with results obtained by electrophoretic methods (discussed later) [13, 16, 17].

Globulin concentration

Calculated globulin concentration

The serum total protein and albumin concentrations are measured routinely as part of serum biochemical profiles. The globulin concentration as reported on these profiles is not measured, however, but rather is calculated by subtracting the serum albumin concentration from the total protein concentration.

Serum protein electrophoresis

Both serum albumin and globulin concentrations can be determined by serum protein electrophoresis (see Chapter 1). Electrophoresis is performed by placing a small amount of serum near one end of a supporting substance such as cellulose acetate or agarose gel. An electrical current is applied, causing the serum proteins to migrate at variable rates as determined by the net negative charge and size of each type of protein. Staining of the gel reveals the various protein bands, which are then scanned by a densitometer to produce an electrophoretogram (i.e., a hard copy depiction of the distribution of the proteins) (Figure 30.1).

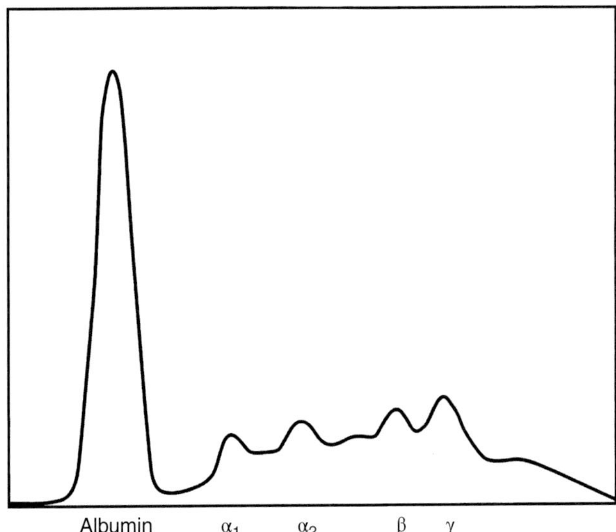

Figure 30.1 An electrophoretogram from a serum protein electrophoresis separation.

Modern scanning densitometers also calculate the concentration of protein in each fraction after the operator inputs the total protein concentration of that sample. This method separates globulins into several fractions, including alpha, beta, and gamma globulins. Albumin and globulin concentrations that are derived using this method do not necessarily match those obtained using spectrophotometric methods. The number of fractions separated by serum protein electrophoresis varies both with the species and with the type of supporting substance used; high resolution agarose gels are capable of resolving more protein fractions than low resolution agarose or cellulose acetate gels. Albumin and the alpha, beta, and gamma globulin fractions can be separated in specimens from all species with all types of support substances. In some species, the alpha, beta, and gamma globulins are separated into $alpha_1$ and $alpha_2$, $beta_1$ and $beta_2$, or $gamma_1$ and $gamma_2$ fractions, respectively. (Causes for altered concentrations of these protein fractions are discussed later.)

A relatively new type of electrophoresis, capillary zone electrophoresis, is now being used with animal sera [18–20]. In this method protein fractions are separated in solution within a narrow-bore capillary exposed to high voltage. No staining of proteins is required; protein fractions are detected and quantified by ultraviolet light absorbance. Potential advantages of capillary zone electrophoresis include smaller sample size, better resolution and reproducibility, and the ability to automate the procedure. The visual appearance of the electrophoretogram produced by this method differs from that of traditional methods, and quantitative results may also differ. In particular, peaks that appear polyclonal with agarose gel electrophoresis may appear monoclonal or biclonal with capillary zone electrophoresis [21]. Thus experience and method-specific reference intervals are necessary for proper interpretation of results [22].

Qualitative and semiquantitative estimation of immunoglobulin concentrations

Several different types of rapid screening tests for the estimation of immunoglobulin concentrations are available. These tests can be performed in clinical practice, and they can provide qualitative or semiquantitative estimates of immunoglobulin concentrations. They primarily are used to screen neonates (especially calves, foals, and crias) for possible failure to ingest colostrum or to absorb immunoglobulins from colostrum; this failure results in increased susceptibility to infection and is referred to as failure of passive transfer (FPT). These tests are not as sensitive or specific as more sophisticated tests such as radioimmunodiffusion (RID; considered the gold standard), but the results are usually available immediately and allow for treatment decisions to be made without delay. Results are most valid as indicators of adequate passive transfer or FPT when tests are performed within a few days of birth. General guidelines have been established for minimum IgG concentrations that that indicate adequate passive transfer; >800 mg/dL for foals and >1000 mg/dL for calves and crias [23–25].

Total protein measurement by refractometry

Immunoglobulins absorbed from colostrum are the major determinant of the total serum protein concentrations in neonates. Total protein concentrations in calves increase by approximately 2 g/dL after the ingestion of colostrum [26]. Measurement of the total protein concentration by refractometry, therefore, has been evaluated as an indicator of serum immunoglobulin concentration and as a gauge for the adequacy of passive transfer.

In calves, use of the serum total protein concentration as an indicator for the serum immunoglobulin concentration has been evaluated using different cutoff values or decision thresholds. A serum total protein concentration of 5.2 g/dL correlates with an IgG concentration of 1000 mg/dL and adequate passive transfer [24]. A decision threshold of either 5.0 or 5.5 g/dL classifies >80% of calves correctly, however sensitivity and specificity of these thresholds are different [24]. Sensitivity and specificity of the 5.0 g/dL threshold are 0.59 and 0.96, respectively, indicating few normal calves would be incorrectly classified as FPT (false positives). Sensitivity and specificity of the 5.5 g/dL threshold are 0.94 and 0.74, respectively, indicating few calves with FPT would be incorrectly classified as normal (false negatives). Because many sick calves with FPT are also dehydrated, which results in a relative hyperproteinemia, the higher decision threshold may be more appropriate for those individuals [27].

In crias, one study found that serum total protein concentrations of <4.5 g/dL measured by refractometer indicated FPT, and concentrations >5.5 g/dL indicated adequate passive transfer; however, concentrations between those values could not be accurately interpreted [28].

In foals, using the serum total protein to estimate IgG concentrations appears to be unreliable and is not recommended as a sole indicator of FPT [23]. The poor performance of serum total protein might result, in part, from wide variations in precolostral protein concentrations in foals.

Turbidity and coagulation assays

These tests are based on the ability of different substances to either precipitate or form insoluble complexes with serum immunoglobulins. Solutions used in these assays can be made in the clinic or purchased in kit form from several different manufacturers. In general these are inexpensive and rapid assays that are easy to perform, but sensitivity and specificity for the diagnosis of FPT varies considerably when different cutoff values are used. Additionally, because assessment of the degree of turbidity or coagulation present is subjective, results can vary between users.

• *Sodium sulfite precipitation test* [29]. The sodium sulfite precipitation test is based on the fact that immunoglobulins can be selectively precipitated from serum using concentrations of anhydrous sodium sulfite ranging from 14% to 18%. A higher sodium sulfite concentration is required to cause precipitation in serum containing lower immunoglobulin concentrations. Sera with very low immunoglobulin concentrations do not undergo precipitation when mixed with any sodium sulfite solutions in the 14–18% range. Fibrinogen also is precipitated by these concentrations of sodium sulfite; thus serum, rather than plasma samples, should be used. This test is useful for calves and crias but does not work well for foals [24, 25, 30, 31]. A procedure for performing the sodium sulfite precipitation test in ruminants is presented in Appendix 30.1; test kits are also commercially available (Bova-S and Llama-S, VMRD, Inc. Pullman, WA). In this test, the immunoglobulin concentration is determined by judging the presence or absence of precipitation in three concentrations of sodium sulfite: 14%, 16%, and 18%. The test can distinguish three ranges of immunoglobulin concentrations: <500 mg/dL, 500–1500 mg/dL, and >1500 mg/dL. Using the <500 mg/dL limit makes the test more specific for detecting FPT (e.g., calves negative for precipitation are likely to have FPT) but less sensitive for detecting FPT (e.g., will miss some calves with FPT). Using the 1500 mg/dL limit makes the test more sensitive for detecting FPT but reduces the specificity (e.g., will indicate FPT in calves with adequate transfer of immunoglobulin). Using the <500 mg/dL limit appears to correctly predict the highest percentage of calves with FPT (~86%); thus some recommend using only the 18% sodium sulfite solution [27].

• *Zinc sulfate turbidity test* [31, 32]. Immunoglobulins are precipitated from serum by zinc sulfate over a wide range of zinc sulfate concentrations. This test is most useful in calves; a procedure is presented in Appendix 30.2. Like the sodium sulfite precipitation test, a positive reaction (i.e., turbidity) in sera with low immunoglobulin concentrations occurs when a solution with a high zinc sulfate concentration is used, but not when a solution with a low zinc sulfate concentration is used. In sera with high immunoglobulin concentrations, turbidity occurs when zinc sulfate solutions of lower concentrations are used. Thus, different sensitivities and specificities for detecting FPT result when different concentrations of zinc sulfate are used (see Appendix 30.2). The highest proportion of calves correctly classified as having FPT (i.e., true immunoglobulin concentration <1000 mg/dL) occurs when either 350 or 400 mg/L concentrations of zinc sulfate are used (83% and 88% correctly classified, respectively) [32]. The actual concentrations most appropriate for this test depend on whether high sensitivity or high specificity is most important in the specific situation. A procedure for the zinc sulfate turbidity test in foals is presented in Appendix 30.3; commercial kits are also available (Equi-Z, VMRD Inc., Pullman, WA). Observing any visible turbidity in the reaction solution after 1 hour of incubation is a good indication that the foal has a serum immunoglobulin concentration of >400 mg/dL. This procedure, however, does not distinguish foals with immunoglobulin concentrations of between 400 and 800 mg/dL, which are considered evidence for partial FPT. Correlations between zinc sulfate turbidity results and those of more specific tests for immunoglobulin concentrations in foals are not strong.

• *Glutaraldehyde coagulation test* [33, 34]. The glutaraldehyde coagulation test is based on the ability of glutaraldehyde to form insoluble complexes with immunoglobulins, resulting in coagulation of the test mixture. Glutaraldehyde also forms insoluble complexes with fibrinogen; therefore, serum rather than plasma is preferred. This test has been evaluated in neonatal calves and foals. A procedure for this test in ruminants is presented in Appendix 30.4; commercial kits previously available (Gamma-Check®-B, Plasvacc USA Inc., Templeton, CA) were unreliable when used with whole blood [35]. In neonatal calves, use of a 10% glutaraldehyde solution results in no coagulation in almost all calf sera with immunoglobulin concentrations of less than 400 mg/dL and complete or partial coagulation in almost all calf sera with immunoglobulin concentrations of greater than 600 mg/dL. Calves with immunoglobulin concentrations of between 400 and 600 mg/dL have results that vary from no coagulation to complete coagulation. However, the accepted cutoff limit for adequate passive transfer in calves is 1000 mg/dL, thus this test has poor sensitivity (FPT in calves with immunoglobulin concentrations between 400 and 1000 mg/dL will not be identified). A procedure for performing the glutaraldehyde coagulation test in foals is presented in Appendix 30.5; a commercial kit is also available (Gamma-Check-E, Plasvacc USA Inc., Templeton, CA). In horses, FPT is defined as serum IgG concentrations <200 mg/dL, and partial FPT occurs at serum IgG concentrations of 200–800 mg/dL [23].

The glutaraldehyde coagulation test distinguishes three ranges of immunoglobulin concentrations: >800 mg/dL, 400–800 mg/dL, and <400 mg/dL. Reported sensitivities and specificities for detection of IgG concentrations <400 mg/dL have ranged from 95% to 100% and 80% to 89%, respectively [23, 36]. For detection of IgG concentrations <800 mg/dL, sensitivities and specificities have ranged from 93% to 100% and 59% to 94%, respectively [36, 37]. Lower test specificity using the 800 mg/dL cutoff value indicates a greater chance of false-positive results (diagnosing FPT in a normal foal), suggesting the need for additional confirmatory tests prior to treatment.

Antibody-based detection kits

A number of manufacturers have developed commercial kits for detection of FPT in foals and calves that use antibody-based methods (e.g., latex agglutination, enzyme-linked immunoassays). Examples include the Quick Test® calf or foal IgG kits (Midland Bio-Products, Boone, IA), Foalcheck® (Centaur, Overland Park, KS), and SNAP® Foal test (IDEXX Laboratories, Westbrook, ME). Accuracy, sensitivity, and specificity of these assays vary with the individual test and cutoff values [23, 37, 38]. These commercially available tests are not necessarily superior to the screening tests described earlier. To minimize false-negative results and ensure detection of a high percentage of animals with FPT, screening tests should have high sensitivity. In foals, the glutaraldehyde coagulation test may be equal or superior to commercially available semiquantitative tests in terms of sensitivity (depending on the cutoff value used) [36, 37]. However, more specific confirmatory tests may be desired in some situations.

Measurement of immunoglobulin concentrations by reference laboratories

Reference laboratories offer more sophisticated antibody-based methods for quantitating specific immunoglobulins (e.g., radial immunodiffusion, immunochemistry). Use of these methods is indicated when a detailed examination regarding the status of the immune system is desired. These methods are more expensive, however, and the results usually are delayed (incubation periods of 18–24 hours are required) compared with those of the screening methods discussed earlier.

Fibrinogen concentration

Plasma fibrinogen concentrations can be determined by two methods. One assesses the conversion of fibrinogen to fibrin in the presence of thrombin (thrombin time, Clauss method) and requires instrumentation that is somewhat expensive for routine use in clinical practice. Such measurement of plasma fibrinogen concentrations also requires citrated plasma that has been harvested from a mixture of nine parts fresh, whole blood and one part 3.8% sodium citrate anticoagulant. Special evacuated blood collection tubes containing sodium citrate anticoagulant are available for this purpose; these tubes draw the appropriate amount of blood to ensure a 9 : 1 ratio of blood to anticoagulant. This method is not routinely used to measure plasma fibrinogen concentrations but may be included in a coagulation profile.

A point-of-care method designed to measure equine fibrinogen using the Clauss method is also available (VetScan VS*pro* fibrinogen test cartridge, Abaxis, Inc.). One study concluded that the accuracy of this test compared to standard laboratory methods was acceptable, but there was greater variability in results when fibrinogen concentrations were increased [39].

In clinical practice situations, the most common method for measuring plasma fibrinogen concentration is heat precipitation. This method is less expensive than the method described earlier and requires minimal equipment; it is summarized in Appendix 30.6. The heat precipitation method provides an estimate of the plasma fibrinogen concentration that is adequate for evaluation of hyperfibrinogenemia but lacks the analytic sensitivity needed for evaluation of hypofibrinogenemia. (The significance of abnormal fibrinogen concentrations is discussed later.)

Abnormal protein concentrations

Both decreased and increased total protein concentrations are commonly detected laboratory abnormalities in animals. These findings may result from alterations in the albumin or globulin concentrations, or both. In plasma, an increased concentration of fibrinogen, which is a globulin, can occasionally produce an increased protein concentration. Interpretation of altered protein concentrations depends on determining which major protein constituents of the serum or plasma are abnormal. A decreased or increased albumin or globulin concentration does not always result in detectable alterations of the total protein concentration. Therefore, albumin and globulin as well as total protein concentrations should be assessed. Causes of decreased or increased total protein, albumin, globulin, and fibrinogen concentrations are summarized here. It is often helpful to consider alterations in albumin and globulin concentrations together for interpretation.

Causes of decreased protein concentrations

Decreased total protein concentrations can result from decreased concentrations of albumin, globulin, or both. A diagnostic algorithm for evaluating variations in these decreases is presented in Figure 30.2.

Hypoalbuminemia with hypoglobulinemia

Concurrent hypoalbuminemia and hypoglobulinemia can result from overhydration (e.g., excessive fluid therapy,

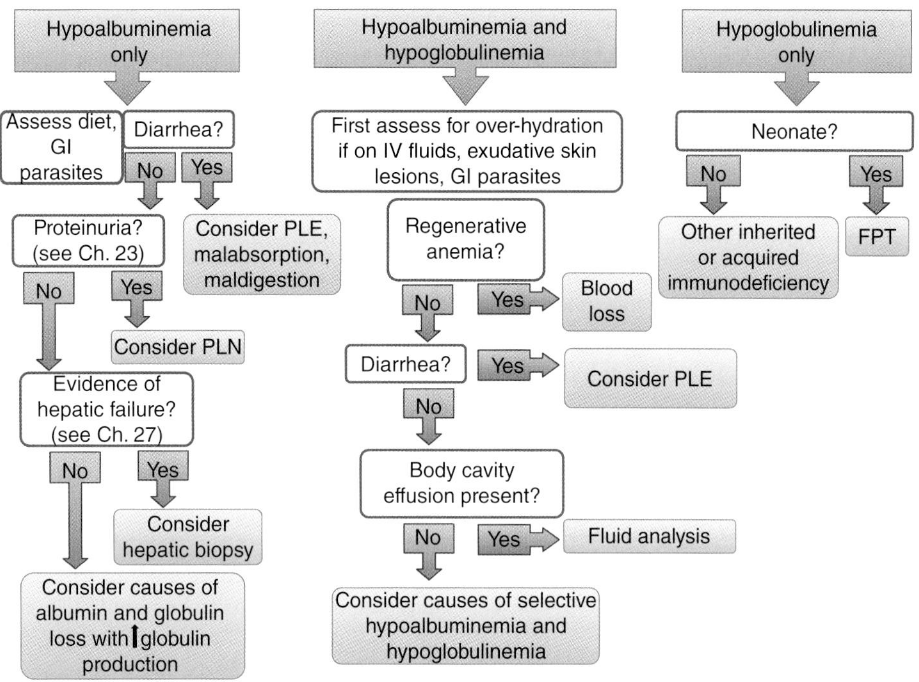

Figure 30.2 An algorithm for evaluation of decreased serum protein concentrations. FPT, failure of passive transfer; PLE, protein losing enteropathy; PLN, protein losing nephropathy. Refer to text for details.

excessive water intake) or from loss of both protein fractions. The latter occurs in the following disorders:

• Blood loss. This results in proportional loss of all blood constituents. Albumin and globulin, therefore, are lost in concentrations equal to their concentrations in the blood. After blood loss, fluid moves from the extravascular space to the intravascular space and dilutes the remaining blood constituents, including the proteins (and erythrocytes). It is important to remember that this water shift takes time to develop, and will not be evident for the first few hours following acute hemorrhage. Hypoproteinemia due to blood loss is generally caused by external (rather than internal) hemorrhage, and may also be caused by blood-sucking parasites (external or internal). Although protein concentrations may decrease with severe internal hemorrhage, such as might occur with a bleeding hemangiosarcoma, in cases of chronic internal hemorrhage the proteins are reabsorbed.

• Protein-losing enteropathy. This may result from a variety of generalized intestinal lesions, including inflammatory bowel disease, lymphangiectasia, infectious diseases, neoplasia, and gastrointestinal hemorrhage [40–42]. Hypoproteinemia can develop whenever protein leakage into the intestinal lumen exceeds the rate of protein synthesis. In some instances a concurrent immune response causes increased instead of decreased globulin concentrations; gastrointestinal lymphoma may also be associated with hyperglobulinemia [43].

• Severe skin disease. Generalized exudative skin disease or burns can result in loss of plasma proteins due to increased vascular permeability [44]. Concurrent immune responses may increase globulin concentrations.

• Effusive disease. This results in the accumulation of body-cavity fluids with high protein concentrations that can result in decreased serum albumin and globulin concentrations [5]. Such decreases depend on the degree of increased vascular permeability accompanying these disorders.

Selective hypoalbuminemia

Decreased albumin concentrations that are not accompanied by decreased globulin concentrations can result from either decreased production or increased loss of albumin. If the globulin concentration is concurrently increased, total protein concentration may be within the reference interval despite hypoalbuminemia.

Decreased production of albumin can occur in the following disorders:

• Hepatic failure. The liver is the site of albumin production. Because of the liver's reserve capacity, most types of liver damage do not result in decreased albumin production. If more than 60–80% of the functional liver mass is lost, however, decreased albumin production and hypoalbuminemia can occur. In such cases, other evidence of hepatic failure is also present (see Chapter 27). Serum globulin concentrations are not usually decreased because immunoglobulin production in lymphoid tissues is not hampered; globulin concentrations may actually be increased in patients with hepatic failure (discussed later).

• Starvation or cachexia. Marked malnutrition or starvation results in less hepatic protein production due to a deficiency of available amino acids. In cachectic states associated with neoplasia or chronic infections, a prolonged negative protein balance causes increased catabolism of body proteins that exceeds protein production. Body fat and muscle mass are lost in both cases, resulting in weight loss. Usually these conditions result in selective hypoalbuminemia; rarely there is concurrent hypoglobulinemia.
• Gastrointestinal parasitism. This can cause hypoalbuminemia by at least two mechanisms. If the parasites absorb significant amounts of nutrients, including amino acids, the animal is deprived of the amino acids needed to produce albumin. If the parasites attach to the gastric or the intestinal wall and consume the host's blood, albumin and globulin are lost. Gastrointestinal parasitism seldom results in a deficiency of amino acids that is severe enough to lead to hypoglobulinemia. Fecal examination for parasite ova is helpful in establishing the diagnosis of this potential cause of hypoalbuminemia.
• Intestinal malabsorption or maldigestion. Decreased albumin production can occur if intestinal malabsorption results in deficient absorption of amino acids. Animals with malabsorption syndrome often have a history of chronic diarrhea or loose stools. If malabsorption syndrome is considered a possible cause of hypoalbuminemia, tests to verify this syndrome should be performed (see Chapter 29).

Inadequate digestion of dietary proteins can result from exocrine pancreatic insufficiency (EPI), in which amino acids are not liberated by protein digestion in the intestine and, therefore, are not available for absorption, thus resulting in amino acid deficiency and decreased albumin production. Animals with EPI often have a history of chronic diarrhea or loose stools. If EPI is suspected, tests to verify this disease should be performed (see Chapter 29).

• Inflammation. Because albumin is a negative APP, albumin synthesis is decreased during acute inflammation. Globulin concentrations are typically mildly increased due to increased positive APP synthesis. Because albumin and globulin concentrations change in different directions, total protein concentrations may be within the reference interval.

Increased loss of albumin can occur in the following disorders:

• Glomerular disease. Because albumin molecules are small and more negatively charged than globulin molecules, they leak more readily through damaged glomerular membranes. Severe glomerular disease, therefore, can result in selective hypoalbuminemia. Both urinary protein concentrations and urinary protein:creatinine ratios will be increased in animals with glomerular disease [45, 46]. Glomerular disease may result in nephrotic syndrome, which is characterized by proteinuria, hypoalbuminemia, hypercholesterolemia, and edema and/or ascites. The combination of hypoalbuminemia and hypercholesterolemia that occurs with nephrotic syndrome (see Chapter 32) contrasts to the hypoalbuminemia and hypocholesterolemia that may be seen with liver failure and protein losing enteropathy (PLE).
• Gastrointestinal parasitism (discussed earlier).
• Diseases listed as being possible causes of hypoalbuminemia with hypoglobulinemia (discussed earlier). Loss of both albumin and globulin typically occurs with these diseases, but a concurrent immune response may cause increased production of globulins resulting in normal to increased globulin concentrations. These diseases also should be considered when hypoalbuminemia with normal to increased globulin concentrations are detected.

Selective hypoglobulinemia

Hypoglobulinemia in the absence of hypoalbuminemia usually results from a decreased beta or gamma globulin concentration. A decreased alpha globulin concentration alone does not result in a decreased globulin concentration. A selective decrease in beta or gamma globulin concentrations is usually due to a decreased immunoglobulin concentration. Such a decrease can occur in the following disorders:

• Failure of passive transfer. Ingestion of colostrum and absorption of immunoglobulins from colostrum are termed passive transfer. Because most animals are born with minimal immunoglobulin concentrations, this process plays an important role in transferring resistance to infection during the neonatal period. Failure to ingest colostrum or to absorb immunoglobulins from colostrum is termed FPT and is well documented in domestic animals [23, 25, 27]. Several screening tests are available to assess the adequacy of passive transfer (discussed earlier).
• Inherited or acquired immune deficiency. Immune deficiency involving B lymphocytes or plasma cells can result in low concentrations of immunoglobulins and, in some cases, hypoglobulinemia. Immune deficiencies resulting in low globulin concentrations have been reported in foals (e.g., severe combined immunodeficiency, selective IgM deficiency, Fell pony immunodeficiency, transient hypogammaglobulinemia, agammaglobulinemia) [23], calves (e.g., selective IgG2 deficiency, severe combined immunodeficiency, transient hypogammaglobulinemia) [5], and puppies (e.g., severe combined immune deficiency, selective IgA deficiency, selective IgM deficiency, selective IgA and IgG deficiency) [5].

Causes of increased protein concentrations

Increased total protein concentrations can result from increased concentrations of albumin, globulin, or both. An increased albumin or globulin concentration, however, does not always produce detectable increases in total protein concentrations. A diagnostic algorithm for evaluating the variations in these increases is presented in Figure 30.3. In clinical practice, serum protein electrophoresis is often

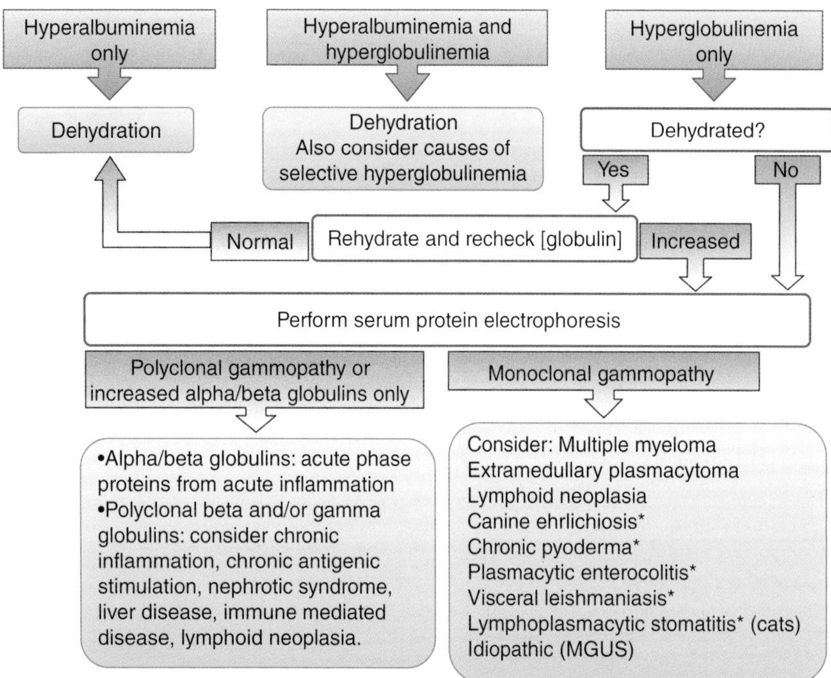

Figure 30.3 An algorithm for evaluation of increased serum protein concentrations. MGUS, monoclonal gammopathy of undetermined significance. *Typically causes polyclonal, not monoclonal, gammopathy. Refer to text for details.

reserved for patients with moderate to severe hyperglobulinemia (>5 g/dL), for which an underlying cause for inflammation or chronic antigenic stimulation has not been identified (discussed later).

Hyperalbuminemia

The primary cause of hyperalbuminemia in clinical patients is dehydration. Loss of plasma water results in a relative increase in albumin, which may be of sufficient magnitude to cause hyperproteinemia. Globulin concentrations also may be increased in some patients with dehydration (discussed later).

Rarely, administration of drugs (glucocorticoids) has been associated with mild transient hyperalbuminemia [47]. A single case report exists of hyperalbuminemia associated with hepatocellular carcinoma in a dog [48].

Hyperalbuminemia with hyperglobulinemia

Concurrent increases in albumin and globulin concentrations most commonly result from dehydration, which causes loss plasma water and a relative increase in both protein fractions. The albumin:globulin ratio is not altered, because both fractions are concentrated equally. The hematocrit is often increased as well (unless there was a preexisting anemia). Other potential causes of hyperglobulinemia should also be considered (discussed later).

Selective hyperglobulinemia

The significance of hyperglobulinemia depends on the magnitude and the type of globulin that is increased, which can be determined by serum protein electrophoresis. No matter what the underlying cause, mild to moderate hypoalbuminemia is often also present. Common disorders and typical electrophoretic patterns are discussed below.

Increased alpha/beta globulin concentrations

Acute/chronic inflammation: During acute inflammation, increased synthesis of APP causes hyperglobulinemia, which is generally mild. The APP are located in the alpha and beta globulin regions of the electrophoretogram (except for fibrinogen, which is absent from serum). There are numerous APP, and generally many of them must be increased in order to visualize an electrophoretic abnormality or result in hyperglobulinemia; however, fibrinogen or haptoglobin alone can be increased to a degree sufficient to cause hyperglobulinemia and an increase in total protein [5]. Because albumin is a negative APP, albumin concentrations usually decrease due to decreased hepatic production during acute inflammation. The magnitude of the decrease is usually <30% [10].

Increased gamma globulin concentrations

The gamma globulin fraction includes immunoglobulins of all types. Increases in gamma globulin concentrations are termed gammopathies. Gammopathies may be monoclonal or polyclonal, which may be distinguished presumptively on the basis of the width of the globulin peak in an electrophoretogram. Polyclonal gammopathies have broad-based peaks (i.e., wider than the base of the albumin peak, with a slope that is less steep than the albumin peak) on the electrophoretogram (Figure 30.4). These polyclonal peaks represent increased quantities of a mixture of immunoglobulin types

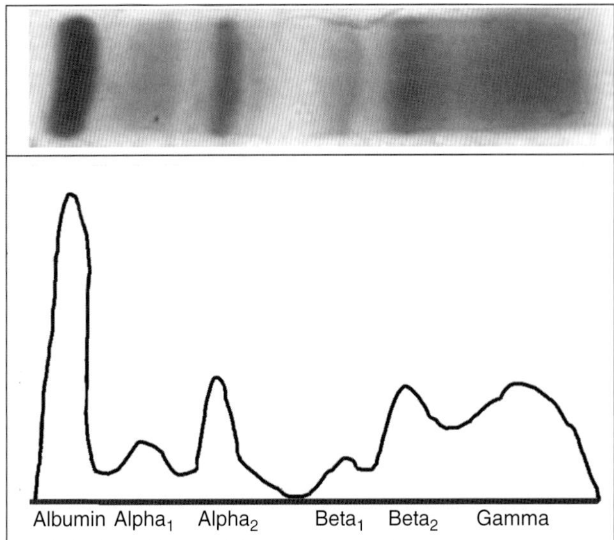

Figure 30.4 An electrophoretogram and corresponding gel from a dog with a polyclonal gammopathy. There is an increase in alpha$_2$-globulins and a broad-based peak in the beta$_2$ and gamma regions.

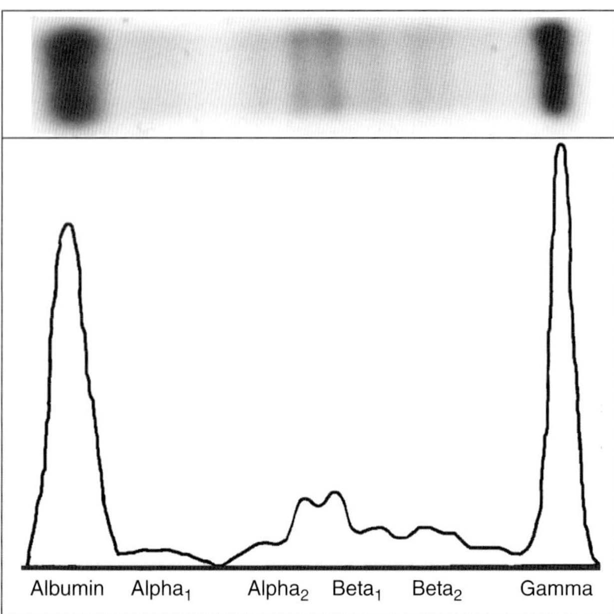

Figure 30.5 An electrophoretogram and corresponding gel from a cat with a monoclonal gammopathy due to multiple myeloma. There is a narrow-based peak in the gamma region; the corresponding monoclonal band is apparent on the gel.

produced by a heterogeneous population of B lymphocytes, plasma cells, or both, each secreting its own immunoglobulin molecule specific for one particular antigen. Monoclonal gammopathies, however, have narrow-based peaks (i.e., similar in width to the base of the albumin peak, with a slope that is as steep or steeper than the albumin peak) on the electrophoretogram (Figure 30.5), and they result from increased production of a single type of immunoglobulin by a single clone of B lymphocytes or plasma cells. Proliferation of a single clone of lymphocyte results in overproduction of its specific immunoglobulin molecule.

Visually determining whether a peak is polyclonal or monoclonal is not always straightforward; peaks may be steep but slightly wider than the albumin peak (Figure 30.6). The term oligoclonal has been used to describe a polyclonal peak with a restricted migration pattern such that it appears narrow and monoclonal on an electrophoretogram [5]. Oligoclonal gammopathies may be difficult to distinguish from monoclonal gammopathies and have been recognized in animals with chronic infectious diseases [5, 20, 21]. When an oligoclonal gammopathy is suspected, characterizing the gammopathy with immunoelectrophoresis may be helpful. If the gammopathy is composed primarily of IgA or IgM, a monoclonal gammopathy due to neoplasia is most likely. If it is composed primarily of IgG, the gammopathy could be monoclonal or polyclonal.

Uncommonly, two narrow-based peaks may be seen on the electrophoretogram; this is termed a biclonal gammopathy (Figure 30.7). Biclonal gammopathies can occur when a single neoplastic clone produces immunoglobulin molecules that migrate separately. Examples include polymerization of

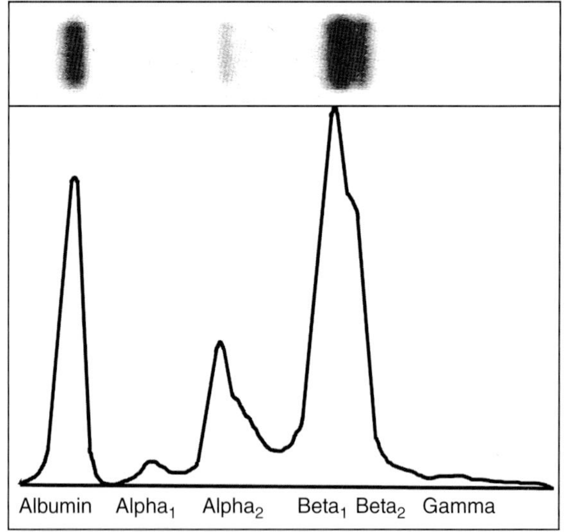

Figure 30.6 An electrophoretogram and corresponding gel from a dog with a suspect oligoclonal gammopathy. There is a steep peak with a narrow shoulder encompassing the beta$_1$ and beta$_2$ regions of the gel. The base is slightly wider than that of the albumin peak. Immunoelectrophoresis demonstrated that the majority of the immunoglobulin was IgA, most consistent with a monoclonal gammopathy caused by lymphoid neoplasia. The narrow shoulder may be caused by the presence of IgA dimers.

immunoglobulin molecules (such as dimer formation), production of incomplete molecules (such as free light chains in addition to intact immunoglobulins), or production of an immunoglobulin that undergoes isotype switching [49, 50].

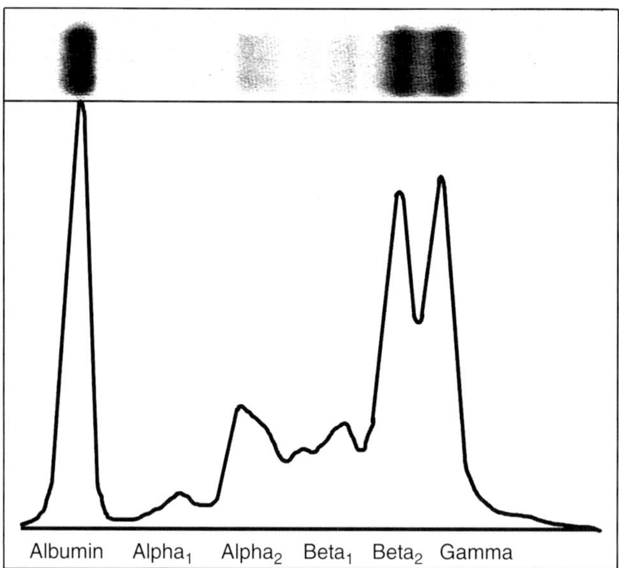

Figure 30.7 An electrophoretogram and corresponding gel from a dog with a biclonal gammopathy. Two distinct tall, sharp peaks are visible, one in the $beta_2$ region and one in the gamma region of the gel. Immunoelectrophoresis demonstrated that the immunoglobulin was predominantly IgA, consistent with lymphoid neoplasia. The second peak in the gamma region most likely resulted from IgA dimer formation.

Rarely, two clones of plasma cells or B lymphocytes may proliferate, resulting in production of two separate, but homogeneous, types of immunoglobulins [51]. It is possible for a monoclonal gammopathy to be obscured by a concurrent polyclonal peak; in these cases, visual inspection of the stained electrophoretic gel may suggest presence of a monoclonal band. More sensitive and specific techniques may be required to confirm presence of a monoclonal gammopathy (i.e., immunoelectrophoresis or immunofixation) [52, 53].

Hyperviscosity of the blood can result from high concentrations of immunoglobulins, especially in association with monoclonal gammopathies. Hyperviscosity syndrome might cause the initial clinical signs observed in animals with monoclonal gammopathies. These signs include epistaxis, ocular abnormalities (e.g., visual impairment, distension and tortuosity of retinal veins, retinal hemorrhage and detachment), cardiovascular abnormalities (e.g., gallop rhythm, left ventricular hypertrophy), and neurologic dysfunction (e.g., disorientation, seizures) [54]. Hyperviscosity syndrome is often associated with monoclonal gammopathies involving IgM (because of their large size) or IgA (because of dimer formation) but can also occur with IgG.

Monoclonal cryoglobulinemia is a rare variation of monoclonal gammopathy that has been reported in dogs, cats, and horses [55]. In this disorder, the monoclonal globulins are soluble at 37 °C but become reversibly insoluble at lower temperatures, causing formation of a gel-like precipitate. To demonstrate cryoglobulins, serum must be harvested from the blood at 37 °C. If blood samples are stored at refrigerator temperature before harvesting the serum, the cryoglobulins are not harvested, and cryoglobulinemia is not detected. Cryoglobulins are rarely associated with polyclonal disorders.

Conditions typically associated with polyclonal gammopathies include:

- Chronic inflammation or antigenic stimulation. As an inflammatory response becomes chronic (>1 week), production of immunoglobulins and complement proteins may be increased; APP may remain increased as well. Chronic antigenic stimulation from any cause, including immune-mediated diseases, can cause similar abnormalities. Immunoglobulins usually migrate in the gamma globulin region, although some (IgA and IgM) occasionally migrate in beta globulin region along with complement proteins. The magnitude of the hyperglobulinemia that occurs with chronic inflammation is variable but can be marked in some cases (>10 g/dL) [56].

Gammopathies associated with chronic inflammation are usually polyclonal, exemplified by canine ehrlichiosis and feline infectious peritonitis. However, exceptions to this rule have been recognized. In particular, apparent monoclonal gammopathies have been reported in dogs with chronic ehrlichiosis, chronic pyoderma, plasmacytic enterocolitis, visceral leishmaniasis, and in cats with lymphoplasmacytic stomatitis [21, 57–61]. In some of these cases, the apparent monoclonal spike was likely oligolonal and not a true monoclonal gammopathy because it consisted of a several subclasses of IgG or heterogeneous light chains [62, 63]. Infection with *Bartonella henselae* has been reported to cause a monoclonal gammopathy (confirmed by immunofixation) in people, and a monoclonal or oligoclonal gammopathy has been described in a dog with *B. henselae* infection [64, 65].

- Liver disease. Especially when chronic, liver disease may lead to increased globulin production, which has been well-documented in horses but also occurs in other species [66]. The globulins are frequently immunoglobulins that migrate in the beta or gamma region of an electrophoretogram and can obscure the border between the beta and gamma regions, known as beta–gamma bridging. It is theorized that mononuclear phagocytes (Kupffer cells) in the diseased liver fail to clear antigens from the portal circulation. The antigens subsequently reach the general circulation, where they stimulate B lymphocytes to mount an immune response. In liver failure, albumin concentrations may be decreased concurrently due to decreased hepatic synthesis. Although historically believed to be pathognomonic for hepatic disease, recent studies have shown that beta-gamma bridging is frequently seen with infectious diseases as well [67].
- Lymphoma and lymphocytic leukemia. Polyclonal gammopathy occasionally occurs with lymphoma and lymphocytic leukemia, sometimes because of increased

production of heterogeneous immunoglobulins by multiple clones of proliferating, neoplastic lymphoid cells [1]. However, monoclonal gammopathies are more commonly associated with lymphoid neoplasia (discussed later). Secondary infectious processes may stimulate immunoglobulin production in animals with lymphoma and lymphocytic leukemia.

***Conditions typically associated with monoclonal gammopathies include*:**

- Multiple myeloma. This is a malignant, proliferative disease of plasma cells that involves the bone marrow at multiple sites and, often, other tissues (e.g., spleen, liver). Infiltration of visceral organs appears to be relatively common in cats [68]. Multiple myeloma typically results from the proliferation of a single clone of plasma cells that produce a homogeneous type of protein that is referred to as paraprotein or M-component. This protein most commonly is IgA or IgG; IgM paraproteinemias occur with lymphoma and lymphocytic leukemia but are rare with multiple myeloma [69, 70]. Primary macroglobulinemia (Waldenström macroglobulinemia) results from neoplastic proliferation of less differentiated B lymphocytes and is an uncommon cause of IgM monoclonal gammopathy; this disease may be difficult to distinguish from multiple myeloma [71]. Multiple myeloma paraproteins can be composed of entire immunoglobulin molecules or of just heavy or light chains of these molecules [50, 72–74]. Paraproteins typically are found as a monoclonal peak in the beta or gamma region and, more rarely, in the alpha region of the electrophoretogram [75]. As discussed previously, biclonal peaks are also possible but rare. Light chains also may be detected in the urine and are referred to as Bence Jones proteins. The diagnosis of this disease is usually established on the basis of finding at least three of the following four features:
  1. Monoclonal gammopathy.
  2. Excessive numbers of plasma cells on a bone marrow film. The percentage of plasma cells that is considered to be suggestive of myeloma varies with different authors (>5% to >20%). Chronic antigenic stimulation also can result in greater than 5% plasma cells on a bone marrow film. Other features that are suggestive of plasma cell neoplasia, such as the presence of plasma cell aggregates, poorly differentiated plasma cells, or both, are helpful in differentiating myeloma from antigenic stimulation in bone marrow films with increased numbers of plasma cells.
  3. Radiographic evidence of osteolytic bone lesions.
  4. Bence Jones proteinuria. Bence Jones proteins are light chains of immunoglobulins that are produced in some gammopathies. Because of their small size, these proteins readily pass the glomerulus. If the concentration of Bence Jones proteins in the urine exceeds the tubular reabsorptive capacity, they are excreted in the urine. Bence Jones proteins rarely are detected by urine dipstick tests for proteins, because dipsticks primarily detect albumin. Bence Jones proteins can be detected by several techniques, including the heat precipitation test, electrophoresis, and immunoelectrophoresis. The heat precipitation test can be performed in a practice laboratory, but this test is difficult to perform and interpret [76]. Bence Jones proteins are detectable in approximately 30% of dogs and cats with multiple myelomas and have been reported in a horse with multiple myeloma [73, 77]. Bence Jones proteins have also been detected in animals with other neoplastic and non-neoplastic monoclonal gammopathies [58, 61, 78, 79].
- Extramedullary plasmacytoma [80]. Extramedullary plasmacytomas are proliferations of plasma cells originating from a site other than bone. They are usually solitary, cutaneous, benign lesions that most commonly occur in dogs but have also been reported in cats. Plasmacytomas that occur in the digestive tract are more likely to be malignant. In cats, there is evidence that extramedullary tumors may progress to multiple myeloma [81]. Monoclonal gammopathies rarely occur in association with these tumors. A biclonal gammopathy has been reported in a cat with two extramedullary plasmacytomas [82].
- Lymphoma and lymphocytic leukemia [83–85]. Monoclonal gammopathies can occur with lymphoma and lymphocytic leukemia. Approximately 5% of dogs with lymphoma and lymphocytic leukemia have monoclonal gammopathies [85]. The incidence appears higher in dogs with chronic lymphocytic leukemia, however, with studies indicating an incidence of greater than 50% in such cases [79]. The immunoglobulin most commonly increased is IgM, especially in cases of chronic lymphocytic leukemia, but IgG and IgA monoclonal gammopathies also have been reported [79].

***Less common causes of apparent monoclonal gammopathies include*:**

- Canine ehrlichiosis [57]. Although polyclonal gammopathies are more common, monoclonal gammopathies have been reported in dogs with ehrlichiosis. Infrequently, polyclonal gammopathies progress to monoclonal gammopathies. Typically, the monoclonal gammopathies are composed of IgG and result from an unexplained proliferation of one plasma cell clone. Monoclonal spikes disappear after treatment for ehrlichiosis. The serum hyperviscosity syndrome (discussed later) has also been reported in these dogs.
- Chronic pyoderma [58]. An IgG monoclonal gammopathy with Bence Jones proteinuria has been reported in a dog with chronic pyoderma. Treatment and resolution of the pyoderma were followed by disappearance of the monoclonal gammopathy.
- Plasmacytic enterocolitis [59]. Monoclonal gammopathy has been reported in a dog with this disease. The monoclonal gammopathy disappeared after treatment and resolution of the inflammation.

• Visceral leishmaniasis (in dogs) [60]. Most dogs with visceral leishmaniasis have polyclonal gammopathies. In a few such dogs, a single clone of plasma cells may proliferate and result in IgG monoclonal gammopathy.
• Lymphoplasmacytic stomatitis (in cats) [61]. Monoclonal gammopathy with Bence Jones proteinuria occurs infrequently in cats with this disease.
• Idiopathic monoclonal gammopathy [78, 86]. Unexplained monoclonal gammopathies among animals in which known causes have been eliminated are termed idiopathic, or monoclonal gammopathy of undetermined significance (MGUS). These animals are asymptomatic and may have stable production of the monoclonal immunoglobulin for a prolonged period of time (i.e., months to years); Bence Jones proteinuria occurs in some of these cases. These gammopathies may relate to antigenic stimulation of a B lymphocyte clone. "Idiopathic" monoclonal gammopathy, however, may precede the onset of overt multiple myeloma.

Hyperfibrinogenemia

Increased plasma fibrinogen concentrations are most often associated with inflammatory conditions and dehydration but have also been recognized pregnancy and neoplasia [5, 87–89].
• Dehydration. With dehydration, fibrinogen increases in proportion to other plasma proteins. To eliminate the effect of hydration status, a plasma protein:fibrinogen ratio (PP:Fib) can be calculated as follows [5]:

$$\text{PP:Fib} = \frac{\text{Plasma protein (g/dL)} \times 1000}{\text{Plasma fibrinogen (mg/dL)}}$$

The PP:Fib should not change with changes in hydration status.

As a general rule, a PP:Fib <10 is considered consistent with hyperfibrinogenemia due to inflammation (discussed later), and a ratio >15 is considered normal or consistent with dehydration [90]. Some authors suggest slightly different cutoff values for horses; <15 for inflammation and >20 for normal or dehydration [5]. These are rough guidelines for use in adult animals, and do not take into account other factors that could influence plasma protein and fibrinogen concentrations.
• Inflammation. Fibrinogen is a positive APP, therefore plasma concentrations increase with inflammation. Although other APP may be better indicators of inflammatory disease, fibrinogen continues to be used because it is easy to measure in practice situations [10, 91, 92]. It is often included in routine equine and bovine complete blood counts. With inflammation in those species, fibrinogen concentrations may sometimes be increased in the absence of an inflammatory leukogram [93]. In dogs, it offers no advantage over leukocyte counts for evaluation of inflammation [94].

Appendix 30.1

A sodium sulfite precipitation test: application in ruminants

1. Prepare three solutions of sodium sulfite (14%, 16%, and 18%) from anhydrous sulfite and distilled water.
2. Place 1.9 mL of sodium sulfite solution into each of three 13 × 100 mm test tubes.
3. Add 0.1 mL of serum into each of the three tubes.
4. Mix immediately, and then incubate at room temperature for 1 hour.
5. After 1 hour, examine the tubes for evidence of precipitation.
6. Interpret as described in Table 30.A.1.

Table 30.A.1 Interpretation of sodium sulfite precipitation test results.

Estimated immunoglobulin concentration (mg/dL)	Sodium sulfite concentration		
	14%	16%	18%
<500	–	–	+
500–1500	–	+	+
>1500	+	+	+

– No precipitation after 1 hour (cloudiness without visible flakes is a negative test).
+ Flakes of precipitation after 1 hour (regardless of flake density).
Source: Adapted from Pfeiffer McGuire TC (1977). A sodium sulfite-precipitation test for assessment of colostral immunoglobulin transfer to calves. *J Am Vet Med Assoc* 170: 809–11.

Appendix 30.2

Zinc sulfate turbidity test: application in ruminants

1. Prepare a solution of zinc sulfate ($ZnSO_4 \cdot 7H_2O$) by mixing 350 mg of zinc sulfate in 1 L of distilled water that has been previously boiled to remove CO_2. Note that lower concentrations of zinc sulfate might be appropriate in some cases. Lower concentrations have a higher sensitivity but a lower specificity; higher concentrations (e.g., 350 mg/L) have a lower sensitivity and a higher specificity (Table 30.A.2).
2. The solution should be stored in an air-tight bottle that is connected to a CO_2 trap to prevent CO_2 absorption.
3. Add 0.1 mL of serum (hemolysis might interfere with the test) to a tube (13 × 100 mm) containing 6 mL of the zinc sulfate solution. Cap the tube to prevent absorption of CO_2, which adds to turbidity.

Table 30.A.2 Zinc sulfate turbidity test performance for detection of FPT in ruminants.

Zinc sulfate concentration (mg/L)	Sensitivity	Specificity
200	100%	25%
250	100%	42%
300	98%	65%
350	94%	76%
400	83%	91%

Source: Adapted from Hudgens KA, Tyler JW, Besser TE, Krytenberg DS (1996). Optimizing performance of a qualitative zinc sulfate turbidity test for passive transfer of immunoglobulin G in calves. *Am J Vet Res* 57: 1711–13.

4. Mix the contents of the tube and incubate at room temperature (23 °C) for 1 hour.
5. After the incubation period, mix the contents of the tube, and then hold the tube in front of newsprint.
6. Cloudiness sufficient to obscure newsprint when viewed through the tube is considered to be a positive reaction.
7. Interpret a negative reaction as being suggestive of the failure of passive transfer.

Appendix 30.3

Zinc sulfate turbidity test: application in horses

1. Prepare a solution of zinc sulfate ($ZnSO_4 \cdot 7H_2O$) by mixing 208 mg of zinc sulfate in 1 L of distilled water that has been previously boiled to remove CO_2.
2. The solution should be stored in an air-tight bottle that is connected to a CO_2 trap to prevent CO_2 absorption.
3. Add 0.1 mL of serum to a 13 × 100 mm test tube containing 6 mL of the zinc sulfate solution. Cap the tube to prevent absorption of CO_2, which adds to turbidity.
4. Mix the contents of the tube and incubate at room temperature (23 °C) for 1 hour.
5. After the incubation period, mix the contents of the tube, and then observe for turbidity.
6. Interpret as follows:
- **A.** Visible turbidity indicates immunoglobulin concentration is at least 400 mg/dL.
- **B.** This test can be made semiquantitative by using a spectrophotometer and reading absorbance at 600 nm, which requires the use of standards.

Appendix 30.4

Glutaraldehyde coagulation test: application in ruminants

1. Prepare a 10% solution of glutaraldehyde (usually prepared via dilution of a 25% solution to a 10% solution).
2. Place 0.5 mL of serum into a 13 × 100 mm test tube.
3. Add 50 µL (0.05 mL) of the 10% glutaraldehyde reagent to the tube.
4. Mix immediately, and then incubate at room temperature.
5. Examine the tube at intervals for as long as 1 hour, looking for evidence of coagulation.
6. Interpret as follows:
- **A.** Complete coagulation indicates immunoglobulin concentration is more than 600 mg/dL.
- **B.** Semisolid gel indicates immunoglobulin concentration is 400–600 mg/dL.
- **C.** No coagulation indicates immunoglobulin concentration is less than 400 mg/dL.

Appendix 30.5

Glutaraldehyde coagulation test: application in horses

1. Perform steps 1 through 4 as outlined in Appendix 30.4.
2. Examine the tube at 5, 10, 15, 20, 30, 45, and 60 minutes.
3. A positive reaction is solid coagulation (i.e., does not move when the tube is tilted).
4. Interpret as follows:
- **A.** Coagulation within 10 minutes indicates immunoglobulin concentration is more than 800 mg/dL.
- **B.** Coagulation by 60 minutes indicates immunoglobulin concentration is 400– 800 mg/dL.
- **C.** No coagulation by 60 minutes indicates immunoglobulin concentration is less than 400 mg/dL.

Appendix 30.6

Fibrinogen determination by heat precipitation

1. Fill two microhematocrit tubes with ethylenediaminetetraacetic acid (EDTA)–anticoagulated blood.
2. Sediment blood in both tubes using a microhematocrit centrifuge.

3. Break one tube at the bottom of the plasma column, apply the plasma to a refractometer, and read the protein concentration.

4. Place the second microhematocrit tube in a water bath at 56–58 °C for 3–5 minutes, which denatures and precipitates the fibrinogen in the sample. Note that hot tap water frequently is in the 56–58 °C range. If so (check with a thermometer), such tap water placed in an insulated container can replace the water bath as an incubation chamber.

5. After incubation, recentrifuge the second microhematocrit tube in the microhematocrit centrifuge to sediment the precipitated fibrinogen.

6. Measure the protein concentration in the second tube using a refractometer.

7. Subtract the protein concentration of the second tube from that of the first tube. The difference is the estimate of the plasma fibrinogen concentration. For example, if the protein concentration in the first tube is 7.1 g/dL and that in the second tube is 6.7 g/dL, then the fibrinogen concentration is 0.4 g/dL.

8. Fibrinogen concentrations usually are converted to mg/dL (e.g., 0.4 g/dL = 400 mg/dL).

31 Laboratory Detection of Muscle Injury

Robin W. Allison

Department of Veterinary Pathobiology, Oklahoma State University College of Veterinary Medicine, Stillwater, OK, USA

Routine laboratory tests that evaluate muscle are primarily aimed at detecting muscle injury. These tests include assays that measure the serum activities of enzymes and other proteins that leak from injured muscle cells and the urine concentrations of myoglobin, which also leaks from injured muscle cells and is excreted via glomerular filtration. Tests that are more specific for cardiac muscle injury measure serum concentrations of proteins or hormones released from cardiac muscle (cardiac biomarkers).

Creatine kinase

Creatine kinase (CK) is an enzyme present in highest concentrations in skeletal muscle, cardiac muscle, smooth muscle, and brain, with lesser amounts present various organs such as intestine, liver, and spleen [1, 2]. CK is found free in the cytoplasm of muscle cells and leaks from these cells when they are damaged. CK is considered a muscle-specific leakage enzyme. Although CK is present in the brain, brain injury causes increased CK activity in the cerebrospinal fluid instead of the blood because of the blood–brain barrier. Increases in CK activity following muscle injury occur rapidly (peaking in 6–12 hours) but also decline rapidly (a day or 2) because CK has a short half-life of about 2 hours (see Figure 31.1) [3]. Thus, persistent increases in CK activity indicate ongoing muscle damage. Although the specificity of CK activity for muscle injury is high, sensitivity is fairly low, likely related to its short half-life [4].

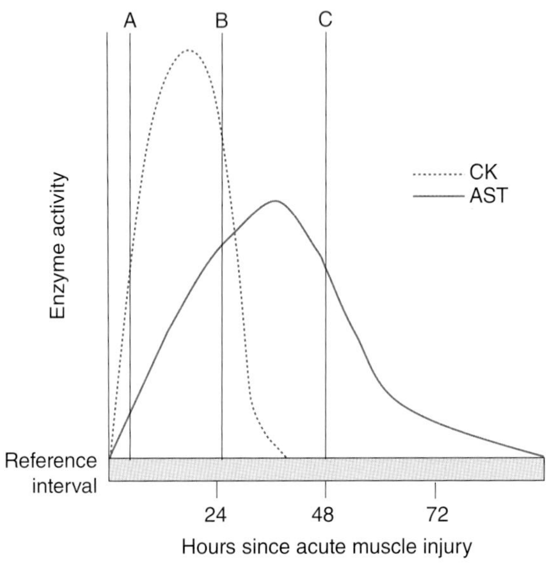

Figure 31.1 Serum activities of both AST and CK increase as a result of muscle injury but rise and fall at different rates. Evaluation of these two enzymes together can help estimate when a muscle injury occurred and indicate whether such injury is still occurring. An increase in predominantly the serum CK activity (line A) suggests very acute muscle injury. Increased serum activities of both AST and CK (line B) suggest active or recent muscle injury. An increase in only the serum AST activity (line C) suggests that muscle injury has stopped and that the serum CK activity returned to normal as a result of the short half-life of CK. An increase in only the serum AST activity may also result from liver injury.

CK exists as a dimer, composed of different combinations of two subunits designated B (brain) and M (muscle). A total of four isoenzymes have been identified. There is some variation by species, but in dogs CK-BB (CK-1) predominates in brain and organs such as spleen and kidney; CK-MB (CK-2) is mainly in intestine, lung, and spleen with a small amount in myocardium; and CK-MM (CK-3) is the major form in skeletal and cardiac muscle [1]. The fourth isoenzyme, CK-Mt, exists within mitochondria of many tissues. The reported distributions of isoenzyme activities in the blood of normal dogs vary, but CK-MM and CK-BB together are responsible for the majority of the CK activity with a small contribution from CK-MB [4]. Because of the different tissue locations, CK isoenzymes have the potential to be tissue specific. In people, increased serum CK-MB activity has historically been considered a reliable marker of myocardial injury but has been replaced by other cardiac biomarkers in recent years (see discussion of cardiac biomarkers) [5]. Measurement of CK isoenzyme activities requires electrophoresis or specifies-specific antibodies, and these assays are not routinely available for animals.

CK activity can be measured in serum or plasma, but the activity is reportedly about 2.5 times greater in serum, most likely due to release of CK from platelets during clot-

Veterinary Hematology, Clinical Chemistry, and Cytology, Third Edition. Edited by Mary Anna Thrall, Glade Weiser, Robin W. Allison and Terry W. Campbell.

Companion website: www.wiley.com/go/thrall/veterinary

ting. In dogs, plasma CK activity is stable for a week when refrigerated and a month when frozen at −20 °C. Serum CK activity has also been reported to be greater in young puppies compared to adult dogs, with four times adult levels found in puppies under a month of age [6]. Marked increases (>20X URL) seen in newborn puppies are suspected to be caused by normal muscle trauma during the birthing process [7]. Moderate increases in CK activity, compared to that of adult dogs, have been demonstrated in puppies up to 2 months of age [7, 8]. A falsely increased CK activity can occur as a result of hemolysis, hyperbilirubinemia and muscle fluid contamination of the blood sample during a difficult venipuncture. Extremely high serum CK activities (>100X URL) occasionally are detected in animals with muscle injuries. These markedly increased CK activities may be greater than the linearity limits for the assay. Technicians analyzing such serum for CK activity may have difficulty reaching an end point in the assay because the serum CK activity continues to increase with serial dilution. Various theories have been postulated to explain this phenomenon, including that dilution of serum CK inhibitors is responsible [9–11]. In these cases CK activity may be reported as greater than the limit of linearity for that particular assay.

Increased serum CK activity results from:

- Skeletal muscle injury. Injury to skeletal muscle is the most common cause of increased CK activity, which may result from such minor procedures as physical restraint and intramuscular injections. Muscle necrosis and ischemia, strenuous exercise or seizures, and trauma during shipping can result in an increased serum CK activity. The underlying causes for muscle injury are numerous and varied, including trauma, toxins, exertional rhabdomyolysis, inflammatory myopathies due to bacterial, viral, or parasitic diseases, and inherited conditions such as muscular dystrophy [4, 12]. So-called "downer" cattle will have increased CK activity due to ischemic muscle necrosis. Increased CK activity has also been reported in dogs with endocrine diseases (hypothyroidism and hyperadrenocorticism) [4]. Depending on the underlying cause, the magnitude of the increase may be mild to marked and correlates somewhat with the extent of muscle injury.
- Cardiac muscle injury. Increases in CK activity can occur with injury to cardiac muscle. In dogs, this is due to increases in both CK-MM and CK-MB activities [13]. Because of the relatively small volume of cardiac muscle compared to skeletal muscle, CK activity increases with cardiac muscle injury are unlikely to reach the magnitude seen with severe injury to skeletal muscle.
- Smooth muscle injury. In theory, injury to tissues containing abundant smooth muscle could cause increased serum CK activity, but this is rarely recognized in practice. However, the bovine uterus has been shown to contain relatively high concentrations of CK, and serum CK increases have been documented in cattle with endometritis [14].
- Muscle catabolism. Increased CK activity can occur in anorexic cats that have diseases not directly involving muscle. A median serum CK activity of 2529 IU/L, with some activities being greater than 10,000 IU/L (reference range = 10–100 IU/L), has been reported in such cats [15]. Muscle catabolism to supply amino acids for protein synthesis and gluconeogenesis is theorized to result in the leakage of CK from muscle cells. The CK activity in these cats decreased rapidly after nutritional support was initiated.

Aspartate aminotransferase

Aspartate aminotransferase (AST), previously known as serum glutamic oxaloacetic transaminase (SGOT), is present at highest concentrations in hepatocytes as well as in skeletal and cardiac muscle cells [1]. AST is present in both the cytoplasm and mitochondria of these cells [2]. Serum AST activity increases not only from muscle injury but also hepatocyte injury and may be mildly increased in dogs due to drug induction (see Chapter 27). Serum AST activity increases more slowly than serum CK activity after muscle injury (Figure 31.1). It peaks at approximately 24–36 hours after acute muscle injury, and it decreases more slowly than serum CK activity after the muscle injury ceases. The half-life of AST in the blood has been estimated between 4 and 12 hours in dogs, 77 minutes in cats, and 7–8 days in horses [1, 3, 16].

The relative serum activities of both CK and AST can be used to estimate when muscle injury occurred and whether active muscle injury is ongoing (Figure 31.1). An increase in only the serum CK activity (Figure 31.1, line A) suggests very acute muscle injury (i.e., there has not been sufficient time since the injury occurred for the serum AST activity to increase). Increased serum activities of both AST and CK (Figure 31.1, line B) suggest active or recent muscle injury. An increase in only the serum AST activity (Figure 31.1, line C) suggests that muscle injury stopped more than 2 days earlier and that the serum CK activity returned to normal as a result of the short half-life of CK. This latter combination of results also can occur with liver injury (i.e., if liver is the source of the AST, the CK activity would be normal).

Alanine aminotransferase

Alanine aminotransferase (ALT), previously known as serum glutamic pyruvic transaminase (SGPT), is a leakage enzyme that is free in the cytoplasm. This enzyme is primarily used to detect hepatocyte injury (see Chapter 27), but it is not totally liver specific [17]. In dogs, the ALT activities in skeletal and cardiac muscles are approximately 5% and 25%, respectively, of the liver ALT activity [1]. In cats, the ALT activities of both skeletal and cardiac muscle are approximately 5% of the liver ALT activity [1]. The situation is different in horses, where liver contains relatively little ALT activity and the ALT activity in skeletal muscle is approximately four times that of liver [1]. Muscle should be considered as a potential source of increased serum ALT activity even in dogs and cats, because the total mass of muscle is much greater than that of liver. Measuring the serum activity of an enzyme with greater muscle specificity (CK) is preferable for detecting muscle damage.

Lactate dehydrogenase

Lactate dehydrogenase (LDH) is located in the cytoplasm of most cells in the body. [1] Injury to most tissues results in leakage of LDH into the extracellular space and the blood; therefore, LDH is a very nonspecific enzyme.

Lactate dehydrogenase isoenzymes

Five LDH isoenzymes exist, which can be identified by electrophoretic separation. Each isoenzyme is present in a limited number of tissues and, therefore is more tissue specific than the serum total LDH activity [18]. LDH molecules are composed of four components, which are either muscle (M) or heart (H) subunits. The five isoenzymes are LDH_1 (H_4), LDH_2 (MH_3), LDH_3 (M_2H_2), LDH_4 (M_3H), and LDH_5 (M_4). The designations H_4, MH_3, and so on refer to the number of each subunit (M or H) in the LDH isoenzyme molecule. Although there is considerable species variation, generally the LDH_1 (H_4) isoenzyme predominates in cardiac muscle and the LDH_5 (M_4) isoenzyme predominates in skeletal muscle [1]. The remaining three isoenzymes are found in variable quantities in several different tissues. Although measurement of specific isoenzyme activities may provide information about skeletal versus cardiac muscle injury, isoenzyme assays are not routinely performed by most veterinary laboratories and more specific serum markers are now available for evaluating myocardial injury (see discussion of cardiac biomarkers).

Cardiac biomarkers

The use of biomarkers in blood to detect cardiac disease is commonplace in human medicine and is the subject of continuing research in veterinary medicine. Two classes of cardiac biomarkers that have received the most attention for use in veterinary species are the troponins (myocardial structural proteins) and the natriuretic peptides (hormones produced by cardiomyocytes).

Cardiac troponins

Troponins are structural proteins of striated muscle. In people, antibody assays developed against cardiac troponins I (cTnI) and T (cTnT) have identified that these proteins are released from injured cardiac muscle and enter the peripheral blood [19]. Assays for cTnI and cTnT have largely replaced assays for CK-MB activity as markers for myocardial injury in people, and are being investigated for similar purposes in animals [5, 20, 21]. Because the cardiac troponins are well-conserved between species, immunoassays designed for use in people have been used to detect these proteins in plasma from a variety of species including dogs, cats, horses, and cattle [21–24]. However, not all commercially available immunoassays have been used successfully in animals [25, 26]. Additionally, values obtained with one type of assay may not be directly comparable to values obtained with another [27].

Although regarded as highly sensitive and specific markers for cardiac disease in people, how cardiac troponin concentrations will correlate with specific diseases in animals is the subject of ongoing investigations. Troponin concentrations in healthy animals are very low or undetectable with many available assays. Increases in serum troponin concentrations are relatively modest in animals with cardiac injury, prompting recent development of assays with lower limits of detection [28]. Several studies have shown that cTnI concentrations are greater in dogs with acquired cardiac diseases compared to normal healthy dogs; conditions included mitral valve disease, dilated cardiomyopathy, and acute myocardial damage secondary to gastric dilatation-volvulus or blunt chest trauma [29–31]. However, cTnI concentrations were also increased in cases of renal failure, noncardiac systemic disease, and noncardiac dyspnea [32, 33].

Breed differences also exist. Greyhound and boxer dogs were shown to have cTnI concentrations significantly greater than those of non-greyhound or non-boxer control dogs [34, 35]. The specificity of cardiac troponins for cardiac injury in animals will depend on development of appropriate decision limits for the particular assay being used. It is important to keep in mind that cardiac injury, and resulting increases in cardiac biomarkers, may occur secondarily to many noncardiac diseases [20]. Serial determinations of cTNI concentrations may provide prognostic information in dogs with known cardiac disease [36]. However, data suggest that intraindividual variability in cTNI values is high and an increase of 112% is needed to be confident that there is a changed clinical status [37].

Natriuretic peptides

Brain naturiuretic peptide (BNP) is a hormone released by cardiomyocytes in response to volume expansion and pressure overload, and has been recognized as a biomarker of systemic hypertension and congestive heart failure in people [38]. Laboratory tests are available to measure plasma concentrations of the C-terminal fragment (C-BNP) in dogs and the N-terminal fragment of proBNP (NT-proBNP) in dogs and cats [39]. A point-of-care SNAP test for NT-proBNP is available for dogs and cats (Cardiopet® proBNP Test, IDEXX Laboratories).

Studies to date have suggested that NT-proBNP may be useful to help distinguish cardiac from noncardiac causes of respiratory abnormalities in dogs and cats [40–43]. Low or normal values are helpful to rule out cardiac disease, but NT-proBNP concentrations should be evaluated in context with clinical findings and other diagnostic tests. Studies have also examined the usefulness of NT-proBNP to detect occult cardiomyopathy. In one study, the combination of NT-proBNP (using the Cardiopet point-of-care assay) and Holter monitoring detected occult dilated cardiomyopathy in Doberman pinschers with 91% accuracy [44]. Measuring NT-proBNP alone, however, has shown low specificity for dilated cardiomyopathy resulting in numerous false-positive results [45]. In cats with risk factors for cardiomyopathy (such as murmur, gallop or dysrhythmia), NT-proBNP reliably identified those with occult cardiomyopathy with relatively high sensitivity and specificity (70–100% and 67–100% respectively, depending on the cutoff values used) [46, 47]. In cats suspected to have heart disease, the point-of-care Cardiopet NT-proBNP test, which reports results as either normal or abnormal, differentiated cats with occult heart disease with an accuracy of 83% [48]. In that study, cats with a normal test result were highly unlikely to have occult heart disease. Echocardiography is recommended for cats with an abnormal result.

Breed differences in NT-proBNP concentrations have been identified in healthy dogs. Breeds with the highest values, Labrador retrievers and Newfoundlands, had median concentrations three times higher than those of some other breeds [49]. The same study found intrabreed differences were pronounced. Similar to cTNI, data have shown high intraindividual variability in NT-proBNP values. If following an individual dog with serial measurements, an increase of 53% has been suggested to be confident that there is a changed clinical status [37].

Myoglobinemia and myoglobinuria

Myoglobin, a red heme protein containing ferrous iron (Fe^{+2}), is released from dead or dying muscle cells into the blood as a result of severe, usually acute muscle injury [50]. Because myoglobin has a low molecular weight (MW = 17,000) and is not significantly bound to proteins in the blood, it quickly passes through the glomerulus and is excreted in the urine [51]. When large amounts of myoglobin enter the renal tubule lumen, it interacts with Tamm-Horsfall protein in acidic urine and precipitates [52].

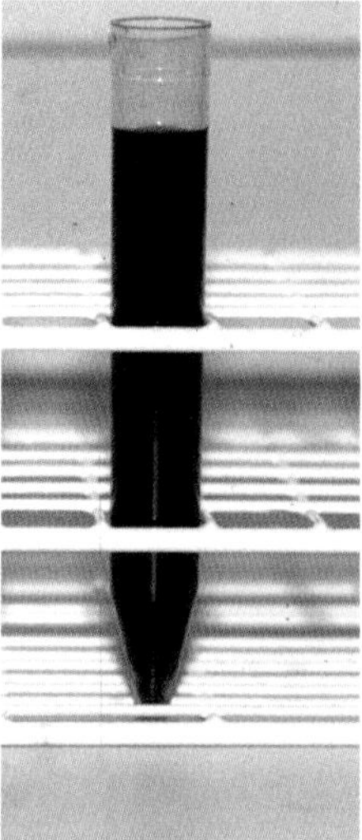

Figure 31.2 Urine from a horse with exertional rhabdomyolysis and myoglobinuria. High concentrations of myoglobin result in brown to red-brown urine.

In addition, reactive oxygen species promote the oxidation of iron to its ferric state (Fe^{+3}), thus generating a hydroxyl radical that can cause renal epithelial cell damage. This is the primary cause for acute kidney injury during myoglobinuria [52]. A higher volume of urine flow helps prevent this damage.

The urine will be brown to red-brown if the urinary myoglobin concentration is high enough (Figure 31.2). Myoglobin is detected as a positive reaction on the urine dipstick test for blood or hemoglobin because of its peroxidase activity. Therefore, myoglobinuria must be differentiated from hemoglobinuria (see Chapter 24 for further discussion of red urine). This differentiation can be aided by observing the packed cell volume and color of the serum. Hemoglobin released into the plasma because of hemolysis is quickly bound to a carrier protein, haptoglobin. Hemoglobin–haptoglobin complexes are large and do not readily pass through the glomerulus. If haptoglobin becomes saturated with hemoglobin, free hemoglobin dimers (MW = 32,000) in plasma are cleared by the kidney, resulting in red urine [51]. Since hemoglobin tends to be retained in the plasma after hemolysis, it imparts a red color to the plasma and serum. Myoglobin, however, is readily excreted by the kidneys, and does not typically cause a color change in the serum. Colorless to yellow serum in animals with evidence of muscle injury (increased CK or AST activity) and a positive reaction for hemoglobin on a urine dipstick test suggests myoglobinuria; red serum in an anemic animal is suggestive of hemolysis and hemoglobinuria.

32 Laboratory Evaluation of Lipids

M. Judith Radin

Department of Veterinary Biosciences, The Ohio State University College of Veterinary Medicine, Columbus, OH, USA

Lipids play diverse roles in normal physiology. The most obvious use is as an energy source that can be stored as triglycerides within adipocytes during times of nutritional plenty and mobilized when needed. Lipid stores within brown fat cells can be rapidly oxidized via uncoupling protein pathways to provide heat (thermogenesis). Fat pads provide thermal insulation and act as shock absorbers. Lipids function as structural components of cell membranes and organelles, as mediators of intracellular signal transduction pathways, as a constituent of surfactant in the lung, and as electrical insulators (myelin in the nervous system). Cholesterol is an important component in cellular membranes of animals and is the precursor for the synthesis of steroid hormones, vitamin D, and bile acids. Cholesterol metabolism also functions as a regulator of both innate and adaptive immunity [1]. Volatile fatty acids (propionate, acetate, and butyrate) are major products of rumen microbial fermentation of carbohydrates and play a significant role in ruminant energy metabolism. While often thought of as indicators of metabolic disturbances, ketones are normally present at low levels in the circulation and are an important energy source during times of negative energy balance.

A variety of lipids are present in the circulation. Alterations in their concentrations reflect energy balance and metabolic disturbances. Lipid abnormalities can contribute to development of serious clinical syndromes such as insulin resistance, hepatic lipidosis, and atherosclerosis. Measurement of different types of lipids is predicated on available test methodologies as well as clinical relevance. Circulating lipids of clinical interest that can be readily assessed include triglycerides, cholesterol, nonesterified fatty acids (NEFA), lipoproteins, and ketone bodies. Prior to discussion of laboratory evaluation and diagnosis of lipid abnormalities, a brief overview of lipid metabolism is presented. More detailed discussions of lipid chemistry and metabolism are available elsewhere [2, 3].

Dietary absorption of lipids

Lipids may be obtained from the diet or by synthesis. Dietary fat entering the small intestine stimulates release of cholecystokinin. Cholecystokinin causes the gall bladder to contract, releasing bile into the intestinal lumen. Bile salts and lecithin in the bile emulsify dietary fat to form micelles that consist of fatty acids, triglycerides, cholesterol, and the fat-soluble vitamins A, D, E, and K. Cholecystokinin also stimulates the exocrine pancreas to secrete lipases that interact with the micelle and break down the lipid into forms that may be absorbed by the intestinal enterocytes. Pancreatic lipase and colipase are responsible for hydrolysis of triglyceride to two fatty acids and a monoglyceride. Dietary cholesterol esters are hydrolyzed by cholesterol esterase to release cholesterol and a fatty acid. Long chain fatty acids (LCFA, fatty acids having more than 12 carbons), monoglycerides, cholesterol, and fat-soluble vitamins diffuse from the micelle across the brush border into the enterocyte, leaving the bile salts within the intestinal lumen (Figure 32.1). Short and medium chain fatty acids having fewer than 12 carbons may be absorbed without the need of micellar emulsification and may be transferred from the enterocyte directly to the portal blood. LCFA must be re-esterified to triglycerides and packaged into lipoproteins called chylomicrons for transport in the lacteals and blood.

Maldigestion and malabsorption of dietary fats can result in steatorrhea and deficiency of essential fatty acids and fat soluble vitamins. If pancreatic exocrine deficiency results in inadequate release of lipases into the intestine, maldigestion will result in high concentrations of triglycerides (also called neutral fats) in the feces. If the stool contains increased fatty acids and glycerol (referred to as split fats), this implies that sufficient lipase is present to hydrolyze triglyceride and that malabsorption of fats is occurring.

Veterinary Hematology, Clinical Chemistry, and Cytology, Third Edition. Edited by Mary Anna Thrall, Glade Weiser, Robin W. Allison and Terry W. Campbell.

Companion website: www.wiley.com/go/thrall/veterinary

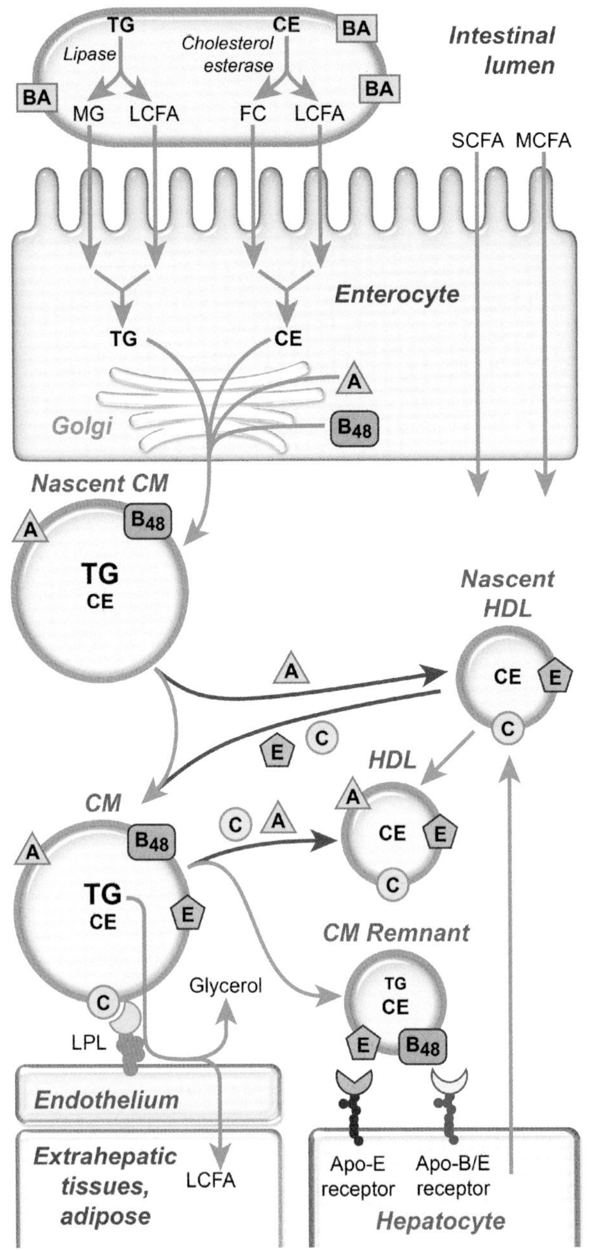

Figure 32.1 Dietary lipids in the intestinal lumen are solubilized by emulsification with bile acids (BA) to form micelles. Pancreatic lipases associate with the micelles and hydrolyze triglycerides (TG) to monoglycerides (MG) and long chain fatty acids (LCFA). Cholesterol esters (CE) are hydrolyzed by cholesterol esterase to free cholesterol (FC) and an LCFA. Short chain fatty acids (SCFA) and medium chain fatty acids (MCFA) do not require micellar emulsification for intestinal absorption. Following absorption by the enterocyte, MG, FC, and LCFA are re-esterified and assembled along with apoprotein-A and apoprotein-B48 into nascent chylomicrons (CM). In the blood, CM exchange apoproteins-A, -C, and -E with high-density lipoproteins (HDL). TG in the CM are hydrolyzed to LCFA and glycerol by lipoprotein lipase (LPL) on the surface of the endothelial cells. This process requires apoprotein-C. LCFA may be used by adipocytes to form TG while glycerol is released into the blood for use by the liver or other extrahepatic tissues. Apoprotein-A and apoprotein-C from CM remnants are transferred back to HDL. Removal of the cholesterol-enriched CM remnant from the blood is mediated by Apo-B/E and Apo-E receptors on hepatocytes.

Lipids present in the blood

Fatty acids

Unesterified fatty acids are referred to as free fatty acids or NEFA. Most mammalian fatty acids contain more than 12 carbon atoms and are referred to as LCFA. Fatty acids may be obtained from the diet or may be synthesized. Because they are hydrophobic, LCFA must be attached to plasma proteins, primarily albumin, for transport in the blood.

In nonruminants, biosynthesis of fatty acids occurs at the highest rates in liver, with lesser amounts produced in adipose tissue and mammary glands. In ruminants, adipocytes are the primary site for fatty acid formation, and the liver plays a less important role in fatty acid synthesis. During lactation, the mammary gland is a major synthetic site. Other tissues are capable of producing fatty acids but at much lower rates. Fatty acids are synthesized from acetyl-coenzyme A (acetyl-CoA) (Figure 32.2). Glucose is the main precursor for acetyl-CoA in nonruminants, while acetate serves this function in ruminants. Amino acids also can be used as precursors for formation of acetyl-CoA. Synthesis of fatty acids is stimulated by insulin and inhibited by glucagon and epinephrine via modulation of activity of acetyl-CoA carboxylase, the rate limiting enzyme of fatty acid synthesis. As a result, the rate of fatty acid synthesis is responsive to diet and metabolic state. For example, fatty acid synthesis is stimulated by high carbohydrate/low fat diets (high insulin and availability of glucose as a precursor). Fatty acid synthesis is decreased by fasting (low insulin, high glucagon), high fat/low carbohydrate diets (increased availability of preformed LCFA), and diabetes mellitus.

Fatty acids are an important energy source for peripheral tissues such as skeletal muscle and are oxidized back to acetyl-CoA as part of this process. Acetyl-CoA produced by mitochondrial β-oxidation of LCFA may be used to generate adenosine triphosphate (ATP) and CO_2 via the tricarboxylic acid (TCA) cycle (Figure 32.2). This process initially requires conversion of acetyl-CoA and oxaloacetate to citrate. If there is inadequate oxaloacetate, such as may occur with a low carbohydrate diet or diabetes mellitus, acetyl-CoA may be directed into ketogenesis. Acetyl-CoA also may be used for production of cholesterol.

Triglycerides

Triglycerides are formed by esterification of three LCFA to glycerol-3-phosphate (Figure 32.3). Triglyceride synthesis occurs in the intestinal mucosal cells, adipocytes, hepatocytes, mammary epithelial cells, and kidneys. Within the intestinal mucosal cell, dietary fatty acids and monoglycerides are re-esterified to form triglycerides. Triglycerides also can be produced by adding dietary LCFA to glycerol-3-phosphate that is newly synthesized from glucose by the enterocyte. Control of triglyceride synthesis by

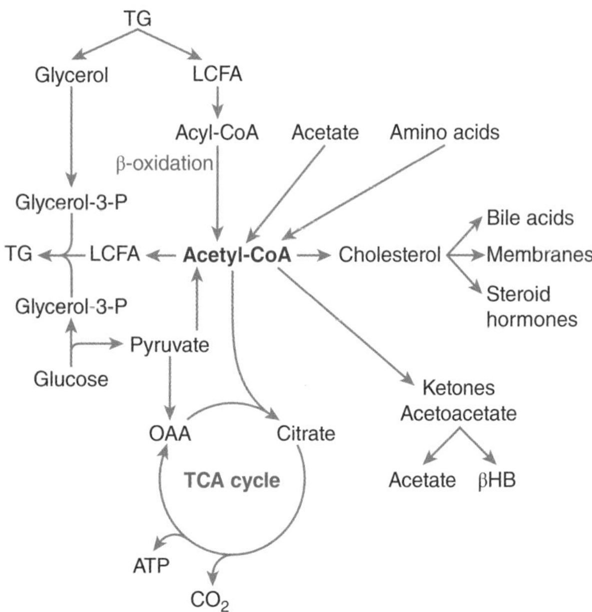

Figure 32.2 Acetyl-coenzyme A (acetyl-CoA) is central to both catabolism and synthesis of long chain fatty acids (LCFA) in the hepatocyte. LCFA derived from lipolysis are converted to acyl-CoA, which undergoes β-oxidation to acetyl-CoA. Other sources of acetyl-CoA include acetate, amino acids, and glucose. Acetyl-CoA may be used in the synthesis of LCFA or cholesterol. Triglycerides (TG) are synthesized by esterification of LCFA to glycerol-3-phosphate (glycerol-3-P) derived from either lipolysis or glucose metabolism. A major route for utilization of acetyl-CoA is for energy production through the tricarboxylic acid (TCA) cycle. This process requires combination of acetyl-CoA with oxaloacetate (OAA) to form citrate. OAA is obtained from glucose metabolism. If there is excess acetyl-CoA and/or insufficient OAA, acetyl-CoA may be shunted into ketogenesis to form acetoacetate. Acetoacetate is then converted to acetone and β-hydroxybutyrate (βHB). This last pathway is stimulated in conditions of negative energy balance characterized by excess lipolysis and undersupply of glucose.

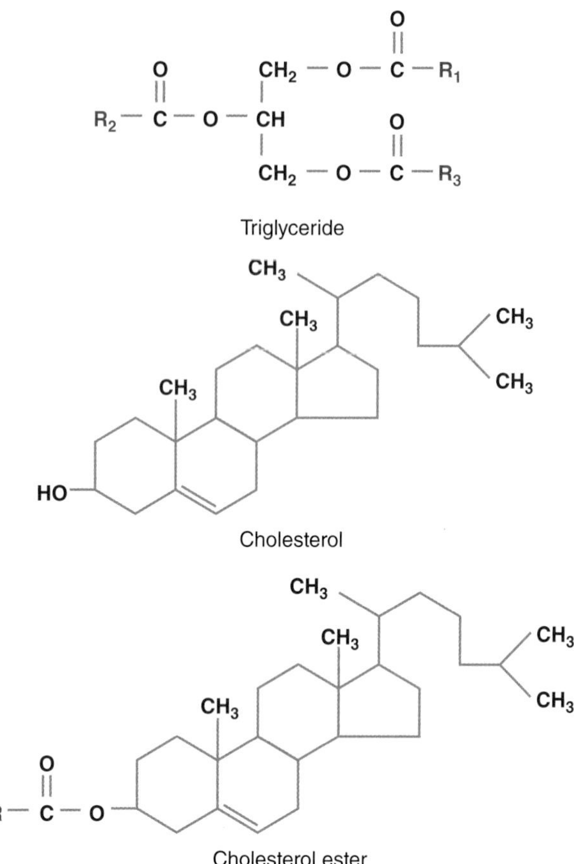

Figure 32.3 The structure of triglycerides, cholesterol, and cholesterol esters. R represents the carbon chain of a long chain fatty acid. The hydroxyl group on cholesterol confers some water solubility, allowing free cholesterol to be part of the outer shell of lipoproteins. Cholesterol esters are hydrophobic and contained within the center of lipoprotein particles.

the enterocytes is largely dependent on dietary availability of fatty acids. Once formed, triglycerides are not stored to any great extent in enterocytes but are packaged into chylomicrons and released into the lacteals.

Hepatocytes use LCFA obtained from the plasma or from de novo synthesis for production of triglycerides. Glycerol may be taken up from the plasma or may be synthesized from glucose. Synthesis of triglycerides by hepatocytes is decreased in conditions with high glucagon and low insulin (fasting, diabetes mellitus) and is stimulated by increased availability of LCFA. Under normal circumstances, triglycerides are released from the hepatocytes into the circulation as a component of lipoproteins called very-low-density lipoproteins (VLDL).

Adipocytes may synthesize LCFA or may obtain them via lipolysis of blood triglycerides present in chylomicrons or VLDL. The enzyme responsible for hydrolysis of chylomicron or VLDL triglycerides is lipoprotein lipase, which is located on the surface of capillary endothelial cells. Unlike hepatocytes, adipocytes lack the enzymes to use glycerol derived from lipolysis. Triglyceride synthesis by adipocytes depends on de novo production of glycerol-3-phosphate from glucose or gluconeogenesis. Insulin is an important regulator of adipocyte triglyceride synthesis through stimulation of activity of lipoprotein lipase (Table 32.1). Insulin also enhances glucose uptake by increasing membrane expression of the GLUT4 glucose transporter, thus increasing intracellular availability of glucose for glycerol-3-phosphate synthesis. Once triglycerides are formed, they are stored for future use as fat droplets in adipocytes.

Mobilization of triglycerides stored in adipocytes is mediated by the enzyme, hormone sensitive lipase (HSL). Hydrolysis of triglycerides results in the release of LCFA and glycerol to the blood for transport to tissues. A variety of hormones directly and indirectly affect lipolysis through modulation of the activity of HSL (Table 32.1). Catecholamines rapidly activate HSL by promoting phosphorylation of the enzyme. This permits a rapid increase

Table 32.1 Effect of hormones on key regulatory steps in lipid metabolism.

	LPL	HSL	Acetyl-CoA carboxylase	HMG CoA reductase	LDL receptors
	Hydrolysis of triglycerides from chylomicrons and VLDL	Lipolysis of triglycerides to LCFA and glycerol	Rate limiting enzyme in the synthesis of fatty acids	Rate limiting enzyme in the synthesis of cholesterol	Clearance of LDL from the blood
Insulin	↑ enzyme activity; ↑ synthesis of the enzyme; ↑ translocation of the enzyme to the endothelium	↓ enzyme activity; ↓ cortisol-induced gene transcription	↑ enzyme activity	↑ activity	↑ synthesis of the receptor
Glucagon		↑ activity	↓ enzyme activity	↓ activity	
Glucocorticoids		↑ gene transcription and synthesis of enzyme		↓ gene transcription and synthesis of the enzyme	↓ synthesis of receptor due to secondary decrease in thyroid hormones
Thyroid hormones		↑ synthesis of adrenergic receptors, which increases the effect of catecholamines		↑ synthesis of the enzyme	↑ synthesis of the receptor
Catecholamines		↑ enzyme activity	↓ enzyme activity		
Growth hormone		↑ enzyme activity			↓ synthesis of receptor due to secondary decrease in thyroid hormones

CoA, coenzyme A; HMG CoA, 3-hydroxy-3-methylglutaryl coenzyme A; HSL, hormone sensitive lipase; LCFA, long chain fatty acids; LDL, low-density lipoproteins; LPL, lipoprotein lipase; VLDL, very-low-density lipoproteins.

in lipolysis to supply fatty acids for energy production. Thyroid hormone acts synergistically with catecholamines by increasing the number of receptors for catecholamines on adipocytes. Glucocorticoids facilitate lipolysis by increasing gene transcription and synthesis of HSL. Insulin and insulin-like growth factor inactivates HSL by promoting dephosphorylation of the enzyme. Insulin also opposes the effect of glucocorticoids on HSL gene transcription.

Cholesterol

Cholesterol may be in the form of free cholesterol or may be esterified with a fatty acid to form a cholesterol ester (Figure 32.3). Because it is not synthesized by plants or microbes, only carnivores or omnivores may obtain cholesterol from the diet. Herbivores must synthesize their own cholesterol. The primary site for cholesterol synthesis is the liver, and the rate limiting enzyme is 3-hydroxy-3-methylglutaryl-CoA (HMG-CoA) reductase. Several hormones modulate HMG-CoA reductase activity and consequently cholesterol synthesis (Table 32.1). HMG-CoA reductase activity is increased by insulin and decreased by glucagon. Thus, cholesterol synthesis increases following a meal (high insulin) and decreases with fasting (high glucagon, low insulin) or with diabetes mellitus. Thyroid hormone increases HMG-CoA reductase activity by increasing synthesis of the enzyme. Glucocorticoids have the opposite effect, decreasing synthesis of HMG-CoA reductase and consequently cholesterol synthesis. Statins, a class of cholesterol lowering drugs, have their effect on serum cholesterol by inhibiting HMG-CoA reductase.

Once formed, cholesterol may be utilized through several routes. The liver can export cholesterol and cholesterol esters to the blood as a constituent of lipoproteins. Cholesterol is a structural component of cell and organelle membranes and is a precursor for vitamin D synthesis. Cholesterol also is used for production of steroid and sex hormones by tissues such as the adrenal gland and gonads. Alternatively, cholesterol may be used by hepatocytes to synthesize bile acids. Bile is a major route for elimination of cholesterol from the body.

Lipid transport in the blood

Because lipids are largely immiscible in water, transport in the blood must be accomplished by binding to carrier proteins. LCFA bind to albumin, while triglycerides, cholesterol, cholesterol esters, and phospholipids are transported by lipoproteins. Lipoproteins consist of a shell of apoproteins, cholesterol, and phospholipids oriented so that amphoteric portions of the molecules are on the outside, facing the aqueous environment of the blood. The hydrophobic ends are oriented toward the center of the particle. Triglycerides and cholesterol esters constitute the hydrophobic core of lipoprotein particles. Lipoproteins are traditionally named based on their density as determined by ultracentrifugation and are further characterized by lipid and apoprotein constituents. Apoproteins may be integrated into the shell of the lipoprotein or be more loosely associated with the surface of the lipoprotein. Integrated apoproteins include apoprotein-B48 (Apo-B48) of intestinal origin and apoprotein-B100 (Apo-B100) of hepatic origin. Peripheral apoproteins such as apoprotein-A (Apo-A), apoprotein-C (Apo-C), and apoprotein-E (Apo-E) are exchanged between lipoproteins in circulation (Figures 32.1 and 32.4).

Enterocytes package fat from the diet into lipoproteins called chylomicrons, which are released into the lacteals with eventual delivery into the blood. Chylomicrons contain mostly triglycerides with lesser amounts of cholesterol, cholesterol ester, fat soluble vitamins, Apo-B48, and Apo-A. In the circulation, Apo-C and Apo-E are transferred from high-density lipoproteins (HDL) to the chylomicron. Chylomicrons are the largest and least dense of the lipoproteins. When present in large quantity, they confer a visible haziness to the serum, contributing to the appearance of lipemia. Apo-C is a cofactor for lipoprotein lipase, which is found on the surface of endothelial cells within tissue beds such as adipose and muscle. Lipoprotein lipase is synthesized by extravascular tissues and transferred to the surface of endothelial cells where it is anchored by heparan sulfate. Injection of heparin can cause release of lipoprotein lipase into the circulation and this technique has been used to clear serum of lipemia. Lipoprotein lipase hydrolyzes triglycerides to LCFA and glycerol for use by extrahepatic tissues. In adipose and muscle, insulin increases lipoprotein lipase activity, facilitating hydrolysis of chylomicron triglycerides and absorption of LCFA. The remaining lipoprotein, now depleted of triglycerides, is called a "chylomicron remnant" and is subsequently removed from the circulation by hepatocytes. Uptake of chylomicron remnants is mediated by binding of Apo-B48 and Apo-E on the chylomicron remnant to either Apo-E or Apo-B/E receptors on the hepatocyte.

Triglycerides synthesized by hepatocytes are packaged into VLDL for transport in the blood (Figure 32.4). VLDL contain a large quantity of triglyceride along with lesser amounts of cholesterol, cholesterol esters, and Apo-B100. Apo-C and Apo-E are obtained from HDL in the circulation. If present in high quantities, VLDL also can contribute to a lipemic appearance of the blood. Like chylomicrons, binding of VLDL to lipoprotein lipase in the tissues is facilitated

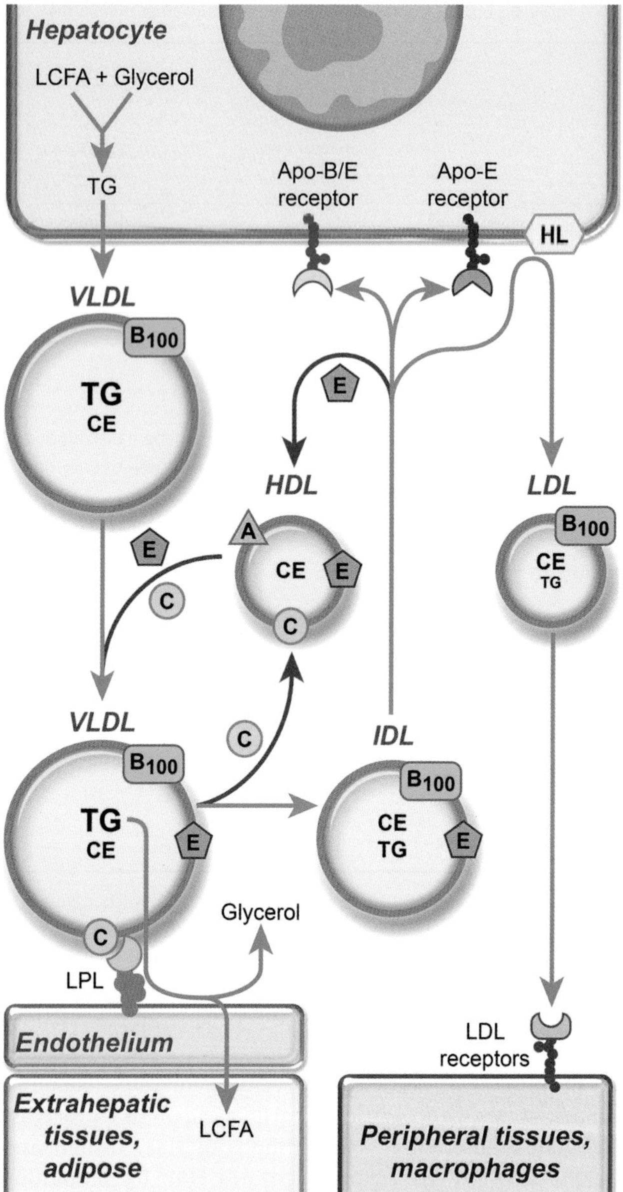

Figure 32.4 Triglycerides (TG) synthesized in hepatocytes are packaged along with cholesterol, cholesterol esters (CE), and apoprotein-B100 into very-low-density lipoproteins (VLDL) for transport in the blood. VLDL pick up apoprotein-C and apoprotein-E from high-density lipoproteins (HDL). TG are hydrolyzed to long chain fatty acids (LCFA) and glycerol by lipoprotein lipase (LPL) on the surface of endothelial cells. LCFA may be used by adipocytes to form TG, while glycerol is released into the blood for use by the liver or other extrahepatic tissues. Depletion of TG results in formation of an intermediate density lipoprotein (IDL) or VLDL remnants. Apoprotein-C and apoprotein-E recirculate back to HDL. IDL may be removed from the circulation by hepatocytes, a process mediated by Apo-B/E and Apo-E receptors. Alternatively, IDL may be further depleted of TG by hepatic lipase (HL) and converted to low-density lipoproteins (LDL). Uptake of LDL by peripheral tissues is mediated by binding of LDL to LDL receptors. Macrophages are also capable of removing LDL from circulation through scavenger receptors.

by Apo-C, and triglycerides are hydrolyzed to LCFA and glycerol for utilization by extrahepatic tissues.

After the VLDL is depleted of triglycerides, the remaining lipoprotein is an intermediate density lipoprotein (IDL) or VLDL remnant, depending on the species [4]. IDL and VLDL remnants may be taken up by hepatocytes, a process mediated by binding of Apo-B and Apo-E to hepatocyte receptors. Alternatively, additional hydrolysis of triglyceride by hepatic lipase converts IDL and VLDL remnants to low-density lipoproteins (LDL). As the lipoprotein loses triglyceride, Apo-C and Apo-E are transferred back to HDL while Apo-B100 is retained. The primary function of LDL is transport of cholesterol to the liver and other tissues. Removal of LDL from circulation is receptor mediated and depends on the presence of Apo-B. LDL receptor expression is stimulated by insulin and thyroxine. Most cells have receptors for LDL and can acquire cholesterol by binding LDL; however the liver plays the major role in LDL clearance.

Cholesterol transport is mediated by HDL. Nascent HDL are synthesized by hepatocytes and contain phospholipids, a small amount of cholesterol, Apo-C, and Apo-E. As previously described, HDL provide a source of Apo-C and Apo-E for exchange with chylomicrons and VLDL. As HDL mature, Apo-A is acquired by exchange with chylomicrons. The small intestine also produces HDL that initially contain Apo-A but lack Apo-C and Apo-E. Intestinal HDL must pick up Apo-C and Apo-E from hepatic-origin HDL in the blood. Importantly, HDL incorporate excess cholesterol from extrahepatic tissues in a process called "reverse cholesterol transport." Cholesterol is then esterified to cholesterol esters by lecithin cholesterol acyl transferase (LCAT) in the HDL, an enzyme that requires Apo-A for activation.

There is species variation in the relative amounts of HDL and LDL (Table 32.2) [5, 6]. In species that typically have high HDL and low LDL in the blood, such as dogs and cats, HDL are the primary transporters of cholesterol and cholesterol esters to the liver. In low HDL/high LDL species such as humans, cholesterol esters may be transferred by cholesteryl ester transfer protein (CETP) to VLDL remnants and LDL for subsequent delivery to the liver. High LDL species are at risk for the development of atherosclerosis because macrophages are capable of scavenger receptor-mediated removal of LDL from the circulation. Accumulation of LDL cholesterol in macrophages results in subendothelial lipid deposits or atherosclerotic plaques. High cholesterol diets can favor increased concentrations of LDL and exacerbate development of atherosclerosis.

Table 32.2 Examples of HDL mammals and LDL mammals [5, 6].

HDL mammals	LDL mammals
Dogs	Guinea pigs
Cats	Hamsters
Ferrets	Pigs
Horses	Camels
Cattle	Rabbits (some strains)
Sheep	Spider monkey
Mice	Humans
Rats	
Chimpanzee	
Most Old World monkeys	

HDL, high-density lipoprotein; LDL, low-density lipoprotein.
HDL mammals are defined as those having HDL as >50% of total lipoproteins, whereas LDL mammals have >50% LDL. Age, strain, breed, and diet may affect the relative distribution of lipoproteins.
Sources: Hollanders et al. [5] and Chapman [6].

Ketones

Ketogenesis is another option available for metabolism of fatty acids by the liver. As described above, LCFA may be repackaged into triglycerides and released as VLDL. Alternatively, LCFA may undergo β-oxidation to acetyl-CoA and subsequently be used for energy production via the TCA cycle, for cholesterol synthesis, or for ketogenesis (Figure 32.2). Under conditions of adequate nutrition, low levels of ketone bodies normally are produced by the liver. The rumen epithelium also appears to be capable of synthesizing β-hydroxybutyrate, which may account for the higher concentrations of ketone bodies in fed ruminants compared to fed monogastric species. The main ketone bodies are acetone, acetoacetate, and β-hydroxybutyrate. Acetyl-CoA is metabolized to acetoacetate, which subsequently is converted to acetone and β-hydroxybutyrate. These small lipids are water soluble and are transported by the blood to other tissues for use as an energy source. Because they are not bound to albumin, ketone bodies easily enter cells and cross the blood–brain barrier and placenta. Tissues such as the heart and brain readily utilize ketone bodies as an energy source.

Ketogenesis increases in conditions of negative energy balance and is a normal response to fasting. As plasma glucose falls, the concentrations of insulin decreases and glucagon increases. This stimulates lipolysis by HSL, mobilizing fatty acids from triglycerides stored in adipocytes. Fatty acids delivered to the liver are converted to acetyl-CoA. At the same time, enhanced gluconeogenesis consumes the available oxaloacetate without which acetyl-CoA cannot enter into the TCA cycle. As a result, acetyl-CoA is directed to ketogenesis.

Transient ketosis may develop following intense exercise and has been seen dogs and horses. During exercise, lipolysis by HSL is stimulated by catecholamines, cortisol and thyroxine, and the released fatty acids are consumed by muscle for energy production. Ketones formed during exercise are rapidly used, and circulating levels remain low to undetectable. In the postexercise period, muscle metabolism switches from oxidation of fatty acids to gluconeogenesis and glycogen synthesis to clear lactate and replenish glycogen stores. Metabolism of acetyl-CoA through the TCA cycle declines as a result of decreased availability of oxaloacetate. Excess circulating fatty acids are cleared by the liver, and the resultant acetyl-CoA may be shunted into ketone production. The degree of post exercise ketosis appears related to intensity and duration of exercise, conditioning of the athlete, and diet.

Measurement of lipids

Because of the technical challenges associated with measurement of lipids, relatively few types of lipids are measured in routine biochemistry panels. Triglycerides and cholesterol can be measured in serum, heparinized plasma, or ethylenediaminetetraacetic acid (EDTA) plasma using spectrophotometric assays that are readily adapted to automated analyzers and are commonly part of biochemical profiles. Measurement of free fatty acids or NEFA in serum or EDTA plasma has been used to assess metabolism in ruminants, horses and camelidae. However, these assays are not as commonly available on routine biochemical profiles. Heparinized plasma or serum obtained using a serum separator tube are not recommended for measurement of NEFA as baseline NEFA concentrations will be higher and concentrations will rise with storage of the plasma [7].

Ketones may be measured on automated analyzers or at the cage side by dry reagent methods such as dipsticks, tablets, or nitroprusside powder. Measurement of ketones in the urine using dipsticks based on the nitroprusside test is frequently used as a less invasive, semiquantitative means to evaluate for accelerated ketogenesis in diabetes mellitus in small animals or in ketosis in cattle. The disadvantage of this method is that these dipsticks are more sensitive to acetoacetate than acetone or β-hydroxybutyrate and may underestimate ketones in some stages of diabetic ketoacidosis. The presence of some drugs or compounds in the urine also may produce a false-positive result. "Point of care" instruments have been evaluated for measurement of blood β-hydroxybutyrate in dogs, cats and cattle [8, 9]. In cattle, test strips are available for measurement of β-hydroxybutyrate in milk, which may prove more practical to obtain than urine.

Measurement of lipoproteins in veterinary species requires more sophisticated methods such as density gradient centrifugation or electrophoresis. Autoanalyzer and "point of care" methods designed to quantitate lipoproteins using precipitation and calculation techniques in humans have not been validated and may not give reliable results in veterinary species [10]. As a result, lipoprotein analyses are not routinely measured in veterinary medicine and require shipment of samples to specialized reference laboratories.

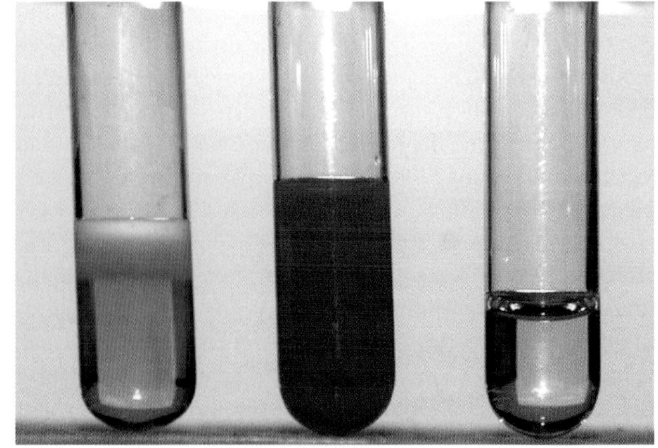

Figure 32.5 Lipemia is characterized by haziness to overt lactescence of a serum sample due to increased triglycerides in the form of chylomicrons and/or very-low-density lipoproteins (VLDL). Formation of a cream-like layer on the top of a sample indicates the presence of chylomicrons (left). Failure of a sample to separate indicates the presence of VLDL (middle). Normal samples are clear (right).

The term "hyperlipidemia" refers to increased circulating lipids. This may be due to hypertriglyceridemia and/or hypercholesterolemia. Lipemia or hyperlipemia refers to a visible haziness (usually when triglycerides exceed 300 mg/dL) to overt latescence of the serum or plasma (triglycerides exceed 600–1000 mg/dL). Lipemia is caused by increased triglycerides in chylomicrons and/or VLDL. Hypercholesterolemia without concurrent hypertriglyceridemia will not cause a sample to appear lipemic. The refrigeration test is a simple means to distinguish between chylomicrons and VLDL as the cause of lipemia (Figure 32.5). To perform this test, a sample is left upright in a refrigerator overnight. Chylomicrons will float to the top of the sample and form a milky or cream-like layer at the top of the sample. If the underlying serum clears, then chylomicrons are the cause of the lipemia. On the other hand, if VLDL are the cause of the lipemia, VLDL will not separate out into a cream layer, and the sample will remain hazy to turbid. If the lipemia is due to increases in both chylomicrons and VLDL, a cream layer will form over a sample that remains turbid.

Clinically relevant changes in serum lipids include hypertriglyceridemia, hypercholesterolemia, hyperketonemia, and hypocholesterolemia. Hypotriglyceridemia is of uncertain clinical relevance and may be most indicative of nutritional state.

Hyperlipidemias

Postprandial hyperlipidemia

Postprandial hyperlipidemia is due to a transient increase in triglycerides in the form of chylomicrons. Hyperlipidemia becomes apparent within 1–2 hours of consuming a meal that contains fat and usually peaks by 6–8 hours. Because postprandial hyperlipidemia is primarily due to increases in triglycerides, blood samples may appear hazy to grossly lipemic. For dogs and cats, fasting for 12 hours should allow sufficient time for clearance of the hyperlipidemia. To evaluate for equine metabolic syndrome, horses should be fasted by confining them to a stall, leaving one flake of hay in the stall after 10:00 p.m. and drawing samples in the morning [11]. Because of continuous rumenal digestion and diet composition, ruminants do not show significant postprandial effects and so need not be fasted prior to sampling.

Persistence of hyperlipidemia after a 12-hour fast in dogs and cats suggests an alternative pathogenesis for the hyperlipidemia. In monogastric animals, consumption of a high fat diet may contribute to higher fasting and postprandial serum lipids compared to normal or low fat diets. The time it takes for serum lipids to decrease to fasting levels may be prolonged following a high fat meal and a 15 hour fast may be needed to establish true fasting lipid levels. As seen in Table 32.1, many key regulatory steps in lipid metabolism are influenced by hormones. It is not surprising that pathologic hyperlipidemia is commonly due to secondary causes such as hormonal or metabolic disturbances. Primary or idiopathic hyperlipidemias are rare and likely have a genetic basis.

Secondary pathologic hyperlipidemias

Secondary pathologic hyperlipidemias are caused by a variety of diseases (Figure 32.6). While described separately below, it is important to realize that there may be overlapping effects promoting abnormalities in lipid metabolism in any given patient. For example, pancreatitis may be complicated by diabetes mellitus due to damage to pancreatic parenchyma. Diabetes mellitus commonly occurs in conjunction with hyperadrenocorticism in cats as a result of corticosteroid-related insulin resistance. Many of these conditions also have an inflammatory component resulting in increased local and systemic release of pro-inflammatory cytokines capable of modulating lipid metabolism.

Hypothyroidism

Hypothyroidism in dogs is a common endocrinopathy and is frequently accompanied by hypercholesterolemia due to

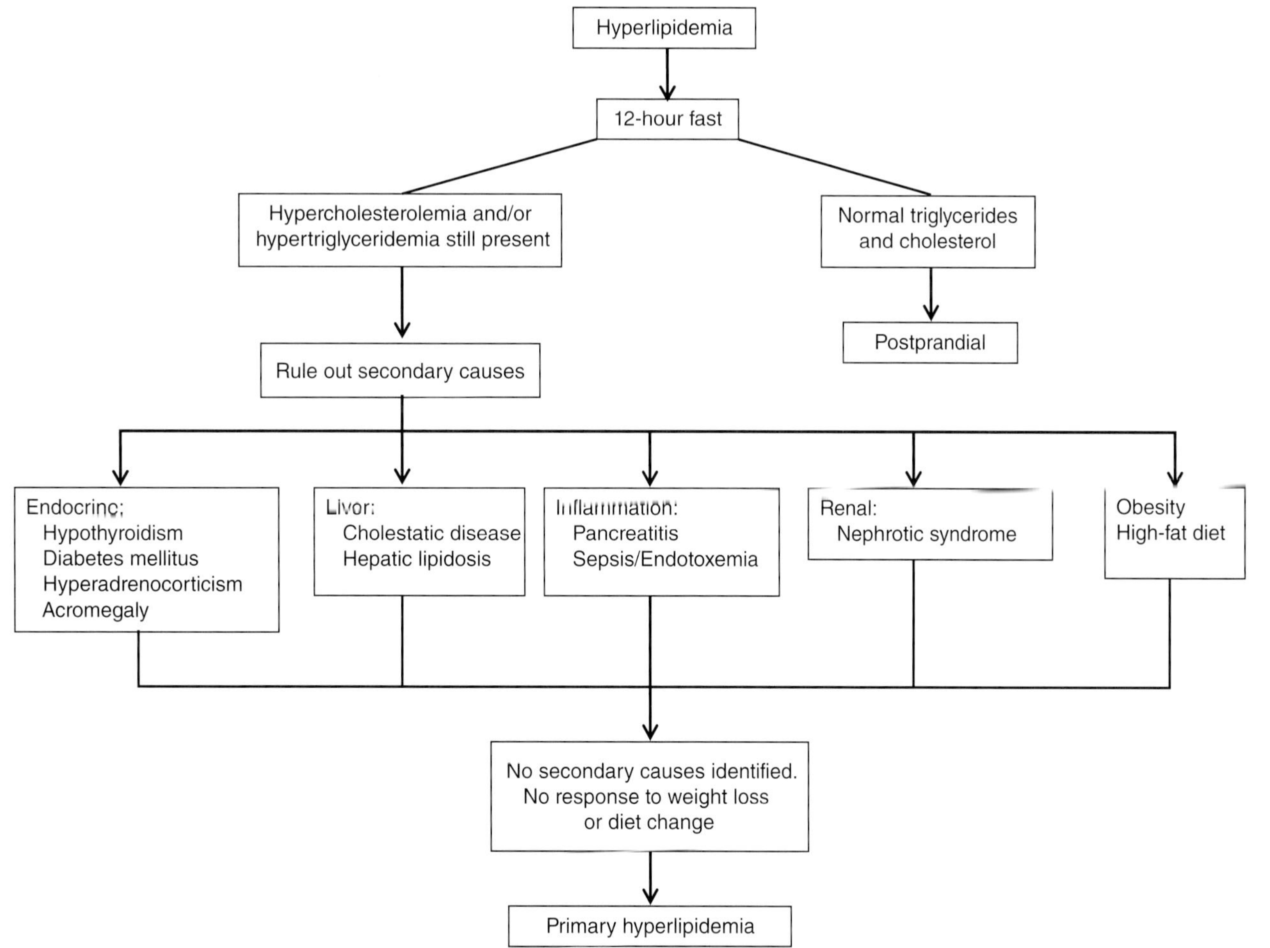

Figure 32.6 Approach to the hyperlipidemic patient.

increases in LDL and HDL [12–15]. Hypertriglyceridemia also is common and is due to increased VLDL and sometimes chylomicrons. In contrast to dogs, spontaneously occurring hypothyroidism is rare in cats but may develop as a sequela to treatment for hyperthyroidism. Congenital hypothyroidism has been described in kittens [16]. Hypercholesterolemia may be a feature of both spontaneous and iatrogenic feline hypothyroidism [16, 17]. In adult horses, the actual incidence of naturally occurring hypothyroidism is very low. Cases initially diagnosed as hypothyroidism may actually be attributable to equine metabolic syndrome or hyperadrenocorticism secondary to a tumor or dysfunction of the pituitary pars intermedia [18]. Experimental ablation of the thyroid glands of adult horses will result in hypercholesterolemia and hypertriglyceridemia characterized by increased LDL and VLDL, respectively [19].

In humans with hypothyroidism, decreased hepatic LDL receptor synthesis and increased receptor catabolism contributes to the hypercholesterolemia by impairing LDL clearance [20]. Biliary excretion of cholesterol also is decreased while intestinal cholesterol absorption is increased. Decreased lipoprotein lipase activity delays clearance of triglycerides from both VLDL and chylomicrons, while decreased hepatic lipase activity slows clearance of cholesterol-enriched chylomicron remnants. Similar mechanisms have not been thoroughly examined in domestic species.

Hyperadrenocorticism

Increased serum concentrations of triglycerides and cholesterol may be observed in dogs with Cushing's disease [15, 21–24]. Hypercholesterolemia also is reported in cats with hyperadrenocorticism [25–27]. As a consequence of corticosteroid-induced insulin resistance, hyperadrenocorticism, especially in cats, is often complicated by concurrent diabetes mellitus that exerts additional effects on lipid metabolism [27]. Horses with pituitary pars intermedia dysfunction (PPID) may develop pituitary-dependent hyperadrenocorticism. Stimulation of lipolysis in these horses results in elevated circulating NEFA as well as increased ketogenesis [28]. Reports vary on the incidence of hypertriglyceridemia in horses with PPID and hyperadrenocorticism [28–31]. Hyperlipidemia can become marked if there is concurrent type 2 diabetes mellitus and metabolic syndrome.

A combination of direct effects of corticosteroids and indirect effects due to steroid-induced insulin resistance contribute to the alterations in lipid metabolism in patients with hyperadrenocorticism [20]. Hypercholesterolemia results from impaired clearance of LDL along with decreased catabolism of cholesterol secondary to steroid-induced hepatopathy and cholestasis. Increased synthesis of VLDL by hepatocytes promotes hypertriglyceridemia.

Diabetes mellitus

Poorly controlled diabetes mellitus due to insulin deficiency (type 1 or insulin dependent diabetes mellitus) is associated with hypertriglyceridemia, increased serum LCFA, and hypercholesterolemia in dogs [12, 32, 33]. Type 1 diabetes mellitus is rare in the horse but may be accompanied by hypertriglyceridemia [34]. Insulin is required for synthesis and activity of lipoprotein lipase, so insulin deficiency results in failure to clear triglycerides from chylomicrons and VLDL. In addition, circulating LCFA are increased due to a combination of increased lipolysis and decreased triglyceride synthesis by adipocytes. A lack of insulin results in increased activity of HSL in adipocytes and subsequent hydrolysis of stored triglycerides and release of LCFA into the circulation. Because adipocytes require glucose for synthesis of glycerol-1-phosphate, impaired insulin-mediated glucose uptake by adipocytes results in decreased availability of glycerol-1-phosphate for esterification of LCFA to form triglycerides. LCFA are released into the blood and are subsequently taken up by hepatocytes, converted to triglycerides, and released as VLDL. If the concentration of LCFA exceeds the ability of hepatocytes to produce and release VLDL or to consume acetyl-CoA through the TCA cycle, acetyl-CoA generated from LCFA may be shunted into synthesis of ketone bodies, contributing to the development of ketoacidosis.

Insulin stimulates production of the LDL receptors so hypercholesterolemia appears to be primarily the result of a decrease in receptor-mediated uptake of LDL. Increased intestinal synthesis of cholesterol also appears to play a role in the genesis of the hypercholesterolemia in the dog.

Obesity, insulin resistance, and metabolic syndrome

Insulin resistance may vary from mild to overt type 2 diabetes mellitus. The pathogenesis of insulin resistance is complex and instigating causes are varied. Conditions associated with insulin resistance include obesity, hyperadrenocorticism, and hypersomatotropism. As a result, the effects of impaired response to insulin are superimposed on the disturbances in lipid profile caused by the original disorder. Type 2 diabetes mellitus is the most common form of diabetes mellitus in cats and horses.

Obesity is a frequently encountered problem in dogs, cats, and horses. Lipid profiles of obese individuals can exhibit a spectrum from normal to marked increases in triglycerides along with variable increases in cholesterol. Plasma NEFA often are increased. The variation observed in lipid profiles in obesity likely relates to the site of excess fat deposition, duration of obesity, and dysfunction of metabolic regulatory hormones such as insulin, cortisol, leptin, and adiponectin. Obesity is now recognized as a pro-inflammatory state, and fat pads are a source of inflammatory cytokines such as interleukin-6 and tumor necrosis factor-α. These inflammatory mediators can have a significant impact on adipocyte and hepatic lipid metabolism (see section below on inflammation) and can promote insulin resistance. Intra-abdominal obesity appears to have more severe metabolic consequences compared to peripheral adiposity and predisposes to the development of insulin resistance and metabolic syndrome.

In addition to increases in absolute concentrations of triglycerides and cholesterol, the composition of lipoproteins may change. Obese dogs show a pattern of increased triglycerides and cholesterol in both VLDL and HDL [35, 36]. In cats, triglyceride and cholesterol content of VLDL are increased while HDL cholesterol is increased [37, 38]. Horses exhibit increases in VLDL-triglyceride and HDL-cholesterol content [11, 39]. Decreases in lipoprotein lipase activity has been documented in obese cats, suggesting that uptake of triglycerides by adipocytes and peripheral tissue beds is impaired [37, 40]. LDL fractions appear unaffected and may account for the relative resistance of these species to development of atherosclerosis even with obesity-related hyperlipidemia.

Hypercholesterolemia has been observed in cats with acromegaly [41]. Acromegaly is the result of increased production of growth hormone. While not specifically explored in cats, there are several mechanisms that may explain the hypercholesterolemia secondary to hypersomatotropism. These cats have metabolic complications from significant insulin resistance to type 2 diabetes mellitus. In addition, growth hormone decreases release of thyroid stimulating hormone resulting in secondary hypothyroidism.

Hepatic lipidosis

Hepatic lipidosis or fatty liver occurs when triglycerides accumulate in hepatocytes. This syndrome may be precipitated by negative energy balance, hormonal or metabolic disturbances, hypoxia, or toxins. It results from an imbalance between hepatic uptake of fatty acids, synthesis of triglycerides, formation of VLDL, and release of VLDL. Hepatic lipidosis may develop in association with conditions such as bovine ketosis, ovine pregnancy toxemia, fasting in obese cats and horses, and a variety of syndromes in camelids. In these syndromes, HSL activity and subsequent adipocyte lipolysis is accelerated, increasing the supply of LCFA. The supply of LCFA outpaces the ability of the liver to oxidize LCFA through the TCA cycle so LCFA are re-esterified to triglycerides. Triglycerides accumulate as the ability to either produce VLDL or transport VLDL out of the hepatocyte is exceeded. Excess fatty acids also may be shunted to ketone body production, and lipidosis is often accompanied by some degree of ketosis. Grossly, the liver appears pale to yellow in color. Microscopically, variably-sized clear fat vacuoles are seen within the cytoplasm of the hepatocytes (Figure 32.7).

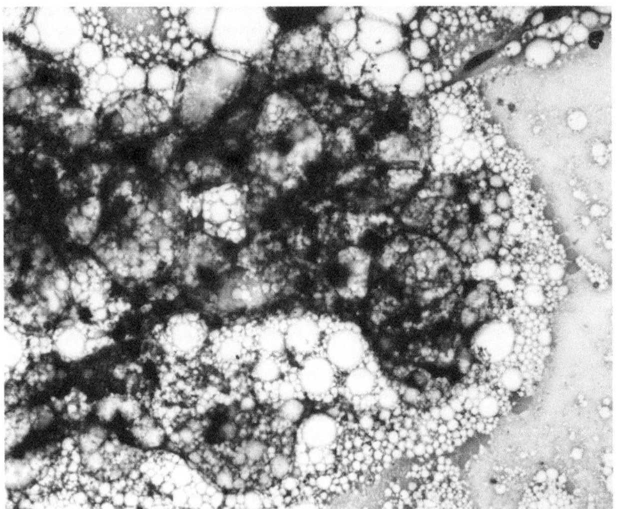

Figure 32.7 Fine needle aspirate of the liver of a cat with hepatic lipidosis. The cytoplasm of the hepatocytes contains variably sized, clear lipid vacuoles. Lipid-laden hepatocytes are often fragile and will break, leaving lipid droplets evident in the background. Wright-Giemsa stain, 400×.

Anorexia in horses, especially if they are obese to begin with, can prompt the development of hyperlipidemia and hepatic lipidosis [11, 39]. Ponies, miniature horses, donkeys, and mares are at increased risk, and the risk may be compounded by pregnancy or lactation. The syndrome in equids is characterized by increased circulating NEFA, triglycerides, and, to a lesser degree, cholesterol [42, 43]. However, ketonemia and ketonuria are not present. Increases in triglyceride concentrations may be marked and are primarily due to increased hepatic production of VLDL. Triglyceride concentrations in anorexic horses have been shown to be inversely related to survival [44, 45].

Obese cats that become anorexic due to illness or are subjected to a rapid weight reduction are at risk for development of hepatic lipidosis as a consequence of increased lipolysis [46]. Hypertriglyceridemia occurs as a result of increased VLDL production as well as impaired peripheral utilization. Although export of VLDL from the liver is increased, this appears insufficient to prevent accumulation of triglycerides in hepatocytes. Hypercholesterolemia is a less consistent finding.

Hepatic lipidosis occurs in camelids secondary to conditions that increase fat mobilization [47, 48]. The syndrome is accompanied by increased NEFA and, in some cases, ketonemia and ketonuria. Like other species, hepatic lipidosis may occur as a sequela to negative energy balance associated with pregnancy or lactation, in which case the dams will be hypoglycemic and ketonemic. In cases not associated with pregnancy and lactation, hyperglycemia may be observed due to the blunted insulin response and excessive gluconeogenesis typical of camelids. Hypertriglyceridemia may develop with severe, terminal lipidosis.

Pancreatitis

Dogs with naturally occurring pancreatitis may have hypertriglyceridemia and hypercholesterolemia, and the serum may exhibit overt lipemia [4, 12, 49, 50]. Hypercholesterolemia also is reported in cats with pancreatitis [51]. Changes in canine lipoprotein patterns include increases in VLDL, chylomicrons, and LDL with decreases in some subtypes of HDL. The hypertriglyceridemia arises from both a decrease in clearance of chylomicrons and VLDL due to decreased lipoprotein lipase activity as well as an increase in VLDL production. Hypercholesterolemia results from decreased biliary excretion due to pancreatitis-associated cholestasis as well as increased hepatic synthesis. Release of inflammatory cytokines likely contributes to the alterations in hepatic lipid metabolism. Pathogenesis of the hyperlipidemia may be further complicated by the comorbidity of diabetes mellitus as pancreatic parenchyma is damaged.

It is speculated that hypertriglyceridemia may contribute to the development of pancreatitis and may help explain the clinical impression that consumption of high fat meals can precede the onset of acute pancreatitis. The theory is that hydrolysis of chylomicron triglycerides by pancreatic lipase within the pancreatic microcirculation results in local release LCFA. LCFA have the potential to damage both the endothelial cells of the pancreatic microvasculature as well as the pancreatic acinar cells. This provides a mechanism for perpetuating a cycle of ongoing release of pancreatic lipase and generation of damaging LCFA as well as release of other potentially harmful pancreatic enzymes into the parenchyma.

Endotoxemia and inflammation

Alterations in serum lipids and lipoproteins may be seen as a response to endotoxin and endotoxin-induced release of inflammatory cytokines [52]. Inflammatory cytokines have been implicated in mediating the changes in lipid metabolism in a number of pro-inflammatory conditions such as obesity and pancreatitis. Response to endotoxin is characterized by increased circulating LCFA, triglycerides, and VLDL. Stimulation of lipolysis by adipocytes and hepatic fatty acid synthesis in concert with decreased fatty acid oxidation results in increased triglyceride and VLDL synthesis. Clearance of triglycerides is impaired due to decreased lipoprotein lipase activity. Decreased lipoprotein Apo-E content blunts receptor mediated removal of lipoproteins from the blood.

Cholesterol levels are more variable and likely depend on species, clinical severity, and time course in the disease. Mild hypercholesterolemia may develop secondary to endotoxin-induced decreases in biliary excretion of cholesterol as well as decreased uptake of LDL secondary to down regulation of LDL receptors. As part of a negative acute phase reaction mediated by inflammatory cytokines, patients may develop mild to moderate hypocholesterolemia due to a decrease in hepatic cholesterol synthesis. HDL may both decrease in concentration and alter in composition. Dogs with parvovirus enteritis exhibit hypocholesterolemia and hypertriglyceridemia that correlated with tumor necrosis factor-α concentrations [53].

Cholestasis

Cholestasis arising from a variety of mechanisms may result in mild to moderate increases in cholesterol with occasional mild increases in triglycerides. This is likely due to a combination of decreased hepatic cholesterol uptake and impaired cholesterol excretion in the bile. Alterations in lipoprotein composition and distribution have been documented in dogs, cats, and horses with natural and experimentally induced cholestasis [54–57].

Protein losing nephropathies and nephrotic syndrome

Nephrotic syndrome may develop as a result of glomerular damage and proteinuria arising from a variety of etiologies. The hallmarks of nephrotic syndrome include proteinuria, ascites, edema, hypoalbuminemia, hypercholesterolemia, and hypertriglyceridemia. Nephrotic syndrome accompanied by hypercholesterolemia and hypertriglyceridemia has been observed in dogs, cats, and horses [58]. While nephrotic syndrome with proteinuria and hypoalbuminemia has been described in cattle, effects on serum cholesterol and triglycerides were not reported [59].

A number of mechanisms have been suggested to explain the altered lipid metabolism secondary to proteinuria and hypoalbuminemia [60]. Experimental studies in human and animal models suggest that proteinuria and hypoalbuminemia are associated with increased activity of hepatic cholesterol synthetic enzymes, resulting in increased production of cholesterol and cholesterol containing lipoproteins. Urinary loss of key enzymes such as LCAT may affect maturation of HDL and impair the mechanism of reverse cholesterol transport. Decreased LDL receptor expression as well as altered binding of LDL to LDL receptors contributes to decreased clearance of LDL. Catabolism of cholesterol and subsequent excretion of cholesterol through the bile also may be impaired due to decreased activity of enzymes involved in bile acid synthesis.

Hypertriglyceridemia results from both increased hepatic synthesis of VLDL and decreased peripheral clearance of VLDL and chylomicrons. Impaired clearance of triglycerides appears to be the result of decreased activity of lipoprotein lipase and hepatic lipase. Loss of activity of lipoprotein lipase is mediated by inhibitors such as angiopoietin-like 4, the production of which by the kidney is stimulated by proteinuria.

Neonates and nursing young

Circulating triglycerides and cholesterol concentrations are higher in healthy young animals compared to adults, so age appropriate reference intervals should be used when possible [61–65]. Higher triglycerides and cholesterol may be due in part to the difficulty in obtaining fasted samples from very young animals that are suckling and the relatively high fat content of a milk diet. Differences in lipid metabolism and enzyme activities between young and adults could also play a role.

Moderate to severe hyperlipidemia, characterized by moderate to marked hypertriglyceridemia and overt lipemia, can be seen in poor doing young kittens and foals. In both species, the syndrome is likely a consequence of negative energy balance due to failure to adequately nurse and, if severe, may result in hepatic lipidosis. Sick foals that become anorexic and fail to nurse often develop hypertriglyceridemia with increased NEFA due to lipolysis [66–68]. This can be accompanied by hypoglycemia that is usually more severe if the foal is septic. Some foals respond to parenteral nutritional therapy with hyperglycemia due to insulin resistance or impaired insulin responses.

A pattern of severe hypertriglyceridemia, hypercholesterolemia and anemia has been reported in 3- to 8-week-old kittens that can resolve in response to supportive therapy [69, 70]. The precipitating circumstances often include causes of negative energy balance such as failure to nurse and flea infestation.

Primary hyperlipidemia

Once other causes of hyperlipidemia have been excluded, a diagnosis of primary hyperlipidemia should be considered. These conditions are rare and usually believed to have a genetic basis, although pathogenesis often remains elusive. In dogs, idiopathic hyperlipidemia is most commonly observed in miniature schnauzers and is characterized by moderate to marked hypertriglyceridemia and moderate hypercholesterolemia [71, 72]. Decreases in lipoprotein lipase activity has been suggested as a mechanism underlying the increases in VLDL with or without increases in chylomicrons observed in this breed [72–74] This syndrome may be an incidental finding or may be associated with clinical signs such as seizures, abdominal pain, pancreatitis or ocular lesions. Proteinuria and renal lesions including glomerular lipid thromboemboli have been associated with hypertriglyceridemia in miniature schnauzers [74, 75]. Idiopathic hyperlipidemia has been reported in other dog breeds as well as sporadically in mixed breeds.

A syndrome of primary hypercholesterolemia and hypertriglyceridemia has been described in Shetland sheepdogs [76, 77] and beagles [78]. Idiopathic hypercholesterolemia with normal triglycerides has been observed in briards [79], while idiopathic hypertriglyceridemia without elevations in cholesterol have been documented in Brittany spaniels [80].

Primary hyperchylomicronemia resulting from a mutation in the lipoprotein lipase gene has been documented in cats [81]. It is suggested that the lipoprotein lipase enzyme cannot bind to the capillary endothelium. These cats have increases in serum chylomicrons, triglycerides, and cholesterol. This condition is associated with overall decrease in body fat mass, development of xanthomata and ocular lipid accumulation [82, 83].

Ketosis and ketoacidosis

Clinically significant ketosis occurs in conditions where energy supply and demand are out of balance. This may be seen in dairy cows in early lactation when high milk production results in a negative energy balance. Clinical bovine ketosis is characterized by increased plasma NEFA, hypoglycemia, hypoinsulinemia, high glucagon, low insulin, and metabolic acidosis [84]. Increased lipolysis supplies LCFA to hepatocytes at a rate that exceeds the ability to produce and export triglycerides or to oxidize them through the TCA cycle. As a result, fatty acids are shunted to ketone production. Hepatic lipidosis usually precedes clinical ketosis due to sluggish export of VLDL. While clinical bovine ketosis is not a fatal disease, it does result in significant loss of milk production and may predispose to other conditions such as displaced abomasum, metritis, and mastitis. Ovine pregnancy toxemia also is a consequence of negative energy balance. In this case, the energy drain is usually the result of late term pregnancy with twins. Ovine pregnancy toxemia is a severe, often fatal disease that may be precipitated by stress. Ewes typically are lethargic with hypoglycemia, severe metabolic acidosis, and ketosis. In sheep with pregnancy toxemia, an inability to either produce VLDL or transport triglycerides out of the hepatocytes occurs and hepatic lipidosis ensues.

Poorly controlled diabetics may develop ketosis and ketoacidosis. Diabetic ketoacidosis is characterized by hyperglycemia, hypercholesterolemia, hypertriglyceridemia, increased NEFA, and metabolic acidosis [32]. Enhanced lipolysis and gluconeogenesis result from a lack of insulin or poor insulin responsiveness. Increased glucagon, cortisol, and norepinephrine also have been implicated in the pathogenesis of diabetic ketoacidosis in dogs [32]. Triglycerides accumulate, resulting in hepatic lipidosis, while excess acetyl-CoA is converted to ketone bodies. Ketone production exceeds the ability to utilize them as an energy substrate and ketone bodies accumulate. Because ketones are strong acids, metabolic acidosis develops as the concentrations of ketone bodies increase.

Hypolipidemias

Table 32.3 lists diseases in which hypolipidemia may occur. Mild decreases in cholesterol and triglycerides alone may be of limited clinical significance and may just reflect a fasting

Table 32.3 Causes of hypolipidemia.

Protein losing enteropathy
Exocrine pancreatic insufficiency
Inflammatory bowel disease
Hepatic insufficiency
Hypoadrenocorticism
Hematopoietic neoplasia
Hyperthyroidism

state. Hypocholesterolemia can be a characteristic of illnesses that result in decreased production, decreased intake such as can be seen with malabsorption and maldigestion, or increased catabolism of cholesterol. Hypotriglyceridemia often is a reflection of inadequate nutrition such as starvation or malnutrition secondary to malabsorption and/or maldigestion.

Protein losing enteropathy, malabsorption, and maldigestion

Conditions resulting in malabsorption and/or maldigestion may be associated with hypocholesterolemia and hypotriglyceridemia, although these findings are inconsistent. Decreased serum cholesterol and triglycerides may occur with exocrine pancreatic insufficiency. In these patients, serum albumin is usually maintained within the reference interval. In contrast, patients that develop protein losing enteropathy may have concurrent hypocholesterolemia and hypoalbuminemia due to loss of both albumin and lipoproteins. Protein losing enteropathy can result from a variety of gastrointestinal pathologies including infectious, inflammatory, or infiltrative intestinal diseases as well as primary or secondary intestinal lymphangiectasia [85]. Five to 30% of cats with idiopathic inflammatory bowel disease (IBD) are reported to have hypocholesterolemia [86]. However, this finding is not consistent, and those same studies indicate that 3–5% of cats with IBD may have hypercholesterolemia. Some breeds of dogs are predisposed to protein losing enteropathy, including the soft-coated Wheaten terrier, Yorkshire terrier, basenji, and Norwegian Lundehund [85]. In soft-coated Wheaten terriers, concurrent protein losing nephropathy and nephrotic syndrome can have counterbalancing effects on serum cholesterol and triglycerides [87].

Hepatic insufficiency

Noncholestatic liver failure may be associated with hypocholesterolemia due to decreased cholesterol production. Hypocholesterolemia has been associated with cirrhosis, toxin-induced parenchymal damage, and portosystemic vascular anomalies. Hypotriglyceridemia also may be present. Hepatic insufficiency can be difficult to distinguish from intestinal diseases resulting in protein losing enteropathy as both may have concurrent hypocholesterolemia, hypoalbuminemia, low blood urea nitrogen (BUN), and gastrointestinal signs. Measurement of bile acids can distinguish between the two disorders.

Hypoadrenocorticism

Hypocholesterolemia is sometimes seen in dogs with hypoadrenocorticism [88, 89]. The incidence of hypocholesterolemia may be more common in atypical Addisonians in which there is a deficiency of glucocorticoid but not mineralocorticoid production [90]. Hypoalbuminemia and hypoglycemia also may be present and can make distinguishing Addison disease from other conditions such as liver or intestinal disease difficult.

Hematopoietic neoplasia

Decreased serum cholesterol is observed in some forms of hematopoietic neoplasia in humans and animals. Hypocholesterolemia was noted in 69% of dogs with hemophagocytic histiocytic sarcoma [91] and cats with multiple myeloma [92]. A recent report indicated that 24% of cats with nasal and nasopharyngeal lymphoma had hypocholesterolemia [93]. The mechanism underlying the hypocholesterolemia is uncertain but may relate to production of inflammatory cytokines such as interleukin-6 and tumor necrosis factor-α. These cytokines suppress hepatic cholesterol synthesis and contribute to the negative acute phase reaction observed with both albumin and cholesterol. Hypoalbuminemia was a relatively common finding in the cats with multiple myeloma and dogs with hemophagocytic histiocytic sarcoma, but not in the cats with nasal and pharyngeal lymphoma. Enhanced catabolism of cholesterol has been suggested as another mechanism to explain hypocholesterolemia in some human cancer patients.

Hyperthyroidism

Hypocholesterolemia and hypotriglyceridemia have been observed in hyperthyroid humans and in some experimental models of hyperthyroidism. While hyperthyroidism is common in older cats, decreases in serum cholesterol and triglycerides are uncommon findings. Concentrations of cholesterol and triglycerides may be near but often do not dip below the lower limit of the reference interval [94]. In one report, hypercholesterolemia was observed in 8% of cases, while hypocholesterolemia was not seen in any of the 131 cats included in the study [95].

33 Laboratory Evaluation of the Thyroid, Adrenal, and Pituitary Glands

Donald Meuten[1] and Saundra Sample[2]
[1]North Carolina State University, Raleigh, NC, USA
[2]University of Missouri College of Veterinary Medicine, Columbia, MO, USA

Clinical endocrinology

Introduction

The endocrine system is unique in that its diseases cause hypofunction or hyperfunction of an endocrine organ. This is in contrast to other organ systems wherein disease causes only hypofunction (e.g., renal, liver, cardiac diseases). Lesions causing disease can be located in any organ within the endocrine axis; however, clinically we evaluate the endocrine gland (primary) and the pituitary gland's respective relationship (secondary). Likewise, an understanding of the normal endocrine physiology and hormone function is essential in identifying the underlying disease, recognizing clinical manifestations, as well as in the selection and interpretation of appropriate diagnostic tests. Before reading any further, let's clarify for the record that there are no perfect diagnostic tests. For diagnostic use, we need tests that distinguish animals with a specific disease from the other differentials that are clinically similar. As veterinarians, we utilize multiple facets of information, including our medical knowledge, the patient's history, clinical signs, and physical exam findings to guide use of diagnostic testing. Endocrinopathies are notorious for being diagnostically challenging, especially if the disease is in the early stages and has not developed fulminate clinical signs or classical laboratory abnormalities. As a result, multiple diagnostic modalities may be required to reach a definitive diagnosis. These include key features in the patient's history, clinical presentation, and physical exam findings along with complete blood count (CBC), serum chemistry, urinalysis results, serologic testing, and diagnostic imaging. Frequently, multiple tests are required to confirm or refute a diagnosis, and they should be performed in logical order. An important principle for almost all diseases and the lab tests used to recognize the disease is that the earlier diagnostic tests are used during the progression of a disease, the more likely that the results can be equivocal. The stages of the patient's disease will influence the clinical signs and laboratory results that are being expressed at that time.

Thus, the general approach to diagnosing an endocrine disorder begins with the same basics used to diagnose all diseases: history, clinical presentation, and physical exam findings. This is followed by routine laboratory evaluation (CBC, chemistry, urinalysis). If endocrine disease is still suspected, appropriate special screening, confirmatory, and differentiating tests are then employed. It is essential to combine all of the data in a case and not rely on single abnormalities. When this is done in logical steps, a definitive diagnosis is obtained.

Endocrine tests are categorized into screening, confirmatory, and differentiating tests. A test's sensitivity (true positive) and specificity (true negative) greatly influence the value of each test. The sensitivity and specificity of lab results can be extreme. For example, an increased serum alkaline phosphatase (ALP) activity, when evaluated in isolation, is extremely sensitive for hyperadrenocorticism (HAC) because >90% of patients with hyperadrenocorticism have an increase in ALP. However, it is not specific for HAC (i.e., many other diseases have an increase in ALP). How we use test results influences their utility. In this example, if a patient has a serum ALP within reference interval (RI/WRI), it is highly unlikely the patient has HAC. Therefore, rule out this differential or at least move it lower on the list of differentials. Nonetheless, when an increased ALP is noted in the presence of other clinical and laboratory signs of HAC, this prompts additional diagnostic testing with screening tests. In HAC, a commonly used screening test is the low-dose dexamethasone suppression test (LDDST). If a dog does not suppress with LDDST, then it supports the diagnosis of HAC. The LDDST is highly sensitive (95% of dogs with HAC will not suppress) but not specific (50% of dogs that do not suppress do not have HAC). Therefore, this test is reliable when negative, and you can rule out HAC with confidence.

Veterinary Hematology, Clinical Chemistry, and Cytology, Third Edition. Edited by Mary Anna Thrall, Glade Weiser, Robin W. Allison and Terry W. Campbell.

Companion website: www.wiley.com/go/thrall/veterinary

However, LDDST is prone to false-positive results, therefore only rule in HAC if other tests agree with LDDST. Similar to routine laboratory testing, when a dog fails to suppress with LDDST, it prompts the use of confirmatory tests. Confirmatory tests have higher sensitivity and specificity values and therefore clinical utility. Ultimately one would like to integrate sensitivity and specificity values with disease prevalence to know the positive and negative predictive values of each test. As a generalization, tests progress from routine lab data to screening tests, and then confirmatory tests. Finally, when an endocrine disorder has multiple pathogeneses, tests that identify the underlying lesion or "differentiating tests" are employed. In the example of HAC, these tests help identify if the lesion is the adrenal gland (primary) or in the pituitary (secondary). This differentiation is critical for HAC in dogs because the treatments are different (e.g., surgical for adrenal dependent and medical management for pituitary).

In this chapter, we will be exploring the clinicopathologic diagnosis of several common endocrinopathies involving the thyroid gland, adrenal glands, and pituitary gland.

Thyroid disorders

Thyrotropin-releasing hormone (TRH) from the hypothalamus stimulates the release of thyroid-stimulating hormone (TSH, thyrotropin) from thyrotropes in the pituitary, which in turn stimulates thyroid gland follicular cell hypertrophy and a cascade of intracellular events that result in the production of thyroxine (TT4, tetraiodothyronine) and smaller amounts of triiodothyronine (TT3), and trace amounts of reverse triiodothyronine (rT3). Approximately 99% of secreted TT4 is bound to plasma proteins and less than 1% is free tetraiodothyronine (fT4). However, fT4 is biologically active, enters cells, leads to intracellular TT3 production, and causes negative feedback to TSH release. Free T4 that passes into cells is metabolized into TT3 or rT3 based on physiologic needs. In normal metabolic states TT3 is produced, and this is the biologically active hormone that stimulates cellular events, but when patients are sick there is preferential conversion to biologically inactive rT3. Reverse TT3 increases in nonthyroidal illness and is responsible for the decrease in TT4 seen in the euthyroid sick syndrome. Increased concentrations of serum rT3, combined with measurement of TT4 and TT3 were used to identify patients with the euthyroid sick syndrome, but measurement of rT3 and TT3 are seldom done anymore. Measurement of rT3 can help identify the euthyroid sick syndrome, or nonthyroidal illness. Although TT3 is the biologically active form of thyroid hormone it is of limited diagnostic value. TT4, the storage form of thyroid hormone, and fT4 are of greater diagnostic value. All of the serum TT4 and fT4 come from the thyroid gland and only a portion of TT3 arises in the thyroid. This may explain the greater utility of TT4 and fT4 as opposed to TT3 to indicate thyroid gland function. The majority of T3 is produced outside of the thyroid glands via deiodination of T4 in nonthyroid cells.

The major diseases of the thyroid gland are neoplasia, hyperthyroidism, and hypothyroidism. Generally, thyroid tumors in cats are benign and thyroid gland tumors that are large enough to be detected clinically in dogs are malignant. Hyperthyroidism is a very common disease of cats but is uncommon in dogs and other species. The majority of thyroid tumors in dogs do not cause hyper or hypothyroidism. Hypothyroidism is very common in dogs and does not occur spontaneously in adult cats. Hypothyroidism in cats is almost always iatrogenically induced following treatment of hyperthyroidism. Hypothyroidism is associated with goiter, or hyperplastic thyroid glands, in ruminants, birds, and horses.

Thyroid tests

TT4

This is an excellent test to rule in hyperthyroidism in cats and rule out hypothyroidism in dogs. Increased serum TT4 in a cat is due to hyperthyroidism until proven otherwise. Serum TT4 concentration within RI rules out hypothyroidism in dogs. TT4 is stable at room temperature for one week, an unusual benefit compared to most hormones that degrade postcollection if not frozen. TT4 can be measured via radioimmunoassay (RIA), chemiluminescent enzyme immunoassay, and ELISA, all of which have similar diagnostic value. Point-of-care ELISA can be used in clinics and provide results within minutes. Numerous drugs and nonthyroid diseases and can suppress serum TT4, the latter being known as euthyroid sick syndrome. It can also be lower in large body size and certain breeds (see Table 33.1). Retesting for the possibility of drug-induced suppression requires cessation of most drugs for 4 weeks. The greater the severity of the nonthyroid disease the greater the suppression of TT4 in both dogs and cats. Low concentrations of TT4 in a dog should prompt consideration of fT4, TSH, and possibly other tests to distinguish primary hypothyroidism, secondary hypothyroidism, and euthyroid sick syndrome.

TT4 <11 nmol/L, with classic clinical signs and routine lab data, may be diagnostic for some cases. When clinical signs and other routine lab data seem inconsistent, measurement of fT4 and TSH may be helpful. Markedly decreased TT4 and fT4 is considered diagnostic for primary or secondary hypothyroidism. Decreased fT4 with increased TSH is diagnostic for primary hypothyroidism. Decreased fT4 with decreased TSH is diagnostic for secondary hypothyroidism.

fT4

Although fT4 is less than 1% of total serum thyroxine, it is of excellent diagnostic value and is suppressed less by nonthyroid diseases and drugs than is TT4. Similar to TT4, the greater the severity of the nonthyroid disease the greater is the suppression of fT4 in dogs and cats. Nonthyroid disease is also associated with increased fT4 in some cats, which

Table 33.1 Summary of thyroid tests.

TT4	Most common test, excellent screening for dogs and cats, used to rule out hypothyroidism in dogs and rule in hyperthyroidism in cats, stable *in vitro*
fT4	Excellent diagnostic utility, use equilibrium dialysis to measure, biologically active hormone; approximately 10% cats false positive
TSH	Endogenous, from thyrotrophs in pars distalis, use with TT4 and/or fT4 to evaluate hypothyroidism, do not use as standalone test
TT4 & TSH	Panel used to diagnose and distinguish type of hypothyroidism
fT4 & TSH	Panel used to diagnose and distinguish type of hypothyroidism
TT3	Most abundant thyroid hormone, biologically active but poor diagnostic value, in some canine thyroid panels but do not use, rely on TT4 and fT4
r′ T3	Used infrequently, helpful to diagnose euthyroid sick syndrome
TRH stim	Substitute for TSH stimulation, GI side effects
TSH stim	Tests thyroid reserve, bovine medical-grade TSH is not available; human TSH is available but expensive; endogenous TSH and TRH stim used if injectable TSH not available
T3 suppression	Used in cats with suspected hyperthyroidism
anti-T3, anti-T4, and anti-thyroglobulin autoantibodies	Antibodies produced in lymphocytic thyroiditis, increased in <5% of cases, used to explain unusual increases or decreases in TT4 or TT3, suggests lymphocytic thyroiditis is present
Thyroid testing by species	
Dog	**Cat**
TT4	TT4
fT4	fT4
fT4 & TSH; TT4 & TSH	
If needed	
Thyroglobulin, T4, and T3 autoantibodies	T3 suppression
TSH, TRH stimulation	TSH, TRH stimulation

could interfere with interpretation when used to evaluate hyperthyroidism. fT4 is useful in dogs and cats in which the concentration of TT4 and the rest of the data are not definitive for a diagnosis. fT4 is not influenced by autoantibodies. Anticonvulsant therapy and glucocorticoids will lower fT4. fT4 within RI rules out hypothyroidism. Decreased values suggest but do not prove hypothyroidism unless other data are supportive. Concentrations of fT4 correlate with the thyroid status at the cellular level and correlate very well with TSH.

Equilibrium dialysis (ED) is the technique of choice for fT4. This means that serum is dialyzed in some manner to separate protein bound from free hormone and remove nonspecific substances in the serum that may interfere with the assay. RIA is performed on the dialysate. It is preferable to measure fT4 by ED if a dog is on levothyroid and results will be used to assess adequate dosage.

TT3 triiodothyronine

TT3 is not recommended for testing in animals. It offers no diagnostic value over TT4 or fT4 in recognizing hyper- or hypothyroidism.

TT3 is often in reference interval in hypothyroid dogs; it is interfered with more by antibodies than is TT4. It is the most abundant and biologically active thyroid hormone, but it has poor diagnostic value perhaps because most is produced outside of the thyroid gland. It is offered in some canine thyroid panels.

r′T3 reverse triiodothyronine

This is used infrequently. It is used to diagnose euthyroid sick syndrome in humans and experimentally in dogs; see euthyroid sick syndrome at end of this chapter. It is available in some labs and clinical investigations for its utility should be done. Anticipated results in euthyroid sick dogs are: decreased TT4, reference interval fT4, reference interval TSH, and increased r′T3 due to preferential conversion of T3 to r′T3.

Thyrotropin, thyroid-stimulating hormone (TSH)

Endogenous TSH is measured in diagnostic labs with various techniques. It is a highly stable analyte, and can be safely stored for up to 8 days at 4, 20, and 37 °C [1]. TSH is used primarily to differentiate primary hypothyroidism, secondary hypothyroidism, and euthyroid sick syndrome (see "screening tests hypothyroidism"). In human medicine TSH is used as a standalone diagnostic test for hypothyroidism [2]. In veterinary medicine standalone TSH has a poor sensitivity. One study suggests that TSH may be within the RI in up to 33% of hypothyroid dogs [3]; however, this study did not account for secondary (pituitary-dependent) hypothyroidism. When interpreted alongside with TT4 and fT4, endogenous TSH has a high specificity. For example, in cases of primary hypothyroidism an increased TSH concentration combined with a decreased TT4 and fT4 results in a specificity of nearly 100% (i.e., very few false positives) and localizes the cause of hypothyroidism to the thyroid gland [4]. There are multiple theories as to why TSH has a low sensitivity in animals including biologic variation, pituitary exhaustion, and assay interference secondary to TSH heterogeneity [2].

Endogenous TSH is produced by the pituitary gland and is regulated primarily by negative feedback effect of thyroid hormones (T3, fT4). Therefore, TSH concentration will vary depending on the site of the lesion (primary vs. secondary hypothyroidism). In principle, TSH is increased in primary, decreased in secondary, and within RI with euthyroid sick cases. However, diseases are in stages of progression with different degrees of severity; therefore, results may not be clear-cut. If TSH is WRI and hypothyroidism is still the best clinical diagnosis, then retesting in several weeks or performing a stimulatory test or imaging studies of the thyroid are options. Additionally, continuing the search for a nonthyroid cause of the decreased TT4, fT4 is prudent.

Hypothyroidism is traditionally treated with a replacement hormone (levothyroid). TSH can be used to monitor treatment of true hypothyroid dogs if TSH was measured in a thyroid panel prior to treatment with levothyroid. Endogenous TSH should decrease by 33% or more post-treatment if the dose of levothyroid being administered is sufficient to break the pituitary thyroid gland axis. Levothyroid treatment of a dog that does not have hypothyroidism will suppress TSH production and cause secondary thyroid atrophy if the dose is large enough. Retesting for this possibility requires cessation of levothyroid for 8 weeks [2].

Most diagnostic labs save serum samples for several days to 1 week. If TT4 is reported as decreased consider contacting the lab to determine if there is sufficient serum for additional tests. If the clinician and owner wish to pursue further diagnostics for hypothyroidism then measure fT4 and TSH in the saved serum sample.

Autoantibodies

These are produced by lymphocytes and plasma cells in the thyroid with lymphocytic thyroiditis. They may be detected in the serum and are used to indicate lymphocytic thyroiditis may be present but are not predictors of thyroid gland function status. These antibodies contribute to the destruction of the gland and are directed against thyroglobulin (aaTg present in 35–50% of hypothyroid dogs), TT3 (35% of hypothyroid dogs), and TT4 (15% of hypothyroid dogs). Thyroglobulin antibodies predominate and thyroglobulin is the protein that TT4 and TT3 are attached to, hence dogs with antibodies against TT4 and TT3 will also have aaTg, but the opposite is not true. Autoantibodies directed against thyroglobulin, TT4, or TT3 may increase or decrease TT4 and TT3 concentrations as measured by RIA depending on methodologies of the separation used. Falsely increased values of TT4 or TT3 are seen if antibody coated tubes are used in a single-step separation technique. However, falsely decreased values of TT4 and TT3 are seen if less specific separation techniques are used such as activated charcoal or ammonium sulfate. Consult the reference lab for clarification of interference.

These antibodies are used primarily to explain unusual increases in TT4 in the serum of dogs being evaluated for hypothyroidism. This happens in some cases of lymphocytic thyroiditis, probably early in the disease while inflammation is present. Results are reported as positive, negative, or inconclusive. A positive result can explain an increased concentration of TT4 in a dog with clinical signs of hypothyroidism. A very infrequent finding is that the antibodies increase the TT4 into reference interval in a dog with true hypothyroidism. A positive antibody test does not prove hypothyroidism, it indicates autoantibodies are in the serum and that lymphocytic thyroiditis is the likely lesion. There may be adequate reserve such that hypothyroidism is not present and may not develop. It is recommended that TT4 and fT4 be repeated some months later if the patient is suspected of developing hypothyroidism. Many of the breeds predisposed to develop hypothyroidism are the breeds with a high prevalence of aaTg. The false-positive rate for aaTg is approximately 6% and transient increases are reported postvaccination. They are not part of initial screens for hypothyroidism and generally are only requested when unusual results for TT4 (or TT3) are obtained.

Stimulation tests: TSH and TRH response tests

TSH stimulation (response) test historically was a gold standard for diagnosis of hypothyroidism. However, exogenous bovine medical-grade TSH is no longer commercially available and endogenous TSH is an alternative as described above. Chemical-grade bovine TSH is not recommended due to life-threatening complications. Recombinant human TSH is available but is expensive. TSH stimulation is used to predict thyroid reserve and differentiate primary hypothyroidism, secondary hypothyroidism, and euthyroid sick syndrome by evaluating the magnitude of increase of TT4 post-TSH administration. In principle TT4 will not increase in primary hypothyroidism because the thyroid gland is destroyed and there are "no" target cells for TSH to stimulate. TT4 values that are less than reference interval (<1.5 µg/dL) pre- and post-TSH are diagnostic. A euthyroid sick dog should increase TT4 normally (twofold or greater increase in TT4, or an increase of TT4 >3 µg/dL). A dog with secondary, pituitary-dependent hypothyroidism will have variable results depending on the degree of atrophy in the thyroid gland, but partial stimulation is expected unless atrophy is severe. Unfortunately, intermediary results occur and it is not known if these represent early stages of the three differentials or mild to moderate lesions.

TRH response test is used in place of TSH to evaluate dogs with potential hypothyroidism and cats with hyperthyroidism when results of other tests are not conclusive or waiting several weeks to months and retesting is not an option. Some euthyroid dogs do not respond to TRH and therefore this dynamic test is less reliable. Both TT4 and TSH can be measured in dogs. Dogs with primary hypothyroidism should have values for TT4 below reference interval, <1.5 μg/dL pre- and post-TRH. Euthyroid dogs should demonstrate an increase of TT4 >2 μg/dL or a doubling of the pre-TT4 value. If TSH is measured there should also be a doubling of the pre TSH value. The principle is similar to the TSH response test in dogs, but distinction of primary and secondary hypothyroidism is not clear. Side effects of TRH are notable and include vomiting, defecation, urination, salivation, tachycardia, and/or tachypnea. They can be reduced by using the lower dose of TRH; see protocols under hyperthyroidism.

In cats suspected of occult hyperthyroidism (TT4 in reference interval) the TRH response test checks for a failure of TT4 to increase post-TRH. Normal cats should double TT4 post-TRH because TRH stimulates release of TSH, which in turn stimulates normal thyroid follicular cells to increase production of TT4. However, hyperthyroid cats do not increase TT4. This is because neoplastic follicular cells do not respond to the increase in TSH caused by the injected TRH and the adjacent non-neoplastic follicular cells are atrophic and cannot respond to the TSH signal. Why the neoplastic thyroid cells do not respond to TRH-TSH has not been determined, but this could be due to lack of TSH receptors.

Thyroid gland biopsy

This is not recommended to diagnose hypothyroidism or hyperthyroidism, but it may prove useful to evaluate thyroid neoplasia in dogs. Fine needle aspiration cytology is recommended for suspected thyroid tumors and biopsy is only needed on those cases in which cytology is not definitive. Approximately 80% of thyroid gland masses in dogs are malignant if an enlarged mass is found clinically, and 40% or less are malignant if necropsy data are used. Size correlates with aggressive behavior and *bilateral* tumors are 16 times more likely to metastasize than unilateral tumors.

Hyperthyroidism

General

Hyperthyroidism or thyrotoxicosis is one of the most common diseases of cats and is the most common endocrine disease of cats. It is caused by adenomas in the thyroid gland. Multinodular adenomatous hyperplasia is another term used to describe the lesion in cats, but the lesions are best explained by neoplasia for the following reasons. A small percentage of cases progress to carcinoma and metastasize. Non-neoplastic tissue is atrophic and is adjacent to neoplastic nodules, whereas functional hyperplasia of endocrine organs produces uniform enlargement of the entire gland. Hyperplastic endocrine lesions respond to stimulatory and suppressive signals, whereas neoplastic lesions generally do not. Cats with these adenomas do not respond to these stimuli. Furthermore, there is overexpression of the c-ras oncogene in the adenomas, and a decrease in inhibitory G protein permitting uncontrolled mitosis and thyroid hormone production. A small percentage of cats will have neoplastic tissue in the anterior mediastinum from rests of thyroid tissue. Some cases have nodules in both thyroid lobes and anterior mediastinum that could suggest multicentric hyperplastic or neoplastic stimuli. Numerous attempts have tried to identify a goitrogenic etiology and none has been found. Attempts to demonstrate antibodies to thyrotropin receptors in hyperthyroid cats, as seen in hyperplastic thyroid disease in humans with Grave's disease, have been negative in multiple studies. Regardless of the term used, 99% of the lesions are benign and they need to be removed surgically, medically, or with radiation if the disease is to be reversed. Approximately 75% of cases have *bilateral* involvement, 20% are unilateral, and 5% have ectopic thyroid proliferation in the anterior mediastinum or thyroid carcinoma.

Hyperthyroidism is uncommon in dogs and when present is due to thyroid adenoma or more likely, carcinoma. Although hyperthyroidism is uncommon, thyroid tumors are relatively common in dogs. Occasionally thyroid tumors may induce hypothyroidism in dogs, but most dogs with thyroid tumors are euthyroid. The size of the thyroid tumor correlates with aggressiveness. Approximately 50% of dogs have rests of thyroid tissue in the anterior mediastinum and occasionally these rests become neoplastic. Even if excessive quantities of TT4 and TT3 are produced, the efficient catabolism and metabolism of thyroid hormones in the dog (up to 20 times the capability of people and cats) leads to rapid degradation of the hormones and a euthyroid status.

Hyperthyroidism is very rare in horses and ruminants. Hyperthyroidism in horses is reported with thyroid tumors and the clinical syndrome and clinical pathology is similar to that seen in hyperthyroid dogs and cats. Horses are hyperactive, have polyphagia, weight loss, and increased serum concentrations of TT4, TT3, and fT4.

Hyperthyroidism summary

Occurs in older cats; adenoma(s); weight loss; polyphagia, hyperactive; one or more liver enzymes (ALP, ALT, AST) increased in 90% of cases; increased TT4 is diagnostic, if fT4 is needed measure by equilibrium dialysis and correlate value with TT4 concentration as fT4 can be falsely increased by nonthyroid diseases (false positive).

Clinical problems

Hyperactivity, weight loss, and polyphagia in a middle aged to old cat is the most common clinical presentation. Weight loss is the most commonly observed clinical problem and may produce cachexia in severe cases. Mean age is 13 years; fewer than 5% of cases are in cats less than 10 years old. Chronic renal failure and cancer look similar, but cats with these diseases will not be polyphagic and hyperactive. Cardiac abnormalities can be detected in more than 50% of hyperthyroid cats, but only 10% are in congestive heart failure. The most common cardiac lesion is left ventricular hypertrophy. Other signs include polydipsia/polyuria, vomiting, tachycardia, patchy alopecia, unkempt hair coat, bulky stools, diarrhea, and apathetic signs such as decreased activity, lethargy, anorexia, and weakness. Apathetic signs may be due to concurrent illnesses in these older cats such as heart failure or renal failure. Due to the incorporation of TT4 in geriatric panels of cats and clinical awareness of this disease, a diagnosis of hyperthyroidism is often established before owners are aware of clinical signs. Clinical signs of hyperthyroidism in dogs are similar to those in cats but are less severe.

Routine lab data

The most consistent lab abnormality is a mild to moderate increase in serum ALP that occurs in approximately 70% of the cats. There may be mild increases in alanine aminotransferase (ALT) and aspartate aminotransferase (AST), and one or more liver enzymes will be increased in 90% of hyperthyroid cats. This nonspecific increase in these liver enzymes is mild to moderate and the pathogenesis is not known. Approximately one-third of the increase in ALP is due to the bone isoenzyme and the rest is liver isoenzyme. Although the increase in ALP is only mild, any increase in ALP should be investigated in cats due to the short half-life of feline ALP. If the ALT is more than 1000 IU/L and TT4 is not markedly increased, pursue other differentials.

Azotemia occurs in 20–50% of hyperthyroid cats and is due to prerenal or concurrent renal disease. If urine specific gravity (SG) is less than 1.025, suspect concurrent renal disease. If it is greater than 1.040 it is probably prerenal. Since cats with hyperthyroidism are geriatric, it is likely that some will have concurrent chronic interstitial nephritis. Hyperthyroid cats that are not azotemic may have decreased serum creatinine concentrations. The mechanism is not known but may be due to muscle cachexia and decreased production of creatinine. Prevalence of concurrent urinary tract infections in hyperthyroid cats is 10–20%. Most of these cats are asymptomatic for this problem, but urinalysis will reveal pyuria and culture will yield *Escherichia coli* in the majority of infections.

Hyperphosphatemia without azotemia is seen in 25–40% of hyperthyroid cats and the mechanism is not known. Total serum calcium is usually in the reference interval, but a mild decrease in ionized serum calcium without associated clinical signs is observed in up to 50% of hyperthyroid cats. Increased concentrations of parathyroid hormone are also reported in hyperthyroid cats. Hypocalcemia, hyperphosphatemia, hyperparathyroidism, and renal problems are a common series of events. The parathyroid hyperplasia may help explain why some cats do not develop postsurgical hypocalcemia and may help explain why postsurgical hypocalcemia is usually not permanent. Although hypercalcemia has been reported for dogs with hyperthyroidism, it is mild and the mechanism is not known.

Nonspecific hematologic abnormalities may occur in about half of cats with hyperthyroidism. Reported abnormalities include mild polycythemia and a stress leukogram. Less frequently, lymphocytosis and eosinophilia are observed, perhaps secondary to a decrease in cortisol due to increased thyroid hormones. Heinz bodies are often present, as they are in many diseases in cats.

Serum fructosamine is decreased in hyperthyroid cats secondary to the increased protein turnover (high metabolic rate, cachexia) and presumably a decrease in available proteins to bind with glucose. Therefore, fructosamine should not be relied upon to assess long-term glucose status in hyperthyroid cats being evaluated for diabetes mellitus.

Screening tests: TT4, if TT4 in reference interval fT4

When this disease was first recognized essentially 100% of the hyperthyroid cats tested had increased serum TT4. Now, basal concentrations of TT4 are increased in 90–95% of the cases. Some (5–10%) of cases have TT4 within the RI. False-positive increases in TT4 are not reported in cats; specificity is 100%. Decreased concentrations of TT4 or concentrations at the low end of reference interval rules out hyperthyroidism with 99% confidence. fT4 is increased in 98% of hyperthyroid cats and it is increased in 6–12% of cats that do not have hyperthyroidism. False positives are 6–12%; therefore the specificity is 88–94%. If a cat has some of the physical and clinical laboratory abnormalities characteristic of hyperthyroidism, and an increased TT4 concentration, it is diagnostic of hyperthyroidism and fT4 or any additional tests are not needed. This will account for the majority of cats with characteristic clinical signs. However, because the disease is common and up to 10% of hyperthyroid cats have TT4 in the reference interval, a considerable effort is placed in correctly identifying this population.

Concentrations of TT4 in the middle to high end of reference may be hyperthyroid, especially if some of the clinical signs and lab data characteristic of hyperthyroidism are present. This is the diagnostically challenging group. Below are some examples of correlation of TT4 with other data.

Examples

- TT4 >4.0 µg/dL rule in hyperthyroidism, if clinical signs and lab data are supportive.
- TT4 3.0–4.0 µg/dL favor hyperthyroidism, if clinical signs and lab data are supportive.
- TT4 2.5–3.0 µg/dL gray zone; perform another test if clinical signs and lab data are supportive.
- TT4 2.0–2.5 µg/dL probably not hyperthyroidism, especially if no other data are supportive; request additional tests if still suspicious.
- TT4 <2.0 µg/dL rule out hyperthyroidism unless other evidence is compelling.

The top two and the bottom two examples above are easy to interpret and will explain TT4 results for the majority of situations. It is the middle gray zone that is difficult and where fT4 can be then be measured as an aid. This scenario is being recognized more frequently. This may be due to more widespread testing that detects cats early in the disease progression. Wellness exams often include TT4 on chemistry panels of geriatric cats, hence we may see clinical chemistry evidence of the disease before signs are easily recognized. When faced with conflicting lab data while trying to confirm a diagnosis of hyperthyroidism, consider approaches in this order, depending on the urgency of a diagnosis:

1. Measure free fT4 (via equilibrium dialysis).
2. Repeat the TT4 concentration at some other time, i.e., 1–2 weeks or later.
3. Palpate and/or image the thyroid gland and find nodule(s)
4. Find the nonthyroid disease that is concurrently suppressing the concentrations of thyroid hormones (euthyroid-sick syndrome just like in dogs).
5. Perform a TT3 suppression test.
6. Perform TRH stimulation; see protocols at end of this section.

Concurrent illness will suppress TT4 in dogs and cats and the greater the severity of the illness, the greater the suppressive influence. Concurrent illness in a hyperthyroid cat can suppress mild or moderate increases of TT4 into the reference interval and therefore explain some of the cases of hyperthyroidism that have concentrations of TT4 within the RI. This suppression also occurs with fT4, but the effect is not as great and therefore measuring fT4 is a logical step to determine if a cat with a normal TT4 is hyperthyroid. However, fT4 may actually be increased in some cats with concurrent illness. Sampling during a pulsating period when not much hormone is being released can also explain TT4 concentrations within the RI. Repeat sampling for this possibility should be delayed for 1–2 weeks or longer because degrees in fluctuations of thyroid hormone secretion are seen over days rather than hours.

Dogs

Routine laboratory data are similar to that in cats, but this is less characterized because of the much lower incidence of hyperthyroidism in dogs. TT4, fT4 are increased. TSH is decreased due to negative feedback on thyrotrophs. Increased TT4 in a dog with a cervical mass and clinical signs of hyperthyroidism is sufficient for diagnosis. The cause will be a thyroid tumor. Therefore palpation, imaging of the neck and thorax, and aspiration cytology of the cervical mass are important diagnostic steps in dogs with suspected hyperthyroidism. Cytology is a preferred step as these tumors are highly vascularized and biopsy procedures will have considerable hemorrhage. Although hypercalcemia has been reported, it may not be due to hyperthyroidism.

Increased TT4 in a dog without a cervical mass and with or without clinical signs of hypothyroidism should be tested for thyroid antibodies that may falsely increase TT4. An increase in TT4 or especially TT3 may be due to cross-reactivity of autoantibodies. Antibodies to various thyroid antigens are attributed to lymphocytic thyroiditis, some of these dogs progress into hypothyroidism and some do not. TT4, fT4, and TSH on the same serum sample should be requested to confirm hypothyroidism.

Confirmatory tests: fT4, T3 suppression, TRH or TSH stimulation, fT4

Usually TT4 is all that is needed to diagnose hyperthyroidism in cats. If the serum TT4 is increased in a cat with clinical signs of hyperthyroidism, then there is no need to measure fT4, as it will also be increased in 100% of these cats. If results of TT4 are not clear-cut, then measure fT4 via equilibrium dialysis and *correlate* with TT4 concentration and *clinical signs*. However, some cats with nonthyroidal disease may have high serum concentrations of fT4, therefore do not diagnose hyperthyroidism based only on the serum fT4.

Endocrine tests should be integrated with all of the laboratory and clinical data.

Serum fT4 is not suppressed by nonthyroidal illnesses to the same degree as is TT4, and therefore fT4 is valuable when concurrent illnesses are suspected to be lowering TT4 into the reference interval. However, nonthyroidal illnesses may increase the serum fT4 concentrations. In a study of more than 900 hyperthyroid cats, 205 were categorized as mildly hyperthyroid, and of these, 125 (61%) had increased TT4 and 191 (93%) had increased fT4. However, increased fT4 concentrations are also present in some cats with nonthyroidal diseases that do not have hyperthyroidism (false positives), and this can confuse interpretation of fT4. The false-positive rate for fT4 is about 10%, but false positives are not seen with serum TT4 (Table 33.2; Figure 33.1). Therefore, it is important to correlate fT4 with TT4 and all of the other lab and clinical data for correct interpretation. The increase in fT4 seen with concurrent diseases is the reason that fT4 should not be relied on solely to diagnose

Table 33.2 Summary of test results in cats with hyperthyroidism.

TT4:

- 90–95% of hyperthyroid cats increased concentrations; sensitivity 90–95%.
- 5–10% of hyperthyroid cats have results within RI = false negative; explanations:
  1. Early in the disease.
  2. Fluctuations in secretion of TT4.
  3. Concurrent nonthyroid diseases that decrease TT4.

"Solutions"

1. Repeat TT4 (1–2 wk, 2 mo, whatever owner will tolerate).
2. Measure fT4 via equilibrium dialysis.
3. Examine thyroid for nodules: palpate, US, radioactive imaging.
4. Find concurrent nonthyroid disease.
5. T3 suppression test.
6. TRH, TSH stimulation test.

freeT4:

- 98.5% of hyperthyroid cats have increased fT4.
- 6–12% false positive = increased fT4 with nonthyroid disease.
- Correlate fT4 with TT4, do not diagnose just on fT4.
- If fT4 is increased, highly probable hyperthyroidism.

TT3:

- Approximately 25% of hyperthyroid cats have TT3 within RI.
- Do not use; better tests are available.

hyperthyroidism and why the fT4 concentration should be correlated with TT4. The greater the increase of both fT4 and TT4, the more likely the diagnosis is hyperthyroidism. However, if TT4 is not increased or is decreased, then the increase in fT4 may be due to nonthyroidal illness.

T3 suppression test

Suppression and/or stimulation tests are recommended when repeat testing for TT4 and fT4 have not provided a diagnosis. Usually, finding the concurrent illness and treating it or repeating the TT4 and fT4 at different time intervals are easier ways to confirm hyperthyroidism than is performing functional thyroid tests. If a functional test is desired, try T3 suppression first as it has fewer side effects and is easier to interpret than the others.

The T3 suppression principle is to administer TT3 orally and see if this decreases serum TT4 by suppressing the secretion of TSH. Normal cats will suppress and hyperthyroid cats do not suppress. Oral TT3 will suppress the secretion of TSH from thyrotrophs, which in turn decreases production and release of TT4 (and TT3) from the thyroid gland in normal cats because the thyroid pituitary axis is intact and the thyroid follicular cells are normal. Hyperthyroid cats already have increased thyroid hormones in their serum from the secreting thyroid tumors, and therefore they already have decreased TSH. Adding more TT3 cannot suppress this axis any further. The neoplastic thyroid follicular cells will continue secreting TT4 independent of TSH and therefore there is no decrease in TT4.

This suppression test is accomplished by administering TT3 orally for six doses; some protocols use three doses. At the start of the study, take a blood sample for a basal TT4, fT4, TT3 and 6–8 hours after the last dose of TT3 take another sample for the same measurements. TT3 determines if the cat successfully received TT3. The concentration of TT4, fT4 after the administration of TT3 should decrease in a euthyroid cat and they do not suppress in hyperthyroidism. If there is no suppression, even if the concentrations of TT4, fT4 are still within the RI, it supports hyperthyroidism.

Thyrotropin releasing hormone response test – TRH response

Principle

Exogenous TRH administered to euthyroid cats will stimulate release of TSH, which stimulates increased TT4 production and secretion. This response will be blunted in hyperthyroid cats because the neoplastic follicular cells are not responding to normal physiologic stimuli and the adjacent atrophic cells are incapable of responding.

Interpretation guidelines

Increase TT4 60% or more from basal = euthyroid.
Increase TT4 50–60% of basal = nondiagnostic.
Increase TT4 <50% to 0 = hyperthyroid.

Side effects can be significant, occur within minutes of administration, and are transient for a few hours. Side effects include vomiting, defecation, salivation, and tachypnea.

Thyroid-stimulating hormone response test – TSH response

Principle

Same as the TRH response test.

Interpretation

Increase TT4 60% or > from basal = euthyroid.
Increase TT4 50–60% of basal = nondiagnostic.
Increase TT4 <50% to 0 = hyperthyroid.

Human recombinant TSH is expensive but can be used in place of bovine medical-grade TSH. Hyperthyroid cats with values in mid to low range of TT4 have a response to TSH that is the same as normal cats.

It is recommended to consult with your reference laboratory to obtain specific suppression and stimulation protocol information and interpretation guidelines.

Endogenous TSH

Assays for feline specific TSH are not yet available, but assays used for dogs and humans are. Consult the reference lab for which antibodies are used and more importantly the

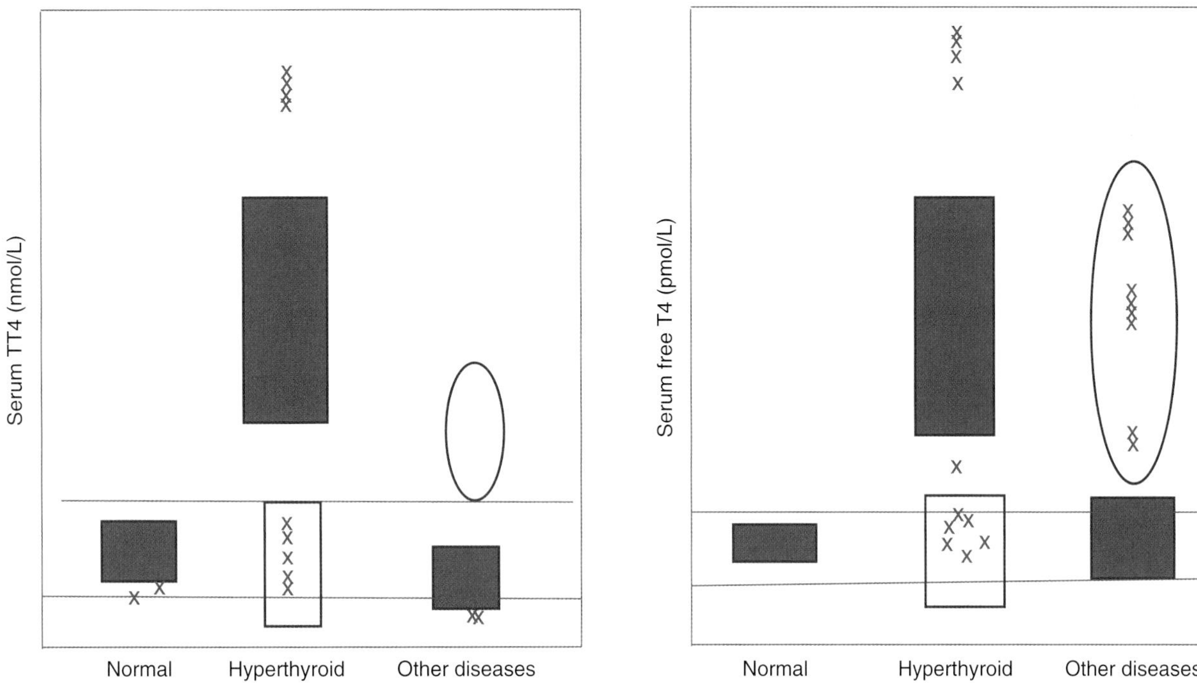

Figure 33.1 Blue boxes represent serum thyroid hormone concentrations expected in cats that are "normal," hyperthyroid, or have a variety of other diseases. Horizontal lines approximate reference intervals. "X" represents outliers; cats with concentrations of TT4 and fT4 not expected for the three classifications. A small percentage of hyperthyroid cats will have serum concentrations of TT4 and fT4 that are not increased – false negatives, open rectangles. Ovals represent false-positive results; there are none for TT4 but there are false-positives value for fT4 (approximately 10%). These cats are not hyperthyroid but fT4 is increased. All tests have false negatives and positives; tests should be integrated with all of the data on a case; no test should be used as a standalone.

reference interval values and cutoff values used to interpret results. Measurement of TSH is not needed when TT4 is increased and is only used in dogs when TT4 and fT4 results are not definitive. When TT4 is normal to high normal, TSH that is decreased and/or below the detectable limit is diagnostic for hyperthyroidism.

Hypothyroidism

General considerations

Hypothyroidism is a common disease in dogs. About 95% of the cases are due to a primary lesion in the thyroid gland defined as lymphocytic thyroiditis and/or idiopathic follicular collapse. These lesions are part of the same disease. It starts as lymphocytic thyroiditis and ends as follicular collapse, with a continuum in between. A dog with primary hypothyroidism late in the disease will have decreased TT4 and fT4 and increased concentrations of TSH. Increased TSH is in response to decreased thyroid hormones and loss of negative feedback on the pars distalis. Other lesions in the thyroid gland that cause hypothyroidism are uncommon. These include thyroid neoplasia, aplasia, hypoplasia, and dyshormonogenesis. Secondary hypothyroidism, due to a structural or biochemical lesion in the pituitary gland that decreases TSH production, is uncommon, 5% or less of cases. A dog with secondary hypothyroidism will have decreased TT4, fT4, and TSH. Decreased TSH is due to the pituitary lesion (tumor) that is destroying or crowding out thyrotrophs. Lesions associated with this are pituitary tumors, pituitary cysts, hypoplasia, dysfunctional thyrotrophs, and an apparent deficiency of TSH production in giant schnauzers. The lack of TSH results in atrophy of the thyroid gland, which theoretically could be reversed if the primary lesion in the pituitary could be corrected. Tertiary hypothyroidism due to a lesion that decreases TRH has not been reported in veterinary medicine. An increased concentration of TSH with concurrent decreases in TT4 and fT4 confirms primary hypothyroidism.

Lymphocytic thyroiditis is an immune-mediated destruction of the thyroid gland directed at thyroid follicular cells, sparing C-cells. It is nonreversible and affected dogs require life-long thyroid replacement therapy. Clinical signs develop gradually over several years and are detected when approximately 75% or more of the gland is destroyed. Lymphocytes and plasma cells produce antibodies directed at thyroid follicular cells, with antigens including thyroglobulin (most common), colloid, TT3, and TT4. There is a genetic component to this disease, and the list of dog breeds that have an increased prevalence of thyroid antibodies in their serum is long. These antibodies and the inflammation gradually destroy the follicular cells. Over time, the inflammation evidenced by inflammatory cells subsides. Histologically, the gland at this point appears as idiopathic follicular collapse.

Autoantibodies directed against thyroglobulin, TT4, or TT3 may increase or decrease TT4 and TT3 concentrations as measured by RIA depending on methodologies. Falsely increased values of TT4 or TT3 are seen if antibody-coated tubes are used in a single-step separation technique. Increased concentrations of TT4 in a dog with clinical signs of hypothyroidism can confuse interpretation of the results. This is uncommon, occurring in less than 5% of the cases and can be confirmed by measuring the different antibodies. Furthermore, the clinical signs of hyperthyroidism versus hypothyroidism are very different. Even more confusing is the situation where the antibodies "raise" the TT4 and/or TT3 into the reference interval. In either situation, if hypothyroidism is the likely differential, then the next step is to consult with the reference lab and to measure antibodies for thyroglobulin, TT3, and/or TT4. If any of these are increased then antibody interference is the most likely explanation for the confounding data. Free T4 is interfered with less than TT4 or TT3, so it is hoped that in these uncommon situations the fT4 will be decreased while TT4 is increased, which further supports antibody interference. This pattern is rarely observed (<5% of cases) and when seen is probably in an early or active phase of the disease when inflammation and antibody production are occurring. The key is to correlate clinical suspicion with the laboratory data. Recent vaccination can also produce antibodies to thyroglobulin, but there is no association with hypothyroidism.

Other causes of hypothyroidism in dogs are rare: neoplastic destruction of the gland, iodine deficiency, iatrogenic destruction (surgery, radioiodine), dyshormonogenesis, pituitary cysts (dwarfism), and congenital – giant schnauzer and an autosomal recessive form in toy fox terriers, in which there is a deficiency of thyroid peroxidase. A genetic test can recognize the carrier trait in fox terriers.

Spontaneous hypothyroidism is very rare in adult cats. An autosomal recessive form of congenital hypothyroidism is reported in Abyssinian cats. Decreased concentrations of TT4 in a cat are much more likely to be due to nonthyroidal illness than true hypothyroidism. Iatrogenic causes from surgical, chemical, or radiation-induced thyroidectomy for the treatment of hyperthyroidism is the most common cause in cats. Disproportionate dwarfism occurs in kittens and causes polyendocrinopathies including growth hormone (GH) defects and hypothyroidism. Other rare causes in kittens are defects in thyroid hormone synthesis, dysgenesis, and an autosomal recessive form of congenital hypothyroidism in Abyssinians. Iodine deficiency may cause hypothyroidism and goiter in kittens fed all meat or home designed diets.

Hypothyroidism in large animals (horses and small ruminants) is almost always due to the intake of some exogenous substance that interferes with the production of TT3 and TT4. Many substances can do this, and they interfere with the production of thyroid hormones at various stages. A few of the more common and/or high-profile substances are sulfa compounds, decreased iodine intake, increased iodine intake, plants (kale, seaweed), and various chemical substances (thiouracil). The decreased production of TT3 and TT4 due to these substances, results in reduced or no negative feedback to the hypothalamus and pituitary gland and, therefore increased TSH production. The increased TSH stimulates follicular cell hypertrophy and hyperplasia, resulting in an enlarged, goitrogenic thyroid gland. These animals have goiter, mild to massive thyroid gland enlargement, and hypothyroidism indicated by decreased TT3 and TT4. Goiter in neonates is the most common thyroid disorder in the horse and small ruminant. In small ruminants it is usually due to iodine deficiency during pregnancy and is associated with dead fetus, poor suckling, weak, hypothermia, and abnormal wool or hair coat. In foals it is associated with prolonged gestation, poor ossification, ruptured tendons, contracted tendons, prognathism, and unthrifty weak foals. It is seen in northwestern USA and western Canada. The etiology is not known, but it is associated with lush pastures. The thyroid gland is not grossly enlarged, but it is hyperplastic microscopically. In weanlings to 2-year-olds hypothyroidism is due to ingestion of excess iodine (supplements, kelp, etc.).

Hypothyroidism is uncommon to rare in adult horses but is often diagnosed in overweight horses and fat ponies with "cresty" necks; it is not usually confirmed with lab data. The horses may have decreased TT4 and TT3, but rarely is endogenous TSH measured or stimulatory tests performed before the horses are empirically placed on thyroid supplements. Most of these horses probably have equine metabolic syndrome (EMS) and are resistant to insulin from being overweight, a form of type 2 diabetes mellitus. Horses with EMS test negative for hypothyroidism and equine Cushing's disease. Furthermore, drugs such as phenylbutazone and food deprivation are known to lower serum thyroid hormones in the horse.

Signalment

Canine breeds

Golden retrievers, Doberman pinschers, dachshunds, Irish setters, miniature schnauzers, Great Danes, miniature poodles, boxers, Shetland sheepdogs, Newfoundland dogs, chows, English bulldogs, Airedales, cocker spaniels, Irish wolfhounds, toy fox terriers, giant schnauzers, Scottish deerhounds, and Afghan hounds may be regarded as high-risk breeds for hypothyroidism. The disease may also occur in all other breeds regarded to be at lower risk. High-risk breeds may present as early as 2 years of age and low-risk breeds after 5 years of age. Both sexes may be equally affected.

History and physical examination abnormalities

These are numerous and some combination of problems may be detected in hypothyroid dogs. These include weight gain to obesity without increased feed consumption, lethargy, dull haircoat, cold intolerance detected as heat-seeking behavior, decreased libido, reproductive failure, alopecia usually at wear points with no pruritus, and hyperpigmentation in areas of alopecia. Secondary skin diseases such as seborrhea, dry coat, and pyoderma may be observed. Uncommon clinical signs include keratoconjunctivitis sicca, polyneuropathy, vestibular disease, and facial nerve paralysis. Myxedema is uncommon but is considered pathognomonic. Thyroid hormones stimulate the immune system and there is decreased T-cell immunity in hypothyroidism that may predispose to the secondary skin infections such as pyoderma, Malassezia, generalized demodicosis, and otitis externa.

The majority of dogs with lymphocytic thyroiditis present as just hypothyroidism, but other immune-mediated diseases and/or endocrinopathies may appear concurrently. These may include lymphocytic adrenalitis, lymphocytic diabetes mellitus, hypoparathyroidism, and lymphocytic orchitis. Most of these will be detected as one endocrinopathy. However, in some cases a second or third endocrine disease is recognized months or years later.

Clinical signs in cats are similar to those in dogs. Clinical signs in dwarf kittens include disproportionate growth, large head, short broad neck, lethargy, retained deciduous teeth, and retained kitten hair coat.

Routine laboratory data

Routine laboratory test abnormalities are nonspecific and may include the following. Mild nonregenerative anemia (30% of cases) due to decreased responsiveness to erythropoietin is recognized in about 30% of cases. More cases may have a decreased hematocrit, but it is still in the reference interval. Increased liver enzymes are attributed to hepatic lipidosis that is often present in these dogs. Increases in muscle enzymes (CPK, LDH) are reported but are not consistent. Hypertriglyceridemia and hyperlipidemia occur in a majority of cases. Hypercholesterolemia is seen in approximately 80% of hypothyroid dogs and a serum cholesterol concentration greater than 500 mg/dL is very suggestive of hypothyroidism. A concentration >600 mg/dL in a dog with appropriate clinical signs is essentially diagnostic. Perhaps as many as 20% of the cases can be diagnosed based on sufficient clinical signs in a middle-aged dog combined with a cholesterol >500 mg/dL and a TT4 <2 µg/dL. This will be enough for many veterinarians to diagnose and start treatment. "Confirmation" with a panel of TT4, fT4, and TSH may not be needed in cases this fully developed. The need to confirm the diagnosis of hypothyroidism with additional tests depends on how advanced the disease is.

Screening tests TT4, fT4; panel TT4 and TSH or fT4 and TSH on same sample

Basal concentration of TT4 should be the initial endocrine diagnostic test utilized when hypothyroidism is suspected. For convenience, TT4 is included in some routine chemistry panels. About 95% of hypothyroid dogs have decreased concentrations of TT4, resulting in a sensitivity 95%. Approximately 20% of dogs without hypothyroidism may also have decreased TT4, resulting in a false-positive rate of 20% or specificity of 80%. Euthyroid sick dogs will account for most or all of these false positives. Therefore, TT4 is an excellent screening test to rule out hypothyroidism because only 5% of hypothyroid dogs will have TT4 in the reference interval. If a panel is selected, choose TT4, fT4, and TSH performed on the same sample, fT4 by equilibrium dialysis (see Table 33.3). Interpretive guidelines are:

fT4 > 1.5 ng/dL or 20 pmol/L

= typical of euthyrid in dogs

fT4 < 0.5 ng/dL or 7 pmol/L

= typical of hypothyroidism in dogs

A dog with primary hypothyroidism late in the disease should have the following abnormalities (see Table 33.4): decreased TT4 and fT4, increased concentration of TSH, and failure to increase TT4 in response to a TSH or TRH stimulation test, if performed. Ninety percent of these dogs will have lymphocytic thyroiditis or idiopathic follicular collapse. The glands will never regenerate and the dog will need lifelong medication. A dog with secondary hypothyroidism will have decreased TT4, fT4, and TSH. Decreased TSH results from the pituitary lesion that is destroying or crowding out thyrotrophs, resulting in thyroid gland atrophy due to the

Table 33.3 Expected results for canine thyroid profiles.

Reference intervals	TT4 nmol/L 20–55	fT4 pmol/L 10–45	TSH ng/mL <0.5	TT4 µg/dL 1.5–4.3
Hypothyroid likely	<11	<10		<1
Hypothyroid unlikely	>20	>15		>2
Gray zone	12–20			
Primary hypothyroid	<15	<10	>1.0	<1
Primary hypothyroid	<15	<15	>1.0	<1
Secondary hypothyroid	15	<10	UD	<1

UD, undetectable, below limit of detection, <0.03 ng/mL; if a lower limit of reference is set, then values below this number are also confirmatory.

Reference intervals and cutoff values used should be from the laboratory performing assays.

Table 33.4 General considerations for interpreting canine thyroid profiles.

Diagnosis/test	T4	fT4	TSH	TSH stimulation
Rule out hypothyroidism	WRI	WRI	WRI	Not performed
Primary late	Decreased	Decreased	Increased	None to suppressed
Primary early	WRI	Decreased	Increased	None to suppressed
Euthyroid sick	Decreased	WRI	WRI	Increased; mild illness
Euthyroid sick	Decreased	Decreased	Variable	Increased; severe illness
The above scenarios cover most cases; the number of tests selected will depend on the veterinarian's experience and how characteristic the clinical signs and routine lab data are. Not all cases require all tests. The following are less commonly observed results that we spend considerable effort trying to understand and diagnose.				
Primary early	WRI	Decreased	WRI	None to suppressed
Primary early	WRI	WRI	Increased	None to suppressed
Primary <2%	Increased	Decreased	Increased	None to suppressed
Autoantibodies[a]	Increased	WRI	WRI	
Secondary	Decreased	Increased	Decreased	Pituitary lesion
Euthyroid sick	Decreased	WRI	WRI	Mild illness
Euthyroid sick	Decreased	Decreased	Variable	Severe illness
False positive inc of TSH	WRI	WRI	Increased	Increased, doubles or >
Drugs	Decreased	Depends on drug and mode of action		If excessive ingestion
Iodine intake	Decreased	Decreased	Increased	
Sight hounds	Normally decreased to half of RI; they need their own RI			
Obese	Increased			
Young	2–5×	Increased		

WRI, within reference interval.
[a]Autoantibodies are not a thyroid function test; they may falsely increase TT4; they indicate lymphocytic thyroiditis is likely; some of these dogs progress into the hypothyroid state and many do not.

absence of trophic hormone. Findings supportive of secondary hypothyroidism include decreased TSH, indications of other endocrine diseases, and visual or central nervous system (CNS) signs.

It is important to not diagnose hypothyroidism on one endocrine test result in isolation. The test(s) must be combined with signalment, history, physical exam, and routine lab data to determine the likelihood of hypothyroidism (Tables 33.4 and 33.5). The more pieces of the puzzle that fit with hypothyroidism, the fewer tests are needed to diagnose and start treatment. If multiple abnormalities are present, especially if the results are marked, then a diagnosis can be made with confidence. The lower the concentration of TT4 and fT4, the greater the likelihood of hypothyroidism. For example, if the TT4 and fT4 are <10 nmol/L (<0.5 μg/dL) and <7 pmol/L (<0.5 ng/dL) respectively, the best diagnosis is hypothyroidism. If cholesterol is markedly increased and TT4 and fT4 are both decreased, and the dog has multiple signs, then this is sufficient for a diagnosis without further testing.

More challenging diagnostic scenarios

The guidelines above are for classic cases that are fully developed. However, use of thyroid hormone tests to confirm hypothyroidism can be frustrating because the disease can be in various stages of development and there are situations in which the test results present conflicting or ambiguous findings. Breed, superimposed disease, drug, and age variables influence results. However, in more than 80% of situations the results are definitive and it is possible to rule out or rule in hypothyroidism. A minority of cases requires more extensive testing evaluation, perhaps over a period of weeks to months. These challenging cases may require more intensive diagnostic procedures such as measurement of antibodies to thyroid antigens, repeat testing in 4 weeks, removal of concurrent drug therapy followed by repeat testing in 4 weeks, stimulation tests (TSH or TRH), imaging of the neck (ultrasound, magnetic resonance imaging [MRI], technetium pertechnetate), and response to T4 trial replacement therapy. Sometimes, there is merit in trial therapy in place of extensive, complex testing. Unlike Cushing's disease, hypothyroidism is a disease that can be misdiagnosed, missed and/or treated for when it does not exist and the consequences are not great. Missing a diagnosis of hypothyroidism is not life-threatening and sometimes repeat testing in a month or more will yield clearer results as the disease progresses. Treating a dog with levothyroid that does not have hypothyroidism also does not have serious

Table 33.5 Examples – use all of the case data; here are some key components.

Cases	Cholesterol mg/dL RI 130–350	TT4 nmol/L RI 20–55	fT4 pmol/L RI 10–45	TSH ng/mL RI <0.5	Other tests	Diagnosis
1 alopecia	>500	<10	NN	NN	NN	Hypothyroid
2 alopecia	>500	<15	<10	NN	NN	Hypothyroid
3 alopecia	>400	<20	<5	NN	NN	Hypothyroid
4 alopecia	400	<25	<15	Increased	NN	Primary hypothyroid
5 alopecia	400	<20	<15	?	?	Hypothyroid
6 alopecia	>300	<20	<10	WRI	TSH	Stim needed
7 lethargy	>300	>25	NN	NN	NN	Rule out
8 lethargy	>300	<20	>20	WRI	NN	Rule out
9 lethargy	>300	12	20	WRI	NN	Rule out
10 lethargy	>400	<15	<10	Decreased	Imaging?	Pituitary lesion
11 alopecia	>500	>55	<10	Increased	Antibodies	Primary hypothyroid
12 vague	WRI	8	7	NN	NN	Normal for saluki
13 vague	WRI	WRI	WRI	WRI	Positive for antibodies	

WRI, within reference interval; consult laboratory doing measurements for RI and recommended cutoff values used for diagnostic, gray zone, etc.
NN. not needed, this is the veterinarian's decision; the more characteristic the clinical signs and routine lab data are for hypothyroidism, the fewer tests are needed.
Examples 1–4 = hypothyroidism confident of diagnosis but have not distinguished primary vs. secondary; primary much more likely, both treated the same.
Example 5 = hypothyroidism likely; additional testing discretion of the veterinarian.
Example 6 = hypothyroidism likely, TSH did not help recommend TSH stim.
Examples 7–9 = rule out hypothyroidism; if clinical signs or other data were strongly suggestive of hypothyroidism, consider a TSH stim. Examples 8 and 9 are consistent with euthyroid sick syndrome; the decrease in TT4 is disproportionately lower than the expected change in fT4.
Example 10 = hypothyroidism, secondary ruled in; consider imaging.
Example 11 = primary hypothyroidism with increased TT4 due to antibodies; <2% of cases have this profile.
Example 12 = TT4 and fT4 diagnostic for hypothyroidism unless a sight hound breed, then a profile like this is normal; diagnostic ranges for sight hounds are approximately half that of other breeds.
Example 13 = dog likely has lymphocytic thyroiditis; dog is euthyroid at this time; some develop hypothyroidism and most do not; repeat testing recommended especially if from a breed with increased prevalence of hypothyroidism.

biologic consequences. In fact, the term "thyroid responsive disease" has evolved to categorize dogs that respond well to levothyroid but actually do not have hypothyroidism. Thyroid hormones may benefit sick patients similar to the nonspecific stimulatory effects of steroids. Perhaps accepting some of the above before testing panels are begun will make the 10–20% of gray zone cases less frustrating. Furthermore, primary and secondary hypothyroidism are treated the same, with synthetic thyroxine (T4), levothyroid supplementation. This supplement is inexpensive and a fat dog may benefit from a little T4 regardless of their thyroid status. The important clinical distinction is to differentiate hypothyroidism from the euthyroid sick syndrome and recognize the correct concurrent disease that is suppressing thyroid hormones. Differentiating primary and secondary hypothyroidism can be done as well. Summary findings of a study of endocrine tests in 108 dogs are shown in Table 33.6. The effects of some variables on thyroid hormone testing are presented in Table 33.7.

A relatively common diagnostic challenge is to determine if a dog with a decreased TT4 is really hypothyroid when only some of the physical and laboratory abnormalities of hypothyroidism are present. This is the syndrome known as "euthyroid sick." The laboratory tests are abnormal, but function of the thyroid gland and the biologic activity of the thyroid hormones is considered normal or "euthyroid." This is a syndrome that occurs in dogs and cats in which a non-thyroid disease causes the suppression of measured thyroid hormones (Figure 33.2). The decrease in thyroid hormones is a physiologic adaptive response stimulated by a variety of cytokines that lower the basal metabolic rate and reduce cellular metabolism in times of illness. There are a variety of mechanisms postulated to decrease the thyroid hormones and some of these may even decrease TSH secretion. These animals will have decreased concentrations of TT4 but are euthyroid. A variety of illnesses can cause this syndrome and the more severe the illness the more pronounced is the decrease in TT4. Approximately 20% of sick dogs that do not

Table 33.6 Thyroid hormones in hypothyroid and euthyroid dogs.

	Hypothyroid		Euthyroid	Sensitivity/specificity
TT4 (n = 108 dogs)	n = 54 dogs Decreased: 48 (90%) WRI: 3 (5%) Increased: 3 (5%)	**Good**	n = 54 dogs Decreased: 10 (18%)	90%/82%
TT3 (68 dogs)	n = 31 dogs Decreased: 3 (10%) WRI: 23 (74%) Increased: 5 (16%)	**Not good**	n = 37 dogs Decreased: 3 (8%)	
freeT4 (n = 108 dogs)	n = 54 dogs Decreased: 53 (98%) WRI: 1 (2%) Increased: 0	**Great**	n = 54 dogs Decreased: 4 (7%)	98%/93%
TSH (n = 108 dogs)	n = 54 dogs Increased: 41 (76%) WRI = 13 (24%) Low normal = 5 (9%)[a]		n = 54 dogs Increased: 4 (7%)	76%/93%

	Sensitivity %	Specificity %	Accuracy %
free T4	98	93	95
TT4	89	82	85
TSH	76	93	84

WRI, within reference interval.
In this study, only one euthyroid sick dog had low T4, low fT4, and increased TSH = false positive.
Author comment: The more fully developed a disease, the easier it is for diagnostic tests to "recognize" the disease.
[a]Some of these five dogs may have had secondary hypothyroidism.

Table 33.7 Interpretation of thyroid hormones in dogs with unique situations.

Consideration	Effect
Body size	
<10 kg	Higher TT4; median 31.5 nmol/L
>30 kg	Lower TT4; median 25 nmol/L
Breed	
Sight hounds	Decrease TT4 and fT4 50% less than other dogs
Nordic breeds	No effect on TSH
Age	
<3 mo	Increase TT4 2–5 times adult
>6 yr	Decrease TT4
Nonthyroidal illness	Decrease TT4 dogs and cats; the greater the severity of illness the greater the decrease
Nonthyroidal illness	fT4 influenced less but can decrease in dogs and cats; can also increase fT4 in cats
Drugs	Decrease TT4 and fT4: glucocorticoids, sulfonamides, propylthiouracil, aspirin, phenobarbital, carprofen, methimazole
	Decrease TT4, little or no effect on fT4: furosemide, phenylbutazone, progestagens
	Sulfonamides may decrease TT4 and fT4 and increase TSH and cause hypothyroidism

Obese dogs have mild increases in serum TT4 concentrations; 50–75% higher.
Sight hounds have TT4 and fT4 much lower than other breeds; normal concentrations for sight hounds would be hypothyroid values for other breeds.
Pregnancy and diestrus will increase TT4.
An age-related decline occurs in serum total TT4 concentrations and response to TSH stimulation in dogs.

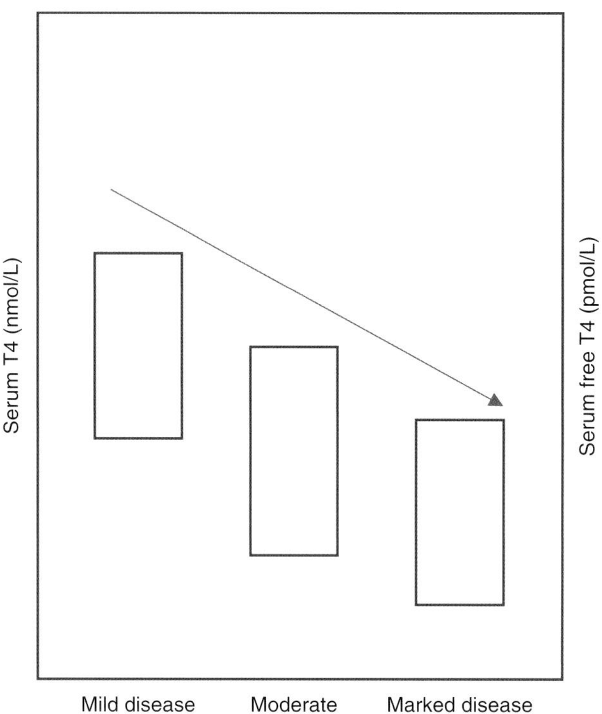

Figure 33.2 Relative serum concentrations for total T4 and free T4 are indicated by open boxes for dogs and cats that have nonthyroid diseases. Nonthyroid diseases cause the serum concentrations of TT4 and fT4 to decrease, and the more marked the disease the greater the decrease in both thyroid hormones. In dogs this phenomenon is relatively common and can lead to misdiagnosis of hypothyroidism if stimulation tests are not performed. Interestingly, nonthyroid disease can increase the serum fT4 in some cats (Figure 33.1).

have hypothyroidism will have decreased concentrations of TT4, a false-positive test result for hypothyroidism. Free T4 is only decreased in 5–10% of these dogs, but similar to TT4, the more severe the illness the more the suppression in fT4. If the decrease in TT4 is disproportionately greater than the decrease in fT4 then it favors the interpretation of euthyroid sick syndrome. The key feature for considering euthyroid sick is decreased TT4 without supporting changes in fT4 and TSH. Another helpful assessment is that dogs with euthyroid sick syndrome are not expected to have the more specific clinicopathologic features of hypothyroidism such as hypercholesterolemia, alopecia, and weight gain. It is important to recognize this group in order to correct the primary disease that is suppressing thyroid hormones.

The euthyroid sick syndrome is also recognized in cats, but the challenge presented is in the diagnosis of hyperthyroidism. The dilemma is recognizing hyperthyroidism when the secondary disease has suppressed TT4 into the reference interval. The severity of the nonthyroid disease is proportional to the decrease in TT4. This happens in older cats with concurrent diseases such as chronic interstitial nephritis, cancer, and debility. Serum fT4 is not suppressed as much as TT4, so that measurement may be helpful. However, fT4 is actually increased in some severely sick cats, which adds a new diagnostic challenge. If TT4 is in reference interval, fT4 is increased it is either true hyperthyroidism or the euthyroid sick syndrome. Distinguishing these two differentials requires correlation of all of the data and perhaps additional testing. See hyperthyroidism discussion for these approaches. Hopefully the clinical expression of these nonthyroid diseases is such that they are recognized or suspected.

Another diagnostic challenge occurs is when the clinical presentation and clinical lab abnormalities support hypothyroidism, but TT4 is increased or perhaps within the mid to upper RI. This creates endocrine testing data that is inconsistent with the clinical picture. It's more likely such a dog is in an early or mid-phase of primary hypothyroidism with lymphocytic thyroiditis and increased concentrations of antibodies directed against thyroid antigens. The way to solve this problem is to measure antibodies for aaTg and possibly TT4 or TT3. The antibodies cross-react with reagents in the *in vitro* measurement of T_4 and T_3, and therefore, cause a "false increase" in T_4 and T_3. These dogs are hypothyroid yet will "appear" to have increased measurable concentrations of T_4 and T_3 but, most importantly, increased concentrations of T_4 and T_3 antibodies.

Diagnostic challenge may occur as a result of ongoing drug therapy. Most of the problems caused by drugs are interference with assays, and usually this is observed as a decrease in TT4 and/or fT4; see Table 33.7. Sulfonamides, however, can cause hypothyroidism characterized by decreased TT4, fT4 and increased TSH. Sulfonamides block iodination of thyroglobulin and prevent production of thyroid hormones if the dose is high enough and given 4 weeks or longer. Cessation of the sulfonamides reverses the effects. Glucocorticoids affect metabolism of thyroid hormones and inhibit TSH secretion resulting in variable combinations of decreased or normal concentrations of TT4, fT4, and TSH. Phenobarbital does not cause hypothyroidism but does decrease TT4 and fT4 and may cause a slight increase in TSH. It is beyond the scope of this chapter to review all of the influences of therapy on thyroid hormones. A general recommendation is to discontinue medications that affect the thyroid gland for 4 weeks before measuring thyroid hormones or doing dynamic testing. Levothyroid should be discontinued for 8 weeks before retesting the thyroid pituitary axis.

It is occasionally useful to determine if the hypothyroidism is secondary to a pituitary lesion. The determination is somewhat academic because thyroid replacement therapy is the same, but documentation of a pituitary lesion may uncover additional endocrinopathies and have longer term case management and prognostic implications.

Sight hounds such as Salukis, greyhounds, whippets, Scottish deerhounds, Irish wolfhounds, Sloughs, and Basenjis have low serum TT4 that is physiologic and considered normal. Salukis and greyhounds also have low fT4 that are in the range of hypothyroidism for other breeds. TT4 may be below the lower limit of reference intervals for normal dogs in 90% of greyhounds and below the limit of detection in up to 33%. Therefore, the diagnosis of hypothyroidism in one of the sight hound breeds should include tests other than TT4. For sight hound breeds it may be more important to measure TSH and fT4 concurrently no matter how low the TT4 concentration is. However, hypothyroidism can be ruled out in a sight hound breed with confidence if TT4 is within the RI used for all dogs. Cutoff values for TT4, fT4, and TSH for hypothyroidism in the sight hound breeds are not established. The cause for low thyroid hormones in sight hound breeds is not known.

Diagnosis in cats

Spontaneous or naturally occurring hypothyroidism is almost nonexistent in cats. Congenital hypothyroidism, lymphocytic thyroiditis, and secondary hypothyroidism are reported but are rare. The most common cause of true hypothyroidism is iatrogenic from treatment of hyperthyroidism. The most common cause of decreased TT4 and/or fT4 in a cat is euthyroid sick syndrome. For true hypothyroidism, essentially all adult cats should have a history of thyroidectomy, radiation, or methimazole treatment. In most of these, thyroid hormones are being assessed periodically to gauge success of treatment. Nonregenerative anemia and hypercholesterolemia are expected if the cat is hypothyroid. TT4 is the initial step and if in the reference interval the cat is euthyroid sick. If it is decreased and the history has an iatrogenic cause, then it is hypothyroid. These cats probably just need their medications adjusted. If TT4 is decreased and there is no history of thyroidectomy, it is either true hypothyroidism or more likely the euthyroid sick syndrome. The most common cause of a decreased TT4 in a cat that has not undergone thyroidectomy is a concurrent illness. Now consider finding the nonthyroid disease and/or evaluate fT4 and TSH via a canine assay. The canine assay for TSH has been validated for cats. If fT4 is decreased and TSH is increased and the clinical signs and laboratory fit then it is hypothyroid. If in doubt consider a TSH or TRH stimulation test or a trial response to levothyroxine, followed with removal of levothyroxine to see if clinical and laboratory abnormalities return.

Horses and small ruminants

Hypothyroidism in large animals is almost always due to the intake of some exogenous substance that interferes with the production of TT3 and TT4. These animals have goiter, characterized as a mild to massive thyroid gland enlargement with decreased TT3 and TT4 and associated hypothyroidism. Many substances can do this, and they interfere with the production of thyroid hormones at various stages. A few of the more common and/or high-profile substances are sulfa compounds, decreased iodine intake, increased iodine intake, plants (kale, seaweed), and various chemical substances (thiouracil). The decreased production of TT3 and TT4 due to these substances results in reduced or no negative feedback to the hypothalamus and pituitary gland and, therefore, increased TSH production. The increased TSH stimulates follicular cell hypertrophy and hyperplasia, resulting in an enlarged, goitrogenic thyroid gland. Goiter in neonates is the most common thyroid disorder in the horse and small ruminant. In small ruminants it is usually due to iodine deficiency during pregnancy and is associated with dead fetus, poor suckling, weakness, hypothermia, and abnormal wool or hair coat. In foals it is associated with prolonged gestation, poor ossification, ruptured tendons, contracted tendons, prognathism, and unthrifty, weak foals. It is seen in northwestern USA and western Canada. The etiology is not known, but it is associated with lush pastures. The thyroid gland is not grossly enlarged, but it is hyperplastic microscopically. In weanlings to 2-year-olds, hypothyroidism is due to ingestion of excess iodine (supplements, kelp, etc.). It is uncommon to rare in adult horses. It is often clinically diagnosed in overweight horses with "cresty" necks but is not usually confirmed with lab data. The horses may have decreased TT4 and TT3, but TSH measurement or stimulatory tests are rarely performed before the horses are placed on thyroid supplements, reduced feed intake, and increased exercise. It is difficult to know which of these treatments is responsible for clinical improvement.

Adrenal gland disorders

Hypoadrenocorticism: Addison's disease

Primary

Lymphocytic adrenalitis – destroys all three zones of adrenal cortex; accounts for 90% or more of cases. The result is mineralocorticoid- and glucocorticoid-deficient hypoadrenocorticism (MGDH).

Secondary

This is caused by pituitary neoplasm or prolonged exogenous steroid administration. Either decreases adrenocorticotrophic hormone (ACTH) causing *bilateral* adrenocortical atrophy of zona fasciculata (ZF) and reticularis. The result is glucocorticoid-deficient hypoadrenocorticism (GDH).

Hyperadrenocorticism (HAC): Cushing's syndrome

Primary AT

Adrenal-dependent HAC is due to a functional adrenal cortical neoplasm resulting in one large adrenal and atrophy of contralateral adrenal. There is also atrophy of zona fasciculata in the ipsilateral adrenal. The cortisol from the adrenal neoplasm provides negative feedback to the pars distalis resulting in decreased production of ACTH and therefore decreased ACTH in the serum.

Secondary PDH

Pituitary-dependent HAC is due to a functional pituitary neoplasm that secretes ACTH stimulating cells in zona fasciculata to undergo hyperplasia and hypertrophy, resulting in *bilateral* adrenal gland enlargement. ACTH is increased in the serum. This accounts for 80% or more of HAC cases in dogs. Pathogenesis is different in horses.

Adrenal gland background

The adrenal gland has a cortex and a medulla. The outer most region of the cortex is the zona glomerulosa (ZG). It produces the mineralocorticoid aldosterone that helps regulate the serum concentration of sodium and potassium, extracellular fluid volume, and blood pressure. The major regulation mechanism is via serum potassium concentrations and by the renin-angiotensin system, with a minor contribution from ACTH. Hyperkalemia will stimulate the release of aldosterone from the ZG to increase potassium excretion via many epithelial cells including renal, salivary, intestinal, and sweat glands. Concurrently aldosterone stimulates renal sodium reabsorption that may increase blood pressure. Renin is released from the juxtaglomerular apparatus near glomeruli in response to decreased blood pressure, decreased sodium, and several other factors. Renin then stimulates a cascade of events that leads to increased angiotensin II that stimulates vasoconstriction and release of aldosterone. The majority of the stimulus to release aldosterone comes from the steps outlined above. Approximately 10% of the overall stimulus to release aldosterone comes from ACTH, and in the absence of ACTH, there is mild atrophy of the ZG but severe atrophy of ZF. The major disease of the ZG is hypoadrenocorticism, or Addison's disease, due to lymphocytic adrenalitis. An uncommon disease is hyperplasia of the ZG, primary hyperaldosteronism that increases aldosterone production.

Subjacent to the ZG is the largest region of the cortex, the ZF, producing many hormones of which glucocorticoids are the most clinically important. Corticotrophs in the pituitary adenohypophysis produce ACTH that stimulates ZF to release glucocorticoids immediately. Glucocorticoids complete the regulatory loop by providing negative feedback to (i) corticotrophs, which decreases ACTH secretion, and (ii) receptors in the paraventricular nuclei in the hypothalamus to decrease corticotrophic release hormone. The major disease of the ZF is HAC or Cushing's disease. This is usually secondary to a pituitary adenoma that secretes excessive amounts of ACTH. HAC may also be caused by an adrenal cortical tumor that autonomously produces glucocorticoids or iatrogenically by the exogenous administration of glucocorticoids. Regardless of the cause, all of the clinical signs and laboratory abnormalities of HAC are due to increased serum cortisol. The inner most region of the adrenal cortex is the zona reticularis (ZR) that produces glucocorticoids and sex hormones. In dogs, cats, and horses this zone has a minor role in HAC. In ferrets, this zone has a significant contribution because most of the clinical abnormalities are due to increased sex steroids.

The medulla is in the middle of each adrenal gland, it produces epinephrine and norepinephrine. The major disease is neoplasia of the adrenal medulla or pheochromocytoma that causes increased serum epinephrine production and resultant hyperactivity, hypertension, and tachycardia.

Hypoadrenocorticism: Addison's disease

The following is an outline of the two types of hypoadrenocorticism with expected major abnormalities and associated diagnostic test findings (Table 33.8).

Table 33.8 Major laboratory findings in various forms of hypoadrenocorticism.

	Primary	Atypical	Secondary
Lesion	Lymphocytic adrenalitis: ZG ZF ZR	Early?	Atrophy ZF
Basal cortisol	Decreased	Decreased	Decreased
ACTH stimulation	No response, post-stimulation cortisol <2 μg/dL for all types		
Plasma ACTH	Increased	Increased	Decreased
Na	Decreased	Within RI	Within RI
K	Increased	Within RI	Within RI
Cl	Decreased	Within RI	Within RI
Na:K ratio	<23 : 1	>25 : 1	>25 : 1
Glucocorticoids	Decreased	Decreased	Decreased
Mineralocorticoids	Decreased	Not affected	Not affected
Outcome	Irreversible	Progressive?	Reversible

Primary

Typical: lymphocytic adrenalitis that destroys the ZG, fasciculata and reticularis; there is decreased mineralocorticoids and glucocorticoids (MGDH). The decrease in aldosterone results in the major electrolyte abnormalities hyponatremia and hyperkalemia. The sodium: potassium ratio (Na:K) is decreased, which is one of the most helpful diagnostic clues. A rare variant is *atypical primary hypoadrenocorticism; glucocorticoid-deficient hypoadrenocorticism*. This may be an early form of primary, but one in which most of the manifestations are related to glucocorticoid deficiency. Some of these cases will develop mineralocorticoid deficiency, but some do not.

Secondary

The cause is either a pituitary lesion ablating ACTH release or prolonged exogenous steroid administration that results in atrophy of zona fasciculata and reticularis resulting in inability of adrenal response to ACTH when steroid administration is abruptly stopped. Glucocorticoids are decreased, but mineralocorticoids and sodium potassium ratio are not affected. GDH is a difficult disease to diagnosis. Fortunately, it is uncommon, accounting for <10% of Addison's cases.

Primary

Primary hypoadrenocorticism accounts for approximately 90–95% of Addison's disease in the dog. The two most common lesions, lymphocytic adrenalitis and idiopathic collapse, represent different stages of the same disease. Early, the lesion is an immune-mediated lymphocytic adrenalitis and in the late stage, it is severe atrophy, similar to primary hypothyroidism. The adrenal cortex cannot regenerate from these destructive lesions and therefore these patients require lifelong replacement therapy. Lymphocytic thyroiditis, parathyroiditis, adrenalitis, and lymphocytic destruction of islets are processes that occur in dogs usually as separate diseases. It is rare that they occur in the same animal and produce polyglandular failure. Failure of multiple endocrine glands is more likely due to pituitary destruction. Infrequent other causes of primary hypoadrenocorticism include neoplasia, granulomatous inflammation, infarction, and iatrogenic chemotherapy (mitotane, trilostane). Mitotane (lysodren) is used in the treatment of HAC and it selectively causes necrosis of zona fasciculata and reticularis. In about 5% of treated dogs, or in overdosed dogs, destruction of the ZG may occur. In the majority of these dogs the necrosis is permanent. The cortical zones do not regenerate and the dogs subsequently require lifelong therapy with mineralocorticoids and glucocorticoids. This is a separate situation from transient glucocorticoid deficiency associated with induction or maintenance therapy with Mitotane. Farm animals may have herpesvirus induced cortical necrosis or bacterial emboli from neonatal septicemia that destroy sufficient adrenal cortex to produce hypoadrenocorticism. Additionally, there is a condition referred to as relative adrenal insufficiency (RAI) syndrome that is diagnosed in weak and/or septic foals.

Approximately 75–90% of both adrenal cortices must be destroyed before clinical signs are observed. Partial deficiency is probably the early stage of lymphocytic adrenalitis and is one explanation for primary atypical cases when there is cortical reserve, but the reserve is inadequate to cope with stresses such as shipping, boarding, and fights. Like all diseases it can be difficult to establish a definitive diagnosis while the disease, the clinical signs, and clinical pathology data are evolving. Eventually the lesions progress and the clinical signs and laboratory data become fully developed and more clearly diagnostic.

Atypical – glucocorticoid-deficient hypoadrenocorticism

These cases could represent either secondary hypoadrenocorticism in which the cause of the decrease in ACTH is not known or is an unusual form of primary hypoadrenocorticism. In the latter possibility they most likely represent early phases of lymphocytic adrenalitis when there is adequate cortical reserve such that some, but not all manifestations of primary hypoadrenocorticism are present. It is also associated with drugs that selectively attack zona fasciculata (mitotane and trilostane) and concurrent diseases that mask the characteristic electrolyte abnormalities. These dogs initially do not have serum sodium and potassium abnormalities. Some of these dogs will progress and have a decreased sodium potassium ratio while others do not develop electrolyte abnormalities even after a year or more of follow up. Because of increased awareness of this subtype of hypoadrenocorticism, ACTH stimulation is performed on dogs with vague clinical signs coupled with suspicion of the disease. Failure of ACTH stimulation to increase cortisol >2 µg/dL is diagnostic of hypoadrenocorticism even if sodium and potassium concentrations are normal.

Secondary

The lesion of secondary hypoadrenocorticism is atrophy of zona fasciculata. Naturally occurring cases are caused by a primary pituitary lesion such as a tumor or cyst that destroys corticotrophs in the pars distalis resulting in decreased ACTH production (Figure 33.3). Probably the most common cause of secondary hypoadrenocorticism is iatrogenic from the sudden withdrawal of exogenous steroid therapy. Prolonged exogenous cortisol therapy causes negative feedback to corticotrophs, decreased serum ACTH, and subsequent atrophy of zona fasciculata. In contrast to irreversible lymphocytic adrenalitis, the adrenal cortex will regenerate if steroids are either gradually stopped or if the pituitary tumor is successfully surgically removed. Atrophy is in ZF and ZR, therefore

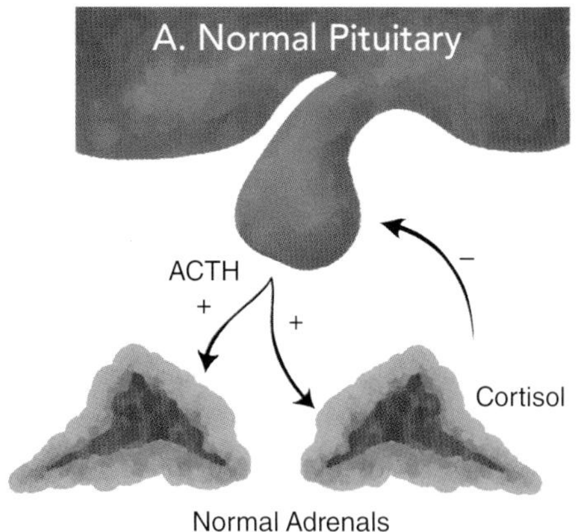

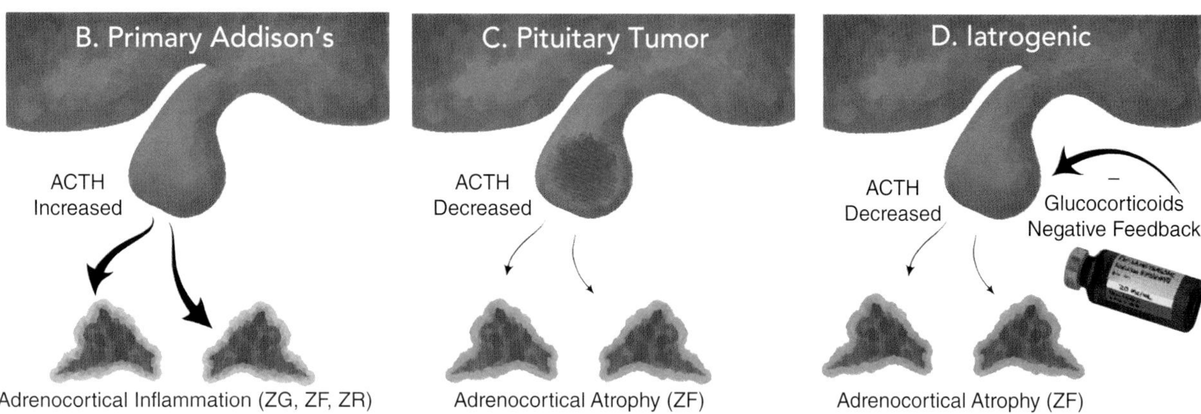

Figure 33.3 Mechanisms of hypoadrenocorticism (Addison's). Arrows represent relative amounts of hormones being secreted with a normal pituitary-adrenal axis and in three disease states. Adrenal gland sizes are relative for normal (A), primary Addison's caused by lymphocytic adrenalitis (B), and two types of secondary Addison's disease (C, D). The medulla is dark brown and is the same size in all of the diseases depicted here. In lymphocytic adrenalitis (B), an immune-mediated process destroys all three zones of the adrenal cortex (ZG, ZF, ZR), resulting in decreased production of mineralocorticoids and glucocorticoids. The decreased glucocorticoid production stimulates corticotrophs in the pars distalis to produce and secrete ACTH, a fruitless effort because the adrenal glands lack the target cells to be stimulated. The end stage of adrenalitis is "idiopathic collapse." A pituitary tumor (C) is an example of a corticotroph-destroying lesion in the pars distalis. As corticotrophs are destroyed, ACTH production and secretion declines and cells in the adrenal ZF are not stimulated. This drives *bilateral* atrophy of the ZF and results in decreased glucocorticoid production. The ZG is spared; mineralocorticoid production is not affected. Iatrogenic Addison's (D) is due to exogenous glucocorticoids that cause negative feedback to the pituitary, resulting in decreased ACTH and *bilateral* adrenocortical atrophy (ZF). These patients may appear Cushingoid on physical examination and laboratory analytes (stress leukogram, increased ALP) due to excess steroids. If the glucocorticoids are stopped too abruptly, the atrophic adrenal glands cannot respond rapidly enough to stress, and the patient may have an Addisonian crisis.

there is glucocorticoid deficiency, but ZG and mineralocorticoids are spared. Atrophy may be secondary to injectable, oral, or topical administration of glucocorticoids. Cortical function usually returns approximately 2–4 weeks after these medications are stopped. Longer-acting steroids are potent suppressants and may suppress the adrenal pituitary axis for 6 weeks or longer.

Clinical signs

Usually dogs are young to middle aged, 3–6 years. It can occur in dogs and cats as early as 2–3 months of age. Seventy percent are females, and intact females have a greater prevalence other than for standard poodles, Portuguese water dogs, and bearded collies. There are multiple breeds associated with this disease; several with a higher risk are standard poodles, Great Danes, Rottweilers, West Highland white terriers, Saint Bernards, Nova Scotia duck trolling retrievers, bearded collies, and Portuguese water dogs. Inheritance of the disease is established for standard poodles, Portuguese water dogs, Nova Scotia duck trolling retrievers, and bearded collies. Chromosomes and loci locations have even been identified in Portuguese water dogs. The disease is rare in cats and therefore no age or sex predisposition has been recognized. Some of the clinical signs are due to deficiency in glucocorticoids and some are due to mineralocorticoids and electrolyte abnormalities. Some may have clinical signs referable to both. Lethargy, weakness, vomiting, diarrhea, abdominal pain, and anorexia are due to glucocorticoids. Bradycardia is due to hyperkalemia and therefore decreased mineralocorticoids. Polyuria and polydipsia is due to chronic hyponatremia leading to renal medullary washout. Microcardia is due to hypovolemia and hypotension from the hyponatremia, as are decreased blood pressure, lethargy, nausea, and depression.

The history often indicates the dog has periodic bouts of vaguely not feeling good, vomiting, anorexia, lethargy. Over time they may either recover spontaneously or benefit by symptomatic treatment with fluids and steroids. A history reporting some of the problems listed above, especially if they recur and respond to symptomatic therapy of cage rest, fluids, and steroids is "classic" for chronic hypoadrenocorticism. Symptomatic treatment of a sick vomiting dog often includes fluid therapy and steroids, which in the case of an Addisonian is an ideal symptomatic treatment. A differential diagnosis for dogs that appear to have renal disease, gastrointestinal upset, and/or a "garbage hound syndrome" should include hypoadrenocorticism, especially if clinical symptoms are vague and recurring. Addison's and renal disease mimic each other clinically and in much of the routine lab data: 90–95% of dogs with Addison's are azotemic. The majority have hyperphosphatemia, and many cannot adequately concentrate urine due to medullary washout. Therefore, these Addisonian patients may be clinically indistinguishable from patients with chronic renal failure. Other signs seen in hypoadrenocorticism include weakness, muscle tremors, intestinal and gastric bleeding, shaking, and hypoglycemic seizures.

Some cases present as a medical emergency in an "Addisonian crisis." Features include total collapse, weak pulse, dehydrated, shocky, hypothermic, and marked bradycardia. The paradoxical combination of bradycardia and shock should trigger the differential of hypoadrenocorticism.

Dogs and cats with a pituitary lesion will have nonspecific signs and lab data referable to decreased glucocorticoids because mineralocorticoids are spared. However, patients on steroid therapy may have clinical signs and laboratory data that look like HAC due to the excess cortisol they were receiving. These dogs may have alopecia, pot belly appearance, and prominent cutaneous blood vessels due to the cortisol as well as increased serum ALP and dilute urine. If steroids are stopped abruptly the patient may collapse, have hypoglycemia, and signs of decreased cortisol. The atrophic ZF cannot respond quickly enough to produce sufficient cortisol to prevent the crisis. Although steroid usage has stopped, and cortisol has decreased, it will take some time before the corticotropes in the pars distalis produce ACTH. Even under the influence of ACTH there is a further delay in glucocorticoid production as the ZF must regenerate. During this phase the dog or cat is susceptible to a crisis should a stressful event happen.

Table 33.9 Laboratory abnormalities of hypoadrenocorticism.

Lab abnormality	% of dogs	Related to or caused by
Hyponatremia	60–80	Aldosterone decreased
Hyperkalemia	95	Aldosterone decreased
Na:K <23:1[a]	95	Aldosterone decreased
Hypochloremia	50–75	Aldosterone decreased
Hyperphosphatemia	90	Dehydration
Hypercalcemia	33	Obscure
Hypocalcemia	10	Hypoalbuminemia
Azotemia	90–95	Prerenal
Hypoglycemia	20–30	Glucocorticoids
Increased albumin	50	Dehydration
Increased serum protein		Dehydration
Decreased albumin	10+	Unknown
Urine SG variable; <1.030	60	Medullary washout
No stress leukogram	90	Glucocorticoids decreased
Anemia	10–30	Glucocorticoids; GI bleeding
Polycythemia		Dehydration

[a]Na:K <15 : 1; when ratio is this low Addison's is the most likely diagnosis, but it is still not pathognomonic and may be seen with other diseases.

Routine clinical laboratory data

A summary of expected routine laboratory findings is presented in Table 33.9.

Some of the laboratory data are caused by glucocorticoid deficiency, while others are caused by mineralocorticoid deficiency. Therefore, dogs with a pure glucocorticoid deficiency (secondary) or those with atypical Addison's do not exhibit the classical problems of mineralocorticoid deficiency such as reduced Na:K ratio and associated hypovolemia and bradycardia.

CBC

Absence of a stress leukogram or a totally normal leukogram in a sick/stressed dog may be the first indicator but is often overlooked. Eosinophilia and mild lymphocytosis can be attributed to decreased glucocorticoids and therefore may be present in both primary and secondary cases. Red blood cell parameters can vary from a mild nonregenerative anemia to a low-normal packed cell volume (PCV) that then enters the anemic range after fluid therapy. The anemia is attributed to lack of steroid stimulus to the bone marrow and possible gastrointestinal bleeding. If the anemia is more severe, look for gastrointestinal bleeding or a second disease. Less frequently there may be polycythemia (PCV 60–70) associated with marked dehydration. There is no direct effect from mineralocorticoids on the CBC.

Urinalysis

The urine SG is expected to be increased due to dehydration, but in about 60% of cases it is <1.030. Infrequently it is even hyposthenuric in primary Addison's due to "medullary washout" from chronic hyponatremia. The renal medulla is not saturated adequately with sodium ions and therefore tubules cannot passively reabsorb water from the glomerular filtrate. Dogs with medullary washout may not be able to concentrate their urine adequately even with concurrent dehydration. Dilute urine or at least urine with a SG of 1.020 or less while the patient is dehydrated, coupled with azotemia and hyperphosphatemia leads to a logical, but erroneous, diagnosis of chronic renal failure. If fluid therapy rapidly reverses the azotemia the patient did not have true renal failure, it had prerenal azotemia. Prerenal azotemia was not recognized because the urine was dilute due to concurrent medullary washout. The remainder of the urinalysis in cases of primary hypoadrenocorticism usually has no abnormalities and if abnormalities are detected, they are unrelated to hypoadrenocorticism. Long-term steroid administration leading to secondary hypoadrenocorticism in dogs may predispose them to development of cystitis and associated inflammatory elements in the urinalysis.

Clinical chemistry

Results for clinical chemistry vary depending on if it is primary (MGDH) or secondary (GDH) hypoadrenocorticism (Table 33.9). Hyperkalemia and hyponatremia are the classical abnormalities and the hallmark of primary hypoadrenocorticism. A Na:K ratio <23 : 1 is the key abnormality to indicate primary hypoadrenocorticism and is present in up to 95% of the cases. If the ratio is <15 : 1 it is very suggestive for hypoadrenocorticism, but by itself is not pathognomonic. Other ratios reported include <27 : 1 or <25 : 1; normal ratios are 27 : 1–40 : 1. Most of the ratio shift is due to hyperkalemia, present in 95% of cases rather than hyponatremia, present in 80% of the cases. Any condition that causes hyperkalemia may result in a Na:K ratio consistent with hypoadrenocorticism. Cases of secondary hypoadrenocorticism and early primary ("atypical" hypoadrenocorticism) should not have decreased Na:K ratios. Therefore, some estimate that up to 25% of all types of canine Addisonians will not have abnormal Na:K ratios. Hypochloremia is also present and may be below 100 mEq/L.

Azotemia is reported in up to 95% of cases and is almost always due to dehydration and prerenal azotemia. Dehydration is due to hypovolemia, fluid loss, and decreased aldosterone. Renal failure is an obvious differential diagnosis and must be ruled out via urinalysis, UN:Ct ratio, and response to fluid therapy. Hyperphosphatemia is also due to dehydration, decreased GFR, and prerenal azotemia. The differentiation of prerenal versus renal azotemia is critical in these patients and is best done by examination of urine SG and response of the azotemia to fluid therapy. If the urine SG is >1.030 in a dog and 1.035 in a cat that is azotemic it indicates adequate concentrating ability and prerenal azotemia. Renal azotemia is associated with urine SG in the 1.007–1.016 range. However, many cases of hypoadrenocorticism have urine SG in the 1.010–1.030 range and if the patient is also azotemic it may be difficult to distinguish renal failure vs hypoadrenocorticism. The decreased ability to concentrate urine is due to chronic hyponatremia and medullary washout. If the serum UN is disproportionately increased compared to serum creatinine, a UN:Ct ratio >25, it suggests prerenal azotemia rather than renal azotemia. Last, if azotemia is corrected rapidly by fluid therapy this indicates prerenal azotemia.

Hypercalcemia is seen in approximately one-third of dogs with hypoadrenocorticism. When present with azotemia and a decreased Na:K ratio the hypercalcemia helps favor the diagnosis of hypoadrenocorticism over renal failure. The pathogenesis of hypercalcemia is not clear. It is considered multifactorial due to increased calcium absorption from the GI tract and urine filtrate in the absence of glucocorticoids (cortisol promotes calciuria). Increased serum citrate permits more calcium to be complexed in the serum and the cortisol effect of inhibition of osteoclastic bone resorption is not present. Ionized calcium was increased in five of seven dogs that had increased total serum calcium and there were no consistent increases in PTH, PTH rp, or 1,25 di-hydroxyvitamin D concentrations to explain the hypercalcemia. The hypercalcemia seen with hypoadrenocorticism is moderate, 12–15 mg/dL as compared with the more marked hypercalcemia characteristic of hyperparathyroidism or hypercalcemia of malignancy. Hypoglycemia is present in about 10–30% of the cases and is due to decreased glucocorticoids. Hypoalbuminemia or hyperalbuminemia can be seen. Hyperalbuminemia is due to dehydration; hypoalbuminemia is difficult to explain in light of hypovolemia and hemoconcentration but is reported to be present in 10–40% of the cases. Possible causes of hypoalbuminemia may include intestinal hemorrhage, concurrent protein losing enteropathy, or chronic hepatopathy. Mild to moderate increases in liver enzymes in 30–50% of dogs with primary hypoadrenocorticism is also difficult to explain and is probably nonspecific. They resolve post-treatment of the hypoadrenocorticism. Total carbon dioxide and bicarbonate concentrations are decreased due to decreased tissue perfusion and decreased tubular excretion of hydrogen ions secondary to decreased aldosterone. The metabolic acidosis contributes to hyperkalemia because potassium shifts out of cells in exchange for movement of hydrogen ions into cells in an attempt to buffer acidosis.

An increase in the activity of serum corticosteroid isoenzyme of alkaline phosphatase (CiALP) is present in >90% of dogs with hypoadrenocorticism. However, an activity for this isoenzyme is within the RI and is not useful to diagnose hypoadrenocorticism (Borin-Crivellenti).

Addison's disease is nicknamed the *great pretender* because it mimics so many other diseases. These include GI disturbances, liver disease, and in particular renal failure. As mentioned, more than 90% of dogs with Addison's have azotemia, and some have a concurrent urine SG suggestive of renal failure. A "clue" to support hypoadrenocorticism rather than renal failure is hypercalcemia, which is present in about one-third of the dogs with Addison's. Hyperkalemia can occur with acute renal failure, but concurrent hyponatremia is seen much more frequently with hypoadrenocorticism than acute renal failure. Urethral obstruction in male cats will produce azotemia and a low Na:K ratio that is due to marked hyperkalemia, but these cats are not hyponatremic and the diagnosis of a urethral obstruction is obvious from physical examination. Uroabdomen will produce hyponatremia and hyperkalemia, Na:K ratios <23, and azotemia. Identification of uroabdomen is done by concurrent measurement of creatinine in peritoneal fluid and blood. The concentration of creatinine will be greater in the peritoneal fluid than blood. Differential diagnoses for these electrolyte abnormalities and tests to help differentiate diagnoses are presented in Table 33.10.

Table 33.10 Differential diagnosis (DDx) for Na:K less than 25 : 1.

- Hypoadrenocorticism.
- Uroabdomen.
- Urethral obstruction with intact bladder.
- Renal failure – acute or chronic.
- GI disease – whipworms, salmonella; calves and foals with diarrhea.
- Spurious – due to failure to separate serum and cells.

Practical DDx are listed above; a more complete list is below. Most of these cause the ratio shift by inducing hyperkalemia:

- Severe acidosis.
- Chlyothorax – especially with repeated drainage.
- "Third space" expansion by any cause: pregnancy, pleuritis, ascites (with or without drainage).
- Spurious – from RBCs and/or platelets and leukocytes.
  Unique breeds and species have potassium-rich RBCs:
  - Dogs – Akita, Shiba, and others; potassium-rich RBCs
  - Horses – young RBCs; certain breeds
  - Sheep – certain breeds; potassium-rich RBCs

  If there is hemolysis or if the RBCs are not separated from the plasma, then K will leach out of the RBCs, increasing the concentration of K in the plasma/serum. Separate serum from RBCs to prevent this event.
- Leukocytosis >100,000/μL.
- Thrombocytosis >1,000,000/μL.
- Phosphofructokinase deficiency – springer spaniels with respiratory alkalosis.
- Variety of GI diseases – diarrhea; gastric dilation volvulus.
- Release of potassium: crush injury, aortic thrombosis, rhabdomyolysis, heat stroke.
- Diabetes mellitus.

Tests to perform to rule in or rule out the common differentials:

Differential Dx	Test to rule in/rule out
Hypoadrenocorticism	Basal cortisol; ACTH stimulation
Uroabdomen	Compare serum and abdominal creatinine
Urethral obstruction	Male, cat, history, anuria, palpation
Renal failure	All data, urinalysis and response to fluids
GI disease	Fecal for parasites and culture
Spurious	Separate serum from blood

Screening tests – ACTH stimulation and basal cortisol

Summary: ACTH stimulation is flat line and <2 μg/dL rule in hypoadrenocorticism. Basal cortisol decreased: if <1 μg/dL 100% there is sensitivity 98% specificity, rule in hypoadrenocorticism. If <2 μg/dL there is 100% sensitivity and 78% specificity (if Na:K ratio is also decreased Addison's is likely). Basal cortisol is an excellent screening test to rule out hypoadrenocorticism. A basal cortisol >2 μg/dL rules out Addison's.

Basal cortisol and ACTH stimulation screening tests are performed after a diagnosis of hypoadrenocorticism is suspected. Recently a model was developed to aid in the screening and final diagnosis of Addison's disease by using results from routine lab requests. These include the Na:K ratio, eosinophil count, UN, albumin, creatine kinase, and CiALP. Authors developed multiple models but indicated that their calculations may not replicate when reference intervals from different labs are used. The combination of these parameters had high sensitivity and specificity and the authors concluded that the models were practical and could obviate the need for an ACTH stimulation test (Borin-Crivellenti).

Basal cortisol is decreased and is a good screening test for primary and secondary hypoadrenocorticism due to a pituitary lesion. However, if the cause of secondary hypoadrenocorticism is exogenous steroids then basal cortisol may be increased if the steroid cross-reacts with the assay (hydrocortisone, prednisone, and prednisolone) or decreased if the steroid used does not cross-react with the assay (dexamethasone). Depending on the dose and duration of the exogenous steroid the patient may appear clinically like a Cushingoid dog and the lab data will be more consistent with HAC. If glucocorticoids are being given to treat a suspected Addisonian patient they should be stopped for at least 24–48 hours before cortisol is measured and it is preferable to use dexamethasone as it does not cross-react with assays for cortisol. One dose of dexamethasone at 5 mg/kg causes only mild decreases in cortisol post-ACTH stimulation.

Basal cortisol will be less than 1 μg/dL in 85% of canine cases and less than 2 μg/dL in 90+% of cases. A basal cortisol <1 μg/dL has 100% sensitivity and a specificity of 98% in dogs, therefore it is a very good screening test for hypoadrenocorticism. If the Na:K ratio is also decreased, a diagnosis of hypoadrenocorticism can be ruled in. A basal cortisol <2 μg/dL still has a 100% sensitivity, but the specificity is reduced to 78%, indicating there will be some dogs that have serum cortisol <2 µg/dL that do not have hypoadrenocorticism and therefore are false positives, about 22%. If the basal cortisol is >2 µg/dL (>60 nmol/L), it is highly unlikely the dog has hypoadrenocorticism and the differential can be ruled out. The gray zone for basal cortisol is 1–2 µg/dL and when values fall in this range ACTH stimulation is needed. In cats the cortisol concentrations pre- and post-ACTH administration should be <2.0 µg/dL to confirm hypoadrenocorticism. Only primary hypoadrenocorticism and iatrogenic hypoadrenocorticism have been observed in cats. An important consideration is that the dog or cat was not given steroids, mitotane, ketoconazole, or other drugs that interfere with steroid production. Samples should be collected for basal cortisol and routine lab data before treatment is started. Based on the results of these tests decide if ACTH stimulation is needed. If there are inconsistent clinical findings or laboratory data, then ACTH stimulation should be performed.

The gold standard to confirm an equivocal diagnosis of hypoadrenocorticism is the ACTH stimulation test. Both primary and secondary Addisonians fail to respond to exogenous ACTH by either doubling their cortisol or increasing post-stimulation cortisol beyond 2 µg/dL (Tables 33.11 and 33.12).

Secondary hypoadrenocorticism, glucocorticoid deficiency (GDH) with normal Na:K ratio, should be confirmed with ACTH stimulation. Although basal cortisol will be decreased in cases of secondary hypoadrenocorticism caused by a pituitary lesion, the clinical signs and laboratory data are too nonspecific to rely on just a basal cortisol. The model described above was successful in recognizing GDH. Secondary hypoadrenocorticism due to iatrogenic use of steroids requires ACTH stimulation and knowledge of the type of steroid used. Depending on the steroid used, the basal cortisol measured could be decreased or increased.

ACTH stimulation is expensive, but it is the gold standard and the case management decision at stake is lifelong therapy with mineralocorticoid and glucocorticoid medications. Consider using the low-dose ACTH stimulation test to reduce costs (protocol below). ACTH stimulation requires a basal sample and samples at 30, 60, 90, or 120 minutes post-ACTH administration depending on the protocol used. Failure of ACTH stimulation to either double the basal cortisol or to increase it above 2.0 µg/dL is diagnostic of hypoadrenocorticism in dogs and cats. It is recommended to consult the reference lab used for the diagnostic guidelines they use for pre and post-ACTH cortisol values for diagnostic purposes. Common protocol recommendations include the following. Collect a serum/plasma sample for prestimulation basal cortisol. For a high-dose ACTH procedure, administer 0.25 mg (250 µg) of synthetic ACTH IV to dogs and cats >5 kg and 0.125 mg IV if <5 kg. Collect a second sample for cortisol in 30–60 minutes post-ACTH for dogs. For cats collect two samples post-ACTH, one at 60 minutes and again at 90–120 minutes.

A low-dose ACTH stimulation protocol uses synthetic ACTH (cosyntropin) at 5 µg/kg IV in dogs. Collect a basal sample and the second sample 60–90 minutes later. The low dose of 5 µg/kg of cosyntropin will maximally stimulate the adrenal cortices of normal dogs and dogs with hyperadrenocorticism and can be used as a screening test for hyperadrenocorticism. False positive or increased cortisol post-stimulation in dogs without hyperadrenocorticism is seen in about 15% of dogs.

Protocols for intramuscular ACTH that are used to diagnose hyperadrenocorticism may not be as reliable in Addisonian suspects as ACTH absorption may be impaired due to hypovolemia and poor hydration. For intramuscular protocols collect a serum sample for prestimulation basal cortisol, administer 2.2 U/lb of ACTH IM, and 2 hours later collect a sample for post-stimulation cortisol. Newer reagents use a one hour stimulation protocol; consult the reference lab and/or package insert with the ACTH. In cats inject 125 µg of cosyntropin IM and collect samples at 0, 30 and 60 minutes.

Multiple ACTH stimulation protocols are available and all work well. An advantage of low-dose ACTH stimulation protocol is reduced costs. Clinical trials have demonstrated that any dose of synthetic ACTH greater than 5 µg/kg will maximally stimulate the adrenal cortices 60 minutes postadministration and therefore higher doses are not needed. It distinguishes dogs with hypoadrenocorticism from dogs with nonadrenal illnesses that appear clinically similar to hypoadrenocorticism. If repetition of the ACTH stimulation test was needed because of sample mishandling or other causes, then

Table 33.11 ACTH response test: A baseline measurement of cortisol is obtained, then inject ACTH, measure cortisol 60–90 minutes later.

Pre ACTH stimulation:

- Basal cortisol, healthy dog (reference interval [RI]): 0.5–6 µg/dL or 10–160 nmol/L.
- Basal cortisol: >2.0 µg/dL; rule out hypoadrenocorticism.

Post ACTH stimulation:

- Post-stimulation cortisol (RI): 6–18 µg/dL; 2–3× increase from basal cortisol is a normal response (dogs).
- Post-stimulation cortisol: <2.0 µg/dL; consistent with hypoadrenocorticism (flat line).

ACTH stim does not differentiate primary from secondary hypoadrenocorticism. Endogenous ACTH will aid this differentiation:

- Adrenal dependent (common) = increased ACTH.
- Pituitary dependent (rare) = decreased ACTH.
- Iatrogenic = decreased ACTH.

Hypoadrenocorticism patients fail to increase cortisol in response to exogenous ACTH.

Table 33.12 Expected results for primary and secondary hypoadrenocorticism.

	Na:K Ratio	ACTH stimulation Cortisol μg/dL			Adrenal lesion
		Basal	Post	e-ACTH	
Primary	<25 : 1	<1.0	<1.5	>300 pg/mL (>40 pmol/L)	Adrenalitis ZG, ZF, ZR
Secondary Pituitary lesion	>27 : 1	<1.0	<1.5	<20 pg/mL (<2 pmol/L)	Atrophy ZF
Secondary Iatrogenic	>27 : 1	<1.0[a]	<1.5	<20 pg/mL (<2 pmol/L)	Atrophy ZF
Reference interval	27 : 1 to 40 : 1	0.5–6	6–18	20–100 pg/mL (2.2–20 pmol/L)	Normal

Either basal cortisol less than 1.5–2.0 μg/dL and/or post-stimulation cortisol of <1.5–2.0 μg/dL are findings indicative of hypoadrenocorticism. Consult with the reference lab for specific recommended cutoff values. Consult with the reference lab for reference intervals and cutoffs for eACTH, as these vary with the methodology.

[a]This value could be increased if the steroid used cross-reacted with the assay for cortisol, e.g., prednisone, prednisolone, hydrocortisone.

the low-dose ACTH or the high dose of 0.25 mg/dog can be repeated in 24 hours with reliable results.

Confirmatory tests

Endogenous ACTH (eACTH) is increased in primary and decreased in secondary hypoadrenocorticism.

Basal cortisol and ACTH stimulation are used to diagnose hypoadrenocorticism, but they do not distinguish primary from secondary hypoadrenocorticism. Measuring the endogenous concentration of ACTH is an easy way to distinguish these two diseases. Dogs with primary hypoadrenocorticism have eACTH > than the reference interval (typically 40–1250 pmol/L) and dogs with secondary hypoadrenocorticism have eACTH < reference interval (typically 1–2 pmol/L) (Table 33.12). Dogs with primary hypoadrenocorticism have markedly increased concentrations of eACTH, dogs with atypical primary hypoadrenocorticism have increased concentrations, and dogs with secondary hypoadrenocorticism have decreased or undetectable concentrations of eACTH. Absolute statements such as this are dependent on the disease being fully developed. As the lesions develop, the concentrations of basal cortisol and eACTH are in transition. The earlier diagnostic tests are used during the progression of a disease, the more likely that the results may be equivocal. The stages of the patient's disease development will greatly influence the clinical signs and laboratory results that are being expressed at that moment. Primary hypoadrenocorticism has increased eACTH because the entire adrenal cortex is being destroyed and serum cortisol is decreasing. Eventually there is no negative feedback to the pars distalis and corticotrophs will secrete ACTH in attempt to stimulate cortisol production. This cycle continues unabated until treatment is started. Serum concentration of eACTH can be marked in these cases, >300 pg/mL to >500 pmol/L depending on the laboratory. Although helpful in the distinction of primary and secondary hypoadrenocorticism the collection, shipment, and measurement of eACTH is delicate. It is recommended that the laboratory be consulted regarding sample handling protocol and interpretation.

If there are the characteristic electrolyte abnormalities, primary hypoadrenocorticism is most likely. Greater than 90% of the cases are primary. When the Na:K ratio is <23 : 1 and basal cortisol and/or ACTH stimulation results indicate hypoadrenocorticism, measurement of eACTH may be optional or not needed. Secondary hypoadrenocorticism will have decreased to undetectable eACTH. The pituitary lesion destroys corticotrophs and therefore ACTH production is decreased. Alternatively, the steroids being administered cause negative feedback to corticotrophs that then decrease the production and secretion of eACTH.

Other species

Hypoadrenocorticism occurs rarely in cats and the information provided above is essentially the same for cats. An exception is that only primary hypoadrenocorticism and iatrogenic hypoadrenocorticism have been observed in cats.

It is rare in all other domestic animals and when present in calves and foals it is usually due to diarrhea or septicemia with an embolic shower to the adrenal gland, as well as other organs. Calves and foals develop hyponatremia and hyperkalemia with hypoadrenocorticism similar to dogs, but these electrolyte abnormalities are much more likely to occur with infectious diarrhea or sepsis than primary hypoadrenocorticism. Calves with *E. coli* septicemia are an animal model for the Waterhouse Friderichsen syndrome, characterized as an endotoxin-induced hypoadrenocorticism. Herpesvirus will produce adrenal cortical necrosis in fetuses and neonates such as piglets, calves, and foals.

There are reports that weak and/or septic foals may have a RAI syndrome, as reported in people. The concept is there is inadequate production of cortisol during critical illnesses, especially with sepsis. One report indicated that the mean ACTH to cortisol ratio was significantly higher in septic foals that did not survive than in septic foals that did survive. In a more recent report, the authors did not confirm this correlation. They also found that the majority of ill foals had adequate responses to cosyntropin administration. Only a small group had low cortisol, low ACTH concentrations, and low responses to cosyntropin indicating a dysfunctional hypothalamic-pituitary-adrenal axis. However, the authors did not conclude this subgroup actually had RAI or that the endocrine status contributed to the illness in these foals. In fact, some foals with septicemia had markedly increased concentrations of ACTH. Endotoxin and the cytokines interleukin-1 and tumor necrosis factor alpha have been shown to cause an increase in ACTH in various species. They also reported that foals that survived had a higher concentration of cortisol in response to low-dose cosyntropin stimulation than did foals that did not survive. This finding suggested that an ACTH stimulation test may be useful to establish a prognosis in these cases. Approximately 50% of critically ill foals will have decreased basal cortisol and an inadequate response to ACTH. It would be beneficial to resolve these conflicting data in foals with sepsis and formulate a consensus to know if steroids should be administered to ill foals and which endocrine tests may be of use in case management.

Paired low-dose (10 µg) and high-dose (100 µg) protocols have been developed to evaluate normal and critically ill foals. Basal samples for cortisol are collected, 10 µg of cosyntropin is given IV as a bolus, and a sample is collected 30 minutes later to assess peak response. Ninety minutes after the 10 µg dose a basal sample is collected and 100 µg of cosyntropin is given IV as a bolus and samples are collected 30 and 90 minutes later for peak cortisol response. Other protocols inject cosyntropin intravenously at 0.1 µg/kg, and measure plasma cortisol concentrations before (baseline), and at 30 and 60 minutes after cosyntropin. Plasma ACTH concentration can be determined via an automated analyzer by enzyme based immunometric assay with chemiluminescent detection. This has been validated for use with equine samples.

Other tests

Plasma to aldosterone, aldosterone to renin, and cortisol to ACTH ratios have been used to help diagnose hypoadrenocorticism in a limited number of dogs. As clinical studies progress these tests may help differentiate primary, atypical, and secondary Addisonians and replace or supplement ACTH stimulation testing.

Primary hyperaldosteronism

Primary hyperaldosteronism (Conn's syndrome) is a rare disease in veterinary medicine but has been reported in dogs, cats, and ferrets. The lesion is hyperplasia or neoplasia of the adrenal cortex that involves the ZG. Cells in the ZG produce excess aldosterone, which causes hypokalemia and hypernatremia along with increased blood pressure and other effects. Aldosterone binds to mineralocorticoid receptors on cells in the distal convoluted tubules and collecting ducts stimulating increased production of Na-K ATPase and an increased number of sodium pumps in the nephron resulting in potassium excretion and sodium reabsorption. Confirmation requires measurement of serum aldosterone and renin combined with physical examination to rule out congestive heart failure and other possible causes of increased blood pressure. Secondary hyperaldosteronism is a normal reaction to decreased blood pressure and activation of the renin-angiotensin-aldosterone system to retain sodium and increase blood pressure. The laboratory differentiation of primary and secondary hyperaldosteronism requires concurrent measurement of aldosterone and renin.

Primary hyperaldosteronism has increased serum concentrations of aldosterone and decreased renin.

Secondary hyperaldosteronism has increased concentrations of aldosterone and renin.

Reference intervals for aldosterone are best obtained from the laboratory analyzing the samples. A guideline is 14–957 pmol/L for dogs and 194–388 pmol/L for cats.

Hyperadrenocorticism – HAC – Cushing's disease, syndrome

There are several causes of hyperadrenocorticism that are described below (Figure 33.4). All will have similar clinical signs and basic laboratory data. Special endocrine tests are useful in distinguishing the cause and this is useful for targeted therapy in case management.

Pituitary-dependent hyperadrenocorticism (PDH)

The primary lesion is a pituitary tumor that secretes ACTH autonomously and stimulates *bilateral* adrenal gland hypertrophy and cortisol secretion. Serum ACTH is increased. Pituitary-dependent hyperadrenocorticism (PDH) is the cause of HAC in more than 80% of dogs and 100% of cats. It is also the cause in 100% of horses with a tumor being in the pars intermedia that secretes various intermediary substances.

Adrenal-dependent hyperadrenocorticism (AT or ADH)

The primary lesion is an adrenal cortical tumor that autonomously secretes cortisol. Serum ACTH is decreased. This cause is responsible for 10–15% of HAC cases in dogs. It is rare in most other species. About half of functional adrenal cortical tumors are benign. In ferrets, adrenal cortical tumors are the most common cause of hyperadrenocorticism and these tumors secrete both sex hormones and cortisol.

Iatrogenic

Exogenous steroids produce the same clinical signs and routine laboratory abnormalities seen in spontaneous cases. Basal concentrations of cortisol will vary with the type of steroid used. It can be increased or decreased depending

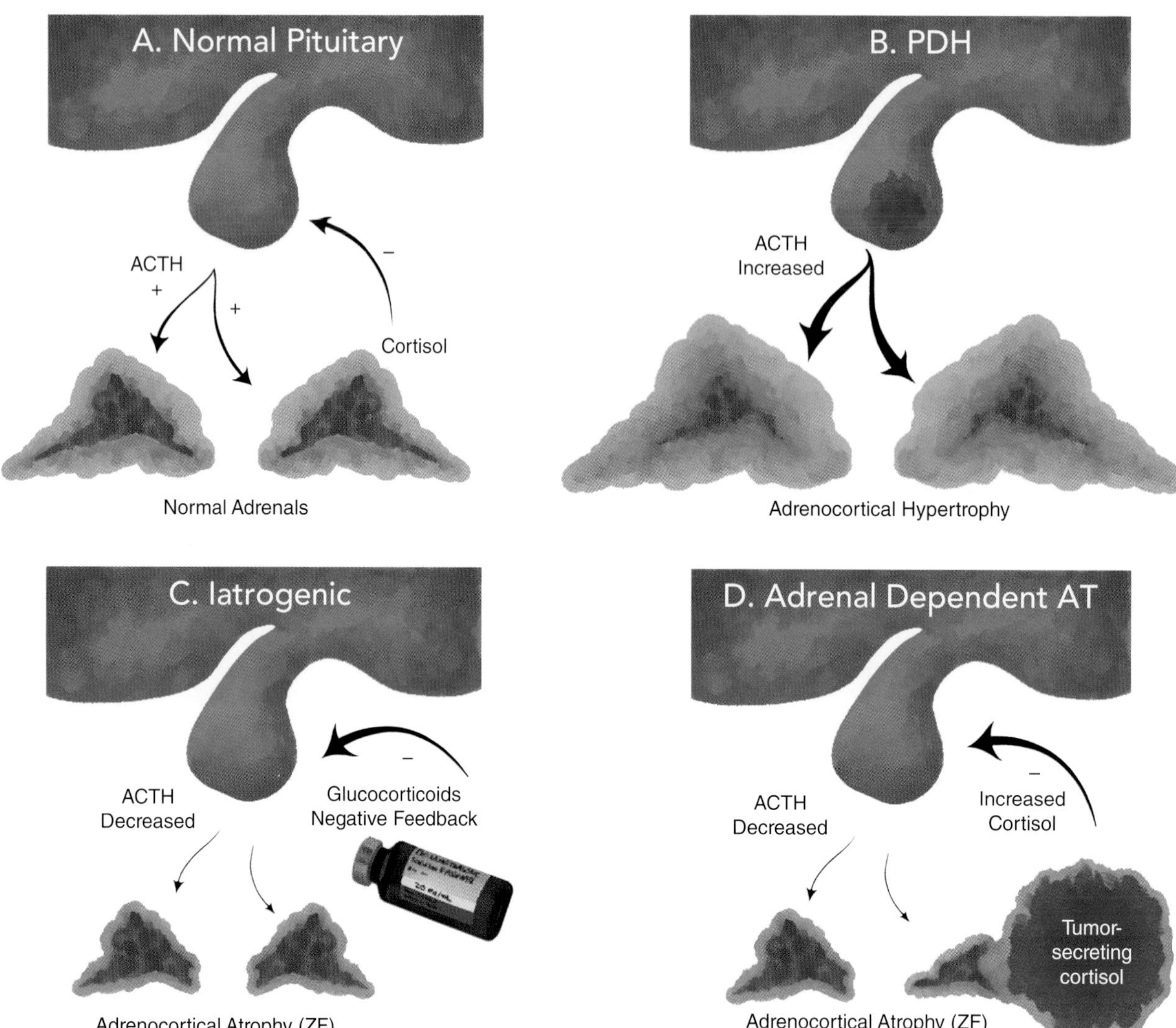

Figure 33.4 Mechanisms of hyperadrenocorticism (HAC) (Cushing's). Arrows represent relative amounts of hormones being secreted with a normal pituitary-adrenal axis and in three disease states. Adrenal gland sizes are relative for normal (A), two types of secondary hyperadrenocorticism (B, C), and primary hyperadrenocorticism (D). The medulla is dark brown and the same size in all of the diseases depicted here. Pituitary-dependent hyperadrenocorticism (PDH) (B) is caused by a functional ACTH-secreting pituitary tumor. PDH produces excessive ACTH, which stimulates bilateral adrenocortical hypertrophy and hyperplasia of the ZF. Iatrogenic HAC (C) is due to an exogenous steroid. The excess glucocorticoid causes negative feedback to the corticotrophs in the pars distalis. This results in decreased ACTH production and secretion. Decreased ACTH secretion leads to *bilateral* adrenocortical atrophy confined to the ZF and decreased endogenous glucocorticoid production. Adrenal-dependent AT (D) is due to a functional cortisol-secreting adrenal tumor. The increased cortisol secretion from the tumor increases negative feedback to the pituitary corticotrophs. The result is a decrease in ACTH production and secretion. Decreased ACTH leads to atrophy of ZF in the contralateral and non-neoplastic ipsilateral adrenal gland. The common feature of all three disease states is increased glucocorticoids, which produce "all" of the physical and clinical pathologic features of HAC.

on cross-reactivity with the cortisol assay. Serum ACTH is decreased. ACTH stimulation is the confirmatory test of choice.

Others

There are a few reports of ACTH ectopically produced by nonadrenal tumors and one report due to food-dependent hypercortisolemia in the dog. These mechanisms are very rare. Ectopically produced ACTH is much more common in human beings because they have a neuroendocrine lung tumor, oat cell tumor, that produces this syndrome. Perhaps because this tumor is rare in veterinary medicine, we do not see this paraneoplastic syndrome.

General considerations

This is primarily a disease of dogs and ferrets, but it also occurs less frequently in horses and rarely in cats. In dogs, the distinction of primary (adrenal dependent

10–15%) from secondary (pituitary dependent 80–85%) is important because primary hyperadrenocorticism is usually treated by surgical removal of the adrenal tumor, and pituitary-dependent hyperadrenocorticism is treated chemotherapeutically or by surgical removal of the pituitary. Mitotane (Lysodren, op'DDD) is capable of selective cytotoxicity of the adrenal cortex. If chemotherapeutic adrenalectomy is the preferred treatment option, it is still important to differentiate the cause of HAC because the dose of mitotane is increased when used on an adrenal tumor. The cause also has bearing on discussion of the prognosis related to treatment. First, the fact that about half of the adrenal tumors are malignant affects prognosis. Second, efficacy of chemotherapy is more variable in AT than in PDH. Furthermore, drugs that inhibit cortisol synthesis do not work as well if the cause is an AT.

Approximately 80% of the dogs with pituitary-dependent HAC disease have a microadenoma in the pituitary that autonomously produces excess ACTH. The increased ACTH stimulates *bilateral* adrenal gland hypertrophy and hyperplasia and increased secretion of cortisol. Only about 10–20% of PDH cases are due to a macroadenoma or a pituitary carcinoma. The tumor in these dogs is larger, invasive, and, therefore, may cause visual defects (pressure or invasion into optic chiasm) or other endocrinopathies due to compression of trophic cells in the pituitary (secondary hypothyroidism) and possibly central nervous system signs if the tumor invades the brain. If some of these problems are detected in a Cushingoid dog then a malignant pituitary tumor is more likely. These cases can be challenging to diagnose as the suppressive tests can respond similar to the results obtained in dogs with adrenal tumors.

Another 10–15% of HAC cases in dogs are due to adrenal cortical tumors that secrete cortisol autonomously. Approximately half of the tumors are benign the other half may metastasize into the vena cava, liver, regional lymph nodes, and lung. *Bilateral* tumors are present in 10% or less of the dogs with HAC; they may be cortical or medullary in origin. Not all adrenal cortical tumors secrete cortisol; some tumors are nonfunctional as is possible for any endocrine tumor. Adrenal cortical tumors do not respond as well to the suppressive and stimulatory tests used to diagnose HAC and these differences can be used to help distinguish PDH from AT.

The distinction of pituitary- versus adrenal-dependent HAC in cats is not as critical because both forms of the disease are treated by surgical adrenalectomy. Feline adrenal glands are less affected by chemotherapy. In cats the pituitary tumor is proportionally much larger than in dogs, however, they are benign. Most cats, 90–100%, with hyperadrenocorticism will have concurrent diabetes mellitus. Concurrent diabetes mellitus in dogs with Cushing's disease is variably reported as 10–33%. However, if resistance to insulin is discovered in either species then investigations for concurrent HAC is a recommended case management consideration.

In horses, Cushing's disease or *pituitary pars intermedia dysfunction* (PPID) is caused by a pituitary tumor or hyperplasia present in the pars intermedia. The pathogenesis and the clinical problems in horses are different from dogs and are discussed later in this chapter under pituitary disease.

About 80–85% of Cushingoid dogs, 90% of cats, and nearly 100% of horses should have a pituitary tumor. These expected results should be considered when trying to interpret the results of endocrine tests. Before the least common cause of HAC is ruled in, an adrenal tumor in a dog and especially an AT in a cat, the test results should be unequivocal. Any equivocal test results should be reconciled by performing multiple tests. Imaging studies to visualize the adrenal tumor and possibly the pituitary tumor have become viable options and should be considered in cases that have confounding endocrine data.

Clinical problems

Almost all of the clinical signs and lesions in dogs and cats are due to the increased concentration of glucocorticoids. Therefore, iatrogenic Cushingoid dogs look identical to spontaneous Cushingoid dogs. There are numerous abnormalities in dogs and cats with HAC. These include alopecia, polyphagia, polyuria/polydipsia, potbelly, muscle wasting, prominent cutaneous blood vessels, comedomes, calcinosis cutis, anestrus, decreased libido, bronchopneumonia, cystitis, and possible pulmonary thromboembolism (Table 33.13). If the cortisol concentration can be reduced, the clinical problems recede, even if a pituitary tumor remains. If blindness or other signs referable to the central nervous system are present, then a large pituitary tumor compressing the optic chiasm and the brain should be suspected. Cats and ferrets have many of the clinical problems seen in dogs with HAC.

Routine laboratory data

Complete blood count (CBC)

A stress leukogram is expected in dogs and is characterized by leukocytosis, mature neutrophilia, lymphopenia, eosinopenia, and monocytosis. Lymphopenia and eosinopenia are the most constant of these. This is present frequently in Cushingoid dogs but is obviously not specific. An increased PCV is seen in a small percentage of cases and some dogs exhibit nucleated red blood cells without regeneration, which is inappropriate and is suggestive of HAC or microangiopathies. Thrombocytosis is often present.

Cats receiving steroids may have a stress leukogram, but cats with naturally occurring HAC do not consistently exhibit a stress leukogram. Erythroid and platelet determinations are normal.

Ferrets may have anemia and/or leukopenia and thrombocytopenia late in the disease due to secretion of estradiol.

Table 33.13 Clinical signs of HAC and approximate percentage of dogs and cats with these abnormalities.

	Dogs	Cats
Polyuria and polydipsia	80–90	90
Alopecia	60–75	60
Fragile skin		50
Polyphagia	50–60	70
Potbelly	70	85
Hepatomegaly	50–70	35
Lethargy	80	50
Anestrus	55	
Calcinosis cutis	10, but considered pathognomonic	
Pyoderma		40
Hyperpigmentation	33	
Comedomes	33	
Concurrent diabetes mellitus depending on report	10–33	90

Others: Muscle wasting, prominent cutaneous blood vessels, testicular atrophy, decreased libido, bronchopneumonia, pulmonary mineralization, cystitis, facial nerve paralysis, and pulmonary thromboembolism.

Table 33.14 Laboratory abnormalities seen with HAC and approximate percentage of dogs and cats with these abnormalities.

	Dogs	Cats
Alkaline phosphatase increased	85–95	15
Alanine aminotransferase increased	50–80	40
Hyperglycemia, fasting	30–40	95
Urea nitrogen decreased	30–50	
Hypophosphatemia	20–40	
Hyperlipidemia	50–80	
Cholesterol increased	50	40
Urine SG <1.020	80	Infrequent, usually concentrated
Urinary infection[a]	50	Infrequent
Proteinuria	75	Common
Glucosuria	10	90
Stress leukogram	Common	Infrequent
Nucleated RBCs	Common	Infrequent
Thrombocytosis	85	
Decreased thyroxine	50	
Decreased free T4	25	
Alkaline phosphatase steroid isoenzyme	85–90	Does not exist

[a]Some canine cases will have bacteriuria, dilute urine, and no or few white blood cells.

The estrogen-induced bone marrow toxicity may cause pancytopenia similar to that induced by persistent estrus in intact female ferrets.

Clinical chemistry (Table 33.14)

ALP is increased in more than 90% of dogs with HAC (sensitive), but it is also increased with many other diseases (not specific). If serum ALP is not increased it is a good indicator that HAC is not present. The increase in ALP is mild, moderate, or marked. Mild and moderate increases are not very helpful to the diagnosis, but marked increases (e.g. 2000–10,000 IU/L) are very suggestive of HAC. However, there is no correlation between the magnitude of the increase and severity of the disease or predicting response to treatments. The increase in ALP in dogs is due to hepatic and a species-unique steroid-induced isoenzyme. Although the corticosteroid-induced isoenzyme (CiALP) activity increases in almost all dogs with HAC (sensitivity 95%) it is also increased in the serum of dogs with nonadrenal illnesses. Therefore, the low specificity (about 18%) limits the diagnostic value of CiALP. An activity for this isoenzyme within RI is not useful to diagnose hypoadrenocorticism (Borin-Crivellenti). Even small increases in serum cortisol, such as those occurring with exogenous steroid administration in ocular preparations, can induce CiALP. Gamma glutamyltransferase (GGT) parallels the increase in ALP in dogs. ALP has a short half-life in cats and therefore does not increase frequently or to the same magnitude as it does in dogs with HAC. Any increase in ALP is significant in cats and should be investigated. Cats and horses do not have a steroid isoenzyme.

Other liver enzymes may also be increased due to hepatomegaly caused by glycogen accumulation that produces hepatocellular vacuolation (not lipid). Glycogen accumulation in hepatocytes is characteristic of HAC, and lipid accumulation is characteristic of diabetes mellitus. Cats therefore will have a fatty liver or a mixture of fat and glycogen. The increases in ALT and AST are mild to moderate and are seen in the majority of dogs. Serum bile acids are increased in about one-third of the dogs and are a nonspecific change that is likely due to hepatomegaly caused by the glycogen hepatopathy. Total bilirubin should not be increased in dogs or cats with HAC. If it is increased look for concurrent diseases, e.g., diabetes mellitus or primary hepatopathies. Mild hyperglycemia is due to the effects of cortisol. If serum glucose is greater than 300 mg/dL in a dog or a cat with HAC consider concurrent diabetes mellitus. Consider HAC in any dog or cat in which it is difficult to regulate serum glucose with insulin as steroids are an insulin antagonist. The majority of feline cases are diagnosed after discovery of insulin resistance. Serum fructosamine may be increased due to chronic hyperglycemia in dogs and an increase is expected in cats. Cholesterol is increased in about half of the dogs and cats. Triglycerides are increased in nearly 90% of dogs but are not increased in cats.

Serum phosphorus is decreased in dogs. The mechanism is not clear but is attributed to the phosphaturic stimulus of glucocorticoids. Urea nitrogen and creatinine may be low due to diuresis in approximately 33–50% of the dogs.

Thyroid status

Approximately 50% of dogs with HAC have decreased total thyroxine (TT4) and 15–50% will have decreased free thyroxine (fT4). Endogenous TSH is normal or decreased in most of these dogs, which means they do not have primary hypothyroidism. If TT4, fT4, and endogenous TSH are decreased they should have secondary hypothyroidism due to the ACTH-secreting pituitary tumor that is compressing thyrotrophs; this is a rare situation. Increased fT4 is seen in about one-third of the dogs and may be similar to the increase seen in cats with nonthyroidal illness. Glucocorticoids may also suppress the release of TSH from the pituitary. If endogenous TSH is in the reference interval, then the decrease in TT4 is attributed to drug interference. Similar abnormalities in thyroid hormones are seen with exogenous steroids and iatrogenic Cushing's. Steroids should be stopped for at least 4 weeks before thyroid profiles are performed to critically evaluate thyroid status.

Dogs with hyperadrenocorticism or hypothyroidism share many clinical problems such as alopecia, obesity, lethargy, and enlarged liver. They also share similar clinical chemistry abnormalities such as increased hepatic leakage enzymes, cholesterol, and triglycerides. Furthermore, TT4 is often included in geriatric panels and is therefore observed early in the evaluation of these cases. Testing to rule in or rule out HAC should be done prior to thyroid profiles when these two diseases are differential diagnoses. Thyroid hormone therapy is not needed in dogs that are successfully treated for HAC as thyroid values return to reference intervals.

Urinalysis

Dilute urine, 1.004–1.020; cystitis, bacteriuria with or without inflammation, proteinuria with or without inflammation.

Dilute urine is due to interference with antidiuretic hormone (ADH) and/or its receptors by the increased cortisol, resulting in a "biochemical nephrogenic diabetes insipidus." Urine SG <1.020 is seen in 85% of dogs with HAC. Polyuria and polydipsia are compensatory responses and are seen in more than 85% of the dogs. If water is withheld, these dogs can usually concentrate into the 1.025 range. Glucosuria is uncommon in dogs, present in 10% of the canine HAC cases, but is present in 90% + of feline cases. Ketonuria does not occur in HAC. If ketonuria is present it should alert one to the possibility of concurrent diabetes mellitus. Persistent glucosuria and/or moderate to marked hyperglycemia are more consistent with diabetes mellitus. Proteinuria is seen in up to 75% of the dogs and in many dogs this is due to cystitis. Proteinuria is also seen in the absence of cystitis, and in these cases it may be due to concurrent glomerulonephritis, which is common in dogs more than 9 years old. It could also be due to steroid-induced glomerular lesions. Urine protein:creatinine ratios range from 1 to 6 (normal <1.0), and successful treatment of HAC does not always reverse proteinuria; therefore, concurrent glomerulonephritis seems likely in some dogs with HAC. Typically, there is not concurrent hypoalbuminemia or other features of nephrotic syndrome if the dogs only have HAC.

Bacterial urinary tract infections are present in half of the dogs with HAC. Bacterial infections are attributed to the compromised immune state due to the corticosteroids. Some dogs will have bacteria in their urine without inflammatory cells. Dilute urine and bacteria without inflammation is an unusual combination and when observed is suggestive for Cushing's disease. Consider urine culture in dogs even if no inflammation or bacteria are observed.

Screening tests – low-dose dexamethasone suppression (LDDS), urine cortisol:creatinine ratio (UCCR), and ACTH stimulation

If the history, clinical signs, and routine laboratory data are suggestive for HAC then the diagnosis at this stage is a two-step process: first rule in or rule out HAC with screening tests and then try to differentiate PDH and AT with confirmatory tests. Differentiation is critical because they are treated differently: chemotherapeutic destruction of the hypertrophic adrenal cortex for PDH and adrenalectomy for adrenal tumors. If surgical correction is not an option and the AT will also be treated with mitotane, differentiation is still appropriate as the dose of mitotane selected is generally higher for an AT than for PDH. Since approximately half of the adrenal tumors are carcinoma, the correct identification of the cause of HAC has prognostic implications. Regardless, this first step is critical. Obtain a correct diagnosis of HAC because either treatment is rigorous.

Each of the screening tests has value. LDDS is the most popular test and is the test of choice if the dog has characteristic signs and lab data of HAC. It also has the highest false-positive rate and should therefore not be used, or used cautiously, if clinical signs and lab data are not classical of HAC. If surgical adrenalectomy of an adrenal tumor is not an option, then LDDS is the test of choice. ACTH stimulation has the lowest false-positive rate and should be used when clinical signs and lab data are not classical of HAC. UCCR is an inexpensive and easy screening test to rule out HAC but should not be used to rule in HAC. When these tests are used in combination very few cases are misdiagnosed. These tests must be used in conjunction with routine clinicopathologic data. They are not stand-alone diagnostic tests used in isolation.

UCCR (urine cortisol:creatinine ratio)

Depending on the study, 90–100% of dogs with HAC will have excess quantities of cortisol in the urine (high sensitivity). However, urine cortisol has low specificity (20%) because it is increased in 80% of dogs with nonadrenal diseases that look like HAC. Therefore, it cannot be used to rule in HAC. More than 90% of dogs that have urine cortisol in the reference interval or below do not have HAC. Therefore, this is a very good, easy, and inexpensive screening test to rule out HAC. If a dog has an increased UCCR then LDDS or ACTH stimulation is required before HAC is diagnosed. The greatest ratios for UCCR are seen in dogs with PDH as opposed to dogs with AT. If UCCR is >100 the dog is very likely to have PDH. A UCCR is the least expensive screening test.

It is imperative to perform this test on urine collected at home in the morning when physiologic stress is at a minimum. Urine for this test should not be collected during a visit to the veterinary hospital as the stress of visitation will produce increased concentrations of serum and urine cortisol that produce false-positive results. Dogs that visit a veterinary hospital, especially if an orthopedic examination is performed, will have moderate increases of UCCR that are in the range seen with Cushing's. Have the owners collect a midstream urine sample, deliver it to the office, and submit at least 1 ml of centrifuged urine to the laboratory. The lab measures cortisol and creatinine and reports a number without units. A UCCR $>20 \times 10^{-6}$ is consistent with a diagnosis of HAC, depending on the lab and the techniques used to measure cortisol. Reference interval values vary with the laboratory. Cortisol may be present in the urine in free form or as metabolites and the assays used will vary in what they recognize, and therefore so will the reference intervals. Creatinine is used in the denominator as it is excreted at a relatively constant rate in the urine and therefore adjusts for differences in urine volume and degree of urine concentration. UCCR permits the use of spot urine or single point determinations as opposed to 24 hour collections of urine.

A good way to utilize this test is the following. If HAC is a differential on initial examination or after the CBC and chemistry panel are reviewed, then avoid returning the dog to the hospital. Instead, have the owner(s) collect a morning urine sample for UCCR. If it is within RI, then rule out HAC, and if it is increased, continue to pursue HAC.

Summary – UCCR

Good estimate of cortisol production for last 24 hours.

- >90% of dogs with normal UCCR do not have Cushing's, ruling out HAC.
- >95% of dogs with Cushing's have increased UCCR (sensitivity 95%)
- 80% of sick dogs with nonadrenal disease have increased UCCR, specificity 20%; false positives (80%). This is too high to rule in HAC.
- UCCR is sensitive to detect increased cortisol in dogs with Cushing's and in dogs with other nonadrenal diseases (stressed).
- If a dog with undiagnosed polyuria/polydipsia (PU/PD) has a UCCR in reference interval and serum ALP is not increased, then HAC is highly unlikely and can be ruled out.

Reference interval

$0.5–17.7 \times 10^{-6}$ check with lab that performed assay.
<15 rule out HAC.
≥20 consistent with HAC.
15–19 gray zone.

Low-dose dexamethasone suppression (LDDS) test

Patients with HAC will not suppress and "non-Cushingoid" patients will suppress.

The principle of the LDDS test is that dogs or cats that have HAC (PDH or AT) will not decrease their serum cortisol in response to the administration of a low dose of dexamethasone. Dexamethasone will cause a decrease in serum cortisol in "non-Cushingoid" dogs that are normal and in about 50% of dogs with other diseases. In normal dogs dexamethasone is recognized by receptors in the pituitary/hypothalamus resulting in a decreased release of ACTH. The decrease in ACTH results in decreased release of cortisol from the adrenal cortex that is interpreted as suppression. This suppression is used to rule out HAC. In normal dogs, LDDS will decrease serum cortisol in 2–3 hours and cortisol will remain decreased for 24–48 hours. LDDS is an excellent test to distinguish normal dogs from Cushingoid dogs, but it is not entirely reliable to distinguish Cushingoid dogs from sick, stressed dogs that have a variety of other diseases.

The concentration of cortisol at 8 hours post-dexamethasone administration is used to determine HAC. Dexamethasone sodium phosphate or dexamethasone in polyethylene glycol can be used. The recommended dosage is 0.01 mg/kg intravenously for the low-dose protocol. Samples are collected before (basal) the administration of dexamethasone and at 4 and 8 hours postadministration. Use the eight-hour sample to rule in or rule out HAC, use the four-hour sample to differentiate PDH from AT. Reagents used to measure cortisol do not cross-react with or recognize dexamethasone. Therefore, there is no "false," cross-reactive increase from the administration of dexamethasone. Because of cross-reactivity, prednisolone or prednisone cannot be used as the suppressing steroid. Dexamethasone is approximately 40 times as potent as cortisol, hence it can suppress ACTH when the concentration of endogenous serum cortisol cannot.

The reference interval for plasma (serum) cortisol is 0.4–6.0 μg/dL (10–160 nmol/L). However, dogs suspected of having HAC or other nonadrenal causes of increased cortisol will have a cortisol concentration at the high end or above this range. Reference intervals and suggested cutoffs for interpretation should be provided by the reference laboratory used. LDDS will decrease serum cortisol to <1.5 μg/dL (<30 nmol/L) at 4 and 8 hours postdexamethasone in normal dogs. If a dog has PDH or AT the eight-hour postdexamethasone sample will be >1.5 μg/dL (>40 nmol/L). Some labs use greater than or equal to 30 nmol/L or 1.4 μg/dL. If a dog has PDH, the low dose of dexamethasone will not decrease ACTH secretion from the pituitary tumor sufficiently to suppress cortisol secretion from the hyperplastic adrenal glands. If a dog has an AT the concentration of ACTH is already suppressed, the AT continues to secrete cortisol independent of ACTH. If the eight-hour cortisol is equal to or greater than 1.5 μg/dL (>40 nmol/L) then there was no suppression. The patient has HAC, either PDH or AT, or the test result is a false positive. All dogs with AT fail to suppress and 90–95% of dogs with PDH fail to suppress.

Many veterinarians prefer this test because 95% of the dogs with Cushing's disease do not suppress, which is similar to the high sensitivity of UCCR. LDDS is a test that recognizes 95% of the dogs with the disease that is being looked for, a very positive feature. However, it "recognizes" another 50% of dogs that do not have the disease, but the results of the test suggest that they do. The specificity of LDDS is between 75% and 44% depending on the study, which means the false-positive rate is 25–56%. Sick, stressed dogs with a variety of illnesses may have hyperplastic adrenals that do not suppress cortisol secretion in response to LDDS and the more severe the nonadrenal illness, the more likely there will be a false-positive test result.

An additional use of LDDS is to differentiate PDH from AT in a dog that has classical signs and lab data of Cushing's, see confirmatory or differentiating tests, below.

Summary – LDDS

- An 8-hour cortisol <1.5 μg/dL is suppression, rule out HAC.
- An 8-hour cortisol >1.5 μg/dL is no suppression, rule in HAC.
- 95% of dogs with HAC do not suppress, 95% sensitivity.
- 25–56% of dogs without HAC do not suppress, false positives; 44–75% specificity; therefore could rule in HAC when the dog does not have HAC.
- 5% of dogs with HAC suppress; false negative; may miss the diagnosis.
- Excellent test to rule out Cushing's when suppression occurs. If UCCR is not increased and a dog suppresses with LDDS, rule out HAC.
- LDDS can also be used to differentiate PDH and AT in about 25% of dogs.
- Popular test, but the false-positive rate is 25–50%. Therefore, signs and lab data must be characteristic of Cushing's before this test is used to rule in HAC.

ACTH stimulation test

The principle of the ACTH stimulation test (ACTH stim) is that dogs or cats with HAC will have an exaggerated increase in the concentration of serum cortisol in response to an injection of ACTH. Normal dogs will increase their serum cortisol approximately twofold; but remain at less than 15 μg/dL. Dogs with hypoadrenocorticism will not increase their serum cortisol (<2 μg/dL). Dogs with PDH or AT will have increases of serum cortisol greater than 2–5 times the basal concentration and greater than 22 μg/dL (>500 nmol/L); see Table 33.15. The protocols for this test require 1 or 2 hours depending on the product used. This test will recognize approximately 80–85% of dogs with PDH but only 60% of dogs with AT. Dogs with PDH have hyperplastic adrenal cortices that are primed to respond to exogenous ACTH. The AT dogs have neoplastic cells that are functioning independent of endogenous ACTH and therefore may not respond to exogenous ACTH. However, only 10% of dogs with HAC have AT and AT is rare in cats. So, although this test only recognizes 60% of dogs with AT, this is an uncommon cause of HAC and therefore few HAC cases are missed. This negative fact is offset by one its best features: it has the lowest false-positive rate of any of the screening tests, only 15%. A false-positive test result for HAC has serious case management consequences. Therefore, this test may be the test of choice in a dog that only has a few of the problems associated with HAC and the clinician is searching for a diagnosis. A reasonable first step in cases that have limited features of HAC is to perform UCCR as it is inexpensive, easy, and does not require a new office visit. If UCCR is in the reference interval, and especially if serum ALP is not increased, then rule out HAC. If UCCR and ALP are increased, then follow up with an ACTH stimulation test. ACTH stim is a relatively expensive diagnostic test due to the cost of ACTH.

There are other uses for the ACTH stimulation test. It recognizes iatrogenic HAC. It is the test of choice to monitor response to therapy and provides a baseline response for monitoring therapy. Last, it may identify rare and unusual cases of HAC that have increases in precursors to cortisol (17-hydroxyprogesterone) but normal concentrations of the end product, cortisol.

Patients that look Cushingoid but have low UCCR, low basal cortisol, and a flat line response to ACTH stimulation may have iatrogenic HAC when the steroid being used does not cross-react with the cortisol assay, e.g., dexamethasone. Patients that look Cushingoid and have a high UCCR, high basal cortisol that remains high, and in a flat line response to ACTH stimulation have iatrogenic HAC and the steroid being used cross-reacts with the cortisol assay, e.g., prednisone. If a LDDS was performed on this latter group, they would react like an AT with high basal cortisol that does not suppress at 4 or 8 hours postdexamethasone.

Table 33.15 Expected responses to ACTH stimulation test in dogs.

	Cortisol µg/dL
Normal basal	0.5–6 µg/dL; 10–160 nmol/L
Normal post-stim	6–18 µg/dL; >220–560 nmol/L; 2–5 times basal
HAC diagnostic	>22 µg/dL
Gray zone	18–22 µg/dL
Iatrogenic HAC	<5 if product does not cross-react
Basal Addison's	<1.5
Post-stim Addison's	<1.5 flat line response

ACTH stimulation protocols:
Easy, done in 1–2 hours; several types of products
2.2 U/kg IM ACTH aqueous porcine gel
Basal sample and 2 hours post-ACTH dog or cat and 8 hours horse
or
Cosyntropin IM or IV 250 µg (one vial)
5 µg/kg will maximally stimulate adrenal cortex
Basal sample and 60 minutes post-ACTH for dog; two post-ACTH samples for cats, at 60 and 90 min
Store reconstituted ACTH in plastic syringes at −20 °C for 6 mo
Results: cortisol µg/dL reference interval (RI)

Cortisol	Dog	Cat	Horse
Basal normal (RI)	0.5–6 µg/dL	0.5–4	3–6

False positive or increased cortisol post-stimulation in dogs without HAC is seen in about 15% of dogs.

When both ACTH stim and LDDS were used on a group of approximately 65 dogs with HAC, no dog had normal results for both tests. Results of any test are not always clear-cut and therefore tests may need to be repeated at different times or used in combination, especially when investigating endocrine diseases. Multiple ACTH stimulation protocols are available for dogs, cats, and horses and all work well (Table 33.15). The protocols are presented in this chapter under discussion of hypoadrenocorticism. An advantage of the low-dose ACTH stimulation protocol is reduced costs, at least for smaller dogs. The low dose of 5 µg/kg of cosyntropin will maximally stimulate the adrenal cortices of normal dogs and dogs with hyperadrenocorticism and can be used as a screening test for both hyperadrenocorticism and hypoadrenocorticism.

Summary – ACTH stim

- Approximately 80–85% of dogs with PDH will stimulate abnormally high.
- It has the highest specificity (85%) and therefore lowest false-positive results of the screening tests.
- It is affected less by nonadrenal illnesses than the other screening tests.
- It recognizes iatrogenic HAC and atypical HAC and is used to monitor treatment.

Various attributes and comparisons of screening tests are presented in Tables 33.16–33.18.

Confirmatory-differentiating tests: endogenous ACTH, HDDS, LDDS, oral dexamethasone, UCCR, and ultrasonography

These tests are designed to distinguish AT from PDH. This will aid in the selection of treatment and providing a prognosis (Table 33.19).

Endogenous ACTH (eACTH)

Pituitary dependent = increased eACTH.
Adrenal dependent = decreased eACTH.
Iatrogenic = decreased eACTH.

Pituitary tumors that cause HAC synthesize and secrete ACTH and therefore plasma from these dogs will have high concentration of eACTH. AT secretes cortisol, which suppresses ACTH synthesis and release, and therefore these dogs will have decreased or undetectable plasma eACTH. Like all tests this works well on advanced cases or cases that are classical, but there will be cases that fall into the gray zone of equivocal results. Reference intervals should be generated by the lab performing the eACTH assay and the assay must be validated for dogs. Reference interval for eACTH via RIA is approximately 20–100 pg/mL. Values <20 indicate AT, values in the 20–45 range are nondiagnostic or equivocal, and values >45 are consistent with PDH. Some cases of PDH may have values greater than 200 µg/dL. Approximately 90% of dogs with PDH will have eACTH >45 pg/mL, 70% of dogs with AT will be <20 pg/mL. There is some overlap of each category with each other and with reference intervals. These latter cases require another differentiating test or resubmission for eACTH at a later time. Approximately 80% of samples tested from 245 dogs had concentrations of eACTH that were diagnostic for PDH or AT. When new samples were analyzed from dogs in which the initial result was equivocal, 235 out of the 245 dogs, or 96%, had diagnostic results. Although there may be overlap with reference intervals, eACTH is being used to distinguish PDH from AT after HAC has been ruled in. It is not used to distinguish normal dogs from dogs with HAC. Endogenous ACTH is a differentiation test and is not to be used as a screening test to rule in HAC.

Endogenous ACTH concentration measured via a two-site solid-phase chemiluminescent immunometric assay (immunoluminometric assay) was very discriminating in 109 dogs with HAC separated into two groups, 91 with PDH and 18 with AT. The reference interval was determined to be 6–58 pg/mL and a threshold for diagnosis was set at 5 pg/dL. For example, adrenal-dependent hyperadrenocorticism was <5 pg/mL and pituitary-dependent hyperadrenocorticism was >5 pg/mL. The limit of detectable ACTH is 5 pg/dL, and the working range of the assay is 5–1250 pg/mL. All 18 dogs

Table 33.16 Screening tests for hyperadrenocorticism in dogs.

Test	Use	Interpretation		Cortisol µg/dL	Comment
UCCR	RO HAC	RO HAC if <15 × 10^{-6}			
			Basal	*Post-stim*	1- and 2-hour protocols
ACTH stim	Dx HAC	RO HAC	2–10	8–19	
		RI HAC	2–10	>24	15% false positive
		Favor HAC	2–10	18–24	
		Iatrogenic	<8	<8	
			4 h	*8 h*	
LDDS	Dx HAC	RO HAC	—	<1.5 µg/dL	
		RI HAC	—	>1.5 µg/dL	25–50% false positive

Consult reference laboratory for reference intervals and interpretation.
RO, rule out; RI, = rule in; HAC, hyperadrenocorticism.

Table 33.17 Comparison of screening tests for HAC.

Screening test	Positive (sensitivity)	False positive	False negative
UCCR	95%	75–85%	0–5%
LDDS	95% at 8 h	55% at 8 h	0–5%
ACTH (when PDH)	80–85%	15%	10–25%
ACTH (when AT)	60%	—	40%
Basal cortisol	Do not use	35%	25–35%

Some dogs with nonadrenal disease will have false-positive test results; therefore it is essential to correlate results with clinical signs, lab data, and more than one screening test when needed. The percentages summarized above change depending on the cutoff values used for abnormal test results.

Table 33.18 Comparison of LDDS and ACTH stimulation.

ACTH stimulation	LDDS
Good features	
Fewest false positive	Popular
Easy, 1–2 h	95% sensitivity
Recognize iatrogenic	May differentiate AT vs. PDH
Used for atypical HAC	Rules out HAC
Provides baseline for treatment	
Not so good features	
60% sensitive for AT	High false positive 25–55%
Expensive	8+ hours

with adrenal-dependent HAC had concentrations of ACTH below the limit of detectability and all dogs with PDH had detectable ACTH that ranged from 6 to 1250 pg/mL with a median concentration of 30 pg/mL. Using a cutoff of 5 pg/mL there was no overlap between dogs with AT and dogs with PDH. However, there is considerable overlap of eACTH between dogs with PDH and normal dogs. The reference interval is 6–58 pg/mL and therefore many dogs with PDH had concentrations of ACTH within RI.

This is perhaps the easiest and most straightforward way to differentiate PDH and AT; however, sample collection requires attention to details. It is recommended that samples be collected in the morning, between 8 and 9 a.m., but different studies reporting on eACTH have not adhered to this time frame but still achieved diagnostic results. ACTH is best measured in plasma, heparin or EDTA as anticoagulant, and the sample should never be in contact with regular glass tubes as this will bind the ACTH and artifactually decrease ACTH. Use only plastic syringes and tubes for the collection and the storage of samples that are used to measure eACTH. Silicon-coated EDTA tubes can also be used to collect blood. Then use plastic tubes for all other steps to harvest plasma. Most EDTA tubes are silicone coated. Try to collect in chilled tubes. Centrifuge chilled right after collection and transfer plasma to plastic tubes for freezing at −20 to −70 °C. Pack samples on dry ice for over-night shipping to the lab. ACTH is very unstable at room temperature. The most critical event to avoid is freeze thawing, as this will degrade almost all proteins, especially hormones. Aprotinin (Trasylol) is a proteinase inhibitor that blocks trypsin, plasmin, and kallikrein and greatly prolongs activity of ACTH. It is used as a preservative that can be added to the blood as soon as it is collected and it will help prevent *in vitro* decay from time and temperature. It is available from diagnostic labs or the manufacturer. Follow directions supplied; add 500 units per mL of blood collected. With this preservative the activity of ACTH is preserved at 4 or −20 °C for 4 days. Samples are acceptable if shipped in a container with frozen packs for

Table 33.19 Differentiating tests for hyperadrenocorticism in dogs.

Test	Interpretation	Cortisol µg/dL	ACTH pmol/mL
e-ACTH	AT		<20
via RIA	PDH		>100
	Gray zone		20–100
e-ACTH via immunometric	AT <5 µg/dL > PDH		
LDDS		*4 h*	*8 h*
	RO HAC	—	<1.5
	PDH	<1.5	>1.5
	PDH	<50% basal	>1.5
	PDH	—	>1.5 and <50% basal
	PDH or AT	>1.5	>1.5
HDDS		*8 h*	
	PDH	<1.5	Suppression
	PDH	<50% basal	Suppression
	PDH 25% of cases	>1.5 or >50% basal	No suppression
	AT	>1.5 or >50% basal no suppression	
		UCCR postdexamethasone	
Oral DS	PDH	<50% basal	
	PDH or AT	≥50% basal	

Consult reference laboratory for reference intervals and interpretation.

4 days. Loss is approximately 10% activity at 22 °C in 4 days. Avoid freeze–thaw cycles. However, do not use aprotinin if the assay for ACTH is immunoluminometric as aprotinin causes a negative bias that may result in inability to quantitate ACTH. It is best to follow all instructions provided by the laboratory where the samples are sent.

ACTH can be measured via RIA, immunoradiometric and immunoluminometric assays. Reference intervals and units will vary with the assay used therefore use a reference lab that has validated the assay for animals and that provides reference intervals and expected values for AT versus PDH for their methodology.

Examples of interpretation guidelines for eACTH measured via RIA:

	eACTH[a]
Reference interval	20–100 pg/mL
Adrenal tumor	<20 pg/mL; seen in approximately 75% of cases
Gray zone	20–45 pg/mL; repeat in a few weeks or perform another test
Pituitary tumor	>45 pg/mL; seen in approximately 90% of PDH, and often markedly increased, e.g., >200

[a]Consult reference lab that performs the assay for their recommended values to interpret results.

Example of interpretation guidelines for eACTH measured via immunoluminometric assay:

	eACTH[a]
Reference interval	6–58 pg/mL
Adrenal tumor	<5 pg/mL
Pituitary tumor	>5 pg/mL

[a]Consult reference lab that performs the assay for their recommended values to interpret results and where they set the threshold for diagnosis: e.g., adrenal-dependent hyperadrenocorticism <5 pg/mL and pituitary-dependent hyperadrenocorticism >5 pg/mL. Do not use aprotinin for ACTH measured via immunoluminometric assay.

High-dose dexamethasone suppression test

75% of dogs with PDH suppress. 100% of dogs with AT and 25% of dogs with PDH do not suppress. Dogs that suppress have PDH and dogs that do not suppress have either AT or PDH; this latter group is small overall and will require another test to differentiate, such as eACTH and/or abdominal ultrasound.

A high-dose dexamethasone suppression test (HDDS) can identify approximately 75% of the dogs that have PDH, but it cannot definitively identify an AT. The principle of HDDS is that when the concentration of dexamethasone gets high enough, it will decrease the release of ACTH from pituitary microadenomas and the decrease in ACTH will cause a decrease in serum cortisol that is interpreted as suppression. This decrease in cortisol post-HDDS also occurs if the dog is normal, or if the dog is sick and stressed by a nonadrenal disease. This has important diagnostic implications because if a HDDS is performed on a dog with a false-positive LDDS result, this dog would now suppress with HDDS and lead to an erroneous diagnosis of PDH. HDDS should not be performed on dogs in which the clinical diagnosis is uncertain and it should never be used as a screening test. Dogs with an adrenal tumor secrete cortisol independent of ACTH. These dogs already have low concentrations of ACTH (decreased by the negative feedback of cortisol secreted from the adrenal tumor), therefore the administration of dexamethasone has no observable effect on ACTH and cortisol secretion continues from the adrenal tumor, hence there is no suppression in the serum concentration of cortisol. However, approximately 25% of dogs with PDH also do not suppress. This latter group may have pituitary macroadenomas or carcinomas or the tumor may be arising from the pars intermedia, which does not respond to negative feedback from corticosteroids. Differentiation of the dogs that are resistant to dexamethasone suppression requires eACTH and/or ultrasonography. Dexamethasone resistance means the dog has either PDH or AT and the odds are about 50 : 50. There is also some data to suggest that a HDDS only provides a clearer interpretation of the 4- and 8-hour LDDS in about 10% of the cases.

This test is performed similar to the LDDS except the dose of IV or IM dexamethasone is now 0.1–1.0 mg/kg or 10 times greater than LDDS. Basal, 4-, and 8-hour samples are collected. An alternate protocol omits the four-hour sample. Suppression indicates PDH and is defined as:

- Cortisol less than 1.4 µg/dL (40 nmol/L) at 4 or 8 hours.
- Cortisol <50% of basal cortisol at 4 or 8 hours.

If a portion of the IV injection becomes extravascular cancel and repeat the procedure after 72 hours or longer.

LDDS as a differentiating test

An additional use of LDDS is to differentiate PDH from AT in a dog that has classical signs and lab data of Cushing's. If suppression is detected, the diagnosis is PDH. If there is no suppression, the diagnosis may be either AT or PDH. Suppression is defined as any of the following in a dog that has an 8-hour cortisol >1.4 µg/dL:

- 4-hour cortisol <1.4 µg/dL (consult reference lab for cutoff value they use).
- 4-hour cortisol <50% of basal cortisol (4-hour could still be >1.4 µg/dL).
- 8-hour cortisol <50% of basal, but >1.4 µg/dL.

Critical to correct interpretation is that there is no suppression at 8 hours, they "all" have a value of cortisol >1.4 µg/dL, consistent with HAC. Overall, approximately 60–80% of dogs with PDH meets one or more of the above criteria and therefore demonstrates a type of suppression with LDDS. These results make the LDDS a useful adjunct to distinguish PDH and AT. However, approximately 20–40% of dogs with PDH do not demonstrate suppression via these criteria. Similarly, 25% of dogs with PDH also do not suppress with HDDS. There are data to suggest that the dogs with PDH that do not suppress, those that are resistant to dexamethasone, have larger pituitary tumors, macroadenomas or carcinomas. It is logical that the pituitary tumor could be so large that a low dose of dexamethasone would not totally suppress the secretion of ACTH or that the tumor lacks receptors for cortisol or is located in the pars intermedia. One hundred percent of dogs with AT do not suppress with LDDS, therefore when no suppression is observed with a LDDS the dog has either an AT or PDH, perhaps a large pituitary tumor. Abdominal ultrasonography or eACTH may help differentiate these. The pattern of suppression at 4 hours followed by an increase at 8 hours is called a "rebound" response and is considered diagnostic of PDH. Critical to the correct interpretation of all of the confirmatory tests is that the patient meets clinical and laboratory criteria for a diagnosis of HAC.

Oral dexamethasone at high dose and UCCR

Urine is collected at home in the morning for 2 consecutive days and stored individually in the refrigerator in closed containers. After urine is collected on day two, dexamethasone is given orally by the owner at 0.1 mg/kg every 8 hours (three doses). Urine is collected on the third morning and all urine samples are analyzed for cortisol and creatinine and UCCR determined. The UCCR on the first two samples is averaged for a baseline value. A baseline value in reference interval will rule out HAC. If the baseline value is increased, then compare this value with the postdexamethasone ratio. If the UCCR postdexamethasone is <50% of baseline it indicates suppression occurred and the diagnosis is consistent with PDH. If the postdexamethasone sample is >50% of basal it indicates suppression did not occur and this is consistent with an AT or PDH, similar to the HDDS test when suppression does not occur. Since there is a high false-positive rate with spot UCCR, it is recommended that a positive test result be correlated with a poster card ideal case of Cushing's and that one other screening test confirm HAC is present.

Diagnostic imaging: US, CT, MRI

These are obviously not clinical pathology tests, but they are procedures used in conjunction with laboratory data. Abdominal ultrasonography can differentiate AT from PDH. However, it is not sensitive enough to differentiate hyperplastic adrenal glands secondary to PDH from other causes of adrenal hyperplasia or even some normal adrenal glands. Therefore, it is not a screening test to diagnose HAC. Furthermore, not all adrenal tumors can be found. Some are missed because the tumor is too small to be visualized or the affected adrenal gland could not be located. If present, adrenal mineralization is a strong indicator of HAC and is seen in hyperplastic and neoplastic adrenal glands in plain radiographs as well as other imaging techniques. Approximately half of the adrenal tumors have mineralization. Ultrasonography may identify invasion of blood vessels or masses in the liver, but it cannot differentiate adenomas from carcinomas unless there is evidence of metastasis such as vascular invasion, masses in the liver, or enlarged regional lymph nodes. The larger the adrenal mass the more likely it is malignant. Diagnostic accuracy of abdominal ultrasonography is dependent on the experience of the ultrasonographer and confounders in the patient such as abdominal fat, large body size, hepatomegaly, gastrointestinal distension, renal mineralization, nodular adrenocortical hyperplasia of old dogs, small size of normal adrenals, and their position in the abdominal cavity. Similar to endocrine testing abdominal ultrasonography is used to distinguish PDH from AT after there is a diagnosis of Cushing's disease. Also similar is that there are false-positive and false-negative results.

Computed tomography (CT) can be used to look for characteristic abdominal lesions or visualize the pituitary. It is more discriminating than abdominal radiographs or ultrasonography, but it also has limitations and conflicting reports as to its discriminating capabilities. CT and MRI are used to visualize a pituitary tumor, especially if a large tumor is suspected. They are more useful in the cat due to the larger size of pituitary neoplasms in cats with HAC or acromegaly. They do not replace endocrine testing as they can only visualize about half of the pituitary tumors in dogs because the tumors are so small. Imaging cannot differentiate a functional versus nonfunctional pituitary mass. However, if the endocrine data suggests a large pituitary tumor versus an AT, then CT or MRI are useful techniques to separate these differentials. If neurologic signs exist then CT or MRI may identify a large pituitary tumor.

Newer technology will continue to improve diagnostic imaging and eventually they may be sensitive enough to accurately distinguish PDH from other forms of adrenal hyperplasia and to visualize pituitary microadenomas. Just like the suppression and stimulatory tests, there will be false-positive and false-negative test results with imaging studies. Clinical pathology and especially clinical endocrinology have done a good job reporting false negatives, positives, sensitivities, and specificities.

Summary of endocrine testing

Dogs and cats that have classical signs for HAC are relatively easy to identify based on clinical signs and laboratory results. However, it can be a diagnostic challenge to recognize HAC in animals that only have some of the signs of HAC or are early in the development of the disease. These are the cases that laboratory testing is needed the most. Each test has its advantages and disadvantages. UCCR is a good first screening test to rule out the differential of HAC as it is easy. The sample can be collected at home, it does not require another office visit, and it is relatively inexpensive. The test's high sensitivity and low specificity mean that most of the time the result is increased (positive). So if it is normal or decreased, it is very unlikely the patient has HAC. A negative UCCR combined with a reference interval ALP is sufficient evidence to rule out HAC. LDDS is the test of choice when the patient looks Cushingoid because of its high sensitivity of 95%. Like the UCCR there are numerous false positives (up to 55%), so avoid LDDS if the pet does not have multiple clinical signs or lab data characteristic of HAC. Because an animal may be stressed by its primary disease, its LDDS can be falsely "positive"; that is, it does not suppress, but it does not have HAC. If HDDS is used in this situation, the results will show suppression that indicates PDH. This is a false-positive diagnosis with serious consequences. Never use HDDS as a screening test. In patients that do not look typical for HAC and may only have a few of the lab data characteristic of HAC, then ACTH stimulation is preferred as it has the fewest false positives, 15%. In patients that look typical for HAC and that have multiple laboratory results characteristic of HAC, then LDDS is preferred. Phenobarbital therapy infrequently produces abnormal results for LDDS, but it does not induce abnormalities for ACTH stimulation tests or e ACTH.

Clinical pathology does a good job of telling its users what the sensitivity and specificity are of lab tests. For endocrine testing, this has led to clarification and some confusion because the ranges provided and cutoff values for diagnoses may vary due to different methodologies. If the reference intervals are wider, the lab tests are less discriminating. Where the cutoff is set for diagnostic values changes sensitivity and specificity. Therefore, use reference intervals and cutoff values from the lab providing results. No test can be 100% positive or negative, or 100% sensitive and specific because there are too many biologic and methodologic variables.

Summary ideas

- If serum ALP is not increased, HAC is very unlikely.
- If UCCR is not increased, rule out HAC. If both ALP and UCCR are not increased, rule out HAC. Consider retesting in future if HAC remains a differential.
- UCCR is a good test to rule out HAC; never use to rule in HAC.
- UCCR avoids a visit; easy first step.
- If characteristic signs and lab data are present, use LDDS.
- If limited signs and lab data are present, use UCCR to rule out, follow with ACTH stim if UCCR is increased. Avoid LDDS as false-positive rate is too high.

- If a nonadrenal illness is more likely than HAC, use UCCR and then ACTH stim if needed.
- PU/PD with characteristic other signs, use LDDS.
- PU/PD with few signs of HAC, use UCCR to rule out and follow with ACTH stim if needed.
- Suspect an adrenal tumor, use of LDDS is preferred. ACTH stim has lower sensitivity for AT. Consider imaging to search for AT.
- Suspect iatrogenic HAC, use ACTH stim and evaluate history.
- Suspect hypoadrenocorticism, measure basal cortisol and then ACTH stim if needed.
- How long to withdraw steroids before retesting: It is difficult to be certain when the pituitary adrenal axis will return to normal. It ranges from 2–8 weeks depending on dosages and duration of steroid administration.
- Unit conversion: To convert cortisol to μg/dL (mcg/dL) from nmol/L, divide cortisol reported in nmol/L by 27.6.

Differentiating tests

- eACTH: It is easy, just submit one sample. It differentiates PDH and AT.
- LDDS: This can rule in HAC and identify 60–80% of dogs with PDH.
- HDDS: This is a traditional test to differentiate AT and PDH. Dogs that suppress have PDH and dogs that do not suppress have either AT or PDH.
- HDDS: An HDDS may successfully identify the only 10% of the cases that LDDS did not distinguish.
- 100% of AT do not suppress with HDDS or LDDS.
- If resistant to dexamethasone consider imaging to look for AT and/or measure eACTH.
- If suspecting a large pituitary tumor, consider imaging by CT or MRI.

Unusual cases

Most dogs that look Cushingoid but that do not test positive with ACTH stim and LDDS do not have HAC. However, some of these dogs could have "atypical or occult HAC." This form of HAC may have increased concentrations of one or more precursors of cortisol. The most diagnostically important precursor is 17-hydroxyprogesterone (17-OHP). If dogs with this atypical form have a deficiency in one of the enzymes needed to convert precursor molecules into cortisol, then the molecule before this enzyme deficiency will increase. For example, 17-OHP will increase if the enzyme 21 beta hydroxylase is deficient or 11-deoxycortisol will increase if the enzyme 11 beta hydroxylase is deficient. If atypical HAC is suspected, then the test of choice is ACTH stimulation. The protocol is modified to measure both cortisol and 17-OHP pre and post-stimulation and comparing both concentrations to reference intervals provided by the laboratory. Post-stimulation cortisol that is not out of the reference interval combined with an increased concentration of 17-OHP is consistent with what is called atypical or occult HAC.

Although increases in 17-OHP can be measured in dogs, it is not clear if this hormone causes lesions or if the "syndrome" actually causes clinical disease. Dogs without adrenal disease can have increased serum 17-OHP just as they have increased serum cortisol due to stress of a concurrent disease. There also are reports of cases treated with trilostane that improved despite continued increase in serum 17-OHP. Furthermore, others have observed that as adrenal function is stimulated by a true adrenal disease or nonspecifically by stress that the production of all hormones increase, cortisol and sex hormones. Other sex hormones that can be measured are progesterone, estradiol, testosterone, and androstenedione, basal and post-ACTH stimulation. This has led to "steroid hormone profiles" or measurement of the parent products, cortisol and estradiol, as well as their various precursors. In ferrets these profiles are diagnostically helpful. If measured, estradiol is often increased in dogs being investigated for HAC. However, studies that correlate these hormone profiles with clinical disease, as well as determination of sensitivity and specificity, are needed for dogs and cats. If 17-OHP can increase post-ACTH in dogs that do not have adrenal disease it seems reasonable that other sex hormones would increase as well, further weakening the concept that occult HAC causes clinical disease. Additional studies are needed before the syndrome of occult HAC is recognized widely.

21-Hydroxylase deficiency does cause prolonged gestation in Holstein cattle because the adrenal gland cannot produce sufficient cortisol to stimulate delivery. The result is a fetal giant.

Ferrets

Hyperadrenocorticism is a common disease in ferrets and produces many of the clinical signs and lab abnormalities described for dogs and cats. The most striking physical abnormality is baldness. The adrenal lesion and the hormones that cause the disease, however, are very different. The lesion is in the adrenal gland. Approximately half of the lesions are hyperplasia and half are neoplastic. About 80% of the lesions involve the left adrenal gland and about 15% are *bilateral*. Unilateral adrenalectomy provides successful treatment for those cases with proliferations in the left adrenal. The principle hormone that causes the clinical signs is estrogen. Serum cortisol is rarely increased. If the disease exists for a long enough period the increased estrogens will cause bone marrow suppression leading to anemia and thrombocytopenia. Diagnosis is confirmed by measurement of estradiol or estradiol precursors (17-hydroxyprogesterone and/or androstenedione). The precursors to estradiol contribute to the disease and if estradiol is not increased, then the precursors should be measured. Commercial assays for these hormone profiles are available.

Most of the neoplastic adrenal lesions are considered carcinomas based on histologic features. However, very few metastasize and therefore their biologic behavior is similar to an adenoma. Some cases have life-threatening hemorrhage from necrosis within the tumor.

Pheochromocytoma – tumor of adrenal medulla, increased epinephrine and norepinephrine

Pheochromocytoma is the most common tumor of the adrenal medulla, but it is rare. It occurs in all species, probably most frequently in cattle, dogs, rats, and a few horses. In bulls and people, it is associated with concurrent tumors of C-cells and is part of multiple endocrine neoplasia (MEN). A concurrent tumor in ectopic adrenal locations is seen in about half of the dogs with a pheochromocytoma. Clinical signs are attributed to the increased catecholamines in the blood, but they may also be due to direct effects of the tumor or concurrent neoplasia. Signs reported in dogs and horses include tachycardia, arrhythmias, tachypnea, panting, weakness, collapse, and seizures. Polyuria and polydipsia are reported frequently in cats with pheochromocytomas. Routine clinical pathology is usually of little help. Nonspecific observations include increased liver enzymes in 10–50% of dogs, mild proteinuria in 50% perhaps secondary to increased blood pressure–induced glomerular leakage, and dilute urine due to inhibition of vasopressin by the increased catecholamines. Approximately half of the dogs will have a stress leukogram and 75% will have increased ALP. A few of these dogs have concurrent HAC. Sometimes the initial consideration of pheochromocytoma is when abdominal ultrasonography reveals a mass in the adrenal region and/or masses in the vena cava. Metastases in dogs are reported in 20–50% of the cases.

Norepinephrine is the principal catecholamine secreted from pheochromocytomas in dogs. Urinary vanillylmandelic acid and free unconjugated catecholamines are increased in bulls with pheochromocytoma. Stimulatory and inhibitory tests are used but have side effects, and the measurement of catecholamines in these tests should be coordinated with a lab that will perform assays and provide reference intervals. Cytology of the suspected tumor reveals "naked nuclei" or nuclei with very little cytoplasm, but this cytologic description is nonspecific.

Pituitary disorders

The pituitary gland is composed of the adenohypophysis (pars distalis or anterior lobe), neurohypophysis (pars nervosa or posterior lobe), pars intermedia (intermediate lobe), and pars tuberalis (infundibular stalk). The adenohypophysis is formed by the differentiation of embryonic oral ectoderm, Rathke's pouch, into trophic secretory cells producing GH or somatotropin, prolactin, TSH, follicle-stimulating hormone (FSH), luteinizing hormone (LH), and ACTH. The most common disease and lesion from the pars distalis is hyperadrenocorticism due to an adenoma secreting ACTH (Table 33.20). Neoplasms that produce other trophic hormones and that cause disease are rare. An example is a GH producing adenoma that causes acromegaly. Nonsecretory neoplasms, inflammation, and embryonic cysts that destroy the pituitary gland are uncommon and result in panhypopituitarism, dwarfism, or selective decrease in specific trophic hormones. Hypoadrenocorticism and hypothyroidism are the most common diseases due to pituitary destruction. These diseases are described in the adrenal and thyroid sections of this chapter.

The neurohypophysis is composed of axons that originate within the supraoptic and paraventricular nuclei of the hypothalamus. Separate neurons within both nuclei synthesize vasopressin (ADH) and oxytocin. These hormones migrate through the infundibular stalk in axons as precursor proteins to be stored in secretory granules in the neurohypophysis, pars nervosa, and are released under appropriate stimuli. Oxytocin stimulates uterine contraction and milk secretion. ADH stimulates water reabsorption in the distal and collecting tubules.

Various pituitary disorders are described below.

Equine Cushing's-like syndromes

Pituitary pars intermedia dysfunction (PPID)

Equine Cushing's disease is more appropriately called PPID. This term is deemed more appropriate because the pituitary lesion does not have to be neoplastic. It is located in the pars intermedia. There are dysfunctional biochemical events and it stimulates a unique pathogenesis with a different profile of pituitary hormones that do not result in marked adrenal cortical hypertrophy. The pituitary lesions range from hyperplasia to large tumors. Clinical disease, hormone profiles, and biochemical changes may occur without overt pituitary adenoma formation. Rare causes of Cushing's in the horse is a neoplasm in the pars distalis or in the adrenal cortex. Nodular

Table 33.20 Regions in the pituitary gland and associated lesions and the most common diseases.

Pars distalis	Neoplasia	Hyperadrenocorticism; acromegaly – cat
Pars distalis	Cyst	Dwarfism
Neurohypophysis	Varied	Diabetes insipidus
Pars intermedia	Neoplasia	Pituitary pars intermedia dysfunction – horse
Pars tuberalis	Obstruction	Diabetes insipidus

adrenocortical hyperplasia does not cause clinical disease and is similar to the lesion in older dogs.

Classical signs such as an aged horse (mean age 24 years, range 15–32) with swayback, hirsutism, laminitis, muscle atrophy, lethargy, abnormal fat distribution, hyperhidrosis, polyphagia, intermittent fever, and secondary infections are adequate to diagnose many cases and start treatment with pergolide. Owners often complain that each year the horse sheds hair later or not at all and the excessive sweating leads to the characteristic long curly coat that mats and persists in warm months. Hirsutism is a unique abnormality present in 80–100% of horses with PPID and it is considered pathognomonic. It probably is a manifestation that occurs late in the course of the syndrome. PU/PD is reported, but owners do not consistently observe it. Secondary skin infections and poor wound healing are observed in 25–50% of horses. Up to 80% of horses with PPID develop laminitis, apparently from carbohydrate intolerance. The hypothalamus is the primary control center for cyclic shedding of hair, appetite control, and temperature regulation. One proposal is that pressure on the hypothalamus from the expanding tumor in the pituitary is responsible for the clinical signs of polyphagia, hypertrichosis, and fever. Tumors may compress the hypothalamus due to their relatively large size and an incomplete sella turcica in the horse. Pressure on the hypothalamus and increased concentrations of intermediary substances and cortisol produce the characteristic physical abnormalities that are diagnostic of this syndrome. Despite large pituitary tumors in some horses, neurologic or visual signs are infrequent and variably reported at 5–50%. PPID is also seen in horses with small pituitary lesions that are hyperplastic. Therefore, size is not the major reason for the disease, but larger lesions correlate with older age of affected horses and more fully developed clinical signs that have characteristic endocrine profiles. PPID is a progressive disease and identification of the starting point is vague. Early disease recognition is difficult because the lab tests and physical characteristics are not definitive in the early stages.

The pars distalis processes the precursor peptide pro-opiomelanocortin into ACTH. Melanotrophs in the pars intermedia synthesize pro-opiomelanocortin and cleave it into ACTH and further processes it into α-and β-melanocyte stimulating hormone (MSH), β-endorphins, and corticotrophin-like intermediate lobe peptide (CLIP). Plasma and tumor concentrations of ACTH are only mildly increased in horses with this syndrome, but the tumor and plasma concentrations of the intermediary peptides listed above are markedly increased. These data help explain the mild to moderate increases in ACTH and cortisol combined with modest adrenocortical hyperplasia versus the marked increases in plasma concentrations of MSH, CLIP, and beta endorphin seen in horses with PPID. Measurement of these peptides is more useful in the diagnosis of PPID in horses than is the measurement of basal cortisol or ACTH. Cortisol strongly inhibits ACTH secretion from the pars distalis but has little effect on peptides secreted by the pars intermedia because melanotrophs do not express glucocorticoid receptors. Hence the dexamethasone suppression tests (DSTs) used in dogs are less useful in horses and require modifications.

Physical and historical data are more helpful to the diagnosis than are routine clinical pathology abnormalities that are common in small animals. Urine SG ranges from 1.022 to 1.047, which helps explain why PU/PD is infrequently reported in horses. This seems paradoxical given that cortisol can be increased and large pituitary tumors could interfere with function of the pars nervosa and ADH release.

When PPID is fully developed, the horse has marked hypertrichosis and the diagnosis is easy to confirm with endocrine tests. It is the early cases that are problematic to diagnose. The standard method of testing is the 19-hour (overnight) DST when confirmation is desired in a horse with hypertrichosis. Normal horses should suppress and failure to suppress is diagnostic for PPID. Inject dexamethasone IM at a dose of 40 μg/kg. Serum cortisol should be <1 μg/dL (27.6 nmol/L) 19 hours later in 97% of normal horses. Horses with PPID do not suppress. Cortisol is >1.0 μg/dL, at least when the disease is fully developed. Confounding factors of the DST include concurrent laminitis, time of the year, and stage of the disease. Therefore, test results should be correlated with all of the other clinical and laboratory information. DST may fail to suppress normal horses and ponies in the fall (false positives). Steroids may induce laminitis and early on in the disease horses with PPID may suppress with DST, which is a false negative. A concern of DST is that it may exacerbate laminitis in horses with a history of current or past laminitis. However, in a study of 43 PPID horses in which DST was used, this was not observed. There are no other diseases that look similar to PPID in its late stages and therefore the main distinction is to separate horses with PPID from horses with normal aging changes. DST is successful in distinguishing these two groups. However, recognizing PPID early in its development, when the pituitary lesion is small and the clinical signs mild, requires tests other than DST.

Other tests that have value are endogenous ACTH, α-MSH, TRH (thyrotropin-releasing hormone response test), combined hormone response tests, and measurement of ACTH after oral administration of domperidone. These tests may prove helpful in recognizing PPID in its early stages. DST is useful for more advanced cases and it is easy to perform. Basal cortisol is not diagnostic and loss of diurnal secretion of cortisol is controversial. ACTH stimulation is not a useful test as it recognizes <20% of the cases. This lack of stimulation is likely because adrenocortical hyperplasia is not a prominent feature of PPID. Endogenous ACTH is also used to diagnose PPID. Using a 10–50 pg/mL reference interval and a cutoff of >55 pg/mL indicates PPID with a disease range of 104–1000 pg/mL. Variables include where the cutoff value is set (critical), time of day, and different reference intervals for ponies versus horses. It is critical to use values set by the reference lab that analyzes the samples. Although this is a simple one-collection procedure, it does not recognize horses in the early stages of PPID and misses some horses in the late stages of the disease. Therefore, basal ACTH is not ideal, and provocative testing is recommended. Assays for ACTH should be validated for equine and collection procedures for ACTH outlined for dogs should be followed.

Measurement of α-MSH may be better than ACTH in horses because MSH is produced primarily in pars intermedia and ACTH is primarily secreted from pars distalis. Plasma α–MSH hormone concentration >91 pmol/L is considered diagnostic of PPID. However, there is seasonal variation in mean concentrations and ranges: fall = 50–60 pmol/L + 65 pmol/L, spring, summer, winter = 11 pmol/L + 4 pmol/L. Therefore, additional guidelines considered diagnostic for PPID are if either plasma α-MSH is >19 pmol/L of mean concentration in spring, summer, winter or if plasma α – MSH is >148 pmol/L of mean concentration in the fall. Plasma α-MSH and ACTH concentrations increase as daylight decreases, from maximum daylight hours to 12 hours of daylight (September), but serum insulin does not fluctuate. This occurs in normal horses and ponies and in horses and ponies with PPID, hence the season of the year should be considered when interpreting results. Ambiguous results can be repeated at a later time, even in a different season. Horses and ponies receiving pergolide, dopamine antagonists have a significantly less increase in α-MSH and lower plasma ACTH. Another diagnostic approach is to measure α-MSH after a DST. A α-MSH >90 pmol/L post-DST is the cutoff value between normal horses and horses with PPID.

CHAPTER 33

The pars intermedia is partially regulated by dopaminergic input from neurons in the hypothalamus and loss of dopaminergic inhibition is hypothesized to stimulate the pars intermedia causing the hyperplastic lesions that lead to neoplasia and PPID syndrome. Domperidone is a synthetic benzimidazole used to treat fescue endophyte agalactia in mares and it blocks dopamine receptors. Therefore, the correct dose of domperidone should block dopamine receptors, thereby permitting melanotrophs to release the pars intermedia peptides α-MSH, β-endorphin, CLIP, and ACTH, and the concentrations of these substances should be greater in horses with PPID than in normal horses. A recent study tested this theory on 33 horses and discovered that horses with histologic lesions in the pars intermedia characteristic of PPID had increased concentrations of ACTH in response to domperidone that distinguished them from aged horses without pituitary lesions. Samples were collected before oral administration of domperidone, 3.3 mg/kg and at 4 and 8 hours postadministration (see below):

Pituitary grade	ACTH (pg/mL)	Lesion, n; mean age (yr); 33 total horses
Grade 1	20.0	Normal 3, 7.5 yr
Grade 2	27.1	Focal lesion of hyperplasia 9, 14.5 yr
Grade 3	64.4	Diffuse hyperplasia 5, 21.0 yr
Grade 4	128.0	Microadenoma 12, 23.3 yr
Grade 5	720.5	Adenoma 4, 25 yr
Reference interval	10–59	

This study used horses without hirsutism or obvious signs of advanced PPID. It found that although basal ACTH was not consistently increased in horses with pituitary lesions, ACTH postdomperidone was increased consistently in horses with pituitary lesions characteristic of PPID. Horses categorized as grade 3 and above had pituitary lesions and mean ACTH concentrations greater than twofold above horses without significant pituitary lesions and were consistent with a diagnosis of PPID. However, approximately 25% of the horses in grade 3 and 4 did not increase ACTH postdomperidone beyond the upper limit of the reference interval. Although horses were tested in all seasons of the year, the authors suggested the need to perform these evocative tests on a greater number of normal and affected horses to determine if there is any seasonal effect or any effect from repeated testing. It is known that season of the year influences concentrations of α-MSH, although it seems unlikely that repeat testing could interfere with the utility of evocative tests. Blood for ACTH is collected into silicon coated, EDTA tubes or plastic tubes with EDTA, plasma harvested, and kept frozen until assayed. The chemiluminescent immunoassay, Immulite ACTH has been validated for the horse.

Horses with PPID have increased basal concentrations of insulin: 35–260 μU/mL, reference interval 27–53 μU/mL. This is not a diagnostic test for PPID as insulin will be increased for other reasons, but it may help explain carbohydrate intolerance, obesity, and propensity for laminitis. The increase in insulin may be due to a combination of the antagonistic effects of cortisol and increased concentrations of CLIP that can stimulate release of insulin. The UCCR reference interval is reported as $4.7–16 \times 10^{-6}$ and a cutoff of $>20 \times 10^{-6}$ is consistent with PPID. However, additional studies are needed.

Horses that have classical signs for PPID are easy to identify from the results of physical examination and laboratory test results. However, it can be a diagnostic challenge to recognize PPID in older horses that only have some of the signs of PPID. These are the cases for which laboratory testing is most needed. Increased awareness of this disease and medications to treat the disease has resulted in increased testing for PPID when the disease is still developing. Horses can be treated medically with low doses of pergolide (0.0017 mg/kg/d) divided in two oral doses or 0.75 mg/d for a 450 kg horse, cyproheptadine (anti-serotoninergic) and bromocriptine (dopaminergic agonist).

Peripheral Cushing's syndrome or equine metabolic syndrome (EMS)

This is a metabolic disorder of older horses (8–18 years) that have hyperinsulinism, activation of cortisol in peripheral tissues, obesity, and laminitis. The disease develops in genetically susceptible horses (Morgan and Spanish breeds) that are overfed and under-exercised. These horses will be overweight, have excess fat in the rump region, "cresty necks," and laminitis that is often attributed to hypothyroidism or PPID. However, DST is negative for PPID and thyroid stimulation tests are negative for hypothyroidism even though there may be a low TT4 concentration on single point determinations. Owners report the horses are "easy keepers" and they maintain their weight despite dietary attempts to reduce it. Fat cells in the abdominal region are important in the pathogenesis of obesity as apparently adipocytes in the abdomen are hormonally different from fat cells in other locations and compound the effects of obesity.

Horses with EMS have hyperinsulinemia and a resistance to the action of insulin that results in increased serum glucose and glucose intolerance or delayed reduction of glucose similar to type 2 diabetes. The mechanism of the insulin resistance is unknown. Substances released or produced in fat cells that lead to insulin resistance are free fatty acids, tumor necrosis factor, leptin, cortisol, and resistin. Resistin is an adipocyte hormone that may be pivotal in this syndrome. Apparently, there is conversion of inactive cortisone to cortisol in peripheral tissues with excess cortisol activity in skin, fat, and laminar tissue of horses with EMS. The enzyme 11 beta-hydroxysteroid dehydrogenase-1 converts inactive cortisone to active cortisol in adipocytes and other tissues. Equine diets rich in grains are referred to as having a high glycemic index because they stimulate increased serum glucose and insulin for sustained periods. Feeding adult horses excess grain for the amount of exercise performed leads to obesity and may start the cascade of events in susceptible individuals. Typically, fasting blood glucose in the horse is 60–90 mg/dL and insulin is <5–20 uIU/mL. Glucose >250 mg/dL and insulin >200 uIU/mL are clearly abnormal.

Diabetes insipidus

Central diabetes insipidus (CDI) may manifest as partial or complete forms. They are characterized by decreased concentration of ADH, PU/PD, and low urine SG ranging from 1.002 to 1.012. They may be dehydrated in the face of dilute urine. They have few to no abnormalities in the CBC or chemistry panel. Typically, there is no renal disease and the patient responds to exogenous ADH by gradually increasing urine SG. The main differentials are nephrogenic diabetes insipidus (NDI) and psychogenic polydipsia. Polydipsia is usually water consumption of >100 ml/kg/d and polyuria is urine production >50 ml/kg/d in dogs and cats.

General

ADH is released or retained under appropriate stimuli from osmoreceptor neurons located in the hypothalamus that sense changes in plasma osmolality. As plasma osmolality increases beyond 310 mOsmo/kg these osmoreceptors stimulate the release of ADH that binds to specific V2 receptor sites and stimulate cellular events leading to the creation of channels in the renal distal tubular and collecting duct epithelial cells to transport water from the glomerular filtrate into the medulla and then into blood vessels. Failure to produce or release ADH results in excretion of dilute urine with a SG less than 1.012, but typically much lower.

CDI is due to inadequate release and/or production of ADH (vasopressin). Idiopathic is the most common "cause," either because a structural lesion cannot be found or one is not looked for. Known causes include tumors, inflammation, head trauma, parasitic, cysts, and pituitary surgery. CDI secondary to surgery on the pituitary may be transient or permanent. Tumors are usually of pituitary origin but can be neural in origin. In dogs and cats there are two forms of CDI, partial and complete. Complete is essentially no ADH and is associated with little to no increase in urine osmolality with increasing plasma osmolality. Animals with complete CDI will have persistent hyposthenuria, severe urine diuresis, and urine specific gravities of 1.005 or less, even if dehydrated. Partial diabetes insipidus is associated with a small,but insufficient increase in urine osmolality with increasing plasma osmolality. These animals can concentrate urine into the isosthenuric range of 1.008–1.015 but cannot increase the SG beyond 1.020 even if dehydrated.

Inhibition of adequate quantities of ADH at the level of renal tubules is referred to as NDI and can be due to decreased tubular cells or compounds in the blood that interfere with the action of ADH. These include corticosteroids, hypercalcemia, *E. coli* toxin in pyometra, and hypokalemia. A rare congenital form occurs in Siberian huskies and cats and may be due to a receptor defect.

Measurement of ADH in serum has not been applied to these diseases because assays are not readily available or used. As assays become available and affordable they may be used to define the syndromes and aid diagnoses. Until then the diagnoses will be established via formulation of differential diagnoses, rule in/rule out tests for each, and use of water deprivation studies to distinguish CDI, NDI, and psychogenic polydipsia. The other causes of PU/PD are identified without water deprivation studies (Table 33.21).

Table 33.21 Causes of polyuria (polydipsia) and dilute urine via associated mechanisms.

Decreased ADH – central diabetes insipidus (DI/CDI)
Pituitary (hypothalamic rare) tumor, abscess, idiopathic, congenital
Inadequate response of tubular cells to adequate ADH – nephrogenic DI
Hypercalcemia, steroids, hypokalemia, pyometra *Escherichia coli* endotoxin, congenital lack of response of tubular cells to ADH
Decreased renal mass = lesions in kidneys, loss of tubular cells
With azotemia = >75% involvement; especially if lesions in medulla and pelvis
Without azotemia = 66% to 75% involvement of total renal mass
Excess fluid intake
Psychogenic polydipsia
Fluid overload diuresis
Medullary washout – medullary interstitium not saturated with sodium and urea
Addison's – prolonged hyponatremia
Liver failure – decreased urea nitrogen (other lab data also); congenital and acquired shunts; end stage liver disease
Psychogenic polydipsia
Fluid overload diuresis
Solute overload
Diabetes mellitus, acromegaly, Fanconi's syndrome, salt toxicity
Diuretics – many; they act on different regions of the tubules
Others, poorly understood mechanism
Hypoparathyroidism, hyperthyroidism, polycythemia, myeloma without hypercalcemia

History, signalment, and routine laboratory data

There is no age, breed, or sex predilection for CDI, but young adults are most commonly affected. The disease has been recognized in dogs ranging range 8 weeks to 14 years, with a mean of 5 years. In cats the observed age range is 8 weeks to 6 years, with a mean of 1.5 years. The major clinical signs of DI are moderate to marked polyuria (up to 100 ml/kg/d) and a nearly constant demand for drinking water, polydipsia. Neurologic signs are infrequent and if present are associated with neoplasms of the CNS or pituitary. The severity of clinical signs varies if CDI is partial or complete. In severe cases nocturia may be hourly and incontinence may be of sudden onset or of several months duration. Weight loss occurs because drinking is so excessive it interferes with eating. The Brattleboro rat has a hereditary form of complete DI such that it will exceed 70% of its body in water consumption and urine output daily.

Routine CBC and serum biochemical panel are normal in animals with CDI. Persistent low urine SG of <1.012 is often the only abnormality detected in routine clinical pathology data. If plasma osmolality is measured it is often high (>310 mOsm/L) due to mild dehydration. They cannot drink sufficient water to keep up with urinary water loss. Mild hypernatremia may be observed in a chemistry panel and is secondary to the dehydration. If water is withheld from dogs with the complete form of CDI they can develop marked hypernatremia, >170 mEq/L, marked hyperosmolality, >380 mOsmol/kg, and lethal hypertonic encephalopathy within hours of water restriction. The combination of hyposthenuria and hypernatremia favors DI. When abnormalities such as slightly increased hematocrit or hypernatremia are present at initial evaluation, they usually are secondary to dehydration from water restriction by the owner. Animals with primary polydipsia have low plasma osmolality (<290 mOsm/L) as a result of overhydration. The reference interval for plasma osmolality in normal dogs and cats is 280–310 mOsm/L.

At the time of initial presentation, the majority of dogs with DI will have urine SG <1.006 and many will be 1.001–1.003 if unlimited water is available. If the urine SG can go below 1.005 then occult renal disease is unlikely because a SG this low implies the kidneys function sufficiently to remove solutes, diluted the glomerular filtrate to the 1.005 range, but then had inadequate ADH to remove water in the collecting tubules. Urine SG of 1.007–1.013, proteinuria, and white blood cells in the urinalysis favor renal failure. This is often due to chronic pyelonephritis in which there is fibrosis in the renal medulla.

Examples of urinalysis findings useful for disease differentiation are:

Patient	A	B	C	D	E
Urine SG	1.003	1.016	1.011	1.002	1.010
Proteinuria	Neg	++	Neg	Neg	+
Glucosuria	Neg	+	Neg	Neg	Neg
Cells	Neg	++	Neg	Neg	Neg
Interpretation	CDI	Renal	Renal	CDI	Renal

A and D: Severe hyposthenuria with no abnormalities in urinalysis favor complete CDI. The urine SG is lower than expected for renal disease. Other differentials are partial CDI, psychogenic polydipsia, and NDI caused by interfering substances such as hypercalcemia or steroids.
B: Urine SG is higher than expected for CDI. The combination of proteinuria, glucosuria, and cells favor nephritis, structural lesion, or possible pyelonephritis. Recommend culture of urine and do not perform a water deprivation study. Partial CDI can concentrate into this range if water is restricted. This type of renal failure patient may not be azotemia (<75% nephron loss) but may be polyuric (>66% nephron loss).
C: If urine SG is persistent in this range it is isosthenuric. With no other abnormalities in urinalysis (UA), then chronic renal disease is most likely, with or without azotemia. Partial CDI can concentrate into this range if water is restricted.
E: If the urine SG is persistent in this range, then the patient has isosthenuria. Proteinuria at one plus in dilute urine is abnormal. Recommend protein:creatinine ratio, microalbuminuria determination, and periodic UA to confirm urine SG range and persistence of proteinuria. If cellular abnormalities develop consider urine culture. This pattern favors chronic renal insufficiency, therefore consider fractional excretion of sodium, creatinine clearance and/or palpation, visualization studies of kidneys before a water deprivation study is recommended.

Diagnostic tests

Table 33.21 lists the causes of PU/PD, and most of these are diagnosed from history, physical examination, routine lab data, and appropriate diagnostic tests. The first step is to determine urine SG at several times during the day. One of these must be a morning collection when concentration is usually at its maximum. The main differentials that have few to no abnormal diagnostic results other than dilute urine are central DI, nephrogenic DI, and psychogenic polydipsia. The test used to differentiate these is one of the water-deprivation tests or response to ADH supplementation. The modified water-deprivation test is indirect evidence of ADH responsiveness designed to determine whether endogenous ADH is released in response to dehydration and whether the kidneys respond by concentrating the urine. However, the more common causes of PU/PD should be ruled out before this procedure is performed. Failure to recognize azotemia before water is restricted is a major clinical error. NDI is due to a structural lesion that decreases renal tubular cells or a biochemical lesion such as substances in the blood that interfere with the action of ADH. These include corticosteroids, hypercalcemia, *E. coli* toxin in pyometra, and severe hypokalemia. These inhibitory factors are ruled out by diagnostic procedures for each substance or the disease that causes them. That leaves the possibility of an occult renal lesion that has resulted in loss of greater than 66% of the renal mass, hence polyuria and dilute urine before enough mass is lost to result in appreciable azotemia. This situation is easier to diagnose or at least suspect if the history indicates the patient survived a previous bout of renal azotemia, but PU/PD have persisted or are now present. If the patient had a prior diagnosis of pyelonephritis, then this scenario is even more likely. An inherent risk of a water deprivation study is the possibility of exacerbating renal problems in these patients. They have renal failure (polyuria, dilute urine) and a structural renal lesion, but they are not yet azotemic. The diagnosis of occult renal lesions should be suspected if there is proteinuria (increased protein:creatinine ratio), isosthenuria, and/or white blood cells in the urine. If these are present avoid a water deprivation study and perform fractional excretion of sodium or creatinine clearance study to rule in/rule out structural renal lesions. If the urine SG can go below 1.005 then occult renal disease is unlikely. If the urine SG can increase beyond 1.020 then occult renal disease and CDI are unlikely and psychogenic polydipsia is more likely. Another risk of a water deprivation study is induction of marked hypernatremia, hyperosmolality, and hypertonic encephalopathy within hours of water restriction in patients with complete CDI. For these reasons patients must be evaluated frequently during water deprivation studies.

The water deprivation principle is to stimulate endogenous ADH production and release by withholding water and inducing mild dehydration of less than 5%. If an animal can start to concentrate urine with water withdrawal then psychogenic polydipsia is the diagnosis. If the patient does not concentrate until exogenous ADH is administered, then central DI is diagnosed. If water withdrawal and exogenous ADH administration do not stimulate urine concentration, then renal disease is diagnosed. Never perform this test on an azotemic patient. Before the study is started the bladder is emptied and baseline urinalysis data are gathered. Urine is then evaluated and recorded every 1–3 hours, depending on the severity of the PU/PD until the study is stopped. The bladder is emptied at each collection period and body weight, skin turgor, PCV, plasma protein, UN, urine SG, and osmolality of plasma and urine are optimal parameters to monitor. Osmolality does not have to be measured, but it is ideal if immediately available. Urine SG and body weight are usually more practical substitutes. Three to 5 % weight loss is maximum stimulus to release endogenous ADH. If the urine is not concentrating at this point in the study, then it is time to administer exogenous ADH. Another means to determine it is time to give ADH is if urine SG has increased less than 10% for three consecutive collections. If plasma osmolality is known during the study, then administer ADH when plasma osmolality is >310 mOsm/kg because this is adequate stimulus to release endogenous ADH. When urine SG is in the 1.025–1.035 range it indicates the kidneys can concentrate urine and the study can be stopped. The urine SG may not increase rapidly in a water deprivation study. The urine SG may sometimes increase in a stepwise fashion due to medullary washout (Figure 33.5). The prolonged polyuria and rapid transit of the tubular filtrate has resulted in dilution of the medullary interstitium sodium and urea concentrations. Until the interstitium is resaturated with solutes, the kidneys can only concentrate the glomerular filtrate a limited amount. Depending on the severity of the medullary washout it may take up to 24 hours or longer of complete or partial water restriction for dogs with primary polydipsia to concentrate into the 1.030 range. Monitor the UN and if azotemia develops stop the study. Serum UN and/or creatinine should not increase in a water deprivation study. The renal failure patient has between 2/3 and 3/4 decreased renal mass and the closer the reduced mass is to the 3/4 mark the easier it will be to induce azotemia via dehydration.

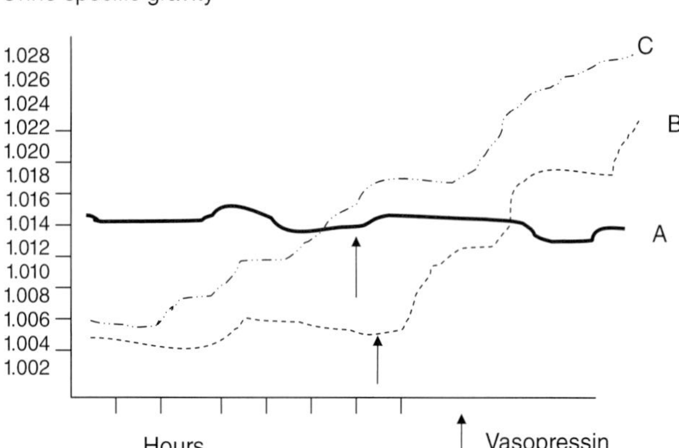

Figure 33.5 Water deprivation study results for dogs with renal insufficiency (A), central diabetes insipidus (B), and psychogenic polydipsia (C). All three dogs are not azotemic. The dog with renal insufficiency has urine SG that starts and remains in the isosthenuric range, even after administration of vasopressin (ADH). The dog with CDI has more dilute urine than the dog with renal insufficiency because the tubules can function and therefore have diluted the glomerular filtrate. This dog has urine SG that starts in the hyposthenuric range and starts to concentrate only after the administration of ADH. A dog with psychogenic polydipsia (C) should have a urine SG in the hyposthenuric range that starts to concentrate after water is withheld and before it is necessary to give ADH. The dogs with CDI and psychogenic polydipsia increased urine SG in a gradual or stepwise fashion because the concentration gradient in the medulla had been "washed out" and needed to reestablish.

If the urine SG increases beyond 1.025 with just water restriction, then primary polydipsia is the diagnosis. If urine remains nonconcentrated after several hours with concurrent mild dehydration, then the disease present is either CDI or NDI (Figure 33.5). The NDI patient will not concentrate urine in response to ADH. The CDI patient that has a complete form of the disease will increase urine SG by approximately 50% and the partial form will increase SG by 15–20% in response to exogenous ADH. The time it takes to lose 3–5% of the body weight (dehydration) is also a clue to the diagnosis. CDI patients often attain this weight loss in less than 6 hours while partial CDI and psychogenic polydipsia dogs will take 8–10 hours or longer.

Pituitary dwarfism and acromegaly

General

GH, or somatotropin, is a single-chain protein that is species-specific in its activity. It is produced by acidophilic somatotrophs. Hypothalamic GH-releasing hormone stimulates production and release of GH, while somatostatin inhibits release. Further inhibition is caused by insulin-like growth factors (IGFs) that stimulate somatostatin release from the hypothalamus and directly inhibit GH in the adenohypophysis. Canine mammary gland epithelial cells produce GH that is identical to pituitary GH. Administered progestins stimulate production of mammary GH, increase plasma GH concentrations, are not inhibited by somatostatin, and can cause acromegaly. The luteal phase of the estrous cycle of healthy bitches has high serum progesterone concentrations that also increase serum concentrations of GH. This progesterone-induced production of mammary GH is important in stimulating lactational mammary tissue and in the development and progression of mammary tumors in the bitch. GH concentration in colostrum is hundreds of times greater than in plasma and may stimulate neonatal gastrointestinal development.

GH stimulates the production of IGFs (IGF-1 or somatomedin) from the liver that in turn stimulates protein synthesis, chondrogenesis, and longitudinal and appositional bone growth. GH may also stimulate these events directly. Absence of GH during the period of growth results in pituitary dwarfism and excessive amounts of GH in adults causes acromegaly. GH also inhibits the action of insulin and therefore increases the serum glucose concentration via reduced glucose transportation into cells, increased gluconeogenesis, and lipolysis leading to insulin resistant diabetes. This form of diabetes mellitus is transitory if associated with the estral cycle or pregnancy. However, diabetes can be permanent if a pituitary tumor secretes GH and these antagonistic effects on insulin are prolonged. Beta cells will increase insulin production in an attempt to balance the hyperglycemia. If transitory, there is glucose stabilization, but if prolonged, this can result in beta cell exhaustion, vacuolation, degeneration, and permanent diabetes mellitus.

Diseases caused by increased concentrations of GH are acromegaly, diabetes mellitus, and mammary neoplasms. Dwarfism is caused by decreased concentrations of GH.

Acromegaly (hypersomatotropism)

Increased serum GH may be due to a GH-secreting pituitary tumor in cats or endogenous or exogenous progesterone that stimulates GH production from the mammary gland in dogs. Measurement of increased IGF-1 is a screening test. Clinical features include soft tissue proliferation, thick coarse facial features, hyperglycemia, and insulin-resistant diabetes mellitus.

Chronic excessive GH causes insulin resistance and acromegaly in adult dogs and cats. Canine acromegaly is due to increased progesterone from the luteal phase of the estrous cycle or the administration of progestational compounds for suppression of estrus in intact female dogs. Both of these cause excessive secretion of GH from mammary epithelial cells. The GH producing pituitary tumor in cats is rare or at least infrequently recognized. They are of acidophilic origin, large, grow slowly, and may be present for a long period of time before the onset of clinical signs. Feline acromegaly occurs in older male cats (8–14 years of age).

Initial signs in dogs are usually changes in their physical appearance. This may include soft tissue proliferation of the neck, head, tongue, mouth, gingiva, and pharynx, with abnormal respiratory noises. Characteristic enlargement of extremities, body size, jaw, tongue, gingival hyperplasia, widened interdental spaces, thick folds of facial skin-subcutis, and inspiratory stridor from proliferation of laryngeal soft tissue (50% of cats) are characteristics of the disease. Visceromegaly, including enlarged kidneys, liver, and endocrine organs, may result in abdominal enlargement. Cardiomegaly, hypertrophic cardiomyopathy, murmurs, and congestive heart failure develop late in the course of disease in cats. Neurologic signs in cats, if present, are due to the large pituitary macroadenoma. Physical changes are not as dramatic in cats and therefore most of the easily recognized signs are related to diabetes mellitus. PU/PD and polyphagia are common problems in cats with acromegaly and these will also occur in some dogs. Acromegaly is most often tested for in cats when insulin resistance cannot be explained via other mechanisms.

Routine clinical pathology

Laboratory tests may reveal hyperglycemia and increased liver enzymes, but there are no specific abnormalities. The more common causes of hyperglycemia and increased liver enzymes must be ruled out before acromegaly is considered. Dogs tend to have hyperglycemia without glucosuria. Cats have hyperglycemia with glucosuria but are not usually ketotic. Hypercholesterolemia and mild increases in serum liver enzymes activities are attributed to hepatic lipidosis from the diabetic state. ALP may be increased due to bone or liver production. Hyperphosphatemia without azotemia is reported but was absent in another study. Increased serum phosphorus may be due to GH-stimulated bone growth. Urinalysis is unremarkable, except for glucosuria and persistent proteinuria. There is usually increased serum protein in the range of 8–9.5 g/dL. Azotemia develops late in the course of disease in approximately 50% of acromegalic cats. Azotemia may be caused by chronic interstitial nephritis, concurrent dehydration, or unregulated diabetes. Measurement of endogenous insulin reveals increased serum insulin concentrations. Resistance to insulin (insulin requirement >2–3 U/kg/BID; or >20 U/d) is common in diabetic cats and consideration of a concurrent pituitary tumor inducing hyperadrenocorticism or acromegaly is done after more common causes of insulin resistance are ruled out.

Establishing a definitive diagnosis of acromegaly in an animal with characteristic signs is accomplished by one or more of the following: cessation of exogenous progestogen in dogs, staging the estral cycle, response to ovariohysterectomy in dogs, measurement of increased plasma GH, and measurement of increased IGF-1. All of the endocrine assays are infrequently performed and some may not be commercially available. The reference laboratory used should be consulted for protocol. Basal GH concentration greater than 6 μg/L is consistent with acromegaly if appropriate signs are present. Concentrations of GH greater than the upper limit of reference interval are considered diagnostic, >5 μg/L dogs, >7 μg/L cats, especially if other data are corroborative. Like any endocrine disease concentrations of GH may not be increased early in the progression of the disease. The diagnosis of acromegaly in dogs is centered on response to treatment rather than hormone assays. Physical examination abnormalities may be a clue to consider acromegaly. Diabetes mellitus in dogs is usually transitory and therefore hyperglycemia and glucosuria are reversed and can be used to monitor response.

The diagnosis in cats uses a combination of insulin resistance increased IGF-1, physical characteristics of acromegaly, and if available imaging of the pituitary region and GH values. It is very difficult to regulate insulin and hyperglycemia in acromegalic cats. Insulin rates >2–3 U/kg/BID or >20 U/d should prompt consideration of concurrent acromegaly. Often the main reason these cats are seen is resistance to insulin and the only clinical pathology abnormalities are referable to diabetes mellitus. Imaging studies of the pituitary are not 100% accurate but are very useful. Cats with hyperadrenocorticism or acromegaly have insulin resistance, and both have macroadenomas of the acidophils. Therefore, imaging studies of the pituitary do not distinguish these differentials. Serum IGF-1 combined with stimulatory and inhibitory tests of the pituitary adrenal axis (LDDS, ACTH stimulation) should be used to screen for these differentials.

Serum IGF-1 or somatomedin C is increased by GH and can be used as a screening test for acromegaly in cats. It has a sensitivity of 84% and a specificity of 92%. IGF-1 is not a species-specific assay. Therefore, assays designed for humans can be used. The reference interval for cats is 208–443 ng/mL. Concentrations >1000 ng/mL are suggestive of acromegaly and can be used to screen for this disease. However, increased IGF-1 has been reported in diabetic cats unrelated to acromegaly and the concentrations of IGF-1 can vary widely. Administration of large doses of insulin, particularly in poorly perfused sites such as the back of the neck, can cause a cross-reaction with the IGF-1 assay. Additionally, cats with hyperadrenocorticism have weight loss in acromegalics as opposed to weight gain. Cats with hyperadrenocorticism may have fragile skin that tears easily as opposed to thick, coarse soft tissue proliferation and skeletal abnormalities of acromegaly. Some individuals consider acromegaly more common than previously thought and is an underdiagnosed endocrinopathy in cats.

Pituitary dwarfism

Major features include decreased GH, cystic Rathke's pouch, proportionate dwarfism, and panhypopituitarism.

Pituitary dwarfism results from failure of the embryonic ectoderm to differentiate into trophic secretory cells of the adenohypophysis. There is a cyst of Rathke's pouch that is primary or secondary to the failed differentiation. It is seen most frequently in German shepherd littermates or related litters and has a simple autosomal recessive mode of inheritance. Affected German shepherds have a deficiency of GH, TSH, and prolactin but adequate ACTH secretion. There is a panhypopituitarism in Carnelian bear dogs associated with decreased production of TSH, ACTH, LH, FSH, and GH. Other affected breeds include spitz, miniature pinschers, Labrador retrievers, and Weimaraner dogs. It may also occur in cats. Pups with pituitary dwarfism are indistinguishable from littermates until 2–4 months of age when reduced growth rate is noticed and mental retardation is manifested as difficulty in house-training. Two diagnostic physical examination findings are proportionate dwarfism and retained puppy hair coat. The hair coat is wooly due to retention of puppy or lanugo hairs, which epilate easily. Therefore, a gradual alopecia is seen that may involve the total body but sometimes spares the limbs. Other clinical problems are delayed dental eruption, alopecia, cutaneous hyperpigmentation, skin infections, infantile genitalia, cryptorchidism, and anestrus. Craniopharyngioma is a very rare tumor of remnants of craniopharyngeal duct that also can produce dwarfism in dogs.

Results of CBC, serum biochemistry panel, and urinalysis are usually normal. Eosinophilia, lymphocytosis, mild normocycitic normochromic anemia, and occasionally hypoglycemia are seen if ACTH is deficient. GH deficiency is associated with abnormal development of glomeruli, decreased glomerular filtration rate, and azotemia. Secondary hypothyroidism occurs in most forms of pituitary dwarfism, therefore TT4, fT4, and TSH are decreased. Response tests for TSH, ACTH, and GH are decreased and can be used to establish a diagnosis. Basal GH and IGF-1 (somatomedin) are decreased. In pituitary dwarfs, GH fails to increase two to fourfold after administration of intravenous stimulants such as GH-releasing hormone (1 μg/kg), clonidine (10 μg/kg), or xylazine (100 μg/kg). Samples are collected basal and at 20 or 30 minutes after the stimulant is given. A GH value <10 μg/L is an inadequate response.

Other diseases of the pituitary

Other diseases of the pituitary gland are prolonged gestation in Jersey and Guernsey cattle due to inherited aplasia of the adenohypophysis in the fetus. Gestation may be prolonged by >200 days. The fetus is underdeveloped, often hairless, and looks like development stopped at 6–7 months. It may have alopecia and short legs, and it will have hypoplasia of all endocrine organs that are dependent on the pituitary for trophic stimulation. Holstein and Ayrshire cattle have prolonged gestation due to an inherited autosomal recessive enzyme deficiency in the adrenal cortex of the fetus such that cortisol is not produced. In the absence of cortisol, there is stimulation to secrete ACTH, which in turn causes marked *bilateral* adrenal cortical hypertrophy with fetal giants of up to 225 lb with long shaggy hair. The cycle of decreased cortisol, increased ACTH and adrenal cortical hypertrophy continues because of the inherited enzyme deficiency. Sheep grazing the teratogenic plant *Veratrum californicum* at 9–14 days of gestation will have fetuses that have an abnormal pituitary gland or a pituitary that functions autonomously from the hypothalamus. The result is prolonged gestation, cyclopia, facial abnormalities, and other musculoskeletal malformations.

34 Parathyroid Glands and Calcium and Phosphorus Metabolic Pathology

Donald Meuten
North Carolina State University, Raleigh, NC, USA

General introduction

A change in the serum calcium concentration of as little as 5–10% can stimulate or inhibit the secretion of parathyroid hormone (PTH). Hypoparathyroidism caused by lymphocytic parathyroiditis and hyperparathyroidism due to a parathyroid adenoma are the two primary diseases of the parathyroid gland.

The parathyroid gland is a simple endocrine organ with intricate cellular events that closely regulate the serum concentration of calcium. The parathyroid or chief cells primarily respond to calcium. Low calcium stimulates the parathyroid cells to undergo hypertrophy and hyperplasia as well as increasing the production and release of PTH. High calcium inhibits these events, resulting in decreased secretion of PTH and, eventually, atrophy of the glands. A change in the serum calcium concentration of as little as 5–10% (total calcium 0.25–0.5 mg/dL, or ionized calcium 0.1 mmol/L) can stimulate or inhibit the secretion of PTH within minutes. Therefore, calcium does not need to be out of reference interval before it changes the production and secretion of PTH. This concept is important when interpreting serum concentrations of PTH and calcium. Calcium-sensing receptors (CaSRs) in parathyroid chief cells and other CaSR-expressing cells detect changes in the concentration of ionized calcium and make adjustments to PTH secretion that rapidly normalize serum calcium. CaSR in the kidney stimulates cellular events that influence calcium and water homeostasis, and these pathways may play a pivotal role in the development of hypercalcemia seen in some animals with renal failure.

PTH rarely needs to be measured. The only time it is "required" is to confirm primary hypoparathyroidism and in some cases of primary hyperparathyroidism. In these diseases, it seems logical the concentration of serum PTH would be decreased or increased, respectively. However, PTH is often within reference intervals in each of these diseases, which seems paradoxical, but the PTH value is *inappropriate* for the serum concentration of calcium. These situations happen regularly because of the close regulation of PTH, calcium, and CaSR. A serum calcium concentration of 15 mg/dL (increased) should trigger the parathyroid gland to decrease and/or stop the secretion of PTH. Therefore, if the concentration of PTH is within reference interval it is "inappropriately high" and diagnostic of hyperparathyroidism. In fact, 75% of dogs with hypercalcemia due to primary hyperparathyroidism have serum concentrations of PTH within the reference interval.

What is equally or more important to parathyroid chief cells than the absolute concentration of serum calcium is the delta in calcium as the CaSR and parathyroid chief cells can reset their signals based on the change of calcium in the blood or at the receptor. For example, in nutritional hyperparathyroidism, the serum concentration of calcium is often in the reference interval, which also seems paradoxical given the pathogenesis of the disease and the marked bone resorption (fibrous osteodystrophy or "rubber jaw"). Even though a dietary imbalance of calcium and phosphorus are constantly lowering the serum and cellular concentration of calcium, the compensatory parathyroid hyperplasia and secretion of PTH are normalizing the serum concentration of calcium, at the expense of decreasing bone mass.

This chapter will discuss the laboratory tests related to basic blood calcium and phosphorus concentrations as well as the less frequently measured parathyroid regulatory peptides. This is followed by discussion of primary parathyroid disorders that affect calcium metabolism. Lastly, numerous causes of calcium and phosphorus metabolic pathology are outlined. Because of the frequency of calcium metabolic pathology, serum calcium and phosphorus are measured in all routine chemistry panels. This practice is established convention because hypocalcemia and hypercalcemia usually provide clues to diagnosis of underlying disorders that affect calcium metabolism.

Veterinary Hematology, Clinical Chemistry, and Cytology, Third Edition. Edited by Mary Anna Thrall, Glade Weiser, Robin W. Allison and Terry W. Campbell.

Companion website: www.wiley.com/go/thrall/veterinary

Background on relevant laboratory tests

Summary

Total serum calcium

This is an excellent screening test and therefore integral on chemistry panels. It is the most common way serum calcium is measured and reported to veterinarians. Total serum calcium consists of ionized (biologically active fraction), complexed (minor fraction) and protein bound (approximately 50% of total calcium).

Ionized calcium

Ionized calcium is the biologically active fraction in blood. Ideally, it is measured in critical care patients no matter what their primary disease or total calcium concentration is. It is excellent for STAT needs and can now be measured by point of patient care instrumentation. It is more useful in hypocalcemic than hypercalcemic patients. Special sample handling is required (see Chapter 1). If ionized calcium is needed it must be measured. Total calcium adjusted for albumin concentration was never intended to estimate ionized calcium and newer adjustment formulae have not been validated.

Adjusted calcium

This calculation should be used because hypoalbuminemia explains the most common cause of hypocalcemia. This is not needed for hypercalcemia or if patient is hyperalbuminemic. It cannot be used to estimate ionized calcium.

The adjustment formula for calcium is used to determine if a decrease in total serum calcium is due to hypoalbuminemia. The adjusted calcium is not a real number; the real and important concentrations of calcium in the blood are the measured total or ionized.

Use and interpretive guidelines

- Calcium disorders are usually discovered by the routine chemistry panel. There are very few clinical signs referable to hypercalcemia. Tetany may be seen with hypocalcemia in dogs, and paresis is seen in cows.
- Differential diagnoses for hyper- and hypocalcemia are the same if either total or ionized calcium is used.
- Examine Ca and P together, then albumin, azotemia, and lipase. Determine the Ca × P product to predict risk of soft-tissue mineralization (use total serum Ca; not ionized Ca).
- Hypercalcemia and hypophosphatemia – two differential diagnoses are (i) hyperparathyroidism, which is rare, and (ii) hypercalcemia of malignancy (HCM), which is common. This finding occurs with renal failure in some horses.
- PTH is rarely needed; it may be measured in a panel with parathyroid hormone related protein (PTH rp) and total or ionized calcium.
- Veterinarians can now select total serum calcium and ionized calcium, and they can use an adjustment formula for hypoalbuminemia if total serum calcium is low. The determination of total serum calcium will remain the screening test on routine chemistry panels to detect abnormalities in serum calcium, predict soft-tissue mineralization, and formulate differential diagnoses. Measurement of ionized calcium is now available in practice. It can be used to formulate differential diagnoses just as well as using total calcium. It is the test of choice for monitoring hypocalcemia in critically ill patients.
- Adjustment formula for calcium is used to help determine if a decrease in total serum calcium is due to hypoalbuminemia, which is the most common cause of hypocalcemia. Only use a formula if the serum concentration of albumin is low; it is not needed if the serum albumin is normal or increased or if hypercalcemia is present.

Calcium and phosphorus metabolism measurements

Total serum calcium

Of the body's calcium 99% is in bones, 1% is intracellular, and only 0.1% is in extracellular fluid. It is this small latter fraction that is measured in the blood. Positively charged calcium ions in the blood are bound to anionic sites on proteins (primarily albumin) or nonprotein anions (citrate, phosphate, lactate) and as an unbound free ionic form. These are listed as protein-bound calcium, approximately 40–50% ionized calcium 35–50% and complexed calcium (citrate, phosphate, etc.) approximately 5–10%. The latter two fractions are freely diffusible, stimulate cellular events, and the ionized fraction is the most prevalent of the two and biologically active. Each fraction can be measured individually. However, total calcium concentration is the only serum measurement routinely needed for screening in animals. Total serum calcium is stable *in vitro*. It can be determined in chemistry panels by various methodologies and reference intervals from different labs are fairly similar. Interfering substances depend on the methodology. For example, hemolysis may artifactually increase total serum calcium by some methods, but not others. Always consult with the lab or procedure documentation about possible interference or sample handling concerns. If an abnormality in total calcium is detected, the concentrations of calcium and phosphorus should be compared to help formulate differential diagnoses. The total serum calcium value multiplied by the phosphorus value should be calculated to predict the risk of soft-tissue mineralization, especially when there is hyperphosphatemia. Then examine albumin, urea nitrogen, and lipase and make a decision if ionized calcium is needed. Ionized calcium is of value if hypocalcemia is detected and is also more useful in critically ill patients. The list of differential diagnoses for hyper- and hypocalcemia are the same if either the total or ionized calcium is used. The magnitude of hypercalcemia for ionized or total serum calcium does not predict a disease, but in general HCM and hyperparathyroidism have the highest concentrations of either total or ionized serum calcium. Hypoparathyroidism and lactational tetany are associated with the lowest calcium concentrations.

Interpretive discrepancies between abnormal total and abnormal ionized calcium concentrations may occasionally occur. Notable discrepancies are that some dogs and cats with renal failure may have increased total serum calcium, but the ionized calcium is in reference interval or mildly decreased. However, this is not absolute as some dogs and cats in renal failure will have both increased ionized calcium and total calcium. In fact, if ionized calcium is used to rank diseases that cause hypercalcemia, then renal failure is the second most common cause in dogs. The total serum calcium is increased in 100% of dogs with primary hyperparathyroidism, and ionized calcium is increased in 90–95%. If primary hyperparathyroidism is a differential diagnosis, then measure total serum calcium. Some hyperthyroid cats have a mild decrease in ionized calcium and normal total calcium. Urinary obstructed cats may have a more pronounced decrease in ionized calcium as compared to the decrease in total calcium. If hypocalcemia is marked or there are clinical signs of tetany, then measure ionized calcium. If it is not available, then treatment decisions are made from total serum calcium and/or tetany. Ionized calcium is preferable to total calcium in critically ill patients, hypocalcemic patients, and animals with sepsis. These differences point out some of the situations when having both the total and ionized calcium values are beneficial. Perhaps if total and ionized were measured in the same sample, or on the same day, there would be better interpretive concordance.

Ionized and total serum calcium measurements result in the same list of differential diagnoses for hypocalcemia or hypercalcemia (Tables 34.2 and 34.3).

Ionized calcium

Ionized calcium and other electrolytes are now easily measured in practice (Chapter 1). Ionized calcium is not measured in serum chemistry profiles, it requires a second sample. For routine screening the total serum calcium will remain the sample of choice. It is important to follow specific sample handling instructions when measuring ionized calcium. Ionized calcium is reported in two different units (Table 34.1). Interpret the values compared to appropriate reference intervals exactly as total serum calcium is interpreted.

Ionized calcium is more valuable if hypocalcemia is detected, especially if total serum calcium is less than

Table 34.1 Example reference intervals and conversion factors for calcium measurements.

To convert mmol/L to mg/dL multiply by 4; mEq/L to mg/dL multiply by 2. Do not convert ionized to total calcium or vice versa; ionized Ca is approximate half of the total calcium when the same units are used.

To convert from mg/dL to mmol/L multiply by 0.25; convert from mg/dL to mEq/L multiply by 0.5; convert from mEq/L to mmol/L multiply by 0.5.

Reference intervals (RIs) of serum calcium in dogs and cats and expected problem ranges; consult with reference lab performing determination.

		Total serum calcium mg/dL	Ionized calcium mmol/L	Ionized calcium mEq/L
Dogs	RI	9–11	1.2–1.5	2–3
Dogs	RI	8.7–11.2	1.12–1.40	2.5–3.0
Dogs	RI		1.25–1.45	2.3–2.8
Dogs	RI	9.2–11.3	1.12–1.32	
Clinical problems may be detected:				
Hypocalcemia		<6.5	<1.0	<2
Hypercalcemia		>12	>2	>4
Cats	RI	8.3–10.5	1.15–1.35	2.2–2.6
Cats	RI	9.2–10.3	1.15–1.40	2.1–2.7
Clinical problems may be detected:				
Hypercalcemia		>11	>1.5	
Horses	RI	11.5–13.5	1.45–1.75	
Horses	RI		1.53–1.61	
Horses	RI		1.61–1.85	

Young dogs: 0.2–1.0 mg/dL higher in total calcium, with concurrent mild hyperphosphatemia; horses and rabbits have the highest RIs for total and ionized calcium of any species, up to 13 mg/dL total serum calcium.

Table 34.2 Differential diagnoses for hypercalcemia.

↑ Ca and N or ↑ P	↑ Ca ↓ P
Hypercalcemia of malignancy	Hypercalcemia of malignancy
Primary hyperparathyroidism	Primary hyperparathyroidism
Idiopathic – cats	Renal failure – only horses
Hypoadrenocorticism	
Renal failure – chronic more common than acute acute – grapes and currant toxicities	
Vitamin D toxicosis – rodenticides, plants, iatrogenic	
Granulomatous diseases – blastomycosis, other fungi, FIP, schistosomiasis, mycobacterium, toxoplasmosis	
Iatrogenic – calcium supplements	
Young, rapid growing, esp. large breed dogs and horses	
Xylitol toxicity – concurrent hypoglycemia can be severe	
Hyperthyroidism – uncommon in dogs vs. decreased calcium in cats	
Hypothermia – rare, may not be cause and effect	
Spurious – lipemia, hemolysis, type of heparin, methodology dependent	
Acidosis – ionized calcium increased	
Osteolytic bone lesions – doubtful; cases of hypertrophic osteodystrophy are probably due to young age of affected dogs	
Bone metastases – probably humoral and not just the osteolysis from local tumor	

With the exception of primary hyperparathyroidism, entities listed above the first solid line are common and entities listed below are physiologic, spurious, or the hypercalcemia may not be caused by the entity listed.

7.0 mg/dL. Decreased ionized calcium is important in the care of critically ill patients. Ionized hypocalcemia has been shown to be a predictor of longer duration of care in the intensive care unit (ICU) and hospital stay of critically ill dogs but is not associated with decreased survival. This study did not examine the same variables for total serum calcium to determine if it was predictive. Septic foals and cattle appear to have calcium aberrations as well. Determining the serum concentration of ionized calcium could be very beneficial during and postsurgery of thyroid glands for hyperthyroidism or parathyroid adenomas. However, even knowing the ionized calcium does not predict clinical signs. For example, within hours post-treatment of hypocalcemia in lactational paresis of cattle the concentrations of ionized calcium have returned to pretreatment concentrations, yet no clinical signs are observed. Similarly, some of the indicators used to determine if calcium and vitamin D supplementation is needed post-thyroidectomy or postparathyroidectomy in cats and dogs are not only the concentration of total or ionized calcium but if clinical signs are present. Like any laboratory test, correlation of calcium and phosphorus with clinical signs is vital.

Shifts in ionized calcium happen with shifts in acid/base balance. Acidosis shifts calcium to the ionized compartment and alkalosis decreases ionized calcium. Alkalosis will increase the available negatively charged binding sites on albumin and lead to increased calcium bound to albumin. These compartmental shifts in calcium may have clinical importance. Acidotic animals with hypocalcemia may not show clinical signs because more calcium is in the ionized compartment, whereas alkalotic animals with the same serum calcium theoretically could have clinical signs of hypocalcemia. Correcting acidosis rapidly in a patient with hypocalcemia could produce tetany. This would warrant calcium supplementation in IV fluids. This could happen when correcting the acidosis seen in ethylene glycol toxicity or neonatal diarrhea in calves, both of which may have severe acidosis with total and ionized hypocalcemia. Because large acid-base changes may occur during critical care, it is prudent to monitor both ionized calcium and blood gases if any clinical signs of tetany are present.

Recently formulae have been created to calculate the ionized calcium in dogs and cats through a cumbersome mathematical calculation that uses creatinine, UN, albumin, total Ca, K, Cl, gamma glutamyltransferase (GGT), and cholesterol. In this author's experience and guidance, use of such a formula may be possible but is too difficult to be reduced to practice and is difficult to validate in a universally applicable way. For example, each of the primary measurements are subject to individual routine systematic measurement variability and can have variation in reference intervals across the employed methodologies. There may also be other unmeasured pathologic biochemical factors that could alter the reliability of the calculation. In addition, and more importantly, adjusting total calcium for albumin was never intended to estimate the ionized calcium. It is recommended that only direct measurement of ionized Ca be used when the ionized fraction is indicated. The ubiquitous availability of this measurement in point of care analyzer technology makes direct measurement more practically implemented and reliable.

Protein adjusted calcium

The majority of the calcium bound to serum proteins is bound to albumin. As the concentration of albumin decreases, the protein-bound fraction of calcium as well as the total calcium decreases. Therefore "adjust" a low total serum calcium concentration if hypoalbuminemia is present. If the adjusted calcium concentration is within the reference interval, then the cause of hypocalcemia is hypoalbuminemia. There is a limit to this relationship; if serum calcium is <7.0 mg/dL in a hypoalbuminemic animal there probably is a second cause of hypocalcemia. Depending on the species, approximately 20–30% of the decrease in total calcium is due to changes in serum albumin. If ionized calcium is desired it must be directly measured. The correction formula does not predict ionized calcium. The real calcium in the

Example 34.1.

Measured calcium 7.8 mg/dL. Measured albumin 1.5 g/dL.
Adjusted calcium = 7.8 + (3.5–1.5) = 9.8

patient is the value that is measured, ionized or total. The adjusted calcium is not a real number. It simply helps the clinician determine that a decrease in total serum calcium is due to hypoalbuminemia. If serum albumin is normal or increased do not use any correction and investigate the cause of hypocalcemia; it is not due to a protein abnormality.

The most common cause of hypocalcemia in animals is hypoalbuminemia. This cause of hypocalcemia is asymptomatic, likely because ionized calcium is within the RI. Hyperalbuminemia does not cause hypercalcemia. The relationship between albumin, total protein and calcium has resulted in "correction formulas" that adjust the measured total serum calcium concentration for the degree of hypoalbuminemia, or hypoproteinemia. These formulas are most reliable in dogs are somewhat helpful in cats and are less reliable in horses and cows. While other formulae exist, the recommended, commonly used correction formula is:

$$\text{Adj. calcium} = \text{measured calcium} + (3.5 - \text{measured albumin})$$

In the example above, the hypocalcemia was corrected for the hypoalbuminemia and the adjusted calcium is now in reference interval (8.8–11.2 mg/dL). Therefore, the cause of the hypocalcemia in this case has been determined. It is important to now determine the cause of the hypoalbuminemia.

Calcium – phosphorus product (Ca × P)

Calcium and phosphorus should be interpreted together in a chemistry panel as the list of differential diagnoses will vary depending on their concurrent values. Additionally, the product of these two electrolytes is predictive of soft-tissue mineralization. A product of Ca × P >70 indicates soft-tissue mineralization is possible and a product >90 indicates mineralization is occurring. Phosphorus and vitamin D are more important in the process of mineralization than is calcium. If phosphorus is increased, the likelihood of mineralization is greater than if calcium is increased. If they are both increased and/or if the product is greater than 90, mineral is being deposited in characteristic locations such as blood vessels, kidney, stomach, lung, heart, intercostals, and intestinal submucosa. If mineralization is severe it can be seen in radiographs and induce or amplify renal failure via nephrocalcinosis. Use total serum calcium in the product formula. See example 34.2.

Example 34.2. Total serum Ca × P

1. Ca 10.2 mg/dL × P 14 mg/dL = 143
2. Ca 8.1 mg/dL × P 21 mg/dL = 170
3. Ca 15.5 mg/dL × P 1.8 mg/dL = 28

1. Normocalcemia and hyperphosphatemia with an increased product is common in renal failure. Soft-tissue mineralization is occurring and making the renal failure worse because kidneys are one of the most common tissues to become mineralized. The mineralization starts in basement membranes and mitochondria of tubular cells and progresses to glomeruli and interstitium.

2. Hypocalcemia and marked hyperphosphatemia with a product of 170. Despite hypocalcemia, the Ca × P product is markedly increased, leading to predictable soft-tissue mineralization. These values can occur with renal failure, and the uremia will hasten soft-tissue mineralization.

3. Hypercalcemia and hypophosphatemia and a normal Ca × P product may be seen in dogs with primary hyperparathyroidism and HCM. Despite hypercalcemia, soft-tissue mineralization is not occurring at this time. However, there can still be side effects from hypercalcemia (dilute urine, paresis, blood pressure changes).

Clinical signs

The most critical signs of imbalances in calcium relate to synaptic neural signal transmission, skeletal muscle contraction, and cardiovascular muscle function. Ionized and complexed calcium are critical to the development of clinical signs. Tetany and seizures are classical signs of hypocalcemia in small animals and horses, but paresis is the predominant sign in cattle. The signs referable to hypocalcemia are distinctive but are generally only seen with severe hypocalcemia. Therefore, signs are usually only seen with lactational hypocalcemia or primary hypoparathyroidism. Clinical signs and history are so obvious with lactational tetany or paresis (milk fever) that measurement of serum calcium is seldom performed. The rapidity in a shift in calcium and the acid base status at that moment will influence development of impending clinical signs. Rapid onset hypocalcemia, especially with alkalosis, may produce tetany or paresis, while a comparable concentration of total or ionized would not if the onset was slower and/or the blood gas status was acidotic.

The clinical signs referable to hypercalcemia are paresis and polyuria/polydipsia (PU/PD). Both are mild and often unapparent to owners. In many cases there are no detectable clinical problems. Therefore, with both hypo- and hypercalcemia there are relatively few clinical signs that cause suspicion of calcium abnormalities. In the majority of cases, the abnormality in calcium homeostasis is found from routine chemistry panels. Primary hypoparathyroidism and primary hyperparathyroidism are two diseases in which the results from a chemistry panel are the clue to the diagnosis in the absence of physical examination findings.

Parathyroid hormone

Ionized calcium is the key signal to calcium receptors on chief cells of the parathyroid gland. Minor contributions come from other factors such as the following. Calcitriol decreases production and secretion of PTH. Hypomagnesemia decreases production and secretion of PTH. Epinephrine has a minor influence on PTH secretion. Phosphorus directly or indirectly stimulates the opposite effects of calcium. PTH is a peptide hormone; it has a half-life that is so short it is measured in minutes and PTH reacts within minutes to changes in the serum concentration of calcium. The chief cells use a CaSR to recognize the serum concentration of ionized calcium and adjust the secretion and production of PTH. This relationship is sigmoid such that at high and low concentrations of calcium the secretion of PTH flattens. A continued increase or decrease in calcium does little to change the amount of PTH secreted. However, in the linear part of the curve a small change in the serum concentration of calcium will change the secretion of PTH in minutes so that physiologic adjustments can be made to keep the serum calcium in a tight physiologic reference interval. This is referred to as the calcium set point and the set point of ionized calcium is approximately 1.2 mmol/L for dogs, 1.37 mmol/L for horses, and 1.0 mmol/L for humans. Acquired and familial diseases may change this set point and/or CaSR. PTH stimulates an immediate rise in serum calcium via multiple steps, one of which is the osteocytic osteolysis pump. PTH also stimulates a sustained increase in serum calcium by stimulating osteoblasts and osteocytes to secrete cytokines that in turn stimulate osteoclastic osteolysis for long-term calcium homeostasis. It is these latter steps that lead to lesions in bones associated with renal and nutritional hyperparathyroidism and HCM. PTH exerts its effect primarily through the binding and activation of PTH receptors, PTH1R.

Receptors for PTH reside on osteoblasts and osteocytes and activation triggers an interaction between these cells and development/activation of osteoclasts. PTH causes the release of calcium and phosphorus from bone, increasing both into the serum. In the kidney, PTH increases the reabsorption of calcium and decreases the maximum renal reabsorption of phosphorus, thereby promoting urinary phosphorus excretion. Ionized and complexed calcium, but not albumin-bound calcium, passes freely into the glomerular filtrate. 99% of the calcium that enters the urinary filtrate is reabsorbed from various locations within the tubules. Hence hyperparathyroidism is associated with hypercalcemia because of bone and renal factors (indirectly through the gastrointestinal [GI] tract and calcitrol). Hypophosphatemia occurs because of the strong phosphaturic stimulus of PTH that exceeds phosphorus resorption from bone. PTH rp, operative in HCM, uses the same PTH1R receptors. Therefore, it acts identically to native PTH and produces hypercalcemia and hypophosphatemia as seen in HCM. Primary hyperparathyroidism and HCM are the only two diseases that cause hypercalcemia and hypophosphatemia in dogs and cats. Due to the phosphaturic effect of PTH the fractional excretion of phosphorus in the urine can be used to estimate an increased serum PTH. If the fractional excretion of phosphorus is greater than reference interval in a nonazotemic animal, then PTH (or PTH rp) is increased. This can be determined on the day serum and urine are sampled, while waiting for the return of PTH measurements. This is clinically useful when distinguishing between primary or nutritional secondary hyperparathyroidism. Serum PTH measurement should complement fractional excretion studies.

PTH also stimulates 1-alpha hydroxylase located in renal proximal tubular epithelium. This enzyme is the rate limiting step in the synthesis of the most potent form of vitamin D, calcitriol or 1,25-dihydroxycholecalciferol. Calcitriol stimulates the production of calcium and phosphorus binding proteins in the intestinal tract to increase the absorption of calcium and phosphorus. Calcitriol also inhibits the production of PTH and has a minor effect on the kidney to increase calcium and phosphorus reabsorption. It stimulates osteoclastic osteolysis releasing calcium and phosphorus into the serum. Only PTH and PTH rp have phosphorus lowering effects hence only primary hyperparathyroidism and HCM are associated with hypercalcemia and hypophosphatemia. Vitamin D toxicity is associated with hypercalcemia and hyperphosphatemia. Calcitonin is secreted from C cells in the thyroid gland and acts to decrease the serum concentration of calcium. Calcitonin may prevent postprandial hypercalcemia, but its effect otherwise is relatively weak compared with PTH. C cells can form medullary carcinomas but reports of tumor-induced hypocalcemia in animals are rare.

The only other cells in the parathyroid gland that can produce lesions are remnants of the duct that connected the thymus and the thyroid. These cells and the ductular remnants can become cystic, referred to as a "Kursteiner cyst." They are of no clinical significance. The only time they may cause problems is during exploratory neck surgery, or imaging of this area, if they were confused with a parathyroid adenoma. These cysts will be fluctuant and light gray in color. A tumor of parathyroid cells will be solid and tan-red in color. It is much more likely that the cysts would be identified microscopically; in fact, they are present in approximately 75% of histological sections of the thyroid and parathyroid glands of dogs. They can be located in the parathyroid gland, thyroid gland, or in the adjacent tissues. Occasionally they even have remnants of thymus with them.

PTH and PTH rp assays

Reference labs have assays for PTH and PTH rp that can be used on plasma or serum from dogs, cats, and horses.

Because of peptide stability factors, it is critical to consult the reference lab for specific sampling procedures, handling and interpretive guidelines.

The most diagnostic information is gained when PTH, PTH rp, and calcium are measured in the same sample or in samples collected at the same time. Usually the final diagnosis is not established when these substances are being measured so request all three as a mini-panel. This will avoid resubmission and delays if the primary differential is not confirmed. Furthermore, clinical interpretation depends on the relative concentration of each compared to the others. Heparinized plasma is preferred for PTH and PTH rp, but serum can be used.

Assays for PTH can measure the amino-terminus (biologically active fragment), mid-region, carboxy-terminus (biologically inactive but immunologically detectable), the entire 1–84 amino acid sequence of PTH, or large fragments of PTH. Studies have not been done in animals to compare which assay is the most diagnostically useful. It would seem the biologically active terminus, amino fragment, would be best, but studies in humans have shown the carboxy-terminal assays have equal or better diagnostic relevance. A two-site assay is available and has been validated to measure serum PTH in dogs, cats, and horses. This is useful when the cause of hypercalcemia or hypocalcemia cannot be determined by other diagnostic aids. The principle of this assay is to use two antibodies. One is specific for the carboxy-terminal region and the other for the amino-terminal region. The assay requires that both bind the respective epitope. It is designed such that the final assay recognizes only intact PTH or at least only large fragments of PTH. The sample can be measured via immunoradiometric (IRIA) technique, which is what most commercial labs use, or via a chemiluminescent technique (Immulite) that is a 20-minute rapid assay. This latter technique can be used to measure PTH during surgery at a veterinary center to determine when all of the hyperactive parathyroid tumor(s) has been removed. The antibody reagents developed to date are not species specific, but they cross-react sufficiently to make meaningful assays. This may explain some of the ambiguous or gray zone results obtained when these assays are used in animals.

If the patient is azotemic, PTH should not be measured, as it will be increased. PTH increases in renal failure due to hypocalcemic-induced parathyroid hyperplasia, hyperphosphatemia, decreased degradation of PTH, and decreased renal clearance of PTH fragments.

Assays designed for humans to measure the complete molecule of PTH rp use an IRIA technique and have been used in dogs, cats, and horses. PTH rp shares a nearly identical amino acid sequence at its amino terminal end as native PTH. Since the amino terminal end is the biologically active fragment, both molecules are recognized by and stimulate the same receptors (PTH1R) and therefore produce the same biological responses. The mid-valent and carboxy regions of native PTH and PTH rp molecules are sufficiently different that antibodies directed at each molecule will recognize one, but not the other, and therefore can be used in diagnostic assays. The ranges for interpretation should be obtained from the laboratory. Example guideline interpretations for PTH and hypercalcemia are shown in the following. It is important to correlate the PTH value with the total or ionized calcium and PTH rp value.

	PTH independent	Equivocal	PTH dependent
Cat hypercalcemic	<2.3	2.3–4.6	>4.6 pmol/L
Dog hypercalcemic	<2.0	2.1–8.0	>8 pmol/L

The coefficient of variation for a measured substance is a number that indicates the expected variability with repeat measurements. For hormone assays the coefficient of variation can be as high as 20%. A much lower percent is preferred, <2% is the approximate coefficient of variation for a hematocrit. This indicates there is considerable variability for hormone assays independent of any real change in the concentration of the hormone measured in the patient. Assays for PTH and PTH rp report coefficient of variations <10%, which is good for hormone assays. The practical application is that the value reported actually has a range; do not take it as an absolute number as there can be considerable variability within assay runs and especially between assay runs. When performing mini-panels of hormones from one patient, whether it is cortisol, thyroid hormones, or PTH and PTH rp request they be placed in the same assay run. If comparisons are to be done, try to send all of the samples together and request all of the samples from one animal be analyzed in the same assay run to decrease interassay variability. Stand-alone absolute values of hormones are rarely diagnostic. They need to be correlated with other laboratory and clinical findings.

Primary parathyroid disorders

Hypoparathyroidism

Lesions and pathogenesis

Spontaneous hypoparathyroidism is due to lymphocytic plasmacytic destruction of parathyroid tissue, which eventually leads to fibrosis, absence of inflammatory cells, and few if any parathyroid cells (sometimes called idiopathic atrophy). The damage is permanent and requires life-long treatment with calcium and/or vitamin D. Do not try to biopsy as very little of the glands remain and they are extremely difficult to visualize during surgery. The histologic lesion is similar to immune mediated destruction of the thyroid or adrenal glands. The disease is uncommon to rare in dogs, extremely rare in cats, and not reported in other animals.

Iatrogenic hypoparathyroidism is due to thyroidectomy in cats with hyperthyroidism. The inadvertent removal or damage of parathyroid tissue results in surgical hypoparathyroidism. If this is recognized during surgery the excised parathyroid tissue can be reinserted in adjacent muscles and it may establish blood supply and function. Despite the removal of the parathyroid glands, these cats rarely require calcium and/or vitamin D supplementation beyond the first month after surgery. Transitory hypocalcemia is expected postoperatively, but most cats stabilize long term and do not require life-long calcium supplementation. Regeneration of damaged parathyroid tissue may explain this. The mechanism for compensation in others is not known. Studies to investigate the possible role of ectopic parathyroid tissue producing PTH or the production of PTH rp by other tissues are inconclusive. Since most animals eventually normalize their serum calcium it is important not to "overtreat" with calcium and vitamin D. Supplements administered in excess may induce hypercalcemia that will prevent damaged parathyroid glands from regenerating. Many animals with total serum calcium and ionized calcium that are decreased do not exhibit clinical signs. It is nice but not necessary to have calcium in the reference interval similar to regulating serum glucose in a diabetic. However, if there are no signs of hypocalcemia try not to overtreat because the hypocalcemia is a stimulus for parathyroid hypertrophy.

Animals with lactational tetany or milk fever do not have hypoparathyroidism. If PTH is measured in cattle with milk fever it is secreted and responding to the stimulus of hypocalcemia. This is discussed under differentials for hypocalcemia.

Signalment

Lymphocytic parathyroiditis is seen most frequently in young to middle aged spayed female dogs. A few sporadic cases are reported in cats.

Signs

Tetany, seizures, fever (due to seizure activity), cataracts, stilted gait, vomiting, diarrhea, panting, and facial pruritus that results in chewing, rubbing, and licking are reported. However, in most cases hypocalcemia is not suspected on initial examination and hypocalcemia discovered in a routine chemistry panel is often the first clue to the diagnosis. The only hypocalcemic disease that is consistently associated with clinical signs is lactation hypocalcemia, tetany in bitches and mares, and paresis in cattle. If the hypocalcemia goes on long enough even dogs will become paretic.

Routine clinical pathology abnormalities

Moderate to severe hypocalcemia and mild hyperphosphatemia with normal albumin, urea nitrogen, creatinine and lipase is essentially diagnostic. If the serum calcium is less then 6 mg/dL and the patient is not azotemic and not lactating, then primary hypoparathyroidism is the most likely diagnosis. Ionized calcium can be measured to confirm hypocalcemia (<1.0 mmol/L; <2.5 mEq/L) and monitor treatment. Total serum calcium can be <6.5 mg/dL in animals with ethylene glycol toxicity but these patients are very sick and are azotemic or will develop azotemia and markedly increased phosphorus shortly. Of all of the causes of hypocalcemia, lymphocytic parathyroiditis, parathyroidectomy, and lactational tetany result in the lowest observed concentrations of calcium. Serum phosphorus is decreased in cattle with milk fever.

Serum phosphorus is greater than the serum total calcium in some animals with hypoparathyroidism. Hyperphosphatemia is expected due to decreased PTH. However, the magnitude of the increased phosphorus is usually mild and if phosphorus is not increased do not rule out hypoparathyroidism. Renal failure causes hypocalcemia and hyperphosphatemia, but these patients will be azotemic, have dilute urine, and the hyperphosphatemia is much greater than the mild hyperphosphatemia of hypoparathyroidism. The distinction of these two diseases is clear. Pancreatitis is associated with hypocalcemia and hyperphosphatemia, but lipase will be increased three- to fivefold. The pancreatitis patient may be icteric, have increased liver enzymes, and the clinical signs are very different.

Any cause of hypocalcemia if severe enough can be associated with hyperglycemia. In addition to the stress induced by the primary disease, calcium is required for microfilament and microtubular contraction, which is needed for the intracellular transportation and secretion of neurosecretory granules containing insulin. Inability to secrete insulin results in hypoinsulinemia and hyperglycemia.

Confirmatory test

Concurrent PTH and ionized or total calcium is measured on the same sample or collected at the same time.

Serum PTH will be decreased or undetectable depending on the stage of the disease. When all of the parathyroid tissue is destroyed, PTH will be undetectable. However, depending on when the disease process is recognized, there may be viable foci of chief cells, in which case, if the concentration of PTH was measured in the serum, it may be detectable. However, if PTH is in the reference interval and especially at the low end of reference interval while there is concurrent and severe hypocalcemia this is an inappropriate response and is still diagnostic of primary hypoparathyroidism.

Examples that are all consistent with primary hypoparathyroidism:

Case	Total Ca	P	PTH
1	5.5	6.6	2.6
2	6.1	7.4	0
3	4.4	6.8	1.3
4	5.8	8.1	0.8
5	5.2	4.7	3.9
Reference interval	9–11 mg/dL	3–5 mg/dL	2–13 pmol/L

Eventually all of the parathyroid gland tissue will be destroyed, in which case, the concentration of PTH in the serum will be undetectable (case 2). In each case above, hypocalcemia is severe and the concentration of PTH is "inappropriately" low for the serum concentration of calcium and therefore each case is diagnostic for hypoparathyroidism even though some PTH was detected in cases 1, 3, 4, and 5. Hypocalcemia of these magnitudes should be associated with increased concentrations of PTH in an attempt to increase serum calcium. Concentrations of PTH below the lower limit of reference interval should be regarded as undetectable (zero). When the serum concentration of PTH is very low the assay may not be measuring true PTH. Every test has a limit of detectability. When a sample contains so little of the substance being measured that the value is below the level of detectability or linearity, then the lab should report "undetectable."

Primary hyperparathyroidism (primary HPTH) – parathyroid adenoma (hyperplasia, carcinoma)

HPTH is due to functional, autonomous secretion of PTH resulting in persistent hypercalcemia and hypophosphatemia. Parathyroid adenomas account for >90% of canine cases of HPTH, carcinoma for less than 5%, and the remainder are considered hyperplasia because a nodule is in more than one gland. These latter cases may represent multiple adenomas, especially if only two glands contain nodules. Rarely are three or more parathyroid glands enlarged in dogs. Histologic and molecular distinction of adenoma versus hyperplasia is not always easy. The tumors can be found via ultrasonography, but they are small, 4–10 mm in diameter, and are unilateral in most cases. If a large neoplastic mass is found it is more likely of thyroid origin. Kursteiner cysts are present in or near the parathyroid thyroid glands microscopically in more than 75% of dogs and occasionally are macroscopic and could be confused with an adenoma. These cysts will be fluctuant and light tan to gray in color and contain fluid. A tumor of parathyroid cells will be solid, tan-red in color and do not contain fluid. The prognosis for full recovery following surgical removal is excellent with a recurrence rate of less than 10%. Postsurgical hypocalcemia is expected because the adjacent non-neoplastic parathyroid glands are atrophic.

The disease is much less common in cats. Most lesions in cats are benign adenomas, but hyperplasia of all four glands may occur. Most tumors are small, 3–5 mm, but they can be >4 cm and may be localized with ultrasonography and less frequently via palpation.

Clinical signs are generally vague, mild, and nonspecific. They may include weakness, PU/PD (50–80%), hematuria, stranguria, crystalluria, urolithiasis, urinary tract infections, lethargy, inappetence, and signs referable to the nervous system. Weakness and PU/PD are due to hypercalcemia and are seen with regularity in dogs. PU/PD is seen less frequently in cats with hypercalcemia. However, many dogs and cats are asymptomatic. The diagnosis is first considered when hypercalcemia and hypophosphatemia are observed in a routine chemistry panel submitted during an annual wellness exam. Clinical signs such as lethargy may be so gradual and mild that owners either do not recognize them or attribute them to aging.

Most dogs, 75%, will have no abnormalities on physical examination. Dogs are older, mean 11 years, with no sex or breed predilection. It also occurs in the cat. The disease is inherited as an autosomal dominant trait in keeshonds, and genetic testing is available. There is one report of a hereditary form in German shepherd pups. Most cases do not have detectable bone lesions clinically or radiographically. If the mandible or maxillas are enlarged, have osteolysis and new bone formation, then the diagnosis is more likely to be secondary hyperparathyroidism. Urinary calculi, crystalluria, and hematuria are reported in approximately 30% of cases. If urinary calculi or crystals are identified as calcium oxalate or calcium phosphate, then consider a diagnosis of primary HPTH or idiopathic hypercalcemia.

Laboratory abnormalities are fairly characteristic. Total serum calcium will be increased in all dogs with primary HPTH. Serum phosphorus is decreased in 90% of dogs and is expected based on the inhibition of phosphorus reabsorption by PTH in the kidneys. There are only two differentials for a dog or cat with hypercalcemia and hypophosphatemia: primary hyperparathyroidism and HCM (Table 34.2). There are many causes of hypercalcemia and the concentration of serum phosphorus is usually increased or within the reference interval in other causes. The serum concentration of calcium and phosphorus should always be compared and not interpreted individually. Horses can have hypercalcemia and hypophosphatemia with renal failure, but dogs and cats with renal failure-induced hypercalcemia have concurrent hyperphosphatemia. Hypophosphatemia is expected in more than 90% of the cases of primary hyperparathyroidism; however, if the animal develops azotemia, the serum phosphorus may be within the reference interval because of reduced glomerular filtration and retention of phosphorus. Hypercalcemic renal injury and hyperphosphatemia is much more likely with HCM than primary HPTH.

Hypercalcemia is constant and is of variable magnitude. Most cases in dogs will be in the 12–16 mg/dL range, but some will exceed 18 mg/dL and infrequently greater than 20 mg/dL. Of all of the differentials for hypercalcemia, the highest concentrations of serum calcium are seen with primary HPTH and HCM. Total and ionized calcium concentrations are increased and are due to PTH stimulated bone resorption, renal reabsorption of calcium, and indirectly from calcitrol stimulated intestinal absorption of calcium. The total serum calcium is increased in 100% of dogs with primary hyperparathyroidism, yet ionized calcium is increased in 90–95% of these dogs. If primary hyperparathyroidism is a differential diagnosis, but ionized calcium is in reference interval then measure total serum calcium.

Despite marked hypercalcemia, less than 5% of primary HPTH cases have azotemia. They rarely develop soft-tissue mineralization. Because of concurrent hypophosphatemia, the Ca × P product is typically less than 70. The concept that hypercalcemia is a medical emergency should probably be modified based on the Ca × P product as chronic hypercalcemia with mild or no symptoms is typical of primary HPTH in dogs, cats and people. Renal injury and azotemia is seen with more regularity in dogs with HCM.

Animals with primary HPTH often have dilute urine and PU/PD due to the inhibitory effect of calcium on ADH. The urine specific gravity will be less than 1.020 in 95% of the cases and the average urine specific gravity is 1.012. Calcium oxalate crystaluria is a diagnostic tip to consider hypercalcemia. Approximately one-third will have urolithiasis and a similar percentage will have urinary tract infections. The calculi are usually calcium oxalate or calcium phosphate. Approximately 20% of the cases will require surgical removal of calculi.

The approach to the diagnosis involves use of screening and confirmatory tests. By way of screening tests, it is recommended to repeat the serum calcium and phosphorus to be certain there is hypercalcemia and hypophosphatemia. If they persist, then there are only two diagnoses, primary hyperparathyroidism (relatively rare) and HCM (relatively common). The easiest way to distinguish these two differentials is to find the tumor in dogs with HCM. Lymphoma is the most common tumor and adenocarcinoma of the anal sacs is next most likely, although any tumor can produce this syndrome. In cats the cancer is usually a carcinoma followed by lymphoma, myeloma, and others. However, the HCM syndrome is uncommon in cats. If a nonparathyroid tumor cannot be localized, then consider confirmatory tests such as measuring PTH, PTH rP, and calcium and/or performing ultrasonography of the neck to search for the parathyroid tumor. PTH, PTH rP, and calcium should be measured in the same sample or samples collected concurrently. It is important to measure both PTH and PTHrp and compare results because there can be overlap of the values for both hormones in dogs with primary HPTH and HCM.

Expected findings

Ca	P	PTH	PTH rp	Diagnosis
Inc	Dec	RI to inc	Dec	Primary HPTH
Inc	RI	RI	Dec	Primary HPTH
Inc	Dec to RI	Dec to RI	Inc	HCM
RI	Inc	Inc	–	Secondary HPTH
Inc	Inc	Dec	Dec	Vitamin D toxicity

See discussion of hypercalcemia for results seen with granulomatous disease, Addison's, etc.

If PTH and serum calcium are increased, and the patient is not azotemic then the diagnosis of primary hyperparathyroidism is easy. However, increased PTH is only present in about 30% of dogs and the majority of dogs (75%) with primary HPTH will have a concentration of PTH within the reference interval: mean = 11.3 pmol/L; reference interval 2.0–13.0, 210 dogs. In fact, 45% of the cases had serum PTH concentrations in the low to middle range, 2.3–7.9 pmol/L. Increased PTH is more typical in humans with primary HPTH probably because of better crossreactivity of the antibody used to measure PTH. Increased concentrations of PTH are the exception in dogs, but if PTH is detectable in an animal that is hypercalcemic and not azotemic, then this combination is inappropriately abnormal because PTH should be decreased or undetectable in response to nonparathyroid-induced hypercalcemia. If PTH is within the reference interval (RI), it is inappropriately high in the face of hypercalcemia, and therefore diagnostic for primary HPTH. It indicates the parathyroid gland is secreting PTH at a time when secretion should be suppressed. It is critical to measure PTHrp concurrently as many dogs with HCM will have detectable PTH. Measure PTH, PTHrp, and calcium as a mini-panel and compare results of each for the best interpretation. It is not recommended to measure PTH or PTH rP if the patient is azotemic because PTH is degraded and excreted via the urinary system and may be increased due to delayed clearance. Increases in PTH can be enormous in dogs with chronic renal failure, >10 000 pg/dL, especially in assays that measure the carboxy-terminus of PTH. However, even mid-valent and amino terminal assays will measure an increased PTH and confuse interpretation. These marked increases are due to concurrent secondary HPTH and decreased clearance of PTH.

Cats with primary HPTH usually have concentrations of PTH within the RI, which is inappropriate for their hypercalcemia. Consult the reference laboratory about validity of the assay for cats and RIs, which are usually considerably lower than dogs, 0–4.6 pmol/L; PTH rp <1.5 pmol/L. Assays for PTH and PTH rp have been validated for cats.

Primary HPTH is rare in horses, as is HCM. However, PTH and PTH rp can be used to establish a diagnosis in horses, but only if hypercalcemia and hypophosphatemia are not due to renal failure.

Ultrasonography of the neck region may clarify ambiguous hormone data and localize the site of the tumor. If HCM is ruled out in a dog with hypercalcemia and hypophosphatemia, then ultrasonographic identification of a mass in the neck region is equally as diagnostic as or better than serum assays for PTH. Based on positive imaging findings, treatment can be started before results of hormone assays are returned. Furthermore, this technique localizes the site for surgery or ethanol or heat ablation. Of dogs with primary HPTH in which ultrasonography was performed, 129 of 130 had one or more masses detected in the parathyroid region.

Hyperparathyroidism: summary

- Hypercalcemia – 100%, hypophosphatemia – 90%.
- 100% if total serum calcium is measured; 90% if ionized calcium is used.
- Azotemia occurs in less than 5% of the canine cases.

The total serum calcium is increased in 100% of dogs with primary hyperparathyroidism, but ionized calcium is increased in 90–95% of these dogs. If primary hyperparathyroidism is a differential diagnosis, then measure total serum calcium.

Laboratory tests are helpful during and following treatment. Measurement of PTH during surgery can now be performed via a rapid assay that helps determine when all neoplastic, hyperfunctioning parathyroid tissue is removed. The half-life of PTH in a nonazotemic animal is only 5–10 minutes. Therefore, serum or plasma PTH will decline within minutes of removal of a secreting parathyroid lesion. The remaining atrophic parathyroid glands will not start secreting PTH for hours to days depending on the severity of their atrophy. If plasma PTH does not decrease within minutes of parathyroidectomy, then continued surgical exploration for additional hyperfunctioning parathyroid tissue is indicated. Ideally a new baseline plasma PTH is measured just prior to the start of surgery, during anesthesia and without palpating the thyroid-parathyroid area (avoids spiking secretion of PTH). After the tumor is removed, 5–10 minutes are lapsed, and postremoval PTH is measured to determine if there is a >50% decrease in PTH, indicating successful removal of the offending lesion. While waiting the 10–20 minutes for the assay results exploration should be performed to search for other enlarged parathyroid tissues. This is essential in keeshonds, and cats in which more than one enlarged parathyroid gland is expected. Excision is considered successful when the plasma concentration of PTH decreases by >50%. However, if a second enlarged gland was found while waiting for the results of PTH it should be removed even if PTH decreases. This latter situation was found in three of five dogs with multiglandular parathyroid disease indicating the necessity to continue surgical exploration and not rely entirely on the change in PTH to determine successful removal of all hyperactive tissue. Whether these tissues would have caused subsequent hyperparathyroidism is not known. If a third sample is required, wait 5–10 minutes from the last sample. This technique is used in our university teaching hospital approximately six times a year. Measurement of PTH is via the chemiluminescent rapid assay, Immulite.

Calcium is monitored postoperatively. If serum calcium does not return to the RI following parathyroidectomy, then there was a second parathyroid tumor, or excessive vitamin D was used preoperatively, or there is a different diagnosis than primary HPTH. Measurement of PTH, PTH rp, calcium, and phosphorus should clarify these possibilities. Recurrence of primary HPTH happens in 5–10% of dogs and takes months to a year.

Postoperative hypocalcemia occurs in about one-third of the dogs following parathyroidectomy. It is usually asymptomatic and may happen immediately or take up to 1 week to develop. Ionized calcium is the ideal fraction to monitor because it can be determined rapidly and is biologically active, but total calcium can be used as well. The atrophic parathyroid glands cannot produce and secrete sufficient PTH rapidly enough in some patients to prevent hypocalcemia after the parathyroid tumor is removed. Hypocalcemia may be dependent on the severity and chronicity of the hypercalcemia and therefore the severity of parathyroid gland atrophy. If the remaining parathyroid glands are not too atrophic, they will start to secrete PTH in response to the declining calcium and prevent postoperative hypocalcemia. The higher the serum calcium prior to parathyroid surgery the more likely there will be postoperative hypocalcemia. The duration of hypercalcemia, if known, may be predictive as well.

Therapy for hypocalcemia postsurgery can induce hypercalcemia and delay the return of the normal Ca–PTH axis. Vitamin D requires several days before it exerts its effects on calcium. If the dose of oral calcium is increased during this time or additional vitamin D is given, then these will work in concert and may increase the serum calcium into the hypercalcemic range. Overzealous treatment with calcium and vitamin D is the correct interpretation for hypercalcemia that occurs in the first week postsurgery rather than recurrence of tumor if normocalcemia was confirmed after surgery. Treating the symptoms of endocrine diseases may be more important than treating the absolute values of hormones or their end products. If clinical signs referable to hypocalcemia are not present, supplementation should be avoided.

There is a report of concurrent hyperparathyroidism in dogs with hyperadrenocorticism. Individual data are not provided, but observations from averaging values from these dogs are the following. There is increased PTH in 92%, threefold increase in PTH in 34%, and no differences or consistent pattern in ionized and total calcium. Serum phosphorus is higher than controls, but the actual incidence of hyperphosphatemia was not reported. Dogs with renal failure were not included in data sets. The authors concluded there is unexplained hyperparathyroidism in dogs with adrenal and pituitary dependent hyperadrenocorticism. Measuring PTH in dogs with hyperadrenocorticism did not change clinical decisions. The status of adrenal function should be considered when interpreting increased concentrations of PTH in dogs.

Disorders of calcium and phosphorus metabolism

There are a number of diseases that disturb calcium metabolism to a degree that cannot be managed by functional parathyroid gland regulation (Tables 34.2 and 34.3). These diseases result in either hypocalcemia or hypercalcemia that occasionally is recognized by clinical signs but is more often detected by routine biochemical test results.

Hypocalcemia

Hypocalcemia – differential diagnoses, summary

Causes of hypocalcemia that are more much common than primary hypoparathyroidism include hypoalbuminemia, hypoproteinemia, renal disease, ethylene glycol toxicity, pancreatitis, and eclampsia/"milk fever." Most of these differential diagnoses are easy to establish without knowledge of serum calcium. Serum calcium is rarely measured for a diagnosis of lactational tetany, and if measured is usually done as confirmation after symptomatic treatment. A complete list of differentials is provided in Table 34.3. The list of differential diagnoses for hypocalcemia is much shorter if hyperphosphatemia is present. Most cases of hypocalcemia are easy to diagnose. Some situations are diagnosed from signalment and presentation without measurement of serum calcium or any other analytes. These include lactation in any species, endurance horses, and grass tetany. If a pet had neck surgery and was not hypocalcemic prior to surgery but is so postsurgery, then trauma to the parathyroid glands is the cause.

Table 34.3 Differential diagnoses for hypocalcemia.

Ca decreased, P variable	Ca decreased, P increased
Hypoalbuminemia intestinal, liver, renal	Azotemia – prerenal, renal, or postrenal Hypoparathyroidism – P mild increase
Renal failure – any cause	Secondary hyperparathyroidism renal or nutritional
Ethylene glycol – severe decrease in Ca	
Pancreatitis; diabetic ketoacidosis	Phosphate enemas – P marked increase
Lactation – eclampsia, milk fever	Tumor lysis syndrome
Critically ill / sepsis	

Hypomagnesemia – dogs; cattle – grass tetany; horses – blister beetle
Cantharadin toxicity – horse; blister beetle
Thyroidectomy – damage and/or removal of parathyroid glands
Hyperthyroidism – ionized decrease, unknown mechanism
Parathyroid atrophy secondary to hypercalcemia
Nutritional hyperparathyroidism – dietary imbalances Ca:P
Oxalate-rich plants
Endurance racing – horses
Myopathies – exertional, hyperthermia
Sick patients – all species; critically ill, sepsis, unspecified illness
Urinary tract obstruction – azotemia
Preparturient hypocalcemia – cats, severe hypocalcemia
Hypovitaminosis D – rickets; GI disease, exocrine pancreatic deficiency
Hyperadrenocorticism – uncommon, unknown mechanism
Metaboloic alkalosis
Tumor lysis syndrome
Soft-tissue trauma
Healing long bone fractures – mild, first 20 days of callus formation
Medullary carcinoma C cell of thyroid – rare
Pseudohypoparathyroidism – not reported in animals
Chelation
  EDTA, oxalate – if *in vitro* = calcium is zero
  Citrate – anticoagulant used in blood transfusions
Iatrogenic: anticonvulsants, furosemide diuretics, IV phosphate solutions; calcium-free IV solutions; transfusions with citrate as anticoagulant; excess bicarbonate infusions, bolus infusion tetracycline

Diseases above the line are common and account for the majority of cases of hypocalcemia. Whenever phosphorus is increased, there is potential for calcium to be decreased.

If the signalment and history are not diagnostic and a chemistry panel reveals hypocalcemia, then examine albumin and urea nitrogen (or creatinine). If albumin is decreased apply the correction formula. If the patient is azotemic that is the most likely explanation for hypocalcemia. If serum calcium is <7 mg/dL in a patient with acute renal failure, test for ethylene glycol toxicity. If these do not identify the cause of hypocalcemia, then examine lipase to rule in or rule out pancreatitis. The only hypocalcemic disease that serum PTH may be required to confirm is primary hypoparathyroidism. Ruling out other causes of hypocalcemia usually rules in this diagnosis, but it can be confirmed by measuring PTH, which should be undetectable or markedly low and therefore is inappropriate for the degree of hypocalcemia. The determination of ionized calcium is of value in critically ill patients no matter what their primary disease or total calcium concentration is.

Artifactual hypocalcemia due to use of calcium binding anticoagulants such as EDTA or oxalate is often listed. Although this is possible, the serum concentration of calcium is usually "zero." Nothing else will do this and therefore there is no confusion as to the diagnosis. If in doubt repeat the measurement and be sure to use a serum sample. The purpose of anticoagulants such as EDTA (purple top tubes) or oxalate (black top) is to chelate calcium as the means of anticoagulation.

Hypocalcemia disorders

The following is a more in-depth discussion of various causes of hypocalcemia.

Hypoalbuminemia

This is the most common cause of hypocalcemia by a large margin in all species. Because hypoalbuminemia is associated with a decrease in the protein-bound fraction of calcium, there are no clinical signs associated with this hypocalcemia. "Adjust" the total serum concentration of calcium for the hypoalbuminemia and if the adjusted-calcium concentration is within the RI, then other causes of hypocalcemia do not need to be pursued. There is a limit to this relationship and if serum calcium is <6.5 mg/dL in a hypoalbuminemic animal there may be a second cause of hypocalcemia and measurement of ionized calcium is recommended. If ionized calcium is desired it must be measured, the correction formulas do not predict ionized calcium. They simply provide an index of how much the decrease in total calcium is due to hypoalbuminemia. The real calcium in the patient is the value that is measured, ionized, or total. The adjusted calcium is not a real number it simply helps the veterinarian determine that the decrease in total serum calcium is due to hypoalbuminemia. Diagnostic efforts are now directed at the cause of hypoalbuminemia. The adjustment formula for total protein can also be used but is not necessary. Just use albumin correction. If serum albumin is normal or increased do not use any correction and investigate the cause of hypocalcemia; it is not due to a protein abnormality. If gastrointestinal disease is the cause of the hypocalcemia there may be multiple mechanisms involved such as hypoalbuminemia, malabsorption, hypomagnesemia, and/or abnormalities of vitamin D absorption and metabolism. Similarly, if there is pancreatic atrophy or pancreatitis there may be multiple mechanisms working in concert to produce hypocalcemia. These include maldigestion, malabsorption, hypomagnesemia, decreased vitamin D, and hypoalbuminemia.

Renal disease

This is the second most common cause of hypocalcemia. Renal failure may be associated with hyper, normo, or hypocalcemia. Most animals with renal failure are normocalcemic. Most cases follow the same pattern for total and ionized calcium, but there are examples where total and ionized concentrations disagree. The stage of renal failure is important in predicting the serum calcium. In compensated renal failure (early or mild) the serum concentrations of total or ionized calcium are usually in the RI. However, as renal failure advances into the uncompensated stages and finally end stage renal failure, hypocalcemia is expected. An exception occurs in some horses where hypercalcemia may be seen.

The diagnosis of renal failure is obvious when there is concurrent hyperphosphatemia (often marked), azotemia, and urine that is not concentrated, especially if isosthenuric. With chronic renal failure there will be marked parathyroid gland hyperplasia and hypertrophy, accompanied by marked increases in the serum concentration PTH. This is a result of the parathyroid response to a decreasing serum calcium that may still be in the RI as well as decreased renal excretion of PTH due to the renal failure. The decrease in calcium happens first and this induces parathyroid hypertrophy, hyperplasia, and secretion of PTH in attempt to compensate for the urinary loss of calcium and raise the serum calcium. In end stage renal failure there are radiographic and microscopic bone lesions (osteoclastic osteolysis), but only a small percent of chronic renal failure animals will have bone lesions severe enough to produce clinically detectable disease (fibrous osteodystrophy = "big head," rubber jaw). Bone lesions are more common in dogs than cats, horses, or ruminants. The most sensitive areas to detect these bony changes in radiographs are teeth, calvarium and "flat" bones that are more metabolically active in the adult than the long bones. Cases of "rubber jaw" or fibrous osteodystrophy still occur in all species, but only with chronic renal failure, not acute.

The hypocalcemia of renal failure is due to (i) decreased reabsorption of calcium from tubules due to loss of tubular cells, (ii) decreased concentration of vitamin D due to destruction of renal cells that produce vitamin D, (iii) increased concentration of phosphorus that reciprocally decreases calcium, (iv) soft-tissue deposition of Ca × P (mineralization), (iv) hypoalbuminemia, if present, and (vi) if the cause of renal failure is ethylene glycol toxicity the calcium will be "complexed" with oxalate. Renal failure-induced hypocalcemia is accompanied by moderate (9 mg/dL) to marked (>15 mg/dL) hyperphosphatemia. When the Ca × P product is greater than 70 the possibility of soft-tissue mineralization is likely and when it is greater than 100 it is occurring, even if hypocalcemia is present. Phosphorus and vitamin D are major precipitators of mineralization and are more important for mineralization than calcium. Mineralization is enhanced with renal failure due to uremic-induced vasculitis and tissue damage (dystrophic mineralization).

The following are examples of TCa × P in dogs with renal failure and azotemia:

Case	Total Ca	P	Ca × P
1	8	10	80
2	7	15	105
3	9	18	162
4	7.4	16.6	123
RI	9–11 mg/dL	3–5 mg/dl	

Soft-tissue mineralization is occurring in all of these examples even though serum calcium is decreased or within the RI. There are no studies that predict soft-tissue mineralization using an ionized calcium × phosphorus product.

Although it is easy to explain the hypocalcemia associated with renal failure, most cases of renal failure are normocalcemic and some are hypercalcemic. This is true if the calcium status is determined via either total or ionized calcium. Emphasis is placed on examples of increased total serum calcium while the ionized calcium is normal or decreased in dogs and cats with renal failure. Ionized calcium can also increase with renal failure and if ionized calcium is used to classify hypercalcemia in dogs then renal failure is the number two cause. The diagnosis of renal failure is usually straightforward. What is clinically more important than the serum calcium is determination of why the patient is in renal failure and what the Ca × P product is. However, dogs in renal failure that have a total serum calcium <8.6 mg/dL have a poorer prognosis for survival and discharge from a hospital than do dogs with higher serum calcium concentrations. This probably reflects the severity of the renal failure and associated magnitude of hyperphosphatemia.

Hypocalcemia is also seen with prerenal and postrenal azotemia, probably secondary to the increase in serum phosphorus. Anytime serum phosphorus is increased there is potential for hypocalcemia due to the physiologic balance of calcium phosphorus homeostasis, soft-tissue mineralization, increased renal excretion of phosphorus anion and therefore calcium cation, and phosphorus inhibition of vitamin D production.

Obstructed tom cats have hyperphosphatemia, hyperkalemia, and azotemia that is associated with hypocalcemia. The decrease in ionized calcium may be disproportionately greater than the decrease in total calcium. For example, more obstructed cats have a decrease in ionized calcium as compared to total calcium. Tetany is not typically observed even when ionized calcium is as low as 1.10 mEq/L or total calcium less than 5 mg/dL. Fluid therapy that rapidly corrects acidosis, thereby decreasing the ionized fraction, may precipitate tetany.

Secondary hyperparathyroidism

This is a chronic parathyroid response secondary to one of two disorders of calcium–phosphorus metabolism. In secondary hyperparathyroidism, either renal disease or a nutritional calcium-phosphorus imbalance problem initiates absolute or relative hypocalcemia and hyperphosphatemia. Parathyroid hypertrophy and hyperplasia occurs in all of the glands as a secondary response to the hypocalcemia caused by the underlying disease. Serum calcium does not need to decrease below the RI to produce this syndrome. The decreasing serum calcium is recognized by CaSRs that trigger parathyroid secretory and cellular responses in an attempt to raise the serum calcium via usual actions in bone, intestines, and kidneys. Until the primary renal or nutritional problem is corrected, these cyclic events continue and eventually produce clinical disease. Both nutritional and renal secondary HPTH will produce bone lesions that range from mild osteolysis only detected radiographically to fractured bones to enlarged bones from excess fibrous tissue deposition.

Examples of expected calcium and phosphorus values are as follows:

Serum	Ca	P	PTH
1° Hyperparathyroidism	↑	↓	↑ or N
2° Hyperparathyroidism	↓ N	↑	↑
Renal	↓ N	↑↑↑	↑↑↑
Nutritional	N ↓	↑	↑↑↑

N, normal value, within RI.

Renal secondary hyperparathyroidism is usually easy to diagnose. It is associated with hypocalcemia, hyperphosphatemia, and in severe chronic renal disease there is marked azotemia, inability to concentrate urine, and nonregenerative anemia. Measurement of ionized calcium and/or repeat measurements of total and ionized calcium may detect a nadir of hypocalcemia, but there will be wide fluctuations if calcium is measured frequently. Younger animals are more likely to develop bony abnormalities that are associated with soft flexible "rubber" bones that result in lameness, bowing of the limbs, and mild to marked facial swellings and distortions. The increase in size of bones is due to excessive fibrous tissue deposits in response to the bone resorption and probable cytokine driven fibroplasia. If radiographs are taken, especially of the head, severe loss of bone can be seen around the teeth and in the calvarium. Radiographically detectable bony lesions are observed rarely with primary hyperparathyroidism or HCM although, osteolysis is present microscopically in both diseases. The most significant clinical problem is the renal failure, which is always chronic and usually severe.

Nutritional secondary hyperparathyroidism is a disease of carnivores, exotics (iguanas, etc.), and horses. Ruminants are more likely to have osteoporosis or rickets (vitamin D or phosphorus deficiency). In the majority of cases, the serum concentration of calcium is within the RI and there is mild to moderate hyperphosphatemia. It is associated with diets that either have insufficient calcium or too much phosphorus, or that have a calcium: phosphorus imbalance, such that the ratio of calcium: phosphorus in the diet is no longer 2 : 1. Diets associated with this disease include all meat diets for carnivores and excessive grain diets (high phosphorus, low calcium) in horses and high grains/nuts diets for reptiles (high phosphorus, low calcium). Horses and reptiles need less grain/nuts and more hay, legumes, or green leafy vegetables to balance dietary Ca:P. It can also be seen in herbivores that graze pastures with oxalate containing plants that chelate and lower serum calcium. The low dietary intake of calcium and/or the reciprocal lowering of calcium by the high dietary phosphorus intake lower the serum calcium concentration resulting in PTH production and release and parathyroid hypertrophy and hyperplasia. To stimulate these events, the ionized serum calcium need only change by 0.1 mmol/L or the total calcium by 0.25–0.5 mg/dL. It is not necessary for the serum calcium concentration to be reduced below the RI to trigger PTH production and release; e.g., serum calcium decreases from 9.7 to 9.2 mg/dL, and the 0.5 mg/dL decrease in serum calcium will stimulate PTH production and secretion. Ionized calcium is the biologically active trigger and it is decreasing as the total serum calcium decreases. The release of PTH stimulates the mechanisms to normalize serum calcium by increasing calcium absorption and resorption. In nutritional HPTH this will continue until the dietary imbalance is corrected. Therefore, when total serum calcium is measured diagnostically it is usually "normal," but at the lower end of the RI. Phosphorus, on the other hand, is not regulated as well as calcium. It may be high in the diet and it is also being released from bone, therefore serum phosphorus is usually increased, and this is a key to the diagnosis. As always examine serum Ca and P concurrently. The increased PTH will stimulate compensatory increased P excretion in the urine. This compensatory mechanism is usually not enough to prevent hyperphosphatemia but can be used to help establish the diagnosis by measuring the fractional excretion of phosphorus, an indirect indicator of PTH activity.

Fractional excretion of electrolytes, measurements of PTH, and dietary evaluation with measurements of calcium and phosphorus in feed are usually the best ways to screen and confirm the diagnosis of nutritional secondary hyperparathyroidism.

Fractional excretion (Fx Exc) of electrolytes:

$$\frac{\text{Serum creatinine}}{\text{Urine creatinine}} \times \frac{\text{Urine electrolyte}}{\text{Serum electrolyte}} \times 100$$

A key to the diagnosis of nutritional secondary hyperparathyroidism is an increased serum PTH that results in an increased Fx Exc of phosphorus.

Dietary analysis should demonstrate a calcium to phosphorus imbalance, with increased phosphorus or decreased calcium. Often the history of the diet is helpful to establish the final diagnosis. As described above, the diagnosis of renal secondary hyperparathyroidism is easy because of chronic azotemia. A Fx Exc Na of >1% indicates renal impairment. Fractional excretion studies of calcium or phosphorus are not indicated when there is azotemia.

Ethylene glycol toxicity

This can result in marked hypocalcemia, <7.0 mg/dL, because of the mechanisms associated with renal failure. Severe hypocalcemia is due to the chelation of calcium with oxalate. However, these dogs and cats rarely have tetany, probably because they are severely acidotic and sick (uremic). The acidosis will preferentially shift calcium to the ionized compartment and therefore make more "biologically active" calcium available, thus preventing tetany. The possibility exists that if the acidosis was corrected rapidly the calcium would shift away from the ionized compartment and tetany could be induced, especially if calcium was not added to the IV fluids. Diagnosis of ethylene glycol toxicity is described in Chapter 24.

Pancreatitis

This is associated with mild hypocalcemia, often in the 8 mg/dL range. All of the clinical problems are referable to pancreatitis and not hypocalcemia. The mechanism of the low serum calcium is unknown. Investigations that evaluated ionized calcium, PTH concentrations, and precipitation of calcium in the areas of fat necrosis, have not established a definitive pathogenesis. Correction of the pancreatitis results in normalization of the serum calcium concentration. The diagnosis is usually obvious because the hypocalcemia is associated with history, clinical signs, and other laboratory abnormalities that are consistent with pancreatitis. If hyperphosphatemia is present it is due to concurrent prerenal azotemia. Ionized calcium is also decreased. Ionized hypocalcemia is also present in about half of the dogs with diabetic ketoacidosis and is associated with a higher likelihood of death.

Lactation tetany

This is the most common cause of hypocalcemia that has associated clinical signs.

Eclampsia, or puerperal tetany, is most commonly recognized in the dog. The hypocalcemia associated with eclampsia is not a diagnostic mystery. The patient is usually a bitch that is approaching peak lactation, approximately 3 weeks postparturient. It is more common in smaller breeds of dogs and seen less frequently in large dogs, cats, ewes, and horses. The hypocalcemia is often severe, <6.0 mg/dL, and is one of the few hypocalcemic disorders associated with tetany. If the condition remains untreated the tetany will progress to paresis. If examined the pupils are often dilated and respond slowly to light. Other signs include tachycardia, fever, salivation, restlessness, and muscle spasms that may progress to seizures. Treatment is usually started before results of serum calcium are known. An ionized calcium measurement is ideal to rapidly confirm the diagnosis and monitor treatment. Symptomatic treatment of the hypocalcemia coupled with reduced lactation and/or supplementation (calcium + vitamin D) to the bitch usually corrects the problem.

Preparturient hypocalcemia has been reported in queens. The condition appears to be rare. The hypocalcemia can be severe, with total calcium <5.0 mg/dL. Similar to cows with milk fever, cats tend to be hypothermic. Ewes may also develop signs prior to parturition, usually in the last month of gestation. This may be part of the pregnancy toxemia syndrome of sheep and is associated with stress and decreased food intake.

Milk fever is the common name for lactation hypocalcemia in cattle. The clinical diagnosis is easy. It is a cow, 1–4 days postparturient. A Channel Island breed is most common (Jersey or Guernsey, but it can occur in any breed). It is much less frequent in beef cows. The affected cow is recumbent, head and neck often folded toward flank, and has bradycardia with possible arrhythmias. Fever is a misnomer as affected cows have a normal or subnormal temperature. Serum calcium is rarely measured. Treatment is started based on classical presentation. If serum is sampled total and ionized calcium are markedly decreased, phosphorus is mildly decreased, and magnesium and glucose will be increased. Total serum calcium can be <4.0 mg/dL and ionized calcium <2.0 mEq/L, <1 mmol/L. The relatively high calcium in the diet during the dry period (not lactating) has resulted in suppression of the parathyroid gland, which in turn has decreased the osteoclastic pool. At and shortly after parturition there is a combination of events that result in the syndrome. These include anorexia, estrogen surge, and increased milk production and secretion. As a result, serum calcium rapidly decreases. The parathyroid gland recognizes the decreasing serum calcium and secretes an adequate amount of PTH. However, the bone pool of osteoclasts is so suppressed that they cannot respond to the PTH rapidly enough to mobilize sufficient calcium to prevent paresis. Calcium continues to exit into milk and there is inadequate influx of Ca from bone, renal, and intestinal sources so hypocalcemia progresses to the point the cow collapses with paresis. If serum total or ionized calcium is measured at this time they will be markedly decreased. However, if measured several hours after successful treatment the serum total and ionized calcium has often returned to pretreatment levels, but there are no signs of paresis. There is more to this disease than simply the serum concentration of total or ionized calcium and acid-base status. Hyperglycemia is common and is due to stress and decreased insulin due to the hypocalcemia.

Ionized and complexed calcium, but not albumin-bound calcium, passes freely into the glomerular filtrate, CSF, and aqueous humor. Therefore, the concentration of total calcium in these fluids is normally approximately half of the serum concentration, 4–5 mg/dL. If CSF or aqueous are used postmortem to confirm hypocalcemia, the concentration of total calcium must be less than 4 mg/dL to be compatible with milk fever.

Iatrogenic – thyroidectomy or removal of a parathyroid adenoma

Removal of the thyroid glands to treat hyperthyroidism in cats often results in complete or partial parathyroidectomy. Therefore, hypocalcemia and hyperphosphatemia may occur within 24–48 hours of the surgery but can be delayed for up to 1 week. This also happens in dogs when a parathyroid tumor is excised. In dogs there is usually not damage to the other parathyroid glands, but they are atrophic due to chronic hypercalcemia induced by the parathyroid adenoma. After removal of the parathyroid secreting adenoma the remaining atrophic glands cannot resume synthesis of PTH rapidly enough to prevent postsurgical hypocalcemia. The degree of atrophy is a combination of the severity and duration of the hypercalcemia. Interestingly, this does not occur following surgical or chemical removal of anal sac tumors or with chemotherapy of lymphomas and other tumors associated with HCM.

Cats and dogs with iatrogenic hypocalcemia usually only require treatment with intravenous or oral calcium and/or vitamin D if clinical signs occur or if the total calcium is <7 mg/dL, ionized <3 mEq/L, <1 mmol/L. In dogs the treatment period is short, days to a week, and even in cats oral treatment is usually only necessary for 1–2 months postsurgery. If cats are weaned off the calcium and vitamin D therapy, their serum calcium concentrations usually remain within the RI. The exact mechanism for normalization of the serum calcium is not known. Investigations that tried to determine if there was ectopic parathyroid tissue that hypertrophied and produced PTH in response to postoperative hypocalcemia indicated this is not the case. Even dogs with experimental complete surgical parathyroidectomy will eventually stabilize their serum calcium and not require calcium or vitamin D supplementation. PTH rp could have a role in the normalization of serum calcium in these patients as the hormone is produced by many tissues in adults and fetuses.

Dogs or cats with hypercalcemia due to a parathyroid tumor often develop hypocalcemia postexcision of the tumor. One dilemma of treatment is to provide just enough oral calcium and vitamin D to prevent symptoms but not enough to induce hypercalcemia and continued suppression of the atrophic glands. It is preferable to keep the serum calcium slightly below the RI to stimulate the atrophic parathyroid glands to undergo hypertrophy. If possible, only treat with calcium as it is easier to monitor and change the dose of calcium than it is to regulate serum calcium with vitamin D. Vitamin D requires 3–7 days to reach peak effect. Therefore, it is more difficult to adjust the dose of vitamin D since there is a delayed response before an effect is observed. It is relatively easy to increase the dose of calcium and vitamin D such that therapy induces postoperative hypercalcemia. Treatment related hypercalcemia persists until the vitamin D is metabolized (up to 1 week).

Endurance racing – horses

Hypocalcemia is due to loss of calcium, along with other electrolytes in sweat and insufficient replacement during 50–100 mile races. Contributing to the hypocalcemia may be an alkalosis induced by hypochloremia and rapid respirations. Equine sweat is hypertonic and rich in calcium, potassium, sodium, and chloride. There is greater loss of electrolytes than water in the sweat of horses and therefore electrolytes must be supplemented during races especially in hot and humid weather conditions. Human sweat is isotonic and electrolyte replacement is not as critical as is water replacement. The hypocalcemia seen in endurance horses can be symptomatic and cause tetany, "thumps" or diaphragmatic flutter (tetany in muscles of diaphragm), weakness, cramping, and a variety of neuromuscular dysfunctions including ileus and colic. This can usually be prevented by adequate supplementation with forced electrolytes during the event. High calcium in the prerace diet such as alfalfa hay (regular feed program) could precipitate this condition similar to milk fever in cattle. The most common electrolyte disturbance in endurance horses is hypochloremia.

Cantharidin toxicity

The hypocalcemia of cantharidin toxicity can be severe and is an important clue to the diagnosis of blister beetle toxicosis in the horse. The mechanism of the hypocalcemia is not clear but is possibly related to concurrent hypomagnesemia. Hematuria, hypocalcemia and hypomagnesemia in a colicky horse eating alfalfa is sufficient to diagnose this toxicity. Toxicosis is confirmed via high pressure liquid chromatography that quantifies cantharidin in the urine (20 ml of urine), in gastric contents (one pint of stomach contents), liver, or kidneys of dead horses. Some horses will have increased muscle enzymes and myoglobinuria. Tetany, diaphragmatic flutter, paresis, and facial muscle spasms can be seen. The toxin causes acantholysis of esophageal and gastrointestinal mucosa, myocardial necrosis and renal tubular necrosis.

The blister beetles are found in alfalfa hay near the time of bloom. If hay is cut before the bloom phase it reduces the likelihood of the beetles being present and if crimping is not done it gives the beetles a chance to leave the cut plants. The crimping process crushes the alfalfa stems and any beetle present, leaving them in the hay to be ingested. Crimping is done to crush the stems, squeeze out water and speed drying of hay in eastern U.S. states. Alfalfa hay produced in the arid West is not crimped and the beetles simply walk out of the cut hay. The toxin is secreted by males, given to the female during mating and the female covers her eggs with it as a defense against predators. Horses are highly sensitive to cantharidin; the lethal dose-50 for horses is approximately 1 mg/kg body weight.

Hypomagnesium

Hypomagnesemia results in impaired PTH release and calcitriol resistance leading to secondary hypocalcemia. This is an uncommon or uncommonly recognized problem. Hypomagnesemia and hypocalcemia are associated with protein-losing enteropathy (PLE) in small animals, grass tetany in cattle, and cantharidin toxicity in horses. If PLE is present, then the most likely cause of hypocalcemia is hypoalbuminemia. Contributing factors may be intestinal loss, malabsorption, and/or abnormalities of vitamin D and PTH metabolism. If the concentration of ionized calcium is decreased there are other factors involved than just hypoalbuminemia, such as hypomagnesemia and decreased PTH. Electrolyte replacement may be required to avoid neurologic and metabolic problems. It is reported to be more common in Yorkshire terriers.

Hypomagnesemia causes grass tetany in beef and dairy cattle when they graze lush grass pastures. Animals are usually recumbent and generalized tetany is present or is especially obvious in cervical muscles. Tetany is preceded by an uncoordinated gait, "grass staggers," and an agitated behavior. Lush grass predominant pastures tend to be deficient in magnesium. Adequate serum concentrations of magnesium are dependent on adequate dietary intake. Cattle tend to be hypocalcemic and treatment includes calcium and magnesium preparations. Tetany versus paresis in cattle with hypocalcemia is most easily explained by examination of serum magnesium. If magnesium is decreased as in grass tetany, they will be tetanic and if increased as in milk fever they will be paretic. If hypocalcemia goes untreated long enough even dogs with lactational tetany may become paretic. The serum glucose may be increased due to stress and hypocalcemia-induced hypoinsulinemia.

Oxalate

Plants rich in oxalates may lower serum calcium in herbivores. In chronic cases this has been associated with nutritional secondary hyperparathyroidism and fibrous osteodystrophy. Example plants with excess oxalates are halogeton, dock, rhubarb, greasewood, and soursob.

Critically ill animals – measure ionized calcium, total, and ionized hypocalcemia

Measurement of ionized calcium in critically ill patients, regardless of the primary disease may influence therapy and prognosis. A mild decrease may not be important, but moderate to marked decreases could influence treatments, especially those aimed at stabilizing cardiovascular deterioration. Serum ionized hypocalcemia in critically ill dogs is associated with a longer duration in ICU and total days in the hospital but is not associated with decreased survival. Critically ill dogs with renal failure, diabetic ketoacidosis, or pancreatitis were more likely to have ionized hypocalcemia, but diseases associated with hypocalcemia were not ranked. The study in dogs did not look at total serum calcium to determine if it was associated with predictive outcomes. Previously it has been shown that dogs in acute renal failure with total serum calcium <8.6 mg/dL have a poorer prognosis for survival and discharge from a hospital than do dogs with higher serum total calcium concentrations.

Critically ill adult horses with endotoxemia and gastrointestinal disease may have hypocalcemia, hypomagnesemia and parathyroid gland dysfunction. Decreased total and ionized calcium can cause or be associated with ileus and colic. Nearly 90% of horses with colic had decreased ionized calcium at the time of admission. Horses with very low ionized calcium were 12 times more likely to develop ileus. A fatal outcome was nine times more likely for horses in the very hypocalcemic group. Ionized calcium and response to calcium replacement was used to predict prognosis. Endurance horses with marked hypocalcemia and hypochloremia can have an ileus that is so severe that it is erroneously diagnosed as a surgical colic. Septic foals were reported to have ionized hypocalcemia, hyperphosphatemia, and increased serum PTH but no differences in magnesium, PTH rp, or calcitonin. However, in this study it is impossible to determine if these changes were related to renal function because creatinine (or urea nitrogen) and PTH concentrations were not reported for individual animals. Therefore, comparisons of Ca to PTH, or PTH to azotemia cannot be made. Calves with severe neonatal diarrhea will have hypocalcemia, but due to concurrent acidosis, the ionized hypocalcemia may not be as severe. With fluid therapy and correction of the acidosis both total and ionized calcium will decrease further. Tetany may develop during therapy as alkalinization shifts calcium from ionized to protein bound.

Sick patients

Hypocalcemia is seen in a variety of illnesses in small and large animals in which the pathogenesis is not known. It becomes difficult to know if there is cause and effect or simply an association. Pancreatitis, ketoacidosis, critical illness, sepsis, colic, endotoxemia, inflammatory diseases, protein abnormalities, cantharidin toxicity, and others could fit in this category of associated problems. There may be a mechanism that is reasonable, such as hypomagnesemia, cytokines or it may represent overlap of common problems. Hypocalcemia is seen in sick cattle with a wide variety of conditions including retained placenta, rumen overload, lymphoma, neonatal calf diarrhea, foot diseases, and abomasal ulcers, to list a few. There may be specific diseases to be aware of or it may be that the severity of the disease/illness in animal and human patients correlates better with the degree of hypocalcemia than the specific disease.

Feline hyperthyroidism

There is a calcium, phosphorus, and parathyroid imbalance in some cats with hyperthyroidism that is not understood. Hyperphosphatemia without azotemia is seen in 25–40% of hyperthyroid cats and total serum calcium is usually in the RI. However, a mild decrease in ionized serum calcium, without clinical signs is observed in approximately 30% (4 of 15) but the mechanisms are not known. The number of cats studied was small. Increased concentration of PTH is reported in up to 77% of hyperthyroid cats studied (small numbers) and hyperparathyroidism and hyperthyroidism are listed as coexistent problems in cats. These abnormalities could be due to concurrent renal disease, which is common in geriatric cats. However, urea nitrogen and creatinine are usually in the RI. Another possibility is the growing association of hypocalcemia with or without an increase in PTH in a variety of concurrent illnesses. The parathyroid hyperplasia may help explain why some cats do not develop postsurgical hypocalcemia and may help explain why postsurgical hypocalcemia is usually not permanent. Humans with hyperthyroidism tend to have the opposite pattern: increased bone turnover, hypercalcemia, and decreased PTH. Hypercalcemia has been reported for dogs with hyperthyroidism. It is mild, the mechanism is not known, and it may not be related to hyperthyroidism. Although the phosphorus, ionized calcium, alkaline phosphatase (ALP), and bone relationship is an interesting paradox in hyperthyroid cats, it is clinically insignificant.

Iatrogenic

Various treatments such as anticonvulsants, intravenous phosphate solutions, calcium-free IV solutions, transfusions with citrate as anticoagulant, excess bicarbonate therapy, tetracycline, and furosemide diuretics can be associated with hypocalcemia. Furosemide inhibits sodium and chloride reabsorption in the loop of Henle and secondarily inhibits calcium reabsorption that can lead to hypocalcemia. Furosemide can be used to lower serum calcium in hypercalcemic patients with adequate hydration. Tetracycline will chelate calcium and rapid intravenous boluses may decrease calcium. Hypocalcemia induced by transfusions is only associated with massive transfusions; e.g., open heart surgery, transfusion equal to 50% of blood volume in a 3-hour period, or transfusion equal to total blood volume over 24 hours can decrease ionized calcium by 1.2 mg/dL (0.3 mmol/L).

Hypercalcemia

Causes of hypercalcemia are outlined in Table 34.2. If ionized calcium is used to classify and rank the frequency of causes of hypercalcemia in dogs they are: HCM (58%), renal failure (17%), hyperparathyroidism (13%), hypoadrenocorticism (5%), miscellaneous diagnoses (4%), and vitamin D toxicity (3%). Cats and horses have the same differentials. Following is discussion of various causes of hypercalcemia that are not related to autonomous PTH hypersecretion. A general diagnostic approach for evaluation of the hypercalcemic patient is outlined in Table 34.4.

HCM is the term used to describe a common syndrome in which a nonparathyroid tumor produces a substance that acts like PTH and causes hypercalcemia and hypophophatemia. There are a variety of substances produced by tumors and the one that is most important from a clinical diagnostic perspective is PTH rp. Total and ionized calcium are increased, but concurrent hypophosphatemia, when present, is the major diagnostic clue because the only two diseases of dogs and cats that do this are HCM and primary HPTH. Historically, HCM was called pseudohyperparathyroidism because the disease resembled primary HPTH. The reason for this is that many tumors produce the protein PTH rp, which shares a nearly identical amino acid sequence at the amino terminal end of the molecule to native PTH. Since the amino terminal end is the biologically active fragment, both molecules are recognized by and stimulate the same receptors (PTH1R) and therefore produce the same biological responses. Many cells throughout the body produce PTH rp, but the only disease associated with this molecule in veterinary medicine is HCM. PTH rp is important for fetal calcium regulation, transplacental calcium transportation, calcium homeostasis of the fetus, important in milk, and no doubt will be linked to other physiological functions and diseases. It can be identified via immunohistochemistry in tumors that cause hypercalcemia and in tumors from normocalcemic animals. In addition to PTH rp, a group of less commonly recognized substances can be produced by tumors and act individually or in concert to amplify this syndrome. These include interleukin-1, interleukin-6, tumor necrosis factor, prostaglandin E2 (PGE_2), fibroblast stimulating factor, epidermal growth factor, transforming growth factor, PTH, and vitamin D derivatives. Some of these factors are important in the hypercalcemia associated with lymphomas and may act synergistically. The only two substances on this list that are diagnostically practical in veterinary medicine are PTH and PTH rP. However, if a malignant tumor was present and both PTH and PTH rp were decreased, then one of these other humoral/local osteolytic substances may be causing the hypercalcemia.

HCM is the most common cause of hypercalcemia in dogs and it has been associated with numerous tumors. The two most common tumors are lymphoma (by a wide margin) and apocrine gland adenocarcinoma of the anal sac. Lymphoma associated with hypercalcemia in dogs is usually a T-cell lymphoma, as it is in people. Approximately 50% of the dogs will have a mass in the anterior mediastinum. Only 6% are leukemic and osteolytic bone lesions are seen rarely in conventional radiographs. If neither of these tumors are present search for multiple myeloma, mammary carcinoma, pulmonary tumor, and histiocytic sarcomas in that order. If a tumor cannot be found, then measuring PTH and PTH rp are helpful diagnostic tests as is ultrasonography of the thyroid region and possibly the abdominal cavity to search for less physically obvious neoplasia.

HCM is not as common in cats when compared with dogs, but HCM is the number one or two cause of hypercalcemia in cats. It is associated with carcinomas, especially squamous cell carcinoma (SCC), lymphoma, feline leukemia virus (FeLV) with or without lymphoma, myeloma, and rarely with a variety of other malignant tumors. Anal sac tumors are rare in cats and only a few are associated with hypercalcemia. Most cats with this tumor are normocalcemic. Ferrets also have this anal sac tumor, but hypercalcemia is not seen. HCM is rare in horses and has been associated with lymphoma, myeloma, ameloblastoma, and gastric SCC. Although lymphoma is common in cattle, there have been no reported cases associated with hypercalcemia. Interstitial cell tumors of the testes are associated with HCM in rats and an integumentary carcinoma will produce the disease in rabbits. There are multiple animal models in rabbits, rats and mice.

In most cases of HCM, the diagnosis is easy and is based on physical examination and/or laboratory findings of neoplasia in the categories described above. Essentially any tumor could produce this syndrome, most are malignant, but some are benign. Aspirational cytology of enlarged lymph nodes or the perineal mass or other tumors can easily confirm the diagnosis. Measurement of PTH and PTH rp is not needed if a tumor can be identified. Glucocorticoids are useful in lowering the serum concentration of calcium but avoid their use until a diagnosis is established. Steroids will cause lymphocytolysis, which will greatly interfere with interpretation of any lymph node aspirates examined via cytology. If an injection of steroids corrected hypercalcemia in a dog with enlarged lymph nodes, then the diagnosis was very likely lymphoma. Aspiration of lymph nodes at this time will probably be nondiagnostic, but when hypercalcemia returns, cytologic confirmation of lymphoma is indicated.

Most clinical signs are referable to the cancer, but some are due to hypercalcemia. These are weakness and PU/PD.

Table 34.4 Evaluation of a hypercalcemic patient.

1. Consider age of patient, compare calcium and P, examine for azotemia.
2. If increased calcium is not due to young age, then consider repeating serum calcium to confirm hypercalcemia; consider ionized calcium if available; if P is decreased, there is no need to repeat serum calcium.

If **hypercalcemic and hypophosphatemic: HCM vs. primary hyperparathyroidism:**

1. If a horse and it is azotemic, done, renal failure is the cause of hypercalcemia, pursue causes of renal failure; more likely to be chronic and have a poor prognosis.
2. If dog or cat, pursue HCM first followed by primary HPTH.
3. Hypercalcemia of malignancy (number one cause of persistent hypercalcemia in dogs and cats); perform a cancer search, do not measure PTH or PTH rp initially.

   Lymphoma most likely; #1 tumor associated with HCM

      Evaluation of lymph nodes, anterior mediastinum, bone marrow, FeLV; 50% of dogs have an anterior mediastinal mass; <10% leukemic; determination of hepatosplenomegaly; aspirational cytology of enlarged lymph nodes and/or organs

   Adenocarcinoma apocrine glands of anal sac, #2 tumor associated with HCM in dogs

      Thorough rectal-perirectal examination; metastases in pelvic canal and/or sublumbar present at time of initial diagnosis; 50% do not protrude caudally and therefore are not visible but can be palpated

   Myeloma

      Markedly increased total protein, monoclonal gammopathy; multiple lytic bone lesions; aspirational cytology; Bence Jones proteinuria

   Other tumors

      Mammary, pulmonary, malignant histiocytosis, squamous cell carcinoma any tumor possible, perform search

      Horse – squamous cell carcinoma of stomach; endoscopy; paracentesis; lymphoma search

If one of the tumors above is found, that is the cause of hypercalcemia; if further confirmation desired, then measure PTH and PTH rp concurrently

4. If a cancer cannot be found or only a benign skin cancer is found, then consider primary hyperparathyroidism: ultrasound the thyroid-parathyroid complex and/or measure PTH and PTH rp concurrently. Small mass in thyroid region with hypercalcemia and hypophosphatemia is usually sufficient evidence for diagnosis and localizes the tumor to left or right; if further confirmation desired, measure PTH and PTH rp concurrently.

Hypercalcemia and hyperphosphatemia:

1. Rule in or out malignancy first as outlined above; HCM much more likely to be hyperphosphatemic than patients with primary HPTH; <5% of dogs with primary hyperparathyroidism are hyperphosphatemic; it is "practical" to rule out hyperparathyroidism if hyperphosphatemic; exceptions always exist.
2. Examine for azotemia, which is likely, and assess degree of azotemia; the higher the azotemia the greater likelihood of primary renal; attempt to rule in/rule out acute vs. chronic renal failure; if a young dog, especially purebred, then progressive familial renal nephropathy is most likely; if acute renal failure consider grape toxicity.

If azotemia is mild to moderate, then the order of differential diagnoses are Addison's, renal disease, and vitamin D toxicity; all are likely to have dilute urine: <1.025 while azotemic.

   90% of Addison's are azotemic, rule in with basal cortisol <2 μg/dL and Na:K <23, decide if ACTH stimulation needed; rule out with cortisol >2 μg/dL.

   Rule in/out renal failure: response to fluids; acute vs. chronic; imaging of kidneys; Fx Exc Na; etc.

   Differentiation of renal causing vs. caused by hypercalcemia: >P more likely primary renal and > calcium more likely hypercalcemia came first; if total calcium increased and ionized normal or decreased renal more likely; but ionized can be increased in renal failure in dogs and cats.

   Consider vitamin D toxicity from history, possible exposure, soft-tissue mineralization, assay for vitamin D; plants unlikely in carnivores, more likely in herbivores.

Table 34.4 *(continued)*

3. If all above ruled out, pursue idiopathic in cats; granulomatous diseases: blastomycosis, other fungi, FIP, schistosomiasis, mycobacterium, toxoplasmosis; iatrogenic.

Hypercalcemia and normophosphatemia – consider all of above

- Patients with HCM – cancer search more practical than PTH PTH rp determinations. Lymphoma first, followed by anal sac, lung, mammary, malignant histiocytosis.
- Hypoadrenocorticism: Na:K <23 : 1; basal cortisol; ACTH stimulation test.
- Renal disease – azotemia, very rare to have normophosphatemia if they are also hypercalcemic; evaluate renal size; acute vs. chronic.
- Primary hyperparathyroidism: serum PTH PTH rp; ultrasound, exploratory surgery of cervical region.
- Idiopathic – cat; rule out others, calcium crystalluria; steroid responsive.
- Bone lesion – other mechanisms besides direct osteolyis are involved.
- Granulomatous – aspirational cytology is test of choice, find etiologic agent.
- Ionized calcium – if desired measure; same list of differential diagnoses and diagnostic approaches; ionized calcium more important to measure in hypocalcemic than hypercalcemic situations.
- Do not use adjustment formulae for protein or albumin if hypercalcemia is present.

Animals with HCM have more dramatic clinical signs than animals with primary HPTH due to the malignancy. These include cachexia, mass lesions, pulmonary metastases, generalized ill health, and azotemia. Hypercalcemia and hypophosphatemia are the key diagnostic laboratory abnormalities. Apocrine adenocarcinomas are one of the best examples to demonstrate how the tumor induces these electrolyte abnormalities. In the following example of an 8-year-old female spayed German shepherd dog, there is hypercalcemia and hypophosphatemia at the time of diagnosis that is rapidly corrected following the first surgical removal of the malignant tumor. When the tumor recurred, so did hypercalcemia and hypophosphatemia, and this cycle repeated itself until the dog's death.

Serum	Total calcium	Phosphorus
Initial diagnosis	21.2	2.4
24-hour postsurgical removal	10.4	3.9
Recurrence 13 months later	16.8	1.8
24-hour postsurgical removal	9.6	4.2
Recurrence 13 months later	18.1	3.4
RI	9–11 mg/dL	3–5 mg/dL

Hypercalcemia can be used as a marker of tumor recurrence and/or metastases. These sequential changes in serum calcium and phosphorus associated with surgical removal of tumors and their recurrence was part of the initial evidence that tumors were producing humoral factors that acted like PTH. In the preceding example, the serum concentration of PTH was appropriately undetectable prior to surgical removal of the tumor and increased rapidly after surgery, preventing postoperative hypocalcemia. Despite the malignant behavior of anal sac tumors, they spread slowly, and surgical resection or chemotherapy often gives affected patients months or even years of life postdiagnosis. Only about half of the tumors protrude caudally to be visible in the perineum, but all can be detected on rectal palpation. They tend to enter the pelvic vault and sublumbar lymph nodes before spreading to liver and/or lungs. This tumor is distinct from benign circumanal or perianal gland adenomas that are common in male dogs and are visible in the perineum.

The hypophosphatemia in dogs, cats, horses, lab animals, and people with HCM is due to the phosphaturic effect of PTH rp on the renal tubules. Causes of hypercalcemia other than HCM and primary HPTH do not stimulate renal phosphorus excretion; hence the serum phosphorus is normal or increased in other diseases. Given time, dogs with HCM often develop normophosphatemia or hyperphosphatemia. This is likely due to concurrent dehydration and prerenal azotemia. Other contributing factors include lymphoma involvement of the kidneys or renal mineralization after the phosphorus increases. Animals with HCM are much more likely to be hyperphosphatemic or normophosphatemic and azotemic than are animals with primary HPTH. This is probably due to the more frequent development of renal complications and subsequent phosphorus retention. Once the Ca × P product is over 90, soft-tissue mineralization is likely, and one of the common tissues that is predisposed to this is the kidney. Hence, nephrocalcinosis is a frequent complication, which further contributes to renal problems.

Urine specific gravity is dilute due to hypercalcemia inhibiting the action of ADH. The triad of azotemia, dilute urine, and hypercalcemia produces the diagnostic challenge of what came first, either renal failure or hypercalcemia. This raises the challenge to determine the cause of hypercalcemia. There are multiple ways to solve this. First, it is much more likely that the hypercalcemia is due to a tumor than renal failure. Second, the physical examination finding of a malignant tumor (particularly lymphoma or anal sac adenocarcinoma) establishes a cause for the hypercalcemia. Next, the greater the serum calcium the more likely it is HCM and not primary renal failure. The lower the serum P, the more likely it is HCM, while the higher the phosphorus, the more it favors primary renal disease. Lastly, if a primary renal disease can be diagnosed then that it is the cause. Since both diseases tend to be in geriatric patients, they may have both HCM and chronic renal failure.

Following the use of screening tests such as physical findings, calcium, and phosphorus, confirmatory tests may be used. Measurement of PTH and PTH rp are the best laboratory methods for confirmation. Use these if an obvious cancer cannot be found. Request PTH, PTH rp, and calcium on the same sample or samples drawn concurrently in a nonazotemic patient. Ideally PTH will be decreased or undetectable and PTH rp will be increased in patients with HCM. The increase in PTH rp is usually diagnostic, but other substances may cause HCM. Therefore, a decreased value of PTH rp does not rule out HCM. The PTH concentration could be within the RI making interpretation difficult because PTH is often in the RI in primary hyperparathyroidism. However, PTH rp will be decreased or undetectable in patients with primary hyperparathyroidism while PTH is normal or increased. There is overlap of the absolute values for each disease and that is why both hormones should be measured concurrently, and the results compared to each other and the serum calcium concentration. If just one hormone is measured, interpretation is difficult and may necessitate repeat sampling.

The easiest and more practical way to differentiate primary HPTH from HCM, however, is simply to find the cancer associated with HCM and then perform aspirational cytology. If a cancer cannot be located, then consider performing ultrasonography of the thyroid region to search for a parathyroid adenoma. The measurement of serum/plasma PTH and PTH rp may be useful adjuncts when physical examination and ultrasonography are not conclusive. Identification of the other humoral factors associated with HCM is difficult and is a research and/or investigative situation.

Examples of interpretation of PTH and PTH rp results for hypercalcemia include:

PTH	PTH rp	Diagnosis
Inc	Dec	Primary HPTH
RI	Dec	Primary HPTH
RI	Inc	HCM
Dec	Inc	HCM
Inc	Inc	Primary HPTH and HCM
Inc	Inc	Renal
Dec	Dec	Other causes of hypercalcemia
Dec	Dec	An ectopic substance other than PTH rp
Dec	Dec	*In vitro* decay

If both PTH and PTH rp are increased, check the serum UN, creatinine, and phosphorus as a likely explanation is decreased clearance due to renal failure.

Interestingly, hypocalcemia does not happen after surgical resection of a tumor associated with HCM or after chemotherapy for tumors causing HCM, which has significant clinical application. PTH secretion is suppressed for several days following the removal of a parathyroid adenoma in dogs with primary HPTH and hypocalcemia develops in some of these dogs. However, PTH is secreted rapidly following surgical removal of anal sac gland adenocarcinomas, preventing postsurgical hypocalcemia. Following removal of anal sac tumors, the concentration of serum calcium returns to normocalcemic ranges in less than 24 hours as serum PTH, which was decreased or undetectable before surgery, now increases. Apparently, the suppression and atrophy of parathyroid glands is greater in primary hyperparathyroidism than in HCM. An explanation for this observation is not clear.

Renal disease with hypercalcemia

In cats this is the number one or number two cause of hypercalcemia. In horses it is the number one cause. It is a relatively common cause in dogs. If ionized calcium is used to classify causes of hypercalcemia in dogs, renal failure is the number two cause. Dogs with renal failure are usually normocalcemic, but hypocalcemia is common, and hypercalcemia may be present in about 10%. Chronic renal failure is more commonly associated with hypercalcemia than acute renal failure, although grape and currant toxicities are examples of acute renal failure that may be associated with hypercalcemia. The cause of hypercalcemia with renal failure is not known. It is referred to as tertiary hyperparathyroidism. Increases in total and ionized calcium are usually mild compared to the hypercalcemia seen in HCM or primary HPTH, e.g., total calcium 11.5–13 mg/dL for renal failure versus >16 mg/dL for HCM or primary

HPTH. Examine the phosphorus and determine the Ca × P product. The product is often increased with renal failure. The pathogenesis probably involves an abnormality with the calcium receptor for PTH located on the parathyroid chief cells and other cells. CaSR controls PTH secretion and arms parathyroid chief cells and other CaSR-expressing cells to detect changes in the concentration of calcium and to make adjustments that normalize serum calcium. Several disorders in humans are due to inherited or acquired abnormalities of these CaSR pathways such that the receptor is reset at a serum calcium concentration that disrupts normal regulation and there is resulting hypercalcemia or hypocalcemia. These pathways may play a pivotal role in the development of hypercalcemia seen in some animals with renal failure. Acquired abnormalities in this receptor may result in a failure of an increasing concentration of calcium to decrease the production and release of PTH. It is as if the thermostat was turned up and it no longer shuts off production of PTH at a high concentration of calcium. Therefore, PTH continues to be produced and secreted even though the present concentration of calcium (high) would normally inhibit the release of PTH. PTH concentrations are increased in patients with renal failure due to hypocalcemia (relative or absolute), hyperphosphatemia, parathyroid hyperplasia, and decreased clearance and degradation of PTH as kidneys excrete PTH. PTH is considered one of the "uremic toxins."

When hypercalcemia is present in dogs with renal disease, it is usually seen in younger dogs that have progressive familial renal dysplasia. This includes breeds such as Lhasa Apso, elkhound, Doberman, Wheaten terrier. Nearly all of these patients will also have hyperphosphatemia and be azotemic. Patients with hypercalcemia and hyperphosphatemia are very prone to the formation of soft-tissue mineralization. Attempts to lower the serum phosphorus and azotemia should be vigorous because renal mineralization will compound the renal failure and may make it irreversible. The differentiation of hypercalcemia due to renal failure from azotemia caused by another hypercalcemic disease is problematic. A generalization is the higher the serum phosphorus, the more likely the cause is renal disease, and the higher the serum calcium, the more likely the cause is not renal. If renal failure is causing the hypercalcemia, the serum phosphorus concentration is usually in double figures in dogs and cats, e.g., 10–25 mg/dL. The lower the concentration of serum phosphorus, the more likely the cause of the hypercalcemia is something other than renal failure. For example, there is a substance in circulation that is both increasing calcium and decreasing phosphorus, such as PTH or PTH rp. These substances have a phosphaturic effect and if phosphorus is decreased or even if in RIs while a patient is azotemic that is strong evidence that the patient has increased PTH or PTH rp. If the total serum calcium is increased but ionized calcium is in the RI or decreased, this pattern is more characteristic of primary renal failure.

Patients with hypercalcemia and renal failure are expected to be hyposthenuric. This is due to either the renal disease or the action of calcium blocking the function of ADH on the collecting ducts. Approximately one-third of horses in chronic renal failure develop the unusual combination of hypercalcemia and hypophosphatemia. This is unique to the horse. The mechanism for hypercalcemia and hypophosphatemia in horses is unknown. Other horses have the traditional hyperphosphatemia expected with azotemia and either hypocalcemia or normocalcemia.

Addison's disease

Approximately one-third of dogs with hypoadrenocorticism will have hypercalcemia. The mechanism is not entirely known, but postulated components are increased complexed calcium to citrate, an absence of glucocorticoids, and therefore absence of corticoid calciureic effects. Steroids promote calciuria and block osteoclastic osteolysis. In the absence of steroids, these two physiologic events may contribute to hypercalcemia. Ionized calcium was increased in five of seven Addisonian dogs that all had increased total serum calcium, but there were no consistent increases in PTH, PTH rp, or 1,25 dihydroxyvitamin D concentrations to explain the hypercalcemia. Almost all dogs with hypoadrenocorticism are azotemic, many do not concentrate their urine beyond 1.020, and most are hyperphosphatemic. Because renal failure and Addison's disease can have similar electrolyte abnormalities, these diseases can appear similar. If hypercalcemia is present with the above laboratory abnormalities it favors hypoadrenocorticism. If the Na:K ratio is <23 in an azotemic patient it favors hypoadrenocorticism, although this lowered ratio may be seen in renal failure and uroabdomen.

Vitamin D toxicity

This usually produces hypercalcemia and normo- or hyperphosphatemia since vitamin D stimulates both calcium and phosphorus absorption from the GI tract and resorption from bone, without a direct phosphorus lowering effect on the kidneys. The combination of hypercalcemia and hyperphosphatemia can produce lethal soft-tissue mineralization. Mineralization of muscles, tendons, heart, lungs, gastrointestinal tract, and blood vessels is expected and is the cause of death. Sources of vitamin D include dietary supplements, rat poisons, and plants (*Cestrum diurnum* or day blooming jasmine, *Solanum malacoxylon, Trisetum flavescens*). Plant toxicities are more common in herbivores. Rodenticides are more common in dogs and cats. Day blooming jasmine is a house plant and has been reported to cause hypercalcemia in pets that eat it. Overzealous treatment of hypocalcemia with vitamin D and calcium products can cause hypercalcemia. This happens with some regularity in the postoperative treatment of hypocalcemia following removal of a parathyroid tumor. Production of one or more metabolites of vitamin

D is involved in the pathogenesis of some cases of HCM and granulomatous diseases (fungi, parasitic). Ingestion of a topical cream used to treat psoriasis in people, calcipotriene, tacalcitol, or Dovonex is another source of vitamin D that has caused hypervitaminosis D in dogs. Calcipotriene is a synthetic derivative of calcitrol that was used to treat osteoporosis in people, and it is not detected by assays for 25-hydroxyvitamin D. Assays for vitamin D are available and include precursors or 1,25 di-hydroxycholecalciferol. Most assays detect 25-hydroxylated forms of vitamin D2 or D3. Consult the reference lab for sample handling, RIs, and interpretation guidelines.

Granulomatous diseases

Hypercalcemia has been associated with granulomatous diseases caused by a variety of organisms in dogs and cats. Blastomycosis is a fairly well-known cause of hypercalcemia, but very few dogs with blastomycosis are hypercalcemic. Blastomycosis may involve bones. However, increased production of vitamin D by macrophages in the granulomas is a more likely mechanism than direct osteolysis from granulomas in bone. Macrophages and some cancer cells can convert vitamin D precursors into calcitrol. Eleven of 22 dogs infected with the flatworm *Heterobilharzia americana* that causes canine schistosomiasis were hypercalcemic. Resolution of hypercalcemia required treatment with praziquantel. Increased serum PTH rp was demonstrated in two dogs with schistosomiasis. Feline infectious peritonitis (FIP), tuberculosis, toxoplasmosis, cryptococcosis, and actinomyces are other granulomatous diseases associated with hypercalcemia infrequently in cats. These “causes” should be viewed as “associated with” until studies confirm a mechanism.

Diagnosis is established by ruling out other causes of hypercalcemia, by confirming the etiologic agent by serology and/or cytology, and by response to treatment.

Young animals

Young, rapidly growing dogs may have mild asymptomatic hypercalcemia and hyperphosphatemia. The increase is seen more frequently in giant breeds but may occur in any breed. The total serum calcium is seldom over 12 mg/dL in young dogs, and by 6 months of age the total serum calcium should be in the RI for adult dogs. Serum concentrations of calcium and phosphorus that are slightly greater than the RI in young growing animals should be interpreted as normal for their age. This pattern is not seen in kittens or foals.

Idiopathic

Idiopathic hypercalcemia is one of the more common causes of hypercalcemia in cats and it may be on the rise. This disorder is unique to cats. It has been suggested that the increased use of acidifying diets introduced in the 1990's for the control of struvite urolithiasis is a contributing factor. Fractional excretion of calcium is increased and urolithiasis (calcium oxalate or struvite) is expected in 50–75% of these cats. Taken together, the data suggests that some susceptible cats develop hypercalcemia, hypercalciuria, and calcium oxalate urolithiasis while on acidifying diets. However, many cats on acidifying diets do not develop this syndrome, or at least it is not recognized. Presence of calcium crystals in the urine should prompt consideration to measure serum calcium. Diagnosis is established by ruling out other causes of hypercalcemia and a test trial of steroids.

Cats with this syndrome are normophosphatemic and hypercalcemic (total and ionized). Treatment with prednisone (5–12 mg/cat/day) seems to reverse the hypercalcemia. Hypercalcemia may be increased for years in some cats with or without clinical signs. FeLV and feline immunodeficiency virus are not causative. Individuals do not believe it is caused by hyperparathyroidism, because the concentrations of PTH are not increased and because subtotal parathyroidectomy only corrects the hypercalcemia temporarily. However, others could interpret the normal concentration of PTH as inappropriately high for the degree of hypercalcemia. Increased and decreased concentrations of PTH rp are reported, but neither PTH rp nor vitamin D is believed to be causative. Another possible undocumented cause could be a congenital or acquired defect in the calcium-regulating receptor.

Xylitol toxicity

This is reported naturally and experimentally in dogs, most of these describe severe hypoglycemia and/or liver failure. Hypercalcemia is reported as are increases in liver enzymes, hypokalemia, and hyper- and hypophosphatemia. Xylitol is a sugar substitute found naturally in trees, vegetables, and fruits and is used as a sweetener in sugar-free gum, candy, baked goods, desserts, oral care products, and in granulated forms for baking. It is lower in calories than sugar and has low impact on serum glucose, but it stimulates rapid insulin release and causes severe hypoglycemia in dogs. Xylitol's effects on glucose are clinically more important than hypercalcemia.

Bone lesions

Osteolytic bone lesions caused by bone metastases, hypertrophic osteodystrophy, or osteomyelitis have been associated with hypercalcemia, but it is unlikely these are a true cause of hypercalcemia. Or at least the mechanism is more complicated then direct osteolysis by a focal lesion and instead involves one or more humoral components. Any increased release of calcium into the blood from bone resorption around a localized lesion will be normalized by renal excretion. Bone metastases associated with hypercalcemia are more likely due to production of tumor factors that act locally to resorb bone and also stimulate renal calcium reabsorption and phosphorus excretion. Dogs with hypertrophic osteodystrophy may have increased serum calcium. It is likely due to their young age and not the infection in the bones, unless cytokines work locally and in the kidneys. These "causes" of hypercalcemia should be viewed as "associated with" until additional studies confirm a mechanism.

V

Clinical Chemistry of Common Nondomestic Mammals, Birds, Reptiles, Fish, and Amphibians

35 Clinical Chemistry of Mammals: Laboratory Animals and Miscellaneous Species

Terry W. Campbell

Department of Clinical Sciences, College of Veterinary Medicine and Biomedical Sciences, Colorado State University, Fort Collins, CO, USA

Blood biochemistry profiles are commonly used to assess the health of nondomestic, mammalian patients. The reason is that diseases are usually associated with specific changes in the blood and urine that are detected using specific analytical techniques. In general, biochemical panels used by most laboratories include glucose, blood urea nitrogen (BUN), creatinine, total protein (TP), albumin (Alb), globulin (Glob), calcium (Ca), phosphorus (P), sodium (Na), potassium (K), chloride (Cl), and total cholesterol. In addition, these panels generally include two or more hepatocellular functions tests, such as alanine aminotransferase (ALT), aspartate aminotransferase (AST), sorbitol dehydrogenase (SDH), lactate dehydrogenase (LD), or total bile acids [1]. The panels will also include two or more hepatobiliary function tests, such as alkaline phosphatase (AP), gamma glutamyltransferase (GGT), total bilirubin, or bile acids [1]. Additions to the biochemical panels may include creatine kinase (CK), triglycerides, magnesium (Mg), and protein electrophoresis. The results of these tests are compared to the reference values that are either produced in the same laboratory conducting the testing or with published normal values for the same or similar species. Biomedical research involves use of laboratory animals such as mice, rats, and rabbits, resulting in a large amount of information concerning the interpretation of biochemical profiles in these species. Fewer clinical chemistry studies, however, have been performed on other nondomestic mammals, such as ferrets, sugar gliders, and hedgehogs. In general, interpretation of clinical chemistry results in nondomestic mammals is the same as that described for domestic species.

It should be noted that many parameters of the patient as an individual, such as age, gender, hydration, and nutritional status, affect biochemical test results. Environmental conditions such as photoperiod, temperature, and husbandry as well as the sampling and analytic methods and the instrumentation used are other sources of variation. Sampling variables include restraint methods, type of anesthetic used, time of day when sampled, anticoagulant used, site of sample collection, and sample processing and storage. For example, a 16–18-hour fast is required in rats to obtain nonlipemic plasma samples, whereas a 16-hour fast in rabbits results in decreased plasma glucose and insulin concentrations but increased glucagon and fatty acid concentrations [2, 3]. Release of epinephrine related to excitement of transportation and blood collection in rabbits results in increased plasma glucose and free fatty acid concentrations. Blood collected by cardiocentesis may be contaminated with muscle enzymes such as CK, AST, LD, and ALT, which are found at high concentrations in cardiac muscle. In rodents, plasma biochemistry results tend to vary in samples obtained from the orbital sinus compared with those obtained by cardiocentesis [4–6].

Results of clinical chemistry analyses performed on identical serum or plasma samples often vary significantly among laboratories; thus, published reference values exhibit considerable variation for many analytes. Therefore, reference ranges obtained by differing methods are not necessarily useful for the veterinary in-house laboratory [7]. Instead, in-house analyzers require their own specific reference ranges. Possible reasons for the differences in reference ranges of the compared studies may be due to undetected subclinical diseases and the use of differing chemical or statistical methods.

Sample collection and handling

Blood samples for biochemical studies can be collected using the same techniques as those described from hematologic studies (see Chapter 19). Many modern analyzers can

Veterinary Hematology, Clinical Chemistry, and Cytology, Third Edition. Edited by Mary Anna Thrall, Glade Weiser, Robin W. Allison and Terry W. Campbell.

Companion website: www.wiley.com/go/thrall/veterinary

perform as many as 20 tests on as little as 50 µl of serum or plasma. Heparinized plasma is routinely used for clinical chemistry evaluations in small rodents such as mice, hamsters, and gerbils; because collection of serum commonly results in hemolysis and a larger sample volume can be obtained with plasma than with serum. The aqueous form of lithium heparin is the preferred anticoagulant for plasma biochemical analysis. As a general guideline, a blood sample volume comprising 10% or less of the total-body blood volume (or 1% of the body weight) can be safely taken from a healthy mammal.

Hemolysis or prolonged contact between serum and blood cells produces changes in the analyte concentrations. Increases in the potassium, phosphorus, LD, and bilirubin concentrations as well as decreases in the glucose concentration may be observed. Serum samples from guinea pigs and rabbits have greater LD and GGT activity compared with that in plasma samples produced by leakage of these enzymes from erythrocytes during the clotting process [3, 8]. In mice, serum CK activity decreases with freezing [9]. Because of the cryoprecipitation of some proteins in serum or plasma samples from rats, protein concentrations may decrease during freezing [9].

Plasma biochemical analyte reference intervals for common small mammals are provided in Tables 35.1–35.4. Tables 35.5 and 35.6 compare serum or plasma hormone concentrations of rodents and rabbits, respectively.

Rodents

Laboratory evaluation of the kidneys

Laboratory evaluation of rodent kidneys is the same as that for domestic mammals, and it involves evaluation of blood parameters, such as urea nitrogen, creatinine, and electrolytes, and urinalysis. The plasma urea nitrogen is influenced by diet, liver function, gastrointestinal absorption, and hydration. Increases in plasma urea nitrogen and creatinine concentrations only occur when more than 75% of renal function is compromised; therefore, these tests lack sensitivity for renal disease. Common causes of renal azotemia in rodents, especially mice, include amyloidosis, immune complex diseases, and polycystic disease. Serum or plasma urea nitrogen concentrations increase with high protein diets because of increased nitrogen metabolism rather than renal disease. Age should be considered when evaluating plasma urea nitrogen in rodents; aged hamsters demonstrate increased plasma urea nitrogen concentrations. Other laboratory abnormalities that may be associated with renal disease are hyperphosphatemia, resulting from decreased glomerular filtration, and hypoproteinemia, resulting from glomerular disease and urinary protein loss.

γ-Glutamyltransferase, N-acetyl-β-D-glucosaminidase, and AP have high tissue activity in the kidney, and measurement of these enzymes in urine may improve the sensitivity of clinical chemical testing for renal disease in rodents. Testing of endogenous creatinine clearance may provide a specific and sensitive test for decreased glomerular filtration before plasma urea nitrogen and creatinine concentrations are increased.

Urine may contain artifacts if proper attention is not paid to the collection technique. The urine should be collected on a clean, dry surface. Without use of commercially available metabolism cages, urine commonly is contaminated with feces, food, hair, bedding, or drinking water. Rodents often spontaneously urinate when handled, thereby providing a clean sample for those who are prepared to collect this urine. Cystocentesis eliminates much of the artifact associated with voided urine but may result in blood contamination. Urinalysis should be performed within 2 hours of collection; otherwise, urine may be refrigerated at 4 °C for as long as 48 hours. Refrigerated urine should be warmed to room temperature before testing.

The urine of normal rodents usually is yellow, but it may vary in both shade and transparency depending on the hydration status of the animal. Urinary pH is influenced by diet. Diets that are high in animal proteins contain high concentrations of sulfates and phosphate precursors, which produce more acid urine; cereal protein–based diets tend to produce a neutral to slightly alkaline urine. Rodents tend to have alkaline urine because of the bacterial conversion of urea to ammonia. The urine pH is helpful in determining the acid-base status of the animal. Rodents suffering from catabolic conditions such as starvation, ketosis, or fever commonly have acidic urine.

Urine specific gravity and osmolality are used to evaluate the ability of the kidneys to concentrate or dilute urine. A water-deprivation test for detecting renal disease in rodents can be conducted by withholding water for 24 hours, after which the urinary specific gravity is determined. Those animals that are unable to concentrate their urine to a specific gravity greater than 1.030 either have significant renal disease with the inability to concentrate their urine or suffer from diabetes insipidus. The urine specific gravity value obtained from a refractometer will be erroneous if the urine contains significant quantities of glucose, protein, or other metabolites that normally are not found in urine. Urine osmolality is the definitive method for measuring the concentrating ability of the kidneys; it depends on the number of particles in solution and is not affected by the degree of ionization or the mass of molecules and ions that are present. The normal urine osmolality of rats and hamsters ranges from 331 to 445 and 307 to 355 mOsm/kg, respectively [4, 13, 14].

The urine of normal rodents may contain a trace amount of glucose. Large amounts of ascorbic acid normally are found in mouse urine and may interfere with urine chemical strips

Table 35.1 Plasma biochemical values in rodents.

	Mouse	Rat	Hamster	Gerbil	Guinea pig	Chinchilla
Glucose (mg/dL)	196–278	114–143	65–144	—	89–95	—
	73–183	74–163	60–160	47–137	60–125	60–120
Urea nitrogen (mg/dL)	21–26	16–19	14–30	—	22–25	—
	18–31	12–22	14–27	17–30	9.0–31.5	10–25
Creatinine (mg/dL)	0.5	0.5–1.4	0.5–0.6	—	1.4	—
	0.48–1.1	0.38–0.8	0.4–1.0	—	0.6–2.2	—
Uric acid (mg/dL)	—	1.3–2.8	1.3–5.1	—	—	—
	—	—	—	—	—	—
Total protein (g/dL)	5.0–7.0	6.4–8.5	1.3–5.1	—	4.8–5.6	—
	5.9–10.3	5.9–7.8	5.5–7.2	4.6–14.7	4.2–6.8	5–6
Albumin (g/dL)	3.0–4.0	4.1–5.4	3.2–4.3	—	2.4–2.7	—
	2.5–4.8	3.3–4.6	2.0–4.2	1.8–5.8	2.1–3.9	2.5–4.2
Calcium (mg/dL)	7.9–10.5	10.5–13.0	10.4–12.4	—	9.6–10.7	—
	4.6–9.6	7.6–12.6	8.4–12.3	3.7–6.1	8.2–12.0	10–15
Phosphorus (mg/dL)	5.6–9.2	5.0–13.0	5.0–8.0	—	5.0	—
	5.2–9.4	5.3–8.4	4.0–8.2	3.7–11.2	3.0–7.6	4–8
Sodium (mEq/L)	138–186	143–150	128–145	—	122–125	—
	143–164	142–150	124–147	143–147	120–152	130–155
Potassium (mEq/L)	5.3–6.3	5.3–7.5	4.7–5.3	—	4.9–5.1	—
	6.3–8.0	4.3–6.3	3.9–6.8	3.6–5.9	3.8–7.9	5.0–6.5
Chloride (mEq/L)	99–108	85–102	94–99	—	92–97	—
	105–118	100–109	92–103	93–118	90–115	105–115
Cholesterol (mg/dL)	—	36–100	94–237	—	—	—
	59–103	44–138	65–148	90–141	16–43	40–100
Total bilirubin (mg/dL)	—	0–0.6	0.2–0.5	—	0–0.9	—
	0.3–0.8	0.2–0.5	0.2–0.7	0.8–1.6	0–0.9	—
Alkaline phosphatase (IU/L)	66–262	70–132	8–202	—	66–74	—
	43–71	40–191	6–14.2	—	55–108	3–12
Alanine aminotransferase (IU/L)	40–189	26–37	28–107	—	39–45	—
	44–87	52–144	22–63	—	25–59	10–35
Aspartate aminotransferase (IU/L)	77–383	40–53	53–202	—	46–48	—
	101–214	54–192	43–134	—	26–68	15–45
Lactate dehydrogenase (IU/L)	—	63–573	94–237	—	—	—
	366	225–275	134–360	—	—	—
Creatine kinase (IU/L)	155	6–309	469–1553	—	—	—
	155	111–334	366–776	—	—	—

Top row of data in each column is compiled from the ranges of mean values without consideration of stain, age, gender, and method of blood collection as published in Loeb and Quimby [10], pp. 417–509.
Second row of data in each column is obtained from Quesenberry and Carpenter [11], pp. 243 and 290.

that use glucose oxidase, thus resulting in a false-negative glucose determination.

Proteinuria is common in normal mice and rats. The semiquantitative urine chemical strips detect large-molecular-weight proteins such as albumin but not the low-molecular-weight glycoproteins of renal origin that are found in the urine of rodents. The normal proteinuria of rodents is associated with a variety of urinary proteins, which include a- and b-globulins, uromucoid protein, and prealbumin. The degree of proteinuria increases with age, and male mice tend to be more proteinuric than female mice.

Rodent urine sediment normally contains fewer than five erythrocytes and leukocytes per high-power field. Increases in the concentration of these cells are suggestive of urinary tract inflammation, calculi, or neoplasia. If urinary casts containing erythrocytes and leukocytes are concurrently present, cells are likely of renal origin, whereas increased numbers of cells without casts are suggestive of lower urinary tract inflammation, such as cystitis and urethritis. Interpretation of rodent urine sediment findings is the same as that described for domestic mammals.

Table 35.2 Plasma biochemical values in rabbits.

	a	b
Glucose (mg/dL)	89–144	75–155
Urea nitrogen (mg/dL)	14–23	13–29
Creatinine (mg/dL)	0.8–2.9	0.5–2.5
Uric acid (mg/dL)	1.1–1.2	—
Total protein (g/dL)	5.0–8.5	5.4–8.3
Albumin (g/dL)	3.0–3.4	2.4–4.6
Calcium (mg/dL)	13.0–15.0	5.6–12.5
Phosphorus (mg/dL)	5.6–9.2	4.0–6.9
Sodium (mEq/L)	114–156	131–155
Potassium (mEq/L)	4.4–7.4	3.6–6.9
Chloride (mEq/L)	89–120	92–112
Cholesterol (mg/dL)	22–69	10–80
Total bilirubin (mg/dL)	0–0.7	0–0.7
Alkaline phosphatase (IU/L)	<120	4–16
Alanine aminotransferase (IU/L)	<100	48–80
Aspartate aminotransferase (IU/L)	<100	14–113
Lactate dehydrogenase (IU/L)	<200	34–129
Creatine kinase (IU/L)	<275	—

[a]Data compiled from the ranges of mean values without consideration of stain, age, gender, and method of blood collection as published in Loeb and Quimby [10], pp. 417–509.
[b]Data from Quesenberry and Carpenter [11], p. 151.

Table 35.3 Plasma biochemical values in ferrets.

	All ferrets[a]	Albino[b]	Fitch[b]
Glucose (mg/dL)	67–124	94–207	63–134
Urea nitrogen (mg/dL)	17–32	10–45	12–43
Creatinine (mg/dL)	0.2–0.6	0.4–0.9	0.2–0.6
Total protein (g/dL)	5.3–7.2	5.1–7.4	5.3–7.2
Albumin (g/dL)	3.3–4.1	2.6–3.8	3.3–4.1
Calcium (mg/dL)	8.5–11	8.0–11.8	8.6–10.5
Phosphorus (mg/dL)	3.3–7.8	4.0–9.1	5.6–8.7
Sodium (mEq/L)	146–160	137–162	146–160
Potassium (mEq/L)	3.7–5.4	4.5–7.7	4.3–5.3
Chloride (mEqLl)	112–129	106–125	102–121
Cholesterol (mg/dL)	60–220	64–296	119–209
Total bilirubin (mg/dL)	0.0–0.3	<1.0	0–0.1
Total Co_2 (mmol/L)	17–23	16.5–28	16–28
Alkaline phosphatase (IU/L)	30–120	9–84	30–120
Alanine aminotransferase (IU/L)	30–100	82–287	78–149
Aspartate aminotransferase (IU/L)	15–40	28–120	57–248
Creatine kinase (IU/L)	60–300	—	—

[a]Data from Thrall et al. [12], p. 471.
[b]Data from Quesenberry and Carpenter [11], p. 20.

Table 35.4 Plasma biochemical values in sugar gliders and hedgehogs.

	Sugar gliders	Hedgehogs
Glucose (mg/dL)	130–183	89+/−30
Urea nitrogen (mg/dL)	18–24	13–54
Creatinine (mg/dL)	0.3–0.5	0–0.8
Total protein (g/dL)	5.1–6.1	4.0–7.7
Albumin (g/dL)	3.5–4.3	1.8–4.2
Calcium (mg/dL)	6.9–8.4	5.2–11.3
Phosphorus (mg/dL)	3.8–4.4	2.4–12.0
Sodium (mEq/L)	135–145	120–165
Potassium (mEq/L)	3.3–5.9	3.2–7.2
Chloride (mEq/L)	—	92–128
Cholesterol (mg/dL)	—	86–189
Total bilirubin (mg/dL)	0.4–0.8	0–1.3
Alkaline phosphatase (IU/L)	—	8–92
Alanine aminotransferase (IU/L)	50–106	16–134
Aspartate aminotransferase (IU/L)	46–179	8–137
Lactate dehydrogenase (IU/L)	—	57–820
Creatine kinase (IU/L)	210–589	333–1964
γ-Glutamyl transferase (IU/L)	—	0–12

Data from Quesenberry and Carpenter [11], pp. 335 and 345.

Electrolytes and acid-base

Interpretation of serum or plasma electrolyte and acid-base changes in rodents is the same as that described in domestic mammals. Normal serum and plasma sodium concentrations in mice (174 ± 23 mEq/L or mmol/L) tend to be slightly greater than those reported for other mammals. Hypernatremia resulting from neurogenic diabetes insipidus occurs as a hereditary disorder in some strains of rat. Nephrogenic diabetes insipidus, which usually is associated with renal amyloidosis, frequently occurs in certain strains of mice and aged Syrian hamsters. Chronic nephropathies causing abnormal retention of sodium in rats may cause hypernatremia, which in turn results in myocarditis. Renal amyloidosis alters the renal tubular permeability to water, thereby resulting in hyperchloremia. Increased serum and plasma phosphorus concentrations occur in younger rodents compared with concentrations in adults. Serum or plasma magnesium concentrations increase in hamsters during hibernation.

Laboratory evaluation of the liver

Serum or plasma enzymes commonly used to detect liver disease in rodents include AP, GGT, AST, ALT, LD, and SDH. Serum or plasma concentrations of these enzymes increase with increased production, increased release, or decreased clearance. Other biochemical tests to detect liver disease in rodents include serum or plasma total bilirubin, bile acid, and cholesterol concentrations.

Table 35.5 Plasma concentrations of the major hormones in rodents.

	Rats	Mice	Hamsters	Guinea pigs
Triiodothyronine (ng/dL)	30–100	30–100	30–80	20–60
Free triiodothyronine (ng/dL)	—	—	—	0.20–0.32
Thyroxine (μg/dL)	3–7	3–7	3–7	2–4
Free thyroxine (μg/dL)	—	—	—	0.9–2.0
Thyroid-stimulating hormone (ng/mL)	400–600	300	300	40–100
Adrenocorticotropic hormone (pg/dL)	30–100	2.6–5.5	40[a]	23[a]
Corticosterone (μg/dL)	15–23[b] 1–6[c]	9[a, d] (males) 40[a d] (females) 5[a e] (males) 13.5[a e] (females)	2.75[e] (males) 0.33[e] (females)	—
Cortisol (μg/dL)	—	—	—	5–30
Free cortisol (μg/dL)	—		—	0.6–5.8
Parathormone (pg/mL)	70–700 (males) 0–400 (females)	—	—	—
Calcitonin (pg/mL)	200–500 (6–8 mo-old males) 450–1100 (6–8 mo-old females) 400–900 (12–14 mo-old males) 700–1800 (12–14 mo-old females)			
1,25-dihydroxy-vitamin D (pg/mL)	72–86 (males) 79–113 (females)			

[a]Average concentration.
[b]Mean maximum value.
[c]Mean minimum value.
[d]Start of dark period.
[e]End of dark period.

Table 35.6 Plasma concentrations of the major hormones in rabbits.

Triiodothyronine (ng/dL)	130–143
Thyroxine (μg/dL)	1.7–2.4
Thyroid-stimulating hormone (μU/mL)	40–100
Protein-bound iodine (nmol/L)	400 (adults)
Adrenocorticotropic hormone (pg/dL)	25[a]
Cortisol (μg/dL)	2.6–3.8 (early morning)
Aldosterone (ng/dL)	20[a] (early morning) 50[a] (late afternoon)
Calcitonin (pg/mL)	1125–1200
1,25-dihydroxy-vitamin D (pg/mL)	27–47

[a]Average concentration.

AP is a membrane-bound enzyme with highest activity in osteoblasts, biliary epithelium, and epithelial cells of the kidneys and intestines. Young rodents have higher plasma AP activity than adults because of osteoblastic activity, and male rats tend to have higher plasma AP activities than female rats. Hepatic AP of rodents is heat labile at 56 °C and sensitive to levamisole inhibition [5]. Significant increases in serum or plasma AP activity occur in rodents with hepatic cholestasis. Ligation of the bile duct in rats produces elevation of both hepatic and intestinal AP isoenzymes. Plasma or serum AP activity is a more sensitive test than bilirubin or ALT for detection of hepatic disease in hamsters [14, 15]. Drugs that increase AP synthesis and plasma activity in rats include cortisol, phenobarbital, and theophylline [7]. Increased plasma AP activity occurs in zinc- and manganese-deficient guinea pigs [16].

Plasma GGT activity is significantly increased in hamsters and rats with experimentally induced hepatic injury resulting in cholestasis. Guinea pigs have higher hepatic GGT activity than rats and demonstrate higher plasma GGT activities with cholestasis. Serum GGT activity is increased in guinea pigs after *in vitro* blood clot formation, which can be avoided with use of plasma for enzyme testing. The kidneys of rodents have the highest GGT activity, but the enzyme is nondetectable in the plasma or serum of most rodents. The kidneys of rats have 200–300-fold the GGT activity of the liver.

AST is a mitochondrial and cytosolic enzyme with high activity in the liver, heart, skeletal muscle, and kidney and low activity in the intestines, brain, lung, and testes. Increases in plasma or serum AST activity usually are associated with hepatic, cardiac muscle, or skeletal muscle injury.

In rats and mice, the activity of ALT, which is a cytosolic and mitochondrial isoenzyme, is highest in the liver. The ratio of the cytosolic to mitochondrial ALT isoenzymes in the liver and heart muscle of rats is 5 : 1 and 50 : 1, respectively. In rodents, the intestines, kidneys, heart, skeletal muscle, brain, skin, and pancreas also have ALT activity. In guinea pigs, ALT activity in the heart is almost equal to that in the liver. Plasma and serum ALT activity increases with hepatocellular damage in most rodents, and the enzyme appears to be liver specific in rats and mice. Plasma ALT, however, does not appear to have diagnostic value for hepatic disease in guinea pigs, which have only half the hepatic ALT activity of rats and mice. Increases in serum ALT activity correlate with the degree of hepatic necrosis in rats. A threefold increase in plasma ALT activity occurs in mice that are restrained by holding the body compared with those that are restrained by the tail.

LD is a cytosolic enzyme with the highest activity in skeletal muscle, followed by cardiac muscle, liver, kidney, and intestines, respectively. In the mouse, LD is characterized by five isoenzymes: LD-1 and LD-2 are found in cardiac muscle, LD-5 in the liver and skeletal muscle, and LD-3 in most other tissues. Serum or plasma LD activity elevates with hepatocellular disease in rodents; however, normal values are highly variable and depend on the analytic method used.

SDH is a cytosolic enzyme that is found in the liver, kidney, and seminal vesicles of mice but is liver specific in rats. Increases in serum or plasma SDH activity occur with hepatic disease in rodents and is a more sensitive test than ALT for detection of hepatocellular disease in rats. SDH assays usually are not performed by veterinary laboratories.

Serum and plasma total bilirubin concentration increases in rodents with primary hepatobiliary disease, extra hepatic biliary obstruction, or hemolysis. Increases in plasma or serum total bilirubin concentration should be evaluated by determining the erythrocyte mass and performing other tests that evaluate the liver or biliary system.

The total serum and plasma bile acid concentration is a sensitive and specific test for hepatobiliary disease and disorders of the enterohepatic circulation. Plasma bile acid concentration has an excellent potential for detecting hepatobiliary disease in rodents, especially rats with a high concentration of circulating bile acids.

The plasma cholesterol concentration may increase in rodents with extrahepatic biliary obstruction. Normal plasma cholesterol concentration varies between strains of mice. Hypercholesterolemia often is associated with fatty infiltration of many tissues. In guinea pigs, the intestine, rather than the liver, is the primary site of cholesterol production [8]. Normal plasma cholesterol concentration (112–210 mg/dL or 2.90–5.43 mmol/L) of hamsters is higher than that of other rodents and decreases during short photoperiods but increases with cold temperatures [4, 14].

Laboratory evaluation of proteins

The normal plasma protein concentration in mice varies among strains. In mice, hyperproteinemia often is associated with severe dehydration and often occurs with loss of urinary protein from renal disease. The major classes of serum or plasma proteins in rodents are evaluated using electrophoresis. The major globulins of rats are α_1- and β-globulins, with lower concentrations of α_2- and γ-globulins. In hamsters, albumin concentrations decrease during the first year of life, α_2-globulins increase during the first 6 months of age, and β-globulins decrease at 8 weeks of age [4, 14, 17]. Fibrinogen migrates into the γ-globulin peaks in hamster protein electrophoretic scans. Amyloidosis is a common disease of hamsters older than 18 months and results in hypoalbuminemia and hyperglobulinemia.

Laboratory evaluation of glucose metabolism

Cells must be quickly separated from the serum or plasma of rodents, or fluoride added to the collection tube, to prevent decreased glucose concentration because of *in vitro* glycolysis (a decrease by 7% is expected if the sample sits for 1 hour at room temperature). The plasma glucose concentration in rats and mice decreases with age, with an average decrease of 2 mg/dL per month in the latter. Blood glucose concentrations are also affected by nutrition/diet, hormonal changes, hibernation, restraint, fasting, and anesthesia.

Many strains of mice are used as animal models for diabetes mellitus; therefore, glucose tolerance tests have been developed for mice [18]. A 1-hour glucose tolerance test compares the preinjection plasma glucose concentration to the glucose concentration obtained 1 hour after an intra peritoneal injection of glucose at a dose of 2 mg/g body weight. A 4-hour oral glucose tolerance test compares the baseline plasma glucose concentration with a plasma glucose concentration obtained 4 hours after the oral administration of a 10% glucose solution at a dose of 10 ml/kg. Certain strains of rodents, such as ob/ob obese mice, Zucker fatty rat (fa/fa), and the LA/N corpulent rat, are used as animal models for noninsulin-dependent diabetes mellitus. The Chinese hamster and Wistar BB rat are animal models for insulin-dependent diabetes mellitus. Insulin-dependent diabetes may result in guinea pigs from an infectious agent that causes fatty degeneration of the pancreas and affects both exocrine and endocrine pancreatic functions; affected guinea pigs have hyperglycemia, glucosuria, ketonuria, and beta-cell hypoplasia. Immunoassays for the determination of insulin in rats can be calibrated to measure plasma insulin in mice, but guinea pig insulin is immunologically different and cannot be determined using rat antibodies. Rat glucagon is measured using human immunoassay techniques; however, guinea pig glucagon, like insulin, is immunologically different and cannot be determined with human antibodies.

Laboratory detection of muscle injury

CK is a dimeric cytosolic enzyme that is composed of M and B subunits. Skeletal muscle contains MM subunits, and cardiac muscle contains MM, MB, and BB subunits. Brain contains BB subunits. As in domestic mammals, plasma CK activity is a useful marker for muscle injury in rodents. Nutritional myopathies, such as those resulting from hypovitaminosis E and selenium deficiency, cause increased plasma CK activity in rats and mice.

Laboratory evaluation of endocrine disorders

The major hormones of rodents are secreted into the peripheral blood in a circadian rhythm that may vary among species. Hormonal secretion also is influenced by environmental factors, such as light-dark cycle. An ultradian rhythm, in which hormones are secreted in an episodic or pulsatile manner with a periodicity of less than 24 hours, can be superimposed on the normal circadian secretion of a hormone. Suggested ranges for the major plasma hormones in rodents are provided in Table 35.5.

Normal male rats have higher plasma thyroid-stimulating hormone (TSH) concentrations with use of reference preparation-1 standard from the National Hormone and Pituitary Program compared with normal female rats. Plasma TSH concentrations of normal female rats peak at the onset of the light cycle. Mice and hamsters have lower normal plasma TSH concentrations compared with rats (according to the same assay method used for rats). A bioassay method using radio-labeled iodine also can be used to obtain plasma TSH concentrations in rodents.

Plasma or serum thyroxine (T_4) and triiodothyronine (T_3) concentrations in rodents can be measured by radio immunoassay. Transport proteins and binding affinity for T_4 and T_3 vary among species. In rats and mice, approximately 80% of the bound T_3 and T_4 are bound to albumin and 20% to T_4-binding prealbumin. Approximately 0.05% of plasma T_4 and 0.25% of T_3 in rats is the free, physiologically active form. Normal plasma total T_4 and T_3 concentrations in rats and mice vary between different strains but generally range between 3 and 7 μg/dL and 30 and 100 ng/dL, respectively. Plasma T_4 and T_3 concentrations exhibit a diurnal rhythm, in which peak concentrations occur during the light phase and minimum concentrations during the dark phase.

Normal plasma adrenocorticotropic hormone (ACTH) concentrations in rodents have been determined using either radioimmunoassay or bioassay techniques. The plasma ACTH concentration in normal mice exhibits a normal circadian rhythm, in which minimal concentrations occur during the morning and peak concentrations during the afternoon.

Corticosterone, which is the primary glucocorticoid in the plasma of mice and rats, exhibits a marked diurnal variation that is affected by the light cycle. In mice, maximum plasma corticosterone concentrations occur at the start of the dark period and minimum concentrations at the end of the dark period. Male mice have lower plasma corticosterone concentrations compared with female mice. Maximum plasma corticosterone concentrations occur late during the light period in rats, and minimum concentrations occur during the end of the dark period. In rats, approximately 80% of plasma corticosterone is bound to transcortin and 10% to albumin, thereby leaving 10% or less in the free, unbound state. Both corticosterone and cortisol are found in the plasma of normal hamsters. The total plasma glucocorticoid concentration 5.5 hours after onset of the light period in hamsters averages 1.8 μg/dL, with an average corticosterone : cortisol ratio of 3.5. The plasma corticosterone concentration is greater in male hamsters than in female hamsters. Cortisol is the primary glucocorticoid in the plasma of normal guinea pigs. Guinea pigs demonstrate maximum plasma cortisol concentrations late in the light period and, again, late in the dark period. Minimum concentrations occur early during the light period and, again, during the middle of the dark period. The stress of restraint or removal of a cagemate significantly increases plasma glucocorticoid concentrations. A twofold increase in plasma corticosterone concentration occurs in rats with 2 minutes of restraint, and a 12-fold increase results after 20 minutes of restraint.

In rodents, plasma concentrations of the calcium-regulating hormones parathormone, calcitonin, and 1, 25-dihydroxyvitamin D_3 are influenced by dietary calcium, age, gender, photoperiod, and strain. Using radio immunoassay techniques, the normal plasma parathormone concentration in male rats tends to be greater than that in female rats.

Normal plasma calcitonin concentrations of rats are extremely variable because of age, stage of light cycle, strain, and gender. Plasma calcitonin concentrations also are influenced by the stage of estrus in females, in which maximum concentrations occur during proestrus. Six- to 8-month-old male Wistar rats have lower plasma calcitonin concentrations compared with 12–14-month-old Wistar rats. Male Wistar rats also have lower plasma calcitonin concentrations than female rats. Plasma concentrations of 1, 25-dihydroxyvitamin D vary in rats with strain, gender, and dietary calcium intake. Normal male Wistar rats have lower plasma 1, 25-dihydroxyvitamin D concentrations than females.

Cholesterol and triglycerides are the most commonly measured lipids, and significant interspecies differences in normal values are expected. High levels of lipids cause lipemia, which interferes with other biochemical assays using photometric analytics. Because cholesterol typically peaks following a meal, fasting is required to improve accuracy of the test.

Lipoproteins are macromolecules that transfer lipids and cholesterol and are classified by a density value that varies inversely with molecular size. Low-density lipoproteins (LDL), also known as beta lipoproteins, carry cholesterol from the liver to the tissues. High-density lipoproteins (HDL), also known as alpha lipoproteins, carry cholesterol from the tissues to the liver. Very-low-density lipoproteins (VLDL) are primarily made up of triglycerides, glycerol bound to three fatty acids, which are broken down by pancreatic lipase.

Rabbits (*Oryctolagus cuniculus*)

Laboratory evaluation of the kidneys

Laboratory evaluation of the kidneys in rabbits is the same as that for rodents and domestic mammals. Plasma urea nitrogen (BUN) and creatinine commonly are used as markers for renal function in rabbits. In general, the normal BUN of rabbits lies between 10 and 30 mg/dL (3.57–10.71 mmol/L) and the normal creatinine between 0.5–2.5 mg/dL (44.2–221 μmol/L). However, the normal plasma urea nitrogen of rabbits is influenced by breed, strain, and gender. Protein catabolism associated with high dietary protein intake, vigorous exercise, dehydration, or urinary tract disease (such as urolithiasis, obstruction of urine flow, urethral ligation, and kidney disease) increases plasma urea nitrogen concentration. Decreases in BUN may be associated with hepatic insufficiency and wasting of body mass caused by dental disease. The time of day when the blood sample is taken also influences the plasma urea nitrogen concentration in rabbits, in which peak concentrations occur between 4.00 and 8.00 p.m. Plasma urea nitrogen and creatinine are insensitive tests for renal disease in rabbits, however, requiring a 50–75% loss of function before plasma concentrations increase. Renal failure in rabbits is often associated with increased plasma BUN, creatinine, calcium, phosphorus, and potassium concentrations. Renal failure rabbits may also exhibit isosthenuria and depending upon the cause (i.e., nephritis) may exhibit proteinuria, ketonuria, pyuria, and urinary cast formation.

Calcium and phosphorus

The normal plasma calcium concentration of 13–15 mg/dL (3.24–3.74 mmol/L) of rabbits is higher than that of most other mammals. The mean urinary fractional calcium excretion of rabbits is 45–65%, compared with less than 2% in other mammals. Excess dietary calcium is absorbed and excreted in the urine of rabbits compared to other animals where it is excreted in the bile. This predisposes rabbits to urinary calculi. Increases in calcium concentration may be associated with renal disease and decreases may be associated with poor diet, hypoalbuminemia, diarrhea, chronic renal disease, and hyperparathyroidism.

The normal plasma phosphorus concentration of rabbits is 2.3–6.7 mg/dL (0.74–2.16 mmol/L). An increase is often associated with renal disease but can be artificially elevated with hemolysis. A decrease can be associated with urinary calcium excretion [1].

Electrolytes and acid-base

Normal plasma electrolyte concentrations of rabbits vary with the breed and strain. The normal plasma sodium concentrations of rabbits generally range between 131 and 155 mEq/L (mmol/L). Because sodium values vary significantly between breeds, it is often not a useful diagnostic indicator in rabbits [1]. Increased sodium concentrations are expected with dehydration, fluid loss with diarrhea, excess dietary salt, peritonitis, and burns. Decreased sodium concentration is seen with acute and chronic renal failure, polyuria, and polydipsia.

Normal plasma chloride values of rabbits generally range between 92 and 120 mEq/L (mmol/L). Increased chloride values are expected with dehydration and excess dietary salt and decreased values are expected with diarrhea and low dietary salt.

Normal plasma potassium concentrations of rabbits generally range between 3.5–6.9 mEq/L (mmol/L). Hyperkalemia is seen with acute renal failure, obstructed urine flow, metabolic acidosis, and severe tissue trauma. Hypokalemia is associated with renal failure, starvation, low dietary potassium, and stress-induced increase in catecholamines.

Normal plasma magnesium concentrations of most rabbits are between 2.0 and 4.5 mg/dL. Magnesium is excreted mainly in the urine of rabbits compared to excretion in the bile by other mammals [1]. Increased magnesium values can be associated with dehydration, hyperthyroidism, tissue trauma, and adrenocortical insufficiency.

The normal bicarbonate concentration in the plasma of rabbits generally ranges between 16.2 and 38.0 mEq/L (mmol/L). Because the kidneys of rabbits have a weak ability to correct acid-base imbalances, these animals are susceptible to electrolyte abnormalities [1].

The serum iron- and total iron-binding capacity of normal rabbits vary with the time of day when the blood was collected, with the lowest concentrations occurring at 8:00 a.m. and the highest at 8:00 p.m. Serum iron concentrations of normal rabbits range between 165 and 250 μg/dL (29.6–44.8 μmol/L) [2].

Laboratory evaluation of the liver

Plasma enzymes used to detect liver disease in rabbits include ALT, AST, LD, glutamate dehydrogenase, AP, and GGT. In rabbits, ALT activity is equal in the liver and cardiac muscle; however, increased plasma ALT activity (normally 14–80 IU/L) is considered by some to be a specific indicator of liver disease in rabbits. The degree of hepatic necrosis correlates positively with the increase in plasma ALT activity.

Interestingly, the rabbit liver ALT activity (approximately 5 hours) is less than half that of the dog causing some to find this enzyme not to be a useful indicator of liver damage in rabbits. Significant AST activity occurs in the liver, heart, skeletal muscle, kidney, and pancreas of rabbits. Therefore, increases in plasma AST activity (normally 14–113 IU/L) are suggestive of injury to one or more of these tissues. Increased plasma AST activity can be associated with liver damage, hepatic coccidiosis, heat stress, or muscle cell damage or excursion (associated with restraint). Increases in plasma AST activity may be associated with cardiac or skeletal muscle injury during blood collection by cardiocentesis or use of restraint methods that cause exertion. LD activity is present in a wide variety of tissues, with each demonstrating a different isoenzyme composition that corresponds with isoenzymes 1 through 5 in humans. Isoenzyme LD-1 and LD-2 predominate in the liver and skeletal muscle. Because erythrocytes have high LD activity, hemolysis may result in high plasma LD activity. The plasma LD activity (normally 30–140 IU/L) can be used to detect liver disease in rabbits, but because of its wide tissue distribution and the effect of handling and hemolysis on plasma activity, it is not commonly used. Plasma glutamate dehydrogenase activity (range, 5.5–7.0 IU/L) and SDH (range, 170–177 IU/L), although not commonly measured in veterinary laboratories, may be useful in the evaluation of hepatocellular injury in rabbits.

The normal plasma AP activity (range, 10–140 IU/L) of rabbits varies with age, breed, and strain. Young rabbits are expected to have two to four times the plasma AP activity of adult rabbits. Rabbits are unique in having three AP isoenzymes. Rabbits have an intestinal and two liver/kidney forms, compared with the intestinal and liver/kidney/bone forms found in mammals other than primates. The predominant liver/kidney isoenzyme of rabbits is similar to the intestinal form and the minor liver/kidney isoenzyme to the liver/kidney/bone isoenzyme of other mammals. The predominant liver AP isoenzyme is not inhibited by levamisole or heating to 56 °F, as the hepatic AP isoenzyme of other mammals is. The plasma GGT activity of normal rabbits is less than 8 IU/L (mmol/L), is derived primarily from bile duct epithelial cells, and increases significantly in rabbits with hepatobiliary obstruction (lipidosis, hepatic coccidiosis, liver lobe torsion, hepatic abscesses, and neoplasia).

Rabbit bile contains approximately 70% biliverdin and 30% bilirubin, of which 90% is conjugated as a mono conjugate. Normal rabbit plasma lacks biliverdin, however, and the normal bilirubin concentration (range, 0–0.8 mg/dL or 0–13.68 μmol/L) is low. A marked increase in plasma bilirubin concentration is expected in rabbits with biliary obstruction (hepatic coccidiosis, hepatic neoplasia, lipidosis, liver lobe torsion, hepatic fibrosis).

The normal plasma cholesterol concentration of rabbits varies with age, breed, strain, and gender. In general, the normal plasma cholesterol concentration will range between 10 and 80 mg/dL (0.26–2.07 mmol/L). At birth, the plasma cholesterol concentration is approximately that of adults, increases by 25 days of age, and then returns to the adult concentrations by 60–80 days of age. Normal adult male rabbits have twice the plasma cholesterol concentration of adult female rabbits. A diurnal variation in plasma cholesterol occurs as well, with peak concentrations being seen between 4:00 and 8:00 p.m. This may be associated with cecotrophy. The plasma cholesterol concentration may increase in rabbits with extrahepatic biliary obstruction. Rabbits are used extensively as animal models for cholesterol metabolism studies because of their ability to rapidly develop cholesterolemia with high-cholesterol diets. Daily feeding of 1 g of cholesterol increases the serum cholesterol concentration to greater than 1000 mg/dL. The Watanabe heritable hyperlipemic rabbit, which primarily exhibits LDL cholesterol, is an animal model for familial hypercholesterolemia in humans.

Increased plasma cholesterol concentration may be associated with anorexia and representing end stage hepatic lipidosis; pancreatitis; diabetes mellitus; nephrotic syndrome; and chronic renal failure. Decreased cholesterol may be associated with liver failure, malnutrition, or pregnancy.

The normal serum lipoprotein distributions of adult female rabbits are 46–58% HDL, which transports approximately two-thirds of the total cholesterol; 9–15% pre- or intermediate-density lipoprotein or VLDL; and 30–42% LDL. High-cholesterol diets fed to rabbits lead to a 20–40-fold increase in VLDL and a four to fivefold increase in LDL. Pregnant rabbits show a decrease in HDL and an increase in LDL [1].

Liver function tests that evaluate plasma disappearance and biliary excretion of dyes, such as sulfobromophthalein (BSP) and indocyanine green (ICG), have been characterized for rabbits. The overall rate of BSP clearance for rabbits has been reported as 1.8 mg/min per kg, in which 75% of the BSP is excreted in the conjugated form. Intravenous BSP dosages of 30, 60, and 120 mg/kg result in 32-minute plasma concentrations of 1, 2, and 20 mg/dL, respectively [19]. ICG is excreted in the bile in the unconjugated form. Rabbits have a curvilinear plasma ICG clearance curve, with a greater capacity to remove ICG from the circulation than either dogs or rats. Rabbits that are given intravenous ICG dosages of 8, 16, and 32 mg/kg demonstrate disappearance rates of 46%, 20%, and 10% per minute, respectively [2].

The normal plasma bile acid concentration of rabbits generally ranges between 0 and 40 mmol/L, but comparison of pre- and postprandial values in healthy rabbits is difficult because of cecotrophy. Persistent high bile acid concentrations may be associated with liver disease.

Laboratory evaluation of proteins

The normal plasma total protein concentration in rabbits (range, 5.4–8.3 g/dL or 54–83 g/L) varies slightly with breed, strain, and gender. Approximately 40–60% of the total plasma protein is albumin (range, 2.4–4.6 g/dL or 24–46 g/L). The normal plasma globulin concentration generally ranges between 1.5–2.8 g/dL or 15–28 g/L. The normal protein electrophoretic components of rabbit serum also include 5–10% α_1-globulin, 5–10% α_2-globulin, 5–15% β-globulin, and 5–15% γ-globulin. The normal albumin to globulin ratio ranges between 0.5 and 1.2. Female rabbits tend to have higher plasma albumin concentrations than male rabbits. Severe renal and hepatic diseases are responsible for most disorders that result in hypoproteinemia and hypoalbuminemia in rabbits. Hyperproteinemia commonly occurs with dehydration, shock, and hyperthermia. Increased globulin concentrations may be associated with coronavirus infections [1].

Laboratory evaluation of glucose metabolism

The normal plasma glucose concentration of rabbits is influenced by genetics, age, and diet. Pre- and postprandial plasma glucose variation occurs, in which the lowest plasma glucose concentrations are found 1 hour before feeding and the highest 3 hours after a meal. Healthy rabbits can maintain normal plasma glucose concentrations during short periods of fasting (e.g., <16 hours). Extreme hyperglycemia (values greater than 500 mg/dL or 27.76 mmol/L) occurs with diabetes mellitus. Hyperglycemia and increased plasma urea nitrogen concentration occur with the increased protein catabolism associated with hyperthermia. Hyperglycemia resulting from glycogenolysis because of stress occurs early in the course of mucoid enteropathy. This common digestive tract disorder of the rabbit causes anorexia, and when glycogen stores become depleted, the rabbit develops hypoglycemia. Hypoglycemia can also be associated with acute sepsis, liver failure, or other chronic disease. It should be mentioned that the use of the human portable blood glucose meters are acceptable for point-of-care testing of blood glucose concentration in rabbits when laboratory analyzers are not available; however, the use of the veterinary portable blood glucose meters often result in overestimation of glucose concentrations in some rabbits [20].

Laboratory detection of muscle injury

Laboratory detection of muscle injury in rabbits follows the same methods as that in rodents and domestic mammals, in which plasma CK, AST, and LD activities are sensitive to muscle injury. Blood collected by cardiocentesis contains CK-MB isoenzyme activity that is not found in serum collected from the ear vein. Blood collected by jugular venipuncture also contains CK-MB activity. Plasma CK activity (normal range, 150–5000 IU/L), primarily the CK-MM isoenzyme, is a rapid, sensitive, and specific indicator of muscle disease in rabbits, and it increases more rapidly than AST and LD activities after muscle injury (which could be associated with restraint). Nutritional-related myopathies, such as those caused by hypovitaminosis E and selenium deficiency, result in increased plasma CK activity.

Laboratory evaluation of endocrine disorders

Laboratory evaluation of endocrine disorders in rabbits follows the same methods as that in rodents and domestic mammals. The TSH concentration in rabbit serum can be obtained using a bioassay method that measures the percentage increase in blood levels of radiolabeled iodine. Serum T_4 and T_3 concentrations from normal rabbits are listed in Table 35.6. The serum protein-bound iodine concentration, as an indicator of thyroid function in rabbits, increases by 20 days of age before decreasing to adult concentrations by 60 days of age. The serum protein-bound iodine concentration varies with strain, gender, and time of day. The plasma ACTH concentration of rabbits as determined by bioassay is subject to circadian variation. The major plasma glucocorticoid of rabbits is cortisol. Evidence is suggestive that genetics and circadian rhythms influence the plasma aldosterone concentration of rabbits, but little information is available regarding the plasma concentration of parathyroid hormone in rabbits.

Laboratory evaluation of amylase

The normal plasma amylase activity of rabbits generally ranges between 200 and 500 IU/L. Increases are associated with pancreatitis, pancreatic duct obstruction, peritonitis, renal failure, and treatment with corticosteroids [1].

Ferrets (*Mustelus putorius furo*)

Laboratory evaluation of the kidneys

Laboratory evaluation of renal function in ferrets involves blood biochemical tests, such as plasma urea nitrogen, creatinine, protein, bicarbonate, and electrolyte concentrations, and urinalysis. Interpretive considerations for the biochemical tests used to evaluate the kidneys are the same as those in domestic carnivorous mammals such as cats and dogs. In normal and azotemic ferrets, the plasma creatinine concentration is lower than that in dogs and cats. The mean plasma creatine concentration of healthy ferrets is 0.4–0.6 mg/dL (35.4–53.0 μmol/L) with a range of 0.2–0.9 mg/dL (17.7–79.6 μmol/L) [21]. As a result, a moderate increase in the plasma creatinine concentration (i.e. 1–2 mg/dL or 88.4–176.8 μmol/L) in a ferret is significant and suggestive of renal disease [22]. Insulin and exogenous creatinine clearance are sensitive tests for measuring glomerular filtration in ferrets; however, delayed clearance may occur before significant increases in plasma urea nitrogen or creatinine concentrations.

Electrolytes and acid-base

Interpretations of plasma electrolyte and acid-base disturbances in ferrets are the same as those in dogs and cats.

Disorders that commonly result in electrolyte disturbances in dogs and cats, hypoadrenocorticism, hyperaldosteronism, primary hyperparathyroidism, pseudohyperparathyroidism, hypoparathyroidism, and hypercalcitonism, have been poorly documented in ferrets.

Laboratory evaluation of the liver

Evaluation of the livers in ferrets by laboratory testing is the same as that for those in dogs and cats. The ferret liver has 3–10-fold more ALT activity than any other tissue, and the plasma ALT activity is a sensitive and specific test for hepatocellular disease in ferrets. Ferrets with hepatocellular disease commonly have increased AST and LD activities as well. Those with cholestasis likely have increased plasma AP and GGT activities. Ferrets rarely become icteric or have plasma bilirubin concentrations greater than 2.0 mg/dL, even when hepatobiliary disease is severe [22, 23].

Laboratory evaluation of proteins

The causes of hypoproteinemia and hyperproteinemia in ferrets are the same as those in dogs and cats. Ferrets with Aleutian disease typically demonstrate hypoalbuminemia and hyperglobulinemia, in which more than 20% of the total protein is γ-globulins [22].

Laboratory evaluation of glucose metabolism

A high incidence of insulin-secreting pancreatic neoplasms (i.e., insulinomas) resulting in hypoglycemia occurs among domestic ferrets in North America. The normal plasma glucose concentration of ferrets varies with the genetic type. A 4–5-hour fasting plasma glucose level often is used to screen ferrets for insulinomas. It should be noted that significant underestimation of blood glucose concentrations has been detected with use of portable blood glucose meters, which will have a substantial impact on clinical decision making; therefore, verification of blood glucose concentrations in ferrets with a laboratory analyzer is highly recommended [24]. Fasting plasma glucose concentrations less than 60 mg/dL (3.33 mmol/L) are supportive of a presumptive diagnosis of insulinoma, whereas concentrations between 60 and 90 mg/dL (3.33–5.0 mmol/L) merely are suggestive of an insulinoma. Concentrations greater than 90 mg/dL (5.0 mmol/L) usually are considered to be normal. Normal serum reference intervals for serum immunoreactive insulin and the insulin:glucose ratio have been reported as being 4.6–43.3 μU/mL (SI units, 33–311 pmol/L) and 3.6–34.1 μUmg (SI units, 4.6–44.2 pmol/mmol), respectively [1]. To compare immunoreactive insulin and the insulin: glucose ratio results from other laboratories using different radioimmunoassay kits to these reference intervals, however, one must validate the results by demonstrating a high correlation between the two assay methods. Although rarely utilized because measurement of a fasting plasma glucose concentration provides the most reliable method for establishing a strong presumptive diagnosis for insulinoma in the ferret, calculation of an amended insulin:glucose ratio (AIGR) may aid in establishing the diagnosis of hyperinsulinism where

$$\text{AIGR} = \text{insulin}\ (\mu\text{U/mL}) \times 100/\text{fasting glucose}\ (\text{mg/dL}) - 30$$

in which AIGR values greater than 30 are suggestive of hyperinsulinism [25]. Other occasional causes for hypoglycemia in ferrets include delayed separation of plasma from erythrocytes, starvation, chronic hepatic disease, septicemia, and endotoxemia.

Other than a postprandial increase in plasma glucose concentration, hyperglycemia in ferrets may result from glucocorticoid excess (e.g., stress induced, exogenous corticoids, and hyperadrenocorticism), epinephrine release related to exertion, and diabetes mellitus. Diabetes mellitus in ferrets usually is iatrogenic and associated with surgical removal of pancreatic insulin-secreting neoplasms or with drugs, such as megestrol acetate, that affect insulin production and secretion.

Laboratory detection of muscle injury

Detection of muscle injury in ferrets follows the same methods as those described in dogs and cats. Increases in the nonspecific plasma enzymes AST and LD and in the specific muscle enzyme CK are to be expected with muscle injury.

Laboratory evaluation of endocrine disorders

The mean basal plasma T_4 concentration as reported for ferrets ranges between 0.99 and 2.63 μg/dL (12.7–33.8 nmol/L) [26]. A thyroid function test using 1 IU of TSH given intravenously to a ferret and measuring changes in the plasma T_4 concentration is preferable to use of thyrotropin-releasing hormone and measuring changes in the plasma T_3 concentration. The plasma T_4 concentration increases significantly as early as 2 hours after TSH stimulation in normal ferrets, whereas no increase in the plasma T_3 concentration is observed. Plasma T_4 concentration should at least double after TSH stimulation; failure to do so is suggestive of hypothyroidism.

Cortisol is the predominant circulating glucocorticoid in ferrets. The mean basal plasma cortisol concentration as reported for ferrets ranges between 0.45 and 2.13 μg/dL (12.4–58.8 nmol/L) [27]. Intravenous or intramuscular injection of ACTH at a dose of 0.5–1.0 mg/kg to a normal ferret results in a three to fourfold increase in plasma cortisol by 30 minutes that persists for as long as 1 hour. A threefold decrease in plasma cortisol concentration occurs in normal ferrets after intravenous injection of 0.2 mg of dexamethasone. This dexamethasone suppression continues even after 5 hours, when plasma cortisol concentrations demonstrate a four to fivefold decrease.

Domestic ferrets in North America experience a high incidence of adrenal gland neoplasms that produce a number of hormones. Excessive production of estradiol is a common occurrence with adrenal gland neoplasms of ferrets, but excessive cortisol production also can occur. The ACTH stimulation and dexamethasone suppression tests have not been useful in establishing the diagnosis of hyperadrenocorticism associated with adrenal neoplasia in domestic ferrets. Also, primary hyperaldosteronism should be considered as a possible cause in ferrets with hypokalemia, hypertension, and an adrenal gland mass [28].

Less common small mammal pets

African hedgehogs (*Atelerix albiventris*) and sugar gliders (*Petaurus breviceps*) are often presented for veterinary care and blood is often sampled for biochemical testing [15, 24]. Little is known about interpretation of plasma biochemical testing in these omnivorous animals; therefore, results are interpreted in the same manner as domestic nonherbivorous mammals.

Blood for plasma biochemical evaluation can be collected from hedgehogs and sugar gliders by puncture of the jugular vein or cranial vena cava. Both structures cannot be visualized; however, knowledge of their anatomical location should guide one's approach. Jugular venipuncture is performed by inserting a small gauge needle (i.e. 25 gauge) on the ventral aspect of the neck midway between the point of the shoulder and the ramus of the mandible avoiding the trachea and esophagus. Puncture of the cranial vena cava is performed by inserting the needle at the thoracic inlet (sternal notch) using a 30° angle and pointing the needle in the direction of the opposite hip.

36 Clinical Chemistry of Birds

Terry W. Campbell

Department of Clinical Sciences, College of Veterinary Medicine and Biomedical Sciences, Colorado State University, Fort Collins, CO, USA

Sample collection and handling

A blood sample representing 1% of the bird's body weight is generally accepted to be a safe volume of blood that can be obtained from nonanemic and dehydrated birds. Avian veterinarians often collect the blood sample into a syringe that contains sodium heparin; however, this is not necessary because a quality sample can be collected in a nonheparinized syringe as long as the blood is immediately transferred into a microcollection tube containing lithium heparin, which must be filled to the appropriate volume. Adding heparin to the syringe has the risk of causing sample dilution and interference with analytical testing of sodium and protein. Once the sample has been collected into a syringe, it should not be passed through the needle a second time, especially small bore needles (25 gauge or smaller); the needle should be removed before blood is dispensed into collection tube to minimize hemolysis of the sample.

Most chemical analyses are conducted on plasma, although testing could also be performed on a serum sample. The reason for this is that collection of serum from birds frequently yields a very small sample size compared to what can be obtained from plasma. This is especially important when collecting blood from very small birds. Also, avian serum often clots once it has been harvested, and the gelled sample is difficult to analyze. Therefore, based on higher sample yield and lack of clinically relevant differences from serum, plasma is a better sample choice for clinical chemistry analysis in birds.

The method by which blood samples are collected and handled during processing has a significant effect on the test results. Blood should be collected rapidly, immediately transferred into the lithium heparin collection tube, and mixed well with the anticoagulant. Hemolysis of the sample during collection and handling should be avoided. Hemolysis results if blood is placed into tubes too quickly, agitated too vigorously while mixing with an anticoagulant, or improperly stored. Blood that is stored at room temperature for a period of greater than 1 hour, kept at too high a temperature, or frozen will hemolyze. In general, the significant changes that occur with hemolysis in the avian sample involve the analysis of potassium, phosphorus, albumin, and lactate dehydrogenase (LD) [1].

Fasting samples are not often obtained from birds, because withholding food from birds that are sick is not advisable. Also, considering the nature of their digestive physiology and anatomy, a fasting state may be difficult to achieve safely. As a result, plasma samples obtained from birds are often lipemic, which can interfere with many biochemical tests. In some avian species, it is normal for the plasma to be yellow because of carotenoid pigments from the diet. It is important to note that such samples do not represent icterus and the pigment does not interfere with biochemical testing.

Reference intervals and decision levels

Published reference intervals for biochemical tests for a few of the common species of birds seen in veterinary practices traditionally have been established to produce a 95% confidence interval for each analyte. Establishment of normal reference intervals for a given species of bird depends on many factors, including age, state of health, and nutrition. Because of the avian patient's ability to mask illness, it is often difficult to guarantee that a given bird is free of disease for inclusion into a population of normal healthy birds. Likewise, because the nutritional requirements for most birds are unknown, it is difficult to determine if their nutritional needs are being met. Both environmental factors and the physiologic status of the birds should be considered when establishing reference values. Factors such as gender, age, temperature, humidity, photo period, season of the year, and time of day may influence the results of a particular analyte [2]. Also, methodology often varies among veterinary laboratories, which can create difficulty when comparing laboratory data obtained from one center with reference values provided by another. For these reasons, reference

Veterinary Hematology, Clinical Chemistry, and Cytology, Third Edition. Edited by Mary Anna Thrall, Glade Weiser, Robin W. Allison and Terry W. Campbell.

Companion website: www.wiley.com/go/thrall/veterinary

values should be established for an individual bird during health, and the same laboratory should be used so that subtle changes in the blood biochemistries can be detected.

Use of a point-of-care analyzer has proven to be useful in avian medicine because of the ability to perform a basic avian biochemistry panel on 0.1 ml of whole blood or plasma. Other advantages of this technology include a short turnaround time of obtaining results, the small size of the analytical instrumentation, affordability, minimal requirement technical training to perform the analysis, and acceptable clinical performance with avian samples for some analytes. The results obtained from point-of-care analyzers when compared to those obtained from reference laboratory analyzers (considered to be the gold standard) has often shown that the two methods are not analytically equivalent [3]. These studies have generally involved small sample sizes, healthy birds, and just a few species. Therefore, use of heterogeneous data to assess the agreement between the two methods in a wide analytic range require larger studies on a widely varying sampling of birds is required to properly investigate the clinical adequacy of the point-of-care analyzer technology in avian blood biochemistry [3].

Because of the difficulty in obtaining meaningful reference intervals for each species of bird that may be presented to a veterinary hospital, many avian clinicians use decision levels when assessing avian biochemical profiles. Although variations associated with factors such as seasonal variability, circadian rhythm, and gender may be significant, they may be too small to influence the clinical decision making process. Decision levels are threshold values above or below which a decision is made to respond to the abnormality. The response may vary from repeating the test, ordering additional tests, or treatment of the patient. Decision levels may be obtained by using published reference intervals and by applying these values to those obtained by the laboratory. Decision levels may vary among avian clinicians depending on their experience and the laboratory results. Values suggested in this text for each analyte in the avian blood profile are simply guidelines that can be used as decision levels. Obtaining a set of normal values from the healthy individual bird housed in a stable environment with a consistent husbandry protocol can refine the process of evaluating that avian patient later when it becomes ill. Therefore, when the bird becomes ill, it has its own set of normal reference values for comparison.

Laboratory evaluation of the avian kidney

Normal anatomy and physiology of the avian kidney

The avian urinary system consists of paired kidneys that are located in the renal fossa of the synsacrum. Each kidney is composed of three divisions: cranial, middle, and caudal. In turn, each division is composed of lobules that contain poorly demarcated, large cortical areas and smaller medullary areas. A ureter transports urine from each kidney to the urodeum of the cloaca. Unlike mammals, birds lack a renal pelvis and a urinary bladder.

Birds have two types of nephrons [4]. The superficial cortical or reptilian-type nephron has a glomerulus with a tubular system that is devoid of loops of Henle and is located entirely in the cortex. Cortical nephrons radiate around the central efferent veins to form lobules, and they empty at right angles to the collecting ducts. The deeper medullary or mammalian-type nephron has a glomerulus with a tubular system that contains loops of Henle. Therefore, medullary nephrons are involved in the countercurrent multiplier and osmotic gradient process to form urine as in mammalian kidneys. The glomeruli of birds are smaller with lower filtration rates (glomerular filtration rate [GFR]) compared to those of mammals; however, they more numerous and as a result the overall GFR of birds is similar to that of mammals [4]. The loops of Henle and the collecting ducts that drain both types of nephrons are bound by connective tissue to form a medullary cone, and each cone ends as a branch of the ureter.

Birds have a juxtaglomerular apparatus but only a rudimentary macula densa. The juxtaglomerular apparatus consists of an afferent arteriole, secretory juxtaglomerular cells that produce renin, and extaglomerular mesangial cells. Renin leads to the formation of angiotensin I and II, which are vasoconstrictors that stimulate the release of aldosterone. In turn, aldosterone stimulates NaCl and water reabsorption by the distal convoluted tubules and collecting ducts.

Blood is supplied to the kidney by the renal arteries, which eventually supply the afferent glomerular arterioles. Avian kidneys also receive blood from a renal portal system, in which the renal veins behave as arteries and supply blood to the kidney tubules; however, the amount of blood supplied in this manner varies with species, stress, and temperature [4]. The cranial and caudal portal veins, which receive blood from the pelvic limbs, intestines, and oviduct, form a vascular ring around the kidney. Valves at the junction of the bifurcation of the external iliac veins control the renal portal blood supply; these valves are controlled by both adrenergic and cholinergic nerves. The renal portal system facilitates tubular secretion by the cortical nephrons by supplying blood to the peritubular capillary plexus, which supplies the cortical nephron and the proximal and distal tubules of the medullary nephron.

The avian kidney plays a major role in osmoregulation by maintaining water homeostasis and electrolyte balance. The avian kidney filters large volumes of water that is later resorbed by the tubules. The medullary nephron concentrates urine by the counter current multiplier mechanism; however, it is less efficient than mammalian kidneys, perhaps because urea does not play a role in medullary hypertonicity among birds. Filtration occurs in the glomeruli, in which crystalloids and substances of small and medium molecular size pass into the glomerular filtrate. Electrolytes, glucose, uric acid, urea, and creatinine are a few of the substances that are removed from blood by glomerular filtration. Some filtrates (e.g., glucose) are reabsorbed by the tubules. The GFR of birds is more variable than that of mammals because of intermittent filtration by avian glomeruli. The GFR, as measured by inulin clearance, varies between 1.2 and 4.6 ml/kg per minute and is affected by the state of hydration. Arginine vasotocin, like mammalian vasopressin, decreases the GFR and increases water reabsorption in response to dehydration or increases in plasma osmolality [5]. The avian kidneys respond to a decrease in the GFR as occurs with dehydration by shunting blood from the reptilian-type nephrons to the mammalian-type nephrons because of the latter's ability to concentrate urine. This urine concentration ability varies between species and appears to be related to the size of the bird; smaller birds have a greater ability to concentrate urine than do large birds.

The intestinal tract and salt glands of birds also aid the kidneys in their osmoregulatory function. Urine that makes its way to the urodeum of the cloaca can retropulse into the rectum via the coprodeum where water can be resorbed. This retropulsion can have a profound effect on the urinalysis.

Other important functions of the avian kidneys include excretion of metabolic wastes and toxins, metabolism of vitamin D, and production of erythropoietin.

Blood chemistry evaluation

Uric acid, produced by the liver and kidneys, is the major end product of nitrogen metabolism in birds. Uric acid is excreted primarily by renal tubular secretion and is largely independent of tubular water resorption; however, decreased GFR from severe dehydration may result in stasis of uric acid movement through the tubules [5]. The principal site of uric acid secretion appears to be in the proximal tubules of the cortical nephrons. Approximately 90% of blood uric acid is removed by the kidneys [4]. Therefore, evaluation of the serum or plasma uric acid concentration has been widely used in the detection of kidney disease in birds. In general, a blood uric acid concentration greater than 13 mg/dL (750 Umol/L) is suggestive of impaired renal function from a variety of causes, including nephrotoxins such as lead or aminoglycoside antibiotics, urinary obstruction, nephritis, nephrocalcinosis, and nephropathy associated with hypovitaminosis A. The blood uric acid concentration is influenced by species, age, and diet. Juvenile birds tend to have lower blood uric acid values than adults, and carnivorous birds tend to have higher concentrations than granivorous birds. Increases in blood uric acid may be observed in birds shortly after consumption of a high-protein meal [6]. This is especially apparent among raptors, in which 24-hour fasting is required to avoid postprandial increases in plasma uric acid concentration. The uric acid concentration may also increase with severe tissue necrosis or starvation because of increased catabolism of nitrogenous compounds such as proteins and nucleic acids.

When the plasma uric acid concentration exceeds the solubility of sodium urate, uric acid (in the form of monosodium urate monohydrate crystals) precipitates in tissues, which is a condition known as gout. Birds with gout exhibit precipitation of urate crystals especially in the synovial joints and on the visceral surfaces. Blood uric acid concentrations are extremely increased (e.g., fivefold greater than normal) in birds with gout and result from severe renal dysfunction.

Uric acid is not a sensitive test for renal disease in birds, because a significant loss (approximately 75%) of renal function is required to increase the blood concentrations of this analyte. Uric acid is also not a specific test for renal disease, because increases can occur after ingestion of a high-protein meal, during starvation, or with severe tissue necrosis. Therefore, whereas the blood uric acid can be used as an indicator of renal function in birds, it does not provide a diagnosis, nor do normal values guarantee an absence of renal disease. Blood uric acid concentration when used as a sequential evaluation can be useful in monitoring treatment or progress of disease.

Because birds are uricotelic, they possess only very small quantities of urea in plasma. Urea is formed in the liver as a product of protein catabolism, and higher concentrations are present in carnivorous than in granivorous birds because of differences in dietary protein intake. The normal blood urea nitrogen (BUN) concentration of normal, noncarnivorous birds ranges between 0 and 5 mg/dL (0–1.8 mmol/L). Urea is generally considered to have limited diagnostic value in the detection of renal disease in birds compared with that of uric acid. Unlike uric acid, which is generally excreted independently of hydration, BUN may be a sensitive test for prerenal azotemia in some avian species because it is eliminated by glomerular filtration, which depends on the hydration status of the bird. Therefore, an increased BUN concentration may be useful in the detection of reduced renal arterial perfusion in some birds. Like the uric acid concentration, the plasma urea nitrogen concentration increases in birds, especially raptors, after ingestion of a high-protein meal. Plasma BUN and uric acid values are often evaluated together in an effort to differentiate prerenal azotemia, renal pathology, and postprandial effects.

Severe renal disease may result in an increased plasma creatinine concentration; however, creatinine is usually considered to have poor diagnostic value in birds. One reason for this is that in birds, creatine is excreted by the kidney before it is converted to creatinine. Therefore, physiologic creatinine concentrations of birds are below the limit of quantification of commonly used creatinine assays [7]. Thus, the measurement of plasma creatinine concentration in birds does not provide a useful assessment of the GFR as it does in mammals. Plasma creatine rather than the creatinine concentration may better detect a decreased GFR in birds.

Unfortunately, veterinary laboratories do not routinely provide creatine analysis.

Potassium is filtered and actively excreted by the kidneys. Birds with severe renal disease may retain potassium and develop hyperkalemia.

Sodium is filtered by the glomerulus and, depending on the osmotic needs, may be resorbed into the plasma or secreted by the kidney tubules for elimination. Birds with chronic renal disease may lose the ability to retain sodium, thereby resulting in hyponatremia.

Hyperphosphatemia can occur in birds with severe renal disease. However, it is not a consistent finding with decreased GFR.

The presence of upper gastrointestinal hemorrhage in mammals leads to a disproportionate increase in BUN concentration relative to reductions in the GFR resulting in a greater BUN:creatinine ratio. This does not appear to occur in birds where it has been demonstrated that plasma BUN, creatinine, and uric acid concentrations are unaffected by the presence of blood in the digestive tract.

Urinalysis

A urinalysis, which routinely is applied to mammalian urine, also can be performed on avian urine. Indications for performing a urinalysis on an avian patient include polyuria, azotemia, and abnormal appearance of the urinary component of the dropping. The urinalysis includes notation of the gross appearance, measurement of the specific gravity or osmolality, chemical evaluation, and microscopic examination.

Urine is collected by aspirating the liquid part of the dropping into a pipette or syringe once the dropping has been deposited onto a nonabsorbable surface (e.g., aluminum foil or wax paper). Aspiration of fecal material or urates along with the liquid urine should be avoided. Ureteral urine enters the cloaca and is forced into the colorectum by antiperistaltic activity, thereby allowing reabsorption of water and electrolytes to occur. For this reason, exposure of urine to cloacal membranes and the large intestine cannot be prevented; however, this exposure is presumed to be minimal when urine is produced at moderate to high rates. Catheterization of the ureter is possible but not routinely performed because it requires general anesthesia and is technically difficult.

Normal avian urine is the clear fluid component of a bird's droppings. The amount of urine produced varies with species, diet, and environmental factors, such as temperature and humidity. Generally, avian urine is hyperosmotic to plasma (362–2000 mOsmol/L), especially in birds that have adapted to arid environments; however, this is affected by the hydration status of the bird. The normal specific gravity of avian urine ranges from 1.005 to 1.020 depending on the species, hydration status, and osmolality [5]. Osmolality is a direct measure of the number of solute particles in the urine, whereas the specific gravity is a crude index of renal tubule function and is affected by the number, size, and weight of solute particles in the urine. The two determinations are related, however, and both can be used to determine the loss of concentrating ability in birds with renal disease. A urine osmolality of 450 mOsmol/kg represents the normal renal concentrating ability in the pigeon (*Columbia livia*) and can be used as a guide for water-deprivation studies in that species.

The color of avian urine can be helpful in detection of certain diseases. For example, a biliverdinuria represented by green urine is suggestive of severe liver disease or hemolysis in birds. Yellow urine is observed in some species such as macaws with liver disease, and this most likely represents bilirubinuria. Hematuria or hemoglobinuria is represented by red urine that changes to brown on standing. Polyuric birds produce liquid urine that may appear to be cloudy if contaminated with urates or containing large concentrations of cells, mucus, fat, or bacteria. Microscopic examination can determine the cause of the cloudy appearance. Green bile pigment from the feces and dietary pigments can stain the urine especially if the dropping is held in the cloaca for a prolonged period of time. A positive urobilinogen on the test strip is supportive of fecal contamination of the urine sample.

The principle difference in the nitrogenous components of avian urine compared with those of mammalian urine is the large amount of uric acid and creatine. Uric acid in avian urine typically occurs as a thick, mucoid, white to cream-colored colloidal suspension containing the small spherical conglomerates of insoluble sodium and potassium urates and protein. This semisolid material is not part of the specific gravity measurement of the urine supernatant.

Commercially available test strips for biochemical examination of mammalian urine can be used for avian urine as well [8]. These test strips usually indicate a negative to trace amount of protein in the urine of normal birds. Protein not reabsorbed from the proximal tubules becomes part of the urate conglomerate, which is not measured in the supernatant. For this reason, renal loss of protein may be difficult to detect by urinalysis; however, detection of significant proteinuria in the absence of hematuria, hemoglobinuria, and fecal contamination of the sample is suggestive of the renal proteinuria that occurs with abnormal glomerular permeability, such as that which occurs with glomerulonephritis. Alkaline urine (pH >8) can produce a false-positive reading in the protein portion of the test strip. Therefore, other methods for testing urine protein should be employed with alkaline urine. Postrenal proteinuria is associated with inflammation of the lower urinary tract and cloaca.

The pH of avian urine varies from 4.7 to 8.0 and depends primarily on the diet. Carnivorous birds that ingest large amounts of animal protein have acidic urine, whereas granivorous birds have more alkaline urine. Increased urine acidity (pH <5.0) may result from acidosis or increased protein catabolism, such as that which occurs during starvation. Increased urine alkalinity (pH >8.0) may be associated with alkalosis. The urine pH also can vary with physiologic state. For example, in poultry, acidic urine is observed in laying hens that are depositing calcium into developing egg shells.

Urine from normal birds contains no glucose, because glucose is completely reabsorbed by the tubules after glomerular filtration. Glucosuria occurs when the renal threshold for glucose is exceeded. In most birds, this threshold is approximately 600 mg/dL. Birds with diabetes mellitus, however, often exhibit blood a glucose concentration of greater than 800 mg/dL and significant glucosuria.

Normal avian urine is devoid of ketones. Excessive ketone formation and ketonuria occurs with increased oxidation of fatty acids as an energy source. This may explain the ketonuria found in migratory birds following migration. Ketonuria may be expected with severe malnutrition or diabetes mellitus, but this has been poorly documented in birds. One explanation for negative ketones in avian urine may be a result of the urinalysis test strips that do not test for the major ketones produced by birds.

Biliverdin is the major bile pigment of birds; therefore, bilirubin is not normally present in the urine. Biliverdin does not react with the bilirubin portion of the urine test strip. Biliverdinuria is indicated by a green coloration of the urine and is suggestive of hepatobiliary disease or hemolysis in birds. The normal urinary urobilinogen concentration in birds ranges from 0 to 0.1 mg/dL. In general, this test has limited diagnostic value in birds and when positive suggests fecal contamination of the sample.

Occult blood in the urine of a normal bird measures negative to trace on the urinary test strips. A positive occult blood reaction is suggestive of erythrocytes, free hemoglobin, or myoglobin in the urine. Microscopic examination of the urine sediment can determine the presence of erythrocytes. A positive test of the supernatant after centrifugation is suggestive of hemoglobinuria, and increased plasma creatine kinase (CK) values may be supportive of myoglobinuria. Hematuria is indicative of hemorrhage originating from either the urinary, reproductive, or gastrointestinal tracts or the cloaca. Hemoglobinuria is suggestive of the intravascular destruction of erythrocytes or, perhaps, the lysis of erythrocytes in hypotonic urine. Hemoglobinuria has been reported in psittacine birds with heavy metal toxicity, especially lead poisoning.

Urinary nitrite tests are designed to detect bacteriuria. This test has limited diagnostic value, however, in the urine of birds.

Microscopic examination of urine is an important part of urinalysis. Whereas 5 ml of urine is suggested to provide a uniform semiquantitation in mammalian urine, this amount rarely is achieved in most avian samples. Microscopic examination, however, can still provide valuable information.

Normal avian urine contains few cells. As many as three erythrocytes and three leukocytes per high-power field (40×) are considered to be normal in direct smears of the urine. Epithelial cells are rare in normal avian urine samples and can originate from the urinary tract, gastrointestinal tract, reproductive tract, or cloaca. Increased cell numbers are a cause for concern.

Casts in the urine of birds are indicative of renal disease, because casts are formed within the renal tubules. Granular casts are the most common and are suggestive of renal tubular epithelial cell degeneration (i.e., tubular nephrosis). Cellular casts also may be present, and the types of cells that are observed reflect the renal pathology. Casts containing epithelial cells are suggestive of acute tubular damage that results in sloughing of the cells that line the tubules. Leukocytes in the casts are indicative of renal inflammation (nephritis). Erythrocytes within the casts are indicative of renal hemorrhage and, typically, occur after trauma to the kidneys.

Crystals in avian urine sediment are primarily sodium and potassium urates. These are round crystals with a spoke-like appearance that are refractile under polarized light. The needle-shaped uric acid crystals may also be present in avian urine. A few drops of sodium hydroxide can be added to the urine sample to dissolve the uric acid crystals to facilitate the examination of the cellular components in the urine.

Microorganisms in urine sediments usually originate in the intestinal tract or cloaca, and represent contamination of the sample. Large numbers of bacteria, however, may be indicative of a urinary tract infection, especially when they occur as a uniform population of a single morphologic type and when casts are present. Because bacteria frequently contaminate avian urine samples and multiply during storage, resulting in artificially high bacterial numbers, fresh samples should be examined.

Electrolytes and acid-base balance

Water consumption in birds is influenced by species, age, size, environmental temperatures, and both the type and amount of food that is consumed. Water intake often relates inversely to body size and ranges between 5% and 50% of body weight per day [4]. Young birds tend to consume more water than adults. Carnivorous birds as well as those that have evolved in arid environments normally drink little water.

Water deprivation, hemorrhage, or administration of hypertonic saline produces thirst in birds, which is caused by the release of angiotensin II [4]. Angiotensin II induces the release of arginine vasotocin (i.e., antidiuretic hormone [ADH]), aldosterone, and corticosterone. Arginine vasotocin increases the reabsorption of water in the renal tubules and collecting ducts; other neurohormonal factors also play a role in the hypothalamic regulation of water intake. Disorders of the hypothalamus and deficiency of ADH from the posterior pituitary result in diabetes insipidus, thereby causing polydipsia and polyuria. These conditions have been reported in chickens and a few other species. A water-deprivation test or administration of exogenous ADH can be performed to differentiate polyuric disorders of birds. In chickens, water deprivation increases the plasma osmolality from 315 to 325 mOsm/L after 24 hours and to 340 mOsm/L after 72 hours. During dehydration and 24-hour water deprivation, the urine osmolality of normal birds is greater than 450 mOsm/L.

The ability of the avian kidney to conserve and excrete water has a wider range than that of mammals. The fractional excretion of water in birds can be as high as 33% during hydration and as low as 1% during dehydration. Cessation of renal water loss during dehydration results partially from shutdown of the cortical nephrons; it is not strictly a function of the tubular resorption of water.

Electrolyte metabolism in birds is similar to that of mammals. Therefore, predominate extracellular and intracellular anions and cations are similar in both types of animals.

Although point-of-care devices are commonly used to assess electrolyte, blood gas, biochemical, and hematologic values in humans and companion mammal critical care settings, few studies have assessed their use in birds. Studies suggest that these devices appear to be acceptable clinical tools in avian critical care, although reference ranges for each analyzer have been recommended [9].

Sodium

Sodium is the primary osmotically active electrolyte in the plasma and urine of birds. Dietary sodium is absorbed in the intestines and carried to the kidneys, where it is excreted by glomerular filtration. Depending on the need for sodium by the bird, sodium may be resorbed into the plasma or secreted by the renal tubules and then excreted.

Birds having salt (i.e., nasal) glands can excrete large amounts of sodium by an extrarenal route. The paired salt glands are located just above the orbits in most marine birds. Ducts from these glands deliver secretions into the nasal cavity, which flow through the nares and drip off the tip of the rhinotheca (i.e., beak). Nasal secretion of sodium occurs not only in marine species but also in at least two orders of terrestrial birds (falconiforms and cuculiformes) [4]. Salt glands also are found in ducks and geese. The typical concentration of sodium in the salt-gland secretions of most species that have been studied ranges between 500 and 1000 mEq/L (mmol/L) [4]. The rate of sodium secretion by the salt glands varies among species, however, as do the degrees of hydration and salt loading. The primary stimulus for salt-gland secretion is plasma osmolality, but hormonal influences also affect nasal secretion, which is increased by adrenal corticosteroids and aldosterone. Holopelagic species of birds whose physiologic regulation of salt depends upon the salt glands, gastrointestinal tract, and renal systems demonstrate significant decreases in serum sodium and chloride concentrations (as much as 72% of the normal reference values) when house in freshwater [10].

Hyponatremia in most species occurs when the plasma sodium concentration is less than 130 mEq/L (mmol/L). Diseases affecting the kidneys, gastrointestinal tract, or perhaps, the salt gland can be associated with excessive sodium loss. Excessive hydration because of polydipsia or iatrogenic delivery of low-sodium intravenous fluids (e.g., 5% dextrose in water) also can result in hyponatremia. Hyponatremia can be corrected by addressing the cause of the sodium loss, control of overhydration, or use of fluid therapy with an appropriate electrolyte balance.

Hypernatremia occurs when the plasma sodium concentration exceeds 160 mEq/L (mmol/L) and may be due to excessive dietary salt intake, decreased water intake, or increased water loss. After salt loading, hypernatremia occurs more rapidly in birds without functional salt glands. Marine birds that are given freshwater over a period of time exhibit atrophy of the salt glands, thereby resulting in hypernatremia after the ingestion of salt water. Hypernatremia associated with salt loading can be associated with excessive dietary sodium or administration of intravenous fluids containing excessive sodium. Hypernatremia associated with excessive free-water loss occurs with diarrhea, renal failure, or rarely, diabetes insipidus.

Chloride

Chloride is the anion of highest concentration in the extracellular fluid. Chloride and sodium represent the primary osmotically active components of plasma. For most species, hypochloridemia is indicated by a plasma chloride concentration of less than 100 mEq/L (mmol/L), whereas hyperchloridemia is indicated by a plasma chloride concentration greater than 120 mEq/L (mmol/L). These conditions rarely are reported in birds. Hyperchloridemia can be associated with dehydration and salt loading.

Potassium

Potassium is the major intracellular cation. Therefore, an artifactual increase in the serum or plasma potassium concentration occurs with hemolysis. Artifactual hyperkalemia or hypokalemia may occur with delayed separation of the cells in the sample, and these changes are species specific. For example, a 30% increase in plasma potassium occurs in macaws (*Anodorhynchus* sp.) following a four-hour delay in plasma separation, whereas a 30% decrease was found in chickens (*Gallus gallus*) following a two-hour delay in plasma separation [5]. True hyperkalemia in most species is indicated by a plasma potassium concentration of greater than 4.0 mEq/L (mmol/L). Hyperkalemia results from renal failure with decreased secretion of potassium, acidosis, and severe tissue necrosis. Hypokalemia in most species of birds is indicated by a plasma potassium concentration of less than 2.0 mEq/L (mmol/L). Hypokalemia can be associated with chronic diarrhea, prolonged anorexia, and alkalosis. Hypokalemia has also been reported in birds with renal disease, which may be associated with chronic loss of potassium in the urine. Use of potassium-poor fluids during fluid therapy in chronically anorectic birds may dilute the plasma potassium to a hypokalemic level, which may enhance the renal loss of potassium. Diuretic therapy rarely is used in birds, but it may enhance renal potassium loss as well. Imbalances of plasma potassium may result in muscle weakness, serious cardiac disturbances (e.g., sinus bradycardia and arrest), or both. Hypokalemia can be corrected with the addition of potassium to supportive fluids.

Calcium

Control of calcium metabolism is mediated by parathormone (PTH), calcitonin, and vitamin D3 (i.e., 1,25-dihydrocholecalciferol, calciferol). Other hormones, such as estrogens, corticosteroids, thyroxine (T_4), and glucagon, also influence calcium metabolism. The primary function of PTH is to maintain normal plasma calcium concentrations by its action on bone, kidney, and intestinal mucosa. When plasma concentrations of ionized calcium decrease, the parathyroid glands are stimulated to release PTH. The primary effect of this is to mobilize calcium from bone; however, increased calcium absorption by intestinal mucosa and calcium reabsorption by renal tubules also aid in the restoration of normal plasma ionized calcium concentration. Parathormone also enhances the renal excretion of phosphorus to maintain a normal calcium:phosphorus ratio.

Calcitonin is produced by the ultimobranchial glands of birds. Avian C cells, which are the calcitonin-secreting cells, migrate from the sixth pharyngeal pouch during embryonic development to form the ultimobranchial gland. In some species of birds, C cells also can be found in parathyroid or thyroid tissue. Calcitonin has the opposite action from that of PTH. Therefore, as the plasma calcium concentration increases, calcitonin is released to inhibit calcium reabsorption from bones.

Calciferol, which stimulates calcium and phosphorus absorption by the intestinal mucosa, increases the sensitivity of bone to the effects of PTH and is important for bone mineralization. The kidney is involved with the conversion of vitamin D_3 to its hormonally active state, 1,25-dihydroxycholecalciferol (calciferol). Renal synthesis of 1,25-dihydroxycholecalciferol is regulated at least partially, by PTH.

Birds differ from mammals by the increased development of medullary bone in the long bones (of hens) before egg laying, hypercalcemia in response to estrogen (and reproductive activity) in females, and the ability of hens to use 10% of their total body calcium stores for egg production on a daily basis for extended periods without detrimental physiologic consequences. Calcium deposition occurs in the medullary spaces of the femur, tibiotarsus, and other nonpneumatic long bones in female birds during the first 10 days before oviposition (egg-laying). This is referred to as medullary bone formation, and it is under the influence of the ovarian hormones, estrogen and testosterone. Medullary bone formation occurs 1–2 weeks before the increase in total plasma calcium concentration and renal hydroxylase activity that increases formation of the hormonally active vitamin D_3. During the ovulation-oviposition cycle, periods of medullary bone formation alternate with periods of medullary bone depletion.

Prolactin and sex hormones influence the 1-hydroxylation of 25-hydroxyvitamin D_3 in the kidney, which in turn plays an important role in calcium metabolism. This activity increases just before egg laying and corresponds to the increase in total blood calcium concentration. Therefore, the renal vitamin D endocrine system is involved in the increased intestinal calcium absorption during the ovulation-oviposition cycle of laying hens.

The total blood calcium concentration of a laying hen ranges from 20 to 30 mg/dL (5.0–7.5 mmol/L). Total calcium consists of ionized calcium, which is the biologically active form, and calcium bound to anionic proteins and nonprotein anions. Estrogen stimulates the production of calcium-binding proteins such as vitellogenin and albumin; therefore, the total plasma calcium concentration increases because of an increase in protein-bound calcium. This occurs several weeks before oviposition in chickens. The ionized calcium level remains unchanged.

Calcium for egg formation is derived from intestinal absorption and bone mobilization. If the dietary calcium is adequate, then most of the eggshell calcium is derived from intestinal absorption. Bone is an important source of eggshell calcium during the night, when food is not being consumed, or if the dietary calcium intake is inadequate.

The normal plasma concentration of calcium in most nonlaying birds ranges from 8.0 to 11.0 mg/dL (2.0–2.8 mmol/L). Approximately one-third to one-half of the plasma calcium is bound to albumin. Therefore, the total plasma calcium concentration is affected by the plasma albumin or total protein concentration; however, this may vary with species. In general, the total plasma calcium concentration usually decreases with hypoalbuminemia and increases with hyperalbuminemia. A significant correlation between total calcium and albumin has been determined for African Gray parrots (*Psittacus erithacus*) with the following correlation formula:

$$\text{Adjusted Ca (mmol/L)} = \text{Ca (mmol/L)} - 0.015 \times \text{Albumin (g/L)} + 0.4$$

A significant correlation was found between total calcium and total protein in the ostrich (*Struthio camelus*) and

Peregrine falcon (*Hierofalco peregrinus*) with correlation formulae for the ostrich:

$$\text{Adjusted Ca (mmol/L)} = \text{Ca (mmol/L)} - 0.09 \times \text{Total protein (g/L)} + 4.4$$

And for the Peregrine falcon:

$$\text{Adjusted Ca (mmol/L)} = \text{Ca (mmol/L)} - 0.02 \times \text{Total protein (g/L)} + 0.67$$

These examples indicate that the total calcium, albumin, and total protein concentrations have a linear relationship that varies between species of birds [5]. These formulae may not be clinically useful when dealing with other avian species.

Evaluation of ionized calcium would be more clinically useful because it is the most physiological active fraction of the total calcium concentration; however, there have been few studies evaluating ionized calcium to disease states in birds and reference values have not been established. Ionized calcium concentration of birds that have been studied suggest that normal concentrations range between 1.0 and 1.6 mmol/L. The concentration of ionized calcium is affected by the acid-base balance. The ionized calcium level will increase during acidosis and decrease during alkalosis.

Most species of birds are considered to be hypocalcemic when the plasma total calcium concentration becomes less than 8.0 mg/dL (2.0 mmol/L), and hypocalcemia has been associated with dietary calcium and vitamin D_3 deficiency, excessive dietary phosphorus, alkalosis, and hypoalbuminemia. African Gray parrots often exhibit a hypocalcemic syndrome with a plasma calcium concentration of less than 6.0 mg/dL (1.5 mmol/L) that results in seizure disorders. The pathophysiology of this condition is unknown, but it has been considered to be a form of nutritional hypoparathyroidism or, possibly, a result of hypovitaminosis D_3. Secondary nutritional hyperparathyroidism commonly is observed in birds that are fed calcium-poor diets (e.g., all-seed or all-meat diets). Affected birds have a decreased plasma calcium concentration, normal plasma phosphorus concentration, and increased plasma alkaline phosphatase (AP) activity.

Hypercalcemia in most species of birds is indicated by a plasma calcium concentration of greater than 11 mg/dL (2.7 mmol/L). Hypercalcemia has been associated with hypervitaminosis D_3, osteolytic bone lesions secondary to neoplasms, and hyperalbuminemia. Causes of hypercalcemia in mammals, such as primary and pseudohyperparathyroidism, certain plant toxicities, and hypoadrenocorticism, have not been documented in birds but should also be considered as possible causes of this condition.

Phosphorus

Plasma phosphorus is primarily regulated via renal excretion stimulated by PTH. Young, growing birds tend to have higher plasma phosphorus concentrations compared with adult birds.

Hypophosphatemia in birds is indicated by plasma phosphorus concentrations of less than 5 mg/dL (1.6 mmol/L). This may occur with hypovitaminosis D_3 (hypocalcemia also occurs), malabsorption, or starvation. Long-term corticosteroid therapy also may result in hypophosphatemia in birds; other disorders in mammals that result in hypophosphatemia have not been reported in birds but should also be considered as possible causes.

Hyperphosphatemia in birds is indicated by plasma phosphorus concentrations of greater than 7.0 mg/dL (2.3 mmol/L), and may occur with severe renal disease because of reduced glomerular filtration, hypervitaminosis D_3 resulting in increased intestinal phosphorus absorption, and excessive dietary phosphorus. Hypoparathyroidism also may be considered in some cases of hyperphosphatemia in birds. Improper sample handling can cause artifactual hyperphosphatemia because erythrocytes contain a higher concentration of phosphorus than is present in plasma. Therefore, hemolysis or delayed separation of plasma from erythrocytes, which allows intracellular phosphorus to leak out, will increase the plasma phosphorus concentration.

Acid-base balance

The normal pH of birds is maintained between 7.33 and 7.45, and the buffering systems that regulate blood pH in mammals appear to be present in birds. The bicarbonate/carbonic acid buffer system is the most important because of the rapid rate of CO_2 elimination by the lungs after conversion from H_2CO_3. Therefore, alterations in plasma bicarbonate and CO_2 content are useful in the detection of acid-base disturbances in birds. Because most CO_2 in plasma is derived from bicarbonate, the clinical interpretation of the total CO_2 concentration is the same as that of the bicarbonate concentration. The total CO_2 concentration rarely is reported, but concentrations between 20 and 30 mmol/L are considered to be normal for most species. Increases in the total CO_2 concentration are suggestive of a metabolic alkalosis or a compensation for a respiratory acidosis, whereas decreases are suggestive of a metabolic acidosis or compensation for a respiratory alkalosis, as occurs with excessive ventilation. During active shell formation in laying hens, the plasma bicarbonate concentration decreases, thereby resulting in a metabolic acidosis.

Blood gases rarely are determined in birds. Avian erythrocytes continue to be metabolically active after blood collection, and alterations in blood gas values *in vitro* can occur quickly. These alterations are influenced by temperature; therefore, blood gas analysis should be performed as quickly as possible after sample collection. Portable blood gas analyzers that are designed for bedside monitoring of human patients may provide a quick, reliable method for monitoring blood gases in birds.

Laboratory evaluation of the avian liver

Liver enzymes

Interpretation of liver enzyme activity, as commonly used in mammalian medicine, has been applied to birds. However, experimental studies evaluating the sensitivity and specificity of these enzymes for detecting liver disease have been limited to only a few avian species. Because the specificity and sensitivity of these enzymes may vary with the species and the type of hepatic disease, only general statements regarding alterations in enzyme activity can be made. Alterations in the plasma activity of enzymes used to detect hepatic disease in birds can reflect either hepatocellular injury or increased enzyme production.

Aspartate aminotransferase

High aspartate aminotransferase (AST) activity has been reported in the liver of birds. High AST activity has also been found in skeletal muscle, heart muscle, brain, and kidney. The distribution of AST among tissues varies with the species, thereby making interpretation of increased plasma AST activity challenging. In general, increases of plasma AST activity in birds are suggested when such activity is greater than 275 IU/L. Increases result from either hepatic or muscle injury, which allow the leakage of intracellular AST into the blood. Plasma AST activity is considered to be markedly increased when the activity is greater than 800 IU/L. Activity of this magnitude is suggestive of severe hepatic insult, especially in the presence of biliverdinuria or biliverdinemia. However, increased AST activity does not provide information about hepatic function. It is useful to evaluate CK activity (see Laboratory Detection of Muscle Injury) in conjunction with AST activity to differentiate between muscle and liver injury.

Alanine aminotransferase

Alanine aminotransferase (ALT) activity has been reported in the liver, skeletal muscle, and many other tissues of birds, and leaks into blood when such tissues are injured. Plasma ALT activity is considered to be neither a specific nor a sensitive test for hepatocellular injury in birds. Plasma ALT activity in most species of normal birds ranges from 19 to 50 IU/L and may be more useful for the detection of hepatic disease in carnivorous birds. Plasma ALT activity increases with significant liver or muscle injury in birds (especially carnivores) and has no advantage compared with AST as a test for hepatocellular disease.

Lactate dehydrogenase

Plasma LD activity is nonspecific for hepatocellular disease in birds. LD isoenzymes are found in nearly all avian tissues. Specific LD isoenzymes could be helpful in determining the source of increased plasma LD activity; however, verification studies evaluating LD isoenzymes in various avian tissues would be required for a large number of avian species.

Plasma LD activity is less than 1000 IU/L in normal birds, and increased activity has been associated with hepatocellular disease. Compared with plasma AST and ALT activity, plasma LD activity increases and declines more rapidly after injury to liver or muscle. The short mean elimination half-life of LD (0.48 hours) compared to that of CK (3.07 hours) makes LD a valuable test in differentiating between muscle and liver disease in the pigeon. Determination of the plasma LD activity has no diagnostic advantage compared with plasma AST activity, especially because the former typically has a wide normal reference interval in birds and its low specificity for liver disease in birds. In addition, avian erythrocytes have high LD activity; therefore, hemolysis results in increased plasma LD activity.

Glutamate dehydrogenase

Although not commonly offered by most veterinary laboratories, plasma glutamate dehydrogenase (GLDH) activity appears to be a specific test for hepatocellular disease in birds; however, sensitivity is low. Because GLDH is a mitochondria-bound enzyme, it is released when severe cell injury has occurred. Significant GLDH activity has been found in the liver, kidney, and brain of pigeons, chickens, ducks, turkeys, and budgerigars. In general, plasma GLDH activity of greater than 10 IU/L is considered to be increased and indicative of hepatic necrosis. The degree of increase in the plasma GLDH activity reflects the severity of the hepatocellular injury. Plasma GLDH activity does not appear to increase with muscle injury, as do the activities of AST, ALT, and LD, thereby making GLDH the most liver-specific plasma enzyme among those species of birds that have been evaluated. Plasma GLDH appears to have a shorter mean elimination half-life (0.68 hours) than does AST (7.66 hours) and ALT (5.69 hours), and it can be used to evaluate not only the severity of the hepatocellular injury but also the duration (if the insult is not ongoing).

Sorbitol dehydrogenase

Sorbitol dehydrogenase (SD) appears to be a liver-specific cytosolic enzyme, and it may be useful in establishing the diagnosis of hepatocellular injury in birds. Plasma SD has a short half-life, and its activity may remain increased for shorter periods of time than those of AST and other enzymes. Plasma SD assays are usually unavailable at most veterinary laboratories. Plasma SD appears to have no diagnostic advantage compared with plasma GLDH.

Alkaline phosphatase

AP activity occurs in multiple tissues including bone and intestine, and increased plasma AP activity results not from leakage of the enzyme but from increased cellular production. Plasma AP activity in birds results primarily from osteoblastic activity. Therefore, increases in the plasma AP activity are suggestive of skeletal growth, nutritional secondary hyperparathyroidism, healing fractures, and the preovulation condition of medullary calcification in hens. Plasma AP activity is not useful in the detection of hepatobiliary disease in birds. Aflatoxin B_1-induced liver necrosis and bile duct hyperplasia have not significantly increased the serum AP activity in the pigeon, cockatiel (*Nymphicus hollandicus*), great horned owl (*Bubo virginianus*), and red-tailed hawk (*Buteo jamaicensis*). Plasma AP activity appears to be a sensitive indicator of intestinal diseases, such as coccidial infections in the duodenum, jejunum, and cecum.

Gamma glutamyltransferase

Plasma γ-glutamyltransferase (GGT) activity does not predictably increase in birds with hepatobiliary disease. Similar to AP, increased plasma activity of GGT is due to increased cellular production rather than leakage. Measurable GGT activity occurs in the kidney, brain, and intestines of birds; however, disorders of these tissues do not increase the plasma GGT activity. The highest GGT activity is found in the kidney of birds. The plasma activity does not increase with renal disease, however, because the enzyme is excreted in the urine. Increased serum GGT activity has increased in some cases of birds with liver disease, but not others, suggesting that the plasma GGT activity may increase in some species of birds depending on the nature of the hepatic insult. Plasma GGT activity is not routinely measured in birds with hepatobiliary disease; therefore, the usefulness of this enzyme in detection of avian liver diseases has not been fully determined.

Biliverdin and bilirubin

CHAPTER 36

Because the avian liver generally lacks the enzyme biliverdin reductase, which is required to convert biliverdin to bilirubin, the primary bile pigment in birds is biliverdin, which is a green pigment. In spite of the fact that birds produce little to no bilirubin, clinical icterus with an increased plasma bilirubin concentration has been reported in ducks and macaws (*Ara* sp.). Presumably, some biliverdin may be reduced to bilirubin by nonspecific extrahepatic enzymes or bacteria; however, bilirubin is considered to be a poor indicator for hepatobiliary disease in most birds. The healthy avian kidney is efficient in clearing bile pigments from the blood; therefore, green-colored urine and urates are suggestive of biliverdinuria and significant liver disease in birds. The presence of biliverdinemia is indicated by green sera or plasma, which reflects severe hepatobiliary disease in birds, and is associated with a poor prognosis for survival. Most veterinary laboratories do not offer biliverdin testing. Biliverdin is an unstable bile pigment that is sensitive to light degradation. The yellow color of the plasma in many avian species may be associated with carotenoid pigments from the diet and should not be misinterpreted as bilirubinemia.

Bile acids

Because plasma enzymes are neither sensitive nor specific for the detection of liver disease in birds and also do not reflect the degree of liver disease, other blood biochemical tests are necessary to evaluate avian liver metabolism and excretion. Moreover, biliverdin and bilirubin concentrations in the blood are either not available or applicable to the detection of liver disease. Bile acid determination, however, is a sensitive test for liver function in some species of birds [11]. Bile acids are produced in the liver, excreted in the bile, reabsorbed by the intestines into the portal circulation, and removed from the blood by the hepatocytes. This process is referred to as the enterohepatic circulation.

Bile acids normally occur in very small amounts in the peripheral blood of healthy birds. The primary bile acids in birds vary among species and may not be the same as those found in dogs, cats, and humans [5]. Fasting plasma bile acid concentrations are lower than postprandial concentrations. The length of required fasting varies between species. For example, plasma bile acid concentrations demonstrate a postprandial peak at 2 hours in Goffin cockatoos (*Cacatua goffini*), 4 hours in African Gray parrots (*P. erithacus*), and more than 8 hours in Amazon parrots (*Amazona* sp).

Increases in fasting plasma bile acid concentrations are suggestive of abnormal hepatic function, and may be due to failure of the liver to uptake bile acids from the portal blood, abnormal bile acid excretion caused by blockage or leakage, or portal circulation abnormalities. When measuring the bile acid concentration, a 12-hour fast is recommended because of the digestive physiology of birds. The emptying time of the ingluvies or crop varies both with diet and among species of birds; thus, the timing of postprandial sampling for bile acid testing is difficult. Moreover, ill birds often have a slow gastrointestinal transit time – or even stasis. Conversely, increased gastrointestinal motility may interfere with bile acid release from the liver and absorption from the intestines. Because fasting is better tolerated in carnivorous birds, such as raptors, and postprandial concentrations remain higher for longer periods of time, a 24-hour fast is recommended for bile acid testing for those species. Both the enzymatic and the radioimmunoassay (RIA) methods have been used for determination of bile acids in birds [12]. Results of the two methods correlate well in plasma samples obtained from six species of birds. The RIA method is linear to 50 μmol/L, whereas the enzymatic method is linear to 200 μmol/L. Lipemia and hemolysis interfere with bile acid testing using the enzymatic method but do not interfere with the RIA method. Variable results have been reported using the RIA method, which is designed for use with human serum samples. Potential explanations include differences in the binding of antibodies to different binding sites in avian bile acids; the tendency of avian samples to have higher bile acid concentrations than are found in humans; and the different predominating bile acids in various species of birds. Others have reported that both methods have adequate precision and accuracy.

Reference intervals for fasting plasma bile acid concentrations have not been determined for many species of birds. Overall, the plasma bile acid concentration of normal birds is greater than that of mammals; therefore avian samples often require dilutions, especially with RIA methods, to stay within the linear parameters of the assay. In general, bile acid concentrations determined by the enzymatic method are considered to be normal if they are less than 75 μmol/L [5]. Assay-specific and species-specific reference intervals for normal fasting bile acid concentrations are recommended.

Cholesterol

The normal plasma cholesterol concentrations of most species of birds range between 100 and 250 mg/dL. Because cholesterol is eliminated in the form of bile acids, increases in the plasma cholesterol concentration may be associated with extrahepatic biliary obstruction, hepatic fibrosis, and bile duct hyperplasia. Hypercholesterolemia also can be associated with conditions other than liver disease, such as hypothyroidism, high-fat diets, lipemia, and during egg production. A hypercholesterolemia occurs during vitelogenesis in female birds preparing to lay eggs. Postprandial increases in cholesterol may occur as well. Hypocholesterolemia may occur with end-stage liver disease, maldigestion or malabsorption, and starvation.

Iron

Excessive iron storage (hemochromatosis) is a common hepatic disorder of ramphastids (toucans), hill mynahs (*Gracula religiosa*), and sturnids (birds of paradise) and occurs less commonly in psittacine birds and other species. It has been suggested that these species of birds develop this disorder because they are more efficient in absorbing iron form their intestines compared to other birds and like humans, some birds (i.e., mynahs) may have a genetic predisposition for the disorder. Birds with this condition may exhibit increased plasma AST activity because of iron-induced hepatocellular damage. Usefulness of serum iron concentration, total iron-binding capacity, and unsaturated iron-binding capacity testing for excessive hepatic iron storage have not been fully evaluated in birds. Studies in toucans with this condition suggest that these tests do not appear to correlate with hepatic iron concentrations. The disease is currently diagnosed based upon histopathology and tissue iron levels.

Other tests

Other abnormalities that may be suggestive of hepatic insufficiency in birds include hypoalbuminemia, hypoglycemia, hyperammonemia, and decreased levels of coagulation factors. Hypoglycemia and hypoalbuminemia could result from chronic liver disease in birds but rarely are reported. An increased plasma ammonia concentration with hepatic encephalopathy resulting from severe hepatic disease has not been documented in birds. Coagulation studies are performed only rarely in birds but could be used to help establish the diagnosis of hepatic insufficiency.

Laboratory evaluation of plasma and serum proteins

The normal plasma protein concentration in birds is less than that in mammals, generally ranging from 2.5 to 4.5 g/dL (25–45 g/L). Albumin, which represents 40–50% of the total plasma protein in birds, is produced in the liver. Other plasma proteins also produced in the liver include transport proteins, proteins of coagulation, fibrinogen, enzymes, and hormones. Immunoglobulins produced by B lymphocytes and plasma cells represent a significant component of the total plasma protein concentration. The normal plasma protein concentration is essential to the maintenance of the normal colloidal osmotic pressure, which preserves normal blood volume and pH. Hens demonstrate a marked increase in plasma total protein concentration just before egg production. This estrogen-induced hyperproteinemia is associated with an increase in vitellogenin and lipoproteins, which are necessary for yolk production. These proteins are produced in the liver, transported in the blood, and incorporated into the oocytes of the ovary.

The biuret method is the method of choice for determining plasma or serum total protein concentration in birds. This method provides accurate and repeatable results when the total protein concentrations fall between 1 and 10 g/dL (10–100 g/L). Because proteins in the serum are primarily responsible for changes in the refractive index, a refractometer commonly is used to obtain a total plasma or serum protein concentration in birds. Temperature-compensated refractometers, as well as those that are not temperature compensated, tend to overestimate the total protein concentration. The high glucose concentration and chromogens in the plasma of birds as well as lipemia and hemolysis affect the accuracy of the refractometric method, which frequently is used for a rapid estimate of the plasma protein concentration. The biuret method, however, is more accurate.

The plasma albumin concentrations generally range from 0.8 to 2.0 g/dL (8–20 g/L) in normal birds. These values may not be accurate, however, because most analyzers determine albumin spectrophotometrically using the bromcresol green

(BCG) dye-binding method using human albumin standards and controls that may have different binding affinity for the dye compared to that of avian albumin. Thus, the BCG method has not been validated in avian plasma samples and may be inaccurate at the low albumin concentrations found in avian plasma [5].

Protein electrophoresis provides a more accurate measure of the albumin concentration as well as those of other plasma proteins; however, there are species differences in albumin migration on gel electrophoresis [13]. Avian protein electrophoresis is typically performed on plasma samples, which is appropriate as it has been shown that there are negligible differences in electrophoretic patterns when using plasma versus serum. The total protein concentration as obtained by the biuret method combined with electrophoretic separation of plasma proteins provides an accurate absolute concentration of the plasma proteins. The primary plasma protein fractions include albumin, alpha globulins (alpha-1 and alpha-2), beta globulins (beta-1 and beta-2), and gamma globulin. A transthyretin (prealbumin) fraction may be present in some species (e.g., psittacines) and absent in others (e.g., waterfowl and raptors). Normal concentrations for transthyretin, albumin, alpha globulin, beta globulin, and gamma globulin as obtained by protein electrophoresis from birds vary. Prolonged refrigeration, repeated freeze-thawing, hemolysis, and lipemia will alter the results [14]. Established species-specific reference intervals are necessary to the interpretation of avian protein electrophoretic patterns and values as well as the knowledge of variations associated with sample handling and conditions.

Protein electrophoresis is a useful test for analyzing the relative distribution of protein fractions in the plasma and has become part of the normal diagnostic workup for many captive and free-ranging birds. Because these protein fractions often change before biochemical or hematological parameters, electrophoresis can be used as prognostic indicator in birds.

The normal albumin: globulin (A:G) ratio for most psittacine birds is between 1.2 and 3.6 when transthyretin is included with the albumin fraction, or 0.6–2.2 if it is not. Transthyretin can be considered to be an acute-phase reactant, which is reason not to include it with the albumin fraction. β-globulin predominates in the globulin electrophoretic fraction in psittacine birds; whereas α-1 globulin predominates in waterfowl and raptors. Acute-phase proteins (APPs) in cases of inflammation typically result in increases of the alpha (specifically α-2 globulins) and total globulin fractions of the electrophoretic tracing. Increases in α-2 globulins may also signal hepatic disease in psittacine birds. Chronic inflammatory disorders such as aspergillosis, sarcocystosis, and chlamydophilosis are often associated with increases in β-globulins. The γ-globulin fraction is composed of immunoglobulins such as IgA, IgM, IgG, and IgE, which increase with a humoral immune response. Some of the immunoglobulins (e.g., IgM and IgA) may migrate into the beta globulin fraction. A polygammopathy is indicative of active chronic inflammatory diseases, especially those associated with infectious agents such as *Chlamydophila*, *Aspergillus*, and *Mycobacterium* spp. The higher γ globulin concentrations demonstrated in wild birds versus captive birds of the same species are likely associated with increased antigenic exposure and immune stimulation [15]. Decreased γ-globulin fractions may be indicative of immunodeficiency.

Hyperproteinemia in most birds is indicated by plasma total protein (biuret) concentrations of greater than 4.5 g/dL (45 g/L). Hyperproteinemia is usually the result of dehydration, acute or chronic inflammation, or a preovulatory condition in hens. Increased albumin and globulin concentrations with a normal A:G ratio are commonly associated with dehydration. Hyperproteinemia caused by hyperglobulinemia with hypoalbuminemia results in a decreased A:G ratio and is frequently associated with chronic inflammatory diseases in birds, especially with diseases such as Chlamydophilosis, aspergillosis, tuberculosis, and egg-related coelomitis. A decreased A:G ratio with a normal total plasma protein concentration may also occur with these chronic disorders. Hyperproteinemia associated with normal albumin and elevated globulin concentrations is suggestive of acute inflammatory diseases or preovulatory conditions in egg-laying hens. With acute inflammation, electrophoretic patterns typically demonstrate increased concentration of alpha and/or beta globulins; however, gamma globulin increases may also be observed. Hens undergoing active folliculogenesis will exhibit a hyperproteinemia with a decreased A:G ratio as a result of estrogen-induced production of yolk proteins that migrate with globulins on electrophoresis. Hyperproteinemia associated with hyperalbuminemia and hypoglobulinemia results in an increased A:G ratio and suggests dehydration in birds with low plasma globulin concentrations. Dehydrated birds subjected to chronic stress or other immunosuppressive conditions may demonstrate this type of plasma protein profile.

Hypoproteinemia in birds can be associated with hypoalbuminemia and hypoglobulinemia. This can occur with overhydration during fluid therapy or a proportional loss of albumin and globulins. The latter can be associated with severe blood loss, effusions (especially birds with heart failure resulting in large volumes of intracoelomic effusion), and protein-losing enteropathies (e.g., intestinal parasitism and bacterial enteritis).

Hypoproteinemia in birds associated only with a hypoalbuminemia occurs with starvation, malnutrition, intestinal malabsorption, and gastrointestinal parasites leading to amino acid deficiencies. Hypoproteinemia also occurs with liver failure resulting in a decreased production of albumin or renal disease resulting in an increased loss of albumin in the urine.

Fibrinogen concentration is often evaluated in raptors to detect the presence of inflammatory diseases, especially those associated with bacterial infections. A plasma total protein/fibrinogen ratio in raptors that is less than 1.5 is indicative of inflammation and possible bacterial infection, whereas a ratio greater than 5 indicates dehydration [5].

Quantitation of APP via protein electrophoresis and specific assays has become a valid indicator of inflammation, both acute and chronic, and as a prognostic indicator in veterinary medicine. These proteins with their short half-life exhibit a rapid increase following inflammation. Some (positive APPs), such as serum amyloid A (SAA), haptoglobin, and α and β globulins increase in concentration in response to inflammation, while others (negative APPs), such as albumin, decrease in concentration in response to inflammation. Because these proteins respond differently among various species of animals, they must be validated for each species. Avian APPs have been studied in chickens, raptors, and psittacines. Measurement of individual APPs, such as haptoglobin that increases after tissue damage, has become common in veterinary medicine and been documented as a diagnostic tool to detect inflammation in birds, such as raptors. Birds do not actually express haptoglobin but instead express a homologous protein (PIT54) that is similar enough that it is referred to as haptoglobin in veterinary literature [16, 17].

Laboratory evaluation of glucose metabolism

In general, the blood glucose concentration in normal birds ranges from 200 to 500 mg/dL (11.10–27.76 mmol/L). The plasma glucose concentration varies according to a circadian rhythm; however, this variation is clinically insignificant in healthy birds. The normal blood glucose concentration is maintained by hepatic glycogenolysis during short-term fasting. Specifically, short-term fasting (e.g., 1–8 days) in birds does not decrease glucose utilization per unit body weight, as it does in fasted mammals. During fasting, the greatest energy loss is associated with fat depletion and protein mobilization, thereby resulting in the loss of body weight in birds, which is seen as a reduction in the pectoral muscle mass. The blood glucose concentration remains remarkably stable during short-term fasting in birds, and it is more stable in carnivorous birds during prolonged periods of fasting compared with granivorous birds.

Blood glucose regulation varies with avian species. Whereas insulin plays a key role in mammalian and carnivorous bird glucose homeostasis, glucagon plays a major role in the maintenance of normal blood glucose concentrations in granivorous birds. This idea is supported by the relative abundance of alpha cells in the pancreas of granivorous birds while the distribution of the pancreatic islet cells of carnivorous birds resembles that of mammals. Granivorous birds also have a lower insulin:glucagon ratio compared with that of mammals. Their pancreas insulin content is less than 20% of the insulin content of a mammalian pancreas while the glucagon content is two to five times greater. Also, pancreatectomy induces hypoglycemia in granivorous birds but hyperglycemia in carnivorous birds.

Glucagon is produced by pancreatic alpha cells that maintain normal plasma concentrations of 1–4 ng/mL, which is 10–50-fold greater than the normal mammalian concentrations. The blood glucagon concentration increases by 100–200% in birds during a 24–48-hour fast. As a result, the blood glucose concentration increases along with an increase in free fatty acids, insulin, and cholecystokinin. On the other hand, glucose decreases the release of pancreatic glucagon. A significant increase in glucose stimulates the release of insulin from pancreatic beta cells.

Hypoglycemia in most birds is indicated by blood glucose concentrations of less than 200 mg/dL (11.10 mmol/L) and results from prolonged starvation, severe liver disease (e.g., Pacheco disease), septicemia, enterotoxemia, or endocrine disorders (e.g., hypothyroidism). Delayed separation of serum or plasma from avian blood cells does not significantly decrease the glucose level in the sample, as it does in mammalian blood, because avian erythrocytes use fatty acids rather than glucose for energy. Hypoglycemia-induced seizures is a common disorder of falcons in which their blood glucose can fall as low as 80 mg/dL (4.44 mmol/L) with sudden exercise following prolonged food restriction during flight training [5].

In general, hyperglycemia in most birds is indicated by blood glucose concentrations of greater than 500 mg/dL (27.76 mmol/L). Hyperglycemia occurs with diabetes mellitus, catecholamine release, and glucocorticosteroid excess, such as occurs with stress or administration of corticosteroids. Excess glucocorticosteroids result in a mild to moderate increase in the blood glucose concentration (≤600 mg/dL [33.31 mmol/L]) in birds. Exertion, excitement, and extreme temperatures stimulate the release of catecholamines, which also results in a mild to moderate increase in the blood glucose concentration. Glucose concentrations of greater than 700 mg/dL (38.86 mmol/L) are suggestive of diabetes mellitus in most birds. The pathophysiology of diabetes mellitus in birds varies among different species and may result from increased glucagon secretion or hypoinsulinemia. Although glucagon appears to have a major role in glucose metabolism in granivorous birds, those with diabetes mellitus have been shown to respond to insulin therapy. Birds with diabetes mellitus have polyuria and urinary glucose concentrations exceeding 1 mg/dL (0.055 mmol/L). Pancreatic islet cell tumors and pancreatitis (bacterial and viral etiologies) have been suggested as being causes of diabetes mellitus in psittacine birds. Detection of pancreatitis by increased serum amylase activity has been occasionally reported in birds. In some species (e.g., toucans, Ramphastidae), diabetes mellitus occurs commonly and appears to be related to a fruit diet. Excessive iron storage, another common disorder of toucans, can also be associated with diabetes mellitus in birds.

Plasma fructosamine and β-hydroxybutyric acid concentrations appear to be useful when monitoring the avian patient being treated for diabetes mellitus. It has been demonstrated that both analytes increase in diabetic birds with prolonged hyperglycemia and decrease following the correction of the hyperglycemic state with insulin therapy. Based on euglycemic psittacine birds, reference intervals for fructosamine are 113–238 μmol/L and intervals for β-hydroxybutyric acid are 450–1422 μmol/L. It has been demonstrated that blood glycated hemoglobin (HbG) can also be an indicator of the blood glucose status of the ostrich (*S. camelus*) and kestrel (*Falco sparverius*) [18]. The glycated hemoglobin of these birds is 1.2 ± 0.20% of the total hemoglobin compared to 3–6% in most mammals. The relatively low normal HbG of birds appears to be related to the lower permeability of the avian erythrocyte membrane to blood glucose. Blood glycated hemoglobin reflects the glucose status of the patient for a longer period of time than does fructosamine concentration because it reflects the blood glucose concentration during the lifespan of the erythrocyte. Although measurement of glycated hemoglobin may be useful in monitoring recovery from the hyperglycemic state, it takes longer to detect changes than does measurement of fructosamine because of its long life span in erythrocytes.

Laboratory evaluation of lipid metabolism

The lipoprotein panel, a standard diagnostic tool in human medicine, is rarely used and therefore, poorly understood, in avian medicine. Many types of captive birds (especially *Amazona* spp. and *P. erithacus*) fed high-fat diets and leading sedentary lifestyles are prone to obesity and atherosclerosis. In human medicine, these conditions are typically correlated with abnormalities in the lipoprotein panel. The components of the typical lipoprotein panel are the lipids cholesterol and triglyceride, as well as three lipoproteins: high-density lipoprotein (HDL), low-density lipoprotein (LDL), and very low-density lipoprotein (VLDL). Measurement of total cholesterol levels includes both free cholesterol and cholesterol esters. The normal serum lipoprotein distributions for birds are likely to vary among species. Reference intervals established for the normal lipoprotein panel in Amazon parrots (*Amazona* spp) indicated a significant difference in HDL values between males and females but no differences associated with diet, body condition score, and age [19].

A high correlation with the prevalence of atherosclerosis in birds has been shown with increasing HDL but not LDL [20]. Dietary management of birds with atherosclerosis has been shown to decrease total and LDL cholesterol but not HDL cholesterol or even mortality; which is likely associated with the severity of the atherosclerotic lesions at time of the dietary changes [21]. However, feeding low-fat diets and monitoring the lipid profile may have long-term beneficial effects in the prevention of atherosclerosis, a condition where obesity and dyslipidemias are among the known risk factors. Daily exercise has also been shown to improve the lipid metabolism of pigeons, parrots, and chickens under varying experimental conditions. In birds, like humans and other mammalians, an increase in HDL cholesterol is the most consistent effect of exercise on circulating lipid and lipoprotein parameters [22].

Laboratory detection of exocrine pancreatic insufficiency

Exocrine pancreatic insufficiency is a disorder resulting from an insufficient secretion of pancreatic digestive enzymes. Clinical signs associated with this disorder result from digestive malabsorption and include voluminous feces with a chalklike appearance, polyphagia, and weight loss. This disorder is a result of a severe progressive loss of pancreatic acinar tissue, either from atrophy or destruction associated with an inflammatory disease (pancreatitis). A presumptive diagnosis can be obtained based upon clinical signs and response of affected birds to oral pancreatic enzyme supplementation. In birds there has been limited use of plasma assays for the activities of pancreatic digestive enzymes such as amylase and lipase that may leak from injured pancreatic cells into the blood. Reference values for pigeons indicate normal plasma amylase activity to be between 382 and 556 IU/L and lipase activity between 0 and 5 IU/L [23].

Laboratory detection of muscle injury

CK is a muscle-specific enzyme in birds that can be used to detect muscle cell damage [24]. The normal plasma CK activity in most species ranges from 100 to 500 IU/L. Increased plasma CK activity can result from muscle cell injury or marked exertion and is frequently observed in birds with seizure disorders or birds that are struggling against restraint during blood collection. Muscle tissue damage can occur with traumatic injury, intramuscular injections of irritating fluids, or systemic infections that affect the skeletal or cardiac muscle.

Skeletal muscle injury should also be considered when plasma AST activity is increased. Measurement of plasma CK activity can be useful for determining if muscle injury versus hepatocellular injury is the cause of increased plasma AST activity. Thus, an increased plasma AST activity without an increased plasma CK activity is suggestive of hepatocellular disease in birds; however, other tests should also be employed to fully evaluate the presence of hepatic disease in birds. (See discussion under Laboratory Evaluation of the Avian Liver.) Severe skeletal muscle injury often results in marked increases of the plasma CK activity and moderate increases of the plasma AST activity. Plasma AST appears to have a longer half-life (mean of 7.10 hours from muscle) than CK (mean of 3.07 hours from muscle), and after a single insult to muscle, as may occur with an intramuscular injection of an irritating drug, the CK activity may return to normal before the AST activity. Regarding situations in which the plasma CK activity has returned to normal after muscle injury but the plasma AST activity remains increased, an erroneous diagnosis of hepatobiliary disease may be made if those two enzymes are the only analytes examined. Unlike plasma CK activity, plasma AST activity does not usually increase significantly with normal capture and restraint of struggling birds, but under these conditions, a bird with a preexisting hepatocellular injury may have increases in both the AST and the CK activity.

Increased plasma ALT activity may occur with muscle injury. Plasma ALT appears to have a longer half-life (mean of 11.99 hours from muscle) compared with plasma CK (mean of 3.07 hours from muscle); therefore, activity of ALT remains increased longer than does CK after muscle injury.

Plasma LD activity also increases with muscle injury. Because the plasma half-life of LD (mean of 0.48 hours from muscle) is shorter than that of CK (mean of 3.07 hours from muscle), the two enzymes can be evaluated concurrently to differentiate hepatocellular damage from muscle injury. In most birds, increased plasma LD activity with normal CK activity is suggestive of hepatocellular disease. Validation and evaluation of LD isoenzymes may be helpful in differentiating hepatic versus muscle disorders; however, most veterinary laboratories do not routinely offer LD isoenzyme determination.

Capture myopathy in Sandhill cranes (*Grus Canadensis tabida*) was associated with increased plasma activity of CK, AST, and LD within 1 hour of capture [24]. The peak activity of these enzymes occurred 3 days following capture and by 10–17 days, CK and LD activities had returned to normal; however, plasma AST activities were still two to five times higher than normal reference values.

Laboratory evaluation of endocrine disorders

Thyroid

Both thyroxine or tetraiodothyronine (T_4) and triiodothyronine (T_3) have been isolated from birds [25]. Most of the secreted hormone is T_4, whereas T_3 is formed peripherally by deiodination of T_4 and in comparison to mammals, birds contain less T_4 but similar T_3 concentrations. The plasma or serum T_4 concentration of adult birds of many species ranges between 5 and 15 ng/mL (6–19 pmol/mL) and the T_3 concentration ranges between 0.5 and 4 ng/mL (0.7–1.5 pmol/mL) [25]. Circulating T_4 and T_3 are bound to protein. A T_4-binding globulin is absent in birds; therefore, most of the thyroid hormones are bound to albumin. These hormones also are bound secondarily to other proteins (e.g., transthyretin [prealbumin] and alpha globulin). The binding of thyroid hormones to albumin and other blood proteins is weak, however, thereby resulting in greater free-T_4 percentages in the blood of birds compared with those in mammals [25]. Compared with T_4, T_3 is more metabolically active at the cellular level. The ratio of T_4 to T_3 in blood varies with the species, however. Thyroid hormones are excreted primarily in the bile and urine. In birds, T_3 and T_4 have relatively short half-lives compared with those in mammals, and a significant diurnal rhythm is more easily demonstrated in birds compared with mammals. In chickens, plasma T_4 concentrations decrease during the light phase and increase during the dark phase of the light cycle. Plasma T_3 concentrations behave in the opposite manner. The pattern of food intake may influence this rhythm.

Competitive protein binding and RIA are sensitive methods used to measure the plasma or serum T_4 and T_3 concentrations in birds. Protein-bound iodine determination is not a sensitive test for iodine-containing hormones in birds, primarily because avian blood contains a large amount of nonhormonal iodo-proteins compared with mammalian blood.

Secretion of thyroid hormones by the thyroid gland is governed by the concentration of circulating thyroid hormones. A decrease in the circulating concentration of thyroid hormones stimulates the pituitary gland to release thyrotropin-releasing hormone, which stimulates the release of thyrotropin (thyroid-stimulating hormone [TSH]) via neuroendocrine-controlled mechanisms. In turn, the release of TSH stimulates the secretion of thyroid hormones.

A TSH-stimulation test has been used to evaluate thyroid function in a variety of birds. In general, a prestimulation plasma T_4 concentration is obtained to compare with a poststimulation sample, which is obtained 4–6 hours after the intramuscular administration of TSH. A dosage of 1 IU of TSH per bird, regardless of the body weight, is typically used. A normal response is indicated by a 2.5-fold or greater increase in the T_4 level after TSH stimulation. Responses of lesser magnitude are suggestive of hypothyroidism. Measurements of T_3 concentrations appear to be inconsistent and unreliable. Low baseline total T_4 concentrations are poor indicators of hypothyroidism in birds, because many healthy birds normally have low T_4 concentrations. This may, however, reflect diurnal variation. Also, other conditions (e.g., stress and systemic disease) can decrease plasma T_4 concentrations. Therefore, TSH-stimulation testing provides a more reliable method for detecting hypothyroidism in birds.

Other blood biochemical abnormalities often associated with hypothyroidism in birds include increases in cholesterol, triglycerides, uric acid, AST, and LD. Hypothyroidism in birds may also result in a mild normocytic, normochromic nonregenerative anemia.

Hyperthyroidism is rare in birds. An increased plasma concentration of T_4 and T_3 is suggestive of hyperthyroidism.

Parathyroid

The primary function of parathyroid hormone (PTH), secreted by the parathyroid gland, is maintenance of the normal plasma calcium concentration by its action on bone, kidney, and intestinal mucosa. Unfortunately, plasma PTH analysis in birds is commercially unavailable. Therefore, detection of disorders associated with abnormal blood PTH concentrations (e.g., hyper- and hypoparathyroidism) depends on the evaluation of blood calcium and phosphorus concentrations in birds. Hypoparathyroidism has not been reported in birds.

Adrenal

Corticosterone is the primary glucocorticoid that is produced by the avian adrenal gland. Corticosterone secretion in birds is regulated by adrenocorticotropic hormone (ACTH), which is released from the pituitary gland in response to corticotropin-releasing factor. In birds given an intramuscular injection of ACTH, plasma corticosterone concentrations peak in 3 hours followed by a sharp decrease at 4 hours. The plasma corticosterone concentration increases during times of stress. Corticosterone also has mineralocorticoid activity. Plasma corticosterone concentrations exhibit a diurnal rhythm as well, with maximum concentrations occurring at the beginning of the day. Plasma corticosterone concentrations are also influenced by other physiologic factors, such as the ovulatory cycle of hens and changes in the seasons.

Plasma corticosterone concentrations in birds can be determined by RIA. Single baseline corticosterone determinations may have little value in establishing the diagnosis of hyperadrenocorticism in birds. An ACTH stimulation test may be more valuable, however, when pre- and 60- to 90-minute post–ACTH stimulation corticosterone concentrations are compared. Normal birds should demonstrate a greater than 10-fold increase in post–ACTH stimulation plasma corticosterone concentration compared with pre–ACTH stimulation concentration. Stimulation dosages of 50 and 125 mg of ACTH have been used in birds for this test.

Hyperadrenocorticism in birds is usually iatrogenic, caused by excessive administration of exogenous glucocorticosteroids; excess endogenous corticosterone is rare. The effects of glucocorticosteroid administration are variable and dependent on both dose and duration. Hematologic changes include lymphopenia, leukocytosis, and heterophilia. Blood biochemical changes include hypercholesterolemia and mild hyperglycemia, with blood glucose concentrations ranging between 500 and 600 mg/dL (27.76–33.31 mmol/L). Glucosuria should also be expected.

Adrenal insufficiency (i.e. Addison disease) is also rare in birds. The decreased production of corticosterone or aldosterone (or both) in this condition results in a decreased plasma sodium:potassium (Na:K) ratio. A Na:K ratio of less than 27, hypoglycemia, hypercalcemia, and low urine specific gravity are suggestive of adrenal insufficiency. Because hyperkalemia from other causes (e.g., delayed separation of plasma from cells, acidosis, hemolysis, and renal disease) may result in a decreased Na:K ratio, an ACTH stimulation test may be helpful in confirming the presence of adrenal insufficiency.

37 Clinical Chemistry of Reptiles

Terry W. Campbell
Department of Clinical Sciences, College of Veterinary Medicine and Biomedical Sciences, Colorado State University, Fort Collins, CO, USA

The clinical chemistry of reptiles has not attracted the same level of attention as for mammals, and normal reference values for specific blood biochemical tests have been established for only a few of the 7500 or so reptilian species. Environmental conditions, such as temperature, season, geographic area, ecological habitat, and wild versus captive status as well as physiologic factors, such as species, nutritional status, reproductive status, sex, and age affect the blood analytes of reptiles [1–5]. It is well recognized that significant metabolic disorders occur in captive reptiles exposed to unhealthy conditions, such as inadequate nutrition, improper environment, and overcrowding. These factors often have not been considered when establishing reference intervals, thereby making those intervals less meaningful. Methods of sample collection, handling, and biochemical analysis are additional sources of variation in the published reference values. Sample collection and handling are specifically problematic for blood biochemical studies of wild reptile populations. Therefore, published reference intervals are best used as a broad guide to the interpretation of blood biochemical results in reptiles. Because of the difficulty in obtaining meaningful reference intervals for each reptilian species seen in clinical practice, most clinicians use decision limits or common ranges when assessing such patients. As discussed with the interpretation of avian blood biochemical results (see Chapter 36), decision limits may vary among clinicians dealing with reptiles depending on laboratory results and experience. The values suggested in this text are general guidelines that can be used as decision limits when evaluating each analyte in the reptilian blood biochemical profile. As suggested with valued avian patients, the process of evaluating the blood chemistries of reptilian patients can be refined by obtaining a set of normal values from that patient when housed under a given set of environmental and nutritional parameters. When that patient becomes ill, a more meaningful set of reference values, which are specific for that individual patient, can be used to evaluate the chemistry results.

Blood biochemistry profiles are frequently used to assess the health of reptilian patients; however, controlled studies designed to clarify the meaning of changes in the blood chemistries of reptiles compared with those of domestic mammals generally are lacking. Therefore, reptilian clinical chemistry has not received the same critical evaluation as that in domestic mammalian medicine.

Activities of diagnostically important enzymes have been examined in the serum and tissue lysates of reptiles in an effort to determine tissue specificity of these tests. Plasma or serum along with lysates of liver, kidney, skeletal muscle, heart, intestine, lung, and pancreatic tissues have been analyzed for alkaline phosphatase (ALP), lactate dehydrogenase (LD), aspartate aminotransferase (AST), alanine aminotransferase (ALT), γ-glutamyltransferase (GGT), and creatine kinase (CK) activities in a few reptile species including the green iguana (*Iguana iguana*), yellow rat snake (*Elaphe obsoleta quadrivitatta*), and loggerhead sea turtle (*Caretta caretta*) [6–8]. Low ALP and ALT and moderate LD and AST activities were found in the majority of the tissues in all of the reptile studies. Little to no plasma or serum and tissue activities of GGT were found in the reptiles. High CK activitiy was present in skeletal and cardiac muscle and moderate (in the turtle) to low activity in gastrointestinal samples. Plasma and tissue activities of glutamate dehydrogenase were low or undetectable in the lizard. Amylase and lipase showed the greatest tissue specificity, with activity found only in pancreatic samples in the lizard and turtle (this was not evaluated in the snake). The results of these studies indicate that the plasma enzymes commonly included in clinical chemistry panels have tissue distributions similar to those of mammals and birds.

In general, interpretations of reptilian blood biochemistries are considered to be the same as those for domestic mammals, with the consideration that external factors (e.g., environmental conditions) have greater influence on the normal physiology and health of ectothermic vertebrates compared with endotherms. As stated above, reptilian blood

Veterinary Hematology, Clinical Chemistry, and Cytology, Third Edition. Edited by Mary Anna Thrall, Glade Weiser, Robin W. Allison and Terry W. Campbell.

Companion website: www.wiley.com/go/thrall/veterinary

biochemistries are influenced by species, age, sex, nutritional status, season, and physiologic status, thereby making the interpretation of results challenging.

Sample collections and handling

Blood samples for biochemical studies can be collected from reptiles using a variety of methods; the choice depends on the species, needed volume, size of the reptile, physiologic condition of the patient, and preference of the collector (see Chapter 21). Depending on the collection site, blood samples from reptiles, especially chelonians, are often contaminated with lymphatic fluid. It has been suggested, based upon evaluation of plasma and lymph samples in red-eared sliders (*Trachemys scripta elegans*) that most of the analytes in lymph (i.e., glucose, calcium, phosphorus, sodium, urea, and enzymes) are comparable with those of plasma or serum in reptiles, while a few others (i.e., total protein and potassium) have a significantly lower concentrations in lymph compared with blood. The same comparisons, however, may not be true for all species of reptiles. Therefore, the amount of lymph contamination in the blood sample should be considered when interpreting the blood biochemical parameters of reptiles. The best results are obtained from blood samples that are uncontaminated with lymph.

Many clinicians prefer to collect blood using an anticoagulant (e.g., lithium heparin) for plasma biochemical testing of reptiles, primarily because a greater sample volume can be achieved for plasma compared with serum. Collection of blood into lithium heparin also allows for evaluation of both the hemogram and blood biochemistries using one sample. Plasma is preferred over serum because clot formation in reptilian blood is unpredictable and often prolonged, thereby producing significant changes in some of the chemistries (e.g., serum electrolytes). Reptilian blood clots slowly because of a low intrinsic thromboplastin activity and a strong natural circulating antithrombin factor, which compensates for the sluggish flow of blood. Therefore, based on higher sample yield and lack of clinically relevant differences from serum, plasma is a better sample choice for clinical chemistry analysis in reptiles.

The ideal sample for biochemical testing is obtained by separating the cells from the plasma by centrifugation immediately after blood collection. This may be difficult to achieve in field studies. The reason for immediate separation is that prolonged contact between the plasma and the cells may cause an artifactual decrease in plasma glucose due to cellular metabolism and an increase in plasma potassium due to leakage from the cells. Also, as erythrocytes age, the cell membranes become increasingly porous resulting in hemolysis, which affects biochemical testing of the blood. In mammals, hemolysis may, depending upon the specific assay used, result in increases in potassium, calcium, phosphorus, magnesium, glucose, AST, ALT, LD, CK, total bilirubin, total protein, lipase, and amylase with decreases in creatinine, ALP, and bile acids. In the green iguana (*I. iguana*), however, hemolytic plasma samples revealed no change in sodium, calcium, uric acid, or CK but did reveal an increase in potassium, phosphorus, total protein, albumin, and AST. Increased storage time or temperature resulted in a decrease in plasma sodium in two species of tortoises with variable effects on potassium. Blood from loggerhead turtles (*C. caretta*) stored up to 24 hours at 4 °C (39 °F) before the cells were separated from the plasma did not reveal significant changes in the majority of the biochemical analytes (only plasma γ-glutamyltransferase demonstrated significant decreased activity) [9]. In the same study, there were also no significant differences in plasma biochemistries between blood collected in lithium heparin or sodium heparin.

The plasma of most reptiles is colorless; however, it may be orange to yellow because of carotenoid pigments in the diets of herbivores such as the green iguana (*I. iguana*). The plasma of some snakes, such as pythons, may be a greenish yellow because of dietary carotenoids and riboflavin. Some lizards normally have green plasma because of high concentrations of biliverdin.

Depending upon the analytic method, the sample collected from small reptiles is often of sufficient volume for only a few tests and not for a complete panel. Therefore, the clinician must decide which tests are most beneficial in the evaluation of the reptilian patient. Blood biochemical tests that appear to be most useful include total protein, glucose, uric acid, AST, CK, calcium, and phosphorus. Other tests that may be helpful include creatine, LD, sodium, potassium, chloride, total CO_2, and protein electrophoresis. Modern blood chemistry analyzers can perform many of these tests using a small sample volume (10–30 μl). Commercial veterinary laboratories often offer chemistry profiles that require a minimal volume of serum or plasma (0.5 ml). Blood chemistry analyzers that use dry reagents and reflectance photometry for "in-house" testing may be used for reptilian samples and often require smaller sample volumes. The use of point-of-care analyzers has become popular in reptile medicine because of the ability to perform a basic biochemistry panel on 0.1 ml of whole blood or plasma. Other advantages of this technology include the short turnaround time of obtaining results, the small size of the analytical instrumentation, affordability, minimal technical training to perform the analysis, and acceptable clinical performance with avian samples for some analytes. However, comparisons of results obtained from reference laboratory analyzers (considered the gold standard) with those from point-of-care analyzers have shown considerable differences for many analytes [10, 11]. Therefore, it is important to identify the specific methodology used when reporting and interpreting biochemical data.

Laboratory evaluation of reptilian kidneys

The paired kidneys of many reptilian species are located within the pelvic canal. The elongated kidneys of snakes are located in the dorsal caudal part of the coelomic cavity, with the right kidney being cranial to the left. The ureters of snakes empty into the urodeum of the cloaca, as they do in birds. Most species of lizards and chelonians (i.e., turtles, tortoises, and terrapins) have a urinary bladder; however, it differs from that of mammals in that the ureters of these reptiles do not empty directly into the bladder but empty into the urodeum of the cloaca [12]. Terrestrial chelonians and, possibly, lizards use the urinary bladder primarily for water storage.

The reptilian renal cortex contains only simple nephrons (i.e., cortical nephrons) with a tubular system devoid of loops of Henle. Therefore, reptiles cannot concentrate their urine. Nitrogenous wastes excreted by the reptilian kidney include variable amounts of uric acid, urea, and ammonia, depending on the animal's natural environment. Freshwater turtles that spend much of their lives in water excrete equal amounts of ammonia and urea, whereas those with amphibious habits excrete more urea. Sea turtles excrete uric acid, ammonia, and urea. Alligators excrete ammonia and uric acid. Terrestrial reptiles such as tortoises must conserve water, and ammonia, urea, and other soluble urinary nitrogenous wastes require large amounts of water for excretion. Therefore, to conserve water, terrestrial reptiles produce more insoluble nitrogenous waste in the form of uric acid and urate salts, which are eliminated in a semisolid state.

Blood biochemical detection of renal disease in reptiles is more difficult than in mammals because of the physiologic differences in their kidneys. Blood urea nitrogen (BUN) and creatinine concentrations generally are poor indicators of renal disease in reptiles; however, plasma urea nitrogen concentrations may be more useful in the evaluation of renal disease among aquatic reptiles that primarily excrete urea. Because terrestrial reptiles are primarily uricotelic, the normal urea nitrogen concentration in these species is less than 15 mg/dL (<5.36 mmol/L), with the exception of terrestrial chelonians (especially desert species), which typically have plasma urea nitrogen concentrations that vary from 30 to 100 mg/dL (10.71–35.70 mmol/L). This is considered to be a mechanism to increase the plasma osmolarity and reduce water loss from the body. The plasma osmolarity of freshwater turtles and crocodilians is approximately the same as that of common domestic mammals, but it is higher in terrestrial reptiles. An increase in plasma urea nitrogen concentration in reptiles may be suggestive of severe renal disease, prerenal azotemia, or a high dietary urea intake; however, it does not reliably increase under these conditions.

Free-ranging desert tortoises (*Gopherus agassizii*) demonstrate a "water metabolism strategy" whereby BUN, uric acid, and osmolality values respond to the amount of available forage and water as determined by rainfall. Free-ranging tortoises that exhibit increased plasma uric acid, sodium, and potassium concentrations with decreased osmolality and urea nitrogen concentration are considered to be actively consuming water along with protein and electrolyte rich forage [3]. This is in contrast to the same population of tortoises that were not consuming significant amounts of food or water, as suggested by increased plasma osmolality and urea nitrogen along with decreased uric acid concentration. Increased urea nitrogen concentration was considered to be a reflection of increased protein catabolism and perhaps dehydration. Increased uric acid concentration was considered to be an indication of increased dietary protein intake. Tortoises that were feeding with restricted water intake revealed higher plasma osmolality with decreased BUN and increased uric acid concentrations. During wet seasons, plasma osmolality and uric acid, urea nitrogen, potassium, and sodium concentrations were lower than other seasons due to increased rates of water consumption and bladder emptying. Plasma concentrations of these analytes in captive tortoises having constant access to water are expected to resemble free-ranging tortoises in wet years.

Creatinine is a normal constituent of mammalian urine, but the amount formed in most reptiles is negligible (<1 mg/dL or 88.4 μmol/L) [1]. The blood creatinine concentration is generally considered to be of poor diagnostic value in the detection of renal disease in reptiles. By contrast, the blood creatine concentration may have diagnostic value in the detection of renal disease in some reptilian species, but the test is unavailable from most veterinary laboratories.

Uric acid is the primary catabolic end product of protein, nonprotein nitrogen, and purines in terrestrial reptiles, and it represents 80–90% of the total nitrogen excreted by the kidneys. The normal blood uric acid concentration in most reptiles is less than 10 mg/dL.

Hyperuricemia is indicated by uric acid values of greater than 15 mg/dL, and is usually associated with renal disease. Renal diseases that are associated with hyperuricemia include severe nephritis, nephrocalcinosis, and nephrotoxicity. Hyperuricemia is not sensitive or specific for renal disease in reptiles. Hyperuricemia associated with renal disease most likely reflects the loss of two-thirds (or more) of the functional renal mass. Hyperuricemia in reptiles can also be associated with gout or recent ingestion of a high-protein diet. Carnivorous reptiles tend to have higher blood uric acid concentrations than herbivorous reptiles, and their plasma uric acid concentrations generally peak the day after a meal, thereby resulting in a 1.5–2.0-fold increase in uric acid.

Xanthine oxidase and hydrolytic enzymes act upon proteins to form uric acid, which in the reptile is further converted into urate, the salt form of uric acid (sodium and potassium urates). Therefore, because urates are an end product of nitrogen metabolism, gout is commonly seen in reptiles. Gout can result from an overproduction of uric acid (i.e., primary gout) or from an acquired disease that interferes with the normal production and excretion of uric acid (i.e., secondary gout). Conditions that result in secondary gout among reptiles include starvation, renal disease (especially tubular damage), severe and prolonged dehydration, and excessive dietary purines (i.e., herbivorous reptiles fed diets rich in animal proteins). Abnormalities seen in the plasma biochemical profile of reptiles with gout included a markedly increased uric acid concentration and moderate hyperglycemia (owing to the stress response) [13].

Although the kidney of some reptiles has high ALT and ALP activity, significant increases in the plasma activities of these enzymes do not occur with renal disease. The reason for this is that most of the enzymes released from damaged renal cells are pass directly into urine and are excreted and do not pass into plasma [7].

Reptiles rarely exhibit polyuria with renal disease. Therefore, urinalysis rarely is performed to assess renal disease because of a lack of available urine to perform the tests.

The normal glomerular filtration rate (GFR) based upon iohexol clearance has been established for the green iguana (*I. iguana*) and can be used to evaluate kidney function in that species [14, 15]. Reported values are 14.78–18.34 ml/kg/hr (mean and standard deviation of 16.56 ± 3.90 ml/kg/hr).

Electrolytes and acid-base balance

Water balance

Species, diet, and environmental conditions such as temperature and humidity influence the water consumption of reptiles. Desert species require less water than temperate and tropical species. Some reptiles have developed methods for conserving water. For example, tortoises and some lizards store water in the urinary bladder. Many reptiles can achieve water uptake through the cloaca by soaking. Water also is conserved in reptiles by the elimination of nitrogenous waste in the form of uric acid and urate salts, which are excreted in a semisolid state.

Sodium and chloride

Dietary sodium is absorbed in the intestines and transported to the kidneys where it then is excreted or resorbed, depending on the reptile's need for sodium. Some reptiles have nasal salt glands that participate in the regulation of sodium, potassium, and chloride concentrations in the blood. Therefore, disorders of the salt gland may affect the electrolyte balance.

The normal serum or plasma sodium concentration ranges between 120 and 170 mEq/L (mmol/L). The normal plasma sodium concentrations of tortoises and freshwater turtles range between 120 and 150 mEq/L (mmol/L). Sea turtles tend to have higher normal sodium plasma concentrations, which range between 150 and 170 mEq/L (mmol/L). The normal plasma sodium concentrations of lizards range between 140 and 170 mEq/L (mmol/L), and those of snakes, such as boas and pythons, range between 130 and 160 mEq/L (mmol/L). Hyponatremia can result from excessive loss of sodium associated with disorders of the gastrointestinal tract (i.e., diarrhea), kidneys, or possibly, the salt gland. Iatrogenic hyponatremia can occur with overhydration when administering intravenous or intracoelomic fluids that are low in sodium. Hypernatremia results from dehydration, either from excessive water loss or inadequate water intake, or from excessive dietary salt intake.

The normal serum or plasma chloride concentration of reptiles varies among species but generally ranges between 100 and 130 mEq/L (mmol/L). Plasma chloride concentrations of turtles tend to range between 100 and 110 mEq/L (mmol/L), whereas those of most lizards and snakes range between 100 and 130 mEq/L (mmol/L). The blood chloride concentration provides the least clinically useful information regarding the electrolytes. Hypochloremia in reptiles is rare and, when present, is suggestive of excessive loss of chloride ions or overhydration with fluids that are low in chloride ions. Hyperchloremia is associated with dehydration and, possibly, renal tubular disease or disorders of the salt glands.

Potassium

Normal serum or plasma potassium concentrations vary among reptilian species, but they generally range between 2 and 6 mEq/L (mmol/L). The normal plasma potassium concentration of most turtles, lizards, and snakes ranges between 2 and 6, 3 and 5, and 3 and 6 mEq/L (mmol/L), respectively. The amount of potassium in erythrocytes also differs among reptiles; therefore, the potential for artifactual hyperkalemia due to hemolysis varies with species. Common imbalances of serum or plasma potassium include inadequate dietary potassium intake or excessive gastrointestinal potassium loss (i.e., hypokalemia) or decreased renal secretion of potassium (i.e., hyperkalemia). Hypokalemia can also be associated with severe alkalosis. Hyperkalemia can also result from excessive dietary potassium intake or severe acidosis.

Acid-base

The normal blood pH of turtles and most other reptiles ranges between 7.5 and 7.7 at 23–25 °C. The normal blood pH of some snakes and lizards may fall below 7.4. The blood pH of reptiles is labile, however, and it changes with fluctuations in temperature. An increase in temperature or excitement may cause the blood pH to decrease. Cold-stunned sea turtles (turtles exposed to a wide range of temperatures and physiologic stressors) are initially affected by metabolic and respiratory acidosis [16]. The blood pH of most reptiles may increase to 7.7–7.8 during anesthesia. As in mammals, the oxygen dissociation curve for reptilian hemoglobin shifts to the left as the pH increases, thereby producing an increased affinity of hemoglobin for oxygen but a decreased release to tissues. The buffering systems that regulate blood pH in mammals are most likely the same in reptiles, with the bicarbonate/carbonic acid buffer system being the most important because of the rapid rate of CO_2 elimination via the lungs after conversion from H_2CO_3. Total plasma CO_2 or bicarbonate concentrations are rarely reported in reptiles; however, normal total CO_2 values for most reptiles are expected to range between 20 and 30 mmol/L. A marked fasting physiologic metabolic alkalosis occurs in postprandial alligators because of an anion shift, with bicarbonate replacing chloride in the blood as chloride is lost (as HCl) via gastric secretions. Therefore, a postprandial decrease of chloride and increase of bicarbonate concentrations are seen in alligators and perhaps other reptiles.

Calcium

Both blood calcium metabolism and the amount of ionized calcium in reptilian plasma are mediated by parathormone (PTH), calcitonin, and activated vitamin D_3 (1,25-dihydroxycholecalciferol). Other hormones, such as estrogen, thyroxin, and glucagon, may also influence calcium metabolism in reptiles. The primary function of PTH is to maintain normal blood calcium concentration by its action on bone, kidneys, and intestinal mucosa. Low blood concentration of ionized calcium stimulates the release of PTH, which results in calcium mobilization from bone, increased calcium absorption from the intestines, and increased calcium reabsorption from the kidneys.

The exact role of calcitonin in reptiles is unknown, but it most likely has a physiologic role opposite that of PTH (i.e., inhibiting calcium resorption from bone). Increases in the blood calcium concentration stimulate the release of calcitonin from the ultimobranchial gland.

The active form of vitamin D_3 stimulates the absorption of calcium and phosphorus by the intestinal mucosa. Photochemical production of the active form of vitamin D_3 by exposure to ultraviolet radiation (wavelength, 290–320 nm) is believed to be essential for normal calcium metabolism in reptiles, especially basking species.

The calcium metabolism of female reptiles during egg production is similar to that of birds. During egg development, female reptiles exhibit hypercalcemia in response to estrogen and reproductive activity. The increase in total plasma calcium is associated with an increase in protein-bound calcium during follicular development before ovulation, and the total plasma calcium level may increase by two- to fourfold or more.

The normal plasma calcium concentration for most reptiles ranges between 8 and 11 mg/dL (2.0–2.7 mmol/L), and it varies both with the species and the physiologic status of the reptile. For example, some species of tortoises have low blood calcium concentrations (<8 mg/dL or 2.0 mmol/L) [1]. Sex-related differences have been reported for plasma calcium concentration in free-ranging populations of reptiles where females exhibit significantly greater calcium concentrations than males. This difference is likely to be associated with reproductive activity (vitellogenesis) at the time of sample collection. Regardless of age and sex, plasma ionized calcium concentrations remain consistent in healthy reptiles. The normal plasma ionized calcium concentration for healthy green iguanas (*I. iguana*) has been determined to be 1.47 ± 0.105 mmol/L (5.9 mg/dL ± 0.42) [17].

In most reptiles hypocalcemia occurs when the plasma calcium concentration is less than 8 mg/dL (2.0 mmol/L). Hypocalcemia can occur with dietary calcium and vitamin D_3 deficiencies, excessive dietary phosphorus, alkalosis, hypoalbuminemia, or hypoparathyroidism. Secondary nutritional hyperparathyroidism is a common disorder of herbivorous reptiles such as green iguanas (*I. iguana*) [18]. Diets fed to captive herbivores are often deficient in calcium and contain excessive amounts of phosphorus. In addition, dietary deficiency in vitamin D_3 or lack of proper exposure to ultraviolet light predisposes reptiles to hypocalcemia. Juvenile reptiles (especially green iguanas) with secondary nutritional hyperparathyroidism commonly develop metabolic bone disease with fibrous osteodystrophy and bone fractures. Adult reptiles often develop muscle tremors, paresis, and seizures with hypocalcemia. Carnivorous reptiles that are fed all-meat, calcium-deficient diets also develop hypocalcemia associated with nutritional imbalances in calcium and phosphorus. Secondary renal hyperparathyroidism may result in hypocalcemia as well.

Hypercalcemia in reptiles is indicated by a plasma calcium concentration of greater than 20 mg/dL (5.0 mmol/L). Typically, this is an iatrogenic condition that is associated with oversupplementation with oral or parenteral calcium and vitamin D_3. Other differentials for hypercalcemia include primary hyperparathyroidism, pseudohyperparathyroidism, and osteolytic bone disease; however, these disorders are rarely reported in reptiles.

Pseudogout is a joint disease that occurs due to accumulations of substances other than urate crystals, such as basic calcium phosphate (hydroxyapatite) in turtles and lizards. This condition must be considered a differential when crystal deposition is observed in joints as pseudogout is a disorder of calcium metabolism that clinically mimics gout [13].

Phosphorus

The normal plasma phosphorus concentration for most reptiles ranges between 1 and 5 mg/dL (0.3 and 1.6 mmol/L). Differences between sexes have been reported for plasma phosphorus concentration in free-ranging populations of reptiles where females exhibit significantly higher concentrations than males. This difference is likely to be associated with reproductive (vitellogenesis) activity at the time of sample collection.

Hypophosphatemia may result from starvation or a nutritional deficiency of phosphorus. Hyperphosphatemia is indicated by a plasma phosphorus concentration of greater than 5 mg/dL (1.6 mmol/L). Disorders resulting in hyperphosphatemia include excessive dietary phosphorus, hypervitaminosis D_3, and renal disease. Rare causes of hyperphosphatemia include severe tissue trauma and osteolytic bone disease. In mammalian blood samples, an artifactual hyperphosphatemia can occur when serum or plasma is not promptly separated from the clot, thereby allowing phosphorus to be released from erythrocytes. A few studies have suggested this may be less likely with reptilian blood samples; however, hyperphosphatemia has been related to hemolysis in reptilian blood samples. The ideal sample for biochemical testing is obtained by the immediate separation of the cells from plasma with no hemolysis.

Laboratory evaluation of the reptilian liver

Liver enzymes in reptiles appear to be similar to those in birds and mammals. The LD and AST activities are high in reptilian liver tissue, and although few critical studies have examined the biochemical testing of reptilian blood to evaluate hepatic disease, increases in the plasma activities of these enzymes may suggest hepatocellular disease. The plasma AST activity is not considered to be organ specific because activity for this enzyme can be found in many tissues. In general, normal plasma AST activity for reptiles is less than 250 IU/L. Increased plasma AST activity suggests hepatic or muscle injury. Generalized diseases such as septicemia or toxemia, however, may damage these tissues, thereby producing increased plasma AST activity. Increased AST activity in the plasma of healthy free-ranging tortoises may be related to muscle activity and injury due to increased male aggression during the breeding season.

LD is considered to have a wide tissue distribution in reptiles. Therefore, increases in the plasma LD activity (>1000 IU/L) may be associated with damage to the liver, skeletal muscle, or cardiac muscle. Hemolysis also may result in increased plasma LD activity.

Like AST, plasma ALT is not considered to be organ specific in reptiles. The normal plasma ALT activity for reptiles is usually less than 20 IU/L. Although ALT activity occurs in the reptilian liver, increases in the plasma ALT activity may not be as reliable in the detection of hepatocellular disease compared with increases in the plasma AST or LD activity. However, it has been suggested that elevated plasma ALT activity can be associated with a prolonged diet of unnatural foods that causes liver disorders in captive tortoises.

ALP is also widely distributed in the reptilian body, and the plasma activity of this enzyme is not considered to be organ specific. Little information is available concerning the interpretation of increased plasma ALP activity in reptiles; however, increased activity may reflect increased osteoblastic activity rather than hepatobiliary disease. Increased plasma ALP has been associated with hyperparathyroidism and bone diseases, such as Paget's disease.

Biliverdin, a green bile pigment, is generally considered to be the primary end product of hemoglobin catabolism in reptiles. Green plasma results from the accumulation of biliverdin in reptilian blood, which is usually a pathologic finding that suggests hepatobiliary disease in these animals. A nonpathologic accumulation of biliverdin can occur in the blood of some reptilian species, such as arboreal scincid lizards (Scincidae) of the southwestern Pacific, which are rarely presented for clinical evaluation. The physiologic advantage of this is not known. Biliverdin appears to be less toxic to tissues compared with bilirubin, and the normal biliverdin concentration in the plasma of some species of lizards (i.e.,, *Prasinohaema*, green-blooded skinks) can be greater than 1000 µmol/L.

Laboratory evaluation of plasma and serum proteins

The plasma total protein concentration of normal reptiles generally ranges between 3 and 7 g/dL (30–70 g/L) depending on sex, species, collection technique, specimen storage, and method of analysis. Female reptiles demonstrate marked increases in their plasma total protein concentration (primarily globulin concentrations) during active folliculogenesis. This estrogen-induced hyperproteinemia is associated with increased levels of the proteins (primarily globulins) necessary for yolk production. The plasma total protein concentration returns to normal after ovulation. Captive reptiles may exhibit greater plasma total protein concentrations when compared to the same free-living species due to prolonged high-protein diets [2].

The biuret method is the most accurate for determining the plasma or serum total protein concentration. The refractometer method, however, is commonly used to rapidly estimate the plasma protein concentration in reptilian blood. Although the refractometric method tends to overestimate the total protein value, it is useful for clinical decisions.

Serum/plasma protein electrophoresis, a standard technique in veterinary medicine to investigate dysproteinemias, provides an accurate assessment of the albumin and globulin concentrations in reptilian blood [19]. Using this technique, absolute concentrations of the various plasma proteins are obtained by determining the total protein concentration using the biuret method in conjunction with electrophoretic separation of the proteins. Difficulties arise, however when performing protein electrophoresis with samples obtained from reptiles. Whereas protein separation has been optimized for human and domestic mammals, no criterion for the identification of different protein fractions in reptiles has been defined. Therefore, the albumin peak is often identified arbitrarily as the first main peak of each study. Agarose gel electrophoresis (AGE) is recommended because of its higher resolution when compared to cellulose acetate electrophoresis (CAE). For example, in one study, a-globulins could usually be separated into α-1 and α-2 fractions when using AGE, but separation was more difficult with CAE [20]. Because difficulties in the identification of the main globulin subfractions (α1, α2, β1, β2) are frequently encountered in some samples, it is recommended to report only one α and one β globulin fraction when calculating minimum–maximum reference intervals [21]. Also, considerable variation in results occurs between species and among individuals within a species associated with environmental factors such as habitat, season, and diet, which create difficulty in the comparison of results with published reference intervals. In general, because globulins behave similarly in vertebrate metabolism regardless of the species, the interpretation of the changes in the different globulin fractions are considered to be comparable to the protein fraction changes in mammals.

Changes in serum and plasma proteins in chelonians have been reported with regard to sex, season, location, and diseases [22]. Albumin was reported to be higher in postprandial turtles in one study [23]. Higher albumin and globulin concentrations are expected to occur before hibernation in chelonians. The higher globulins are likely related to the abundance of α2 macroglobulin and lipoproteins (high- and very-low-density lipoproteins) as seen with hibernating mammals. The increased α2 macroglobulin is likely associated with an important circulating protease inhibitor involved in regulating a number of steps in the clotting cascade and in complement activation, which would prevent clot formation when the heart rate decreases and blood viscosity increases during hibernation as seen in hibernating mammals [24]. Other alpha globulins include lipoproteins. In mammals, α1-lipoprotein (HDL) is responsible for transporting cholesterol from peripheral tissues to the liver, and very-low-density lipoprotein (VLDL) is responsible for triglyceride delivery to peripheral organs [25]. The abundance of α2 macroglobulin in hibernating chelonians likely indicate a switch to a lipid-based metabolism, as reported for hibernating mammals [21]. In another study, significant differences were observed with total protein, α-1 globulins, α-2 globulins, β globulins, γ globulins, with regard to sex, season, and location [26]. Differences in β globulin fractions also occurred with regard to age.

Limited studies have been conducted on serum and plasma protein in lizards. A double peak with a migration rate similar to that of albumin was detected in healthy and diseased Green Iguanas (*I. iguana*) indicating that many of these animals have bisalbuminemia [20, 27]. Bisalbuminemia has been reported in certain salamanders (subspecies of *Salamandra*) as well as hereditary or acquired disorder of humans. In iguanas, bisalbuminemia probably has a genetic origin, based on the symmetric shape of the double peak and its lack of association with a specific disease or pharmacological treatment [20]. Studies also indicate the β-globulin fraction generally accounts for 28% of the total protein concentration in healthy green iguanas (*I. iguana*) [20]. Seasonal changes in albumin (between March and December) and γ globulins (between June and September) were also noted in this species [27].

There have been few attempts to establish reference intervals for protein electrophoretic fractions in snakes [28–30]. Variation in results occurs between species and among individuals within a species associated with age, sex, and environmental factors, such as habitat. For example adults have been shown to have higher gamma globulin fractions (0.47 g/dL) than juveniles (0.28 g/dL) and male snakes have higher α-2 globulins (0.98 g/dL) than females (0.85 g/dL) [28]. Total protein, albumin, and globulin concentrations may also vary with the location of snakes within the same species.

In most reptiles, hyperproteinemia is indicated by total protein values of greater than 7 g/dL (70 g/L); common causes include dehydration or hyperglobulinemia associated with chronic inflammatory diseases. The alpha, beta, and gamma globulins may increase with infectious diseases. A significant increase in total protein as measured by chemical analyzers can occur with hemolysis.

Hypoproteinemia, as indicated by a total protein value of less than 3 g/dL (30 g/L), is commonly associated with chronic malnutrition in reptiles. Other causes, however, such as malabsorption, maldigestion, chronic malnutrition, protein-losing enteropathy (usually associated with parasitism), severe blood loss, and chronic hepatic or renal disease, should also be considered.

Laboratory evaluation of glucose metabolism

In general, the normal blood glucose concentration of most reptiles ranges between 60 and 100 mg/dL (3.33–5.55 mmol/L), but this is subject to marked physiologic variation. The blood glucose concentration of normal reptiles varies with species, nutritional status, and environmental conditions. For example, an increase in temperature produces hypoglycemia in turtles but hyperglycemia in alligators. In aquatic reptiles, hypoxia associated with diving results in a physiologic hyperglycemia because of anaerobic glycolysis. Normal oral glucose tolerance curves in reptiles differ both among species and with temperature. A significant sex-related difference in plasma glucose concentration has been observed in free-ranging tortoises where males have higher concentrations than females [31]. The reason for this is not known.

Common causes of hypoglycemia in reptiles include starvation and malnutrition, severe hepatobiliary disease, and septicemia. Clinical signs associated with hypoglycemia in reptiles include tremors, loss of righting reflex, torpor, and dilated, nonresponsive pupils.

In mammals, prolonged exposure of the serum to erythrocytes results in a glucose concentration that decreases at a rate of approximately 10% per hour. Limited studies have shown that this does not occur in reptiles. A significant decrease in plasma glucose concentration may not occur until erythrocytes have been in contact with the plasma for 96 hours [20]. This is likely a result of slower reptilian erythrocyte metabolism compared to that of mammals.

Hyperglycemia in reptiles often results from the iatrogenic delivery of excessive glucose. A persistent, marked hyperglycemia and glucosuria are suggestive of diabetes mellitus, which is a rarely reported disorder of reptiles. Hyperglycemia also may occur with glucocorticosteroid excess [32, 33].

Laboratory evaluation of lipid metabolism

The normal serum cholesterol concentration of reptiles varies depending upon the natural diet. In general, healthy herbivorous reptiles are expected to have lower normal cholesterol concentrations (77–270 mg/dL or 2–7 mmol/L) compared to that of omnivores and carnivores. Low-density lipoprotein (LDL) is the major carrier of cholesterol in the serum of tortoises (*Agrionemys horsfieldi, Testudo graeca,* and *Testudo hermanni*) with high-density lipoprotein (HDL) representing a minor carrier [34].

Seasonal and sex-related variation in the plasma lipid profile can occur in reptiles. For example, serum lipid concentrations tend to be higher in males than females. In one study, cholesterol represented 21% of the total lipid content in male Asian tortoises (*A. horsfieldi*) and only 14% in females [34]. Triglycerides and phospholipids are the major serum lipids in both sexes of these tortoises during reproduction (vitellogenesis). The lipid content of free-ranging tortoises changes immediately prior to hibernation as indicated by phospholipids and low-density lipoprotein cholesterol (LDL-C) being the major lipid fractions in serum, whereas triglycerides are very low [34].

Laboratory detection of muscle injury

CK is considered to be a muscle-specific enzyme and is used to test for muscle cell damage. Increases in the plasma CK activity can result from muscle cell injury or exertion. Increased plasma CK activity is frequently observed in reptiles that are struggling to resist restraint during blood collection, or that are exhibiting seizure activity. Increased plasma CK activity resulting from muscle cell damage occurs with traumatic injury, intramuscular injections of irritating drugs or fluids, and systemic infections that affect skeletal or cardiac muscle. Brain tissue generally has high CK activity; however, whether brain lesions contribute significantly to plasma CK in reptiles is not known.

Muscle injury also results in mild to moderate increases in plasma AST and LD activities. These enzymes are not organ specific for muscle, however, and their activities could increase with hepatobiliary disease. Increased plasma AST and LD activities associated with normal CK activity suggests hepatobiliary disease. Damage to both liver and skeletal muscle can occur simultaneously, such as occurs with trauma and septicemia, which would result in elevated plasma AST, LD, and CK activities.

Laboratory evaluation of endocrine disorders

Laboratory evaluation of reptilian thyroid and adrenal function is uncommon. Because of the ectothermic nature of reptiles, their physiologic status, which includes endocrine physiology, is highly dependent on the external environment. Therefore, correction of environmental and nutritional deficits usually results in restoration of normal physiologic health.

The hypothalamo-pituitary-adrenal axis of reptiles appears to be typical of most vertebrates; therefore, a reptile's response to stress has an influence on glucose utilization and other metabolic activities modulated by the adrenal gland. Use of plasma corticosterone concentration as the sole measurement of stress is not recommended due to physiological variations. For example, there is a circadian and seasonal variation in plasma corticosterone concentrations in free-ranging reptiles, which tend to have higher concentrations than do captive reptiles of the same species. Because a twofold increase in corticosterone is expected to occur in one hour following capture with peak increases in 3 hours, it is recommended that baseline concentrations be obtained within 10 minutes of capture.

38 Clinical Chemistry of Fish and Amphibians

Terry W. Campbell

Department of Clinical Sciences, College of Veterinary Medicine and Biomedical Sciences, Colorado State University, Fort Collins, CO, USA

Fish

Blood biochemical evaluation is not routinely part of the clinical assessment of piscine patients most likely owing to the expense involved and lack of meaningful reference intervals. As a result, much of the blood biochemical studies have focused on economically important (either as a food source or for exhibit) species, such as salmonids (salmon and trout), catfish, and cyprinids (carp, goldfish, and koi) [1–7]. Routine assay methods for the biochemical evaluation of mammalian blood appear to be useful for fish blood; however, interpretation of the results can be difficult. Many endogenous (i.e., species, age, nutritional status, gender, reproductive status) and exogenous factors (i.e., environmental conditions, population density, time of day [diel cycle], and method of capture) influence the plasma biochemistry results of fish.

Because the physiology of fishes is influence by the aquatic environment, the "normal" reference intervals for one group of fish from one environment may be considered "abnormal" from those of the same species living in a separate environment. Therefore, established reference intervals for each species of fish should include as many variables as possible. These should include sex, age, nutrition, water-quality parameters, stocking density, and sampling techniques [8].

Sample collection and handling

Blood samples for biochemical studies of fish are collected in the same manner as that described for hematologic studies (see Chapter 22). When collecting blood, emersion, and handling of fish for as little as 30 seconds can elicit changes in plasma biochemical analytes such as electrolytes and ammonia [9, 10]. Changes in plasma electrolyte concentrations resulting from transmembrane shifts of H^+, Na^+, Cl^-, and H_2O also may continue until the erythrocytes and plasma are separated. The magnitude of these changes varies directly with the handling time and with the time that elapses between blood collection and analysis. In sturgeon and presumably other fish, storage at 4 °C limits serum glucose decline for at least 4 hours: however, at 25 °C, serum-clot contact time should not exceed 2 hours [11]. *In vitro* changes after blood collection can be minimized by separating plasma from the erythrocytes as soon as possible after the specimen is obtained.

Capture stress is unavoidable when dealing with wild-caught fish or removal of fish from large exhibits. The stress response will have a significant effect on some plasma biochemistry analytes [9, 10, 12, 13]. For example, lactic acidosis may occur after 5 minutes of capture involving strenuous muscle activity as a result of lactate released from the white muscle of fish. The resulting intracellular fluid shift affects the majority of plasma constituents. Complete recovery of the blood parameters may require 2 weeks following 2-minute handling stress. Chemical restraint of captive fish may also affect plasma biochemical results. For example, tricaine methanesulfonate, a commonly used anesthetic for fish, can cause increases in plasma glucose and potassium and urinary electrolyte loss is teleost fish.

Biochemical evaluations on piscine blood can be performed using either serum or plasma [14]. Blood may be collected into an anticoagulant such as lithium heparin to harvest a plasma sample. Plasma is preferred over serum in some species of fish owing to the long time required for clot formation that may produce significant changes in some of the blood biochemical values. Furthermore, a larger sample volume can usually be obtained when performing biochemical tests on plasma versus serum; an important consideration when testing small fish. Collection of blood into lithium heparin also allows for evaluation of the hemogram and plasma chemistry parameters with use of only a single sample.

The sample size is often small, especially when blood is collected from small fish. Therefore, the clinician must decide which tests would be most beneficial in the evaluation of piscine patients. Blood biochemical tests that may be useful include those for total protein, glucose, aspartate

Veterinary Hematology, Clinical Chemistry, and Cytology, Third Edition. Edited by Mary Anna Thrall, Glade Weiser, Robin W. Allison and Terry W. Campbell.

Companion website: www.wiley.com/go/thrall/veterinary

aminotransferase (AST), ammonia, creatinine, calcium, sodium, chloride, potassium, and bicarbonate.

Laboratory evaluation of the piscine kidney

Both grossly and histologically, the anatomy of the piscine kidney varies among species [15, 16]. Freshwater species have larger and more numerous glomeruli compared with those of marine species, some of which have aglomerular kidneys. When present, fish glomeruli resemble those of mammals. Fish kidneys lack a loop of Henle, and collecting ducts occur only in freshwater species. Fish also lack a true urinary bladder, although an enlargement of the distal ureter, which is of mesothelial rather than endothelial origin, resembles a bladder in some species. The primary urinary function occurs in the caudal kidney.

Normal renal physiology of freshwater fish

The kidney of freshwater teleosts (bony fish) have well-developed glomeruli, proximal and distal tubules, and collecting ducts. The proximal tubule has two subunits. The first (segment I) is homologous to the proximal tubule of tetrapod vertebrates, and the second (segment II) is found only in fish. Freshwater bony fish faced with a water volume load and salt loss maintain a high glomerular filtration rate (GFR) and urine production rate to counteract the marked osmotic uptake of water, whereas they conserve sodium chloride (NaCl) by reabsorption in the renal tubules and collecting ducts. The final processing of urine occurs in the water-impermeable "urinary bladder," where ion reabsorption is substantial.

Normal renal physiology of saltwater fish

The kidneys of marine teleosts have fewer and smaller glomeruli compared to those of freshwater species, and the distal tubule is usually missing. Glomeruli and proximal tubules also are missing in some marine species. Marine teleosts face water volume depletion and salt loading. In these fish, some reabsorption of urine occurs in the tubules and the "urinary bladder," which is permeable to water.

Normal renal physiology of sharks and rays

The kidneys of elasmobranchs (i.e., cartilaginous fish such as sharks, skates, and rays) are extremely complex and composed of glomeruli, proximal tubules, and distal tubules that are divided into segments, and collecting tubules and ducts. The GFR of marine elasmobranchs approaches that of freshwater teleosts to balance the osmotic influx of water across the gill [17]. The proximal tubules of these fish can secrete NaCl, and both fluid and salt are reabsorbed in the distal tubule to establish an osmotic gradient, thereby facilitating a tubular countercurrent system to promote the passive reabsorption of urea. The high urea concentration of marine elasmobranchs causes the plasma to be slightly hyperosmotic to the surrounding seawater. Thus, marine elasmobranchs face a net osmotic influx of water, because their gill epithelium is permeable to water but not to NaCl. The high plasma urea concentration of these fish would be fatal without the presence of trimethylamine oxide (TMAO), which, when present at 50% of the urea concentration, counteracts the toxic effects of urea. Both plasma urea and TMAO are derived from hepatic biosynthesis, and the concentrations are maintained by low branchial (gill) permeability and renal tubular reabsorption. Freshwater rays have lost the ability to reabsorb urea and actually excrete urea to lower the plasma osmolarity; therefore they produce dilute urine similar in composition to that of freshwater teleosts with the exception that urea is the primary osmolyte [18, 19].

Plasma urea, uric acid, creatine, and creatinine

Piscine kidneys primarily are involved in ion excretion and osmoregulation [20]. Because these kidneys contribute little to the excretion of nitrogenous wastes, interpretation of the plasma concentrations of urea nitrogen, uric acid, and creatinine may not be useful in the evaluation of renal disease in fish. Urea is derived primarily from degradation of purines via uric acid. Most fish produce small amounts of urea with the exception of marine elasmobranchs, a few ureogenic teleosts, and coelacanths that produce urea as the major end product of nitrogen metabolism. Little is known concerning factors that regulate urea metabolism in teleosts. The gills, however, appear to predominate over the kidneys as the major organ of urea excretion in most fish (except perhaps marine elasmobranchs). Therefore, increases in the plasma urea concentration may be more indicative of branchial epithelial disease than of renal disease in teleost fish [21]. Freshwater teleosts living in alkaline lakes with high pH have high plasma urea concentrations because of a possible interaction of acid-base with urea production. Plasma urea concentrations increase in species such as the lungfish (*Protopterus* sp.), which can survive out of water (i.e., estivation) for extended periods. These fish primarily are ammoniotelic when living in water, but during estivation, the plasma ammonia concentration decreases to negligible levels and the urea concentration increases to avoid ammonia toxicity. The plasma urea concentration also increases in cyprinids (carp, goldfish, and koi) exposed to high environmental levels of ammonia.

The normal plasma urea concentration of freshwater and marine teleosts is less than 10 mg/dL (3.57 mmol/L) and 5 mg/dL (1.79 mmol/L), respectively. Marine elasmobranchs (sharks and rays) have a normal mean plasma urea concentration that ranges between 350 (125 mmol/L) and 1000 mg/dL (357 mmol/L) or higher. Decreases in the plasma urea concentration, especially in marine elasmobranchs, suggest decreased production consistent with hepatic disease or starvation. Captive individuals typically have higher blood urea nitrogen (BUN) concentrations compared to those of the same species living in the wild [22]. Renal disease in marine elasmobranchs also may produce a decreased plasma urea concentration owing to reduced reabsorption.

Fish produce small amounts of uric acid, creatine, and creatinine, but little is known regarding their physiologic role. Uric acid, a degradation product of purine nucleotides and protein catabolism (via purines), produced primarily in the liver and white muscle of fish is generally converted to urea for excretion. Creatine, an end product of glycine, arginine, and methionine metabolism primarily in white muscle, represents more than 50% of the nitrogenous waste that is excreted through the kidney. Therefore, the plasma creatine concentration may be valuable in the assessment of renal disease among fish. Unfortunately, studies have not been performed to evaluate the use of creatine as an indicator of such renal disease, and most veterinary laboratories do not offer creatine assays.

Creatinine is formed from creatine and it also is secreted by piscine kidneys. The normal plasma creatinine concentration is low in most fishes, 0.11 (9.7 µmol/L) to 0.88 mg/dL (77.8 µmol/L) [8]. In the English sole (*Parophrys vetulus*), increases in the plasma creatinine concentration have been associated with renal disease, although the urea concentrations remained normal [23].

Divalent ions

Excess divalent and monovalent ions are excreted in marine teleosts by different routes after the oral ingestion of seawater. The kidneys excrete divalent ions such as magnesium and sulfate, and increases in the plasma concentrations of these ions may indicate renal disease in these fish.

Laboratory evaluation of electrolytes and acid-base balance

Electrolytes are indicative of a fish's ability to osmoregulate and are the best understood biochemical analytes in fishes. Values are compromised by stress, disease, or gill lesions that increase permeability of the gills to ions.

Osmoregulation

Teleost (bony fish) plasma is hyperosmotic to freshwater but hypoosmotic to seawater. Freshwater teleosts are hyperregulators, and they face hyperhydration and ion losses by diffusion. They maintain osmotic and ionic homeostasis by active uptake of ions across the intestinal and branchial epithelium. Because plasma sodium and chloride concentrations are more commonly measured than plasma osmolarity, the formula $Osm_{NaCl} = [Na^+ + Cl^-] \times 0.91$ is frequently used as a measurement of osmolarity in the literature [20]. Marine teleosts (Osm_{NaCl} greater than 300) are hyporegulators and maintain plasma osmolality at approximately one-third that of seawater and slightly greater than that of freshwater teleosts (Osm_{NaCl} = 195–252) [17]. The resulting osmotic water loss compensated for by drinking seawater. A $Na^+/K^+/Cl^-$ co-transporter drives the water uptake in the intestinal epithelium, and the high uptake of monovalent ions is compensated for by excretion of these ions via the gills. Therefore, marine teleosts ingest saltwater to balance the osmotic loss of water across the gills, and freshwater teleosts excrete large volumes of dilute urine to balance the osmotic uptake of water.

Whereas plasma sodium chloride contributes to greater than 75% of the osmolarity of teleost fish, it contributes to only 50% or less in elasmobranchs (sharks, rays, and skates). Nonprotein nitrogen, primarily urea, makes up most of the balance in marine elasmobranchs to raise the osmotic pressure to slightly greater than that of the ambient seawater. Therefore, marine elasmobranchs, unlike marine teleosts, do not lose water across the gills; instead, they gain small amounts that allow for urine formation. Thus, marine elasmobranchs do not drink seawater. A decrease in plasma urea concentration and osmolarity occurs in marine elasmobranchs during fasting because of a decrease in urea biosynthesis. These decreases also occur when marine elasmobranchs move to environments with lower salinity because of increases in renal urea clearance.

Some freshwater elasmobranchs have higher plasma osmolarity (Osm_{NaCl} approximately 380) compared to that of other freshwater fish and yet maintain a high urea concentration, although it may be 50% that of marine elasmobranchs [18, 19]. These fish are considered to be more recent emigrants to the freshwater environment. Freshwater rays, known to be long-term inhabitants of freshwater habitats, have a lower osmolarity (Osm_{NaCl} approximately 281) with urea having negligible participation.

Osmoregulation of marine elasmobranchs involves the kidneys, rectal glands, gills, and diet. A high level of urea is maintained by renal tubular reabsorption. In freshwater, urea is excreted to lower the osmolarity. Rays adapted to living in freshwater have lost the ability to reabsorb urea. The rectal gland of marine elasmobranchs is a salt secreting organ. When exposed to freshwater, these fish exhibit regression of the gland. Freshwater rays have no functional rectal gland. Two-thirds of the total sodium and chloride excreted by elasmobranchs occurs in the gills. Their gills have low permeability to urea. Finally, metabolic urea is directly related to food availability.

Sodium chloride

Na^+ and Cl^- are the major ions in the blood of all fish [20]. Marine teleosts display a higher branchial permeability to salt; therefore, the unidirectional Na^+ and Cl^- fluxes are

10- to 50-fold greater than those of freshwater teleosts. Ionic gradients across the gill epithelium are of the same magnitude as those of freshwater fish, but they are reversed in direction. Because the kidney of marine teleosts cannot produce urine, which is hyper-osmolar relative to plasma, extrarenal salt secretion must occur. The mitochondria-rich chloride cells of the gills are most likely the sites of ionic and/or acid-base regulation involving Na/H [NH_4] and Cl/HCO_3 exchanges in fish.

The rectal gland is the site of extrarenal salt secretion in marine sharks and rays [24]. This gland produces a solution that is iso-osmotic to the plasma but that contains more NaCl than seawater (in a manner similar to the NaCl transport system in the thick, ascending limb of the loop of Henle in mammals). An increase in plasma volume, rather than in NaCl concentration, appears to stimulate rectal gland secretions in marine elasmobranchs [17].

Fish have adapted to marine or freshwater environments by using osmotic and ionic regulating mechanisms allowing them to maintain a relatively constant plasma and intracellular salt concentration as well as cellular volume. Whereas the kidney is the primary osmoregulatory organ of terrestrial vertebrates, fish use organs such as the gills, intestines, rectal glands, and to a lesser extent, the kidneys to regulate fluid volume and salt concentration.

The normal plasma sodium and chloride concentrations of freshwater teleosts and marine teleosts are approximately 150 mEq/L (mmol/L) and 130 mEq/L (mmol/L), respectively. Plasma sodium and chloride concentrations are affected by changes in ambient salinity, gill function, and stress. Within a few minutes of capture and handling trauma, catecholamines, and cortisol are released along with lactic acid release from muscles. Stress-induced release of catecholamines causes an increase in blood pressure resulting in an increased electrolyte permeability of the gills that causes a rapid decrease in sodium and chloride in freshwater teleost fish and increase in those ions in marine teleost fish. Hyponatremia and hypochloremia in freshwater fish can be associated with gill and renal disease or with acidic or soft-water environments.

Influx of Na and Cl in marine elasmobranchs from the environment is compensated for by efficient salt excretion mechanisms in both the kidney and the specialized rectal gland [24]. Variability seen in plasma and serum Na and Cl ion concentrations between wild-caught and captive elasmobranchs may relate to differences in environmental salinity and diet and subsequent alterations in ion regulation or may reflect normal variability [22].

Potassium

The normal plasma potassium concentration of freshwater fish is approximately 2–4 mEq/L (mmol/L). Less than 2% of the total body potassium is found in extracellular fluids; therefore, plasma levels are unaffected by changes in gill electrolyte permeability [20]. Greater than 95% of the potassium ingested by marine fish is absorbed in the intestines, and the excess is excreted extrarenally as part of the slime coat. Variability seen in plasma and serum K ion concentration between wild-caught and captive elasmobranchs may relate to differences in environmental salinity and diet and subsequent alterations in ion regulation or may reflect normal variability [22]. Hypokalemia may be associated with alkalosis, gastrointestinal or cutaneous potassium loss, or nitrite toxicity. Hyperkalemia may be associated with acidosis, such as occurs following strenuous muscle activity during capture and handling, and decreased renal secretion of potassium in freshwater teleosts. Hemolysis will also cause an artificial increase in plasma potassium.

Calcium

The normal plasma calcium concentration of teleosts is approximately 8–10 mg/dL (2–2.5 mmol/L). Because water is a readily available source of calcium, the plasma calcium concentration is influenced by the environmental calcium concentration. Fish have access to a continuous supply of calcium, so they must limit their calcium intake (unless the environmental calcium levels are low). In freshwater teleosts, calcium is transported by the chloride cells in the gills to the blood. Calcium ions enter these cells passively along the electrochemical gradient via calcium channels in the apical cell membrane. Stanniocalcin is a hormone that is unique to certain fish (e.g., teleosts) and that acts as a calcium-channel blocker to prevent the development of hypercalcemia [20]. Fish do not have parathyroid glands or a parathormone-like hormone. How fish that do not produce stanniocalcin regulate their blood calcium concentrations is not yet known.

In contrast to tetrapods, calcitonin whose role is to correct excessive calcium levels does not play a prominent role in calcium regulation in fish. Calcitonin is produced by the ultimobranchial bodies of fish and has a role in protecting the skeletal system during periods of increased demand for Ca^{2+} during active oogenesis.

In male and nongravid female freshwater teleost fish, 30–40% of the total plasma calcium is bound to protein. Approximately 22% of the total calcium is bound to protein in marine teleosts. Therefore, changes in plasma protein will affect the plasma total calcium concentration. For example, during vitellogenesis, a greater than threefold increase in total protein and calcium will be expected; however, free Ca^{++} concentration remains constant.

Both stress and circadian fluctuations have negligible effects on plasma calcium concentrations in freshwater fish [8].

Phosphorus

In general, the normal plasma phosphorus concentration of fish is approximately 3.5–8.9 mg/dL (1.1–2.9 mmol/L).

However, variations in diet, water quality, and age can lead to alterations in phosphorus concentrations [2, 4, 25].

Magnesium

The plasma magnesium concentration of freshwater fish and marine elasmobranchs is generally lower than the calcium concentration; however, marine teleosts have magnesium concentrations that are greater than calcium. In general, inorganic ions, such as Na, Cl, and Ca, are kept below levels found in the ambient marine water. Approximately 25% of the plasma magnesium concentration is bound to protein; however, the mechanism of magnesium regulation is unknown. Because magnesium concentration within erythrocytes is nearly 10 times that of plasma, hemolysis would be expected to produce an artificial increase in plasma magnesium concentration.

Acid-base balance

Acid-base regulation in fish is more challenging compared with that of terrestrial animals, because the composition of water varies to a greater degree than that of air. Large and rapid changes in oxygen and carbon dioxide (CO_2) levels, electrolyte concentrations, and temperature are significant challenges to acid-base regulation. The branchial epithelium is the site of gas exchange and principal ion regulation in fish; ions readily transfer across the gill surface. Therefore, changes in the water ionic composition affect the ionic transfer process across the branchial epithelium, which in turn affects osmotic and acid-base regulation.

Fish have a low blood CO_2 concentration compared with that of terrestrial animals [26]. This results from the high rate of gill ventilation and the much larger capacity of water for carbon monoxide (CO) dissolution. The small environmental CO_2 and arterial CO_2 differences limit the ability of fish to compensate for changes in arterial CO_2 by hyper- or hypoventilation. Therefore, changes in CO_2 are too small to contribute significantly to the acid-base balance in fish. However, even though respiratory regulation contributes little to acid-base balance, fish have a larger epithelial ionic transfer capacity than that of air-breathing mammals, and they also have the capacity for a net gain of bicarbonate from the environment to facilitate normalization of the acid-base status [27]. This epithelial ionic transfer is a function of the chloride cells located in juxtaposition to the secondary circulatory system of the central venous gill sinus. Ionic transfer for acid-base regulation also occurs, although to a lesser extent, across the skin and kidney of fish.

Laboratory evaluation of branchial epithelium

Because the gills of fish are important organs for osmotic, ionic, and acid-base regulation as well as for removal of nitrogenous waste, changes in the blood biochemistry may reflect damage to the branchial epithelium. Injury to gill tissue may result in thickening of the branchial epithelium and an increased distance for diffusion from blood to water. In turn, this may lead to an increased plasma concentration of analytes normally excreted by the branchial epithelium. Therefore, acid-base disturbances, electrolyte imbalances, and increases in the blood ammonia and urea concentrations may occur with damage to the branchial epithelium of fish.

Ammonia

Ammonia is the major end product of nitrogen metabolism in most fish except marine elasmobranchs. Ammonia is the most reduced and energy-efficient nitrogenous waste product of the biologic oxidation of dietary or structural proteins. The primary mechanism of ammonia excretion in freshwater teleosts is branchial excretion. The skin also contributes to ammonia excretion, especially in marine teleosts. The kidneys excrete less than 15% of ammonia.

The mechanism of branchial ammonia excretion primarily involves diffusion along a concentration gradient from blood to water and an electro-neutral Na^+/NH_4^+ exchange located on the apical membranes of the branchial epithelial cells [15, 21]. Electro-neutral H^+/NH_4^+ exchange also may occur in the gill membranes of fish. Marine teleosts excrete ammonia by NH_4^+ diffusion along an electrochemical gradient from blood to water.

The inflammation, swelling, and mucinification that occur with gill damage result in an increased diffusion distance between blood and water, thereby creating an increased blood ammonia concentration. Environmental toxins, changes in the environmental pH and ammonia concentrations, or infections can damage the gills of fish, thus resulting in increased blood ammonia concentrations. Increases in the environmental pH and ammonia concentration also can increase the blood ammonia concentration by the inhibition of ammonia diffusion, thereby reversing the blood-to-water gradient.

Plasma total ammonia is highly variable and rarely used in diagnostic testing of piscine patients. Both the site of blood collection and the duration of restraint affect the blood ammonia concentration in fish. Total plasma ammonia concentration is higher in samples obtained by caudal venipuncture (prehepatic blood) compared to samples obtained by cardiocentesis (posthepatic blood). Venous blood contains 50–60% more ammonia than arterial blood. During restraint, the release of ammonia from hypoxic muscles and the interference with branchial excretion also can increase the blood ammonia concentration in fish. Plasma ammonia levels increase with feeding, exhaustive exercise, exposure to air, and under certain water quality parameters, such as an increase in water temperature, increase in ammonia concentration, and alkaline pH.

Laboratory evaluation of the piscine liver

Little information is available regarding laboratory evaluation of the liver in fish. The liver tissue of teleosts appears to be rich in AST and possible alanine aminotransferase (ALT). Therefore, plasma activity of these enzymes may elevate with severe hepatocellular disease in some piscine species.

There is a general lack of information regarding the influence of nonpathogenic factors on the activities of these enzymes in the plasma of fish; however, a few studies have suggested that plasma enzyme evaluation in fish may not be as straightforward as it is in mammals. For example, the high ammonia levels of fish may lead to high transaminase activities; therefore, the increase in activities may be associated with liver disease or changes in plasma ammonia concentration. High activities of AST and creatine kinase (CK) also occur in muscle of fish; therefore, elevated plasma activities of these enzymes will increase following muscle injury or strenuous muscle activity associated with capture and restraint. Temperature changes have been reported to affect plasma enzyme activity of alkaline phosphatase (AP). The method of blood collection influences plasma lactate dehydrogenase (LDH) and CK activities in fish leading to the recommendation that blood collected by cardiocentesis be used for enzyme studies. Plasma LDH activity is also influenced by feeding and activity levels resulting in lower LDH values starvation and inactivity. It has also been shown that plasma LDH activity is positively correlated with water temperature and pH.

Bile pigments in most fish include both bilirubin and biliverdin; however, the percentages of these pigments vary between species. The serum usually is a light yellow color because of the presence of bilirubin. Hepatic disease in fish may not reliably cause an increased plasma bilirubin concentration. The serum from some fish (e.g., certain eels) is bluish green because of the presence of biliverdin.

There is little information about the normal bile acid metabolism in fish. Fish may continuously secrete bile acids into the intestines resulting in no change in plasma bile acid concentration associated with feeding.

Glucose

Plasma glucose concentration in fish is variable and can be as low as 30 mg/dL (1.67 mmol/L) in some species. The source of plasma glucose in fish is hepatic glycogen metabolism; therefore depletion of hepatic glycogen reserves may result in hypoglycemia. Plasma glucose concentration in fish is highly dependent upon the activity level of the fish. For example, sluggish benthic species have lower plasma glucose concentrations compared to the more active pelagic species. Plasma glucose concentration also varies with age, nutritional and reproductive status, and stress. The duration and magnitude of postprandial hyperglycemia in fish depends upon dietary carbohydrate intake. The effect of starvation on plasma glucose concentration is species and time dependent because many species of fish exhibit normal blood glucose concentrations (up to 150 days) following prolonged starvation. The mechanism allowing for maintenance of normal blood glucose concentrations with prolonged starvation is not known. Variation in blood glucose concentration also occurs with the reproductive status of fish were lowest blood glucose values in males and females are associated with spawning.

Stress-induced hyperglycemia is a common occurrence in fish and the extent and duration is influenced by the severity of stress. The increased plasma concentrations of catecholamines and adrenocorticosteroids associated with stress changes the muscle and hepatic glycogen reserves in fishes. Catecholamines mobilize glycogen stores and corticosteroids induce glycogen synthesis. Therefore, the plasma hyperglycemia associated with marked glycogenolysis in liver and muscle is likely due to stress-induced increases in catecholamines. Fluctuations in blood glucose concentrations appear to be linked to cortisol and thyroid hormone variations [28].

Cholesterol

It is not known whether changes in the plasma cholesterol concentration have significant meaning in regards to hepatic disease. Most fish, except for elasmobranchs, normally have higher blood cholesterol concentrations than do mammals. The majority of the blood cholesterol (60–90%) of fish is carried by high-density lipoproteins (HDL). The blood cholesterol concentration of elasmobranchs is lower than that of teleosts and varies with gender and reproductive status. Males undergoing active spermatogenesis have higher cholesterol values compared to inactive males. Females have lower blood cholesterol concentrations compared to males were females undergoing active egg production have the lowest values. Although the role of cholesterol is not well understood in elasmobranchs, the higher blood cholesterol concentration noted in captive elasmobranchs compared the same species caught in the wild may reflect a difference in nutritional plane between the two groups [22].

Protein

The total plasma protein concentration of fish ranges between 2 and 8 g/dL (20–80 g/L) when using the refractometric method. The normal plasma albumin concentration of fish ranges between 1.0 and 2.4 g/dL (10–24 g/l = L). The normal albumin: globulin ratio of fish is expected to be lower than that of mammals. Albumin and globulins are the major blood proteins in fish, with globulin levels being greater than those for albumin. These serum proteins play a large role in innate immunity, thus higher concentrations, in particular of globulins, in serum may be reflective of enhanced nonspecific immune responses in fish. Total plasma protein is expected to have a higher value when determined by refractometry as compared to spectrophotometry. The use of the refractometer is often preferred because of its greater practicality compared to the more labor intensive and expensive spectrophotometer method. Protein is a major contributing factor of plasma refractive index, but nonprotein components such as glucose, cholesterol, and chloride can interfere with measurements in the refractometer. Due to these discrepancies, there should be awareness of the elevated values when using refractometry for estimating total plasma protein in fish. Plasma protein concentrations increase significantly with age in some species of freshwater fish [29]. The increase, mainly due to an increase in the globulin fraction, indicates that separate reference intervals for this analyte should be generated with respect to age in fish.

Changes in plasma protein can be an indicator of an underlying systemic infection or subclinical organ pathology. In veterinary medicine, plasma protein electrophoresis has been shown to be an important diagnostic tool when recognizing disease in various terrestrial species; however, there have been few studies involving its use in fish. The automated cellulose acetate electrophoresis and densitometry method, used widely in human and veterinary clinical biochemistry laboratories, is a practical method for estimation of serum protein fractions in freshwater teleost fish [30].

Gel electrophoresis was used to establish reference intervals for the following protein fractions: total protein, prealbumin, albumin, a-1 globulin, a-2 globulin, β globulin, c globulin, C-reactive protein, serum amyloid A, and haptoglobin in Whitespotted bamboo sharks (*Chiloscyllium plagiosum*) [31]. A significant difference was found in regard to sex, whereby females had higher β fractions and total protein concentrations when compared to males.

Laboratory evaluation of endocrine disorders

The neuroendocrine system of fish is similar to those of other vertebrates. Because fish have a very close interaction with the ambient aquatic environment, their endocrine system may differ functionally from those of terrestrial animals. For example, hormones such as prolactin, growth hormone, cortisol, glucagon, and somatostatin have important ionic regulating functions in fish that are not observed in terrestrial vertebrates. Fish also have unique hormones, including somatolactin, melanophore-concentrating hormone, urotensin, and stanniocalcin. Parathormone and aldosterone are not found in fish, however, and this implies the absence of a requirement for these hormones because of their close association with their aquatic environment.

Commercial kits for the measurement of hormones in mammalian plasma have been used successfully in the determination of hormones that are common to both types of animals [32]. Homologous radioimmunoassays (RIA) have been developed to assay the blood hormones of a few species of fish (salmonids and cyprinids).

Thyroid

Fish thyroid tissue appears to behave similarly to that of terrestrial mammals. It is stimulated by a thyroid-stimulating hormone to release thyroxine (T_4), which is de-iodinated to triiodothyronine (T_3) in target organs such as the gills and liver. There are species differences associated with blood thyroid hormone concentrations. The plasma concentration of thyroid hormones may be influenced by plasma protein concentration as they are bound to transport proteins. Increases in plasma T_3 and T_4 concentrations are associated with significant physiologic functions in fish, such as the adaptation of salmonids to seawater. Decreases in T_4 concentration indicate either decreased thyroid secretion or increased conversion of T_4 to T_3. In general, both hormones are elevated during growth and decreased during conditions such as stress, starvation, and vitelogenesis.

Adrenal (inter-renal tissue)

The inter-renal tissue of fish is homologous to the adrenal tissues of higher vertebrates. The major corticosteroid produced by this tissue in most jawed fish is cortisol. The major corticosteroid in elasmobranchs is 1α-hydroxycorticosterone. Plasma cortisol concentration is cyclic and affected by the photoperiod (diel cycle) and time of feeding with peak concentrations occurring prior to the onset of light and increased locomotory activity. Cortisol is involved in energy metabolism, ion regulation, and response to stress. Cortisol secretion is stimulated by the stress response (i.e., capture, handling, crowding, transport, rapid changes in water quality, and other physical disturbances) mediated by adrenocorticotropic hormone (ACTH) resulting in a rapid hyperglycemia. The corticosteroid stress response of elasmobranchs is small compared to that of teleost fish.

Amphibians

Blood samples for use in biochemical studies of amphibians are collected in the same manner as that described for hematologic studies (see Chapter 23). Blood to be evaluated for hematology and plasma biochemistry generally is collected into an anticoagulant (e.g., lithium heparin). Plasma is preferred to serum, because a larger sample volume usually can be obtained when collecting plasma.

Blood biochemical evaluation is not routinely part of the clinical assessment of amphibian patients. Routine assay methods for the biochemical evaluation of mammalian blood appear to be useful for amphibians. Interpretation of the results is difficult, however, because little information

Table 38.1 Normal serum biochemistry reference values for American bullfrogs (*Rana catesbeiana*) kept at 20–25 °C.

Urea (mg/dL)	3.00 ± 1.00[a]
Creatinine (mg/dL)	0.99 ± 0.20
Uric acid (mg/dL)	0.06 ± 0.05
Total protein (g/dL)	4.40 ± 0.30 (females)
	3.70 ± 0.80 (males)
Albumin (g/dL)	1.60 ± 0.30
Aspartate aminotransferase (IU/L)	45 ± 21
Lactate dehydrogenase (IU/L)	33 ± 20
Calcium (mg/dL)	8.7 ± 0.6 (females)
	7.4 ± 0.6 (males)
Phosphorus (mg/dL)	3.3 ± 0.7
Sodium (mEq/L)	111 ± 3.0 (females)
	105 ± 4.0 (males)
Potassium (mEq/L)	2.7 ± 0.4
Chloride (mEq/L)	77 ± 6.0
Total carbon dioxide (mmol/L)	25 ± 4.5
Anion gap (calculated)	9.9 ± 6.5

[a]All values represent mean +/− standard deviation.
Source: Modified from Cathers et al. [38].

is available regarding plasma or serum chemistry values. Table 38.1 demonstrates the expected normal serum biochemical values in bullfrogs (*Rana catesbeiana*). Extrinsic factors such as environmental temperature and humidity, photoperiod, season, water-quality parameters, diet, and population density likely affect the normal plasma biochemistries. Intrinsic factors such as gender and age also likely influence the variation in plasma biochemistry values. As an example, female bullfrogs have higher plasma total protein, calcium, and sodium concentrations than male bullfrogs.

Significant morphological and physiological changes take place during metamorphosis that is accompanied by biochemical changes that occur during organ differentiation and maturation. One important change during this period is an increase in total protein. Increased total protein serves to increase the osmotic pressure of the blood to improve its water carrying capacity as the aquatic larval form transforms into the postmetamorphic terrestrial adult. Albumin (which exerts 2–3 times the osmotic pressure per unit as does globulin) increases proportionately more than globulins during metamorphosis. During this period, serum proteins more than double and at least 20% of the increase is associated with an increase in albumin, which increases more than 10 times. In amphibian species where the adult remains aquatic, there is no change in serum protein. An increase in the serum albumin concentration has also been seen as an adaptation of amphibian species to a more arid environment. Therefore, because adult newts and salamanders and gilled aquatic amphibian larvae are more fishlike than adult toads and frogs, the interpretation of changes in their plasma biochemistry profiles may be more like those in fish. The plasma biochemical changes in adult toads and frogs may be more like those of reptiles.

Few biochemical reference intervals for wild and captive amphibians have been established. Higher serum concentrations of protein, cholesterol, glucose, urea, and uric acid have been found to be higher in female frogs compared to males; however, serum creatinine concentrations were higher in males [33]. Serum concentrations of calcium, total protein, albumin, HDL, amylase, potassium, carbon dioxide (CO_2), and uric acid were found to be significantly higher in aged frogs compared to young frogs [34]. Parameters found to be significantly lower in aged frogs included glucose, AST, ALT, cholesterol, BUN, phosphorus, triglycerides, low-density lipoprotein (LDL), lipase, sodium, chloride, and anion gap. These findings indicate that chemistry reference intervals for young amphibians may be inappropriate for use with aged frogs. Studies have also shown that wide interspecies and seasonal variations also occur, especially in wild populations [35]. These findings indicate the need to establish species-, season-, age-, and sex- specific reference intervals for amphibians.

Increases in serum gamma glutamyltransferase and alkaline phosphatase activities along with an increase in total cholesterol concentrations have been found useful in the detection of hepatic injury in amphibians exposed to cadmium toxicity [36]. Indicators of renal dysfunction, such as BUN, creatinine, and calcium were also useful in that same group of animals.

The pathogen *Batrachochytrium dendrobatidis* (Bd), which causes the skin disease chytridiomycosis, is one of the few highly virulent fungi in vertebrates and has been implicated in worldwide amphibian declines. Because the skin is critical in maintaining amphibian homeostasis, disruption to cutaneous function produces morbidity and mortality in these animals.

The electrolyte transport across the epidermis of amphibians with chitridiomycosis can be inhibited by greater than 50% resulting in a reduction of plasma sodium and potassium concentrations by 20% and 50%, respectively [37]. This results in death by asystolic cardiac arrest. Electrolyte depletion has been the most consistent finding in studies designed to determine the physiological effects of chytridiomycosis.

VI

Cytopathology of Common Domestic Animals

39 Cytology of Inflammation and Infectious Agents

Robin W. Allison

Department of Veterinary Pathobiology, Oklahoma State University College of Veterinary Medicine, Stillwater, OK, USA

Inflammation may be encountered in any cytologic sample and is, therefore, important to recognize. Inflammation is characterized by the types of inflammatory cells present, which may give clues to the underlying cause (Table 39.1). Inflammatory cells exfoliate readily, resulting in highly cellular cytologic samples. Inflammation can have noninfectious or infectious causes, and infectious agents may be visualized in cytologic specimens. Some infectious agents are morphologically distinct, allowing specific identification, while others may require additional diagnostics (culture, histopathology with special stains, polymerase chain reaction [PCR]) for identification.

Inflammatory cell types

Neutrophils

Inflammatory lesions characterized by a predominance of neutrophils are termed suppurative, purulent, or neutrophilic inflammation. Neutrophils are further characterized as nondegenerate or degenerate. Nondegenerate neutrophils appear similar to those in peripheral blood; nuclei have dense chromatin with distinct segmentation (Figure 39.1). Degenerate neutrophils have nuclear changes reflective of a toxic environment, most often associated with bacterial infections. Degenerate neutrophils have swollen nuclei that lose segmentation and stain pale pink (Figure 39.1). Such cells may eventually disintegrate and become unrecognizable (Figure 39.2). Neutrophils may appear degenerate in some microenvironments even in the absence of infection (i.e., airway or gastrointestinal tract samples, exposure to urine). Neutrophils may also lyse because of trauma from improper slide preparation or because of poor-preservation caused by improper sample handling. Neutrophils that are undergoing normal aging and cell death may be hypersegmented or pyknotic. Pyknotic neutrophils have nuclei that have become dense, dark purple spheres (Figure 39.1).

Underlying causes of suppurative inflammation include a wide variety of infectious and noninfectious disorders. Noninfectious causes include tissue inflammation secondary to neoplasia, necrosis, trauma, and immune-mediated disease. Many different types of infectious agents, especially bacteria, may cause predominantly suppurative inflammation. Neutrophils are phagocytic cells, thus microorganisms (most frequently bacteria) may be visualized within neutrophils, signifying septic, suppurative inflammation (Figure 39.2). If bacteria are only extracellular, potential contamination of the sample or presence of normal flora must be considered.

Macrophages

Inflammation characterized by a predominance of macrophages is termed histiocytic, granulomatous, or macrophagic inflammation. A mixed inflammatory cell population composed predominantly of neutrophils and macrophages may be termed either mixed or pyogranulomatous (Figure 39.3). Some pathologists prefer the term mixed, because a true pyogranulomatous process is an architectural arrangement that is best visualized by histopathology. Such mixed inflammatory processes may also contain small numbers of lymphocytes and plasma cells. Macrophage morphology can vary considerably in cytologic samples, causing confusion for even experienced cytologists. They may appear similar to peripheral blood monocytes but typically are large round cells with oval to indented nuclei and abundant lightly basophilic cytoplasm (Figure 39.4). Activated macrophages are vacuolated and often contain phagocytized cells or cell debris, erythrocytes or hemosiderin (evidence of previous hemorrhage), or microorganisms. Epithelioid macrophages are nonvacuolated and tend to cluster, mimicking epithelial cells. In chronic inflammatory conditions macrophages may fuse to become multinucleated inflammatory giant cells (Figure 39.5). Macrophages are capable of proliferating in tissues, in which case mitotic figures may be observed

Veterinary Hematology, Clinical Chemistry, and Cytology, Third Edition. Edited by Mary Anna Thrall, Glade Weiser, Robin W. Allison and Terry W. Campbell.

Companion website: www.wiley.com/go/thrall/veterinary

Table 39.1 Inflammatory cells and associated conditions.

Type of inflammation	Predominant cell types	Commonly associated conditions
Suppurative (purulent, neutrophilic)	Neutrophils	Bacterial infections, immune-mediated disorders, necrosis, neoplasia, trauma
Histiocytic (macrophagic, granulomatous)	Macrophages	Foreign body reactions, mycobacterial infections
Lymphocytic/plasmacytic	Lymphocytes and plasma cells	Immune-mediated disorders, chronic inflammation, vaccine reactions
Eosinophilic	>10% eosinophil (± mast cells)	Eosinophilic granuloma, hypersensitivity reactions, parasite migration, some infections (*Pythium*, some fungal infections), neoplasia (mast cell tumor, lymphoma)
Mixed (pyogranulomatous)	Neutrophils and macrophages (± lymphocytes)	Foreign body reactions, fungal infections, some bacterial infections (*Mycobacteria*, filamentous bacteria), sterile panniculitis, chronic tissue injury, vaccine reactions

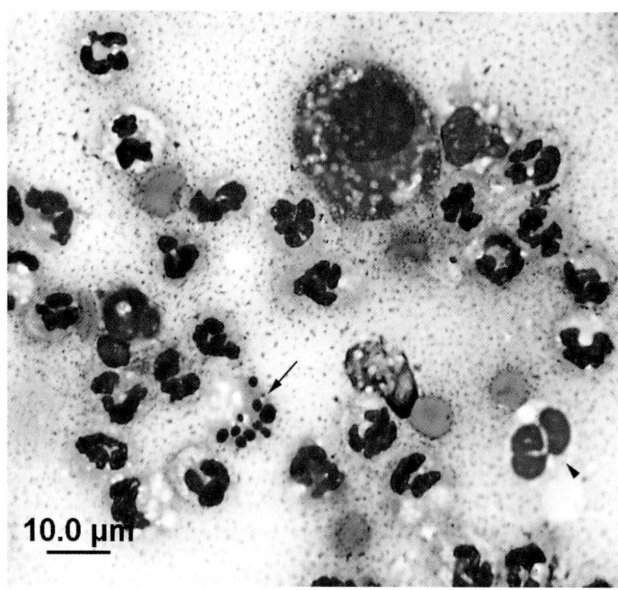

Figure 39.1 Suppurative inflammation. Most neutrophils are nondegenerate with distinct segmentations and dark chromatin. One cell has become pyknotic (arrow), with chromatin condensed into small dark spheres. One degenerate neutrophil (arrowhead) has swollen, pale-staining chromatin. One macrophage is present (large cell top center, round nucleus and cytoplasmic vacuoles). Aqueous Romanowsky stain.

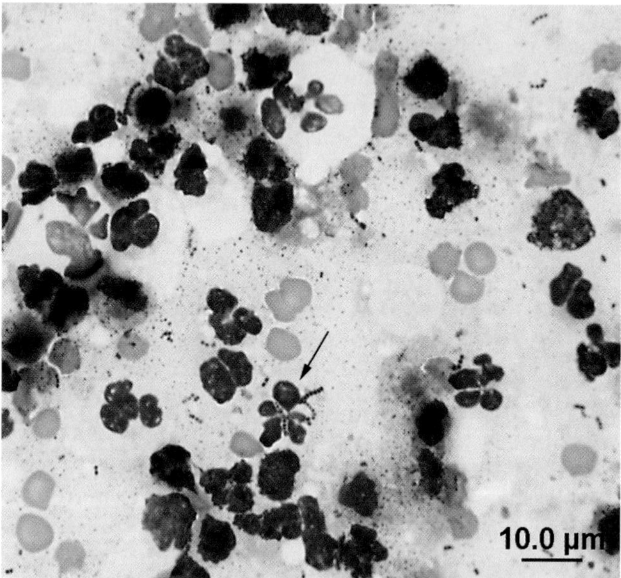

Figure 39.2 Septic, suppurative inflammation. Neutrophils are degenerate and barely recognizable; many have lysed. Dark blue bacterial cocci, most in chains, are present in the background and phagocytized by one neutrophil (arrow). There are also pink protein precipitates in the background. Aqueous Romanowsky stain.

(Figure 39.6). Because macrophages can normally have features that are considered criteria of malignancy (anisocytosis, bi- or multinucleation, prominent nucleoli, mitotic figures; see Figures 39.4–39.6), extreme caution is warranted when considering an interpretation of malignant neoplasia in the face of inflammation.

Lesions that typically contain moderate to large numbers of macrophages include chronic inflammation caused by foreign body reactions, sterile panniculitis, mycobacterial infections, fungal infections, infections caused by filamentous bacteria, and vaccine reactions. Vaccine reactions typically contain a mixture of macrophages, lymphocytes, plasma cells, and neutrophils. Vaccine adjuvant may be identified in cytologic samples from these lesions [1]. Adjuvant appears as magenta or blue (depending on the type of adjuvant) amorphous material that is often phagocytized by macrophages (Figures 39.7 and 39.8).

Lymphocytes and plasma cells

Lymphocytic inflammation is characterized by a mixed population of small and intermediate sized lymphocytes, often admixed with plasma cells and other inflammatory cells (neutrophils and macrophages). Lymphocyte

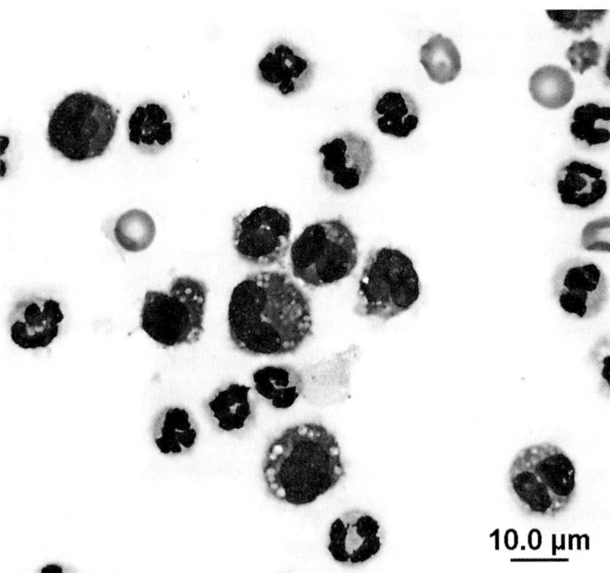

Figure 39.3 Pyogranulomatous inflammation. Neutrophils are nondegenerate. Macrophages vary from resembling blood monocytes to larger cells with indented nuclei and cytoplasmic vacuoles. Aqueous Romanowsky stain.

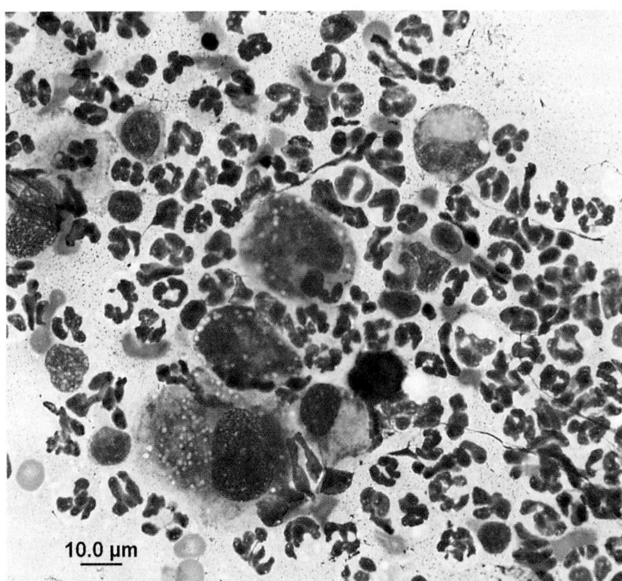

Figure 39.4 Pyogranulomatous inflammation. Neutrophils are a mixture of nondegenerate and degenerate cells. Macrophages are pleomorphic with variably sized nuclei, visible nucleoli, and cytoplasmic vacuolation. The pink granular proteinaceous background should not be confused with bacteria, which would stain blue. Aqueous Romanowsky stain.

and plasma cell morphology is similar to that found in hyperplastic lymph node aspirates (see Chapter 45). Lymphocytic/plasmacytic inflammation occurs with immune reactions (i.e., lymphocytic stomatitis and enteritis), vaccine reactions (Figure 39.7), and chronic inflammation.

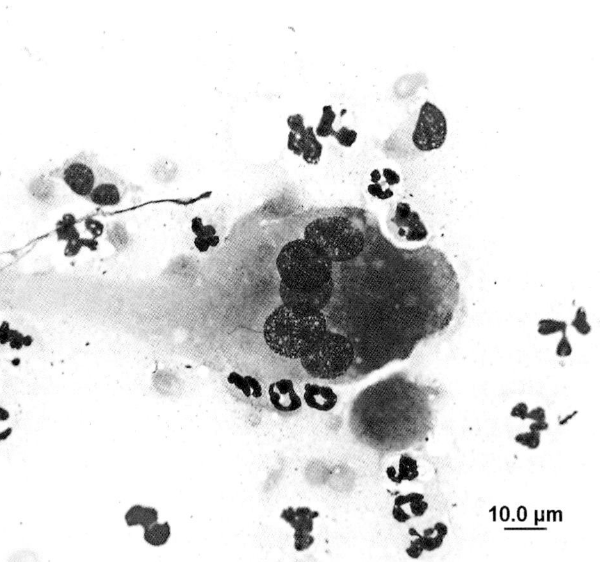

Figure 39.5 Pyogranulomatous inflammation. One large multinucleated inflammatory giant cell (center) contains five nuclei with coarse chromatin and prominent nucleoli. Aqueous Romanowsky stain.

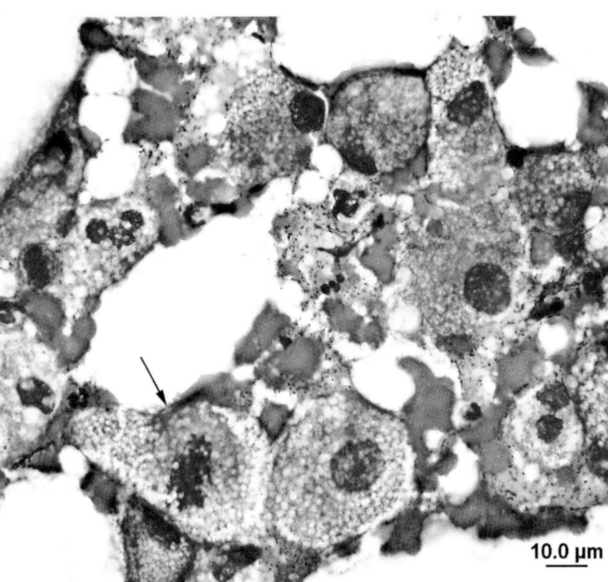

Figure 39.6 Histiocytic inflammation, steatitis. Large, vacuolated macrophages predominate. Macrophages are moderately pleomorphic and one mitotic figure is present (arrow). Aqueous Romanowsky stain.

Eosinophils and mast cells

An inflammatory process is considered to have an eosinophilic component if eosinophils comprise >10% of inflammatory cells. Eosinophils appear similar to those in peripheral blood, with abundant eosinophilic cytoplasmic granules (Figure 39.9). Mast cells are round cells containing round nuclei and moderately abundant cytoplasm that contains abundant dark purple (metachromatic) granules

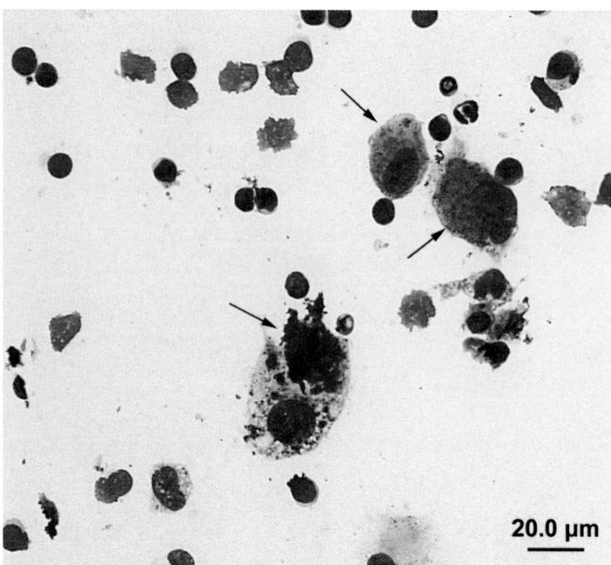

Figure 39.7 Vaccine reaction. Inflammatory cells are a mixture of small lymphocytes and macrophages, with fewer neutrophils. Amorphous magenta material is present within macrophages (arrows), consistent with vaccine adjuvant. Aqueous Romanowsky stain.

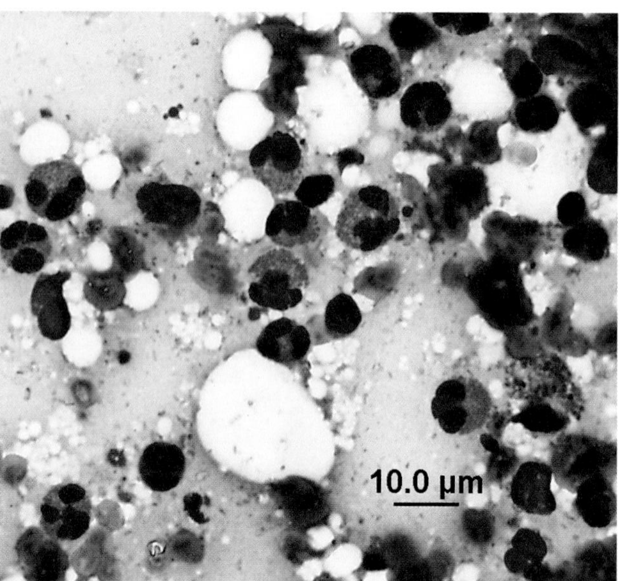

Figure 39.9 Eosinophilic inflammation, cat. Numerous eosinophils containing pink cytoplasmic granules are present in a background of erythrocytes and pale blue tissue fluid. Free eosinophil granules from lysed cells can also be seen. Aqueous Romanowsky stain.

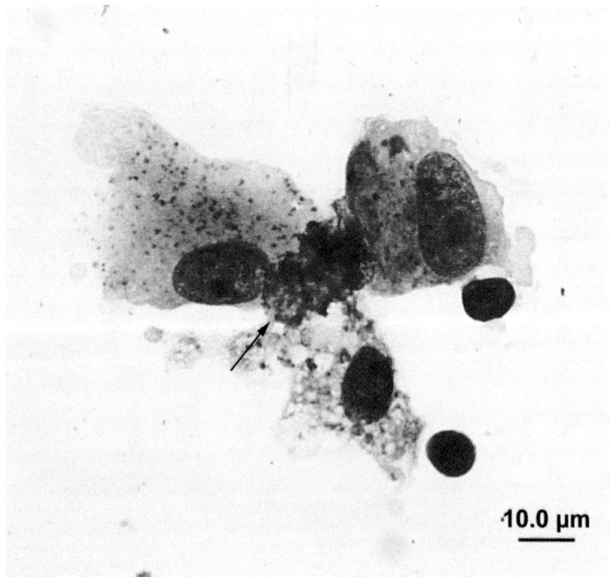

Figure 39.8 Vaccine reaction. Three macrophages and two small lymphocytes are present. Amorphous magenta material consistent with vaccine adjuvant is seen extracellularly (arrow) and is also present within the macrophages. Aqueous Romanowsky stain.

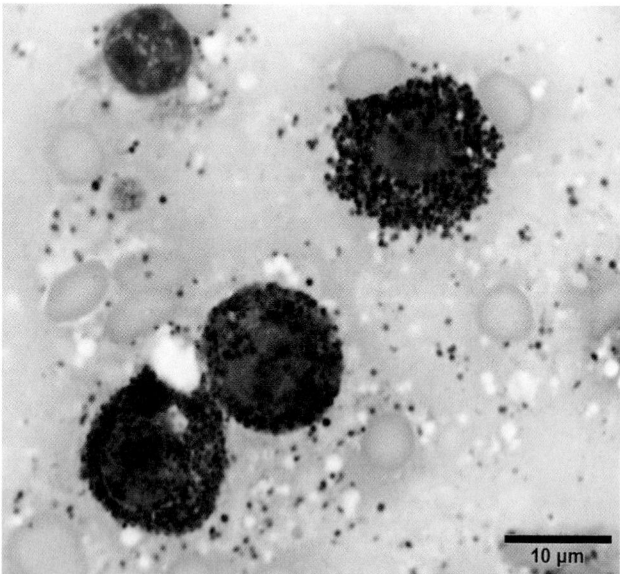

Figure 39.10 Mast cells. These mast cells have abundant dark purple (metachromatic) cytoplasmic granules that sometimes obscure the nucleus. Free granules from lysed cells are in the background and should not be confused with bacteria. Aqueous Romanowsky stain.

(Figure 39.10). Granules may stain poorly or not at all with aqueous Romanowsky stains (Figure 39.11) [2]. Low numbers of mast cells often accompany eosinophils in inflammatory conditions. If mast cells are numerous and/or have criteria of malignancy, mast cell tumor should be considered (see Chapters 40 and 41). Presence of significant numbers of eosinophils in addition to other inflammatory cells occurs with hypersensitivity reactions, parasitic migration, some fungal infections and pythiosis. Numerous eosinophils may also accompany neoplastic conditions, such as lymphoma and mast cell tumor (see Chapters 40 and 41).

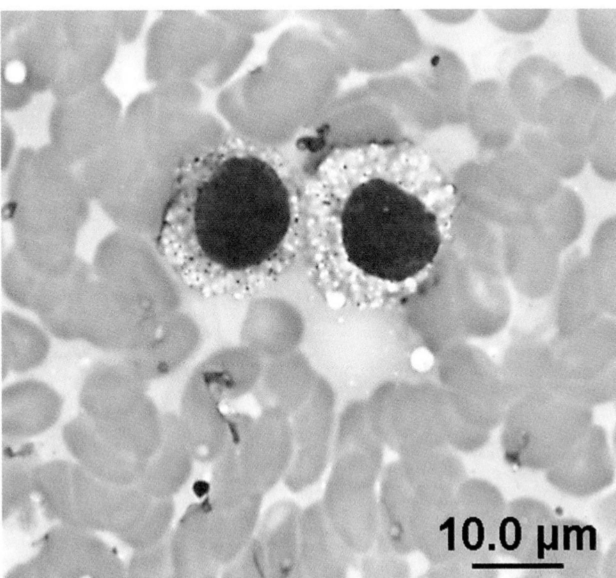

Figure 39.11 Mast cells. The cytoplasmic granules in these two mast cells failed to stain adequately, resulting in a vacuolated appearance. Aqueous Romanowsky stain.

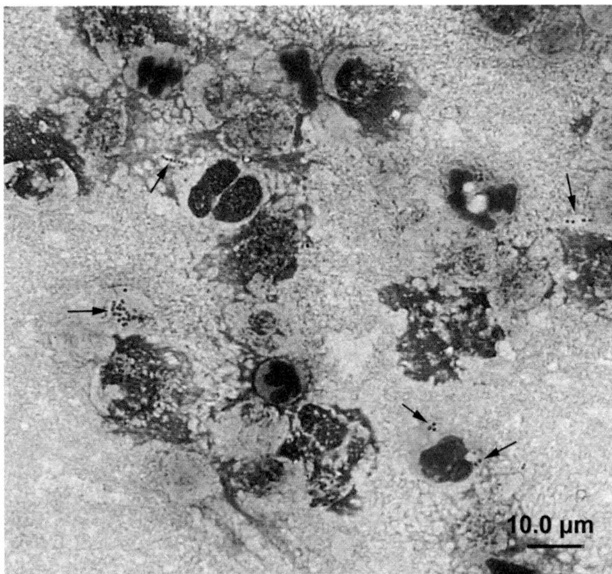

Figure 39.12 Septic, suppurative inflammation, horse abscess. Numerous small bacterial cocci are present in small clusters and short chains (arrows) and are both extracellular and intracellular. Neutrophils are degenerate and disintegrating, creating a thick background of debris that makes bacteria difficult to see. Culture identified the bacteria as *Streptococcus zooepidemicus*. Wright stain.

Selected infectious agents

Microorganisms may be present in cytologic samples for multiple reasons; the challenge is to recognize when they may be a significant finding and not part of normal flora or a result of contamination. Generally, some type of inflammatory reaction is expected if the microorganisms are part of a pathogenic disease process. Finding intracellular (phagocytized) organisms is considered evidence of pathogenicity. If only extracellular organisms are seen, contamination or presence of normal flora must be considered.

Bacteria

Bacteria stain blue with Romanowsky stains, with the exception of *Mycobacteria* spp. that do not stain at all. Phagocytized or dying bacteria may stain less intensely. Types of bacteria commonly identified include bacterial cocci, rods, filamentous bacteria, and spirochetes. Bacterial culture (aerobic and anaerobic) is required for definitive identification of bacteria observed in cytologic samples, and sensitivity testing is recommended to guide antibiotic selection.

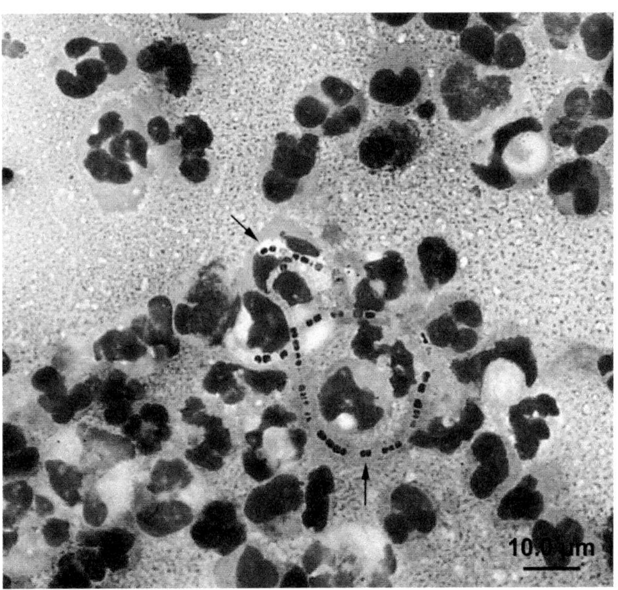

Figure 39.13 Septic, suppurative inflammation, horse abscess. Inflammatory cells consist of degenerate and nondegenerate neutrophils in a thick, stippled, pink proteinaceous background. One long winding chain of bacteria cocci is present (arrows). Wright stain.

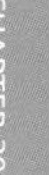

Cocci appear round and may be individualized, in small clusters, or in chains (Figures 39.12 and 39.13). Cocci are usually Gram-positive organisms that may be aerobic (i.e., *Streptococcus* and *Staphylococcus* spp.) or anaerobic (i.e., *Peptostreptococcus* spp.). Bacterial rods may be seen individually or in chains and sizes are variable (Figures 39.14 and 39.15). Bacterial rods that are small are typically Gram negative (i.e., *Escherichia coli*, *Klebsiella* spp., *Pseudomonas* spp.), but some pleomorphic rods are Gram positive (i.e., *Rhodococcus* spp.). Large bacterial rods may be Gram positive (i.e., *Bacillus* spp.) or Gram negative (i.e., *Clostridium* spp.). Gram staining may be attempted on cytologic samples but results are not reliable; Gram staining is best performed on organisms grown in culture. Filamentous rods (i.e., *Actinomyces* and *Nocardia* spp.) grow in long, slender chains that may

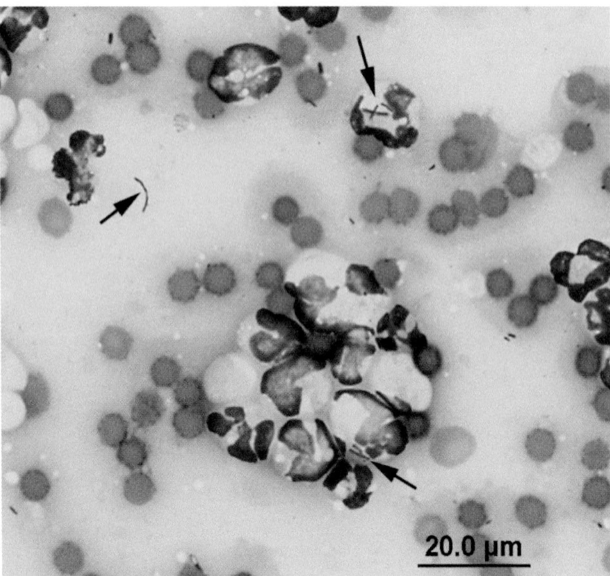

Figure 39.14 Septic, suppurative inflammation, dog toe lesion. Inflammatory cells are predominantly degenerative neutrophils. Bacterial rods are present individually and in short chains (arrows) and are both extracellular and intracellular. Aqueous Romanowsky stain.

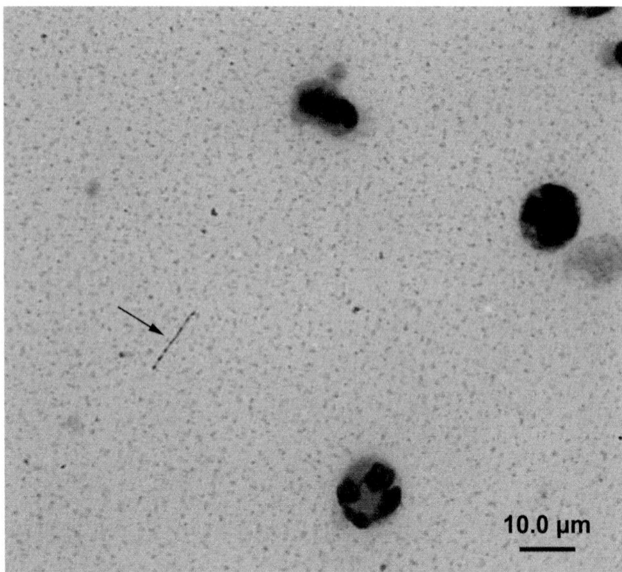

Figure 39.16 Filamentous rod bacteria (arrow), extracellular, bovine. The prominent proteinaceous background makes this thin, beaded filamentous organism difficult to see. Filamentous bacteria are usually considered pathogenic even when only visualized extracellularly. Wright stain.

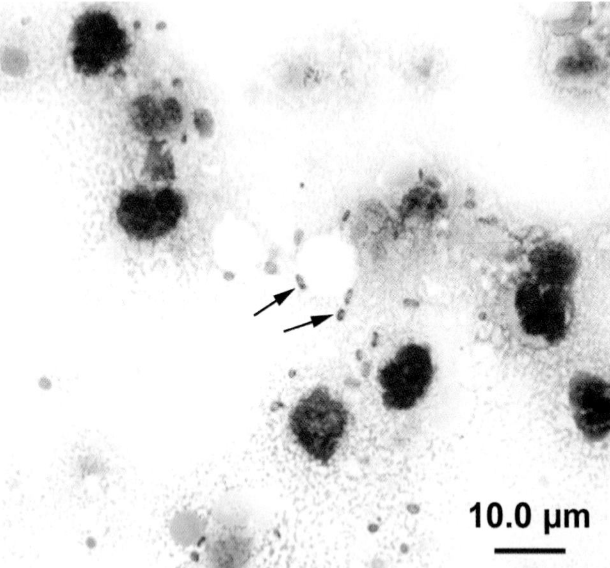

Figure 39.15 Septic, suppurative inflammation, cat abscess. Numerous plump bipolar bacterial rods (arrows) and coccobacilli are present extracellularly. The purple smudges are degenerating nuclei from lysed cells, presumably neutrophils. These organisms were identified as *Yersinia pestis*, the causative agent of plague. Wright stain.

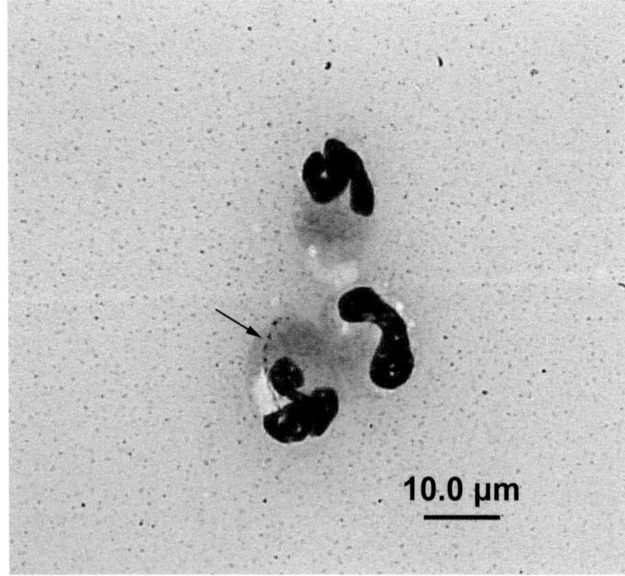

Figure 39.17 Filamentous rod bacteria (arrow), intracellular, bovine. Long, thin bacteria with this beaded appearance are suggestive of *Actinomyces* or *Nocardia* spp. Wright stain.

have a beaded appearance (Figures 39.16–39.19). These organisms can be exceedingly difficult to see, particularly if there is background debris present. Filamentous bacteria require special culture conditions, so it is useful to notify the microbiology laboratory when these organisms are seen in cytologic samples. Large, nonpathogenic rods that grow in parallel rows (*Simonsiella* or *Conchiformibius* spp.) are part of the normal oral flora and thus can be evidence of oropharyngeal contamination (Figure 39.20). Spirochetes can also be part of the normal oral and gastrointestinal flora, and thus may be found along with other bacteria in lesions caused by bite wounds or gastrointestinal leakage [3]. *Helicobacter* spp. may be found in gastric samples from

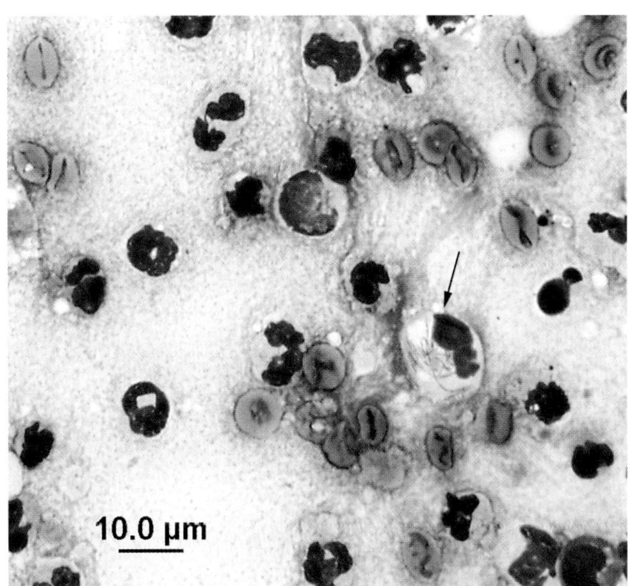

Figure 39.18 Septic, suppurative inflammation, toe lesion, dog. Inflammatory cells are predominantly neutrophils. One degenerate neutrophil contains multiple long, thin filamentous bacteria (arrow). Aqueous Romanowsky stain.

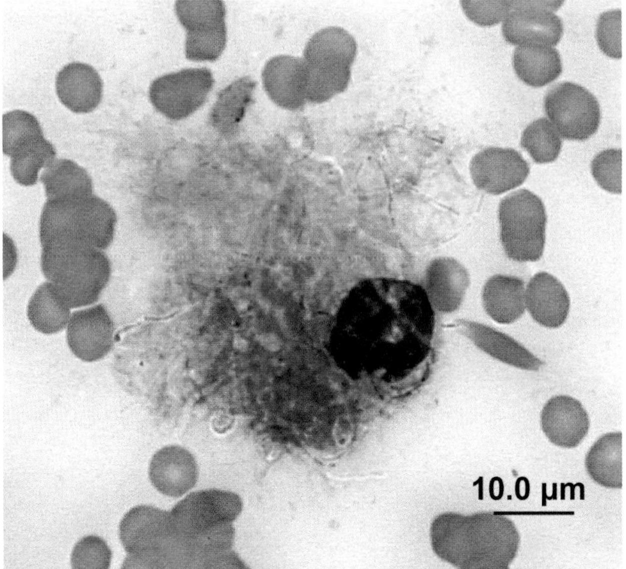

Figure 39.19 Filamentous rod bacteria within a macrophage, cat neck lesion. The inflammatory cells were predominantly macrophages, many of which were multinucleated giant cells. Numerous fine, filamentous bacteria, a few with bulbous ends, are present within this macrophage. Culture identified the organism as *Nocardia paucivorans*. Wright stain.

normal animals but have also been implicated as a cause of gastritis (Figure 39.21) [4, 5].

Typically, most bacterial infections are associated with predominantly suppurative (neutrophilic) inflammation. However, pyogranulomatous inflammation is expected with infections caused by filamentous organisms, and some

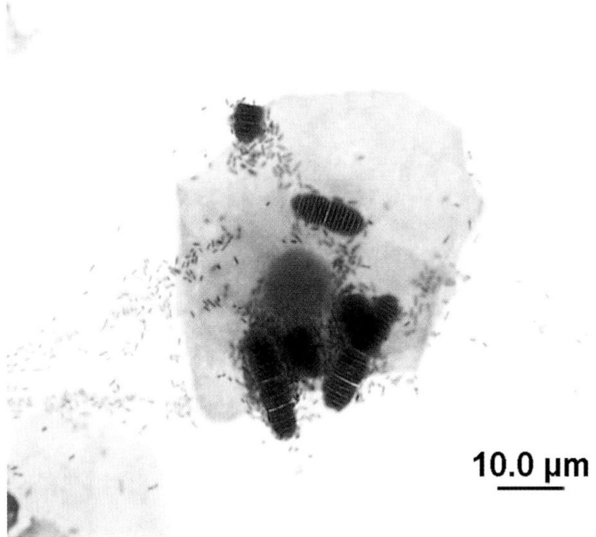

Figure 39.20 Nonpathogenic *Simonsiella* spp. bacteria attached to a squamous epithelial cell. These bacteria grow in distinctive parallel rows and are common oral flora. Numerous individualized rod bacteria are also present. Aqueous Romanowsky stain.

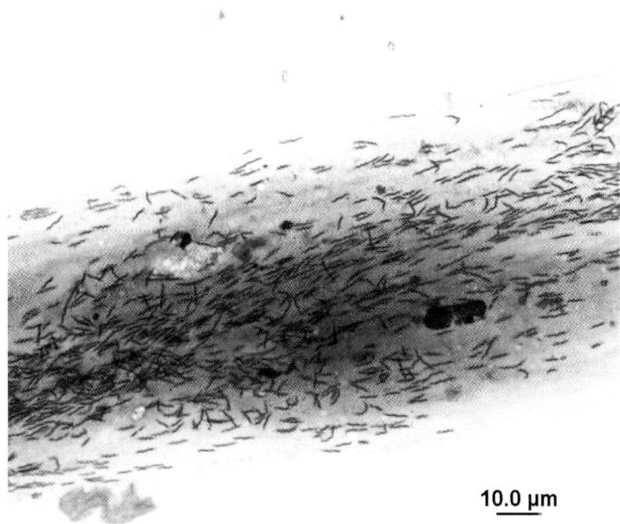

Figure 39.21 Numerous spiral bacteria (*Helicobacter* spp.) in a gastric biopsy imprint from a dog with chronic vomiting. Aqueous Romanowsky stain.

bacteria (such as *Rhodococcus* spp.) are often phagocytized by macrophages instead of neutrophils (Figure 39.22) [6]. Mycobacterial organisms are also associated with predominantly granulomatous (macrophagic) inflammation, but these bacteria do not stain blue with Romanowsky stains. Instead, they appear as slender negative images in the cytoplasm of macrophages, and may be easily overlooked (Figures 39.23 and 39.24).

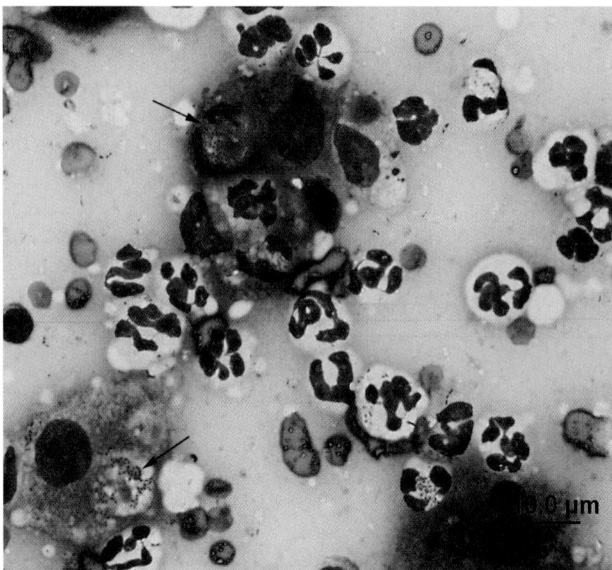

Figure 39.22 Septic, pyogranulomatous inflammation, submandibular lesion, cat. Small, pleomorphic coccobacilli are present in large numbers within macrophages (arrows) and in fewer numbers within neutrophils. Culture identified the organism as *Rhodococcus equi*. Wright stain.

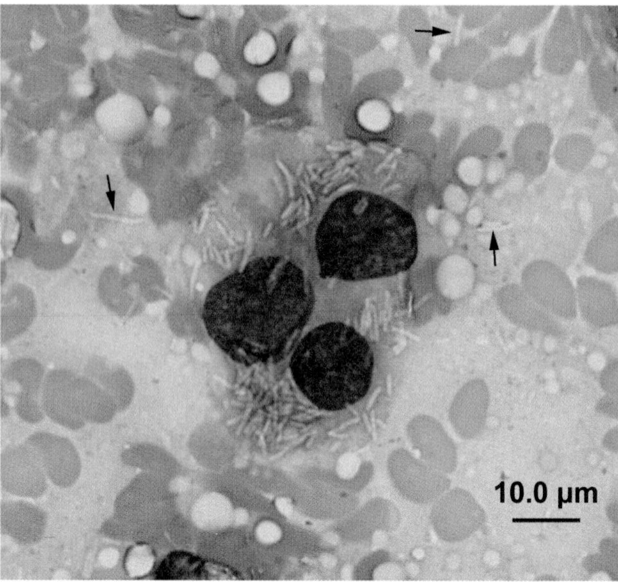

Figure 39.24 Multinucleated macrophage containing many mycobacterial organisms, ferret. Negative images of the bacteria are visible within the macrophage and also in the background (arrows), highlighted by the proteinaceous fluid. Wright stain.

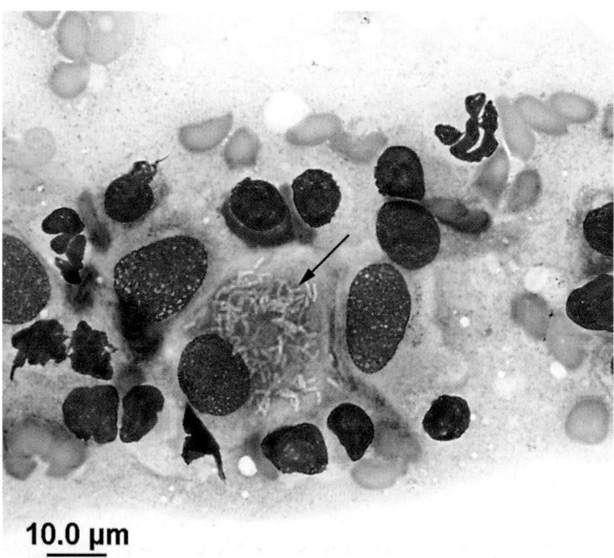

Figure 39.23 Septic, pyogranulomatous inflammation, ear lesion, dog. Negative images of nonstaining, elongated bacterial rods consistent with *Mycobacteria* spp. are visible within one macrophage (arrow). Aqueous Romanowsky stain.

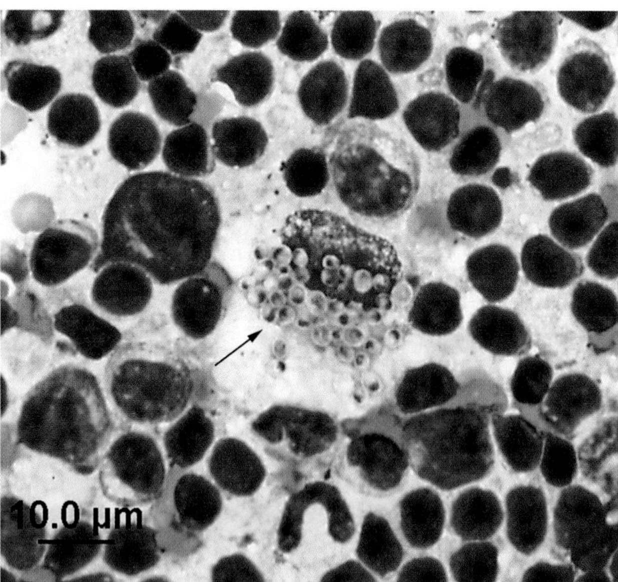

Figure 39.25 Histoplasmosis, lymph node, cat. One macrophage (arrow) contains numerous small fungal yeasts that have a crescent-shaped, eccentric nucleus, pale cytoplasm, and a narrow clear halo. Aqueous Romanowsky stain.

Fungi

Dimorphic fungi

The dimorphic fungi capable of causing systemic infections exist as yeasts at body temperature but can form hyphae in the environment. The morphologies of the yeast forms are distinctive, often allowing definitive cytologic identification.

- *Histoplasma capsulatum* is a small (2–4 μm diameter), round to oval yeast that replicates by narrow-based budding. They stain pale blue with an eccentric, magenta nucleus that is often crescent-shaped (Figure 39.25). There is usually a thin, clear halo surrounding the organism. The associated inflammation is usually pyogranulomatous, with organisms

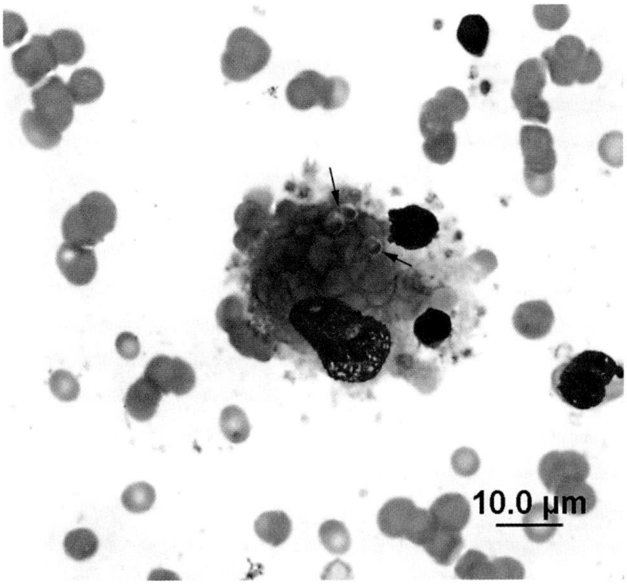

Figure 39.26 Histoplasmosis, kidney, cat. One macrophage contains three small fungal yeasts (arrows) as well as numerous erythrocytes (erythrophagocytosis). Aqueous Romanowsky stain.

phagocytized by both neutrophils and macrophages. In cats with histoplasmosis, erythrophagocytosis by macrophages is a common cytologic feature (Figure 39.26). Dead or dying yeast may be present in samples from animals undergoing treatment, and appear as faded or negative images (Figure 39.27). *Histoplasma* has a wide geographic distribution, thriving in nitrogen-rich organic matter in temperate regions. Disseminated disease often follows inhalation of organisms. Almost every body system may be infected, but dogs typically show clinical signs related to the gastrointestinal tract, while cats more often show respiratory signs [7].

- *Sporothrix schenkii* is a small, oval to elongated yeast with an appearance that is similar to *Histoplasma* [8]. The elongated, fusiform shape is distinctive, and the nucleus may be central to eccentric (Figure 39.28). The numbers of yeast organisms typically seen within skin lesions varies considerably. Cats and horses tend to have numerous organisms, but organisms are rare in lesions from dogs (Figure 39.29). There is generally marked suppurative to pyogranulomatous inflammation with yeast phagocytized by both neutrophils and macrophages. *Sporothrix* is widespread in nature, existing in decaying organic matter. Sporotrichosis is a zoonotic disease, and precautions should be taken especially when handling infected cats.
- *Blastomyces dermatiditis* is a medium-sized (8–20 μm diameter) round yeast that replicates by broad-based budding. Yeasts have a thick wall and are deeply basophilic (Figure 39.30). The associated inflammation is pyogranulomatous, and yeast are usually extracellular but may occasionally be seen phagocytized by macrophages. *Blastomyces* is endemic in river valleys of the midwestern and eastern United States and Canada, and may be expanding its distribution [9]. Canine infections are more common than feline infections, and dogs frequently develop disseminated

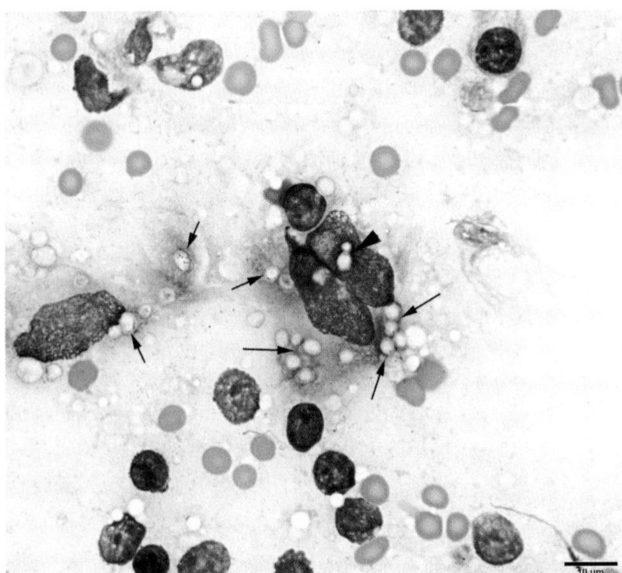

Figure 39.27 Histoplasmosis, lymph node, cat undergoing systemic antifungal therapy. Yeasts are still present within macrophages and in the background but appear faded or as negative images without clear internal structure (arrows), indicating they are dead or dying. One negative image of a budding yeast is seen (arrowhead). Aqueous Romanowsky stain.

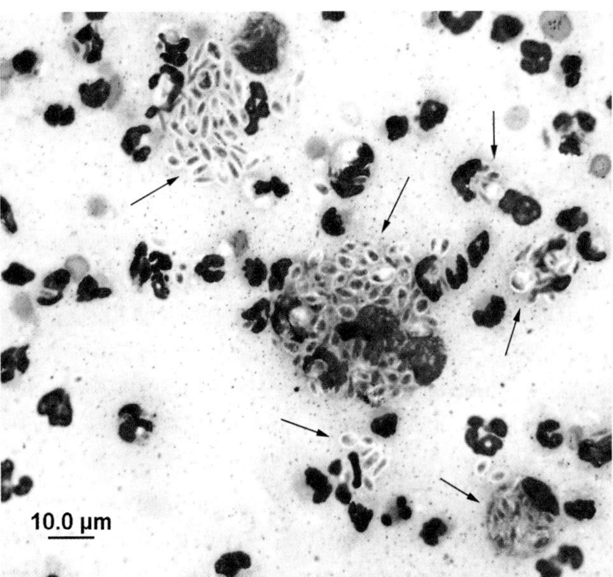

Figure 39.28 Sporotrichosis, skin lesion, cat. Numerous small fungal yeasts are present within macrophages, neutrophils, and free in the background (arrows). The elongated, fusiform shape of some organisms differentiates *Sporothrix* spp. from *Histoplasma* spp. Aqueous Romanowsky stain.

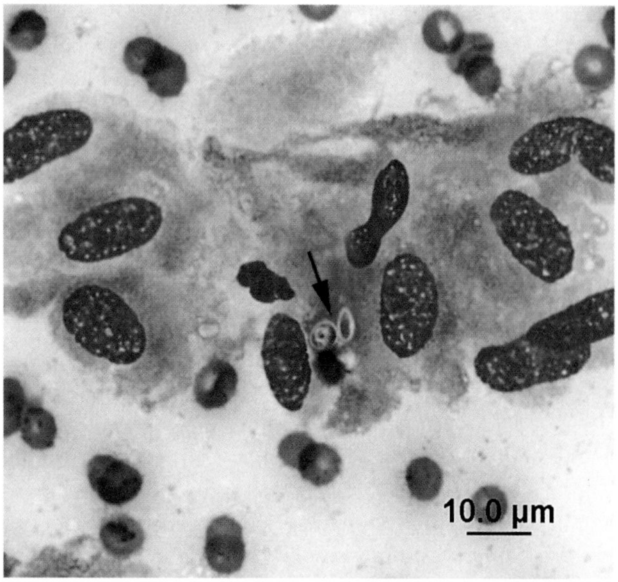

Figure 39.29 Sporotrichosis, skin lesion, dog. Epithelioid macrophages (nonvacuolated, clustered) are present. Fungal yeasts were rare; one round and one elongated yeast are visible here (arrow). Aqueous Romanowsky stain.

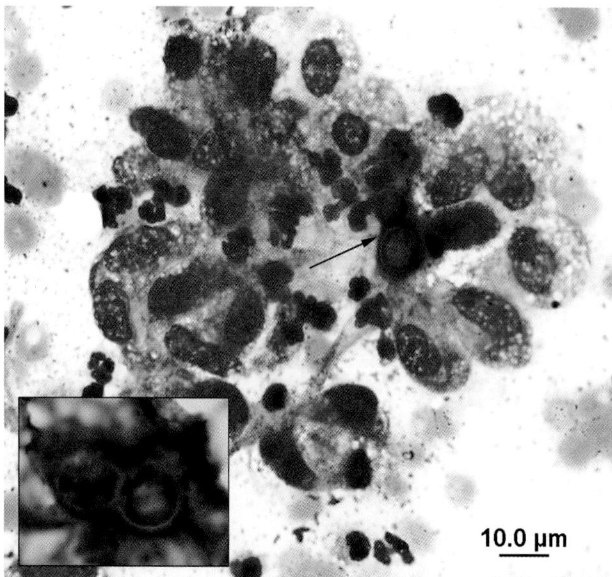

Figure 39.30 Blastomycosis, skin lesion, dog. There is pyogranulomatous inflammation with one deeply basophilic, budding fungal yeast present embedded within the inflammatory cells (arrow). Inset shows details of the broad-based budding typical of *Blastomyces* spp. Aqueous Romanowsky stain.

disease following inhalation of organisms [10]. *Blastomyces* may revert to the mycelial phase when skin lesions are bandaged, causing a health risk to veterinarians and technicians. Culture is not recommended except by specialized laboratories.

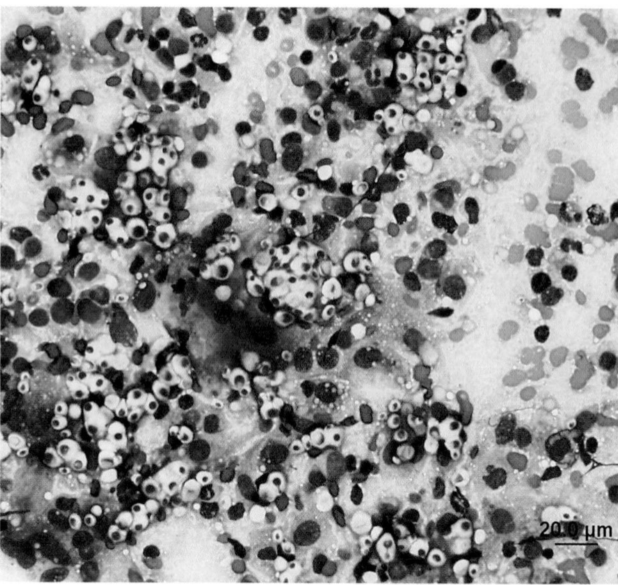

Figure 39.31 Cryptococcosis, lymph node, dog. Thick nonstaining capsules surrounding the yeast create a soap-bubble appearance from low power. Inflammatory cells are predominantly macrophages, some multinucleated, with fewer neutrophils. Lymphocytes and plasma cells are the normal resident population. Aqueous Romanowsky stain.

- *Cryptococcus spp.* are medium-sized, pleomorphic round to oval yeast that replicate by narrow-based budding (Figures 39.31 and 39.32). They frequently have a thick nonstaining capsule, but poorly capsulated forms also exist. Their size varies from 4 to 15 µm in diameter, excluding the capsule. The yeast stain variably from blue to magenta. The associated inflammation usually consists predominantly of macrophages and multinucleated giant cells (granulomatous) with low numbers of eosinophils, but inflammation may be minimal. *Cryptococcus neoformans* proliferates in bird droppings, while *Cryptococcus gattii* is an emerging pathogen in the northwestern United States and California that appears to be associated with tree bark [11, 12]. Cats tend to have respiratory signs and nasal lesions, and dogs more frequently have disseminated disease [11, 13].
- *Coccidioides* spp. are the largest organisms of this group, forming a round spherule measuring 10–200 µm in diameter. The larger, mature spherules contain endospores that are 2–5 µm in diameter (Figure 39.33). Spherules are blue to clear and may have a crumpled surface. The associated inflammation is granulomatous to pyogranulomatous; larger numbers of neutrophils are observed when free endospores are present. *Coccidioides* is endemic to desert regions of the American southwest, causing disease in people and animals following inhalation, and frequently resulting in disseminated disease in dogs [14]. The mycelial phase is highly infectious, so culture is not recommended.

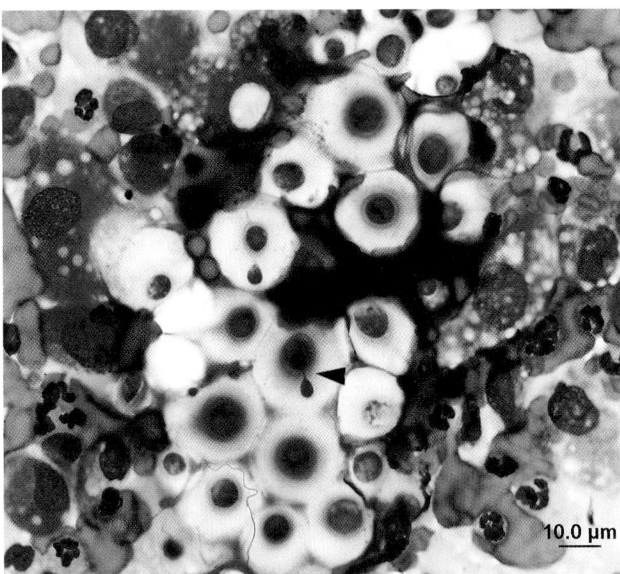

Figure 39.32 Cryptococcosis, cat. Numerous variably sized fungal yeasts possessing thick, nonstaining capsules are present. One yeast demonstrates narrow-based budding (arrowhead). The surrounding inflammation is pyogranulomatous. Aqueous Romanowsky stain.

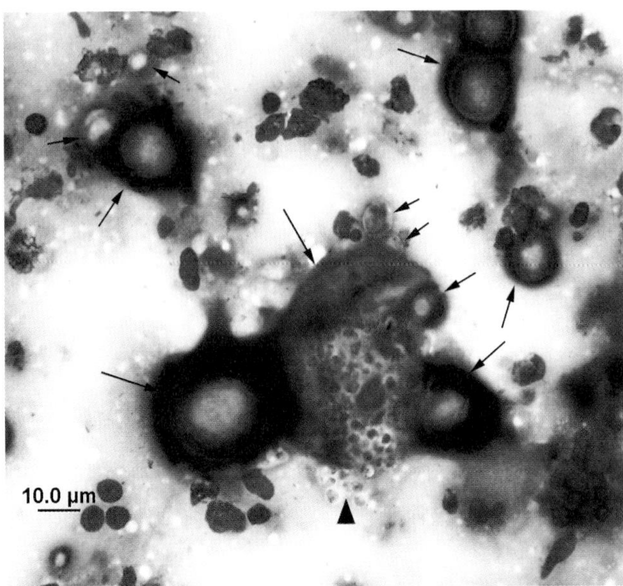

Figure 39.33 Coccidioidomycosis, dog. Spherules of *Coccidioides* vary markedly in size (arrows). The larger spherules have a visible internal structure. One mature spherule has broken to release small endospores (arrowhead). Most of the surrounding inflammatory cells are lysed and cannot be identified. Aqueous Romanowsky stain.

Hyphae-forming fungi

There are numerous hyphae-forming fungi capable of causing local or systemic infections in veterinary species, and fungal hyphae are occasionally encountered in cytologic specimens. Examples include the agents that cause candidiasis, aspergillosis, hyalohyphomycosis, and phaeohyphomycosis [15]. Hyphae are often present within thick aggregates of macrophages and can have variable shapes and sizes (Figures 39.34 and 39.35). Complicating recognition, fungal hyphae do not always stain well and may appear as negative images (Figures 39.36 and 39.37). The histochemical stain GMS can be helpful to highlight

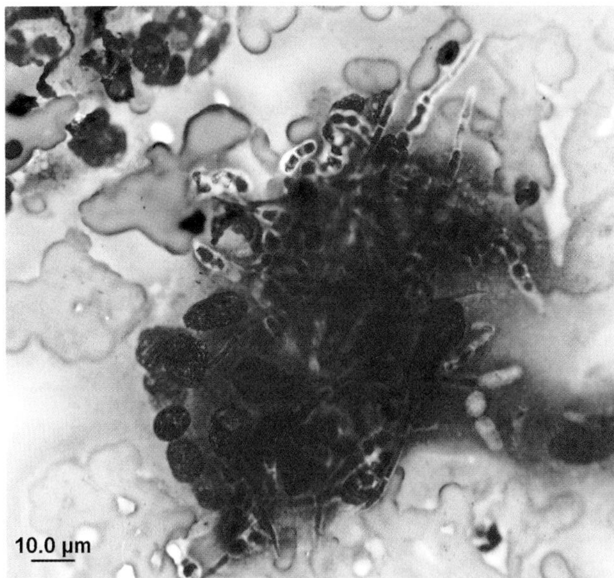

Figure 39.34 Fungal hyphae, lymph node, dog. A thick mat of fungal hyphae are present embedded within macrophages. Hyphae are pleomorphic; some are narrow and septate while others have rounded dilations. This fungus was identified using molecular methods as *Paecilomyces* spp. (hyalohyphomycosis). Aqueous Romanowsky stain.

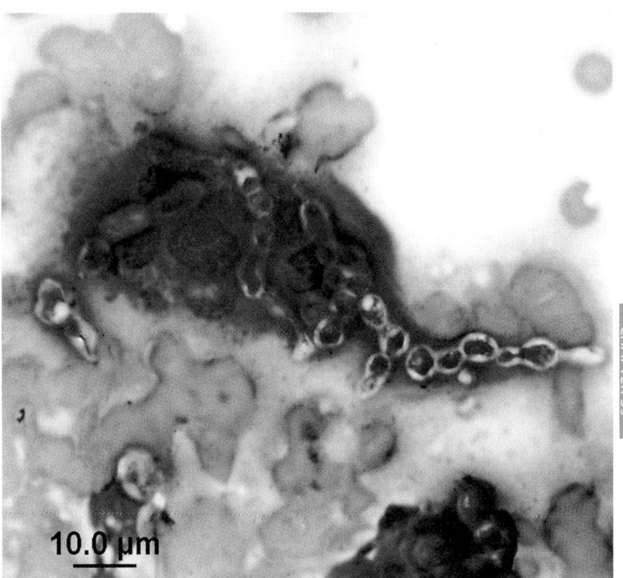

Figure 39.35 Fungal hyphae, same sample as Figure 39.34 (hyalohyphomycosis). The fungal hyphae seen here within a large macrophage have dilated, bulbous segments. Aqueous Romanowsky stain.

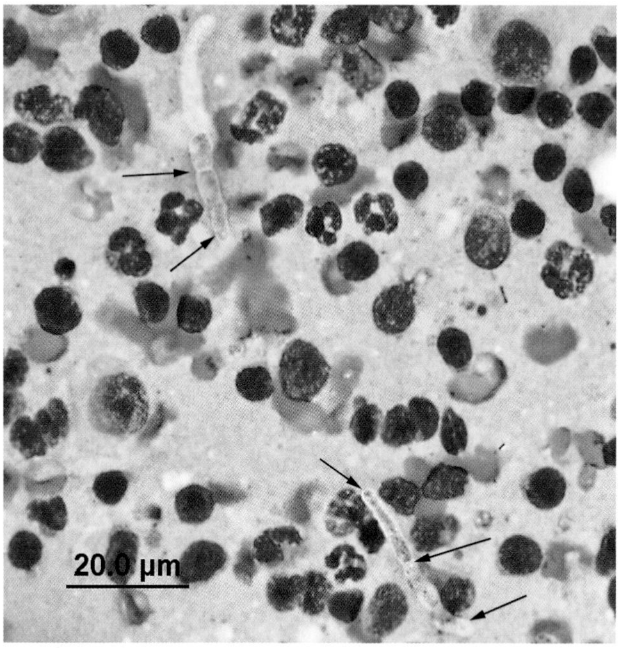

Figure 39.36 Fungal hyphae, lymph node, dog. Two long, septate pale-staining fungal hyphae are visible extracellularly (arrows). Aqueous Romanowsky stain.

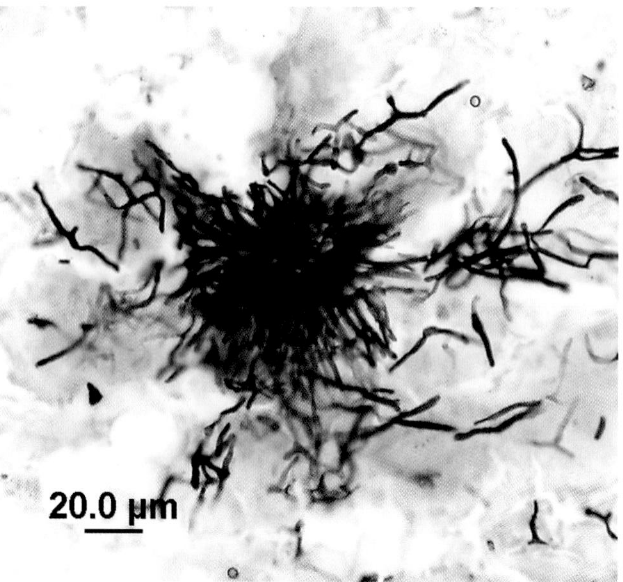

Figure 39.38 Fungal hyphae, same sample as Figure 39.36. The fungal hyphae stain black with GMS, which makes it easier to appreciate the numbers of organisms present. Gomori methenamine silver stain.

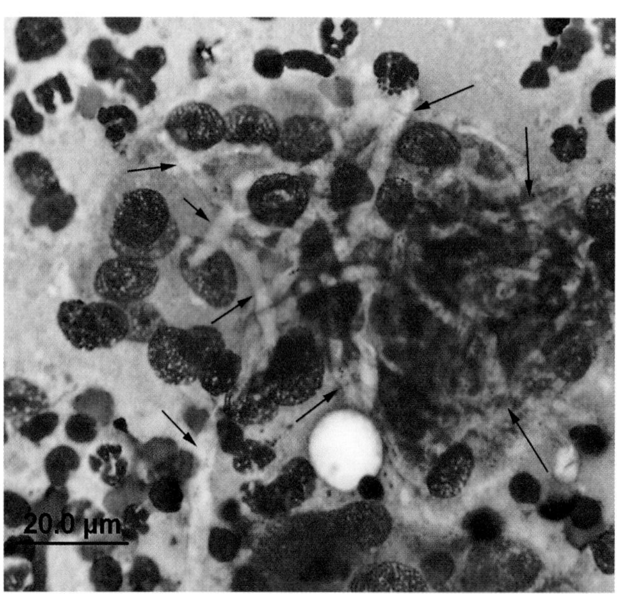

Figure 39.37 Fungal hyphae, same sample as Figure 39.36. A mat of nonstaining fungal hyphae can be seen as negative images (arrows) embedded within epithelioid macrophages. Aqueous Romanowsky stain.

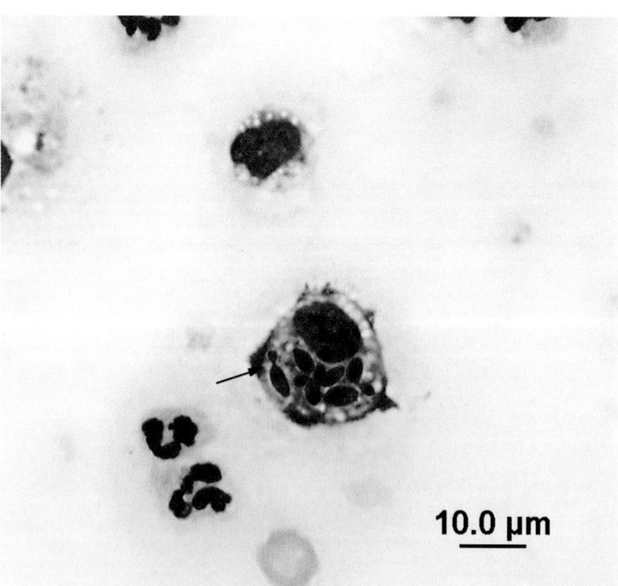

Figure 39.39 *Candida* peritonitis, dog. Multiple *Candida* yeasts are present within a vacuolated macrophage, and one demonstrates narrow-based budding (arrow). Aqueous Romanowsky stain.

fungal hyphae (Figure 39.38). Although there are differences in morphology that may suggest a particular group of fungi (presence or absence of septae and pigmentation, size and shape of hyphae), generally culture or molecular techniques are required for definitive identification [15]. *Candida* spp. can have multiple morphologies in cytologic samples including small yeast, yeast with germ tube formation, pseudohyphae, and true hyphae (Figures 39.39 and 39.40, also see Chapter 42) [16]. Some pseudofungal organisms that grow as elongated hyphal structures are actually aquatic pathogens of the class Oomycetes (i.e., *Pythium* and *Lagenidium*, discussed later).

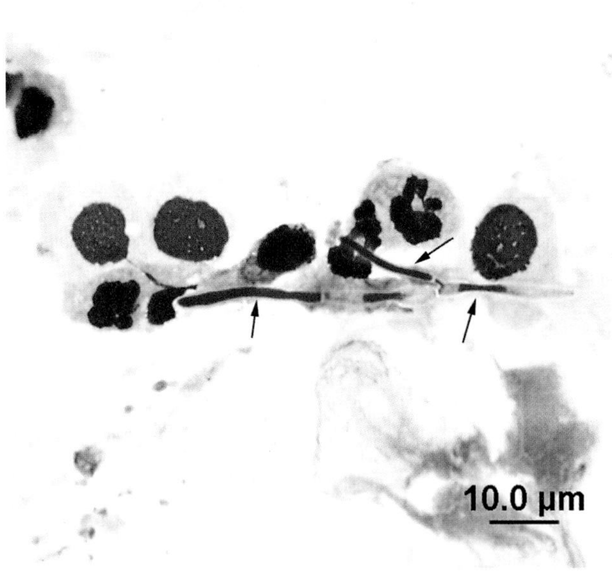

Figure 39.40 *Candida* peritonitis, dog, same sample as Figure 39.39. The fungus is present as true hyphae in this image (arrows). Aqueous Romanowsky stain.

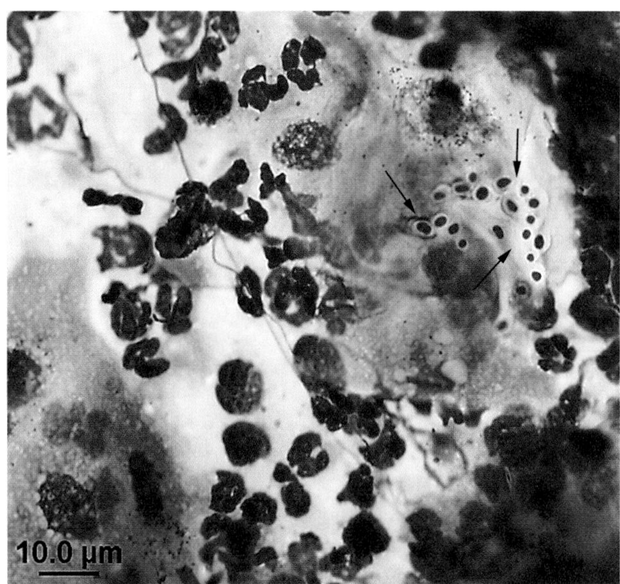

Figure 39.41 Dermatophytosis, skin scraping, dog. Multiple small, dark blue round to brick-shaped arthrospores are present (arrows). There are several squamous epithelial cells present and numerous inflammatory cells (neutrophils and eosinophils). Aqueous Romanowsky stain.

Dermatophytes

Dermatophytes (*Microsporum* and *Trichophyton* spp.) cause scaly hairless skin lesions (dermatophytosis or ringworm) and may be identified in deep scrapings taken from the edge of active lesions. Scrapings should be deep enough to result in oozing of tissue fluid or blood in order for the sample to adhere to a glass slide for staining. Heat-fixing of these samples is neither required nor recommended. Small, brick-shaped arthrospores appear dark blue with Romanowsky stains and may be seen free in the background or adhered to epithelial cells or hair shafts (Figures 39.41 and 39.42). There is usually a mixed inflammatory cell population present. Fungal culture is necessary for specific identification. Dermatophytosis is a zoonotic disease.

Malasezzia spp.

Malasezzia spp. are small budding yeasts that are normal inhabitants of skin. Overgrowth is associated with dermatitis and otitis externa. The yeast have a characteristic peanut or shoe-print shape and stain dark blue (Figure 39.43).

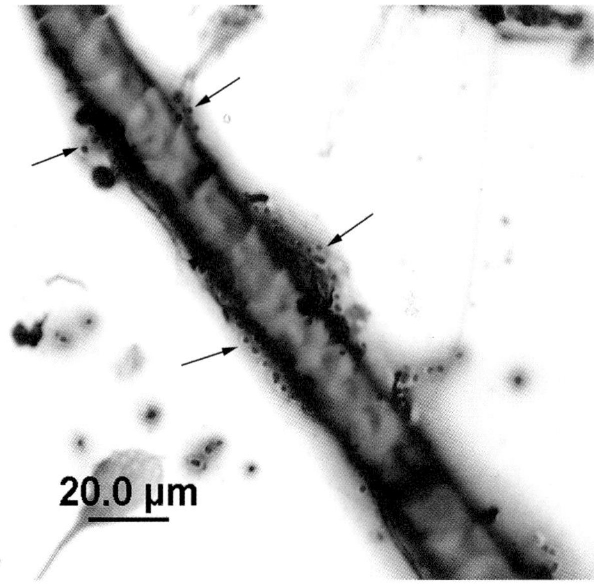

Figure 39.42 Dermatophytosis, skin scraping, cat. Arthrospores are visible attached to a hair shaft (arrows) and free in the background. Aqueous Romanowsky stain.

Protozoa

Cytauxzoon felis

C felis causes severe and often fatal disease in domestic cats [17]. The erythrocytic stage (piroplasm) is often the basis for diagnosis, which typically is made from a blood film (see Chapter 9). The tissue phase of the parasite (schizont) may be encountered in cytologic specimens from infected cats (i.e., aspirates of lymph node, spleen, lung, etc.). Schizonts develop within macrophages, which become enlarged with distended cytoplasm and large, prominent nucleoli (Figure 39.44). The appearance of the schizont varies depending on the stage of development, transforming from a poorly defined basophilic mass to circular blue merozoites with a purple nucleus (Figure 39.45). Schizonts develop in tissues prior to the appearance of piroplasms in peripheral blood.

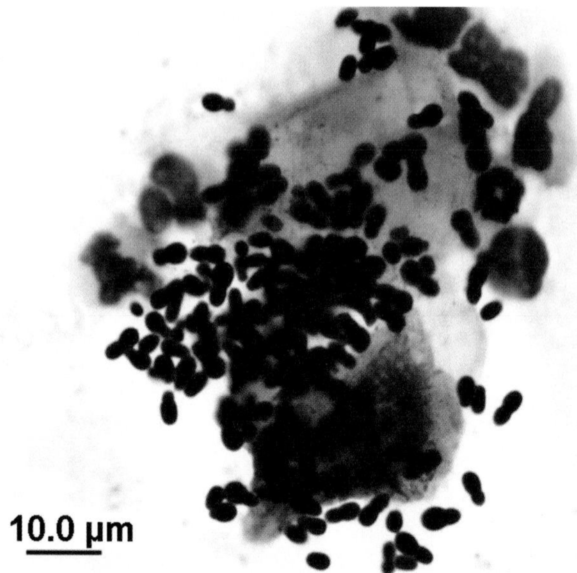

Figure 39.43 *Malassezia* spp., ear swab, dog. Numerous dark blue peanut-shaped *Malassezia* yeasts are present adhered to squamous epithelial cells. There are neutrophils out of focus in the background. Aqueous Romanowsky stain.

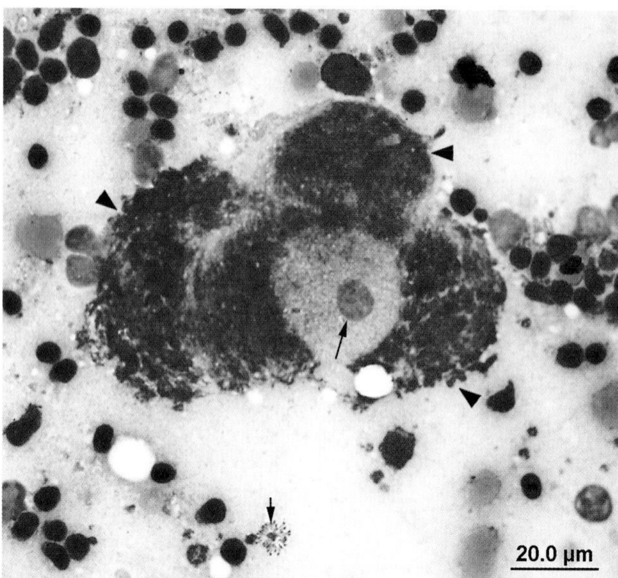

Figure 39.45 *Cytauxzoon felis* schizont, lymph node, cat. This macrophage is disrupted allowing better visualization of merozoites (arrowheads). The prominent nucleolus (long arrow) is as large as the surrounding small lymphocytes. One cluster of extracellular, nearly mature merozoites (short arrow) is present. Aqueous Romanowsky stain.

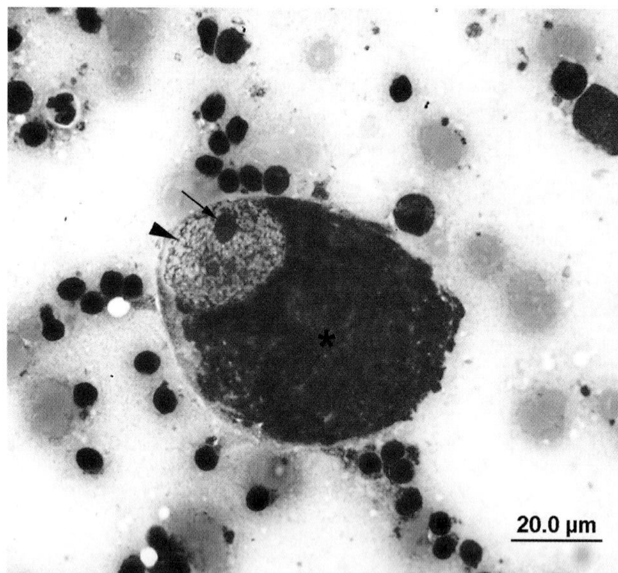

Figure 39.44 *Cytauxzoon felis* schizont, lymph node, cat. The enlarged macrophage contains a pale nucleus (arrowhead) with a large prominent nucleolus (arrow). The cytoplasm (*) is distended with ill-defined, dark blue developing merozoites. Surrounding cells are predominantly small lymphocytes and erythrocytes. Aqueous Romanowsky stain.

Toxoplasma and *Neospora* spp.

Tachyzoites of *Toxoplasma gondii* or *Neospora caninum* are occasionally encountered in cytologic specimens and have an identical microscopic appearance; molecular methods (PCR) can be used to differentiate them. The associated inflammation is often mixed. Tachyzoites typically are 2–4 µm long, crescent- or banana-shaped, with pale blue cytoplasm and a central purple nucleus (Figure 39.46). Toxoplasmosis can affect both dogs and cats and tachyzoites may be found in a variety of samples including tissue aspirates (lung, lymph nodes) and body fluids (respiratory washes, ocular fluids, cerebrospinal fluid [CSF], and cavity effusions) [18, 19].

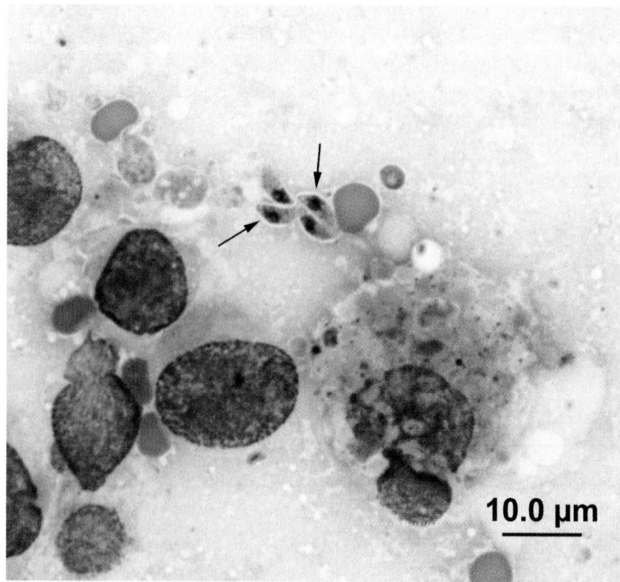

Figure 39.46 Toxoplasmosis, lymph node, cat. Four small, banana-shaped protozoal tachyzoites (arrows) are present extracellularly. The macrophage on the right contains phagocytized debris. Wright stain.

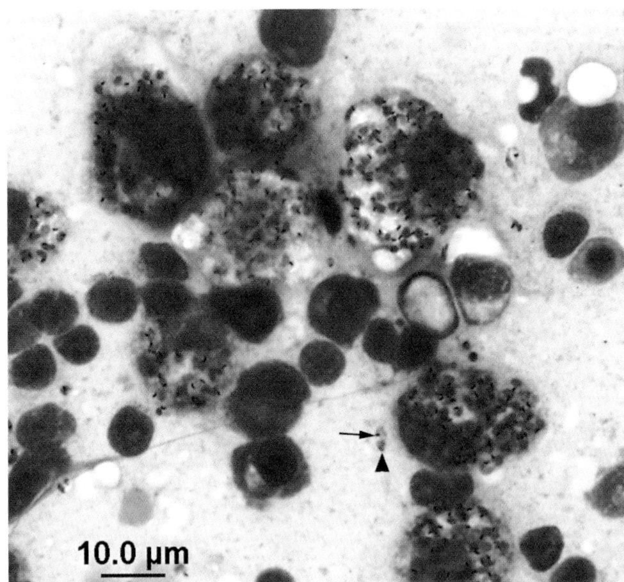

Figure 39.47 Leishmaniasis, lymph node, dog. Multiple macrophages contain numerous small protozoal amastigotes. The internal structure of the amastigotes can be visualized best in the extracellular organisms, which have a light purple nucleus (arrowhead) and dark purple, rod-shaped kinetoplast (arrow). Other cells present include lymphocytes and plasma cells. Wright stain.

Toxoplasmosis is a zoonotic disease; people are infected transplacentally or following ingestion of sporulated oocysts (cat feces) or tissue cysts (undercooked meat). Neosporosis is recognized most often as a cause of polymyositis and paralysis in dogs under a year of age. Similar to toxoplasmosis, a wide range of body tissues may harbor tachyzoites.

Leishmania spp.

Leishmaniasis causes visceral and cutaneous disease in animals and people worldwide, and has become a problem in the United States since 2000 [21]. Organisms (amastigotes) may be found in cytologic samples from infected dogs and are often present phagocytized by macrophages. They are 2–4 µm, oval, and pale with an oval purple nucleus and rod-shaped dark purple kinetoplast (Figure 39.47). The kinetoplast distinguishes this organism from the similarly sized *Histoplasma* yeast. Amastigotes of *Trypanasoma cruzi*, the cause of American trypansomiasis in dogs, have an identical appearance but are uncommon in cytologic samples [22]. The associated inflammation is pyogranulomatous to mixed. Leishmaniasis is a zoonotic disease that relies on the sandfly vector for transmission. However, human exposure to infected open wounds should be avoided.

Other

Pythium, *Lagenidium*

These organisms mimic fungi in cytologic samples, in which they appear as broad, poorly septate hyphae that often stain poorly (Figures 39.48 and 39.49). The histochemical stain GMS can be used to highlight the organisms (Figure 39.50). They are actually aquatic pathogens (class Oomycetes) that typically affect animals with frequent exposure to lakes or ponds in warm climates [15]. Horses may develop cutaneous mass lesions [23]. Canine pythiosis is often gastrointestinal or cutaneous; lagenidiosis may be cutaneous, locally

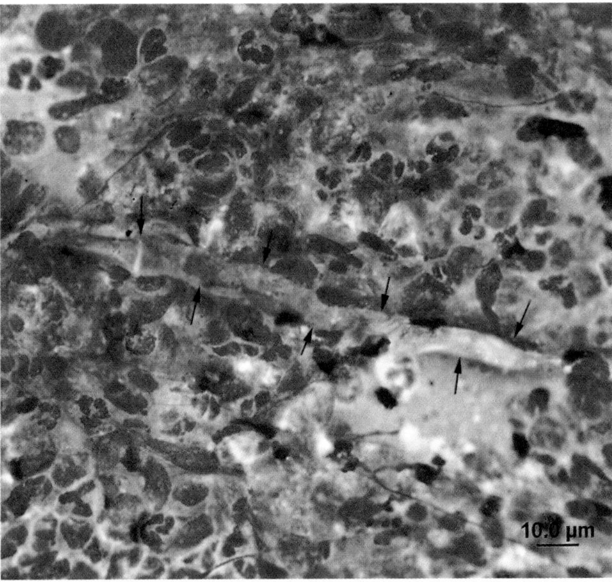

Figure 39.48 Pythiosis, mesenteric mass, dog. Buried within a thick aggregate of mixed inflammatory cells (neutrophils, macrophages, eosinophils) is the negative outline of a broad, poorly septate hyphal structure (arrows). Aqueous Romanowsky stain.

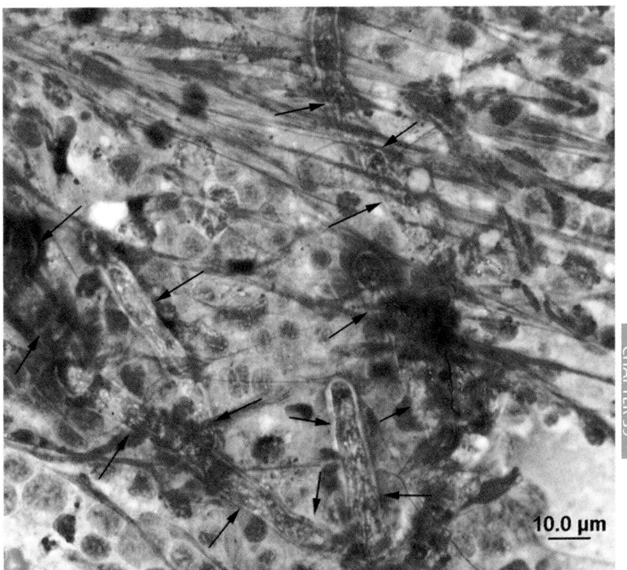

Figure 39.49 Pythiosis, same case as Figure 39.48. Multiple broad, branching, poorly septate, lightly staining hyphae are present (arrows). There is mixed inflammation with an eosinophilic component. Aqueous Romanowsky stain.

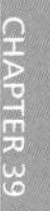

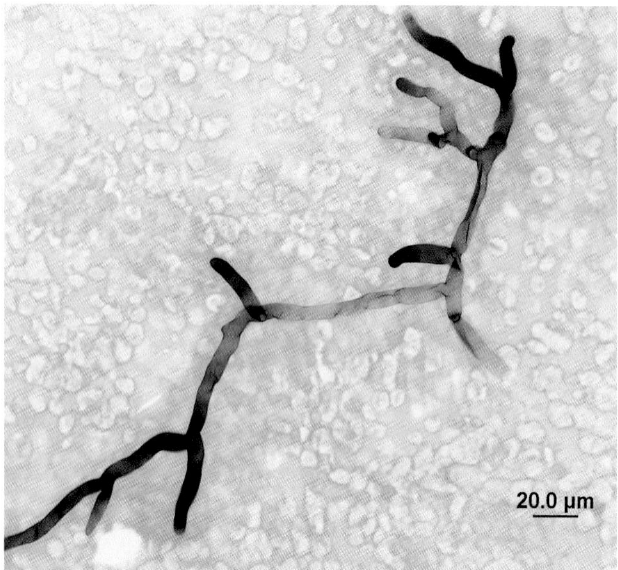

Figure 39.50 Pythiosis, same case as Figure 39.48. A large, branching hyphal structure is easily visualized when stained black with GMS. Gomori methenamine silver stain.

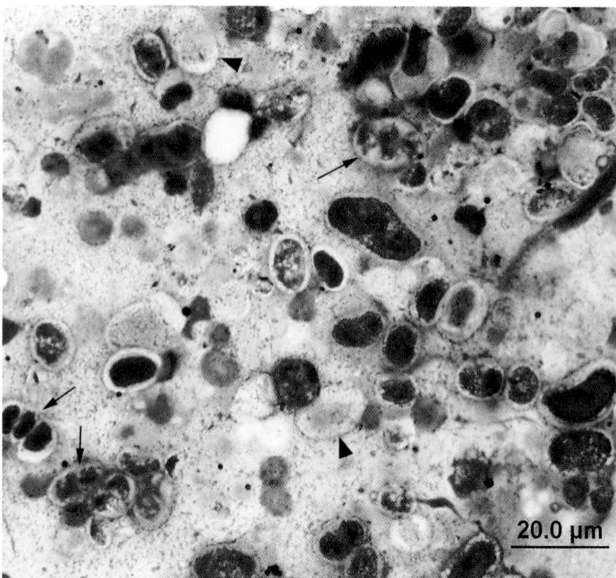

Figure 39.51 Protothecosis, vitreous, dog. Numerous oval *Prototheca* organisms are present and have variable staining qualities. Most are basophilic with a granular appearance. Internal endospores can be seen (arrows) and clear empty theca are also present (arrowheads). Aqueous Romanowsky stain.

invasive and occasionally disseminated. Associated inflammation is pyogranulomatous and may have an eosinophilic component.

Prototheca

These organisms are single-celled algae ubiquitous in nature, with canine infections occurring in warm, moist climates [25]. Cutaneous infections may be secondary to trauma, and disseminated disease is thought to be associated with immunosuppression. Dogs with disseminated disease often have involvement of the intestinal tract. The organisms are round to oval and 5–20 μm in diameter. Internal septation produces endospores. *Prototheca* stains variably basophilic with a granular appearance and a narrow clear halos; clear empty theca are often present (Figure 39.51). The associated inflammation is pyogranulomatous, occasionally mixed with lymphocytes and plasma cells.

Rhinosporidium

Rhinosporidium seeberi is an unusual aquatic protistan organism that exists near the animal-fungal divergence, classified as Mesomycetozoea [26]. *R seeberi* causes nasal mucosal polypoid masses in people and animals (dogs, horses, rarely cats) that live in warm, humid climates. The organism forms large sporangia in tissues, but the form most commonly identified in cytologic samples is the mature endospore (Figures 39.52 and 39.53). The endospores are round to oval, 8–15 μm in diameter, with a thick cell wall. Visible internally are numerous spherical, dark pink globular structures that are distinctive. Smaller, developing immature endospores, similar in size to *Histoplasma*, have also been described [27]. The associated inflammation is pyogranulomatous.

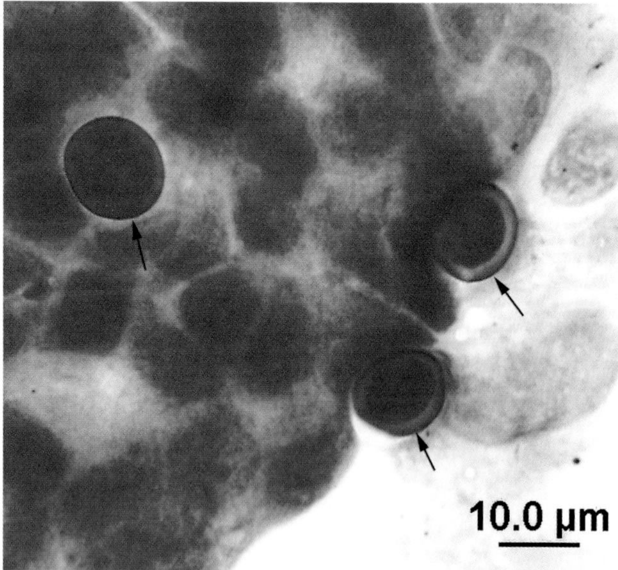

Figure 39.52 Rhinosporidiosis, nasal lesion, dog. Three round to oval, thick-walled endospores of *R seeberi* (arrows) are associated with a cluster of epithelial cells. The pink spherical internal globules are distinctive. Aqueous Romanowsky stain.

Neorickettsia helminthoeca

N helminthoeca is the cause of canine salmon poisoning disease in dogs that consume uncooked salmon infected with the trematode vector *Nanophyetus salmincola* [28]. The

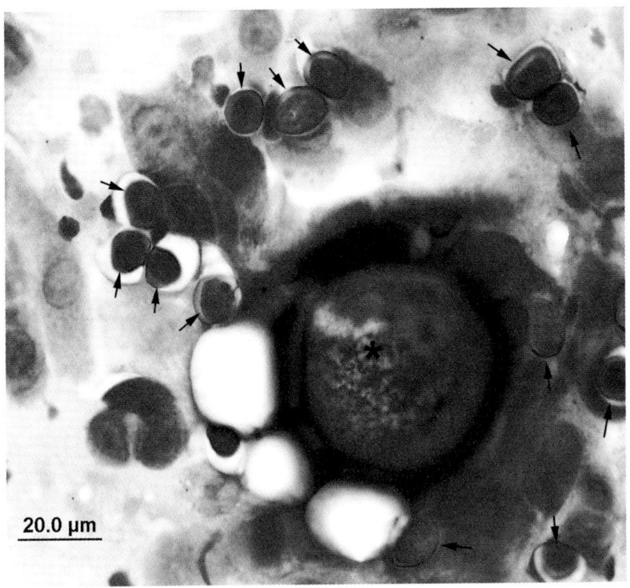

Figure 39.53 Rhinosporidiois, same case as Figure 39.52. One large, deeply basophilic, granular immature sporangium (*) and multiple endospores (arrows) are present with normal epithelial cells. Aqueous Romanowsky stain.

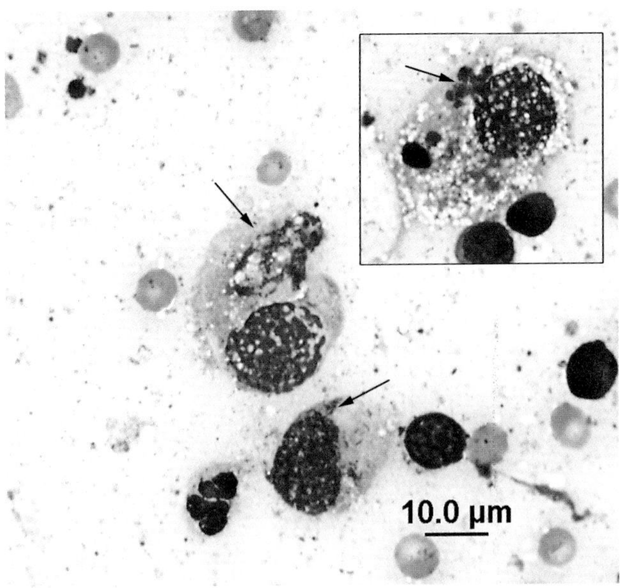

Figure 39.54 *Neorickettsia helminthoeca*, lymph node, dog. Rickettsial organisms that cause salmon poisoning disease are small, basophilic, and tend to occur in indistinct aggregates (arrows) within macrophages rather than distinct morulae. Aqueous Romanowsky stain.

rickettsial organism may be found in lymph node aspirates from infected dogs, where it replicates within macrophages. Cytologically, the organisms are pleomorphic, appearing individually and in diffuse clusters rather than distinct morulae (Figure 39.54) [29].

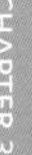

40 Cytology of Neoplasia

Donald Meuten[1] and Kristina Meichner[2]

[1]North Carolina State University, Raleigh, NC, USA
[2]University of Georgia, Athens, GA, USA

Introduction

Cancer is an uncontrolled proliferation of cells due to nonlethal mutation(s) in the genome (genetic makeup of a species). Mutations are a constant event in DNA and RNA. There are genes that repair these mutations and genes that stimulate the mutations, and each can contribute to the formation of cancer. Etiologic agents such as viruses, chemicals, and radiation can cause tumors in animals, but for many tumors an etiology is not yet known, so we use the term *spontaneous*. The pathogenesis of cancer is complicated, and there are textbooks and review manuscripts that describe the many details required for a neoplasm to form, evade host defenses, transform into a malignant tumor, invade regionally, invade blood or lymphatic vessels, and spread (metastasize) [1, 2].

There is a considerable amount of jargon that accompanies cancer and the cytology of cancer. The jargon is less important than recognizing the cellular abnormalities associated with cancer. In this chapter the words *cancer, tumor,* and *neoplasm* will be used synonymously. Strict definitions reserve cancer for a malignant proliferation of cells, tumor for any swelling (one of the four components of inflammation), and neoplasm as an abnormal growth that usually results in a mass. The term *neoplasm* is derived from "neo" = new and "plasm" = formation. The neoplastic transformation of normal resident cells results in the proliferation of a new cell population. If host defenses cannot control those cells, then they proliferate and form a mass. The larger the mass the more likely it is neoplastic. Exceptions: there are some cancers that do not form masses, e.g., leukemia, and there are some cancers that proliferate within an organ and make the organ diffusely enlarged without forming a discrete mass, e.g., lymphoma in the liver or spleen.

Neoplasms can arise in any system in the body. In histopathology we identify a cancer by the organ in which it arose and then name the specific cell type, e.g., hepatocellular carcinoma, cholangiocarcinoma. In cytology we often separate cancer into three main groups: epithelial, mesenchymal, and round cell (Figure 40.1). Some cytologists add a fourth category, neuroendocrine; these tumors are uncommon but will be included in this discussion. Cytological diagnoses also attempt to name the specific tumor, but many times this is not possible. Histopathology uses histologic organization and cytology uses cellular features to identify cancer. There is no individual cytologic or histologic feature that identifies a cell as neoplastic. There are no histochemical, immunohistochemical, or molecular markers that identify a cell or a mass as neoplastic. These techniques are aids used to help diagnose cancer when the diagnosis is not clear. There are molecular markers that characterize specific human and animal tumors. The false-positive and false-negative rates are usually not known for these markers, nor are positive and negative predictive values known (based on prevalence). It is important to know the molecular marker(s) for a specific tumor and then what percent of those tumors express that marker (well differentiated? poorly differentiated?) as well as whether the marker can be present in other tumors, hyperplasia, or dysplasia. Research in the molecular fields of veterinary pathology and oncology is evolving rapidly, and results need to be integrated with clinical, cytologic, and histologic features and, most importantly, with accurate long-term outcome assessments [3–6]. A diagnosis of neoplasia is made by interpreting the overall cytologic and/or histologic findings and integrating these with clinical information such as species, age, and location. Do not separate the microscopic findings from the clinical information.

For the majority of cancers, histopathology provides a more definitive diagnosis than does cytology, but there are advantages and disadvantages of both techniques (Table 40.1).

There are some cancers or locations of cancer in which cytology is the preferred technique to establish a diagnosis and treatment plan: mast cell tumor (MCT), circumanal tumors, lipoma, lymphoma, leukemias, osteosarcoma, urothelial carcinoma (UC), transmissible venereal cell tumor (TVT), histiocytoma, plasma cell tumor, histiocytic

Veterinary Hematology, Clinical Chemistry, and Cytology, Third Edition. Edited by Mary Anna Thrall, Glade Weiser, Robin W. Allison and Terry W. Campbell.

Companion website: www.wiley.com/go/thrall/veterinary

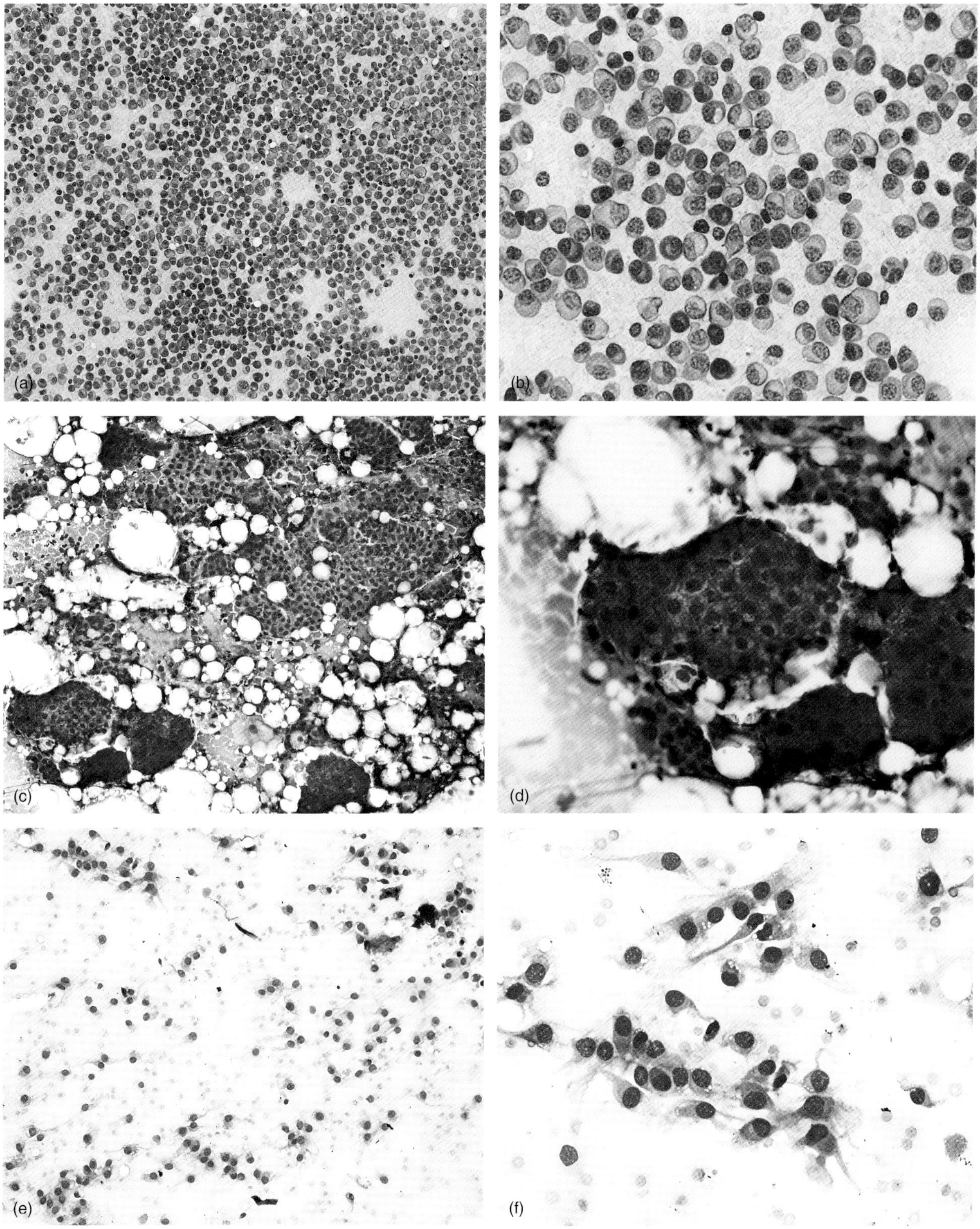

(a) (b) (c) (d) (e) (f)

Figure 40.1 Cytologic patterns of neoplasia. Left column (a, c, e): 20× objective (low power). Right column (b, d, f): 50× objective (high power). (a, b) *Round cell*: high cellularity, individual cells, round shape. (c, d) *Epithelial*: high cellularity, cells adhered in aggregates. (e, f) *Mesenchymal*: low cell numbers, spindle-shaped cells with elongated cytoplasmic ends. Shape of nuclei is not reliable to estimate cell shape as they are round in all patterns; oval-shaped nuclei can be seen in some mesenchymal tumors. *Neuroendocrine* tumors are uncommon (see Figure 40.11). Wright-Giemsa stain.

Table 40.1 Comparison of cytology and histopathology for the diagnosis of neoplastic lesions.

Cytology	Histopathology
Noninvasive	Gold standard for tumor diagnosis
Grading being developed	Grades for many tumors aid prognosis
Margins cannot be evaluated	Margin evaluation and invasion by tumor
Preferred technique for lymph node, bone marrow, body cavity fluids, vaginal cytology	
Short turnaround time; if sample is inadequate can resample while patient is still in hospital	Allows application of histochemistry or immunohistochemistry to get additional diagnostic or prognostic information, e.g., immunophenotyping of lymphoma
Fast diagnosis to initiate treatment, determine if additional tests and/or staging is needed; e.g., mast cell tumor, majority of lymphomas	Definitive diagnosis when cytology is inconclusive, e.g., poorly exfoliative tumors, inflamed tumors
Evaluation of cellular details that is difficult to achieve with histopathology, e.g., bone marrow aspirates, diagnosis of large granular lymphocyte (LGL) lymphoma, infectious agents	Evaluation of tissue architecture, which is required for diagnosis of certain subtypes of lymphoma, to differentiate granulation tissue from fibroma, fibrosarcoma, or sarcoid, etc.
Targeted aspiration of lesions via ultrasound guidance	Evaluation of invasion, e.g., blood or lymphatic vessels, adjacent tissues, basement membrane
Less expensive	Higher costs
Light sedation, if at all, usually sufficient	General anesthesia may be required

Histology or other diagnostic tests may be requested by clinicians if they or the owner want additional information and are willing to pay for them; e.g., PARR, immunohisto- or immunocytochemistry, staging, etc. Tumors that can be reliably diagnosed from cytology, with histology or other tests being optional, include lipoma, perianal gland adenoma, adenocarcinoma of anal sac, lymphoma, leukemias, mast cell tumor, TVT, histiocytoma, plasma cell tumor, histiocytic tumors, transitional cell carcinoma (TCC)/urothelial carcinoma (UC), osteosarcoma.

tumors, and neoplasms in body cavity fluids. Using ultrasound guidance, almost any organ or location in the body can be sampled with fine needle aspirational cytology (FNA). Furthermore, cytology is much less expensive than histopathology, can be performed in-practice, which allows assessment while the patient is still in the hospital and available for reaspiration if needed, is less invasive, does not require general anesthesia (depending on location), and the turnaround time for results is short – immediate or less than 3 days. Cytology slides can be examined by the in-practice veterinarians and/or sent to a diagnostic lab or photographed via cell phone or other means and the images sent to referral centers for preliminary reports (Figure 40.2). Not everyone should try to diagnose lesions from cytology. Cytology is like all specialties: there are individuals certified in each specialty that have advanced training and expertise. However, many veterinarians perform procedures associated with a specialty because of their competence and sometimes because owners do not want to pay for a specialist. The information in this chapter is targeted for individuals not already certified in clinical pathology. An excellent time to use cytology is presurgery on masses in which excision for local cure is intended. Results of cytology can be used by the clinician to plan the surgical dose (i.e., extent and depth of resection) required for the type of tumor. Surgical dose will vary if the tumor is determined to be benign, malignant, round cell, epithelial cell, or mesenchymal. Note: each of these is a general category, yet knowing this information before surgery is one of the better uses of cytology.

Do not overlook the importance of the steps necessary to perform FNA, prepare good-quality slides, avoid artifacts, stain the slides, and adjust the microscope. An inadequate number of cells (QNS – quantify not sufficient), lysed cells, preparations so thick and smeared across the glass that they look like a hit-by-car, excessive amounts of blood, artifacts, understained slides, and using a poorly maintained and adjusted microscope will prevent a diagnosis and frustrate the diagnostician. If poor-quality slides are sent to a referral lab a diagnosis is unlikely, and the same charge is rendered as for good-quality slides that yield a diagnosis. Only attempt to interpret or send to a diagnostic lab slides that are of good quality. It is preferable to designate one microscope in the hospital for cytology and use another microscope of lesser quality for urinalysis and fecal examinations.

Throughout this chapter the authors will generalize. Please accept this approach and understand this is biology; therefore, there will always be exceptions. When the exceptions are important we will point these out; however, including every exception confuses the big picture. The chapter is an overview of how cytology is used to diagnose cancer and determine if it is benign or malignant. Benign means the tumor is indolent; it will not spread or directly result in the death of the patient. Malignant means the tumor is aggressive, and if the pet lives long enough, the tumor will likely lead to the death of the pet. There are other chapters

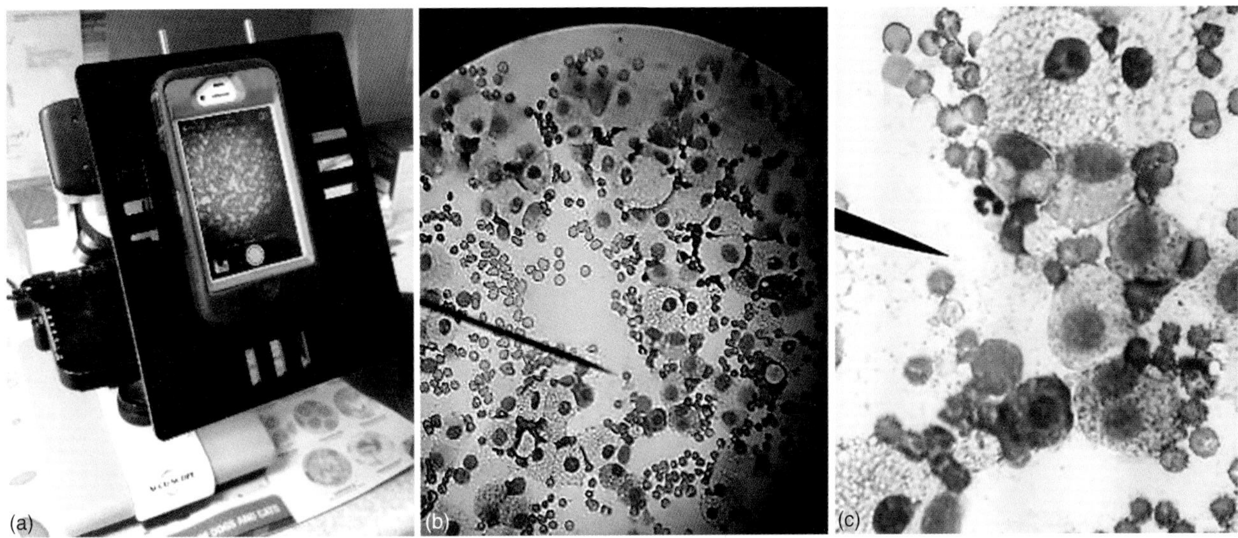

Figure 40.2 (a) Holsters are available that fit on microscopes, and a cell phone can then be attached and used to take a photograph of the fine needle aspirate. An internet search using "cell phone holsters for microscope" will give you options that can be used for different types of smartphones. (b) The central image was captured via this method and the image to the right (c) is enhanced sufficiently to diagnose a round cell tumor that contains cytoplasmic granules: mast cell tumor. Low granularity and binucleation (arrow) suggest aggressive behavior. Aqueous Romanowsky stain.

or sections in this book that describe how to diagnose cancer by where it is located: the organ system, body cavity fluid, lymph node, bone marrow, etc. Location of the suspected neoplasm is an absolutely critical piece of information, as the differential diagnoses for tumors and masses that look like a tumor will change based on organ location. For example: masses in the spleen or liver could be nodular hyperplasia, but this diagnosis is not even a consideration for masses in the skin or subcutis. Similarly, hyperplasia can cause lymphadenomegaly and splenomegaly, but hyperplasia does not produce skin masses. Therefore, the distinction of hyperplasia and hypertrophy from neoplasia is important when examining FNA from organs, but if a nodule or a mass is present in the skin it is most likely inflammatory, a cyst or a neoplasm, and hyperplasia and hypertrophy are not possibilities. Of course, there are exceptions: collagenous hamartoma, fibroadnexal dysplasia, nodular fasciitis, and nodular dermatofibrosis are non-neoplastic lesions of skin or subcutis and each may produce a mass.

Initial examination

Answers to the following clinical questions are part of interpreting the results of FNA. Is there a discrete mass, what is the size, and what is the consistency? Tumors form nodules and masses of various sizes, and they are solid on palpation, not flat, not cystic or fluid filled (exceptions: hemangioma, hemangiosarcoma, myxoma, leukemia, mammary tumors). Is the patient of "cancer age"? Generally, this means the pet is older (exceptions: histiocytoma occurs in young dogs and lymphoma can be seen in young animals of any species). Differential diagnoses for the mass will be formed based on species, history, breed, and location of the mass. Readers should consult specific sections of this book that describe cytological diagnoses by the organ in which the lesion is located. For purposes of this section, the authors will describe how to interpret cytology of a mass in the skin or subcutis, because lesions in this system are the most frequently aspirated, and there are fewer confounders compared to lesions in organs. The principles in this approach can be used in all other systems.

Prepare good-quality slides stained with a Diff-Quik type stain. If neoplasia is a differential diagnosis, do not use wet mounts stained with new methylene blue (NMB) because NMB preferentially stains nuclei and nucleoli. The enhanced staining of DNA and RNA by NMB will make the nuclei in non-neoplastic cells appear neoplastic. First, look at the slide to find regions that are stained and position the slide so these regions are under the 4× objective. Place a dry coverslip on top of the stained slide and examine at low to medium magnifications searching for an area free of artifacts and with an adequate number of cells. When that area is identified, scan with the 20× objective and then proceed to 40×. Avoid using the 100× objective and immersion oil during these first steps. Once oil is placed on the glass slide it is difficult to search for different areas to examine without coating the 40× objective with oil. Almost all diagnoses can be made with the 40× objective and a dry coverslip (exception: microorganisms). The 40× objective is manufactured such that a coverslip is required for uniform in focused view. If a coverslip is not applied to the glass slide, then the field of view will be hazy and appear as if immersion oil is on the objective of the 40× lens (Figure 40.3).

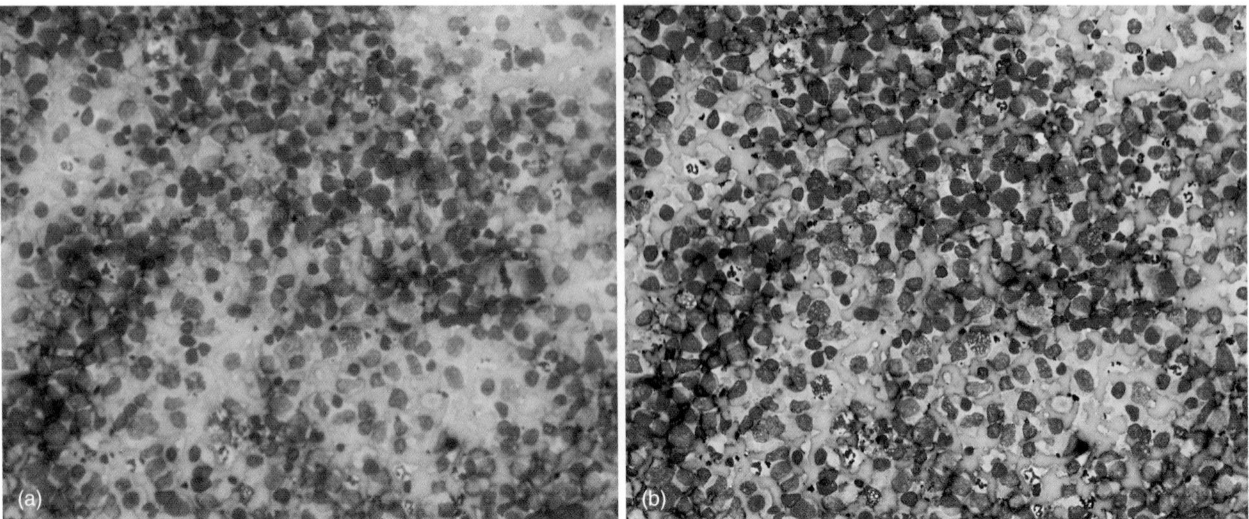

Figure 40.3 Both images (a, b) are as seen with the dry 40× objective. They are the exact same field but the image on the right (b) has a dry coverslip placed on the glass slide over the cells. The image on the left (a) is hazy because there is no coverslip. A fuzzy field of view that appears out of focus with 40× is usually due to the lack of a coverslip. A similar appearance happens if oil contaminates the 40× objective. If the cells are fuzzy and appear out of focus with lower power objectives, the glass slide may be upside down (just flip it over). Avoid oil immersion for the diagnosis of tumors. Wright-Giemsa stain.

For most cases, the critical distinction is inflammation vs. neoplasia. This is accomplished with the 10–40× objectives by determining if the most prevalent cell population is neutrophils. If neutrophils are the number one population, the diagnosis is an inflammatory lesion and not cancer (Figure 40.4 algorithm). Exception: body cavity fluids. Cancer within body cavities often stimulates an inflammatory response and neutrophils can be more prevalent than the neoplastic cells. Lymphoma in body cavities is one of the few neoplasms in which the neoplastic lymphocytes are usually the predominant cells in the fluid (see Figure 42.20). If neutrophils predominate, then determine if they appear healthy or degenerate, which is an indirect way to estimate the likelihood of sepsis. If other inflammatory cells (eosinophils, macrophages, small lymphocytes) are the predominant cells present, then consider inflammation, and refer to Chapter 39 for specific considerations associated with different types of inflammatory cells. If neutrophils are absent or only a few are seen and there are numerous mononuclear cells, then the likely diagnosis is neoplasia. This is relatively straightforward if the mass is in the skin, but in organs the diagnostician must also be able to recognize *normal resident cells* of that organ, which are also mononuclear.

Do not worry about identifying specific cells at this point. Focus on identifying the process: cancer vs. inflammation. Find an area with the most cells for that slide and in which the cells are in a thin monolayer (Figure 40.5). Decide if the cells are individualized or aggregated. The goal now is to decide if most of the cells are round, epithelial, or mesenchymal (spindle shape) (Figure 40.1). This is accomplished by assessing overall cellularity, organization of the cells, amount of cytoplasm per cell and shape of the cells. This can be done using the 20× and 40× objectives; oil immersion is not needed to classify the tumor. Relative size of cells can be estimated by finding red blood cells (7 µm, canine) and neutrophils (approximately 15 µm). Almost all neoplastic cells are larger than both cells. The smallest tumor cells are probably small T-cell lymphoma, and the largest are likely squamous cell carcinoma (SCC) and histiocytic sarcoma (HS). There is no specific size that predicts a cell is neoplastic and measuring cell sizes has little benefit. Exception: cell size as determined by flow cytometry is used to assess biologic behaviors of some lymphomas (see Chapter 45) [6].

Round cell tumors usually exfoliate a large number of cells. The cells are individualized (discrete); they may contact adjacent cells but do not pile together (unless preparation is thick and highly cellular). Volume of cytoplasm is low to moderate and the shape of the cell is round or oval. Do not consider the shape of the nuclei as most nuclei are round, even in mesenchymal cells. Round cell tumors are MCT, histiocytoma, plasma cell tumor, lymphoma, and TVT (Figure 40.6). The last two differentials rarely produce tumors on the skin; they are usually in lymph nodes (lymphoma) or on external genitalia (TVT). If lymphoma is in the skin the lesions are usually multiple hyperemic plaques (not a singular mass). The first three tumors are described in greater detail in the section on skin tumors. The most common skin tumor in dogs is MCT and it is usually easy to recognize because the tumor cells exfoliate readily and have numerous purple cytoplasmic granules. Granularity varies widely from barely visible to obscuring the nucleus (Figure 40.7). Although preparations from round cell tumors usually have high cellularity,

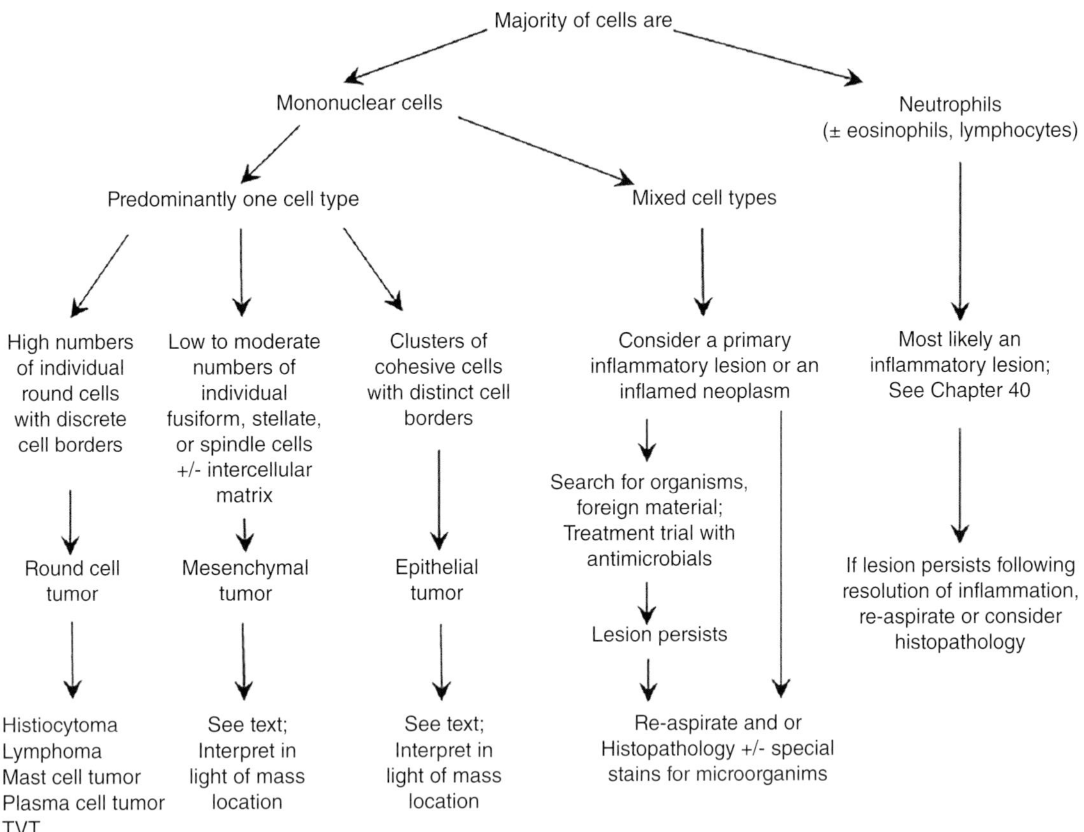

Figure 40.4 Cancer vs. inflammation algorithm.

the exception is histiocytoma, which may have a paucity of cells on the slide.

Epithelial cell tumors generally exfoliate numerous cells. The cells can be individualized, but the important feature is the presence of cohesive clusters of cells piled together (Figures 40.1 and 40.8). Search at low to medium magnifications for these cohesive units as they are the key to the correct diagnosis. Proceeding to high magnification before searching for these may result in a missed diagnosis. Generally, epithelial cells have abundant cytoplasm and cell shapes are cuboidal, columnar or polygonal. The shape of the cell is not critical to the diagnosis and shape may be difficult to discern in the aggregates. Epithelial cells are often organized into groups that form clusters, morula, or acini. These histologic structures form due to desmosomes that connect epithelial cells. It is rare, and not needed for the diagnosis, that an epithelial tumor yields distinct acini with a central lumen, as seen in histology. A few epithelial tumors are so distinct that their origin can be determined from cytological features: UC (transitional cell carcinoma [TCC]), sebaceous, circumanal, (perianal gland) tumor, anal sac apocrine gland adenocarcinoma, thyroid follicular carcinoma, etc. (Figure 40.8). Therefore, epithelial tumors are generally identified by knowing the organ from which they were aspirated: urinary bladder, mammary, prostate, etc.

Mesenchymal tumors usually exfoliate a low to moderate number of cells, the cells are individualized or may appear adhered but will not form circular acini, and cytoplasm is elongated such that the cells have a spindle shape, which is critical to the correct diagnosis (Figures 40.1 and 40.9). Most of the nuclei will be round, but if they are oval-shaped or elongated, it makes cell identification easier. Mesenchymal tumors have a wide range of appearances depending on their origin. They tend to yield few cells because the collagenous intercellular matrix holds the neoplastic cells within the tumor tightly. However, osteosarcoma and perivascular wall tumor (PWT) usually yield numerous cells (Figure 40.9). PWT is a term used for a group of spindle-shaped tumors that arise from cells in the wall of blood vessels, and histology and immunohistochemistry are required to accurately identity subtypes: *hemangiopericytomas, myopericytomas, angioleiomyomas, angiofibromas, adventitial tumors* [7, 8]. PWT is the most common mesenchymal tumor in the skin and subcutis of dogs, and they are rarely malignant. The intercellular matrix of mesenchymal tumors is seldom seen in FNA cytological

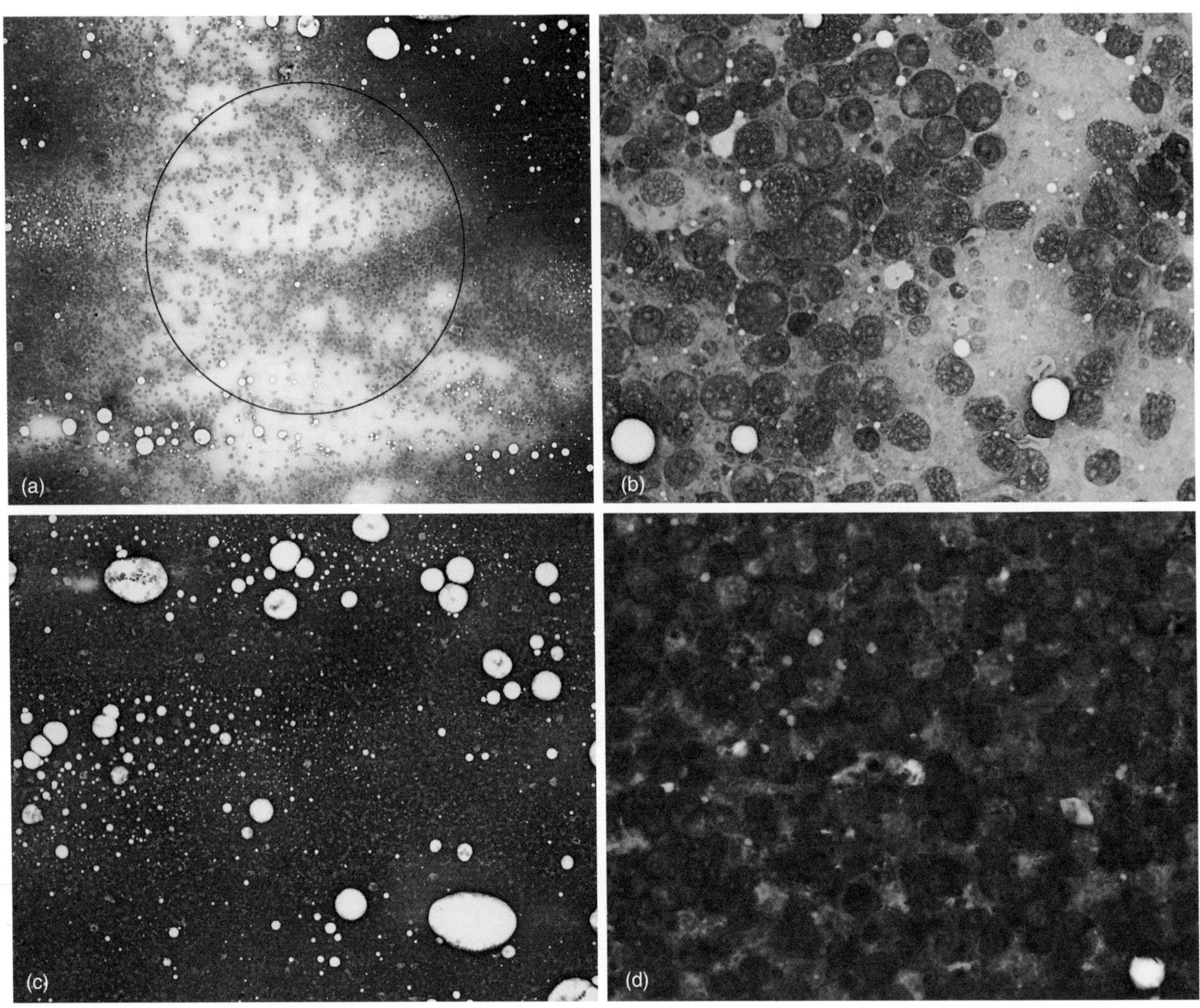

Figure 40.5 Thin monolayer (a, circle, 10× objective) will provide diagnostic regions (b, 100× objective) vs. thick areas outside of circle that are nondiagnostic. Search the slides with 10 or 20× objectives and no coverslip, then proceed to a higher magnification when the thinner regions are located. Two lower panels (c, d), are too thick, even at 100× (d); a diagnosis is not possible. Do not try to make diagnoses on poor-quality slides. Wright-Giemsa stain.

preparations but occasionally is found in osteosarcoma (Figure 40.9) and chondrosarcoma. HSs are so unique in their origin and cytological and histological appearances that they are described separately in this section; they do not have a visible intercellular matrix.

Melanocytic tumors are mesenchymal, but their cytological appearance can be a mixture of spindle, round and epithelial-like aggregates. Cytoplasmic pigment is the key to the diagnosis, and it ranges from green to black and from a light dusting to so heavily pigmented that nuclei cannot be seen (Figure 40.10). When no pigment is observed, they are sometimes referred to as amelanotic. Rarely is pigment truly absent. It may require extensive searching but almost always a few cells with pigment will be present. Histochemical stains (Fontana-Masson) and immunohistochemistry (Melan A, PNL-2) or immunocytochemistry can be requested if pigment is not identified to confirm the diagnosis of melanoma. Names for melanocytic tumors are quite varied: melanoma, melanosarcoma, melanocytic melanoma with benign histologic features; melanoma with low malignant potential; melanocytoma; well differentiated melanoma. The name is unimportant; predicting biologic behavior is important (see end of this chapter).

Endocrine/neuroendocrine tumors is a fourth category of cytologic tumor classification. Neuroendocrine tumors exfoliate moderate to high number of cells; however, the cells are often not intact and bare nuclei devoid of encompassing cytoplasm or embedded in a sea of cytoplasm are present. Apparently, these cells are fragile and cell membranes are easily broken during preparation, therefore cell borders are usually indistinct. If the slide is searched well, intact cells with a small to moderate amount of lightly stained cytoplasm can be found (Figure 40.11). Nuclei are round and uniform. Biological behavior of neuroendocrine tumors

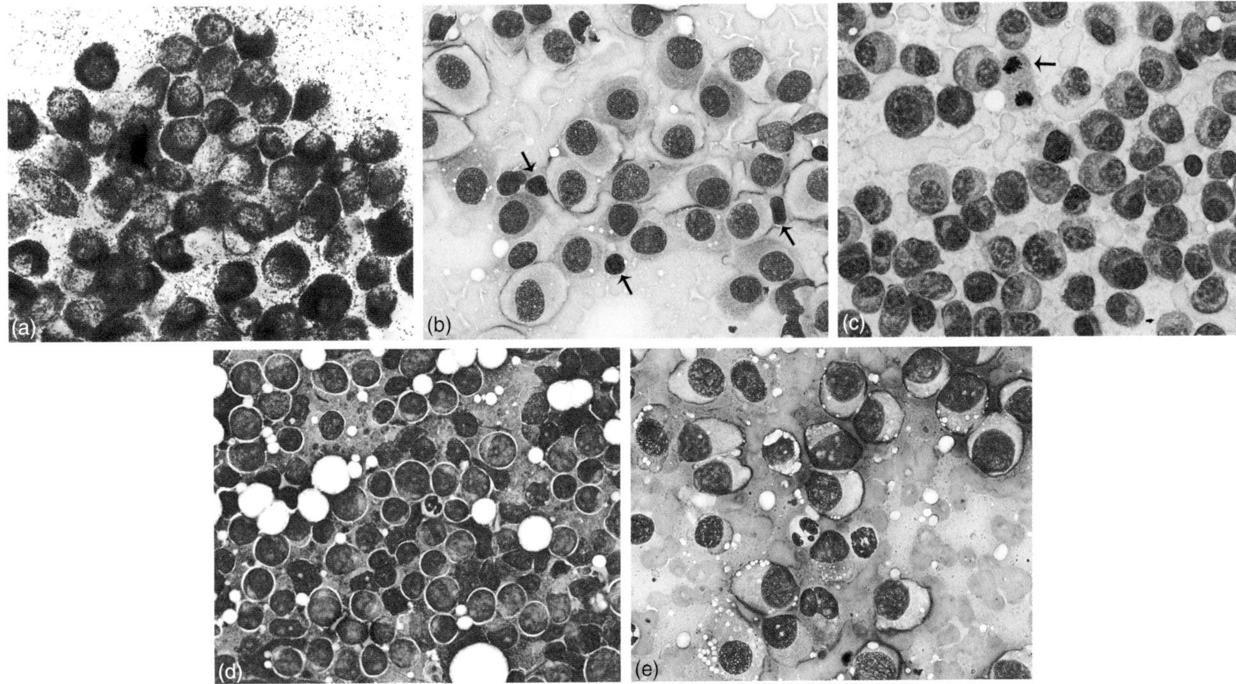

Figure 40.6 Round cell tumors. (a-e) 50× objective; common feature is individual round cells. (a) Mast cell tumor – numerous cells, obvious purple granules. (b) Histiocytoma – low number of cells, pale cytoplasm; the few dense nuclei with scant cytoplasm (arrows) are lymphocytes. (c) Plasma cell tumor – eccentric nuclei and pale paranuclear zone (Golgi) are diagnostic, arrow points to a mitotic figure (anaphase). (d) Lymphoma – high cellularity, uniform round cells with minimal cytoplasm and single large nucleus that fills the cytoplasm; note neutrophil in center for size comparison. (e) TVT – resembles histiocytoma but cytoplasmic vacuoles aid distinction and location on genitalia confirms diagnosis. Histopathology is not needed to establish diagnosis for any of these examples. Wright-Giemsa stain.

is better predicted from historical data and not from cellular and nuclear characteristics.

Neuroendocrine tumors are diagnosed infrequently in primary care centers due to their location in the abdominal (adrenal, pancreas) or thoracic cavities (aortic body tumors). They are also located at the carotid bifurcation in the jugular furrow (carotid body tumor), and therefore may be aspirated easily from this location. Another possible site is thyroid; however, most thyroid tumors in dogs and cats are of follicular origin, and these are epithelial (although these cells typically have a neuroendocrine appearance). C-cell tumors are neuroendocrine and are in or expanding from the thyroid gland. The distinction of follicular tumors from C-cell tumors usually requires histopathology and often immunohistochemistry or immunocytochemistry. Follicular tumors are more common than C-cell tumors in dogs and cats; they are aggressive in dogs and benign in cats. They usually do not cause functional thyroid problems in dogs but cause hyperthyroidism in cats. Nodular adenomatous hyperplasia in cats is a misnomer; the lesion is adenoma. Merkel cell tumors are neuroendocrine tumors found in the skin and are exceedingly rare.

Histiocytic sarcoma is a mesenchymal tumor, but the tumor cells are not spindle-shaped; in fact, they look cytologically like a pleomorphic round cell tumor (Figure 40.12). A malignant plasma cell tumor (poorly differentiated) and HS may look similar microscopically. Both tumors yield highly cellular preparations. Cells are individualized and large with abundant cytoplasm that contains one to numerous nuclei. Nuclei and nucleoli are highly variable in number, size, and shape. If giant cells, multinucleation, bizarre nuclei, and nucleoli are numerous, then favor HS over plasma cell. The most definitive way to distinguish these two tumors is to use the antibody MUM-1, which will stain plasma cells positively but not histiocytic cells [9]. Immunohistochemical stains that recognize histiocytic cells require special handling and expertise. Less technical ways to distinguish these tumors use clinical criteria: *breed of dog*: Bernese mountain dogs, flat-coated retrievers, Rottweilers, and golden retrievers are predisposed to develop HSs, but they can occur in any breed; *location*: articular joints, widely disseminated, or pulmonary favors histiocytic; oral, rectal favors plasma cell; *serum total protein*: very high concentration, especially with monoclonal gammopathy, favors plasma cell, but this and intratumor amyloid are uncommon to rare.

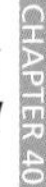

HSs are a disease complex with designated subtypes. The majority arise from interstitial dendritic cells that are present in perivascular tissues in many organs [10]. However, hemophagocytic histiocytic tumors arise from macrophages in the spleen. The distinctive microscopic

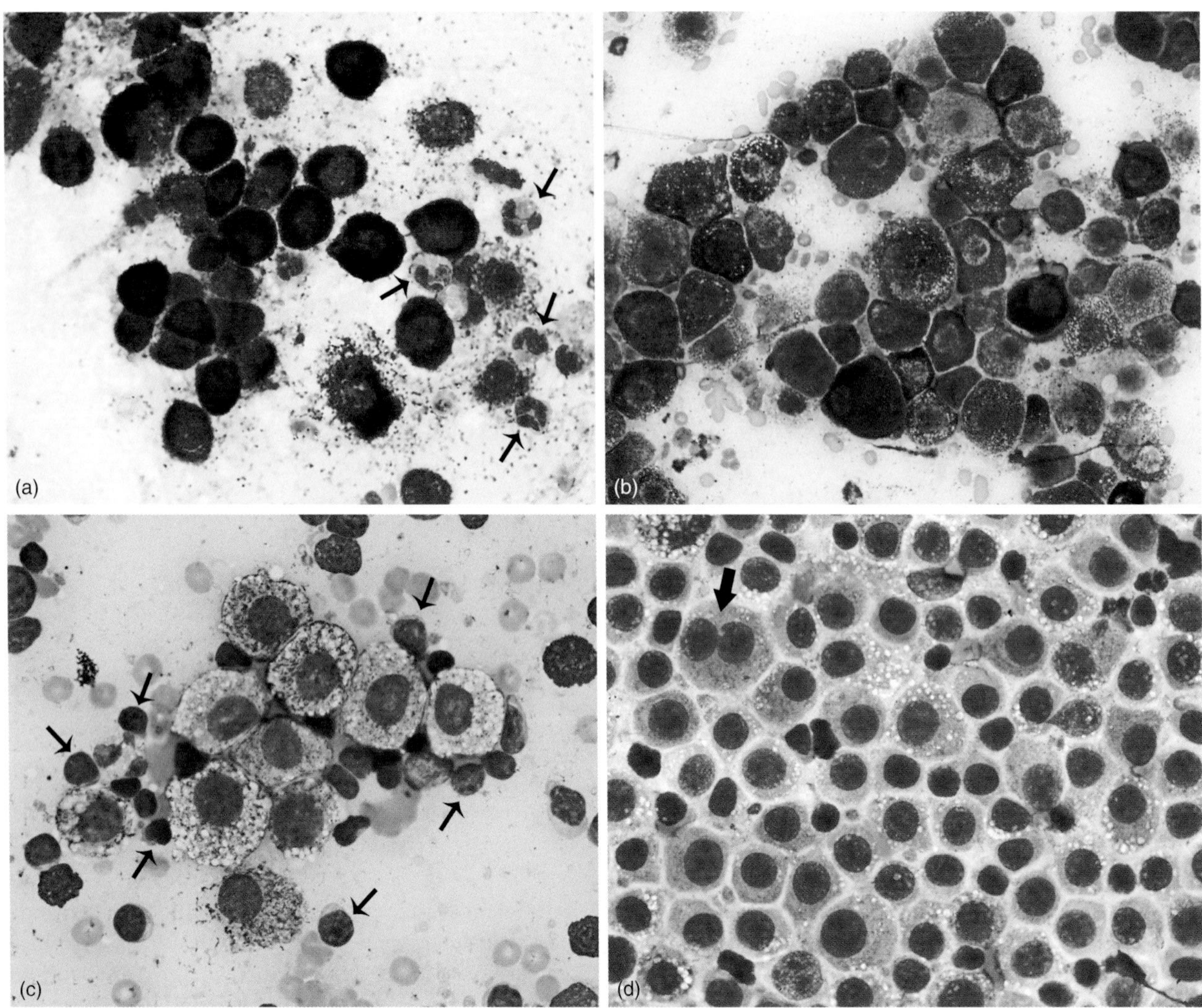

Figure 40.7 This collage is from four different canine cutaneous MCTs and demonstrates how tumors can have a range of cytological (and histological) appearances. Cytologic grading of canine MCT is based on the variability of cells and nuclei. Less aggressive MCTs are heavily pigmented (a, b) and cells are relatively uniform. Note the numerous eosinophils in (a) (arrows) and lymphocytes in (c) (arrows). More aggressive MCTs have less cytoplasmic pigment that may be faint (c) to absent (d). They also exhibit variability in cell and nuclear sizes and shapes including binucleation (arrow, d), as well as multinucleation and mitotic figures. Cytological grading schemes will estimate these features in a determined number of mast cells seen on the preparation. (a, c, d) 100× objective; (b) 50× objective. Wright-Giemsa stain.

feature for this subtype is the presence of erythrophagocytosis (Figure 40.12). The tumor complex can be highly malignant but there are localized diseases as well. There are no definitive criteria to diagnose synovial cell sarcoma in dogs, and tumors previously classified as such are HSs. Deletion of tumor suppressor genes CDKN2A/B, RB1, and PTEN are part of the pathogenesis of HS in dogs [11].

Combine all known clinical facts with microscopic observations to identify the tumor categories, but the most important cytological features within each category are *round cell tumors* – individualized cells with a round shape; *epithelial tumors* – large cells adhered in clusters, morulae; *mesenchymal tumors* – spindle-shaped cells; *neuroendocrine* – uniform nuclei often without surrounding cytoplasm.

Benign vs. malignant

After the cytologist establishes a tumor is present, the next most important determination for an owner and clinician is to determine if the pet's tumor is benign or malignant. The cytological features associated with each are summarized in Table 40.2.

These criteria are standard in publications about cytology and neoplasia, but they should not be relied on too heavily

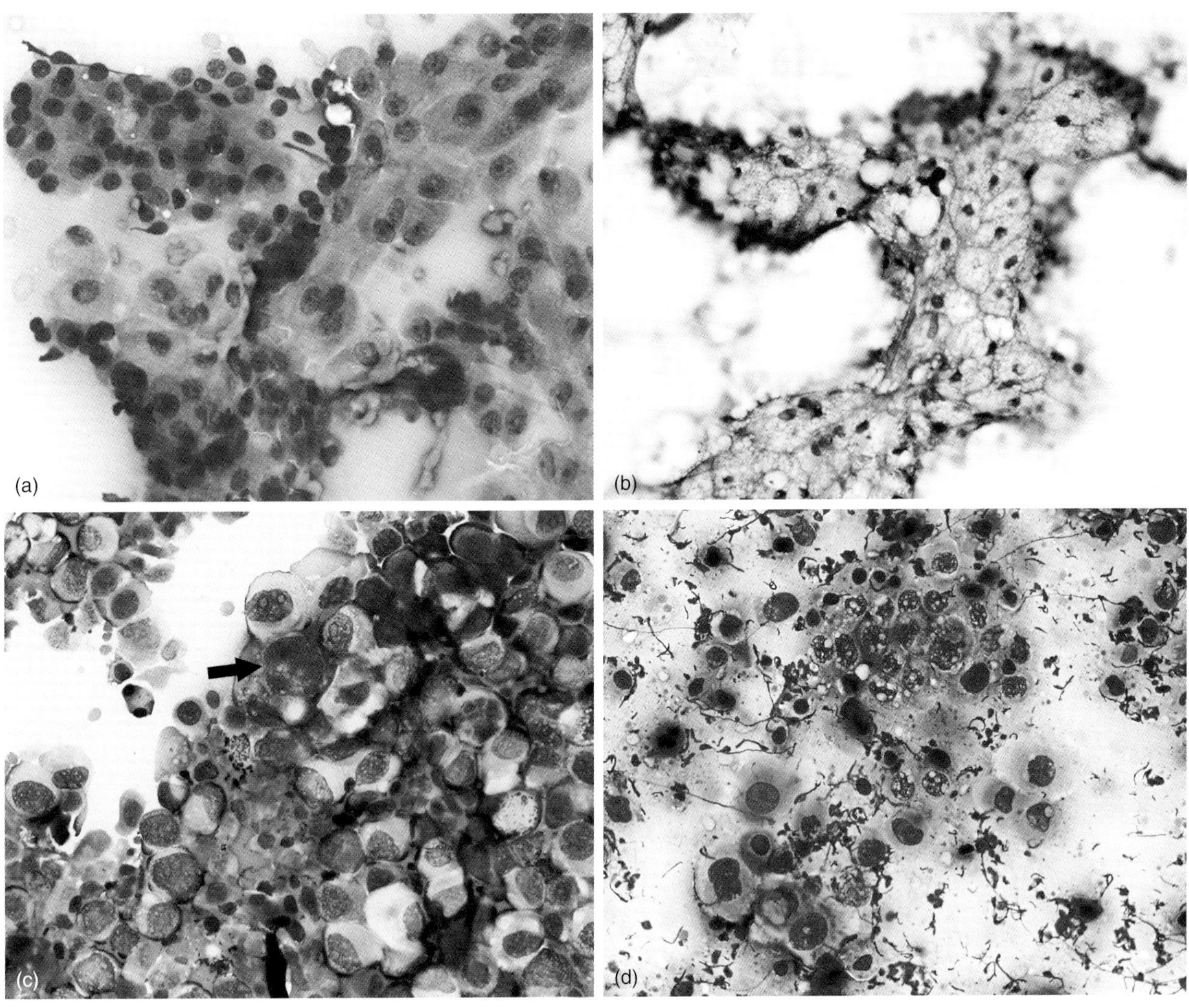

Figure 40.8 Epithelial tumors – the common feature in each image is large cells adhered together. (a, c, d) 50× objective; (b) 40× objective. (a) and (b) have numerous cells that overlap such that some regions are out of focus. Cytological features help name the tumor, but the key to each diagnosis and predicted behavior is location of the tumor. (a) Perineum, perianal gland tumor, benign. (b) Eyelid (or any location on skin) – sebaceous gland adenoma (typical abundant clear to vacuolated cytoplasm), benign. (c) Urinary bladder – urothelial carcinoma (TCC), malignant, arrow points to a Melamed-Wolinska inclusion body, which is diagnostic for urothelial cell origin. (d) Ear, eye, oral, or genitalia – squamous cell carcinoma, malignant. Epithelial cells are extremely pleomorphic; the numerous smaller cells in the background are neutrophils, many of which have degenerated. Neutrophils are a common finding in SCC. Biologic behavior of each tumor is based on diagnosis and location rather than cytological criterion. Wright-Giemsa stain.

→

Figure 40.9 Fine-needle aspirates of mesenchymal tumors. (a–f) 50× objective. (a, b) Perivascular wall tumor (PWT) or hemangiopericytoma; histopathology and ancillary tests are needed to subtype these tumors, but a clinical diagnosis and behavior can be provided from cytology and size of tumor. A blood vessel, characteristic of PWT, is indicated by arrows. Spindle shape is seen at higher magnifications but will not be seen in all cells. (c) Fibrosarcoma (injection-site sarcoma) from a cat; large subcutaneous mass located on the left thoracic wall. Note pleomorphic spindle cells exhibiting anisocytosis, anisokaryosis, binucleation (thick arrows), micronuclei (satellite nuclei, thin arrow), and macronucleoli (arrowhead); cells are surrounded by pink, fibrillar matrix. Such matrix is not always seen nor this abundant. (d) Hemangiosarcoma (spleen, dog); low numbers of highly pleomorphic spindle cells with punctate clear cytoplasmic vacuoles (arrows), large nuclei (compare size to surrounding neutrophils), and macronucleoli (arrowheads). It is uncommon to retrieve neoplastic cells in HSA with FNA because the majority of the mass is composed of blood vessels with large regions of hemorrhage and necrosis. (e, f) Osteosarcoma – distal radius, large-breed dog, lytic bone lesion. No neutrophils and numerous mononuclear cells with eccentric nuclei. There is variability in sizes of cells and nuclei. Spindle shape is only apparent in a few cells. Osteoid matrix (pink, white arrow) is present. Several mitotic figures are indicated by arrows, and the thick arrow is directed at a cell with a macronucleolus. The cells inside the circle are osteoblasts, which resemble plasma cells due to their eccentric nuclei, blue cytoplasm, and pale Golgi. Osteoblasts will stain positively for alkaline phosphatase. Histopathology is not needed when the cytological features and clinical data are this classic.

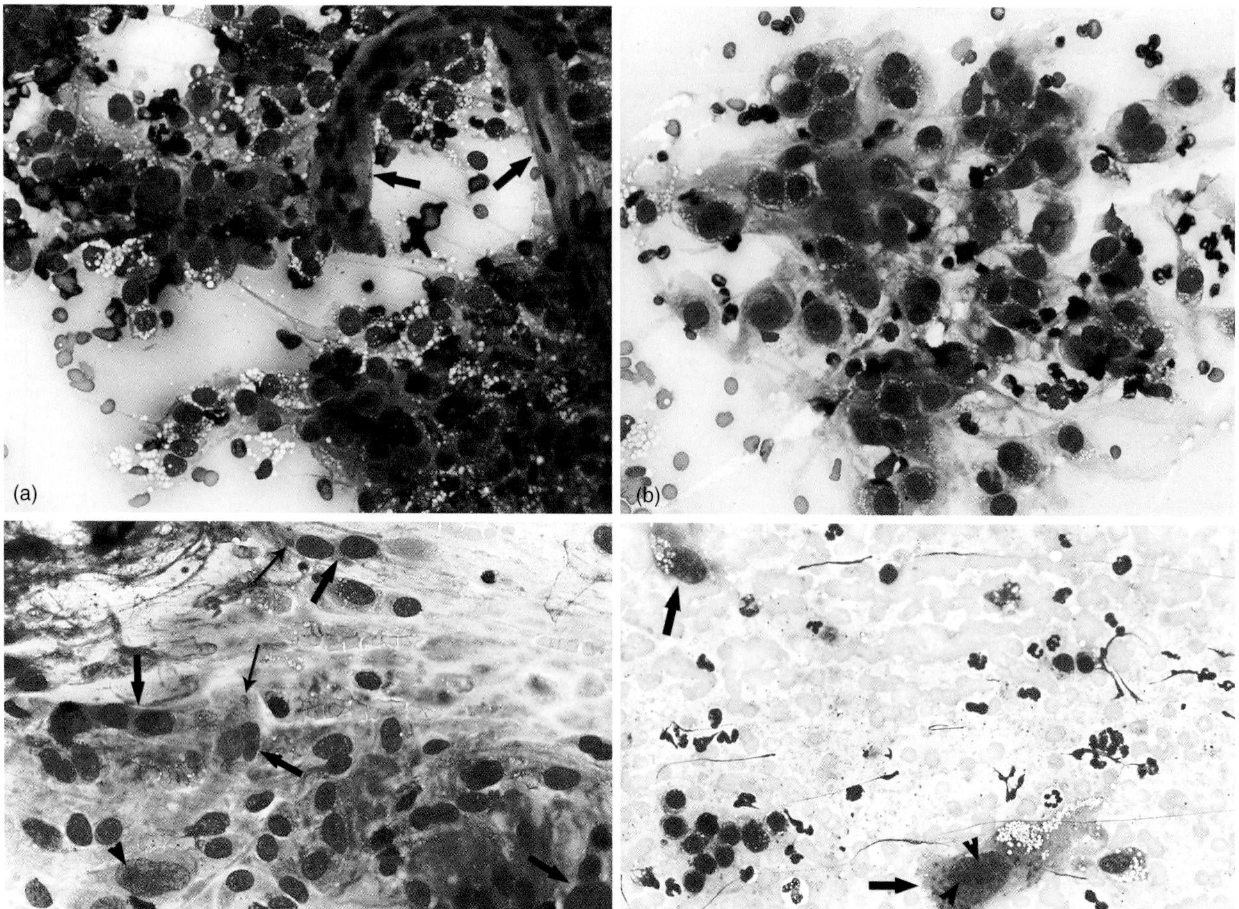

(a)

(b)

(c)

(d)

(e)

(f)

osteoid

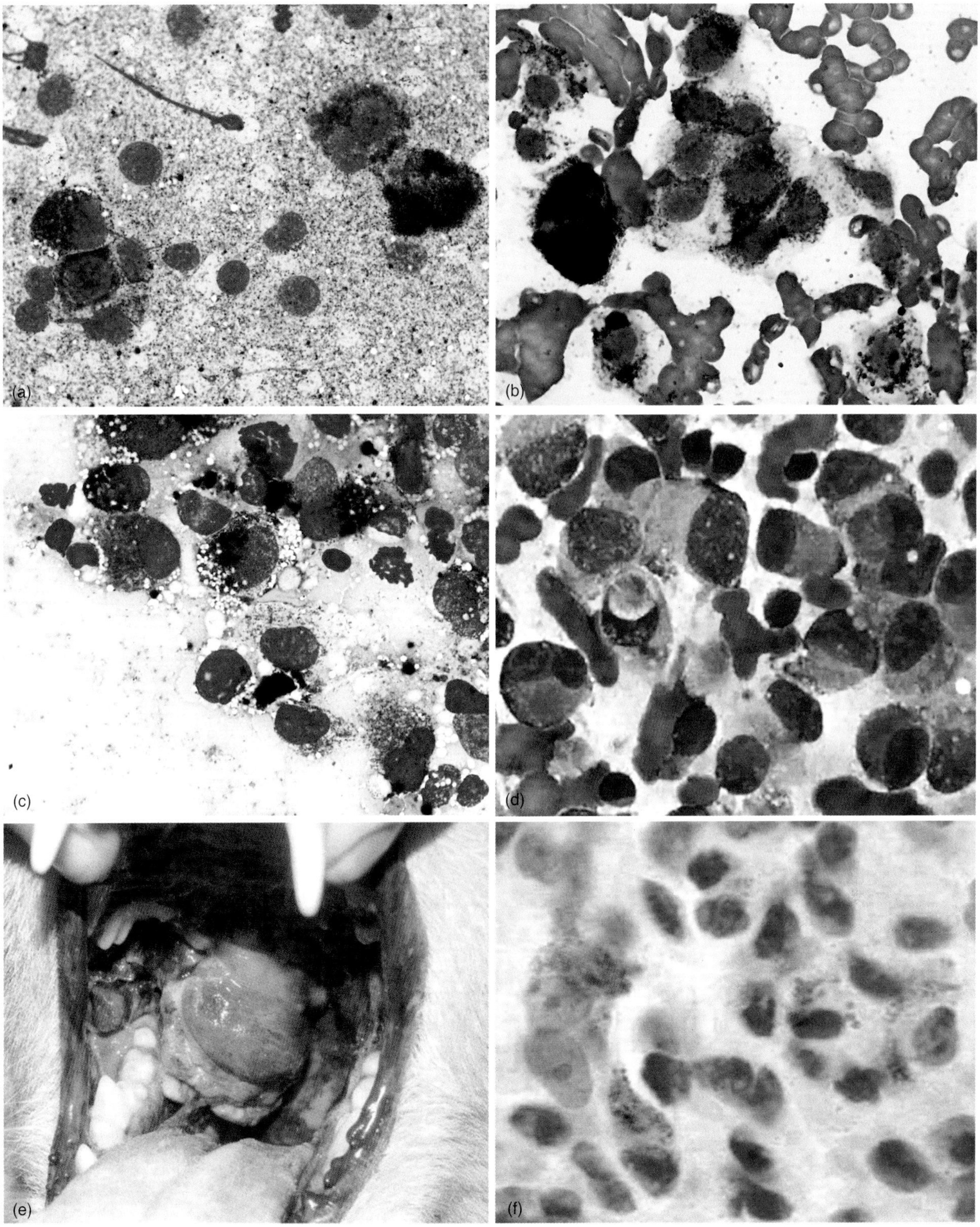

(a) (b) (c) (d) (e) (f)

Figure 40.10 Canine melanocytic tumors, range of cytological patterns. (a, b, d, f) 100× objective. (c) 50× objective. (a) Cutaneous melanoma/melanocytoma, heavily pigmented individual cells, round nuclei; abundant pigment in background will make the slide black on gross inspection. Histology is needed to assess biological behavior. (b) Digit melanoma, aggregate of cells in middle are epithelial-like, arrow points to a spindle-shaped cell. (c) Metastasis in regional lymph node from an oral malignant melanoma; binucleated cell, moderate to marked variability in cell and nuclear morphology; amount of pigment is highly variable (large black globules, small black granules, and some cells are devoid of pigment). (d–f) Oral malignant melanoma, amelanotic; note the absence of visible melanin pigment in these pleomorphic cells (d); cells stained positive (brown) with a melanocytic marker (Melan A) on histopathology (f). (e) A pale gray mass is protruding from the soft palate in this dog. Touching the surface of tumors is futile; FNA into the mass is needed to yield cells that represent the tumor.

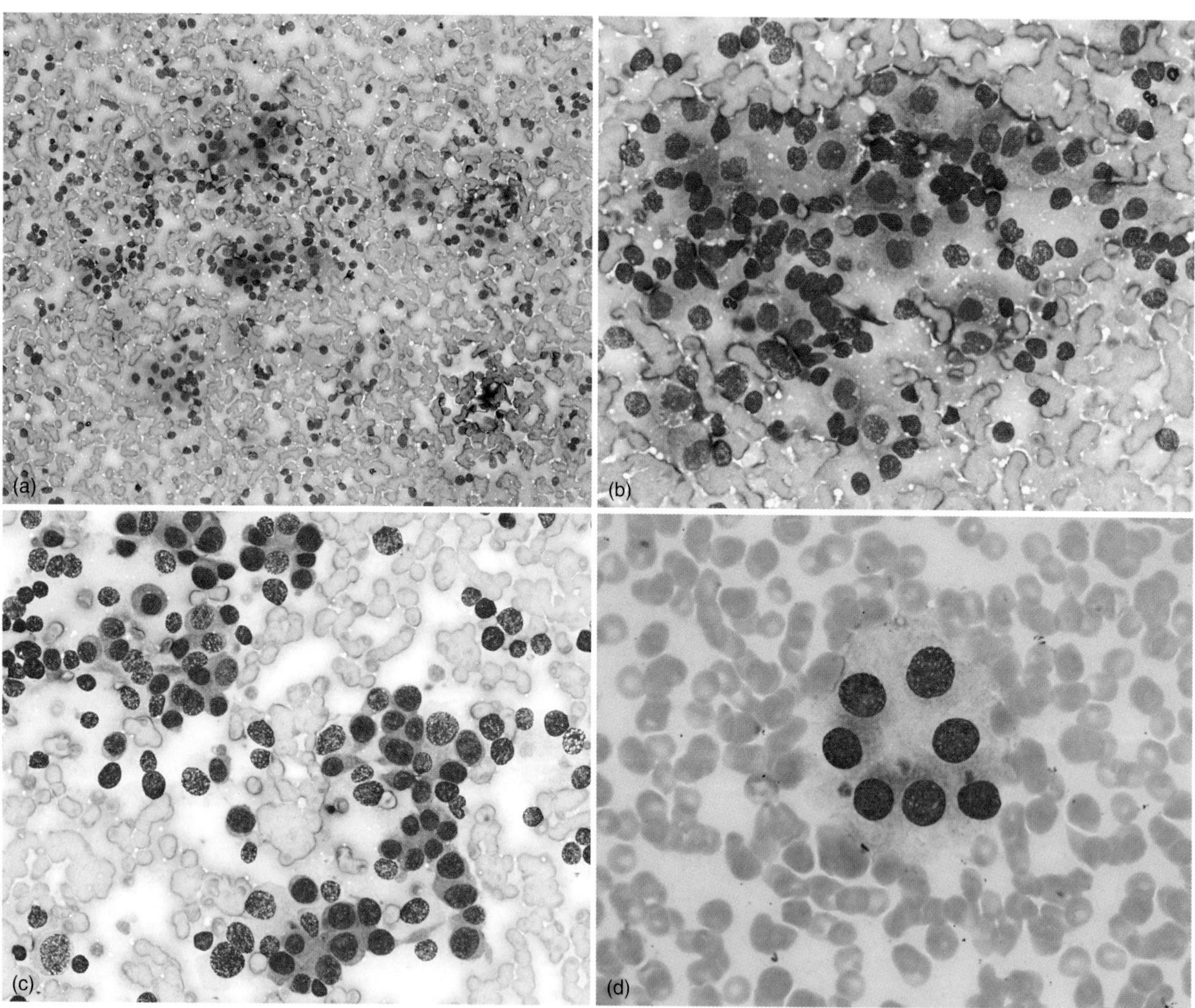

Figure 40.11 Neuroendocrine/endocrine – this is a fourth pattern of neoplasia that can be recognized by cytological examination. These tumors are seen infrequently in primary care facilities as most are located in the abdominal or thoracic cavities. Top panel is an insulinoma (a: 20× objective, b: 50× objective); the tumor cells were aspirated from the liver, which is a frequent metastatic site. Bottom panel is a thyroid tumor (c: 20× objective, d: 100× objective), likely follicular in origin, due to the circular or acinar pattern seen at higher magnification (d). Common features in both examples are uniform round cells that are in close proximity and appear to be adhered; pale cytoplasm and/or naked nuclei. The uniformity of cells and nuclei would suggest benign behavior, but both tumors metastasize readily: 90% of insulinomas will metastasize and thyroid follicular tumors that are palpable metastasize to lungs.

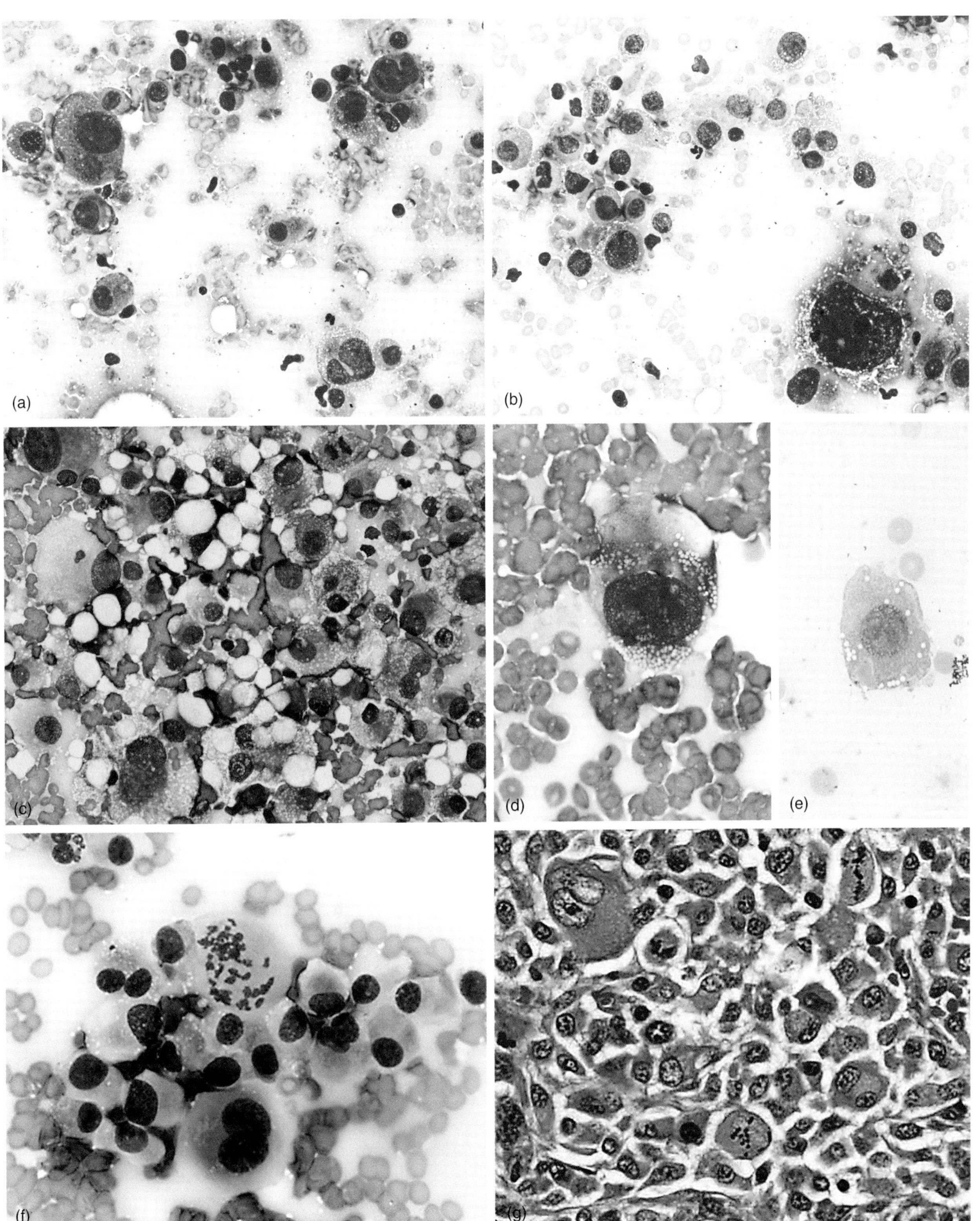

Figure 40.12 Histiocytic sarcoma. Tissue source in top two panels is lymph node (a, b: 50× objective); there are no neutrophils or lymphocytes but pleomorphic mononuclear cells predominate, indicating metastatic neoplasia. There is marked variability in the size of tumor cells and their nuclei. Image (c) (50× objective) is from the lung and images (d) and (e) (100× objective) are from the spleen. Each image contains at least one incredibly large cell with abundant cytoplasm. The nuclei in these cells are as large as three to six red blood cells. The tumor cells in (d) and (e) exhibit erythrophagia; although other tumor cells can be phagocytic, this feature is characteristic of histiocytic tumors. Images (f) (50× objective) and (g) (40× objective) are from the joint of a retriever dog, and they demonstrate the marked pleomorphism of this tumor on cytology (f) and histopathology (f, g; Source: Images courtesy of Keith Thompson). See text for other ways to diagnose this tumor and cells of origin. (a–f) Wright-Giemsa stain. (g) H&E stain.

Table 40.2 Criteria to help predict benign vs. aggressive (malignant) behavior.

General
Historical data about a specific tumor type and location are better than cytological criteria
Single-cell type, no inflammation, uniform cells and nuclei favor benign[a]
Small well-delineated mass (<2 cm) favors benign; large (>6 cm) poorly delineated or infiltrative/ulcerated favors aggressive
Cellular and nuclear pleomorphism – aggressive
Cells exfoliate in high numbers (especially for mesenchymal tumors) – aggressive, vs. low number of cells – benign
Variation in cell size (anisocytosis) and/or irregular cell shape – aggressive
Variation in nucleus-to-cytoplasmic (N : C) ratio – aggressive
Nuclear criteria of malignancy = *"variability" – pleomorphism*
Variation in nuclear size (anisokaryosis)
Irregular nuclear shape, sizes, giant nuclei
Multinucleated cells, binucleation – note: non-neoplastic monocytes/macrophages have these same features
Nuclei and cells that pile together with no respect to cell or nuclear borders
Micro-/satellite nuclei, fragmented nuclei
Large nucleoli, macronucleoli (exceeding the size of a red blood cell)
Multiple nucleoli of variable size and/or irregular shape
Increased mitoses with abnormal (bizarre) mitotic figures

[a] Notable exceptions are lymphoma, insulinoma, thyroid tumors, some carcinomas that appear uniform but are aggressive; other exceptions are described in the text of this chapter.

because there are no studies that correlate these features with outcome assessments, and exceptions to the predicted behavior patterns are numerous. The term "criteria of malignancy" in cytopathology implies a tumor is malignant when these features are present. Yet a tumor may have these features and not be malignant. Furthermore, inflammatory cells and reactive fibroblasts and young blood vessels can possess the nuclear features listed as criteria of malignancy (see "Confounders in Interpretation"). Alternatively, a tumor may not possess any of these cytologic criteria of malignancy, but it is aggressive: invades adjacent tissues, is present in blood or lymphatic vessels, and/or metastasizes. The term criteria of malignancy is better considered *criteria of neoplasia*.

If cytological criteria are imprecise, then what should be used at this juncture? Known historical data about the behavior of a type of tumor are more useful than trying to predict how an individual tumor will behave from the cytological criteria. For example: MCT in cats are benign, 90% of cutaneous MCT in dogs are benign, histiocytoma is benign, sebaceous tumors are benign, lymphoma is malignant, osteosarcomas are malignant, injection site sarcoma in cats is invasive, insulinoma in dogs appears cytologically benign but greater than 90% metastasize (see end of this chapter).

There are no cytological grading schemes for tumors in pets that have been shown to have statistical significance to predict prognosis, and there are few histologic grading schemes and no molecular markers that have been validated with robust cohorts in animals. Cytological grading schemes will be developed, and they will be plagued by problems inherent in our present studies: an absence of standardized parameters (microscopic, molecular, immunohistochemistry, outcome assessment), excessively subjective microscopic evaluations, limited number of cases, different stages of disease at enrollment, different therapies, weak or inaccurate follow-up data, and lack of concordance between pathologists. Outcome assessment determines if a test is predictive of treatment or prognostic of tumor behavior. Outcome assessment data must be collected as carefully and accurately as the cytological, histological, or molecular techniques used to assess tumors. Yet survival times and even disease-free intervals are heavily influenced by owners' decisions about euthanasia. Owner decisions are influenced by personal factors including the value of pets in a family, finances, and/or nursing care. These factors are part of but difficult to separate from the tumor's behavior or the host's defenses.

The best cytological feature to estimate behavior is uniformity vs. variability (pleomorphism) in cells, nuclei, and nucleoli (Table 40.2). The more uniform the cell size and shape, the more likely the tumor is benign (indolent). Uniformity is associated with benign behavior, whereas variable sizes, numbers, and shapes of nuclei and nucleoli are used to predict aggressive behavior (Figures 40.13 and 40.14). Nuclear and nucleolar pleomorphism are more important to assess than cellular features. Multiple nucleoli of various sizes is a widely used cytological feature associated with aggressive tumors. All living cells have nuclei and nucleoli; it is their variability that must be evaluated, not just their presence. Names can be applied to the cellular and nuclear features observed, but more important than the name is the recognition of the abnormality: anisocytosis, anisokaryosis, karyomegaly, abnormal mitotic figures, multinucleation, etc. The determination of uniformity vs. variability is done by evaluating many cells and recognizing a pattern, not just finding one large cell or nucleus with an abnormality.

Generally, the greater the nucleus to cytoplasmic ratio (N : C), the more aggressive the tumor. Cells with a paucity of cytoplasm and large nuclei that nearly fill the entire cell are often aggressive, e.g., lymphoma. These generalizations are guides; they should be used in concert and integrated with all of the other clinical data available, especially location and size of tumor. An obvious exception to the generalization that uniformity is associated with benign behavior is lymphoma, as most lymphomas are fairly uniform in appearance

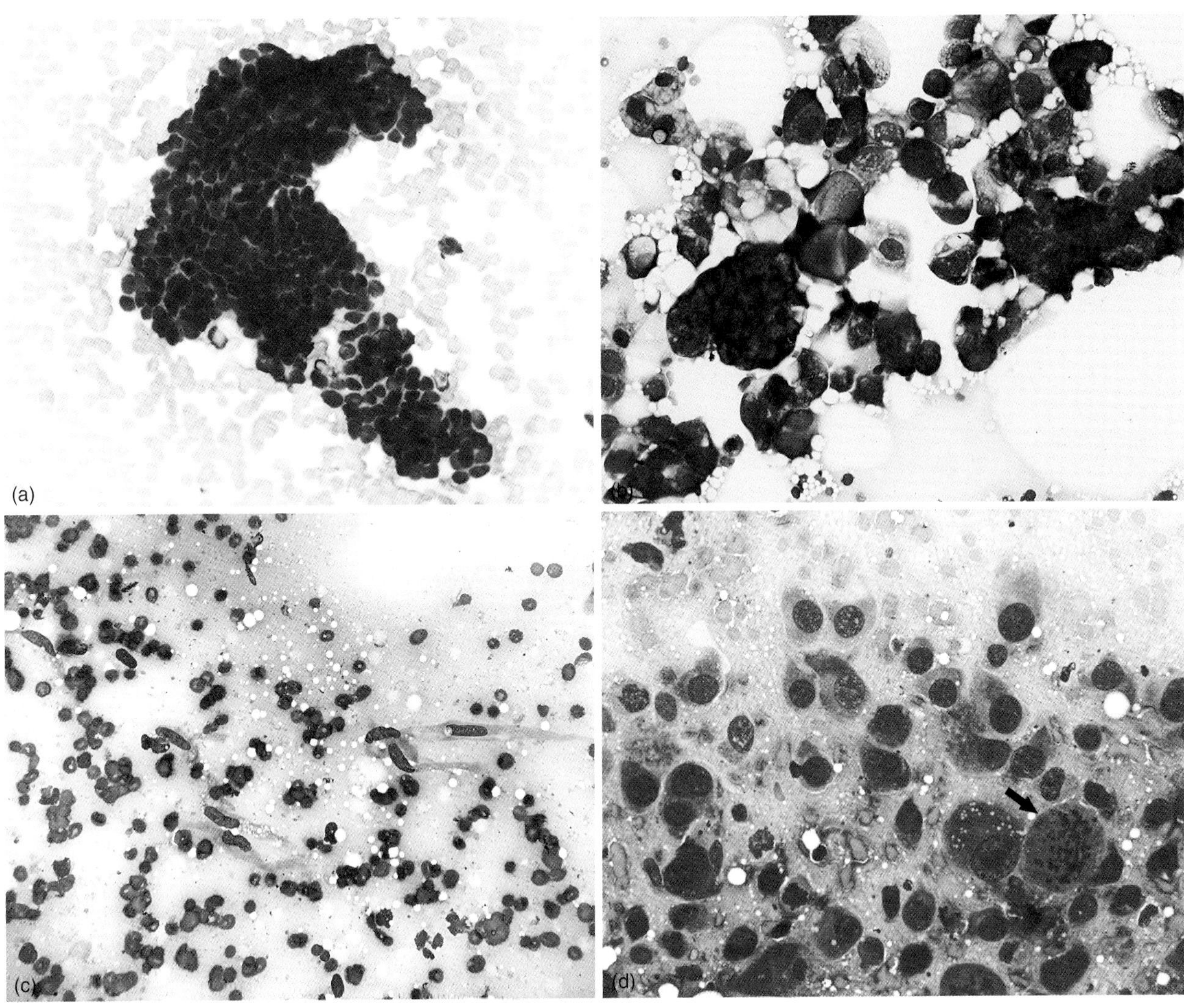

Figure 40.13 Cytological criteria to predict benign vs. malignant behavior are not precise but include uniform vs. pleomorphic patterns of cells, nuclei, and nucleoli. (a–d) 50× objectives. The left-hand images are benign tumors: (a) an epithelial tumor (basilar epithelial cell), and (c) a mesenchymal tumor (leiomyoma). The right-hand images are of malignant tumors: (b) carcinoma of the prostate and (d) an osteosarcoma. The malignant tumors have pleomorphic cells and nuclei. Aggressive tumors also tend to exfoliate numerous cells. The arrow in (d) points to a mitotic figure in which the chromosomes are so dispersed (abnormal) that they could be confused for an infectious organism. (a–d) Wright-Giemsa stain.

but are clinically aggressive. Lymphoma is not one tumor, it is an umbrella term; there are many types of lymphomas in animals. The chapter on lymph nodes provides details of how flow cytometry, B- vs. T-cell origin, and cell size can be used to predict survival times in dogs and cats with lymphoma. Other tumors that are cytologically uniform in appearance but behave aggressively are listed earlier and at the end of this chapter.

Mitotic figures are associated with neoplasia and linked to more aggressive tumors (Figure 40.15). However, mitoses are part of normal cell lines as they are required for cell replication. Certain tissues proliferate at faster rates, and therefore mitotic figures are expected in samples from non-neoplastic bone marrow, lymph nodes, and intestines. Young granulation tissue with proliferating fibroblasts and endothelial cells (neovascularization) will contain mitotic figures in histological and cytological preparations. Therefore, just finding a mitotic figure does not confirm a lesion is neoplastic. However, if multiple mitotic figures are found along with other microscopic and clinical information that suggest neoplasia, then they are a convincing piece of data. They are found regularly in lymphomas, HSs, TVT, and histiocytomas. The latter is the best example in veterinary medicine of a benign tumor that contains numerous mitotic figures. Abnormal mitotic figures (Figure 40.15) are a definite indicator of neoplasia, and even malignancy, but like many "abnormalities" they can be created artefactually. The process of cells drying and collapsing on a glass slide may distort chromosomes and the spindle apparatus producing what look like abnormal mitotic figures [12]. There are a

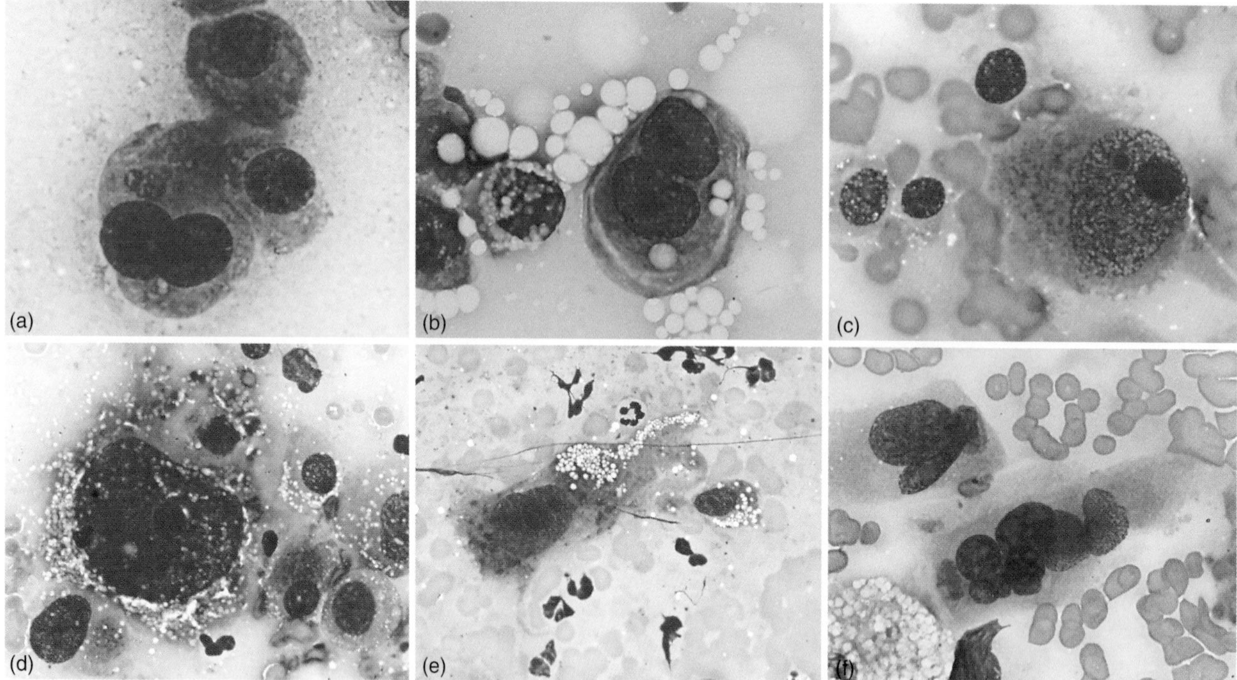

Figure 40.14 These images demonstrate nuclear and nucleolar pleomorphism (variability), which are features associated with malignancy (all oil immersion 100x objective). (a) Binucleation and presence of micro-/satellite nuclei in a pleomorphic variant of a plasma cell tumor (dog). (b) Binucleation and macronuleoli in a cell from a prostatic carcinoma (dog). (c–e) (dogs) Cell gigantism and macronucleoli (histiocytic sarcoma, spleen (c) and lymph node (d); hemangiosarcoma, spleen (e). (f) Bi- and multinucleated cells with marked anisokaryosis from an injection-site sarcoma (cat). Regenerating muscle cells can look identical, which is a good example of why cytological features associated with malignancy are not pathognomonic and require integration with all data available. In this case there were cells in adjacent fields consistent with sarcoma.

variety of names for abnormal mitoses: polar asymmetry, lagging chromosomes and anaphase bridging. Most of these names refer to "Y" shapes (tripolar) rather than a single dense line (metaphase), and chromosomes that are "lagging," which is a form of "dangling chads," reflect loose chromosomes in the cytoplasm that appear as dots adjacent to the dense spindle (Figure 40.15).

Identification of abnormal mitoses is probably best left for board-certified pathologists. Mitotic figures and abnormal mitoses are powerful observations to support the diagnosis of neoplasia. They will only be present when there is other compelling microscopic evidence of neoplasia. Counting mitotic figures in 10 high-power fields (2.37 mm^2) to predict behavior of a tumor is used commonly in histological preparations, but comparable methods for cytological preparations are not standard [13]. Methods have been described for using cytology to grade MCT in dogs [14, 15].

The color of tumor cell cytoplasm cannot be used to predict biological behavior. Basophilic cytoplasm means there is increased RNA and likely the cell is "young," but it does not mean the cell is neoplastic. As all cells mature, they tend to lose cytoplasmic RNA, develop other subcellular organelles, and become more eosinophilic. For example, as red blood cells mature their cytoplasm goes from deeply basophilic, to lighter blue, finally becoming blue gray in metabrubricytes, because even at this late stage of maturation they still have RNA on retained ribosomes. Similarly, hyperchromatic nuclei simply means there is increased color, i.e., darker nuclei, and it is not a criterion of malignancy. In fact, pyknotic and karyorrhectic nuclei are dark, have condensed hyperchromatic nuclei that indicate the cell is dead. Chromatin is nuclear DNA and is seen cytologically and histologically in two forms: *heterochromatin* has small, darkly staining, irregular particles or granules, often at periphery of the nucleus, and *euchromatin* (parachromatin) is loosely packed and appears uniformly lightly stained. Young nuclei tend to be large and have more euchromatin and these are referred to as vesicular or open nuclei. This can be seen in neoplastic and non-neoplastic cells. However, irregular clearing of chromatin forms by an abnormal distribution of heterochromatin granules with large uneven, clear areas of euchromatin between granules and this is a criterion of malignancy. Nuclear and nucleolar features are likely the best cytological evidence of neoplasia; however, rather than trying to identify the type of chromatin, look for variability of sizes, shapes, and number of nuclei and nucleoli per cell. These features are easier to recognize and indicate the lesion is likely neoplastic and aggressive; the more uniform nuclei appear the more likely the lesion is benign.

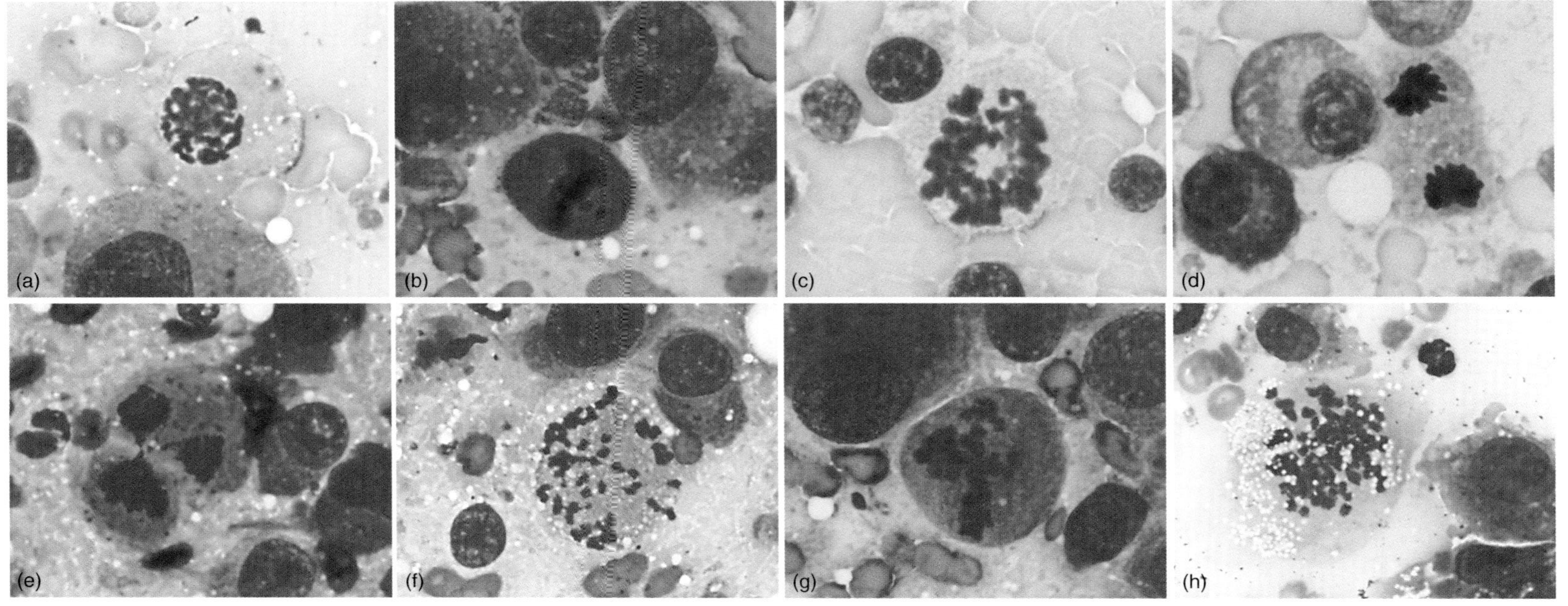

Figure 40.15 Mitotic figures. In all of these images the nuclear membrane is absent (all oil immersion 100× objective). Dissolution of the nuclear membrane is the first step in the process of nuclear division and is part of the definition of a mitotic figure. Naming the stage of mitosis is not as important as recognizing mitotic figures. (a) *Prophase/prometaphase* – chromosomes are a circular group of rope-like aggregates of similar sizes; this stage is often overlooked. (b) *Metaphase* – dark linear band of chromosomes are aligned perpendicular to the long axis of the spindle apparatus; this pattern is seen most frequently in histological preparations. (c) This is also *metaphase*, but the chromosomes are parallel to the spindle apparatus and form a circular pattern; this form can be confused with an abnormal mitosis. (d) *Anaphase* – recognized easily by chromosomes that form two distinct clumps, but the cell has not divided and a nuclear membrane is not present around either nucleus. (e) *Telophase* – two clumps with nuclear membrane forming and cytoplasm dividing into two cells. (f–h) Abnormal mitotic figures (sometimes referred to as "bizarre") with dispersed, unorganized chromosomes and lagging chromosomes.

Very few grading schemes based on cytological criterion have been developed and none have been validated in a large cohort. A cytological grading scheme is described in the skin chapter for cutaneous MCT in dogs. A publication also describes how to assess regional lymph nodes in dogs with MCT [16]. Molecular profiles of MCT, urothelial tumors and lymphomas are used to assess biological behavior in dogs, help direct therapies, monitor progress, or substantiate a diagnosis [3–5, 11, 17, 18]. In human oncology molecular characteristics of tumors is used extensively to diagnose, predict behavior, monitor and select treatments. These methods are employed on tumors in pets but primarily in research centers that use the tumors in pets as models for similar tumors in humans. For some tumors, for example soft-tissue sarcoma (STS), a histological grading scheme can be offered to owners to help predict biological behavior of the tumor or select treatment options, as these tumors cannot be graded from cytology. There are tremendous opportunities to integrate cytological, histological, and molecular parameters to assess tumor behavior, or validate prior studies, if there are accurate long-term outcome assessments (RESIST, PERSIST, CASS) to determine which test(s) may be predictive of prognosis or predictive of treatment efficacy [19, 20].

Table 40.3 Tumors that can have concurrent inflammation.

Tumor type	Inflammatory cells
Squamous cell carcinoma	Neutrophils, can be numerous
Feline injection site sarcoma	Lymphocytes ± plasma cells ± neutrophils ± eosinophils ± macrophages/multinucleated giant cells ± mast cells; lesion may be predominantly or start as inflammatory; multinucleated giant cells can be numerous and the number of nuclei/cells 20–100.
Mast cell tumor	Eosinophils common in dogs, rarely eosinophils may be predominant cells present on slide; few lymphocytes
Histiocytoma	Lymphocytes ± plasma cells, neutrophils – indicates regression
TVT	Lymphocytes, plasma cells, low numbers
Seminoma, dysgerminoma	Lymphocytes, few
Fibrosarcoma	Lymphocytes, eosinophils – eotaxin production by fibroblasts
Neoplastic body cavity fluids	Neutrophils, macrophages, reactive mesothelial cells; note – lymphoma can be 100% lymphoid cells (see Chapters 42 and 43).

Note: Any skin or gastrointestinal tumor that is ulcerated can have secondary inflammation near the ulcer. Therefore, do not touch the ulcerated surface with glass slides. Instead perform FNA some distance from the ulcer and penetrate deep below the surface. Figure 40.14 is a panel that demonstrates some of the tumors that may contain concurrent inflammation. Remember, before making a diagnosis of a tumor with inflammation, rule out granulomatous or pyogranulomatous inflammation.

Confounders in interpretation

If inflammatory cells are numerous, the lesion is more likely to be primary inflammation. When inflammatory cells are absent and FNA of a skin mass contains numerous mononuclear cells, the diagnosis of neoplasia is straightforward. However, if mononuclear cells predominate and there is a mixture of neutrophils, the distinction of neoplasia vs. primary inflammation is difficult. The mononuclear cells seen could be tumor cells, resident tissue cells, plasma cells, lymphocytes, monocytes, or macrophages (histiocytes). The presence of neutrophils in this cell mix suggests inflammation, likely pyogranulomatous. A generalization is to favor inflammation rather than neoplasia, because although many tumors contain areas of necrosis, inflammation within the neoplastic mass is uncommon. Table 40.3 lists tumors in which inflammation can be present and the type of inflammatory cells expected. This inflammation is seen more frequently in histologic sections than cytological specimens (Figure 40.16). In these ambiguous cases, consider additional approaches such as biopsy and histopathology, treatment for inflammation and/or infection, and reevaluation following clearance of the inflammation. If the mass persists, offer repeat FNA and/or biopsy.

The biggest confounder is granulomatous or pyogranulomatous inflammation vs neoplasia. Either of these types of inflammatory lesions will have macrophages (histiocytes), multinucleated giant cells and granulation tissue. Some of the macrophages and giant cells will exhibit the cytological features that are characteristic of the "criteria of malignancy": large nuclei, prominent nucleoli, and multinucleation (Figure 40.17). Examining these suspect cells under oil immersion will not clarify the diagnosis; this simply enlarges the nuclei and nucleoli. A better approach is to drop to lower magnifications and search the entire slide for pattern recognition by answering these simple questions: are more neutrophils present than large cells? Search for etiologic agents associated with granulomatous and pyogranulomatous inflammation: fungi, protozoa, acid fast bacteria, microaerophilic bacteria (*Nocardia, Actinomyces,* etc.) and foreign material. (Note that oil immersion is usually needed to identify microorganisms.) Also consider location of the lesion and size of the lesion. Flat, ulcerated lesions, especially if located where trauma is possible (legs), are more likely to be inflammation. Masses >6 cm, especially if there is no skin ulceration, are more likely neoplastic.

The two neoplasms that could be confused with granulomatous inflammation are HSs and SCC. Therefore, consider facts about each tumor: breed of dog (HS has strong breed

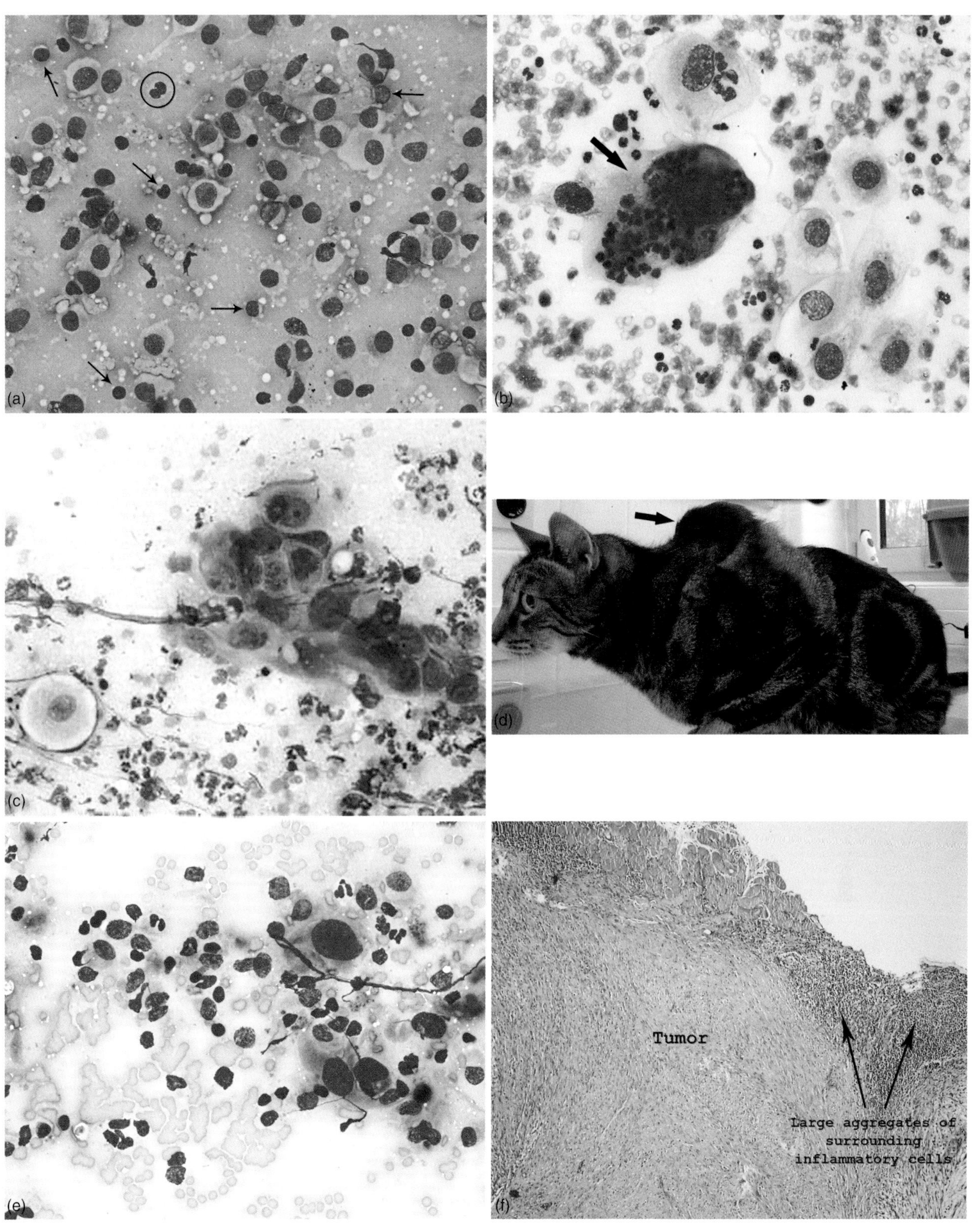
(a)
(b)
(c)
(d)
(e)
(f)
Tumor
Large aggregates of surrounding inflammatory cells

Figure 40.16 Tumors with inflammation. Large tumors may have regions that are necrotic, but most do not have inflammation and, when present, it is a minor component. (a–c and e) 50x objective; (f) 10x objective. (a) Young dog, skin nodule – histiocytoma with lymphocytes (arrows) and neutrophils (circle); concurrent inflammation suggests this tumor is regressing. (b, c) Squamous cell carcinoma (SCC) – this neoplasm often has considerable inflammation, which is due to the tumor's location (skin, genitalia, oral, stomach) and the tendency for ulceration. The large cells are neoplastic, and the small dots are nuclei of neutrophils. One very large tumor cell (b, arrow) appears to have numerous neutrophils within the cell (emperipolesis) but these could also be on the cell surface. (d–f) Cat – injection site sarcoma. (d) Cat with a large interscapular injection-site sarcoma (arrow). (e) The three large nuclei are in tumor cells and the other nuclei are in inflammatory cells. Injection-site sarcomas often have inflammation, and the inflammatory reaction may precede the transformation into a neoplasm. (f) Histopathology of the mass shown in (d). Note the large tumor surrounded by aggregates of inflammatory cells (mainly lymphocytes, arrows).

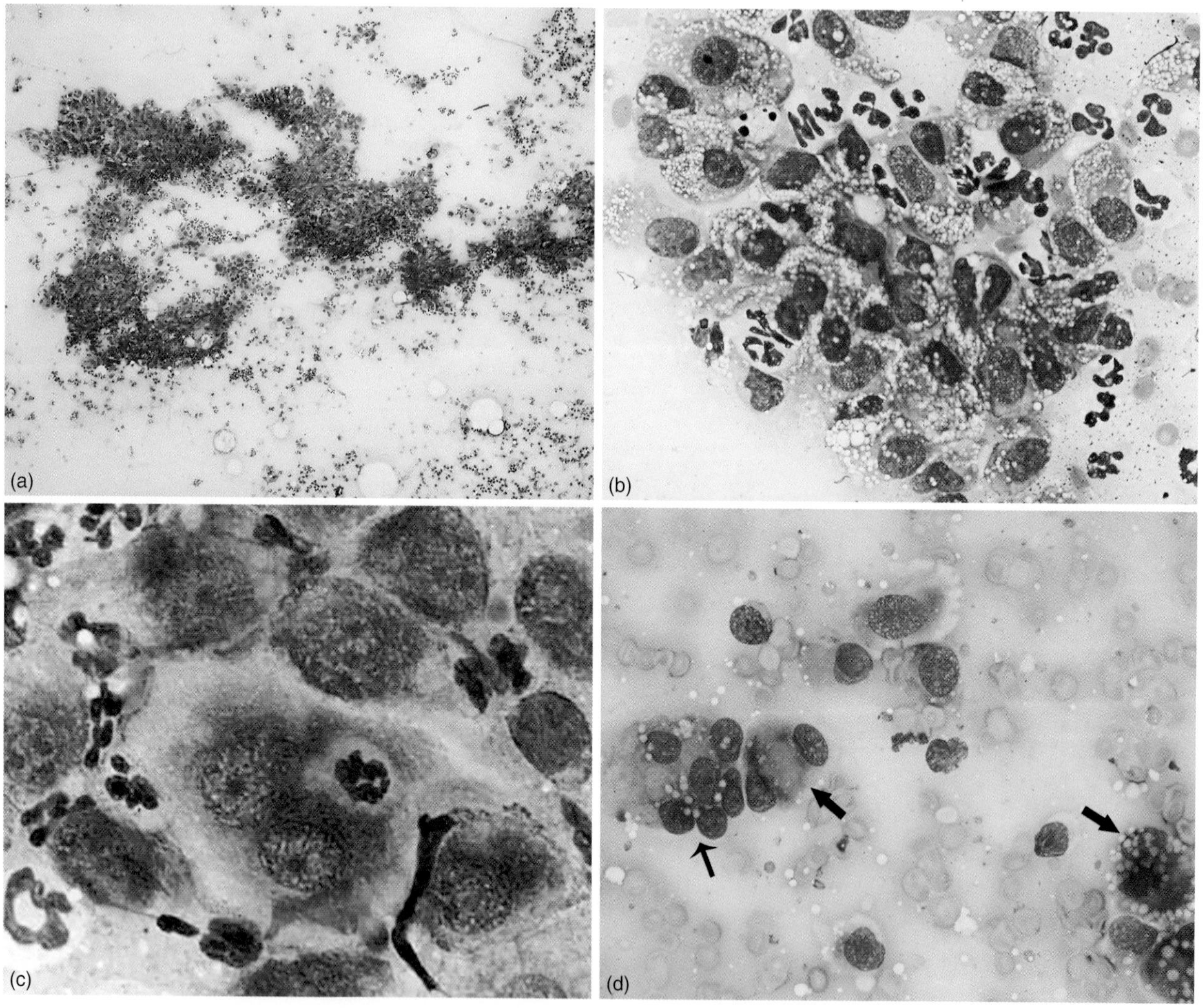

(a) (b) (c) (d)

Figure 40.17 Pyogranulomatous/granulomatous inflammation, four different magnifications. (a) 20x objective; (b) 50x objective; (c) 100x objective; (d) 40x objective. This type of inflammation is sometimes misdiagnosed as a neoplasm with inflammation. At low magnification (a), there appear to be groups of cohesive epithelial cells. Higher magnifications (b–d) reveal large cells, some containing vacuoles in the cytoplasm (b). The large cells are macrophages, which are called histiocytes when in tissues. When macrophages are this large, they are also called "epithelioid macrophages" (c) to indicate how they resemble epithelial cells. They can get very pleomorphic (b–d), with binucleated (d, thick arrows) and multinucleated (d, thin arrow) forms; therefore be careful not to confuse them with a neoplastic population. The numerous neutrophils scattered in background are key to the correct diagnosis of pyogranulomatous inflammation. Search for fungi, yeast forms, foreign material, and protozoa when this pattern is seen.

associations), if location is a site where SCC is expected favor SCC (white cat with mass on ear or eye; vagina, etc.) or probe for foreign material (splinters, fox awn). Lesions and cases are puzzles, and the key is to put all of the pieces together (integrate) and do not rely too heavily on one piece of data (i.e., large cells with cellular and nuclear abnormalities). A clinician has an advantage in these cases vs. a diagnostic pathologist; the former can try a week or more of antibiotics to determine if the lesion regresses or expands. A diagnostic pathologist has the advantage of special stains such as acid fast, gram, and fungal stains (GMS, PAS), therefore the best approach is for the clinician and pathologist to work together! There is no stain or molecular test that can determine if the large cells are neoplastic. The diagnostic pathologist can employ markers for histiocytes, but both neoplastic and non-neoplastic histiocytes will be positive. Similarly, markers for epithelial cells will label both neoplastic and non-neoplastic epithelial cells. There are no *neoplastic markers* that can be applied to cytological or histological specimens to identify the process as neoplastic. Polymerase chain reaction (PCR) for antigen receptor rearrangement (PARR) identifies clonality of lymphoid populations, not neoplasia. The presence of a monoclonal pattern favors neoplasia, but this can also be present with a few infectious diseases (ehrlichiosis, leishmania, feline infectious peritonitis, and others) as well as regressing histiocytoma and hepatitis [21]. Like all tests, there are false-positive and false-negative results with PARR, and insufficient prevalence data are known to be able to report positive and negative predictive values. PARR is only one test and results must be integrated with all of the other case data.

Certainly, if mitotic figures are seen the lesion must be neoplastic. NO, absolutely not. Mitotic figures can be seen in reactive fibroblasts in proliferating granulation tissue, they can be seen in young endothelial cells entering an area of inflammation (angiogenesis) and any cell that proliferates locally could leave the fingerprints of mitotic figures (hematopoiesis). However, just like clonality detected by PARR or nuclear abnormalities, the observation of numerous mitotic figures favors neoplasia. One mitotic figure does not equal neoplasia. Nothing new has been said in these sentences; mitotic figures are just one more piece of the puzzle, and the more confusing the case the more pieces that must be integrated. A single test result does not replace the ability to think.

Prognosis

If an owner and clinician want additional information to help predict biologic behavior, cytology is useful to help direct the next level of testing. The two most common "tests" are staging (especially assessment of regional lymph nodes and imaging of lungs) and histopathologic grading. Below are examples, based on a cytological diagnosis of a specific tumor, of what other test could be offered as well as a general guide to the biologic behavior of that tumor. Knowledge of tumor type, host species, size, and location of tumor are critical to predicting behavior. These patterns of behavior are based on studies published in journals and textbooks as well as the authors' experiences. More detailed information is published in multiple resources; however, it should be noted that grading schemes and other tests used to help predict behavior of a tumor or select treatments are based on a specific study population, and it is not known how well that information will extrapolate when used on different groups of dogs, owners, and treatments. Furthermore, these studies predict how a tumor, purportedly to be of the same type, might behave in a *population* of dogs. There are no tests (yet) that will predict how an *individual tumor* will behave in an *individual pet*. For all tumors, there is no single parameter or combination that is 100% predictive; this is biology and exceptions and inconsistencies exist.

Round cell tumors

- MCT – cytological and histological grading schemes [14, 15, 18]; tumors in cats generally benign, in dogs 80–90% of cutaneous tumors are benign, 100% of subcutaneous tumors are benign; cytologic assessment of mast cells in regional lymph nodes of dogs has been correlated with survival times; increased numbers of mast cells is associated with shorter survival, but this may be a self-fulling prophecy (euthanasia) and dogs with MCT in regional nodes have been treated and determined to have long survival times [22]. Very few MCTs in dogs and cats cause cachexia or metastasize widely. MCTs have a wide range of clinical and cytologic appearances (Figure 40.18).
- Lymphoma – see Chapter 15, determine B vs. T vs. null cell, determine size of cells via cytometry. The most important step may be to determine if the lymphoma is small T cell because these tumors are indolent with survival times of years regardless if treated or not; an estimate of this lineage can be provided by observing cytoplasmic extensions (mirror handle cells; cone heads), but more sophisticated tests are available. Large-cell lymphomas are malignant.
- Plasma cell tumor – MUM-1 immunoreactivity helps identify. Cytology or histopathology to assess uniformity vs. variability; if single cutaneous tumor, no further staging required. If multiple cutaneous tumors, or located in other organs (e.g., spleen), screening for osteolytic bone lesions (radiographs), serum and urine protein electrophoresis to identify paraproteins, and bone marrow assessment for presence of plasma cells can be considered.
- TVT – no further testing as cytology is diagnostic; no tests to predict the relatively few cases that become malignant; consider staging.

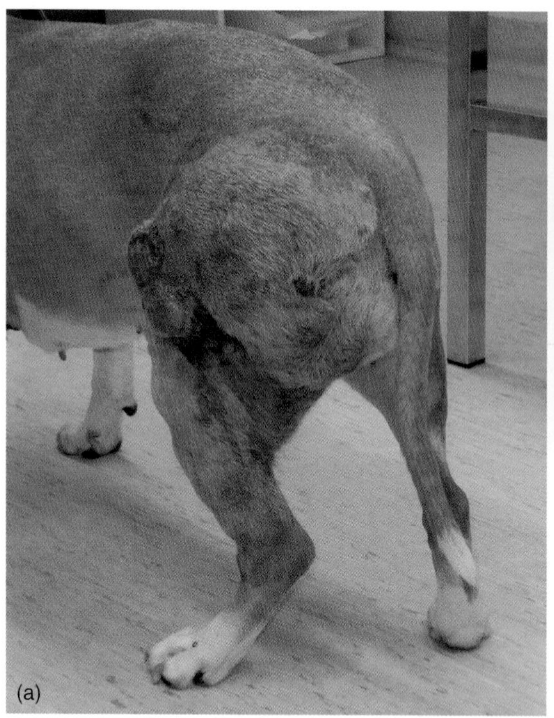

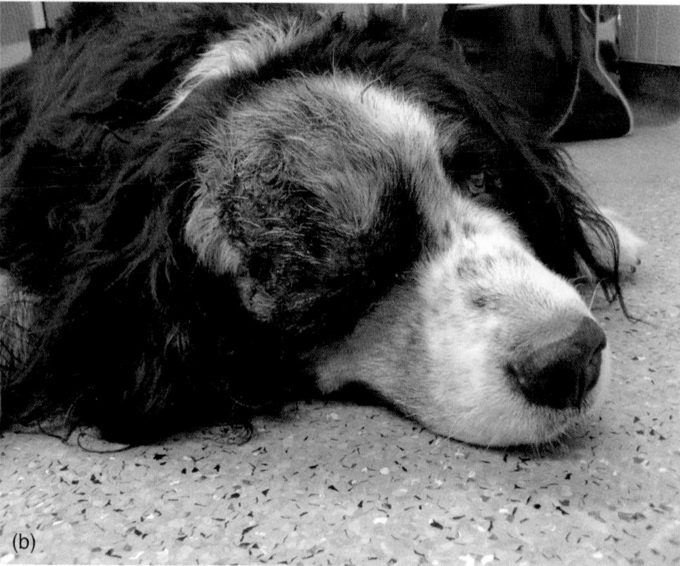

Figure 40.18 Correlate cytological findings with all of the other data. Neoplasia is the most likely differential in both of these dogs based on size of lesion and gross appearance. If cytological examination suggests inflammation, then repeat FNA until you are absolutely certain there are no neoplastic cells. If neoplastic cell are not found, then consider biopsy for histopathology and special stains if needed (histochemistry, immunohistochemistry). (a) Tumor on rear leg was MCT. (b) Sedated dog had a fibrosarcoma.

- Histiocytoma – the majority are benign, may regress spontaneously; important to differentiate from HSs and intraepithelial lymphomas.

Epithelial tumors

- Additional tests and prognosis depend on location.
- Bladder – UC (TCC) – malignant 100%; one of the most aggressive tumors in veterinary medicine; additional tests include BTA [23], FISH [3].
- Mammary – histologic grade for dogs and cats; do not rely on cytological criteria to determine behavior.
- Circumanal – benign, generally male dogs, difficult to identify the rare malignant subtypes even with histopathology.
- Anal sac – malignant but cytologic appearance in primary and metastatic locations is benign; they are epithelial tumors but look "neuroendocrine"; cause hypercalcemia.
- Thyroid – cats benign; dogs – size is linked to behavior, if tumor is large enough to be palpated it is likely to be malignant; tend to spread to lung rather than regional node.
- Prostate – malignant; benign forms not seen in dogs.
- Nose – malignant; nasal adenomas not seen in dogs or cats; polyps are benign.
- Note: Benign tumors do not exist in the prostate or nose of dogs or have not yet been confirmed, and benign epithelial tumors in the urinary bladder are rare. Therefore, when reviewing samples from these tissues, the key is to differentiate hyperplasia and dysplasia from neoplasia. Inflammation in these organs will stimulate hyperplasia and dysplasia. Knowledge about tumors in specific locations is a tremendous help in predicting what to expect cytologically and what the behavior of a tumor will be.

Mesenchymal tumors

- In the skin these tumors are often referred to as STS; however, soft-tissue mesenchymal tumor (STMT) is a preferred name because the vast majority are not aggressive. Histological grading schemes exist but none have been validated. PWT is the most common subset of STMTs; previously most were classified as hemangiopericytoma. Histologic recognition of PWT provides prognosis: <5% metastasize, clean margins predict no recurrence, greater likelihood of recurrence if tumor is large (>5 cm) and infiltrates muscle [7].
- HS complex – as a group aggressive; localized and disseminated subtypes.
- Osteosarcoma – no validated grading schemes, >90% malignant, infrequent reports of less aggressive variants.
- Melanocytic tumors (Figure 40.10) – although these tumors are mesenchymal, the cytological appearance can be a mixture of spindle cells, round cells, and

CHAPTER 40

epithelial-like aggregates. The amount of melanin pigment is variable. Oral tumors are usually malignant, but benign oral forms can be recognized with histopathology [24]; pedunculated oral or skin melanoma are benign; location in skin favors benign course. Mitotic counts in histological slides are predictive of behavior; other tests that can be requested are Ki67 immunoreactivity, nuclear atypia scores, etc. No test or combination of tests is 100% correct [18, 25].

Neuroendocrine tumors

- Prognosis varies with endocrine organ and tumor type; islet cells tumors appear cytologically benign (uniform) but invariably will metastasize. Aortic, carotid body, and C-cell tumors do not usually metastasize but can cause serious clinical problems; pheochromocytoma and adrenal cortical tumors are difficult to predict.

41 Cytology of Skin and Subcutaneous Masses

Donald Meuten[1], Kristina Meichner[2], and Mary Anna Thrall[3]

[1] North Carolina State University, Raleigh, NC, USA
[2] University of Georgia, Athens, GA, USA
[3] Department of Biomedical Sciences, Ross University School of Veterinary Medicine, Basseterre, Saint Kitts and Nevis

Introduction

Neoplasms (tumors) are classified into three main groups: epithelial, mesenchymal, and round cell (Figure 40.1). A fourth category, neuroendocrine, are common in endocrine organs but are rare in the skin (Merkel cell tumor). Chapter 40 details these types of tumors and how to diagnose neoplasia; Chapter 39 describes inflammatory lesions – those chapters complement the information in this chapter. The diagnosis of neoplasia (cancer) is made by integrating cytologic and/or histologic findings with clinical information (species, age) and appearance of the mass including location on the body. Cytological diagnoses attempt to name the specific tumor type, but many times this is not possible and often is not needed to plan treatment options.

Cytology uses cellular and nuclear features to identify cancer and histopathology uses histologic organization. Each discipline has its benefits, and they are discussed in Chapter 40. Various techniques are used to help diagnose the type of cancer, but the diagnosis of cancer is made by *integrating cytologic, histologic, and clinical features.*

This chapter emphasizes tumors in the skin and subcutaneous tissue. Other chapters or sections in this book describe how to diagnose cancer in different locations. Location of the suspected neoplasm is a critical piece of information, as the differential diagnoses for tumors and masses will change based on organ location.

Throughout this chapter the authors will generalize. Please accept this approach and understand this is biology; therefore, there will always be exceptions. When the exceptions are important, we will point these out; however, including every exception confuses the big picture.

Chapter 2 explains how to perform fine-needle aspiration (FNA), prepare good-quality slides, avoid artifacts, stain the slides, and adjust the microscope. Do not overlook the importance of each of these steps. An inadequate number of cells (QNS – quantity not sufficient), lysed cells, preparations that are too thick and smeared across the glass, excessive amounts of blood, artifacts, understained slides, and using a poorly maintained and adjusted microscope will prevent a diagnosis and frustrate the diagnostician. If poor-quality slides are sent to a referral lab a diagnosis is unlikely, and the same fee is charged as is for good-quality slides that yield a diagnosis. Diagnostic labs have pathologists with advanced training and expertise. However, many veterinarians perform procedures associated with a specialty because of their competence and sometimes because owners do not want to pay for a specialist. The information in this chapter is targeted for individuals not already certified in clinical pathology.

Numerous skin and subcutaneous diseases can result in mass formation, including inflammation, dysplasia, and neoplasia, as well as cyst, seroma, and hematoma formation. The distinction of hyperplasia and hypertrophy from neoplasia is important when examining FNA from organs and lymph nodes, but if a nodule or a mass is present in the skin, then hyperplasia and hypertrophy are unlikely. Of course, there are exceptions; collagenous hamartoma, fibroadnexal dysplasia, nodular fasciitis, and nodular dermatofibrosis are non-neoplastic lesions of skin or subcutis, and each may produce a mass, but they are not neoplasms. Fortunately, all of these are uncommon cytologic diagnoses.

Adnexal dysplasia occurs in dogs, is benign, and should be confirmed with histopathology. A common skin mass is a sebaceous adenoma, and sometimes these are determined to be hyperplastic by histopathology, but the distinction is unimportant because both lesions are benign. Cysts, seromas, and hematomas have fluid that is sometimes admixed with inflammation. If the mass is solid and cellular the critical distinction is *inflammation vs. neoplasia*. In most cases this will be straightforward, as inflammatory lesions are composed of numerous inflammatory cells, usually predominantly neutrophils, and neoplastic lesions are predominantly composed of either *round, epithelial, or spindle cells*, usually with no or minimal inflammatory cells (see Figure 40.1).

Veterinary Hematology, Clinical Chemistry, and Cytology, Third Edition. Edited by Mary Anna Thrall, Glade Weiser, Robin W. Allison and Terry W. Campbell.

Companion website: www.wiley.com/go/thrall/veterinary

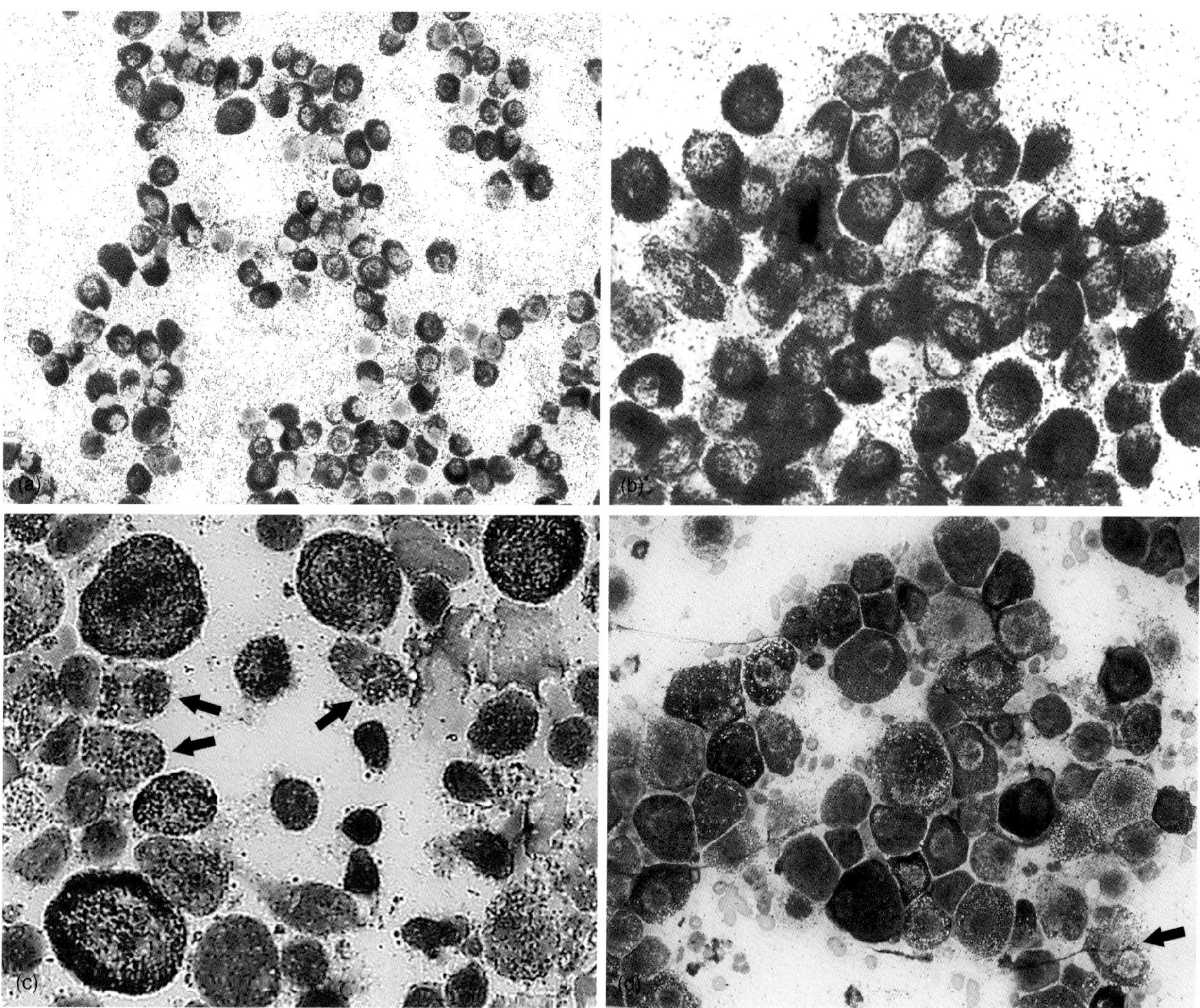

Figure 41.1 Canine cutaneous mast cell tumors. (a) 50× objective, (b–d) 100× objective. (a, b) Example of a low-grade (grade I) mast cell tumor. Mast cells are relatively uniform and packed with cytoplasmic granules that obscure cellular details. Numerous free mast cell granules are present in the background. (c) Note numerous eosinophils (arrows) in this mast cell tumor. (d) A high-grade (grade III) mast cell tumor. Neoplastic mast cells are variably granulated. Compare to (a) and (b), in which all of the mast cells are uniform and heavily granulated. Also note the presence of anisocytosis, anisokaryosis, binucleation (arrow), and nuclei with prominent nucleoli. Wright-Giemsa stain.

The classification of an inflammatory lesion and what etiology might produce that type of inflammatory cell response is located in Chapter 39. Hematomas, seromas, sialoceles, cysts, abscesses, mycotic granulomas, etc. can produce masses in the skin or subcutaneous tissues that have an inflammatory component, and examples are provided in different plates in this chapter and throughout this book (Figures 39.5, 39.6 and 40.16). A general rule is that skin lesions that are predominantly neutrophilic are inflammatory, and skin lesions that have no or only a few neutrophils are usually neoplastic. These patterns are recognized at low magnification (10–20× objectives) while you are assessing the cellular density and searching for regions to scrutinize. At higher magnifications you will examine the organization of cells and the shape of cells and their nuclei to decide if they are round (Figures 41.1–41.6), epithelial (Figures 40.1 and 40.8), or mesenchymal cells (Figures 40.1 and 40.9). Chapter 40 provides an overview of each general category of tumor. Identification of *intracellular pigment* commonly allows a specific diagnosis of tumor type. If intracellular pigment is seen, the diagnosis is usually easy to make. Purple granules are characteristic of *mast cells* (Figures 41.1 and 41.2) and black or green granules are features of *melanomas* (Figure 41.15).

The following descriptions for skin tumors are organized by clinical and cytologic characteristics. The cytologic observations are outlined by what you see at low through high magnifications. The descriptions are generalities, and of course there are a range of patterns for each tumor. All of these diagnoses can be made at 40–500× magnifications; higher magnification (1000×) using an oil immersion

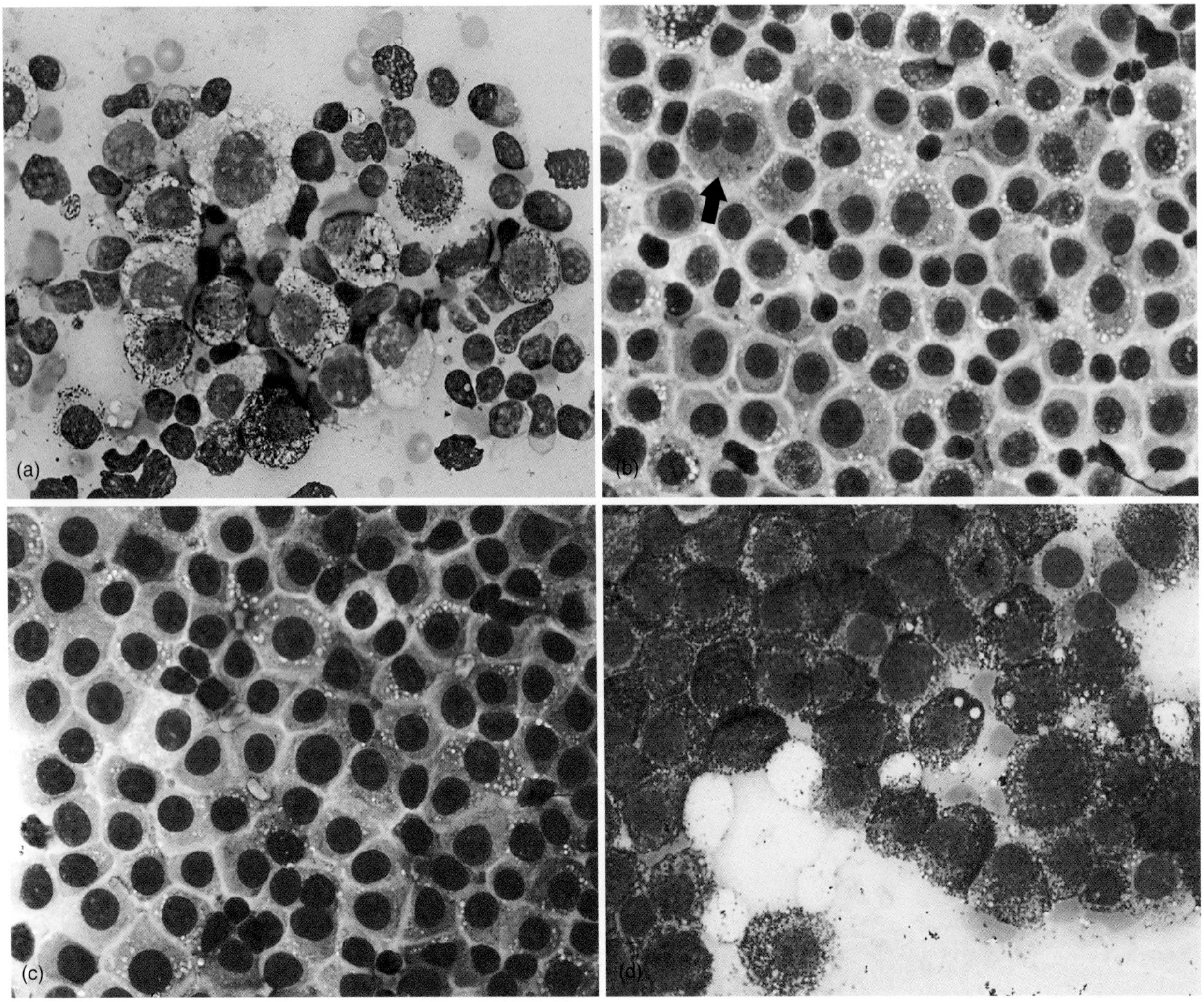

(a) (b) (c) (d)

Figure 41.2 Canine mast cell tumors. (a) Poorly granulated, neoplastic mast cells and a few mature lymphocytes and plasma cells in a lymph node from a metastatic cutaneous mast cell tumor. Note the presence of cytoplasmic vacuoles, which are usually obscured by mast cell granules in heavily granulated mast cells. (b) Very poorly granulated mast cells in this tumor. Also note the variability in cell size and the presence of a binucleated cell (arrow). Cytological grading schemes will estimate these features in a determined number of mast cells seen on the preparation. (c) Fine-needle aspirate cytology from a cutaneous mast cell tumor stained with an aqueous Romanowsky stain (Diff-Quik). Cytoplasmic mast cell granules do not stain adequately compared to (d). (d) Same aspirate as in (c), stained with a methanolic Romanowsky stain (Wright-Giemsa). Cytoplasmic mast cell granules are evident. It would be easy to miss the diagnosis of a mast cell tumor in (c) with only Diff-Quik stain. (a–d) 100× objective. (a, b, d) Wright-Giemsa, (c) aqueous Romanowsky stain.

objective is usually unnecessary for diagnosis of neoplasia, although high magnification is needed to identify bacteria and other infectious agents.

Round cell neoplasms

Lymphoma, histiocytoma, transmissible venereal tumor (TVT), and plasma cell and mast cell tumors (MCTs) are considered round cell tumors. Basal cell tumor is an epithelial cell tumor but cytologically they may appear as round cells, especially if the groups of basal cells are small or one does not appreciate their organization. Systemic histiocytosis and malignant histiocytosis (MH) (histiocytic sarcoma, HS) may also mimic a round cell tumor. Some aggressive-appearing plasma cell tumors and poorly granulated MCTs can be confused with malignant histiocytosis.

Mast cell tumor (MCT)

Clinical features

MCT is one of the most common tumors in dogs; they may be cutaneous or subcutaneous. They are not common in cats and most of the following discussion refers to MCT in dogs. Well-granulated MCTs are easy to diagnose, and

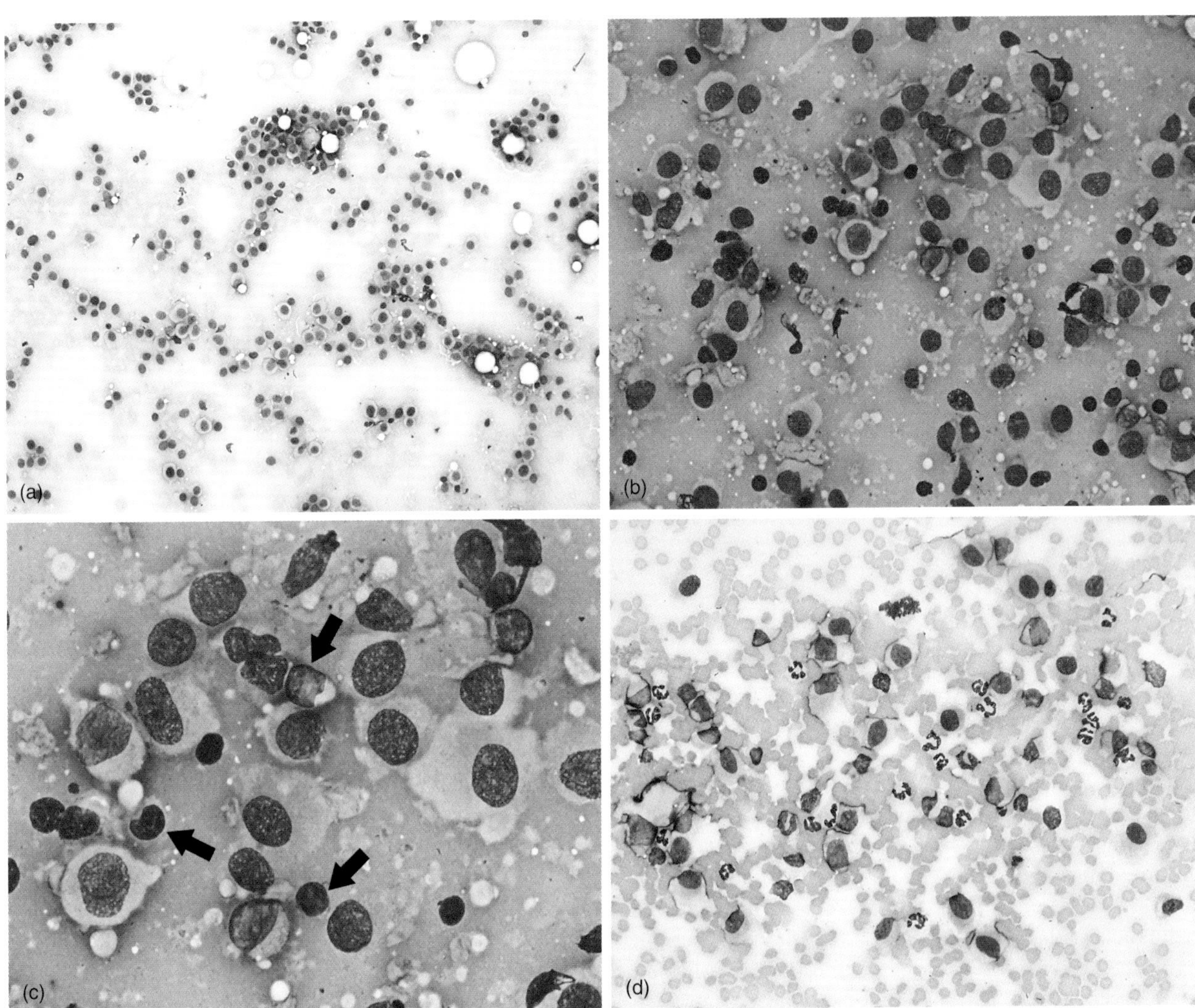

Figure 41.3 Cutaneous histiocytomas from dogs. (a) Note the moderate numbers of individual round cells on low power (20x objective). Histiocytomas exfoliate low numbers of cells. (b, c) Histiocytes have moderate amounts of gray-basophilic cytoplasm, which can have ruffled borders. Also note the blue proteinaceous background (b, 50x objective; c, 100x objective). (c) Small, mature lymphocytes (arrows) are a common finding in histiocytomas, especially during regression. (d) (50x objective) Another example of secondary inflammation of a canine histiocytoma, here indicated by the presence of neutrophils. Wright-Giemsa stain.

there is no need to consult with referral labs (diagnose these in clinic/hospital). MCTs produce one or more skin lesions that are often ulcerated and bulge outwards. They are overrepresented in boxers and Boston terriers. In dogs these tumors can be graded using histopathology; these grades are used to predict survival time (ST) and help make treatment selections. Grading using cytologic specimens is being evaluated.

Nodules identified as MCTs via cytology should be widely excised. Histopathology can be offered to owners for grading and to help ascertain a prognosis. Most MCTs are grade I or II, which carry a good prognosis. Using the two-tier system approximately 90% are low grade. Grades I and II predict the tumor will not recur, that it is not aggressive, and a good prognosis can be offered. However, approximately 5% of MCT do not behave as predicted by histopathology. If a grading scheme is not correlated with clinical outcomes it is useless. Completeness of surgical excision can be determined on histopathology. However, 90% of low-grade MCT do not recur even if the tumor extends to the surgical margin. Furthermore, a "histologic tumor free margin" that predicted nonrecurrence could not be determined for high-grade MCT in previous studies [1]. Grade of tumor is a more important predictor of recurrence than is evaluation of margins and is discussed in detail below.

MCTs usually exfoliate many cells and are one of the easiest tumors to diagnose via cytology, if the cytoplasmic granules stain. However, the staining intensity of the cells range from abundant deep purple granules that obscure nuclei (common), to lightly stained uniform granules

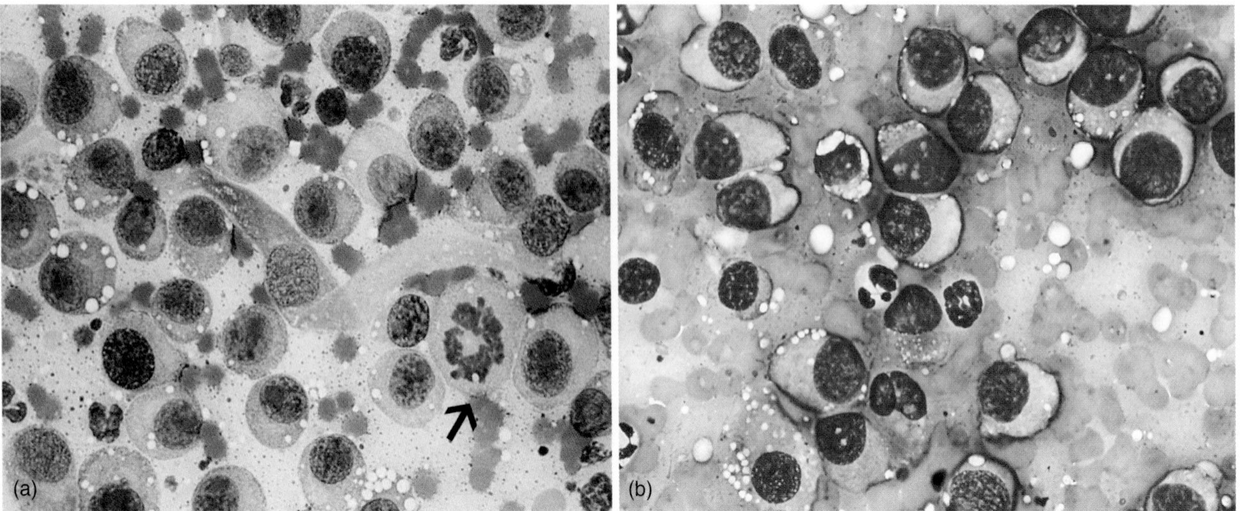

Figure 41.4 Transmissible venereal tumor (TVT). These tumors look very similar to histiocytoma (compare Figure 41.4b and Figure 41.3c). Location of the mass is critical to the correct diagnosis. However, TVT usually exfoliates numerous cells, cytoplasm tends to be more abundant with much deeper blue color, and clear, discrete cytoplasmic vacuoles are more prominent (a, b). A mitotic figure (arrow) is present in (a). (a) Source: Meuten DJ Tumors in Domestic Animals Ed 5, Wiley Blackwell 2017 p. 953–960; p. 957–959. (a and b, 100x objective). Wright-Giemsa stain.

(relatively common), to an absence of staining (uncommon to rare) (Figures 41.1 and 41.2). These latter cases can be problematic, but if you request a special stain for MCTs from a referral lab or if you recognize eosinophils scattered among the round cells that appear neoplastic, then you will be able to confirm your suspicion. Quick, dip-type stains are aqueous-based (e.g., Diff-Quik) and do not stain mast cell granules as well as alcohol-based stains such as Wright-Giemsa (Figure 41.2c, d). This is especially true for MCT in cats. Therefore, consider requesting or using an alcohol-based stain when you suspect a poorly granulated MCT. Lack of staining intensity is a cytologic and histologic criterion for higher-grade MCT.

Cytologic features

MCTs can often be correctly identified at 100–2000× (final magnification) by recognizing numerous, large, purple cells with barely discernible nuclei. A variant is numerous large cells with lightly violet to weakly stained cytoplasm and prominent round nuclei (Figures 41.1 and 41.2).

At medium (200×) to high (400–500×) magnification the tumor cells are numerous and large. Cytoplasmic granules range from poorly stained to deeply purple. Visualization of nuclei depends on the staining intensity of the granules. In densely stained cells nuclei may not be seen because they are obscured by the granules. Cells with lightly stained cytoplasmic granules have round nuclei with or without visible nucleoli. Tumors with well-stained purple granules usually have free purple granules in the background. Eosinophils are visible in the background of canine MCTs but are rare in feline MCTs. Eosinophils tend to be unilobed or bilobed rather than multilobed, cytoplasm is stained eosinophilic to red-brown to green-gray with variably sized granules in dogs and small uniform rod-shaped granules in cats. It is easy to overlook eosinophils in tissue preparations stained with aqueous Romanowsky stains such as Diff-Quik because the granules often do not stain brightly eosinophilic. Once eosinophils are recognized, the index of suspicion for MCT should markedly increase.

The following observations are for those MCTs that do not stain intensely. The cells are round or polygonal. A classic pattern is a round or oval-shaped cell with a centrally positioned round nucleus that gives a "fried egg" appearance (neuroendocrine tumors have a similar pattern). Few cells may be bi- or multinucleated. Nuclei are round to oval and contain prominent nucleoli and lightly vesiculated chromatin. Lymphocytic inflammation is infrequently seen in these neoplasms. More commonly, non-neoplastic spindle-shaped cells are seen admixed with the round mast cells. These are supporting stromal cells and are not neoplastic. Poorly differentiated MCTs may appear similar to histiocytic tumors or plasma cell tumors.

Tumor cells that stain intensely purple are not a diagnostic challenge. The staining intensity of the cytoplasmic granules varies with the type of stain used, the maturity of the cells and their granules and on the concentration of heparin in the cytoplasmic granules. It is heparin that accounts for the metachromasia (purple) characteristic of these cells. The quick-type stains *may not stain* the cytoplasmic granules of mast cells, especially in cats. Therefore, large round cells with abundant cytoplasm that completely encases the nucleus ("fried egg") with numerous eosinophils in the background is probably a MCT and should be confirmed by staining other slides with Wright-Giemsa, Giemsa, or toluidine blue stains.

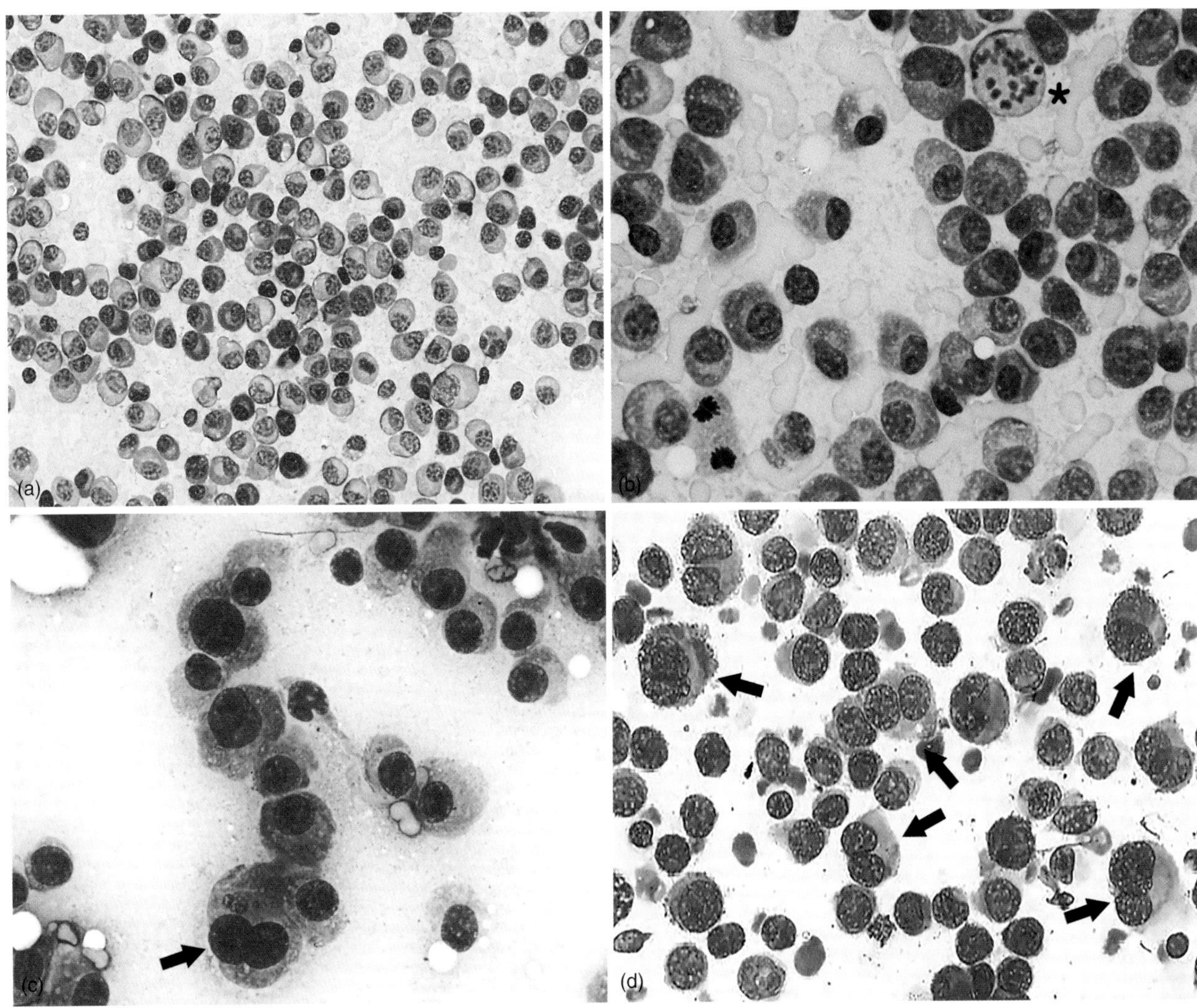

Figure 41.5 Plasma cell tumor. (a, b) A monomorphic population of round cells with very characteristic features of plasma cells: abundant deeply basophilic cytoplasm, a Golgi apparatus (pale paranuclear zone), eccentrically located nucleus with condensed and aggregated chromatin. An abnormal mitotic figure is also present (b, star). (c, d) Poorly differentiated, pleomorphic neoplastic plasma cells: these cells lack a Golgi zone, binucleation (thick arrows) is frequent, and nuclei in (c) contain prominent, bizarre nucleoli. Pleomorphic plasma cell tumors can be difficult to differentiate from histiocytic sarcoma or a high-grade poorly granulated mast cell tumor. Look at many fields and request immunocytochemical staining with MUM-1 (a, 50× objective; b–d, 100× objective). (d) Source: Meuten DJ Tumors in Domestic Animals Ed 5, Wiley Blackwell 2017 p. 953–960; p. 957–959. Wright-Giemsa stain.

Grading

Grading schemes are only established for canine cutaneous MCT. Subcutaneous and oral-perioral canine MCTs and feline MCTs do not have grading schemes, but there are gross and histological features used to predict outcomes for each [2]. Grading canine cutaneous MCT via histopathology is well established, and grading via cytology is being evaluated. Several studies used the two-tier histopathology system to develop a comparable grading scheme for cytology [3, 4]. Granularity of tumor cells, mitoses, and multinucleation were the three best cytologic features to determine grade. Nuclear pleomorphism, the fourth criterion in the histopathology scheme, was not reliable. Greater than 100 cells/tumor were evaluated, and slides must be stained with methanolic Romanowsky-type stains rather than an aqueous-based quick stain for grading. Cytoplasmic mast cell granules (and granules in large granular lymphocytes) do not stain adequately with water-based stains, even if fixed in methanol. A cytological diagnosis of low-grade MCT had a 98% likelihood of being low grade via histopathology; however, the correlation was not as good for high-grade MCT. Follow-up data that correlate cytologic grade with outcome assessment need to be done, as do validation studies of histopathology and cytology grading schemes. Grading via cytological criteria is subjective and should be done by experienced cytologists.

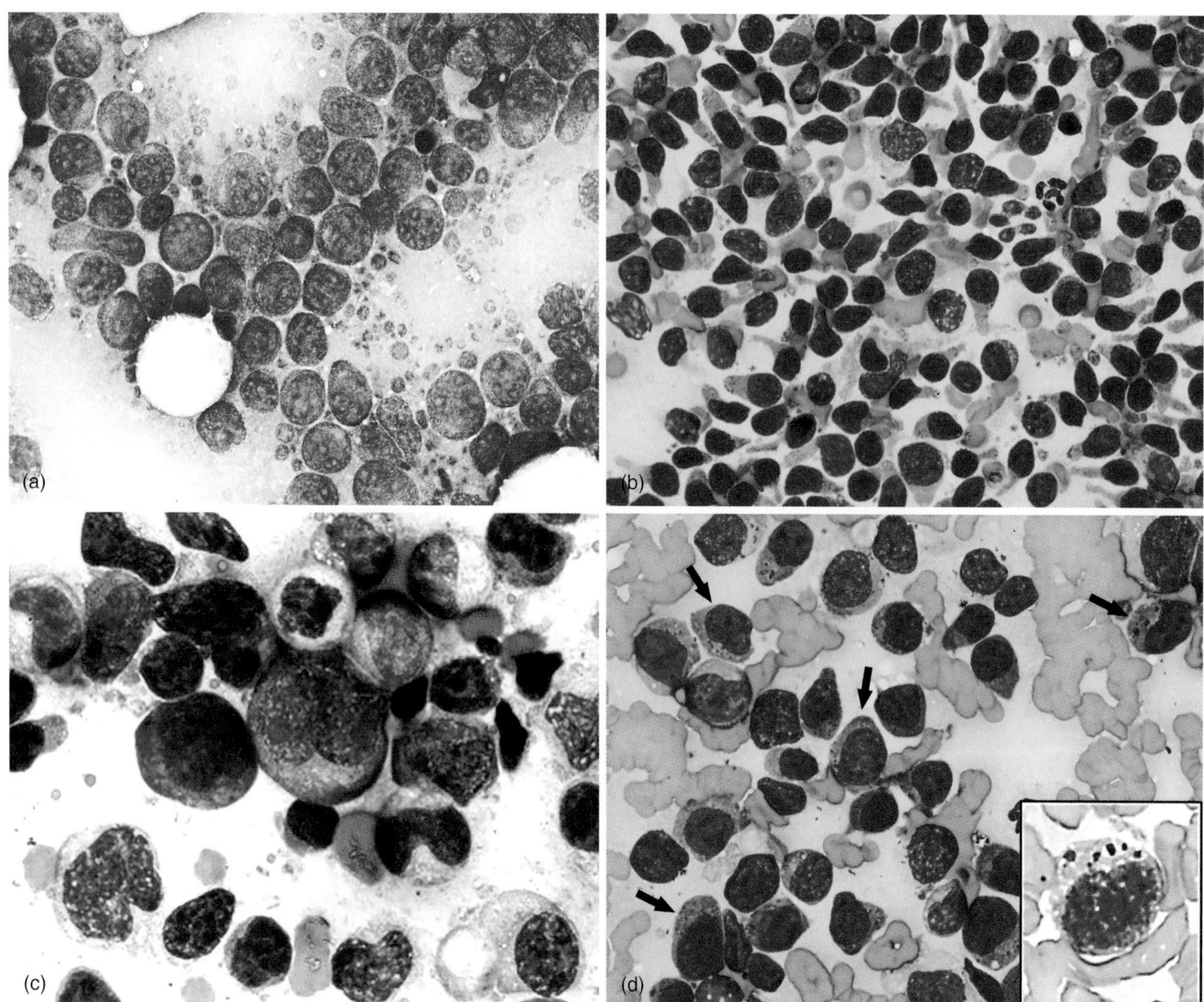

Figure 41.6 This collage is from different types of lymphomas. Most lymphomas are in lymph nodes or organs. (a) Lymph node aspirate from a dog. A monomorphic population of large lymphocytes with small amounts of cytoplasm and nuclei with stippled chromatin and prominent nucleoli indicate large-cell lymphoma; the most common cytologic type in dogs. The numerous fragments in the background with similar tinctorial properties to the cytoplasm of lymphocytes are lymphoglandular bodies. (b) T-zone lymphoma (TZL), aspirate from the submandibular lymph node, dog. The "hand mirror" appearance of the cytoplasm is readily apparent. The hand mirror feature is suggestive of TZL but not diagnostic and not present in all TZL. (c) Neoplastic lymphocytes from a dog with cutaneous epitheliotropic lymphoma. Nuclei of these tumors are often more pleomorphic with indentations, and a few horseshoe-shaped nuclei are present. (d) Large granular lymphocyte (LGL) lymphoma from a cat. Note the large lymphocytes with few cytoplasmic magenta granules (arrows and insert). This sample was from a liver aspirate. LGL lymphoma in cats is an aggressive tumor that arises from the small intestine. In advanced disease, many other organs can be affected. However, skin involvement is usually not seen. (a–c) Source: Meuten DJ Tumors in Domestic Animals Ed 5, Wiley Blackwell 2017 p. 953–960; p. 957–959. (a–d) 100x objective. Wright-Giemsa stain.

Approximately 85–90% of canine cutaneous MCT are low grade via histopathology and approximately 95% are benign: they will have STs greater than 4 years, and more than 95% are cured by complete surgical removal alone [5]. Between 75% and 90% of low-grade MCTs do not recur even if margins are incomplete or narrow (<1 mm) and 95% do not recur if margins are free of tumor cells. Dogs with higher-grade MCTs have STs of 6–12 months; however, the decisions to euthanize influence survival data, and the total number of dogs evaluated is small. Around one-third of high-grade MCTs will recur even if the histologic margins are free of tumor cells [1]. The histologic tumor-free margin distance that will prevent local recurrence of high-grade MCTs is not known and the majority of indolent MCTs will not recur even if tumor cells are at the margin [6]. It appears the biology of the MCT and/or host are more important predictors of recurrence than is margin evaluation. There is no grading scheme that provides 100% correlation with outcomes. Some MCTs that are predicted to behave in a benign or malignant manner will not behave as predicted and identifying these subsets of MCT is problematic [2]. Fortunately, this is a small percentage (estimate <5%) of canine cutaneous MCTs.

Lymph node evaluation for potential metastatic MCT

Cytology is used more frequently than histopathology to evaluate regional lymph nodes in dogs with MCT. However, no markers or cellular features distinguish neoplastic from non-neoplastic mast cells. Mast cells can be found throughout the body, including lymph nodes, bone marrow, buffy coats, and organs such as liver, spleen, and reproductive tract of normal dogs that do not have MCT. Therefore, the diagnosis of regional metastasis is based on numbers of mast cells seen and if the mast cells are aggregated. The subjective nature of this assessment means considerable experience is needed. Greater risk of lymph node metastasis is seen in high-grade MCT, tumors larger than 3 cm diameter, ulcerated tumors, tumors located on the digit, Shar-Pei dogs, and dogs with substage b disease (dogs are clinically ill) [2, 4, 7].

Diagnosis of MCT in regional lymph nodes can alter prognosis, treatments and staging [4, 7, 8]. If a patient with MCT has metastasis to a regional lymph node (regardless of grade), then further staging, including additional lymph node evaluation and abdominal ultrasound, is often recommended. The likelihood of additional lymph node or visceral metastasis in a patient with regional lymph node MCT metastasis ranges from 10% to 20%. In a series of 220 dogs with MCT who underwent complete staging, none of the dogs with nonmetastatic regional lymph nodes had clinically detectable metastasis in other areas [9]. All dogs with distant metastasis had metastasis in the regional lymph node; pulmonary metastases were not seen and are not expected in dogs with MCT. Approximately 30% had lymph node metastasis and 7% of dogs had distant metastases. MCTs rarely cause malignant cachexia. Euthanasia attributed to MCT is more likely due to recurrence, nursing care decisions, concurrent diseases and owners' elective choices than tumor metastases that erode health.

A study reported ST of approximately 8 months in dogs with cytologically confirmed lymph node metastasis (stage 2 disease) as compared to 6 years for dogs with normal or reactive lymph nodes [8]. However, once owners are informed that the prognosis is not as good due to regional node involvement, this information may influence decisions to treat, which in turn affects survival data (self-fulfilling prophecy). Additional studies examining treatment outcome in dogs with stage 2 MCT have reported prolonged ST. Long ST (years) and disease-free intervals can be seen in dogs with low-grade cutaneous or subcutaneous MCTs that have metastasized to a regional lymph node [2]. Multiple treatments can be offered.

Histiocytoma

Clinical features

The cell of origin is a dendritic cell in the epidermis, not a histiocyte or monocyte. These tumors are usually easy to diagnose because of the signalment (usually young), location of tumor (commonly on the ear, head, or neck), and appearance of tumor (one or more round, raised ulcerated hairless masses). However, they can occur in middle aged and geriatric dogs and can be located on parts of the body other than head and neck. The button-shaped mass is often "pink-tan colored," hairless and protrudes through the skin, may be ulcerated, and some tumors regress spontaneously.

Cytologic features

Histiocytoma cells do not exfoliate well, and therefore preparations are usually of low cellularity. Cells are round, individualized and have small amounts of lightly basophilic to blue-gray cytoplasm that may contain a few vacuoles (Figure 41.3). Cell borders are often distinct because of the basophilic proteinaceous material in the background of the slide (Figure 41.3). Tumor cells have round to oval nuclei that may be eccentric and have minimal anisocytosis (size variability). Nuclear chromatin condensation is variable, sometimes becoming ropey. There may be mature small lymphocytes or other inflammatory cells in low numbers admixed amongst the larger neoplastic cells. The lymphocytes are usually present in large numbers when the tumor is in the regression stage due to cellular immunity.

Differential cytologic diagnoses are lymphoma, TVT and plasmacytoma. Histiocytomas have more cytoplasm than lymphoid cells, the cytoplasm is less blue than lymphoma and inflammation is associated with histiocytoma. They can be difficult to differentiate from TVT without a history, although usually TVT cells have more abundant, more basophilic cytoplasm that contains many small discrete clear vacuoles, as well as more malignant nuclear features. TVTs typically exfoliate more cells than do histiocytomas. Although TVTs can be in many different locations on the body, if the tumor is found on the genitals and it is a round cell then TVT is the most likely diagnosis by far.

Transmissible venereal tumor (TVT)

Clinical features

TVTs, a tumor only seen in canids, are more common in areas where dogs run free and are not neutered, such as the Caribbean islands and in a few areas of the southern and midwest United States. The tumor cells contain 59 chromosomes, unlike the normal canine karyotype of 78 chromosomes [10]. The tumor cell has been shown to have been present in canids for at least 6000 years, during which time it has mutated approximately 38,000 times resulting in the marked difference in karyotype [10].

TVTs are usually located on the genitals of male or female dogs and less frequently on the skin, mucous membranes of the nose, mouth, and eyes, and more rarely in other areas such as lymph nodes, abdominal cavity, and brain, due to expansion into those tissues or metastasis [11]. It is transplantable from dog to dog, and does so readily via social or sexual activity.

When on the vaginal wall or penis, the tumor begins as a nodule beneath the mucosa; they then break through the overlying mucosa where they appear as an ulcerated friable mass.

These tumors can appear cytologically similar to histiocytomas. They exfoliate easily and therefore numerous cells will be in the preparations. Location of the mass is usually helpful in making the correct diagnosis. In comparing TVT's to histiocytomas, the following features of TVTs can be used to differentiate the tumors: location, presence of many cells, abundant cytoplasm, a slightly more blue color than that of histiocytomas, and clear distinct discrete cytoplasmic vacuoles, which are much more common in TVTs (Figure 41.4). Nuclei of TVT cells tend to be larger, distinct and lightly basophilic as compared to histiocytomas. Nucleoli are usually readily visualized. In aspirates of histiocytomas the inflammatory cell component is mild, if present at all, although regressing tumors may contain numerous lymphocytes. Conversely, imprints of TVTs usually contain many inflammatory cells, predominantly neutrophils. TVTs are one of the few tumors for which imprints or swabs of the tumor surface are diagnostic.

The three primary differentials with which TVT can be confused are histiocytoma, plasmacytoma, and lymphoma. If the preparations appear similar to that of lymphoma but are from the vagina or penis, then the diagnosis is much more likely to be TVT. Lysozyme is a nonspecific cellular marker that positively stains most cases of TVT and approximately 60% of histiocytomas. When they are extra-genital or cytologically difficult, TVTs can be definitively diagnosed using polymerase chain reaction (PCR) to detect a unique long nuclear element upstream of the myc gene [12]. TVTs rarely spontaneously regress, but regression almost always occurs after therapy with vincristine.

Plasma cell tumor

Clinical features

Cutaneous plasma cell tumors are common in middle-aged dogs and are rare in cats. They can occur any place on the dog's skin/subcutaneous tissues and mucous membranes (oral, rectal). Plasma cell tumors appear as discrete nodules that are hairless and are often ulcerated. The majority are benign, and are not associated with bone marrow involvement and paraneoplastic syndromes (monoclonal gammopathy, hypercalcemia, amyloidosis) commonly associated with multiple myeloma, a separate and malignant entity (see Chapter 16).

Cytologic features

Diagnosis can usually be made from low magnification based on the presence of round cells with abundant deeply basophilic cytoplasm and a Golgi apparatus, which is a pale paranuclear zone visible in some cells (Figure 41.5). The nucleus is usually eccentrically located. The nuclear chromatin is condensed and aggregated. The classic "clock-face" or "spoke-wheel" pattern in the nuclear chromatin is only present in a minor population of the tumor cells and is much more visible on histopathology than on cytology. Some tumors contain neoplastic cells that have one or more intracytoplasmic globules that can be clear, pale blue or eosinophilic. These cells are called Mott cells; the cytoplasmic vacuoles are Russell bodies and they represent packets of immunoglobulin. If seen, they help confirm the diagnosis as plasma cell tumor, although Mott cells may be seen in non-neoplastic accumulations of plasma cells. A proteinaceous magenta or blue background color may be present due to the large amount of immunoglobulin that may be secreted by the tumor cells.

Some tumors produce a monomorphic population of round cells with very characteristic features of well-differentiated plasma cells that allow for a quick cytologic diagnosis (Figure 41.5a, b). Other tumors can be heterogenous and are predominated by more atypical cells with binucleation, multinucleation, lobated, bizarrely shaped nuclei; only on searching throughout the preparation can the more recognizable plasma cells be found (Figure 41.5c, d) that provide the clue to a correct diagnosis. Tumors with pleomorphic cellular and nuclear features as just described need to be differentiated from malignant histiocytosis.

Pleomorphic plasma cell tumors can be confused with histiocytic sarcoma, malignant histiocytosis (MH), histiocytoma, poorly stained MCT and osteosarcoma. Plasma cell tumors can usually be distinguished from these differential diagnoses by searching for well-differentiated plasma cells amongst all of the tumor cells. Examining the multinucleated or bizarre nuclei is interesting but does not help identify the cell of origin. Plasma cell tumors tend to be singular; malignant histiocytosis tends to have multiple tumors, may involve internal organs and/or joints, and has breed predispositions. The MH cells have more pleomorphic features than do plasma cells, are usually larger, and erythrophagocytosis is a characteristic, but sometimes difficult to find, cytologic feature.

Lymphoma

Clinical features

Although lymphoma is a common tumor in dogs and cats, it is uncommon in skin and therefore is the least common round cell tumor in skin or subcutaneous tissues. Lymphoma very rarely occurs as a solitary skin mass. If lymphoma is present in the skin it appears as multiple skin and subcutaneous lumps, or flat plaques located anywhere on the body; some have a mucocutaneous distribution (T-cell lymphoma). Regional or peripheral lymph nodes are often involved at presentation. Dogs are usually middle aged to older and have weight loss. Cats often have weight loss, anemia, and are commonly feline leukemia virus (FeLV) positive with enlarged abdominal lymph nodes. It is rare for lymphoma to be confined to one system in the body; it is usually in multiple locations and lymph nodes (see Chapter 45).

Cytologic features

Lymphoid tissue exfoliates very well; aspirates of neoplastic lymphoid tissue are usually very cellular and may be too thick in some areas of the slide. The cells are round and discrete, often appearing close to each other due to the marked cellularity. The cells have uniform nuclei and typically a minimal amount of basophilic cytoplasm (Figure 41.6). The amount of cytoplasm will vary from a thin rim to a bulge, almost always off to one side. Distinct cytoplasmic protrusions, like mirror handles or cone heads are seen with a fairly indolent type of T-cell lymphoma (Figure 41.6b) [2]. The nucleus: cytoplasm ratio is high, usually 1 : 1, and rarely 1 : 2. The most characteristic cytologic feature of lymphoma is the uniformity and high nucleus: cytoplasm ratio. Many cytoplasmic fragments, commonly referred to as "lymphoglandular bodies," are usually present (Figure 41.6a). These cytoplasmic fragments may be confused with platelets. Nuclei usually have fine chromatin and nucleoli are often prominent. Intermediate (prolymphocytic) variants have nuclear chromatin that is clumped or marginated along the outer nuclear membrane. Cytoplasm is usually scant and moderately to deeply basophilic. For those lymphomas that differentiate toward the plasma cell line there is more cytoplasm, the cytoplasm is more basophilic and sometimes a pale perinuclear zone (Golgi apparatus) can be seen. Small-cell variants of lymphoma consist of well-differentiated normal-appearing lymphocytes and are very rarely, if ever, seen in the skin or subcutis. If large numbers of small lymphocytes are seen in a mass, it is likely normal lymphoid tissue or lymphocytic inflammation. The diagnosis of small-cell lymphoma should be confirmed by a pathologist. Most cases of cutaneous lymphoma consist of large cells with stippled chromatin and prominent nucleoli (features of immature cells) and are relatively easy to diagnose. All of the other round cell tumors will have more cytoplasm and nuclei will have more condensed chromatin than seen in lymphoma.

Cutaneous lymphoma can be further classified to subtype using immunophenotyping, flow cytometry, or PCR (see Chapter 15). There are numerous subtypes of lymphomas but one of the most important determinations for prognosis and treatment plans is to identify T vs. B immunophenotype. T-cell lymphoma is the most common immunophenotype for cutaneous lymphoma. Histopathology showing tissue architecture is required for the recognition of intraepithelial lymphomas (mycosis fungoides).

Epithelial cell tumors

Basal cell neoplasm (basilar epithelial neoplasm)

Clinical features

Basal cell neoplasm is one of the most common skin tumors of dogs and cats, and they are usually benign in behavior. They produce one or more bulging skin nodules, often located on the head and neck, and they are usually ulcerated.

Cytologic features

Although they are epithelial, they often exfoliate as round cells, individually or in groups, and can be confused with round cell tumors. Preparations are usually of low to moderate cellularity and consist of small individual cells as well as cells in clumps, aggregates, and ribbons (Figure 41.7a, b). Recognizing these patterns of cell organization is the key to the correct diagnosis of epithelial tumor. Inflammation is not present unless the tumor is ulcerated or is producing keratin, which can induce a neutrophilic or pyogranulomatous inflammatory response. Tumor cells are polygonal, oval or round with round to oval uniform nuclei; however, around the edges of the clumps some cells may be spindeloid. The amount of cytoplasm in basal cells is minimal to moderate and light blue to gray.

A pure basal cell neoplasm consists of just the polygonal/round cells that represent the basal epidermal cells. However, these tumors may differentiate toward secretory sebaceous cells and can have large areas that are pigmented. If cells are differentiating into sebaceous cells the cytoplasm can be abundant and vacuolated. Moderate numbers of vacuolated lipid-filled sebaceous cells and scattered melanin-laden cells may be present. Multicellular sheets composed of homogenous basal cells or a mixture of basal cells, sebaceous cells and melanin-filled basal epithelial cells may be present.

It is important to not confuse pigmented basal epithelial cells with melanocytes, as one could mistakenly make a diagnosis of melanoma.

Histopathology is usually necessary to definitively diagnose differentiated basal cell tumors, such as pigmented basal cell tumors, as well as determine malignant potential. The vast majority are benign. There are other groups of tumors that have a similar lineage such as trichoepithelioma, keratoacanthoma and calcifying epithelioma. These are recognized on histopathology based on how the cells are organized, what structures and products they produce. They cannot be classified as such on cytologic examination. They are all epithelial cell neoplasms that have a similar origin but different differentiation.

Sebaceous cell adenoma

Clinical features

Sebaceous cell adenoma is one of the most common skin tumors in dogs and is seen frequently in cats, as well. They

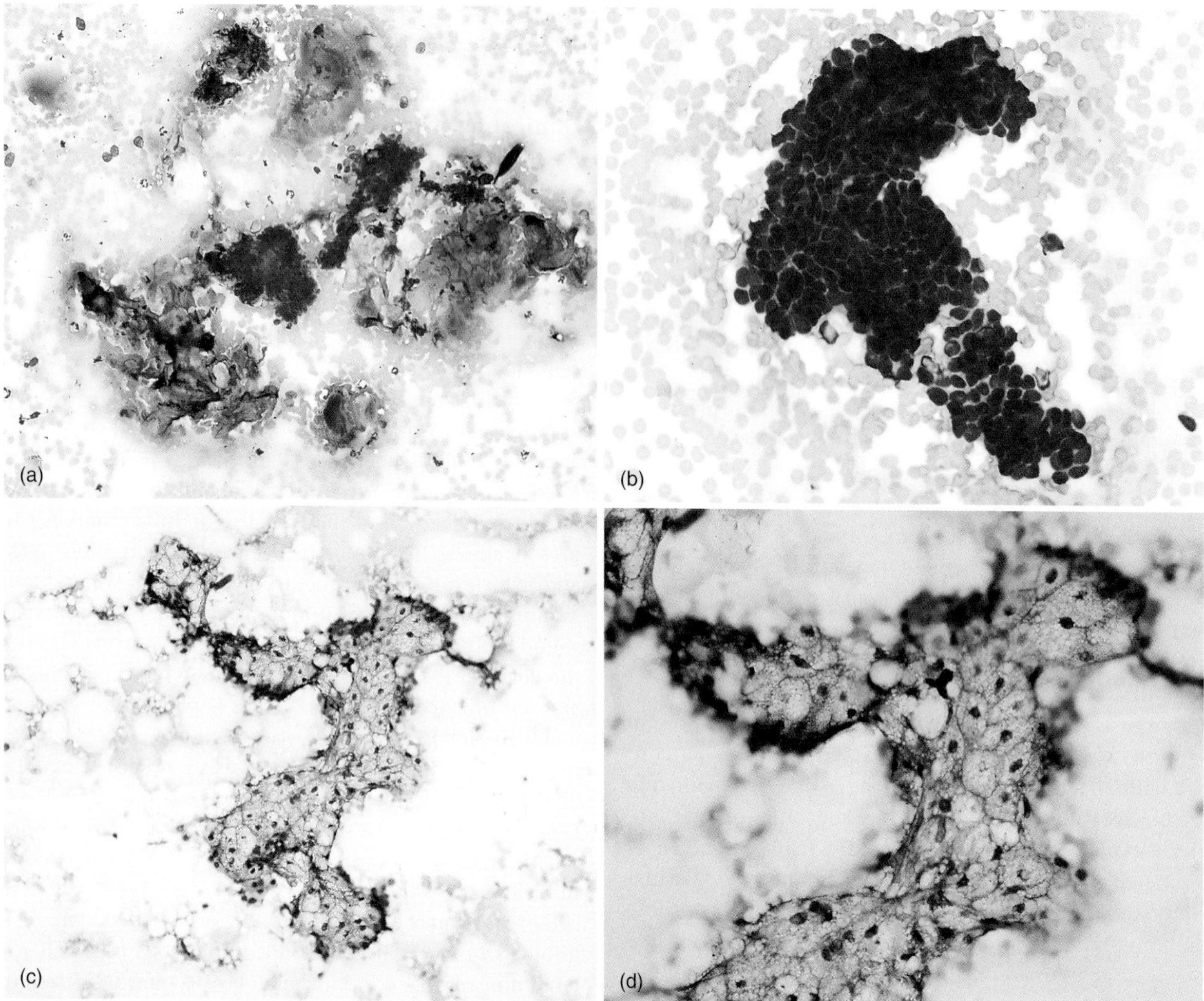

Figure 41.7 Cutaneous basilar cell tumor (a, b). Ribbons and clusters of uniform, cohesive epithelial cells with scant amount of cytoplasm, central round nuclei, and indistinct nucleoli. Some of these tumors can produce keratin (a). In addition to true basal cell tumors, trichoblastoma, trichoepithelioma, keratoacanthoma, and calcifying epithelioma can have the same basilar epithelial cell appearance on cytology, and their distinction would require histopathology. However, the vast majority of these tumors are benign. Sebaceous cell adenoma (c, d). Cohesive epithelial cells with marked amounts of vacuolated, foamy cytoplasm and a central round nucleus. Pleomorphism is absent. Sebaceous cell hyperplasia will look identical to an adenoma. However, their distinction is not clinically relevant. Basal cell and sebaceous cell tumors are easy to identify at medium magnifications due to cell-to-cell adhesions that form distinct clusters or aggregates. (a, c) 20× objective, (b) 50× objective, (d) 40× objective. Wright-Giemsa stain.

are overrepresented in cocker spaniels and poodles. These neoplasms are often on the head, neck, and especially the eyelids. Sebaceous adenomas may have a "wart-like" appearance on gross examination.

Cytologic features

Microscopically these tumors, and their hyperplastic counterparts, consist of numerous cells with a large amount of cytoplasm that is markedly vacuolated or foamy (Figure 41.7c, d). The cytoplasmic vacuoles vary in size; they are smaller than erythrocytes. Cells are usually in aggregates or groups that identify their epithelial heritage. Nuclei are usually positioned in the center or slightly eccentrically. They are benign in their appearance cytologically and benign in their biologic behavior. Sometimes they have numerous round cells scattered through them, which may be basal cells that are proliferating along with the sebaceous cells. Differentiation of sebaceous adenoma from sebaceous gland hyperplasia is clinically inconsequential.

Sebaceous cell carcinoma

Sebaceous cell carcinomas are uncommon. They resemble sebaceous adenomas but carcinomas have cellular and nuclear pleomorphism. The more differentiated tumors resemble sebaceous adenomas and the more undifferentiated have marked variability in nuclear and cellular morphology. These tumors often shed cells individually and in clusters, adhered by desmosomes and hemidesmosomes. Some cells or groups of cells will have relatively little cytoplasm and the cytoplasm is basophilic due to the presence of increased RNA. Other cells will be much larger, the cytoplasm lighter, faintly blue or lightly eosinophilic and they will contain cytoplasmic vacuoles (lipid). Nuclei are often two to five times the size of neutrophils.

Liposarcoma is the primary differential diagnosis. Liposarcoma yields individual fat-laden cells (vacuolated) and sebaceous carcinoma produces fat-laden cells in clusters, aggregates or morulae. Liposarcoma is a rare tumor in animals; lipomas are common in dogs (see "Mesenchymal/Spindle Cell Tumors").

Squamous cell carcinoma (SCC)

Clinical features

Squamous cell carcinoma is a common tumor of the skin and epithelial tissue of older domestic animals and they occur in various locations including the nose, nasal cavity, ears (especially in white cats), gingivae of dogs and cats, tonsils of dogs, tongue of cats, stomach, vagina, prepuce, penis, and lungs.

Cytologic features

Touch imprints or FNA contain large cells, greater than 60 μm in diameter, with abundant basophilic to gray cytoplasm and central to eccentric round nuclei (Figure 41.8). Very few other neoplastic cells are as large as neoplastic squamous epithelial cells. SCCs are often so well differentiated that the diagnosis is relatively easy. Usually there are numerous neutrophils present because the tumors have an ulcerated

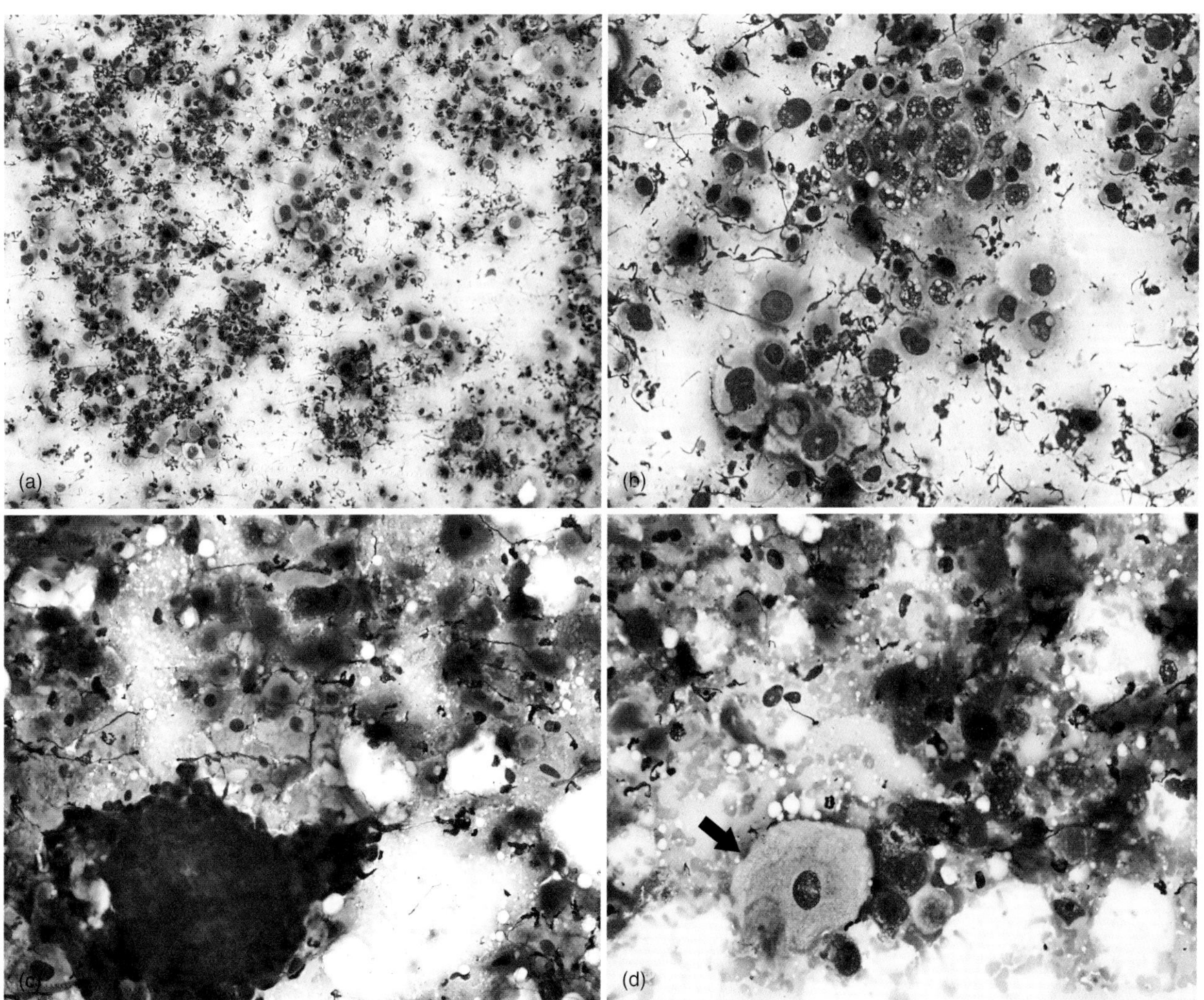

Figure 41.8 Squamous cell carcinoma from a cat (a, b) and a dog (c, d). Individualized cells and cells in large aggregates. Note the marked variation in cell size and shape. There are some very large squamous epithelial cells with angular cell borders and glassy, basophilic (keratinized) cytoplasm (d, arrow). Secondary inflammation is very common in these tumors, due to epidermal ulceration (a, b). (a) 20× objective, (c) 40× objective, (b, d) 50× objective. Wright-Giemsa stain.

surface, or because they produce keratin that induces an inflammatory response.

Some cells are individualized, and others are in cellular aggregates of 10–50 or more cells. Cell sizes and shapes are variable. Some cells are deeply basophilic, others lightly basophilic or gray and others pink due to keratinization. Nuclei and nucleoli are equally as pleomorphic. Nuclei are 2–10 times the size of neutrophils. Nucleoli will be variable in number and are prominent. Features that help make a diagnosis of SCC include characteristic location, gross appearance and marked variability in cellular clusters, cell size, nuclear size and nucleolar size.

Preparations made from non-neoplastic preputial exudates will contain numerous large well-differentiated squamous epithelial cells surrounded by many neutrophils. The cells will not be in clumps, and they will be uniform in morphology, a characteristic pattern of balanoposthitis and not SCC.

Perianal/circumanal gland tumors

Clinical features

Perianal gland tumors are very common tumors in the perineum of intact male dogs but can occur in castrated males and intact or spayed females. In male dogs they are hormonally (testosterone) responsive and regress, or at least decrease in size, after castration. If they occur in cats they are extremely rare. Circumanal glands are modified sebaceous glands. Adenomas and hyperplasia look similar cytologically and both are benign. These tumors rarely become malignant and there are no reliable criteria to recognize their malignant counterparts using cytology or histopathology of the primary lesion. The only way to be completely certain a malignant form is present is to find recognizable circumanal cells in a regional lymph node.

Cytologic features

Characteristic organization and cytologic features of individual tumor cells make this tumor easy to recognize at low and medium magnifications (Figure 41.9). Cells are individualized or in cohesive clusters of 8 to 50 or more cells. Large cells have abundant light blue, to blue-gray to lightly eosinophilic cytoplasm with a low N : C ratio of 1 : 3 to 1 : 5. The cells resemble hepatocytes and the nuclei are often central and completely encircled by cytoplasm. This cytologic feature has led to the nickname "hepatoid tumor" or "hepatoid cells." There is no associated inflammation. Higher magnification is not needed to confirm diagnosis.

No cytologic criterion predicts malignancy. However, if cells are smaller than usual, the N : C ratio is higher than usual (1 : 2) and there is variability in cellular and nuclear features, then the tumor may be malignant. Malignant circumanal tumors are rare. Female dogs are more likely to have a neoplasm arising from the apocrine gland adenocarcinoma (see next section).

Apocrine gland adenocarcinoma (AGAC) of anal sacs

Clinical features

Apocrine gland adenocarcinoma of anal sacs is the most common malignant tumor in the perineum of female and male dogs. It is more common in female dogs. Approximately half of the tumors bulge caudally and are readily visible. The other half are occult, lie beneath haired skin but are readily found on palpation of the perineum. The easiest way to diagnose this tumor is via rectal palpation and then FNA of the mass. Approximately 50–80% of these patients will have hypercalcemia and approximately one third of affected

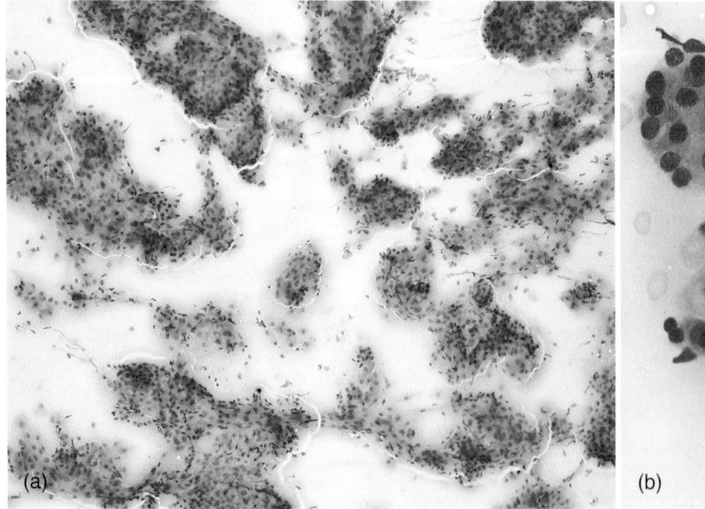

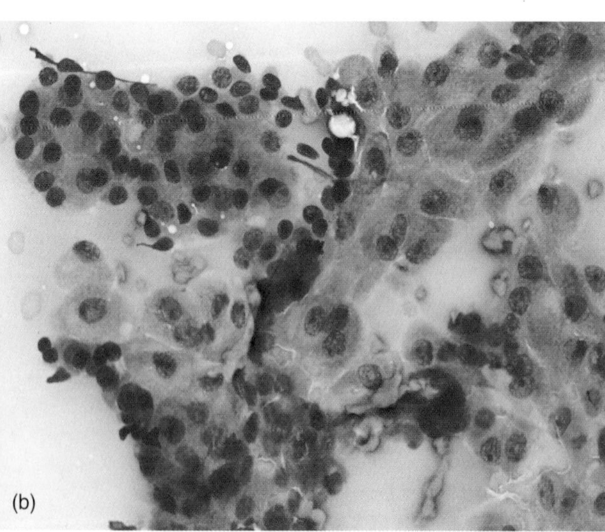

Figure 41.9 Perianal/circumanal ("hepatoid") gland tumor from a dog. (a) Clusters and morulae of uniform epithelial cells. (b) Large cells with abundant light blue to blue-gray to lightly eosinophilic (amphophilic) slightly granular cytoplasm with a low N : C ratio (lots of cytoplasm and a small nucleus). The cells resemble hepatocytes ("hepatoid"). Location in perineum is key to this diagnosis and for anal sac tumors, Figure 41.10. (a) 10× objective, (b) 50× objective. Wright-Giemsa stain.

dogs present for problems referable to their hypercalcemia, such as polyuria, polydipsia, lethargy, and weakness.

Cytologic features

These tumors exfoliate easily but the cells seldom remain intact. Therefore, numerous nuclei with a minimal amount of, or no, visible cytoplasm (naked nuclei) are usually present. Cells will be individualized and in clumps of various sizes indicating their epithelial origin (Figure 41.10). If cytoplasm is seen, it is a light blue-gray or lightly eosinophilic, and only a small amount is present, such that the N : C ratio is approximately 1 : 1 or 1 : 2 at the most (much less than that seen with circumanal tumors). The nuclei are characteristically uniform, round to oval and the chromatin pattern is usually fine with some visible nucleoli. Inflammation is not present.

The tumor cells have very few features of malignancy. However, almost all dogs who are diagnosed with these adenocarcinomas already have metastatic disease. Metastases occur first via direct extension into the pelvic vault, followed by systemic spread into sublumbar lymph nodes and, much later in the course, pulmonary and organ metastases. Sublumbar lymphadenopathy is a common finding on radiographs of the abdomen. Some dogs can survive for 1–2 years with repeated excisions of the primary and recurring masses. Removal of the tumor is followed by remission of hypercalcemia and hypophosphatemia; recurrence is followed by a return of the serum abnormalities (see case

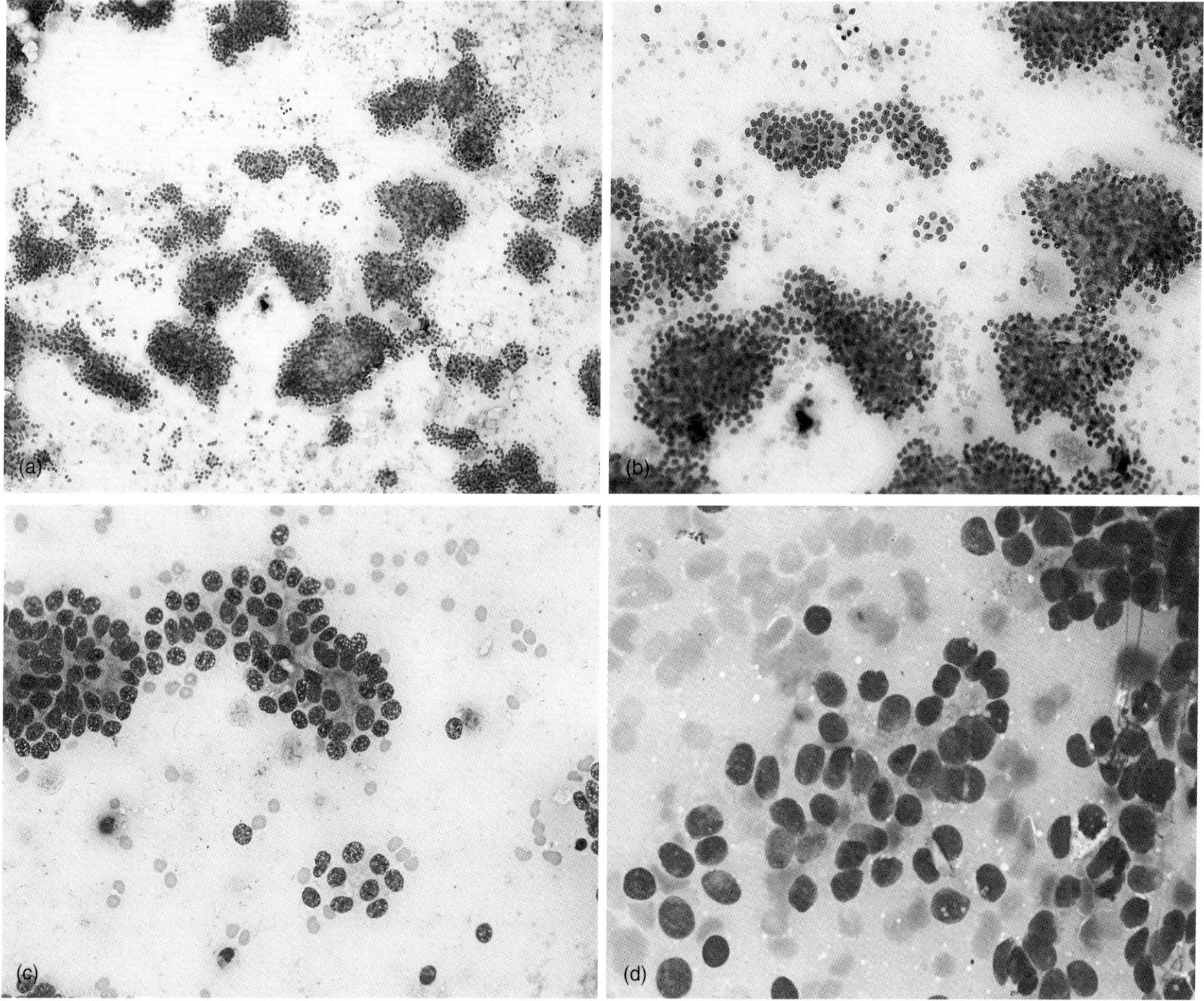

Figure 41.10 Anal sac apocrine gland adenocarcinoma from a dog. These tumors exfoliate easily and in high numbers, but the cells seldom remain intact. Therefore, numerous nuclei in a pool of cytoplasm or no visible cytoplasm (naked nuclei) is a common finding. The amount of cytoplasm and N : C ratio is much less than that seen with perianal gland tumors (Figure 41.9). Nuclei are uniform, round to oval in shape, with fine chromatin and some visible nucleoli. Despite the relatively uniform cytologic appearance, this is a malignant tumor with a high rate of metastasis to local lymph nodes at the time of diagnosis. More than 50% of dogs will also have paraneoplastic hypercalcemia. (a) 10× objective, (b) 20× objective, (c) 50× objective, (d) 100× objective. Wright-Giemsa stain.

example). Only primary hyperparathyroidism and hypercalcemia of malignancy are characterized by hypercalcemia and hypophosphatemia in dogs. If renal failure develops, often because of mineralization of the kidney, the serum phosphorus concentration will increase.

Diagnosis of this neoplasm may require integrating signalment, clinical signs, laboratory findings, and cytologic findings. For example, a female dog presenting with polyuria polydipsia, hypercalcemia, hypophosphatemia (unless there is concurrent decreased glomerular filtration rate), mass in the perineum, and aspirate consisting of the typical cytologic pattern described above would be relatively easy to diagnose.

Case example:

	Serum total Ca (mg/dL)	Serum P (mg/dL)n
Presentation	18.5	1.5
Removal of tumor	10.1	3.4
Recurrence (6 months)	16.2	2.0
Removal	9.0	4.2
Recurrence (16 months)	21	1.8

Postoperative hypocalcemia does not occur in these patients, unlike postoperative hypocalcemia associated with removal of a parathyroid adenoma. This is interesting in that the parathyroid glands are inactive to atrophic because of the prolonged hypercalcemia and therefore hypocalcemia would be expected.

Summary of expected features with circumanal tumors and AGAC:

	Circumanal tumor	AGAC
Sex	Male[a]	Female
Calcium	Within reference interval	Increased
Phosphorus	Within reference interval	Decreased
Perineum	Mass visible	Mass may be occult
Rectal	No masses in pelvic vault	Tumor in pelvic vault
Biologic behavior	Benign	Malignant

[a]These are generalities; certainly male dogs can develop AGAC and females can develop circumanal tumors.

Apocrine sweat gland tumors

Clinical features

Apocrine sweat gland tumors occur in dogs and cats but not as frequently as sebaceous gland or basal cell tumors. They can be benign or malignant.

Cytologic features

Cytologic features of apocrine sweat gland tumors overlap with those of sebaceous tumors, basal tumors and AGAC; thus they cannot be specifically identified via cytology. Nevertheless, cytology can be helpful in telling if it is an epithelial tumor and if it is more likely an adenoma or carcinoma.

Mammary gland tumors

The primary reason to perform FNA cytology of a mammary lump is to distinguish neoplasia from inflammation (mastitis). One should not use cytology to distinguish a benign from a malignant mammary tumor, although if the aspirate has many cytologic characteristics of malignancy, it is likely that the tumor is malignant. Once one has determined that the lesion is neoplastic, an excisional biopsy should be performed to determine the lesion's biologic behavior. Even with histopathology it can be difficult to distinguish benign from malignant tumors.

Mastitis, on the other hand, is characterized by nearly 100% neutrophils, and most neutrophils are degenerative. There is usually considerable extracellular, eosinophilic, amorphous material (milk) that prevents the formation of a good monolayer. Bacteria can often be identified intracellularly. Usually the animal is lactating and one or more glands are enlarged, red, tender, and inflamed.

Neoplastic lesions are predominated by mononuclear cells with few or no inflammatory cells. The cells vary greatly from case to case depending on the histologic type of tumor as well as the presence or absence of malignancy. Cells are individual and in groups, clusters, aggregates or acini to indicate their epithelial nature. Cells may contain one or more large cytoplasmic vacuoles. Cytoplasm is usually abundant with a high nucleus: cytoplasm ratio (up to 1 : 5). There can be considerable cellular and nuclear variability in terms of size and shape. Cells with markedly variable nuclear and cytologic features are more likely to be malignant. Aggregates of cells that pile together into disorganized, irregularly shaped morulae are more likely to be malignant. However, one should not rely on cytology alone to determine biologic behavior.

In dogs the ratio of benign to malignant mammary tumors is approximately 2.3 : 1 and in cats it is 0.25 : 1. In other words, mammary tumors are much more likely to be malignant in cats than in dogs. In summary, cytology is a useful tool to differentiate inflammation of the mammary gland from mammary gland neoplasia, but it is not very useful in determining degree of malignancy or tumor type.

Thyroid tumors

Clinical features

Around 80–90% of palpable thyroid masses in dogs are malignant and 98% of palpable thyroid lesions in cats are benign. Thyroid tumors tend to metastasize to the lungs before they spread to regional lymph nodes. Dogs with thyroid tumors are generally euthyroid, but thyroid tumors in cats often cause hyperthyroidism. The clinical distinction of thyroid adenoma, hyperplastic nodules, and adenomatous hyperplasia is inconsequential in cats because they all have benign behavior. The clinical syndrome is usually seen in cats over 10 years of age and is distinctive. Some of the features are hyperactivity, weight loss, polyphagia, EKG abnormalities, increased serum alkaline phosphatase activity (70% of cats have a mild to moderate increase), increased serum alanine aminotransferase (ALT) activity, and polycythemia (20%) (see Chapter 33). Hyperthyroidism is uncommon in dogs.

The distinction of benign vs. malignant is better made by clinical criteria than cytologic criteria. All palpably enlarged thyroid nodules in dogs should be considered malignant even if the cytologic pattern appears benign, and thyroid masses in cats should be considered benign. In cats thyroid tumors are follicular but in dogs they can be follicular (multiple subtypes further classified) or medullary (C-cell). Follicular vs. medullary origin in dogs requires immunocytochemistry or immunohistochemistry to be certain of origin and should be considered as medullary tumors are less aggressive.

Cytologic features

Tumor aspirates yield few to numerous usually uniform cells that have distinct cell borders and round nuclei (Figure 41.11). Cells are in clumps or small rafts of 10–50 cells. Tumors with benign cytologic features have uniform cellular and nuclear characteristics. Cells are usually well-spaced and do not appear in piles or clumps. Cytoplasm is not abundant, is lightly eosinophilic to gray-blue, and on careful inspection at 400 or 1000× green-blue intracytoplasmic granules may be observed (Figure 41.11c, d). These granules stain for lipofuscin, although others have reported them to be thyroglobulin, or a thyroglobulin precursor (personal observations, confirmed with histochemistry). Their presence helps in the identification of thyroid cells if the tissue of origin is a ventral neck mass. Nuclei are uniformly round or slightly oval, central or basilar. Some cells may be organized in rows or clusters, and rarely are organized in acinar formation with colloid preserved. Cytoplasm is often missing, leaving free, round nuclei, a characteristic often associated with neuroendocrine tumors.

Tumors with more aggressive cytologic features are characterized by some of the above observations but coupled with moderate to marked cellular and nuclear variability, multinucleation, high nucleus: cytoplasm ratio, cytoplasmic vacuolation, and cellular piling.

Neuroendocrine tumors

Clinical features

The only neuroendocrine tumor of the skin, the Merkel cell tumor, is very rare. This diagnosis should not be made from cytologic examination of the aspirate alone. However, neuroendocrine tumors are common in other locations including the jugular groove (carotid body tumor), the base of the heart (aortic body tumors), or in the adrenal glands (cortical tumors or pheochromocytoma). Carotid body tumors can produce clinical problems and visible bulges from their location in the jugular groove at the ramus of the mandible in dogs. They are a differential diagnosis for a palpable mass in the ventral neck region of middle aged to older dogs. Brachycephalic breeds tend to have more carotid body tumors than other breeds. Biological behavior of these tumors varies with their location. Tumors in the carotid artery region rarely metastasize and aortic body tumors vary in their metastatic capability, but they may be lethal due to their location. Despite their somewhat benign cytologic appearance they are capable of invading blood vessels and metastasizing.

Cytologic features

Cytologically, neuroendocrine cells have uniform round nuclei with indistinct or no visible cytoplasm. Cytoplasm, if present, is lightly basophilic to dusty-gray. Nuclei and cells are individualized and rarely to never form true aggregates or clumps of cells. This pattern of uniform nuclei with little to no visible cytoplasm ("naked nuclei") is highly characteristic of neuroendocrine tumors (Figure 40.11; Figure 41.11). For unknown reasons these cells are fragile and rarely remain intact. A similar pattern is seen in apocrine gland tumors of the anal sac. Cells may have a "fried egg" appearance (centrally placed nucleus surrounded by cytoplasm) similar to MCT cells. Mild variation in nuclear size (anisokaryosis) may be noted at higher magnifications. Nuclear chromatin is fine, and a single nucleolus is often visible.

Neuroendocrine tumors can usually be diagnosed at lower magnifications because of the characteristic uniform appearance of numerous round nuclei and the clinical information of where the mass is located. Cytoplasmic neuroendocrine granules are not typically visible. There are no definitive cytologic criteria to differentiate malignant vs. benign tumors.

Mesenchymal/spindle cell tumors

Introduction

The mesenchymal tumors include fibroma, fibrosarcoma, hemangioma, hemangiosarcoma, hemangiopericytoma, neurofibroma, peripheral nerve sheath tumor, myxoma, myxosarcoma, rhabdomyoma, rhabdomyosarcoma, undifferentiated sarcoma, vaccine-induced sarcoma, and vaccine-induced lesion. Examples of this group of tumors are found in this chapter as Figures 41.12–41.14, and Figures 40.1 and 40.9.

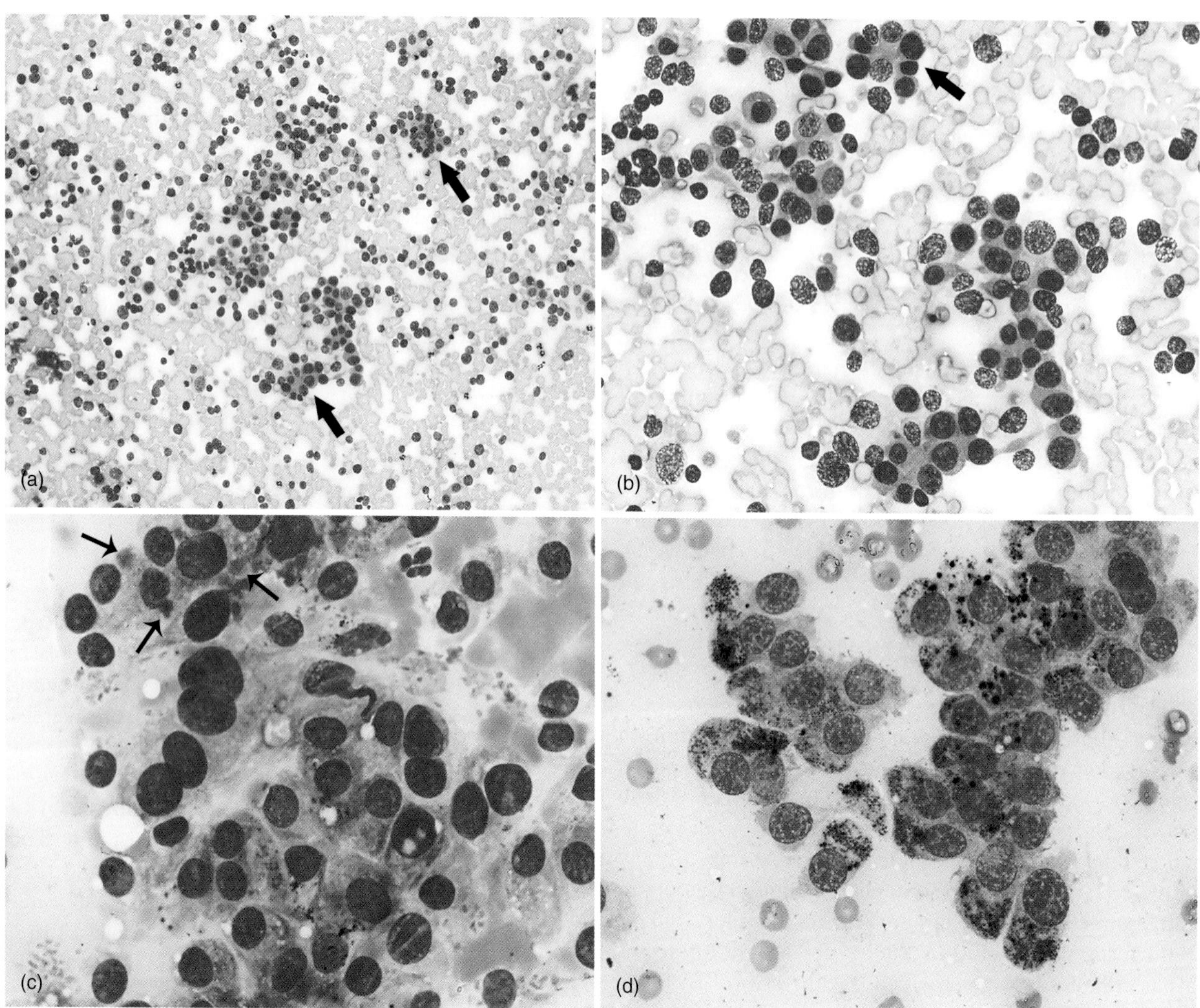

Figure 41.11 Thyroid tumor from dogs. Cells are organized in rows and clusters with acinar-like formation (a, b; arrows and Figure 40.11). Cytoplasm is often missing, leaving free, round nuclei (a, b). The small to moderate amount of cytoplasm stains lightly eosinophilic to grayish blue, and there may be green-blue intracytoplasmic granules consistent with lipofuscin (c, d). This lipofuscin pigment is positive to Schmorl's stain and is often mislabeled as thyroglobulin. Central or basilar nuclei are uniformly round or slightly oval. Colloid can be preserved between the cells (c, thin arrows). Despite their uniform appearance on cytology, all clinically detectable thyroid masses in dogs should be considered malignant. The tumor in (c) demonstrates more pleomorphic cytologic features characterized by variation in nuclear size and binucleation. The cells in (d) would be difficult to differentiate from normal thyroid cells, therefore look at many fields and use clinical data, e.g., mass is present in thyroid region. If a mass is palpable in the thyroid of a dog it is likely aggressive; the opposite is true for cats. (a) 20× objective, (b) 50× objective, (c, d) 100× objective. Wright-Giemsa stain.

Determining the exact identity of each of these tumors may not be possible using cytology. All available information should be considered when establishing a diagnosis. Tumors of mesenchymal origin tend to exfoliate poorly or at least yield fewer cells than do the round cell or epithelial tumors. This is attributed to their low cellularity and the presence of extracellular matrix that holds the cells together. However, less differentiated variants (more anaplastic) tend to have less extracellular matrix and more cells, and therefore may yield very cellular preparations. The key to placing cells in this category is to find cells or nuclei that are elongated. It is difficult to differentiate spindle cell tumors from fibroplasia (granulation tissue) with cytology alone. The quickest clue to identification is the absence of inflammatory cells and the predominance of oval or spindle-shaped nuclei. Several slides may need to be searched before enough cells can be found to evaluate. These tumors may require surgical excision and the "scrape" technique to produce enough cells to establish a diagnosis. The cells are individualized, and though they may be close together they do not form clusters, morulae or acini characteristic of epithelial cell tumors. When cells are closely opposed their true cell borders are rarely seen. Individual cells have distinct to barely discernible cell borders and their spindle shape is

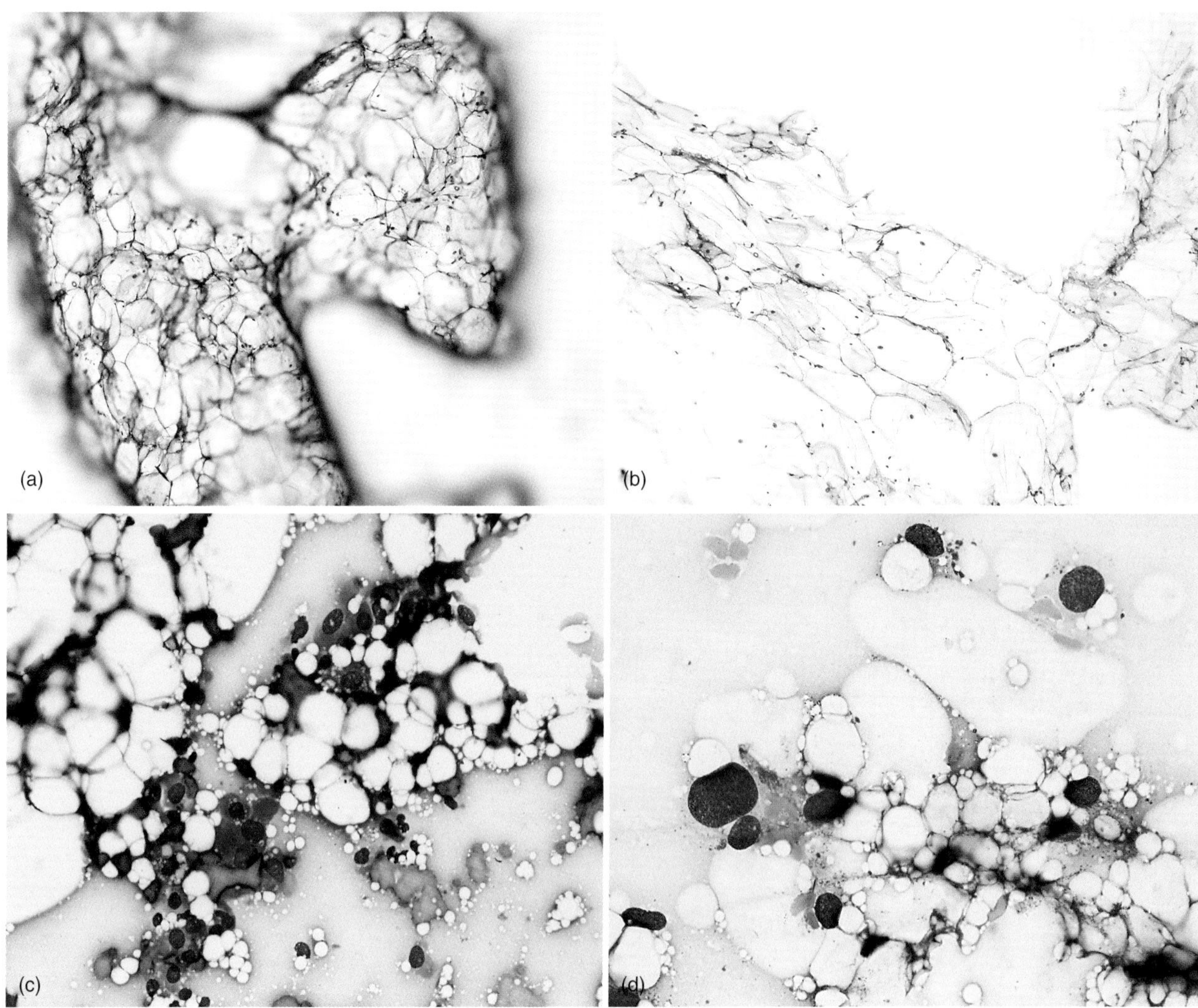

Figure 41.12 Lipoma (a, b) and liposarcoma (c, d) from dogs. (a, b) Lipoma: clumps of uniform adipocytes with large amount of cytoplasm and a small eccentric nucleus. Aspiration of subcutaneous fat will yield cells with a similar appearance. Therefore, the distinction must be made based on clinical findings, e.g., a mass is palpable in the subcutis. Histopathology is not needed to diagnose lipoma if the aspirate was taken from a soft subcutaneous mass. (c, d) Liposarcoma. This is a very rare tumor in animals yet is one of the most common soft-tissue mesenchymal (sarcoma) tumors in humans. The background contains numerous large and small, clear vacuoles of extracellular fat. Admixed are spindle cells with marked anisokaryosis, round to oval nuclei with finely stippled chromatin, and multiple, prominent nucleoli. There is no inflammation. (a, b) 10× objective, (c) 50× objective, (d): 100× objective. Wright-Giemsa stain.

usually easy to appreciate. The cytoplasm is light blue to gray or lightly eosinophilic; it follows the contour of the nucleus and therefore is elongated, oval-shaped, or streams at both ends to form points or a "tail." Sometimes the cells are plump with an angular, pointed cellular end that streams outward. Nuclear chromatin arrangement and nucleoli vary considerably. More cellular tumors tend to have multiple nuclei, multiple nucleoli and varying shapes and sizes to nuclei and nucleoli (features of malignancy). Multinucleation is a characteristic of more aggressive tumors.

Most of these tumors are relatively easy to classify as of mesenchymal origin but determination of malignant **vs.** benign is speculative as is their exact histologic origin. The following descriptions for the specific tumor types are subjective and are based on combining clinical and cytological features. Some cytologists believe lesions predominated by spindle cells should be described as "spindle cell tumor, spindle cell proliferation, fibroplasia or spindle cell tumor" and add the comment: "histopathology necessary for differentiation."

Histologic classifications of these tumors are in Table 41.1; however, as mentioned above, recognition of these individual types of tumors cannot be achieved with cytology. Histopathologic distinction of each of these tumors can also be difficult, requiring histochemical or immunohistochemical

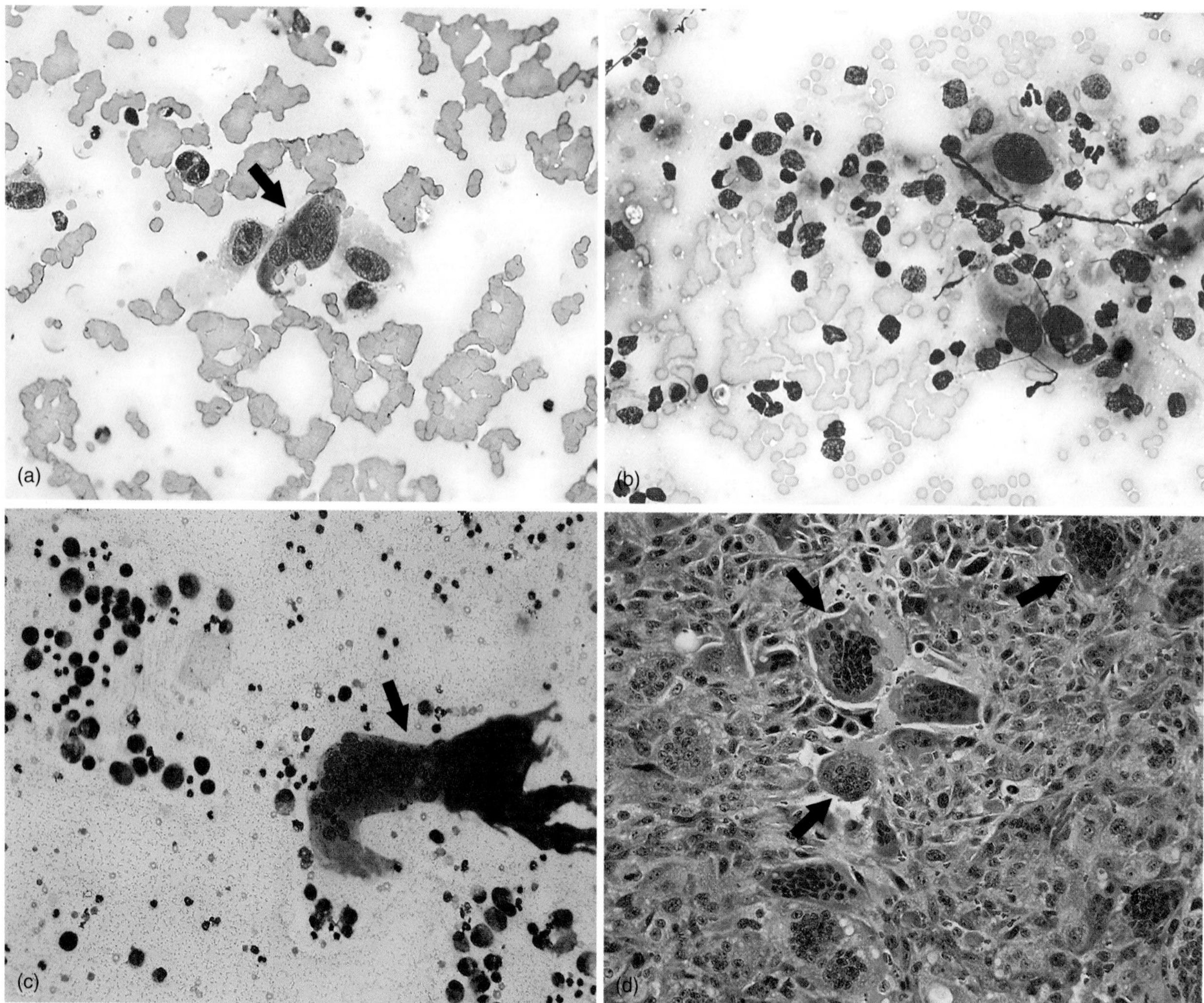

Figure 41.13 Fibrosarcoma (injection-site sarcoma) from cats. Note pleomorphic spindle cells exhibiting anisocytosis, anisokaryosis, and nuclei with multiple, large nucleoli. (a, c, d) These tumors can contain very large, multinucleated (>10–15 nuclei) cells (thick arrows). (b, c) Secondary inflammation, here indicated by the presence of lymphocytes, macrophages, and neutrophils, is a characteristic finding in these tumors. (a, b) 50× objective, (c, d) 40× objective. (a–c) Wright-Giemsa stain, (d) H&E stain.

stains [2, 6, 13]. Despite these generalizations some spindle tumors can be definitively diagnosed as far as subtype, and tumor behavior can be predicted. For example, lipomas are easy to recognize cytologically. Perivascular wall tumor (PWT, previously called hemangiopericytoma), is the most common spindle cell tumor in dogs and it has characteristic cytological features. Fibrosarcoma can also usually be diagnosed, especially in cats. All of the others can be categorized as spindle cell tumors, but recognition of the specific histologic type is not reliable. Therefore, a reasonable series of goals from cytologic evaluation of a mesenchymal tumor in the skin or subcutaneous tissues would be to first identify the process as neoplastic, then categorize it as spindle cell, then benign vs. malignant when possible, then a specific diagnosis (name of tumor), if possible.

Lipoma

Clinical features

Lipomas are very common subcutaneous tumors of middle aged to older dogs. They produce a bulging, nonulcerated mass in the subcutaneous tissues that is soft on palpation, although if they are in an area that is constricted by other tissue, they may feel firm. Tumors can be large, exceeding 12 cm in diameter and are often along the sides of thoracic and abdominal walls. They are uncommon to rare in cats.

A tentative diagnosis of lipoma can be made from how the mass palpates, and when material is squirted onto a glass slide numerous clear fat droplets can usually be observed.

Cytologic features

Initial interpretation at low magnification might be that nothing was aspirated as the slide appears devoid of cells.

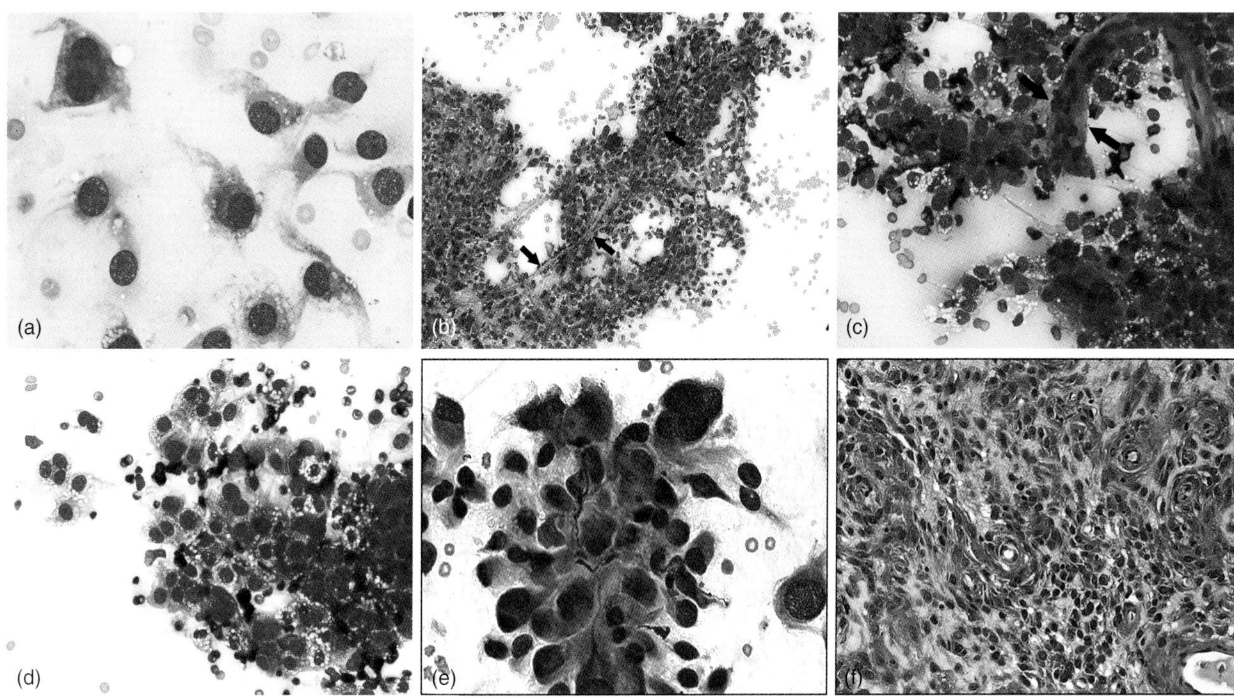

Figure 41.14 Soft-tissue mesenchymal tumors. (a–e) Fine-needle aspirates, (f) tissue biopsy and histopathology. (a) A spindle cell tumor from a subcutaneous mass from a dog. (b–f) Perivascular wall tumor (PWT). Unlike many other spindle cell tumors, fine-needle aspirates of these tumors yield very cellular preparations (b). Sometimes, vascular structures (capillaries) are aspirated as the tumor originates from cells lining the outer wall of blood vessels (arrows, b, c). Neoplastic spindle cells have long cytoplasmic "tails," often with "bipolar" pointed cellular ends (d, e). The cytoplasm can contain a few, small, discrete, clear lipid vacuoles (c, d). (f) Whorls of spindle-shaped cells are the most diagnostic feature of perivascular wall tumor (previously called hemangiopericytoma), best appreciated in biopsy specimens. (e) Source: Meuten DJ Tumors in Domestic Animals Ed 5, Wiley Blackwell 2017 p. 953–960; p. 957–959. (a, e) 100× objective, (b) 20× objective, (c, d) 50× objective, (f) 40× objective. (a–e) Wright-Giemsa stain, (f) H&E stain.

Table 41.1 Benign and malignant (aggressive) mesenchymal (spindle cell) tumors.

Benign	Malignant
Lipoma	Liposarcoma
Fibroma	Fibrosarcoma
Perivascular wall tumor	
Hemangioma	Hemangiosarcoma
Myxoma	Myxosarcoma
Leiomyoma	Leiomyosarcoma
	Undifferentiated
[a]Nerve sheath tumors (NSTs)	

[a]Schwannoma, neurolemmoma, and neurofibroma are now lumped together as NST. Differentiation of these individual tumors is generally not needed and cannot be done cytologically or with routine histology.

By looking at areas that may look like debris, large vacuoles, and perhaps adipocytes may be observed. Adipocytes are very large cells with a nucleus that could be round or simply compressed over to the side of the cell and difficult to see (Figure 41.12a, b). In comparison to lipid-laden sebaceous cells (Figure 41.7c, d), the vacuoles in adipocytes are 5–20 times the size of the vacuoles in sebaceous adenoma cells. Adipocytes may appear as one large vacuole. Nuclei when seen are usually eccentric in adipocytes, unlike in sebaceous adenoma cells, where they are usually central in location. There is no inflammatory cell component with these tumors, although they sometimes contain numerous capillaries that are lined with cells that appear spindeloid. Histopathology is not needed for confirmation of the cytologic diagnosis, although if subcutaneous fat is aspirated, it can appear similar to a lipoma aspirate.

Liposarcoma

This is a rare tumor in all animals but one of the most common spindle cell sarcomas in humans. There are no unique clinical features.

Cytologic features

Numerous large and small clear lipid vacuoles within spindle-shaped cells are characteristic. Cell borders may not be readily discernible. Nuclei are round to oval to spindle-shaped. The cellularity is greater than that of a lipoma aspirate and nuclei have anaplastic feature (Figure 41.12c, d). Cytologic diagnosis of a liposarcoma should be confirmed with histopathology. Differential cytologic diagnoses are sebaceous tumor or panniculitis. However, the tumor cells are not in clumps as is seen with sebaceous tumors, and there is no evidence of inflammation, as is seen with panniculitis.

Fibroma/fibrosarcoma

Fibromas exfoliate poorly and few cells will be on the slide. This is because the tumors do not contain many cells per unit area and those cells are firmly embedded in abundant collagenous matrix that connects the tumor cells. The cells are elongated, cytoplasm is light blue and nuclei are oval-shaped to round and are devoid of nucleoli (benign features). Aspirates of fibrosarcomas consist of numerous spindle cells with moderate to marked cellular and nuclear variability, including multinucleation. Fibrosarcoma aspirates are more cellular than aspirates of fibromas because the tumors do contain many cells per unit area and much less collagenous matrix. There may be a small amount of extracellular amorphous pink to eosinophilic material that resembles osteoid. This material is collagen (glycosaminoglycans). On careful inspection, eosinophilic to purple granules may be seen in a few cells.

Fibrosarcomas are more common in cats than dogs. They can be associated with injection sites as well as feline sarcoma virus in FeLV-positive cats.

Injection-site sarcoma/vaccine-induced lesion

Clinical features

Injection site sarcomas or lesions are recognized frequently in cats (Figures 40.9, 40.16, and 41.13). Originally, they were associated with vaccines but now are known to be associated with any injection, as well as chronic irritation and trauma. In fact, trauma-induced sarcomas have been reported in the eyes of cats. Most are in sites where injections are common, including the dorsum of the neck, between the shoulder blades, flank, rear limb, or chest wall.

Cytologic features

Lesions have a wide range of patterns that include pure inflammation to inflammation with preneoplastic changes, sarcoma, fibrosarcoma, and may or may not have accompanying inflammation (Figures 40.9c and Figure 41.13). When spindle cells with inflammatory cells are seen especially with extracellular, amorphous pink material that may be vaccine adjuvant, one should suspect a lesion of injection origin, with or without the historical information of location. The combination of anaplastic spindle-shaped cells, extracellular amorphous material, and location at the dorsum of the neck are very suspicious for this lesion.

Early lesions may contain only inflammatory cells with predominantly neutrophils but also numerous lymphocytes, plasma cells, macrophages and occasionally eosinophils; a few multinucleated giant cells and reactive fibroblasts may also be present. The lesions seem to then proceed through stages in which the inflammatory components decrease and the neoplastic changes increase, culminating in a clearly recognizable sarcoma. At the latter stage the lesions exfoliate numerous cells with a wide variety of cellular and nuclear abnormalities. Sometimes there are multinucleated giant cells with so many nuclei that they defy the pathologist's ability to count them all (hundreds in one extremely large cell) (Figure 41.13). Even at this latter state some inflammatory cells, especially lymphocytes and macrophages may remain (Figure 41.13b, c). The extracellular amorphous pink to purple, acellular material is interesting and highly suggestive of these vaccine-/injection-induced lesions. The composition of the extracellular material is unknown, but it may be of adjuvant origin. It is nonbirefringent and it resembles the cytologic appearance of ultrasound gel.

Predicting biologic behavior is best done by recognizing what the lesion is, and then relying on published case series that report they are deeply infiltrative, difficult to entirely excise and are notorious for recurrence but seldom metastasize to distant sites. Imaging studies sometimes demonstrate long fibrils that extend into deeper muscle layers and into vertebrae.

Hemangioma/hemangiosarcoma

FNA cytology of these lesions is frustrating as they tend to produce lots of blood and relatively few to no neoplastic cells (Figure 40.9d). If you are lucky to find any spindle-shaped cells it will be after carefully reviewing several slides and searching through a background of blood. The cells are spindle-shaped and plump but have no unique identifying features. Although these tumors are found in the skin, they are also commonly seen in the spleen and heart. Histopathology is a requirement for confirmation of this cytologic diagnosis.

Perivascular wall tumor/hemangiopericytoma/neurofibroma/peripheral nerve sheath tumors

These are different neoplasms that can be categorized under the terms *soft-tissue mesenchymal tumor (STMT)* or *soft-tissue sarcoma (STS)* (Figure 41.14). The latter term is popular but somewhat of a misnomer in that most tumors in this group are not aggressive and therefore are not sarcomas. Do not rely on cytology to distinguish these spindle cell tumors; even histopathology may require immunohistochemistry for definitive identification.

The most common canine STMT are the PVTs and 90% of these are not aggressive and do not metastasize [2, 6, 13]. They were previously diagnosed as hemangiopericytomas. They are found frequently on thoracic or pelvic limbs and occur in the subcutis on body walls. FNAs of these tumors yield preparations of relatively high cellularity, composed of distinctly spindle- or banana-shaped cells with long cytoplasmic "tails" (Figure 41.14b–e). They tend to have bipolar pointed cellular ends rather than only one pointed cellular pole. They will be individual and in aggregates or whorls of 10–30 cells. Sometimes capillaries are aspirated as the tumor contains numerous blood vessels (Figure 41.14b, c). Whorls of spindle-shaped cells are the best diagnostic feature but are better appreciated in biopsy specimens (Figure 41.14f).

Cytology is very useful to establish a diagnosis of STMT and plan surgical removal. These tumors should be excised widely; they tend to recur but rarely metastasize. If treatment beyond surgical excision is planned or an estimate of survival is desired, then the excised tumors should be graded histologically. Excisional rather than core biopsy should be used for grading. However, the best predictors of behavior for PWT are size of tumor and depth of invasion of primary tumor. PWTs greater than 5 cm in diameter and/or tumors that have penetrated into deeper tissue layers are associated with more aggressive behavior, regardless of grade. Grading with histopathology uses mitotic count, percent necrosis and degree of differentiation to assign a grade of low or high. These grading schemes should be considered estimates of behavior as they are fraught with errors.

Low grade: recurrence rate of 25% after surgical excision, median ST of 118 weeks, 2% metastatic rate.

High grade: Recurrence rate of 62% after surgical excision, median ST of 49 weeks, 15% metastatic rate; however, the number of dogs in high-grade group with accurate follow-up information was very small [2].

Myxoma/myxosarcoma

These are uncommon tumors, found on the feet or legs of dogs. The best diagnostic feature is abundant background matrix (glycosaminoglycans or mucin) that is light blue, sometimes eosinophilic stippled (like joint fluid) or forming crescents and streams. The cellularity will be low and the cells may not spread into a monolayer due to the myxomatous stroma that adheres to the cells. This mucoid material may even cause the cells to align in rows (rowing). Rowing happens frequently in other viscous fluids such as normal synovial fluid or effusions due to feline infection peritonitis.

Differential diagnoses would include any of the other spindle cell neoplasms. Benign vs. malignant varieties cannot be determined cytologically and therefore should cytologic assessment should be confirmed with histopathology.

Rhabdomyoma/rhabdomyosarcoma

These are tumors of skeletal muscle, and occur on the legs, back and in somewhat other unusual locations including the dorsal laryngeal area, urinary bladder and tongue. Some tumors yield spindle-shaped cells and others have plump polyhedral cells that look epithelial or histiocytic. Rarely the tumor exfoliates elongated cells in which the cross-striations are still visible. Aspiration of normal skeletal muscle will produce broad muscle fibers in which cross-striations are seen easily. The nuclear density is less and the muscle fibers are wider in normal muscle. Benign vs. malignant behavior cannot be predicted cytologically and is difficult to impossible to accurately predict histologically. There are few long-term studies that have followed dogs with muscle tumors to determine their biologic behavior.

Undifferentiated sarcoma

This differential diagnosis is made frequently for STMT that are too undifferentiated to identify tissue of origin. Many of the features already described apply to this diagnosis. The preparations will vary from low to high cellularity, but the latter is more likely. The cells are individualized and in various shapes and forms, but some are clearly spindeloid. Plump cells that are polygonal, but with pointed streams of cytoplasm at one cellular pole, are enough for this designation. There will be moderate to marked cellular and nuclear variability or atypia. Binucleation and multinucleation are present, and various sizes, shapes and numbers of nuclei and nucleoli will further attest to the tumor's malignant nature.

Melanoma

Clinical features

Melanomas are common in the skin, toes, and oral cavity of dogs (Figure 41.15) and the perineum of gray Arabian horses. They are not as common in the skin of cats but are found with regularity in the eyes of cats. Most canine oral melanomas are malignant, but benign tumors, or at least tumors with low malignant potential, can be recognized with histopathology [14]. Skin melanomas in dogs and cats can be graded via histopathology to help predict malignancy and STs [15]:

Canine melanoma			
Location	Skin	Skin	Oral
Mitotic count (MC)	<3	≥3	≥4
2-year survival	90%	25%	10%
Median survival	104 weeks	30 weeks	<4 months
Eventual death due to tumor	10%	45%	90%

MC was performed in 10 high-power fields (400× magnification but size of fields was not defined).

Cytologic features

Pigmented tumors are easy to diagnose; nonpigmented types are problematic. An interesting feature of melanomas is that they exfoliate in epithelial and mesenchymal patterns. If one sees both epithelial clusters and single spindle-shaped cells, or even round discrete cells, one should be suspicious of melanoma. If pigment is obvious the diagnosis is straight forward, and wide surgical excision with evaluation of margins via histopathology should be done. Pigment is intracellular

CHAPTER 41

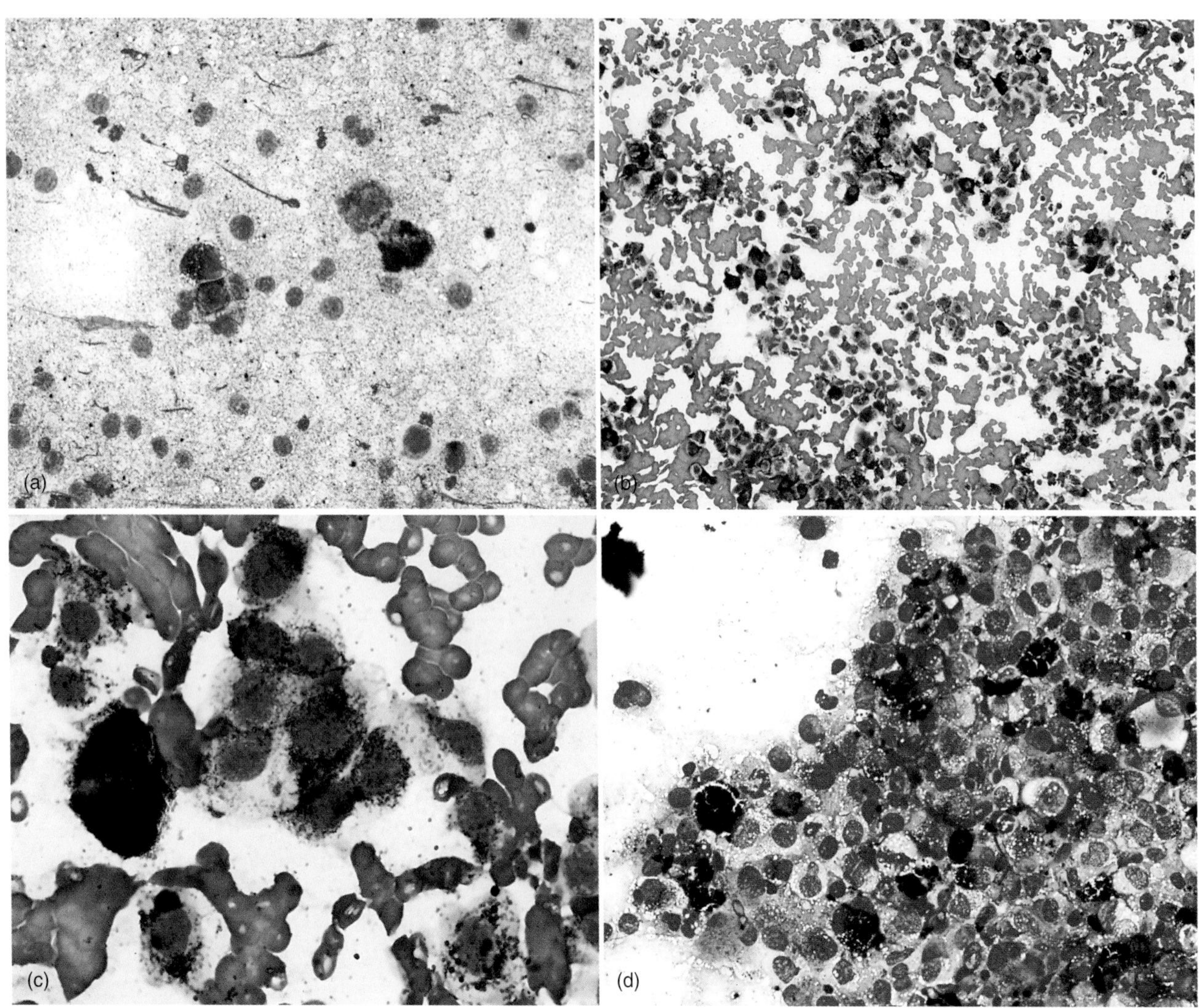

Figure 41.15 Canine melanocytic tumors, range of cytological patterns. (a) Cutaneous melanoma/melanocytoma, heavily pigmented individual cells, round nuclei; abundant pigment in background will make the slide black on gross inspection and the diagnosis easy. Histology is needed to assess biological behavior. (b, c) Digit melanoma, individual cells and aggregate of spindle-shaped cells with variable amounts of melanin pigment. (d) Metastasis in regional lymph node from an oral malignant melanoma; moderate to marked variability in cell and nuclear morphology; amount of pigment is highly variable (large black globules, small black granules, and some cells are devoid of pigment). (a) 50× objective, (b) 20× objective, (c) 100× objective, (d) 40× objective. Wright-Giemsa stain.

and is green to black (Figure 41.15). The granules can be uniform, small and needle like or can be globular and of variable sizes and shapes. If pigment is abundant it will also be extracellular. Tumors with abundant cytological pigment are usually black on gross inspection and the slides may be black. Hemangiomas may look red or black on gross examination as well. Place a cut surface of the tumor on a white paper towel and if the paper turns red it most likely is a hemangioma; if it turns black it is likely melanoma. True amelanotic melanomas are uncommon. Pigment can almost always be found but it may require diligent searching at higher magnifications 400× (40× objective) or with oil immersion (1000×). Poorly pigmented tumors will have a small amount or dusting of light green/yellow/brown pigment in a few tumor cells. Slides can be stained histochemically (Fontana Masson) and immunohistochemically (Melanin-A) at referral labs. If one sees large round cells with very large and distinct nucleoli ("owl eye" pattern) but no pigment, one should consider amelanotic melanoma and request special stains from the diagnostic lab.

Histiocytic sarcoma

This tumor is rare in cats; it can occur in any breed of dog, but Bernese mountain dogs, flat-coated retrievers, Rottweilers, and golden retrievers are breeds in which histiocytic sarcoma (HS) is most commonly seen [16] (see also Chapter 40).

There are molecular diagnostic tests for HS based on deletion of tumor suppressor genes CDKN2A/B, RB1, and PTEN [17]. Histiocytic sarcomas are a disease complex with multiple subtypes: malignant histiocytosis, systemic histiocytosis, disseminated histiocytosis, hemophagocytic syndrome, histiocytic sarcoma, etc. The majority of these tumors arise from interstitial dendritic cells that are present in perivascular tissues; however, hemophagocytic histiocytic tumors arise from splenic macrophages [11]. The distinctive microscopic feature for this subtype is the presence of erythrophagocytosis (Figure 40.12d, e). A unique location for this tumor is in joints. Many previous diagnoses of synovial sarcoma are likely to have been HS. Skin and subcutaneous are the most common sites and the tumor may be singular or multiple and occasionally is widely disseminated. These latter varieties are highly malignant. Some dogs will be hypercalcemic.

Although HS is a mesenchymal tumor, the tumor cells are not spindle-shaped; in fact, they look cytologically like a pleomorphic round cell tumor (Figure 40.12). Most HS are easy to diagnose because the tumor cells exfoliate in large numbers and the neoplastic cells have abundant cytoplasm that contains one to numerous nuclei. Multinucleated giant cells are characteristic. Nuclei and nucleoli are highly variable in number, size, and shape. Aggressive plasma cell tumor (Figure 41.5d) is a differential diagnosis but if giant cells, multinucleation, bizarre nuclei and nucleoli are numerous, then HS is more likely than plasma cell *tumor*. A definitive way to distinguish these two tumors is to request immunocytochemistry with antibody to MUM-1, which will stain plasma cells positively but not histiocytic cells [18]. Immunohistochemical stains that recognize histiocytic cells require special handling and expertise.

Non-neoplastic skin and subcutaneous lesions

Abscess

Aspirates of abscesses consist of predominantly neutrophils, and usually a few macrophages. Neutrophils are degenerative and, depending on the degree of sepsis, the bacteria may be infrequent or numerous, both intracellular and extracellular. Sometimes the degenerative features are so severe the neutrophils appear to be macrophages. The nuclei may be markedly swollen and round and cell and nuclear features are indistinct. Inflammatory lesions are discussed in detail in Chapter 39.

Hematoma and seroma

Clinical features

Hematomas present as a soft, fluctuant, nonpainful swelling in a location that is easily traumatized such as the ear. Aspirated fluid may be red, pink, orange, or yellow in color. Recent hematomas contain blood that appears similar to venous blood. As the blood in the hematoma is resorbed and the erythrocytes are phagocytized by macrophages, the color changes from red to yellow (seroma) and the transparency goes from cloudy to clear (seroma). The viscosity of the fluid increases as the hematoma is resorbed.

Cytologic features

The microscopic pattern varies as the lesion progresses from a hematoma into a seroma (Figure 41.16). Aspirates of recently formed hematomas appear similar to venous blood except that no platelets are seen and erythrophagocytosis by macrophages and occasionally neutrophils can be observed (Figure 41.16a, b). The platelets are activated during the bleeding process, are then incorporated into clot formation, and will not be visible cytologically. The presence of platelets, often found in clumps at the feathered edge of the film and lack of evidence of erythrophagocytosis indicates peripheral blood contamination, rather than a hematoma (Figure 41.16f). As the lesion ages, erythrophagocytosis will be more obvious, and the erythrocytes will be degraded. The iron complex (hemosiderin) resulting from the erythrocyte degradation appears as green, blue or yellow granules of varying sizes in the cytoplasm of the macrophages (Figure 41.16c). Hematoidin, a hemoglobin degradation product similar to unconjugated hemoglobin, forms later in the process and consists of intra- or extracellular yellow crystals that have a straight edge and are often in the shape of diamonds or rhomboids. Hematoidin is birefringent when viewed with polarized light and hemosiderin is not (Figure 41.16d, e). The nucleated cells will be a mixture of neutrophils and macrophages. Erythrophagocytosis can be in either cell but is predominantly in macrophages, especially in older hematomas.

As the lesion progresses into a seroma the gross color changes from red to yellow and it contains fewer cells. The macrophages may be inactive (blue gray cytoplasm with few to no vacuoles) or activated with increased amount of cytoplasm with foamy, vacuolated cytoplasm containing cellular debris. Seromas may develop independent of hematoma formation as a result of constant pressure. For example, seromas occur in dogs at sites subjected to constant bruising of tissues (elbow). The seroma fluid is high in protein and typically low in cell numbers. Macrophages are the principal nucleated cell found in seromas.

If the location, history and cytology are classic for a hematoma, such as on the ear, other differential diagnoses likely need not be considered. However, if you are suspicious that the cause of the hematoma could be neoplasia, then search for neoplastic cells, and consider excision or biopsy and histopathology.

Epidermal inclusion cyst (follicular cyst)

Clinical features

Epidermal inclusion cysts occur predominantly in dogs. The cysts arise from epidermal and adnexal structures. They vary

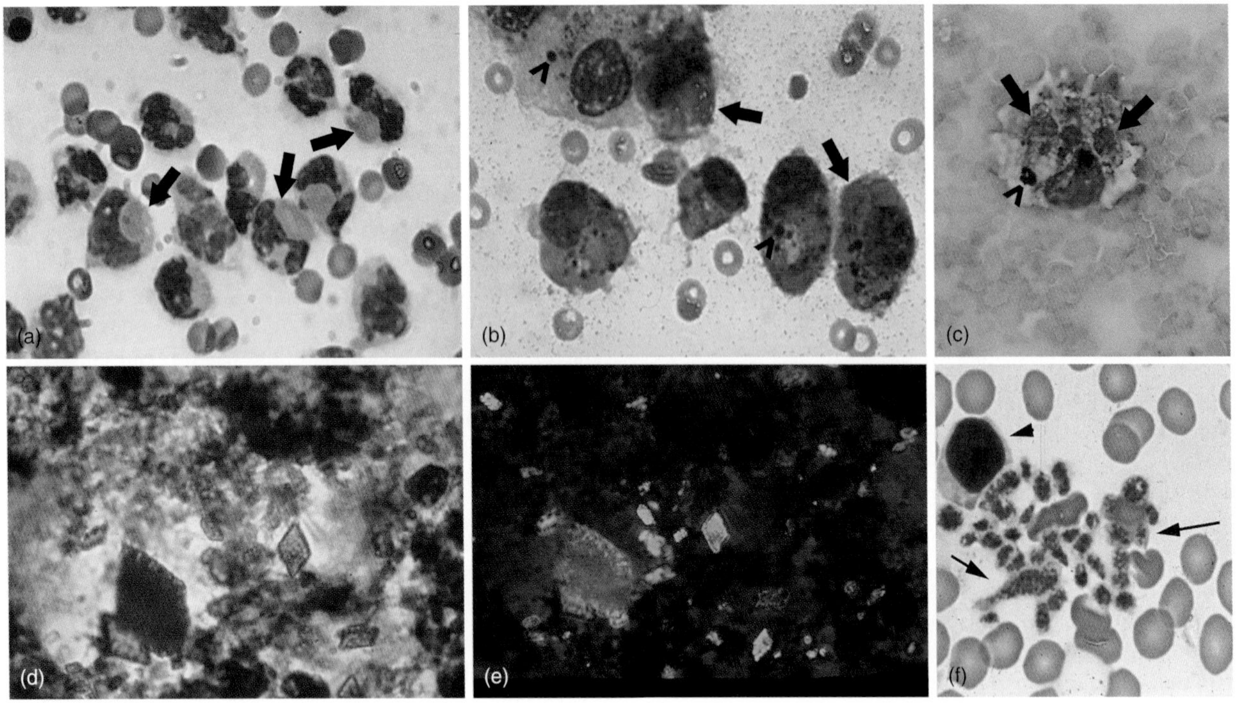

Figure 41.16 Hemorrhage (hematoma); early to later, starting with erythrophagocytosis (a–c, thick arrows) in neutrophils and monocytes in early lesions (a), followed by the presence of erythrophagia and hemosiderin (b, c; green-bluish globular pigment in macrophages, arrowheads). Hematoidin (d, e) forms after hemosiderin, and these golden, rhomboid crystals are birefringent when viewed with polarized light (e). Platelets (f, arrows) are *not* seen in hematomas, even in very early stages. They indicate aspiration of a blood vessel but not true hemorrhage. (a–f) 100× objective. Wright-Giemsa stain.

in size and consistency but often are 1–3 cm in diameter and are soft on palpation. Yellow-white to gray-tan "tooth-paste" like material oozes from them or can be expressed through a pore or can be aspirated into a syringe. Expressing the material through a pore may push the contents into the adjacent tissues resulting in an inflammatory reaction and causing the lesion to expand. The pasty and caseous accumulations range from white, gray to black in color, and may be oily in consistency. Lesions that are traumatized (spontaneous or iatrogenic) can be inflammatory and painful. The cysts are lined by squamous epithelium; the cells cornify, slough into the center and the lumen is filled with keratin (Figure 41.17). Pigmented epithelial cells cause the accumulations to become discolored, even black, like that of comedomes. The cyst fluid or cellular accumulations that degenerate are rich in lipids. Cholesterol crystal formation is common to these lesions (Figure 41.17).

Cytologic features

Cytologic samples from these lesions range from cellular to hypocellular. Key to the correct diagnosis is the recognition of cholesterol clefts and plates, accompanied by numerous keratin bars, squamous epithelial cells, and sometimes macrophages with hemosiderin or hematoidin. The keratin and cholesterol crystals in these preparations occasionally do not stain well but can be better visualized by reducing the size of the iris diaphragm or lowering the condenser. The cholesterol crystals are best seen using the 10 or 20× objectives; they appear as large, semiclear plates with straight edges. At 200 or 400× you will see numerous keratin bars or keratinocytes. These cells usually stain deeply blue but can be gray and vary in number from few to numerous. The cells have sharp, linear borders, are often folded and nuclei are not visible. Some nucleated, viable squamous epithelial cells may be present, with or without intracellular melanin. Macrophages with phagocytosed material and hemosiderin can also be present. Lesions that rupture may have numerous neutrophils but cysts that are still intact contain few or no neutrophils. Once these cysts rupture, they are associated with a moderate to marked pyogranulomatous cellulitis.

Sialocele/mucocoele

Clinical features

Sialoceles are soft swellings located where there are salivary glands or salivary drainage ducts such as the ramus of mandible, intermandibular space, or under the tongue, and are quite common in dogs. They are formed from saliva that has leaked into the adjacent tissues or accumulated as a result of a blocked salivary duct. The aspirated fluid is usually quite viscous.

Cytologic features

These lesions can be diagnosed at low magnification (4–10× objective) by observing fairly large amorphous areas of

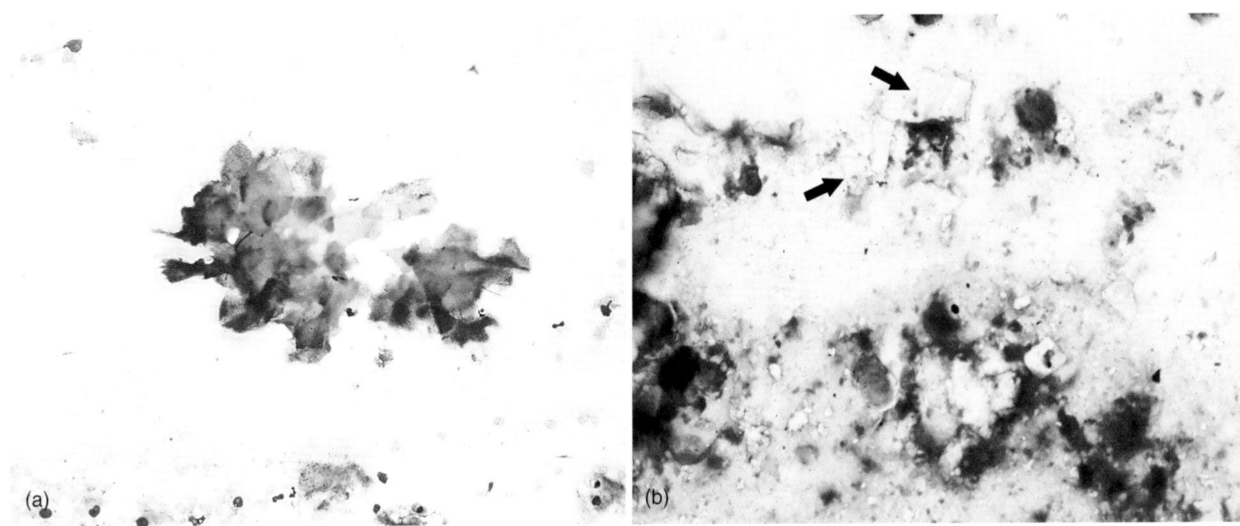

Figure 41.17 Epidermal inclusion cyst ("follicular cyst") from a dog. (a) Aggregates of superficial, anucleate squamous epithelial cells (keratinocytes, "keratin bars") are characteristic for these lesions. (b) Keratin is often accompanied by cholesterol crystals (arrows), which result from cellular degeneration. When these cysts rupture, they may stimulate granulomatous inflammation. (a) 20x objective, (b) 50x objective. Wright-Giemsa stain.

acellular, homogenous, pink to blue-gray material, sometimes having a cloud-like formation. These "clouds" likely consist of salivary fluid that has congealed. The presence of this background material should not be overlooked as it is helpful in making a diagnosis. The material is sometimes better visualized by reducing the iris diaphragm. The cellular response is typically modest to low and consists primarily of macrophages and mucin-containing epithelial cells, as well as a few erythrocytes and neutrophils (Figure 41.18a, b). The fluid stimulates a variable inflammatory response. Fluid may gravitate into unusual locations, including the mediastinum. The cells observed are usually macrophages exhibiting marked phagocytic activity. Salivary epithelial cells may resemble macrophages but will have more cytoplasm and no cytophagia. The high viscosity of the fluid may prevent cells from laying flat and therefore the neutrophils may appear as dense blue mononuclear cells. Examination of the preparation in thinner areas will help with the identification of neutrophils. The salivary epithelial cells have abundant cytoplasm with numerous clear vacuoles and variable numbers of distinct purple granules (mucous). The nucleus: cytoplasm ratio is low, often as low as 1 : 5. Macrophages are not as large, they are also vacuolated and often phagocytic, sometimes containing erythrocytes, neutrophils, or hemosiderin. Hematoidin crystals are products of intracellular digestion of rbcs that appear after hemosiderin and are commonly seen in aspirates of sialoceles (Figure 41.18b).

Sialodenosis

Clinical features

Sialodenosis is a clinical entity characterized by noninflammatory, non-neoplastic, idiopathic, usually bilateral enlargement of the mandibular salivary glands in dogs [19]. The salivary glands are sometimes clinically mistaken for enlarged lymph nodes. Clinical signs may include retching and gagging that is responsive to phenobarbital therapy.

Cytologic features

Aspirates of the enlarged salivary gland consist of normal-appearing salivary gland epithelial cells. The salivary epithelial cells are arranged in sheets, are very uniform, and have abundant vacuolated cytoplasm.

Salivary gland infarction

Clinical features

This is either an uncommon lesion or it is diagnosed incorrectly. Salivary gland infarction is more common in younger than older dogs.

Cytologic features

The glands will contain squamous cell metaplasia of the ducts, which has been misinterpreted as SCC. The squamous cells will be large and dysplastic and it is easy to assume they are part of a SCC. Invariably there will be considerable inflammation. Additionally, dead, necrotic material will be admixed with the viable squamous epithelial cells and neutrophils. The main differential is neoplasia; however, salivary gland neoplasia is not common in dogs and cats. Therefore, one should be certain the cellular changes are highly consistent with neoplasia before diagnosing a salivary gland SCC or salivary adenocarcinoma, as the lesion may actually be a salivary gland infarct with squamous metaplasia. The squamous cells in an infarct will be in clusters or sheets but the cells will not have the marked cellular and nuclear pleomorphism that characterize SCC. Many cells are

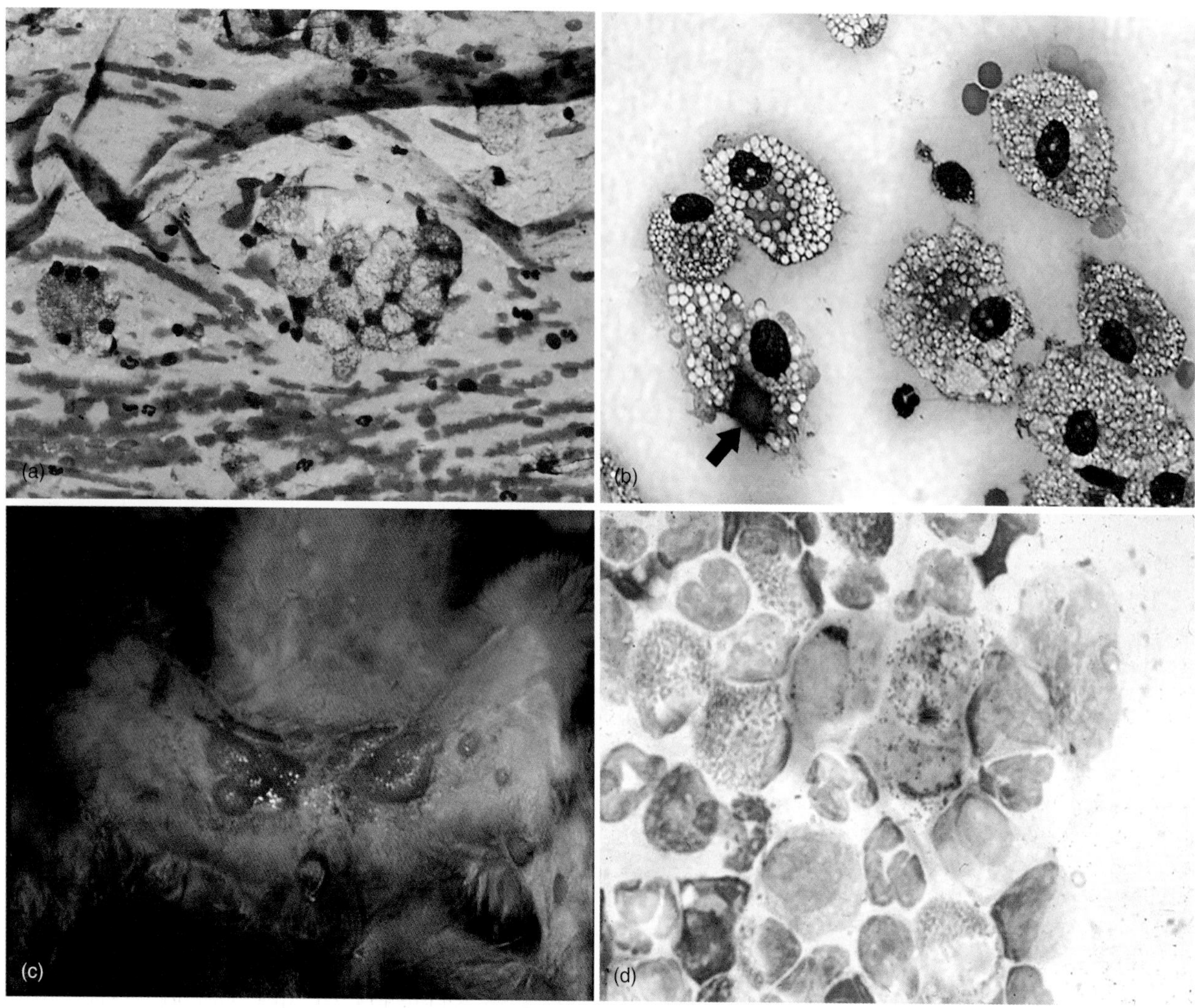

Figure 41.18 (a) Small clusters of uniform salivary gland epithelial cells from a dog with sialocele. Note the abundant, foamy cytoplasm of the epithelial cells, the pink stippled, mucinous background, and lining-up of erythrocytes ("rowing") indicating the presence of thick, viscous fluid (saliva in this case). Mildly increased numbers of neutrophils are consistent with inflammation. (b) Golden, rhomboid hematoidin crystal (arrow) in a macrophage is associated with prior hemorrhage and a frequent finding in sialoceles. (c, d) Cat with eosinophilic granuloma complex. Note the lavender granules within feline eosinophils (d) aspirated from the lesion in (c). Compare to green-black melanin pigment present in pigmented epithelial cells in the center of the image. (a) 50× objective, (b, d) 100× objective. Wright-Giemsa stain.

necrotic. Treatment is surgical excision; histopathology can be used to confirm the diagnosis.

Eosinophilic granuloma

Clinical features

Eosinophilic granulomas occur in the oral cavity and the skin of cats. They are most commonly located on the lips, abdomen, groin and along the pelvic limbs (Figure 41.18c). A similar oral lesion is seen in Siberian huskies.

Cytologic features

Eosinophils will make up greater than 25% of the nucleated cells and may predominate (Figure 41.18d). Mast cells can be numerous but will not be more common than eosinophils. Other cells present in smaller numbers include macrophages and lymphocytes. Fibroblasts may be present in low numbers and some may appear anaplastic. MCT is the main differential; however, eosinophils will not be as plentiful in MCT as they are in eosinophil granulomas (Figures 40.7 and 41.18d). Furthermore, eosinophils are not as prevalent in feline MCT as they are in canine MCT. Other differentials are hypersensitivity reactions secondary to insect bites/stings and parasites.

The diagnostic features of eosinophilic granuloma are that the patient is a cat, location of lesion, and numerous eosinophils present in cytologic preparations.

42 Cytology of Body Cavity Effusions

Robin W. Allison

Department of Veterinary Pathobiology, Oklahoma State University College of Veterinary Medicine, Stillwater, OK, USA

Effusions that develop in the peritoneal or pleural cavities are generally considered indicators of an underlying pathologic or physiologic process rather than a primary disease. Effusions are easily sampled, allowing for analysis that may provide a specific cause for the effusion or, more commonly, categorize the effusion such that a list of differentials can be prioritized. Healthy dogs and cats have a small amount of fluid present in the peritoneal and pleural cavities that is of insufficient quantity to sample. It is possible, however, to obtain a fluid sample from the peritoneal or pleural cavities of healthy horses and cattle.

Sample preparation

Fluid samples should be collected using aseptic technique and an aliquot placed into two tubes: a purple top blood collection tube containing EDTA and a sterile red top blood collection tube. Fluid from the EDTA tube is best for cytologic evaluation, obtaining nucleated cell counts and total protein estimation. Fluid from the sterile red top tube may be used for bacterial or fungal culture and ancillary biochemical testing, if needed. Slides should be prepared and the remaining fluid should be refrigerated if sample processing is not immediate.

Smears for cytologic evaluation should be made shortly after fluid collection. Slides should be air-dried completely, kept at room temperature, protected from formalin fumes, and stained within 3 days to prevent cell deterioration and staining artifacts. Direct smears are made from a well-mixed fluid sample using the same technique used for making blood films. Direct smears are usually adequate if the fluid has at least moderate cellularity (approximately 10,000 cells/μL); such fluid often appears cloudy. Fluids with low cellularity may be clear or hazy, in which case both a direct smear and a concentrated preparation should be evaluated. Many laboratories use a cytocentrifuge to concentrate fluid samples, but fluid samples can be processed in-clinic by centrifuging an aliquot of fluid in a conical tube, removing the supernatant, resuspending the cell pellet, and making a smear from the sediment (the same method used for processing urine samples). The concentrated preparation is best for evaluating various cell populations, while the direct smear is useful for estimating total nucleated cellularity.

Fluid analysis

Physical characteristics

The color and transparency of the fluid can be helpful to classify the effusion. For example, a clear, colorless sample typically has low nucleated cellularity and low total protein concentration, consistent with a transudate. Cloudy, red or pink samples frequently contain blood, which may indicate intracavitary hemorrhage or contamination during sampling. Opaque, tan or beige samples are generally highly cellular, often containing numerous inflammatory cells consistent with an exudate. Samples with a white or milky appearance may contain high concentrations of lipoproteins suggestive of chyle; these samples will continue to appear milky after centrifugation (Figure 42.1).

Total protein concentration

The fluid total protein concentration is used in conjunction with the total cell count to help classify the effusion as to potential etiology (Table 42.1). Fluids with low total protein concentrations and low nucleated cell counts are consistent with transudates, while exudates will have higher total protein concentrations and higher nucleated cell counts. Total protein is usually estimated using a refractometer. If the fluid is cloudy, the fluid should be centrifuged and the protein measured on the supernatant. Chylous effusions, containing high concentrations of lipoproteins that increase the refractive index, will often have artifactually increased total protein measurements.

Veterinary Hematology, Clinical Chemistry, and Cytology, Third Edition. Edited by Mary Anna Thrall, Glade Weiser, Robin W. Allison and Terry W. Campbell.

Companion website: www.wiley.com/go/thrall/veterinary

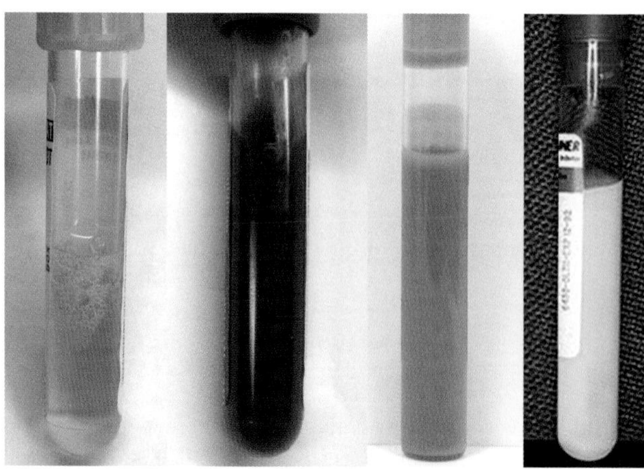

Figure 42.1 Physical characteristics of effusions may provide useful information. From the left, effusions shown here are (a) clear and pale yellow, consistent with a transudate; (b) cloudy and red, as seen with hemorrhage; (c) opaque and tan, consistent with an exudate; (d) milky white, suggestive of a chylous effusion.

Cell counts

Effusions may contain cells other than leukocytes, so it's preferable to refer to the nucleated cell count rather than leukocyte count. Nucleated cell concentrations can be determined with automated hematology instruments or by manual hemacytometer methods. If the fluid contains visible debris or clumped or clotted material, an automated method should not be used as tubing in the electronic cell counter may become clogged. Any clumping of cells will result in an artifactually decreased nucleated cell count. Often, however, estimation of nucleated cell numbers from microscopic evaluation of a direct smear is sufficient for clinical diagnostic interpretation. Erythrocyte concentrations will also be reported by automated analyzers, and a spun packed cell volume (PCV) is helpful to determine if a hemoabdomen or hemothorax is present.

Ancillary testing

In specific situations, additional tests can provide important diagnostic information. For example, if uroabdomen is suspected, creatinine and/or potassium concentrations can be measured in abdominal fluid and compared with serum concentrations. A summary of useful ancillary biochemical tests is provided in Table 42.2.

Cell types found in effusions

Mononuclear cells

This category includes macrophages, lymphocytes and mesothelial cells. These cell types are commonly present in low concentrations in cavitary effusions. Macrophages may appear quiescent, resembling large monocytes, or activated with abundant cytoplasmic vacuoles that may contain phagocytized cells, microorganisms or debris (Figure 42.2).

Table 42.1 Classification scheme for peritoneal and pleural effusions.

Classification	Total protein (g/dL)	Total nucleated cells/µL	Typical cell types	Comments
Transudate (protein-poor)	<2.5	<1500	Neutrophils, macrophages	Reactive mesothelial cells may be present.
Transudate (protein-rich)	>2.5	<5000	Neutrophils, macrophages	Reactive mesothelial cells may be present.
Exudate	>2.5	>5000 (dogs, cats) >10,000 (horses)	Neutrophils, macrophages, reactive mesothelial cells	Neutrophils may be degenerate. Microorganisms may be present. Mixed bacteria and plant material may be seen with gastrointestinal tract leakage.
Bile peritonitis	>2.5	>5000	Neutrophils, macrophages, reactive mesothelial cells	Bile pigment or mucinous material may be present.
FIP	>4	<5000	Neutrophils, macrophages	Prominent proteinaceous background present.
Chylous	>2.5	Variable	Small lymphocytes, finely vacuolated macrophages	Neutrophil numbers increase with time. Total protein often artifactually increased.
Uroperitoneum	<2.5	Variable	Neutrophils, macrophages, reactive mesothelial cells	Neutrophils may appear degenerate. Bacteria absent unless urinary tract infection exists.
Hemorrhagic	>2.5	Variable	Erythrocytes, leukocytes from peripheral blood	Platelets absent unless hemorrhage is acute or ongoing.
Neoplastic	Variable	Variable	Neoplastic cells (lymphocytes, mast cells, epithelial cells, mesothelial cells)	May have concurrent inflammation and reactive mesothelial cells.

Table 42.2 Selected ancillary tests for peritoneal and pleural effusions.

Parameter	Suspected condition	Expected results
α_1-acid glycoprotein (AGP)	FIP	Effusion AGP >1500 µg/mL
Albumin-globulin ratio (A : G)	FIP	Effusion A : G <0.9
Creatinine	Uroperitoneum	Effusion creatinine ≥2× serum creatinine
Potassium	Uroperitoneum	Effusion potassium >1.4× serum potassium
Total bilirubin	Bile peritonitis	Effusion bilirubin ≥2× serum bilirubin
Triglyceride	Chylous effusion	Effusion triglyceride > serum triglyceride Effusion triglyceride >100 mg/dL

Normal small to intermediate sized lymphocytes have a similar appearance to lymphocytes in peripheral blood, and are often the predominant cell type in chylous effusions. Reactive lymphocytes with more abundant deeply basophilic cytoplasm may be present as part of an inflammatory process. If lymphocytes are predominantly large cells containing nuclei with dispersed chromatin and nucleoli, lymphoma should be suspected (see Chapter 45).

Mesothelial cells, which line the peritoneal and pleural cavities and cover the viscera, frequently exfoliate into effusions. They are large round cells with a round nucleus and moderately abundant basophilic cytoplasm. Cytoplasmic borders may show a distinct pink fringe or cytoplasmic blebs

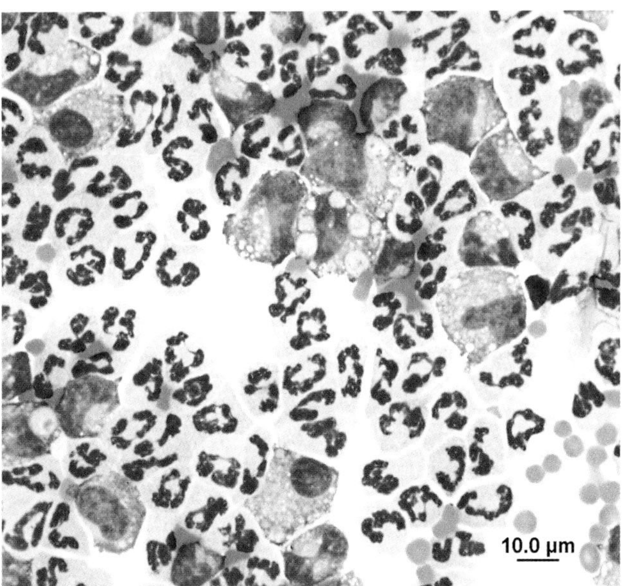

Figure 42.2 Nondegenerate neutrophils and macrophages, peritoneal effusion, horse (concentrated preparation). Neutrophils have dense chromatin and distinct segments; a few have become hypersegmented (an aging change). Macrophages have oval to indented nuclei with variable cytoplasmic vacuolation. Several macrophages contain phagocytized cell debris. Low numbers of erythrocytes are present in the background. Aqueous Romanowsky stain.

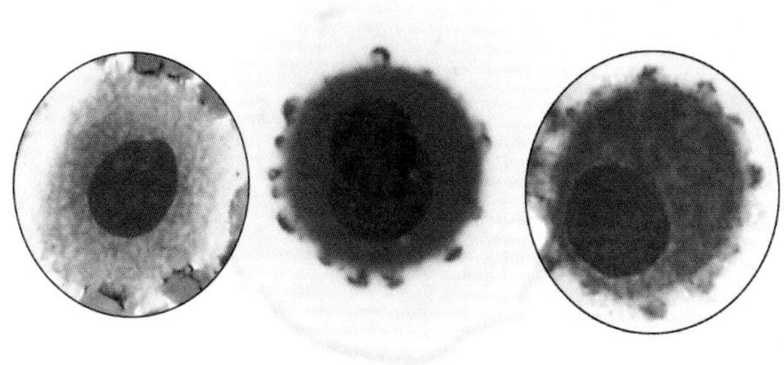

Figure 42.3 Mesothelial cells, pleural and peritoneal effusions, dog. Mesothelial cells have round to oval nuclei, may be binucleated, and often have a pink cytoplasmic fringe or cytoplasmic blebs. Aqueous Romanowsky stain.

(Figure 42.3). They are usually arranged individually or in small cohesive clusters. Mesothelial cells become hyperplastic and reactive whenever fluid accumulates in the pleural or peritoneal space, and especially when inflammation is present. Reactive mesothelial cells may be present in larger clusters and can sometimes be confused with neoplastic cells when they develop significant criteria of malignancy, including prominent nucleoli, deeply basophilic cytoplasm, anisocytosis, and anisokaryosis (Figure 42.4). Cells in mitosis may also be observed. Reactive mesothelial cells, when present in large numbers, may be difficult or impossible to distinguish from carcinoma or mesothelioma (discussed later). Fortunately, mesothelial cells are usually present in small numbers.

Neutrophils

A few neutrophils are often present in effusions, but the concentration can increase dramatically with inflammation.

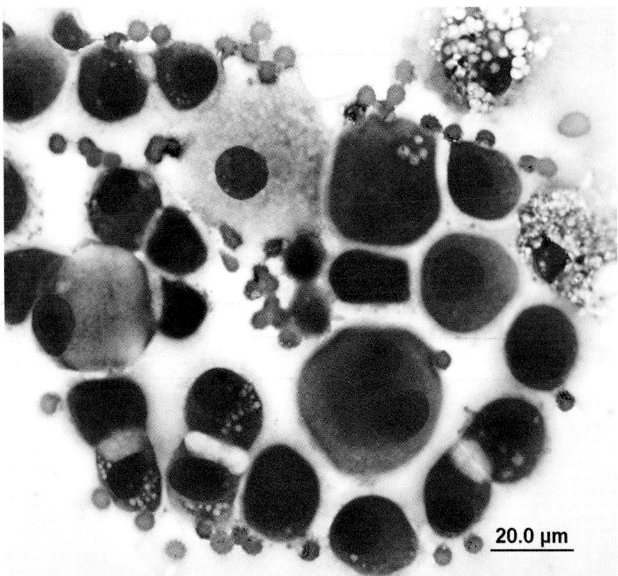

Figure 42.4 Reactive mesothelial cells, peritoneal effusion, dog (concentrated preparation). These reactive mesothelial cells are present individually and in small cohesive clusters. The cells have multiple criteria of malignancy including anisocytosis, anisokaryosis, and binucleation with prominent nucleoli, which raise suspicion for neoplasia. Two highly vacuolated activated macrophages are present in the upper right corner, and there are low numbers of erythrocytes in the background. Aqueous Romanowsky stain.

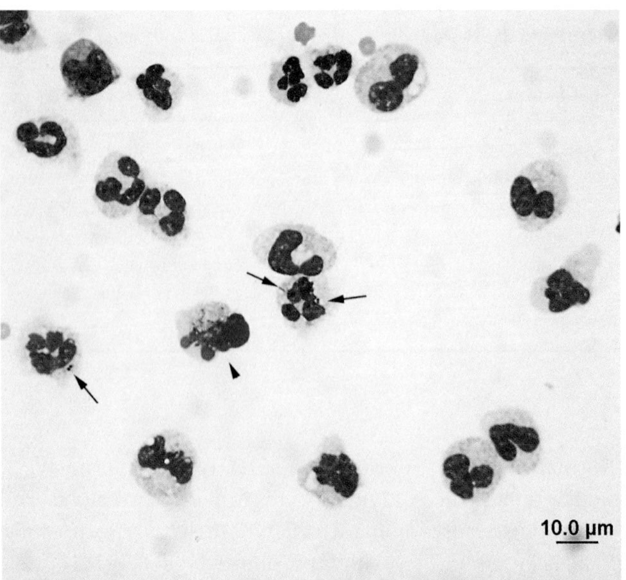

Figure 42.5 Degenerate neutrophils, peritoneal effusion, horse. Most of these neutrophils are degenerate with swollen nuclei that lack distinct segmentation. One nucleus has lysed (arrowhead). Two cells contain phagocytized bacteria (arrows), making this a septic exudate. Aqueous Romanowsky stain.

The morphology of normal, nondegenerate neutrophils in effusions is similar to that of neutrophils in peripheral blood. Nuclear chromatin is dense and segmentation is distinct (Figure 42.2). When neutrophils undergo normal aging within an effusion they become hypersegmented and pyknotic, and are eventually phagocytized by macrophages (cytophagia). Degenerate neutrophils have swollen nuclei that lose segmentation and stain pale pink; these cells may go on to disintegrate and become unrecognizable (Figure 42.5). Degenerate neutrophils suggest the presence of bacterial toxins. Neutrophils can also degenerate *in vitro*, and for this reason it is important to make smears of effusions prior to shipping to a diagnostic laboratory.

Eosinophils and mast cells

Eosinophils in effusions have the same morphology as those in peripheral blood and are usually few in number. The nuclei of aged eosinophils usually lose segmentations and become round. Increased eosinophil concentration (>10% of cells) may occur with a variety of underlying conditions including hypersensitivity disorders, parasitic infections, lung lobe torsion, heart failure, mast cell neoplasia, and some types of lymphoma (Figure 42.6) [1–3]. Mast cells have round nuclei and abundant cytoplasmic granules that stain dark purple with alcohol-based Romanowsky stains. Granules sometimes stain poorly or not at all with water-based (aqueous) Romanowsky stains (Figure 42.7) [4, 5]. Mast cells

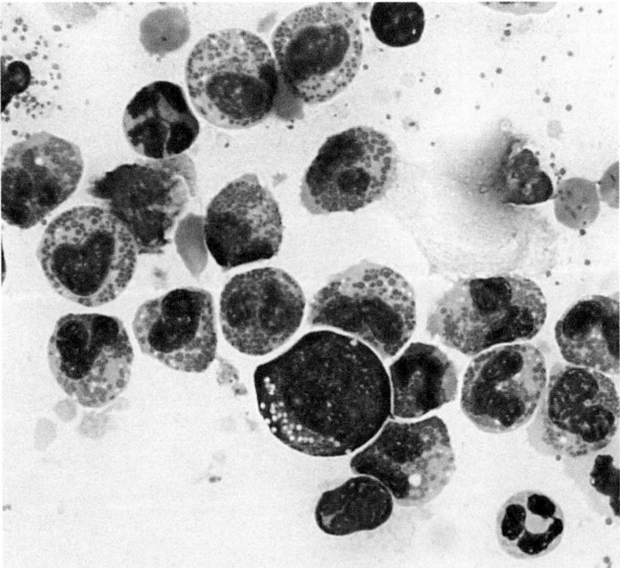

Figure 42.6 Eosinophils, peritoneal effusion, dog. Numerous eosinophils containing round, pink cytoplasmic granules are present. Granules are also seen free in the background, with few erythrocytes. A single large neoplastic lymphocyte contains a round nucleus with multiple nucleoli and has deeply basophilic cytoplasm containing a few vacuoles. This dog had lymphoma involving the mesenteric lymph nodes, liver, and intestine. Wright stain.

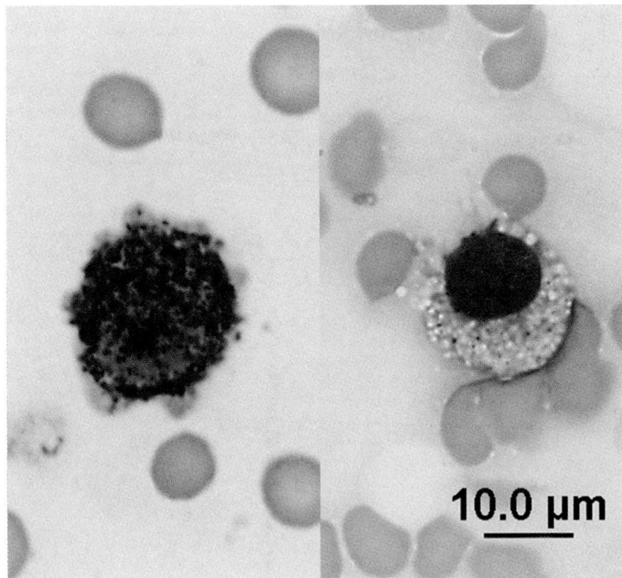

Figure 42.7 Mast cells, alcohol-based Romanowsky stain (left) and aqueous Romanowsky stain (right). Mast cells often contain abundant cytoplasmic granules that obscure the nucleus. These granules stain dark purple with alcohol-based Romanowsky stains but may stain poorly or not at all with aqueous Romanowsky stains.

may accompany many types of inflammatory conditions, but concentrations are generally low in effusions. Mast cell tumors within a body cavity can exfoliate large numbers of mast cells into an effusion, and cell morphology may be atypical (see Chapters 40 and 41).

Erythrocytes

Erythrocytes may be seen in large numbers whenever there is hemorrhage into a body cavity or when there is iatrogenic blood contamination at the time of sampling. Differentiating these situations is important and discussed in the section on hemorrhagic effusions. Inadvertent aspiration of the spleen will also result in a sample containing abundant blood.

Neoplastic cells

Tumors within the pleural or peritoneal cavities frequently cause effusions but do not always exfoliate neoplastic cells into the effusion. Tumor types most likely to exfoliate cells, and therefore be identified by cytologic evaluation, include lymphoma, mast cell tumor, carcinoma/adenocarcinoma, and mesothelioma. Details are discussed in the section on neoplastic effusions.

Effusion classifications and cytologic findings

Table 42.1 presents a classification scheme for peritoneal and pleural effusions that is based on total nucleated cell counts, total protein concentrations, and cytologic findings. Cutoff values used for total nucleated cell counts and total protein concentrations in the various categories of effusions vary by author [2, 6, 7]. Historically, the term "modified transudate" has been used to describe effusions that don't fit neatly into the transudate or exudate category based on nucleated cell counts and protein concentrations, but describing an effusion as a modified transudate has limited utility because of the wide variety of potential underlying disorders. It is preferable to use all of the effusion characteristics, including cytologic findings, to classify such effusions as specifically as possible.

Transudates

Transudates form secondary to decreased vascular oncotic pressure, increased hydrostatic pressure, or decreased lymphatic drainage [7]. Transudates can be further characterized as protein-poor or protein-rich.

- Protein-poor transudates (pure transudates): The most common cause is severe hypoalbuminemia, which may be associated with diseases such as protein-losing nephropathy or enteropathy and hepatic insufficiency or failure. Other potential causes include portal hypertension (presinusoidal or sinusoidal), portosystemic shunt and early cardiac insufficiency. Protein-poor transudates are clear and colorless with a low total protein concentration (<2.5 g/dL) and low total nucleated cell count (<1500/µL). Cytologically, the nucleated cells consist of mononuclear cells (macrophages, small lymphocytes, and mesothelial cells), and nondegenerate neutrophils. Mesothelial cells may become reactive if the effusion is long-standing.
- Protein-rich transudates: These effusions have also been referred to as modified transudates. They most commonly form secondary to congestive heart failure and portal hypertension (postsinusoidal). Increased hydrostatic pressure causes high-protein fluid to escape vessels in the lungs or liver. Protein-rich transudates may be clear to hazy with an increased total protein concentration (>2.5 g/dL) and low to moderate numbers of nucleated cells (<5000/µL) consisting of mononuclear cells and nondegenerate neutrophils. Mesothelial cells may be reactive.

Exudates

Exudative effusions form when inflammation alters capillary permeability. The underlying inflammation may be caused by infectious or noninfectious disorders such as bacterial, fungal, protozoal or viral infections, parasites such as *Mesocestoides*, pancreatitis, bowel or biliary tract rupture, organ necrosis and neoplasia. Exudates are hazy, cloudy or opaque with an increased total protein concentration (>2.5 mg/dL) and large numbers of nucleated cells (>5000/µL in dogs and cats or >10,000/µL in horses [8]). Nucleated cells are usually predominantly neutrophils, which may be degenerate, with variable numbers of macrophages and mesothelial cells (Figure 42.8). Cytology may allow differentiation of

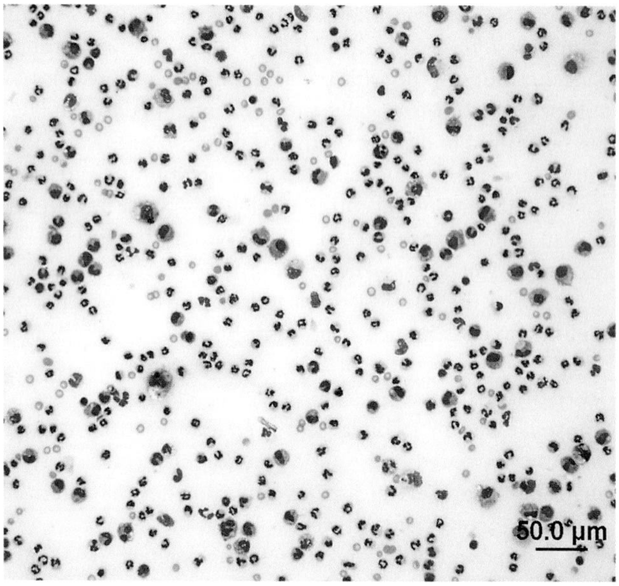

Figure 42.8 Exudate, pleural effusion, dog. This direct smear has high nucleated cellularity consisting predominantly of neutrophils with moderate numbers of macrophages, low numbers of small lymphocytes, and moderate numbers of erythrocytes. Some of the neutrophils are degenerate, so bacterial and fungal cultures would be recommended even in the absence of visible microorganisms. Aqueous Romanowsky stain.

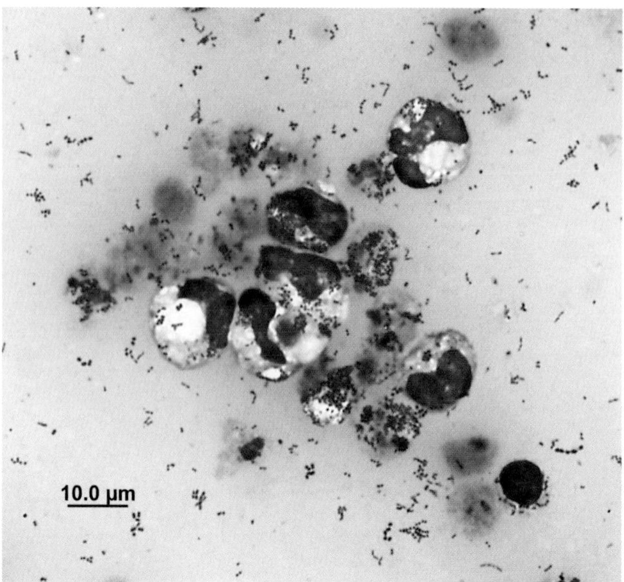

Figure 42.9 Septic exudate, pleural effusion, horse. Many bacteria are visible free in the background and phagocytized by leukocytes that are markedly degenerate (likely neutrophils). Bacterial culture identified two populations of bacteria (*Streptococcus zooepidemicus* and *Arcanobacterium pyogenes*). The nucleated cell count was 73,000/µL, and total protein was 5.5 g/dL. Aqueous Romanowsky stain.

specific types of exudates, discussed below. Bacterial and/or fungal cultures may be needed to identify specific infectious agents and may be useful to rule-out infectious causes when microorganisms are not visualized.

Septic exudates

Neutrophils are often degenerate, which should prompt close evaluation for the presence of microorganisms. In some cases, neutrophils may be so degenerate that most cells lyse, resulting in lower than expected total nucleated cell counts. Bacteria may be observed extracellularly or intracellularly, phagocytized by neutrophils and/or macrophages (Figure 42.9). Phagocytized bacteria must be seen in order to refer to an effusion as septic. In cases of infections secondary to penetrating foreign bodies or gastrointestinal leakage, a mixed population of bacteria (cocci, rods, spirochetes) may be evident. In addition to bacteria, other microorganisms that may be identified include yeast or fungi (such as *Histoplasma* spp., *Candida* spp., *Blastomyces* spp.) and protozoa (*Toxoplasma* spp., *Neospora* spp.) (see Chapter 39). Peritonitis related to *Candida* spp. has been recognized in dogs that had gastrointestinal or biliary tract leakage (Figure 42.10) [9]. In cases of gastrointestinal tract rupture or leakage, plant material (ingesta) and other fecal debris may be present in addition to a mixed bacterial population (Figures 42.11 and 42.12). Large ciliated protozoa (normal gastrointestinal tract flora) may be observed in peritoneal effusions from horses with gastrointestinal tract leakage (Figure 42.13).

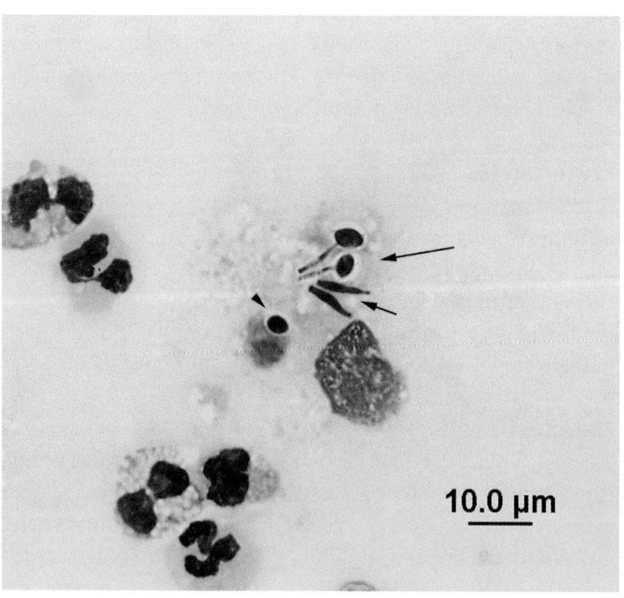

Figure 42.10 Fungal peritonitis, dog. Two hyphal structures (short arrow), two germ tubes emerging from yeast (long arrow), and one yeast form (arrowhead) are present extracellularly. Organisms were also seen phagocytized. Fungal culture grew *Candida albicans*, which was confirmed by polymerase chain reaction. This dog developed a fungal peritonitis following dehiscence of a previous intestinal resection site. Aqueous Romanowsky stain.

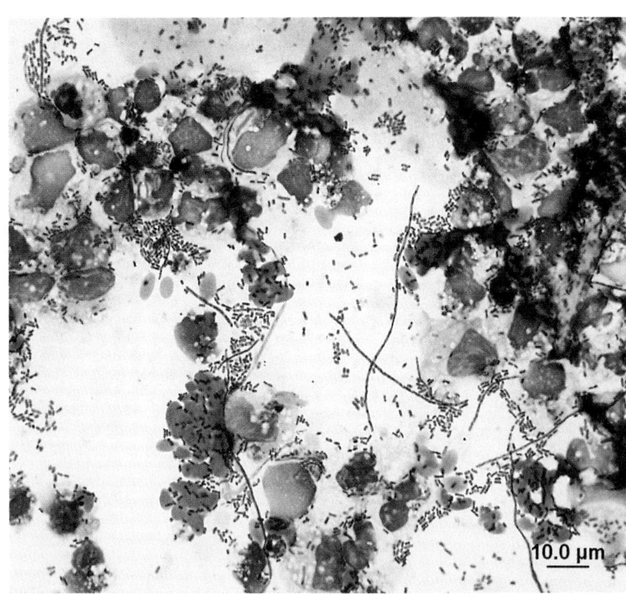

Figure 42.11 Septic exudate, peritoneal effusion, alpaca (concentrated preparation). Large numbers of mixed bacteria are present extracellularly and phagocytized by leukocytes. Leukocytes are degenerate and lysed, which makes them difficult to identify, but are most likely neutrophils. Low numbers of erythrocytes are present. The total protein was 2.7 g/dL, and the total nucleated cell count was 3000/µL, which is lower than expected likely because lysed neutrophils were not counted. This alpaca had an intestinal tract rupture resulting in septic peritonitis. Wright stain.

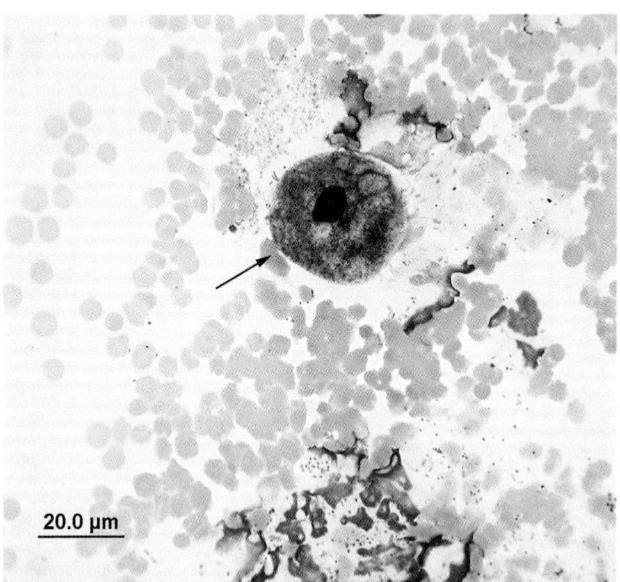

Figure 42.13 Ciliated protozoan, peritoneal effusion, horse (concentrated preparation). The arrow points to a large ciliated protozoal organism, which is a normal inhabitant of the intestinal tract. Neutrophils are degenerate and lysed, and there are numerous bacteria present intra- and extracellularly, with many erythrocytes in the background. These findings indicate septic peritonitis caused by intestinal tract leakage. The total protein was 4.7 g/dL, but the nucleated cell count was only 800/µL, probably because most of the neutrophils were lysed and couldn't be counted. Wright stain.

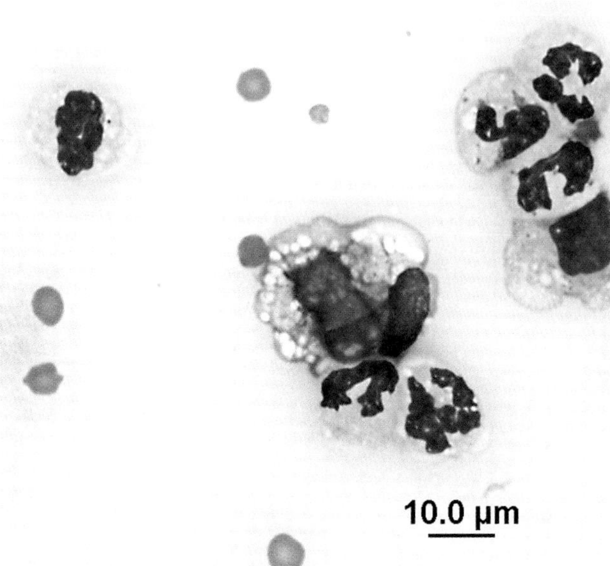

Figure 42.12 Plant material, peritoneal effusion, horse. The vacuolated macrophage in the center contains a large blue fragment of phagocytized plant material. Total nucleated cellularity was high, estimated at >200,000/µL from the direct smear. Neutrophils represented 74% of cells and were often degenerate. This horse had septic peritonitis caused by intestinal tract leakage. Aqueous Romanowsky stain.

Accidental enterocentesis may also be a cause for the presence of mixed bacteria and ingesta in cytologic samples.

Bile peritonitis

Bile is a chemical irritant in the peritoneal cavity that causes inflammation. Bile leakage can occur because of damage to the gallbladder or bile duct, which may be secondary to underlying disorders such as bile duct obstruction, cholecystitis or cholangitis, mucocele formation, trauma, and biliary neoplasia. Grossly, the effusion may be orange, brown or green tinged from the bile pigments. Neutrophils are typically most numerous with variable numbers of macrophages. Bacteria or fungal organisms (*Candida* spp.) may also be present. Bile pigment may be visualized on cytologic preparations as amorphous blue-green to yellow-green extracellular material (Figure 42.14); such material may also be seen phagocytized by macrophages. Phagocytized bile pigment can be difficult to differentiate from hemosiderin in some cases. When bile peritonitis is suspected, measurement of effusion total bilirubin concentration may be useful; effusion total bilirubin concentration that is at least two times greater than the serum total bilirubin concentration supports biliary tract leakage (Table 42.2) [10, 11].

So-called "white bile" has been described in cases of biliary mucocele or bile duct ruptures [11]. This material is mucinous and does not contain the greenish bile pigment. Instead

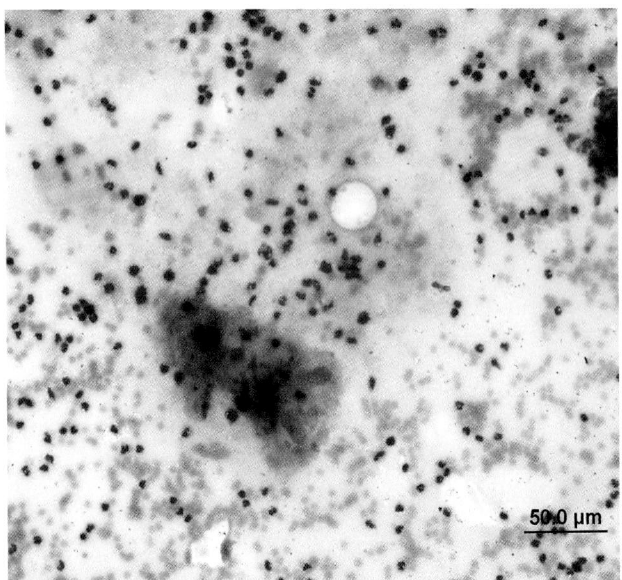

Figure 42.14 Bile peritonitis, dog. Nucleated cellularity is high and consists predominantly of neutrophils with many erythrocytes in the background. The green-yellow material is consistent with bile pigment, and the pale blue amorphous material is typical of mucinous "white bile." Aqueous Romanowsky stain.

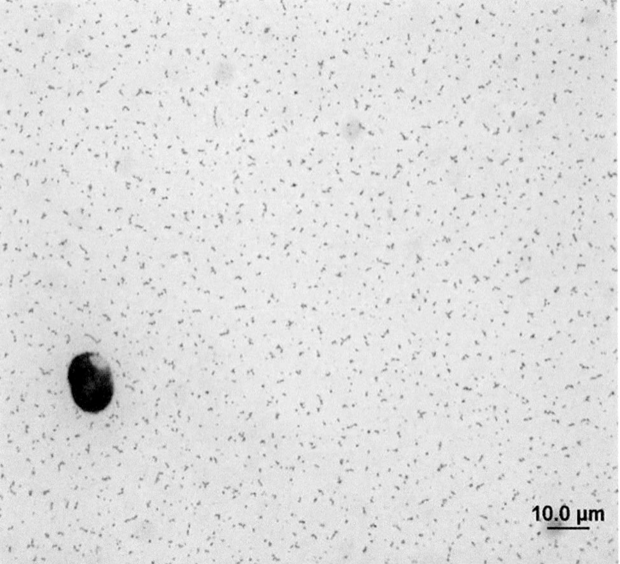

Figure 42.15 FIP, abdominal effusion, cat. One macrophage is present in a prominent pink, stippled background consistent with a high protein concentration. The pink protein precipitates should not be confused with bacteria, which stain blue with routine cytologic stains. The total nucleated cell count was 300/µL, the total protein was 6.0 g/dL, and the A : G ratio was 0.3. Aqueous Romanowsky stain.

it appears as lakes of pale basophilic amorphous material, usually seen in the background of the smear (Figure 42.14). The effusion is typically exudative, but effusion total bilirubin concentration is not always greater than the serum total bilirubin concentration. Measuring effusion bile acid concentration may still be helpful in these cases [12].

Feline infectious peritonitis (FIP)

Peritoneal and pleural effusions caused by FIP are somewhat unique. Grossly the effusion is usually yellow and clear to hazy, viscous, and may contain small flecks of fibrin. Although the effusion is caused by inflammation (vasculitis), nucleated cell counts are typically lower than the 5000/µL threshold for an exudate. Nucleated cells are a mixture of nondegenerate neutrophils and macrophages. Total protein concentration is high, frequently exceeding 4 g/dL [13]. These proteins are visible on cytologic preparations as pink, granular precipitates in the background (Figure 42.15). Measuring the effusion albumin and globulin concentrations may be useful (Table 42.2). Globulins are expected to dominate, so an albumin to globulin ratio (A : G) less than 0.9 is consistent with FIP [14]. Acute phase protein concentrations can also be measured in effusions and are expected to be high in cats with FIP. In one study, an effusion α_1-acid glycoprotein (AGP) concentration of >1550 µg/mL had a 93% sensitivity and specificity for diagnosing FIP [15]. The Rivalta test is a relatively simple in-clinic procedure that involves adding effusion fluid to a dilute acetic acid solution and observing if a white protein precipitate forms (positive test). Although it has long been popular for its low cost, the predictive value of a positive test is only 58.4%, and there is considerable subjectivity in determining a positive test result [16, 17].

Chylous effusions

Chylous effusions form when lymph containing a high concentration of chylomicrons leaks from lymphatic vessels, most often in the pleural cavity. Underlying causes for such leakage include trauma and many different disorders that may obstruct lymphatics, including heart disease, lung lobe torsion, diaphragmatic hernia, neoplastic masses, and other mass lesions such as granulomas. Some cases are idiopathic. Chylous effusions are usually milky white and opaque (Figure 42.1), and do not clear with centrifugation. Total protein concentration is artifactually increased by the presence of lipoproteins (chylomicrons), which increase the refractive index. Nucleated cell concentrations are variable but consist predominantly of small lymphocytes and macrophages; neutrophil concentrations may increase with chronicity because of inflammation associated with fluid accumulation or repeated thoracocentesis. Macrophages frequently contain numerous fine clear vacuoles consistent with lipid (Figure 42.16). Chylomicrons contain a high concentration of triglycerides, so comparing triglyceride concentrations with that of serum is helpful to confirm chylous effusion (Table 42.2). Chylous effusions will have higher triglyceride (typically >100 mg/dL) concentrations relative to serum [18, 19].

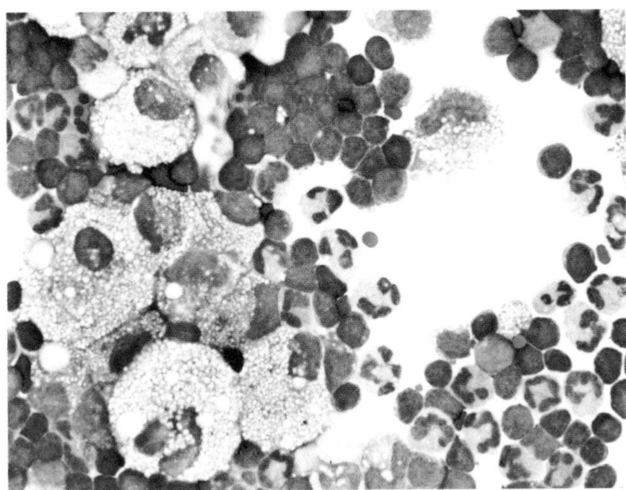

Figure 42.16 Chylous pleural effusion, cat (concentrated preparation). Lymphocytes, small to intermediate in size, predominate (77% of cells) with lower numbers of nondegenerate neutrophils (20%) and macrophages (3%). Macrophages contain numerous fine, distinct cytoplasmic granules suggestive of lipid. In chylous effusions, neutrophil numbers often increase with chronicity of the effusion. Wright stain.

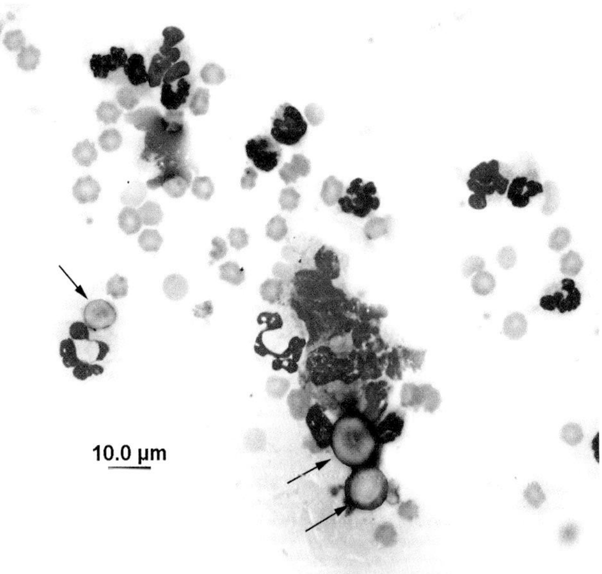

Figure 42.17 Uroperitoneum, horse (concentrated preparation). Arrows point to three crystalline structures that are consistent with calcium carbonate urinary crystals. Degenerate and nondegenerate neutrophils are present with few erythrocytes. The total nucleated cell count was 4300/μL, total protein was <2.5 mg/dL, and effusion creatinine concentration was 44 mg/dL. Wright stain.

Uroperitoneum

Urine may leak into the peritoneal cavity because of a variety of underlying disorders (such as trauma, neoplasia and urolithiasis) involving the urinary bladder, urethra, ureters, and kidneys. Urine is usually sterile unless there is a urinary tract infection, but urine acts as a chemical irritant causing inflammation. Nucleated cell concentrations and types of cells present will vary depending on duration of the effusion and the dilutional effect of the urine volume present, but cell concentrations are generally low to moderate and total protein concentration is low. Mononuclear cells predominate early and the neutrophil concentration increases with chronicity. Neutrophils may appear degenerate even in the absence of bacteria because of the inhospitable environment caused by urine. Occasionally, urinary crystals can be observed on the smear, confirming the diagnosis (Figure 42.17). When uroperitoneum is suspected, measuring creatinine or potassium concentration in the effusion and comparing to the serum concentration is helpful (Table 42.2). Creatinine is preferred to urea (BUN) because urea diffuses faster from the effusion back into blood. Generally, if uroperitoneum is present, the creatinine concentration in the effusion is expected to be greater than twice that of serum in samples obtained concurrently [20–22]. An abdominal fluid to serum potassium concentration ratio of >1.4 : 1 is also predictive of uroabdomen, with a sensitivity and specificity of 100% in one study [22]. However, stomach secretions are also high in potassium, and high abdominal fluid potassium concentration with a fluid to serum ratio of greater than 2.67 : 1 has been reported with gastric perforation [23].

Hemorrhagic effusions

Hemorrhagic effusions are caused by underlying disorders that result in bleeding into the thoracic or peritoneal cavities, such as trauma, neoplasia, and hemostatic defects. The effusion characteristics vary depending on the amount of blood present and the duration of hemorrhage, but a fluid PCV >3% suggests hemorrhage is contributory [7]. Total protein concentration is often >2.5 g/dL and nucleated cell numbers are low to moderate, consisting mainly of leukocytes, the distribution of which is reflective of peripheral blood. If neoplasia is the underlying cause, neoplastic cells may or may not be identified on the smear; hemangiosarcoma is frequently associated with hemorrhage but neoplastic cells are rarely recognized in the effusion. When hemorrhage is acute or ongoing, platelets may be present, but platelets rapidly aggregate and disappear from body cavities. Macrophages are frequently present and may contain phagocytized erythrocytes if the hemorrhage duration is greater than 24 hours. With chronicity, red cell breakdown products (hemosiderin, hematoidin) become evident within macrophages (Figures 42.18 and 42.19). Hemosiderin is usually blue-green but can be quite variable (yellow, green, blue) [24]. Since it contains iron, hemosiderin can be confirmed with an iron stain such as Prussian blue. Hematoidin does not contain iron but has a distinct golden yellow to amber crystalline appearance.

Iatrogenic hemorrhage during the sample collection process must be differentiated from true pathologic hemorrhage.

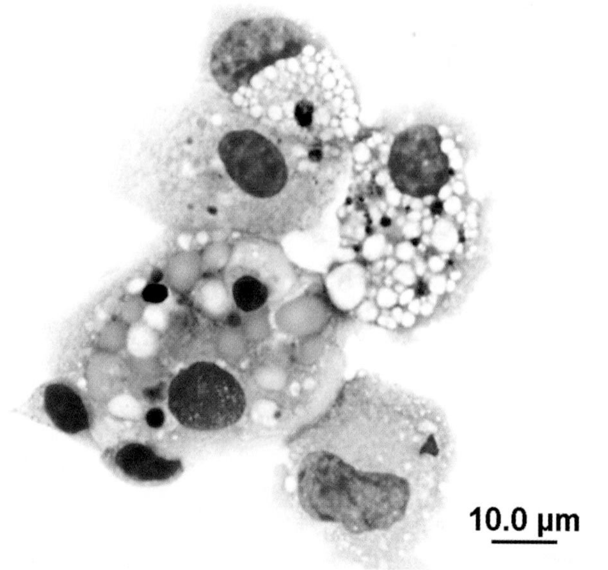

Figure 42.18 Evidence of previous hemorrhage, horse. Macrophages contain phagocytized erythrocytes (lower left) and/or dark blue-green globular pigment consistent with hemosiderin, a red-cell breakdown product containing iron. Aqueous Romanowsky stain.

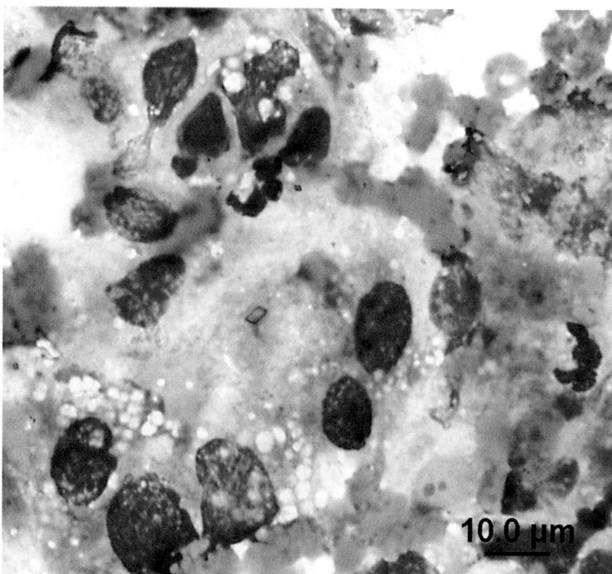

Figure 42.19 Evidence of previous hemorrhage, dog. Vacuolated macrophages contain crystalline golden to amber hematoidin, a red-cell breakdown product lacking iron. The amorphous yellow material is likely hemosiderin. Aqueous Romanowsky stain.

Many samples contain small numbers of erythrocytes as a result of minor contamination, and this does not cause a diagnostic challenge. When marked blood contamination is suspected, it is useful to consider presence or absence of platelets and red cell breakdown products as presented in Table 42.3. Inadvertent aspiration of the spleen may also result in a grossly bloody sample. In that case the effusion PCV may be greater than that of peripheral blood, platelets will be present, and hematopoietic precursors may be seen on the smear if extramedullary hematopoiesis is present in the spleen, which is common.

Neoplastic effusions

An effusion is characterized as neoplastic if there are identifiable neoplastic cells present. Many different types of tumors can exfoliate cells into an effusion, but in general, round cell tumors (such as lymphoma or mast cell tumor), carcinomas, and mesotheliomas do so much more readily than do mesenchymal tumors (sarcomas). Lack of identifiable neoplastic cells does not exclude neoplasia as the underlying cause of an effusion. Effusion characteristics are variable; there may be inflammation or hemorrhage present in addition to the neoplastic cells, which may be rare or numerous.

Neoplasia is easiest to recognize when there are large numbers of neoplastic cells with marked criteria of malignancy and there isn't concurrent inflammation or significant hemorrhage (see Chapter 40). Additionally, the presence of numerous reactive mesothelial cells may be confounding.

Lymphoma

Neoplastic lymphocytes in effusions look similar to those in other cytologic samples (see Chapter 45), and may be present individually in small to large numbers. Typically, neoplastic lymphocytes are larger than neutrophils, have high nucleus:cytoplasm ratios, and contain nuclei with a fine chromatin pattern (Figures 42.6 and 42.20). Nuclear outlines may be irregular, and large, prominent nucleoli are often evident. Lymphoma may involve large granular lymphocytes, which have distinct magenta cytoplasmic granules (Figure 42.21). Gastrointestinal lymphoma may cause a bowel perforation, in which case there may be a confusing mixture of inflammatory cells with phagocytized mixed bacteria (septic peritonitis) and variable numbers of neoplastic lymphocytes (Figure 42.22).

Mast cell tumor

Neoplastic mast cells may exfoliate from intracavitary mast cell tumors in large numbers. Mast cells have round nuclei and contain variable numbers of metachromatic (dark purple) cytoplasmic granules that can obscure the nucleus (see Chapter 41). In effusions, mast cell granules may have a packeted appearance in the cytoplasm. Cells from high grade tumors have more criteria of malignancy (anisokaryosis, karyomegaly, multinucleation) and may contain fewer granules (Figure 42.23) [25]. Mast cell granules may stain poorly or not at all with commonly used aqueous Romanowsky dip stains (Figure 42.7) [4, 5].

Carcinoma

Intracavitary carcinomas or adenocarcinomas may exfoliate neoplastic cells in small to large numbers. In contrast to lymphoma and mast cell tumors, neoplastic epithelial cells

Table 42.3 Distinguishing causes of hemorrhagic effusions.

Cytologic findings	Possible processes	Comments
Platelets present No erythrophagocytosis No hemosiderin, hematoidin	• Iatrogenic hemorrhage • Acute hemorrhage	Iatrogenic hemorrhage (blood contamination during sampling) is most common.
No platelets present Erythrophagocytosis and/or hemosiderin, hematoidin present	• Previous hemorrhage	Following hemorrhage, platelets disappear rapidly, erythrophagocytosis may occur within hours, hemosiderin or hematoidin may appear within a couple days.
Platelets present Erythrophagocytosis and/or hemosiderin, hematoidin present	• Ongoing hemorrhage • Previous hemorrhage combined with iatrogenic hemorrhage	Platelets are observed most often with blood contamination but may also be present if hemorrhage is acute or ongoing.

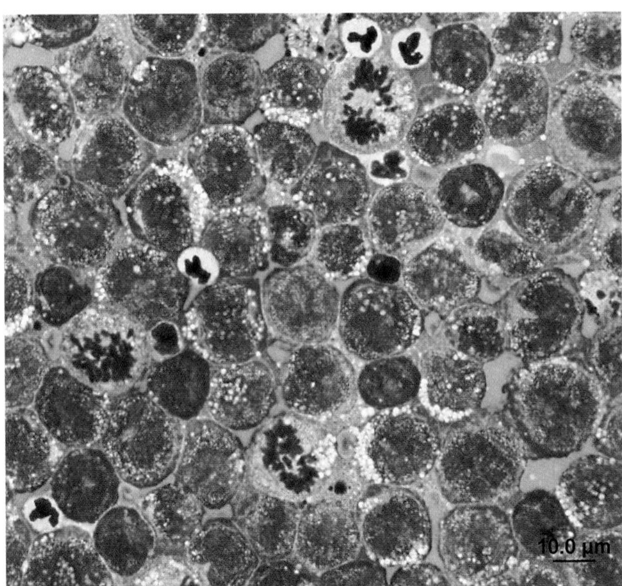

Figure 42.20 Neoplastic pleural effusion, lymphoma, dog (concentrated preparation). Neoplastic lymphocytes predominate and are large cells with high nucleus:cytoplasm ratios, dispersed chromatin, and prominent nucleoli. Nuclear outlines are irregular, and many mitotic figures are present. In this case, many of the lymphocytes have small cytoplasmic vacuoles. Few nondegenerate neutrophils and erythrocytes are also present. Aqueous Romanowsky stain.

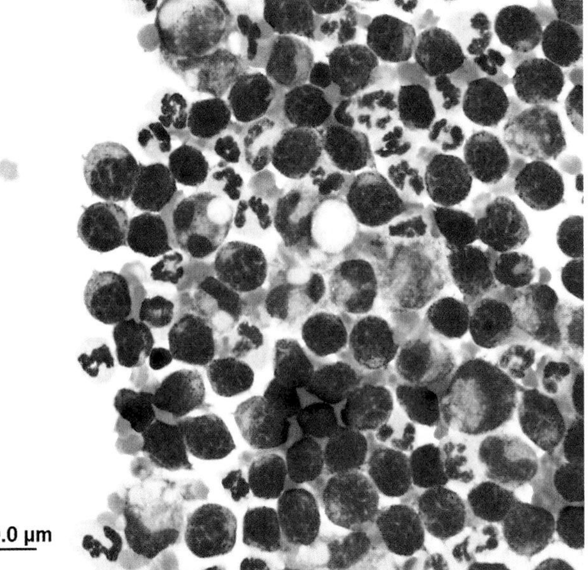

Figure 42.21 Neoplastic peritoneal effusion, large granular lymphocyte (LGL) lymphoma, horse (concentrated preparation). Most of the cells are large atypical lymphocytes containing coarse chromatin and distinct magenta cytoplasmic granules, consistent with LGLs. Other cells include nondegenerate neutrophils, macrophages, and erythrocytes. This horse had LGL lymphoma affecting the intestine. Aqueous Romanowsky stain.

tend to form cohesive clusters and are sometimes present in large sheets (Figures 42.24 and 42.25). Acinar structures may be recognized (Figure 42.26). Individualized cells may also be present and are typically large cells with rounded cell borders, easily confused with reactive mesothelial cells. Neoplastic epithelial cells often have marked nuclear criteria of malignancy including anisokaryosis, macrokaryosis, multinucleation, and coarse chromatin with large bizarre nucleoli (Figures 42.25 and 42.27). Mitotic figures and atypical mitoses may be observed (Figure 42.25). Cytoplasm is usually deeply basophilic and may be vacuolated or contain secretory material that pushes the nucleus to one side (Figures 42.25 and 42.28). There may be significant inflammation present concurrently. When carcinoma is suspected, differential diagnoses that should be considered include mesothelioma and markedly reactive mesothelial cells (discussed below).

Mesothelioma and reactive mesothelial cells

The distinction between reactive or hyperplastic mesothelial cells, mesothelioma and carcinoma is difficult and often

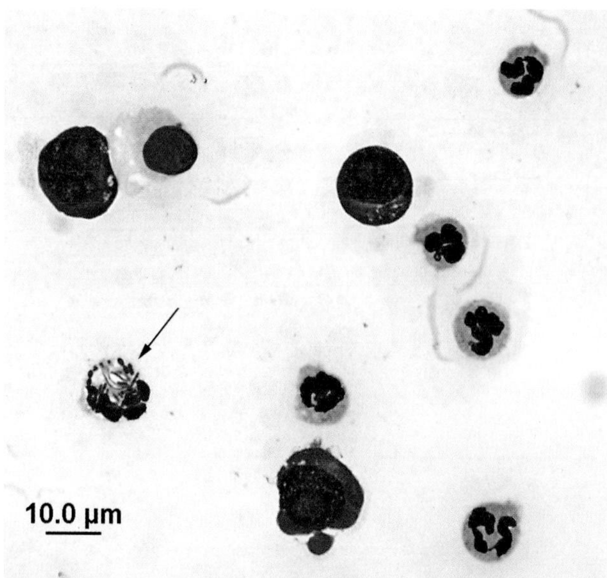

Figure 42.22 Neoplastic peritoneal effusion (lymphoma) with septic inflammation, cat. Three large neoplastic lymphocytes have dispersed chromatin with prominent nucleoli and deeply basophilic cytoplasm. Neutrophils are also present and one (arrow) contains phagocytized mixed bacteria. The nucleated cell count was 44,600/μL, with neutrophils predominating, and the total protein was 4.7 g/dL. This cat had intestinal lymphoma that caused an intestinal perforation and septic peritonitis. Aqueous Romanowsky stain.

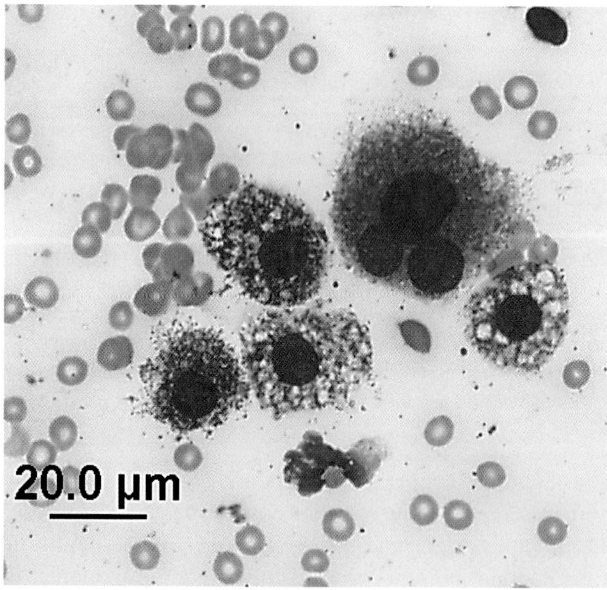

Figure 42.23 Neoplastic peritoneal effusion, mast cell tumor, dog. The neoplastic mast cells have variable cytoplasmic granulation, and one large trinucleated cell has anisokaryosis with large nucleoli. Free granules from lysed mast cells are seen in the background. There are numerous erythrocytes and platelets present, indicating either blood contamination during sampling or acute/ongoing hemorrhage. Aqueous Romanowsky stain.

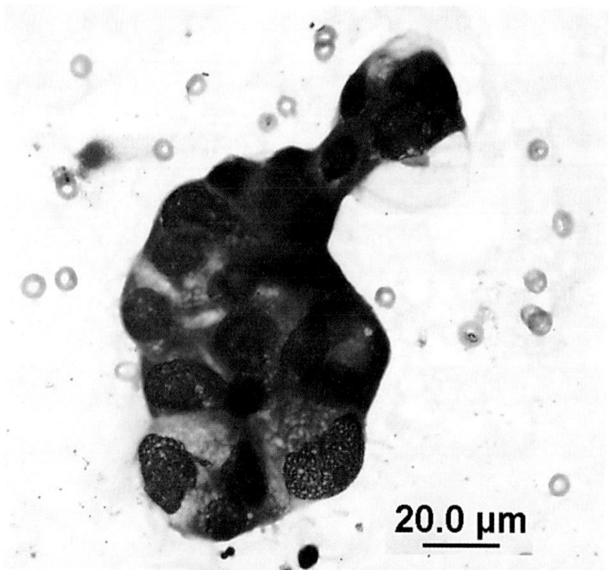

Figure 42.24 Neoplastic pleural effusion, carcinoma, dog. A tightly cohesive cluster of neoplastic epithelial cells have multiple criteria of malignancy including anisokaryosis, binucleation, coarse chromatin, and prominent nucleoli. The total nucleated cell count was 7500/μL and the total protein was 5 g/dL. This dog had a mammary gland anaplastic carcinoma that metastasized to the lungs. Aqueous Romanowsky stain.

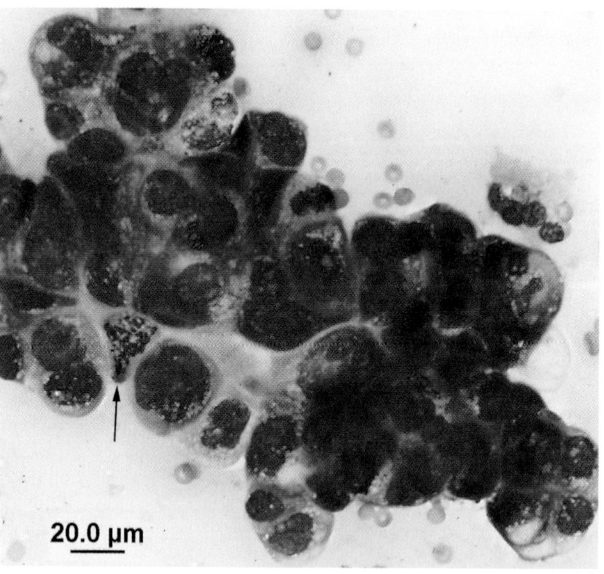

Figure 42.25 Neoplastic pleural effusion, carcinoma, dog. Same case as Figure 42.24. Many neoplastic epithelial cells are present in disorganized cohesive clusters. One abnormal mitotic figure is seen here (arrow). Cells have marked criteria of malignancy (anisokaryosis, binucleation, coarse chromatin with large, abnormal nucleoli), and some cells contain cytoplasmic vacuoles. Aqueous Romanowsky stain.

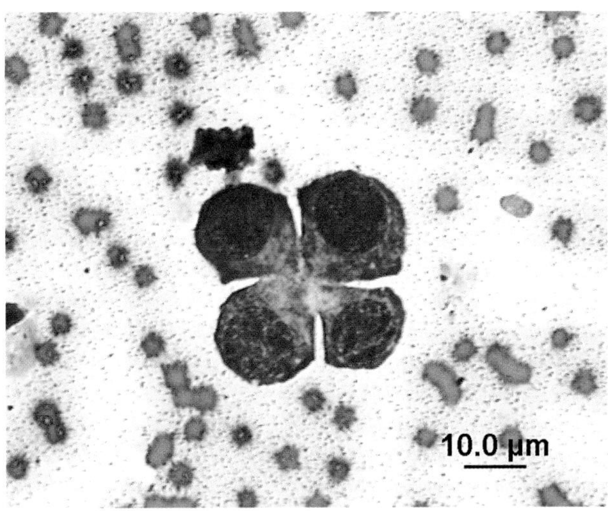

Figure 42.26 Acinar structure, adenocarcinoma, horse. The background contains protein precipitates and erythrocytes. Aqueous Romanowsky stain.

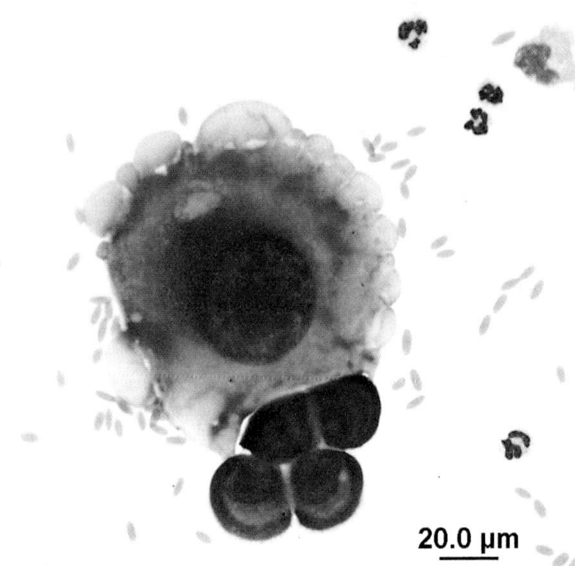

Figure 42.27 Neoplastic peritoneal effusion, carcinoma, llama. Five neoplastic epithelial cells are present; four smaller cells are deeply basophilic and appear cohesive. One karyomegalic cell has coarse nuclear chromatin and a huge, bizarre nucleolus. The total nucleated cell count was 500/μL, and the total protein was 2.7 g/dL. This llama had bicavitary neoplastic effusions secondary to metastatic mammary carcinoma. Wright stain.

impossible to make with cytology alone, even for experienced cytologists. In some cases, even histopathology may be inconclusive without the use of immunohistochemistry or ultrastructural studies [26]. Because mesothelial cells become reactive and exfoliate into any effusion, regardless of underlying cause, and frequently develop criteria of malignancy, extreme caution in interpretation is warranted, especially if there is concurrent inflammation (Figure 42.4).

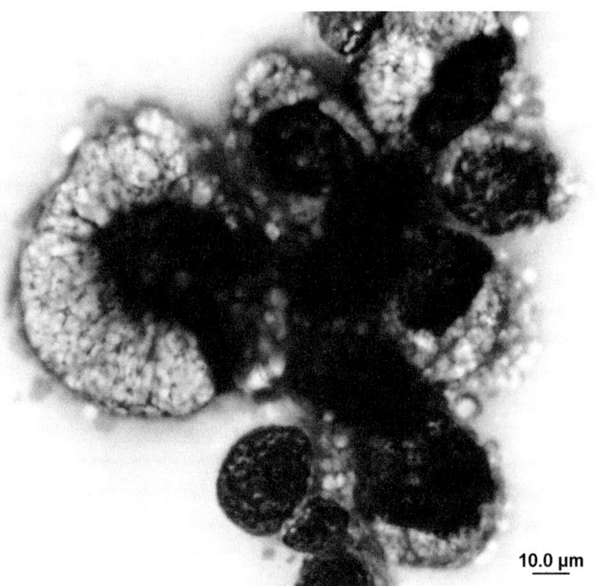

Figure 42.28 Neoplastic peritoneal effusion, adenocarcinoma, dog. Tightly cohesive neoplastic epithelial cells are vacuolated and have multiple criteria of malignancy (anisokaryosis, coarse chromatin, multiple large nucleoli). This dog had a pancreatic adenocarcinoma. Wright stain.

Cells from mesothelioma may develop the same criteria of malignancy as described for carcinomas, and are frequently present in large papillary clusters with irregular outlines (Figures 42.29 and 42.30) [27]. When an effusion contains

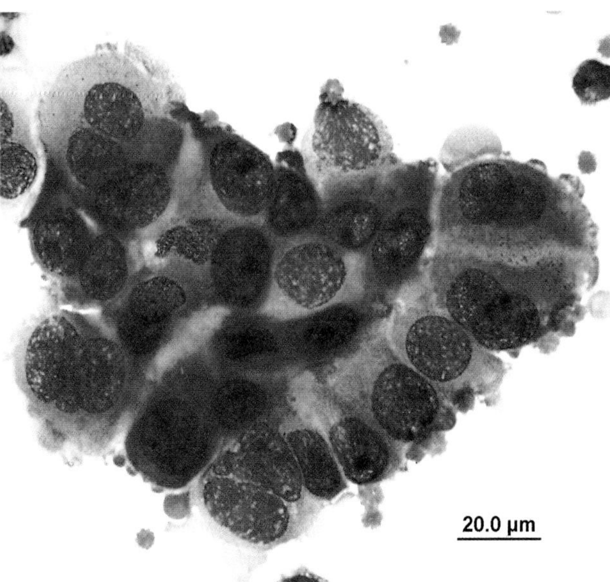

Figure 42.29 Neoplastic pleural effusion, mesothelioma, dog. A large cluster of cohesive neoplastic cells has marked criteria of malignancy including bi- and multinucleation, anisokaryosis, coarse chromatin, large prominent nucleoli, and nuclear molding. Cytologic differentials include carcinoma or mesothelioma. Histopathology confirmed mesothelioma in this case. Aqueous Romanowsky stain.

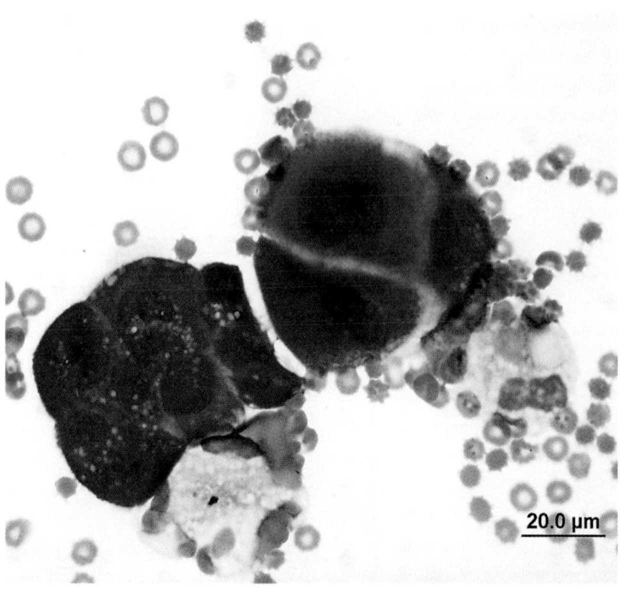

Figure 42.30 Neoplastic pleural effusion, mesothelioma, dog. Same case as Figure 42.29. Two clusters of cohesive neoplastic cells are present with two vacuolated macrophages and few erythrocytes. Criteria of malignancy include anisocytosis, anisokaryosis, binucleation, prominent nucleoli, deeply basophilic cytoplasm that is occasionally vacuolated. Aqueous Romanowsky stain.

many large clusters of markedly atypical cells, the abdominal or thoracic cavity should be evaluated thoroughly for mass lesions. In many cases, direct sampling of a mass for cytologic evaluation enables a more definitive interpretation.

Sarcomas

Sarcomas rarely exfoliate sufficient numbers of neoplastic cells into an effusion to allow diagnosis. Hemangiosarcoma, a common sarcoma of the spleen, is composed of neoplastic endothelial cells. These tumors frequently rupture and bleed, causing hemorrhagic effusions, but tumor cells are almost never seen on cytologic evaluation of the effusion.

43 Cytology of Synovial Fluid

James Meinkoth

Department of Veterinary Pathobiology, Oklahoma State University, Stillwater, OK, USA

Synovial fluid analysis is a fundamental part of the database in animals presenting with either monoarticular or polyarticular joint effusion. Additionally, it may provide useful information in animals with generalized lameness, generalized pain, or fever of unknown origin in an attempt to localize disease. The exact parameters measured and ancillary tests performed may vary between labs and will depend on the volume and nature of the sample acquired. However, the vast majority of clinically relevant information that can be derived from synovial fluid samples can be obtained by cytologic assessment of well-made, well-stained direct smears of synovial fluid. With experience, this can be performed in-clinic as long as the clinician has access to routine hematologic stains and a good-quality microscope. The results obtained can help determine the need for additional testing or direct treatment in a timelier manner than awaiting results from an outside lab.

There are a limited number of changes that can be seen in synovial fluid, despite a variety of potential disease processes. The downside to the clinician is that synovial fluid analysis rarely gives a definitive etiologic diagnosis. More often, it identifies a general process for which there are differential diagnoses. This must then be correlated with information from the history, physical exam findings, and additional tests to arrive at a specific diagnosis. The benefit to the clinician is that it is easier to gain competency in interpretation since, compared to other cytologic samples, the majority of synovial fluid samples have a very narrow spectrum of possible findings with which to become familiar. The main information to glean from examination of synovial fluid is to know the features of normal synovial fluid and then be able to identify and differentiate the following main processes:

1. *Inflammatory arthropathies:* These may also be termed *neutrophilic* or *suppurative* arthropathies and are usually the result of either infectious or immune-mediated diseases.
2. *Noninflammatory arthropathies:* These are also termed *degenerative joint diseases* (DJDs) and can result from a variety of congenital and acquired structural defects.
3. *Hemarthrosis:* This indicates hemorrhage into the joint space and must be differentiated from blood contamination during sample collection.

The goals of this chapter are to familiarize the reader with the various test results that may be received as part of synovial fluid analysis and their interpretation, optimal sample handling procedures (especially when limited sample is obtained), proper procedures to make and examine direct smears of synovial fluid, and the cytologic features of the above three main disease processes.

Parameters evaluated: normal and abnormal findings

Volume

The volume of joint fluid that can be obtained varies between species and the joint involved. Typically only a few drops to ~0.5 ml can be collected in dogs and up to 0.25 ml collected in cats [1, 2]. Several milliliters can be collected from normal joints in large animal species [3, 4]. Depending on the type of disease present, the volume may increase significantly. Increased volume of synovial fluid is best assessed by the person collecting the sample.

Physical properties

The color and relative viscosity of the sample should be noted. Normal synovial fluid is clear to pale yellow and extremely viscous [2, 5]. Viscosity can be assessed subjectively by the length of a strand that is formed before breaking if a drop of sample is gently expelled from the needle tip onto a slide and then the needle is slowly lifted away. Alternatively, a drop can be placed between the operator's fingers, which are then slowly pulled apart. Normal joint fluid should form a strand of a least 2.5 cm before breaking apart [2, 5]. Viscosity can be reduced with synovial effusion of any cause but is most significantly reduced in samples with a markedly increased concentration of neutrophils.

Veterinary Hematology, Clinical Chemistry, and Cytology, Third Edition. Edited by Mary Anna Thrall, Glade Weiser, Robin W. Allison and Terry W. Campbell.

Companion website: www.wiley.com/go/thrall/veterinary

Normal synovial fluid does not clot as it lacks a significant concentration of fibrinogen, although it may gel to a semisolid state if left standing at room temperature. This property is termed *thixotropy*. This can be easily differentiated from clot formation since the sample will return to a fluid state with warming and mixing. Clotting may occur if there is either gross blood contamination or marked inflammation present. In these cases, if sufficient sample is obtained for cell counts, some should be placed into an anticoagulant tube to prevent clot formation. EDTA is the best anticoagulant to both prevent clot formation and to preserve cell morphology. Heparin can also be used if a mucin clot test is desired (discussed later); however, this is not a permanent anticoagulant and cell counts can decrease significantly in 24 hours [6].

Turbidity of the synovial fluid usually results from increased cellularity, which would be reflected either as an increased cell count, if measured, or as a subjective increase in cellularity of a well-made direct smear. A reddish tinge or grossly bloody color results from addition of blood, either through bleeding into the joint (hemarthrosis) or blood contamination of the sample during collection. The cytologic distinction between these two is discussed later in the section on hemorrhagic samples, but it is often best assessed by the person collecting the sample. True hemarthrosis is likely if the sample was equally discolored throughout collection. Conversely, with blood contamination during collection, the sample is often initially clear and then becomes discolored over time. In this event, collection should by stopped immediately to minimize further contamination of the sample.

If a hemodilute sample is suspected a small amount of the sample can be spun down to examine the color of the supernatant. If sample volume is limited, this can be done with a microhematocrit tube. A clear supernatant suggests either acute hemarthrosis or sample contamination during collection. With chronic hemarthrosis, the red cells are broken down and the hemoglobin is metabolized to pigments, which may impart a yellowish discoloration termed *xanthochromia*.

Mucin quality

The *mucin clot test* assesses the quality of hyaluronic acid in a sample and is performed by adding a small amount of synovial fluid to a tube of glacial acetic acid and assessing the quality of the clot that forms. Normal synovial fluid forms a tight, ropey clot, leaving the remainder of the acetic acid clear. With degradation of the hyaluronic acid in the sample, this clot becomes less tightly condensed or may fail to form altogether. The mucin clot test is typically subjectively graded as "good," "fair," or "poor". A mild decrease in quality of the mucin clot can be seen with any severe joint effusion due to dilution of hyaluronic acid. Marked decreases in mucin clot quality are most often seen with neutrophilic inflammation owing to the action of proteolytic enzymes present in neutrophils, which can degrade hyaluronic acid.

EDTA can break down polymerized hyaluronic acid, affecting results of this test. For this reason, the mucin clot test should be run on either a sample with no anticoagulant or on a sample collected in a lithium heparin tube.

The mucin clot test was historically used in the assessment of synovial fluid but is no longer run by most labs. The presence of inflammation within the joint is better assessed by cell count or simple direct examination of direct smears of synovial fluid.

Total nucleated cell count (TNCC)

Cellularity of synovial fluid, which is normally very low, is one of the major parameters assessed in determining the type of pathologic change present. The TNCC of synovial fluid can be determined by (i) use of an automated hematology analyzer, (ii) manual counts done on a hemocytometer, or (iii) subjective assessment of cellularity based on examination of direct smears. Several studies have shown good correlation between hemocytometer counts and those obtained from automated analyzers, supporting the use of automated methods for generating cell counts [7–10]. However, it should be noted that cell counts generated by either automated analyzers or hemocytometers can be falsely decreased due to cell clumping in the diluent due to the viscosity of the synovial fluid [7, 10]. With either method, more accurate cell counts may be obtained if the sample is pretreated with hyaluronidase to break down the viscosity of the sample and allow for more even distribution of the cells within the sample and analyzer diluent [7, 10]. Hyaluronidase treatment also reduces the incidence of error flags from automated analyzers and prevents clogging of the flow cells [8, 10]. Hyaluronidase treatment is not typically available for use with in-clinic analyzers and may not be available in many smaller reference laboratory settings. Therefore, clinicians must be aware that cell counts may suffer from this artifact. The TNCC obtained from either of these methods should be confirmed by comparing it to the subjective assessment of cellularity as determined by microscopic evaluation of direct smears. Often, subjective assessment of cellularity is the only parameter available when sample volume is scant, and it is usually sufficient for clinical assessment if done by experienced observers.

Cell counts of normal synovial fluid in all species are extremely low, typically less than 1000/μL [1, 4, 5]. In dogs, some joint may have cell counts as high as 3000/μL and there may be variability between joints [2].

In addition to pathologic increases in cellularity, TNCC may also be affected by gross hemodilution of the sample since the white blood cell (WBC) concentration of peripheral blood is much higher than that of normal synovial fluid. If the nucleated cell count is increased in a hemodilute sample, a subjective assessment should be made and reported as to whether the increase in nucleated cells appears proportional to what would be expected for the amount of hemodilution or if there is likely an underlying pathologic process in addition to the hemodilution. This is best achieved by examining a direct smear and comparing the number and type of leukocytes present with what would be expected form peripheral blood contribution given the amount of erythrocytes present.

Erythrocyte concentrations are not typically reported other than a description of the sample color and a subjective comment on the amount of background blood on the smear.

Protein concentration

Protein concentration is most often estimated by refractometry. Published references list normal synovial fluid protein as assessed by refractometry to be less than ~2.5 g/dL [4, 5]. Increases in protein concentration are typically associated with inflammation. However, refractometry can significantly overestimate the protein concentration if an insufficient amount of sample is placed in an EDTA tube, as happens when there is limited sample obtained, because of the high refractive index of EDTA. Therefore, increased protein concentration alone should not be relied upon to determine inflammation in a sample and this should be confirmed by evaluating the cellularity and type of inflammatory cells seen on cytologic evaluation of direct smears.

A more accurate measurement of protein concentration would require a true protein to be determined using a colorimetric assay as is done on serum samples. However, this is not done for most routine diagnostic samples.

Cytologic evaluation

Cytologic examination of the specimen is the single most important part of synovial fluid analysis [5]. When sample volume is limited, cytologic examination of a direct smear is typically sufficient to obtain all clinically relevant information that can be obtained from the sample [11]. Conversely, without cytologic examination the interpretation of any other data is severely limited.

Preparation of cytologic slides

A direct smear will allow for both an estimation of the cellularity of the sample and a determination of the type of cells present [11]. If the cellularity of the sample is extremely low and sufficient sample is available, the preparation of either a cytocentrifuged sample (in a reference lab) or a sediment smear will yield a more cellular preparation and allow for assessment of a greater number of cells. However, when the cellularity of a synovial sample is this low there is generally little information to be gained from the cytomorphology of the cells. Most diagnostically important findings related to cellular morphology or presence of infectious organisms are associated with highly cellular samples.

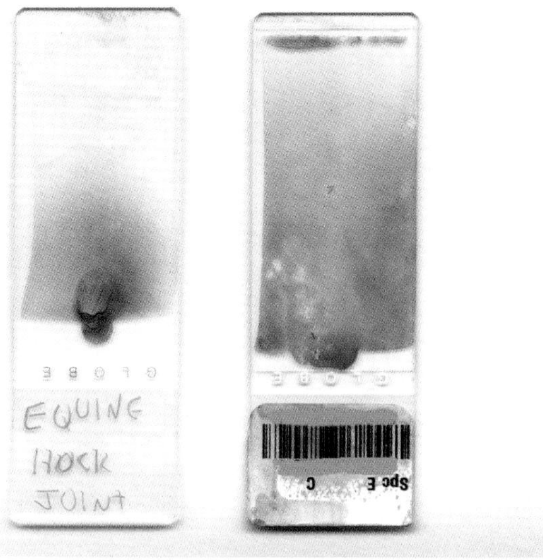

Figure 43.1 Two direct smears made from synovial fluid. The slide on the left has a feathered edge that will allow for visualization of cells in a well-spread-out area. On the slide on the right, the sample extends to the edge of the slide and has a thick abrupt end. This may not have a sufficiently thin area to evaluate.

Direct smears of synovial fluid are made by placing a small drop of well-mixed sample at one end of a glass slide. A second spreader slide is then used to spread out the sample similar to making a blood film [11]. Alternatively, if the sample is viscous and will not spread out along the spreader slide, a slide over slide preparation can be made similar to a standard cytology smear from a fine needle biopsy (see Chapter 39). The high viscosity of synovial fluid will often prevent cells from spreading out sufficiently to evaluate in thick portions of smears [12]. So, it is extremely important to have a thin area on the smear and thus a feathered edge should be present rather than allowing the sample to extend all of the way to the edge of the slide [11] (Figure 43.1). It is wise to make at least two to three slides per sample to ensure at least one diagnostic slide.

Estimation of cellularity

The cellularity of the sample can be estimated from a thin portion of the direct smear. Generally, only a few cells (0–5) will be seen per 20× objective field (200× magnification) *in thin areas* of smears from normal animals. As a general rule of thumb, the white cell count can be estimated by taking the average number of cells seen per 20× objective field and multiplying by 500. The goal is not to get a precise number of cells/μL but to differentiate normal cellularity, mildly increased cellularity and markedly increased cellularity. With practice, the cellularity can be estimated by "eyeballing" the number of leukocytes seen at low magnification and comparing that to a comparable white cell concentration on a blood film with a known WBC count. Since cells are often unevenly distributed or may be present in clumps, evaluation of the entire smear including thinner portions may give a better overall assessment than counting the averaging the number of cells in a limited number of fields. Estimation does require experience and estimates can vary among observers but with practice can be done reliably [11, 12].

The number of cells seen per field will vary with the thickness of the smear made, and this can be quite variable due to the viscosity of synovial fluid. It is important to be in a thin area that would be equivalent to the monolayer of a blood film when estimating cellularity. This area can often be determined by the density of the background and by how well the individual leukocytes have spread out. In the thicker areas of the smear near where the sample was applied, the background if often diffusely proteinaceous with or without a stippled eosinophilic nature (Figure 43.2). In this area, the cells will not be well spread out and it is often not possible to clearly see the demarcation between the nucleus and the cytoplasm of the cell (Figure 43.2). As you move toward the feathered edge of the smear, the background will lighten and eventually the cells will spread out to where a clear demarcation can be seen between the border of the nucleus and the cytoplasm (Figure 43.3). In this area, the numbers of cells per field will be most representative of true cellularity of the sample and the estimate should be performed.

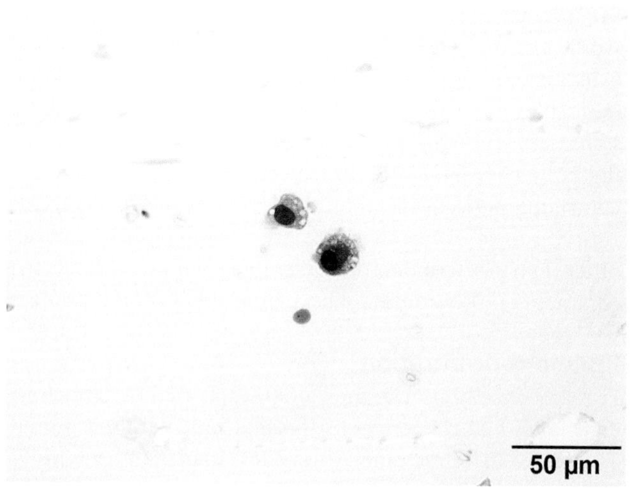

Figure 43.3 Thinner area of same smear. The background is clear. In this area, cells have spread out as evidenced by the demarcation between purple nucleus and basophilic cytoplasm being more distinct. This is the area where differential counts should be performed and where estimations of cellularity are likely to be more accurate. Aqueous Romanowsky stain.

Estimation of viscosity/proteoglycan layer

The viscosity of the sample is typically assessed grossly by its physical properties. The viscosity of the sample and the quality of the hyaluronic acid may also be apparent on the cytologic preparation. If there are either erythrocytes or leukocytes present, these may be lined up in single file rows if the viscosity of the sample is high. This is termed *windrowing* and can be seen in normal synovial fluid as well as other viscous samples such as salivary aspirates (Figure 43.4). In addition, normal joint fluid often has a characteristic stippled eosinophilic background resulting from the presence of hyaluronic acid (Figure 43.5). It should

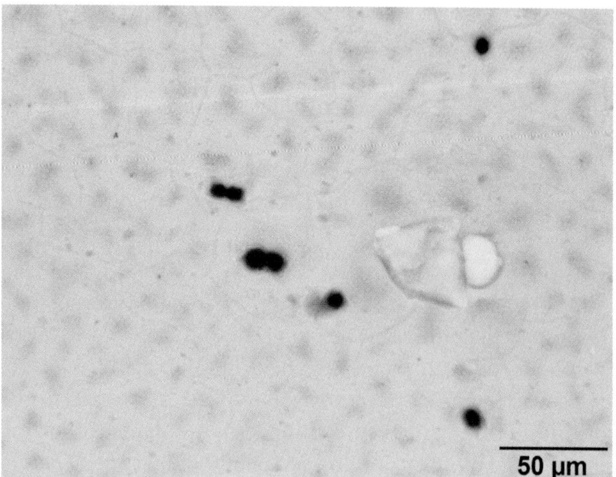

Figure 43.2 Thicker area of a direct smear shows a variably dense eosinophilic background. In this area, cells are not well spread out. Seven dark spheres representing nucleated cells can be seen, but cell type cannot be determined. In this area of the smear cellularity may appear artificially increased. Aqueous Romanowsky stain.

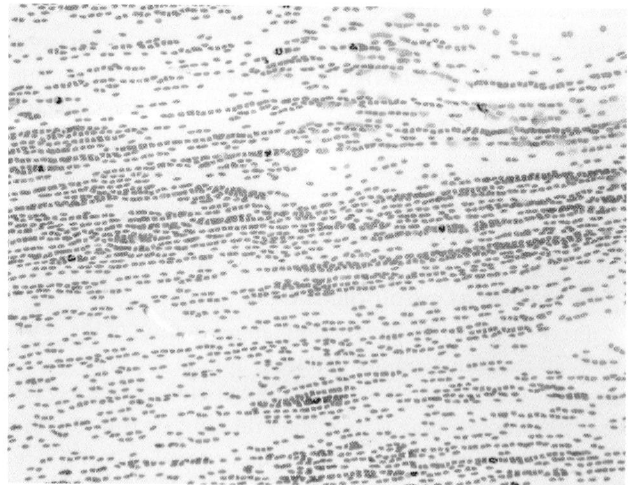

Figure 43.4 Low-magnification images of a direct smear of synovial fluid with blood contamination. The erythrocytes are lined up in a single-file manner termed "windrowing" typical of any highly viscous sample. There are a few neutrophils present, but they are in numbers that would be expected from peripheral blood contribution based on the amount of hemodilution present rather than suggesting inflammation. Aqueous Romanowsky stain.

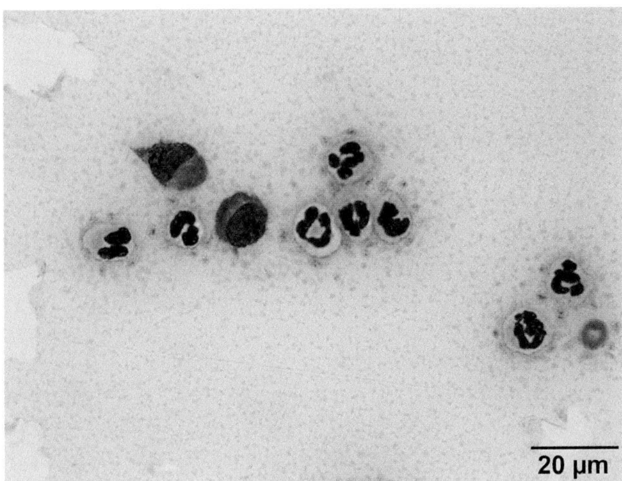

Figure 43.5 Direct smear of synovial fluid from a dog. Note the pink, stippled background, which is typical of synovial fluid. There is evidence of neutrophilic inflammation in this joint based on many neutrophils with no hemodilution. Aqueous Romanowsky stain.

be noted that this stippled background may be absent from some normal samples [1].

With marked neutrophilic inflammation, this stippled background may break down and be less prominent or absent, although this is not a consistent finding.

Differential count

In addition to a low nucleated cell count, normal synovial fluid is typically composed predominantly of various mononuclear cells and very few neutrophils. "Mononuclear" cells really refer to "mono*morpho*nuclear" cells rather than cells with one nucleus. This includes any cell without the nuclear segmentation characteristic of neutrophils, eosinophils and basophils. These can be small lymphocytes, macrophages or even synovial lining cells (Figure 43.6). The percentage of the different mononuclear cells present is variable and generally not of diagnostic significance, so they are all combined together and contrasted to the percentage of neutrophils present. Neutrophils (Figure 43.5) generally make up a low percentage of cells in synovial fluid, typically less than ~10% [1, 2, 4, 5]. Original publications report a slightly higher percentage of neutrophils in some samples [1]. However given the very low WBC counts of normal synovial fluid, consideration must be given to the potential effect that even a small amount of peripheral blood contamination could have on the differential count.

Most of the macrophages in normal synovial fluid do not have distended, vacuolated cytoplasm or show evidence of phagocytosis of other material [2]. Vacuolated macrophages may be present in a higher percentage in animals with inflammatory or degenerative arthropathies. However, this type of change may also occur in the tube if there is a delay between sample collection and preparation of cytologic

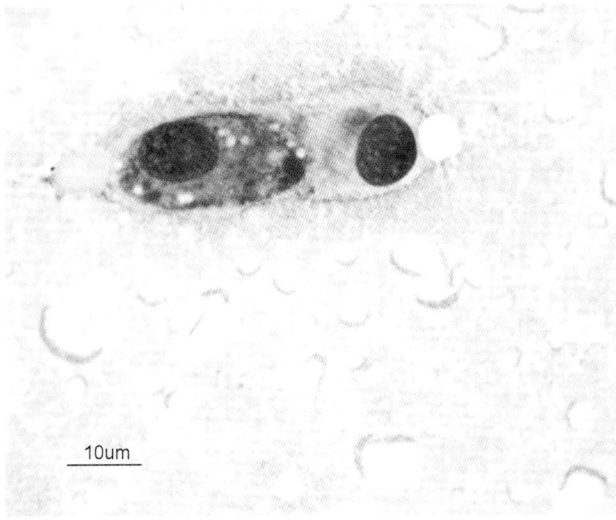

Figure 43.6 Two mononuclear cells in a direct smear of synovial fluid from a dog. The cell at the right is likely an unstimulated macrophage (also termed Type B synovial cell). The cell on the left, with the pink cytoplasmic granules, is likely a secretory or Type A synovial cell. Distinguishing between the various types of mononuclear cells in fluid is generally not of diagnostic significance. Wright-Giemsa stain.

slides. It is best to make smears immediately upon collection to avoid any artifacts associated with cellular aging.

With septic or immune-mediated arthropathies, there is typically a dramatic increase in both the absolute number and percentage of neutrophils present (Figure 43.7). Modest increases in neutrophils can be seen with inflammation resulting from trauma/inflammation of periarticular tissues, chronic hemarthrosis or secondary to intra-articular injections.

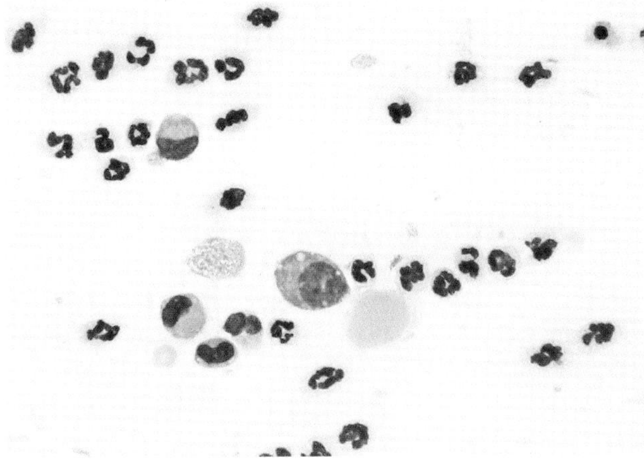

Figure 43.7 Direct smear of synovial fluid from a dog with septic arthritis. The cellularity is markedly increased with a predominance of neutrophils. The neutrophils appear nondegenerate despite a septic process. This is common with synovial fluid. Aqueous Romanowsky stain, 500x original magnification.

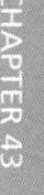

Any time there is significant blood contamination during sample collection, there is the potential for an increased percentage of neutrophils. The magnitude of this increase will depend on both the amount of contamination and the leukocyte count of the peripheral blood (more would be expected if the patient had a significant neutrophilia).

Samples submitted and triage of samples of limited volume

The amount of sample that can be collected is often limited, so it is important to consider which tests are most important to run given the suspected disease. Generally, the top priority is to make one or more well-made, thin, direct smears with a feathered edge. This is generally sufficient both to estimate the cellularity of the sample and then determine the cytologic abnormalities present, if any. Preparation of either cytocentrifuged or sediment smears uses significantly more sample, often does not add significant information, and should be done only if sufficient sample is available and other testing needs such as culture are met first.

If infectious joint disease is considered clinically likely, some sample should immediately be inoculated onto culture media or a culture transport system. Studies have shown improved recovery by using blood culture medium enrichment [13, 14]. Samples placed in EDTA are not appropriate for culture, since this anticoagulant can inhibit bacterial growth. Samples placed in sterile tubes may be used for culture, but organisms in these tubes may die during transit to the lab. Inoculation of microbial culture system is best done immediately after sample collection rather than after submission to the lab to maximize diagnostic yield.

If sufficient sample remains after making direct smears and inoculating culture systems (if needed), the remaining sample can be placed into either a serum tube (red top tube) or EDTA tube (purple top tube) that can be used to obtain a TNCC. Normal synovial fluid will not clot, so a cell count can often be obtained from a serum tube. However, if there is significant blood contamination or evidence of inflammation (turbid, less viscous sample) then synovial fluid should be placed into EDTA to prevent clot formation. The only limitations of an EDTA compared to a serum tube or other anticoagulant is that it may cause an artifactual increase in total protein (TP) as measured by refractometry if the tube is not adequately filled and it may alter the mucin clot test results. The former is not a problem if an appropriate sized EDTA tube is used considering the sample volume and the latter test is no longer run by most labs.

Heparin tubes can be used to obtain cell counts, and will not interfere with the mucin clot test. However, samples in heparin are not as stable as those in EDTA tubes. Significant decreases in cell counts can be seen by 24 hours when samples are collected in heparin [6]. So, unless cell counts can be obtained in a timely fashion, heparin is not the best choice.

Abnormal synovial fluid cytology

As previously described, normal synovial fluid will be clear to pale yellow and noted to be viscous when making direct smears. The cellularity is extremely low and nucleated cells present should be predominantly mononuclear cells. These can be a mixture of small lymphocytes, macrophages and synovial lining cells although the varying percentages of these is generally not clinically relevant. Relatively few (<10%) of the mononuclear cells should be highly vacuolated macrophages or contain phagocytized material [2]. Neutrophils should be less than ~10% of the nucleated cells. Departures from this appearance can generally be grouped into one of major categories below. Table 43.1 presents a summary of synovial fluid findings from both normal joints and each of the major classifications of abnormality.

Noninflammatory/degenerative arthropathies

This category encompasses a variety of conditions in which there are noninflammatory, degenerative changes to articular surfaces from a variety of underlying causes. These may be variably referred to in different publications as either *degenerative arthropathies, nonsuppurative arthropathies*, or *noninflammatory arthropathies*.

These conditions result in relatively mild changes in synovial fluid parameters [15–17]. There may be a mildly increased TNCC, typically not more than about ~5000 to 10,000/µL [5, 15, 17]. Nucleated cells still comprise >90% mononuclear cells with very few neutrophils. In some cases, there may be increased numbers of macrophages that appear "activated," having increased amounts of vacuolated cytoplasm and sometimes containing phagocytized material. If the articular damage is severe enough, multinucleated osteoclasts may be present. Because of the lack of neutrophilic inflammation, viscosity is normal to only mildly reduced and the normal stippled eosinophilic background is present. The mucin clot, if performed, is usually "fair" or "good."

This type of synovial fluid pattern can be seen with any form of osteoarthritis, which must be defined by clinical findings. Osteoarthritis can be either *primary* (due to a primary defect in articular cartilage) or *secondary* (resulting from an underlying joint disease leading to abnormal stresses on the articular surface) [18]. Secondary osteoarthritis may result from osteochondrosis, hip dysplasia, elbow dysplasia, joint trauma, or joint instability due to ligament damage (e.g., cruciate rupture).

Inflammatory (suppurative) arthropathies

Inflammatory arthropathies are also referred to as *suppurative arthropathies*, because they are usually characterized by a

Table 43.1 Summary of typical synovial fluid findings in various conditions.

Condition	Gross appearance	Viscosity	TNCC	Cytologic findings	Other considerations
Normal	Pale yellow	Highly viscous	Low <1000/μL <3000/μL in dogs	Predominantly mononuclear cells <10% nondegenerate neutrophils	Even mild hemodilution may affect differential count.
Degenerative arthropathy	Pale yellow	Normal to mildly decreased	Mildly increased (<~10,000/μL)	Predominantly mononuclear cells <10% neutrophils	May see increased % of vacuolated macrophages. May see osteoclasts if severe.
Inflammatory articular sepsis[a]	Turbid, opaque	Markedly decreased	Markedly increased (>~50,000/μL)	Marked predominance of neutrophils (>90%)	Bacteria often not evident or in very low numbers. Neutrophils often nondegenerate. Inoculate culture material directly upon collection. Typically monoarticular. May be oligo- to polyarticular in cases of hematogenous spread.
Inflammatory immune-mediated	Clear to turbid, depending on cellularity	Mildly to markedly decreased	Mildly to markedly increased	Neutrophils >10% but variable (20% to >90%)	LE cells may be present but rare. Typically polyarticular disease. Clinically normal joints may show inflammatory changes cytologically.
Hemarthrosis	Pink to dark red throughout collection	Mildly to markedly decreased	Normal to mildly increased	Many erythrocytes May see erythrophagia Neutrophils may be mildly increased disproportionately	May see erythrophagia. Platelets typically absent unless ongoing hemorrhage.
Iatrogenic blood contamination	Initially clear then bloody	Mildly to markedly decreased	Normal to mildly increased	Many erythrocytes Neutrophils increase in proportion to amount of blood No erythrophagia Platelets present	Erythrophagia may form *in vitro*. Make slides immediately. May still be possible to detect underlying inflammation if hemodilution is mild.

[a]Referring only to true infection of joint. Findings with infectious diseases of other tissues that result in immune-complex-mediated joint disease are similar to other immune-mediated diseases.

predominance of neutrophils in the synovial fluid. This type of response is most common with either infectious or immune-mediated disease. Often, the cytologic findings in these two classes of disease are virtually identical and they must be differentiated based on clinical findings and other tests results.

With inflammatory arthropathies, the TNCC typically is moderately to markedly increased, usually much higher than with degenerative arthropathies. Cell counts commonly range from ~20,000/μL to >100,000/μL [19–22]. A defining characteristic is that neutrophils comprise significantly more than 10% of the nucleated cells present. In most cases neutrophils are the predominant cell type (>50%) and it is not uncommon for them to comprise >90% of the nucleated cells present [19–22]. There may also be a concurrent increase in the absolute number of mononuclear cells and this may include large vacuolated macrophages. TP as assessed by refractometry is typically increased, ranging from 4.5–7.5 g/dL [19, 20, 22]. Because of the proteolytic enzymes released from these neutrophils, the viscosity of the sample is often markedly reduced, the typical stippled eosinophilic background may be absent and the mucin clot test, if performed, is often poor.

Infectious conditions

Pathogenesis

Infectious diseases can result in a suppurative arthropathy by one of two mechanisms. The first and most intuitive mechanism is true *septic arthritis* in which there is an infectious agent colonizing the articular tissues, which may be recoverable by culture. Such infectious arthritis can result from either direct inoculation of the joint (i.e., penetrating wound, surgical complication) or hematogenous spread. Direct inoculation will result in monoarticular disease while hematogenous spread may result in either monoarticular or polyarticular disease.

A second mechanism involves infectious diseases affecting distant tissues, often systemic infections. Not true "joint infections," these most likely result in suppurative arthritis via a Type III hypersensitivity reaction. Circulating immune complexes formed outside the joint are nonspecifically trapped within synovial membranes, similar to what happens with immune complex glomerular disease. Deposited immune complexes incite a suppurative response that in turn causes damage to the joint. This mechanism is essentially immune-mediated disease induced by an infectious agent (see later discussion of immune-mediated conditions).

Rhodococcus equi infection in foals most characteristically manifests as bronchopneumonia but affected foals may have many extrapulmonary disorders (EPD) as well. About one-third of the cases will show polyarticular joint swelling, which may be a prominent clinical finding [23–26]. Affected animals are not typically lame, joint swelling resolves with resolution of the pneumonia, and they have no lasting joint damage. Synovial fluid may show a neutrophilic inflammatory response without identifiable bacteria cytologically or by culture [25, 26]. However, some foals may have a true septic arthritis, osteomyelitis or both with organisms cultured from the joints [26]. Thus, the distinction between infectious arthritis and immune-mediated arthritis secondary to infectious disease is not clear cut in all cases.

Synovial fluid findings

Arthritis caused by infectious diseases typically results in a TNCC >50,000/μL and often >100,000/μL [19–22]. Septic arthritis of the joint itself is unlikely if the cell count is only mildly increased (<~20,000/μL), even if there is a neutrophilic predominance. The neutrophils in bacterial arthritis are often uncharacteristically nondegenerate because the viscosity of the synovial fluid is protective to cell morphology (Figure 43.7) [21, 22]. While not common, if degenerative change of the neutrophils is observed, then bacterial sepsis should be strongly suspected and a diligent search for infectious organisms on the slides should be performed (Figure 43.8).

If intracellular bacteria, or other infectious agents, can be found on cytology then septic arthritis is confirmed. However, in most cases bacteria are either not evident in the smears or are present in extremely low numbers, making direct visualization of bacteria in smear an insensitive method to confirm sepsis [19, 21]. If clinical and/or cytologic findings are suggestive of bacterial infection, culture should be performed by directly inoculating culture systems at the time of sample collection [27]. Even with properly performed culture, bacteria are not always isolated from cases of septic arthritis [27, 28]. Certain organisms, such as anaerobes and *Mycoplasma* spp., require specific culture conditions and the microbiology lab should be consulted for specific sample handling recommendations if these are suspected. *Mycoplasma* spp. is a significant cause of septic arthritis in cattle and specific culture should be considered in all cases of septic arthritis from this species [29].

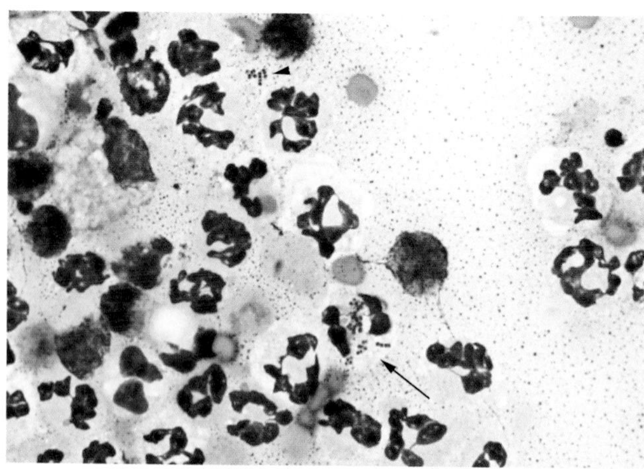

Figure 43.8 Direct smear of synovial fluid from a horse with septic arthritis. Bacterial rods are seen both within neutrophils (arrow) and extracellularly (arrowhead) in the presence of a marked suppurative response. Bacteria are often not present in cytologic preps in cases of septic arthritis, and culture should always be performed if clinical findings are suggestive. Aqueous Romanowsky stain, 1000x original magnification.

Various organisms involved in infectious arthritis

Bacteria are the most common infectious agents in septic arthritis in all species [27, 29–31]. In adult animals, these are usually monoarticular infections resulting from direct inoculation of the joint from a puncture wound or other traumatic injury. Polyarticular disease may occur secondary to septicemia, such as in cases of bacterial endocarditis in adults or navel infection in neonates. In some cases, the site of hematogenous spread is not apparent [32].

Certain rickettsial diseases commonly induce a neutrophilic polyarthritis. Lameness and neutrophilic polyarthritis are common findings in dogs infected with either *Ehrlichia ewingii* or *Anaplasma phagocytophilum* and should be considered in geographically endemic areas [33, 34]. Synovial fluid cell counts range from 15,000/μL to >100,000/μL. Neutrophils predominate and morulae are commonly found within neutrophils in acute infections (Figure 43.9). Unlike monocytic ehrlichiosis, morulae are often readily identifiable in neutrophils in the peripheral blood of acutely infected animals as well. Conversely, infection with *Ehrlichia canis* has not been reported to cause polyarthritis [35]. Early reports of such noted the morulae to be in neutrophils and likely represented infections with either *E. ewingii* or *A. phagocytophilum* prior to the characterization of these organisms. The inflammation seen with rickettsial organisms may be related to immune complex deposition rather than true infection of the joint. The presence of organisms within the synovial fluid may result simply because they are in peripheral blood neutrophils. Clinical signs of lameness and joint swelling are reported with cases of Rocky Mountain spotted fever in

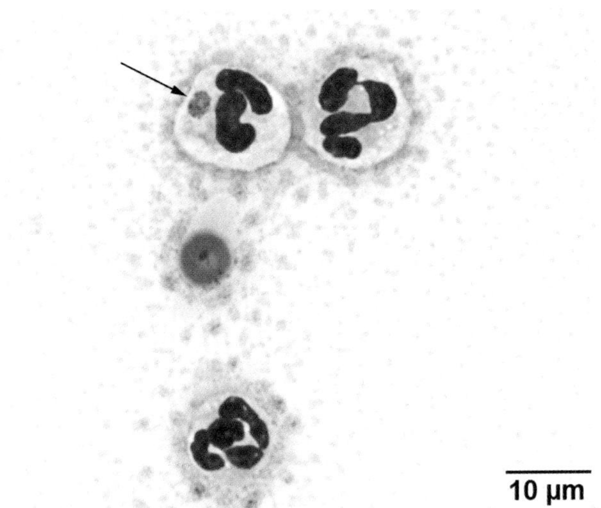

Figure 43.9 Direct smear of synovial fluid from a dog infected with *Ehrlichia ewingii*. Unlike monocytic ehrlichial (e.g., *Ehrlichia canis*) infections, morulae are often present within neutrophils (arrow) in either peripheral blood or synovial fluid in acute infections. Aqueous Romanowsky stain, 1000x original magnification.

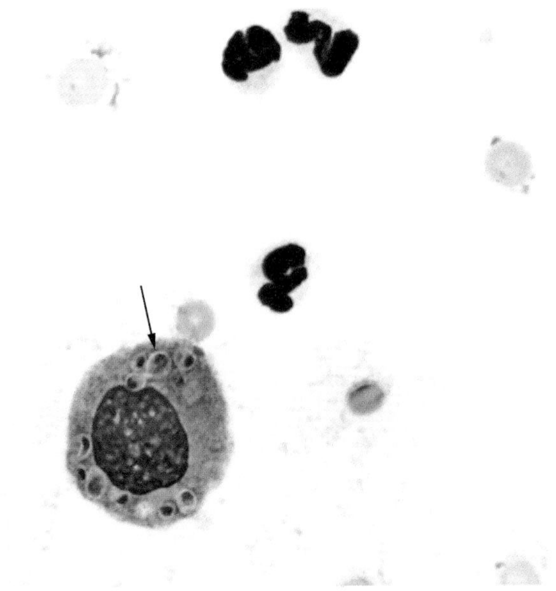

Figure 43.10 Direct smear of synovial fluid from a cat with histoplasmosis. Pyogranulomatous inflammation is typical. Organisms are seen within a macrophage (arrow). In some cases of feline histoplasmosis, lameness may be the primary, and sometimes sole, presenting complaint. Aqueous Romanowsky stain, 1000x original magnification.

dogs, but descriptions of synovial fluid analysis are lacking [27].

Arthritis involving one or several joints is a prominent finding in Lyme borreliosis in dogs. One or several joints are affected and the joint(s) affected may shift over time [36, 37]. Reports of synovial fluid analyses from experimentally affected animals showed an increase in TNCC that ranged from ~2500 to 40,000/μL with neutrophils comprising from ~20% to 90% of the total cells in affected joints of lame dogs [37]. Synovial fluid from unaffected joints in the same animal did not show significant changes.

Fungal diseases are rarely reported as causative agents of arthritis, typically occurring as an extension of fungal osteomyelitis [27]. One notable exception in endemic areas is erosive arthritis induced by histoplasmosis in cats (personal observations). In the author's experience, this is the most common cause of inflammatory joint disease in cats in Oklahoma. Organisms are found in synovial fluid cytology in many cases (Figure 43.10) but may be present in extremely low numbers. Diagnosis is often confirmed via urine antigen measurements. In people, infection of joints with *Candida* spp. has been reported in neonates, secondary to immunosuppression, and following joint implant surgery [38–40]. Rare cases have also been reported in veterinary medicine (Figure 43.11) [41, 42].

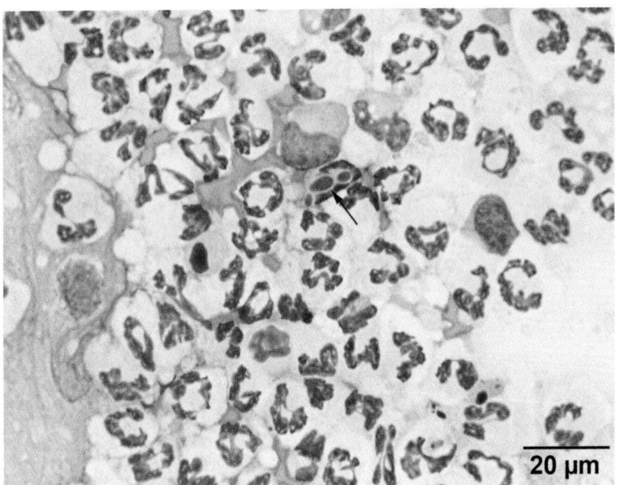

Figure 43.11 Direct smear of synovial fluid from a horse with fungal arthritis following joint surgery. Three fungal yeasts are seen in center (arrow). A thin clear halo is visible surrounding the organisms. *Candida tropicalis* was cultured from the fluid and confirmed via polymerase chain reaction of the isolate. Aqueous Romanowsky stain.

Immune-mediated conditions

Immune-mediated diseases are most common in dogs but have been reported in other species as well. They typically present as polyarticular disease. Different joints may be affected with varying severity and the joint(s) most affected may change over course of disease. In suspected cases it can be beneficial to sample multiple joints, even those that may not appear clinically affected, to confirm the polyarticular nature of the disease as a neutrophilic response is often detected in joints with minimal joint effusion.

The synovial fluid findings are generally similar, or identical to, those seen with arthropathy caused by infectious

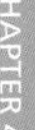

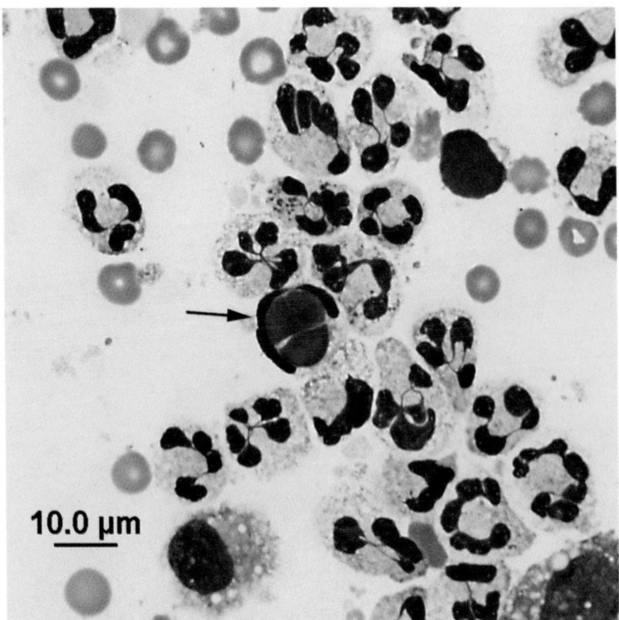

Figure 43.12 Direct smear of canine synovial fluid from a dog with immune-mediated polyarthritis. A lupus erythematosus cell (LE cell) is seen in the central neutrophil, which contains a single large, hyalinized, pink ("ground glass") inclusion (arrow) representing opsonized nuclear material from other cells that have lysed. This material displaces the nucleus of the neutrophil to the periphery. Aqueous Romanowsky stain. Source: Photo courtesy of Dr. Robin W Allison.

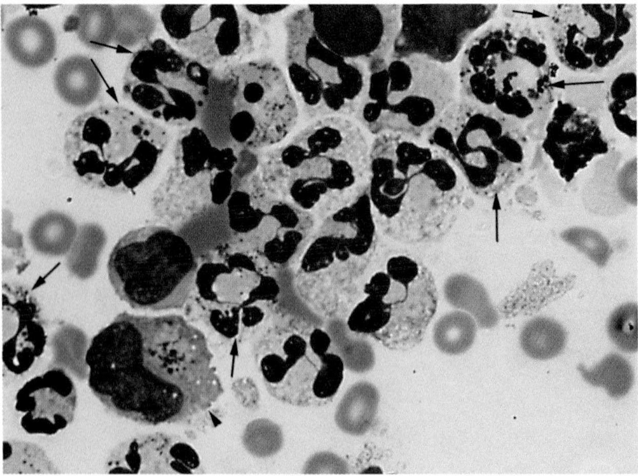

Figure 43.13 Cytospin preparation of synovial fluid from a dog. There is a suppurative inflammatory response present. Many of the neutrophils (arrows) and one macrophage (arrowhead) contain small, purple basophilic inclusions thought to be nuclear material. LE cells were seen in other fields along with these cells. These inclusions resemble bacteria in size and color but are generally more pleomorphic, lacking the distinct shape of bacterial rods or cocci. Aqueous Romanowsky stain, 1000x original magnification.

disease. TNCC may be mildly to markedly increased, depending on the joint sampled, and consist of a predominance of nondegenerate neutrophils. In rare cases, neutrophils may be found that have phagocytized opsonized nuclear material from other cells. These neutrophils are referred to as "LE cells" (lupus erythematosus cells). In the classic LE cell, the nucleus of the neutrophil is often displaced peripherally around a large mass of hyalinized, bright pink to pink-purple material (Figure 43.12). Oftentimes, neutrophils will contain smaller fragments of phagocytized material that stain dark purple, the more typical color of nuclear material. This material is thought to be phagocytized nuclear fragments and must be differentiated from neutrophils containing phagocytized bacteria (Figure 43.13). These cells have been termed "ragocytes," although this name is erroneous and should be discontinued. Finding these cells is suggestive of an immune-mediated pathogenesis, particularly systemic lupus erythematosus (SLE) (discussed later).

Since the cytologic findings in most immune-mediated diseases are similar, the differentiation of specific disease process present relies on clinical findings and additional testing. Table 43.2 lists the various reported conditions and a brief overview is given below. Immune-mediated diseases may be broadly categorized into erosive and nonerosive conditions based on presence of absence of bone lysis evident on imaging. Nonerosive conditions are more numerous, more

Table 43.2 Immune-mediated causes of arthropathy.

Erosive
• Rheumatoid arthritis
• Feline progressive polyarthritis (periosteal proliferative polyarthritis)
Nonerosive
• Idiopathic polyarthritis
Type I
Type II (associated with infections at other body sites)
Type III (associated with enteric inflammation)
Type IV (association with neoplasia)
• Associated with affectation of other tissues
Steroid-responsive meningitis-arteritis
Polymyositis
• Systemic lupus erythematosus
• Postvaccination
• Drug associated
• Breed-specific
Shar-Pei
Akita

common and generally associated with a better prognosis [27, 43].

Erosive immune-mediated conditions

The two erosive diseases described in veterinary medicine are rheumatoid arthritis (RA) and feline progressive polyarthritis.

RA has been described in both dogs and cats, although relatively infrequently compared to the incidence of this disease in humans [43–45]. In people, clinical findings and rheumatoid factor (RF) testing are standard to define this disease. Compared to humans, only a low percentage of dogs suspected as having RA based on clinical findings are positive for RF, and then only at a low titer [43, 45]. Furthermore, positive RF tests are actually seen more frequently in animals with other immune-mediated diseases (SLE) and inflammatory conditions (heartworm disease, pyometra) than in animals with RA [45]. This has led to recommendations that RF not be relied on as a diagnostic test for this disease [27].

A chronic erosive polyarthritis of cats has been described as either *feline progressive polyarthritis* or *periosteal proliferative polyarthritis* [44, 46, 47]. Cats are mostly young to middle aged and the disease most commonly affects hocks and carpi, but any joint may be affected. In one report, about half the cats were euthanized and most others had persistent lameness despite continuous immunosuppressive therapy [44]. At our institution, we have seen a similar clinical presentation eventually attributed to histoplasmosis, with organisms identified in synovial fluid but sometimes not until after several months of immunosuppressive therapy.

Nonerosive immune-mediated conditions

Nonerosive polyarthritis is much more common in veterinary medicine than erosive arthritis. Of these, the majority of cases are idiopathic and this designation requires first excluding the other defined disorders, which are listed in Table 43.2 and briefly described below. Idiopathic immune-mediated polyarthritis (IMPA) itself has been classified into four subtypes. Type I, which is most common, occurs in patients in which there are no inflammatory or neoplastic conditions identified at other sites in the body. The other types are also referred to as *reactive polyarthritis* as they are associated with other conditions. Type II IMPA is defined as polyarthritis associated with an infectious process occurring in any distant tissue (i.e., not articular infections). Type III IMPA, also called *enteropathic*, is associated inflammatory disease of the gastrointestinal tract. Type IV IMPA is defined as polyarthritis associated with underlying neoplasia.

Polyarthritis can also be an uncommon complication of vaccination or administration of certain drugs. Polyarthritis associated with vaccination typically occurs within 5–7 days after inoculation and resolves spontaneously within 1–2 days. This is likely the result of transient circulating immune complex formation induced by the immunization [27]. A temporal association between onset of polyarthritis and administration of any drug therapy should prompt consideration of a causal relationship. Polyarthritis has been described in Doberman pinscher dogs following TMS therapy [48]. Clinical signs began between 10 and 21 days after initiation of treatment and rapid resolution was noted following withdrawal of the offending drug [48]. Repeated exposure to the drug resulted in relapse of signs.

Breed-specific polyarthritis has been reported in Shar Pei dogs associated with amyloidosis ("Shar Pei fever") and in young Akita dogs. In Shar Pei dogs, the hock joints are most commonly affected but carpal joints may also be involved. Usually only one or few joints are affected at a time, but joints affected can vary between episodes in a single individual. There are rare reports of synovial fluid findings [49, 50]. One dog showed a marked nonseptic, neutrophilic inflammation during acute disease, with normal joint fluid cytology seen during remission [49]. Another report demonstrated normal synovial fluid findings from several clinically affected as well as unaffected joints [50]. Joint pain and swelling is usually short-lived and resolves either without treatment or with administration of nonsteroidal anti-inflammatory drugs [49]. By contrast, Akita dogs seem to have a guarded prognosis and poor response despite treatment with immunosuppressive drugs [51]. Affected dogs usually first show clinical signs at a young age (<8 months) and have recurrent episodes of profound pain, which are often associated with fever and peripheral lymphadenopathy. Some affected dogs may also have suppurative meningitis [51].

Polyarthritis has also been associated with immune-mediated diseases concurrently affecting other tissues. Some dogs that present with steroid-responsive meningitis-arteritis (SMRA) also have IMPA [52]. Most cases are in young, medium- to large-breed dogs and clinical signs are often predominantly related to the meningitis, such as pain on flexion of neck. Lameness and joint effusion may not be evident despite inflammatory synovial fluid. Reported cases have responded well to immunosuppressive therapy. Polyarthritis has also been reported in association with polymyositis, predominantly in spaniel breeds [52, 53]. Myositis was confirmed on biopsy of at least two muscles in each case. Antinuclear antibody (ANA) testing was negative in all cases. The response to immunosuppressive therapy was more variable leading to the suggestion of worsened prognosis when polymyositis and arthritis occur concurrently compared to idiopathic IMPA alone [53].

SLE is a true autoimmune disease in which there is formation of antinuclear antibodies, in addition to autoantibodies against other cellular constituents [54]. Cases have been reported in both dogs and cats, although this disease is much less common than idiopathic IMPA. SLE should be considered when there are multiple, characteristic abnormalities present. Nonerosive polyarthritis is the most common clinical manifestation, but most affected animals also have glomerular protein loss and dermatologic lesions [54]. Immune-mediated cytopenias of any hematologic cell line may also be seen but are much less common than the previously mentioned features. Measurement of antinuclear antibodies is the most commonly performed "specific" test, although diagnosis of SLE is not based on any one finding or test result. One feature of note in some cases of SLE is identification of so-called "LE cells" (lupus erythematosus cells) in synovial fluid or other body fluids (Figure 43.12). These cells form when neutrophils phagocytize opsonized nuclear material that has been released from other cells in the fluid. The neutrophil nucleus is displaced peripherally by the phagocytized material, which has a characteristic, hyalinized pink appearance. While these cells are uncommon, when seen they are strongly suggestive of SLE. In addition to the characteristic LE cells, neutrophils may also contain small, dark fragments of material presumed to also be phagocytized nuclear material. These often lack the characteristic, smooth, pink appearance of the material in LE cells and must be differentiated from bacteria (Figure 43.13).

Other causes of suppurative arthropathy

While immune-mediated and infectious disease are the most common causes of a neutrophilic arthropathy, other possibilities need to be considered.

Repeated arthrocentesis at 3-week intervals did not induce a significant increase in synovial fluid neutrophil numbers in nine healthy dogs [55]. Likewise, arthrocentesis repeated at either weekly or 10-day intervals in normal horses did not result in significant changes in TNCC or percentage of neutrophils [56]. However, a study of normal calves did show an increase in both TNCC (mean 14,000/μL) and absolute neutrophil count (mean 7920/μL) in repeat samples collected 24 hours after initial sample [57]. Similar increases in TNCC have been noted 24 hours after initial arthrocentesis in horses [58], so caution should be exercised in interpretation if repeated samples are collected in this short of a time interval.

Intra-articular injections (antibiotics, local anesthetics, corticosteroids) can often incite a rapid neutrophilic inflammatory response, the magnitude of which can vary depending on the degree of irritation incited by the injected agent [5]. TNCCs greater than 30,000/μL have been observed. Even lavage of the joint with saline can result in a moderate neutrophilic inflammatory response [58]. Marked inflammation of periarticular tissues may also be associated with a neutrophilic response within the synovial fluid itself [15]. Mild neutrophilic inflammatory response sometimes occurs following chronic hemarthrosis.

General considerations in differentiating infectious from immune-mediated arthropathies

If there is no history suggesting administration of intra-articular injections, lavage, or joint trauma in a case with suppurative arthritis, then a distinction between infectious and immune-mediated disease must be made.

The only potential relevant findings from the fluid cytology itself regarding this decision would be either the presence of (i) infectious organisms (bacteria, morulae, yeast) or markedly degenerate neutrophils, which would support infectious causes, or (ii) LE cells or neutrophils with other phagocytized nuclear material, which would support immune-mediated causes. These are uncommon to rare findings but should be specifically considered and searched for in such cases. Other factors to consider are the cell count and percentage of neutrophils present. Most cases of septic arthritis have markedly increased cell counts (typically >50,000/μL and often >100,000/μL). By contrast, with immune-mediated disease, including those induced by systemic infections resulting in immune-complex disease, TNCC may vary from mildly to markedly increased. Additionally, with true septic arthritis neutrophils usually comprise the vast majority (>90%) of the nucleated cells. By contrast, with immune-mediated diseases the neutrophil percentage may vary from 20% to >90% of all nucleated cells. Thus, in cases with only a mild increase in cellularity or percentage of neutrophils, immune-mediated disease is more likely. If there is a marked increase in cellularity and marked predominance of neutrophils, septic or immune-mediated are equally likely. It is important to realize that in many cases, the above findings will not differentiate the two processes and distinction must be made by the clinician based on other clinical considerations.

Monoarticular involvement is more likely to be related to an infectious cause since most immune-mediated diseases result in a polyarthropathy [21, 27]. Sampling of several joints may help detect polyarticular involvement even if joints are seemingly unaffected based on physical findings. Prior surgery, intra-articular injections, or a traumatic wound near the affected joint would be common potential sources of infection [21, 27].

Polyarthritis is typical of immune-mediated diseases but can also be seen with infectious disease resulting from hematogenous spread rather than a penetrating wound [27]. Immune-mediated disease is more common in dogs than in other species and is the most common cause of polyarthritis in that species. Hematogenous spread of bacteria is most common with neonatal sepsis or bacterial endocarditis [27]. Regionally endemic systemic infections appropriate for the species of the patient (e.g., neutrophilic ehrlichiosis in dogs, histoplasmosis in cats, post-*Rhodococcus* infection in foals) must also be considered and ruled out via infectious disease testing.

Hemorrhagic or hemodilute samples

Samples that are hemodilute result from either (i) true hemarthrosis, (ii) blood contamination during sample collection, or (iii) diapedesis of red cells (transmigration across intact capillaries) that is often seen in association with inflammatory arthropathies. These can typically be differentiated based on a combination of the characteristics noted during collection and the cytologic findings.

Hemarthrosis

In true hemarthrosis, the sample is typically noted to be bloody from the very beginning of collection rather than

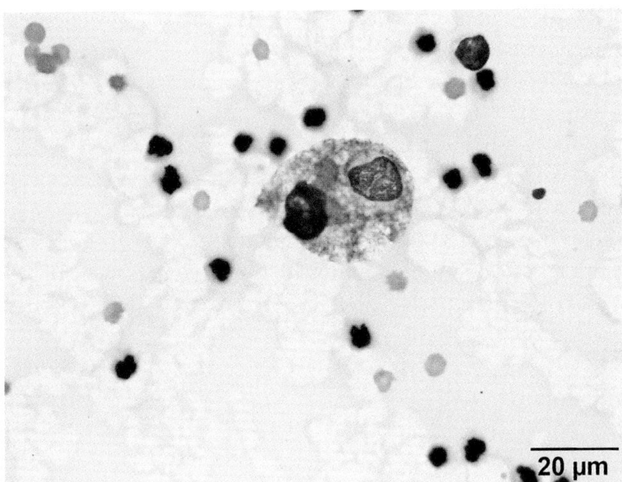

Figure 43.14 Direct smear of feline synovial fluid. A macrophage in the center displays phagocytosis or erythrocytes (erythrophagia). This finding suggests either hemarthrosis or diapedesis of erythrocytes secondary to inflammation rather than blood contamination during sample collection. In this case, there are many poorly spread out neutrophils surrounding the macrophage as well as relatively few erythrocytes, suggesting inflammation-induced diapedesis rather than frank intra-articular hemorrhage. Aqueous Romanowsky stain.

starting out clear. Cytologically, erythrocytes and leukocytes are generally present in numbers proportional to those seen in peripheral blood, after accounting for the patient's peripheral WBC count. This is subjectively assessed and is easy to do with experience. The sample may be compared to a blood film prepared from peripheral blood if there is any doubt.

With true hemarthrosis, macrophages may either display *erythrophagia* (phagocytosis of erythrocytes) or contain dark cytoplasmic pigment representing hemosiderin formed as a result of metabolism of erythrocyte hemoglobin (Figure 43.14). It is important to realize that erythrophagia is not found in every case since the amount of blood present may dilute out macrophages and make them difficult to find.

Even with blood contamination, *in vitro* erythrophagia may occur in the tube within a few hours. Therefore, direct smears should always be made immediately upon collection. Following bleeding into any body cavity such as the synovial space, platelets will aggregate and be removed. Thus, neither platelets nor platelet clumps will be seen unless the hemorrhage is active and ongoing. With chronic hemarthrosis, xanthochromia, a yellowish discoloration that forms from production of pigments from hemoglobin metabolism, may be noted in the supernatant formed following synovial fluid centrifugation.

Blood is cleared rapidly from the joint after a single bleeding event, at least in dogs. An *in vivo* study in dogs showed clearance of 71% of red cells at 24 hours and 96% at 48 hours [59]. The experimental hemorrhage was associated with an apparent inflammatory response as the TNCC increased from a baseline of <5000/µL to between ~5000 and 10,000/µL at 15 minutes and further increased to ~10,000 to 20,000/µL at 24 hours before returning to ~5000/µL at 48 hours. Unfortunately, differential leukocyte counts were not reported in this study. However, given the magnitude of the increase, this was likely a neutrophilic response. Experimental hemarthrosis in horses was noted to cause a "mild to moderate" increase in total WBC, neutrophils and mononuclear cells at 24 hours, which had resolved by 30 days, although the magnitude of the increases was not listed [60].

Hemarthrosis most often results from an acute traumatic injury to the joint. Recurrent hemarthrosis may also occur in animals with a hemostatic defect. Abnormalities of coagulation factors (hemophilia, vitamin K antagonism) are more likely to result in hemarthrosis than are platelet disorders such as thrombocytopenia. Intra-articular neoplasia is a much less common potential cause of hemarthrosis.

Contamination during collection

Blood contamination during sample collection can range from a minor increase in erythrocytes, only noted via microscopic examination, to a grossly blood sample. Compared to hemarthrosis, the collector may notice the sample be initially clear and then become bloody. Erythrophagia will be absent if smears were made immediately and platelets and/or platelet clumps will typically be found (Figure 43.15).

Direct smears should be examined even if there is blood contamination from sample collection to see if there is any evidence of leukocyte changes beyond what would be expected by the amount of hemorrhage. This is accomplished

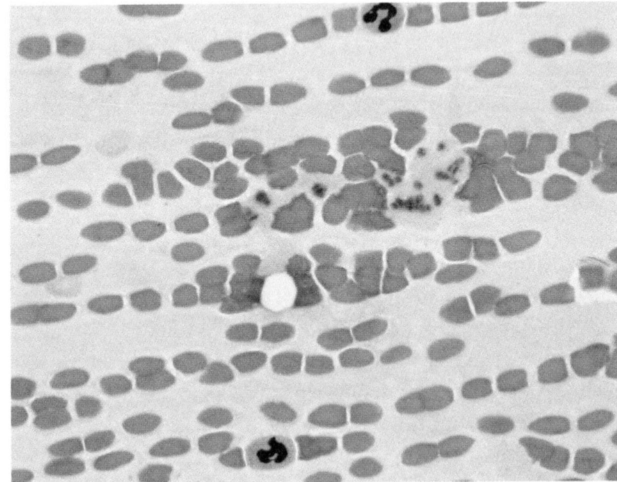

Figure 43.15 Iatrogenic blood contamination during sample collection in a direct smear of canine synovial fluid. Platelets are present in the center of the image amidst numerous erythrocytes exhibiting windrowing. Since platelets are removed quickly following intra-articular hemorrhage, this finding suggests either blood contamination during collection or ongoing hemorrhage. Aqueous Romanowsky stain, 500x original magnification.

by finding either (i) increased numbers of cells that would not be expected to come from peripheral blood (i.e., large, vacuolated macrophages) or (ii) a subjectively greater total number of neutrophils than would be expected from the amount of blood present. The former situation would suggest underlying degenerative joint disease. The latter situation may be seen in cases of infectious or immune-mediated joint disease. Since suppurative arthropathies are typically associated with dramatically increased neutrophil counts, detecting underlying inflammation may be possible despite significant blood contamination.

Blood contamination will have a significant effect on the *percentage* of neutrophils present, since normal synovial fluid has few neutrophils while neutrophils are the most prevalent leukocyte in peripheral blood. However, the effect on TNCC or TP is often minimal. One study examined the effects of blood contamination on synovial fluid results by adding autologous peripheral blood to normal synovial fluid *in vitro* in volumes up to 50% of the sample. While there were *statistically significant* increases in both TNCC and TP, the highest TNCC reported was 5000/μL and the highest TP found was 3.2 g/dL, even with addition of 50% blood [61]. Thus, even gross blood contamination is not likely to result in TNCCs suggestive of inflammatory arthropathies.

Hemorrhage/diapedesis secondary to DJD/inflammation

Minor hemorrhage or diapedesis of erythrocytes may occur secondary to either DJD or inflammatory arthropathies but is more common with inflammation. In these cases, the leukocyte changes related to the underlying condition are typically most prominent, but there may be mild to moderate increases in the numbers of erythrocytes in the background. Unless the sample is grossly discolored, the blood is unlikely to have a clinically significant effect on the TNCC. There may be an increased percentage of neutrophils present, especially if the baseline total cell count is low, since neutrophils will be the most common leukocyte added by the peripheral blood.

Neoplasia

Diagnosis of neoplasia via synovial fluid analysis is extremely rare. Certain primary neoplasms can involve the synovial membrane itself. The most common of these are synovial histiocytic sarcoma and synovial myxoma, but a variety of other sarcomas may less commonly arise from synovial tissue [62]. The histogenesis of the neoplasm previously termed "synovial cell sarcoma" is controversial. Many reported cases were likely misclassifications of histiocytic tumors prior to the widespread use of immunohistochemistry. The analogous tumor in humans is now thought to arise from a mesenchymal stem cell rather than truly being of synovial origin, even though the name has not changed [62]. Regardless, the diagnosis of these tumors is typically based on either histologic biopsy or fine needle aspiration biopsy of the lesion itself rather than from examination of synovial fluid.

Certain carcinomas have a propensity to metastasize to joint spaces. There are sporadic reports of patients presenting with a primary complaint of lameness and a diagnosis of metastatic carcinoma made by finding neoplastic cells via cytologic evaluation of synovial fluid (Figures 43.16 and 43.17) [63, 64].

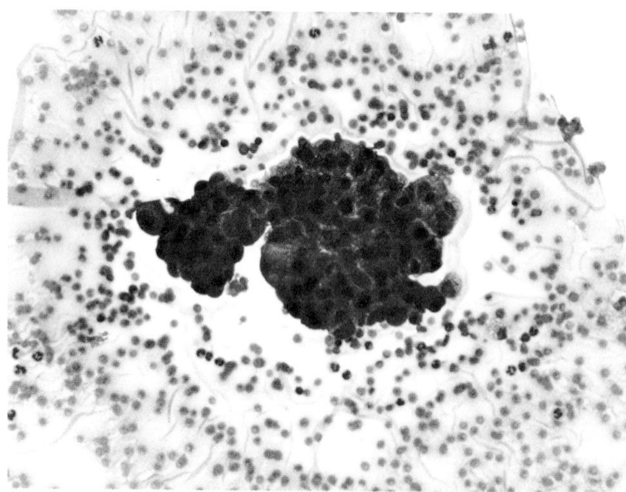

Figure 43.16 A large cluster of epithelial cells in a direct smear of synovial fluid of a dog with metastatic transitional cell carcinoma causing lameness. Epithelial cells are poorly spread out, which obscures cellular detail, but they are an atypical finding in synovial fluid. Aqueous Romanowsky stain, 200x original magnification.

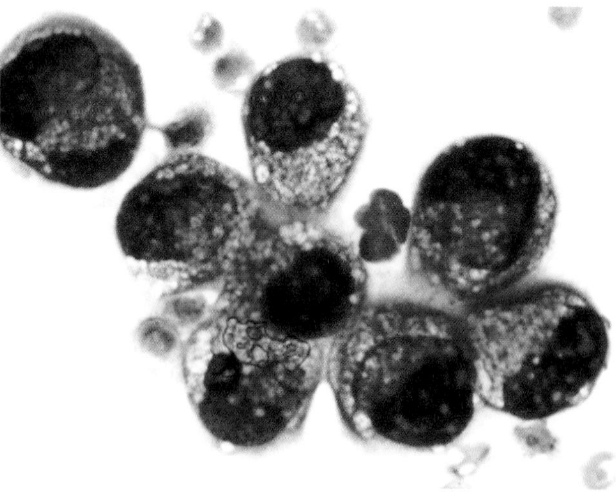

Figure 43.17 Higher magnification of cells from the same case as in Figure 43.16. Atypical epithelial cells are well spread out, allowing identification of cellular atypia. The cells have a high N : C ratio and significant anisokaryosis. Aqueous Romanowsky stain, 1000x original magnification.

44 Cytology of Abdominal Organs

Mary Anna Thrall[1] and Andrea A. Bohn[2]

[1]Department of Biomedical Sciences, Ross University School of Veterinary Medicine, Basseterre, Saint Kitts and Nevis

[2]Department of Microbiology, Immunology and Pathology, College of Veterinary Medicine and Biomedical Sciences, Colorado State University, Fort Collins, CO, USA

This chapter is a relatively brief introduction to cytology of selected organs, with emphasis on the liver and spleen. The reader is referred to other books such as *Veterinary Cytology* edited by Sharkey et al. (Wiley-Blackwell, 2021) for more detailed information. Examination of cytologic material that has been aspirated from enlarged abdominal organs and abnormal masses within the abdominal cavity is commonly used as a diagnostic aid. While aspiration can sometimes be accomplished using palpation, ultrasonography is almost always utilized in localizing specific organs and masses. This diagnostic tool has introduced an artifact in cytologic preparations: the presence of ultrasound gel on the slide, which is amorphous and stains a magenta color (Figure 44.1). To avoid contamination of the slide with gel, a minimum amount should be used, and the gel should be wiped from the biopsy site with gauze and alcohol prior to aspiration and removed from fingers if present. An excellent review of preferred techniques for obtaining cytologic samples has been published (see Liffman and Courtman 2017 in "Suggested Reading" under "General").

The discussion below is categorized by organ. The general principles of cytology apply to the interpretation when examining material from any abdominal mass or organ. One is generally attempting to determine if the tissue is normal, and if not, if inflammation or neoplasia is present. If inflammation is present, one then tries to determine the cause of the inflammation. Non-neoplastic, noninflammatory lesions may also be diagnosed, such as cystic structures, and depending on the organ involved, other abnormalities may be detected. Examples of specific causes of abdominal organ enlargement not due to inflammation or neoplasia would include hepatic lipidosis, extramedullary hematopoiesis (EMH) in the spleen, etc.

Liver

Indications

Hepatomegaly and nodular lesions identified by ultrasonography are the primary reasons for liver aspiration. Other indications include the suspicion of neoplasia or inflammation within the liver, suspicion of hepatic lipidosis, and increases in liver enzyme activity and/or bile acids in blood. The primary contraindications are abnormal hemostasis, caused by either thrombocytopenia (<30,000/μL) or decreased coagulation factor activity, and the suspicion of hemangiosarcoma, which could potentially rupture if lacerated during aspiration. In dogs with normal or mild coagulation abnormalities, hemorrhage as evidenced by decreased packed cell volume occurred in 42% of dogs in which ultrasound-guided percutaneous liver biopsies were obtained (see Reece et al. 2020 in "Suggested Reading" under "Liver"). However, fine-needle aspiration is much less likely to result in hemorrhage, which is one of the advantages of fine-needle aspiration over biopsy. In general, if tissue architecture is needed for the diagnosis, a biopsy is indicated, as cytology will not be diagnostic.

Technique

Unguided liver aspirates are usually taken from the left side, with the animal in right lateral or dorsal recumbency or standing. More commonly, cytologic samples are taken using ultrasound guidance. More cellular samples with less blood contamination are obtained using a nonaspiration technique, in which a 22-gauge needle of varying length (2.5–8.9 cm) is attached to a 12-mL syringe via a 30-in. flexible extension line normally used for IV sets. The syringe is filled with air, then hung over the shoulder to keep it out

CHAPTER 44

Veterinary Hematology, Clinical Chemistry, and Cytology, Third Edition. Edited by Mary Anna Thrall, Glade Weiser, Robin W. Allison and Terry W. Campbell.

Companion website: www.wiley.com/go/thrall/veterinary

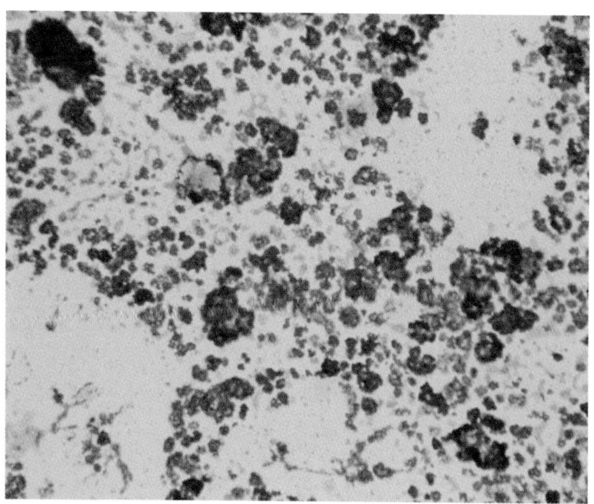

Figure 44.1 Ultrasound gel on a cytologic preparation. Wright stain.

of the way, and the needle is held like a pen to enhance manipulation. Visualization of the needle point is enhanced by orienting the bevel toward the transducer. The transducer is pointed directly toward the target that is to be aspirated, and the needle is maintained in the center of the ultrasound beam. To avoid tissue trauma–induced clotting, the needle tip is positioned in the area to be aspirated within 10 seconds. Once within the target, the needle tip is moved rapidly back and forth 5–10 times without using negative pressure. The back-and-forth motion of the needle detaches cells, and the lack of negative pressure decreases the chance of blood contamination. The needle is removed from the animal, and the biopsy material within the lumen of the needle is expelled onto one or two glass slides using the syringe that was prefilled with air. The slides are then prepared using the pull technique described in Chapter 2, air dried, and stained. Three separate aspirates from different areas of the lesion should be obtained to improve the chances of making a correct cytologic diagnosis. This technique is described in more detail elsewhere (see Menard and Papageorges 1995 in "Suggested Reading" under "Liver"). When compared to aspirates using negative pressure, aspirates without negative pressure such as described above have greater cellularity, less blood contamination, and fewer broken cells (see Fleming et al. 2019 in "Suggested Reading" under "Liver").

Interpretation of liver aspirates

A significant amount of variability has been reported regarding the diagnostic accuracy of liver cytology when compared to histopathology. Quality of the samples and expertise and experience of the cytologists and histopathologists likely contribute to this reported variability. In general, cytology of focal lesions is more sensitive and has a higher positive predictive value for the diagnosis of vacuolar change and neoplasia, and is less sensitive and has a lower positive predictive value for the diagnosis of inflammation, necrosis, and hyperplasia (see Bahr et al. 2013 in "Suggested Reading" under "Liver"). Even though the cytologic findings may not exactly match those of histopathology, numerous liver diseases can often be accurately diagnosed using cytology, including (i) increased cytoplasmic vacuolation due to hydropic degeneration, accumulation of glycogen, or accumulation of lipid; (ii) increased copper in the cytoplasm; (iii) cholestasis; (iv) inflammation; (v) metastatic and primary liver neoplasia; and (vi) fibrosis. Cytologic descriptions of aspirates of normal and abnormal liver are presented below.

Normal

Normal hepatocytes are uniform, large, round cells with abundant amphophilic, somewhat granular cytoplasm. Cells contain a round centrally located nucleus with a single prominent pale blue to lavender nucleolus. Cells sometimes contain two nuclei. Normal hepatocytes often contain a small amount of dark blue-black pigment (Figure 44.2). This pigment is lipofuscin, a type of lipid within lysosomes that is commonly seen in older animals and typically is a slightly lighter and bluer color than is bile pigment or hemosiderin. The presence of lipofuscin can be confirmed by numerous lipid-staining methods such as Sudan III, oil red, and ferric ferricyanide (Schmori method I). Bile is rarely seen within hepatocytes and appears as dark green-blue or blue-black and can be identified with certainty by using a bile stain. Hemosiderin may also be seen within hepatocytes and is usually a more golden-brown to dark brown color and can be confirmed by an iron stain such as Prussian blue. Increased amounts of hemosiderin are seen in hepatocytes and macrophages of animals with hemolytic anemia.

Hepatocytes may occur singly or in clusters. Very infrequently, rectangular crystalline clear to pink-colored inclusions may be seen in the nuclei of some hepatocytes and are of no known significance (see Richter et al. 1965 in "Suggested Reading" under "Liver"). Biliary epithelial cells (cholangiocytes) may also be seen occasionally in normal

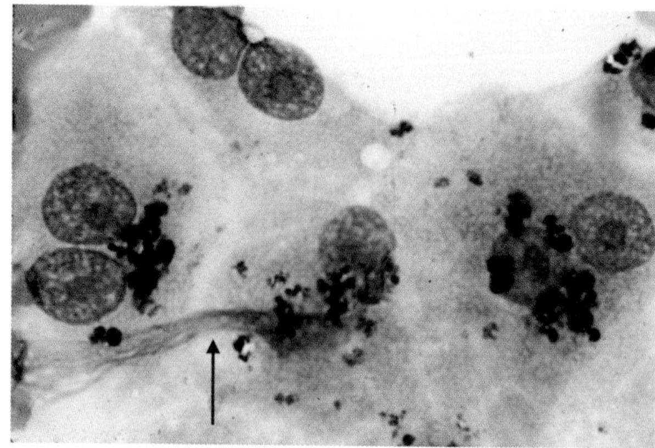

Figure 44.2 High magnification of normal binucleate hepatocytes. Note the single prominent nucleoli. One of the nuclei has ruptured and is streaming to the left (arrow). Lipofuscin granules within the hepatocytes are normal. Wright stain.

CHAPTER 44

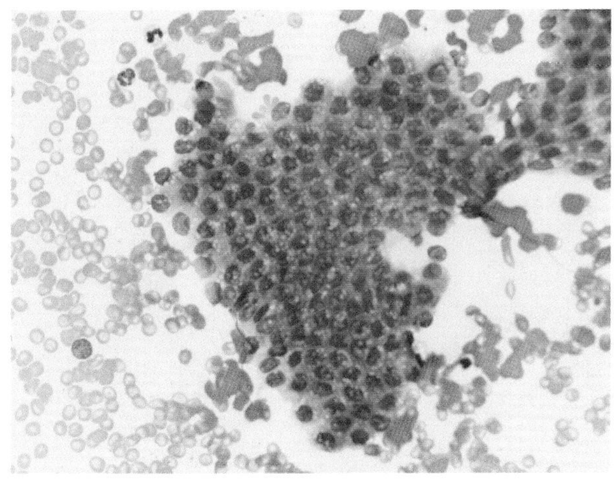

Figure 44.3 A cluster of biliary epithelial cells (cholangiocytes). Wright stain.

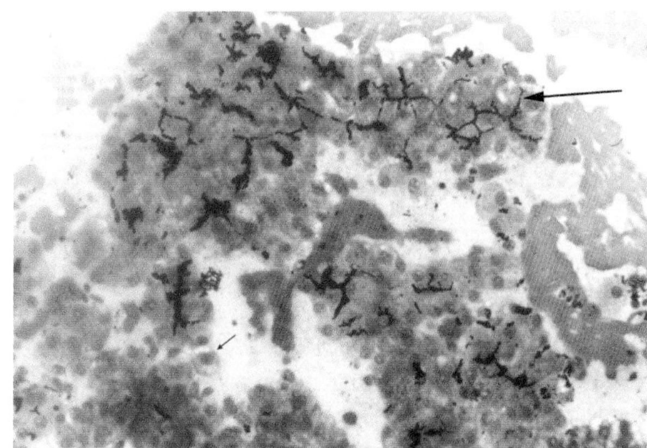

Figure 44.4 Aspirate of liver with marked cholestasis. Bile pigment is in canaliculi, exhibiting a linear appearance (large arrow). Most hepatocytes appear relatively normal, with a few showing vacuolar change (small arrow). Wright stain.

aspirates. They are small and uniform in size with round nuclei and a relatively small amount of pale blue cytoplasm (Figure 44.3). Other cells occasionally observed in small numbers in aspirates from normal livers include mast cells, macrophages (Kupffer cells), lymphocytes, and neutrophils. Hepatic stellate cells (Ito cells) are rarely observed. They are round and contain clear globules of lipid within the cytoplasm. Mesothelial cells from the surface of the liver are occasionally seen in liver aspirates and should not be confused with neoplastic epithelial cells or fibroblasts. Occasionally hematopoietic precursors can be seen in aspirates of normal liver. Although aspirates of the liver of normal kittens are usually not indicated or performed, the hepatocytes of normal kittens often contain vacuoles that appear to be lipid.

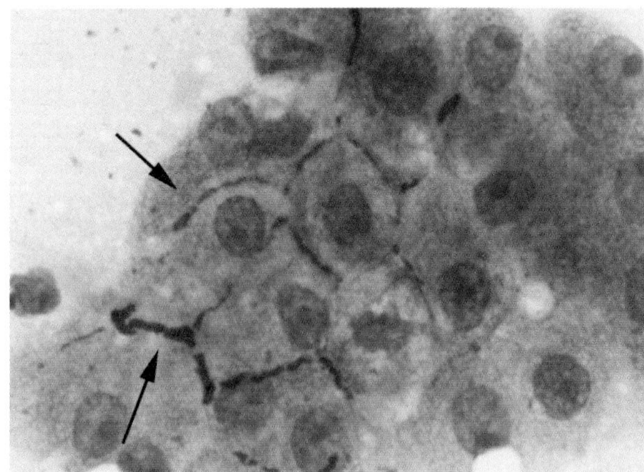

Figure 44.5 High magnification of bile pigment in canaliculi between hepatocytes (arrows). Wright stain.

Cholestasis

In animals with either intrahepatic or extrahepatic cholestasis, an increased amount of bile pigment may be observed within hepatocytes. Much more significantly, extracellular canalicular casts of bile, representative of the biliary tree, may be seen between hepatocytes (Figures 44.4 and 44.5).

Inflammation

Inflammation is evidenced by the presence of neutrophils, macrophages, lymphocytes or eosinophils, or some mixture of inflammatory cells. Inflammation may be suppurative (neutrophils) or nonsuppurative (lymphocytes or macrophages). The cytologic presence of inflammation should trigger biopsy and histologic examination, since the distribution of the inflammation cannot be determined unless an abscess visualized by ultrasonography was aspirated. The presence of inflammatory cells may indicate chronic hepatitis, acute hepatitis, cholangitis, cholangiohepatitis, or could accompany neoplasia. Liver inflammation in dogs is usually idiopathic or copper-related but can also be secondary to infectious diseases or neoplasia. In cats, cholangitis may be associated with the liver fluke *Platynosomum fastosum*, the incidence of which is very high in tropical and subtropical regions of the world such as the Caribbean and Brazil (Figure 44.6). In one study, eggs of *P. fastosum* were seen from 81% of stray cats in St. Kitts (see Krecek et al. 2010 in "Suggested Reading" under "Liver"). Centrilobular congestion, cholestasis, fibrosis, and liver failure may also be associated with this parasite, which is acquired by eating infected lizards.

Finding leukocytes within clusters of hepatocytes usually is indicative of hepatitis (Figures 44.7–44.10). Macrophagic inflammation may be indicative of an infectious disease that is typically associated with that type of inflammation, such as those caused by *Mycobacterium* spp., fungal diseases such as histoplasmosis, or protozoal diseases caused by *Leishmania* spp. or *Cytauxzoon* spp. (Figure 44.11). Ehrlichia morulae have been reported in lymphocytes within liver aspirates from a dog with hepatitis secondary to canine monocytic ehrlichiosis (see Mylonakis et al. 2010 in "Suggested

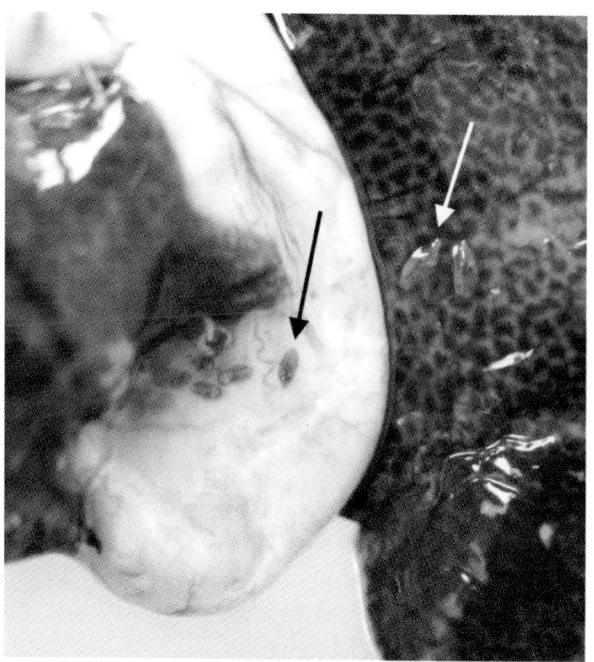

Figure 44.6 Cat liver fluke *Platynosomum fastosum* (arrows) on the surface of the liver after dissecting the gall bladder, bile ducts, and liver at autopsy of an adult St. Kitts cat. Note the enhanced reticular pattern of the liver due to congestion. The multiple lancet-shaped trematodes are approximately 5–12 mm long and 1 mm wide with a brown uterus and white vitellaria visible through the semitransparent tegument. Source: Courtesy Dr. Pompei Bolfa, Ross University School of Veterinary Medicine, St. Kitts, West Indies.

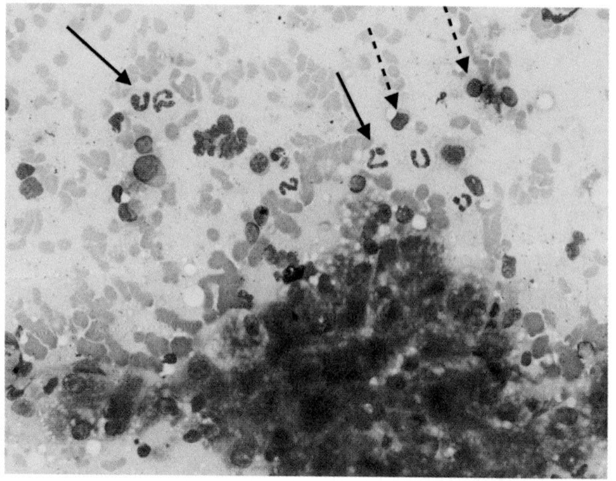

Figure 44.7 Liver aspirate from a dog with mixed inflammation. Lymphocytes are indicated by dashed arrows and neutrophils by solid arrows. Note the vacuolar change in the hepatocytes. Wright stain.

Reading" under "Liver"). Rarely viral inclusions of canine infectious hepatitis may be seen in hepatocyte nuclei; they appear as magenta-colored bodies of various sizes, surrounded by chromatin. If neutrophils or lymphocytes are seen in a liver aspirate, one should consider if they are from blood contamination of the sample and check the complete blood count for the presence of neutrophilia or lymphocytosis.

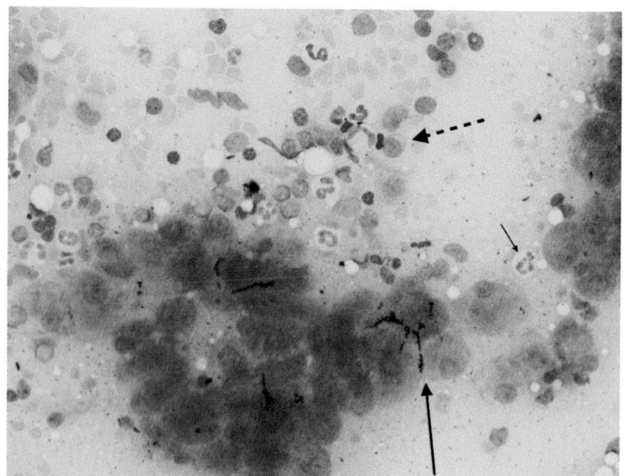

Figure 44.8 Liver aspirate from a dog with marked mixed inflammation. Many lymphocytes (dashed arrow) and neutrophils (small solid arrow) are present. Note the linear bile pigment within canaliculi between hepatocytes (large arrow) indicating cholestasis. Wright stain.

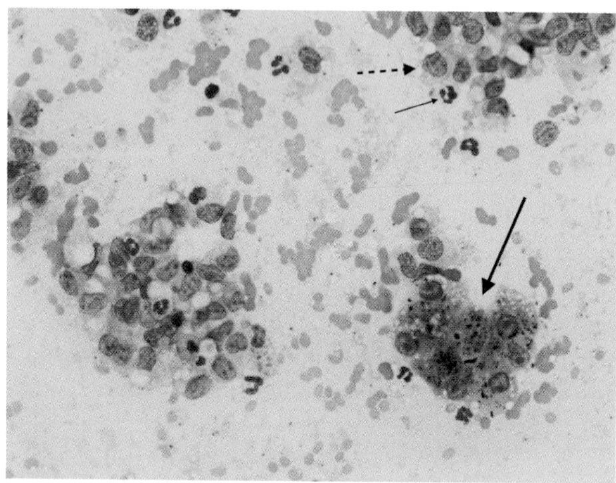

Figure 44.9 Liver aspirate from a cat with chronic inflammation of the liver. A cluster of hepatocytes (large arrow) with mild to moderate vacuolar change and pigment (likely lipofuscin) within the cytoplasm are shown in the center of the image. Neutrophils (small arrow) are scattered throughout, and an aggregate of macrophages is shown by the dashed arrow. Wright stain.

Vacuolar change

Vacuoles within the cytoplasm of hepatocytes are usually due to hepatic lipidosis, increased glycogen content, or hydropic degeneration. The presence of clear round discrete vacuoles is usually suggestive of lipid; the vacuoles may vary in size from small to large ballooning vesicles that distend hepatocytes, pushing the nucleus to the side, making them appear similar to small adipocytes (Figures 44.12 and 44.13). The clear staining areas are categorized by their size as either microvesicular or macrovesicular but on cytology often seem quite variable. Poorly delineated, light-colored, lacy-appearing areas in the cytoplasm are usually suggestive of increased glycogen content or hydropic degeneration (Figure 44.14). Special stains, such as periodic acid-Schiff (PAS) for glycogen or Sudan III for lipid, may be helpful

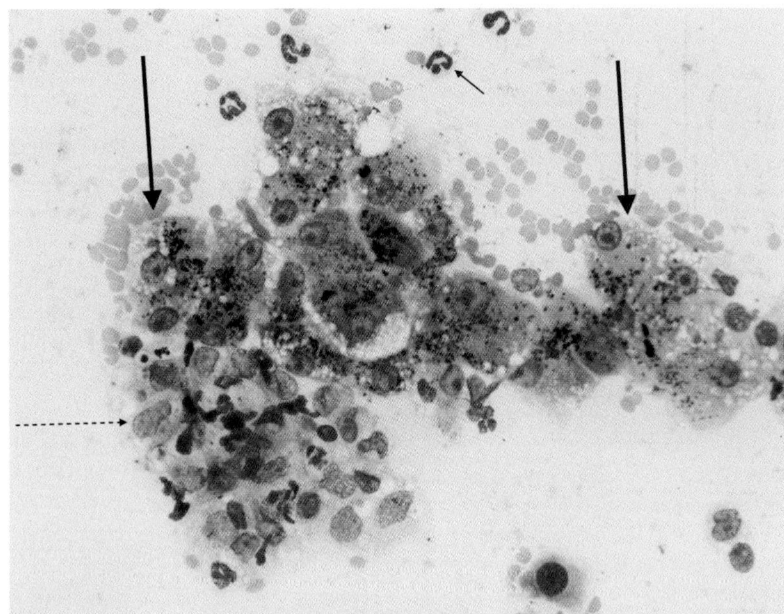

Figure 44.10 Same aspirate as shown in Figure 44.9. Large arrows indicate hepatocytes with vacuoles and lipofuscin, small arrow indicates neutrophil, and dashed arrow indicates macrophage. Wright stain.

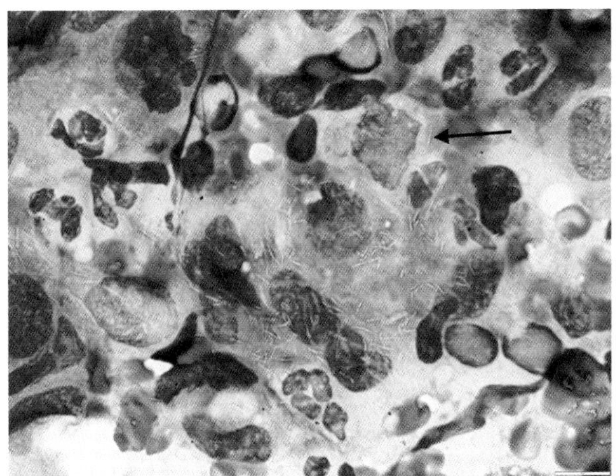

Figure 44.11 Aspirate of the liver of a dog. Pyogranulomatous inflammation is present as shown by the neutrophils and macrophages. Within the macrophages are clear nonstaining rods consistent with *Mycobacteria spp* (arrow). Wright stain.

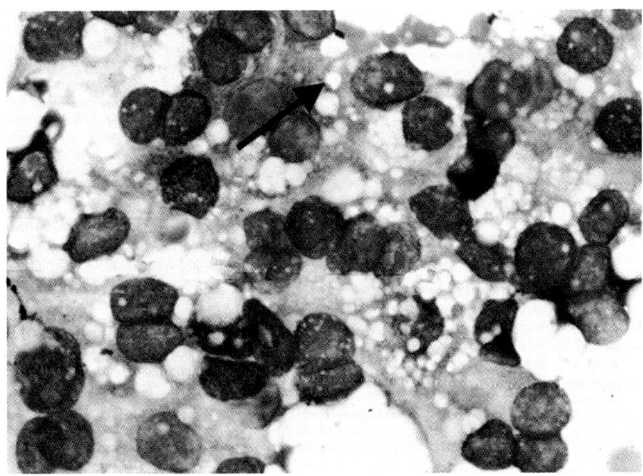

Figure 44.12 Aspirate of an enlarged liver from a patient with hepatic lipidosis. Note the numerous clear vacuoles within the cytoplasm of the hepatocytes (arrow). Wright stain.

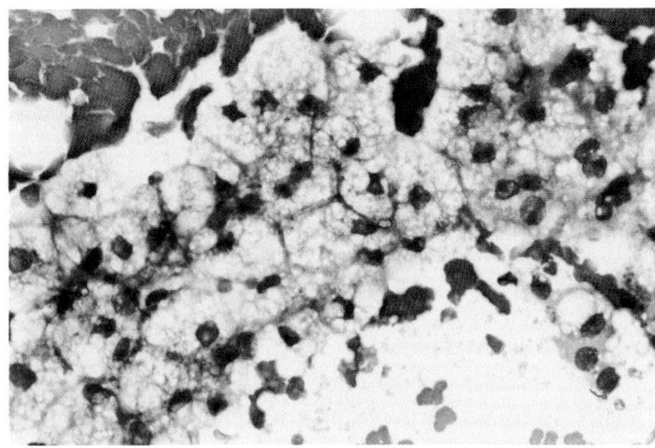

Figure 44.13 Aspirate of an enlarged liver from a patient with hepatic lipidosis. Hepatic vacuolization is marked, making the hepatocytes appear somewhat similar to adipocytes. Wright stain.

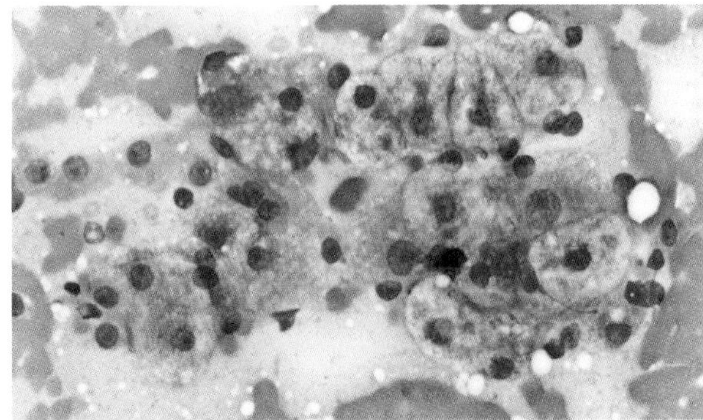

Figure 44.14 Aspirate of an enlarged liver from a dog with steroid hepatopathy. Note the lacy appearance of the cytoplasm compatible with increased glycogen. Wright stain.

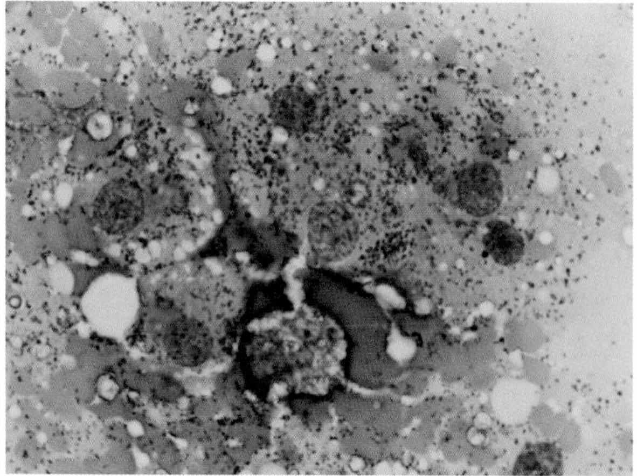

Figure 44.15 Liver aspirate from a cat with mucopolysaccharidosis VI. Note the numerous azurophilic granules within the cytoplasm and free in the background that consist of abnormally stored glycosaminoglycans (dermatan sulfate) resulting from inherited arylsulfatase B deficiency. Wright stain.

in differentiating the cause of vacuolar change. Hepatic lipidosis is more commonly seen in cats, whereas increased glycogen content and hydropic degeneration is more commonly seen in dogs. Steroid hepatopathy is a common cause of increased glycogen content. Although rare, lysosomal storage disorders may result in either granules (the mucopolysaccharidoses) (Figure 44.15) or vacuoles (lipid storage disorders) (Figure 44.16) in hepatocytes as a result of abnormal accumulation of substrate in lysosomes.

Nodular hyperplasia

Nodular hyperplasia is common in old dogs and may appear similar to primary or metastatic neoplasia by ultrasonography. Hyperplastic hepatocytes from these nodules usually appear much like normal hepatocytes. More binucleate hepatocytes may be observed, but the cells usually do not have features of malignancy. Cytologic abnormalities may

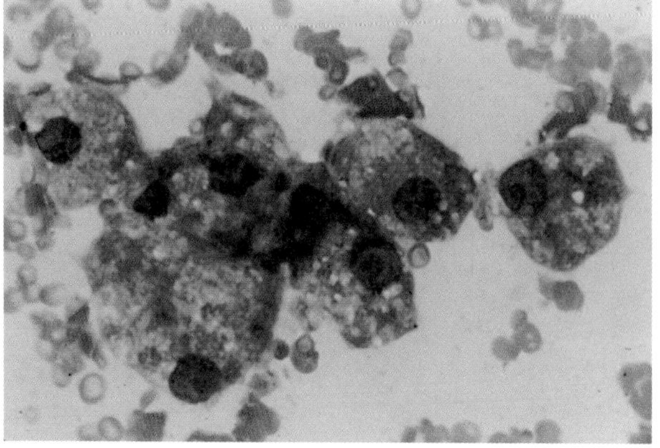

Figure 44.16 Liver aspirate from a cat with the lysosomal storage disease Niemann–Pick C, a cholesterol storage disorder. The vacuoles within the cytoplasm are representative of cholesterol. Wright stain.

include subtle increases in cell and nuclear size and slight variation in cell and nuclear size. Increased basophilia and vacuolization can also be seen.

Extramedullary hematopoiesis

EMH is commonly observed in liver aspirates of animals with increased hematopoiesis due to either inflammation, anemia, or hypoxia (Figure 44.17). Cells are those encountered in a bone marrow aspirate (erythroid and myeloid precursors and megakaryocytes). Progression of maturation is orderly, thus distinguishing EMH from a myeloproliferative disorder (Figure 44.18) (see Chapter 16).

Copper accumulation

Inherited copper-associated hepatopathy has been recognized in numerous breeds, including Bedlington terriers, West Highland white terriers, and Labrador retrievers. Increased copper in the liver can also be seen in Doberman pinschers with chronic hepatitis and may have a genetic predisposition. Increased copper in hepatocytes can also be seen in other breeds of dogs with cholestasis and inflammation. Copper is sometimes visible within the cytoplasm of hepatocytes and appears as pale green or turquoise crystalline granules with Wright stain (Figure 44.19). The presence of copper can be confirmed by staining for copper with rhodanine (Figure 44.20). De-staining cytology slides for special staining works well and is described in Marcos et al. 2009 in "Suggested Reading" under "General."

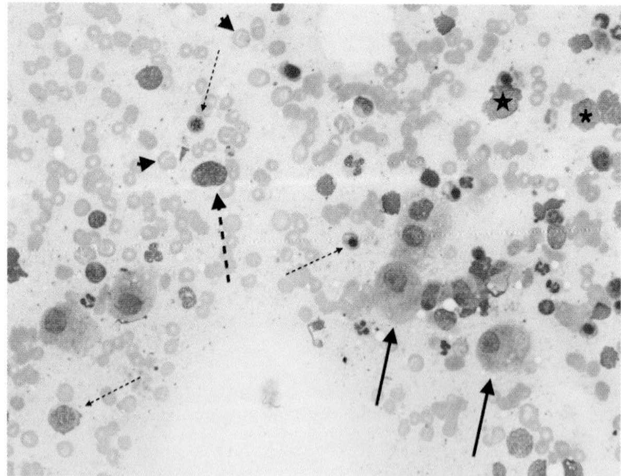

Figure 44.17 Liver aspirate from a dog with hepatomegaly, regenerative anemia, and marked extramedullary hematopoiesis with erythroid predominance. Maturation is orderly with marked polychromasia (arrowheads). Normal-appearing hepatocytes (large arrows), rubriblasts (large dashed arrow), and rubricytes and metarubricytes (small dashed arrows) are present. It is important not to confuse rubriblasts with lymphoblasts; the presence of more mature erythroid precursors helps differentiation. Broken nuclei likely from hepatocytes are indicated by stars. Wright stain.

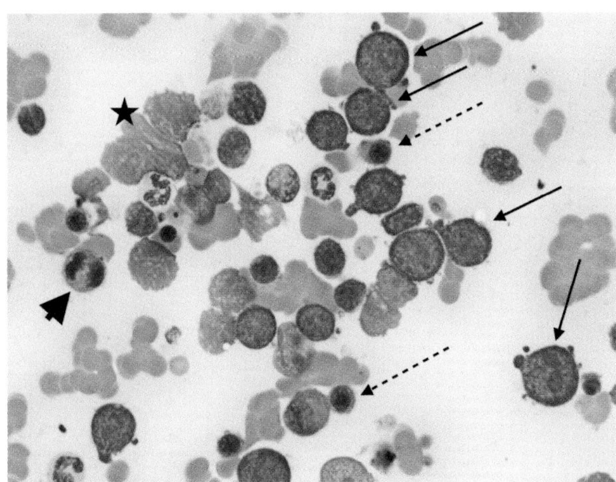

Figure 44.18 Liver aspirate from a cat with myeloproliferative disorder involving erythroid cell line (red cell leukemia). Note the disorderly maturation. Most of the erythroid precursors are rubriblasts (arrows). More mature metarubricytes are indicated by dashed arrows. An erythroid precursor in mitosis is also present (arrowhead). Broken cells are indicated by star. Wright stain.

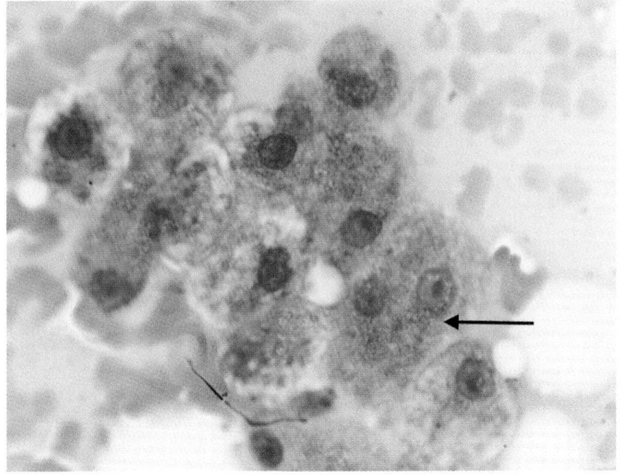

Figure 44.19 Liver aspirate from an 8-year-old dog with copper-associated hepatopathy. The alanine aminotransferase (ALT) activity in the serum was >1000 IU/L (normal = <125) on presentation, and alkaline phosphatase (ALP) activity was 549 IU/L (normal = <212). Note the turquoise-colored crystalline material within the cytoplasm of hepatocytes (arrow). Wright stain. Source: Courtesy Dr. Russell Moore, Colorado State University.

For additional information on copper-related hepatopathy, see Moore et al. 2016 and 2019 in "Suggested Reading" under "Liver."

Hepatic fibrosis

Hepatic fibrosis is a wound-healing response to chronic hepatitis, usually either idiopathic or copper-associated in the dog, that leads to deposition of fibrillar extracellular matrix components in the liver that are made of collagen. Fibrosis may lead to portal hypertension and acquired portosystemic shunts. Damaged hepatocytes and cytokines cause hepatic stellate cells (Ito cells) to transform into myofibroblasts that are thought to be the primary source of the matrix formation. Other cells that may play a role include resident fibroblasts, bone-marrow-derived fibrocytes, smooth muscle cells around vessels, and epithelial cells that transform to mesenchymal cells. Advanced fibrosis may lead to discrete nodule formation. Progressive replacement of hepatic parenchyma by fibrosis eventually results in hepatic synthetic failure, in which the liver fails to produce albumin, urea, cholesterol, and coagulation factors (see Chapter 27). Fibrosis can sometimes be diagnosed by aspiration cytology by the increase in spindle cells and mast cells, with at least 1 spindle cell per 10 hepatocytes and 4 mast cells per 100 hepatocytes considered increased enough to suggest fibrosis (see Masserdotti and Bertazzolo 2016 in "Suggested Reading" under "Liver"). However, for a definitive diagnosis, histologic examination of biopsy samples from several liver lobes is recommended, although in animals with liver failure secondary to fibrosis, biopsy could result in hemorrhage. A coagulation panel should be performed prior to biopsy.

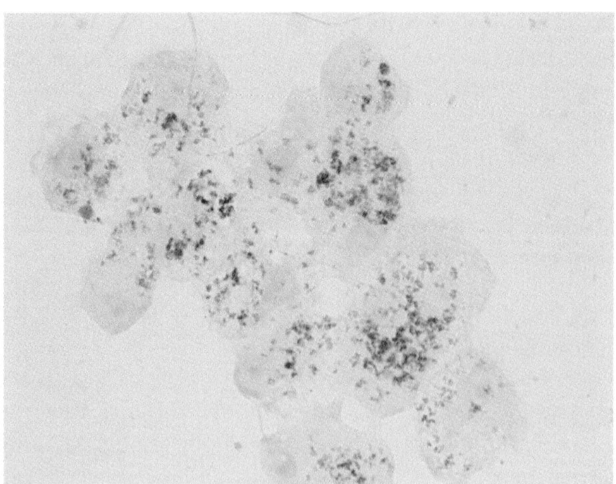

Figure 44.20 Same aspirate as shown in Figure 44.19. The presence of copper is confirmed by using a stain specific for copper, which stains an orange-brown color. Rhodanine stain. Source: Courtesy Dr. Russell Moore, Colorado State University.

Primary neoplasia

Hepatomegaly and increased bilirubin are common findings in dogs and cats with hepatobiliary neoplasia. Depending on the extensiveness of the neoplasia, other laboratory findings may include hypoalbuminemia, hyperglobulinemia, increased serum bile acids, and increased serum liver enzyme activity. Primary hepatocellular tumors are hepatocellular adenomas or carcinomas. Neoplasms of the liver can also originate from bile duct epithelium (biliary adenoma or carcinoma), cells of neuroendocrine origin (hepatic carcinoid), and mesenchymal cells (sarcoma).

Hepatocellular adenoma

Hepatocellular adenomas are more common in cats than dogs and are usually singular, often large tumors. They are difficult to distinguish from hyperplasia on cytology, as the hepatocytes usually appear quite normal. Cytologic features, however, may include mild anisocytosis, anisokaryosis, increased nucleus:cytoplasm ratio, and mild increased cytoplasmic vacuolation (Figure 44.21).

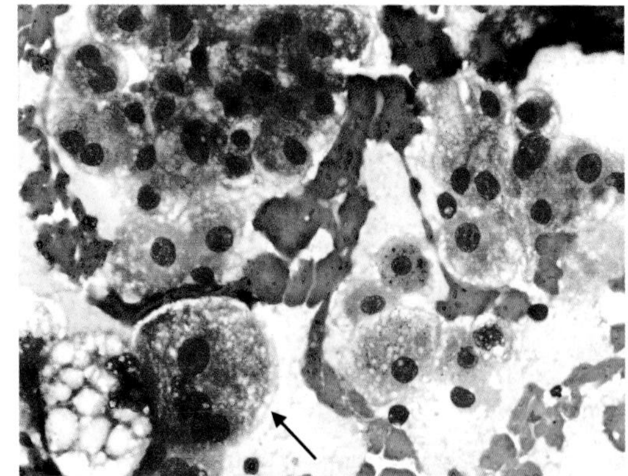

Figure 44.21 Liver aspirate from a dog with hepatocellular adenoma. Many of the hepatocytes appear relatively normal. Abnormal features include cytomegaly, increased vacuolation, and multinucleated hepatocytes (arrow). Wright stain.

Hepatocellular carcinoma

Hepatocellular carcinomas are more common in dogs than in cats and are usually single large tumors, although they may be nodular or diffuse. Neoplastic hepatocytes often resemble normal hepatocytes to some extent, in that they typically have abundant basophilic cytoplasm. They usually have features of malignancy, however, such as cell crowding or piling, multiple nucleoli, variation in nuclear size, increased nucleus:cytoplasmic ratio, and variation in cell size, unless they are very well differentiated (Figure 44.22). Definitive diagnosis of well-differentiated hepatocellular carcinomas often requires large biopsies for histologic examination because hepatic structure is necessary to differentiate these tumors from hyperplasia or adenomas. Highly malignant hepatocytes are usually distinguishable from hyperplastic hepatocytes. Cytologic evidence of necrosis may also be present.

Occasionally hepatocellular carcinomas are so poorly differentiated that they cannot be distinguished from metastatic carcinoma (Figure 44.23).

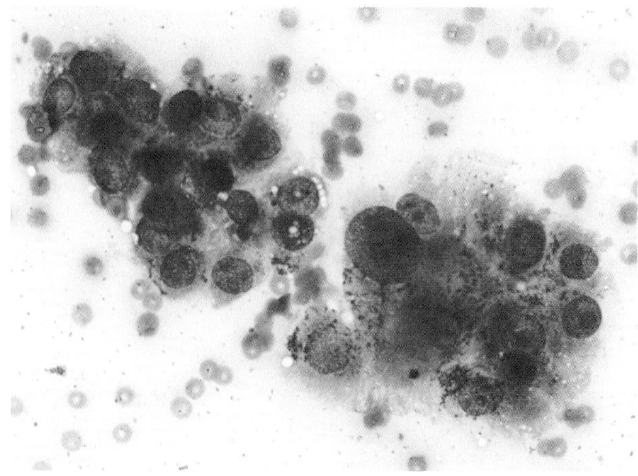

Figure 44.22 Liver aspirate from a dog with hepatocellular carcinoma. Note that the cells maintain some features of hepatocytes, but numerous criteria of malignancy are present including anisokaryosis, prominent large multiple nucleoli, and anisocytosis. Granules in the cytoplasm have been reported with hepatocellular carcinoma. Wright stain.

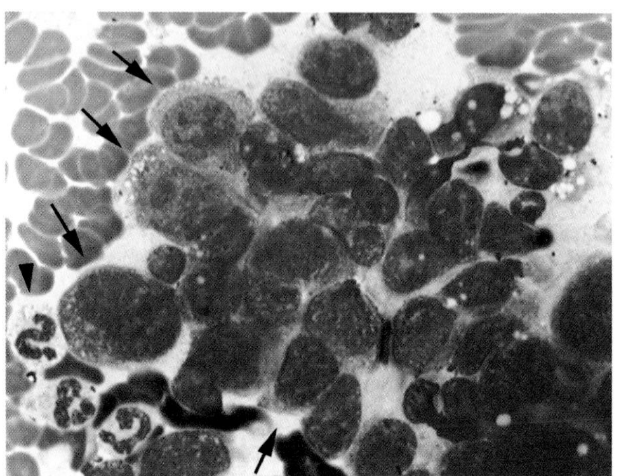

Figure 44.23 Liver aspirate from a dog with poorly differentiated hepatocellular carcinoma in which the neoplastic cells would be difficult to differentiate from a metastatic carcinoma by cytology. Note the numerous features of malignancy including high nucleus:cytoplasm ratio, multiple prominent nucleoli, and nuclear molding (arrows). A few neutrophils are present (arrowhead). Wright stain.

Biliary adenoma and biliary cystadenoma

Biliary adenomas are rare, and whether biliary cystadenomas are neoplasms or a developmental anomaly is controversial. Biliary cystadenomas are more common in cats, can become large, and when aspirated, the material usually contains cyst contents and a scattering of normal-appearing biliary epithelial cells.

Biliary carcinoma (cholangiocarcinoma) and biliary cystadenocarcinoma

Biliary carcinomas are common liver tumors in cats and dogs and are typically aggressive with metastasis. Biliary carcinomas are tubular structures lined with cuboidal or columnar biliary epithelial cells. Biliary cystadenocarcinomas are similar but contain cysts. Malignant biliary epithelial cells have scant cytoplasm and may exhibit marked nuclear

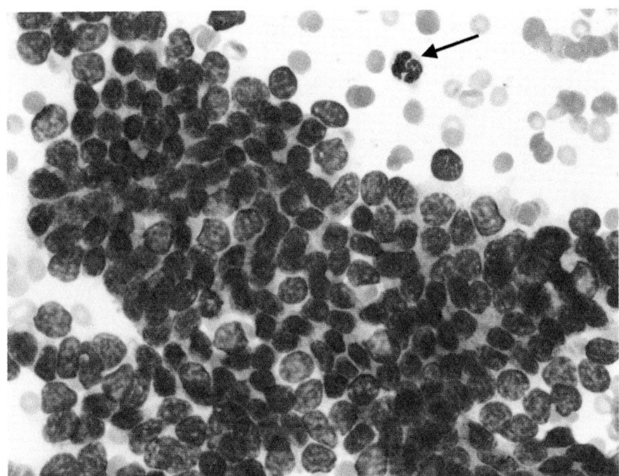

Figure 44.24 Liver aspirate from a dog with a well-differentiated cholangiocarcinoma. Note the cellular piling and mild anisocytosis. A neutrophil is indicated by the arrow, for size comparison. Wright stain.

atypia such as prominent nucleoli and clumped chromatin (Figure 44.24). Cells in mitosis may be seen.

Neuroendocrine tumors (carcinoids)

Intrahepatic neuroendocrine tumors are usually nodular or diffuse. These tumors are derived from the APUD (amine precursor uptake and decarboxylation) cells of the biliary system. The cells are similar to other neuroendocrine tumors and are usually quite fragile, thus numerous naked or bare nuclei are seen. Intact cells are small with round central nuclei. Chromatin is usually condensed, nucleoli are indistinct, and the cytoplasm is moderate to abundant and usually pale in color. Cytoplasmic vacuoles may be present. Cellularity is usually abundant in aspirates of these tumors, and they are difficult to differentiate from metastatic endocrine tumors.

Metastatic neoplasia

The liver is a common site for metastasis of tumors, which may occur as a single mass, multiple masses, or diffusely throughout the liver. These are briefly discussed in the following sections. Metastatic carcinomas could be from any epithelial tissue, including pancreas, gastrointestinal tract, bladder, mammary glands, etc. The most common metastatic sarcoma is hemangiosarcoma from the spleen. Metastatic round cell tumors include lymphoma, plasma cell neoplasia (usually multiple myeloma), mast cell neoplasia, and malignant histiocytic cells (histiocytic sarcoma or malignant histiocytosis).

Metastatic carcinoma and neuroendocrine and endocrine tumors

Metastatic carcinomas are detected cytologically by seeing epithelial cells that are not consistent with hepatocytes. Carcinoma cells usually can be recognized by their cell-to-cell relationship and commonly have malignant features, including large size, variability in cell size, variability in nuclear size, prominent nucleoli, basophilic cytoplasm, and perinuclear cytoplasmic vacuoles, especially in secretory cells (see Chapter 40). Commonly, the tissue of origin cannot be determined. Metastatic endocrine and neuroendocrine tumors appear as described above.

Sarcomas

Although sarcomas may originate in the liver, they are more commonly metastatic. Sarcoma cells are spindle-shaped with oval nuclei and prominent nucleoli (Figure 44.25). The cytoplasm is basophilic and may be vacuolated. They may be uniform or vary in size and shape. They may not exfoliate as readily as carcinoma cells, but they are readily observed on imprints of surgical biopsies. These cells should not be confused with fibroblasts, which may be present in animals with hepatic fibrosis. Hemangiosarcomas are the most common sarcomas and have usually metastasized from the spleen. Evidence of previous hemorrhage (erythrophagocytosis and hemosiderin-laden macrophages) and polychromatophilic erythrocytes may be observed, as may the abnormally shaped erythrocytes (acanthocytes) sometimes observed in blood films from dogs with hemangiosarcoma.

Lymphoma

Lymphoma is a relatively common neoplasm within the liver and is usually easily diagnosed by cytology. Neoplastic lymphocytes are usually diffusely distributed among normal-appearing hepatocytes (Figures 44.26 and 44.27). Liver aspirates containing large numbers of small lymphocytes can be more difficult to interpret, as the lymphoid population may be representative of an inflammatory process or small cell lymphoma. Surgical biopsy and histopathology,

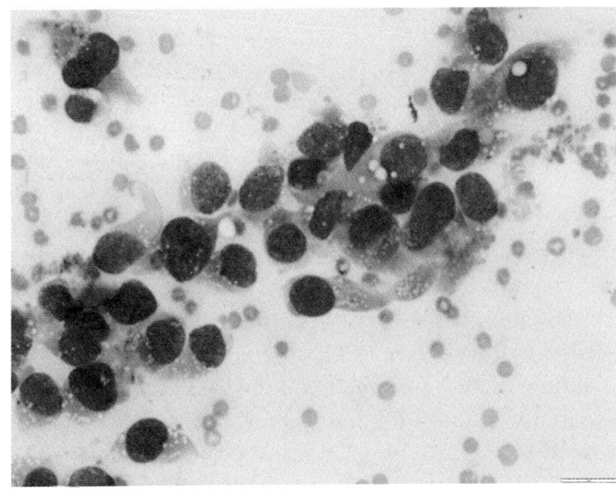

Figure 44.25 Liver aspirate from a dog with sarcoma in liver. Note the numerous spindle-shaped cells with punctate vacuoles within the cytoplasm. No hepatocytes are in this image. Wright stain.

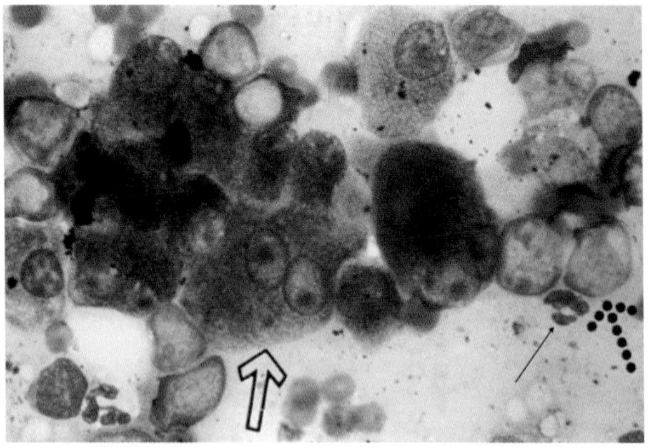

Figure 44.26 High magnification of a liver aspirate from a dog with disseminated lymphoma. Normal hepatocytes are indicated by open arrow, lymphoblasts by dotted arrow, and a neutrophil for size comparison by the small solid arrow. Wright stain.

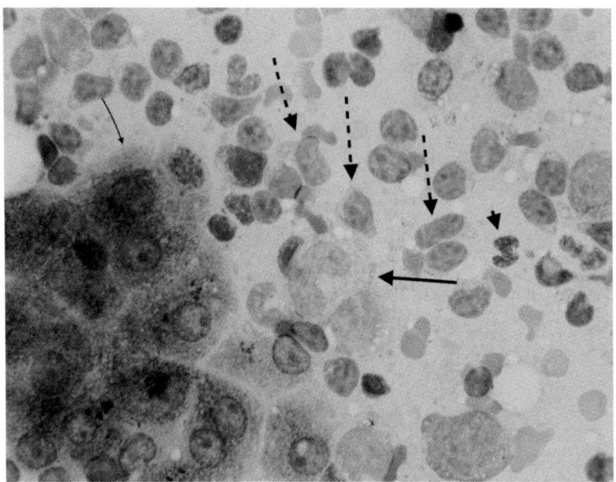

Figure 44.27 Liver aspirate from dog with large granular lymphocyte lymphoma (T-cell). Normal hepatocytes are indicated by small solid arrow, small to intermediate-sized large granular lymphocytes by dotted arrows, a neutrophil for size comparison by an arrowhead, and a probable myeloid precursor by the large solid arrow. Wright stain.

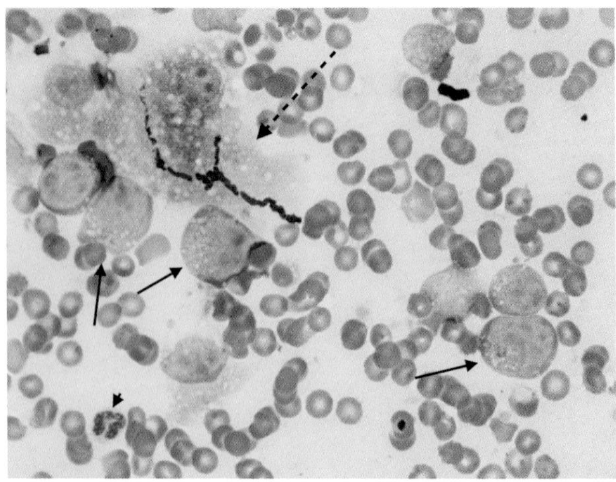

Figure 44.28 Liver aspirate from dog with large granular lymphocyte lymphoma (T-cell). Numerous immature T cells are indicated by arrows. Evidence of canalicular bile stasis around a normal hepatocyte is indicated by dashed arrow. Note neutrophil (arrowhead) for size comparison of lymphoid cells. Wright stain.

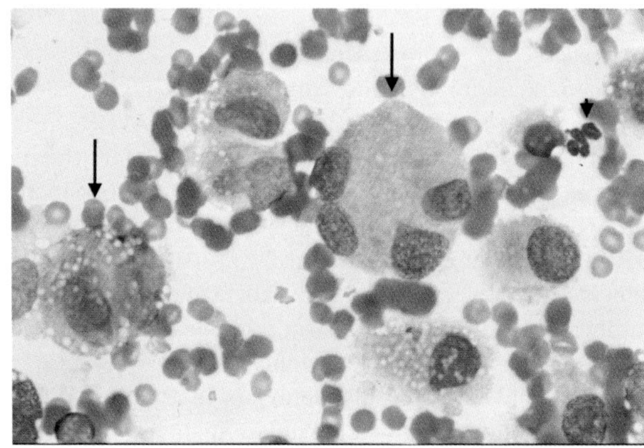

Figure 44.29 Liver aspirate from dog with disseminated histiocytic sarcoma. Numerous malignant histiocytes are present. Multinucleated cells are indicated by arrows. A neutrophil for size comparison is indicated by arrowhead. Wright stain.

as well as blood, bone marrow, lymph node cytology, immunophenotyping, and polymerase chain reaction (PCR) should distinguish the two processes. Lymphoma may originate in the liver or may metastasize from other areas. T-cell lymphoma that involves the liver in the absence of peripheral lymphadenopathy is usually either hepatosplenic T-cell lymphoma, which is very aggressive, or hepatocytotropic T-cell lymphoma (see Keller et al. 2013 in "Suggested Reading" under "Liver") (Figure 44.28). Hepatosplenic lymphoma is also discussed in the "Spleen" section of this chapter.

Disseminated histiocytic sarcoma

Disseminated histiocytic sarcoma, previously referred to as malignant histiocytosis, is often characterized by the systemic proliferation of large, pleomorphic, single and multinucleated histiocytes with moderate amounts of lightly basophilic vacuolated cytoplasm. Neoplastic histiocytic cells can appear fairly well differentiated but often exhibit marked cellular atypia. Features of malignancy include marked anisocytosis and anisokaryosis, prominent nucleoli, bizarre mitotic figures, and occasional phagocytosis of erythrocytes and leukocytes. The presence of multinucleated giant cells supports the diagnosis (Figure 44.29). Disseminated histiocytic sarcoma is a rapidly progressive, ultimately fatal, disorder that has been described in adult dogs, including Bernese mountain dogs; an increased incidence of the disorder is also seen in the golden retriever and flat-coated retriever breeds.

Myeloproliferative disease

Neoplastic myeloid cells commonly infiltrate the liver (see Chapter 16). If they are somewhat differentiated, recognizable progranulocytes with pink cytoplasmic granules will aid in the diagnosis. If they are undifferentiated, they may resemble lymphoblasts, and immunophenotyping may be necessary to accurately determine cell type.

Mast cell neoplasia

Large numbers of mast cells are present on the aspirate, and/or mast cells with atypical morphologic features are present. Although a few mast cells can be seen in normal liver, and increased mast cell numbers are seen with fibrosis, the number of mast cells with metastatic neoplasia is usually markedly increased, and they often appear in aggregates.

Gall bladder

Normal gall bladder aspirates are characterized by amorphous granular material and are usually acellular, although a few biliary epithelial cells may be seen (Figure 44.30). Bilirubin crystals may be seen and are usually needle-shaped and golden brown in color. In infected and/or inflamed gall bladders, bacteria may be seen and sometimes identified; however, culture should be performed for definitive identification. Inflammatory cells may include neutrophils, macrophages, and lymphocytes. Fluke eggs, yeast, and protozoa have been occasionally observed in aspirates. If the gall bladder is distended due to obstruction, or the wall is necrotic, gall bladder rupture may occur during aspiration, but this complication is very rare.

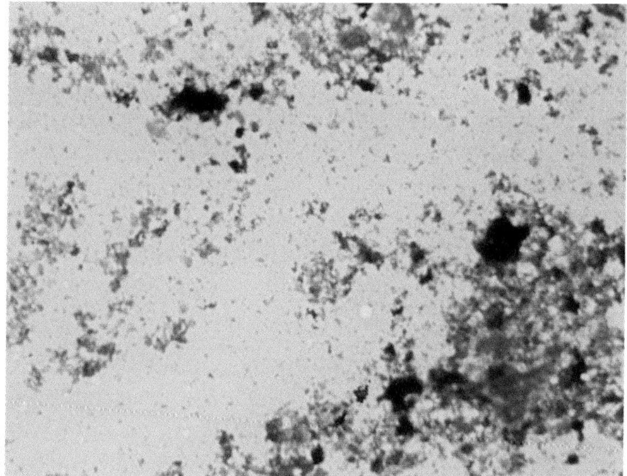

Figure 44.30 Aspirate of normal bile from the gall bladder of a dog. Note the granular amorphous material. No inflammatory cells or bacteria are present. Wright stain.

Spleen

Aspiration cytology of the spleen has been performed in humans since at least 1932. Splenomegaly, the presence of a splenic mass or nodule, an abnormal appearance on ultrasound examination, and staging of multicentric neoplasia, such as lymphoma or mast cell neoplasia, are the most common indications for aspiration of the spleen. In one study of 370 small dogs undergoing splenectomy for nodular splenic lesions, 44% of the lesions were benign and 56% were neoplastic, and the presence of hemoabdomen was usually associated with malignancy (see Fernandez et al. 2019 in "Suggested Reading" under "Spleen"). In another study of 105 dogs with incidentally detected non-ruptured splenic masses, 70% of the lesions were benign, and 30% were malignant, the most common malignancy being hemangiosarcoma (see Cleveland and Casale 2016 in "Suggested Reading" under "Spleen").

As with liver, a nonaspiration technique is usually better than aspiration techniques. Nonaspiration techniques result in less blood contamination and higher cellularity. Also as with liver, if the diagnosis depends on architecture, cytology is not diagnostic.

In most studies, cytologic diagnoses correlated reasonably well with histologic diagnoses. Complications are rare, even in thrombocytopenic patients.

Normal

Specimens from normal spleen usually contain a large amount of blood since one of the functions of the spleen is to store blood. However, the presence of blood should not be considered diagnostic of a normal spleen, since blood can also be aspirated from tumors, hematomas, and congested spleens. Nucleated cells are primarily lymphoid cells, most of which are small lymphocytes. Small numbers of lymphoid cells are intermediate or large with nucleoli (see Chapter 45 for guidelines for lymphoid cell sizing). Numerous well-differentiated mast cells may be present, as well as small numbers of plasma cells and hematopoietic precursors. Splenic stromal tissue is commonly present, consisting of small uniform mesenchymal (spindle-shaped) cells. Numerous macrophages containing hemosiderin may also be seen.

Non-neoplastic lesions of the spleen

Non-neoplastic cytologic diagnoses of the spleen can include splenic hyperplasia, inflammation, EMH, and hemosiderosis.

Splenic hyperplasia

Splenic hyperplasia may be nodular or diffuse and is proliferation of the normal components of the spleen in response to antigenic stimulation, inflammation, or neoplasia. Hyperplasia may involve stromal elements and macrophages or

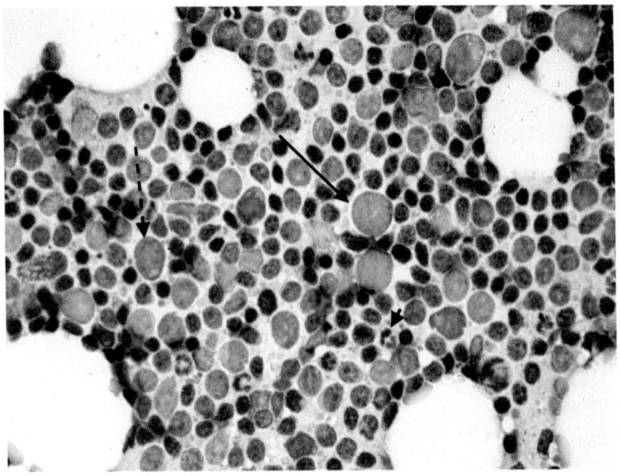

Figure 44.31 Aspirate of a spleen with lymphoid hyperplasia. Most of the cells are small lymphocytes. A large immature lymphoid cell is indicated by the arrow. An immature plasma cell is indicated by the dashed arrow, and a neutrophil for size comparison is indicated by the arrowhead. Wright stain.

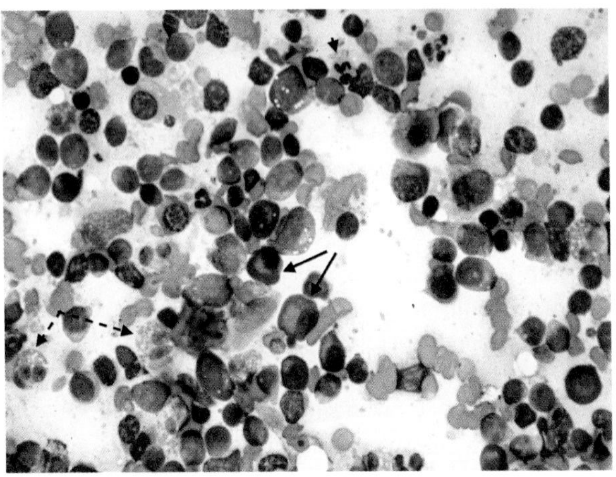

Figure 44.32 Spleen aspirate from a dog with evidence of antigenic stimulation. Normal-appearing plasma cells are increased in number (arrows). Also note the numerous eosinophils (dashed arrows). A neutrophil is indicated by an arrowhead. The majority of the cells are small normal-appearing lymphocytes. Wright stain.

consist of primarily lymphoid hyperplasia with increases in immature lymphoid cells and plasma cells. Cellularity is usually high (Figure 44.31). Increased splenic plasma cell concentration may be marked in some diseases associated with chronic antigenic stimulation (Figure 44.32). Canine splenic lymphoid nodules are typically classified as indolent lymphomas (marginal zone lymphoma [MZL] and mantle cell lymphoma [MCL], which are discussed in the lymphoma section below) or nodular lymphoid hyperplasia. Splenic hyperplasia involving the lymphoid component may be difficult to distinguish from lymphoid or plasma cell neoplasia, in which case flow cytometry or PCR for antigen receptor rearrangement (PARR) is usually helpful (see Chapter 14).

Macrophagic (histiocytic) hyperplasia may be seen in association with increased phagocytosis of abnormal erythrocytes, due to immune-mediated disease, Heinz body formation, or the presence of microorganisms in or on erythrocytes. Hemophagocytic syndrome, a benign histiocytic proliferative disorder that can occur in response to inflammation or neoplasia, primarily affects the bone marrow but may also involve the spleen and will also result in increased macrophages. With any type of histiocytic hyperplasia, numerous macrophages containing erythrocytes and hemosiderin are usually observed.

Inflammation (splenitis)

As with other organs and tissues, inflammation may be neutrophilic, macrophagic, eosinophilic, lymphocytic, plasmacytic, or mixed, and be septic or nonseptic. Examples of infectious organisms that may result in splenitis include fungi and yeasts such as *Cryptococcus* spp., *Candida albicans*, *Aspergillus* spp. and *Penicillium* spp. Protozoan organisms that have been reported in the spleen include *Neospora caninum*, *Hepatozoon canis*, *Leishmania* spp., *Trypanosoma cruzi*, and *Cytauxzoon felis*. Reported bacteria include organisms that cause anthrax (*Bacillus anthracis*), listeriosis (*Listeria monocytogenes*), tuberculosis (*Mycobacterium* spp.), salmonellosis, and tularemia. *Neorickettsia helminthoeca* and *Stellanchasmus falcatus* are neorickettsial organisms that may cause granulomatous or lymphoplasmacytic splenitis (see Chapters 39 and 45).

Hemosiderosis and siderotic nodules

Hemosiderosis, an increased amount of iron in the form of hemosiderin, can occur in the spleen resulting from excessive erythrophagocytosis associated with hemolytic anemia and with localized hemorrhage. Siderotic plaques and nodules have been associated with trauma, neoplasia, and advanced age. Aspirates of nodules contain macrophages, usually containing hemosiderin, as well as lymphocytes and hematopoietic precursors. Gamna-Gandy bodies, calcium–iron complexes, may be seen in areas of previous hemorrhage (see Ryseff et al. 2014 in "Suggested Reading" under "Spleen"). These complexes can be confused with fungal hyphae or other foreign material due to the formation of negative-staining, branching structures with septal-like divisions along the branches (Figure 44.33). Stains for iron or calcium are helpful in their identification.

Extramedullary hematopoiesis

A few hematopoietic precursors, including megakaryocytes, can be seen in normal splenic aspirates. When EMH is increased, often resulting from anemia-related hypoxia, it may be diffuse or nodular, and erythroid precursors usually predominate. The hematopoietic precursors appear identical to those found in the bone marrow (see Chapter 15).

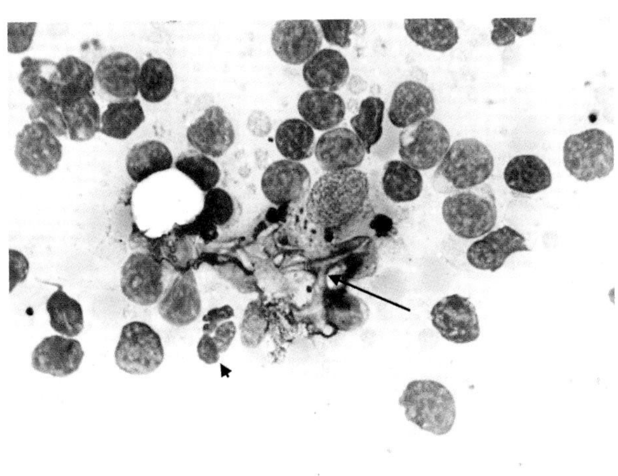

Figure 44.33 A Gamna-Gandy body in a splenic aspirate (arrow). Note the branching septate appearance, making it possible to confuse the calcium–iron complex with a fungal hypha. Most of the cells are small normal-appearing lymphocytes. Neutrophil indicated by arrowhead. Wright stain. Source: Courtesy Dr. Christina Jeffries, Colorado State University.

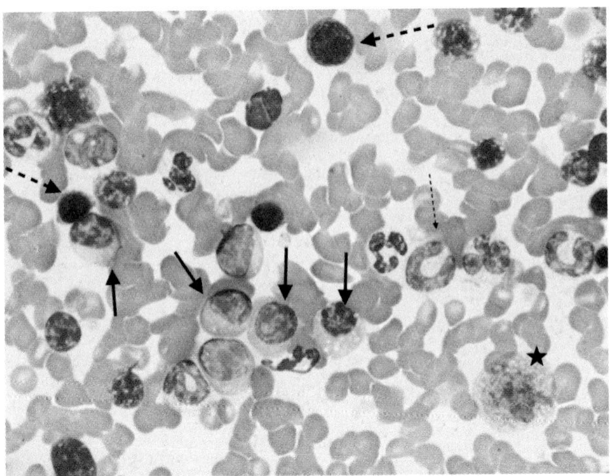

Figure 44.34 Aspirate of the spleen from a domestic ferret. Numerous plasma cells are present, indicated by arrows. Although plasma cells appear moderately well differentiated, the ferret had disseminated multiple myeloma. Extramedullary hematopoiesis is also present. Large dashed arrows indicate red cell precursors, and small dashed arrow indicates a band neutrophil. A broken nucleus is present (star). Wright stain.

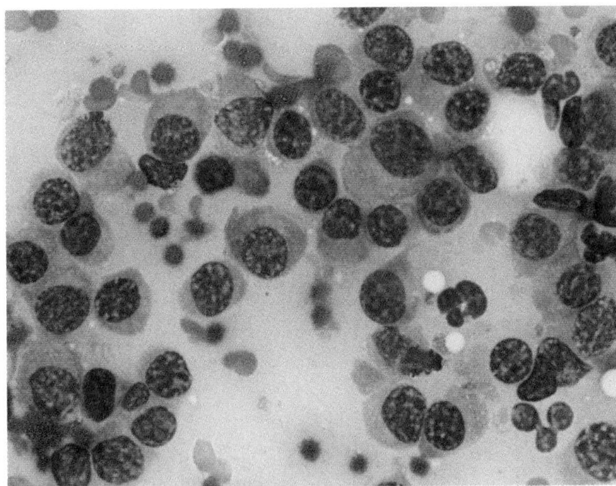

Figure 44.35 Disseminated plasma cell myeloma in the spleen. Numerous poorly differentiated plasma cells are seen. Wright stain.

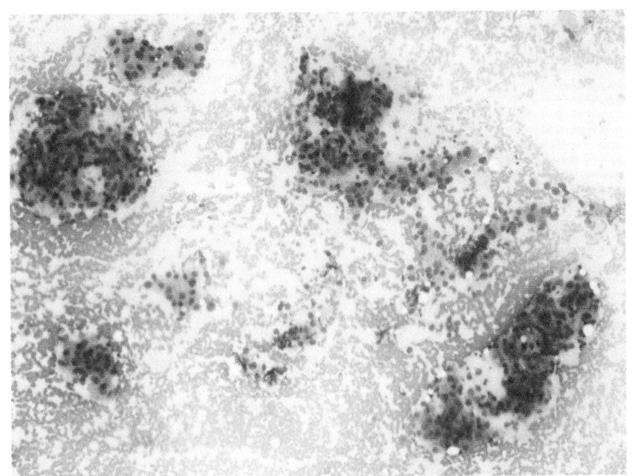

Figure 44.36 Splenic aspirate in a dog with metastatic apocrine gland anal sac adenocarcinoma. Note the abundant small, fairly uniform cohesive cells. No normal components of the spleen are present. Wright stain.

Splenic neoplasia

Neoplasia in the spleen may be primary or metastatic. Round cell tumors such as lymphoma, plasma cell neoplasia (Figures 44.34 and 44.35), and mast cell neoplasia, carcinomas, neuroendocrine tumors, and sarcomas may metastasize to the spleen (Figure 44.36). More common types of splenic neoplasia are discussed in the following section.

Lymphoma

Splenic lymphoma may be primary (arising in and confined to the spleen) or secondary (splenic involvement as part of multicentric disease) and is relatively common in dogs and cats. Multicentric lymphoma is also discussed in Chapters 40 and 45. As with lymph nodes, aspirates of spleens with lymphoma usually have greater than 40–50% large lymphoid cells containing nucleoli, although small cell lymphomas may also occur in the spleen. Three types of primary splenic lymphoma have been described in dogs. Two are indolent B-cell lymphomas and the third is hepatosplenic T-cell lymphoma; splenic MZL, MCL, and hepatosplenic lymphoma are described briefly below.

Splenic MZL (SMZL) is an uncommon form of lymphoma and is one of three subtypes of MZL (the others are nodal MZL and mucosal-associated). SMZL is an indolent small-cell B-cell lymphoma characterized by splenic infiltration and bone marrow involvement and little or no lymph node involvement. The majority of splenic MZL cases are solitary splenic lesions identified on routine abdominal ultrasound examination.

MCL is an indolent B-cell lymphoma that is very rare in dogs, comprising approximately 1% of all cases of lymphoma. MCL primarily affects the spleen with occasional visceral node involvement. Peripheral node involvement is minimal if any, and bone marrow involvement is very uncommon. Mantle cells are in the cuff surrounding lymphoid follicles of the spleen. The neoplastic cells are small to intermediate in size and have a small amount of cytoplasm and inconspicuous nucleolus. For both types of indolent B-cell lymphoma, prognosis is good following splenectomy if the disease is confined to the spleen. Chemotherapy may not improve survival.

Hepatosplenic T-cell lymphoma has been described in humans and rarely in dogs, cats, and horses. Neoplastic lymphoid cells are intermediate to large with a moderate amount of pale blue cytoplasm, pink to magenta cytoplasmic granules, and prominent nucleoli. Peripheral lymph nodes are not involved. Clinical course is aggressive and response to therapy is poor. Neoplastic lymphoid cells occasionally are phagocytic (Figure 44.37).

Hemangioma and hemangiosarcoma

Hemangioma and hemangiosarcoma are connective tissue tumors arising from the vasculature (see Chapter 40). They are relatively common in dogs, especially large-breed dogs, and are the most common primary splenic tumor in dogs; they are relatively rare in cats. The spleen is a common site of occurrence in dogs; in one study of 370 small-breed dogs, 27% of splenic lesions were hemangiosarcomas (see Fernandez et al. 2019 in "Suggested Reading" under "Spleen"). Hemangiomas are significantly less common in dogs and are also uncommon in cats. Rupture of hemangiosarcoma may occur with aspiration but is quite uncommon. Because large areas of the tumor are filled with blood, one commonly only sees blood on aspirates of hemangiosarcomas, making the lesions difficult to distinguish from hematomas or hemangiomas. Evidence of previous hemorrhage (erythrophagocytosis and hemosiderin) is often present. Hemangiosarcoma cells are occasionally aspirated and are often spindle-shaped and usually show features of malignancy (Figure 44.38). It is not possible, based on cytology alone, to definitively differentiate hemangiosarcoma cells from other types of sarcomas that may have metastasized to the spleen (Figure 44.39).

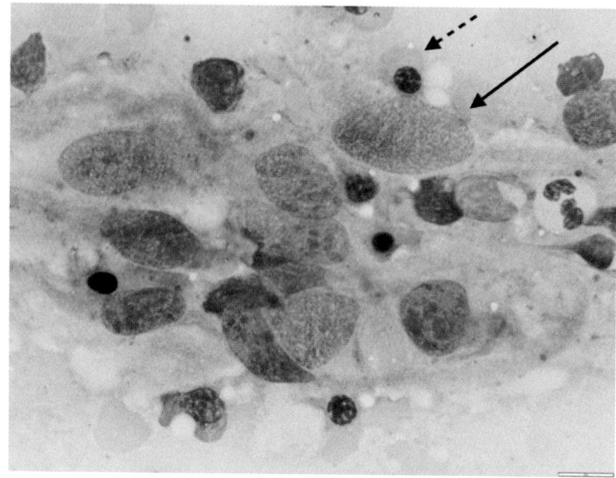

Figure 44.38 High magnification of a splenic aspirate from a dog with hemangiosarcoma. Note the large spindle-shaped sarcoma cells (arrow) that exhibit several criteria of malignancy, including nuclear molding and multiple prominent nucleoli. Extramedullary hematopoiesis is evidenced by the multiple erythroid precursors. A metarubricyte is indicated by the dashed arrow. Wright Stain.

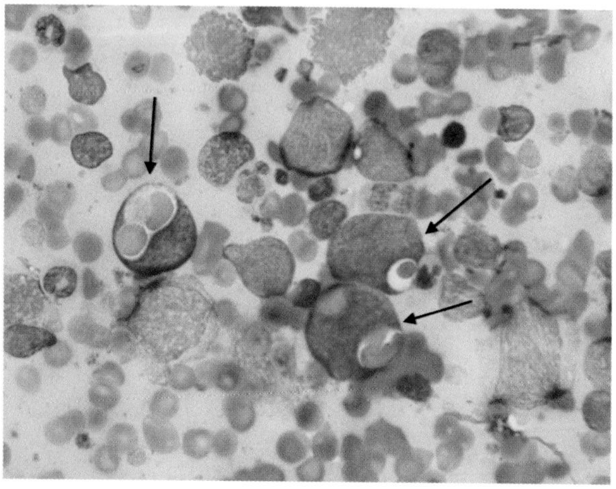

Figure 44.37 Aspirate of the spleen of a hedgehog with lymphoma. Neoplastic lymphoid cells have phagocytized erythrocytes (arrows). Wright stain.

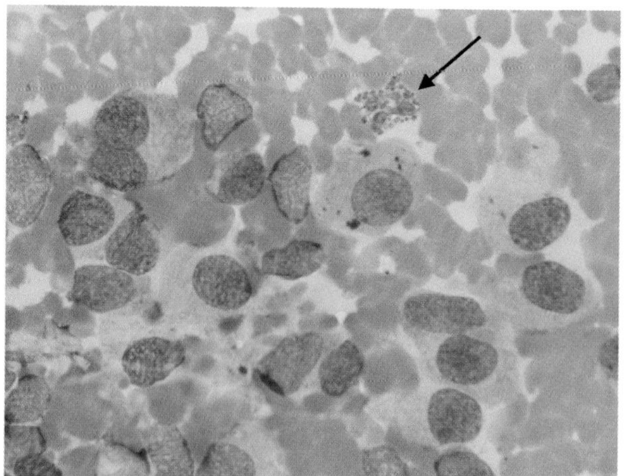

Figure 44.39 Splenic aspirate from a dog with metastatic osteosarcoma. Note the large spindle-shaped cells, a few of which have pink glycosaminoglycans in the cytoplasm. An eosinophil is indicated by the arrow, for size comparison. Wright stain.

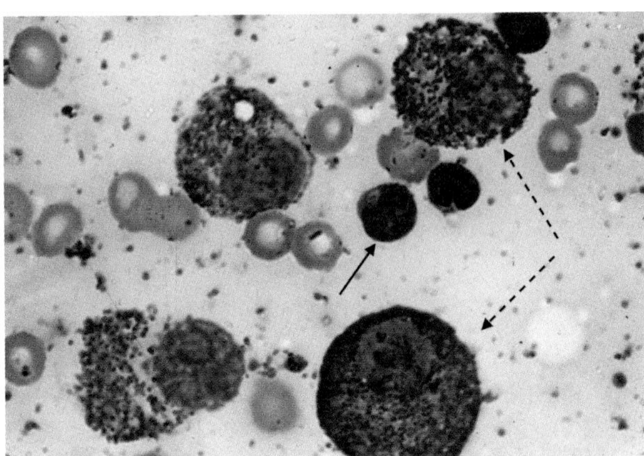

Figure 44.40 Splenic aspirate from dog with metastatic mast cell neoplasia. Mast cells are indicated by dashed arrows, and small normal-appearing lymphocyte by arrow. Note the numerous free mast cell granules in the background from broken mast cells. Wright stain.

Splenic mast cell neoplasia

Mast cell tumors are the most common splenic disorder of cats. Mast cell neoplasia of the spleen is much less common in dogs. Mast cells are round, discrete cells with numerous dark blue to purple cytoplasmic granules (Figure 44.40). Anaplastic mast cells tend to have fewer granules. However, occasionally mast cell granules do not stain with the quick Romanowsky stains, and these poorly staining cells (Figure 44.41) should not be confused with anaplastic mast cells. Because mast cells may be found in normal spleens, and increased numbers may be seen with reactive hyperplasia, benign mastocytosis may be difficult to differentiate from mast cell neoplasia. Mast cell tumors are also discussed in Chapters 40 and 41.

Histiocytic sarcoma

Histiocytic sarcoma is classified into three forms: localized, disseminated, and hemophagocytic histiocytic sarcoma.

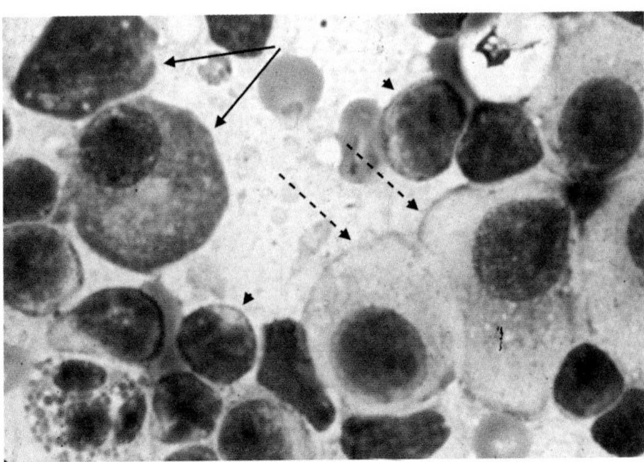

Figure 44.41 Mast cell tumor stained with a quick Romanowsky stain (Diff-Quik). Poorly staining mast cells are indicated by dashed arrows, plasma cells by arrows, and normal small lymphocytes by arrowheads. Wright stain.

Localized histiocytic sarcoma arises from dendritic cells and presents as discrete lesions in one tissue such as the spleen, skin, lymph nodes, joints, lung, and bone marrow. Disseminated histiocytic sarcoma, previously referred to as malignant histiocytosis, also arises primarily from dendritic cells and is characterized by multicentric disease. Hemophagocytic histiosarcoma is aggressive, primarily arises from splenic or bone marrow macrophages, and is characterized by neoplastic macrophages that exhibit erythrophagocytosis. Splenic histiocytic sarcoma can be any of the three subtypes. Splenic involvement is usually characterized by marked splenomegaly, often with numerous coalescing nodules. Cytological description of malignant histiocytes is discussed in this chapter under "Liver" and also discussed in Chapters 40 and 45. If localized to the spleen, splenectomy is indicated, and survival time can be longer than 1 year.

Myelolipoma

Myelolipomas are rare, benign tumors composed of adipose tissue and normal hematopoietic cells. Aspirates consist of well differentiated adipocytes and normal-appearing hematopoietic precursors.

Kidney

As with other organs, cytology is not useful if architecture is required to make a diagnosis. Suspected necrosis, inflammation, and neoplasia of the kidney are indications for cytology. Cytology of the kidney is particularly useful for diagnosing lymphoma. While diffuse lesions can be aspirated without ultrasound guidance, ultrasound-guided aspiration is recommended for focal lesions and to avoid puncturing major blood vessels. Detailed technique is discussed in other publications (see Borjesson 2003 and McAloney and Sharkey 2021 in "Suggested Reading" under "Kidney"). An excellent review of urinary tract cytology was published by Wycislo and Piech 2019 (see "Suggested Reading" under "Kidney").

Normal

As with other tissues, one needs to recognize the normal cytologic features to recognize abnormalities. The primary cells seen in renal cytologic samples are renal tubular epithelial cells, which exfoliate either individually or in small clusters. Cells are uniform, round to polygonal with abundant lightly basophilic cytoplasm. Dark blue to black granules may be seen occasionally in the cytoplasm, consistent with cells in the descending loop of Henle or distal tubules (Figure 44.42). In cats, the cytoplasm commonly contains clear lipid vacuoles (Figure 44.43). Occasionally glomerular tufts are aspirated.

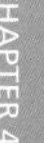

Inflammation

Inflammatory lesions in the kidney are similar to those described for other tissues. Infectious agents such as bacteria, yeast, and fungi can usually be accurately identified.

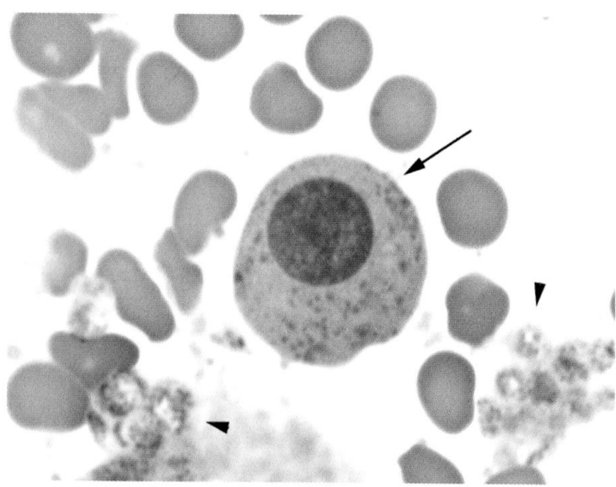

Figure 44.42 High magnification of a normal renal epithelial cell with granules in the cytoplasm, likely from the loop of Henle or distal tubule (arrow). Clumps of platelets from blood contamination are indicated by arrowheads. Wright stain.

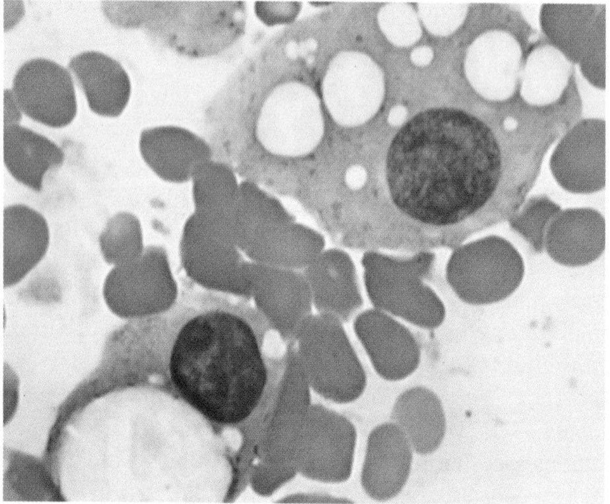

Figure 44.43 High magnification of a normal renal epithelial cell from a cat showing the common lipid vacuoles within the cytoplasm. Wright stain.

Renal toxicosis caused by ethylene glycol and melamine from contaminated pet food have been identified by the characteristic crystals in aspirates. Calcium oxalate crystals are usually the monohydrate form that are elongated with sharp edges (see Chapter 24).

Renal neoplasia

Renal neoplasms usually originate outside of the kidney and metastasize or extend to the kidney. Carcinomas, sarcomas, and nephroblastomas may originate in the kidney. Nephroblastoma cells have been described as large, round, sometimes cohesive cells with scant to moderate basophilic cytoplasm with round nuclei and associated matrix. In one case, the cohesiveness, presence of matrix, and absence of cytoplasmic fragments differentiated them from neoplastic lymphoid cells (see Michael et al. 2013 in "Suggested Reading" under "Kidney"). However, other reports show aspirates that could be easily confused with lymphoma (see Wycislo and Piech 2019 in "Suggested Reading" under "Kidney"). Metastatic tumors include lymphoma, melanoma, and hemangiosarcoma. Cytologic characteristics of these types of tumors are described in Chapter 40.

Pancreas

Pancreatic disease is difficult to definitively diagnose by laboratory evaluation or imaging. Cytology has been shown to be a safe and reasonably effective diagnostic tool. Indications include clinical and imaging findings that suggest the possibility of pancreatic disease, as well as nodular lesions that may be due to hyperplasia or neoplasia. Technique for aspiration is like that described for the liver, although some authors recommend using a smaller-gauge needle to minimize trauma. Several samples should be collected from different locations. Pancreatic cells are reported to exfoliate less readily than those of other organs such as the liver. Complications are reportedly rare compared to pancreatic surgical biopsy.

Normal

The exocrine pancreas is composed of acinar tissue and ducts that drain the acini. The endocrine pancreas is made up of islets within the exocrine pancreas; cells within the islets are morphologically similar, although they have varying functions. Cytology samples from normal pancreatic tissue have low cellularity and consist of epithelial cells that appear in clusters. They have a moderate amount of light blue cytoplasm containing fine pink granules, a round nucleus, and a single prominent nucleolus, similar to that of hepatocytes, although the cells have slightly less cytoplasm than hepatocytes (Figures 44.44 and 44.45).

Necrosis and inflammation

Necrotic pancreatic tissue appears as amorphous basophilic debris, similar to other types of necrotic tissue. Mineralization of the necrotic tissue is commonly seen and appears as colorless refractile small round crystaline material.

Pancreatic inflammation is like inflammation elsewhere and is usually classified as acute or chronic. Acute inflammation is usually neutrophilic, and chronic inflammation is typically mixed or lymphocytic. Granulomatous inflammation is uncommon. The inflammation is typically nonseptic, although bacteria may be seen in association with pancreatic abscesses.

Neoplasia

Benign neoplasia is rare. The most common malignant pancreatic tumor is acinar carcinoma, although ductal carcinoma also occurs. Typical malignant features of neoplastic epithelial cells are seen (see Chapter 40). Lymphoma of

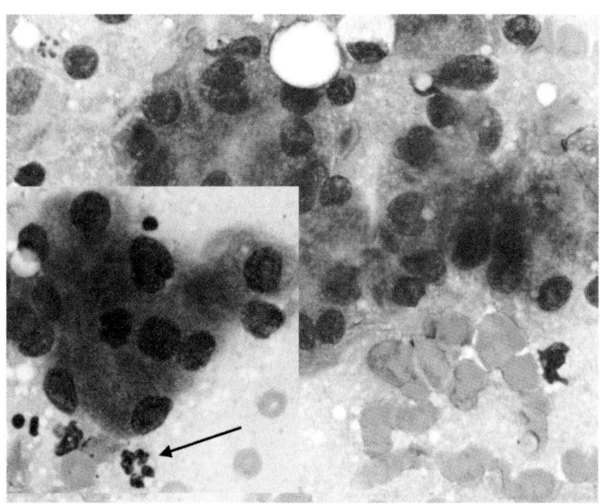

Figure 44.44 Aspirate of the pancreas showing normal pancreatic epithelial cells. Inset, lower left corner, shows a similar aspirate with a neutrophil (arrow) for size comparison. Wright stain.

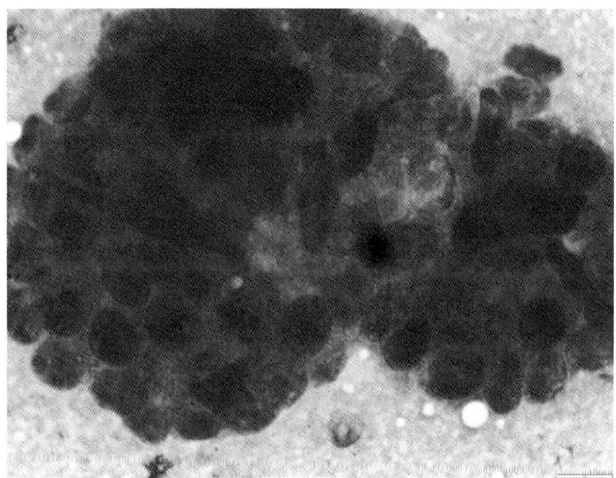

Figure 44.45 Aspirate of a pancreatic nodule from a 12-year-old English bulldog. The cells appear fairly well differentiated but the aspirate was very highly cellular with piling and increased nucleus:cytoplasm ratios, suggesting a possible well-differentiated carcinoma. Other differentials were benign neoplasia and hyperplasia. Histopathology was not performed. Wright stain.

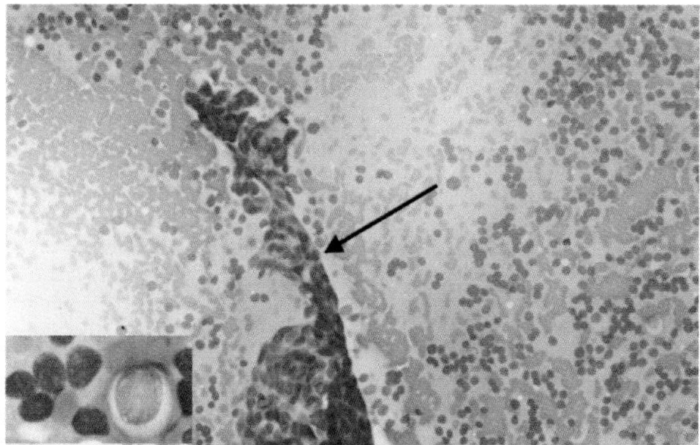

Figure 44.46 Aspirate of the pancreas of a dog with laboratory and clinical signs compatible with insulinoma. Inset in lower left corner shows higher magnification. Note the sheet of mesothelial cells in the center of the field (arrow). Wright stain.

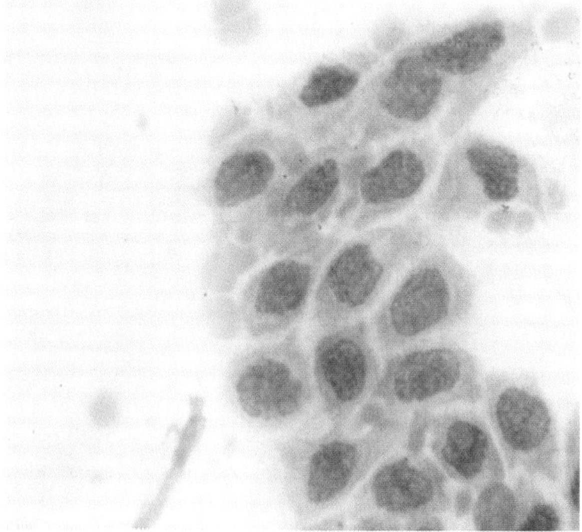

Figure 44.47 Higher magnification of the mesothelial cells that are shown in Figure 44.46. These are sometimes mistakenly confused with carcinoma or sarcoma cells or fibroplasia. Wright stain.

the pancreas has been rarely reported. Insulinoma is the most common tumor of the endocrine pancreas. Cytologic features are those of any endocrine tumor and include many free round nuclei and relatively uniform cells with scant to moderate cytoplasm that may contain fine eosinophilic granules (Figures 44.46 and 44.47).

Adrenal gland

The adrenal glands are located near each kidney and are composed of the medulla and the cortex. Neuroendocrine cells in the medulla produce catecholamines (epinephrine and norepinephrine). The cortex is made up of the glomerulosa, where aldosterone is made, and the fasciculata and reticularis, where cortisol and sex hormones are made. The most common indication for adrenal gland cytology is the detection of an adrenal mass by diagnostic imaging such as ultrasonography, computed tomography, or magnetic resonance imaging. In one study of 50 canine cases identified by imaging in which adrenal gland cytology was performed, the cytological analysis was conclusive in 77% and inconclusive in 23%, and the complication rate was very low, with hemorrhage being the most common complication. Diagnoses included pheochromocytoma (56%), carcinoma (14%), adenoma (12%), hyperplasia (7%), EMH (5%), and granulomatous inflammation from a migrating foreign body

(2%) (see Pey et al. 2020 in "Suggested Reading" under "Adrenal Gland").

Normal

Cortical cells have abundant lightly basophilic cytoplasm containing clear lipid vacuoles and a round central nucleus. Cells from the medulla have a typical neuroendocrine appearance with a small amount of lightly basophilic cytoplasm and a round central nucleus. Like other neuroendocrine cells, they easily lose their cytoplasm, and naked nuclei arranged in rows or rosettes are present.

Inflammation (adrenalitis)

Immune-mediated destruction of the adrenal gland is associated with lymphocytic or plasmacytic inflammation that results in hypoadrenocorticism, often in young dogs (see Section VII, Cases 108 and 109). The lymphocytes have been shown to be CD4+ T cells (see Friedenberg et al. 2018 in "Suggested Reading" under "Adrenal Gland"). While it would be theoretically possible to diagnose the presence of lymphocytic inflammation by cytology, most of these cases present due to clinical signs and laboratory findings associated with hypoadrenocorticism and are definitively diagnosed by baseline cortisol concentration and an adrenocorticotropic hormone (ACTH) stimulation test (see Chapter 33).

Neutrophilic and macrophagic inflammation can also occur in the adrenal glands, usually resulting from bacteria (including mycobacteria), fungi, and protozoa. Most of the organisms seen in cytologic samples have been reported in humans, rather than domestic animals. Eosinophilic infiltration of the adrenal gland has been reported in cats with hypereosinophilic syndrome.

Neoplasia

Primary adrenal neoplasia is common in dogs and ferrets and relatively uncommon in cats. Gonadectomy has been shown to induce sex-steroid-producing adrenocortical tumors in domestic ferrets. Neoplasms of the cortex (adrenocortical tumors) are adenomas or carcinomas, and neoplasms of the medulla are termed pheochromocytomas, a type of neuroendocrine tumor. Many adrenal tumors are functionally active. Adrenocortical tumors in dogs usually secrete cortisol and result in hyperadrenocorticism. Adrenocortical tumors in cats may cause hyperadrenocorticism or hyperaldosteronism. Pheochromocytomas from the medulla produce catecholamines; clinical signs include hypertension and tachycardia (see Chapter 33). The cells in neoplasms of the cortex (Figure 44.48) and medulla appear similar to those in normal adrenal glands and are described above. Whether the tumor is cortical or medullary in origin is usually easily determined by cytology, but because the cells do not exhibit much atypia, benign or hyperplastic tissue cannot usually be differentiated from malignant neoplasms by cytology (see Bertazzolo et al. 2014 in "Suggested Reading" under "Adrenal Gland"). EMH is sometimes seen in association with adrenocortical neoplasms and is reported to be more common in association with adenomas than carcinomas. Other rare primary adrenal neoplasms include myelolipomas, neuroblastomas, ganglioneuromas, and schwannomas.

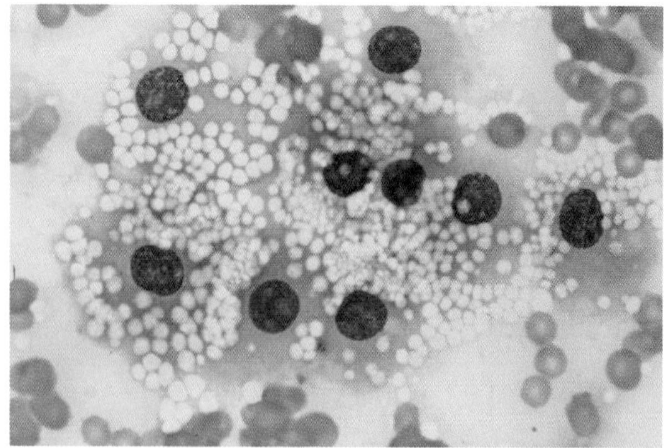

Figure 44.48 Aspirate of the adrenal gland from a dog with an adrenocortical tumor and laboratory evidence of Cushing's syndrome. Note the numerous discrete vacuoles within the cytoplasm. Wright stain.

Various types of neoplasms may metastasize to the adrenal gland and include carcinomas, hemangiosarcomas, and melanomas.

Intestine

The small intestine consists of the duodenum, jejunum, and ilium. Mucosal surface is lined by columnar epithelial cells with long microvilli and goblet cells that secrete mucus. Below the mucosal surface are smooth muscle layers. The large intestine contains more goblet cells. The rectum is lined by simple columnar epithelium. Aspiration of the intestine is typically performed with ultrasound guidance and is usually quite accurate, especially for lymphoma. However, samples can also be taken via endoscopy, usually using a brush passed through the endoscope to obtain samples. The accuracy of that technique is quite good as well and is described in detail in numerous reports (see Jergens et al. 1998 in "Suggested Reading" under "Intestine"). Rectal scrapings using a conjunctival scraper can also be performed to obtain cells (Figure 44.49). In one study of 167 dogs with clinical signs of chronic gastrointestinal disease in which endoscopic cytology was performed, cytologic diagnosis was in agreement with the histologic diagnosis in 81% of cases. For the differentiation between enteritis and lymphoma, endoscopic cytology had a sensitivity of 98.6%, a specificity of 73.5%, a positive predictive value of 72.3%, and a negative predictive value of 98.6%. The following diagnoses in this series of dogs were determined by histopathology: lymphocytic-plasmacytic enteritis in 93,

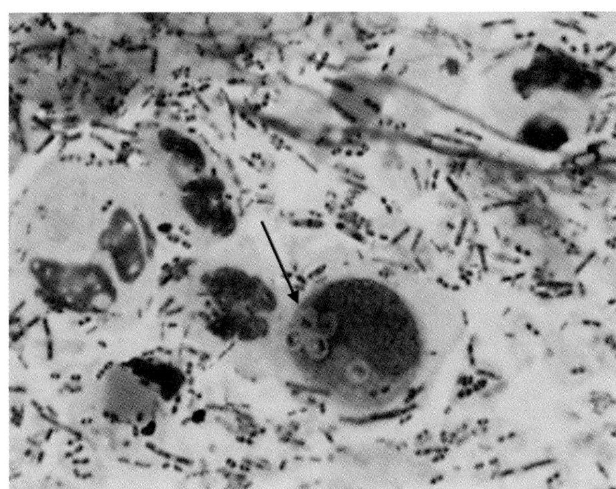

Figure 44.49 Rectal scraping from a dog with disseminated histoplasmosis. Note the multiple *Histoplasma* organisms in the macrophage (arrow). Wright stain.

eosinophilic enteritis in 5, small cell intestinal lymphoma in 45, and large cell intestinal lymphoma in 24 (see Maeda et al. 2017 in "Suggested Reading" under "Intestine").

Normal

Columnar epithelial cells are elongated with lightly basophilic cytoplasm and microvilli on the apical border. The nucleus is round and usually basilar, with an indistinct nucleolus. Goblet cells are also elongated and contain large purple mucin granules in the cytoplasm. Occasional eosinophils, lymphocytes, large granular lymphocytes, and plasma cells may be seen. If lymphoid follicles (Peyer's patches) are aspirated, numerous lymphocytes may be seen.

Inflammation

Inflammation of the intestine may be neutrophilic, lymphocytic-plasmacytic, or eosinophilic. Neutrophilic inflammation is usually caused by bacteria, including *Clostridium perfringens*, *Campylobacter jejuni*, *Salmonella* spp., and *Escherichia coli*. Neutrophils are destroyed rapidly in the lumen of the intestine. Evidence of overgrowth of these bacteria may be seen in fecal cytology, as well (Figures 44.50 and 44.51). Inflammation secondary to neoplasia can be difficult to differentiate from primary inflammatory processes if the aspirate is not fully representative of the lesion.

Lymphocytic-plasmacytic inflammation of the intestine in dogs is most commonly caused by hypersensitivity to food or gut microorganisms and can also be caused by lymphangiectasia and bacterial overgrowth. Differentiating lymphocytic inflammation from small cell lymphoma can be challenging in both dogs and cats. Flow cytometry and PAAR may be helpful in making the distinction (see Chapter 14).

Eosinophilic inflammation may be associated with hypersensitivity to food antigens, or with parasites, or be secondary to T-cell lymphoma or mast cell neoplasia.

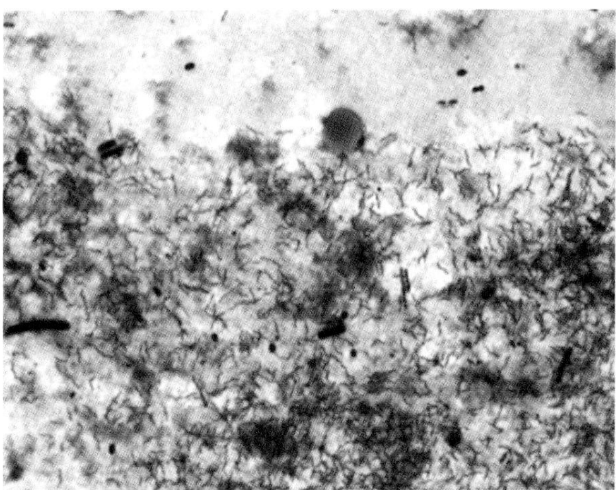

Figure 44.50 Fecal cytology from a dog with an overgrowth of *Campylobacter*. Note the "gull-wing" shaped organisms and the lack of diversity of bacteria. Wright stain.

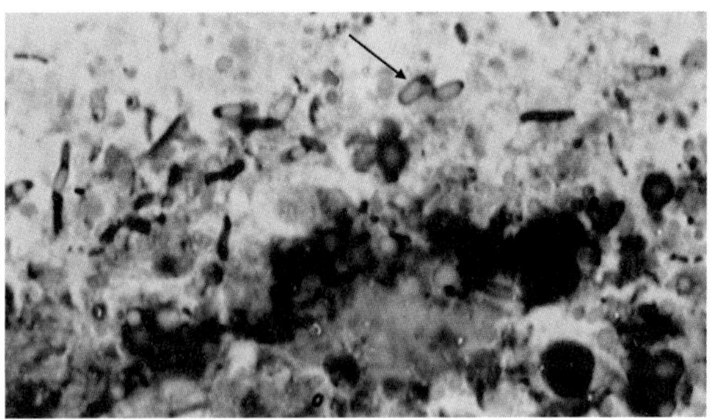

Figure 44.51 Fecal cytology from a dog with an overgrowth of *Clostridium*. Note the numerous safety-pin-shaped sporulated organisms (arrow). Wright stain.

Occasionally microorganisms such as *Giardia lamblia* may be seen on intestinal aspirates, particularly when the lumen of the duodenum is aspirated (Figure 44.52).

Neoplasia

Lymphoma of the gastrointestinal tract is the most common tumor of the intestine of dogs and cats, followed by adenocarcinoma and, least frequently, gastrointestinal stromal cell tumors and leiomyosarcomas. Mast cell tumors of the intestine in cats may also be seen.

Lymphoma

Intestinal lymphoma may be either nodular or diffuse. Intestinal lymphoma is the most common type of lymphoma in the cat but is a relatively rare type of lymphoma in dogs. Various subtypes of lymphoma occur in the intestine, just as in lymph nodes (see Chapter 45). In cats, lymphoma was traditionally classified as small cell or large cell and has more recently been classified as mucosal T cell that

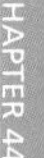

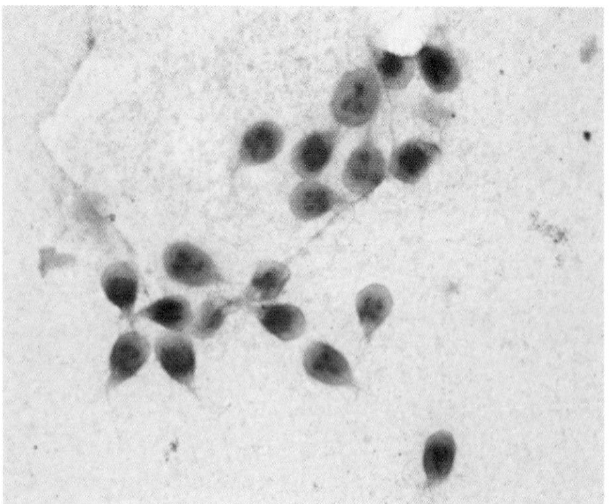

Figure 44.52 Aspirate of the intestine of a dog. The lumen was inadvertently aspirated and numerous *Giardia* organisms are seen. Note the pear-shaped organisms with two nuclei. The flagella are indistinct in this image. Wright stain.

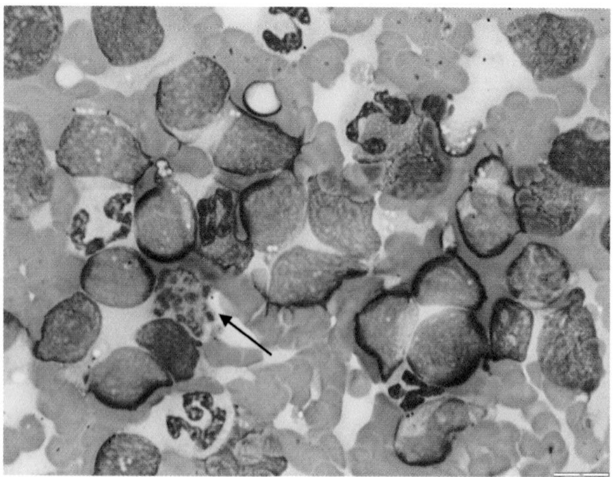

Figure 44.54 Aspirate of the stomach wall of a dog with gastric lymphoma. The numerous lymphoid cells are slightly larger than neutrophils. A platelet clump is indicated by the arrow. Wright stain.

has a relatively long survival time, transmural T-cell lymphoma (usually large granular cell lymphoma) that is less common, usually aggressive, and may be accompanied by leukemia (see Section VII, Case 13), and large B-cell lymphoma, which is also aggressive. Three histologic forms have been described in dogs: diffuse large B-cell lymphoma and enteropathy-associated T-cell lymphoma types 1 and 2, which are more common. Lymphomas that consist of large lymphoid cells with nucleoli are easy to recognize and have been described elsewhere (Figures 44.53 and 44.54). Small cell lymphomas are more common in cats and usually require histopathology or molecular methods to differentiate them from lymphocytic inflammation. Large granular lymphocyte lymphoma (T-cell lymphoma) is quite easy to diagnose cytologically and is described in Chapter 45. What were previously described as large globular leukocytes in the cat are now considered large granular lymphocytes.

Mast cell neoplasia

Mast cell tumors are the third-most-common tumor in the intestine of cats (after lymphoma and adenocarcinoma) and occur occasionally in dogs. Mast cell appearance has been described under "Spleen" in this chapter and elsewhere (see Chapter 40). In the intestine, they may be poorly granulated.

Carcinomas

Intestinal adenocarcinomas appear similar to other adenocarcinomas (see Chapter 40). Cellular piling and numerous other characteristics of malignancy such as anisocytosis and prominent nucleoli are usually present (Figure 44.55).

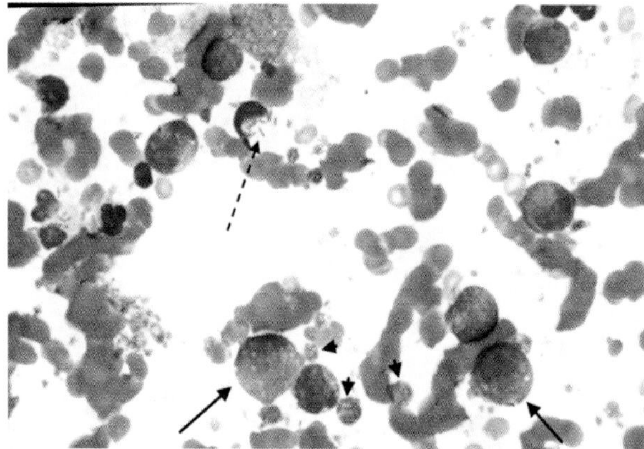

Figure 44.53 Aspirate of the intestine of a cat. Note the large immature lymphoid cells that are indicative of large cell lymphoma (arrows). The tumor had perforated the mucosa, and numerous neutrophils and bacteria can also be seen (dashed arrow). Cytoplasmic fragments indicating lymphoid origin are numerous (arrowheads). Wright stain.

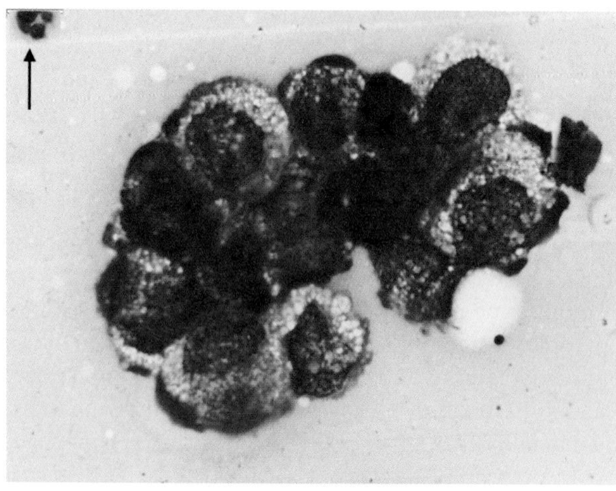

Figure 44.55 Aspirate of the intestine of a dog with intestinal adenocarcinoma. Note the cluster of very large vacuolated epithelial cells exhibiting prominent nucleoli and variability in size. A neutrophil is indicated by the arrow for size comparison. Wright stain.

Necrosis may be present. However, histopathology may be required since tissue architecture is often necessary for differentiating benign from malignant epithelial masses from the intestine.

Carcinoid

Carcinoids in the intestine are rare neuroendocrine tumors arising from enterochromaffin cells. They appear like other neuroendocrine cells and are uniform, in clusters and cord-like arrangements. Numerous naked nuclei are usually present.

Mesenchymal intestinal tumors

Connective tissue tumors of the intestine are referred to as gastrointestinal stromal cell tumors and were previously classified as either leiomyomas or leiomyosarcomas. Cells are spindle-shaped with wispy elongated cytoplasm and elongated nuclei with inconspicuous nucleoli. True leiomyosarcomas are likely less common than previously thought.

45 Cytology of Lymph Nodes

Mary Anna Thrall[1], Donald Meuten[2], Andrea A. Bohn[3], and Kristina Meichner[4]

[1]Department of Biomedical Sciences, Ross University School of Veterinary Medicine, Basseterre, Saint Kitts and Nevis
[2]North Carolina State University, Raleigh, NC, USA
[3]Department of Microbiology, Immunology and Pathology, College of Veterinary Medicine and Biomedical Sciences, Colorado State University, Fort Collins, CO, USA
[4]University of Georgia, Athens, GA, USA

The function of lymph nodes includes filtering of particles and microorganisms, allowing antigens to come into contact with lymphocytes, resulting in subsequent activation of T and B lymphocytes. Lymph nodes were probably the first tissue to be studied by aspiration cytology. In 1904, the technique was used to search for organisms in human patients with trypanosomiasis (sleeping sickness). Aspiration cytology of lymph nodes has been increasingly advocated in both human and veterinary medicine because of the inexpensiveness, small amount of time required, and reasonably good sensitivity and specificity. In humans, cytology has a >90% sensitivity and specificity in differentiating a malignant process from reactive hyperplasia.

Lymph node enlargement, whether localized or generalized, is the primary indication for lymph node aspiration cytology (Figure 45.1). The differential diagnosis for an enlarged lymph node includes antigenic stimulation (reactive hyperplasia), lymphadenitis, lymphoma, and metastatic disease. Even if the node is not enlarged, lymph node cytology is occasionally helpful in determining if neoplastic metastasis to a lymph node has occurred.

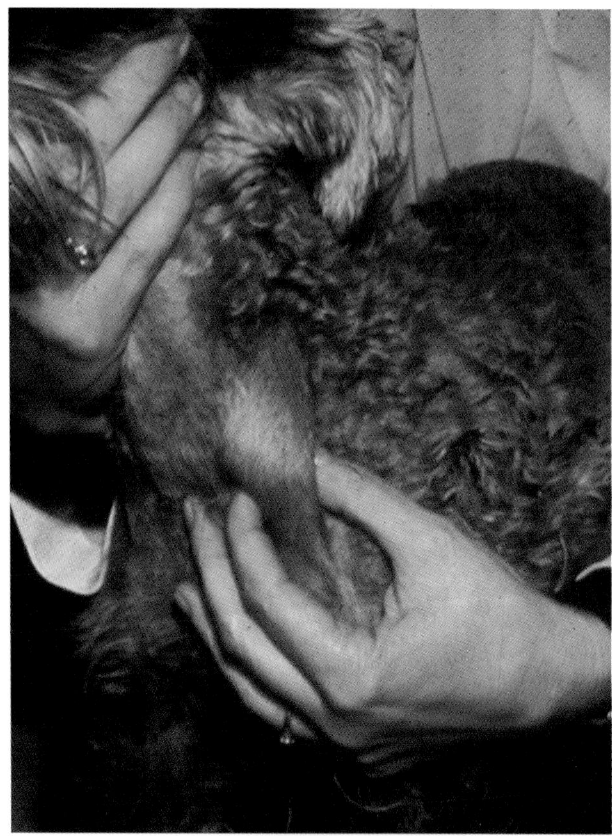

Figure 45.1 Enlarged prescapular lymph node from a miniature schnauzer with generalized lymphadenitis due to *Mycobacteria*.

Because cytology involves the study of aspirated cells, no architectural structures can be observed. However, it is worthwhile to review normal lymph node architecture to better understand the potential variability of the types of cells aspirated in normal and reactive nodes. B lymphocytes that matured in the bone marrow and T lymphocytes that matured in the thymus colonize lymph nodes. A normal node consists of a capsule, a cortex, a medulla, and sinuses (subcapsular, cortical, and medullary sinuses). The cortex contains follicles and parafollicular regions (Figure 45.2). Primary follicles contain primarily B lymphocytes. While T cells are also found in follicles, most are in parafollicular regions. Medullary cords consist of primarily B lymphocytes and plasma cells and are surrounded by sinusoids containing macrophages attached to reticular fibers (reticulum cells) and occasional mast cells. Lymph enters the node via afferent lymphatics and moves through the sinusoids, where antigens

Veterinary Hematology, Clinical Chemistry, and Cytology, Third Edition. Edited by Mary Anna Thrall, Glade Weiser, Robin W. Allison and Terry W. Campbell.

Companion website: www.wiley.com/go/thrall/veterinary

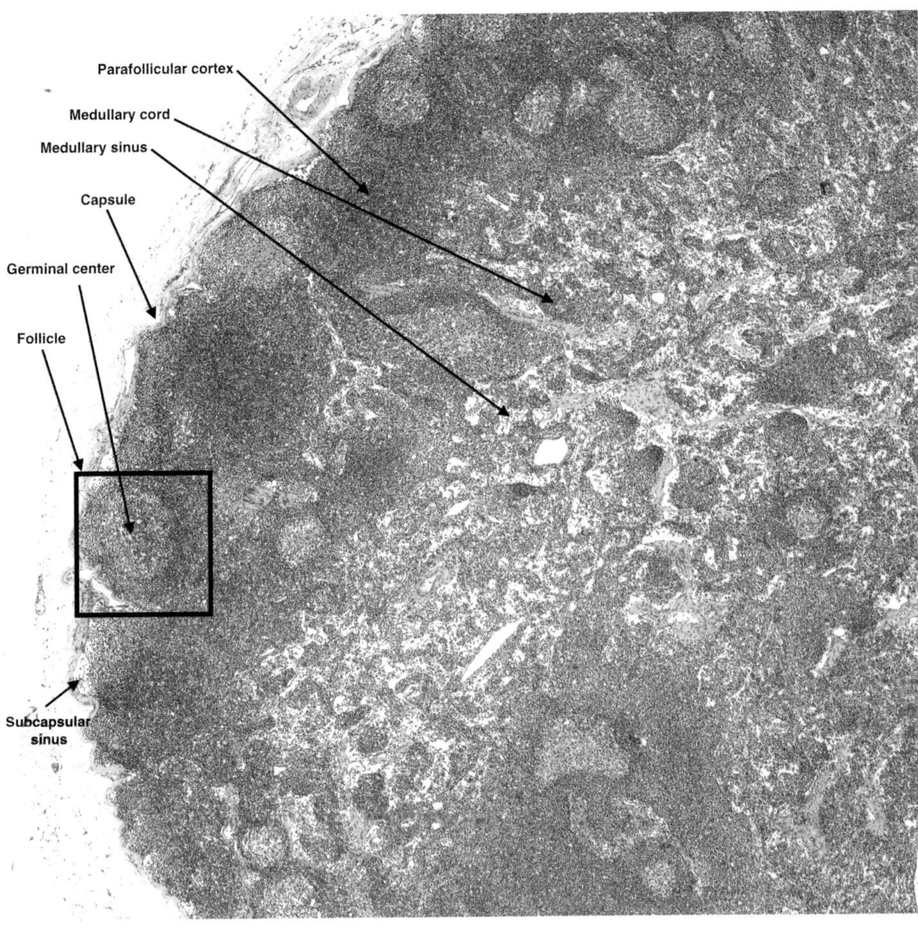

Figure 45.2 Normal lymph node from an African green monkey showing structures in the cortex and medulla. Within the cortex are follicles and parafollicular regions, as well as subcapsular sinuses. The medulla contains medullary cords made up of B lymphocytes and plasma cells, and sinuses containing macrophages. Different populations of cells may be aspirated from various areas of a lymph node. Hematoxylin and eosin (H&E) stain. Source: Courtesy of Dr. Pompei Bolfa, Ross University School of Veterinary Medicine.

are processed by reticulum cells and presented to T and B lymphocytes. Activated B cells enter primary follicles and become centroblasts that then migrate to the peripheral zone of the germinal center and become centrocytes. Centrocytes can reside in the mantle zone around the germinal center or form the marginal zone around the periphery of the mantle zone. Some centrocytes become plasma cells within the germinal centers. Macrophages containing phagocytized dying (apoptotic) B lymphocytes can be found within germinal centers and are sometimes called "tingible (stainable) body macrophages." Activated T lymphocytes in the parafollicular regions become T immunoblasts. Sinuses converge at the hilus of the node, and lymph then exits by the efferent lymphatics.

Technique

Selection of lymph nodes to be aspirated should be made on the basis of clinical findings. In animals with generalized lymphadenopathy, at least two nodes should be aspirated. Lymph nodes draining the oral cavity and gastrointestinal tract tend to be antigenically stimulated under normal conditions and should not be chosen if others are available. Superficial lymph nodes can be aspirated without using a local anesthetic, since the procedure is usually no more painful than venipuncture. Inflamed lymph nodes tend to be more painful than those affected with a neoplastic disorder. Lymph nodes within the thoracic or abdominal cavity should be aspirated using ultrasound guidance. A small-gauge needle (21–23 gauge) is redirected several times without withdrawing the needle from the skin. The needle is then attached to an air-filled syringe, and the material is expressed onto glass slides and "pull" films made, as is done when making films from bone marrow aspirates. One can also attach the needle to a syringe and apply gentle negative pressure to help obtain cells. Negative pressure should be released prior to withdrawing the needle from the tissue. Lymphoid cells, like bone marrow cells, are very fragile. Very little pressure should be placed on the spreader slide when

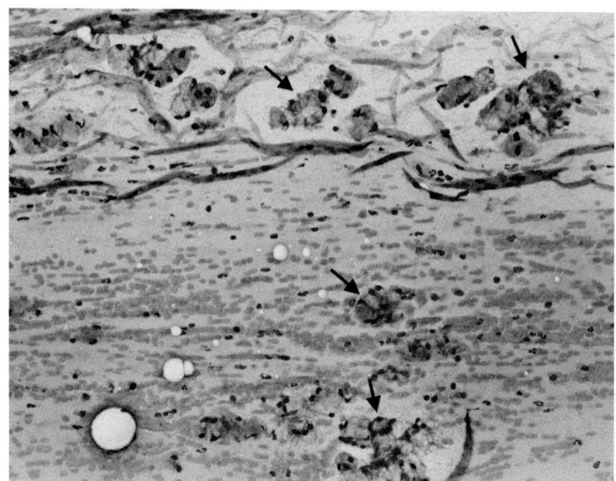

Figure 45.3 Salivary gland mistakenly aspirated when attempting to aspirate submandibular lymph node. Note the clusters of normal-appearing salivary gland epithelial cells (arrows). Background erythrocytes are arranged in a linear pattern ("windrowing") due to mucin within the salivary gland. Wright stain.

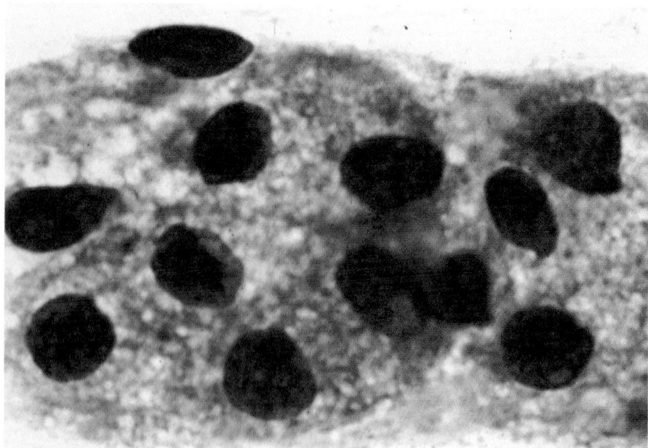

Figure 45.4 High magnification of aspirate of salivary gland from a dog. The enlarged salivary gland was originally thought to be the submandibular lymph node. Note the abundant vacuolated cytoplasm typical of secretory cells. Wright stain.

placing the material on the slide (see "Tissue Aspirates," Chapter 2). Imprints of biopsied nodes can also be made. Lymph node aspirates are often quite cellular, and additional staining time may be needed.

Nondiagnostic samples are usually due to a lack of cellularity or to the presence of many broken cells. Gentle spreading will usually prevent cells being broken. Aspirates of lymph nodes, like other tissue, tend to clot quickly, and if clotted they are nondiagnostic, as the cells are incorporated in the clot. Cells should be spread onto the slide within a few seconds of aspiration to prevent clotting. Sometimes perinodal fat is aspirated, rather than the lymph node itself, resulting in a nondiagnostic sample or a mistaken diagnosis of lipoma. Salivary glands are sometimes aspirated mistakenly when attempting to aspirate the mandibular lymph node, another reason to avoid aspirating that node if multiple nodes are enlarged (Figures 45.3 and 45.4). In some instances, aspiration of the salivary gland occurs because it is the salivary gland that is enlarged due to sialodenosis, and not the lymph node (see Chapter 41, "Sialodenosis").

Identification of cell types and other lymphoid elements

Small lymphocytes

Small lymphocytes are similar in appearance to the small lymphocytes found in blood. Small B and T lymphocytes cannot be distinguished from each other based on appearance. Because various subsets of lymphocytes in lymph nodes can not be identified based on morphology, lymphoid cells are described according to size and the presence or absence of a visible nucleolus within the nucleus. Small lymphocytes are slightly smaller than a neutrophil (7–10 μm), and the nucleus is lightly larger than a red blood cell, with dense chromatin. A nucleolus is not visible within the nucleus, but chromatin clumps can be confused with nucleoli. The cytoplasm is generally scant and consists of a narrow rim around the nucleus (Figure 45.5). Some prefer to use nuclear size, rather than cell size, and consider a lymphocyte small if the nucleus is smaller than a neutrophil. The small lymphocyte is the primary cell type present in normal and hyperplastic nodes.

Intermediate lymphocytes

Intermediate lymphocytes have a nuclear diameter approximately equal to two red blood cells (9–15 μm), the nucleus is slightly larger than a neutrophil, and they have less densely packed nuclear chromatin (Figure 45.5). They are likely follicular centrocytes and marginal zone B cells.

Large immature lymphoid cells with apparent nucleoli (formerly called lymphoblasts)

The nuclear chromatin is fine and diffuse, and one or more nucleoli are observed in the nucleus. They are approximately 2–4 times the size of a small lymphocyte and 1.5–2 times the size of neutrophils. The nucleus is larger than a neutrophil. They may possess a broad or narrow rim of cytoplasm, but it is most commonly narrow (Figure 45.5). Large immature lymphoid cells are present in small numbers in normal nodes and usually do not exceed 20% of the total cell population in reactive lymph nodes. Lymphoid blasts are either follicular centroblasts or B or T immunoblasts from the paracortex and medullary cords and are difficult to classify as to type, based on cytologic appearance. Centroblasts have one to three peripheral nucleoli in the nucleus and scant cytoplasm, whereas immunoblasts have one centrally located nucleolus and a moderate amount of cytoplasm. Historically in veterinary medicine, the term "lymphoblast"

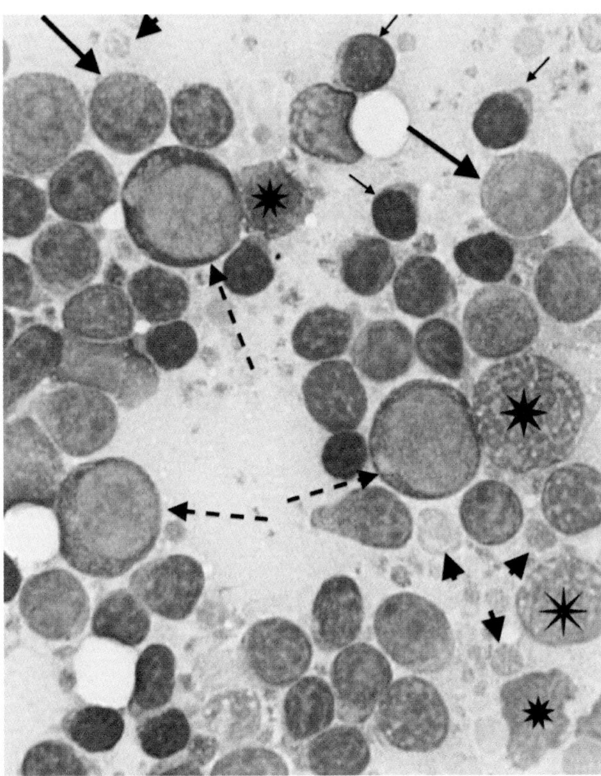

Figure 45.5 Lymph node aspirate from a dog with early antigenic stimulation. Small lymphocytes predominate (small arrows). Intermediate lymphoid cells are also present (large solid arrows). Large immature lymphoid cells are indicated by large dashed line arrows. Numerous cytoplasmic fragments are interspersed between cells (arrowheads). Broken nuclei are common to see in lymph node aspirates and are identified with asterisks. Wright stain.

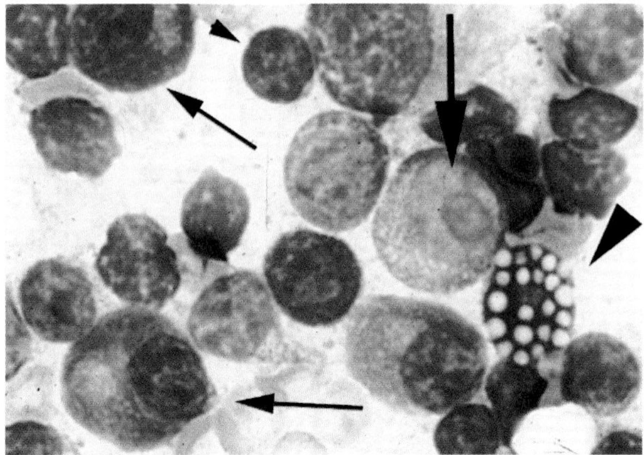

Figure 45.6 Reactive lymph node as evidenced by plasma cells (small arrows), a plasmablast (large arrow), and a Mott cell (large arrowhead). Small lymphocytes are also present (small arrowhead). Wright stain.

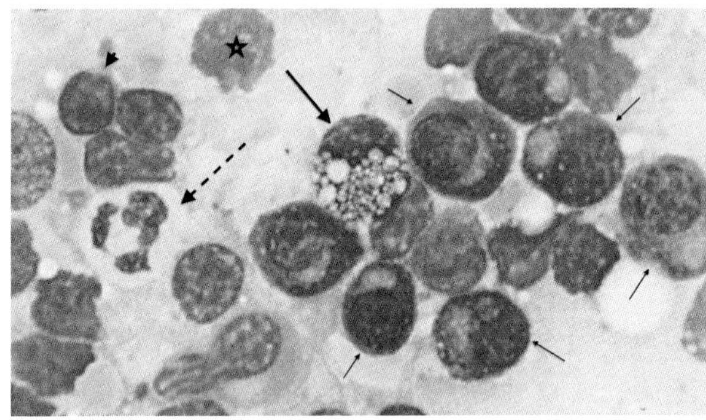

Figure 45.7 Aspirate of very reactive lymph node in a dog. Numerous plasma cells are present (small arrows), as well as a Mott cell (large arrow). The dashed line arrow indicates a neutrophil. Numerous cells are broken, with only nuclear material remaining (star). Wright strain.

was used for all immature lymphoid cells. According to the World Health Organization (WHO) classification of lymphoma, the term "lymphoblast" should only be used when describing specific precursor cells with defined morphologic features that are found in lymphoblastic lymphoma (LBL), a rare subtype of lymphoma arising from precursor cells that are uniform and small to medium in size, with round or convoluted nuclei not larger than the diameter of two erythrocytes and fine chromatin pattern and scant, sometimes vacuolated lightly basophilic cytoplasm. Nucleoli are small to inconspicuous and numerous cells in mitosis are seen; this subtype of lymphoma is discussed in more detail under the lymphoma section in this chapter. Some have suggested that when describing what have been traditionally called "lymphoblasts," the terms "immature large lymphoid cells with nucleoli," "lymphoid blasts," "centroblasts," or "immunoblasts" should now be used.

Plasma cells and plasmablasts

Plasma cells and plasmablasts are derived from antigenically stimulated B lymphocytes. The nucleus of plasma cells is eccentrically placed, the cytoplasm is generally quite basophilic, they may contain vacuoles, and a perinuclear clear area (Golgi zone) is commonly present. Plasma cells that contain many discrete packets of immunoglobulin (Russell bodies) are called Mott cells or Russell body cells and are commonly seen in reactive lymph nodes (Figures 45.6–45.8). Plasmablasts, B cells that have undergone blast transformation, are similar to other immature lymphoid blasts but usually have more cytoplasm that is basophilic and sometimes vacuolated, a Golgi zone may be apparent, and the nucleus may be more eccentric.

Neutrophils

Inflamed nodes will usually contain many neutrophils. These may appear healthy and intact whether the inflammatory process is septic or nonseptic (Figures 45.9 and 45.10), although degenerative changes may indicate septic inflammation. Karyolysis and karyorrhexis may be present. Bacteria are best observed within the cytoplasm of the neutrophils in thin portions of the preparation.

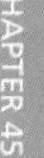

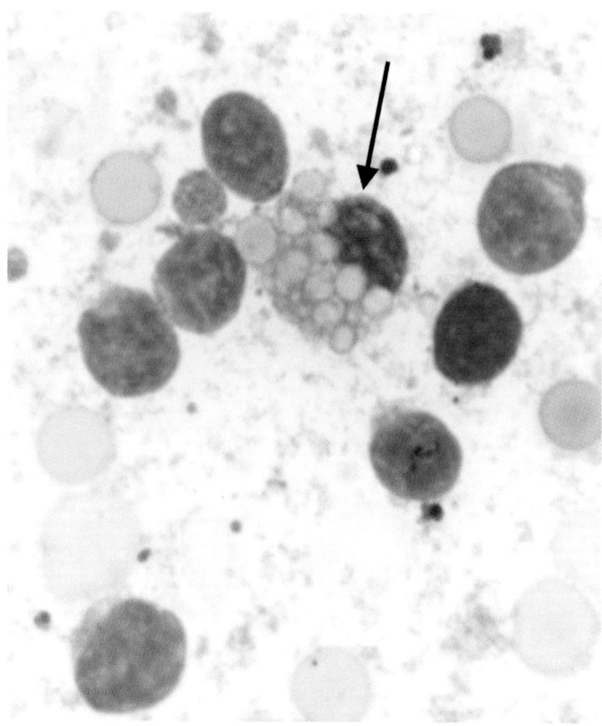

Figure 45.8 A Mott cell is indicated by the arrow. Russell bodies may not stain and appear clear, or the bodies may stain pink or light blue, as shown in this image. Wright stain.

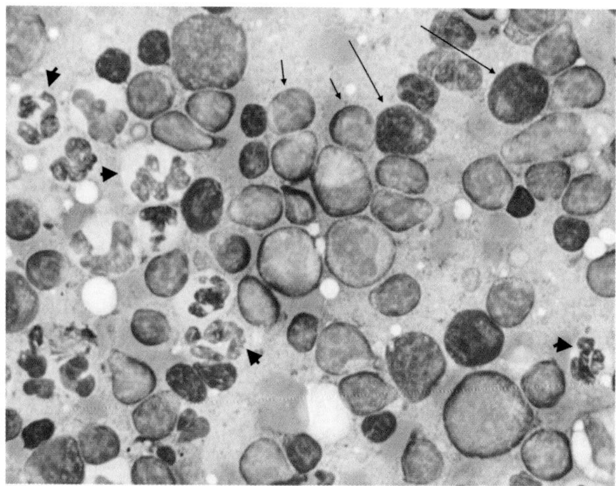

Figure 45.9 Aspirate of a submandibular lymph node of a dog that is both reactive and inflamed. Small lymphocytes are indicated by small arrows, plasma cells by long arrows, and neutrophils by arrowheads. Wright stain.

Macrophages

Macrophages may be observed in some inflammatory conditions. These cells are phagocytic, have abundant, usually vacuolated cytoplasm, and may contain cellular debris. Macrophages are sometimes multinucleated. When macrophages develop some of the characteristics of epithelial cells, such as abundant cytoplasm that lacks vacuoles, they are often referred to as epithelioid cells. Care should be taken not to confuse epithelioid cells with metastatic carcinoma cells (Figure 45.11).

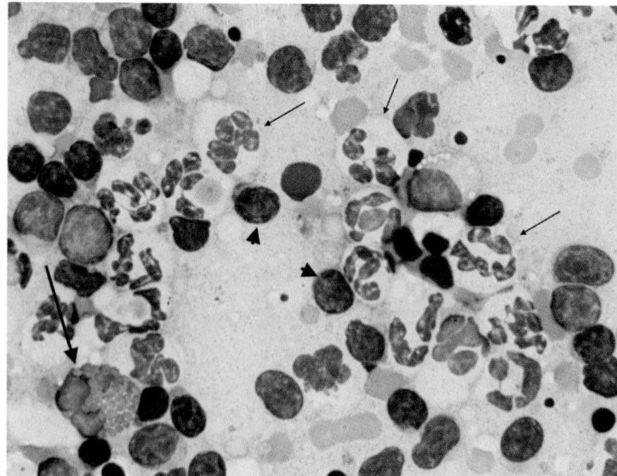

Figure 45.10 Suppurative lymphadenitis in a horse. Note the numerous neutrophils (small arrows), an eosinophil (large arrow), and small lymphocytes (arrowheads). The neutrophils are nondegenerate and no microorganisms are seen. Wright stain.

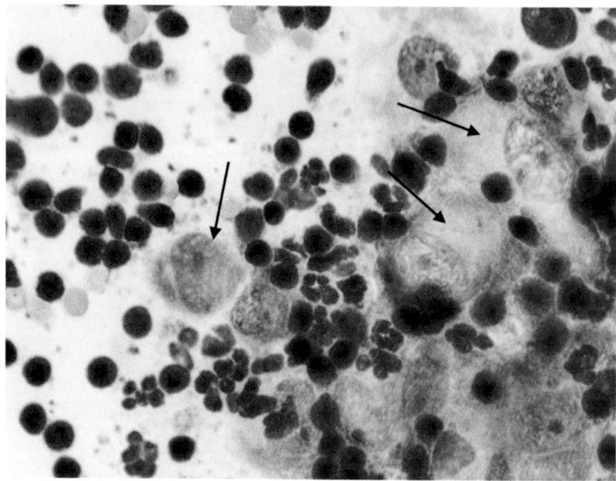

Figure 45.11 Pyogranulomatous lymphadenitis in a cat. Epithelioid macrophages are present in aggregates (arrows) and could be confused with epithelial cells. Numerous small lymphocytes and neutrophils are present as well. Wright stain.

Eosinophils

Eosinophils in lymph nodes appear similar to eosinophils in peripheral blood and are associated with allergic reactions, parasitic diseases, and neoplasms, including lymphoma and mast cell tumors. Eosinophilic inflammation of lymph nodes is commonly seen in patients with dermatitis or flea-bite allergy (Figure 45.12).

Mast cells

Mast cells are round cells with numerous basophilic granules in the cytoplasm. A few may be seen in normal lymph nodes.

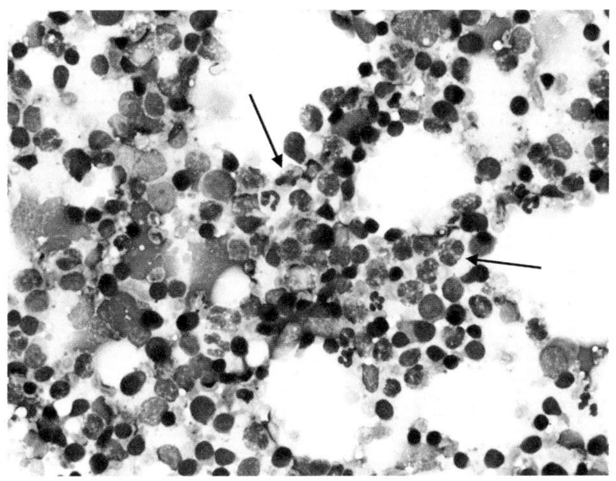

Figure 45.12 Eosinophilic lymphadenitis in a dog. Eosinophils are the predominant cell type (arrows). Numerous small lymphocytes and a few plasma cells are also present. Wright stain.

Lymph nodes draining skin lesions often have increased mast cells. The presence of many mast cells especially in aggregates is suggestive of mast cell neoplasia with metastatic involvement of the lymph node (Figure 45.13).

Neoplastic cells other than lymphoid cells

Neoplastic cells other than lymphoid cells, such as carcinoma cells, may be seen in lymph nodes to which neoplasms have metastasized (Figure 45.14). Cells not belonging to the normal population of the lymph node can usually be seen at low magnification. Malignant epithelial cells are usually quite pleomorphic and large, exhibiting numerous criteria of malignancy (Figure 45.15). Nuclei vary in size and shape and may exhibit nuclear molding. Nucleoli are often prominent and multiple. Occasional mitotic figures and multinucleated cells may be observed. The cytoplasm of malignant epithelial cells (carcinomas) commonly stains quite basophilic and may contain perinuclear vacuoles. Sarcomas metastasize to lymph nodes less frequently than carcinomas. Mast cell tumors commonly metastasize to lymph nodes and must be differentiated from normal mast cells that may be present in small numbers, particularly in inflamed lymph nodes. Malignant melanomas also commonly metastasize to lymph nodes. Metastatic disease in lymph nodes is discussed in more detail in a later section of this chapter.

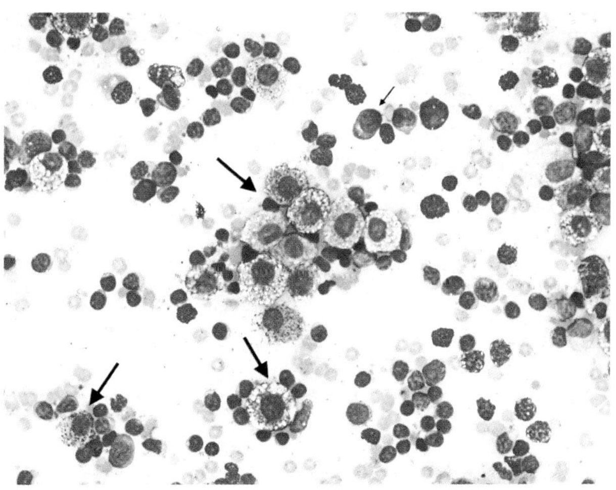

Figure 45.13 Metastatic mast cell tumor in a lymph node of the dog. Aggregates and single mast cells are scattered throughout (large arrows). The lymph node is also reactive (note plasma cell, small arrow). Small lymphocytes predominate, with some erythrocytes in the background. Wright stain.

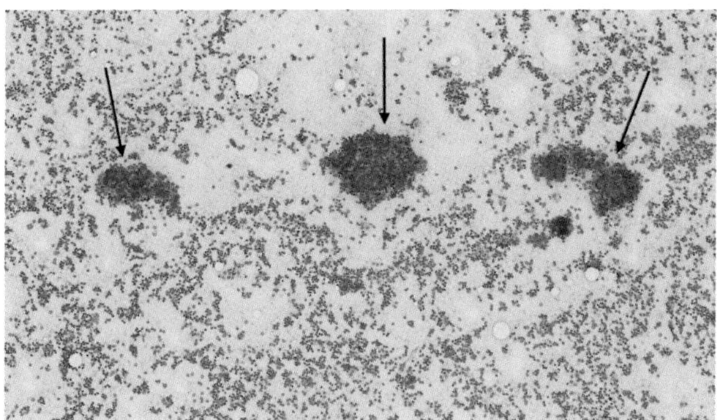

Figure 45.14 Low magnification of a lymph node with metastatic nasal carcinoma. Note the clusters of large cohesive epithelial cells (arrows) among the normal lymphoid population. Wright stain.

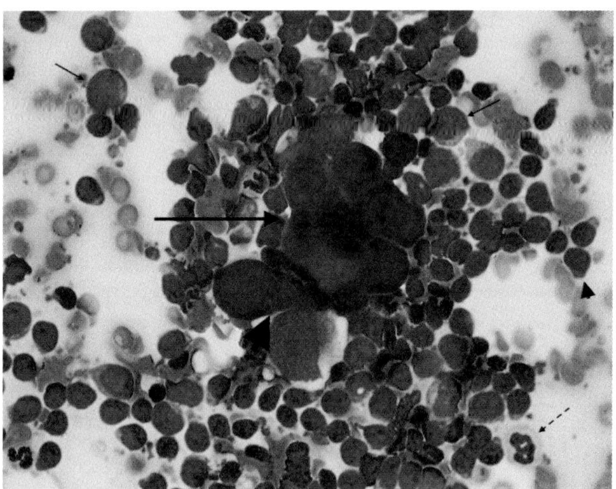

Figure 45.15 Metastatic nasal squamous cell carcinoma in a lymph node of a dog. A large cluster of neoplastic epithelial cells is indicated by the large arrow. Note the variability in size of the cells and the nuclear molding (large arrowhead). Small lymphocytes predominate (small arrowhead), with an occasional large immature lymphoid cell (small arrows), and neutrophils (dashed line arrow). Wright stain.

Cytoplasmic fragments and free nuclei

Small pieces of cytoplasm approximately 1–5 µm in diameter may be observed between cells (Figure 45.5). These fragments have been referred to as lymphoglandular bodies and are a characteristic feature of lymphoid tissue aspirates.

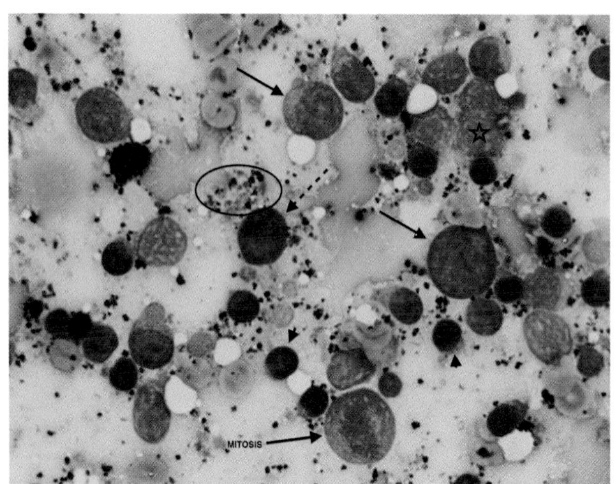

Figure 45.16 A large amount of hemosiderin (oval) is scattered throughout the preparation, indicating previous hemorrhage. The node is reactive, as indicated by plasma cells (dashed line arrow) and plasmablasts (arrows). One plasmablast appears to be in mitosis. Numerous cells are broken (star). A small lymphocyte is indicated by the arrowhead. Wright stain.

They should not be confused with platelets or organisms. Lymphoid cells are fragile and rupture easily, releasing nuclear material. Free nuclei are pink and swollen, and sometimes a light blue nucleolus can be seen within the broken nucleus (Figure 45.5). These broken cells with apparent nucleoli should not be confused with immature lymphoid cells containing nucleoli. If all of the cells are broken, the node should be reaspirated.

Pigment

Hemosiderin, a pigment resulting from red blood cell degradation by macrophages, is frequently seen in lymph nodes and may be intracellular or extracellular (Figure 45.16). Hemosiderin, the insoluble form of storage iron, stains blue-green to black with Wright stain and is usually within macrophages. Melanin is usually golden brown to black but may be confused with hemosiderin. If necessary, a Prussian blue stain can be used to confirm the presence of iron. Melanin may be present within macrophages in nodes draining pigmented lesions or may be seen in melanocytes with metastatic melanoma. It is sometimes difficult to differentiate macrophages that contain melanin from melanocytes; melanin within macrophages usually consists of homogeneous clumps within phagolysosomes, whereas melanin in melanocytes consists of individual melanin granules. Fontana Masson stain can be used to identify melanin.

Interpretation of cytologic findings

Normal lymph nodes

Small lymphocytes are the predominant cell type in normal nodes, comprising 85–90% of the cells observed. Very small numbers of macrophages, medium lymphocytes, large immature lymphoid cells containing nucleoli, plasma cells, and neutrophils may be present. One study of normal canine lymph node cytology reported a median percentage of neutrophils, eosinophils, and macrophages as 1.4%, 2.0%, and 1.4%, respectively. Plasma cells comprise less than 4% of cells in a normal canine lymph node. Intermediate lymphocytes are reported to make up 3–4% of cells in normal canine lymph nodes.

Reactive (hyperplastic) lymph nodes

The term "reactive lymphoid hyperplasia" describes the enlargement of the lymph node secondary to antigenic stimulation, the most common cause of lymph node enlargement. Hyperplasia may occur in follicles, interfollicular paracortical areas, medullary cords (plasma cell hyperplasia), and sinuses (histiocytosis). The cytologic features of antigen-stimulated lymph nodes is variable, depending on the area aspirated and the length of time since antigenic stimulation began. Small lymphocytes predominate in antigenically stimulated lymph nodes. Variable numbers of intermediate lymphocytes and large immature lymphoid cells may be observed. Mature and immature plasma cells are increased and are the key feature of a reactive lymph node (Figure 45.7). Rarely, plasma cells are the predominant cell in reactive lymph nodes, and in those cases, plasma cell neoplasia must be considered as a differential diagnosis. Macrophages, neutrophils, eosinophils, and mast cells may be slightly increased in number. Ultimately, inflammatory cells may be increased to the point that the node is classified as both inflamed and reactive. Aggregates or syncytia of macrophages may be seen and should not be confused with clusters of metastatic epithelial cells. Reactive nodes draining inflamed skin frequently contain increased numbers of eosinophils and mast cells. While some veterinary clinical pathologists distinguish hyperplastic lymph nodes from reactive lymph nodes based on the number of plasma cells present ("reactive" lymph nodes having more plasma cells), this is likely an artificial classification, since the number of plasma cells obtained will vary with the site within the lymph node from which the aspirate was taken. Caution must be taken not to confuse hyperplastic lymph nodes from small-cell variants of lymphoma. When nodes are enlarged and aspirates are very cellular, consisting of a uniform monomorphic population of small lymphocytes, a small-cell variant of lymphoma is more likely than hyperplasia (see lymphoma discussion later in chapter). The cause of the antigenic stimulation is usually not apparent in aspirates, although an exception is leishmaniasis, in which the typical nodal response is reactive hyperplasia, rather than inflammation, and organisms are commonly seen.

Ehrlichia canis

Ehrlichia canis morulae are rarely seen in lymph node aspirates of dogs with canine monocytic ehrlichiosis (CME).

Generalized lymphadenopathy due to antigenic stimulation is seen in the majority of dogs with ehrlichiosis. Increases in plasma cells, intermediate lymphocytes, and plasmablasts are typically seen.

Borrelia burgdorferi

Borrelia burgdorferi, a spirochete transmitted by *Ixodes* spp. ticks and the causative agent of Lyme disease, causes lymphadenopathy in humans and dogs in the acute stage of disease, particularly in the regional lymph node near the site of infection, but generalized lymphadenopathy is common. The lymphadenopathy is primarily due to reactive hyperplasia, and in dogs with experimental Lyme disease, it is characterized by proliferation of follicles, parafollicular B-cell proliferation, and increases in plasma cells in medullary cords. Macrophages, a few neutrophils, and sometimes eosinophils are found within medullary sinuses in variable numbers. Extracellular spirochetes are found persistently in the subcapsular sinus and superficial cortex of lymph nodes in experimentally infected mice. Lymphadenopathy is a hallmark of acute infection but the underlying causes and the functional consequences of this lymph node enlargement have not been revealed. Studies demonstrate that extracellular, live spirochetes accumulate in the cortical areas of lymph nodes following infection of mice with either host-adapted or tick-borne *B. burgdorferi* and that they, but not inactivated spirochetes, drive the lymphadenopathy. The ensuing lymph node response is characterized by strong, rapid extrafollicular B-cell proliferation and differentiation to plasma cells, while germinal center reactions have not been consistently observed.

Leishmaniasis

Leishmaniasis is an infectious cause of reactive lymph node hyperplasia in which the organisms are commonly seen in aspirates. The causal agent of canine leishmaniasis is the protozoan *Leishmania infantum* (also known as *L. chagasi*), which is quite common in Europe and other parts of the world. *Leishmania* is typically transmitted by sand flies and is also seen in the United States in dogs that have a travel history to endemic areas such as Spain. However, leishmaniasis also has been diagnosed in dogs that have no travel history, especially foxhounds in the eastern part of the United States, where the disease has become increasingly common. It is thought to be transmitted vertically or by dog-to-dog mechanisms in these states, because no vectors such as sand flies have been identified. The amastigote form of the parasite reproduces in macrophages, resulting in rupture and spread to numerous organs, including spleen, liver, bone marrow, and lymph node (Figure 45.17). The disease can take several forms, ranging from a mild cutaneous form to disseminated visceral leishmaniasis. Almost all dogs with clinical leishmaniasis have reactive lymph node hyperplasia, although a small percentage may also have a combination of reactive hyperplasia and histiocytic lymphadenitis or histiocytic lymphadenitis only. The amastigote is round with a light purple round nucleus and dark purple rod-shaped kinetoplast, as also shown in Figures 15.21 and 39.47.

Feline immunodeficiency virus

Feline immunodeficiency virus (*FIV*) infection in the early stages will commonly result in generalized lymphadenopathy due to antigenic stimulation. The lymph nodes appear reactive

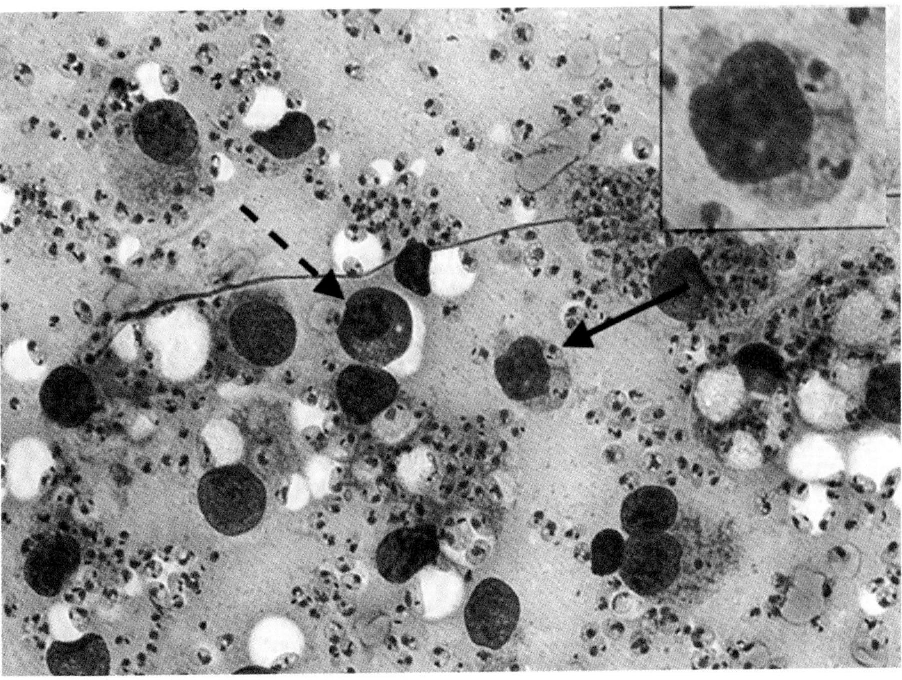

Figure 45.17 Lymph node aspirate from a dog with leishmaniasis. Note the "two-dot" organisms within the cytoplasm of cells (arrow). A plasma cell is indicated by the dashed arrow. Inset, right upper corner shows a higher magnification. Wright stain.

on cytology as a result of increased germinal centers and increased plasma cells in the medulla.

Phenobarbital hypersensitivity

Phenobarbital hypersensitivity is a rare idiosyncratic cause of reactive lymph nodes in dogs and cats. Cytology of the lymph nodes is consistent with reactive hyperplasia, and mixed inflammation is seen in spleen and liver aspirates. This well-recognized syndrome in humans is referred to as pseudolymphoma.

Lymphadenitis

The types of cells present in an inflamed lymph node are variable depending on the cause of inflammation; neutrophils, eosinophils or macrophages may predominate. If the most predominant cell is the neutrophil, the inflammation is classified as neutrophilic inflammation; "purulent" or "suppurative" are commonly used synonyms. If the predominant cell is the macrophage, the inflammatory response is classified as macrophagic, histiocytic, or granulomatous inflammation. Mixed inflammatory reactions may also be seen, in which some combination of inflammatory cells are present. If neutrophils and macrophages predominate, the inflammation is often referred to as pyogranulomatous. The required percentage of inflammatory cells present when describing a node as inflamed is subjective but has been reported to be >5% neutrophils for neutrophilic inflammation, >3% macrophages for macrophagic inflammation, and >3% eosinophils for eosinophilic inflammation. Inflamed lymph nodes may also be reactive, with increased numbers of plasma cells, intermediate lymphocytes, and large immature lymphoid cells containing nucleoli. Neutrophilic inflammation may become so severe that abscessation and necrosis occur, making it sometimes difficult to recognize that the origin of the abscess was a lymph node. Lymphadenitis may be due to multiple causes, but an immune-mediated or, more commonly, an infectious etiology must be considered when numerous neutrophils and/or macrophages are present.

Idiopathic pyogranulomatous lymphadenitis

Idiopathic pyogranulomatous lymphadenitis in dogs is assumed to be immune mediated since it is steroid responsive. It is most common in English springer spaniels. Clinical signs include pyrexia and lymphadenopathy, often accompanied by dermal lesions (nodular panniculitis), lethargy, hyporexia, and gastrointestinal and respiratory signs. Lymph node aspirates show mixed (pyogranulomatous) sterile inflammation. A very similar condition resulting in mandibular lymphadenopathy is *sterile granulomatous dermatitis and lymphadenopathy* (SGDL), also known in young dogs as juvenile cellulitis or puppy strangles, which occurs in both puppies and adult dogs, is reported in multiple breeds including Havanese, Australian shepherds, Irish setters, Dachshund, bichon frise, and Maltese, and is also steroid responsive and assumed to be immune mediated.

Infectious lymphadenitis

Microorganisms eliciting lymphadenitis include bacteria, protozoa, rickettsia, and fungal agents.

Bacterial lymphadenitis

Bacteria that may result in marked lymphadenitis include *Streptococcus equi, Yersinia pestis, Francisella tularensis, Mycobacterium* spp., *Bartonella henselae,* and various other bacteria that may cause regional lymphadenitis, such as *Salmonella*-related and *Listeria monocytogenes*–related mesenteric lymphadenitis, and *Rhodococcus equi*–related lymphadenitis, as shown in Figure 39.22.

- *Streptococcus equi* is the causative agent of "strangles" in horses, a frequently diagnosed infection that is characterized by neutrophilic lymphadenitis followed by abscessation of the lymph nodes of the head and neck. The cocci can be easily seen in lymph node aspirates, similar to what is shown in Figure 39.2. The disease was first described in 1251 and the causative agent was identified in 1888. *Streptococcus zooepidemicus*, a bacterium that is very closely related to *Streptococcus equi,* can also result in lymphadenopathy, appears identical to *Streptococcus equi,* as shown in Figures 39.12 and 39.13, but is less pathogenic and less contagious.
- *Yersinia pestis*, a Gram-negative coccobacillus with a bipolar safety-pin shape, is the causative agent of plague, a relatively rare zoonotic disease of historical significance in Europe (Black Death). The disease is more common in cats than dogs. In the United States, plague is more common in Colorado, California, and New Mexico. It also occurs in semi-arid parts of Asia, Europe, and Africa. Transmission occurs via flea bite or ingestion of infected rodents or rabbits. Cats commonly have bilateral mandibular lymphadenopathy;

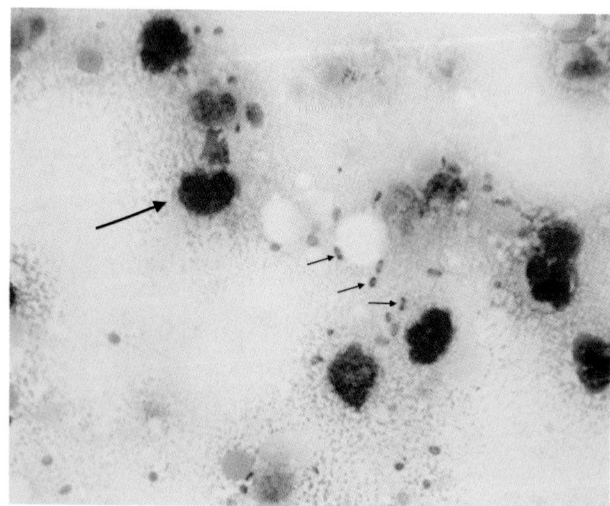

Figure 45.18 Submandibular lymph node aspirates from a Colorado cat with plague. Lymph nodes were abscessed, and neutrophils are very degenerate (large arrow), appearing as nuclear smudges. Numerous free *Yersinia pestis* organisms are present (small arrows). Wright stain. Source: Courtesy of Dr. Kyra Somers and Dr. Robin Allison.

lymphadenopathy is less common in infected dogs. Aspirates of nodes show neutrophilic inflammation as shown in Figure 39.15, and the coccobacilli are typically numerous (Figure 45.18). Neutrophilic lymphadenitis often evolves into abscessation and necrosis. Infected individuals may also develop pulmonary lesions and septicemia. Treatment of choice is gentamycin or doxycycline.

• *Francisella tularensis*, the causative agent of tularemia, also known as "rabbit fever," is a very virulent intracellular Gram-negative bacterium that is usually fatal in rabbits. Infection occurs in dogs and cats most commonly by contact with or ingestion of infected animals, usually rodents or rabbits, but can also be transmitted by arthropod vectors such as ticks or deer flies, inhalation of contaminated dust, or ingestion of contaminated food and water. The disease occurs in dogs, cats, humans, and many other mammalian, avian, piscine, reptilian and amphibian species in the Northern Hemisphere of the world. In the United States, it is most common in Arkansas, Missouri, South Dakota, Oklahoma, Kansas, and between the Rocky Mountains and the Sierra Nevada Mountains; it is reportable in some states. Tularemia is more severe, and probably more common, in cats than in dogs. Clinical signs are similar to those of plague and may include fever, lethargy, anorexia, lymphadenopathy, vomiting, diarrhea, mucopurulent oculonasal discharge, and occasionally skin lesions. Common laboratory findings in dogs include neutrophilia and thrombocytopenia. Lymphadenopathy associated with tularemia in humans is called "glandular tularemia." Lymphadenopathy occurs in approximately 20% of dogs with tularemia and is usually in the head and neck area. Cytologic findings range from reactive hyperplasia in acute disease, to suppurative or mixed inflammation, to necrosis. Lymph node aspirates are diagnostically useful as the organisms can sometimes be seen as well as cultured.

• *Bartonella henselae*, the causative agent of "cat scratch fever" in humans, is a very small (0.3–0.6 × 1.0–1.7 μm), pleomorphic Gram-negative rod. The organism is transmitted by the cat flea, and cats are typically asymptomatic when infected. Bartonellosis has been rarely associated with pyogranulomatous lymphadenitis in dogs. Both peripheral and visceral lymph nodes may be enlarged, and the pattern of inflammation is similar to what is seen in humans.

• *Mycobacterial* infections typically result in macrophagic or granulomatous lymphadenitis. Weight loss, lethargy, and generalized lymphadenopathy are the most common clinical signs. The majority of cells in infected lymph nodes are macrophages, and most macrophages contain nonstaining clear rods within the cytoplasm (Figure 45.19). Mycobacteria may also be seen within neutrophils and free between cells. Mycobacteria appear as nonstaining rods in Wright-stained preparations due to their lipid-rich cell wall that does not stain, as shown in Figures 39.23 and 39.24, but they stain pink with an acid-fast stain (Ziehl-Neelsen) (Figure 45.20). The most common species seen in dogs is *Mycobacterium avium*, an opportunistic non-tuberculous mycobacteria (NTM). The species *Mycobacterium avium* is currently divided into four subspecies including *avium* (MAA), *silvaticum* (MAS), *hominissuis* (MAH), and *paratuberculosis* (MAP). The subspecies *hominissuis* (MAH) is responsible for the majority of infections in dogs and is usually contracted from soil and water in the environment. The disease is usually systemic and commonly fatal, with mycobacteria in numerous locations in addition to lymph nodes, including the small and large intestine, spleen, liver, lungs, and bone marrow. While canine mycobacteriosis is relatively rare, a strong breed predisposition is seen in miniature schnauzers and basset hounds; dogs less than 5 years of age are most commonly affected. An autosomal

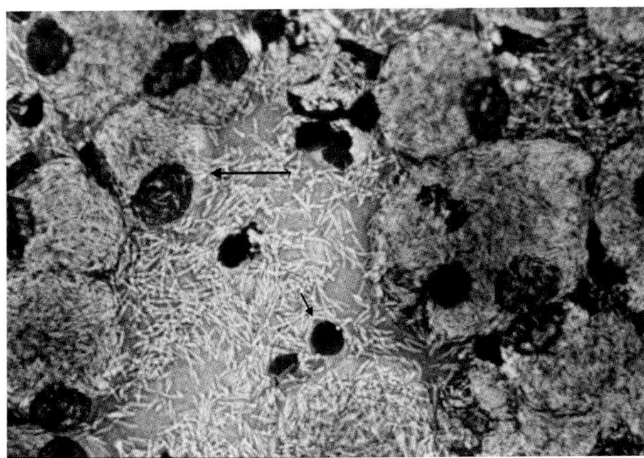

Figure 45.19 High magnification of an aspirate of a lymph node from a miniature schnauzer with generalized lymphadenopathy that was referred with an erroneous diagnosis of lymphoma and had been treated previously with glucocorticosteroids. Macrophages are the predominant cell (large arrow) and are filled with nonstaining large rods that were confirmed as *Mycobacterium avium*. Numerous organisms are also free in the background. A small lymphocyte is indicated by the small arrow. Wright stain.

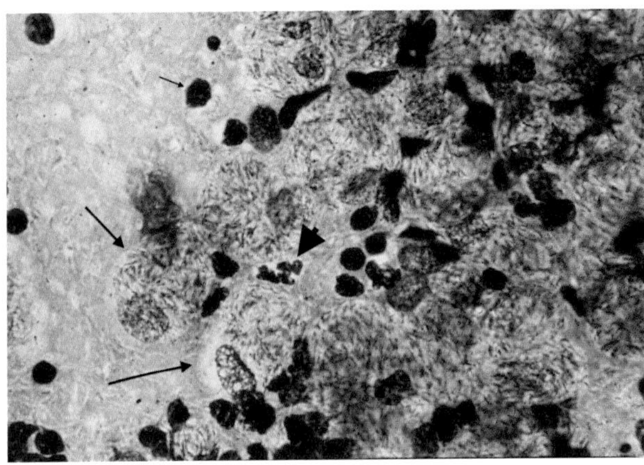

Figure 45.20 Aspirate of the same lymph node as shown in Figure 45.19, shown at a lower magnification and stained with an acid-fast stain. The mycobacteria stain pink. Macrophages predominate (large arrows), with numerous small lymphocytes (small arrow) and occasional neutrophils (arrowhead). Ziehl-Neelsen stain.

recessively inherited defect in the adaptor protein CARD9 (caspase recruitment domain-containing protein 9) has been shown to be responsible for the increased susceptibility in miniature schnauzers. All miniature schnauzers that are homozygous for the CARD9 variant gene develop mycobacteriosis due to *Mycobacterium avium* (see Ghielmetti and Giger 2020 in "Suggested Reading" under "Mycobacterial Lymphadenitis"). The CARD9 signaling pathway is essential in host defense against numerous fungal organisms and intracellular bacteria.

Rickettsial lymphadenopathy

Rickettsia that cause lymphadenomegaly include *Ehrlichia canis, Neorickettsia helminthoeca,* and *Stellanchasmus falcatus.* Lymphadenopathy associated with the rickettsial agent *Ehrlichia canis* is a result of reactive hyperplasia, rather than lymphadenitis, and is discussed in that section. *Neorickettsia helminthoeca* is an intracellular bacterium that causes salmon poisoning disease in dogs, primarily seen in the Northwest United States, Southern California, Western Canada, and Southern Brazil. However, dogs eating undercooked or raw trout or salmon from supermarkets in other areas can also be infected. The term "salmon poisoning" is a misnomer, since no poison is involved. *N. helminthoeca* is carried by the fluke *Nanophyetus salmincola,* the life cycle of which is complex and involves the snail *Juga plicifera* as the first intermediate host, salmonid fishes, primarily trout and salmon, as the second intermediate host, and fish-eating mammals as the definitive host. The ingested immature flukes (metacercaria) mature to adult flukes in the small intestine. Adult flukes begin producing eggs in approximately 1 week. Fluke eggs develop into miracidia that infect snails, thus completing the life cycle. The disease is fatal in approximately 90% of dogs that are not treated, usually within 1 week of showing clinical signs that include fever, weakness, anorexia, vomiting, diarrhea, dehydration, and lymphadenopathy. Histopathology shows granulomatous lymphadenitis, splenitis, enteritis, and hepatitis with necrosis. Diagnosis is made by recognition of clinical signs, the presence of fluke eggs in the feces, lymph node aspiration showing granulomatous inflammation and organisms, and serology or polymerase chain reaction (PCR) for *N. helminthoeca.* Histiocytic lymphadenitis, with numerous *N. helminthoeca* organisms within macrophages, is seen on lymph node aspirates. The rickettsia appear as small basophilic aggregates as shown in Figure 39.54, rather than distinct morulae. Doxycycline and supportive therapy are curative if given early in the course of the disease. A second closely related organism with similar transmission, *Stellanchasmus falcatus,* causes Elokomin fluke fever, a disease with similar clinical signs and outcome in bears but which typically only causes mild disease in dogs. However, *S. falcatus* has been reported to cause severe disease and death in a small number of dogs in the Pacific Northwest, with clinical signs and cytologic findings very similar to those seen in dogs infected with *N. helminthoeca.*

Protozoan lymphadenopathy

• *Leishmania* spp. usually results in reactive hyperplasia of lymph nodes and is discussed in that section. In some patients, however, macrophagic (histiocytic) lymphadenitis is seen, as shown in Figures 45.17 and 39.47.

• *Cytauxzoon felis,* a protozoan haemoparasite of the family *Theileriidae* that infects wild and domestic cats and causes cytauxzoonosis, is discussed in detail in Chapter 9 in the section on hemolytic anemia. This protozoan organism has two phases, one in macrophages (sporozoites and schizonts), and one in erythrocytes (merozoites/piroplasms). Sporozoites infect endothelial-associated macrophages and undergo asexual replication within the macrophages; sporozoites develop into large structures known as schizonts that occlude blood vessels in various organs, resulting in thrombosis, circulatory impairment, and an inflammatory response that leads to organ failure and death within a few weeks of infection. Merozoites are released from ruptured monocytes and macrophages and then infect erythrocytes. The organism can be identified not only within erythrocytes in the merozoite stage but also in lymph node, spleen, and liver aspirates, where schizonts can be observed, as shown in Figures 9.20, 39.44, and 39.45. The large macrophages often have prominent nucleoli, and the cytoplasm is distended with dark blue developing signet ring merozoites that are 1–2 µm in diameter.

• *Toxoplasma gondii* is another protozoan organism that can be found in lymph node aspirates of cats. It is an obligate intracellular coccidian parasite that can infect all mammals, but domestic and wild cats are the natural hosts. Transmission occurs vertically (transplacentally), by ingestion of infective oocysts or ingestion of infected tissue. Cats are usually infected by eating intermediate hosts, usually rodents, that are infected with tissue cysts. Bradyzoites are then released in the stomach and intestine from the tissue cysts and enter epithelial cells of the small intestine and form schizonts. Merozoites, formed and released from the schizonts, eventually form male and female gamonts. A wall is then formed around the fertilized macrogamont to form an oocyst. Oocysts, round to oval structures, 10×12 µm in diameter, are excreted in feces and are not infectious until after they sporulate, which takes 1–5 days. If infective oocysts are ingested, sporozoites hatch in the intestine and enter intestinal cells and form tachyzoites, which then multiply in almost any cell of the body, resulting in rupture of the cell and release of tachyzoites. Tachyzoites then infect additional cells and eventually encyst. Tissue cysts conform to the shape of the infected cell and range in size from 15 to 60 µm. On cytology, tachyzoites can be seen within cells or free, are falciform in shape (sickle or banana-shaped), have a small round nucleus, and are approximately 2×6 µm in diameter, as shown in Figures 15.20 and 39.46. Clinical signs are rare in infected cats, and when they occur are due to inflammation and tissue necrosis as a result of intracellular growth of tachyzoites. Diagnosis can be made by finding the organism in fluids or macrophages of tissue aspirates, most commonly lymph nodes or bronchoalveolar lavage, or PCR to detect organism DNA. Treatment consists of oral clindamycin for 4 weeks.

• *Trypanosoma* spp. are protozoal organisms transmitted by biting flies and other insects that cause trypanosomiasis in domestic large and small animals, humans, and wildlife species worldwide. Lethargy due to anemia and/or central nervous system involvement and lymphadenopathy are common clinical signs. While they are commonly found in blood, they may also be seen in lymph node aspirates. As mentioned earlier in this chapter, lymph nodes were first aspirated in humans more than a century ago to diagnose trypanosomiasis. Trypomastigote forms of *Trypanosoma* spp. are fusiform in shape, contain a nucleus, a kinetoplast, and a flagellum, and are 16–26 µm in length. Cysts containing organisms can be seen in many tissues including muscle and brain.

Fungal lymphadenitis

Whenever a combination of neutrophils and macrophages (pyogranulomatous inflammation) is seen on a lymph node aspirate, fungal infection should be suspected and a search for organisms should be performed. Five dimorphic yeast organisms can cause systemic infections and include cryptococcosis, blastomycosis, histoplasmosis, coccidioidomycosis, and paracoccidioidomycosis. In addition, other fungal organisms with hyphae may be seen in lymph nodes. Some structures can be confused with fungal hyphae and are also briefly mentioned in this section.

• *Cryptococcosis* is a fungal disease that infects mammals, reptiles, and birds and is worldwide (see Chapter 39). Cats are more commonly affected than dogs. The asexual yeast phase of the organism in tissues reproduces by budding, which is very narrow-based. Cryptococcal organisms are round to oval, 4–6 µm in diameter, and surrounded by polysaccharide capsules that vary in size but can be up to 30 µm in diameter. The capsule aids in preventing phagocytosis by neutrophils and macrophages and also prevents neutrophil migration and cytokine production, thus decreasing T lymphocyte-mediated immune responses. The characteristic capsule is very helpful in identifying *Cryptococcus* in tissue aspirates, and because of capsule function, sometimes the organisms will be seen in the absence of any inflammatory cells. The capsule does not stain with Wright stain, giving a clear halo appearance around the organism, as shown in Figures 39.31 and 39.32. Wet mounts using new methylene blue or India ink are particularly useful in aspirates with few inflammatory cells and many cryptococcal organisms (Figures 45.21 and 45.22). When inflammation is associated with the organism, it is usually pyogranulomatous. If lymphadenopathy is present, usually lymph nodes of the head and neck are affected. The genus *Cryptococcus* includes over 37 species, the majority of which do not cause disease in mammals. The disease-producing species are referred to as the *C. neoformans–C. gattii* species complex, the most common of which are *C. neoformans* var. *neoformans*, *C. neoformans* var. *grubii*, and *C. gattii*. Virulence factors include the ability to grow at mammalian body temperature, the size of the capsule surrounding the organism, and the ability to resist oxidative damage.

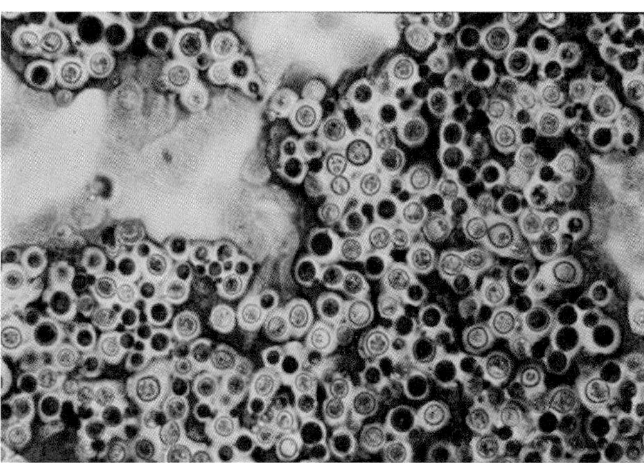

Figure 45.21 Imprint of an ulcer on a cat's paw showing numerous cryptococcal organisms, many of which are budding. Lymph node aspirates from this patient looked similar. Note the lack of inflammatory response. Wet mount using new methylene blue stain.

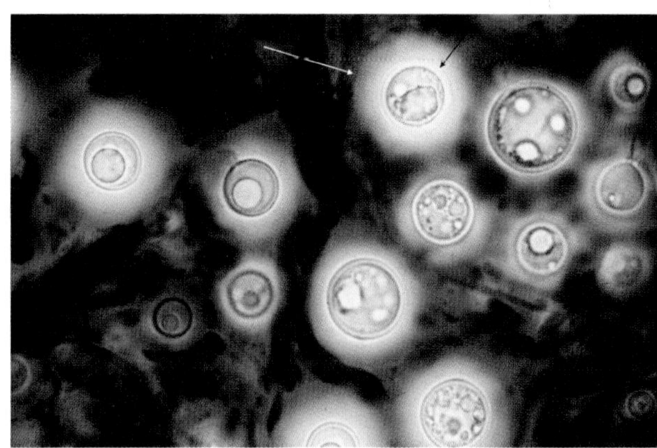

Figure 45.22 Very high magnification of aspirate of lymph node with many cryptococcal organisms and little inflammatory response. A wet mount was prepared by allowing the slide to air-dry, adding a drop of fountain pen ink (India ink is preferred), and placing a cover slip on top. The capsule does not allow the ink to permeate the organisms, producing a negative stain that allows good visualization of the capsule (white arrow), cell wall (black arrow), and cell contents.

• *Blastomyces dermatitidis* and other less common species (*B. gilchristii*, *B. helicus*, and *B. percursus*) are the causative agents of blastomycosis (see Chapter 39). *Blastomyces dermatitidis* is thick walled, 8–12 µm in diameter, does not have a capsule, and reproduces in tissue by broad-based budding (Figure 45.23). Blastomycosis is primarily seen in North America around the Great Lakes and the Ohio, Mississippi, Missouri, and St, Lawrence rivers. It is also

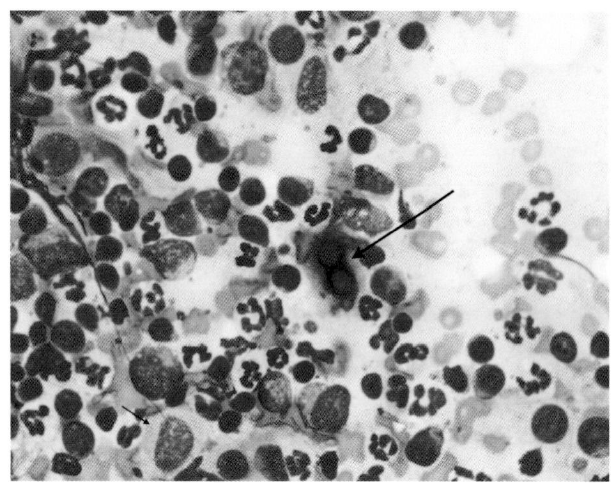

Figure 45.23 Lymph node aspirate from a dog with pyogranulomatous lymphadenitis due to blastomycosis. Note the budding organisms (large arrow). Small lymphocytes and neutrophils predominate, but occasional epithelioid macrophages are present (small arrow). Wright stain.

found throughout most of Africa and has been reported in India and the Middle East. *Blastomyces helicus* is smaller, similar in size to Histoplasma capsulatum, with which it is sometime confused, and is primarily found in western North America. The organism is in the environment and is usually associated with moist, acidic, sandy soils enriched with decaying organic matter and animal feces. Infections are most common in dogs and second most common in humans, but all mammals may be infected, including marine mammals. The conidia of the mold phase are inhaled; in the lungs, temperature-dependent transformation to the yeast phase occurs, and the yeast organisms are phagocytized by macrophages, where they are either eliminated or spread to various organs causing disseminated infection. Pulmonary disease is most common; disseminated infection manifests primarily as skin lesions and osteomyelitis, but many other organs including lymph nodes are commonly infected. Peripheral pyogranulomatous lymphadenitis is seen in approximately 50–60% of dogs with disseminated disease, and organisms are usually found in lymph node aspirates. A few cases of suppurative lymphadenitis and reactive hyperplasia have also been reported.

• *Histoplasma capsulatum* is also a dimorphic soil-borne fungus that is endemic in the Midwest and southern United States, especially along the Missouri, Mississippi, and Ohio River Valleys, and also has been reported in Central and South America, Africa, Asia, and Australia, and may infect all mammals but is most commonly reported in cats, dogs, and humans (see Chapter 39). Microconidia from the environment are inhaled or ingested and convert to the yeast form within the lungs or intestine, where they are either eliminated, cause local infection, or are disseminated within macrophages via the lymphatics and bloodstream to other organs, which may include the liver, spleen, bone marrow, oral cavity and gastrointestinal tract, eye, lymph nodes, skin, bone, and central nervous system. Clinical signs of histoplasmosis are nonspecific and may include fever, lethargy, anorexia, weight loss, respiratory or gastrointestinal signs, and lymphadenopathy. Histiocytic lymphadenitis with multinucleated macrophages and epithelioid cells is typical, and organisms are easily found phagocytized within macrophages, as shown in Figures 15.19, 39.25, 39.26, and 39.27. They are round to oval, surrounded by a narrow capsule, and are very small (2–4 μm) compared to the other dimorphic fungal organisms that cause systemic infections. Diagnosis is made by cytologic or histologic evidence of the characteristic organism, the presence of antigen in urine, or PCR. Treatment consists of long-term oral administration of antifungal agents such as itraconazole.

• *Coccidioides immitis and C. posadasii* are the largest of the pathogenic dimorphic fungi and are responsible for coccidioidomycosis (Valley fever), which is endemic in the southwestern United States and portions of Mexico and Central and South America in semiarid areas (see Chapter 39). The organisms occur in soil and air after soil disturbance, and as with the other potentially pathogenic dimorphic fungi, inhalation of arthroconidia leads to usually benign respiratory disease, but occasionally severe or fatal infections that are systemic. The morphology of *Coccidioides* spp. is dramatically different from *Histoplasma* and *Blastomyces*. Individual arthroconidia adopt a spherical form (spherules) that form an outer shell via synchronous internal division of their nuclei and cytoplasm, and the inner section fills with hundreds of individual (2–4 μm) endospores, as shown in Figure 39.33. Mature spherules are 20–100 μm in diameter and are too large to be phagocytized. When a spherule ruptures, it releases its endospores that then differentiate into new spherules. Dogs are the most severely affected species, with a susceptibility similar to that of humans. However, *Coccidioides immitis* can cause infection in many other species, including cats, horses, cattle, and other livestock. Osteomyelitis is the most common form of disseminated disease in the dog, while skin lesions predominate in the cat. While hilar lymphadenopathy is a common radiographic finding in dogs with coccidioidomycosis, peripheral lymphadenopathy is relatively uncommon in both cats and dogs. The lymphadenopathy is due to pyogranulomatous inflammation, and while infrequent organisms may be seen in lymph node aspirates, quite a bit of searching using low magnification is usually required (Figure 45.24).

• *Paracoccidioides brasiliensis* and *P. lutzii* are the causative agents of paracoccidioidomycosis, another dimorphic fungal infection that is relatively common in people in South America, particularly Brazil, and has also been reported in dogs, cats, and numerous wild mammals, especially armadillos, which are thought to harbor the fungus. Like the other dimorphic fungi, it grows in soil, and aerosolized conidia are inhaled, after which the infection may become systemic,

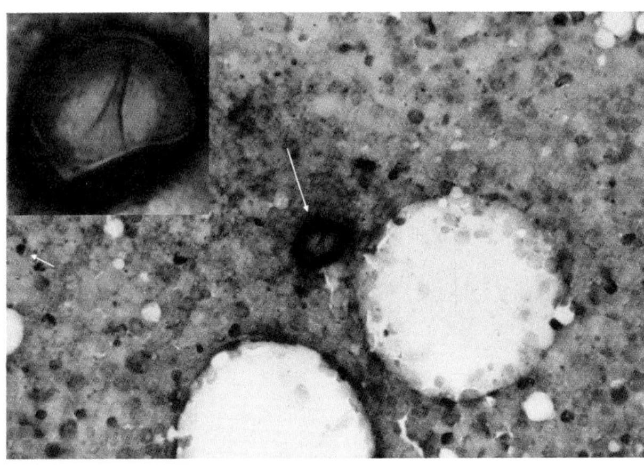

Figure 45.24 Low magnification of a lymph node aspirate from a dog with coccidioidomycosis. Only one *Coccidioidomyces* spherule was present on the entire slide (large arrow) and is in a very thick portion of the preparation. For size comparison, a small arrow is pointing at a plasma cell. Inset in left upper corner shows the spherule at high magnification. Wright stain.

primarily affecting skin, lymph nodes, lungs, and oral, nasal, and gastrointestinal mucous membranes and eliciting marked histiocytic inflammation. The systemic disease can be fatal if not treated. The yeast phase of the organism reproduces in tissue by multiple narrow based budding in which multiple buds will originate from the "mother" yeast, sometimes forming a "Mickey Mouse" appearance, with the mother yeast appearing as the head with two ear-like buds. The mother cells are 20–30 µm in diameter and can produce 10–12 daughter cells, each approximately 2–10 µm in diameter (Figure 45.25). Aspirates of lymph nodes show pyogranulomatous inflammation with numerous budding yeast organisms.

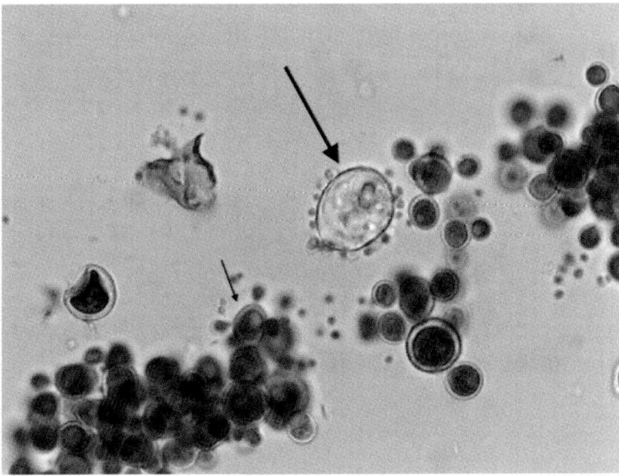

Figure 45.25 Yeast culture (37 °C) of *Paracoccidioides brasiliensis*. Note the "mother yeast cell" with multiple buds (large arrow) and the "Mickey Mouse" appearance of a cell with budding (small arrow). Organisms look similar on cytologic preparations. Wright stain. Source: Courtesy of Dr. Paulo Murillo Neufeld, Federal University of Rio de Janeiro, Brazil.

- *Other fungal organisms* that exist in the environment, such as *Paecilomyces, Penicillium, Aspergillus, Monocillium*, etc. can also cause localized or generalized lymphadenopathy, as shown in Figures 39.34–39.38. They typically elicit a histiocytic or pyogranulomatous lymphadenitis, and the hyphae and associated structures are usually evident in aspirates (see Chapter 39).
- *Pseudofungal structures: Gamna–Gandy bodies*, structures that may be seen in lymph node aspirates that look remarkably similar to fungal hyphae, form as a result of deposition of calcium and hemosiderin complexes on collagenous fibers, usually associated with previous hemorrhage within the lymph node (see Figure 44.33). Due to their similarity to fungal hyphae, periodic acid-Schiff (PAS) or Grocott-Gomori's methenamine silver staining is warranted to rule out fungal infection. Positive reaction with iron and calcium stains is needed for definitive identification.

Oomycosis lymphadenitis

Pythiosis and lagenidiosis are often fatal infectious diseases affecting animals that have exposure to lakes or ponds, primarily in the southeastern United States and other tropical and subtropical areas of the world such as Southeast Asia, eastern coastal Australia, and South America (see Chapter 39). These organisms are not true fungi but are aquatic pathogens in the class Oomycetes ("water mold"). They are more closely related to algae than fungi, but the appearance of the broad hyphae and the histiocytic inflammatory response is very similar to that of fungal infections, as shown in Figures 39.48–39.50. Cutaneous lesions are most common, but animals with systemic disease may have pyogranulomatous lymphadenitis, sometimes with an eosinophilic component; numerous broad hyphae are usually evident in aspirates. Definitive diagnosis can be made by culture or PCR. Treatment consists of early surgical excision of the granulomatous lesions and antifungal antibiotics, but animals are often unresponsive to therapy.

Lymphadenitis due to algae

Protothecosis, caused by members of the genus *Prototheca*, is a disease of humans and animals caused by infection with fungus-like, colorless microalgae that are no longer photosynthetic and have become parasitic. *Prototheca bovis, P. ciferrii, P. wickerhamii*, and *P. zopfii* are pathogenic in dogs and cats. *P wickerhamii* is often associated with cutaneous disease and has been isolated from all affected cats so far. *P bovis* is the most virulent variant and causes the majority of cases of bovine *Prototheca* mastitis cases, as well as most cases of disseminated protothecosis in dogs. Infection is acquired by ingestion or penetrating skin wounds. Clinical signs in dogs are often related to infection of the colon, and include colitis, severe diarrhea with mucus, and hematochezia. Systemic protothecosis may involve the central nervous system, lungs, spleen, liver, eyes, tongue, skin, and lymph nodes and is

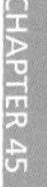

more common in boxers and French bulldogs. In cats, the disease is limited to the skin and subcutis. Aspirates of lymph nodes show pyogranulomatous or histiocytic lymphadenitis, with numerous organisms phagocytized by macrophages or free. The organism has a thick wall, internal septations, and is 3–11 μm in diameter. The large sporangia form a morula, which has endospores that are radially arranged and molded to each other. Small endospores 1–2 μm in diameter may also be seen. Organisms stain deeply basophilic to magenta, sometimes with a clear halo (see Figure 39.51). Diagnosis is usually made by cytologic or histologic examination and confirmed by culture and/or PCR. Antifungal drugs are used to treat disseminated disease, and small lesions may be surgically excised. The prognosis in dogs with disseminated disease is very poor. *In vitro* testing has shown that ravuconazole (RVZ) has higher algaecide effect than other azoles tested against *Prototheca* species. An excellent review of protothecosis in dogs and cats has been published (see Masuda et al. 2021 in "Suggested Reading" under "Algae (Protothecosis)").

Neoplasia in lymph nodes

Lymph nodes are neoplastic either because of primary neoplasia of lymphoid cells or metastatic neoplasia in which other types of tumors are growing within lymph nodes. Primary neoplasia (lymphoma) is much more common than metastatic neoplasia. Cytology has variable sensitivity and specificity that is likely dependent on the expertise and experience of the person who is taking the aspirate, as well as the cytologist. In one study comparing cytology and histopathology findings in 367 canine and feline lymph nodes, of which 110 were neoplastic (including both lymphoma and metastatic neoplasia), cytology had a sensitivity of 66.6%, specificity of 91.5%, and accuracy of 77.2% for neoplasia. Likelihood of malignancy when a positive cytologic diagnosis of neoplasia was made was 93%. False negative findings were primarily found in mesenteric small T-cell lymphoma in cats, metastatic sarcomas, and metastatic mast cell tumors (see Ku et al. 2017 in "Suggested Reading" under "Lymph Node Metastasis"). Diagnostic utility of cytology for lymphoma and metastatic neoplasia is discussed in more detail in the following sections.

Primary lymphoid neoplasia (lymphoma, malignant lymphoma, lymphosarcoma)

Primary lymphoid neoplasia occurs in many species, but of the common domestic species, it occurs most frequently in dogs and is one of the most common types of neoplasia affecting dogs. Peripheral lymph nodes are usually involved in dogs, while this form of lymphoma is relatively rare in cats. Because most dogs with lymphoma present with enlargement of one or more peripheral lymph nodes due to the presence of many large neoplastic cells within the node, aspiration cytology of lymph nodes has very good diagnostic sensitivity and specificity and is much less expensive and invasive than lymph node biopsy and histopathology. A very simple approach to diagnosing primary lymphoid neoplasia is to consider the number of immature lymphoid cells present in the aspirate. Malignancy of lymphoid tissue is almost always characterized by a predominance of immature large lymphoid cells with apparent nucleoli (Figure 45.26), because large-cell lymphoma is by far the most common type of lymphoma. Numerous cells in mitosis may be present. Small lymphocytes and macrophages may be present in variable numbers. Plasma cells are usually quite few to absent, which aids in the differentiation between lymphoma and lymphoid hyperplasia. In general, the more plasma cells that are present, the less likely that lymphoma is the correct diagnosis. While it may be possible to aspirate numerous immature cells from a germinal center of a reactive node, plasma cells would almost always be increased as well. Redirecting the needle will help prevent aspiration of cells from one site in the node, and it is unusual to see more than 20% large immature cells in a reactive node. A mistaken positive diagnosis of lymphoma is very rare, and when erroneous diagnoses are made, it is usually a failure to confirm that lymphoma is present, sometimes due to excessive caution on the part of the cytologist. Infrequently, lymphoid tumors may be composed entirely of small lymphocytes. If an aspirate of an enlarged lymph node consists of a homogeneous population of small lymphocytes with no cytologic suggestion of reactive hyperplasia, a small-cell variant of lymphoma is likely. When a diagnosis of lymphoma cannot be confirmed by cytology, determination of clonality by PCR technology or immunophenotyping using flow cytometry is

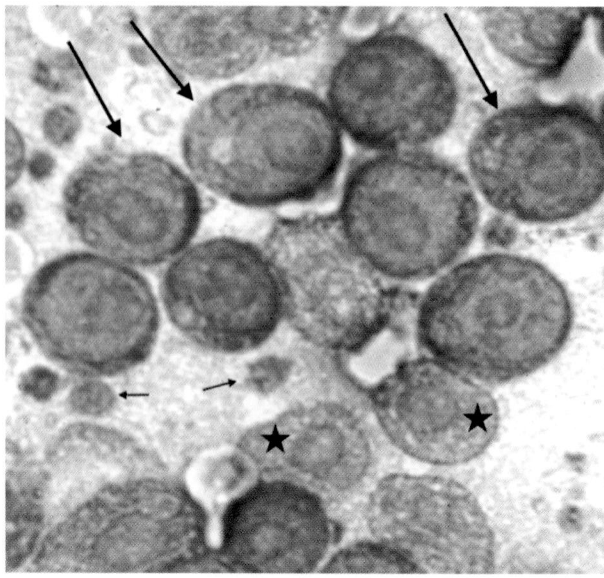

Figure 45.26 Lymph node aspirate from a dog with lymphoma. All cells are large immature lymphoid cells with a single large nucleolus (large arrows). Cytoplasmic fragments (lymphoglandular bodies) are indicated by small arrows. Broken cells with only no cytoplasmic borders are indicated by stars. Wright stain.

CHAPTER 45

very helpful, since clonality is very characteristic of malignant cells, as they are derived from expansion of a single malignant cell. Molecular diagnostic techniques for diagnosis of hematologic malignancies including lymphoma are reviewed in Chapter 14.

Classification of lymphoma

A simple cytologic diagnosis of lymphoma is no longer adequate in many cases because biologic behavior, prognosis, and response to therapy can be quite variable, depending on the type of lymphoma present. Some types of lymphomas, especially T-zone lymphoma (TZL), common in golden retrievers, are very indolent with long survival times, and therapy is usually not indicated until the late stages of the disease. Correct classification of lymphoma is critical so that dogs with indolent lymphomas are not unnecessarily treated or euthanized. Lymphomas have been classified using cell morphology, tissue architecture, immunophenotyping, clinical features, and, in some cases, genetic analysis. These categorizations of lymphomas and other hematopoietic neoplasms are modeled on those already established in human medicine by the WHO, as discussed briefly in reference to leukemia classification in Chapter 16. The WHO classification of lymphoma was first adopted for use in dogs in 2002. Currently at least 20 subtypes of lymphoma in dogs and cats have been recognized, using the WHO classification (see Valli et al. 2011 in "Suggested Reading" under "Lymphoma – Dog").

- **Neoplastic lymphoid cell morphology.** Neoplastic lymphoid cell size is based on nuclear size compared to erythrocyte size when using histopathology, and cells are classified as small (nuclei approximately 1–1.25 times the diameter of an erythrocyte), intermediate (nuclei approximately 1.25–2 times the diameter of an erythrocyte), or large (nuclei same as or greater than 2.0 times the diameter of an erythrocyte). With cytology, lymphoid cell size is usually established by comparison to a neutrophil. Large cells are 1.5–2 times the size of a neutrophil, intermediate-sized cells are slightly larger than neutrophils, and small lymphoid cells are the same size or slightly smaller than neutrophils. Cytoplasmic volume and staining intensity and nuclear shape, chromatin pattern, and nucleolar features are also typically described (see "Identification of Cell Types and Other Lymphoid Elements" earlier in this chapter).
- **Lymphoma architecture.** Lymphomas are classified by histopathology as either diffuse or nodular/follicular. In diffuse lymphoma, lymph node architecture is effaced by the neoplastic infiltrate, whereas in nodular, the neoplastic infiltrate mimics or spares some portion of lymph node tissue.
- **Immunophenotyping of lymphoma.** For determination of immunophenotype, antibodies against lymphocyte markers (antigens called "cluster of differentiation" or "CD") are applied to tissue sections (immunohistochemistry), cytologic preparations (immunocytochemistry), or aspirated individual cells that have been placed in a fluid medium (flow cytometry). T-cell markers include CD3 (pan T), CD4 (helper T), and CD8 (cytotoxic T). B-cell markers are CD79a, CD20, and CD21, although some types of neoplastic T cells express CD21. Other cell markers that can be detected by flow cytometry are CD45, a common leukocyte antigen present in all hematopoietic cells except erythrocytes and plasma cells, the expression of which is sometimes lost in some types of neoplastic lymphoid cells, and CD34, an antigen on precursor cells. The presence or absence of major histocompatibility complex (MHC) class II peptides on lymphocytes is also typically reported when using flow cytometry for classification of lymphoma (see Chapter 14 for more detail).
- **Tumor behavior and prognosis.** Lymphomas are also classified as either indolent or aggressive, which helps predict survival time. Lymphomas with a slow rate of biologic progression are called indolent lymphomas. Many dogs with indolent lymphoma may have a normal lifespan without treatment and die of other disorders. Dogs with lymphoma classified as intermediate or high grade (more aggressive) usually respond better to chemotherapy but may go out of remission early.
- **Aspiration cytology for diagnosis of subtypes of lymphoma.** Although lymph node resection and histopathology in combination with immunophenotyping is the gold standard for classification and grading of lymphoma, aspiration cytology is more commonly used, due to the lack of invasiveness and lower expense. While aspiration cytology has numerous advantages, it is sometimes unsuccessful for certain subtypes of lymphoma, particularly small-cell variants, but when used in conjunction with flow cytometry, a definitive diagnosis of lymphoma, as well as subtype, can usually be made. Determination of lymphoma subtype using cytology alone is usually not possible and is highly dependent on the experience of the cytologist. In one study, agreement between the results of cytology alone and immunocytochemistry as to whether lymphoma was B cell or T cell was made in 90% of 70 cases in dogs (see Sapierzyński et al. 2012 in "Suggested Reading" under "Lymphoma – Dog"). However, cytologic appearance may sometimes be misleading. For example, sometimes T cells may have a plasmacytoid appearance that is usually associated with B cells, particularly in peripheral T-cell lymphoma (PTCL). In general, four broad categories of lymphoma in dogs can usually be determined based on cytology, sometimes with the help of flow cytometry: (i) diffuse large B-cell lymphoma; (ii) CD4+ T-cell lymphoma, including both PTCL and T-cell LBL, (iii) TZL; and (iv) large granular-cell lymphoma. Cytologic features of these types of lymphoma are discussed below. A study to determine if cytologic features were useful to predict survival time in dogs with aggressive lymphoma showed that relatively few cytologic features were useful, other than the presence of binucleated or multinucleated cells, which perhaps suggested a decreased survival time. Also noted

in this study was that the number of cells in mitosis was increased in aspirates made at time of relapse of remission, compared to those seen in aspirates at original diagnosis (see Munasinghe et al. 2015 in "Suggested Reading" under "Lymphoma – Dog").

Nodal lymphoma in cats is quite rare, and classification schemes that have been developed for dogs are lacking in cats. One study suggests that definitive cytologic diagnosis of lymphoma immunophenotype, using histopathology and immunocytochemistry as the gold standard, is likely not possible (see Gelain et al. 2021 in "Suggested Reading" under "Lymphoma – Cat"). Diagnostic accuracy in predicting nodal or mediastinal lymphoma immunophenotype varied from 35% to 75% of cases and did not appear to be correlated with the experience of the cytologists, likely because specific diagnostic criteria have been poorly described due to the low prevalence of this disease. In general, large granular lymphocyte (LGL) T-cell lymphoma in cats is almost always recognizable, B-cell lymphomas are more likely to have vacuolated cytoplasm, and B-cell lymphomas tend to have neoplastic cells that are large.

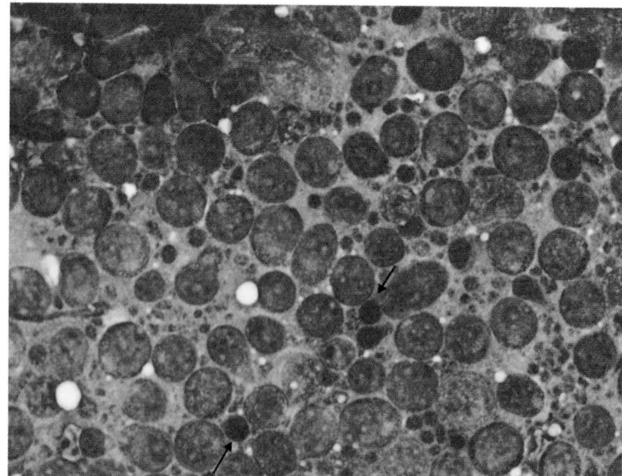

Figure 45.27 Lymph node aspirate from a dog with lymphoma that was confirmed to be diffuse B-cell lymphoma by flow cytometry. Almost all cells are large immature cells with multiple nucleoli. A few small lymphocytes are remaining (arrows). Wright stain.

Lymphoma subtypes in dogs and cats

The five most common types of canine lymphoma, listed in decreasing frequency, are diffuse large B-cell lymphoma (DLBCL), peripheral T-cell lymphoma not otherwise specified (PTCL-NOS), TZL, T-lymphoblastic lymphoma (also called precursor T-cell neoplasia), and marginal zone lymphoma (MZL), which is of B-cell linage. These classifications were established using histopathology and architecture, but as mentioned earlier, flow cytometry in conjunction with cytology can usually establish the type of lymphoma present as relates to cell type and size.

- *DLBCL* makes up about 50% of canine lymphoma cases and may be separated into two distinct subtypes, centroblastic, which is more common in dogs, and immunoblastic, which is more common in cats, although it may be difficult to differentiate the two types of blasts based on cytology. Centroblasts are medium to large (1.5 times the size of a neutrophil) and consist of moderately abundant blue cytoplasm with a round nucleus containing several prominent peripherally located nucleoli (Figure 45.27). Cytoplasm may contain punctate vacuoles. Medium-sized lymphocytes and residual small lymphocytes may be present. The immunoblastic form consists of large immunoblasts with scant darkly basophilic cytoplasm and a single central prominent nucleolus. Neoplastic cells are CD21, CD79a, and CD20 positive. Human DLBCL has been further subdivided into four subgroups according to genetic, immunophenotypic, and molecular findings. Genetic variation correlating with biologic behavior is also likely to exist in canine DLBCL and is currently being explored. Dogs with DLBCL usually present with rapidly progressive, generally painless nodal or extranodal disease and many have leukemia (stage V lymphoma) at the time of presentation. Flow cytometry is more accurate than blood film examination for determining peripheral blood involvement. Depending on the stage of disease at presentation, survival times of 12–24 months can be achieved with chemotherapy. Immunophenotypic characteristics are associated with prognosis. Large cell size and low MHC class II expression are predictive of decreased survival time. Rarely the cells express CD34 while retaining MHC class II expression, but this finding does not affect prognosis, and these cases should not be confused with B-cell LBL.
- *PTCL-NOS* is a relatively common, aggressive variant of lymphoma, often seen in golden retrievers, with a median survival time of 5–6 months, independent of treatment regimen. Cells are somewhat variable in size, ranging from 10 to 20 μm in diameter, with moderate amounts of pale blue cytoplasm that has no granules or vacuoles. Nuclei are variable in shape with fine chromatin, ranging from round to indented to multilobulated or cerebriform (flower-shaped). Nucleoli are multiple and variably prominent, and numerous cells in mitosis are usually seen (Figure 45.28). Few residual non-neoplastic lymphocytes are present, and rare plasma cells may be seen. Sometimes, the blasts may have a plasmacytoid appearance, and thus a plasma cell tumor or a B-cell lymphoma may be mistakenly diagnosed. They typically express CD4 and CD45 and express low amounts of class II MHC. This subtype exhibits a consistent gene expression profile with upregulation of phosphatidylinositol 3-kinase (PI3K) activity. PI3K plays a role in regulation of the cell cycle, leading to increased cell proliferation and survival.
- *TZL* is a relatively common type of indolent canine t-cell lymphoma characterized by clonal expansion of T-zone

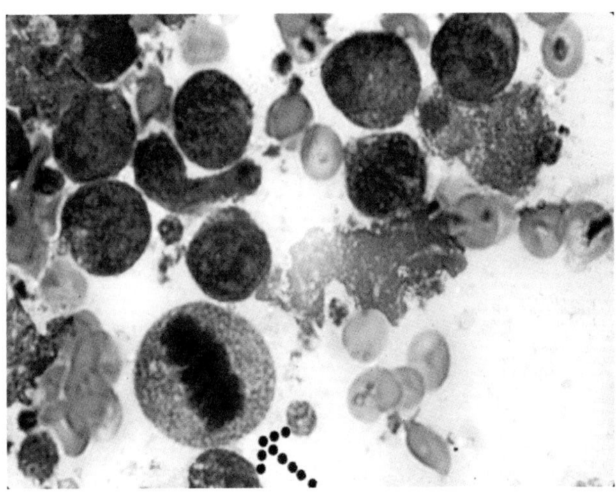

Figure 45.28 Lymph node aspirate from a dog with peripheral T-cell lymphoma. Note the cerebriform nuclei and cell in mitosis (dotted arrow). Wright stain.

lymphocytes that have a unique architectural and cytomorphologic pattern. Median age at onset is 8–10 years, and golden retriever and Shih Tzu breeds are most commonly affected. Mandibular lymph nodes are usually enlarged on presentation. Aspiration of lymph nodes shows predominantly intermediate-sized lymphocytes that range from 12 to 20 μm in diameter. The nuclei are small and round, and nucleoli are usually not evident. Cytoplasm is moderate to abundant and commonly forms unipolar cytoplasmic extensions or pseudopodia, sometimes referred to as "cone-heads" or "mirror-handles" (Figure 45.29). Very few, if any, cells in mitosis are seen. A few plasma cells may be present, as well as residual non-neoplastic lymphocytes, which sometimes

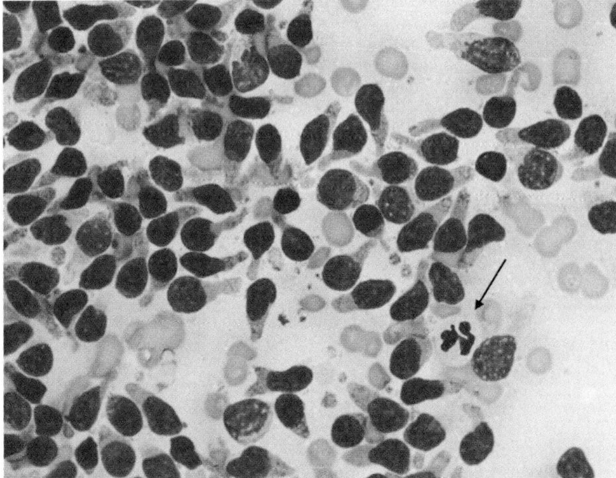

Figure 45.29 Lymph node aspirate from a dog with indolent T-zone lymphoma. Note the small size of the cells and the cytoplasmic extensions ("mirror-handles"). The neutrophil (arrow) is useful for size comparison. Wright stain.

results in cytologic misdiagnosis of these types of lymphoma as reactive hyperplasia or "inconclusive," especially when the cytoplasmic atypia is not present. Diagnosis can be confirmed by immunohistochemistry or flow cytometry, which show a unique loss of CD45 expression in the vast majority of cases, a high expression of class II MHC, and frequently an aberrant expression of CD21 (a B-cell antigen), as well as CD3 and CD5 positivity as expected for T cells. Expression of CD4 and CD8 is variable. Blood and bone marrow are infiltrated in 90% of cases, and about 50% of dogs have neoplastic lymphocytosis (leukemia). T-zone lymphocytes in peripheral blood are about the size of a neutrophil, have a round centrally located nucleus, slight to moderate amount of cytoplasm, and rarely a fairly indistinct nucleolus. Although canine TZL is incurable, it is considered indolent with a good prognosis, with or without treatment, with median survival times of 2–2.75 years. Therapy is not recommended until development of cytopenias or marked lymphocytosis, lymphadenopathy, or hepatosplenomegaly.

- LBL (*precursor neoplasia*) is quite rare, comprising 3–9% of cases of canine lymphoma. LBL and acute lymphoblastic leukemias (ALLs) are of B- or T-cell lineage and arise from precursors in the bone marrow or thymus, respectively. Whether classified as LBL or ALL depends on whether bone marrow or lymph node involvement is dominant. The biologic behavior and prognosis of LBL and ALL is similar, thus the primary tissue of origin is not significant, and both are now considered the same disease. Aspirates of either bone marrow or lymph nodes consist of a homogeneous population of cells that are small to intermediate in size with round to convoluted nuclei containing variable chromatin and faint to indistinct nucleoli and a small, often unipolar, cap of cytoplasm as shown in Figures 16.25 and 16.26. Numerous cells in mitosis may be seen. Despite the homogeneous population of relatively small cells without evident nucleoli, the disease is aggressive, with mean survival times of days to months. The T subtype is more common than the B subtype, occurs most commonly in the boxer breed, and is slightly less aggressive, with a mean survival time of 150 days. Studies have shown that 77% of boxers with lymphoma have the T-cell variant of LBL. The immunophenotype of the T subtype is similar to that of PTCL (CD45+, CD3+, CD4+, MHC II–). The lymphoblasts usually express the precursor marker CD34 when flow cytometry is used on viable cells, thus confirming their immaturity. On archived formalin-fixed tissues, CD34 is usually negative.
- *MZL* is a mature B-cell lymphoma that may affect lymph nodes, the spleen, or extranodal tissues. Cells originate from postfollicular memory lymphocytes of the marginal zone of either the spleen or lymph nodes. Splenic marginal zone lymphoma (SMZL) is an indolent, small-cell B-cell lymphoma characterized by splenic infiltration and bone marrow involvement, little or no lymph node involvement, good prognosis following splenectomy, and is discussed

briefly in the "Spleen" section of Chapter 44. Nodal marginal zone lymphoma (NMZL) accounts for approximately 6–10% of all canine lymphomas and almost always presents as generalized lymphadenopathy. The predominant cell on aspirates is intermediate in size, with round nuclei the size of two erythrocytes containing a large central nucleolus and a moderate amount of pale cytoplasm. Centroblasts and immunoblasts, as well as mitotic figures, are few in number. Few residual normal lymphocytes are usually present. Transformation of NMZL to DLBCL is thought to occur but may actually be a late stage of NMZL, in which the follicles are effaced, leading to a more diffuse appearance, with increased lymphoid blasts and more aggressive clinical disease. Median survival time for NMZL in one study was 259 days.

- *Mantle cell lymphoma* is an indolent B-cell lymphoma that is very rare in dogs, comprising approximately 1% of all cases. Mantle cell lymphoma primarily affects the spleen with occasional visceral node involvement. Peripheral node involvement is minimal, if any, and bone marrow involvement is very uncommon. The neoplastic cells are small to intermediate in size and have a small amount of cytoplasm.
- *Follicular lymphoma* is a mature B-cell lymphoma that is very rare in dogs, representing less than 1% of lymphoma cases. Complete effacement of the nodal architecture by neoplastic follicles of both peripheral and visceral nodes occurs. Distinguishing the neoplastic follicles from benign follicles in reactive hyperplasia may be difficult. Aspirates are composed of small cells that have pale and evenly dispersed chromatin and inconspicuous or small nucleoli. Few mitotic figures are seen. Cytologic diagnosis can be challenging, but numerous small cells, a few centroblasts, and the lack of plasma cells in an aspirate of a large node should trigger flow cytometry or PCR for antigen receptor rearrangement (PARR).
- *Large granular lymphocyte (LGL) lymphoma* is relatively rare and is more common in cats than in dogs. It has also been reported in horses, a cow, and goats. In dogs, LGL lymphoma usually involves the spleen and liver, and in cats the intestine is usually affected; LGL leukemia may be present (see Chapter 16 and Section VII, Case 13). LGL lymphoma has been associated with hemophagocytic syndrome, in which activated macrophages proliferate in various organs such as spleen and bone marrow and phagocytize erythrocytes, leukocytes, or platelets, as shown in Figures 15.16 and 15.17, resulting in pancytopenia or bicytopenia; the syndrome is difficult to distinguish from phagocytosis of cells due to primary immune-mediated disease. LGL lymphoma is rarely seen in peripheral lymph nodes, but mesenteric lymph node involvement is common in cats with intestinal LGL lymphoma. In one report of 109 cats with LGL lymphoma, 73 had abdominal lymph node involvement, 11 had thoracic lymph node involvement, and only two had peripheral lymph node involvement (see Finotello et al. 2018 in "Suggested Reading" under "Lymphoma – Cat"). The cells are intermediate to large in size, with moderate to abundant light blue cytoplasm containing azurophilic granules that are variable in size, ranging from very fine to large globular structures (Figures 45.30 and 45.31). The presence of the granules makes cytologic identification of this type of lymphoma quite easy, although the granules sometimes do not stain distinctly when the quick types of Wright stain are used. Nuclei are round to indented, have smooth to clumped chromatin, and have variably prominent nucleoli. LGLs are also described in Chapters 11 and 16 and shown in Figure 11.4 and Section VII, Case 13. Canine LGL lymphoma is usually composed of CD8+ cells. The disease is poorly responsive to therapy, and patients typically have a very short survival time.

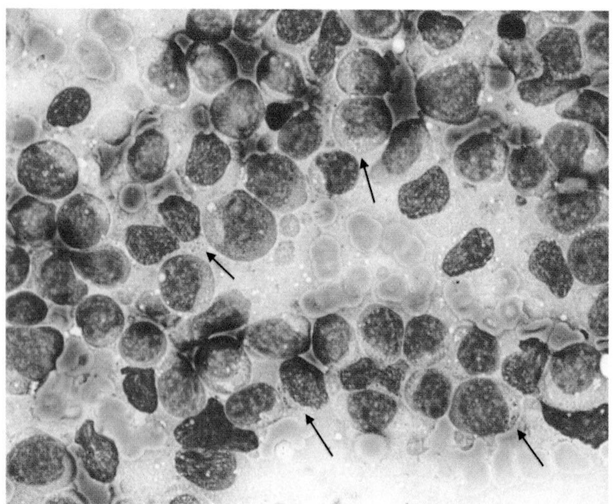

Figure 45.30 Mesenteric lymph node aspirate from a dog with T-cell lymphoma. Notice the very subtle large granular lymphocytes (arrows). Wright stain.

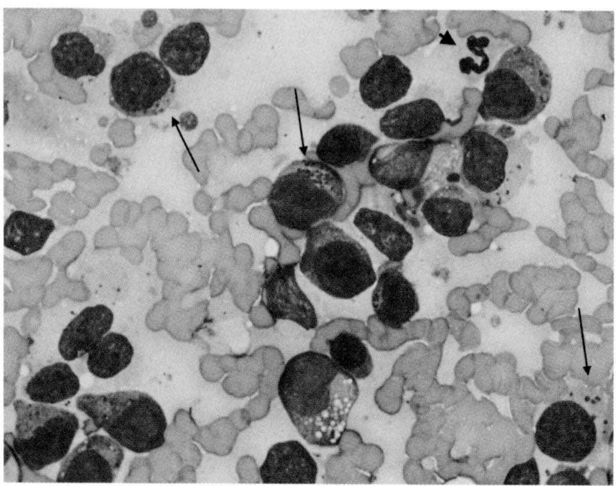

Figure 45.31 Mesenteric lymph node aspirate from a cat with large granular lymphocyte lymphoma. The azurophilic granules in the cytoplasm are quite large (arrows). Note the large size of the LGLs compared to the neutrophil (arrowhead). Wright stain.

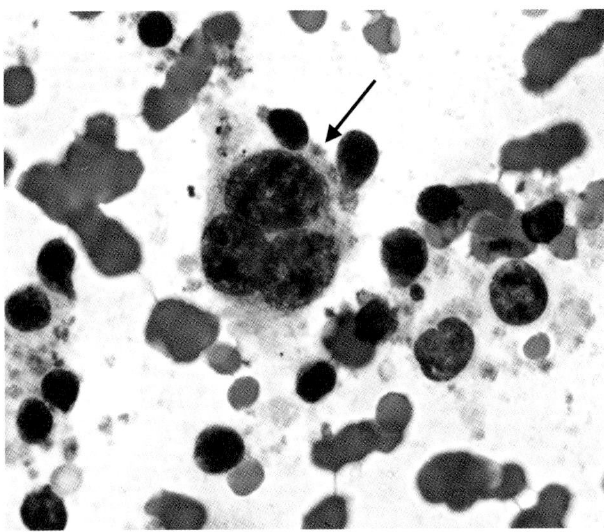

Figure 45.32 Lymph node aspirate from a cat with Hodgkin's-like lymphoma. Note the multinucleated Reed-Sternberg cell. Wright Stain. Source: Courtesy Dr. Jennifer Steinberg, Mid-Atlantic Veterinary Pathology, LLC.

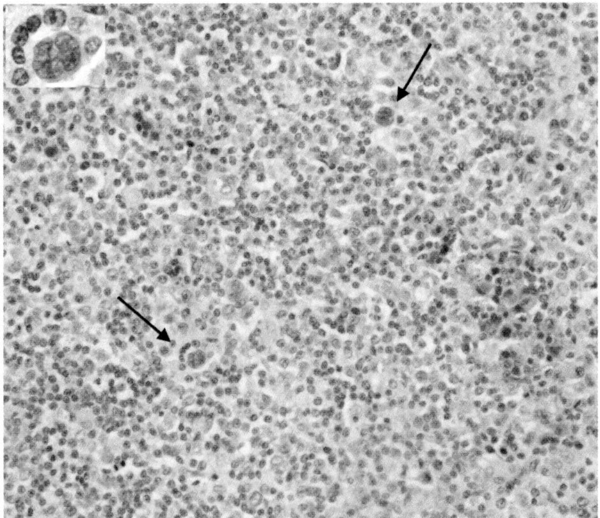

Figure 45.33 Histopathology of a cervical lymph node in a cat with Hodgkin's-like lymphoma. Two Reed-Sternberg cells are present in this image (arrows). Inset upper left: higher magnification of a Reed-Sternberg cell. H&E stain. Source: Courtesy Dr. Jennifer Steinberg, Mid-Atlantic Veterinary Pathology, LLC.

- *Hodgkin's-like lymphoma* is a rare form of lymphoma that has been reported most frequently in the cat and reported sporadically in the dog, ferret, whale, rat, and skunk. Hodgkin's lymphoma in people is very distinct from the other types of non-Hodgkin's lymphoma and is a common neoplasm in young adults that can be cured by chemotherapy and/or radiotherapy in approximately 85% or more cases. In people, it arises from transformed germinal-center or postgerminal center B cells and appears to be of B-cell origin in domestic animals. The tumor usually arises in a single lymph node or chain of lymph nodes and is usually slow growing in both people and cats. A classical diagnostic finding, in either cytologic or histopathologic biopsies, is the presence of the large and atypical malignant Reed-Sternberg cells, which constitute a minority of the cells present. Reed-Sternberg cells are very large (30–40 µm in diameter) and are typically binucleate with a "mirror-image" appearance (Figures 45.32 and 45.33). The other lymphoid population is usually mixed, with another population of large round cells, 20–30 µm in diameter with scant basophilic, sometimes vacuolated cytoplasm, and irregularly round nuclei with single large nucleoli. In addition, numerous small- and intermediate-sized lymphocytes and a few plasma cells and macrophages are usually present. A cytologic misdiagnosis of reactive hyperplasia is sometimes made unless Reed-Sternberg cells are recognized and not all aspirates contain them. Cervical lymph nodes are most commonly affected in cats, although extranodal sites have been reported. Most cats with Hodgkin's-like lymphoma have very long survival times, sometimes up to years, with or without surgical removal or chemotherapy. While affected lymph nodes are sometimes surgically removed in cats, surgical removal is not typically part of the therapeutic regime in humans. One reported cat with extranodal Hodgkin's-like lymphoma had complete remission following surgical incisional biopsy of the tumor.

Lymphoma in horses

Lymphoma is the most common type of malignant neoplasia seen in horses and is classified by anatomic distribution into multicentric, which is most common (41%), cutaneous (19%), and alimentary (11%). In one study, T-cell rich large B-cell lymphoma (TCRLBCL) was the most common histologic subtype seen in horses with lymphoma, and peripheral T-cell lymphoma and diffuse large B-cell lymphoma also were seen relatively frequently. Ages ranged from 2 months to 31 years (mean, 10.7 years). A total of 14 lymphoma subtypes in horses have been identified. Few descriptions of the cytologic appearance of lymph node aspirates have been published, but large B cells, intermediate T cells, small T cells, and LGL T cells have been described and are similar in appearance to those neoplastic cells in dogs.

Lymphoma in cattle

Two broad lymphoma syndromes have been recognized in cattle: enzootic bovine leukosis (EBL) and sporadic bovine leukosis (SBL). EBL is related to infection with *bovine leukemia virus* (BLV) and is a disease of mature cattle (see Chapter 16). Sporadic lymphoma is a disease of younger animals that are not infected with BLV and has been classified as calf, thymic, and cutaneous; the cutaneous form has two subsets, nonepitheliotropic (B cell) and epitheliotropic (T cell). EBL is a B-cell neoplasm, while SBL may originate

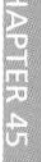

from either B or T lymphocytes. Lymph node involvement may be seen with either type of lymphoma syndrome, and aspirates typically consist of medium to large numbers of lymphoid blasts with scant basophilic cytoplasm and multiple distinct nucleoli.

Lymphoma in goats

One study in goats showed that the median age of disease was 3 years and that 73% had T-cell lymphoma and 27% had B-cell lymphoma. Multicentric distribution was most common. T-cell lymphoma usually involved the neck or thoracic cavity and was further classified as LBLs (27%), LGL lymphoma (9%), diffuse small lymphocytic lymphomas (27%), and PTCL not otherwise specified (36%). B-cell lymphomas were classified as diffuse large B-cell lymphoma (50%) or B-cell lymphocytic lymphoma intermediate type (50%). Only two cytologic descriptions of lymph node aspirates in goats with lymphoma were found in the literature. In a goat with B-cell lymphoma, the aspirate was described as consisting of a monomorphic population of large round cells with a large round nucleus, prominent multiple nucleoli, and a small amount of light blue cytoplasm intermixed with small lymphocytes, and in a goat with T-cell lymphoma, intermediate-sized T-cell lymphoblasts were described. Cell morphology of various subtypes of lymphoma on histopathology is similar to that of dogs.

Lymphoma in ferrets

Lymphoma is the second most common malignant neoplasm in domestic ferrets. Location of lymphoma, in order of decreasing frequency, is nodal, splenic, gastrointestinal, multicentric, and cutaneous. The cytologic appearance of malignant lymphoid cells appears to be similar to that seen in dogs and cats.

Metastatic neoplasia

Malignant tumors commonly metastasize via lymphatics, resulting in proliferation of neoplastic tissue in the lymph node. These neoplasms can often be diagnosed from lymph node aspirates. Diagnostic success is due to the ease with which alien tumor cells can be distinguished from the normal constituents of the node and depends on the degree of node involvement (Figure 45.34). Aspirates may yield only tumor cells, with complete displacement of normal lymphoid elements, when the node has been effaced by metastatic neoplastic cells. While metastasis may be detected by aspiration cytology in nodes that are not enlarged, the probability is decreased.

Some studies have shown that cytology is as accurate as histopathology in diagnosing carcinoma and sarcoma metastasis. However, both aspiration cytology and incisional or excisional biopsy may not always be successful in identifying metastasis. One problem is that the actual sentinel lymph node may not always be accurately identified. The sentinel lymph node is the first lymph node to which a cancer is likely to spread but may be different from the closest regional lymph node to the primary tumor, especially with tumors involving the head. In a study of 20 mast cell tumors in 17 dogs, the sentinel lymph node was different than the regional lymph node in 25% of cases, leading the authors to recommend indirect computed tomographic lymphangiography and sentinel lymph node excision and histopathology as a new standard of care in dogs with mast cell tumors, rather than regional lymph node cytology (see Lapsley et al. 2021 in "Suggested Reading" under "Lymph Node Metastasis").

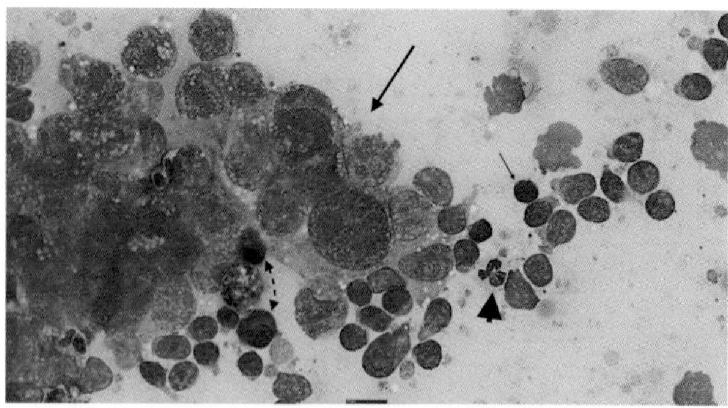

Figure 45.34 Aspirate of a lymph node with metastatic nasal carcinoma in a dog. A very large cluster of highly malignant-appearing epithelial cells is indicated by the large arrow. A normal population of lymphocytes (small arrow), as well as a few plasma cells (dashed line arrow) and neutrophils (arrowhead) are seen. Wright stain.

Also attributing to missed diagnoses of metastasis by both cytology and histopathology is that, in some cases, so few neoplastic cells may be in the lymph node at the time of aspiration or biopsy that they are not detectable by routine methods. Immunohistochemistry, using antibodies directed against the tumor cells, can detect very small numbers of neoplastic cells in aspirates or biopsies but is not routinely used in veterinary medicine.

Accurately predicting metastasis of mast cell tumors using cytology is more difficult than detecting neoplastic epithelial (carcinomas) or mesenchymal cells (sarcomas). Mast cells are commonly present in reactive lymph nodes. Thus, when very few neoplastic mast cells are present in a node, they can be mistaken for normal mast cells. Additionally, many lymph nodes with any type of metastasis are reactive. If the mast cells exhibit atypia, and if numerous mast cells are present in a node that is not inflamed as shown in Figure 45.13, the diagnosis of metastasis becomes less difficult.

Diagnosing melanoma metastasis can also be challenging for several reasons. The primary reason is that macrophages with phagocytized melanin (melanophages) are commonly seen in inflamed lymph nodes, as well as lymph nodes draining melanomas. Melanophages can sometimes be difficult to differentiate from melanocytes, although the melanin in lysosomes of macrophages is usually in aggregates, versus the fine granules seen in melanocytes. Melanocytes

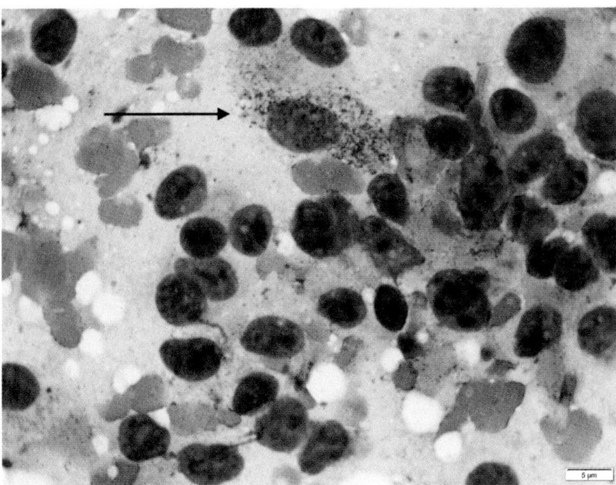

Figure 45.35 Lymph node aspirate from a dog previously diagnosed with a malignant melanoma on a digit. No lymphoid cells are present. Melanocytes without pigment predominate, but one melanocyte in this field contains fine melanin granules (arrow). Wright stain.

can be round, spindle-shaped, or epithelial in appearance (Figure 45.35) (see Chapter 41). Melanocytes from amelanotic melanomas that do not contain pigment can also be difficult to identify. Melanocytes sometimes are round and, if not pigmented, can be mistaken for immature lymphoid cells.

Very rarely, transmissible venereal tumors (TVTs) metastasize to lymph nodes and can be particularly difficult to distinguish from immature lymphoid cells with nucleoli, due to similar appearance and size. One distinguishing characteristic of TVT cells is their punctate vacuoles in moderately abundant cytoplasm, as shown in Figure 40.6e. Other hematopoietic tumors such as granulocytic leukemia may also spread from the bone marrow to such other tissues as lymph nodes, and if poorly differentiated, they are extremely difficult to distinguish from immature lymphoid cells based on cytology, as shown in Figure 16.2.

When attempting to aspirate the mandibular lymph node in the dog, the salivary gland may be mistakenly sampled. Normal salivary gland cells should not be confused with metastatic neoplastic epithelial cells. An extremely rare condition that might be mistaken for metastatic disease in a lymph node is the presence of a choristoma, a mass of normal tissue found in an abnormal location. Choristomas consisting of glandular epithelial tissue have been reported in lymph nodes from cattle, goats, and humans.

VII Clinical Case Presentations

Clinical Case Presentations

Alex Mau
Department of Biomedical Sciences, Ross University School of Veterinary Medicine, Basseterre, Saint Kitts and Nevis

CASES

Introduction

This section presents a number of case studies taken from animal medical records. Each case is presented with its relevant clinicopathologic data. The cases are organized more or less by the primary disease or organ system involved in disease, with the understanding that many of them have multiple system abnormalities. For example, the first 17 cases focus on common primary hematologic disease. However, abnormal hematologic processes are dispersed throughout the remaining cases. The following is a directory of cases classified by the primary system abnormality or disease problem.

Clinical Case Presentations: Contents

Veterinary Hematology, Clinical Chemistry, and Cytology, Third Edition. Edited by Mary Anna Thrall, Glade Weiser, Robin W. Allison and Terry W. Campbell.

Companion website: www.wiley.com/go/thrall/veterinary

CASES

Fluid and Electrolyte and Acid-Base Disturbances

Disorders of electrolytes and acid-base disturbances are not primary disease problems. Therefore, most electrolyte and acid-base disturbances are best considered with their primary disease process(es). For more broad exposure to this category, also see:

Hepatic Disease

Pancreatic and Gastrointestinal Disease and Glucose Metabolism

Endocrine Disorders

Perspective on Use of This Section

Interpretation of laboratory data is an art that is developed through accumulated experience. The interactions and patterns of data related to disease diagnosis are complex. One also must develop an appreciation for magnitudes of abnormality that influence interpretation of each measurement. This case discussion appendix is designed to provide the reader with both experience and guidance in beginning to learn the art of interpretation. This art is then continually cultivated through real-time experience in the clinical setting.

The laboratory data are presented for each case in a form that allows the reader to learn from making his or her own effort at describing and interpreting data. Please note the following formatting:

1. Data in the majority of the cases are presented in conventional units most commonly used in the United States. Data provided in some cases are in the International System of Units (SI), and in a few cases for which both types of units are provided, the SI units are in italics. Reference intervals vary between cases because the tests were performed at numerous laboratories.

2. Laboratory values that are abnormal and central to the interpretation are given in bold type.

Following each data set, an Interpretive discussion is presented. These narratives may be used by the reader for self-assessment of proficiency in interpretation of data.

List of Abbreviations

The following list of abbreviations identifies test results that are typically used in laboratory reports. The user should refer to these as needed while learning the content of laboratory reports.

Alb	Albumin
ALP	Alkaline phosphatase
ALT	Alanine aminotransferase
An. gap	Anion gap
aPTT	Activated partial thromboplastin time
AST	Aspartate aminotransferase
Bands	Band neutrophils
BUN	Blood urea nitrogen
Ca	Calcium
Calc. osmolality	Calculated osmolality
Chol	Cholesterol
CK	Creatine kinase
CL	Chloride
Creat	Creatinine
Eos	Eosinophils
Epith cells	Epithelial cells
GGT	Gamma glutamyltransferase
Glob	Globulin
Gluc	Glucose
Hgb	Hemoglobin
hpf	High-power fields
Lymphs	Lymphocytes
MCHC	Mean corpuscular hemoglobin concentration
MCV	Mean cell volume
Meas. osmolality	Measured osmolality
Metas	Metamyelocytes
Monos	Monocytes
Na	Sodium
NCC	Total nucleated cell count (also commonly called WBC for "white blood cell count")
PCV	Packed cell volume
Phos	Phosphorus
PT	Prothrombin time
RBCs	Red blood cells
Retics	Reticulocytes
SDH	Sorbitol dehydrogenase
Segs	Segmented neutrophils
Sp. gr.	Specific gravity
T. bili	Total bilirubin
TCO_2	Total CO_2
TP	Total protein
TP (P)	Total plasma protein
TP (S)	Total serum protein
Trig	Triglyceride
UN	Urea nitrogen (same as BUN)
WBCs	White blood cells
WRI	Within reference interval(s)

CASES

Case 1

Signalment and history: 11-year-old male cat. Lethargy and polydipsia. One month ago, PCV was 38%.

Hematology		Reference interval
PCV (%)	**13**	25–45
RBC (×10⁶/µL)	**1.55**	5–11
Hgb (g/dL)	**4.0**	8–15
MCV (fL)	**84**	39–50
MCHC (g/dL)	31	33–37
Retics (×10³/µL)	**155**	0–60
NCC (×10³/µL)	**20.6**	5.5–19.5
Metas (×10³/µL)	**0.4**	0
Bands (×10³/µL)	**0.8**	0–0.3
Segs (×10³/µL)	9.9	2.5–12.5
Lymphs (×10³/µL)	**1.4**	1.5–7.0
Monos (×10³/µL)	**3.1**	0–0.8
Eos (×10³/µL)	0.2	0–1.5
Nucleated RBCs (×10³/µL)	**4.8**	0
Platelets (×10³/µL)	Adequate	150–700
TP (P) (g/dL)	**8.9**	6.0–8.5

Hemopathology: Many *Mycoplasma haemofelis* organisms on erythrocytes. Occasional reactive lymphocyte.

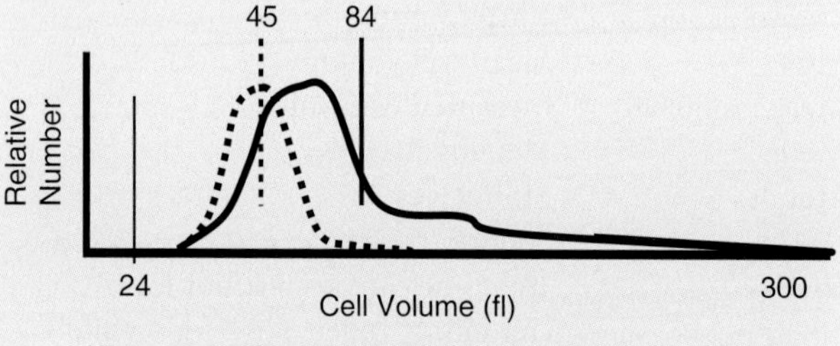

Histogram: Solid line = patient; dashed line = normal.

Biochemical profile		Reference interval
Gluc (mg/dL)	**249**	67–124
BUN (mg/dL)	**96**	17–32
Creat (mg/dL)	**6.6**	0.9–2.1
Ca (mg/dL)	10.2	8.5–11
Phos (mg/dL)	**7.9**	3.3–7.8
TP (g/dL)	**8.4**	5.9–8.1
Alb (g/dL)	3.3	2.3–3.9
Glob (g/dL)	**5.1**	2.9–4.4
T. bili (mg/dL)	0.3	0–0.3
Chol (mg/dL)	**386**	60–220
ALT (IU/L)	53	30–100
ALP (IU/L)	19	6–106
Na (mEq/L)	150	146–160
K (mEq/L)	4.9	3.7–5.4
CL (mEq/L)	127	112–129
TCO_2 (mEq/L)	**10**	14–23
An. gap (mEq/L)	18	10–27
Calc. osmolality (mOsm/kg)	**337**	290–310

Urinalysis (cystocentesis)		Urine sediment	
Color	Yellow	WBCs/hpf	6–8
Transparency	Cloudy	RBCs/hpf	1–2
Sp. gr.	**1.020**	Epith cells/hpf	1–3 transitional
Protein	Negative	Casts/lpf	0
Gluc	**2+**	Crystals	0
Bilirubin	Negative	Bacteria	0
Blood	Negative	Other	fat droplets
pH	5.0		
Ketones	Negative		

Interpretive discussion

Hematology

Packed cell volume, Hemoglobin, Red blood cell count: The cat is severely anemic; all measurements of red blood cell mass are decreased.

MCV: The mean cell volume is increased, which one would expect with a regenerative anemia. However, the increase is greater than can be accounted for by the reticulocytes, suggesting that agglutination is causing the increase, since doublets are being counted as one erythrocyte. This is confirmed by the histogram tailing to the right.

Reticulocytes are increased, indicating that the anemia is regenerative. Regenerative anemia is due to blood loss or blood destruction. The protein concentration suggests hemolysis and tends to rule out blood loss.

Nucleated RBCs are increased due to early marrow release, and are often present in a regenerative anemia.

Erythrocyte morphology: The presence of *Mycoplasma haemofelis* organisms explains the anemia (blood destruction). Agglutination is likely due to the presence of antibodies against the organisms.

Monocytosis and increased immature (band) neutrophils are indicative of an inflammatory leukogram.

Lymphopenia is indicative of a stress component in the leukogram.

Total protein: Total protein is increased. In this patient, it is due to hyperglobulinemia (see biochemical profile interpretation below).

Biochemical profile

The serum glucose concentration is moderately increased. This could be due to stress (glucocorticoid release), as the lymphopenia suggests, but could also be due to diabetes mellitus.

The BUN and serum creatinine concentrations are increased, and in the face of a urine specific gravity of only 1.020, is indicative of renal azotemia.

The serum phosphorus concentration is mildly increased, and is compatible with decreased glomerular filtration rate.

The serum total protein concentration is increased due to an increase in the globulin concentration. The increase in globulin should trigger protein electrophoresis to determine if gammopathy is monoclonal or polyclonal.

The serum cholesterol concentration is moderately increased. This may be due to metabolic disorders associated with diabetes mellitus.

Serum total CO_2 is decreased, suggesting metabolic acidosis.

The increased calculated serum osmolality is primarily due to hyperglycemia and increased BUN.

Urinalysis

As evidenced by the relatively low urine specific gravity in the face of azotemia, the animal is not concentrating adequately, indicating renal dysfunction. The presence of glucose indicates that the renal threshold of glucose has been exceeded.

Summary

This animal had been previously diagnosed with diabetes mellitus and was not being controlled adequately. *Mycoplasma haemofelis* is often an opportunist in cats that are immunosuppressed. The hyperglobulinemia was polyclonal, indicating antigenic stimulation, possibly due to *Mycoplasma haemofelis*.

Case 2

Signalment: 5-year-old spayed female cocker spaniel
History: Acutely lethargic
Physical examination: Pale, slightly icteric mucous membranes

Hematology		Reference interval
PCV (%)	**12**	37–55
Hgb (g/dL)	**3.6**	12–18
RBC (×10^6/μL)	**0.95**	5.5–8.5
MCV (fL)	**114**	60–72
MCHC (g/dL)	**30**	34–38
Retics (×10^3/μL)	**123**	<60
NCC (×10^3/μL)	**96.1**	6–17
Segs (×10^3/μL)	**69.1**	3–11.5
Bands (×10^3/μL)	**6.7**	0–0.3
Metas (×10^3/μL)	**1.0**	0
Monos (×10^3/μL)	**5.8**	0.1–1.3
Lymphs (×10^3/μL)	0	1–4.8
Eos (×10^3/μL)	0	0.1–1.2
NRBCs (×10^3/μL)	**13.5**	0
Platelets (×10^3/μL)	284	200–500
TP (P) (g/dL)	6.8	6–8

Hemopathology: Polychromasia increased, agglutination present, many spherocytes present. Occasional Howell-Jolly body.

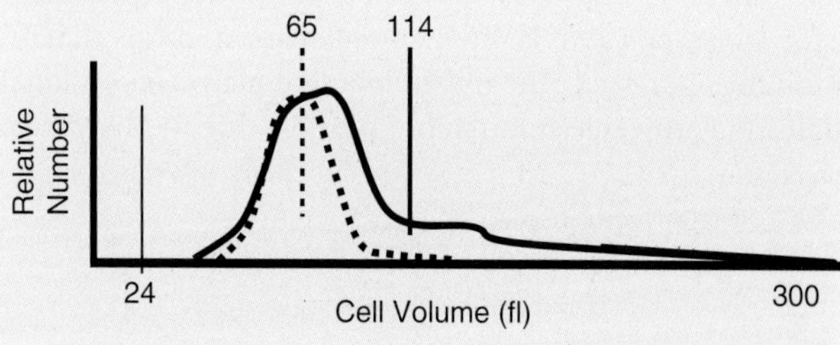

Histogram: Solid line = patient; dashed line = normal.

Biochemical profile		Reference interval
Gluc (mg/dL)	**143**	75–130
BUN (mg/dL)	**39**	7–28
Creat (mg/dL)	1.3	0.9–1.7
Ca (mg/dL)	9.0	9.0–11.2
Phos (mg/dL)	4.4	2.8–6.1
TP (g/dL)	6.5	5.4–7.4
Alb (g/dL)	3.3	2.7–4.5
Glob (g/dL)	3.2	1.9–3.4
T. bili (mg/dL)	**4.7**	0–0.4
Chol (mg/dL)	269	130–370
ALT (IU/L)	32	10–120
AST (IU/L)	30	16–40
ALP (IU//L)	**438**	35–280
Na (mEq/L)	146	145–158
K (mEq/L)	5.0	4.1–5.5
CL (mEq/L)	118	106–127
TCO_2 (mEq/L)	14	14–27
An. gap (mEq/L)	19	8–25

Urinalysis (catheterized)			
Color	Orange	**Urine sediment**	
Transparency	Turbid	WBCs/hpf	0
Sp. gr.	1.038	RBCs/hpf	**10**
Protein	1+	Epith Cells/hpf	0
Gluc	Negative	Casts/lpf	0
Bilirubin	**2+**	Crystals	Numerous **Bilirubin**
Blood	**1+**	Bacteria	0
pH	6.0		

Interpretive discussion

Hematology

Packed cell volume, Hemoglobin, Red blood cell count: The dog is very anemic, as all measurement of red blood cells mass are decreased. The RBC count is likely erroneously decreased, due to erythrocyte agglutination, and groups of red blood cells being counted as one red blood cell.

MCV: The mean cell volume is erroneously increased due to agglutination. Although the anemia is regenerative, the MCV is much higher than can be accounted for by an increase in reticulocytes. As one can see on the histogram, erythrocytes that are agglutinated are being counted as one large erythrocyte (note histogram tailing to right).

Reticulocytes are increased, indicating that the anemia is regenerative, suggesting either blood loss or blood destruction. The protein and RBC morphology findings indicate hemolysis. The decreased MCHC may be attributed to regeneration.

Nucleated RBCs are increased, likely due to early release from bone marrow in response to marked anemia. However, it is also possible that the dog has decreased splenic function secondary to glucocorticosteroid administration.

Erythrocyte morphology: Presence of spherocytes and agglutination, in the absence of a previous blood transfusion, are indicative of immune-mediated hemolytic anemia.

Neutrophilia, increased immature neutrophils, and monocytosis are indicative of a markedly inflammatory leukogram. The absence of lymphocytes is suggestive of stress or corticosteroids. Inflammatory leukograms are commonly seen in association with immune-mediated hemolytic anemia.

Biochemical profile

Glucose is mildly increased. Considering the lymphopenia, this may be due to stress or steroids.

BUN is mildly increased, suggesting decreased GFR or bleeding into the GI tract. Since the creatinine is within the reference interval, and the dog is concentrating urine, this is likely prerenal azotemia, due to GI hemorrhage (high-protein diet) or decreased blood flow to the kidneys.

Bilirubin is increased, indicating either cholestasis or increased red blood cell destruction. Because the dog has immune-mediated hemolytic anemia, increased RBC destruction is most likely the cause.

Serum alkaline phosphatase activity is increased, which could be due to either cholestasis or previous treatment with corticosteroids.

Urinalysis

Bilirubinuria and the presence of bilirubin crystals reflect the increased serum bilirubin concentration. Conjugated bilirubin readily passes through glomeruli and is then excreted in the urine. Blood and protein may be present due to traumatic catheterization. The animal is concentrating, indicating that the increase in BUN is not due to renal dysfunction.

Summary

This is a typical case of immune-mediated hemolytic anemia. Dog was treated with prednisone and recovered. It had been previously treated with corticosteroids, accounting for the stress leukogram, hyperglycemia, and increased serum alkaline phosphatase activity.

Case 3

Signalment and history: 11-year-old DSH spayed female cat presented for anorexia and lethargy

Hematology		Reference interval
PCV (%)	**13**	25–45
RBC ($\times10^6/\mu L$)	**1.84**	5–11
Hgb (g/dL)	**4.2**	8–15
MCV (fL)	**71**	39–50
MCHC (g/dL)	32	33–37
Retics ($\times10^3/\mu L$)	7.4	0–60
Nucleated cells ($\times10^3/\mu L$)	**71.3**	5.5–19.5
Metas ($\times10^3/\mu L$)	**0.7**	0
Bands ($\times10^3/\mu L$)	**2.1**	0–0.3
Segs ($\times10^3/\mu L$)	**33.2**	2.5–12.5
Lymphs ($\times10^3/\mu L$)	2.8	1.5–7.0
Monos ($\times10^3/\mu L$)	**6.9**	0–0.8
NRBCs ($\times10^3/\mu L$)	**24.9**	0
Blasts ($\times10^3/\mu L$)	**0.7**	0
Platelets ($\times10^3/\mu L$)	Adequate	150–700
TP (P) (g/dL)	8.0	6.0–8.5

Hemopathology: Blasts appear to be rubriblasts. Many prorubricytes and rubricytes also present.

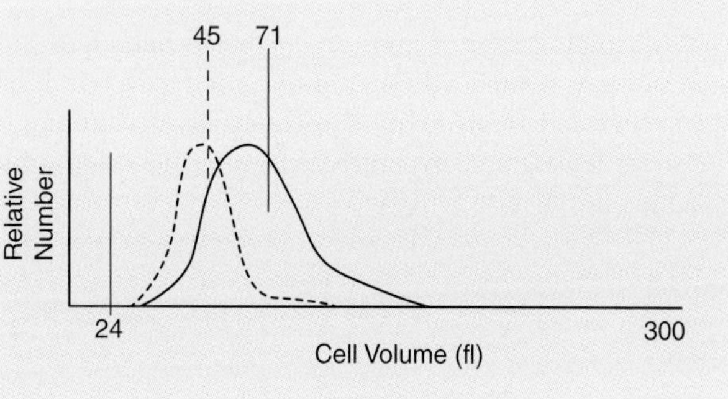

Histogram: Solid line = patient; dashed line = normal.

Interpretive discussion

Hematology

Packed cell volume, Hemoglobin, Red blood cell count: Cat is markedly anemic. Reticulocytes are not increased, indicating that the anemia is nonregenerative.

MCV is markedly increased, in the absence of reticulocytosis or agglutination. In a cat, this should trigger testing for feline leukemia virus, as the MCV may be increased as a result of viral-induced erythrodysplasia. Macrocytosis with widened histogram is often seen in FeLV positive cats with anemia.

Neutrophilia, increased band neutrophils and metamyelocytes, and monocytosis are indicative of inflammation.

Nucleated red blood cells are increased in the absence of reticulocytes. Moreover, many of these are quite immature, indicating that the cat has leukemia involving the erythrocytes.

Summary

Myeloproliferative disorder, red cell leukemia or M6(E).

Case 4

Signalment and history: 17-year-old male cat presented for lethargy and enlarged abdomen. Liver disease suspected, but biochemical profile normal.

Hematology		Reference interval
PCV (%)	**24**	25–45
MCV (fL)	**33**	39–50
MCHC (g/dL)	32	33–37
Retics ($\times 10^3/\mu L$)	ND	0–60,000
Nucleated cells ($\times 10^3/\mu L$)	13.2	5.5–19.5
Bands ($\times 10^3/\mu L$)	**4.5**	0–0.3
Segs ($\times 10^3/\mu L$)	6.6	2.5–12.5
Lymphs ($\times 10^3/\mu L$)	**0.5**	1.5–7.0
Monos ($\times 10^3/\mu L$)	0.5	0–0.8
Eos ($\times 10^3/\mu L$)	0.3	0–1.5
Basophils ($\times 10^3/\mu L$)	**0.8**	rare
Platelets ($\times 10^3/\mu L$)	Adequate	150–700
TP (P) (g/dL)	6.6	6.0–8.5

Hemopathology: Many keratocytes, schistocytes.

Histogram: Solid line = patient; dashed line = normal.

Interpretive discussion

Hematology

Packed cell volume: The cat is mildly anemic.

MCV: The mean cell volume is prominently decreased. Decreased mean cell volume is almost always caused by iron deficiency anemia, which in adults is almost always secondary to chronic external blood loss. The borderline decrease in MCHC is not important diagnostically.

Erythrocyte morphology: Keratocytes are commonly associated with iron deficiency anemia. Iron deficiency anemia is not as common in cats as in dogs, and the few cases we have seen did not have increased central pallor.

The total leukocyte count and the mature neutrophil concentration are within the reference interval, but the increase in band neutrophils is indicative of inflammation. Lymphopenia is indicative of stress or previous corticosteroid administration.

Total protein is within the reference interval. Although one might expect total protein to be decreased with chronic blood loss, animals often compensate for this chronic loss of protein.

Summary

Owner declined further diagnostic evaluation. Chronic GI blood loss secondary to an intestinal tumor would be the most likely diagnosis in this aged patient with iron deficiency anemia.

Case 5

Signalment: 1-year-old pointer
History: Treated for neck or back pain with corticosteroids by referring veterinarian. Dog was thought to have GI parasites due to occult blood in feces and was treated with anthelmintics. The dog returned 1 month later with a PCV of 15% and MCV of 40 fL. At that time the dog had an abdominal effusion.
Physical examination: Painful abdomen, pale mucous membranes

Hematology		Reference interval
PCV (%)	**18**	37–55
Hgb (g/dL)	**3.76**	12–18
RBC (×10⁶/μL)	5.8	5.5–8.5
MCV (fL)	**47**	60–72
MCHC (g/dL)	33	33–38
Retics (×10³/μL)	18	<60
NCC (×10³/μL)	**40.1**	6–17
Segs (×10³/μL)	**36.5**	3–11.5
Bands (×10³/μL)	**0.4**	0–0.3
Metas (×10³/μL)	**0.4**	0
Monos (×10³/μL)	1.2	0.1–1.3
Lymphs (×10³/μL)	1.2	1–4.8
Eos (×10³/μL)	0.4	0.1–1.2
Platelets (×10³/μL)	**623**	200–500
TP (P) (g/dL)	**5.9**	6–8

Hemopathology: Numerous keratocytes, few schistocytes, some RBCs appear hypochromic. Occasional lymphocyte with azurophilic granules.

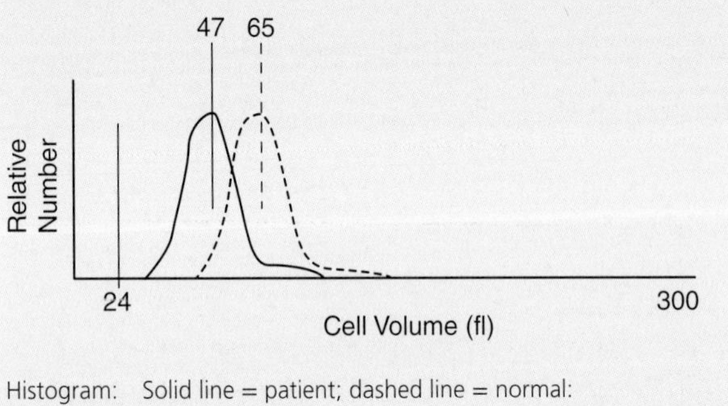

Histogram: Solid line = patient; dashed line = normal:

Abdominal fluid analysis	
NCC (μL)	**90,000**
TP (g/dL)	**4.0**

Cytology: All cells are degenerate neutrophils. Bacteria of various types are present.

Interpretive discussion

Hematology

Packed cell volume, Hemoglobin: Both are decreased, indicating that the dog is anemic. The red blood cell count is within the reference interval, suggesting erythrocytes are small.

MCV: The mean cell volume is decreased. Decreased mean cell volume is almost always caused by iron deficiency anemia, which in adults is almost always secondary to chronic external blood loss.

Reticulocytes are not increased, indicating that the anemia is nonregenerative. While uncomplicated iron deficiency anemia is usually regenerative, this anemia may be nonregenerative due to the presence of inflammation (note inflammatory leukogram).

Erythrocyte morphology: Keratocytes, erythrocyte fragmentation, and increased central pallor are commonly associated with iron deficiency anemia.

Neutrophilia and increased immature neutrophils are indicative of a marked inflammatory leukogram. The inflammatory leukogram is compatible with the presence of inflammation in the peritoneal cavity, although one would usually expect to see more band neutrophils in dogs with peritonitis. The presence of this inflammation may be the explanation for the lack of a regenerative response to the anemia, as an anemia of inflammatory disease may be superimposed on the iron deficiency anemia. The noted occasional granulated lymphocyte is interpreted as an incidental finding.

Platelets are increased. Approximately half of all animals with iron deficiency anemia have increased platelets, probably in response to cytokines and growth factors.

Total protein: Total protein is slightly decreased, probably as a result of chronic blood loss.

Histogram confirms the presence of a population of microcytic cells (normal histogram represented by dashed line).

Abdominal fluid analysis

Supportive septic inflammation. The presence of different types of bacteria suggests a GI source of bacteria.

Summary

The dog died, and on necropsy had an intestinal perforation secondary to an ulcer, chronic diffuse peritonitis, pyogranulomatous lymphadenitis and amyloidosis of the spleen, liver, and kidney. Presumably, the dog had been chronically bleeding from this ulcer, resulting in iron deficiency anemia.

Case 6

Signalment and history: 9-year-old female beagle presented for lethargy and pale mucous membranes. Owner reported that the dog occasionally had blood in feces.

Hematology		Reference interval
PCV (%)	**12**	37–55
RBC (×10^6/μL)	**2.76**	5.5–8.5
Hgb (g/dL)	**3.2**	12–18
MCV (fL)	**40**	60–72
MCHC (g/dL)	**29**	34–38
Retics (×10^3/μL)	**242**	0–60
Nucleated cells (×10^3/μL)	**33.4**	6.0–17.0
Metas (×10^3/μL)	–	0
Bands (×10^3/μL)	–	0–0.3
Segs (×10^3/μL)	**30.7**	3.0–11.5
Lymphs (×10^3/μL)	1.0	1.0–4.8
Monos (×10^3/μL)	1.0	0.2–1.4
Eos (×10^3/μL)	–	0.1–1.2
NRBCs (×10^3/μL)	**0.7**	0
Platelets (×10^3/μL)	Adequate	200–500
TP (P) (g/dL)	6.3	6.0–8.0

Hemopathology: Increased central pallor, occasional keratocyte, giant platelets.

Interpretive discussion

Hematology

Packed cell volume, Hemoglobin, Red blood cell count: The dog is markedly anemic; all measurements of red blood cell mass are decreased.

MCV: The mean cell volume is markedly decreased. Decreased mean cell volume is almost always caused by iron deficiency anemia, which in adults is almost always secondary to chronic external blood loss. The MCHC may be mildly decreased in iron deficiency as it is here. The reticulocytosis may also contribute to the decreased MCHC.

Reticulocytes are increased, indicating that the anemia is regenerative, suggesting blood loss or blood destruction. In this case, the decreased MCV strongly suggests iron deficiency anemia secondary to chronic blood loss. The presence of nucleated red blood cells is compatible with this degree of regenerative response.

Erythrocyte morphology: Keratocytes and increased central pallor are commonly associated with iron deficiency anemia.

Neutrophilia is indicative of inflammation, even though no band neutrophils are present, since the neutrophil concentration is greater than twofold upper reference interval. The lymphocyte count is in the low normal range, indicating that there may be a stress or steroid component to the leukogram.

Total protein is within the reference interval. Although one might expect total protein to be decreased with chronic blood loss, animals often compensate for this chronic loss of protein.

Summary

GI barium series performed and jejunal mass seen. At surgery, a mass in the mid-jejunum was resected and determined to be a leiomyosarcoma with clean surgical margins. The regenerative response in this case is in contrast to the previous case to make the point that iron deficiency anemia may be either regenerative or nonregenerative.

Case 7

Signalment: 5-year-old mixed-breed dog
History: Lethargy
Physical examination: Lethargic, pale mucous membranes

Hematology	1/20[a]	1/28	Reference interval
Packed cell volume (%) (spun)	**14**	**30**	37–55
Hematocrit (%) (calculated)	**12.4**	**21.3**	37–55
Hgb (g/dL)	**4.4**	**9.0**	12–18
RBC ($10^6/\mu L$)	**4.26**	5.77	5.5–8.5
MCV (fL)	**29**	**37**	60–77
MCHC (g/dL)	**35.2**	**42.1**	31–34
RDW	**23.8**	**31.7**	12–15
Platelets($\times 10^3/\mu L$)	**803**	**883**	200–500
Reticulocytes ($\times 10^3/\mu L$)	**102**	**403**	0–60
Total protein (g/dL)	**5.3**	6.2	6–8

[a]Sample moderately lipemic.

1/20 histogram and blood film

VetScan HM2

Sample ID:	1100		
Patient ID:	9818	Doctor:	Gillespie
Name:	Fluffy	Age/Sex:	5 years / Male
Test time:	01.28.2010 09:31 AM	S/N:	270107
Mode:	Dog	Report date:	01.28.2010 09:31 AM

Parameter	Value	Flag	Unit	Low	High
WBC	8.86		10^9/l	6	17
LYM	2.03		10^9/l	1	4.8
MON	0.43		10^9/l	0.2	1.5
GRA	6.40		10^9/l	3	12
LY%	22.9		%	12	30
MO%	4.8	+	%	2	4
GR%	72.3		%	62	87
RBC	4.26	–	10^12/l	5.5	8.5
HGB	4.4	–	g/dl	12	18
HCT	12.39	–	%	37	55
MCV	29	–	fl	60	77
MCH	10.3	–	pg	19.5	24.5
MCHC	35.2	+	g/dl	31	34
RDWc	23.8		%		
PLT	803	+	10^9/l	200	500
PCT	0.67		%		
MPV	8.3		fl	3.9	11.1
PDWc	36.6		%		

WBC: 48, 104, 115, 400
RBC: 14, 200
PLT: 14, 50

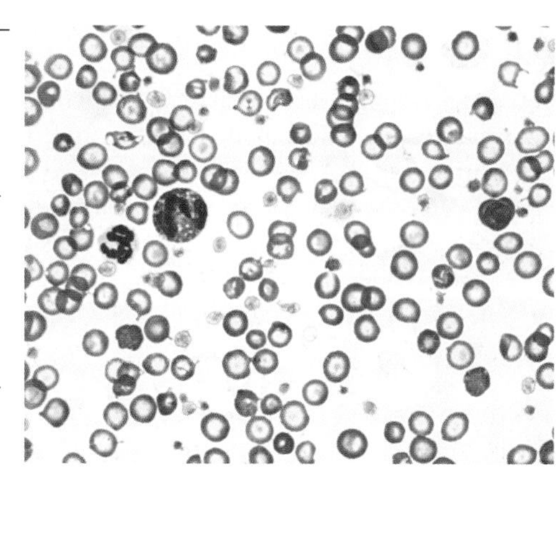

1/28 histogram and blood film

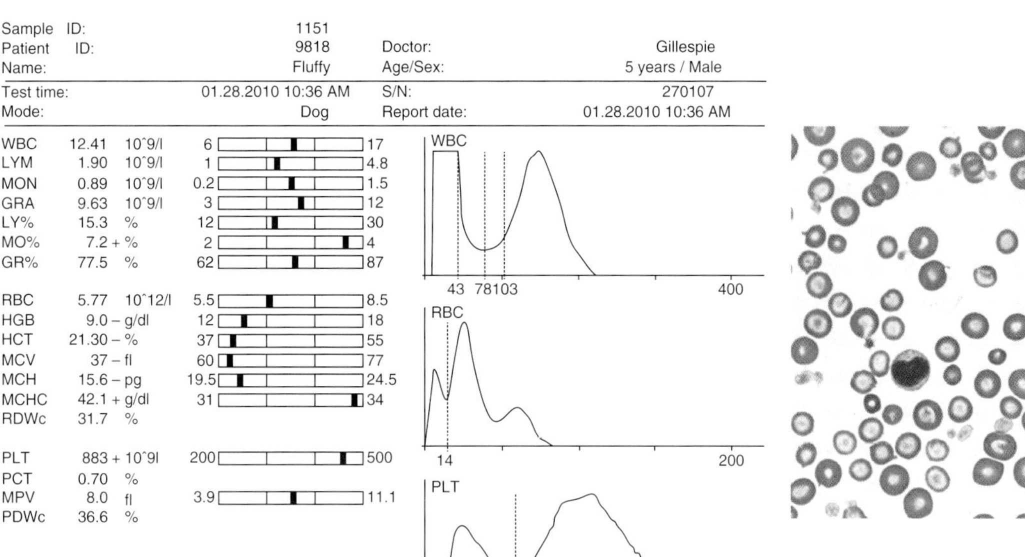

VetScan HM2

Sample ID:	1151		
Patient ID:	9818	Doctor:	Gillespie
Name:	Fluffy	Age/Sex:	5 years / Male
Test time:	01.28.2010 10:36 AM	S/N:	270107
Mode:	Dog	Report date:	01.28.2010 10:36 AM

Parameter	Value	Unit	Low	High
WBC	12.41	10ˆ9/l	6	17
LYM	1.90	10ˆ9/l	1	4.8
MON	0.89	10ˆ9/l	0.2	1.5
GRA	9.63	10ˆ9/l	3	12
LY%	15.3	%	12	30
MO%	7.2 +	%	2	4
GR%	77.5	%	62	87
RBC	5.77	10ˆ12/l	5.5	8.5
HGB	9.0 –	g/dl	12	18
HCT	21.30 –	%	37	55
MCV	37 –	fl	60	77
MCH	15.6 –	pg	19.5	24.5
MCHC	42.1 +	g/dl	31	34
RDWc	31.7	%		
PLT	883 +	10ˆ9l	200	500
PCT	0.70	%		
MPV	8.0	fl	3.9	11.1
PDWc	36.6	%		

Interpretive discussion

Hematology

PCV and Hematocrit: Decreased, indicating anemia. Note the marked discrepancy in the calculated hematocrit (HCT) and the spun packed cell volume (PCV). The HCT is calculated by the instrument using the following formula: (MCV × RBC)/10 = HCT(%). In the case of the sample from 1/28/10, the RBC count may be under-reporting the sample's RBC concentration since some small RBCs are likely appearing in the PLT channel. The lower reported RBC count is also likely due to the fact that two overlapping RBC peaks are now present in the RBC histogram from 1/28/10; the two overlapping peaks will be underestimated since the software expects only one RBC peak to be present and will not apply curve fitting algorithms here. Since the RBC count is underestimated, the HCT calculated here is lower than the reported PCV.

RBC

The RBCs are decreased as a result of anemia, but they are likely undercounted in this patient due to their small size, and are likely being counted in the platelet channel (see the platelet histogram below the erythrocyte histogram).

MCV

The decreased MCV indicates a severe microcytic anemia. The degree of microcytosis is illustrated by the RBC histogram on 1/20. The blood film contained many hypochromic erythrocytes, as well as keratocytes and schistocytes, erythrocyte shape changes and fragmentation that are very characteristic of iron deficient erythrocytes. The dog was treated with iron. Note that 1 week later on 1/28, the MCV increased, and the new normal-sized erythrocytes are evident in the erythrocyte histogram on 1/28. They are represented by the additional curve on the right side of the histogram as well as on the blood film made on 1/28.

MCHC

The MCHC is miscalculated to be high on 1/28 likely as a result of the undercounted RBCs. The MCHC is probably erroneously increased on 1/20 as well. The MCHC is calculated from the hemoglobin concentration and the HCT using the following formula: HGB (g/dL) divided by the HCT (%) × 100 = MCHC (g/dL). It provides an index for the quantity of hemoglobin relative to the volume of packed erythrocytes. It may be erroneously increased due to lipemia, hemolysis, or an erroneously low HCT. On 1/28, it is likely erroneously high due to the erroneously low HCT. On 1/20, it may also be erroneously high due to lipemia artifactually increasing the HGB.

RDW

The increased variation in erythrocyte size (anisocytosis) is represented by the increased red cell distribution width (RDW) on 1/28, a numerical expression (coefficient of variation) that correlates with the degree of anisocytosis and that the instrument determines by dividing the standard deviation of the red cell size by the MCV. Both iron deficient microcytic erythrocytes and young macrocytic erythrocytes can also be seen on the blood film.

Platelets

The platelet concentration is markedly increased, as is often the case in patients with iron deficiency anemia. Some of the platelets are quite large. Also, some microcytic RBC are counted as PLT, falsely increasing the PLT concentration.

Reticulocytes

The reticulocyte concentration is increased, indicating a regenerative anemia.

Total protein

The total protein is slightly decreased on 1/20, likely due to chronic blood loss (protein is lost as well as erythrocytes).

Summary

Iron deficiency anemia as indicated by marked microcytosis.

Outcome

The diagnosis of iron deficiency anemia was confirmed by measuring serum iron, which was 27 μg/dL (Reference interval = 98–220 μg/dL). The source of chronic blood loss is usually the gastrointestinal tract. An occult blood test was performed on the feces on multiple occasions, and was consistently negative. An examination of feces for the eggs of parasites such as hookworms was also negative. Further history revealed that the owner had given the dog an anthelmintic 2 weeks prior to presentation, presumably eliminating a hookworm infestation. The dog was treated with 15 mg/kg iron dextran IM, and the owner was instructed to give him 162.5 mg Ferrous sulfate orally once daily for 4 weeks. The hematocrit and MCV were normal at his follow-up examination 6 months later.

Case 8

Signalment: 5-month-old male Great Dane/Labrador retriever/mastiff cross weighing 23 kg

History: Lethargy, eating dirt (pica), vomited once and a small amount of blood was in vomitus, pruritic. Four of his five littermates died at 4–6 weeks of age. Hookworm eggs were seen on a fecal examination done at 7 weeks of age, and he also possibly had coccidiosis at that time and was treated for both. His sire is also his grandsire.

Physical examination: Pale mucous membranes, skin lesions present that appear to be pustular dermatitis

CASES

Hematology	Day 1	Day 60	Day 90	Day 120	RI
Packed cell volume (%)	**17**	**26**	41	42	37–55
Hematocrit (%)	**15**	**26**	39	38	37–55
RBC ($\times10^6/\mu L$)	**4.70**	7.28	**9.46**	8.17	5.5–8.5
Hgb (g/dL)	**4.4**	**8.0**	13.7	13.4	12–18
MCV (fL)	**32**	**35**	**41**	**47**	60–72
MCHC (g/dL)	**29.3**	31.3	34.8	35	31–36
Reticulocytes ($10^3/\mu L$)	**352.5**	**160.2**	ND	ND	0–60
RDW (%)	**29.7**	**24.6**	**31.7**	**34.7**	12–16
NCC ($10^3/\mu L$)	**23.4**	15.3	16.5	13.6	6.0–17.0
Segmented neutrophils ($10^3/\mu L$)	**17.0**	8.4	8.8	6.2	3.0–11.5
Band neutrophils ($10^3/\mu L$)	**0.5**	0.2	**0.8**	–	0–0.3
Metamyelocytes ($10^3/\mu L$)	–	–	–	–	0
Monocytes ($10^3/\mu L$)	0.5	0.9	0.3	1.4	0.2–1.4
Lymphocytes ($10^3/\mu L$)	4.2	4.7	**5.1**	4.8	1.0–4.8
Eosinophils ($10^3/\mu L$)	1.2	1.1	**1.5**	1.2	0.1–1.2
Platelets ($10^3/\mu L$)	**68**	**183**	318	221	200–500
Plasma protein by refractometry(g/dL)	**5.2**	**5.4**	6.0	6.2	6.0–8.0

Hemopathology Day 1: Hypochromasia, microcytosis, keratocytes, schistocytes, marked polychromasia present, numerous macroplatelets present, some platelet clumping, platelet concentration appears adequate on blood film.

Hemopathology Day 60: Marked hypochromasia and microcytosis. Numerous large and giant platelets seen. Occasional schistocytes and keratocytes. Moderate polychromasia present.

Hemopathology Day 90: Occasional keratocyte seen.

Hemopathology Day 90: A few microcytic and hypochromic erythrocytes seen.

Histogram from Day 60

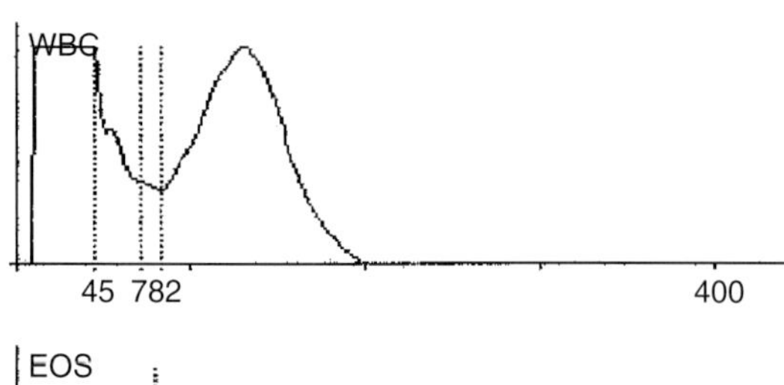

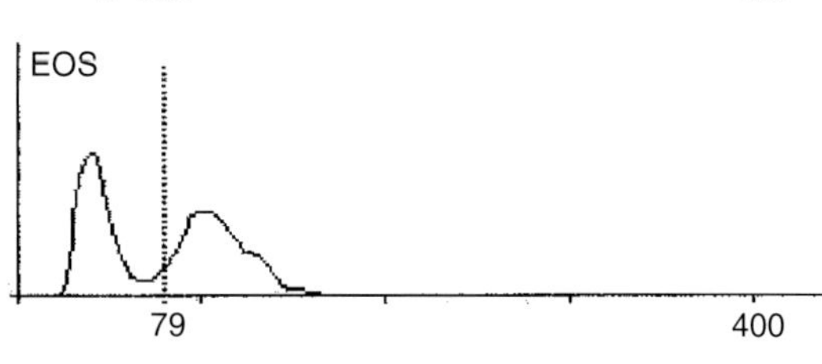

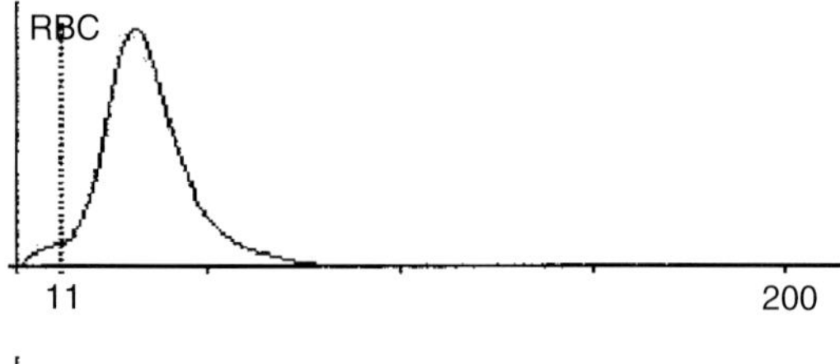

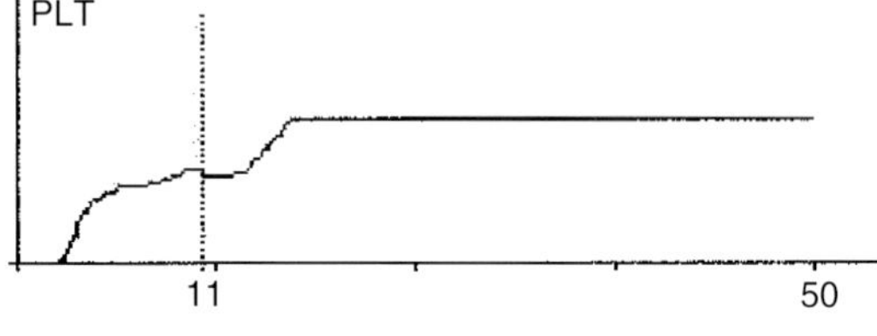

Histogram from Day 90:

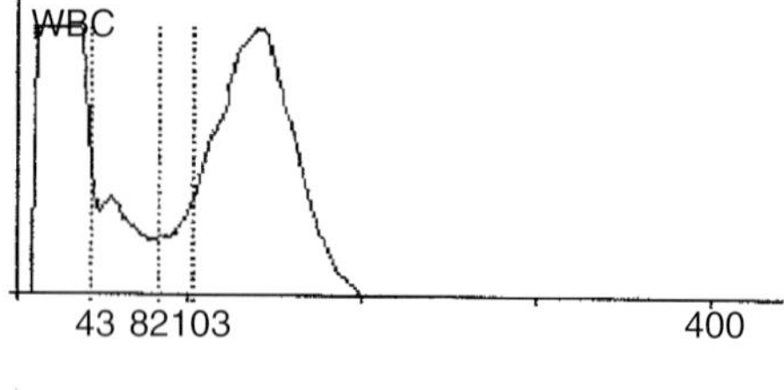

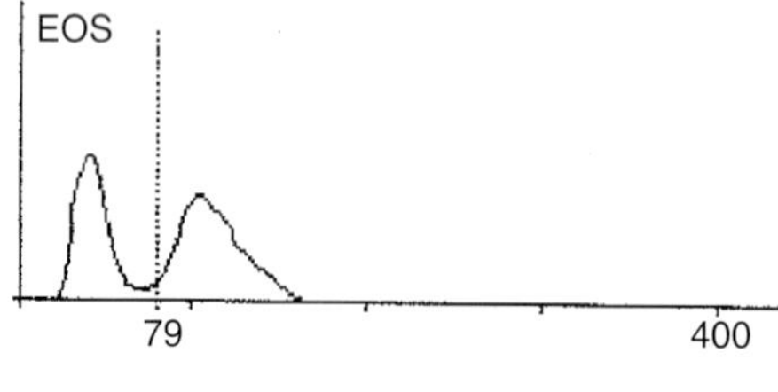

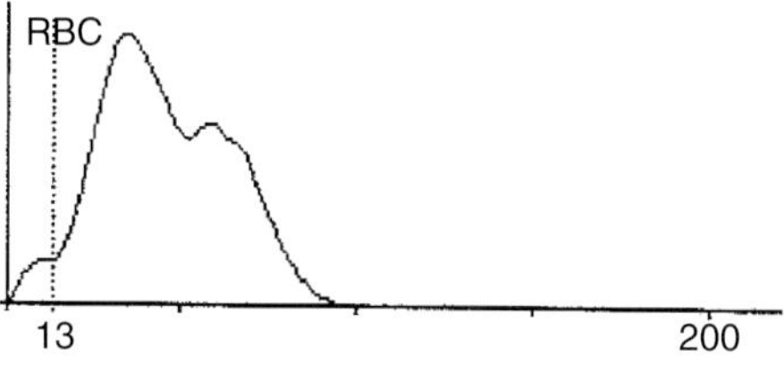

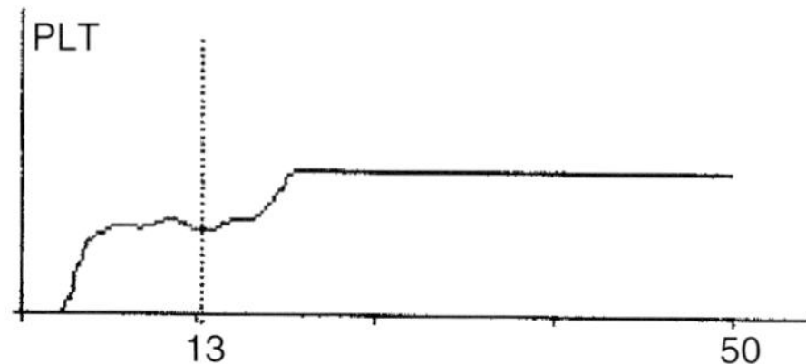

Additional tests

Biochemical profile

Abnormalities are shown below.

Phosphorus (mg/dL)	**7.5**	Reference interval: 2.9–6.6
Total protein (g/dL)	**4.9**	Reference interval: 5.4–8.2
Globulin (g/dL)	**1.4**	Reference interval: 2.3–5.2

PCR for babesia on Day 1– negative.

Fecal examination on Day 60 was negative for parasites, **positive for occult blood,** and **positive for Giardia antigen**.

Coagulation panel (aPTT and PT) on Day 60 was within normal limits.

Interpretive discussion

Hematology

Day 1: Marked anemia is present as evidenced by the decreased PCV, hemoglobin and erythrocyte count. The anemia is extremely microcytic (decreased MCV) and hypochromic (decreased MCHC), indicating iron deficiency anemia secondary to chronic blood loss. Microcytosis occurs with iron deficiency anemia because iron availability determines reticulocyte size. Under normal conditions, hemoglobin concentration in the rubricyte increases to a point that the concentration will trigger nuclear degeneration resulting in inability to undergo further mitosis. Hemoglobin synthesis is delayed when iron is limited, presumably resulting in extra rubricyte divisions and subsequent microcytosis.

Anemia is markedly regenerative as evidenced by the increased reticulocyte concentration. The red cell distribution width (RDW) is increased, indicating an increased variation in erythrocyte size (anisocytosis). The RDW is determined by the following calculation: Standard deviation of the MCV divided by the MCV × 100. RDW is consistently increased in patients with iron deficiency anemia, not only because of heterogenous volumes of erythrocytes but also because of the low MCV.

An inflammatory leukogram is present as evidenced by the increased band neutrophils.

The electronic platelet concentration is erroneously decreased, due to the presence of macroplatelets and platelet clumping.

The plasma protein is decreased, likely due to chronic blood loss or protein loss through the intestine (see below).

Examination of the blood film showed the presence of microcytosis and hypochromasia, which is compatible with the decreased MCV and MCHC. Keratocytes and schistocytes are often associated with iron deficiency anemia due to oxidative membrane changes. The polychromasia seen on the blood film is consistent with the increased reticulocyte concentration.

Day 60: The anemia is slightly less severe. Interestingly, the erythrocyte concentration is within the reference interval, even though the hemoglobin and PCV are decreased. This is likely explained by the fact that the erythrocytes are approximately half normal size, as shown by the MCV, which results in a decreased red cell mass and hemoglobin even though the red cell concentration is normal. Additionally, large platelets are being counted as erythrocytes, which would account for a slight increase in the erythrocyte concentration. Note that the red cell and platelet histograms show that there is no clear demarcation between the large platelets and the small red blood cells. The histogram is unimodal (i.e., all of the erythrocytes are one microcytic population). The anemia is regenerative, but less regenerative than on Day 1, suggesting that iron stores are further depleted. The RDW is still increased, indicating a variation in erythrocyte size. The electronic platelet count is slightly below the reference interval, likely due to large platelets being counted as erythrocytes rather than platelets.

Day 90: The patient is no longer anemic, and the erythrocyte concentration is above the reference interval. As on Day 60, this is likely due to the presence of increased numbers of small erythrocytes, so that the PCV and hemoglobin concentrations are discordant with the erythrocyte concentration. Additionally, large platelets are likely contributing at least slightly to this increased red cell concentration, as they are being counted as small red blood cells. The RDW is markedly increased, indicating a large variation in erythrocyte size. This variation is also evident in the bimodal red cell histogram, in which two distinct populations of red cells can be seen. The microcytic subpopulation consists of the residual cells produced during limited iron availability. There is also a new population of normal sized erythrocytes as a result of iron repletion that makes up approximately 30 to 40% of the erythrocyte population. A histogram from an iron deficient dog that received a blood transfusion of normal sized erythrocytes would look similar, but a transfusion was not given to this patient.

A reticulocyte count was not performed on Day 90, but it is likely that some of the erythrocytes are larger than normal. The MCV is still decreased due to the remaining microcytic cells, but it has increased by 6 fL since the previous CBC on Day 60.

Day 120. The only abnormalities are decreased MCV and increased RDW, due to the remaining microcytic erythrocytes. There is a discrepancy of 4% between the manual PCV and HCT, which is calculated by multiplying the MCV by the RBC count (in this case, $47 \times 8.17 = 38$). Erythrocytes from patients with iron deficiency anemia do not pack within the column of the hematocrit tube as completely as do normal erythrocytes. This may be due to their containing less hemoglobin, or possibly due to increased rigidity associated with membrane oxidation that occurs as a result of iron deficiency. The discrepancy is not as large when the patients are more anemic (see Day 1), because fewer erythrocytes are involved. These mild discrepancies should not alter interpretation or patient management.

Biochemical profile

The phosphorus is slightly increased, which is common in large-breed growing dogs. The total protein is decreased as a result of hypoglobulinemia. It is likely that the hypoglobulinemia was a result of loss of globulins through the inflamed GI tract (see below), although loss as a result of blood loss is likely contributing.

Summary and outcome

The dog was initially treated with oral iron (80 mg ferrous sulfate bid), famotidine, a histamine-2 receptor antagonist that decreases stomach acid, and sucralfate, a gastric protectant, with the assumption that the iron deficiency anemia was a result of chronic blood loss from an inflamed GI tract. He was also given an anthelmintic in case hookworm eggs had been missed on the fecal examination. The patient improved slightly but 2 months later developed obvious melena and was vomiting blood. Ultrasound examination and a duodenal and stomach biopsy by endoscopy were performed on Day 60. The duodenum appeared hyperemic but no ulceration was seen. Ultrasound showed a thickened hyperechoic gastric wall, and biopsies revealed severe eosinophilic plasmacytic lymphocytic gastritis and enteritis. A skin biopsy showing eosinophilic lymphocytic plasmacytic dermatitis was also likely due to hypersensitivity.

The patient was then treated with injectable iron on Day 60 (42 mg iron dextran IM) and every 2 weeks thereafter for the next 2 months. He also received dietary therapy for the inflammatory bowel disease (a digestive prescription diet) and benzimidazole, an anthelmintic with effectiveness against Giardia. Famotidine was discontinued, and omeprazole, a proton pump inhibitor, was initiated. By 90 days post–initial admission, the dog was no longer anemic, although his microcytosis persisted due to the relatively long lifespan of erythrocytes.

In summary, Iron deficiency anemia was a result of the chronic blood loss from the intestine. The most important keys to the diagnosis were the decreased MCV and increased RDW. The intestinal inflammation may have been secondary to giardiasis or a food allergy. An additional cause of iron deficiency anemia in patients with inflammatory bowel disease is decreased ability of enterocytes to absorb iron due to the presence of inflammation. The pathophysiology of this phenomenon is complex and is addressed by Kaitha et al. (see "Suggested Reading"). Additionally, both proton pump inhibitors and histamine 2 receptor antagonists can interfere with intestinal iron absorption. The patient's anemia did not significantly improve until injectable iron therapy was instituted. A serum iron was not performed until Day 60, at which time it was normal (146 μg; reference interval: 98–220), suggesting that oral iron had at least been effective in increasing serum iron. Presumably serum iron on Day 1 would have been found to be decreased, considering the severe microcytosis.

Contributors: Mary Anna Thrall, Patrice Bernier, and Glade Weiser

Case 9

Signalment: 10-year-old castrated male Labrador retriever

History: Four episodes of acute weakness over past 3 months. At time of wellness exam 4 months ago, dog had PCV of 44% and TP of 8.2 g/dL.

Physical examination: Pale mucous membranes, abdomen slightly distended

Hematology		Reference interval
PCV (%)	**16**	37–55
Hgb (g/dL)	**5.3**	12–18
RBC (×10^6/μL)	**2.48**	5.5–8.5
MCV (fL)	63	60–72
MCHC (g/dL)	34	34–38
Retics (×10^3/μL)	**342**	<60
NCC (×10^3/μL)	**39.1**	6–17
Segs (×10^3/μL)	**33.2**	3–11.5
Bands (×10^3/μL)	**1.2**	0–0.3
Monos (×10^3/μL)	**3.1**	0.1–1.3
Lymphs (×10^3/μL)	**0.4**	1–4.8
Eos (×10^3/μL)	0.4	0.1–1.2
NRBCs (×10^3/μL)	**0.8**	0
Platelets (×10^3/μL)	**130**	200–500
TP (P) (g/dL)	6.2	6–8

Hemopathology: Polychromasia increased, numerous acanthocytes and schistocytes. Numerous Howell-Jolly bodies.

Biochemical profile
No abnormalities

Abdominal fluid analysis	
PCV (%)	**24**
NCC (×10^3/μL)	**34**

Cytology: 95% nondegenerate neutrophils; 5% macrophages, many of which have phagocytized erythrocytes.

Interpretive discussion

Hematology

Packed cell volume, Hemoglobin, Red blood cell count: The dog is anemic; all measurements of red blood cell mass are decreased.

MCV: The mean cell volume is normal. However, it is surprising that it is not higher considering that the reticulocyte count is increased.

Reticulocytes are increased, indicating that the anemia is regenerative, and is thus due to blood loss or blood destruction. The borderline low plasma protein suggests blood loss is likely; this will be confirmed by additional findings. Nucleated RBCs are increased due to early marrow release as part of regeneration.

Erythrocyte morphology: Acanthocytes are commonly seen in dogs with hemangiosarcoma. The schistocytes are suggestive of microangiopathy, which may also be associated with hemangiosarcoma.

Neutrophilia, increased immature (band) neutrophils, and monocytosis are indicative of an inflammatory leukogram, although a component of the mature neutrophilia is likely due to stress or corticosteroids. Lymphopenia is indicative of stress.

Platelets are slightly decreased. Considering the presence of schistocytes, the animal may have DIC.

Total protein: Total protein is within the reference interval. However, considering that it was 8.2 g/dL 4 months previously, it is likely decreased due to blood loss within the abdominal cavity.

Abdominal fluid analysis

Hemoabdomen.

Summary

The signalment (large breed, older dog), history (episodes of weakness), regenerative anemia, erythrocyte morphology, and the hemoabdomen are all suggestive of hemangiosarcoma. An exploratory was performed, and the dog had hemangiosarcoma of the spleen and liver, which had ruptured. Previous episodes of weakness were likely due to previous ruptures of the tumor, which had subsequently sealed, then ruptured again.

Case 10

Signalment: 15-year-old Staffordshire terrier
History: Lethargic
Physical examination: Pale mucous membranes

Hematology	January	October	Reference interval
PCV (%)	**30**	**28**	37–55
RBC (×10^6/μL)	**4.70**	**4.44**	5.5–8.5
Hgb (g/dL)	**10.1**	**9.5**	12–18
MCV (fL)	61	64	60–72
MCHC (g/dL)	35	34	34–38
Retics (×10^3/μL)	**178**	13	0–60
NCC (×10^3/μL)	**23.4**	10.2	6.0–17.0
Bands (×10^3/μL)	**0.5**	0.2	0–0.3
Segs (×10^3/μL)	**15.7**	6.2	3.0–11.5
Lymphs (×10^3/μL)	**6.1**	1.5	1.0–4.8
Monos (×10^3/μL)	0.7	**1.7**	0.2–1.4
Eos (×10^3/μL)	–		0.1–1.2
NRBCs (×10^3/μL)	–		0
Platelets (×10^3/μL)	150	**12**	200–500
TP (P) (g/dL)	**8.2**	**5.6**	6.0–8.0
Alb	**1.5**		2.7–4.5
Glob	**6.0**		1.9–3.4

Hemopathology (January): Increased rouleaux, giant platelets, lymphs contain azurophilic granules.
Hemopathology (October): Increased rouleaux, lymphs contain azurophilic granules. Numerous *Mycoplasma haemocanis* organisms present.

Interpretive discussion

Hematology

Packed cell volume, Hemoglobin, Red blood cell count: The dog is anemic; all measurements of red blood cell mass are decreased.

Reticulocytes are increased in January, indicating that the anemia is regenerative, suggesting either blood loss or blood destruction. Although the PCV is further decreased in October, the anemia is no longer regenerative, suggesting bone marrow dysfunction.

Neutrophilic leukocytosis with left shift and monocytosis is indicative of an inflammatory leukogram (January).

Lymphocytosis in January is most suggestive of either lymphocytic leukemia or ehrlichiosis.

Platelets: The animal is markedly thrombocytopenic in October. The combination of thrombocytopenia and nonregenerative anemia should trigger a bone marrow aspirate examination and ehrlichia titer. Common causes of thrombocytopenia include ehrlichiosis, immune-mediated thrombocytopenia, and DIC.

Total protein: Total protein is increased. In this patient, it is due to hyperglobulinemia, which should trigger protein electrophoresis.

The presence of increased rouleaux is compatible with increased globulin. The presence of large granular lymphocytes is suggestive of certain types of antigenic stimulation, commonly ehrlichiosis, or a leukemia of LGL cells. The presence of *Mycoplasma haemocanis* organisms in October suggests either a previous splenectomy or splenic dysfunction, since the erythrocyte parasite is rarely seen in dogs with functional spleens. The anemia is no longer regenerative in the face of anemia and this erythrocyte parasite, suggesting marrow impairment of some type, and a bone marrow aspirate is indicated.

Summary

In January, the anemia was possibly due to blood loss associated with a large hematoma of the spleen, and the dog was splenectomized. The lymphocytosis, hyperglobulinemia, and presence of large granular lymphocytes should have triggered an ehrlichia titer but did not. The animal returned in October, severely anemic and thrombocytopenic. An ehrlichia titer was done at this time, and was strongly positive. The dog was treated for ehrlichiosis and hemoplasmosis, and recovered.

Case 11

Signalment: Three approximately 3-year-old adult intact dogs from St. Kitts that presented as strays

History: No history available

Physical examination: Poorly nourished, rough hair coats

Dog 1

Hematology	Day 1	Day 60	Day 90	Ref range
Packed cell volume (%)	**30**	44	43	36–54
MCV (fL)	**55**	**55**	**59**	60–72
NCC ($10^3/\mu L$)	**19.5**			6.0–17.0
Segmented neutrophils ($10^3/\mu L$)	9.0	11.3	8.1	3.0–11.5
Band neutrophils ($10^3/\mu L$)	–	–	–	0–0.3
Monocytes ($10^3/\mu L$)	0.1	0.6	0.3	0.2–1.4
Lymphocytes ($10^3/\mu L$)	**9.5**	**5.5**	**5.0**	1.0–4.8
Eosinophils ($10^3/\mu L$)	**0.9**	**1.1**	**1.6**	0–0.8
Platelets ($10^3/\mu L$)	**57.5**	257	280	200–500
Plasma protein by refractometry (g/dL)	**9.5**	**11.1**	**9.5**	6.0–8.0

Day 1 hemopathology: Rouleaux present, many large granular lymphocytes seen, marked platelet clumping, neutrophil clumping (leukergy).

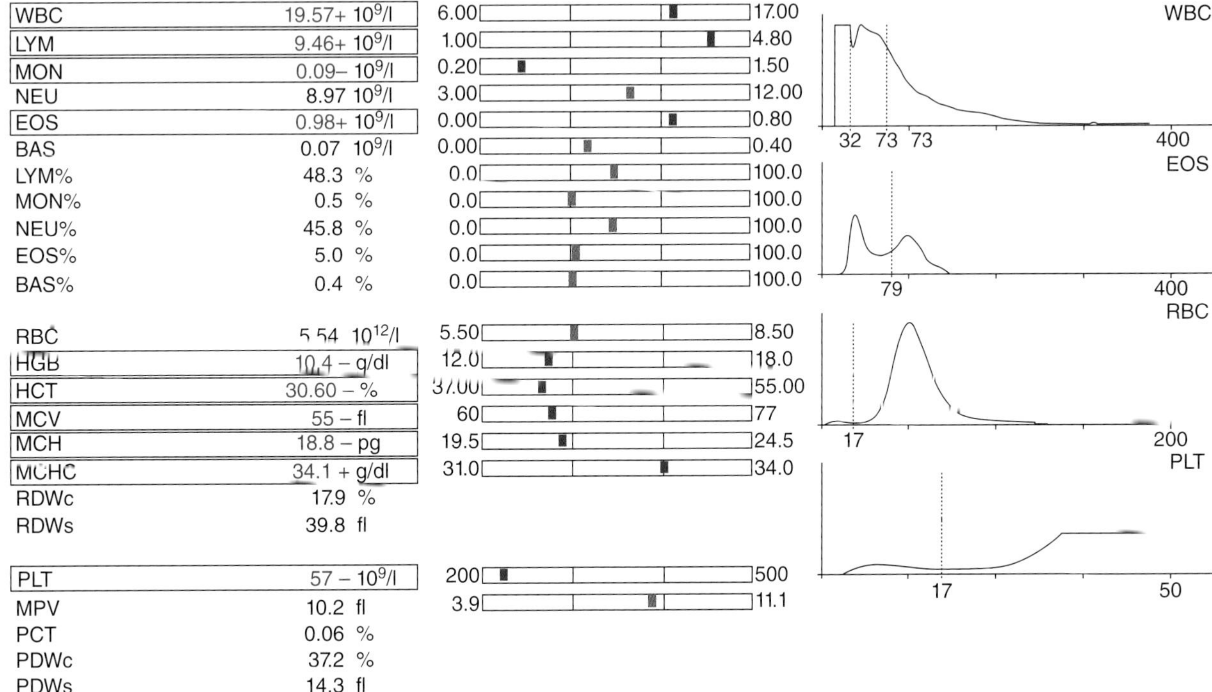

Parameter	Result	Low	High
WBC	19.57+ 10^9/l	6.00	17.00
LYM	9.46+ 10^9/l	1.00	4.80
MON	0.09– 10^9/l	0.20	1.50
NEU	8.97 10^9/l	3.00	12.00
EOS	0.98+ 10^9/l	0.00	0.80
BAS	0.07 10^9/l	0.00	0.40
LYM%	48.3 %	0.0	100.0
MON%	0.5 %	0.0	100.0
NEU%	45.8 %	0.0	100.0
EOS%	5.0 %	0.0	100.0
BAS%	0.4 %	0.0	100.0
RBC	5.54 10^{12}/l	5.50	8.50
HGB	10.4 – g/dl	12.0	18.0
HCT	30.60 – %	37.00	55.00
MCV	55 – fl	60	77
MCH	18.8 – pg	19.5	24.5
MCHC	34.1 + g/dl	31.0	34.0
RDWc	17.9 %		
RDWs	39.8 fl		
PLT	57 – 10^9/l	200	500
MPV	10.2 fl	3.9	11.1
PCT	0.06 %		
PDWc	37.2 %		
PDWs	14.3 fl		

Diagnostic flags
Leukocytosis, Lymphocytosis, Anemia, Microcytosis, Thrombocytopenia

Figure 1 Abaxis HM5 histogram from dog 1.

CASES

Biochemical profile (performed on Day 60)

The only abnormalities are shown below.

		Reference interval
Total protein (g/dL)	**9.6**	5.3–7.2
Globulin (g/dL)	**6.2**	2.0–3.8

Serology and PCR

SNAP 4Dx positive and PCR positive for canine monocytic ehrlichiosis.

Fecal examination

Positive for hookworm eggs.

Dog 2

	Day 1	Day 7	Day 18	Day 30	Reference rang
Packed cell volume (%)	**33**	**34**	**34**	41	36–54
MCV (fL)	**57**	61	62	62	60–72
NCC ($10^3/\mu L$)	15.2	15.5	**23.5**	13.2	6.0–17.0
Segmented neutrophils ($10^3/\mu L$)	5.9	5.9	**15.1**[a]	7.0	3.0-11.5
Band neutrophils ($10^3/\mu L$)	–	–	**3.8**	–	0–0.3
Monocytes ($10^3/\mu L$)	0.9	0.5	**1.6**	0.8	0.2–1.4
Lymphocytes ($10^3/\mu L$)	**7.8**	**7.6**	3.1	**5.3**	1.0–4.8
Eosinophils ($10^3/\mu L$)	0.6	**1.6**	–	0.1	0–0.8
Platelets ($10^3/\mu L$)	304	248	**197**	325	200–500
Plasma protein (g/dL)	**11.1**	**10**	**9.1**	**10**	6.0–8.0

Hemopathology: Rouleaux present, many large granular lymphocytes on all days.
[a] Toxic segmented and band neutrophils observed on blood film on Day 18.

Biochemical profile (performed on Day 1)

The only abnormalities are shown below.

		Reference interval
Total protein (g/dL)	**9.7**	5.3–7.2
Globulin (g/dL)	**7.2**	2.0–3.8

Serology and PCR

SNAP 4Dx positive and PCR positive for canine monocytic ehrlichiosis.

Fecal examination

Positive for hookworm eggs.

Dog 3

Hematology	Day 1	Day 60	Day 90	Day 100	Ref range
Packed cell volume (%)	**23**	**31**	**28**	**33**	36–54
MCV (fL)	**57**	**59**	62	63	60–72
NCC ($10^3/\mu L$)	9.8	13.0	11.6	12.9	6.0–17.0
Segmented neutrophils ($10^3/\mu L$)	3.0	**2.9**	**2.8**	4.5	3.0–11.5
Band neutrophils ($10^3/\mu L$)	–	–	–	–	0–0.3
Monocytes ($10^3/\mu L$)	0.3	0.9	0.7	0.6	0.2–1.4
Lymphocytes ($10^3/\mu L$)	**5.3**	**8.1**	**4.9**	**6.2**	1.0–4.8
Eosinophils ($10^3/\mu L$)	**1.3**	**1.2**	0.3	**1.5**	0–0.8
Platelets ($10^3/\mu L$)	**18**[a]	**58**[a]	**98**[a]	91	200-500
Plasma protein (g/dL)	**10**	**11.5**	**11.1**	**10.6**	6.0–8.0

Hemopathology: Rouleaux present, many large granular lymphocytes.
[a] Platelet clumping on blood film noted on Days 1, 60, and 90.

Biochemical profile (performed on Day 1). The only abnormalities are shown below.

		Reference interval
Total protein (g/dL)	**9.6**	5.3–7.2
Globulin (g/dL)	**6.2**	2.0–3.8

Serology and PCR

SNAP 4Dx positive and PCR positive for canine monocytic ehrlichiosis.

Fecal examination

Positive for hookworm eggs.

Dog 1

Interpretive discussion

Hematology

The dog has a mild microcytic anemia, suggesting iron deficiency anemia secondary to chronic blood loss. Serum iron was not measured. Leukocytosis due to lymphocytosis is present. Persistent lymphocytosis could be due to a neoplastic or benign expansion of lymphocytes, and considering that the dog is positive for ehrlichiosis, this is likely the cause of a benign lymphocytosis. A mild eosinophilia is present, likely due to parasitism, in this case hookworms (see fecal examination).

The electronic platelet count on Day 1 is erroneously low due to platelet clumping, which was observed on the blood film. When platelet clumping is present, the platelet concentration is difficult to estimate, and it is possible that the dog is thrombocytopenic or that the platelet concentration is actually normal. The total plasma protein by refractometry is persistently increased, likely due to hyperglobulinemia (see chemistry section). On Day 60, there is a discrepancy of 1.5 g/dL between the plasma protein estimate by refractometry and the protein concentration on the biochemical profile. Part of the difference is due to the presence of fibrinogen in the plasma, but the discrepancy is significant, and it is likely due to an error on the plasma protein estimate, possibly due to lipemia although that was not noted. On blood film examination, an increase in large granular lymphocytes was seen, which is a common finding in dogs with ehrlichiosis. Rouleaux was observed, which is associated with increased globulin concentration. Leukergy is also associated with high globulin concentrations. The top leukocyte histogram shows the lymphocytosis, and the bottom platelet histogram shows evidence of thrombocytopenia or platelet clumping (Figure 1). Clumped platelets can also be counted as lymphocytes on some hematology analyzers.

Chemistry

The only abnormalities are increased total protein concentration and increased globulin concentration. The hyperglobulinemia is likely due to chronic antigenic stimulation as a result of ehrlichiosis. A protein electrophoresis was not performed, but the gammopathy associated with ehrlichiosis is typically polyclonal.

Dog 2

Interpretive discussion

Hematology

The laboratory data are very similar to that of dog 1 (see above). One significant difference is that on Day 18, the dog had an inflammatory leukogram as evidenced by the neutrophilia and increased band neutrophils; toxicity of neutrophils was seen, which also indicates inflammation and early release of leukocytes, and a lymphocytosis was not present on that day. She had aborted a dead puppy the previous day, and the inflammatory leukogram is likely associated with inflammation in the uterus. The decrease in lymphocytes down to the reference interval is likely due to stress (cortisol) as a result of illness. As in dog 1, there is a significant discrepancy between the plasma protein estimate and the serum protein. The cause is not apparent, but again may have been due to the presence of lipemia if the dog was not fasted prior to sampling of blood.

Dog 3

Interpretive discussion

Hematology

The laboratory data are very similar to that of dog 1 (see above).

One significant difference is that the electronic platelet count is persistently decreased. The electronic count is erroneously low due to platelet clumping on Days 1, 60, and 90. However, the dog is also thrombocytopenic on Day 100 when no platelet clumping was observed. Ehrlichiosis commonly causes a mild to moderate thrombocytopenia, likely due to immune-mediated mechanisms.

Summary

Testing for canine monocytic ehrlichiosis is warranted in dogs with unexplained persistent lymphocytosis, particularly in endemic areas. The list of causes of persistent lymphocytosis in dogs is quite short and with few exceptions is due to either leukemia, thymoma, canine monocytic ehrlichiosis, hypoadrenocorticism, and very rarely, excitement. Gammopathy is also commonly associated with canine ehrlichiosis as seen in these three dogs, and is a result of an ineffective immune response to the organism. Although all dogs were treated with doxycycline for 2 months, the lymphocytosis and gammopathy persisted following therapy.

The gammopathy is typically polyclonal. Canine monocytic ehrlichiosis, first reported in 1935, is caused by *Ehrlichia canis*, a small, cocoid, intracellular Gram-negative bacteria transmitted by *Rhipicephalus sangineus*, a ubiquitous tick. Clinical signs and lesions of canine ehrlichiosis are related to the infection and immune response produced by the host, and frequently include thrombocytopenia and occasionally neutropenia. Anecdotal reports and the experience of some clinicians and clinical pathologists suggest that lymphocyte concentrations up to 30,000 cells/μL are possible in dogs with *E canis* infection. The lymphocyte response usually consists of an increased percentage of cells with a large granular lymphocyte (LGL) phenotype, which have been shown to be CD8+ T cells. Therefore, an important differential for lymphocytosis in dogs is *E canis* infection, and unexplained lymphocytosis should prompt testing for ehrlichiosis. In our experience, approximately 15% of dogs with ehrlichiosis develop lymphocytosis.

Contributor: Dr. Mary Anna Thrall

Case 12

Signalment: 9-year-old male castrated beagle dog
History: Owner complaint of lethargy
Physical examination: Mildly enlarged peripheral lymph nodes, somewhat thin

Hematology		Reference interval
Plasma protein g/dl	7.3	6.0–8.0
PCV (%)	**32**	40–55
Hgb (g/dL)	**11.5**	13.0–20.0
RBC (×10^6/μL)	**4.80**	5.5–8.5
MCV (fL)	69	62–73
MCHC (g/dL)	35	33–36
Reticulocytes (×10^3/μL)	**49**	0–100
NCC (×10^3/μL)	**83.7**	4.5–15.0
Bands (×10^3/μL)	0	0–0.2
Neutrophils (×10^3/μL)	**16.7**	2.6–11.0
Lymphocytes (×10^3/μL)	**64.4**	1.0–4.8
Monocytes (×10^3/μL)	1.6	0.2–1.0
Eosinophils (×10^3/μL)	0.1	0.1–1.2
NRBC (×10^3/μL)	**0.8**	0
Platelets (×10^3/μL)	**139**	200–500
MPV (fL)	**11.4**	7.5–14.6

Hemopathology noted on blood film:
- Many of the lymphoid cells are large with fine chromatin and classified as prolymphocytes and lymphoblasts.
- No platelet clumps found.

Interpretive discussion

There is marked leukocytosis with the predominant abnormality being marked lymphocytosis. Further, the morphology indicates the presence of large lymphocyte forms. The magnitude of lymphocytosis is clearly interpreted as lymphocytic leukemia, with morphologic features of a blastic form that some would term "acute." There is a mild mature neutrophilia and monocytosis that is difficult to interpret. These could be related to steroid release, with neoplastic lymphocytosis masking the expected steroid-induced lymphopenia. Alternatively, there may be a compensated inflammatory stimulus. There is a disproportionate number of NRBC that may be related to either marrow and/or splenic injury associated with lymphoma/Leukemia.

The erythrocyte values indicate mild anemia. The anemia is poorly regenerative as indicated by the reticulocyte concentration. There is mild thrombocytopenia. The presence of two cell lines that potentially have decreased production along with evidence of leukemia suggests that marrow may be involved.

Summary

The pattern present is characteristic of lymphocytic leukemia. Cytometric analysis is recommended if treatment is considered.

CASES

Case 13

Signalment: 8-year-old DSH neutered female cat
History: Lethargy and anorexia for 3 days
Physical examination: Slightly dehydrated

Hematology:		Reference interval
Packed cell volume (%)	35	25–45
RBC ($10^6/\mu L$)	8.39	5–10
MCV (fL)	41	39–50
MCHC(g/dL)	32	32–36
Nucleated cells ($\mu L \times 10^3$)	**32.1**	5.5–19.5
Segmented neutrophils ($\mu L \times 10^3$)	6.4	2.5–12.5
Band neutrophils ($\mu L \times 10^3$)	1	0–0.3
Lymphocytes ($\mu L \times 10^3$)	**25.0**	1.5–7.0
Monocytes ($\mu L \times 10^3$)	**1.5**	0–0.8
Eosinophils ($\mu L \times 10^3$)	–	0–1.5
Nucleated RBCs ($\mu L \times 10^3$)	–	0
Platelets ($\mu L \times 10^3$)	114	150–700

An image of the blood film is shown below (Figure 1).

Biochemical profile (only abnormality is shown below)

Total bilirubin (mg/dL)	1.1	0–0.3

Interpretive discussion

Hematology

A leukocytosis is present due to lymphocytosis. The concentration of lymphocytes is very suggestive of leukemia, assuming that the cat was not excited. An excitement lymphocytosis can rarely result in a lymphocytosis of this magnitude. Examination of the blood film reveals that the lymphocytes range from 8 to 25 um in diameter and have scant to abundant pale to deep basophilic cytoplasm,

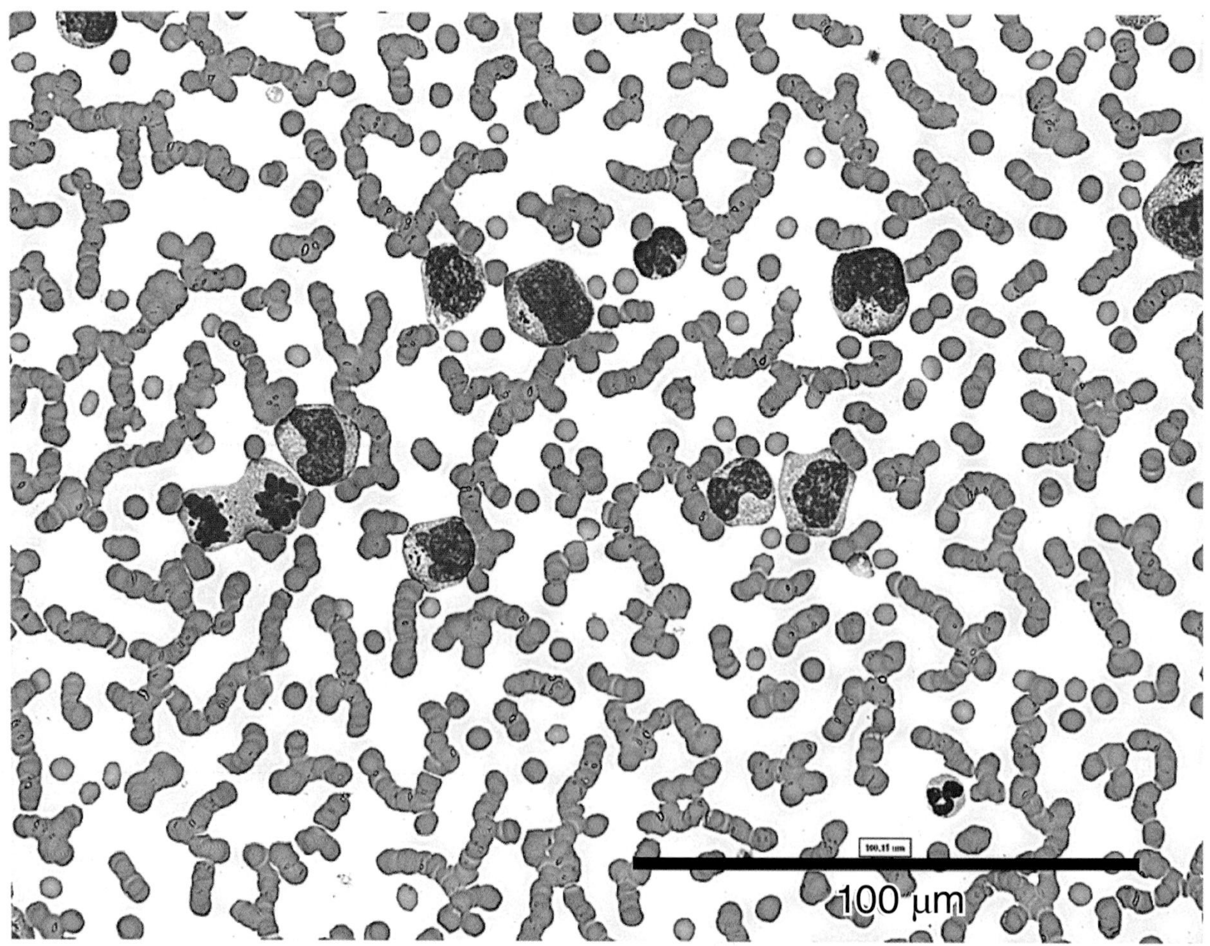

Figure 1 Almost all leukocytes are large granular lymphocytes. Note mitotic figure at left. Marked rouleaux is present.

containing round, small to large azurophilic, irregularly distributed granules, large pleomorphic nuclei with coarsely clumped chromatin and often prominent nucleoli. Cytoplasmic fragments containing azurophilic granules are occasionally observed as well as rare bizarre cells in mitoses. The granules in the lymphocytes are characteristic of those seen in large granular lymphocytes (LGLs).

Rouleaux is increased, which is typically due to increased globulin concentration, but the globulin concentration was normal in this cat.

Biochemical profile

The only abnormality was an increase in bilirubin. This is likely not due to increased erythrocyte destruction, as the PCV is normal. Liver disease or cholestasis remain as differentials, and without any other biochemical abnormalities, it would be difficult to determine which of these are resulting in the abnormality.

Summary and outcome

Flow cytometry of blood revealed that the neoplastic LGLs were CD3 and CD8 positive, indicating that they are T cells. Chemotherapy was instituted, and the lymphocyte concentration decreased for a period of time, followed by an increase to 64 000/μL, at which time severe anemia and thrombocytopenia were present. The patient's condition suddenly declined and the owner elected humane euthanasia. Autopsy was not performed.

Large granular lymphocytes (LGLs) are a morphologically distinct subset of lymphocytes characterized by intracytoplasmic azurophilic granules. LGLs are normally a minor component of blood lymphocytes but are the most common subset of lymphocytes in intestine. LGL expansion in dogs can be reactive and benign, such as seen with canine ehrlichiosis (see cases 10 and 11), or neoplastic, such as is seen in acute or chronic leukemias, and primary lymphomas. In cats, LGL neoplasia is usually aggressive, with a mean survival time of approximately 3 months. Almost all cats with LGL leukemia have neoplastic infiltrates in the intestine, most commonly the jejunum, and most also have infiltrates in the mesenteric lymph nodes and liver, and some have infiltrates in the spleen, kidneys, and bone marrow. The leukemia is usually secondary to the LGL intestinal lymphoma. Approximately 30% of intestinal lymphoma in cats have an LGL morphology, which may be missed on histopathology with H&E stains. The majority of cats with LGL lymphoma have increased serum bilirubin concentration, as did our patient, likely due to liver involvement.

Contributor: Dr. Mary Anna Thrall

CASES

Case 14

Signalment and history: 9-year-old male castrated dog presented for lethargy

Hematology		Reference interval
PCV (%)	**36**	37–55
RBC (×10^6/μL)	**5.42**	5.5–8.5
Hgb (g/dL)	13.2	12–18
MCV (fL)	66	60–72
MCHC (g/dL)	37	34–38
Retics (×10^3/μL)	0	0–60,000
NCC (×10^3/μL)	**96.4**	6.0–17.0
Metas (×10^3/μL)	–	0
Bands (×10^3/μL)	**7.7**	0–0.3
Segs (×10^3/μL)	**82.9**	3.0–11.5
Lymphs (×10^3/μL)	1.0	1.0–4.8
Monos (×10^3/μL)	**4.8**	0.2–1.4
Eos (×10^3/μL)	–	0.1–1.2
NRBCs (×10^3/μL)	–	0
Platelets (×10^3/μL)	**39**	200–500
TP (P) (g/dL)	6.2	6.0–8.0

Hemopathology: Decreased platelets, giant platelets, toxic neutrophils, numerous echinocytes, occasional schistocyte.

Interpretive discussion

Packed cell volume and hemoglobin are slightly decreased, indicating mild anemia.

Reticulocytes are not increased, indicating that the anemia is nonregenerative. Considering the inflammatory leukogram, this is most likely an anemia of inflammatory disease.

Marked neutrophilia with increased immature neutrophils and monocytosis is indicative of a chronic inflammatory leukogram.

Lymphopenia is indicative of a stress or steroid component to the leukogram.

Platelets are decreased. Thrombocytopenia is most commonly due to ehrlichiosis, immune-mediated thrombocytopenia or DIC. This should trigger other coagulation tests. The presence of giant platelets suggests that immature platelets are being released by the bone marrow, and the thrombocytopenia is not due to bone marrow dysfunction.

Summary

Anemia of inflammatory disease. Site of inflammation was a prostatic abscess. DIC was confirmed.

Case 15

Signalment: 4-year-old Doberman
History: Acutely ill, vomiting
Physical examination: Pendulous abdomen

Hematology	Day 1[a]	Day 2	Reference interval
PCV (%)	50	**20**	37–55
Hgb (g/dL)	18.3	**7.5**	12–18
RBC ($\times 10^6/\mu L$)	7.70	**3.11**	5.5–8.5
MCV (fL)	66	66	60–72
MCHC (g/dL)	36	37	34–38
Retics ($\times 10^3/\mu L$)	ND	**124**	<60
NCC ($\times 10^3/\mu L$)	6.6	14.7	6–17
Segs ($\times 10^3/\mu L$)	**0.4**	4.1	3–11.5
Bands ($\times 10^3/\mu L$)	**3.1**	**7.9**	0–0.3
Metas ($\times 10^3/\mu L$)	**0.1**	**1.5**	0
Monos ($\times 10^3/\mu L$)	0.5	0.3	0.1–1.3
Lymphs ($\times 10^3/\mu L$)	2.1	**0.4**	1–4.8
Eos ($\times 10^3/\mu L$)	0.1	0.1	0.1–1.2
Platelets ($\times 10^3/\mu L$)	**193**	**90**	200–500
TP (P) (g/dL)	**5.9**	**4.0**	6–8

Hemopathology: Marked toxic neutrophils on Days 1 and 2.
[a] Had abdominal exploratory surgery the evening of Day 1; treated with fluids between Day 1 and Day 2.

Biochemical profile	Day 1[a]	Day 2	Reference interval
Gluc	**26**	**36**	75–130
BUN (mg/dL)	**45**	**62**	7–28
Creat (mg/dL)	**0.6**	**1.8**	0.9–1.7
Ca (mg/dL)	**8.2**	**7.6**	9.0–11.2
Phos (mg/dL)	5.9	**11.0**	2.8–6.1
TP (g/dL)	**4.5**	**2.6**	5.4–7.4
Alb (g/dL)	**1.8**	**1.0**	2.7–4.5
Glob (g/dL)	2.7	**1.0**	1.9–3.4
T. bili (mg/dL)	0.1	**3.0**	0–0.4
Chol (mg/dL)	145	140	130–370
ALT (IU/L)	20	**328**	10–120
AST (IU/L)	**77**	**775**	16–40
ALP (IU/L)	208	**440**	35–280
GGT	1	1	0–6
Na (mEq/L)	**136**	143	145–158
K (mEq/L)	4.1	5.8	4.1–5.5
CL (mEq/L)	**100**	106	106–127
TCO_2 (mEq/L)	**9.4**	19.4	14–27
An. gap (mEq/L)	**31**	23	8–25

[a] Had abdominal exploratory surgery the evening of Day 1; treated with fluids between Day 1 and Day 2.

Abdominal fluid analysis	
NCC (/µL)	**93 000**
TP (g/dL)	1.5

Cytology: 100% degenerate neutrophils; various types of bacteria phagocytized and extracellular.

Interpretive discussion

Hematology

Packed cell volume, Hemoglobin, Red blood cell count: Within or near reference intervals on Day 1, markedly decreased on Day 2 following blood loss that occurred at the time of surgery. Dog seemed to bleed excessively during the surgery, and given the breed, Von Willebrand disease should be investigated. Anemia may have also 'worsened' with aggressive fluid therapy resulting in hemodilution.

Reticulocytes are increased on Day 2, indicating that the anemia is regenerative. This regenerative response is earlier than is typically seen, in that reticulocytes do not usually increase until 24–72 hours following the onset of anemia.

Neutropenia is present on Day 1, with an increase in immature neutrophils, indicating in this case that the mature neutrophils are being consumed in an inflammatory process, and the marrow is not meeting the consumption demand. On Day 2, the mature neutrophils have increased, as have the immature neutrophils (bands and metamyelocytes). This indicates that the consumptive process has decreased (source of inflammation) or that the marrow has increased production, or both.

Lymphopenia is indicative of a stress or steroid component to the leukogram.

Platelets are mildly decreased on Day 1 and more markedly decreased on Day 2. While some platelets may have been consumed in clotting process secondary to surgery related blood loss, it is also possible that the animal has DIC, particularly with the history of excessive bleeding during surgery. This should trigger additional tests such as FDPs, PT, aPTT, and activated clotting time.

Total protein: Total protein is decreased on Day 1 and Day 2. In this patient, this is likely due to loss into the abdominal cavity on Day 1, compounded by blood loss on Day 2. Fluid administration may also be diluting the PCV and plasma protein on Day 2.

Biochemical profile

The serum glucose concentration is markedly decreased, both on Day 1 and Day 2. In this patient, considering the leukogram, this is most likely due to sepsis. Other differentials should include insulinoma, although this is a relatively young dog for an insulinoma.

The BUN is increased on both Day 1 and Day 2, and the serum creatinine is increased on Day 2. This may be either prerenal azotemia or renal azotemia. A urinalysis was not performed.

The serum calcium is decreased on both Days 1 and 2, due to the hypoalbuminemia.

The serum phosphorus concentration is increased on Day 2 and is compatible with decreased glomerular filtration rate.

The serum total protein concentration is decreased due to hypoalbuminemia on Day 1, and both hypoalbuminemia and hypoglobulinemia on Day 2 (see explanation above).

The serum bilirubin concentration is increased on Day 2, likely due to cholestasis related to septicemia.

The ALT and AST activity on Day 2 indicates hepatocellular injury, possibly related to anemia, shock, surgery, or septicemia.

The ALP activity is increased on Day 2, possibly related to endogenous corticosteroids or cholestasis.

Both sodium and chloride are decreased on Day 1, possibly due to loss of electrolytes into abdominal effusion, or loss due to vomiting.

Serum total CO_2 is decreased on Day 1, suggesting metabolic acidosis. This has been corrected by Day 2, likely due to fluid therapy.

The anion gap is increased on Day 1, likely due to lactic acid.

Abdominal fluid

The nucleated cell count is very high and all of the cells present are neutrophils, indicating suppurative inflammation or peritonitis. The total protein may be low because the serum protein is decreased, or it may he diluted in the large volume of fluid. The presence of different types of bacteria suggests that the source of bacteria is the gastrointestinal tract.

Summary

This dog had a consumptive inflammatory leukogram and hypoglycemia due to sepsis. On exploratory, the abdominal cavity contained 1400 ml of fluid, and a toothpick was found to have perforated the intestine. Dog died on the evening of Day 2 as a result of septic peritonitis.

Case 16

Signalment: 11-year-old female spayed border terrier dog

History: Owner noticed intermittent nose bleeds for a few days

Physical examination: Few petechial hemorrhages noted on mucous membranes, otherwise normal

Hematology		Reference interval
Plasma protein (g/dL)	**6.2**	6.0–8.0
PCV (%)	**24**	40–55
Hgb (g/dL)	**8.4**	12.0–18.0
RBC ($\times 10^6/\mu L$)	**3.34**	5.5–8.5
MCV (fL)	72	62–73
MCHC (g/dL)	35	33–36
Reticulocytes ($\times 10^3/\mu L$)	**149**	<60
NCC ($\times 10^3/\mu L$)	11.5	4.5–15.0
Bands ($\times 10^3/\mu L$)	0.1	0–0.2
Neutrophils ($\times 10^3/\mu L$)	9.0	2.6–11.0
Lymphocytes ($\times 10^3/\mu L$)	1.4	1.0–4.8
Monocytes ($\times 10^3/\mu L$)	0.7	0.2–1.0
Eosinophils ($\times 10^3/\mu L$)	0.1	0.1–1.2
NRBC ($\times 10^3/\mu L$)	0.2	0
Platelets ($\times 10^3/\mu L$)	**7**	200–500
MPV (fL)	**22**	7.5–14.6

Hemopathology noted on blood film:
- Moderate polychromasia.
- No platelet clumps found.
- Few macroplatelets on scanning.

Interpretive discussion

The erythrocyte values indicate moderate anemia. The anemia is regenerative as indicated by reticulocytosis, along with a few nucleated red cells. While the plasma protein concentration is seemingly normal, there is a reasonable probability it is decreased for this patient. The reason is that older dogs tend to have higher protein concentrations and 6.2 is regarded as low normal; the dog may have had a protein between 7 and 8 g/dL before bleeding occurred. The triad of anemia, regeneration, and decreasing protein is classical for blood loss.

The cause of the blood loss is thrombocytopenia. This magnitude of thrombocytopenia is expected to result in both petechial hemorrhages and blood loss that may not be physically visible.

Examination of the data from the bone marrow perspective indicates that the marrow is producing erythrocytes (regeneration) and neutrophils appropriately. The thrombocytopenia present is therefore a selective, specific cytopenia. When present at this magnitude, typically less than $20 \cdot 10^3/\mu L$, immune-mediated thrombocytopenia is by far the most likely cause or diagnosis. Furthermore, the increased mean platelet volume (MPV) corroborated by macroplatelets on the blood film suggests accelerated marrow thrombopoiesis. This is the expected response to a consumptive thrombocytopenia.

Summary

The pattern present is characteristic of immune-mediated thrombocytopenia, with bone marrow response to hemorrhage.

Case 17

Signalment: 14-year-old castrated male mixed-breed dog
History: Polydipsia and polyuria, bloody diarrhea, weight loss
Physical examination: Lethargic, bilateral masses in perianal region

Hematology		Reference interval
Packed cell volume (%)	**33**	37–55
Hemoglobin (g/dL)	**11.1**	12–18
RBC ($10^6/\mu L$)	5.77	5.5–8.5
MCV (fL)	**57**	60–72
MCHC (g/dL)	34	34–38
Total nucleated cell count ($\times 10^3/\mu L$)	5.6	6–17
Segmented neutrophils ($\times 10^3/\mu L$)	4.6	3–11.5
Monocytes ($\times 10^3/\mu L$)	0.7	0.2–1.4
Lymphocytes ($\times 10^3/\mu L$)	**0.6**	1–4.8
Platelets ($\times 10^3/\mu L$)	190	200–500
Plasma protein (g/dL)	**11.4**	6–8
Hemopathology: Marked rouleaux		

Biochemical profile		
Glucose (mg/dL)	93	65–122
Blood urea nitrogen (mg/dL)	19	7–28
Creatinine (mg/dL)	1.2	0.6–1.5
Calcium (mg/dL)	**14**	9.0–11.2
Phosphorus (mg/dL)	6.0	2.8–6.1
Total protein (g/dL)	**12.0**	5.4–7.4
Albumin (g/dL)	**1.7**	2.7–4.5
Globulin (g/dL)	**10.3**	1.9–3.4
Total bilirubin (mg/dL)	0.4	0–0.4
Cholesterol	154	130–300
Alanine aminotransferase (IU/L)	49	10–120
Aspartate aminotransferase (IU/L)	**41**	16–40
Alkaline phosphatase (IU/L)	**249**	18–141
Gamma glutamyltransferase (IU/L)	5	0–6
Sodium (mEq/L)	144	145–158
Potassium (mEq/L)	4.2	4.1–5.5
Chloride (mEq/L)	117	106–127
HCO_3 (mEq/L)	**13.1**	14–27
Anion gap	18	8–25

Urinalysis (cystocentesis)		Urine sediment	
Color	pale yellow	WBCs/hpf	0–1
Transparency	clear	RBCs/hpf	0–1
Specific Gravity	**1.012**	Epithelial cells/hpf	0
pH	5.0	Casts/lpf	0
Glucose	neg	Crystals	few amorphous
Bilirubin	neg	Bacteria	0
Blood	1+		
Protein	**3+**		
Ketones	neg		

Serum protein electrophoresis tracing

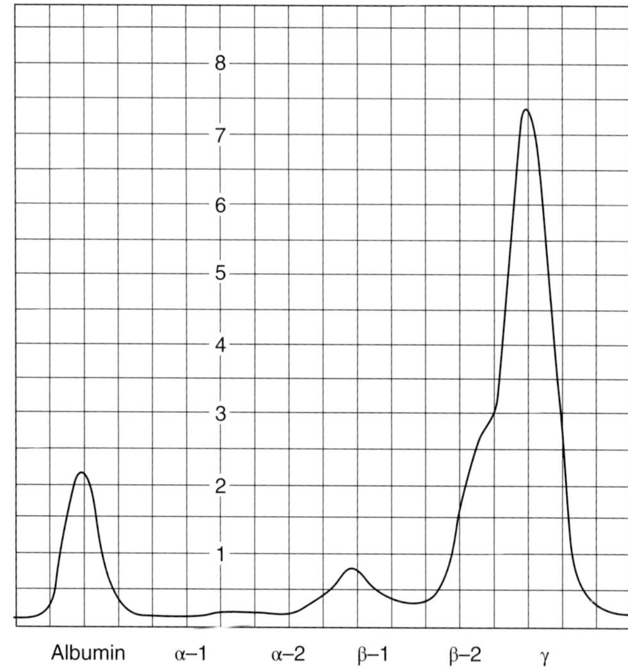

Interpretive discussion

Hematology

There is a mild normochromic, microcytic anemia that appears nonregenerative (no increased polychromasia is noted on the blood film). A reticulocyte count should be done to confirm this. In a sick dog, anemia of chronic disease should be considered; however, anemia of chronic disease is not usually microcytic. Given that the dog has bloody diarrhea, iron deficiency due to GI blood loss should also be considered as a cause of the microcytosis.

The lymphopenia suggests a stress/steroid response, although the expected neutrophilia is not observed. The slight thrombocytopenia is not clinically significant. Marked rouleaux seen on the blood film is related to the markedly increased plasma protein concentration (discussed further below).

Biochemical profile

The increased total protein concentration is due to marked hyperglobulinemia. This degree of hyperglobulinemia is usually caused by lymphoid neoplasia (such as multiple myeloma) but can also be seen with ehrlichiosis in dogs. A serum protein electrophoresis is indicated to evaluate for monoclonal versus polyclonal gammopathy (discussed later), and evaluation for tick-borne diseases should be pursued. The albumin concentration is moderately decreased, which may be from decreased production in response to the hyperglobulinemia. However, there is also evidence for urinary protein loss that may be contributing to the hypoalbuminemia.

The other significant abnormality present is hypercalcemia. Since this dog has palpable perianal masses and adenocarcinoma of the anal sac is a common cause of paraneoplastic hypercalcemia in dogs, aspiration cytology or biopsy of those masses should be performed. Hypercalcemia may also accompany lymphoid neoplasia, which is another possible differential in this dog based on the hyperglobulinemia. Ionized calcium could be measured to confirm the hypercalcemia but was not done in this case.

The slight increase in ALP suggests induction due to cholestasis or steroids. Decreased bicarbonate concentration with a normal anion gap is consistent with a secretional metabolic acidosis, and can be explained by the diarrhea (GI loss of bicarbonate).

Urinalysis

The urine is in the isosthenuric range, which can be explained by the hypercalcemia. Hypercalcemia interferes with ADH action in the renal tubules, preventing adequate urine concentration and causing polyuria with polydipsia. The pH is acid, consistent with the metabolic acidosis. The 3+ protein is significant given the urine specific gravity and inactive sediment. A urine protein: creatinine ratio could have been performed but was not in this case. Possibilities for the proteinuria include a prerenal proteinuria due to glomerular overload (paraproteinuria associated with multiple myeloma) or renal proteinuria due to glomerular disease.

Serum protein electrophoresis

There is a distinct monoclonal peak in the gamma region, suggestive of a neoplastic monoclonal gammopathy. However, some cases of canine ehrlichiosis have apparent monoclonal gammopathies, so further diagnostics are warranted to confirm lymphoid neoplasia.

Summary

The hypercalcemia was consistent with the clinical suspicion of anal sac adenocarcinoma, but the hyperglobulinemia suggested a second pathologic process. Fine needle aspirates of the perianal masses were consistent with anal sac adenocarcinoma, which was later confirmed by surgical removal and histopathology. Radiographs of the thoracic cavity showed no evidence of pulmonary metastases, however pathologic fracture of the right 6th rib was identified. Pending tickborne disease titers, a bone marrow aspirate was performed and was diagnostic for plasma cell myeloma (61% of marrow cells were plasma cells). An immunoelectrophoresis identified the paraprotein as IgA. Ehrlichial titers were negative. This dog was treated with melphalan and prednisone, and did well at home for about 1 year.

CASES

Case 18

Signalment: 14-month-old 23 kg male Belgian Malinois dog

History: Stung by approximately 200 honeybees 30 minutes prior to admission

Physical examination: Ataxia, vomiting, pruritis, and submandibular and ear edema on presentation. On Day 2 the dog exhibited severe ataxia, hematuria, hematemesis, and hematochezia.

Hematology	Day 1	Day 2	Day 4	Reference interval
Packed cell volume (%)	**60**	**36**	**14**	37–55
RBC (×10^6/μL)	7.64	5.59	**2.15**	5.5–8.5
Hgb (g/dL)	**20.3**	13.6	**6.2**	12–18
MCV (fL)	**>77**	69	71	60–72
MCHC (g/dL)	34.4	35	**40.3**	31–36
NCC (10^3/μL)	**28.1**	**52.3**	**21.5**	6.0–17.0
Segmented neutrophils (10^3/μL)	**22.1**[a]	**36.1**	**14.9**	3.0-11.5
Band neutrophils (10^3/μL)	–	**1.0**	**1.9**	0–0.3
Metamyelocytes (10^3/μL)	–	–	**0.4**	0
Monocytes (10^3/μL)	0.8	**3.7**	1.3	0.2–1.4
Lymphocytes (10^3/μL)	3.7	**8.4**	2.6	1.0–4.8
Eosinophils (10^3/μL)	**1.4**	**1.6**	–	0.1–1.2
Platelets (10^3/μL)	**170**[b]	**32**	**20**	200-500
Plasma protein by refractometry (g/dL)	**8.5**	**5.2**	6.0	6.0–8.0

Plasma was red in color every day, indicating hemoglobinemia.
[a] Numerous degenerate neutrophils seen on blood film.
[b] Platelet clumping seen on blood film.

The only serum biochemical abnormality was an increased serum bilirubin on Day 2 (**0.8 mg/dL**; reference interval 0.1–0.6 mg/dL).

aPTT and PT were performed and were within normal limits.

Urinalysis (Day 2)

Color	**Red**
Transparency	**Opaque**
Sp. gr.	1.025
Protein	**2+**
Glucose	Neg
Bilirubin	Neg
Blood	**4+**
Sediment	Normal

Photomicrographs of blood films from Day 1 and 4 are shown in Figures 1 and 2.

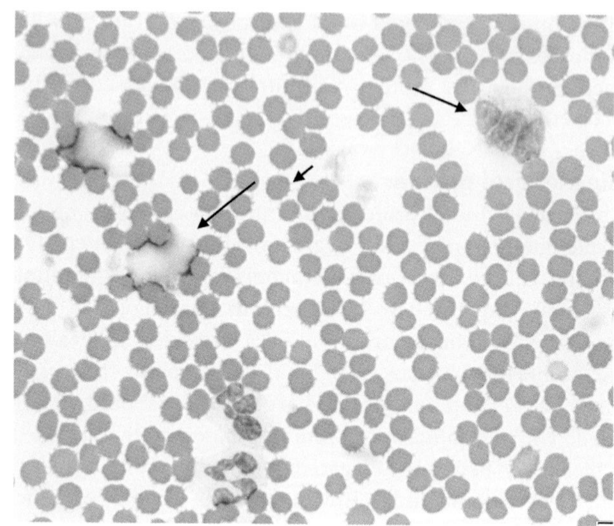

Figure 1 Blood film from Day 1. Note that all erythrocytes are echinospherocytes (small arrow). Degenerate neutrophils were numerous (large arrows).

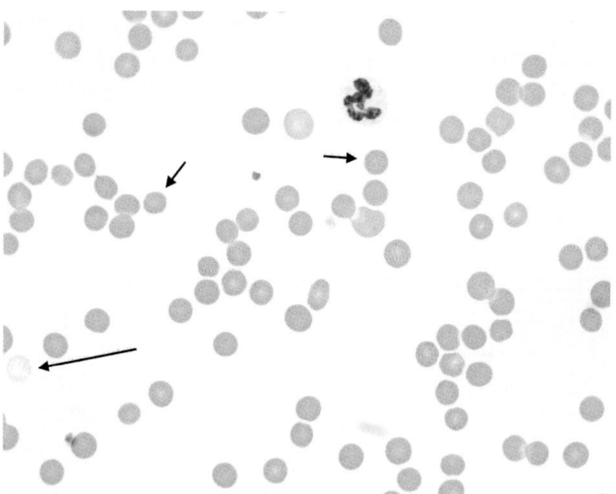

Figure 2 Blood film from Day 4. Note the lack of density of erythrocytes in the counting area, indicating severe anemia. Most erythrocytes are spherocytes (small arrows). Occasional lysed erythrocytes (ghost cells) are present (large arrow).

Interpretive discussion

CBC

The PCV is increased on admission, and echinospherocytes are present on the blood film. By Day 4, a marked hemolytic anemia is present, and spherocytes and lysed erythrocytes are seen. Echinospherocyte and spherocyte formation has been reported with snake envenomation and bee envenomation. While spherocyte formation is usually associated with immune-mediated hemolytic anemia, it is likely that the spherocytosis and hemolysis associated with acute massive bee envenomation are not due to immune-mediated mechanisms. Two of the primary components of bee venom, melittin, and phospholipase A_2 (PLA_2), have been shown to induce hemolysis, both *in vivo* and *in vitro*, through a mechanism associated with echinocyte formation at low doses and spherocyte formation at higher doses. However, delayed hemolytic anemia could be due to antibody formation against altered erythrocyte membranes. The PLA_2 in bee venom is very similar to that found in snake venom and also causes type III echinocytosis and spherocytosis. The decreases in red blood count and hemoglobin concentration on Day 4 are also indicative of severe anemia.

The MCV is markedly increased on Day 1. Polychromasia was not present, suggesting that the increased MCV was due to erythrocyte swelling. The decreased MCV in our patient on Day 2 may have been due to the effects of melittin. In addition to spectrin stiffening, the changes in morphology could be due to leakage of ATP through melittin-induced pores; ATP depletion also triggers echinocytosis and spherocytosis.

The MCHC is erroneously increased on Day 4, likely due to hemolysis.

An inflammatory leukogram is present, as indicated by the neutrophilia on Days 1, 2, and 4, and presence of band neutrophils on Day 2 and 4 and metamyelocytes on Day 4. The monocytosis on Day 2 is also likely due to inflammation. A lymphocytosis is present on Day 2, possibly from antigenic stimulation.

The platelets are markedly decreased on Days 2 and 4. DIC was excluded as a cause based on the normal aPTT and PT. The thrombocytopenia may be immune mediated and has been previously described in dogs, horses, and humans with massive bee envenomation. However, it is also possible that platelet destruction occurs as a direct result of the cytotoxic effects of PLA_2 and melittin, both of which induce mitochondrial breakdown resulting in platelet apoptosis. Autoantibodies can be formed against altered platelet membranes, and an immune-mediated mechanism has been shown to be involved in the removal of apoptotic platelets. Thrombocytopenia is also often associated with rattlesnake envenomation.

The plasma protein is increased on Day 1, likely due to hemoconcentration. It is slightly below normal on Day 2 following fluid therapy.

Chemistry

The hyperbilirubinemia is compatible with increased erythrocyte destruction.

Urinalysis

Abnormalities include the present of protein and blood. Because of the normal sediment, and red coloration of plasma, the positive blood reading is due to hemoglobinuria.

Summary and outcome

Spherocytosis, hemolytic anemia and thrombocytopenia were associated with massive bee envenomation. Over 200 stingers were removed, and the dog was treated with IV fluids, glucocorticoids, antihistamine, a narcotic for pain, epinephrine, an H2 receptor antagonist, an antiemetic, and a cephalosporin antibiotic. The dog made a full recovery and the CBC was normal 1 month later.

Contributor: Dr. Mary Anna Thrall

Case 19

Signalment: 1-month old foal
History: Presented for progressive coughing and pyrexia
Physical examination: Increased respiratory effort, tachypnea and tachycardia

Hematology		Reference range
Packed cell volume (%)	**15**	32–53
RBC (×10^6/μL)	**5.53**	6.8–12.9
Hgb (g/dL)	**5.8**	11–19
MCV (fL)	**27**	37–59
MCHC (g/dL)	**38.7**	31–38.6
NCC (10^3/μL)	**57.9**	5.4–14.3
Segmented neutrophils (10^3/μL)	**50.33**	2.26–8.85
Band neutrophils (10^3/μL)	**2.0**	0.0–0.1
Monocytes (10^3/μL)	**2.0**	0.0–1.0
Lymphocytes (10^3/μL)	3.5	1.5–7.7
Platelets (10^3/μL)	**78**	100–350
Plasma protein by refractometry (g/dL)	**5.6**	5.8–8.7
Fibrinogen (g/dL)	0.4	0.1–0.4

Hemopathology: Moderate neutrophil toxicity.

Biochemical profile		Reference range
Glucose (mg/dL)	84	83–113
Blood urea nitrogen (mg/dL)	**97**	8–23
Creatinine (mg/dL)	**3.3**	0.8–1.8
Calcium (mg/dL)	**10.4**	11.5–13.1
Phosphorus (mg/dL)	**9.5**	1.8–3.6
Total protein (g/dL)	**5.0**	6.3–8.1
Albumin (g/dL)	**1.7**	3.5–4.4
Globulin (g/dL)	3.3	2.4–4.1
Total bilirubin (mg/dL)	2.6	0.2–2.8
AST (IU/L)	**149**	175–394
GGT (IU/L)	**9**	10–22
CK (IU/L)	**573**	109–456
Triglyceride (mg/dL)	**542**	10–63
Sodium (mEq/L)	**121**	134–145
Potassium (mEq/L)	4.4	3.3–4.6
Chloride (mEq/L)	**83**	96–106
Bicarbonate (mEq/L)	**11**	26–35
Anion gap (mEq/L)	**31**	8–16

Hematology

A marked anemia is present with no overt evidence of regeneration. Rather, the MCV is decreased and may be due to analyzer artifact due to the patient's hypo-osmolar state. More likely, the decreased MCV is due to iron deficiency commonly seen in neonates. Foals may remain microcytic up to 1 year of age [1]. An increased MCHC is not physiologically possible and reflects artifact, possibly due to hyperlipidemia. Causes for the anemia are not overt but concurrent hypoproteinemia could suggest blood loss, although a component of anemia of inflammatory disease, chronic renal failure or iron deficiency cannot be excluded. Serum iron is indicated.

An inflammatory leukogram is present and characterized by a marked neutrophilia with left-shift, toxic change and mild monocytosis. The marked neutrophilia is consistent with inflammation. Interestingly, the fibrinogen is within normal limits, which could indicate either excess consumption in DIC or decreased production with hepatic insufficiency, although there is minimal evidence of the latter.

Mild thrombocytopenia could reflect blood loss/hemorrhage or consumption due to severe inflammation (DIC). Consumption is also supported by the seemingly 'normal' fibrinogen considering severe inflammation, raising concern the fibrinogen along with platelets are being consumed in DIC.

Chemistry

A moderate azotemia is present and characterized by an increase in creatinine and disproportionate increase in BUN. This discrepancy may be due to decreased muscle mass (lower creatinine) or gastrointestinal bleeding (increased BUN). Notwithstanding, these changes indicate a decrease in GFR and could reflect prerenal (dehydration) or renal disease in this case. A urine specific gravity would be required to assess concentrating ability. Concurrent hyperphosphatemia is explained by decreased GFR but does not indicate the type of azotemia. Furthermore, in a growing animal such as this, increased phosphorus can be seen with bone growth.

The mild hypocalcemia is most likely due to decreased protein binding (hypoalbuminemia) and an ionized calcium is recommended to confirm this. If ionized calcium is also decreased, differentials to consider include sepsis and gastrointestinal or renal losses. The Ca × P product is calculated to be 99 mg/dL, indicating that soft-tissue mineralization may be occurring.

Hypoproteinemia is characterized by a hypoalbuminemia, which could be due to decreased production (negative acute phase protein), protein losing nephropathy or enteropathy, blood loss, and third spacing (effusions). A urinalysis with a urine protein to creatinine ratio may help rule in or out a protein losing nephropathy. A protein losing enteropathy is made less likely given the globulins are within normal limits, however, concurrent inflammation may be increasing the globulin into the reference range.

Decreased AST and GGT activities are unlikely to be significant. A very mild increase in CK activity is not clinically significant but could indicate mild muscle damage.

The most common cause of hypertriglyceridemia in horses, and the most likely in this case, is a negative energy balance leading to subsequent lipolysis and formation of VLDLs. While not mentioned in the history, this animal may have been anorexic in combination with the increased energy demand associated with massive inflammation.

The corrected chloride is calculated to be 96 mEq/l indicating a proportional hyponatremia and hypochloremia with differentials to consider including gastrointestinal losses (diarrhea), third spacing (cavitary effusion), or excessive free water gain (thirst response). Electrolyte losses through excessive sweating, while possible, are less likely given the potassium is within normal limits.

Decreased bicarbonate and an increased anion gap indicate a titrational metabolic acidosis with increased unmeasured anions. The most likely cause in this patient is accumulation of uremic acids and lactate. A lactate measurement is indicated.

Summary and outcome

Laboratory results reveal anemia, inflammation, possible renal disease and raises concern for DIC and sepsis. Additional testing in this patient should include a coagulation panel, urinalysis, blood gas and lactate measurement.

Despite medical management and aggressive fluid therapy, this patient failed to produce urine and died in hospital. Necropsy revealed necrotizing, suppurative pneumonia and enterocolitis. *Rhodococcus equi* was cultured from the lung abscess. Histopathology failed to reveal abnormalities in the kidneys; however, acute injury was still suspected.

Contributor: Drs. Alex Mau and Saundra Sample

Case 20

Signalment: 10-year-old neutered male mixed-breed dog from Missouri

History: Presented acutely obtunded and laterally recumbent with a markedly edematous and swollen right forelimb with two large puncture wounds

Physical examination: Pale mucus membranes, CRT 2–3 seconds, poor pulses, tachypnea (RR 56 bpm), tachycardia (HR 168 bpm)

Bloodwork provided is after 24 hours of hospitalization

Hematology		Reference range
Sample condition	Moderate icterus	
Hematocrit (%)	**24.5**	37.2–56.4
Hemoglobin (g/dL)	**7.6**	13.3–20.8
RBC ($\times 10^6/\mu L$)	**3.14**	5.29–8.34
MCV (fL)	**78.0**	62.5–72.9
MCH (pg)	24.2	22.4–26.2
MCHC (g/dL)	**31.0**	34.2–37.9
RDW (%)	14.7	12.9–19.4
Abs Reticulocyte ($\times 10^3/\mu L$)	**163.9**	15.1–123.9
Total white blood cell count, corrected ($\times 10^3/\mu L$)	**25.94**	4.08–14.60
Segmented neutrophils ($\times 10^3/\mu L$)	**22.44**	2.27–10.60
Band neutrophils ($\times 10^3/\mu L$)	**1.04**	0.0–0.18
Lymphocytes ($\times 10^3/\mu L$)	1.69	0.83–4.80
Monocytes ($\times 10^3/\mu L$)	0.65	0.05–1.24
Eosinophils ($\times 10^3/\mu L$)	0.13	0.07–1.40
Nucleated RBCs/100 WBC	**14.0**	0.0–1.0
Platelets ($\times 10^3/\mu L$)	**64**	140–350
MPV (fL)	12.1	8.7–12.8
PCT (%)	**0.06**	0.17–0.39
Plasma protein (g/dL)	**3.8**	6.0–7.9

Hemopathology: Moderate polychromasia, moderate anisocytosis, mild codocytosis, marked echinocytosis, moderate neutrophil toxicity, few reactive lymphocytes, few small platelet clumps seen, few giant platelets.

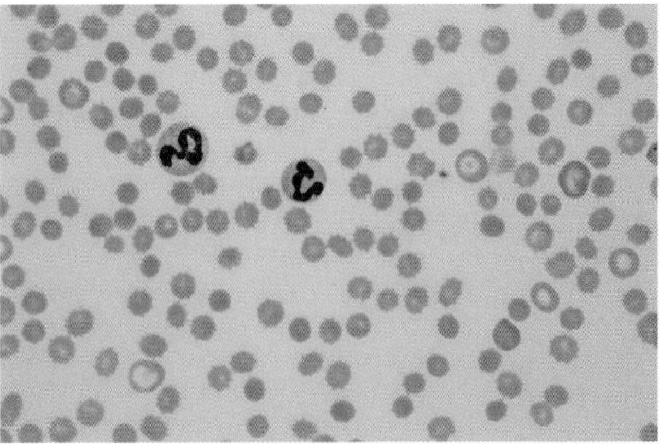

Figure 1 Photomicrograph of the blood smear demonstrating echinocytosis, polychromasia, and toxic change within neutrophils.

Biochemical profile		Reference range
Glucose (mg/dL)	**118**	81–115
Blood urea nitrogen (mg/dL)	**33**	8–29
Creatinine (mg/dL)	1.0	0.7–1.4
Calcium (mg/dL)	**7.9**	9.1–10.8
Phosphorus (mg/dL)	**6.7**	2.3–5.0
Magnesium (mg/dL)	2.0	1.6–2.2
Total protein (g/dL)	**3.2**	5.4–6.9
Albumin (g/dL)	**1.7**	2.7–3.7
Globulin (g/dL)	**1.5**	2.4–3.7
Cholesterol (mg/dL)	**24**	131–320
Total bilirubin (mg/dL)	**3.7**	0.1–0.4
ALT (IU/L)	**193**	14–76
ALP (IU/L)	**149**	12–98
GGT (IU/L)	<3	0–8
Creatine kinase (IU/L)	**27 168**	40–226
Sodium (mEq/L)	**156**	145–151
Potassium (mEq/L)	3.8	3.5–4.9
Chloride (mEq/L)	**127**	110–117
Bicarbonate (mEq/L)	21	17–26
Anion gap (mEq/L)	12	12–20

Additional diagnostics		Reference interval
PT (seconds)	**14.0**	9.3–10.5
PTT (seconds)	**58.7**	9.7–22.1
Condition:	Slight hemolysis	
Cardiac troponin-I (ng/dL)	>**50.00**	0.0–0.05

Interpretive discussion

Hematology

A macrocytic hypochromic regenerative anemia present supported an increased reticulocyte count and the presence of anisocytosis and polychromasia on the blood film (Figure 1). In the presence of a regenerative anemia, the nucleated erythrocytes seen on the blood film are appropriate (i.e., consistent with a regenerative response). Differentials for a regenerative anemia include hemorrhage vs. hemolysis. Hemorrhage may be contributing to the hypoproteinemia in this case, although the hypoproteinemia is more severe than the anemia (see chemistry discussion). Additionally, there may be a hemolytic component in this patient with moderate icterus and only mild increases in ALP. Codocytes (aka. target cells) are increased in regenerative anemia in dogs. Transient echinocytosis occurs in dogs with envenomation of certain species of snakes (e.g., rattlesnake, coral snake, water moccasin, and asp vipers) secondary to the presence of phospholipases in the venom that causes ATP depletion. Other differentials not pertinent in this case include marked electrolyte abnormalities, marked uremia, glomerulonephritis, and some neoplasms.

An inflammatory leukogram is present characterized by a moderate neutrophilia with a regenerative left shift and toxic change. A moderate thrombocytopenia is present. As only a few small platelet clumps are observed, the platelet count is likely mildly to moderately decreased. The presence of a few giant platelets suggests a regenerative bone marrow response. Differentials include vasculitis, phospholipase-mediated aggregation and sequestration in the edematous limb, venom-induced consumptive coagulopathy (VICC), and disseminated intravascular coagulopathy (DIC).

Coagulation

The prolonged prothrombin and partial thromboplastin time in this case may be due to factor consumption secondary to venom-induced consumptive coagulopathy. In VICC the procoagulant clotting pathway is initiated by snake venoms at various places in the pathway (varies by venom), not tissue factor [1]. Additionally, it is not associated with systemic microthrombi and end-organ failure seen in DIC [1]. Thus, IVCC has a pathogenesis, mechanism of initiation, and outcome that is different than what is seen with DIC [1]. It should be noted that there are many hemostatically active toxins in snake venoms, and an individual snake's venom often contains many different toxins [1]. Some toxins are pro-coagulative and others anticoagulative, resulting in complex hematologic changes that may cause hemorrhagic diathesis and/or formation of macro- or microthrombosis that result in end-organ failure [1].

Biochemical profile and additional diagnostics

A severe panhypoproteinemia is present with relatively proportional decreases in both the albumin and globulin fractions. Differentials include hemorrhage, loss of plasma (vasculitis), hemodilution (overzealous IVF administration, use of plasma expanders, edematous disorders such as heart failure).

There is a marked increase in creatine kinase consistent with muscle injury and supports the clinical finding of puncture wounds with limb edema (i.e., recent trauma). Other potential contributors would include myositis and myonecrosis that are sometimes associated with rattlesnake envenomation [1].

A mild hypocalcemia is present and is consistent with hypoalbuminemia, and a mild hyperphosphatemia is present. This pattern has been associated with massive cellular lysis (e.g., myonecrosis, tumor lysis syndrome). The release of intracellular phosphorus drives the hyperphosphatemia. The extracellular phosphorus then binds to calcium, resulting in the pattern of hypocalcemia and hyperphosphatemia. An ionized calcium would be required to determine if a true hypocalcemia is present.

A marked hypocholesterolemia is present in this patient. It is an interesting finding that is associated with rattlesnake envenomation [1]. The mechanism is unknown; however, there are several speculations include lipoprotein leakage through capillaries, changes in lipoprotein transport, and increased lipoprotein metabolism caused by phospholipase activity [1].

There is a mild mixed hepatocellular pattern. The mildly ALT is increased by approximately 2.5× the upper reference interval (URI) indicating hepatocellular damage. In this case, the primary differential is hypoxic injury secondary to anemia. Additionally, a skeletal injury component should also be considered in this case, as the half-life of ALT is approximately 2–3 days in dogs. The ALP is approximately 1.5× the URI and in the presence of a moderate hyperbilirubinemia suggests a cholestatic pattern. The hyperbilirubinemia subjectively seems higher than expected with only mild increases in ALT. In this case, a prehepatic etiology (e.g., hemolysis) is a reasonable differential, especially as some snake venoms include hemolysins.

A mild azotemia is present characterized by a mild increase in BUN. This may represent resolving dehydration, or potentially a mild upper GI bleed.

The mild hypernatremia and hyperchloremia suggests free water loss (panting/hyperventilation, pyrexia), and/or iatrogenic (hypertonic saline administration).

The mild hyperglycemia is likely a glucocorticoid-mediated response to stress (in this case, likely pain).

Ancillary Testing

The marked increase in cardiac troponin-I (cTnI) is a sensitive and specific marker of myocardial injury and necrosis. The marked increase is consistent with myocardial injury. There are two proposed mechanisms, venom-induced myocardial injury (i.e., specific cardiotoxins) and myocardial injury occurring secondary to systemic inflammation [2].

Summary

The patient was admitted into the ICU and received IVF resuscitation (including hypertonic saline administration), multiple doses of antivenom, aggressive analgesia, antibiotics, and multiple transfusions (packed RBCs, fresh frozen plasma, and albumin). Shortly after this bloodwork was collected, the patient had a right forelimb amputation performed. He continued to be hospitalized with aggressive supportive care. Sadly, the dog went into cardiopulmonary arrest and died.

Contributor: Dr. Saundra Sample

Case 21

Signalment: 14-year-old male-neutered domestic short-haired feline

History: Presented for investigation of persistent pancytopenia and progressive anemia. Had received two whole blood transfusions 3 weeks ago and immunosuppressive therapy. PCV initially responded but declined 2–3 days after, and the patient was discharged on symptomatic therapy. A probable hematopoietic (possibly histiocytic based on negative PARR and faint CD204 immunocytochemistry) neoplasm was diagnosed. A two-unit cross-match was performed prior to receiving an additional required transfusion. Both the patient (A) and donors (X and Y) were supposedly Type A.

Interpretive discussion

The results of the two-unit cross-match (Table 1) show compatibility between the recipient (A) and donor X, but not donor Y. Major cross-matching results indicate the recipient's serum does not contain antibodies against the donors' erythrocytes, however, minor cross-matching results between the recipient (A) and donor Y, suggest the presence of preformed antibodies in the serum of donor Y against the recipient's erythrocytes.

The history of prior transfusions is not responsible for this result. Since the major cross-matches were performed several weeks after the first transfusions and results against both donors were negative, the patient was probably not sensitized by prior transfusions. Furthermore, auto agglutination interference is ruled out based on a negative Auto Control result.

Despite the recipients and donors being previously reported as Type A, mis-typings can occur. However, since approximately 30% of Type A cats can have naturally occurring Anti-B antibodies and these tend to be weaker antibodies, the weak positive minor cross-match might suggest the donor Y is Type A and that the other donor, X, and the recipient are Type B. This is an unlikely scenario given the low frequency of Type B cats (<1% in DSH/DLH) [1]. In addition, all Type B cats have strong Anti-A antibodies by the time they are about 3 months old, so one would expect a very strong major cross-match reaction against donor Y.

Assessing both Tables 1 and 2 in conjunction, it is apparent that Donor Y is the animal of concern since there are

Table 1 Two-unit cross-matching results for recipient in question (A) and potential donors (X and Y).

Patient	Donor		Result (Macro)[a]	Result (Micro)[b]	Interpretation	Auto QC
A	X	**Major**[c]	Neg	Neg	Compatible	Neg
		Minor[d]	Neg	Neg	Compatible	
A	Y	**Major**	Neg	Neg	Compatible	
		Minor	Neg	3+	**Incompatible**	

Key:
[a]Macroscopic agglutination reaction.
[b]Microscopic agglutination reaction.
[c]Major cross-match.
[d]Minor cross-match.

Table 2 Historical cross-matching results for unrelated recipients (B and C) and potential donors (X, Y, Z).

Patient	Donor		Result (Macro)	Result (Micro)	Interpretation	Auto QC
B	Z	**Major**	Neg	Neg	Compatible	Neg
		Minor	Neg	Neg	Compatible	
B	Y	**Major**	Neg	Neg	Compatible	
		Minor	1+	2+	**Incompatible**	
C	X	**Major**	Neg	Neg	Compatible	Neg
		Minor	Neg	Neg	Compatible	
C	Y	**Major**	Neg	Neg	Compatible	
		Minor	2+	4+	**Incompatible**	

three different patients cross-matched against donor Y, and minor-side reactions occurred in each of them. The primary differential for this case is the presence of an antibody in the donor's serum against an antigen present on the patient's erythrocytes, such as Mik [2]. The other negative cross-match reactions make a common reagent issue, e.g., phosphate buffered saline (PBS), unlikely. Typing the donor and/or patient for the Mik antigen is no longer available. Human error in this case was unlikely as two different testers obtained similar results when cross-matching against donor Y.

Although donor Y was only minor cross-match incompatible, plasma is still present that might contain sufficient antibodies to agglutinate the patient's RBCs. The *in vitro* reaction was only at the microscopic level so it is not clear if this is strong enough to be clinically significant, however, historical minor cross-matching results did show microagglutination in recipients B and C (Table 1).

Outcome

The recipient received pRBC from donor X and initially tolerated this well but toward the end of the transfusion became febrile and lethargic. The transfusion was discontinued, and fluid therapy was reinstated along with administration of antihistamine. The cat become progressively hypotensive, hypoglycemic and pancytopenic. He also developed hyperbilirubinemia (1.2, then 3.1 mg/dL). Despite supportive care, patient continued to decline and was humanely euthanized 4 days later.

A transfusion reaction may have occurred and laboratory testing to assess this should include checking for data entry errors, examination of patient serum for increased hemolysis and serum icterus index or bilirubin over pretransfusion levels, Coombs testing on a fresh post-transfusion sample, and possibly re-typing and re-cross-matching.

Contributor: Dr. Linda Vap

Case 22

Signalment: 6-month-old ovariohysterectomized female dachshund
History: Lethargy, anorexia, adipsia, diarrhea
Physical examination: Pale mucous membranes
Hematology: Plasma markedly hemolyzed
PCV was 34% on day of entry; a complete CBC was not performed

	Day 2	Reference range
Packed cell volume (%)	**18**	36–54
MCV (fL)	70	60–72
MCHC (g/dL)	38	32–36
NCC ($10^3/\mu L$)	**19.0**	6.0–17.0
Segmented neutrophils ($10^3/\mu L$)	**17.0**	3.0–11.5
Band neutrophils ($10^3/\mu L$)	**0.5**	0–0.3
Monocytes ($10^3/\mu L$)	1.0	0.2–1.4
Lymphocytes ($10^3/\mu L$)	**0.5**	1.0–4.8
Platelets ($10^3/\mu L$)	435	200–500
Antinuclear antibody titer	<1:40	<1:40
Coombs test	Neg	Neg

Biochemical profile	(Serum markedly hemolyzed)	Reference interval
Glucose (mg/dL)	92	70–138
Blood urea nitrogen (mg/dL)	**38**	6–31
Creatinine (mg/dL)	0.8	0.5–1.6
Calcium (mg/dL)	9.5	8.9–11.4
Phosphorus (mg/dL)	5.3	2.5–6.0
Magnesium (mg/dL)	2.4	1.5–2.5
Total protein (g/dL)	6.1	5.0–7.4
Albumin (g/dL)	3.7	2.7–4.4
Globulin (g/dL)	2.4	1.6–3.6
Total bilirubin (mg/dL)	**1.3**	0.1–0.3
Cholesterol (mg/dL)	187	92–320
Triglycerides (mg/dL)	37	29–291
AST (IU/L)	**158**	15–66
ALT (IU/L)	31	12–118
ALP (IU/L)	**614**	5–131
GGT (IU/L)	**17**	1–12
CK (IU/L)	286	59–895
Sodium (mEq/L)	146	139–154
Potassium (mEq/L)	3.6	3.6–5.5
Chloride (mEq/L)	113	102–120
Amylase (IU/L)	**6428**	290–1125
Lipase (IU/L)	**2140**	77–695

Interpretive discussion

Hematology

The PCV decreased rapidly, and that in conjunction with hemolyzed plasma, suggests a hemolytic anemia. A blood film was not examined until later, at which time numerous Heinz bodies and a few spherocytes were seen, explaining the cause of the hemolysis. A Coombs test was performed because a differential at the time was Immune-mediated hemolytic anemia.

The increase in band neutrophils is indicative of an inflammatory leukogram, and the lymphopenia is indicative of a stress or cortisol leukogram. The neutrophilia may be due to both inflammation and stress.

Chemistry

Increased BUN and normal creatinine suggest decreased glomerular filtration rate (GFR) due to prerenal azotemia secondary to dehydration, or the increase could be due to bleeding into the GI tract. A third possibility is that the increase in BUN could be indicative of early kidney damage. A urine analysis was not performed.

Total bilirubin is increased, likely due to increased erythrocyte destruction, but liver disease and/or cholestasis could also be present.

The AST activity is slightly increased, which could be due to hepatic damage or muscle damage. The ALT is normal, suggesting that it is not due to hepatic damage, and the CK activity is not increased, suggesting it is not due to muscle damage. In this case, the increase is likely due to hemolysis, since AST is present within erythrocytes.

Alkaline phosphatase and GGT activities are increased, suggesting cholestasis since the bilirubin is increased, although most of the bilirubin increase is likely due to increased erythrocyte destruction. The cholestasis could be secondary to pancreatitis (see below).

Amylase and lipase activity are both markedly increased, and this increase is likely due to pancreatitis. Although both amylase and lipase are commonly increased in patients that are azotemic, this dog is only mildly azotemic, and the decreased GFR if likely not contributing significantly to the increases. Pancreatic lipase immunoreactivity was not performed in this patient.

Radiographs were taken on Day 2 (Figure 1).

Radiology

In a survey lateral abdominal radiograph there was a round metallic foreign body in the stomach. There is mild gaseous

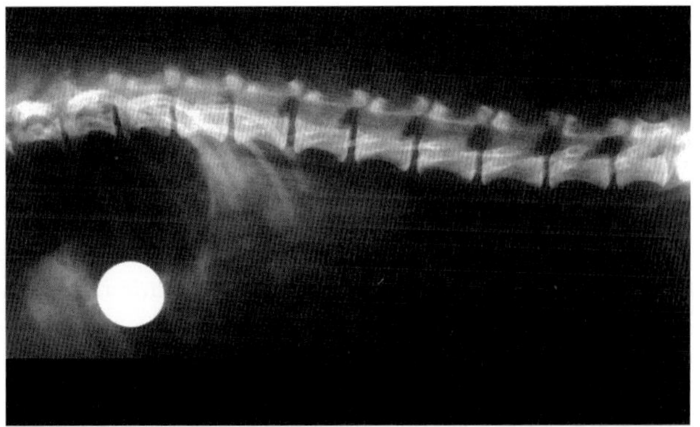

Figure 1 Lateral abdominal radiograph. Note the metallic foreign body in the stomach. Source: Image courtesy of Dr. Krystal Blair.

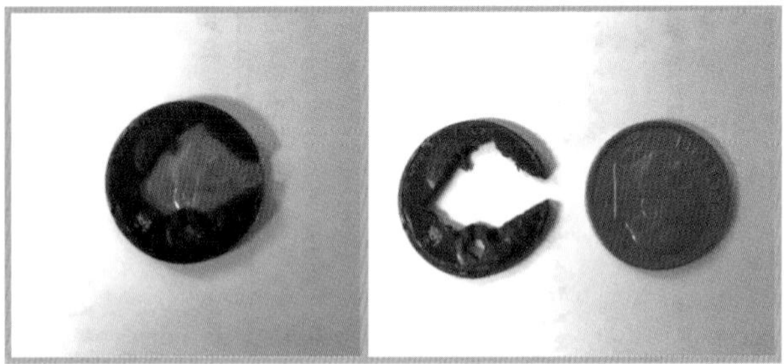

Figure 2 A corroded penny adhered to a dime; this was the origin of the metallic foreign body discovered in the abdominal radiograph. Note the erosion of the penny due to the action of gastric hydrochloric acid. Source: Images courtesy of Dr. Krystal Blair.

distension of the stomach but the degree of distension is not concerning for an obstruction without more fluid accumulation. From one view, it is not possible to determine whether this is a disc, such as a coin, or a sphere, such as a ball bearing. If the foreign body is discoid, a coin is the most likely identity. In DICOM images that are calibrated, it is possible to measure the diameter of a foreign body using the calipers of the viewing software. The approximate diameter of the most commonly used US coins, from small to large, is as follows: 10 cent – 17.9 mm; 1 cent – 19.1 mm; 5 cent – 21.2 mm; 25 cent – 24.3 mm. Measurement can assist in estimating whether the coin is likely to be a one cent piece, under which circumstance removal may be more urgent if the coin is in the stomach. In this dog, it was not possible to measure the coin preoperatively.

Summary and outcome

A penny and dime were surgically removed from the patient's stomach on Day 2 (Figure 2). Since 1983, United States Lincoln pennies are composed primarily of zinc (approximately 2440 mg of elemental zinc per coin) [1]. The LD_{50} of zinc is approximately 100 mg/kg. Acid in the stomach causes the release of free zinc, which is distributed to the liver, kidneys, muscle, bone and pancreas, where it has a direct corrosive effect on tissues. Pancreatitis is present in this patient and has been previously reported in dogs with zinc toxicosis [2]. Zinc has been shown to concentrate in the pancreas and be eliminated in pancreatic secretions. The necrosis and inflammation may be due to activation of intrapancreatic trypsinogen by zinc [3].

The cause of the Heinz body formation is theoretically due to zinc interference with glutathione reductase. Spherocyte formation can also be seen with zinc toxicosis, possibly due to altered antigenicity of erythrocyte membranes, or more likely due to direct damage of erythrocyte membranes by zinc. Zinc has also been reported to interfere with coagulation factor synthesis. An aPTT and PT were not performed in this patient.

Major histopathologic findings include hepatocellular centrilobular necrosis with hemosiderosis and vacuolar degeneration, renal tubular necrosis with hemoglobin casts, and pancreatic duct necrosis with fibrosis of the interlobular fat.

The patient required intermittent hospitalization and IV fluids for several weeks, and eventually made a full recovery. Prognosis for patients with zinc toxicosis is good if a prompt diagnosis is made, the source of zinc is removed immediately, and supportive therapy is instituted. In one series of 19 cases, 89% survived to discharge [4].

Contributors: Drs. Mary Anna Thrall and Donald Thrall

Case 23

Signalment: Holstein Friesian high-producing dairy cow, 15 days postpartum
History: Brown urine, anorexia, decreased milk yield
Physical examination: Tachycardia, dyspnea, and increased jugular pulse

Hematology		Reference range
Packed cell volume (%)	**19**	28–38
RBC ($\times10^6/\mu L$)	**2.2**	5.0–8.5
Hgb (g/dL)	**7.2**	9.8–13.0
MCV (fL)	**86**	41–61
MCHC (g/dL)	**38.4**	30–37
NCC ($10^3/\mu L$)	**2.9**	5.0–9.5
Segmented neutrophils ($10^3/\mu L$)	**0.9**	1.0–4.0
Monocytes ($10^3/\mu L$)	**0**	1.0–7.0
Lymphocytes ($10^3/\mu L$)	2.0	2.2–5.8
Eosinophils ($10^3/\mu L$)	**0**	0.2–1.0
Platelets ($10^3/\mu L$)	200	100–800
Plasma fibrinogen (g/dL)	**0.8**	<0.5

Biochemical profile		Reference range
Non-esterified fatty acids (NEFA) (mmol/L)	**700**	100–600
Beta-hydroxybutirate (BHB) (mmol/L)	**1.2**	<1.0
Cholesterol (mmol/L)	**2.0**	2.7–5.3
Total protein (g/L)	**90**	66–80
Albumin (g/L)	**23**	29–41
Globulin (g/L)	**67**	30–40
Blood urea nitrogen (mmol/L)	**8.0**	2.6–7.0
Phosphorus (mmol/L)	**0.5**	1.1–2.3
Glutathione peroxidase (GPX) (U/gHb)	**90**	>130
Glutamate dehydrogenase (GDH) (U/L)	**150**	<30

Urinalysis

Brown color after centrifugation.

After saturation with ammonium sulfate solution the urine became clear.

Rothera test in urine: positive ++

Interpretive discussion

Hematology

The cow is moderately anemic, with macrocytosis and high MCHC concentration. While no reticulocyte count is available, macrocytosis due to acceleration of erythropoiesis and a regenerative anemia are likely in this case. Considering the increased MCHC, which may be falsely increased due to a false increase in hemoglobin due to the presence of free hemoglobin, one should suspect an intravascular hemolytic anemia.

Neutropenia along with hyperfibrinogenemia in a ruminant suggests acute inflammation, as neutrophils are being consumed in the inflammatory process and fibrinogen is an acute phase protein.

Chemistry

Increased NEFA and BHB, indicating negative energy balance and lipid mobilization, which is a frequently observed during the transition period (less than 21 days before calving until 21 days after calving) of high producing dairy cows. BHB measurement in blood is the gold standard test for diagnosing ketosis and the observed value (1.2) indicates a subclinical ketosis (values within 1.0–2.4 are considered to be subclinical ketosis). Subclinical ketosis is related to decreased milk yields, mastitis, and metritis in dairy cows.

Hypocholesterolemia during the transition period is frequently associated to low dry matter intake, although it can also be related to a liver dysfunction.

Hyperproteinemia due to hyperglobulinemia suggests inflammation and/or active immune response to antigenic stimulation. Hypoalbuminemia is likely related to this protein being a negative acute phase protein, which decreases during inflammation. Hypoalbuminemia can also be observed during the early stages of lactation due to mobilization for milk production.

Blood urea nitrogen increase in dairy cows is frequently associated to negative energy balance, rather than due to decreased glomerular filtration. BUN is part of the rumen degradable protein (RDP) that is digested by the rumen microbiota. Lack of energy prevents the rumen microbiota from digesting the RDP, and consequently the excess of BUN is directed to the blood and milk. An increased BUN in a dairy cow presenting with increased NEFA and BHB should be interpreted as negative energy balance.

Hypophosphatemia is frequently associated with the high demands during lactation in high producing dairy cows, especially if the dietary phosphorus supplementation is not adequate. Phosphate is an essential component of ATP, the energy source of the cell. ATP is required for normal red blood cell membrane integrity. An intravascular hemolysis is the most severe side-effect of hypophosphatemia and occurs when serum concentrations of phosphate are severely decreased, as observed in this case.

The low GPX activity indicates Selenium (Se) deficiency, likely related to insufficient supplementation on the diet. Selenium is found in the soil and taken up by plants at different levels. A continual dietary supply of Se in cattle is essential in areas where the soil is deficient. Se is an antioxidant and a component of the GPX enzyme that inhibits and destroys naturally occurring peroxides that cause cell damage. Se deficiency can predispose to hemolysis and white muscle disease, among other syndromes in cows. Se deficiency is also related to decreased milk production, as observed in this case.

The GDH activity increase is likely related to liver injury due to overload, which is a common finding in high producing dairy cows during the early lactation.

Urinalysis

Brown colored urine can be observed due to hematuria, hemoglobinuria or myoglobinuria. Absence of color change after centrifugation suggests hemoglobinuria or myoglobinuria. The clearance of the brown color after saturation with 80% of ammonium sulfate confirms the presence of hemoglobinuria, as the reaction precipitates the hemoglobin.

A positive result in the Rothera qualitative test in urine indicates the presence of acetone and acetoacetate (ketone bodies), confirming the subclinical ketosis.

Summary

A postparturient hemoglobinuria with intravascular hemolytic anemia due to hypophosphatemia was diagnosed in this dairy cow. The syndrome has been recognized in a few high-producing dairy cows fed low phosphate rations. It is observed sporadically in dairy cows up to 6 weeks postpartum associated with high milk production. It is characterized by an acute intravascular hemolytic anemia with hemoglobinuria. The first sign of the disease is seen when affected animals present a red to brown urine. Its presentation has been associated to diets with low content of phosphorus, although in this case the low concentration of selenium could have worsen the clinical scenario. Deficiency of selenium or copper can also trigger postparturient hemoglobinuria in cows.

Furthermore, some plants have been incriminated on causing postparturient hemoglobinuria, and those include (i) sugar beet roots (mangels) and leaves, (ii) field crops such as green oats, perennial ryegrass, Egyptian clover, and alfalfa, and (iii) members of the genus *Brassica*, often referred to as cruciferous plants. In addition to their low phosphorus content (<0.4% dry matter) or high calcium to phosphorus ratio (>2 : 1), some feeds (e.g., rape, sugar beet, and kale) contain hemolytic substances. Hemolytic saponins from sugar beets or alfalfa may interact with a low serum phosphorus concentration to produce postparturient hemoglobinuria. It has also been postulated that phosphorus deficiency was a necessary predisposing factor and that feeding cruciferous plants precipitated the hemolytic crisis.

Differential diagnosis of hemolytic anemia in ruminants should include infectious causes such as *Babesia* spp., *Theileria* spp., *Anaplasma maginale*, and *Leptospira* spp.

Additionally, this cow presented with subclinical ketosis and liver injury frequently described in high producing dairy cows during the transition period. An acute inflammation is observed and could be a consequence of the hemolytic anemia, the negative energy balance and/or liver injury.

Contributor: Dr. Ananda Muller

Case 24

Signalment: 6-year-old unknown gender Amazon parrot (*Amazona ochrocephala*)
History: Ataxia of 4-week duration
Physical examination: 460 g, bright, alert, response with bilateral leg weakness and hematuria

Hematology	Day 1	Reference range [1]
Packed cell volume (%)	51	45–55
Anisocytosis	<2.0%	(<2.5%)
Polychromasia	2%	(<5%)
Hypochromasia	None	(None)
Poikilocytosis	<2%	(<2.5%)
Erythroplastids	None	(<0.5%)
Immature RBC (rubricytes)	**10%**	(None)
WBC ($10^3/\mu L$)	8.5	6.0–17.0 (8.0–20.0)
Heterophils ($10^3/\mu L$)	6.0	(4.0–11.0)
Heterophils (%)	70.5	30–75
Monocytes ($10^3/\mu L$)	0.2	(0.0–0.7)
Monocytes (%)	2	0–3
Lymphocytes ($10^3/\mu L$)	1.5	(1.5–8.0)
Lymphocytes (%)	17.5	20–65
Eosinophils ($10^3/\mu L$)	0.4	(0.0–0.4)
Eosinophils (%)	5	0–1
Basophils ($10^3/\mu L$)	0.4	(0.0–0.4)
Basophils (%)	5	0–5
Thrombocytes	adequate	1–5/1000x field
Plasma protein (g/dL)	3.5	3.0–5.0

Normal leukocyte and thrombocyte morphology.

Biochemical profile		Reference interval
Glucose (mg/dL)	271	220–350
Blood urea nitrogen (mg/dL)	3	(0–5)
Uric acid (mg/dL)	5.1	2–10
Calcium (mg/dL)	8.4	8.0–13.0
Phosphorus (mg/dL)	5.7	3.1–5.5
Total protein (g/dL)	2.5	3.0–5.0 (2.5–4.0)
Albumin (g/dL)	1.2	
Globulin (g/dL)	1.3	
AST (IU/L)	**430**	130–350
Creatine kinase (IU/L)	**3054**	45–265
Sodium (mEq/L)	158	136–152
Potassium (mEq/L)	2.2	3.0–4.5 (2.0–4.0)
Chloride (mEq/L)	124	(100–120)
Bicarbonate (mEq/L)	29.2	(20–30)

Suggested decision levels when reference values are unavailable or to offer another set of values are in parentheses.

Interpretive discussion

Hematology

The bird has a normal packed cell volume with the normal expected number of polychromatic erythrocytes; however, there is an increased number of immature erythrocytes (rubricytes). An inappropriate release of rubricytes in a nonanemic bird in the absence of a significant polychromasia is suggestive of lead poisoning, myeloproliferation, or myelodysplasia.

Chemistry

The plasma creatine kinase (CK) activity is markedly increased, indicating skeletal muscle injury or exertion. The degree of increased plasma aspartate aminotransferase (AST) activity is also likely associated with skeletal muscle involvement rather than hepatocellular disease. A much higher degree of AST activity would be expected with hepatocellular disease: however, one cannot completely rule out coexisting hepatocellular disease based on plasma CK and AST activities alone.

Whole body radiographs revealed multiple small mineral and metallic objects in the ventriculus. Blood heavy metal analysis revealed a whole blood lead concentration of 1.5 ppm with an expected normal <0.2 ppm and zinc concentration of 0.39 ppm with an expected normal <2.0 ppm. These findings were indicative of lead poisoning and the cause of the inappropriate release of immature erythrocytes in the peripheral blood as well as hematuria, a common finding on physical examination of psittacine birds with lead poisoning.

Chelation therapy for lead poisoning was performed (CaEDTA treatments on 5 days on, 5 days off cycle). Following two treatments the bird's strength returned and it was no longer exhibiting ataxia. After 21 days, the bird's blood profile was normal, and no hematuria was seen.

Heavy metal poisoning is a common disorder of pet birds. Sources of the heavy metals include paint, stained glass, soldered metals, curtain weights, fishing weights, cages (antique, homemade, imported), wine foil, metal pipes, and hardware, such as nuts, bolts, and screws. Clinical signs of acute heavy metal toxicity include weakness, depression, hematuria, abnormal droppings, and central nervous system disorders, such as seizures and ataxia. Clinical signs of chronic heavy metal toxicity include weakness, weight loss, vomiting, hematuria, and central nervous system disorders, such as seizures and ataxia.

Contributor: Dr. Terry W. Campbell

CASES

Case 25

Signalment: 8-year-old spayed female golden retriever
History: Presented for lethargy, anorexia, a mass over the humeroradial joint, and prolonged bleeding at a biopsy site
Physical examination: Fever, icterus, and an enlarged liver and spleen

Hematology		Reference interval
PCV (%)	**23**	37–55
Hgb (g/dL)	**8.5**	12–18
RBC (×10^6/μL)	**3.27**	5.5–8.5
MCV (fL)	71	60–72
MCHC(g/dL)	37	34–38
Retics (×10^3/μL)	**130.8**	<60
NCC (×10^3/μL)	**45.4**	6–17
Segs (×10^3/μL)	**41.8**	3–11.5
Bands (×10^3/μL)	**0.5**	0–0.3
Monos (×10^3/μL)	**3.2**	0.1–1.3
Lymphs (×10^3/μL)	**0.0**	1–4.8
Eos (×10^3/μL)	0.0	0.1–1.2
Platelets (×10^3/μL)	**25**	200–500
TP (P) (g/dL)	**4.6**	6–8

Hemopathology: Increased polychromasia and giant platelets.

Biochemical profile		Reference interval
Gluc (mg/dL)	70	65–122
BUN (mg/dL)	11	7–28
Ca (mg/dL)	**8.2**	9.0–11.2
Phos (mg/dL)	4.0	2.8–6.1
TP (g/dL)	**5.0**	5.4–7.4
Alb (g/dL)	**2.2**	2.7–4.5
Glob (g/dL)	2.8	1.9–3.4
T. bili (mg/dL)	**7.6**	0–0.4
Chol (mg/dL)	329	130–370
ALT (IU/L)	58	10–120
ALP (IU/L)	**775**	35–280
Na (mEq/L)	**144**	145–158
K (mEq/L)	**4.0**	4.1–5.5
CL (mEq/L)	109	106–127
TCO_2 (mEq/L)	16.6	14–27
An. gap (mEq/L)	22	8–25

Urinalysis		Urine sediment	
Color	Yellow	WBCs/hpf	0–2
Transparency	Clear	RBCs/hpf	0–1
Sp. gr.	1.012	Epith cells/hpf	0
Protein	–	Casts/lpf	0
Gluc	–	Crystals	0
Bilirubin	**4+**	Bacteria	0
Blood	Trace	Other	1 + fat
pH	5.5		

Coagulation data		Reference interval
Activated clotting time (seconds)	**>300**	72–86
PT (seconds)	**14.5**	6.4–7.4
aPTT (seconds)	**32.3**	9–11
FDPs (μg/mL)	**>80**	<10

Interpretative discussion

Hematology

There is anemia that is regenerative as evidenced by the significant reticulocytosis and polychromasia. Anemia in combination with low total protein suggests that the cause is blood loss. There is a mixed inflammatory and stress (steroid) leukogram evidenced by the neutrophilia with band neutrophils, monocytosis, and absence of lymphocytes and eosinophils. The thrombocytopenia in conjunction with the large platelets suggests increased consumption and production of platelets.

Biochemical profile

Hypocalcemia corrects into the normal range, and thus is due to hypoalbuminemia. Hypoproteinemia is due to blood loss. The hyperbilirubinemia may result from increased erythrocyte destruction or cholestasis. Increased alkaline phosphatase activity supports cholestasis. Very mild hyponatremia and hyperkalemia are probably insignificant in this case.

Urinalysis

The urine specific gravity is isosthenuric, but the urea nitrogen is normal, so the specific gravity may not be significant. Water deprivation and ensuing specific gravity would determine renal function reserve. Hyperbilirubinuria is a consequence of hyperbilirubinemia.

Coagulation data

Decreased platelets, prolonged ACT, PT, aPTT, and increased FDPs support disseminated intravascular coagulation. Erythrocytes may be destroyed during disseminated intravascular coagulation, thus contributing to elevated total bilirubin.

Summary

The mass was diagnosed as malignant histiocytosis, with nodules in the liver, spleen, mediastinum, and peripheral lymph nodes at necropsy. A likely scenario is that extensive tumor mass developed necrosis and/or inflammation that triggered hypercoagulability leading to disseminated intravascular coagulation. Involvement of liver likely explains the hypoalbuminemia and other liver changes.

Case 26

Signalment: 5-month-old female dog
History: The puppy bleeds excessively when it loses teeth
Physical examination: The mucous membranes were pale. There is moderate bleeding evident at the site of a recent tooth loss.

Hematology		Reference interval
PCV (%)	**19**	37–55
Hgb (g/dL)	**6.1**	12–18
Retics ($\times 10^3/\mu L$)	**188**	<60
NCC ($\times 10^3/\mu L$)	**35.4**	6–17
Segs ($\times 10^3/\mu L$)	**29.7**	3–11.5
Bands ($\times 10^3/\mu L$)	**2.5**	0–0.3
Monos ($\times 10^3/\mu L$)	**3.2**	0.1–1.3
Lymphs ($\times 10^3/\mu L$)	**0.0**	1–4.8
Eos ($\times 10^3/\mu L$)	0.0	0.1–1.2
Platelets ($\times 10^3/\mu L$)	**915**	200–500
TP (P) (g/dL)	6.5	6–8

Hemopathology: Moderate polychromasia and anisocytosis is present.

Coagulation data		Reference interval
Activated clotting time	>**180**	72–86
PT (seconds)	6.8	6.4–7.4
aPTT (seconds)	>**120**	9–11
Fibrinogen (mg/dL)	200	100–400
Bleeding time (minutes)	3	1–5

Interpretative Discussion

Hematology

The anemia is regenerative as the reticulocyte count is increased and there is polychromasia and anisocytosis on the blood film. The cause of anemia is not determined but is likely due to hemolysis or blood loss since it is regenerative. The clinical findings of hemorrhage suggest that blood loss is the cause. Thrombocytosis is common in iron deficiency anemia. Microcytosis is evident in chronic iron deficiency, and may contribute to anisocytosis. Size of erythrocytes is not known, since the MCV is not provided. Serum iron and iron binding capacity would be useful in determination of the cause of anemia. The neutrophilia, left shift, and monocytosis indicate an inflammatory leukogram. Lymphopenia is indicative of a concurrent stress/steroid mediated response.

Coagulation data

The coagulation profile suggests a deficiency of one or multiple coagulation factors in the intrinsic pathway. Platelet concentration is increased in number, and no large forms are seen in peripheral blood. Bleeding time is normal, and in the face of adequate platelet concentration, indicates that platelet function is normal. The most common cause of a severe coagulopathy with normal platelet concentration, normal hepatic enzyme activity, and a prolongation of the aPTT with normal PT is factor 8 deficiency. The occurrence is less common in females, and to have an affected female requires that the sire also be affected.

Summary

This dog was tested for factor 8 plasma activity and was found to have 21% of normal activity, which is diagnostic for factor 8 deficiency or hemophilia A. This is compatible with the major abnormalities in the ACT and aPTT and the clinical description of bleeding in a young dog.

Case 27

Signalment: 7-year-old female Walker hound
History: The owner noticed a swelling on the right front leg on the day of admission
Physical examination: The mucous membranes were pale. There was a subcutaneous swelling in the right ventral thoracic area, with some dried blood on all four legs.

Hematology		Reference interval
PCV (%)	**25**	37–55
Hgb (g/dL)	**8.4**	12–18
RBC ($\times 10^6/\mu L$)	**4.03**	5.5–8.5
MCV (fL)	62	60–72
MCHC (g/dL)	34	34–38
Retics ($\times 10^3/\mu L$)	44	<60
NCC ($\times 10^3/\mu L$)	14.4	6–17
Segs ($\times 10^3/\mu L$)	**12.2**	3–11.5
Monos ($\times 10^3/\mu L$)	**1.6**	0.1–1.3
Lymphs ($\times 10^3/\mu L$)	**0.6**	1–4.8
Platelets ($\times 10^3/\mu L$)	315	200–500
TP (P) (g/dL)	**4.6**	6–8

Hemopathology: 1+ leptocytosis and anisocytosis.

Biochemical profile		Reference interval
Gluc (mg/dL)	88	65–122
BUN (mg/dL)	17	7–28
Creat (mg/dL)	1.1	0.9–1.7
Ca (mg/dL)	10.2	9.0–11.2
Phos (mg/dL)	3.5	2.8–6.1
TP (g/dL)	**4.1**	5.4–7.4
Alb (g/dL)	**2.3**	2.7–4.5
Glob (g/dL)	**1.8**	1.9–3.4
T. bili (mg/dL)	0.3	0–0.4
Chol (mg/dL)	188	130–370
ALT (IU/L)	35	10–120
ALP (IU/L)	40	35–280
Na (mEq/L)	**144**	145–158
K (mEq/L)	**4.0**	4.1–5.5
CL (mEq/L)	107	106–127
TCO_2 (mEq/L)	18	14–27

Coagulation data		Reference interval
Activated clotting time (seconds)	**>180**	72–86
PT (seconds)	**>180**	6.4–7.4
aPTT (seconds)	**>180**	9–11
Fibrinogen (mg/dL)	300	100–400
Bleeding time (minutes)	**4**	1–5

Interpretive discussion

Hematology

The anemia is nonregenerative as the erythrocyte indices are normal and the reticulocyte count is normal. The plasma and serum protein are low, with equal deficiency of globulin and albumin, suggesting blood loss as the cause of anemia. The anemia is likely too acute for there to be a regenerative response. Aspiration of the subcutaneous mass confirmed the presence of blood. Mild neutrophilia, monocytosis, and lymphopenia are indicative of a stress leukogram.

Biochemical profile

The protein changes discussed above indicate subacute blood loss, with fluid shifting and dilution of plasma protein resulting in anemia and hypoproteinemia. The mild decrease in sodium and potassium are insignificant.

Coagulation data

The coagulation data indicates either a deficiency of multiple coagulation factors, or a single factor deficiency of the common pathway. Platelets are normal in number, and, no large forms are seen in peripheral blood. Bleeding time is normal and in the face of normal platelet concentration, indicates that platelet function is also normal. The most common cause of a severe coagulopathy with normal platelets and normal hepatic enzyme activities is vitamin K antagonism.

Summary

This dog was exposed to diphacinone, a rodenticide that is a vitamin K antagonist; coagulation times returned to normal following administration of vitamin K.

CASES

Case 28

Signalment: 2-month-old female horse
History: Off feed
Physical examination: Depressed, evidence of diarrhea

Hematology		Reference interval
PCV (%)	**14**	32–52
Hgb (g/dL)	**6.5**	11–19
NCC ($\times 10^3/\mu L$)	6.5	5.5–12.5
Segs ($\times 10^3/\mu L$)	4.7	2.7–6.7
Monos ($\times 10^3/\mu L$)	0.1	0–0.8
Lymphs ($\times 10^3/\mu L$)	1.6	1.5–5.5
NRBCs ($\times 10^3/\mu L$)	**0.1**	0
Platelets ($\times 10^3/\mu L$)	**14**	100–600
TP (P) (g/dL)	6.3	6–8

Hemopathology: Mod toxic neutrophils, few reactive lymphs, mod Howell-Jolly bodies, few echinocytes, marked anisocytosis.

Biochemical profile		Reference interval
Gluc (mg/dL)	91	70–110
BUN (mg/dL)	**40**	14–27
Creat (mg/dL)	**2.1**	1.1–2.0
Ca (mg/dL)	**9.7**	11.0–13.7
Phos (mg/dL)	**6.3**	1.9–4.1
TP (g/dL)	**4.6**	5.8–7.6
Alb (g/dL)	**2.2**	2.7–3.7
Glob (g/dL)	**2.4**	2.6–4.6
T. bili (mg/dL)	**3.2**	0.6–2.1
AST (IU/L)	280	185–300
GGT (IU/L)	**28**	7–17
SDH (IU/L)	**27**	0–9
CK (IU/L)	169	130–470
Na (mEq/L)	**120**	133–145
K (mEq/L)	3.8	2.2–4.6
CL (mEq/L)	**84**	100–111
TCO_2 (mEq/L)	**11.0**	24–34
An. gap	**28.8**	5–15
Calc. osmolality (mOsm/kg)	**250**	280–310
Amylase (IU/L)	34	0–87
Lipase (IU/L)	534	ND [a]
Grossly lipemic serum		

[a] ND, not determined for foals.

Blood gas data (arterial)		Reference interval
pH	**7.282**	7.38–7.46
pCO_2 (mmHg)	**20.6**	35–47
pO_2 (mmHg)	**60.9**	67–96
HCO_3 (mEq/L)	**9.3**	22–30

Coagulation profile		Reference interval
PT (seconds)	**14.6**	9.5–11.5
aPTT (seconds)	39.8	24–45
Fibrinogen (mg/dL)	500	100–400
FDPs (μg/mL)	>10 and <40	ND [a]

[a] ND, not determined for foals.

Abdominal fluid analysis	
Color	Red
Clarity	**Opaque**
NCC (/μL)	**16 000**
TP (g/dL)	**5.7**
PCV	**13%**

Comments: Erythrophagia and platelets noted in film.

Interpretive discussion

Hematology

There is a marked anemia. While it is not unusual for neonatal animals to have a "congenital anemia" due to iron deficiency, the PCV is much lower than is typically encountered by this physiological change. The presence of anisocytosis leads one to suspect that there may be a regenerative response, for which evaluation of the MCV and RBC histogram would be useful. The presence of nucleated erythrocytes in the peripheral blood is uncommon in horses but occasionally seen in foals with profound regenerative responses, or with damage to the bone marrow endothelium, as might occur with sepsis. Combined decreases in PCV and serum proteins may indicate hemorrhage. There is a marked thrombocytopenia, which may be due to decreased production or increased consumption; thrombocytopenia is severe enough to be resulting in blood loss. Refer to the discussion of the coagulation profile for more on this matter.

Biochemical profile

The BUN, serum creatinine, and phosphorus concentrations are increased, but the nature of this azotemia cannot be definitively differentiated without a urinalysis.

There is hypocalcemia and hyperphosphatemia. This combination of mineral abnormalities may be seen in nutritional secondary hyperparathyroidism due to excessive dietary phosphorus. However, higher serum phosphorus concentrations are commonly observed in growing animals, and hypocalcemia may also be due to uptake by widespread damaged tissues, decreased intake with anorexia, or to an apparent decrease due to hypoalbuminemia.

Serum total protein concentration is decreased, including both hypoalbuminemia and hypoglobulinemia. Low serum albumin may be hepatocellular dysfunction or cachexia and decreased albumin synthesis. Alternatively, there may be pathologic albumin loss due to gastrointestinal or renal disease. Low serum globulin in a 2-month-old foal is not due to failure of passive transfer but may be due to decreased production, malnutrition, or pathologic loss. Loss of all proteins would be expected with hemorrhage, which could also account for the profound anemia. This is the most likely cause.

The serum total bilirubin concentration is increased, with only a mild increase in serum GGT activity. This may reflect hyperbilirubinemia of fasting in an equine anorexic patient. However, SDH activity is increased, indicating hepatocellular damage.

Serum sodium and chloride concentrations are decreased. This is commonly observed in young animals with an enterotoxigenic or secretory diarrhea. This may also be due to gastrointestinal stasis, a third space accumulation in the abdominal cavity, as well as to decreased intake. One would typically expect a hyperkalemia to occur in secretory diarrhea, owing to acidosis-induced intercompartmental exchange. Hypokalemia may be expected in third space syndromes, owing to potassium loss and renal decompensation. It is possible to observe normokalemia with concomitant potassium loss and metabolic acidosis, wherein redistribution of potassium from the intracellular to the extracellular fluid compartment obscures the whole-body potassium deficit. There is evidence in support of abdominal hemorrhage and third spacing due either to acute pancreatitis or a gastric ulcer (see below).

Marked lipemia is often seen in ponies with starvation and metabolic disease but is unusual in horses. In other species, hyperlipidemia may occur due to impaired triglyceride clearance associated with endotoxemia. One should consider other potential causes of hyperlipidemia such as pancreatitis. In this case, serum amylase activity is normal, but lipase activity may be increased. There is evidence of recent hemorrhage into the abdominal cavity, which could be related to acute pancreatitis, but is more often due, in diseased foals, to a bleeding gastric ulcer. The low calculated osmolality would be expected, given the hyponatremia and hypochloremia.

Blood gas data

There is an increased anion gap metabolic acidosis with respiratory compensation. This is consistent with a secretory diarrhea, complicated by hypovolemia and/or sepsis. If there were gastrointestinal stasis, one might expect an alkalosis. If there were a ruptured urinary bladder, one might expect a metabolic acidosis with hyperkalemia. The increased anion gap may result from sepsis, with hypovolemia and lactic acidosis due to reduced tissue perfusion and/or the metabolic effects of endotoxemia. The decreased oxygen tension may indicate respiratory compromise as well.

Coagulation data

The prothrombin time is prolonged slightly, the activated partial thromboplastin time is normal, and the FDP concentration is in an intermediate range. These findings may indicate disseminated intravascular coagulation, particularly in light of the severe thrombocytopenia, wherein Factor VII levels are becoming depleted, thereby prolonging the PT, but other coagulation factor concentrations are adequate to maintain a normal aPTT. The concurrent observation of thrombocytopenia and findings consistent with blood loss anemia support a diagnosis of DIC with pathologic hemorrhage.

Summary

Enterotoxigenic *E. coli* diarrhea, pancreatitis, hepatitis, and DIC were findings confirmed at necropsy. On necropsy, the pancreas was 5 to 6 times normal size and the liver was swollen. Histopathology showed necrosis and inflammation of the pancreas, diffuse mesenteric steatitis, fat necrosis and fat saponification, inflammation of the liver with thrombi in central veins and associated focal ischemic necrosis. Inflammatory disease is often not reflected in equine leukograms.

CASES

Case 29

Signalment: 9-year-old 14 kg male Welsh corgi mix from Wisconsin

History: Stiff joints, shifting leg lameness for 1-week duration, severe pain over shoulder area, anorexia for 1 day

Physical examination: Pale mucous membranes, labored breathing. When sedated for radiographs, hematoma under tongue (see Figure 1) and bruising in axillary region were noted.

Hematology	Day 1	Day 2	Reference range
Packed cell volume (%)	**23**	**24**	37–55
RBC (×10^6/μL)	**3.24**	**3.1**	5.5–8.5
Hgb (g/dL)	**7.1**	**7.8**	12–18
MCV (fL)	73	75	60–77
MCHC (g/dL)	34.5	32.5	31–34
Reticulocytes (10^3/μL)	**74.5**	**409.2**	0–60
NCC (10^3/μL)	**23.8**	**48.6**	6.0–17.0
Segmented neutrophils (10^3/μL)	**12.9**	**31.1**	3.0–11.5
Band neutrophils (10^3/μL)	**4.5**	**5.3**	0–0.3
Monocytes (10^3/μL)	**3.5**	0.5	0.2–1.4
Lymphocytes (10^3/μL)	3.6	**6.8**	1.0–4.8
Eosinophils (10^3/μL)	–	0.4	0.1–1.2
Nucleated RBCs (10^3/μL)	0	**3.4**	0
Platelets (10^3/μL)	**66**	**43**	200–500
Plasma protein by refractometry (g/dL)	**5.4**	7.0	6.0–8.0

Hemopathology: Clumped platelets on Day 1, no platelet clumping seen on Day 2; toxic neutrophils are present on Day 2.

Serology

A 4Dx SNAP test was positive for *Borrelia burgdorferi* (Lyme disease).

Biochemical profile

The only abnormalities are shown below.

		Reverence range
Total bilirubin (mg/dL)	0.6	0.1–0.6
Total protein (g/dL)	**5.2**	5.4–7.4
Albumin (g/dL)	**2.5**	2.7–4.5

Urinalysis

Color	Brown
Transparency	Opaque
Sp. gr.	1.019
Protein	**2+ (100 mg/dL)**
Bilirubin	**3+ (6 mg/dL)**
Blood	**4+**
Sediment	
RBC/hpf	**5**
Bilirubin crystals present	

Coagulation profile

	Day 1	Day 2	Day 23	Reference interval
aPTT (seconds)	**26**	17.5	17.1	14–19
PT (seconds)	**>200**	**194.6**	**107.4**	75–105

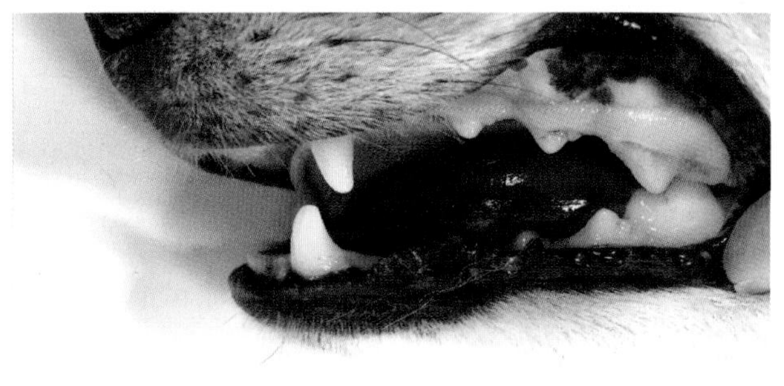

Figure 1 Hematoma under tongue of patient.

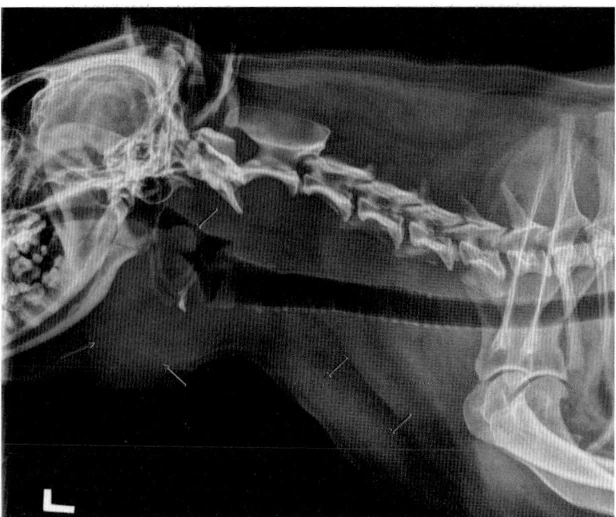

Figure 2 Lateral radiograph of the neck. Abnormal findings are indicated by the arrows.

Interpretive discussion

Hematology

The dog has a normocytic normochromic regenerative anemic on Days 1 and 2, likely due to blood loss. On Day 2, the anemia is extremely regenerative as evidenced by the marked reticulocytosis. All measures of red cell mass are decreased.

An inflammatory leukogram is present, as indicated by the marked neutrophilia and presence of band neutrophils on Days 1 and 2. The monocytosis on Day 1 is also likely due to inflammation. A lymphocytosis is present on Day 2, possibly due to antigenic stimulation.

The thrombocytopenia may be partially due to blood loss, but blood loss would not account for this magnitude of thrombocytopenia. Other considerations should include disseminated intravascular coagulopathy (DIC), since aPTT and PT are prolonged. The dog is antibody positive for Lyme disease, which has infrequently been associated with thrombocytopenia in dogs. Other differentials should include immune-mediated thrombocytopenia. A lack of production of platelets is not likely, considering the bone marrow is functional as indicated by the regenerative anemia and neutrophilia. Warfarin toxicosis (see below) has been associated with mild to marked thrombocytopenia in dogs. The mechanism is not known but is apparently not due to DIC [1].

The plasma protein estimate is slightly decreased on Day 1, likely due to blood loss.

Serology

The dog had antibodies to *Borrelia burgdorferi*. Lyme disease has infrequently been associated with thrombocytopenia and arthropathy [2, 3], and because the dog was from an endemic area, an initial tentative diagnosis of Lyme disease was made. However, the majority of dogs from endemic areas are antibody positive, with a small percentage having active infections [3].

Chemistry

The only abnormalities present were a decreased total protein and albumin, likely due to blood loss in this case. However, proteinuria, while likely from hematuria, could be the cause of the hypoalbuminemia, and a urine protein:creatinine ratio should be considered.

Urinalysis

The urine contains 4+ blood as measured on the dipstick. Erythrocytes were seen on urine sediment, but not as many as would be suggested by the 4+ blood. Proteinuria may be associated with hematuria. Bilirubin and bilirubin crystals were present, more than usual with a serum bilirubin in the reference range. Bilirubin is likely from increased extracellular erythrocyte destruction following hemorrhage into tissues. Hematuria is consistent with bleeding in other areas, such as under the tongue.

Coagulation panel

The aPTT and PT are both prolonged on Day 1, and the PT is markedly prolonged on Days 1 and 2; PT is still slightly prolonged on Day 23. Differentials for prolongation of both the aPTT and PT, indicating defects in both the intrinsic and extrinsic and/or common coagulation pathways, include DIC, liver failure, and a lack of vitamin K dependent factors (II, VII, IX, X). The thrombocytopenia in conjunction with prolonged aPTT and PT could suggest DIC, and additional tests, such as D-dimers or fibrin degradation products, are indicated but were not performed. Liver failure was excluded as a differential because cholesterol, BUN, and bile acids were within the reference interval. Warfarin toxicosis remained a top differential, as it blocks vitamin K epoxide reductase that reactivates vitamin K_1. Without active vitamin K_1, factors II, VII, IX, and X have decreased clotting ability. The PIVKA (proteins induced by vitamin k absence or antagonism) test is sometimes used to confirm warfarin toxicosis [4] but was not performed in this case.

The aPTT and PT are both prolonged on Day 1, and the PT is markedly prolonged on Days 1 and 2; PT is still slightly prolonged on Day 23. Differentials for prolongation of both the aPTT and PT, indicating defects in both the intrinsic and extrinsic and/or common coagulation pathways, include DIC, liver failure, and a lack of vitamin K dependent factors (II, VII, IX, X). The thrombocytopenia in conjunction with prolonged aPTT and PT could suggest DIC, and additional tests, such as D-dimers or fibrin degradation products, are indicated but were not performed. Liver failure was excluded as a differential because cholesterol, BUN, and bile acids were within the reference interval. Warfarin toxicosis remained a top differential, as it blocks vitamin K epoxide reductase that reactivates vitamin K_1. Without active vitamin K_1, factors II, VII, IX, and X have decreased clotting ability. The PIVKA (proteins induced by vitamin k absence or antagonism) test is sometimes used to confirm warfarin toxicosis [4] but was not performed in this case.

Radiology

There is a lobular mass in the pharynx, dorsal to the hyoid apparatus (Figure 2). This in nonspecific, and also unusual, and the considerations would normally be a neoplasm or an inflammatory mass, but in this patient, this was a hematoma. There is also poorly defined swelling in the submandibular region and in the ventral aspect of the neck. These too are nonspecific, and the considerations are cellulitis/abscess and diffuse tumor, such as mast cell tumor, but in this patient, hematomas have to be considered. This is a very unusual distribution of hemorrhage due to a coagulopathy but illustrates that variation is commonly observed.

Summary and outcome

Additional history revealed that the dog had been exposed to diphacinone, a long-acting warfarin rodenticide, and had a previous history of diphacinone toxicosis. The dog was treated with 5 mg/kg vitamin K1 daily, divided in two doses, for 30 days, and recovered uneventfully. He was also treated with doxycycline for 1 month for Lyme disease, although probably unnecessarily. Aspiration to confirm the presence of blood in the joints would have been diagnostically useful to possibly explain the shifting leg lameness, which resolved following vitamin K1 therapy. Bleeding into joints in humans, as a result of warfarin therapy or inherited coagulopathies, has been reported to induce inflammation and joint pain [5, 6].

While an explanation for the marked inflammatory leukogram was not readily apparent, warfarin toxicosis has been reported to cause a leukocytosis and neutrophilia, possibly related to hemorrhage within tissues and resultant inflammation, but in some cases simply due to a stress leukogram [7, 8].

Contributors: Drs. Mary Anna Thrall and Donald Thrall

Case 30

Signalment: 3-year-old spayed female cocker spaniel
History: Left in owner's car in shopping mall parking lot for approximately 3 hours on a hot summer afternoon
Physical examination: Depressed and mildly dehydrated

Hematology		Reference interval
PCV (%)	**58**	37–55
NCC ($\times10^3/\mu L$)	16.0	6–17
Segs ($\times10^3/\mu L$)	**13.4**	3–11.5
Monos ($\times10^3/\mu L$)	**1.6**	0.1–1.3
Lymphs ($\times10^3/\mu L$)	1.0	1–4.8
Platelets ($\times10^3/\mu L$)	Adequate	200–500

Biochemical profile		Reference interval
Gluc (mg/dL)	**142**	65–122
BUN (mg/dL)	**62**	7–28
Creat (mg/dL)	**3.0**	0.9–1.7
Ca (mg/dL)	**8.4**	9.0–11.2
Phos (mg/dL)	4.9	2.8–6.1
TP (g/dL)	**9.4**	5.4–7.4
Alb (g/dL)	**5.4**	2.7–4.5
Glob (g/dL)	**4.0**	1.9–3.4
T. bili (mg/dL)	0.4	0–0.4
Chol (mg/dL)	160	130–370
ALT (IU/L)	**178**	10–120
ALP (IU/L)	60	35–280
Na (mEq/L)	**164**	145–158
K (mEq/L)	5.4	4.1–5.5
CL (mEq/L)	124	106–127
TCO_2 (mEq/L)	14	14–27
An. gap (mEq/L)	**31.4**	8–25
Meas. osmolality (mOsm/kg)	**358**	290–310
Calc. osmolality (mOsm/kg)	**344**	290–310
Osmol gap (mOsm/kg)	**14**	0–10

Blood gas data (arterial)		Reference interval
pH	**7.09**	7.33–7.45
pCO_2 (mmHg)	**46**	24–39
HCO_3 (mEq/L)	**13**	14–24

Urinalysis			
Color	Dk yellow	**Urine sediment**	
		WBCs/hpf	2–3
Transparency	Cloudy	RBCs/hpf	4–5
Sp. gr.	**1.011**	Epith cells/hpf	2–3
Protein	**1+**	Casts/lpf	**2–3 fine granular**
Gluc	Neg		
Bilirubin	Neg	Crystals	2+ Ca oxalate
Blood	Neg	Bacteria	0
pH	5.5		

Interpretive discussion

Hematology

Hemoconcentration is indicated by the increased PCV and physical signs of dehydration. Mild neutrophilia, monocytosis, and borderline lymphopenia is interpreted as a stress leukogram.

Biochemical profile

There is a mild hyperglycemia, which may be due to a catecholaminergic or steroid stress response.

The BUN and serum creatinine concentrations are increased. See discussion of urinalysis below to explain whether the azotemia is likely prerenal, renal, or postrenal.

Hyperalbuminemia with hyperproteinemia indicates dehydration. In this case, hyperglobulinemia is also likely caused by dehydration.

There is a mild hypocalcemia in the face of hyperalbuminemia due to dehydration. Thus, serum calcium concentration is truly decreased. This is often seen in heat stressed animals, subsequent to widespread tissue damage and precipitation of calcium salts in ischemic areas.

The small increase in serum ALT activity may not be significant, or may reflect some hepatocellular damage.

The hypernatremia, in concert with other signs of dehydration, indicates a hypertonic dehydration. This is commonly seen in heat-stressed dogs owing to increased insensible losses of water, in excess of solute, due to hyperventilatory evaporation.

The measured and calculated osmolality values are increased, consistent with hypertonic dehydration. However, the osmol gap is also increased, indicating the accumulation of unmeasured osmotically active solutes in the blood. The anion gap is likewise increased, and given the dehydration and probable tissue hypoperfusion, some degree of lactic acidosis is likely.

Blood gas data

There is a combined metabolic (decreased bicarbonate) and respiratory (increased pCO_2) acidosis. The metabolic acidosis results from lactic acidosis due to tissue hypoperfusion. The respiratory acidosis suggests compromised pulmonary function.

Urinalysis

The presence of 1+ proteinuria with a specific gravity of 1.011 indicates significant urinary protein loss. The fine granular casts indicate tubular epithelial damage. The isosthenuric specific gravity in the face of dehydration and azotemia, yet in the absence of electrolyte depletion, suggests renal disease as well. This is likely a case of acute renal failure secondary to heat stress. The presence of calcium oxalate crystals may have no importance, or may represent one potential route of calcium loss due to renal tubular damage associated with the hypocalcemia.

Summary

Heat stress, hypertonic dehydration, and acute renal failure. If one did not have the history given, or doubted its veracity, laboratory findings like these would strongly suggest antifreeze intoxication. One could analyze serum for ethylene glycol concentration to definitively rule this possibility in or out.

Case 31

Signalment: 4-year-old intact male Cairn terrier dog
History: Experiencing intermittent periods of weakness and lameness
Physical examination: Mild dehydration, foul-smelling breath, teeth covered with tartar

Hematology		Reference interval
PCV (%)	**11**	37–55
Hgb (g/dL)	**4.0**	12–18
RBC ($\times10^6/\mu L$)	**1.64**	5.5–8.5
MCV (fL)	67	60–72
MCHC (g/dL)	36	34–38
Retics ($\times10^3/\mu L$)	13.1	<60
NCC ($\times10^3/\mu L$)	8.7	6–17
Segs ($\times10^3/\mu L$)	7.7	3–11.5
Bands ($\times10^3/\mu L$)	0.1	0–0.3
Monos ($\times10^3/\mu L$)	0.3	0.1–1.3
Lymphs ($\times10^3/\mu L$)	**0.4**	1–4.8
Eos ($\times10^3/\mu L$)	0.2	0.1–1.2
Platelets ($\times10^3/\mu L$)	370	200–500
TP (P) (g/dL)	6.8	6–8

Hemopathology: Slight anisocytosis and slight polychromasia.

Biochemical profile		Reference interval
Gluc (mg/dL)	91	65–122
BUN (mg/dL)	**183 *(65.3)***	7–28 *(2.5–10.0 mmol/L)*
Creat (mg/dL)	**8.1 *(716)***	0.9–1.7 *(79–150 μmol/L)*
Ca (mg/dL)	**8.2 *(2.05)***	9.0–11.2 *(2.25–2.8 mmol/L)*
Phos (mg/dL)	**17.2 *(5.5)***	2.8–6.1 *(0.9–2.9 mmol/L)*
TP (g/dL)	5.8	5.4–7.4
Alb (g/dL)	3.2	2.7–4.5
Glob (g/dL)	2.6	1.9–3.4
T. bili (mg/dL)	0.4	0–0.4
Chol (mg/dL)	180	130–370
ALT (IU/L)	19	10–120
AST (IU/L)	17	16–40
ALP (IU/L)	40	35–280
Na (mEq/L)	146	145–158
K (mEq/L)	5.0	4.1–5.5
Cl (mEq/L)	115	106–127
TCO_2 (mEq/L)	16	14–27
An. gap (mEq/K)	20	8–25

Urinalysis (catheterized)			
Color	Yellow	**Urine sediment**	
Transparency	Clear	WBCs/hpf	3–5
Sp. gr.	**1.008**	RBCs/hpf	2–3
Protein	Trace	Epith cells/hpf	0
Gluc	Negative	Casts/lpf	0
Bilirubin	Negative	Crystals	0
Blood	Negative	Bacteria	0
pH	5.0		

Interpretive discussion

Hematology

The nonregenerative anemia is secondary to chronic renal disease. Decreased erythropoietin production by the kidneys is a major factor leading to anemia in animals with chronic renal disease. The severity of anemia is unusual for chronic renal disease. Such anemias are typically of mild to moderate severity. Other causes of nonregenerative anemia should also be considered in this case.

The cause of the lymphopenia is increased blood steroid concentration associated with stress. The leukocyte response in not a typical steroid-mediated response in that a mature neutrophilia typically accompanies lymphopenia. It is likely that the animal's resting neutrophil concentration was low normal and it has approximately doubled due to the steroid influence.

Biochemical profile

The triad of BUN, creatinine, and phosphorus concentrations is markedly increased indicating decreased glomerular filtration. These products are passively filtered by the glomerulus, and any cause of decreased glomerular filtration will result in retention of these analytes in the blood. In light of the urine specific gravity in the isosthenuric range, primary renal azotemia is interpreted.

At least two mechanisms have played a role in causing the hypocalcemia. The phosphorus concentration is markedly increased, and the Ca · P product is 141. When this product exceeds 70, calcium and phosphorus precipitate in soft tissues, decreasing the serum calcium concentration. In addition, chronic renal disease may result in decreased activation of vitamin D by the kidneys (i.e., conversion of 25-hydroxycholecalciferol to 1,25-dihydroxycholecalciferoL). Decreased activated vitamin D results in decreased absorption of calcium from the intestinal tract.

Urinalysis

A urine specific gravity in the isosthenuric range in an azotemic animal suggests an inability to concentrate urine. Animals with prerenal azotemia due to decreased renal perfusion (e.g., dehydration, cardiac insufficiency, circulatory shock) should be conserving water and concentrating urine. The urine specific gravity is a key to properly interpreting the cause of the azotemia in this case.

Urine sediment—Small numbers of leukocytes and erythrocytes are normal in urine. These numbers must be interpreted in light of the urine concentration and the technique used to concentrate the sediment. Leukocyte numbers may be slightly increased in this case, suggesting minimal inflammation in the urinary tract.

Summary

These data indicate chronic renal failure. Chronicity is suggested by the nonregenerative anemia, which would not be present with acute renal failure. Postmortem diagnosis in this case was chronic interstitial nephritis or end-stage renal disease. No lesions suggesting suppurative inflammation in the urinary tract were found.

Case 32

Signalment: 9-year-old intact female dog
History: Abscess on rear leg 2 months ago. Intermittent vomiting began 2 days ago.
Physical examination: Popliteal and cervical lymph nodes are enlarged

Hematology		Reference interval
PCV (%)	**35**	37–55
Hgb (g/dL)	12.1	12–18
RBC (×10^6/μL)	5.6	5.5–8.5
MCV (fL)	62	60–72
MCHC (g/dL)	36	34–38
Retics (×10^3/μL)	22.4	<60
NCC (×10^3/μL)	13	6–17
Segs (×10^3/μL)	9.4	3–11.5
Bands (×10^3/μL)	0.1	0–0.3
Monos (×10^3/μL)	0.8	0.1–1.3
Lymphs (×10^3/μL)	2.4	1–4.8
Eos (×10^3/μL)	0.3	0.1–1.2
Platelets (×10^3/μL)	250	200–500
TP (P) (g/dL)	6.2	6–8

Hemopathology: Normal.

Biochemical profile		Reference interval
Gluc (mg/dL)	89	65–122
BUN (mg/dL)	**114 *(40.7)***	7–28 *(2.5–10.0 mmol/L)*
Creat (mg/dL)	**3.2 *(283)***	0.9–1.7 *(79–150 μmol/L)*
Ca (mg/dL)	**8.5 *(2.12)***	9.0–11.2 *(2.25–2.8 mmol/L)*
Phos (mg/dL)	**8.8 *(2.84)***	2.8–6.1 *(0.9–2.9 mmol/L)*
TP (g/dL)	**5.2**	5.4–7.4
Alb (g/dL)	**1.2**	2.7–4.5
Glob (g/dL)	**4.0**	1.9–3.4
T. bili (mg/dL)	0.3	0–0.4
Chol (mg/dL)	**582 *(15.1)***	130–370 *(3.4–9.6 mmol/L)*
ALT (IU/L)	18	10–120
AST (IU/L)	20	16–40
ALP (IU/L)	22	35–280
Na (mEq/L)	**142**	145–158
K (mEq/L)	4.7	4.1–5.5
CL (mEq/L)	120	106–127
TCO_2 (mEq/L)	18	14–27
An. gap (mEq/L)	9	8–25
Amylase (IU/L)	**1530**	50–1250
Lipase (IU/L)	**720**	30–560

Urinalysis (catheterized)			
Color	Yellow	**Urine sediment**	
Transparency	Cloudy	WBCs/hpf	0
Sp. gr.	**1.021**	RBCs/hpf	0
Protein	**4+**	Epith cells/hpf	0
Gluc	Negative	Casts/lpf	2–3 granular
Bilirubin	Negative	Crystals	0
Blood	Negative	Bacteria	0
pH	6.0		
protein/ creatinine ratio (UPC)	5.4		

Interpretive discussion

Hematology

A mild nonregenerative anemia (reticulocyte count is in the normal range) is present. This should prompt an evaluation for endocrine disease, renal disease, and chronic inflammatory disease as potential causes. In this case, chronic renal disease is probably the underlying cause. There is no evidence of inflammatory disease in the leukogram.

Biochemical profile

The azotemia indicated by increased concentrations of BUN, creatinine, and phosphorus should be classified as renal since urine concentration is not adequate (i.e., <1.030), suggesting a loss of renal concentrating ability.

The hypocalcemia is probably due to two factors. The calcium · phosphorus product is 75. When this product exceeds 70, precipitation of calcium and phosphorus in soft tissues can occur, and decreased serum calcium concentrations may result. In addition, activation of vitamin D by the kidney is decreased in chronic renal disease, resulting in decreased absorption of calcium from the small intestine.

The hyperphosphatemia is due to decreased glomerular filtration rate (GFR). In this case, glomerular disease has caused decreased GFR and subsequent hyperphosphatemia.

In light of the marked proteinuria, the most likely cause of the hypoproteinemia and hypoalbuminemia is renal protein loss, due to glomerular disease. The hyperglobulinemia most likely resulted from chronic antigenic stimulation. History of a previous abscess and subsequent lymph node enlargement are compatible with such antigenic stimulation (i.e., the original infection may not have been completely eliminated, resulting in chronic antigenic stimulation and hyperplasia in lymphoid tissue). Such chronic antigenic stimulation can predispose to some forms of glomerular disease.

Hypercholesterolemia is interpreted as a component of nephrotic syndrome. Nephrotic syndrome, a group of abnormalities that may be associated with serious glomerular disease, includes hypoalbuminemia, proteinuria, hypercholesterolemia and edema. In this case, edema was not observed; however, presence of the other three components is still suggestive of this syndrome. Edema is not likely to occur until the albumin is below 1.0 g/dl. The mechanism causing hypercholesterolemia in this syndrome has not been identified.

The cause of mild hyponatremia is not certain in this case. Renal Na loss is a possible cause. If edema were present, it is possible that dilution of extracellular Na in this fluid (third-spacing) could result in decreased serum Na concentration. Edema was, however, not evident in this case, and, even in animals with edema, hyponatremia is not common.

Serum amylase and lipase activities are commonly increased in animals with decreased GFR. Although other causes of increased activities such as pancreatitis could be considered in this case, the clinical presentation and other laboratory data are more compatible with decreased GFR resulting in mildly increased amylase and lipase activities.

Urinalysis

Urine concentrating ability is inadequate. If the azotemia in this dog were due to prerenal causes such as dehydration, cardiac insufficiency, or circulatory shock, urine specific gravity should be >1.030. The specific gravity suggests inadequate concentrating ability and primary renal azotemia. Postrenal azotemia is ruled out by the demonstration of a patent urethra via catheterization and by the absence of evidence of urine leakage into tissues or the abdomen. Lack of concentrating ability results from loss of nephrons and/or tubular damage. Both of these alterations are probably occurring in this dog. Although the disease is primarily glomerular, severe damage to glomeruli results in secondary tubular damage and in loss of nephrons.

A 4+ protein in a moderately dilute urine and a urine protein/creatinine ratio (UPC) of 5.4 are evidence of severe proteinuria. In the absence of evidence of hemorrhage or inflammation (i.e., increased erythrocyte or leukocyte numbers in the urine sediment), a UPC >1.0 is abnormal in the dog, and a UPC >5.0 is indicative of glomerular disease. A UPC of >15 is diagnostic for glomerular disease.

Summary

Renal biopsy revealed amyloidosis. Chronic infection resulting in chronic antigenic stimulation probably predisposed the dog to this disease. The lymph node enlargement was most likely due to hyperplasia secondary to chronic antigenic stimulation. The combination of hypoalbuminemia, proteinuria, and hypercholesterolemia suggest imminent onset of nephrotic syndrome.

Case 33

Signalment: 13-year-old castrated male cat
History: Rear leg paralysis, dyspnea, vomiting
Physical examination: Lethargy and dyspnea. Systolic murmur detected.

Hematology	Day 1	Reference interval
PCV (%)	35	24–45
Hgb (g/dL)	11.3	8–15
RBC (×10^6/μL)	8.05	5–11
MCV (fL)	44	39–50
MCHC (g/dL)	**32**	33–37
NCC (×10^3/μL)	18.1	5.5–19.5
Segs (×10^3/μL)	**16.3**	2.5–12.5
Monos (×10^3/μL)	0.5	0–0.8
Lymphs (×10^3/μL)	**0.9**	1.5–7.0
Basophils (×10^3/μL)	0.2	Rare
NRBC (×10^3/μL)	**0.2**	0
Platelets (×10^3/μL)	Adequate	
TP (P) (g/dL)	7.2	6–8

Hemopathology: Normal.

Biochemical profile	Day 1	Day 3	Reference interval
Gluc (mg/dL)	**153 *(8.4)***	**360 *(19.8)***	67–124 *(3.7–6.8 mmol/L)*
BUN (mg/dL)	**46 *(16.4)***	**137 *(48.9)***	17–32 *(6.1–11.4 mmol/L)*
Creat (mg/dL)	**2.9 *(256)***	**9.8 *(866)***	0.9–2.1 *(80–186 mmol/L)*
Ca (mg/dL)	**8.4 *(2.12)***	**4.9 *(1.22)***	8.5–11 *(2.12–2.75 mmol/L)*
Phos (mg/dL)	**8.0 *(2.6)***	**16.1 *(5.2)***	3.3–7.8 *(1.1–2.5 mmol/L)*
TP (g/dL)	6.9	**5.4**	5.9–8.1
Alb (g/dL)	2.8	2.4	2.3–3.9
Glob (g/dL)	4.1	3.0	2.9–4.4
T. bili (mg/dL)	0.2	0.3	0–0.3
Chol (mg/dL)	192	151	60–220
ALT (IU/L)	**158**	**294**	30–100
AST (IU/L)	**461**	**643**	14–38
ALP (IU/L)	54	25	6–106
GGT (IU/L)	0	1	0–1
CK (IU/L)	**45 313**	**350 930**	60–300
Na (mEq/L)	150	**139**	146–160
K (mEq/L)	4.9	**6.6**	3.7–5.4
CL (mEq/L)	119	**99**	112–129
TCO_2 (mEq/L)	19.2	15.9	14–23
An. gap (mEq/L)	17	**31**	10–27

Urinalysis (cystocentesis)	Day 1	Day 3	Urine sediment	Day 1	Day 3
Color	Dark yellow	Light yellow	WBCs/hpf	**15–20**	0–1
Transparency	Hazy	Clear	RBCs/hpf	**35–50**	5–10
Sp. gr.	1.050	**1.010**	Epith cells/hpf	0	0
Protein	**2+**	**1+**	Casts/lpf	**Few granular**	0
Gluc	**4+**	**4+**	Crystals	0	0
Ketones	**2+**	Negative			
Bilirubin	Negative	Negative	Bacteria	0	0
Blood	**4+**	**4+**			
pH	5.5	5.0			

Fractional excretion	Day 1	Reference interval
Na (%)	**7.2**	<1.0
K (%)	**165.1**	5–20
P (%)	**68.6**	<7–21
Ca (%)	**10.5**	<1.0

Coagulation data	Day 1	Day 3	Reference interval
PT (seconds)	10.0	8.9	7–11.5
aPTT (seconds)	**8.2**	16.5	10–18

Endocrine data	Day 1	Day 3	Reference interval
Total T4 (μg/dL)		1.34	1.2–4.8

Interpretive discussion

Hematology

In light of normal values for other erythrocyte measurements, the slightly decreased MCHC is not significant. Mature neutrophilia and lymphopenia are typical of a stress leukogram. The basophils are not significant. Occasionally, nucleated RBCs may be found in the blood of normal animals. In the absence of anemia or other erythrocyte abnormalities, the few nucleated RBCs noted in this cat are not important.

Biochemical profile

The cat is hyperglycemic on Days 1 and 3. This abnormality could be due to severe excitement or stress with resulting increased epinephrine or corticosteroid levels, respectively. The leukogram is suggestive of stress. The presence of ketonuria on Day 1 suggests that diabetes mellitus should also be considered. Although this cat's blood glucose concentration on Day 1 is not above the renal threshold, detection of glucosuria on this day suggests that the cat may have had periods with higher blood glucose concentrations or that this cat has an abnormally low renal threshold for glucose.

The cat has an azotemia that progresses from mild to severe. Since urine specific gravity is high on Day 1, the azotemia on that day appears to be prerenal. Urine specific gravity is in the isosthenuric range on Day 3 and may be of renal origin; however, the cat had received fluid therapy, and this, rather than renal failure, likely caused the low urine specific gravity on this day.

Hypocalcemia progresses from mild on Day 1 to marked on Day 3. While ethylene glycol toxicosis may result in hypocalcemia and causes severe azotemia, rear leg paralysis and increased CK activity are not associated with ethylene glycol toxicosis. The Ca · P product on Day 1 is 67 on Day 1 and 79 by Day 3. Precipitation of Ca and P in the tissues may, therefore, be occurring on Day 3 and may, in part, explain the decreasing Ca concentration. Massive muscle tissue destruction, as evidenced by increased CK activity, may have resulted in calcium precipitation in damaged tissues and subsequent hypocalcemia.

Hyperphosphatemia resulted from decreased glomerular filtration rate. Maintenance of normal serum P concentration depends on normal glomerular clearance of P.

Total serum protein concentration was normal on Day 1 but decreased by Day 3. Although both albumin and globulin concentrations remained within reference intervals, concentrations of both of these proteins decreased due to fluid therapy and subsequent expansion of blood volume. In light of normal serum albumin and globulin concentrations, the significance of the hypoproteinemia is borderline.

Increased serum ALT activity suggests mild hepatocyte injury that progressed to moderate.

The combination of increased serum AST and CK activities indicates muscle injury. Since CK has a short half-life (less than 4 hours), the extremely high CK activity implies active muscle damage. AST is also present in hepatocytes, and hepatic injury is an alternate explanation for the increased serum AST activity, but, in light of the increased serum CK activity, muscle origin is most likely.

Hyponatremia on Day 3 may be due to renal loss (see fractional excretion results). Since hypochloremia is also evident, vomiting could also be a cause of Na loss. Hypochloremia on Day 3 may be due to both renal loss and vomiting.

Hyperkalemia on Day 3 may be due to several different causes. Since the cat is in renal failure, kidneys may not be excreting K normally. This cat also had a significant degree of tissue necrosis that could have resulted in release of K from dead or dying cells.

The increased anion gap suggests increased concentrations of anions such as ketones, uremic acids, phosphate, sulfate, or lactate. Ketones are not present in the urine of this cat on Day 3, and a significant ketosis is, therefore, not likely. Since the cat is severely azotemic, concentrations of uremic acids are probably increased. Serum phosphorus concentration confirms that increased phosphate is contributing to the anion gap. The final diagnosis suggested that this cat had significant tissue damage, and this probably increased serum sulfate concentrations. Hypoxia was also a component of this cat's disease; therefore, lactic acidosis was also occurring.

Urinalysis

The implications of the urine specific gravities were discussed in the interpretation of this cat's azotemia. The cat has proteinuria and hematuria on both days and pyuria on Day 1. These abnormalities suggest urinary tract inflammation. Cystitis or pyelonephritis are possible causes of this inflammation. The protein concentration decreased between Days 1 and 3, but this probably reflects the change in the concentration of the urine with more dilution of protein on Day 3. Both pyuria and hematuria probably contributed to the proteinuria. Other causes of proteinuria such as glomerular or tubular disease cannot be eliminated. The dipstick test for blood was equally increased on Days 1 and 3, but the RBC concentration decreased markedly between these days. This suggests that the positive test is due to either hemoglobinuria or myoglobinuria. In light of the apparent muscle injury (increased CK), myoglobinuria is most likely.

Glucosuria is marked on both days. On Day 3, this reflects a blood glucose concentration that exceeds the renal threshold. The glucosuria is more difficult to explain on Day 1, when the blood glucose is below the renal threshold. While it is possible that this cat has a lowered renal threshold, it is also possible blood glucose concentrations were fluctuating on Day 1 with periods above the renal threshold occurring.

Presence of a few granular cast suggests tubular damage.

The significance of the positive urine ketone reaction is considered in the discussion of hyperglycemia.

Fractional excretions of Na, K, P, and Ca are increased. This indicates abnormal reabsorption of these electrolytes and, in this case, is probably due to acute renal damage.

Coagulation data

The activated partial thromboplastin time (aPTT) is slightly decreased on Day 1 and probably reflects this cat's hypercoagulable condition. The mechanism of this change is not known but may be related to this cat's cardiac problem (see summary). This cat was treated with streptokinase between Days 1 and 3, and this treatment increases aPTT and PT, and return of aPTT to within the reference interval on Day 3 may have resulted from this treatment; however, the absence of a longer PT on Day 1 as compared to Day 3 makes a significant effect of streptokinase treatment less certain.

Summary

Clinical diagnosis was restrictive cardiomyopathy with aortic thromboemboli (saddle and renal thrombosis and pulmonary thromboembolism). Restrictive cardiomyopathy predisposes to thrombosis. In this case, the thrombotic disease involved the kidneys and resulted in acute renal failure. In addition, hypoxia occurred in other tissues including the muscles of the rear legs. This resulted in increased serum activities of AST and CK. Necropsy examination was not performed.

CASES

Case 34

Signalment: 11-year-old FS canine
History: Weight loss and polyuria
Physical examination: Thin, slightly dehydrated

Hematology		Reference interval
PCV (%)	**36.0**	37–55
Hgb (g/dL)	12.5	12–18
RBC ($\times10^6/\mu L$)	**5.38**	5.5–8.5
MCV (fL)	67.0	60–72
MCHC (g/dL)	35.0	34–38
NCC ($\times10^3/\mu L$)	7.0	6–17
Segs ($\times10^3/\mu L$)	6.1	3–11.5
Bands ($\times10^3/\mu L$)	0.1	0–0.3
Monos ($\times10^3/\mu L$)	0.2	0.1–1.3
Lymphs ($\times10^3/\mu L$)	**0.5**	1–4.8
Eos ($\times10^3/\mu L$)	0.1	0.1–1.2
Platelets ($\times10^3/\mu L$)	400	200–500
TP (P) (g/dL)	8.1	6–8

Biochemical profile		Reference interval
Gluc (mg/dL)	112	65–122
BUN (mg/dL)	**216 (77.1)**	7–28 *(2.5–10.0 mmol/L)*
Creat (mg/dL)	**15.6 (1379)**	0.9–1.7 *(79–150 µmol/L)*
Ca (mg/dL)	**12.1 *(3.0)***	9.0–11.2 *(2.25–2.8 mmol/L)*
Phos (mg/dL)	**20.9 (6.75)**	2.8–6.1 *(0.9–2.9 mmol/L)*
TP (g/dL)	6.9	5.4–7.4
Alb (g/dL)	4.0	2.7–4.5
Glob (g/dL)	2.9	1.9–3.4
T. bili (mg/dL)	0.4	0–0.4
Chol (mg/dL)	335	130–370
ALT (IU/L)	73	10–120
AST (IU/L)	25	16–40
ALP (IU/L)	**662**	35–280
GGT (IU/L)	**8**	0–6
Na (mEq/L)	**144**	145–158
K (mEq/L)	**6.2**	4.1–5.5
CL (mEq/L)	**98**	106–127
TCO_2 (mEq/L)	**13.1**	14–27
An. gap (mEq/L)	**39**	8–25
Amylase (IU/L)	866	50–1250
Lipase (IU/L)	386	30–560

Urinalysis			
Color	Yellow	**Urine sediment**	
Transparency	Cloudy	WBCs/hpf	1–2
Sp. gr.	**1.011**	RBCs/hpf	1–2
Protein	**3+**	Epith cells/hpf	5–8
Gluc	Negative	Casts/lpf	**0–1 coarse granular and waxy**
Bilirubin	1+	Crystals	Negative
Blood	Trace	Bacteria	Negative
pH	6.0		
UPC	**11.1**		

Interpretive discussion

Hematology

The PCV is marginally decreased, but without reticulocyte count it is difficult to classify the regenerative response. A marginal normocytic, normochromic anemia is observed in renal failure, for which there are other indications in the laboratory data.

The lymphopenia indicates a steroid response.

Biochemical profile

The serum glucose concentration is normal.

The BUN, serum creatinine, and serum phosphorus values are markedly increased. These findings are consistent with decreased glomerular filtration rate. However, one cannot differentiate the nature of the azotemia (prerenal, renal, or postrenal) based on these findings alone. Refer to the discussion of urinalysis results for further interpretation.

Serum total calcium is mildly increased, for which one should consider hypercalcemia of malignancy, hypoadrenocorticism, renal failure, vitamin D toxicosis, or primary hyperparathyroidism.

A significant increase in serum ALP activity and mild increase in GGT activity is consistent with cholestasis. Because AST and ALT activities are normal, there is not likely any hepatocellular damage. ALP and GGT activities may also be increased by corticosteroids.

Serum Na and Cl are decreased in concentration, while serum K is increased. The Na: K ratio is 23.2, which may indicate hypoadrenocorticism. Alternatively, renal disease may result in a functional hypoadrenocorticism due to inability of the damaged renal tubules to respond appropriately to mineralocorticoids or may be due to a simple loss of sodium and retention of potassium because of renal disease and oliguria. The serum total CO_2 is decreased, indicating a metabolic acidosis, while the anion gap is increased, indicating the accumulation of organic anions. Acidosis may result in hyperkalemia as well.

The serum calculated osmolality is increased, predominantly because of the profound azotemia. Likewise, the increased anion gap is due to retention of urinary metabolic products.

Serum amylase and lipase activities are normal, and while not definitive, lessen the probability for pancreatitis.

Urinalysis

The urinary specific gravity is in the isosthenuric range, and there is 3+ proteinuria in the absence of significant hematuria or pyuria. The urinary protein: creatinine ratio is 11.1, which is significantly increased. The mild bilirubinuria is likely significant considering the low specific gravity. The coarse granular and waxy casts also definitively indicate renal tubular damage. Together with the marked azotemia, these findings support a diagnosis of renal disease.

Summary

Malignant fibrous histiocytoma of both kidneys identified at postmortem examination. This accounted for chronic renal failure.

Case 35

Signalment: 12-year-old quarter horse gelding
History: Losing weight and recently has loose stools
Physical examination: Thin to poor body condition, mild dependent edema all four limbs. Horse developed watery diarrhea during hospitalization.

Hematology		Reference interval
Packed cell volume (%)	**23**	32–52
Hemoglobin (g/dL)	**7.9**	11–18
RBC ($10^6/\mu L$)	**4.41**	6.5–10.5
MCV (fL)	52	36–52
MCHC (g/dL)	34	34–39
Total nucleated cell count ($\times 10^3/\mu L$)	2.5	5.5–12.5
Segmented neutrophils ($\times 10^3/\mu L$)	**0.10**	2.7–6.7
Band neutrophils ($\times 10^3/\mu L$)	**0.025**	0–0.1
Monocytes ($\times 10^3/\mu L$)	0.150	0–0.8
Lymphocytes ($\times 10^3/\mu L$)	2.20	1.5–5.5
Eosinophils ($\times 10^3/\mu L$)	0.025	0–0.9
Platelets ($\times 10^3/\mu L$)	217	150–500
Plasma protein (g/dL)	**4.6**	6–8

Note: Toxic changes in neutrophils

Biochemical profile		Reference interval
Glucose (mg/dL)	**153**	70–110
Blood urea nitrogen (mg/dL)	**254**	14–27
Creatinine (mg/dL)	**23**	1.1–2.0
Calcium (mg/dL)	**16.7**	11–13.7
Phosphorus (mg/dL)	**1.2**	1.9–4.1
Total protein (g/dL)	**4.1**	5.8–7.6
Albumin (g/dL)	**1.7**	2.7–3.7
Globulin (g/dL)	**2.4**	2.6–4.6
Total bilirubin (mg/dL)	**5.2**	0.6–2.1
Aspartate aminotransferase (IU/L)	229	185–300
Alkaline phosphatase (IU/L)	255	90–290
GGT (IU/L)	**23**	7–17
CK (IU/L)	**2341**	130–470
Sodium (mEq/L)	**125**	133–145
Potassium (mEq/L)	**8.5**	2.2–4.6
Chloride (mEq/L)	**95**	100–111
Total CO_2 (mEq/L)	**17**	24–34
Anion gap (mEq/L)	**22**	5–15

Urinalysis voided			
Color	yellow	**Urine sediment**	
Transparency	clear	WBCs/hpf	0–3
Specific Gravity	**1.009**	RBCs/hpf	0–5
Protein	**2+**	Epithelial cells/hpf	None
Glucose	neg	Casts/lpf	Neg
Ketones	neg	Crystals	Calcium carbonate
Blood	neg		

Interpretive discussion

Hematology

The PCV, hemoglobin, and total RBC count are decreased, indicating a moderate anemia is present. It cannot be determined if the anemia is regenerative because reticulocytes are not released from marrow in the horse. Given the biochemistry profile the anemia is likely due to chronic renal failure (CRF). The mild to moderate degree of anemia fits with CRF as severe anemia is not seen with renal failure unless there is a second problem, e.g., blood loss. If this horse is dehydrated the anemia is more severe as are the protein losses. The plasma protein is markedly decreased, likely due to diarrhea and GI loss. There is severe, life-threatening leukopenia, neutropenia with a left shift and toxic changes in neutrophils. This is seen with acute diarrheal disease in horses due to endotoxemia and/or overwhelming sepsis. The bone marrow cannot meet demands and a likely source of the problem is enteric salmonellosis with or without septicemia.

Biochemistry profile

This horse has GI and renal disease, both appear to be severe. Marked azotemia, isosthenuria and hypercalcemia with hypophosphatemia are diagnostic for renal failure in the horse. Suspect chronic renal failure due to poor body condition, history, anemia, hypoalbuminemia, electrolyte abnormalities and an inactive urine sediment. Additionally, chronic renal failure is more common than acute renal failure in horses. UN and Ct are about as high as possible in a living patient; clearly this is not due to a prerenal cause. Isosthenuria confirms renal and postrenal is rare in an adult horse, especially one that is urinating, perhaps even with an increased volume of urine. Lesion in the kidneys is likely to be end-stage, small shrunken kidneys with fibrosis and little to no chance of regeneration or long-term survival. Lesion may have started as glomerulonephritis or amyloidosis as hypoalbuminemia is moderate, but it can also be seen in severe chronic renal failure from any cause that compromises glomerular function. Peripheral edema is attributed to hypoalbuminemia and decreased colloidal osmotic pressure. Horses tend to develop peripheral edema rather than ascites with hypoalbuminemia.

Hypercalcemia and hypophosphatemia are only seen with renal failure in Equidae, all other species develop hyperphosphatemia even if hypercalcemia is present. The only other differentials for hypercalcemia and hypophosphatemia are a malignancy and primary hyperparathyroidism. Hypercalcemia of malignancy (HHM) is uncommon in horses but has been reported in horses with gastric carcinoma and lymphoma. Primary hyperparathyroidism is very rare in horses and would only be pursued if renal failure and HHM are ruled out first. All three differentials are associated with dilute urine due to inhibition of ADH by hypercalcemia. If mild or moderate azotemia is present with dilute urine in a horse with hypercalcemia and hypophosphatemia it can be difficult to distinguish HHM and chronic renal failure. The easiest diagnostic tests are to first search for cancer (enlarged lymph nodes and endoscopy to look for gastric SCC), rectal and/or ultrasound examination of kidneys to determine if they are small and shrunken. If this does not clarify, then consider protein creatinine ratio and/or fractional excretion of sodium, if <1% rule out renal, if >1% rule in renal. Always favor renal failure over HHM in horses.

Hyponatremia and hypochloremia can be attributed to chronic renal failure and/or GI loss; the latter is more likely. The hyperkalemia is severe and life threatening. This is unusual as adult horses tend to develop hypokalemia with GI disease but young horses with diarrhea will have hyperkalemia. The most likely explanation is metabolic acidosis even though it does not appear that severe in this horse. The pattern of hyponatremia and hyperkalemia can be seen with renal failure, urinary bladder rupture and hypoadrenocorticism. Decreased bicarbonate (TCO_2) is due to GI and/or renal loss. Increased anion gap is due to retained uremic acids, shock and anaerobic glycolysis with accumulation of lactic acid. Horses with diarrheal diseases usually have a metabolic acidosis as does this horse. Hypoalbuminemia and concurrent decreased serum globulin are due to GI disease, suspect salmonellosis. Hypoalbuminemia is moderate and more severe than the decrease in globulins, which may be due to renal loss of albumin in addition to the loss in GI tract. Proteinuria without blood is present in the urine and supports renal loss of albumin. Increased bilirubin is due to anorexia, which is the most common cause of icterus in horses. Although hepatic disease and cholestasis are possible explanations, they are too unlikely given all of the clinical and biochemistry data (liver enzymes WRI). The mild increase in GGT may be spurious rather than a true indicator of liver issues. GGT seems to increase in horses easily and is not reliable indicator of hepatic problems if increased without any increases in other hepatic parameters.

Increase in CPK is mild for a horse and is due to recumbency, it is too low to consider a primary muscle disease. The AST is WRI so it is not a muscle problem in which the CPK is decreasing while the AST is still increased. The urine is yellow, no evidence of brown color or blood, rule out myoglobin-induced renal damage with these values. Urine is not concentrated; a second check to confirm isosthenuria is usually recommended but in this case is not needed. Proteinuria with no evidence of hemorrhage or active sediment in an animal with hypoalbuminemia is due to renal loss. The proteinuria is more severe than 2+ since the urine is dilute. A protein to creatinine ratio could help assess the degree of severity but is not needed in this case, given all of the data. The few white and red blood cells are inconsequential, may be due to voided urine and the calcium carbonate crystals are normal for a horse.

Summary

Marked chronic renal failure and salmonellosis

Outcome

Horse was euthanized and chronic renal failure and salmonellosis were confirmed at autopsy. Initially the horse presented primarily for weight loss, while it was being evaluated it developed profuse diarrhea in the hospital. The horse was sick and stressed and likely had a recrudescence of salmonella. The horse may have been a carrier of salmonella.

Both kidneys were small, knobby and looked like irregular bovine kidneys due to marked fibrosis. Microscopically there was severe glomerulonephritis, chronic interstitial nephritis and even oxalate crystals in many tubules. The oxalate crystals were attributed to either being a horse or endogenous formation of oxalates, which happens in chronic renal failure in dogs and other species as well. It was not ethylene glycol toxicity. Glomerulonephritis was considered the primary lesion but it was difficult to determine if it preceded the interstitial nephritis. Pulmonary thrombi were present and one large thrombus was present in the pulmonary artery. These thrombi were likely due to hypoalbuminemia and decreased AT III (not measured), which lead to a state of increased coagulability. Pulmonary thrombosis associated with decreased AT III and glomerular lesions is seen most frequently, or documented most frequently in dogs.

Hypercalcemia and hypophosphatemia are present in some horses with renal failure, empirically, perhaps about one third. The pathogenesis is not known and multiple theories are postulated. These electrolyte changes will even occur with nephrectomy in the horse. Some horses may excrete excess dietary calcium (from alfalfa-rich diet) in the urine and retain phosphorus. Hypercalcemia is then attributed to decreased excretion by the failing kidneys and hypophosphatemia to increased excretion. However, if the kidneys are removed it seems impossible to explain how they would develop hypophosphatemia. Certainly there cannot be increased renal loss because the kidneys have been removed, so it must be increased GI loss, but this is unproven. Many horses with chronic renal failure will have hyperphosphatemia and normo or hypocalcemia, similar to other species.

Case 36

Signalment: 6-year-old MC feline DSH
History: Approximately 1-month duration of intermittent weakness, exercise intolerance, poor hair coat
Physical examination: Cat is near collapse and approximately 10% dehydrated. There is definite cervical ventroflexion.

Hematology		Reference interval
PCV (%)	41.0	24–45
Segs (×10^3/μL)	**18.0**	2.5–12.5
Monos (×10^3/μL)	0.7	0–0.8
Lymphs (×10^3/μL)	**0.5**	1.5–7.0
Platelets (×10^3/μL)	Adequate	150–700

Biochemical profile		Reference interval
Gluc (mg/dL)	98	67–124
BUN (mg/dL)	**68 *(24.3)***	17–31 *(6.1–11.4 mmol/L)*
Creat (mg/dL)	**2.8 *(247)***	0.9–2.1 *(80–186 μmol/L)*
Ca (mg/dL)	10.9	8.5–11
Phos (mg/dL)	6.8	3.3–7.8
TP (g/dL)	**9.3**	5.9–8.1
Alb (g/dL)	**5.3**	2.3–3.9
Glob (g/dL)	4.0	2.9–4.4
T. bili (mg/dL)	0.3	0–0.3
Chol (mg/dL)	180	60–220
ALT (IU/L)	52	30–100
ALP (IU/L)	48	6–106
CK (IU/L)	**2419**	60–300
Na (mEq/L)	157	146–160
K (mEq/L)	**2.0**	3.7–5.4
CL (mEq/L)	114	112–129
TCO_2 (mEq/L)	15	14–23
An. gap (mEq/L)	**30**	10–27

Blood gas data (arterial)		Reference interval
pH	**7.130**	7.33–7.44
pCO_2 (mmHg)	**44.0**	35–42
HCO_3 (mEq/L)	**14.0**	16–22

Urinalysis		Urine sediment	
Color	Yellow	WBCs/hpf	0–2
Transparency	Cloudy	RBCs/hpf	0–2
Sp. gr.	**1.014**	Epith cells/hpf	0–2
Protein	Trace	Casts/lpf	Negative
Gluc	Negative	Crystals	Negative
Bilirubin	Negative	Bacteria	Negative
Blood	Negative	Other	
pH	5.5		

Fractional excretion		Reference interval
Na (%)	0.55	<1.0
K (%)	**37.7**	<20.0

Interpretive discussion

Hematology

There is a mature neutrophilia and lymphopenia, indicating a stress leukogram. Other components of the hemogram are normal.

Biochemical profile

The BUN and serum creatinine concentrations are mildly increased. These findings are consistent with decreased glomerular filtration rate. However, one cannot differentiate the nature of the azotemia (prerenal, renal, or postrenal) based on these findings alone. Refer to the discussion of urinalysis results for further interpretation. The normal serum phosphorus and total calcium concentrations do not contribute to the characterization of renal disease.

Serum total protein and albumin concentrations are increased; this documents marked dehydration or hemoconcentration.

Serum CK activity is increased significantly and is indicative of muscle damage.

Serum Na and Cl concentrations are normal, but serum K concentration is markedly decreased. This is especially significant in light of the acidosis, which results in a shift of potassium from within cells to extracellular fluid and suggests a marked potassium deficit.

Blood gas data

There is prominent acidosis. This is due to a combined metabolic (decreased HCO_3) and respiratory (increased pCO_2) acidosis, with an increased anion gap. It would not be unusual for this degree of dehydration to lead to hypovolemia-induced lactic acidosis. It is also possible that this degree of hypokalemia may have caused sufficient respiratory muscle dysfunction to impair normal ventilation.

Urinalysis

The urinary specific gravity is in the isosthenuric range. Given the azotemia and normal serum Na and Cl concentrations, this indicates probable renal disease. However, hypokalemia can also impair ADH responsiveness by the kidneys, so that urine concentration should be evaluated following rehydration and K repletion.

The urinary FE_{Na} is 0.55%, which speaks against a generalized renal tubular disease. However, the. FE_K is 37.7%, which is markedly increased, especially for a cat with this degree of hypokalemia.

Summary

The combined observations of azotemia, hypokalemia, acidosis, and hyperkaluria in a cat with cervical ventroflexion and evidence of widespread muscle damage support a diagnosis of feline kaliopenic polymyopathy/nephropathy syndrome. In this case, it was completely corrected by dietary change (nonacidifying, higher K diet). This syndrome is no longer seen, as dietary imbalances in commercial cat food were corrected.

Case 37

Signalment: 2-year-old male West Highland white terrier
History: Polyuria, polydipsia

Hematology		Reference interval
PCV (%)	**33.0**	37–55
Hgb (g/dL)	**11.3**	12–18
RBC (×10^6/μL)	**4.45**	5.5–8.5
MCV (fL)	**74.0**	60–72
MCHC (g/dL)	35.0	33–38
NCC (×10^3/μL)	5.9	6–17
Segs (×10^3/μL)	3.9	3–11.5
Monos (×10^3/μL)	0.4	0.1–1.3
Lymphs (×10^3/μL)	1.2	1–4.8
NRBC (×10^3/μL)	**0.4**	0
Platelets (×10^3/μL)	425	200–500
TP (P) (g/dL)	6.7	6–8

Hemopathology: Few acanthocytes and schistocytes.

Biochemical profile		Reference interval
Gluc (mg/dL)	108	65–122
BUN (mg/dL)	**65 *(23.2)***	7–28 *(2.5–10.0 mmol/L)*
Creat (mg/dL)	**2.0 *(176.8)***	0.9–1.7 *(79–150 μmol/L)*
Ca (mg/dL)	**7.2 *(1.8)***	9.0–11.2 *(2.25–2.8 mmol/L)*
Phos (mg/dL)	6.1	2.8–6.1
TP (g/dL)	5.8	5.4–7.4
Alb (g/dL)	3.7	2.7–4.5
Glob (g/dL)	2.1	1.9–3.4
T. bili (mg/dL)	0.3	0–0.4
Chol (mg/dL)	**382 *(9.9)***	130–370 *(3.4–9.6 mmol/L)*
ALT (IU/L)	56	10–120
ALP (IU/L)	137	35–280
Na (mEq/L)	147	145–158
K (mEq/L)	**3.0**	4.1–5.5
CL (mEq/L)	115	106–127
TCO_2 (mEq/L)	22.3	14–27
An. gap (mEq/L)	12.7	8–25
Calc. osmolality (mOsm/kg)	**317**	290–310

Blood gas data (arterial)		Reference interval
pH	7.349	7.33–7.45
pO_2 (mmHg)	80.1	67–92
pCO_2 (mmHg)	39.1	24–39
HCO_3 (mEq/L)	21.0	14–24
ionized Ca++ (mEq/L)	**3.44**	4.5–5.6

Urinalysis		Urine sediment	
Color	Yellow	WBCs/hpf	3–6
Transparency	Clear	RBCs/hpf	3–6
Sp. gr.	1.028	Epith cells/hpf	0–2
Protein	**2+**	Casts/lpf	**Rare fine gran**
Gluc	**3+**	Crystals	Negative
Bilirubin	1+	Bacteria	Negative
Blood	Negative		
pH	5.0		
Ketones	Trace		
osmolality	358 (mOsm/L)		
UPC	**1.75**		

Fractional excretion		Reference interval
Na (%)	**1.62**	<1.0
Ca (%)	**7.47**	<1.0

Interpretive discussion

Hematology

The packed cell volume, erythrocyte count, and hemoglobin concentration are decreased, indicating an anemia. Observed red blood cell morphologic abnormalities include acanthocytes and schistocytes. These may be observed when there is erythrocytic membrane damage due to free radical or lipid metabolic abnormalities, or when there is microangiopathic pathology due to vascular disease or neoplasia. Although a reticulocyte count has not been provided, the increased erythrocyte MCV and nucleated erythrocytes are consistent with a regenerative response. There are no other hematologic abnormalities.

Biochemical profile

Serum glucose concentration is normal, and its importance in the interpretation of the glucosuria is discussed below.

The BUN and serum creatinine concentrations are increased, while the serum phosphorus value is at the upper limit of the reference interval. These findings are consistent with decreased glomerular filtration rate. However, one cannot differentiate the nature of the azotemia (prerenal, renal, or postrenal) based on these findings alone. Refer to the discussion of urinalysis results for further interpretation.

The serum total calcium concentration is decreased. The ionized calcium concentration reported with the blood gas panel is likewise less than normal, indicating a true hypocalcemia. In this case, excessive loss of calcium in the urine is the likely cause (see urinalysis discussion).

Serum total protein, albumin, and globulin concentrations are within the reference interval. This observation suggests that there is not hemoconcentration due to dehydration, although a concurrent protein losing disorder might exist. Thus, the azotemia noted above is less likely due to dehydration, and more likely renal in origin.

Serum cholesterol is increased, whereas other indices of hepatic function are normal. There are no other indicators of a primary metabolic disease like diabetes mellitus, but it is possible, nevertheless, that this dog has hypothyroidism or hyperadrenocorticism.

The serum sodium and chloride concentrations are normal, yet there is hypokalemia. Possible causes in this case might include hyperadrenocorticism, chronic renal disease, or urinary potassium wasting associated with diuresis. Calculated serum osmolality is mildly increased due to the azotemia.

Blood gas data

Indices of acid-base metabolism (pH, pCO_2, HCO_3, and anion gap) are normal.

Urinalysis

Although the urinary specific gravity indicates some concentrating ability, one would expect this to be greater if the azotemia were prerenal in origin. It is also possible for the specific gravity to be increased by the presence of solutes, which do not contribute to renal concentration capacity (glucose, protein, amino acids). Concomitant determination of urinary. Osmolality (358 mOsm/L) confirms that the urine is not being adequately concentrated relative to the calculated osmolality of the serum. Inability to concentrate the urine may be due to central diabetes insipidus (a defect in hypothalamic/pituitary antidiuretic hormone release), or nephrogenic diabetes insipidus (ADH is released, but the kidney is unable to respond). The latter may be caused by anatomic pathology or functional impairment of renal tubular actions necessary to maintain a medullary concentration gradient and water reabsorption. This finding may indicate that the observed azotemia is renal in origin.

The presence of proteinuria on the dipstick was followed by a chemical determination of urinary protein concentration. When indexed to the urinary creatinine value, the urinary protein: creatinine ratio is 1.75. While this value is probably abnormal, it is not sufficiently high to indicate glomerular protein loss. Values in the range of 1.0 to 2.0 have been associated epidemiologically with tubular or inflammatory causes of proteinuria. The absence of significant numbers of leukocytes suggests there is no inflammatory disease. The presence of fine granular casts is indicative of renal tubular damage, and may explain the proteinuria.

Glucosuria concomitant to euglycemia may be explained by three mechanisms. (i) There is a Fanconi's-type syndrome wherein tubular malfunction leads to loss of glucose, protein, and other solutes that would otherwise be reabsorbed from the glomerular filtrate. This is supported by the findings of modest proteinuria and increased urinary fractional excretion of electrolytes. Fanconi's syndromes may be inherited (as reported in Basenjis and Whippets) or acquired (as reported following exposure to nephrotoxicants, including aminoglycoside antibiotics and heavy metals). (ii) There was an earlier episode of hyperglycemia that exceeded the renal threshold for glucose reabsorption, during which time the urine analyzed was produced. Depending on the rate of urine formation, a single void may represent blood chemistry-related changes for many hours prior to specimen collection. (iii) A laboratory error was made in the determination of either the serum glucose (improper preservation of the blood sample or analytical error) or the urinary glucose (cross-contamination of dipstick reaction squares by excess urine or operator error in interpreting the color change).

The FE_{Na} is 1.62%. This may be indicative of renal tubular disease or dysfunction due to mineralocorticoid deficiency or transport malfunction. The FE_{Ca} is 7.47%. This is particularly inappropriate given the hypocalcemia, and may well be the cause of calcium loss from the body. This may be indicative of renal tubular disease or dysfunction due to parathyroid hormone deficiency or transport malfunction. Increased urinary excretion of both of these electrolytes may be observed in renal failure (consider the azotemia and impaired urinary concentrating ability) or in Fanconi's syndrome, wherein proximal renal tubule reabsorptive function is impaired (consider the euglycemic glucosuria).

Summary

This is a case of congenital Fanconi's syndrome that did not resolve following supportive treatment for renal failure. Other tests one should perform include those that evaluate the parathyroid gland.

Case 38

Signalment: 8-year-old male canine
History: Polydipsia
Physical examination: Slightly dehydrated

Hematology		Reference interval
PCV (%)	38.0	37–55
Hgb (g/dL)	12.0	12–18
RBC (×10^6/µL)	5.51	5.5–8.5
MCV (fL)	69.0	60–72
NCC (×10^3/µL)	**18.2**	6–17
Segs (×10^3/µL)	**2.0**	3–11.5
Monos (×10^3/µL)	0.6	0.1–0.3
Lymphs (×10^3/µL)	**13.8**	1–4.8
Platelets (×10^3/µL)	298	200–500
TP (P) (g/dL)	**8.8**	6–8

Hemopathology: Clumped platelets.

Biochemical profile		Reference interval
Gluc (mg/dL)	91	65–122
BUN (mg/dL)	**33 *(11.8)***	7–28 *(2.5–10.0 mmol/L)*
Creat (mg/dL)	**2.9 *(256)***	0.9–1.7 *(80–150 µmol/L)*
Ca (mg/dL)	**15.4 *(3.85)***	9.0–11.2 *(2.25–2.80 mmol/L)*
Phos (mg/dL)	**7.1 *(2.3)***	2.8–6.1 *(0.9–2.0 mmol/L)*
TP (mg/dL)	**7.9**	5.4–7.4
Alb (g/dL)	4.0	2.7–4.5
Glob (g/dL)	**3.9**	1.9–3.4
T. bili (mg/dl)	**1.0 *(17)***	0–0.4 *(0–6.8 µmol/L)*
Chol (mg/dL)	291	130–370
ALT (IU/L)	**152**	10–120
AST (IU/L)	**64**	16–40
ALP (IU/L)	**361**	35–280
GGT (IU/L)	**14**	0–6
Na (mEq/L)	154	145–158
K (mEq/L)	**5.8**	4.1–5.5
CL (mEq/L)	109	106–127
TCO_2 (mEq/L)	**12.1**	14–27
An. gap (mEq/L)	**38.7**	8–25

Urinalysis		Urine sediment	
Color	Straw	WBCs/hpf	2–3
Transparency	Clear	RBCs/hpf	1–2
Sp. gr.	**1.011**	Epith cells/hpf	Negative
Protein	**2+**	Casts/lpf	Negative
Gluc	Negative	Crystals	Negative
Bilirubin	**2+**	Bacteria	Negative
Blood	Negative		
pH	6.5		
UPC	**2.6**		

Fractional excretion		Reference interval
Na (%)	**1.73**	<1.0
Ca (%)	**3.37**	<1.0

Interpretive discussion

Hematology

The nucleated cell count is mildly increased, but there is a neutropenia and marked lymphocytosis. Other hematologic parameters, including cell morphology, are normal. However, the concurrent observation of marked lymphocytosis and neutropenia should alert one to the possibility of lymphocytic leukemia, lymphoma with bone marrow involvement, or ehrlichiosis. The concurrent observation of marked lymphocytosis and hypercalcemia should likewise lead to consideration of lymphoma and humoral hypercalcemia of malignancy.

Biochemical profile

The BUN, creatinine, and phosphorus concentrations are mildly increased. These findings are consistent with decreased glomerular filtration rate. However, one cannot differentiate the nature of the azotemia (prerenal, renal, or postrenal) based on these findings alone. Refer to the discussion of urinalysis results for further interpretation.

The serum total calcium concentration is markedly increased. In light of the lymphocytosis, humoral hypercalcemia of malignancy is most likely. PTH-rp could be measured to support this interpretation. The Ca · P product is increased at 109, indicating likely soft-tissue mineralization.

The serum total protein and globulin concentrations are slightly increased. Increased globulin concentration may occur in dogs with lymphoproliferative disorders.

The total bilirubin concentration is increased, as are the serum ALP and GGT activities. These findings are evidence of cholestasis. There are mild increases in the serum activities of ALT and AST, so there may be some hepatocellular damage as well.

The increase in serum potassium is probably due to redistribution of intracellular potassium to the extracellular space secondary to acidosis. The serum total CO_2 concentration is mildly decreased, indicating a metabolic acidosis. A complete blood gas panel is required to completely evaluate acid-base status.

Urinalysis

The urine specific gravity is in the isosthenuric range. The dog does not appear to be dehydrated, and it is possible for a normal dog to produce urine with a specific gravity in this range. However, this dog is azotemic. Dilute urine in the face of azotemia usually indicates renal disease, but hypercalcemia interferes with concentrating ability by antagonizing the actions of ADH. Hypercalcemia may also cause damage to the kidney, especially when phosphorus is concurrently increased. There is significant proteinuria of 2+ on the dipstick, and a UPC of 2.6. In the absence of significant sediment changes, this is indicative of renal protein loss, probably glomerular in origin. The FE_{Na} is 1.73%, indicating tubular dysfunction. Increased fractional excretion of Ca is expected given the hypercalcemia.

Summary

This is a case of lymphoma with hypercalcemia of malignancy and hypercalcemic nephropathy.

Case 39

Signalment: 9-year-old female dog
History: Polydipsia, polyuria
Physical examination: Mass in pelvic inlet

Biochemical profile		Reference interval
Gluc (mg/dL)	106	65–122
BUN (mg/dL)	8	7–28
Creat (mg/dL)	1.4	0.9–1.7
TP (g/dL)	**7.7**	5.4–7.4
Alb (g/dL)	**5.2**	2.7–4.5
Ca (mg/dL)	**16.4** ***(4.5)***	9.0–11.2 *(2.25–2.80 mmol/L)*
Phos (mg/dL)	3.5	2.8–6.1
T. bili (mg/dL)	0.2	0–0.4
ALT (IU/L)	43	10–120
ALP (IU/L)	**428**	35–280
Na (mEq/L)	155	145–158
K (mEq/L)	3.9	4.1–5.5
CL (mEq/L)	119	106–127
TCO_2 (mEq/L)	21.6	14–27

Urinalysis	
Specific gravity	**1.014**

Interpretive discussion

Biochemical profile

Hyperproteinemia is due to hyperalbuminemia, indicating dehydration. There is marked hypercalcemia and this magnitude of increase is suggestive of hypercalcemia of malignancy or primary hyperparathyroidism. Hypercalcemia of this magnitude may result in renal injury leading to azotemia and loss of concentrating ability. A dehydrated animal should be maximally concentrating its urine, and this dog's urine is nearly isosthenuric. This could be consistent with renal disease (early, prior to development of azotemia), but hypercalcemia alone is sufficient to explain this abnormality (due to antagonism of ADH at the renal tubules).

A slight increase in alkaline phosphatase activity (ALP) suggests cholestasis or drug induction (corticosteroids, anticonvulsants). If cholestasis is present it is not of sufficient magnitude to affect the serum bilirubin. A more likely explanation for the increased alkaline phosphatase is increased bone turnover secondary to increased serum concentration of PTH or PTH-rp, which could be measured.

Summary

The mass in the pelvis was aspirated, and appeared neuroendocrine, rather than lymphoid. The mass was surgically removed and confirmed by histopathology to be an apocrine gland adenocarcinoma of the anal sac. Following surgery, the calcium normalized, but later metastasis to the lungs resulted in return of hypercalcemia. In contrast to the previous case, the hypercalcemia has not resulted in sufficient renal injury to cause azotemia.

Case 40

Signalment: 6-month-old DSH female cat
History: Vomiting, weakness, acute onset
Physical examination: Tachypnea for 24 hours, weakness

CASES

Hematology		Reference interval
PCV (%)	40	24–45
WBC (×10^3/μL)	**21.0**	5.5–19.5
Segs (×10^3/μL)	**20.2**	2.5–12.5
Bands (×10^3/μL)	0	0–0.3
Lymphs (×10^3/μL)	**0.2**	1.5–7.0
Monos (×10^3/μL)	0.6	0–0.85

Biochemical profile		Reference interval
Gluc (mg/dL)	**150 *(8.2)***	67–124 *(3.7–6.8 mmol/L)*
BUN (mg/dL)	**45 *(16.1)***	17–32 *(6.1–11.4 mmol/L)*
Creat (mg/dL)	**2.2 *(194)***	0.9–2.1 *(80–186 μmol/L)*
Ca (mg/dL)	**18 *(4.5)***	8.5–11 *(2.12–2.75 mmol/L)*
Phos (mg/dL)	**9.5 *(3.1)***	3.3–7.8 *(1.1–2.5 mmol/L)*
TP (g/dL)	8.0	5.9–8.1
Alb (g/dL)	**4.2**	2.3–3.9
Glob (g/dL)	3.8	2.9–4.4
T. bili (mg/dL)	0.2	0–0.3
Chol (mg/dL)	120	60–270
ALT (IU/L)	100	30–100
ALP (IU/L)	25	11–210
Na (mEq/L)	159	146–160
K (mEq/L)	**6.4**	3.7–5.4
CL (mEq/L)	112	112–129
TCO_2 (mEq/L)	16.8	14–24
An. gap (mEq/L)	**37**	10–27

Blood gas data (arterial)		Reference interval
pH	**6.926**	7.33–7.44
pCO_2 (mmHg)	**72.1**	35–42
pO_2 (mmHg)	**65**	80–95
HCO_3 (mEq/L)	**14.9**	16–22

Urinalysis	
Sp. gr.	**1.020**
Gran casts/hpf	**2**

Interpretive discussion

Hematology

There is a stress leukogram indicated by mature neutrophilia and lymphopenia.

Biochemical profile

Increased glucose is compatible with stress identified in the leukogram. The BUN and creatinine are mildly increased, indicating azotemia. The urine specific gravity is less than what one would expect in a cat with prerenal azotemia, therefore renal azotemia should be considered. However, hypercalcemia alone can interfere with normal concentrating ability. With a calcium of 18 mg/dl, renal dysfunction is likely occurring due to soft-tissue mineralization. The total protein and albumin are increased, particularly for a young cat, indicating dehydration.

The calcium is markedly increased. Primary causes of this degree of hypercalcemia are hypercalcemia of malignancy, primary hyperparathyroidism, and hypervitaminosis D. Vitamin D toxicosis should be very high on the differential list, due to the age of the cat and the acute onset. Because of acidosis, ionized calcium is likely very high. Phosphorus is mildly increased. This could be in part due to the young age of the cat or may be due to decreased GFR. It is also seen with hypervitaminosis D. The Ca · P product is markedly increased at 171, which will result in calcification of renal tubules, lungs and other soft tissues.

Potassium is increased. This may be due to acidosis and an associated shift of K out of cells or the animal may be becoming oliguric. Increased anion gap indicates increase in unmeasured anions. Possible unmeasured anions are lactic acid or uremic acids. Increased phosphates are also adding to the anion gap.

Blood gas data

The pH is extremely decreased indicating severe acidemia. The pCO_2 is the major abnormality in the balance between bicarbonate and CO_2. Therefore, respiratory acidosis is the major component of the acidosis. The bicarbonate is also decreased indicating a component of metabolic acidosis is superimposed. Hypoxemia is also present. The combined hypoxemia and retention of CO_2 indicate a severe ventilation abnormality, probably due to calcification of lungs. The metabolic acidosis is probably a result of renal failure.

Summary

The cat was diagnosed with renal disease with severe acidemia, both metabolic and respiratory. The respiratory component may be due to calcification of lungs. Cholecalciferol toxicosis was diagnosed, as the cat had an opportunity to ingest a rodenticide containing cholecalciferol.

Case 41

Signalment: 3-year-old male cat
History: Acute lethargy, vomiting, and anorexia
Physical examination: Obese, almost comatose

Hematology		Reference interval
PCV (%)	**50**	24–45
NCC (×10³/μL)	**24.0**	5.5–19.5
Segs (×10³/μL)	**23.0**	2.5–12.5
Monos (×10³/μL)	0.7	0–0.88
Lymphs (×10³/μL)	**0.3**	1.5–7.0
Platelets (×10³/μL)	Adequate	200–500

Biochemical profile		Reference interval
Gluc (mg/dL)	**285**	67–124
BUN (mg/dL)	**110**	17–32
Creat (mg/dL)	**7.5**	0.9–2.1
Ca (mg/dL)	**6.5**	8.5–11
Phos (mg/dL)	**14**	3.3–7.8
TP (g/dL)	**9.0**	5.9–8.1
Alb (g/dL)	**4.9**	2.3–3.9
Glob (g/dL)	4.1	2.9–4.4
T. bili (mg/dL)	0.3	0–0.3
ALT (IU/L)	35	30–100
ALP (IU/L)	45	11–210
Na (mEq/L)	**165**	146–160
K (mEq/L)	**6.8**	3.7–5.4
CL (mEq/L)	**107**	112–129
TCO_2 (mEq/L)	**10**	14–23
An. gap (mEq/L)	**55**	10–27
Calc. osmolality (mOsm/kg)	**394**	290–310
Meas. osmolality (mOsm/kg)	**440**	290–310
Osmolal gap (mOsm/kg)	**46**	>10

Urinalysis (cystocentesis)			
Color	Yellow	**Urine sediment**	
Transparency	Cloudy	WBCs/hpf	2–3
Sp. gr.	**1.016**	RBCs/hpf	2–3
Protein	**1+**	Epith cells/hpf	1–3 transitional
Gluc	**1+**	Casts/lpf	0
Bilirubin	Negative	Crystals	**Calcium oxalate monohydrate**
Blood	**1+**	Bacteria	0
pH	5.0		

Interpretive discussion

Hematology

PCV is slightly increased. This is likely due to dehydration, considering that the albumin is also increased. The mature neutrophilia and lymphopenia are suggestive of a stress or corticosteroid leukogram.

Biochemical profile

The serum glucose concentration is increased. Differentials should include stress or corticosteroids, excitement and diabetes mellitus. Excitement is less likely than the others, since the cat does not have an excitement leukogram and there is glucosuria. (See summary for further discussion of hyperglycemia.)

The BUN and creatinine are increased, and considering that the cat is not concentrating its urine, this is most likely a renal azotemia. Since the cat is dehydrated, a prerenal component to the azotemia may be present as well. Because the cat is not anemic, is obese, and the history is acute, this is most likely acute renal failure. Phosphorus is increased due to decreased glomerular filtration rate.

The serum calcium is decreased. Considering that the cat likely has acute renal failure, the most likely cause of the hypocalcemia is formation of calcium oxalate crystals associated with ethylene glycol toxicosis. Oxalate is one of the metabolites of ethylene glycol and combines with calcium to form calcium oxalate crystals.

Hyperproteinemia is due to hyperalbuminemia, indicating dehydration.

The sodium is increased, likely due to dehydration. Chloride would be expected to increase with sodium but is selectively decreased in this case, probably due to vomiting of gastric HCl. This causes a hypochloremic alkalosis. However, TCO_2 is decreased and the anion gap is increased, suggesting concurrent metabolic acidosis and a mixed acid–base disorder. A blood gas would more fully characterize the acid–base status.

The increased anion gap indicates increased concentrations of anions other than those used in the formula to calculate the anion gap (chloride and HCO_3^-). In this case, uremic acids, phosphate, albumin, and most importantly, metabolites of ethylene glycol are probably contributing to the anion gap and a high-gap metabolic acidosis.

The calculated osmolality is increased, since the substances that are included in the formula to calculate osmolality are increased (glucose, urea, sodium, potassium). However, the measured plasma osmolality is much higher than the calculated osmolality, since a substance is present in the blood that is not used in the formula to calculate osmolality. The most common cause of an increased osmole gap is the presence of ethylene glycol, which contributes to plasma osmolality due to its low molecular weight.

Urinalysis

The urine specific gravity of 1.016 in an azotemic dehydrated cat indicates that the cat is not capable of concentrating urine, and that renal dysfunction is present. The presence of calcium oxalate monohydrate crystals in a cat with acute renal failure is very suggestive of ethylene glycol toxicosis. The renal threshold for glucose has been exceeded, resulting in glucosuria. The 1+ proteinuria is probably significant in light of the low urine specific gravity and probably resulted from tubular damage.

Summary

The cat died, and necropsy revealed renal tubular necrosis and the presence of calcium oxalate crystals in the tubules due to ethylene glycol toxicosis. The cat had access to antifreeze shortly before it became ill. Approximately 50% of dogs and cats with ethylene glycol-induced renal failure have hyperglycemia, probably due to a combination of stress and the formation of aldehyde, a metabolite of ethylene glycol that interferes with glucose metabolism. While diabetes mellitus could cause hyperglycemia and metabolic acidosis, the presence of acute renal failure and calcium oxalate crystalluria should prompt consideration of ethylene glycol toxicosis.

Case 42

Signalment: 9-year-old intact male mixed-breed dog
History: Two-hour history of tremors and seizure-like activity, unable to stand; previously healthy; free-roaming dog
Physical examination: Recumbent, unable to stand, tacky mucus membranes, CRT <2 seconds

Hematology		Reference range
Hematocrit (%)	43.2	37.2–56.4
Hemoglobin (g/dL)	14.7	13.3–20.8
RBC ($\times10^6/\mu$L)	6.24	5.29–8.34
MCV (fL)	69.2	62.5–72.9
MCH (pg)	23.6	22.4–26.2
MCHC (g/dL)	**34.0**	34.2–37.9
RDW (%)	13.8	12.9–19.4
Abs Reticulocyte ($\times10^3/\mu$L)	71.1	15.1–123.9
Total white blood cell count ($\times10^3/\mu$L)	**18.16**	4.08–14.60
Segmented neutrophils ($\times10^3/\mu$L)	**17.43**	2.27–10.60
Band neutrophils ($\times10^3/\mu$L)	0.0	0.0–0.18
Lymphocytes ($\times10^3/\mu$L)	**0.18**	0.83–4.80
Monocytes ($\times10^3/\mu$L)	0.55	0.05–1.24
Eosinophils ($\times10^3/\mu$L)	**0.0**	0.07–1.40
Platelets ($\times10^3/\mu$L)	288	140–350
MPV (fL)	10.4	8.7–12.8
PCT (%)	0.30	0.17–0.39
Plasma protein (g/dL)	7.0	6.0–7.9

Hemopathology: Few reactive lymphocytes, occasional mild neutrophil toxicity, few small platelet clumps seen.

Biochemical profile		Reference range
Glucose (mg/dL)	**77**	81–115
Blood urea nitrogen (mg/dL)	**87**	8–29
Creatinine (mg/dL)	**8.0**	0.7–1.4
Calcium (mg/dL)	**4.1**	9.1–10.8
Phosphorus (mg/dL)	**10.8**	2.3–5.0
Magnesium (mg/dL)	**2.9**	1.6–2.2
Total protein (g/dL)	6.2	5.4–6.9
Albumin (g/dL)	3.0	2.7–3.7
Globulin (g/dL)	3.2	2.4–3.7
Cholesterol (mg/dL)	259	131–320
Total bilirubin (mg/dL)	0.2	0.1–0.4
ALT (IU/L)	75	14–76
ALP (U/L)	69	12–98
GGT (U/L)	3	0–8
Creatine kinase (U/L)	**511**	40–226
Sodium (mEq/L)	151	145–151
Potassium (mEq/L)	4.6	3.5–4.9
Chloride (mEq/L)	**94**	110–117
Bicarbonate (mEq/L)	**11**	17–26
Anion gap (mEq/L)	**51**	12–20

Additional diagnostics		
Venous blood gas pH	**7.1**	(7.31–7.42)
iCa (mmol/L)	**0.53**	(1.12–1.4)
Urine specific gravity	1.009	

Urine sediment: Many calcium oxalate monohydrate crystals.

Interpretive discussion

Hematology

The erythrocyte indices on the CBC and the appearance of the RBCs on the blood film appear within normal limits. There is a mild decrease in the MCHC, which is likely spurious (normal variant). A mild leukocytosis due to a mild neutrophilia with toxic change is consistent with inflammation. The lymphopenia and eosinopenia are likely due to increased endogenous glucocorticoids and are consistent with a stress component to the leukogram. While the mild neutrophilia may be also due to glucocorticoids, the toxic change suggests inflammation. The platelet count is within reference limits and likely slightly higher than the reported value, as a few platelet clumps are seen.

Biochemical profile and additional diagnostics

A severe azotemia due to a marked increase in serum creatinine and BUN is present, alongside poorly concentrated urine (isosthenuria) indicating a renal azotemia. Considering the history and the lack of anemia of renal disease, this is likely due to acute kidney injury (toxins, infectious organisms, ischemic injury). Additionally, it is likely the renal azotemia has a prerenal component. Most animals with isosthenuria are dehydrated as they cannot keep up with renal water losses. Dehydration is further supported by tacky mucus membranes noted on physical exam. The albumin is at the lower end of the reference interval in a dehydrated and may decrease below the reference interval with rehydration therapy. The most common cause of a mild hypoalbuminemia is acute inflammation (albumin is a negative acute phase protein).

A hyperphosphatemia and hypermagnesemia are also present. In the face of a renal azotemia, this is most likely due to a decreased GFR. In this particular case, the hyperphosphatemia may be also due to phosphate rust inhibitors found in antifreeze. A marked total hypocalcemia is noted on the chemistry and confirmed with an ionized calcium. Hypocalcemia has been reported in dogs with kidney disease due to renal loss. Additionally, calcium is being bound to oxalic acid, a metabolite of ethylene glycol, and excreted in the calcium oxalate monohydrate crystals found on urine sediment. The primary differential for calcium oxalate monohydrate crystals in the presence of azotemia and hypocalcemia is ethylene glycol toxicosis.

The patient has a mixed acid-base status. A severe acidemia is noted on venous blood gas. There is a titration metabolic acidosis characterized by a low bicarbonate (metabolic acidosis) with a markedly increased anion gap (unmeasured ions). Common causes of an increased anion gap include lactate, uremic ions, ketones, and ethylene glycol toxicosis. In this particular case, uremic ions are likely a contributing factor; however, this is a substantially high anion gap to assign to kidney insufficiency alone. Ethylene glycol metabolites are probably contributing to the acidosis. Additionally, there is a disproportionate hypochloremia, consistent with a hypochloremic metabolic alkalosis. In dogs, this is commonly associated with gastric vomiting.

A mild hypoglycemia is present, which is unusual in patients with ethylene glycol toxicosis. Approximately 50% of dogs and cats with ethylene glycol toxicosis are hyperglycemic secondary to ethylene glycol metabolites interfering with glucose metabolism. Based on the physical exam findings, and the potential for somewhat prolonged seizure-like activity, an increased metabolic rate (i.e., increased glucose consumption) may be causing the hypoglycemia. Another consideration would be delayed sample separation and processing, as glucose continues to be metabolized by the cellular components of blood.

The mild increase in creatine kinase is reflective of mild muscle injury. In this case, it is likely due to seizure-like activity and tremors, or potentially in-hospital treatments (intra-muscular injection or inadvertent muscle penetration during venipuncture).

Summary

The patient was stabilized with intravenous fluid therapy and a calcium gluconate infusion. Based on the strong clinical suspicion of ethylene glycol toxicosis and an associated poor prognosis, owners elected humane euthanasia.

Contributor: Dr. Saundra Sample

Case 43

Signalment: 3-month-old Saint Bernard
History: Stumbling for 4 hours
Physical examination: Cannot stand, in a stupor
Hematology: No abnormalities

Biochemical profile		Reference interval
Gluc (mg/dL)	**129**	65–122
BUN (mg/dL)	20	7–28
Creat (mg/dL)	1.6	0.9–1.7
Ca (mg/dL)	11.2	9.0–11.2
Ionized calcium (mg/dL)	5.6	4.5–5.6
Phos (mg/dL)	**10.2**	2.8–6.1
TP (g/dL)	5.8	5.4–7.4
Alb (g/dL)	2.9	2.7–4.5
Glob (g/dL)	2.4	1.9–3.4
T. bili (mg/dL)	0.2	0–0.4
Chol (mg/dL)	220	130–37
ALT (IU/L)	60	10–120
AST (IU/L)	30	16–40
ALP (IU/L)	**300**	35–280
GGT (IU/L)	2	0–6
Na (mEq/L)	148	145–158
K (mEq/L)	5.2	4.1–5.5
CL (mEq/L)	105	106–127
HCO_3 (mEq/L)	15.1	14–27
An. gap (mEq/L)	**33**	8–25
Meas. osmolality (mOsm/kg)	**442**	290–310
Calc. osmolality (mOsm/kg)	**330**	290–310
Osmole gap (mOsm/kg)	**112**	0–10
Serum ethylene glycol concentration (mg/dL)	**>250**	0

Blood gas data (arterial)		Reference interval
Blood pH	**7.305**	7.33–7.44
HCO_3 (mEq/L)	**13.7**	16–22
pCO_2 (mm/Hg)	**29**	35–42

Urinalysis	
Urine specific gravity	**1.012**
Urine pH	5

Interpretive discussion

Biochemical profile

The serum glucose concentration is slightly increased. This may be due to stress, although the leukogram is normal. Aldehydes, a metabolite of ethylene glycol (see later discussion), are reported to interfere with glucose metabolism.

The BUN and creatinine are normal in this dog that has a high serum ethylene glycol concentration. In dogs, azotemia begins between 24 and 36 hours following ingestion. The history suggests that this dog ingested antifreeze approximately 5 hours prior to the time of these laboratory data.

Phosphorus is markedly increased. Hyperphosphatemia may be due to the young age of the dog but is somewhat high for this. In this case the serum phosphorus increase was likely due to phosphate rust inhibitors present in most commercial antifreeze.

Serum alkaline phosphatase activity is mildly increased, likely due to the bone isoform that is increased in growing dogs.

The anion gap is increased, likely due to either phosphates or metabolites of ethylene glycol, which are anions. The calculated osmolality is slightly increased. However, the actual (measured) plasma osmolality is much higher than the calculated osmolality, resulting in a large osmole gap, since a substance is present in the blood that is not used in the formula to calculate osmolality. The most common cause of an increased osmole gap is the presence of ethylene glycol, which contributes to plasma osmolality due to its low molecular weight. This was confirmed by measuring serum ethylene glycol concentration.

Blood gas data

The blood pH is slightly low and HCO_3 is decreased, indicating metabolic acidosis. Metabolites of ethylene glycol are acids. Decreased pCO_2 is consistent with a compensatory respiratory alkalosis. The blood gases were determined about 1 hour following the biochemical profile, which probably accounts for the discrepancy between the HCO_3 determined on the biochemical panel, and that from the blood gas machine.

Urinalysis

The urine specific gravity of 1.012 in this patient is likely due to ethylene glycol causing osmotic diuresis. It is also possible that concentrating ability has been impaired, but the animal is not yet azotemic.

Summary

The dog was treated with fomepizole, an alcohol dehydrogenase inhibitor, approximately 7–8 hours following antifreeze ingestion, and did not become azotemic. In contrast to the previous case, the biochemical profile is often not diagnostic in acute ethylene glycol poisoning, and other tests, such as serum ethylene glycol concentration or measured osmolality must be used to confirm the diagnosis. The acute onset of stumbling and stupor triggered suspicion of ethylene glycol toxicosis.

Case 44

Signalment: 5-day-old male foal
History: Foal was fine at birth, now will not eat
Physical examination: Acts colicky, seems constipated

Hematology		Reference interval
PCV (%)	32	28–46
Hgb (g/dL)	11	11–16
TP (P) (g/dL)	**5.6**	6–8

Biochemical profile		Reference interval
Gluc (mg/dL)	80	70–110
UN (mg/dL)	**32**	7–27
Creat (mg/dL)	**4.8**	1.1–2.0
Ca (mg/dL)	**9.6**	11–13.7
Phos (mg/dL)	**10**	1.9–3.6
TP (g/dL)	5.9	5.8–7.6
Alb (g/dL)	3.0	2.7–3.7
Glob (g/dL)	2.9	2.6–4.6
T. bili (mg/dL)	**3.8**	0.6–2.5
AST (IU/L)	229	185–300
ALP (IU/L)	**340**	66–180
CK (IU/L)	237	130–470
Na (mEq/L)	**118**	133–145
K (mEq/L)	**7.1**	2.2–4.6
CL (mEq/L)	**92**	98–103
TCO_2 (mEq/L)	**18**	24–29
An. gap (mEq/L)	15	10–15

Interpretive discussion

Hematology

There is a mild decrease in plasma proteins; concerned about failure of passive transfer of colostrum but globulins on chemistry panel are adequate.

Biochemical profile

Azotemia is present but there is no urine specific gravity to help determine if this is prerenal or renal azotemia. Recommend catheterization to collect urine and determine if the foal can urinate on its own. UN is mildly increased but creatinine (Ct) is moderately increased, the ratio of UN/Ct is 6. This can happen with recent fluid therapy and a more rapid decrease in UN than Ct, but no fluids have been administered. It could happen with a hepatic shunt and decreased synthesis of UN and with noncreatinine chromogens in horses and cattle. The latter is more likely but confuses the interpretation of the severity of the azotemia. The increase in phosphorus is consistent with a decreased GFR; prerenal, renal, or postrenal causes can do this.

The key abnormalities are the hyponatremia, hyperkalemia and hypochloremia. The Na:K ratio is low at 16 (see comments section). In a foal the most likely differentials are diarrhea, ruptured urinary bladder, renal failure, and hypoadrenocorticism due to a septicemia. There is no evidence of diarrhea at this time; renal failure is a possible explanation. To evaluate uroabdomen recommend abdominocentesis and determination of Ct (and/or UN) on the abdominal fluid and in a concurrent serum sample to compare Ct in abdominal fluid to serum; they should be equal if the bladder wall is intact. Ct (and/or UN) will be higher in abdominal fluid than serum if bladder has ruptured. Hypoadrenocorticism is unlikely; only pursue if other differentials are ruled out. Bicarbonate (TCO_2) is decreased, AG is high end of reference interval, and there likely is a metabolic acidosis, possibly due to dehydration and decreased tissue perfusion. ALP is mildly increased probably due to bone (growth) or liver source; does not seem important to pursue at this time. The bilirubin is increased, which could be due to a liver problem, but anorexia is the more likely cause (anorexia is the number one reason for hyperbilirubinemia in horses).

Abdominocentesis	
Clear, slight yellow color	
TNCC 8500/µl 50 : 50 neutrophils and mononuclear cells	
Total protein (refractive index) 2.8 g/dl	
Creatinine (mg/dL)	
Abdominal fluid	9.2
Serum	4.8

Summary and comment

Uroabdomen. There was a hole in the dorsal aspect of the urinary bladder. It was surgically repaired and the bladder wall appeared healthy at surgery. The foal recovered.

Rupture of the urinary bladder is usually caused by an obstruction (calculi) in males or excessive trauma (hit by car) in all species except horses. Typically, the problem is seen in male foals that appeared fine at birth but gradually develop anorexia and other problems. The male urethral lumen is small and apparently does not allow expulsion of urine easily enough during birth, and the back pressure caused by the mare's strong contractions during parturition causes the bladder to rupture. There are no calculi obstructing outflow. Usually there is a history of dribbling urine or that the foal was seen to urinate. The hole is almost always located dorsally due to the musculature of the bladder wall and therefore patients may still urinate. If contrast dyes are used to determine bladder integrity, the dye may still be retained for the same reason. Comparison of abdominal Ct concentration to serum Ct is the diagnostic test of choice. Abdominal Ct does not have to be twice as great as serum Ct to rule in a ruptured bladder, it just needs to be several mg/dl higher than the serum Ct. If the bladder wall is intact the serum and abdominal Ct will be similar or identical. If the patient is not azotemic, then both samples will have Ct concentrations WRI, if the bladder wall is intact. If the patient has renal failure and is azotemic than the abdominal Ct concentration will be increased to a comparable value, if the bladder wall is intact.

The serum electrolytes and Na:K ratio of less than 20 are key to consider this differential diagnosis. In dogs the following are the four most likely differentials and the tests to rule in or rule out each differential for this electrolyte pattern:

Diagnosis	Test of choice
Hypoadrenocorticism	Basal cortisol; ACTH stim
Renal failure	Fluid therapy; complete UA; fractional excretion of Na
Uroabdomen	Compare abdominal and serum Ct concentrations
GI – whipworms, *Salmonella*	Fecal floatation; fecal culture

Case 45

Signalment: 7-year-old male intact mixed-breed canine
History: Presents for icterus, vomiting, diarrhea, and lethargy
Physical examination: Dull but responsive, markedly icteric, and 10–12% dehydrated

Biochemical profile		Reference range
Glucose (mg/dL)	**164**	81–115
Blood urea nitrogen (mg/dL)	**222**	8–29
Creatinine (mg/dL)	**12.4**	0.7–1.4
Sodium (mEq/L)	**137**	145–151
Potassium (mEq/L)	4.2	3.5–4.9
Chloride (mEq/L)	**71**	110–117
Bicarbonate (mEq/L)	20	17–26
Anion gap (mmol/L)	**50**	12–20
Total protein (g/dL)	**7.6**	5.4–6.9
Albumin (g/dL)	3.4	2.7–3.7
Globulin (g/dL)	**4.2**	2.4–3.7
Calcium (mg/dL)	**8.8**	9.1–10.8
Phosphorus (mg/dL)	**24.8**	2.3–5.0
Magnesium (mg/dL)	**3.6**	1.6–2.2
Total bilirubin (mg/dL)	**11.2**	0.1–0.4
Cholesterol (mg/dL)	283	131–320
ALT (Alanine aminotransferase) (IU/L)	**756**	14–76
ALP (Alkaline phosphatase) (IU/L)	**1911**	12–98
Gamma glutamyltransferase (GGT) (IU/L)	**29**	0–8
CK (IU/L)	**701**	40–226

Urinalysis	
Urine specific gravity	**1.016**
Urine pH	5.5
Protein (dipstick)	2+
Bilirubin	3+
Heme	2+

Sediment: Low numbers of erythrocytes, leukocytes, occasional squamous cells and the rare granular cast.

Interpretive discussion

Hematology

A mild microcytosis and hyperchromasia is indicated by the hematology analyzer and is most likely an artifact secondary to hyponatremia or hypochloridemia. The patient is not anemic making iron-deficiency unlikely. A falsely decreased MCV is an artifact of the Sysmex (and potentially other) analyzers, that is caused by a hypo-osmolar environment *in vivo* (hyponatremia) to which red cells adjust by increasing cytoplasmic water content. When put in a diluent, osmosis results in water loss, causing cell shrinkage (low MCV and high MCHC).

Low numbers of codocytes (target cells) are usually a nonspecific finding. They have been reported with liver disease and is the most likely cause in this case with unrelated differentials being iron deficiency, regenerative anemia, and congenital dyserythropoiesis, although target cells can be seen in many conditions, including health.

A mild leukocytosis characterized by a mature neutrophilia, low-normal lymphocyte count, monocytosis and eosinopenia is consistent with a stress response. There is also a likely component of inflammation that is supported by the degree of monocytosis, the presence of reactive lymphocytes, and the mild hyperglobulinemia noted in the chemistry (see below).

The platelet count is within the reference interval; however, a few giant platelets are observed and are suggestive of bone marrow stimulation.

Mild hyperproteinemia by refractometry is discrepant with the biochemistry analyzer and likely secondary to the increased BUN. Proteins will be further discussed in the chemistry. Moderately icteric serum supported by the hyperbilirubinemia is unlikely to be secondary to severe hemolysis as the patient is not anemic.

Chemistry

A mild hyperproteinemia characterized by a mild hyperglobulinemia is present. If the patient is clinically dehydrated, the protein concentration may decrease after restoring fluid balance. Hyperglobulinemia in an adult dog is suggestive of either an inflammatory or neoplastic (lymphoma, multiple myeloma) etiology.

Marked increase in ALT (~10× the upper reference interval) is indicative of hepatocellular injury and differentials to consider include:

- Infectious agents. Leptospirosis is the primary differential in the presence of renal insufficiency. Other potential infectious agents include canine adenovirus-1 (CAV-1), which is typically seen in unvaccinated dogs under the age of 1.
- Hepatotoxins such as NSAIDs, amanita phalloides ("death cap"), psago palm, blue-green algae, aflatoxins, xylitol, etc.
- Hypoxic injury; ischemia secondary to thrombi, congestion.
- Neoplasia.

There is a concurrent marked increase in ALP (~10× over upper reference internal) and moderate-to-marked increase in GGT, which most likely reflects biliary tract disease. Elevation in GGT activity can also be attributed to renal insufficiency as the enzyme is excreted in urine.

The is a marked hyperbilirubinemia with an associated bilirubinuria. Typical pathomechanisms to consider are hepatic and posthepatic causes of icterus with prehepatic being unlikely in the absence of anemia. Given the increased ALT activity, hepatic jaundice is most likely and may be due to defective uptake of unconjugated bilirubin or impaired excretion.

A marked azotemia with inadequately concentrated urine (<1.030) is suggestive of renal azotemia, although a prerenal (dehydration) component is also likely. The marked hyperphosphatemia and a mild hypermagnesemia is consistent with a decreased GFR. Hemolysis may be a minor contributing factor. Mild hypocalcemia may be due to sepsis, decreased vitamin D production, increased renal excretion or tissue mineralization. The Ca × P product is 218 (well above 70) meaning that mineralization of tissues is occurring. Renal injury is also supported by the presence of rare granular casts in the urinalysis. Given the RBC concentration is within reference limits (absence of anemia), acute renal injury is more likely than chronic. Differentials to consider for the acute renal injury include infectious agents (leptospirosis), toxins (NSAIDs, ethylene glycol) and ischemic injury.

There is a hyponatremia and marked hypochloremia that may be due to both renal and gastrointestinal losses. The corrected chloride is 76.7 mmol/l and indicates selective chloride loss due to vomiting in this case. Bicarbonate is within the reference interval; however, there is a markedly increased anion gap consistent with titration acidosis and most like due to uremic ions or lactate. In the presence of diarrhea, loss of bicarbonate may also be contributing to metabolic acidosis. While the potassium is within reference intervals, there may be transcellular shifts out of cells (inorganic acidosis) and into cells (metabolic alkalosis) as well as renal and gastrointestinal losses that are masked by the complex acid-base disturbances.

A mild hyperglycemia is present and could reflect stress (epinephrine or cortisol mediated) or acute pancreatitis.

Urinalysis

Urine specific gravity is inadequately concentrated and is suggestive of renal insufficiency (discussed in chemistry). The aciduria (pH 5.5) in this case is paradoxical (given the hypochloremic alkalosis) and can occur when severe dehydration is present. There is marked bilirubinuria, particularly given the relatively dilute urine and this secondary to hyperbilirubinemia (although bilirubinuria typically precedes hyperbilirubinemia).

The 2+ Heme result in combination with the observed erythrocytes is indicative of hematuria. Differentials to consider include acute hemorrhagic renal injury, inflammation or iatrogenic causes.

A true proteinuria is present and is unlikely to be explained solely by the 2+ Heme result. Typical pathomechanisms to consider for proteinuria are prerenal (hypertension, pyrexia), renal (nephropathy, glomerulopathy), and postrenal (cystitis).

Summary

This patient had a leptospirosis SNAP test, which was negative. Further testing for leptospirosis may have included a microscopic agglutination test (MAT) or PCR.

He was hospitalized with IVF and supportive care for 24 hours and discharged from the hospital with a presumptive diagnosis of leptospirosis.

Contributors: Drs. Saundra Sample and Alex Mau

Case 46

Signalment: 9-week-old, intact male, American bull terrier (canine)
History: 1-day history of lethargy, hyporexia, vomiting, and diarrhea; littermate died a few days prior
Physical examination: Marked jaundice, abdominal distention

Hematology		Reference range
Hematocrit (%)	**18**	37–55
Hemoglobin (g/dL)	**5.7**	12.0–18.0
RBC (×10⁶/μL)	**2.97**	5.5–8.5
MCV (fL)	63	60–77
MCH (pg)	**19.3**	19.5–24.5
MCHC (g/dL)	**30.7**	31.0–39.0
RDW (%)	16.5	14.0–20.0
Total white blood cell count (×10³/μL)	13.34	6.0–17.0
Segmented neutrophils (×10³/μL)	10.5	6.0–17.0
Band neutrophils (×10³/μL)	0.3	0.0–0.3
Lymphocytes (×10³/μL)	1.5	1.0–4.8
Monocytes (×10³/μL)	1.1	0.2–1.4
Platelets (×10³/μL)	**0**	165–600
Plasma protein (g/dL)	6.3	6.0–7.5

Hemopathology: Normal RBC morphology, no platelet clumping, platelets appear markedly decreased.

Biochemical profile		Reference range
Glucose (mg/dL)	**139**	60–110
Blood urea nitrogen (mg/dL)	**167**	7–25
Creatinine (mg/dL)	**3.9**	0.3–1.4
Calcium (mg/dL)	11.2	8.6–11.8
Phosphorus (mg/dL)	**>20**	2.9–6.6
Total protein (g/dL)	**5.2**	5.4–8.2
Albumin (g/dL)	**2.3**	2.5–4.4
Globulin (g/dL)	2.9	2.3–5.2
Total bilirubin (mg/dL)	**7.5**	0.1–0.6
ALT (IU/L)	44	20–150
ALP (U/L)	**497**	20–150
Sodium (mEq/L)	139	138–160
Potassium (mEq/L)	**7.1**	3.7–5.8
Amylase (U/L)	408	200–1200

Peritoneal fluid	
Color	Pale yellow
Clarity	Clear
TNCC (cells/μL)	250
PCV (%)	<1
TP (g/dL)	0.6

Differential: macrophages (58%), lymphocytes (38%), neutrophils (4%)

Interpretive discussion

Hematology

The packed cell volume, hemoglobin, and red blood cell concentration are all proportionally decreased consistent with a moderate anemia. The low-normal MCV and lack of polychromatophilia is consistent with a nonregenerative or preregenerative anemia, despite the mildly decreased MCH and MCHC. The mildly decreased MCH and MCHC is suspected to be a spurious finding in this case. The leukogram is overall unremarkable. There is a marked thrombocytopenia that is supported by findings on the blood film. Differentials include a consumptive process (e.g., DIC, vasculitis), platelet destruction (e.g., ITP), or potentially bone marrow disease as a nonregenerative anemia is also present.

Biochemical profile

There is a marked azotemia characterized by a marked increase in BUN and a moderate increase in creatinine. Although a urine specific gravity is not available, the azotemia is severe enough to be a renal azotemia. Additionally, the BUN is disproportionately increased with respect to the creatinine, suggesting a prerenal component (dehydration). The other potential consideration would be poor muscle mass, which may mask the severity of increase in creatinine.

A marked hyperphosphatemia is present, likely representing a decreased glomerular filtration rate (GFR) in this patient. This marked increase is roughly proportional to the increase in BUN, further supporting the diagnosis of renal disease. The calcium is within reference limits; however, the product of the calcium and phosphorus exceeds 100; therefore, soft-tissue mineralization is occurring and likely accelerating the kidney injury. A marked hyperkalemia is present, and most likely secondary to decreased renal excretion (oliguria or anuria). Puppies have mildly increased phosphorus concentration due to increased growth hormone; however, this is likely only a minor contribution to the marked hyperphosphatemia.

An approximately threefold increase in the ALP enzyme activity alongside a moderate increase in the total bilirubin concentration consistent with cholestasis. A small portion of the increase in ALP is likely due to the bone isoenzyme as this is a young growing animal. Increases in bALP do not cause a hyperbilirubinemia.

A mild hyperglycemia is present. Puppies tend to have higher glucose concentrations, and this result falls comfortably into that general reference range.

There is a mild hypoproteinemia due to a mild hypoalbuminemia. Considering the patient is likely dehydrated, these values will likely mildly decrease with rehydration therapy. It is important to remember that puppies, in general, tend to have lower protein concentrations than adult dogs. This is likely contributing to the hypoalbuminemia. Additional considerations in this case include inflammation (negative acute phase protein), renal loss, or liver insufficiency. A urinalysis would be helpful in assessing if protein is being lost in the urine. The globulin fraction is within the low-end of the adult reference interval, and in the presence of vomiting and diarrhea, GI loss of both albumin globulin cannot be ruled out.

Abdominal fluid analysis

A transudate effusion (TNCC <5000 cells/μL, TP <2.5 g/dL) is present in this patient. Hypoalbuminemia is the classic cause of transudate effusion; however, the albumin is only mildly decreased and probably only a mild contributor. An underlying cause of increased hydrostatic pressure was not identified in this case, so the underlying cause of the effusion is unclear. A vasculitis is a possibility; however, these effusions typically result in a high-protein (modified) transudate or exudate.

Summary

Serum antibody titers for canine leptospirosis were positive. The nonregenerative anemia and thrombocytopenia are common CBC findings in canine leptospirosis. The nonregenerative anemia is likely related to renal injury and possible anemia of inflammatory disease. A thrombocytopenia has been reported in up to 50% of dogs with leptospirosis, and is likely due to vasculitis and/or DIC. The most common biochemical changes are associated with acute kidney injury (AKI) and include azotemia and hyperphosphatemia. Increased serum liver enzyme activity is reported some dogs, and rarely seen without azotemia. Increases in serum ALP activity and total bilirubin, seen in this case, are more common than increases in serum ALT activity. The hyperkalemia is likely caused by decreased renal excretion (oliguria/anuria) and extracellular shifts in response to an inorganic titration acidosis due to uremic ions. Hypoalbuminemia is reported in some cases, and occasionally associated with an effusion.

The clinicians suspected leptospirosis and treated accordingly; however, the patient quickly progressed to anuric renal failure. A positive *Leptospira* spp. PCR and direct florescent antibody test confirmed the clinical suspicion. Findings on necropsy included: marked icterus; multifocal and subcutaneous hematoma; severe multifocal-to-coalescing lymphoplasmacytic interstitial nephritis; hemorrhaging and lymphoplasmacytic cystitis; diffuse hepatopathy with scattered individual hepatocyte necrosis and hepatocellular dissociation. The renal and hepatic findings, icterus, and lesions related to bleeding diathesis (hemorrhagic cystitis and cutaneous hematomas) are classical lesions for the subacute state of leptospirosis.

Contributors: Drs. Saundra Sample, Judit Wulcan, and Alex Mau

Case 47

Signalment: Flock of 9-month-old white Suffolk cross lambs

History: 15 sheep found dead over a period of 3–4 days. Many that are remaining are recumbent and obtunded.

Hematology	Sheep 1	Sheep 2	Reference interval
PCV (%)	43	**62**	21–45
Total protein (g/L)	78	**89**	60–80

Biochemical profile	Sheep 1	Sheep 2	Reference interval
Glucose (mmol/L)	**10.7**	**16.3**	2.4–4.5
BUN (mmol/L)	**50.4**	**56.1**	2.8–7.2
Creatinine (μmol/L)	**774**	**1454**	70–120
Calcium (mmol/L)	**4.37**	**4.54**	2.4–3.2
Phosphorus (mmol/L)	**3.2**	**2.8**	1.61–2.35
Magnesium (mmol/L)	**1.89**	**2.40**	0.50–1.50
Total protein (g/L)	79	**87**	60–82
Albumin (g/L)	38	38	25–40
Globulin (g/L)	41	**49**	30–42
Total bilirubin (μmol/L)	5	7	0–9
AST (IU/L)	118	96	53–153
GLDH (IU/L)	**61**	**64**	0–20
GGT (IU/L)	**68**	39	30–66
CK (IU/L)	**339**	**2153**	69–182
Cholesterol (mmol/L)	1.9	2.1	1.3–2.1
BOHB (mmol/L)	0.3	0.4	0.0–0.9
Sodium (mmol/L)	151	151	139–152
Potassium (mmol/L)	3.6	**5.8**	3.6–5.4
Chloride (mmol/L)	96	102	95–103
Bicarbonate (mmol/L)	**9**	**7**	15–25

Urinalysis	Sheep 1	Sheep 2	Reference interval
Specific Gravity	**1.016**	**1.017**	1.004–1.045
Blood	Trace	3+	Negative
pH	**5.5**	**6**	Alkaline
Protein	3+	3+	Negative

Sediment: Large numbers of casts observed in both samples. RBC >**10/HPF** and WBC >**50HPF**.

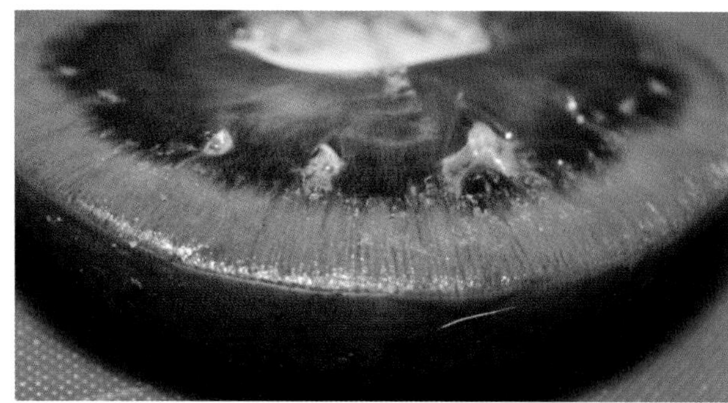

Figure 1 Photograph of a kidney from one of the sheep. The kidneys were diffusely enlarged, bulged away from the capsule on section, and had a pale-tan cortex that was slightly granular.

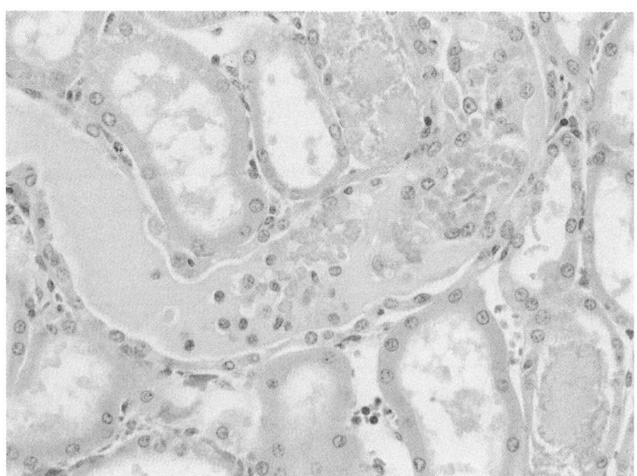

Figure 2 Histological section of the renal tubules, showing shed epithelial cells and debris and the early formation of a cast.

Interpretive discussion

Hematology

The increased PCV and total protein in sheep 2 is suggestive of relative polycythemia (dehydration). Protein will be discussed in the section below.

Chemistry and urinalysis

Both sheep are hyperglycemic, and this is likely a stress (corticosteroid) response.

Azotemia in both sheep is severe and characterized by a marked increase in BUN and creatinine. A prerenal component may be present considering the likely dehydration, but an inadequate USG of 1.016 is supportive of renal dysfunction. Decreased GFR and renal insufficiency also explains the hyperphosphatemia and hypermagnesemia.

Sheep 2 has a hyperproteinemia characterized by a hyperglobulinemia and high-normal albumin, suggestive of dehydration. Increased globulins could also be due to inflammation, although the lack of an inflammatory leukogram makes this less likely.

An ionized calcium is strongly recommended to further characterize the nature of the hypercalcemia present in both sheep. Dehydration and relatively increased albumin binding may be a contributing factor; however, renal disease is also possible as evidenced by the azotemia and USG.

Increased GLDH activity is suggestive of mild hepatocellular injury. The mild increase in GGT observed in sheep 1 may be clinically insignificant, but the possibility of biliary disease should be considered.

An increase in CK activity is indicative of muscle injury and probably due to prolonged recumbency.

A metabolic acidosis is present as evidenced by the moderately decreased bicarbonate. The anion gap for sheep 2 is calculated at 48, indicating the presence of a titration/consumption acidosis. The unmeasured anions present are most likely uremic acids or lactate. Both acidosis (transcellular shifting of potassium) and the likely anuric/oligouric renal failure are likely contributors to the hyperkalemia.

Azotemia and inadequately concentrated urine are strongly suggestive of renal disease. The finding of cellular cast within the urine in this number in these animals is pathognomonic for renal tubular necrosis. Increased numbers of RBCs and WBCs could be an indication of inflammation or hematuria. The acidic pH is secondary to the metabolic acidosis.

Summary and outcome

The clinical pathology findings indicated acute renal tubular necrosis as the likely cause of the renal failure, and the farmer was advised to move the sheep. Necropsy and subsequent histopathology confirmed severe acute tubular necrosis as the cause of renal failure in the affected sheep (Figures 1 and 2). Further investigation of the pasture revealed very little green feed and the presence of Amaranthus spp., commonly referred to as "pigweed," a toxic weed known to cause toxic nephrosis in livestock. The affected sheep were pregnant at the time of intoxication, and in those that survived the subsequent lambing percentage was markedly decreased when compared to unaffected cohorts on the same property. This likely indicates loss of pregnancy in affected sheep secondary to the intoxication.

Contributor: Dr. Allan Kessell

Case 48

Signalment: 21-year-old captive male Southern white rhinoceros (*Ceratotherium Simum simum*)

History: Chronic weight loss, inappetence, and decline in activity

Hematology		Reference range
Packed cell volume (%)	41.5	22–47
RBC ($\times10^6/\mu L$)	6.43	3.33–7.53
Hgb (g/dL)	15.6	7.9–17.3
NCC ($10^3/\mu L$)	**15.8**	3.9–12.7
Segmented neutrophils ($10^3/\mu L$)	**14.8**	1.54–7.5
Monocytes ($10^3/\mu L$)	0.32	0.00–1.42
Lymphocytes ($10^3/\mu L$)	0.63	0.22–4.30
Platelets ($10^3/\mu L$)	316	109–520
Fibrinogen (mg/dL)	**650**	0–401

Biochemical profile		Reference range
Glucose (mg/dL)	**133**	30–121
Blood urea nitrogen (mg/dL)	**40**	11–22
Creatinine (mg/dL)	**4.0**	1.1–2.3
Calcium (mg/dL)	**20.2**	10.1–13.7
Phosphorus (mg/dL)	**0.5**	2.1–5.7
Total protein (g/dL)	**5.3**	7.2–9.5
Albumin (g/dL)	**1.1**	2.1–3.7
Globulin (g/dL)	**4.1**	4.3–6.7
Total bilirubin (mg/dL)	0.1	0.0–0.6
Cholesterol (mg/dL)	**289**	41–139
AST (IU/L)	130	21–111
ALP (IU/L)	36	0–192
GGT (IU/L)	9	0–29
CK (IU/L)	590	N/A
Sodium (mEq/L)	**124**	125–140
Potassium (mEq/L)	4.3	3.7–5.7
Chloride (mEq/L)	88	88–103
Bicarbonate/TCO_2 (mEq/L)	**30.5**	16.5–25.9
Anion gap (mEq/L)	9	N/A

Urinalysis

Urine specific gravity	1.010
Urine pH	8.5
Protein	**2+** (200-300 mg/dL)
Urine Protein: Creatinine ratio	**2.2** Reference interval: <0.4 (if not azotemic; Canine RI)

Sediment: 3+ Calcium carbonate crystals. RBC <5/HPF. WBC <5/HPF

Additional tests	
Parathyroid hormone (pmol/L)	0.00
Ionized calcium (mmol/L)	3.2
Parathyroid related protein (pmol/L)	Not performed

Interpretive discussion

Hematology

The neutrophilia and concurrent hyperfibrinogenemia are suggestive of inflammation.

MCHC is calculated to be 38 g/dl (RI: 32–41 g/dL) and Hgb appears disproportionately high for this HCT. This may be insignificant, but intravascular hemolysis and Heinz bodies should be excluded as possible causes of an erroneous increase in hemoglobin concentration. The severe hypophosphatemia in this patient could also be responsible for intravascular hemolysis.

Chemistry and additional tests

Mild hyperglycemia is likely due to stress (cortisol or epinephrine induced).

Azotemia is present and characterized by mild increased urea nitrogen and creatinine, which combined with isosthenuria, indicates renal insufficiency. The hypercalcemia is a confounder in that it may be the cause or contributing factor for apparent inability to concentrate urine.

BUN/Creatinine ratio is 10; BUN is only mildly increased while creatinine is disproportionately higher, suggesting there may be a decrease in urea synthesis, potentially due to chronic liver failure, which is also supported by the hypoalbuminemia. Alternatively, creatinine may be falsely increased due to noncreatinine chromogens such as vitamin C, bilirubin, and carotene.

Causes of hypercalcemia in rhinoceroses are not widely reported in the literature. Like other mammals, differential diagnoses to consider in this animal include paraneoplastic hypercalcemia, primary hyperparathyroidism, renal disease, granulomatous inflammation, and vitamin D toxicosis. However, phosphorus is markedly decreased and the three differentials for hypercalcemia **and** hypophosphatemia are primary hyperparathyroidism, humoral hypercalcemia of malignancy (HMM), and renal failure in horses. While renal failure usually results in hypocalcemia and hyperphosphatemia, the opposite occurs in some horses. Hypophosphatemia is a more important diagnostic clue in this patient than is hypercalcemia, as there are so many causes of hypercalcemia.

Undetectable levels of PTH make hyperparathyroidism very unlikely. However, it is also possible that the PTH was falsely decreased due to either the lack of cross-reactivity with antibodies, since the test was designed for use in human patients, or improper preservation of the serum sample. Poor preservation may occur if the sample is not frozen **or** if repeatedly freeze-thawed, resulting in denaturation of proteins. With renal failure, a marked increase in PTH is expected and is due to secondary hyperparathyroidism and decreased PTH clearance by the kidneys. PTH-rp was not performed and is needed to rule out HMM. Any animal of this age could possibly have a tumor, such as lymphoma, and HHM is much more common than primary hyperparathyroidism in all domestic animals. There is no indication of enlarged lymph nodes to support lymphoma but a thorough search for concurrent malignant neoplasia such as lymphoma or carcinoma is recommended. PTH and PTH-rp should always be performed simultaneously so a situation just like this does not have to be interpreted. The only time these hormones are needed is when an obvious cause of hypercalcemia and hypophosphatemia cannot be found.

Chronic renal failure leading to hypercalcemia and concurrent hypophosphatemia is a phenomenon observed commonly in horses, contrary to the hypocalcemia and hyperphosphatemia seen in other domestic species. In a retrospective study of chronic renal failure in 99 horses, hypercalcemia and hypophosphatemia was observed in 67% and 47% of cases, respectively. Hypercalcemia due to renal failure can occasionally be seen in other species such as the dog and the cat, but they exhibit hyperphosphatemia with CRF; the concurrent hypophosphatemia with azotemia is rare and only seen in horses. (More typically, dogs and cats with renal failure and hypercalcemia have hypercalcemia due to some other cause, and the renal failure is caused by mineralization of the kidneys.) Interestingly, horses, rhinoceroses and other odd-toed ungulates are taxonomically related, and this could explain physiological similarities. Anorexia and decreased intake may also be contributing to hypophosphatemia.

CPK is 590 IU/L, which could be mildly increased but certainly is not in the range expected for rhabdomyolysis and secondary renal failure. The history of chronic weight loss, combined with proteinuria without evidence of inflammation in UA, and mild azotemia make acute nephrotoxicity unlikely and all point to CRF, especially due to glomerulonephritis.

Hypoalbuminemia is likely multifactorial in this case and the result of inflammation (negative acute phase protein), decreased intake (anorexia) and a protein losing nephropathy. The proteinuria supports the latter, and although guidelines for the interpretation of urine protein: creatinine ratios in rhinoceroses have not been published, a value >2.0 is suggestive of glomerular disease in other species. There is no evidence of inflammation in the urine sediment, suggesting that the proteinuria is not associated with inflammation. The significance of the hypoglobulinemia is uncertain but could reflect a protein losing enteropathy given that blood loss is unlikely. One would expect cholesterol to also be decreased (see below). Decreased albumin and globulin are usually associated with protein losing enteropathy; other causes of hypoalbuminemia being glomerulonephropathy, liver failure, and blood loss. End-stage liver disease is usually associated with hypoalbuminemia and hyperglobulinemia, possibly due to decreased Kupffer cell function, with antigens from the GI tract then gaining access to the immune system.

Hypercholesterolemia in this case is possibly due to nephrotic syndrome since the patient has hypoalbuminemia and proteinuria; hypercholesterolemia is postulated to occur as an attempt to restore oncotic pressure lost due to hypoalbuminemia. Anorexia and subsequent development of a negative energy balance leading to lipolysis may also be factor. Cholestasis is unlikely given that bilirubin and liver enzyme activities are within reference range. It is also important to note that **decreased** cholesterol is typically observed with protein losing enteropathies, making this a less likely differential for protein abnormalities.

On biochemical profiles, bicarbonate is calculated by measuring TCO_2 and as such, an increased bicarbonate is indicative of a metabolic alkalosis. A cause for the increased bicarbonate is not evident in this case, as a corrected chloride of 94 mEqv/L makes alkalosis secondary to H+ loss unlikely. If this animal was receiving fluid therapy, added bicarbonate or lactate in commercially available fluid solutions should be considered. Ultimately, this animal requires a blood gas analysis to assess pH. A urine pH of 8.5 is typical for herbivores in health but having alkaline urine may further evidence the alkalosis, possibly reflecting an increased serum pH.

A mild hyponatremia and proportionately decreased serum chloride may indicate gastrointestinal (diarrhea) or renal losses, or an increase in water intake with fluid therapy or excessive drinking.

A urine specific gravity of 1.010 is likely attributed to CRF. However, increased serum Ca interferes with the action of ADH on tubules and therefore is a likely contributor to isosthenuria. Hydration status is not reported, and interpretation of USG should take this into consideration. If the animal is receiving fluid therapy at the time of urinalysis, the USG is not meaningful. If the animal is dehydrated, and not concentrating urine, it is likely not capable of concentrating. An alkaline urine of pH 8.5 is common with many herbivores and horses, as is the presence of calcium carbonate crystalluria in horses, further implying the physiological similarities between the rhinoceros and the horse.

Summary and outcome

This animal decompensated and was found dead. Postmortem and histopathology revealed: severe interstitial nephritis and chronic glomerulonephritis periglomerular sclerosis (chronic kidney disease). There was no evidence of neoplasia such as lymphoma or gastric squamous cell carcinoma, both of which are associated with humoral hypercalcemia of malignancy in horses. The parathyroid glands were not assessed histologically so primary hyperparathyroidism remains a possibility, however the undetectable concentration of PTH makes this unlikely. Concurrent hypercalcemia, hypophosphatemia, azotemia and isosthenuria all suggest CRF and a pathogenesis of hypercalcemia similar to that seen in horses.

In horses, the kidneys are a major route of excretion for calcium and anything that causes a decreased in GFR, including CRF, can result in hypercalcemia. Many horses in renal failure have calcium and phosphorus concentrations similar to other species, most notably hyperphosphatemia, although some horses have hypercalcemia and hypophosphatemia. Perissodactyla is an order of odd-toed ungulates that includes Equidae (horses, zebras), Rhinocerotidae (rhinoceroses), and Tapiridae (tapirs). Literature regarding the renal physiology of rhinoceroses is sparse, but given the common ancestry and taxonomical relationship between rhinoceroses and horses, it is possible that they share similarities, maybe explaining the hypercalcemia and hypophosphatemia in this case and perhaps the calcium carbonate crystalluria.

The cause of the panhypoproteinemia remains uncertain as there was no evidence of a protein losing enteropathy at postmortem, although autolysis was preset and the small intestine was not closely examined. The cause of the hypoalbuminemia was renal loss but the hypoglobulinemia remains unexplained.

Contributor: Dr. Alex Mau

CASES

Case 49

Signalment: 10-year-old castrated male domestic short hair cat
History: Anorexia, lethargy
Physical examination: Dehydrated

Miscellaneous tests		Reference interval
Plasma glucose (mg/dL)	**328**	67–124
Urinalysis dipstick abnormalities	Glucosuria and ketonuria	
Na (mEq/L)	**130**	146–160
K (mEq/L)	**2.2**	3.7–5.4
CL (mEq/L)	**74**	112–129
pH	**7.28**	7.33–7.44
HCO_3 (mEq/L)	**9.2**	16–20
pCO_2 (mmHg)	**20**	28–34

Interpretive discussion

There is moderate hyperglycemia that exceeds the renal glucose threshold. There is resultant glucosuria. Ketonuria indicates impaired glucose utilization by tissues suggesting insulin deficiency. This establishes a working diagnosis of diabetes mellitus.

There is marked hypokalemia in the face of acidosis (see blood gas discussion), which would be expected to increase potassium due to an intracellular to extracellular shift. It would be suspected that total body potassium is depleted and there should be caution in insulin administration that would drive potassium into cells, resulting in weakness due to even more severe hypokalemia. There is also hyponatremia and disproportionate hypochloremia. The hyponatremia may be due to a combination of urinary and gastrointestinal loss. The disproportionate hypochloremia is of a magnitude that suggests upper gastrointestinal chloride loss due to vomiting.

The acid-base data show a low pH and decreased bicarbonate, consistent with a metabolic acidosis. The decreased pCO_2 is a compensatory response (respiratory alkalosis). There is also a likely hidden component of metabolic alkalosis (hypochloremic alkalosis), resulting in a mixed acid-base disorder. The loss of HCl in gastric fluid will metabolically generate bicarbonate. The generation of ketoacids that require buffering by bicarbonate is judged to be more severe in the balance between bicarbonate utilization and production.

Summary

Diabetic ketoacidosis pattern, largely compensated.

Case 50

Signalment: 5-year-old spayed female Manx cat

History: Decreased appetite of approximately 2 weeks' duration. Fluid draining from a fistula over the terminal coccygeal vertebrae of 8 months' duration.

Physical examination: Approximately 6% dehydrated. Coccygeal vertebrae were noted to terminate cranial to the anal sphincter. The fistula was noninflamed and draining a clear, colorless fluid.

Hematology		Reference interval
PCV (%)	**49**	24–45
NCC (×10^3/μL)	11.6	5.5–19.5
Segs (×10^3/μL)	9.6	2.5–12.5
Monos (×10^3/μL)	0.6	0–0.8
Lymphs (×10^3/μL)	**1.4**	1.5–7.0
Platelets (×10^3/μL)	Adequate	200–500

Biochemical profile		Reference interval
Gluc (mg/dL)	91	67–124
BUN (mg/dL)	**82**	17–32
Creat (mg/dL)	**2.2**	0.9–2.1
Ca (mg/dL)	**7.3**	8.5–11
Phos (mg/dL)	5.2	3.3–7.8
TP (g/dL)	**8.4**	5.9–8.1
Alb (g/dL)	**4.1**	2.3–3.9
Glob (g/dL)	4.3	2.9–4.4
T. bili (mg/dL)	0.1	0–0.3
Chol (mg/dL)	153	60–220
ALT (IU/L)	40	30–100
Na (mEq/L)	**131**	146–160
K (mEq/L)	4.6	3.7–5.4
CL (mEq/L)	**101**	112–129
TCO_2 (mEq/L)	16	14–23
An. gap (mEq/L)	18.6	10–27

Urinalysis	
Color	Straw
Transparency	Clear
Sp. gr.	**1.015**
Protein	Negative
Gluc	Negative
Bilirubin	Negative
Blood	Negative
pH	6.5

Fractional excretion		Reference interval
Na (%)	0.03	<1.0
CL (%)	0.08	<1.0

Interpretive discussion

Hematology

The increased PCV is consistent with hemoconcentration due to dehydration. Other data are unremarkable.

Biochemical profile

The azotemia (increased BUN and serum creatinine concentrations) may be prerenal and/or renal. Refer to the discussion of urinalysis below.

There is hypocalcemia, despite hyperproteinemia due to hemoconcentration, suggesting that serum calcium concentration may be truly decreased. An ionized calcium could be measured for confirmation. Hypocalcemia could have occurred secondary to chloride depletion and loss of the electrochemical gradient needed to support calcium absorption from the glomerular filtrate in the Loop of Henle of the renal tubules.

Serum sodium and chloride are decreased in concentration. This usually reflects increased loss, compounded by reduced intake in sick, anorexic patients. In this case, there is physical evidence of cerebrospinal fluid loss from a draining meningomyelocele. Cerebrospinal fluid contains higher sodium and chloride concentrations than the blood, owing to the active chloride transport mechanism employed by the choroid plexus for secretion. Draining CSF from the body will create electrolyte depletion in excess of water, an otherwise classic scenario for hypotonic dehydration. Although this cat had been losing CSF for some time, the development of anorexia probably precipitated an imbalance between these pathologic losses and replacement of the electrolytes, resulting in the clinical presentation.

Urinalysis

The urinary fractional excretion values for sodium and chloride were well within the normal reference interval, thereby ruling out renal loss as a cause for the electrolyte depletion. The only significant abnormality is a urine specific gravity of 1.015. Dehydration should stimulate antidiuretic hormone release from the hypothalamus, and increased water reclamation by the renal tubules. However, electrolyte loss in this type of hypotonic dehydration often leads to medullary solute depletion and a loss of the renal concentration gradient. Another alternative is that there is renal disease, due to renal hypoperfusion, sepsis, etc., resulting in both azotemia and loss of concentrating ability.

Summary

Sodium chloride depletion in a Manx cat with a fistulated meningomyelocele (Hall JA, MJ Fettman, JT Ingram. Sodium chloride depletion in a cat with fistulated meningomyelocele. J Am Vet Med Assoc 1988;192:1445–1448).

Case 51

Signalment: 10-year-old female horse
History: Abdominal pain
Physical examination: Tense abdomen, slight fever

Hematology		Reference interval
PCV (%)	52.0	32–52
Hgb (g/dL)	18.1	11–19
RBC ($\times 10^6/\mu L$)	11.15	6.5–12.5
MCV (fL)	46.0	36–52
MCHC (g/dL)	34.0	34–39
NCC ($\times 10^3/\mu L$)	**14.2**	5.5–12.5
Segs ($\times 10^3/\mu L$)	**11.8**	2.7–6.7
Monos ($\times 10^3/\mu L$)	0.3	0–0.8
Lymphs ($\times 10^3/\mu L$)	2.1	1.5–5.5
Platelets ($\times 10^3/\mu L$)	162	100–600
TP (P) (g/dL)	7.0	6–8
Fibrinogen (mg/dL)	200	100–400

Biochemical profile		Reference interval
Gluc (mg/dL)	**166**	70–110
BUN (mg/dL)	23	14–27
Creat (mg/dL)	**4.2**	1.1–2.0
Ca (mg/dL)	**10.5**	11.0–13.7
Phos (mg/dL)	**4.5**	1.9–4.1
TP (g/dL)	7.1	5.8–7.6
Alb (g/dL)	3.2	2.7–3.7
Glob (g/dL)	3.9	2.6–4.6
T. bili (mg/dL)	1.1	0.6–2.1
AST (IU/L)	**430**	185–300
GGT (IU/L)	8	7–17
SDH (IU/L)	**99**	0–9
CK (IU/L)	**8422**	130–470
Na (mEq/L)	140	133–145
K (mEq/L)	3.5	2.2–4.6
CL (mEq/L)	**86**	100–111
TCO_2 (mEq/L)	**22.6**	24–34
An. gap	**35**	5–15

Interpretive discussion

Hematology

There is a neutrophilic leukocytosis with low normal lymphocyte numbers, which most likely reflects stress, rather than inflammation. The fibrinogen is within normal limits. The PCV is at the top of the reference interval and serum proteins are normal, suggesting possible splenic contraction.

Abdominal fluid analysis	
Fluid color	Straw
Fluid clarity	Hazy
Supernatant color	Straw
Supernatant clarity	Clear
TP (g/dL)	1.3
NCC (/μL)	300

Cytology: There are approximately equal numbers of neutrophils and large mononuclear cells. Although the overall cellularity and protein are low, some of the neutrophils are degenerate and bacteria are seen extracellularly, predominantly rods. Some of the macrophages and neutrophils contain cytoplasmic material suggestive of bacterial remnants. There are moderate numbers of lymphocytes and rare mast cells seen. There is debris present in the background.

Biochemical profile

There is a mild hyperglycemia, which is consistent with stress. The increases in serum creatinine and serum phosphorus are likely the result of decreased glomerular filtration rate. Creatinine is a more sensitive marker for decreased GFR in horses because of their ability to excrete urea into the GI tract. A urinalysis might help differentiate prerenal from renal azotemia, but the low chloride (discussed later) might affect urinary concentrating ability. There may be a prerenal component (dehydration) to the azotemia since the PCV is at the top of the reference interval. However, the normal albumin does not support dehydration, and there does not appear to be much protein loss into the abdominal effusion (which would lower the serum albumin).

There is a slight hypocalcemia, which may be due to deposition in injured tissue.

Increased CK activity indicates muscle cell damage. The increased SDH activity is specific for hepatocellular injury. The slight increase in AST activity could be from muscle or hepatocellular injury.

There is a selective hypochloremia, indicating a hypochloremic alkalosis. Selective chloride loss can result from upper GI loss or sequestration of CL and excessive sweating in horses. In addition, the decreased TCO_2 and increased anion gap indicates a high-gap metabolic acidosis; thus, there is a mixed acid-base disorder. Uremic acids and lactic acid, secondary to hypoperfusion, are likely contributors to the anion gap. A blood gas profile is needed to fully assess acid-base status in this horse.

Abdominal fluid analysis

Although the quantitative indices are all within normal limits, the presence of degenerate inflammatory cells, bacteria, and debris are all consistent with an acute rupture of the intestinal tract.

Summary

This mare experienced intestinal colic, followed by acute rupture of the involved strangulated intestine. There had not been time for an inflammatory leukogram to develop.

Case 52

Signalment: 7-year-old spayed female DLH cat
History: Attacked by dog in same household
Physical examination: Dehydration, tachypnea, marked bruising, and several small bite wounds on the back of the neck

Hematology	Day 1	Day 4	Day 7	Reference range
Packed cell volume (%)	45	**23**	**21**	24–45
RBC ($\times 10^6/\mu L$)	9.47	5.20	**4.52**	5.0–10.0
Hgb (g/dL)	14.2	**7.6**	**6.2**	8.0–15.0
MCV (fL)	47	45	48	39–55
MCHC (g/dL)	31.7	32.4	**28.8**	30–36
NCC ($10^3/\mu L$)	13.1	15.2	14.4	5.5–19.5
Segmented neutrophils ($10^3/\mu L$)	2.8	10.1	9.5	2.5–14.0
Band neutrophils ($10^3/\mu L$)	0.0	**3.6**	**0.6**	0.0–0.3
Monocytes ($10^3/\mu L$)	0.4	0.6	0.7	0.0–0.9
Lymphocytes ($10^3/\mu L$)	**8.8**	**0.6**	1.6	1.5–7.0
Eosinophils ($10^3/\mu L$)	0.9	0.2	0.7	0.0–0.8
nRBC ($10^3/\mu L$)	**0.3**	0.0	**1.1**	0.0–0.0
Platelets ($10^3/\mu L$)	324	**53**	**65**	300–800
Plasma protein (g/dL)	7.0	6.2	6.2	6.0–8.0
Reticulocytes ($10^3/\mu L$)	–	5.2	**54.2**	0.0–40.0

Biochemical profile	Day 1	Day 4	Day 7	Reference range
Glucose (mg/dL)	104	**165**	81	70–150
Blood urea nitrogen (mg/dL)	23	14	20	10–30
Creatinine (mg/dL)	1.0	0.8	1.0	0.3–2.1
Calcium (mg/dL)	8.4	9.8	9.5	8.0–11.4
Phosphorus (mg/dL)	**2.9**	3.5	6.2	3.4–8.5
Total protein (g/dL)	5.6	6.2	5.7	5.4–8.2
Albumin (g/dL)	2.5	**1.7**	**2.1**	2.2–4.4
Globulin (g/dL)	3.1	4.5	3.5	1.5–5.7
Total bilirubin (mg/dL)	**1.0**	**5.4**	**0.7**	0.1–0.6
ALT (IU/L)	**642**	**425**	**130**	20–100
ALP (IU/L)	19	15	19	10–90
Sodium (mEq/L)	143	146	152	142–164
Potassium (mEq/L)	**8.2**	**5.9**	4.5	3.7–5.8

Urinalysis	Day 1
Color	Brown
Turbidity	Very Cloudy
Specific gravity	1.048
pH	7.0
Protein	**3+**
Hb/Blood	**4+**
Bilirubin	**1+**
Sediment	
RBC/HPF	0–5
WBC/HPF	None seen
Epithelial cells/HPF	Transitional (0–5), squamous (0–5)
Casts/lpf	Coarse granular (0–5), hyaline (0–5)
Crystals	Struvite (4+), bilirubin (1+)
Microorganisms	None seen

Interpretive discussion

Hematology

On Day 1, although erythrocytosis is not observed, the PCV is shifted towards the upper reference interval, possibly due to a combination of dehydration and an epinephrine-mediated response. On Days 4 and 7 the cat has developed a mild anemia. A decreasing PCV combined with increased bilirubin concentration should raise concerns of hemolytic disease. However, given the history and presentation of this case, a combination of inflammatory disease and blood loss from the attack offers a most likely explanation. The slightly increased reticulocyte concentration on Day 7 is indicative of an initial regenerative response.

Even though it is not accompanied by neutrophilia, the mild lymphocytosis observed on Day 1 is most likely the result of an excitement response caused by epinephrine release from being attacked by the dog. On Day 4, a left shift without neutrophilia, and lymphopenia are appreciated, and attributable to inflammation. On Day 7 the left shift still present but the total number of band neutrophils has decreased significantly, indicating that the inflammation is subsiding.

Thrombocytopenia is observed on Days 4 and 7. Excessive consumption/Loss associated with blood loss is a potential explanation. A declining platelet count on a trauma patient could raise concerns of DIC, however, coagulation profiles were within reference intervals in this patient.

Chemistry

Marked hyperkalemia is present on Day 1. Considering the lack of azotemia and the urinalysis results, causes other than lack of renal excretion should be considered. Potassium shifting from the intracellular to the extracellular fluid is a likely explanation, with both tissue necrosis (damage from the trauma) and metabolic acidosis (lactic acidosis induced by the struggle with the dog) being potential contributors to hyperkalemia. Mild hyperkalemia persists on Day 4 and potassium concentration has returned to the reference interval on Day 7.

Hypophosphatemia, observed on Day 1, is not a frequent finding in cats. In this case, it is likely a consequence of hyperventilation inducing respiratory alkalosis, leading to changes in cellular pH that stimulate glycolysis and ATP production depleting serum phosphate concentration.

Total bilirubin and ALT activity were increased on all exams.

ALT is fairly liver-specific and usually associated with hepatocellular damage. However, the history of trauma and other laboratory findings suggests a potential muscle origin for the increased ALT activity.

Hyperbilirubinemia is normally associated with cholestasis and /or hemolytic disease. However, there was no evidence of cholestasis on imaging exams, and although hemolysis cannot be excluded it is more likely that the increased bilirubin concentration is caused by the breakdown of hemoglobin within the hematomas, as well as some contribution of nonblood heme (i.e., myoglobin). CK and AST activities could help to assert if muscle damage was indeed a contributor to these findings. Unfortunately, they were not performed.

Hypoalbuminemia is observed on Days 4 and 7. This is likely an acute phase response to inflammation, as evidenced by the left shift and the increase in the globulin concentration, albeit still within the reference interval, in comparison with Day 1. Blood loss could also have contributed to the hypoalbuminemia.

Urinalysis

Brown-colored urine with a 4+ dipstick result for blood in the absence of compatible hematuria indicates pigmenturia. The dipstick is not capable of differentiating between hemoglobinuria and myoglobinuria. Proteinuria is also observed. Although the dipstick is more sensitive to albumin, it is impossible to rule out the interference of hemoglobin and/or myoglobulin in this result.

The presence of casts is indicative of acute tubular injury, which can be due to ischemic lesions and nephrotoxic substances, such as myoglobin and hemoglobin, among other causes. Although their presence can be suggestive of renal disease, it isn't a reliable indicator of prognosis as it doesn't necessarily correlate with the extent and reversibility of the injury. Although no further urinalysis was performed, gross appearance of the urine was normal on Day 2.

Summary and outcome

The cat suffered severe soft-tissue trauma to the neck, which likely led to muscle injury and local inflammation. Blood loss from the injuries was not considered to be major but it seemed to have contributed to the anemia along with the inflammatory disease. The cat was severely ataxic for the first few days but clinical improvement was observed during the 8 days of hospitalization before being discharged. Follow-up CBC and chemistry panel performed on Day 15 were all within reference intervals and the patient was fully recovered within 3 weeks following the incident.

Contributor: Dr. Pedro Bittencourt

Case 53

Signalment: 11-year-old intact male miniature schnauzer
History: Intermittent vomiting and diarrhea for last 2 weeks
Physical examination: Tense, painful abdomen. Very fat.

Hematology		Reference interval
PCV (%)	38	37–55
Hgb (g/dL)	13.2	12–18
RBC ($\times 10^6/\mu L$)	5.7	5.5–8.5
MCV (fL)	67	60–72
MCHC (g/dL)	35	33–38
NCC ($\times 10^3/\mu L$)	**17.9**	6–17
Segs ($\times 10^3/\mu L$)	**14.2**	3–11.5
Bands ($\times 10^3/\mu L$)	**0.5**	0–0.3
Monos ($\times 10^3/\mu L$)	0.7	0.1–1.3
Lymphs ($\times 10^3/\mu L$)	2.5	1–4.8
Platelets ($\times 10^3/\mu L$)	250	200–500
TP (P) (g/dL)	**9.0**	6–8

Hemopathology: Moderate polychromasia.

Biochemical profile (serum was lipemic)		Reference interval
Gluc (mg/dL)	**124 *(6.8)***	65–122 *(3.5–6.7 mmol/L)*
BUN (mg/dL)	**42 *(15)***	7–28 *(2.5–10.0 mmol/L)*
Creat (mg/dL)	1.2	0.9–1.7
Ca (mg/dL)	9.8	9.0–11.2
Phos (mg/dL)	5.8	2.8–6.1
TP (g/dL)	**7.7**	5.4–7.4
Alb (g/dL)	3.7	2.7–4.5
Glob (g/dL)	**4.0**	1.9–3.4
T. bili (mg/dL)	**10.8 *(184.7)***	0–0.4 *(0–6.8 μmol/L)*
Chol (mg/dL)	**1230 *(32)***	130–370 *(3.4–9.6 mmol/L)*
ALT (IU/L)	**600**	10–120
AST (IU/L)	**540**	16–40
ALP (IU/L)	**660**	35–280
Na (mEq/L)	148	145–158
K (mEq/L)	4.3	4.1–5.5
CL (mEq/L)	110	106–127
TCO_2 (mEq/L)	24	14–27
An. gap (mEq/L)	18	8–25
Amylase (IU/L)	510	50–1250
Lipase (IU/L)	120	30–560

Urinalysis (voided)		Urine sediment	
Color	Yellow	WBCs/hpf	**>50**
Transparency	**Cloudy**	RBCs/hpf	0–1
Sp. gr.	**1.022**	Epith cells/hpf	0
Protein	**3+**	Casts/lpf	0
Gluc	Negative	Crystals	0
Bilirubin	**2+**	Bacteria	**Many bacilli**
Blood	Negative		
pH	7.0		

Interpretive discussion

Hematology

The PCV, hemoglobin concentration, and RBC count are at the lower end of the reference interval, and it is possible that an anemia has been masked by dehydration. With a history of vomiting and diarrhea and an increased plasma protein concentration, it is possible that this animal is dehydrated. However, we have no additional support for dehydration in these data. Because the serum is lipemic, a likely explanation for the high total plasma protein as measured by refractometry is the presence of lipids, which interfere with the reading. The presence of moderate polychromasia suggests a regenerative response. Blood loss may have caused a regenerative anemia in this dog (see summary).

Neutrophilia with a left shift indicates an inflammatory leukogram.

Biochemical profile

The BUN concentration is only mildly increased and the serum creatinine concentration is normal. Urine specific gravity indicates inadequate urine concentrating ability in the face of possible dehydration (if present) and azotemia, suggesting possible renal disease. Increased BUN with normal creatinine also prompts consideration of prerenal azotemia secondary to GI tract hemorrhage (which acts as a high-protein meal).

Both plasma and serum protein concentrations are increased, but the plasma protein concentration is much higher than the serum protein concentration. Because fibrinogen is present in plasma but not in serum, one would expect the plasma protein concentration to be 0.2 to 0.4 g/dl higher than that of serum. However, the difference is often greater because plasma protein concentration is estimated using a refractometer, while serum protein is measured spectrophotometrically. Increased plasma concentration of lipids may falsely increase the protein estimate determined by a refractometer. The increased difference between these protein concentrations in this case is likely due to lipemia.

The hyperglobulinemia may be the result of chronic antigenic stimulation with subsequent increase in antibody production.

The combination of hyperbilirubinemia and increased serum ALP activity is typical of cholestasis. The increased bilirubin concentration in the urine reflects the hyperbilirubinemia; conjugated bilirubin is cleared by the glomerulus and excreted in the urine. Although hypercholesterolemia is a nonspecific problem, cholestasis is a common cause of this abnormality and may be an explanation in this case. The magnitude of the hypercholesterolemia is unusual for cholestasis alone. Since this dog is a miniature schnauzer, and the serum is lipemic, suggesting hypertriglyceridemia and/or chylomicronemia, idiopathic hyperlipidemia is likely.

Increased serum AST and ALT activities indicate hepatocyte injury. Both of these enzymes are leakage enzymes and are present in significant concentrations in hepatocytes. AST is also present in high concentrations and ALT in low concentrations in muscle, but muscle is an unlikely source of these enzymes in this case. In light of the evidence for cholestasis, hepatic origin is most likely for these enzymes in this dog.

Urinalysis

Proteinuria, pyuria, and bacteriuria suggest inflammation in the urinary tract. Since these are found in a voided urine sample, reproductive tract origin must also be considered. Bacteria in a voided urine sample may be contaminants but are more significant when accompanied by pyuria. Culture of this urine sample is indicated.

Summary

This dog had a suppurative cholangiohepatitis, a duodenal ulcer, and pyelonephritis. The cholangiohepatitis resulted in the cholestasis and damage to hepatocytes. The chronic antigenic stimulation caused by both cholangiohepatitis and pyelonephritis resulted in hyperglobulinemia. The mild azotemia could have resulted from pyelonephritis or GI hemorrhage secondary to the duodenal ulcer.

Case 54

Signalment: 6-year-old CM German shepherd
History: Receiving prednisone for inflammatory bowel disease. Losing weight for 6 months.
Physical examination: Thin, with multiple hairless scaly skin lesions. Hepatomegaly.

Hematology		Reference interval
PCV (%)	38	36–60
Hgb (g/dL)	13.1	12–18
RBC ($\times 10^6/\mu L$)	4.9	4.8–9.3
MCV (fL)	79	58–79
MCHC (g/dL)	34	33–38
NCC ($\times 10^3/\mu L$)	**27.8**	4–15.5
Segs ($\times 10^3/\mu L$)	**25.5**	2–10.5
Bands ($\times 10^3/\mu L$)	0	0–0.3
Monos ($\times 10^3/\mu L$)	**2.0**	0–0.9
Lymphs ($\times 10^3/\mu L$)	**0.3**	1–4.5
Eos ($\times 10^3/\mu L$)	0	0.1–1.2
Platelets ($\times 10^3/\mu L$)	374	200–500

Hemopathology: Moderate acanthocytes, few echinocytes, keratocytes, schistocytes.

Biochemical profile		Reference interval
Gluc (mg/dL)	103	70–138
BUN (mg/dL)	11	6–25
Creat (mg/dL)	0.5	0.5–1.6
Ca (mg/dL)	**8.4**	8.9–11.4
Phos (mg/dL)	4.4	2.5–6.0
TP (g/dL)	5.3	5.0–7.4
Alb (g/dL)	**2.3**	2.7–4.4
Glob (g/dL)	3.0	1.6–3.6
T. bili (mg/dL)	**1.6**	0.1–0.3
Chol (mg/dL)	121	92–324
Trig (mg/dL)	102	29–291
ALT (IU/L)	**1041**	12–128
AST (IU/L)	**101**	15–66
ALP (IU/L)	**640**	5–131
GGT (IU/L)	**237**	1–12
CK (IU/L)	174	59–895
Na (mEq/L)	149	139–154
K (mEq/L)	4.9	3.6–5.5
CL (mEq/L)	108	102–120
TCO_2 (mEq/L)	23	15–25

Coagulation profile		Reference interval
PT (seconds)	7.0	6–12
aPTT (seconds)	15.9	10–25

Interpretive discussion

Hematology

There is a moderate leukocytosis characterized by a mature neutrophilia, lymphopenia, and monocytosis. This is most consistent with a steroid/stress leukogram, which is expected given the history of prednisone administration. The magnitude of the mature neutrophilia is slightly greater than that usually seen with a stress response alone, so chronic inflammation should also be considered.

Although there is no anemia present there are significant erythrocyte membrane changes observed. Acanthocytes may be seen with liver disease and hemangiosarcoma. Keratocytes and schistocytes suggest there is some red cell fragmentation occurring.

Biochemical profile

The most significant abnormalities relate to the liver. Increased activities of the leakage enzymes ALT and AST indicate there has been hepatocellular injury. Increased activities of the inducible enzymes ALP and GGT may be due to cholestasis and/or drug induction, given the history of steroid administration. The increased total bilirubin concentration supports cholestasis, since there is no indication of hemolysis, and indicates that hepatic function has been compromised.

Albumin is slightly decreased, most likely due to the ongoing inflammatory bowel disease. Decreased production due to liver failure is less likely since glucose, BUN, and cholesterol are normal. The mild decrease in calcium is likely due to a decrease in protein-bound calcium secondary to hypoalbuminemia. An ionized calcium could be measured to confirm this.

Summary

There is laboratory evidence for hepatocellular injury and cholestasis severe enough to affect hepatic function. Given the history of prednisone administration, a steroid hepatopathy is most likely. Red cell membrane changes may be due to hepatic disease or potentially hemangiosarcoma. A liver aspirate was performed and revealed marked indistinct hepatic vacuolization consistent with glycogen, and numerous bile casts indicating cholestasis. These findings were confirmed on a liver biopsy; there was no evidence of neoplasia or inflammation. Biopsies of the skin lesions revealed pyogranulomatous dermatitis with intralesional pigmented fungal hyphae. Presumably immune suppression due to the prolonged steroid administration predisposed to the fungal infection.

Case 55

Signalment: 5-year-old FS canine
History: On phenobarbital to control seizures for 2.5 years. Vomiting daily and lethargic for about 1 month.
Physical examination: Lethargic, icteric, pendulous abdomen; arthritic, and appears older than stated age

Hematology		Reference interval
PCV (%)	40.0	37–55
Hgb (g/dL)	13.6	12–18
RBC (×10^6/μL)	5.53	5.5–8.5
MCV (fL)	72.0	60–72
MCHC (g/dL)	34.0	33–38
NCC (×10^3/μL)	**47.2**	6–17
Segs (×10^3/μL)	**40.1**	3–11.5
Bands (×10^3/μL)	**0.9**	0–0.3
Monos (×10^3/μL)	**4.7**	0.1–1.3
Lymphs (×10^3/μL)	**0.9**	1–4.8
Eos (×10^3/μL)	0.5	0.1–1.2
Platelets (×10^3/μL)	299	200–500
TP (P) (g/dL)	**5.5**	6–8

Hemopathology: Slightly toxic neutrophils, many echinocytes.

Biochemical profile		Reference interval
Gluc (mg/dL)	69	65–122
BUN (mg/dL)	**5 *(1.78)***	7–28 *(2.5–10.0 mmo1/L)*
Creat (mg/dL)	**0.6**	0.9–1.7
Ca (mg/dL)	**8.1 *(2.02)***	9.0–11.2 *(2.25–2.80 mmol/L)*
Phos (mg/dL)	5.1	2.8–6.1
TP (g/dL)	**4.8**	5.4–7.4
Alb (g/dL)	**2.0**	2.7–4.5
Glob (g/dL)	2.8	1.9–3.4
T. bili (mg/dL)	**4.5 *(77)***	0–0.4 *(0–6.8 μmol/L)*
Chol (mg/dL)	**126 *(3.28)***	130–370 *(3.4–9.6 mmol/L)*
ALT (IU/L)	**348**	10–120
AST (IU/L)	**176**	16–40
ALP (IU/L)	**4503**	35–280
GGT (IU/L)	**426**	0–6
Na (mEq/L)	**142**	145–158
K (mEq/L)	**3.3**	4.1–5.5
CL (mEq/L)	114	106–127
TCO_2 (mEq/L)	14.8	14–27
An. gap (mEq/L)	16.5	8–25
Lipase (IU/L)	**575**	30–560

Urinalysis		Urine sediment	
Color	Orange		
Transparency	**Cloudy**	WBCs/hpf	**8–10**
Sp. gr.	1.015	RBCs/hpf	0–2
Protein	**2+**	Epith cells/hpf	**80–100**
Gluc	Negative	Casts/lpf	Negative
Bilirubin	**4+**	Crystals	Negative
Blood	**3+**	Bacteria	**4+ rods**
pH	6.0		
Ketones	**3+**		

Coagulation data		Reference interval
PT (seconds)	9.8	7.5–10.5
aPTT (seconds)	14.0	10.5–16.5

Interpretive discussion

Hematology

There is a moderate neutrophilia with a mild left shift, monocytosis, and slightly toxic neutrophils were observed in the blood film. This is an inflammatory leukogram, but the lymphopenia indicates a concurrent steroid-induced component. Monocytosis is consistent with the combined leukocyte response.

Biochemical profile

The serum glucose concentration is at the low end of the reference interval and the BUN is decreased. These findings may indicate hepatic functional impairment, particularly in light of the observation of a potential stress leukogram (stress would be expected to increase the glucose concentration). See discussion of serum protein below. Decreased creatinine likely reflects decreased muscle mass.

The serum total protein and albumin concentrations are decreased. Considerations in this case include renal loss (see urinalysis discussion) and, more likely, decreased production secondary to hepatic disease (discussed more later).

There is a mild hypocalcemia that is likely secondary to hypoalbuminemia, and therefore not clinically significant. An ionized calcium could be measured to confirm this.

Serum cholesterol is decreased. While one should not overinterpret decreases in some analytes, this is commonly observed in end-stage liver disease, owing to impaired hepatic lipid synthesis. This is particularly notable given the degree of hyperbilirubinemia and increases in enzyme activities indicative of cholestasis (ALP and GGT). The magnitude of increase in serum ALP activity is large enough to warrant consideration of corticosteroid induction. Likewise, the degree of increase in GGT activity may be related to steroid induction rather than cholestasis alone. The serum ALT and AST activities are moderately increased, indicating hepatocellular damage. Phenobarbital may induce increased production of several liver enzymes.

The serum sodium and potassium are decreased, and one should consider typical causes for electrolyte depletion, including pathologic losses from the gastrointestinal and urinary systems, as well as third space syndromes. Hypokalemia is a frequent observation in hepatic disease, often due to anorexia and vomiting.

Coagulation data

The aPTT and PT are normal. If hepatic disease or end-stage liver failure has progressed sufficiently, as suggested by even lower values for glucose, BUN, albumin, and cholesterol, one might expect these indices of coagulation factor synthesis to become abnormal as well.

Urinalysis

The urinary specific gravity indicates the urine is poorly concentrated and may reflect impaired concentrating ability. This may be due to the decreased BUN, since urea also plays a role in urine concentration. The concentrations of protein, ketones, bilirubin, and blood are particularly notable given this weak urine concentration. The proteinuria is explained by the urinary tract inflammation/infection as indicated by the significant pyuria, bacteriuria, and presence of marked occult blood. The presence of bilirubin is not surprising given the degree of hyperbilirubinemia. The presence of ketonuria in the absence of glucosuria is unusual. Ketosis is a possible sequela to impaired oxidative lipid metabolism by the diseased liver, especially when triglyceride absorption from the GI tract or mobilization from peripheral stores is greater than hepatic functional capacity for processing.

Summary

There is biochemical evidence of chronic liver failure, cholestasis, and hepatocellular injury. Phenobarbital-induced hepatopathy was considered. Ultrasound of the liver showed an enlarged liver with numerous well-defined hypoechoic foci throughout. Masses throughout the cranial mid-abdomen had similar echogenicity as masses within liver. Cytology of a liver aspirate showed vacuolated hepatocytes, bile stasis, and a population of nonhepatic cells with a high nucleus: cytoplasm ratio, most of which were broken. Numerous cells in mitosis were observed, and neoplasia was diagnosed. Biopsy of liver revealed adenocarcinoma that effaced and replaced hepatic parenchyma and glucocorticoid hepatopathy with severe bile stasis. The neoplasm had a neuroendocrine (potentially adrenal) pattern, and was possibly causing the steroid hepatopathy. Endocrine panel was not performed. Dog was euthanized; necropsy was not allowed.

Case 56

Signalment: 6-year-old spayed female dog
History: Struck by car 1 month ago. Not taken to veterinarian. Dyspnea since accident. Anorexia.
Physical examination: Emaciated and lethargic. Intestinal sounds auscultated in thorax.

Hematology		Reference interval
PCV (%)	37	37–55
Hgb (g/dL)	12.3	12–18
RBC ($\times 10^6/\mu L$)	6.1	5.5–8.5
MCV (fL)	61	60–72
MCHC (g/dL)	33	33–38
NCC ($\times 10^3/\mu L$)	16.1	6–17
Segs ($\times 10^3/\mu L$)	**13.5**	3–11.5
Bands ($\times 10^3/\mu L$)	0.2	0–0.3
Monos ($\times 10^3/\mu L$)	1.0	0.1–1.3
Lymphs ($\times 10^3/\mu L$)	**0.6**	1–4.8
Eos ($\times 10^3/\mu L$)	0.8	0.1–1.2
Platelets ($\times 10^3/\mu L$)	330	200–500
TP (P) (g/dL)	**3.3**	6–8

Hemopathology: Normal.

Biochemical profile		Reference interval
Gluc (mg/dL)	77	65–122
BUN (mg/dL)	**3 *(1.07)***	7–28 *(2.5–10.0 mmol/L)*
Creat (mg/dL)	1.5	0.9–1.7
Ca (mg/dL)	**6.3**	9.0–11.2
Phos (mg/dL)	**4.4**	2.8–6.1
TP (g/dL)	**2.9**	5.4–7.4
Alb (g/dL)	**0.6**	2.7–4.5
Glob (g/dL)	2.3	1.9–3.4
T. bili (mg/dL)	**3.0 *(51.3)***	0–0.4 *(0–6.8 μmol/L)*
Chol (mg/dL)	**102 *(2.65)***	130 370 *(3.4–9.6 mmol/L)*
ALT (IU/L)	**170**	10–120
AST (IU/L)	**72**	16–40
ALP (IU/L)	**540**	35–280
Na (mEq/L)	146	145–158
K (mEq/L)	**6.0**	4.1–5.5
CL (mEq/L)	118	106–127
TCO_2 (mEq/L)	**11**	14–27
An. gap (mEq/L)	23	8–25
Plasma ammonia (mg/dL)	**150**	0–90

Urinalysis (catheterized)		Urine sediment	
Color	Yellow	WBCs/hpf	0
Transparency	Clear	RBCs/hpf	0
Sp. gr.	1.035	Epith cells/hpf	0
Protein	Negative	Casts/lpf	0
Gluc	Negative	Crystals	**Bilirubin**
Bilirubin	**1+**	Bacteria	0
Blood	Negative		
pH	5.5		

Interpretive discussion

Hematology

This dog's erythrocyte measurements are near the lower end of their reference intervals, and there is no evidence of a regenerative response. This may be normal for this dog, or it is possible that this dog is developing a nonregenerative anemia secondary to chronic disease.

Leukocyte abnormalities are a mature neutrophilia and lymphopenia, typical of a corticosteroid-mediated leukogram.

Biochemical profile

Decreased BUN concentration can be caused by hepatic failure, diuresis, decreased protein intake, or treatment with anabolic steroids. BUN concentration below the reference interval can also occur in normal animals. In light of other laboratory findings in this case, the decreased BUN concentration is probably due to hepatic failure and resulting failure of hepatocytes to synthesize urea. Anorexia resulting in decreased protein intake may have also contributed to this abnormality.

This dog has hypocalcemia; however, it also has severe hypoalbuminemia. Hypoalbuminemia, and resultant decreased protein-bound calcium, may be the cause for the hypocalcemia, in which case it is not clinically significant. Ionized calcium could be measured to confirm this. While not always necessary, determining the ionized calcium would be recommended in this case because of the magnitude of the hypocalcemia and the critical condition of the patient.

Both plasma and serum protein concentrations are decreased. These decreases are a result of hypoalbuminemia. When interpreted in combination with other laboratory data, this abnormality is probably due to decreased albumin synthesis by the liver. Decreased protein intake can result in hypoalbuminemia and may also have played a role in this case. The albumin concentration is low enough to lead to ascites; however, ascites was not noted in this animal.

In dogs, hyperbilirubinemia can result from hemolysis, failure of hepatocyte uptake and metabolism of bilirubin, or failure to excrete bilirubin due to cholestasis or other disruption of bile flow. In this case, failure of hepatic uptake and metabolism of bilirubin is probably the major abnormality leading to hyperbilirubinemia. It is also probable the bile duct is partially blocked and cholestasis is playing a role in producing this abnormality. The increased serum ALP activity suggests cholestasis is present in this dog.

Hypocholesterolemia is probably another result of hepatic failure. The liver is a major site of cholesterol synthesis and excretion. Abnormalities of these two processes have opposite effects on serum cholesterol concentrations. In this case, synthetic failure is apparently more severe than failure to excrete cholesterol.

Both serum ALT and AST activities are mildly increased. These enzymes leak from injured hepatocytes, and liver injury is the appropriate interpretation in this case. AST is also present in muscle cells, and muscle injury cannot be ruled out, but the mild increase of AST activity in conjunction with the increased ALT activity suggests the AST has leaked from the liver in this case.

Increased ALP activity most often results from either cholestasis or increased blood corticosteroid concentrations. In combination with other laboratory data suggesting hepatic disease, cholestasis is the most important cause of the increased ALP in this case. This dog probably had an increased blood corticosteroid concentration as suggested by the leukogram, and this may have also played a role in increasing the serum ALP activity.

Hyperkalemia may be a result of metabolic acidosis-induced shifting of potassium from within cells to extracellular fluid. In animals with metabolic acidosis, hydrogen ions enter cells in an attempt to equalize their concentrations in the intracellular and extracellular compartments. In order to maintain electrical neutrality, potassium ions must leave the cells. The net result is increased extracellular and, therefore, serum potassium concentrations.

The cause of the decreased total CO_2 is not certain. Since this animal has a compromised respiratory system, it is reasonable to assume that it has a respiratory acidosis. However, the total CO_2 concentration would be expected to increase in compensation for the respiratory acidosis. Since this concentration decreased rather than increased, it is reasonable to assume the dog has another abnormality causing metabolic acidosis. Although the anion gap is normal, the markedly low albumin may be masking an increase in unmeasured anions, thus there could be a hidden high-gap acidosis. Abnormal renal regulation of acid-base balance is another possible cause of decreased total CO_2, but there is no evidence of renal dysfunction in this case. A blood gas analysis would be helpful to further evaluate this dog's acid-base status.

The hyperammonemia is a result of hepatic failure. Ammonia is normally absorbed from the digestive tract and transported to the liver by the portal circulation. The liver is responsible for removing and metabolizing this ammonia. Alterations in blood flow to the liver and/or markedly decreased numbers of functional hepatocytes can result in increased blood ammonia concentrations.

Urinalysis

Bilirubinuria and the presence of bilirubin crystals are the only abnormalities in the urine. These changes reflect the increased serum bilirubin concentration. Conjugated bilirubin readily passes through glomeruli and is then excreted in the urine. The very mild increase in urine bilirubin suggests that most of the serum bilirubin is unconjugated. Interestingly, this dog is concentrating urine in the face of a very low bun.

Summary

Exploratory surgery revealed a diaphragmatic hernia through which the liver and a portion of the GI tract had passed. The liver was decreased in size and firm. Many fibrous adhesions were present. On the surgeon's recommendation, the dog was euthanized.

This dog had hepatic failure due to chronically decreased blood supply to the liver. Decreased BUN, albumin, and cholesterol concentrations suggested decreased synthetic function by the liver. Increased bilirubin and ammonia concentrations resulted from decreased delivery of these substances to the liver and, therefore, decreased removal from the blood as well as due to decreased functional hepatic mass. Cholestasis resulting from partial occlusion of the bile duct also contributed to hyperbilirubinemia. Since this was an end-stage liver disease, leakage of ALT and AST from hepatocytes was minimal due to the small number of hepatocytes remaining, and serum activities of ALT and AST were, therefore, only slightly increased.

Case 57

Signalment: 10-year-old spayed female Doberman dog
History: Lethargy, weight loss, diarrhea, and poor appetite
Physical examination: Depressed, dehydrated, hypotensive, and icteric

Hematology		Reference interval
TP (P) (g/dL)	**4.7**	6.0–8.0
PCV (%)	41	40–55
Hgb (g/dL)	14.6	13.0–20.0
RBC ($\times10^6/\mu L$)	6.07	5.5–8.5
MCV (fL)	67	62–73
MCHC (g/dL)	36	33–36
NCC ($\times10^3/\mu L$)	**26.6**	4.5–15.0
Bands ($\times10^3/\mu L$)	**1.3**	0–0.2
Segs ($\times10^3/\mu L$)	**12.2**	2.6–11.0
Lymphs ($\times10^3/\mu L$)	**11.9**	1.0–4.8
Monos ($\times10^3/\mu L$)	**1.1**	0.2–1.0
Eos ($\times10^3/\mu L$)	0	0.1–1.2
Platelets ($\times10^3/\mu L$)	**90**	200–500
MPV (fL)	13.9	7.5–14.6

Hemopathology noted on blood film:
- Most lymphoid cells are large with fine granular chromatin; interpreted as mostly prolymphocytes with some blasts.
- No platelet clumps found, occasional giant platelets.

Biochemical profile		Reference interval
Gluc (mg/dL)	65	75–130
BUN (mg/dL)	**69**	7–32
Creat (mg/dL)	1.5	0.4–1.5
Phos (mg/dL)	**13.2**	2.1–6.0
Ca (mg/dL)	9.4	9.2–11.7
Mg (mg/dL)	**3.4**	1.8–2.5
TP (g/dL)	**3.9**	5.3–7.2
Alb (g/dL)	**2.4**	2.5–4.0
Glob (g/dL)	**1.5**	2.0–3.8
Chol (mg/dL)	**102**	130–300
T. bili (mg/dL)	**12.6**	0–0.3
ALP (IU/L)	**1717**	20–142
ALT (IU/L)	**590**	10–110
AST (IU/L)	**401**	16–50
GGT (IU/L)	5	0–8
Na (mEq/L)	**138**	142–152
K (mEq/L)	4.3	3.5–5.2
CL (mEq/L)	**100**	108–120
Bicarbonate (mEq/L)	**10.5**	16–25
An. gap (mEq/L)	**32**	13–22

Blood gas analysis–venous		Reference interval
pH	**6.92**	7.33–7.45
pCO_2 (mmHg)	**57.3**	24–39
pO_2 (mmHg)	75.9	67–92
HCO_3 (mEq/L)	**11.3**	15–24
Lactate (mmol/L)	**8.4**	0.2–1.4

Interpretive discussion

Hematology

The hematocrit is low normal, but some degree of anemia is probable given physical dehydration; the baseline hematocrit is not known.

There is moderate hypoproteinemia, to be considered in chemistry interpretation.

The leukogram indicates moderate lymphocytosis. The presence of mostly abnormal lymphocyte forms indicates lymphoproliferative disease that is leukemic. The left shift with mild neutrophilia indicates concurrent inflammatory stimulus. Minimal monocytosis accompanies the inflammatory pattern.

There is thrombocytopenia with some giant platelets, indicating active thrombopoiesis. A consumptive process should be considered.

Chemistry

Renal analytes

The following processes are identified:
- Moderate azotemia indicated by BUN and prominent hyperphosphatemia. The creatinine has likely increased in this individual, within the reference interval. Increased magnesium is due to decreased GFR.
- Likely a prerenal component given dehydration and other evidence of poor perfusion such as lactic acidosis (later). A urinalysis, especially specific gravity, would be helpful.
- Possible renal component requires urinalysis for further characterization.
- The Ca · P is 124 indicating calcification will be occurring.

Liver

The following processes are identified:
- There is hepatocellular injury indicated by increased activities of ALT/AST.
- There is evidence of liver function failure in the form of probable decreased cholesterol synthesis and marked hyperbilirubinemia in the face of near normal HCT.
- Cholestasis and/or steroid-induced ALP are considerations given the ALP magnitude; cholestasis is a likely contributing factor to the hyperbilirubinemia.

• Mild hypoglycemia and hypoalbuminemia may also be related in part to function failure.

Protein

There is marked hypoproteinemia due to panhypoproteinemia. All potential causes of loss should be evaluated, particularly GI given the observation of diarrhea.

Acid-base/electrolyte

The following processes are identified:

• There is severe, life-threatening acidemia. This is a mixed acidosis of two processes.

• There is metabolic acidosis indicated by decreased bicarbonate. This is most likely related to poor tissue perfusion and development of lactate acidemia, as well as uremic acids.

• There is also a component of respiratory acidosis indicated by the prominent increase in pCO_2. The respiratory component is likely related to terminal respiratory failure; this would prompt evaluation of cardiopulmonary function.

• Both the pCO_2 and bicarbonate are counter to any detectable compensation.

• The increased anion gap is attributable to retention of renal-excreted anions such as phosphate and sulfate, and lactate is a contributing factor.

Summary

• Biochemical evidence of liver function failure, with hepatocellular injury and cholestasis. Hepatic infiltrate with lymphoma should be considered given that there is blood evidence of lymphoproliferative disease.

• Azotemia likely prerenal; kidneys should be investigated further.

• Severe mixed acidemia compatible with multiple causes of metabolic acid and respiratory acid formation.

• Lymphoproliferative disorder.

• Marked panhypoproteinemia.

Recommendations for further characterization would include:

• Urinalysis.

• Evaluation of liver and kidney size with sampling for possible infiltrative disease (lymphoma).

• Bone marrow for possible infiltrate.

• Cytometric analysis of blood leukocytes if treatment is contemplated.

As follow-up, the dog was euthanized. Necropsy findings included splenomegaly, hepatomegaly, lymphadenopathy with marked involvement with lymphoma. The severity of this change in liver would explain the biochemical evidence of function failure.

Case 58

Signalment: 9-month-old intact female dog
History: Struck by car 3 weeks ago. Treated for shock and released. Listless since then.
Physical examination: Abdomen distended and fluid-filled

Hematology		Reference interval
PCV (%)	**30**	37–55
Hgb (g/dL)	**10.3**	12–18
RBC (×10^6/μL)	**5.45**	5.5–8.5
MCV (fL)	**55**	60–72
MCHC (g/dL)	34	33–38
Retics (/μL)	42	<60
NCC (×10^3/μL)	16	6–17
Segs (×10^3/μL)	**12.8**	3–11.5
Bands (×10^3/μL)	**0.5**	0–0.3
Lymphs (×10^3/μL)	2.7	1–4.8
Platelets (×10^3/μL)	270	200–500
TP (P) (g/dL)	6.5	6–8

Hemopathology: Slight hypochromasia, moderate number of keratocytes.

Biochemical profile		Reference interval
Gluc (mg/dL)	65	65–122
BUN (mg/dL)	25	7–28
Creat (mg/dL)	1.2	0.9–1.7
Ca (mg/dL)	**8.4 *(2.1)***	9.0–11.2 *(2.25–2.80 mmol/L)*
Phos (mg/dL)	6.0	2.8–6.1
TP (g/dL)	5.8	5.4–7.4
Alb (g/dL)	**2.5**	2.7–4.5
Glob (g/dL)	3.3	1.9–3.4
T. bili	**0.5 *(8.5)***	0–0.4 *(0–6.8 μmol/L)*
Chol (mg/dL)	170	130–370
ALT (IU/L)	23	10–120
AST (IU/L)	28	16–40
ALP (IU/L)	51	35–280
Na (mEq/L)	**139**	145–158
K (mEq/L)	5.2	4.1–5.5
CL (mEq/L)	**105**	106–127
TCO_2 (mEq/L)	15	14–27
An. gap (mEq/L)	24	8–25

Urinalysis (voided)		Urine sediment	
Color	Dark yellow	WBCs/hpf	0
Transparency	Clear	RBCs/hpf	0
Sp. gr.	1.030	Epith cells/hpf	0
Protein	Negative	Casts/lpf	0
Gluc	Negative	Crystals	**Bilirubin**
Bilirubin	**3+**	Bacteria	0
Blood	Negative		
pH	6.0		

Body fluid analysis		Differential	
Color	**Red-brown**	Neutrophils	74%
Transparency	Hazy	Lymphs	5%
TP (g/dL)	**3.8**	Macrophages	21%
NCC (/μL)	**8800**		

Other observations: Neutrophils are nondegenerate. Lymphocytes are uniformly small. Large mononuclear cells are a mixture of reactive mesothelial cells and macrophages. Macrophages contain large amounts of blue-green pigment, suggestive of bile. No micro-organisms are evident. Moderate numbers of erythrocytes are present.

Interpretive discussion

Hematology

This dog has a nonregenerative anemia. The indices reveal that this anemia is microcytic and borderline hypochromic. These abnormalities, in combination with the presence of hypochromasia and keratocytes observed on the blood film, indicate iron deficiency. Serum iron concentration should be measured in this dog. Although the most common cause of iron deficiency is chronic blood loss, there is no history of such blood loss in this case. In most such cases, examination of feces will reveal the presence of blood. GI parasites such as hookworms, should also be considered.

Borderline neutrophilia with a slight left shift suggests a mild tissue demand for neutrophils, and, therefore, a mild inflammatory process. It is likely that the anemia is nonregenerative due to the presence of inflammation (anemia of inflammatory disease).

Biochemical profile

The blood glucose concentration is at the bottom of the reference interval. Decreased carbohydrate intake or decreased hepatic production are possible causes. Since there is little evidence of hepatic failure in this case, decreased intake appears to be the most likely explanation. Alternatively, it may be normal for this dog.

The hypocalcemia may be a result of hypoalbuminemia, in which case it is not clinically significant. An ionized calcium could be measured to confirm this.

The mild hypoalbuminemia is probably due to decreased protein intake or decreased amino acid absorption from the GI tract. Evidence of hepatic failure is not present, and urine protein concentration is normal; therefore, decreased albumin production by the liver and increased albumin loss through the kidneys are unlikely. In light of the anemia and the evidence of iron deficiency, chronic blood loss should be considered as a cause of hypoalbuminemia in this case; however, globulin concentration usually decreases proportionally with albumin concentration during blood loss. The globulin concentration may, however, have been increased in this dog due to chronic antigenic stimulation, and this would explain a normal globulin concentration despite blood loss severe enough to result in hypoalbuminemia.

The combination of increased serum and urine bilirubin concentrations suggests disruption in the hepatic excretion of conjugated bilirubin. The serum bilirubin concentration, while increased, appears inappropriately low in light of the marked increase in urine bilirubin concentration. Dogs have a low renal threshold for bilirubin, and, in dogs with abnormalities of hepatic conjugated bilirubin excretion, urine bilirubin concentration may increase prior to increases in serum bilirubin concentration, or urine bilirubin concentration may be markedly increased while serum bilirubin concentration is only mildly increased.

Hyponatremia and hypochloremia were probably caused by dilution of these electrolytes in an increased volume of extracellular fluid. This increased fluid volume is a result of accumulation of fluid in the peritoneal cavity. This "third-spacing" phenomenon commonly results in hyponatremia and hypochloremia.

Urinalysis

Marked bilirubinuria and presence of bilirubin crystals are the only abnormalities in the urinalysis. These changes probably resulted from increased passage of conjugated bilirubin into the blood with subsequent renal excretion. Either cholestasis or rupture of the bile duct or gall bladder could be an underlying cause.

Abdominal fluid analysis

Based on the total nucleated cell count and on the predominance of neutrophils, the peritoneal fluid should be classified as an exudate. Since neutrophils are nondegenerate and bacteria are absent, this is probably a nonseptic exudate. The pigment noted in macrophages is suggestive of bile and, therefore, gall bladder or bile duct rupture are likely.

Summary

Exploratory surgery revealed a ruptured gall bladder. Due to severe adhesions throughout the peritoneal cavity, the owner was offered a guarded prognosis. The owner opted for euthanasia.

Bilirubin leaking with bile into this dog's peritoneal cavity was reabsorbed through the peritoneal wall. The bilirubin entered the blood and was efficiently excreted by the kidneys. As a result, serum bilirubin concentration increased only slightly while urine bilirubin concentration increased markedly. Serum activities of the hepatic leakage enzymes, ALT and AST, did not increase since there was no direct liver injury. Serum activity of ALP did not increase since there was no cholestasis.

Case 59

Signalment: 2-year-old male mixed-breed dog
History: Weight loss, lethargy
Physical examination: Thin dog, pendulous abdomen
Hematology: Unremarkable

Biochemical profile		Reference interval
Gluc (mg/dL)	**64 *(3.5)***	65–122 *(3.5–6.7 mmol/L)*
BUN (mg/dL)	**6 *(2.1)***	7–28 *(2.5–10.0 mmol/L)*
Creat (mg/dL)	1.0	0.9–1.7
Ca (mg/dL)	**7.4 *(1.85)***	9.0–11.2 *(2.25–2.80 mmol/L)*
Phos (mg/dL)	2.8	2.8–6.1
TP (g/dL)	**4.2**	5.4–7.4
Alb (g/dL)	**1.2**	2.7–4.5
Glob (g/dL)	3.0	1.9–3.4
T. bili (mg/dL)	0.4	0–0.4
Chol (mg/dL)	**65 *(1.7)***	130–370 *(3.4–9.6 mmol/L)*
ALT (IU/L)	**30**	10–120
ALP (IU/L)	260	35–280
Bile Acids (μmol/L)	**30**	3.0–9.0
Na (mEq/L)	146	145–158
K (mEq/L)	4.1	4.1–5.5
CL (mEq/L)	115	106–127

Abdominal fluid analysis	
TP (g/dL)	1.0
NCC (/μL)	1500
Segs (%)	60
Lymphs (%)	22
Macrophages (%)	18

Morphology: Neutrophils nondegenerate

Interpretive discussion

Biochemical profile

A number of factors in the profile suggest liver failure. These include a borderline low glucose, low BUN, hypoproteinemia characterized by severe hypoalbuminemia, and a markedly low cholesterol concentration. Hepatic enzymes are often normal with end-stage liver disease. An alternative, but less likely, possibility for this pattern is severe starvation. The increased bile acids indicate decreased liver function and help confirm end-stage liver disease.

Hypocalcemia may be due to hypoalbuminemia, in which case it is clinically insignificant. An ionized calcium could be measured to confirm this.

Body fluid analysis

The abdominal fluid has the typical features of a transudate. With end-stage liver disease this is due to a combination of hypoalbuminemia and increased portal blood pressure resulting in transudation of fluid into the cavity.

Summary

Hepatic cirrhosis; end-stage liver disease.

Case 60

Signalment: 3-month-old intact female dog
History: Anorexia, depression, and diarrhea of 1-week duration. Poor growth rate.
Physical examination: Severe, diffuse dermatitis with multifocal ulcerative lesions

Hematology		Reference interval
PCV (%)	**13**	37–55
Hgb (g/dL)	**4.5**	12–18
RBC (×10^6/μL)	**2.5**	5.5–8.5
MCV (fL)	**52**	60–72
MCHC (g/dL)	35	33–38
Retic (×10^3/μL)	2.5	<60
NCC (×10^3/μL)	**1.6**	6–17
Segs (×10^3/μL)	**0.5**	3–11.5
Bands (×10^3/μL)	0.1	0–0.3
Monos (×10^3/μL)	0.1	0.1–1.3
Lymphs (×10^3/μL)	**0.9**	1–4.8
Platelets (×10^3/μL)	340	200–500
TP (P) (g/dL)	**3.4**	6–8

Hemopathology: Markedly toxic neutrophils, few RBC fragments.

Biochemical profile		Reference interval
Gluc (mg/dL)	**40 (*2.2*)**	65–122 (*3.5–6.7 mmol/L*)
BUN (mg/dL)	**4 (*1.43*)**	7–28 (*2.5–10.0 mmol/L*)
Creat (mg/dL)	**0.3**	0.9–1.7
Ca (mg/dL)	**7.8 (*1.95*)**	9.0–11.2 (*2.25–2.80 mmol/L*)
Phos (mg/dL)	**2.0 (*0.65*)**	2.8–6.1 (*0.9–2.0 mmol/L*)
TP (g/dL)	**2.9**	5.4–7.4
Alb (g/dL)	**1.7**	2.7–4.5
Glob (g/dL)	**1.2**	1.9–3.4
T. bili (mg/dL)	0.2	0–0.4
Chol (mg/dL)	142	130–370
ALT (IU/L)	15	10–120
AST (IU/L)	22	16–40
ALP (IU/L)	63	35–280
GGT (IU/L)	6	0–6
Na (mEq/L)	**141**	145–158
K (mEq/L)	**3.7**	4.1–5.5
CL (mEq/L)	114	106–127
TCO_2 (mEq/L)	17	14–27
An. gap (mEq/L)	14	8–25
Fasting bile acids (μmol/L)	**88**	<10
Iron (μg/dL)	**50 (*8.95*)**	60–110 (*10.7–19.7 μmol/L*)

Urinalysis (cystocentesis)			
Color	Yellow	**Urine sediment**	
Transparency	Clear	WBCs/hpf	0–2
Sp. gr.	1.029	RBCs/hpf	0
Protein	Negative	Epith cells/hpf	0
Gluc	**2+**	Casts/lpf	0
Bilirubin	Negative	Crystals	0
Blood	Negative	Bacteria	0
pH	5.0		

Interpretive discussion

Hematology

This dog has a severe nonregenerative anemia. The anemia in this dog is microcytic, and the serum iron concentration is decreased, suggesting iron deficiency secondary to chronic blood loss. Alternately, microcytic anemia is also seen in dogs with portosystemic shunt, in which case serum iron may or may not be decreased, and anemia may be secondary to other abnormalities in iron metabolism. Red blood cell fragmentation is a typical finding in iron deficiency anemia. While iron deficiency anemia may be regenerative, this dog's bone marrow is not adequately responding, perhaps due to viral damage or concurrent anemia of chronic disease.

Severe leukopenia has resulted from a combination of neutropenia and lymphopenia. In a young dog with diarrhea as well as neutropenia and lymphopenia, parvovirus infection with virus-induced bone marrow damage should be a strong consideration. Acute bacterial enteritis resulting in endotoxemia may result in a similar leukogram. The presence of toxic neutrophils suggests that the bone marrow is rapidly producing neutrophils, and this may signal early recovery of previously suppressed neutrophil production, or may be a response to loss of neutrophils due to rapid, destruction or emigration into tissues as would occur with endotoxemia or overwhelming tissue demand for neutrophils, respectively.

Platelets are adequate, indicating chronic marrow failure is not present.

Biochemical profile

Hypoglycemia probably resulted from decreased hepatic glucose production. Numerous diseases can result in hypoglycemia, but, in light of other laboratory data, hepatic failure is the most likely cause of hypoglycemia in this dog. The decreased blood supply to the liver that occurs with portosystemic shunts can result in liver atrophy. Such a liver cannot play its normal role in maintenance of blood glucose concentrations. A second possibility, in light of the decreased neutrophil concentration, is that the dog has bacteremia or endotoxemia that may result in hypoglycemia. A third possibility is that glucose is being lost through the urinary tract (see discussion of glucosuria).

Both the BUN and serum creatinine concentrations are decreased. Since there is evidence of hepatic failure, it is likely that the decreased BUN concentration resulted from decreased liver production of urea. Decreased creatinine reflects decreased muscle mass.

This dog has both hypocalcemia and hypoalbuminemia. The hypocalcemia may be caused by decreased protein-bound calcium secondary to the hypoalbuminemia, in which case it is clinically insignificant. An ionized calcium could be measured to confirm this.

Hypophosphatemia occurs most commonly in hypercalcemic disorders such as primary hyperparathyroidism and pseudohyperparathyroidism, but these are unlikely in a 3-month-old dog. Other causes include dietary phosphate or vitamin D deficiency, malabsorption syndrome, diabetes mellitus, and canine Fanconi-like syndrome. This dog appears to have a renal tubular defect (see discussion of glucosuria), and it is possible that this defect is part of a canine Fanconi-like syndrome. In such a syndrome, inadequate tubular reabsorption of phosphate results in excessive loss of phosphate in the urine.

The hypoproteinemia is the result of both hypoalbuminemia and hypoglobulinemia. These abnormalities, in combination with anemia, indicate that blood loss should be considered. In this case, it is likely that chronic liver disease is also contributing to hypoalbuminemia.

This dog's serum bilirubin concentration, serum alkaline phosphatase (ALP) activity, and gamma glutamyltransferase (GGT) activity are normal, suggesting that cholestasis is not occurring. While most forms of liver failure result in some degree of cholestasis, liver failure resulting from a portosystemic shunt usually does not. These normal values, in combination with the history and other laboratory abnormalities, suggest that a portosystemic shunt is likely. Since this is a young dog, a slight increase in ALP of bone origin would not have been unusual. Despite evidence of hepatic disease, serum ALT and AST activities are normal. Serum activities of hepatic leakage enzymes such as ALT and AST may be normal to increased in dogs with portosystemic shunts.

The hyponatremia and hypokalemia may have resulted from diuresis induced by glucosuria, or losses associated with diarrhea. It is also possible this dog's tubular function defect includes abnormal reabsorption of Na and K. Decreased intake likely contributed to the hypokalemia.

Markedly increased fasting bile acid concentration can result from decreased hepatic blood flow, hepatic failure, or cholestasis. In this case, decreased hepatic blood flow and subsequent hepatic failure are the most likely explanations.

Blood loss is the most common cause of decreased serum iron concentration in animals, although nursing animals have low serum iron due to inadequate dietary intake. In this case, however, the decreased serum iron concentration is probably due to the presence of a portosystemic shunt. Decreased serum iron concentration does not always occur in dogs with portosystemic shunts and the cause is not known, but it appears to be related to iron sequestration in tissues such as liver and/or defects in the transport of iron. Some cases also have intermittent gastrointestinal bleeding associated with pica.

Urinalysis

Moderate glucosuria in an animal with a low or normal blood glucose suggests a lowered renal threshold for glucose and, therefore, a renal tubular absorption defect. Such a defect may be confined to glucose absorption only, or may include defective absorption of several substances. As previously noted, this dog may also have defective absorption of phosphate, sodium, and potassium. If this is the case, this is probably a form of canine Fanconi-like syndrome. Measurement of the fractional excretion of phosphate, sodium, and potassium would have helped in assessing this possibility.

Summary

This dog had a portosystemic shunt. Hypoglycemia, decreased BUN concentration, hypoalbuminemia, and increased serum bile acid concentrations resulted from decreased hepatic blood flow and subsequent hepatic failure. Microcytosis has been reported as common in dogs with portosystemic shunts. This dog also has a renal tubular defect. Glucosuria in the presence of hypoglycemia, hypophosphatemia, hyponatremia, and hypokalemia are probably a result of defective tubular reabsorption of these substances. This defect is probably a canine Fanconi-like syndrome. Neutropenia does not typically occur in either portosystemic shunts or canine Fanconi-like syndrome, and this dog may have a concurrent enteric infection, most likely caused by parvovirus or endotoxin-producing bacteria, resulting in this abnormality.

CASES

Case 61

Signalment: 8-month-old German shepherd
History: Lethargic, "poor doer," weight loss

Hematology		Reference interval
PCV (%)	**34**	37–55
MCV (fL)	**52**	60–72
NCC ($\times 10^3/\mu L$)	**44.6**	6–17
Segs ($\times 10^3/\mu L$)	**38.0**	3–11.5
Bands ($\times 10^3/\mu L$)	**2.2**	0–0.3
Lymphs ($\times 10^3/\mu L$)	3.1	1.0–4.8
Monos ($\times 10^3/\mu L$)	0.9	0.2–1.4
Eos ($\times 10^3/\mu L$)	0.4	0.1–1.2
Platelets ($\times 10^3/\mu L$)	Adequate	200–500

Biochemical profile		Reference interval
Gluc (mg/dL)	87	65–122
BUN (mg/dL)	**6 (*2.1*)**	7–28 (*2.5–10.0 mmol/L*)
Creat (mg/dL)	**0.5**	0.9–1.7
Ca (mg/dL)	**8.6 (*2.15*)**	9.0–11.2 (*2.25–2.80 mmol/L*)
Phos (mg/dL)	5.6	2.8–6.1
TP (g/dL)	**4.3**	5.4–7.4
Alb (g/dL)	**2.4**	2.7–4.5
Glob (g/dL)	1.9	1.9–3.4
T. bili (mg/dL)	0.4	0–0.4
Chol (mg/dL)	**75 (1.95)**	130–370 (*3.4–9.6 mmol/L*)
ALT (IU)	**250**	10–120
ALP (IU)	129	35–280
GGT (IU)	**7**	0–6
Na (mEq/L)	154	145–158
K (mEq/L)	4.1	4.1–5.5
CL (mEq/L)	126	106–127
TCO_2 (mEq/L)	22.3	14–27
An. gap (mEq/L)	10	8–26
Bile acids, fasting (μmol/L)	**88.5**	<10
Serum iron (μg/dL)	**22**	60–100

Interpretive discussion

Hematology

The dog has mild anemia that is not characterized by a reticulocyte count. The anemia is microcytic suggesting iron deficiency. Microcytosis should also prompt consideration of a portosystemic shunt in a young dog. Although some dogs with portosystemic shunt will have low serum iron concentrations, marked hypoferremia suggests iron deficiency is the cause of the microcytosis. There is a marked leukocytosis characterized by neutrophilia with a left shift; this is interpreted as an inflammatory leukogram.

Biochemical profile

The decreased BUN suggests reduced biosynthesis of urea by the liver. The same may be interpreted for cholesterol and albumin. There is a slight increase in ALT suggesting a mild degree of hepatocellular injury. The markedly increased bile acid concentration confirms a defect in hepatic function. The bilirubin and ALP do not indicate cholestasis. The slight increase in GGT is of questionable significance.

Hypocalcemia may be due to hypoalbuminemia, in which case it is clinically insignificant. An ionized calcium could be measured to confirm this.

Decreased creatinine reflects decreased muscle mass.

Summary

The findings of reduced hepatic biosynthesis with retention of bile acids in a young dog are highly suggestive of portosystemic shunt.

Case 62

Signalment: 10-year-old Yorkshire terrier
History: Disoriented and vomiting. The referring veterinarian (rDVM) performed a biochemical profile and urine analysis and referred the patient to a specialty hospital, where additional laboratory data were obtained.
Physical examination: Extremely small, even for breed, and very thin.

Initial laboratory data (provided by rDVM)		Reference interval
Glucose (mg/dL)	**45**	(75–130)
ALT (IU/L)	**313**	(<100)
ALP (IU/L)	**312**	(<100)
Urine specific gravity	1.023	
Urine glucose (mg/dL)	**Trace = 50**	(0)

Hematology		Reference range
Packed cell volume (%)	54	36–54
RBC ($\times 10^6/\mu L$)	8.27	5.5–8.5
Hgb (g/dL)	17.5	12–18
MCV (fL)	63	60–72
MCHC (g/dL)	33	32–36
NCC ($10^3/\mu L$)	**23.6**	6.0–17.0
Segmented neutrophils ($10^3/\mu L$)	**21.0**	3.0–11.5
Band neutrophils ($10^3/\mu L$)	0.2	0–0.3
Monocytes ($10^3/\mu L$)	1.0	0.2–1.4
Lymphocytes ($10^3/\mu L$)	1.4	1.0–4.8
Platelets ($10^3/\mu L$)	319	200–500

Biochemical profile		Reference range
Glucose (mg/dL)	**40**	60–110
Blood urea nitrogen (mg/dl)	9	7–25
Creatinine (mg/dL)	**0.2**	0.3–1.4
Calcium (mg/dL)	**7.2**	8.6–11.3
Phosphorus (mg/dL)	4.6	2.9–6.6
Total protein (g/dL)	**4.0**	5.2–7.3
Albumin (g/dL)	**2.0**	3.0–3.9
Globulin (g/dL)	2.0	1.7–3.8
Total bilirubin (mg/dL)	0.3	0.1–0.6
Cholesterol (mg/dL)	143	100–250
ALT (IU/L)	**110**	12–54
AST (IU/L)	**199**	20–120
ALP (IU/L)	**369**	16–140
GGT (IU/L)	**65**	0–6
CK (IU/L)	**647**	43–234
Sodium (mEq/L)	145	138–160
Potassium (mEq/L)	4.3	3.7–5.8

Additional laboratory tests		
Bile acids preprandial (μmol/L)	**33.2**	0–30
Bile acids postprandial (μmol/L)	**391**	0–50
Ammonia (μmol/L)	**159**	10–30
Fasting insulin (IU/mL)	**4.5**	8.1–31.9
Fasting glucose (mg/dL)	**35**	81–118

Urine analysis	
Color	gold
Transparency	flocculant
Urine sp. gr.	1.029
pH	6.5
Protein	**2+ (100 mg/dL)**
Glucose	**1+ (100 mg/dL)**
Ketones	**2+ (40 mg/dL)**
Bili	**2+**
Blood	**1+**
Sediment	
RBCs (hpf)	0–5 (RI: 0–2)
WBCs (hpf)	rare (RI:0–2)
Epithelial cells (hpf)	0–5
Fat droplets	Many
Bilirubin crystals	Rare

Imaging

Initial radiographs and ultrasound findings were normal, without evidence of a portosystemic shunt. The presence of an extrahepatic portosystemic shunt was determined by computed tomography angiography. Areas of hypoperfusion with possible necrosis were seen in the liver. A splenophrenic portosystemic shunt was identified as evidenced by an anomalous vessel that has a leftward and dorsal course after the splenic vein joins the portal vein; it then has a tortuous course before joining the vena cava along the diaphragm. Bilateral renal mineralization and cortical cysts were also observed.

Interpretive discussion

Hematology

The only abnormality in the CBC was leukocytosis due to neutrophilia. The mature neutrophilia may be due to inflammation or possibly stress, since the lymphocyte concentration is toward the lower end of the reference interval.

Most dogs with portosystemic shunts are microcytic; the MCV in this patient is within the reference interval.

Chemistry

Persistent hypoglycemia is present. Hypoglycemia in an older dog is usually a result of an insulinoma, which in this case was excluded as a diagnosis by measuring serum insulin. If an insulinoma were present, insulin concentration would be increased, rather than decreased. The decrease is appropriate in light of the hypoglycemia. The probable cause of hypoglycemia in this patient is severe, possibly end-stage liver disease, as evidenced by the pre- and postprandial increase in bile acids, and the high blood ammonia concentration as a result of a shunt. However, hypoglycemia may also be a result of the loss of glucose in the urine (see below).

The BUN is at the low end of the reference interval, which may be significant, considering the other evidence of severe liver dysfunction. The creatinine is below the reference interval and in this case is likely due to muscle wasting or small muscle mass.

Hypocalcemia is present, and can be primarily explained by the hypoalbuminemia, since approximately half of calcium is bound to albumin. However, other causes of hypocalcemia should be considered, such as hypovitaminosis D or hypoparathyroidism. Ionized calcium, vitamin D concentrations and PTH were not measured. Another possibility, considering the glucosuria in the face of hypoglycemia, is the possibility that the dog has a proximal tubular defect that is resulting in the loss of calcium through the urine. Phosphorus is within the reference interval, and would be expected to be decreased with hypovitaminosis D and likely increased with hypoparathyroidism. Additionally, if a proximal tubular defect is responsible for a loss of calcium in the urine, one would also expect a loss of phosphorus and electrolytes.

Total protein is decreased due to hypoalbuminemia, which in this case is likely due to a lack of production of albumin by the liver. Proteinuria is present, which may be another possible cause of hypoalbuminemia in this patient. A protein:creatinine ratio was not performed.

Serum ALT activity is increased, indicating hepatocellular damage. AST activity is also increased, which may be coming from the liver or from muscle. ALP and GGT activities are moderately increased, indicating cholestasis or induction by glucocorticoids or other drugs. However, bilirubin is not increased, suggesting that cholestasis is not present. CK activity is moderately increased, indicating muscle damage, which could be a result of trauma or intramuscular injections in this small dog.

The marked bile acid increase is indicative of liver disease, and when postprandial bile acids are increased to this magnitude, a portosystemic shunt should be strongly suspected. Imaging confirmed that the dog had a shunt (see below).

Blood ammonia increase is indicative of severe liver dysfunction, since ammonia is cleared from the portal circulation by the liver and converted to urea (see low normal BUN concentration discussion above). The increased ammonia concentration is likely causing the disorientation that the dog is experiencing, since ammonia is toxic to the central nervous system.

Urinalysis

Proteinuria is present, and should trigger a protein:creatinine ratio, which was not performed.

Glucosuria in the face of hypoglycemia is the most significant of the abnormal findings, and indicates a proximal tubular defect in the kidney. Ketonuria is also present and is likely due to hypoglycemia, and resultant mobilization of fat for energy. It also may be due to a lack of tubular resorption of acetoacetic acid. To confirm a Fanconi-like syndrome, fractional excretion of sodium, potassium, calcium and phosphorus can be performed, as well as measurement of amino acids in the urine, which are also not resorbed. The cause of the glucosuria and hypoglycemia was not pursued in this patient, and additional tests were not performed to confirm Fanconi syndrome. One confounding aspect of the case is that the dog received IV glucose to treat the hypoglycemia at some time prior to urinalysis, and it is possible that the renal threshold of glucose was exceeded as a result of glucose therapy. It could not be confirmed whether or not the dog had received IV glucose prior to the urinalysis performed by the rDVM.

It is unusual that the dog did not have ammonium biurate crystals in the urine, considering the high concentration of ammonia in the blood.

Summary and outcome

The patient was diagnosed with an extrahepatic splenophrenic portosystemic shunt. Congenital portosystemic shunts are usually diagnosed in young dogs, but clinical signs may not occur until the dog is old if the shunt is small. The patient was treated medically; therapy included metronidazole, lactulose, a nonabsorbable sugar that traps ammonia, prednisolone, omeprazole, and mirtazapine, an appetite stimulant. The dog was euthanized by the rDVM a short time following diagnosis, and an autopsy was not performed.

Extrahepatic portosystemic shunts are anomalous vessels that join the portal and systemic venous circulation, thus bypassing the liver, at least to some extent. They result in hepatic encephalopathy due to increased blood ammonia concentrations, stunted growth, urate cystic calculi, and sometimes GI signs. They are more common in small-breed dogs, such as the Yorkshire terrier. Laboratory findings are dependent on the stage of liver disease and the degree of shunting of blood away from the liver. Microcytosis is a very common finding, and should trigger suspicion of a shunt if chronic blood loss is excluded. Decreases in blood urea nitrogen and albumin are common, due to a lack of synthesis by the liver, and glucose and cholesterol may be decreased. Serum liver enzyme activity may be increased. Urine specific gravity is often decreased due to low urea concentration, and ammonium biurate crystals are commonly seen in the urine. Serum bile acid concentrations are increased due to the anomalous circulation of the portal vein. Blood ammonia is very commonly increased as well.

Acquired or inherited diseases of the proximal renal tubule are rare in domestic animals. Primary renal glucosuria and congenital and acquired Fanconi syndrome has been described. Fanconi syndrome is characterized by a failure to reabsorb glucose, amino acids, water, bicarbonate, phosphorus, calcium, and other electrolytes. Renal glucosuria in the face of normal or low serum glucose is usually the initial finding. Metabolic acidosis eventually develops and is often the cause of death. Blood gases or total CO_2 were not measured in this dog. The diagnosis is confirmed by the presence of increased amino acids in the urine. Fanconi syndrome is relatively common in Basenjis, and is inherited as autosomal recessive. Up to 10% of Basenjis are affected, with onset of disease usually at the age of 4–7 years. Idiopathic Fanconi syndrome has been described in border terriers, Norwegian elkhounds, whippets, Yorkshire terriers, Labrador retrievers, Shetland sheepdogs, and mixed-breed dogs. Age at diagnosis ranges from 10 weeks to 11 years, with most affected dogs developing clinical signs from about 2–4 years of age. Acquired Fanconi syndrome has been associated with hypovitaminosis D, hypoparathyroidism, and with drugs, such as chemotherapeutic agents and antibiotics including gentamycin and amoxicillin. Toxins found in contaminated dried meat treats have also been reported to induce proximal tubular disease and a Fanconi-like syndrome [1, 2].

There are numerous reports in the literature of dogs with liver disease that have acquired Fanconi syndrome [3]. Several of these were dogs shown to have copper-associated chronic hepatitis. In one series of 30 Labrador retrievers with copper-associated chronic hepatitis, approximately 30% of them had acquired Fanconi syndrome, and the authors suggested that increased ALT activity and glucosuria with normal serum glucose in a Labrador retriever is suggestive of copper-associated hepatopathy. Although increased amount of copper is present in the renal epithelial cells of these dogs, and has been postulated to be the cause of the proximal tubular defect, in some of these dogs the Fanconi syndrome resolved with therapy that did not involve copper chelation, suggesting that the renal defect is related to liver disease, and not copper toxicosis [4, 5]. Concurrent Fanconi syndrome and liver cirrhosis has also been reported in human patients [6]. In summary, this patient had a portosystemic shunt resulting in liver disease, and possible Fanconi syndrome. Also see Case 60 for similar laboratory findings in a puppy with portosystemic shunt and concurrent Fanconi syndrome.

Contributors: Mary Anna Thrall and Crystal Lindaberry

CASES

Case 63

Signalment: 6-month-old intact male dog
History: Struck by a car on Day 1
Physical examination: Pale mucous membranes. Day 1 blood sample obtained 12 hours after accident.

Hematology	Day 1	Day 6	Reference interval
PCV (%)	**29**	**35**	37–55
Hgb (g/dL)	**9.6**	**11.5**	12–18
RBC (×10^6/μL)	**4.7**	**5.1**	55–8.5
MCV (fL)	62	69	60–72
MCHC (g/dL)	33	33	33–38
Retics (×10^3/μL)	**47**	**304**	<60
NCC (×10^3/μL)	**22.7**	**20.0**	6–17
Segs (×10^3/μL)	**22.0**	**12.0**	3–11.5
Bands (×10^3/μL)	0	**2.0**	0–0.3
Monos (×10^3/μL)	0	1.0	0.1–1.3
Lymphs (×10^3/μL)	**0.7**	**5.0**	1–4.8
Platelets (×10^3/μL)	340	460	200–500
TP (P) (g/dL)	**5.4**	6.5	6–8

Hemopathology: No abnormalities on Day 1. Moderate anisocytosis and polychromasia on Day 6.

Biochemical profile	Day 1	Day 6	Reference interval
Gluc (mg/dL)	**125 (*6.9*)**	**105**	65–122 (*3.5–6.7 mmol/L*)
BUN (mg/dL)	9	13	7–28
Creat (mg/dL)	1.1	1.3	0.9–1.7
Ca (mg/dL)	**8.9 (2.22)**	9.3	9.0–11.2 (*2.25–2.80 mmol/L*)
Phos (mg/dL)	5.5	5.6	2.8–6.1
TP (g/dL)	**5.0**	6.0	5.4–7.4
Alb (g/dL)	3.4	4.0	2.7–4.5
Glob (g/dL)	**1.6**	2.0	1.9–3.4
T. bili (mg/dL)	0.3	0.4	0–0.4
Chol (mg/dL)	210	180	130–370
ALT (IU/L)	**1098**	**150**	10–120
AST (IU/L)	**948**	**80**	16–40
ALP (IU/L)	**302**	**295**	35–280
Na (mEq/L)	150	147	145–158
K (mEq/L)	4.8	4.7	4.1–5.5
CL (mEq/L)	120	121	106–127
TCO_2 (mEq/L)	**12**	21	14–27
An. gap (mEq/L)	23	10	8–25

Urinalysis (catheterized) – obtained on Day 1		Urine sediment	
Color	Yellow	WBCs/hpf	1–2
Transparency	Clear	RBCs/hpf	**3–5**
Sp. gr.	1.019	Epith cells/hpf	0
Protein	Trace	Casts/lpf	0
Glucose	Negative	Crystals	0
Bilirubin	Negative	Bacteria	0
Blood	Negative		
pH	6.5		

Interpretive discussion

Hematology

This dog is anemic on both days. The anemia is more severe on Day 1 and is nonregenerative. Since the Day 1 blood sample was obtained 12 hours after the accident, it is likely that the anemia is due to acute blood loss. The concurrent hypoproteinemia (see discussion below) also supports blood loss as the cause of this anemia. Increased polychromasia and reticulocyte count are not evident in blood until 2–4 days following acute blood loss. While the anemia appears nonregenerative on the initial sample, by Day 6, the erythrocyte values have increased, and there is evidence of increased erythrocyte production (increased polychromasia and reticulocyte count). This dog is, therefore, responding appropriately to the blood loss.

Although normal on both days, the MCV increased between Day 1 and Day 6, probably due to increased erythrocyte production resulting in increased number of large, immature erythrocytes.

The dog has a mature neutrophilia and lymphopenia on Day 1. This is compatible with a corticosteroid-mediated leukogram, resulting from stress associated with pain or trauma.

Neutrophilia and a left shift on Day 6 are typical of an inflammatory leukogram. Tissue injury associated with the accident probably incited an inflammatory response. An infectious etiology cannot be excluded, however.

Biochemical profile

Mild hyperglycemia on Day 1 resulted from stress. The presence of a stress leukogram supports this explanation.

Slight hypocalcemia may be normal in this dog since young animals commonly have slightly lower serum Ca concentrations than adults. However, the serum Ca concentration returned to within the reference interval on Day 6, suggesting that this is the more normal value for this dog. It is possible that the hypocalcemia on Day 1 resulted from loss of albumin and albumin-bound Ca during hemorrhage.

Hypoproteinemia and hypoglobulinemia on Day 1 probably resulted from loss of protein during hemorrhage. Although the serum albumin concentration is in the reference interval, this might actually be low for this animal. The serum albumin concentration increased by Day 6, implying that this is the more normal concentration for this dog. All protein concentrations returned to within the reference intervals by Day 6, indicating that compensatory mechanisms had replaced the protein lost through hemorrhage.

Both serum ALT and AST activities are markedly increased on Day 1 but decrease to nearly normal by Day 6. These increases suggest liver and/or muscle injury. High concentrations of ALT are present in the liver and lower concentrations are present in muscle. The marked increase in ALT in this case, therefore, probably resulted from liver injury, but muscle injury may have also contributed. Aspartate aminotransferase (AST) is present in high concentrations in both liver and muscle, and both tissues may be sources of AST in this case. Liver and muscle trauma may explain these increased enzyme activities on Day 1. Shock with subsequent hypoxia and tissue injury can also result in leakage and increased serum activities of both enzymes. Regardless of the underlying cause of their leakage, the decreasing activities of both enzymes by Day 6 imply the damage was acute, and it is no longer active.

Increased alkaline phosphatase (ALP) activities are likely normal for this dog. Young, growing animals commonly have slightly to moderately increased serum ALP activity since, due to active bone growth, increased amounts of ALP are released from osteoblasts.

There is a slight decrease in the total CO_2 on Day 1, suggesting metabolic acidosis. Hypovolemic shock leading to tissue hypoxia may have resulted in production of acid metabolites, and decreased renal blood flow may have interfered with renal acid-base regulation. The anion gap, while still within the reference interval, is higher on Day 1 as compared to Day 6, and this may have resulted from increased blood concentrations of anions such as lactate.

CASES

Urinalysis

In light of the relatively dilute urine (specific gravity = 1.019), the urine concentration of erythrocytes may be slightly increased. Mild hematuria may have resulted from trauma.

Summary

This dog had a dislocated hip and broken femur. Surgery was performed between Days 1 and 6. The dog's recovery was uneventful. This case demonstrates a normal response to acute blood loss. It also demonstrates the importance of serial measurement of serum enzyme activities in animals with increases of these activities. Steady or increasing activities of these enzymes indicates active and continuing damage to the tissue(s) of origin. Decreasing activities usually indicate that the injury has ceased and/or is resolving.

Case 64

Signalment: 5-year-old cocker spaniel
History: Presented for anorexia and dark orange urine and feces. Dog had ITP 2 years previously and has been given phenobarbital (100 mg bid) for epilepsy for several years.

Hematology		Reference interval
PCV (%)	**13**	37–55
RBC (×10^6/μL)	**1.95**	5.5–8.5
Hgb (g/dL)	**4.6**	12–18
MCV (fL)	67	60–72
MCHC (g/dL)	35	33–38
Retics (/μL)	**0**	0–60,000
NCC (×10^3/μL)	**54.9**	6.0–17.0
Metas (×10^3/μL)	**1.1**	0
Bands (×10^3/μL)	**6.0**	0–0.3
Segs (×10^3/μL)	**43.4**	3.0–11.5
Lymphs (×10^3/μL)	1.1	1.0–4.8
Monos (×10^3/μL)	**2.2**	0.2–1.4
Eos (×10^3/μL)	0.5	0.1–1.2
NRBCs (×10^3/μL)	**0.5**	0
Platelets (×10^3/μL)	260	200–500
TP (P) (g/dL)	6.3	6.0–8.0

Hemopathology: Occasional imperfect spheres, slight agglutination.
Coombs test: **Positive.**

Bone marrow aspirate
Megakaryocytes present. Myeloid and erythroid hyperplasia, with normal maturation up to metarubricyte stage. M : E ratio decreased slightly. Rare erythrophagocytosis.

Biochemical profile		Reference interval
Gluc (mg/dL)	**56 (*3.1*)**	65–122 (*3.5–6.7 mmol/L*)
BUN (mg/dL)	**56 (*19.9*)**	7–28 (*2.5–10 mmol/L*)
Creat (mg/dL)	0.6	0.6–1.5
Ca (mg/dL)	**8.5 (*2.1*)**	9.0–1.12 (*2.25–2.80 mmol/L*)
Phos (mg/dL)	**6.4 (*2.1*)**	2.8–6.1 (*0.9–2.0 mmol/L*)
TP (g/dL)	**3.8**	5.4–7.4
Alb (g/dL)	**1.5**	2.7–4.5
Glob (g/dL)	2.3	1.9–3.4
T. bili (mg/dL)	**35.8 (*612.2*)**	0–0.4 (*0–6.84 μmol/L*)
Chol (mg/dL)	**64 (*1.6*)**	130–370 (*3.4–9.6 mmol/L*)
ALT (IU/L)	**70**	16–40
ALP (IU/L)	**566**	18–141
GGT (IU/L)	**15**	0–6
Na (mEq/L)	**160**	145–158
K (mEq/L)	**3.2**	4.1–5.5
CL (mEq/L)	**135**	106–127
TCO_2 (mEq/L)	**9.5**	14–27
An. gap (mEq/L)	16	8–26

Urinalysis	
Color	**Brown**
Transparency	**Cloudy**
Sp. gr.	1.022
Bilirubin	++++

No other abnormal findings.

Interpretive discussion

Hematology

The dog is markedly anemic. Reticulocytes are not increased, indicating that the anemia is not regenerative. The presence of the imperfect spherocytes and agglutination is suggestive of immune-mediated hemolytic anemia, possibly very acute, or with destruction of precursors. An unexplained nonregenerative anemia, when platelets and neutrophils are normal and increased, respectively, triggered a bone marrow aspirate. The bone marrow aspirate findings further substantiated immune-mediated hemolytic anemia with destruction of polychromatophilic cells.

Neutrophilia, increased immature neutrophils, and monocytosis are indicative of inflammation.

If the animal has not received a previous transfusion, a positive Coombs test is suggestive of immune-mediated hemolytic anemia.

Bone marrow

In light of marked erythroid response in marrow, anemia is either very acute, and will respond, or precursors are being destroyed. Because imperfect spherocytes are present on blood film, the latter is more likely.

Biochemical profile

The serum glucose concentration is decreased. Differentials should include insulinoma and, in this patient, end-stage liver disease, since the animal is also hypoalbuminemic and hypocholesterolemic.

The BUN is increased, and although the creatinine is within the reference interval, one would expect the animal to be concentrating greater than 1.022 if the azotemia is prerenal. One should consider if the animal is bleeding into the GI tract, increasing the BUN, or since IMHA is suspected based on the hematology, if the animal has hemolysis with subsequent hemoglobinuric nephrosis. If the animal does have end-stage liver disease, one would expect the BUN to be decreased as well, so the increase in BUN is slightly confusing. The mild increase in serum phosphorus suggests decreased glomerular filtration rate.

The serum calcium is decreased, likely due to hypoalbuminemia. An ionized calcium could be measured to confirm this.

The serum total protein concentration is decreased due to hypoalbuminemia. Since the globulin is within the reference interval, liver failure would be the best differential, since the animal is not proteinuric. Another consideration would be that blood loss is causing the anemia and hypoproteinemia, but there is no clinical evidence of blood loss.

The serum bilirubin concentration is markedly increased and may be due to hemolysis, liver failure, or cholestasis or some combination of the three. The ALT is only slightly increased, indicating mild hepatocellular damage. The ALP activity is increased, as is GGT activity, indicating cholestasis. Alternatively, enzymes may be induced by phenobarbital.

Serum total CO_2 is decreased, suggesting metabolic acidosis. This may be secondary to lactic acidosis associated with marked anemia. Increased sodium and chloride suggest hypertonic dehydration or administration of hypertonic fluid. The hypokalemia in conjunction with metabolic acidosis (which should have caused an increased potassium) suggests whole body potassium depletion.

Urinalysis

The marked bilirubinuria reflects conjugated hyperbilirubinemia. Specific gravity is discussed above.

Summary

Immune-mediated hemolytic anemia, liver failure, and renal dysfunction. The dog died, and necropsy showed severe chronic micronodular cirrhosis and cholestasis, possibly related to phenobarbital. Bone marrow showed myeloid and erythroid hyperplasia. Examination of the kidneys revealed severe hemoglobinemic nephrosis with mild chronic interstitial nephritis.

Case 65

Signalment: 8-year-old male Samoyed
History: Diarrhea
Physical examination: Recumbent, arrested prior to treatment

Hematology		Reference interval
PCV (%)	**18**	37–55
Retics ($\times10^3/\mu L$)	**197 (*7.3%*)**	<60
MCV (fL)	66	60–72
NCC ($\times10^3/\mu L$)	**78.0**	6–17
Segs ($\times10^3/\mu L$)	**44.5**	3–11.5
Bands ($\times10^3/\mu L$)	**14.8**	0–0.3
Metas ($\times10^3/\mu L$)	**3.9**	0
Myelocytes ($\times10^3/\mu L$)	**0.8**	0
Monos ($\times10^3/\mu L$)	0.8	0.1–1.3
Lymphs ($\times10^3/\mu L$)	3.1	1–4.8
NRBC ($\times10^3/\mu L$)	**9.4**	0
Platelets ($\times10^3/\mu L$)	158	200–500

Hemopathology: Increased polychromasia, target cells, giant platelets, toxic neutrophils.

Biochemical profile		Reference interval
Gluc (mg/dL)	**580 (*31.9*)**	65–122 (*3.5–6.7 mmol/L*)
BUN (mg/dL)	**98 (*35*)**	7–28 (*2.5–10.0 mmol/L*)
Creat (mg/dL)	**3.1 (*274*)**	0.9–1.7 (*80–150 μmol/L*)
Ca (mg/dL)	9.6	9.0–11.2
Phos (mg/dL)	**13.1 (*4.2*)**	2.8–6.1 (*0.9–2.0 mmol/L*)
TP (g/dL)	**4.7**	5.4–7.4
Alb (g/dL)	**2.4**	2.7–4.5
T. bili (mg/dL)	**0.6 (*10.3*)**	0–0.4 (*0–6.8 μmol/L*)
Chol (mg/dL)	246	130–370
ALT (IU/L)	**1031**	10–120
ALP (IU/L)	**2500**	35–280
Na (mEq/L)	**130**	145–158
K (mEq/L)	**6.5**	4.1–5.5
CL (mEg/L)	**87**	106–127
TCO_2 (mEq/L)	**10.6**	14–27
An. gap (mEq/L)	**39**	8–26

Urinalysis	
Sp. gr.	**1.017**
Gluc	**2+**
Protein	0
Ketones	0

No other abnormalities present.

Interpretive discussion

Hematology

There is moderate regenerative anemia. Considering the hypoproteinemia, hemorrhage is the most likely cause. The nucleated RBC are interpreted as part of the regenerative response. There is a marked leukocytosis characterized by prominent neutrophilia with toxic change and a left shift to myelocytes indicating inflammation. The mild thrombocytopenia may be caused by hemorrhage, and giant platelets indicate active thrombopoiesis.

Biochemical profile and urinalysis

There is marked hyperglycemia. This is associated with an expected glucosuria. The magnitude of hyperglycemia should prompt consideration of diabetes mellitus. The lack of urine ketones makes the diagnosis more difficult.

Moderate azotemia is indicated by increased concentrations of BUN and creatinine. The specific gravity indicates minimal concentrating ability in the face of azotemia. This suggests an element of primary renal disease. However, electrolyte depletion (see later) may be contributing to the decreased concentrating ability. The increased phosphorus is compatible with decreased glomerular filtration.

The hypoproteinemia along with regenerative anemia is compatible with blood loss.

There is a marked increase in ALT activity indicating hepatocellular injury. Diabetes is associated with fat mobilization to the liver; this may result in modest ALT activity increases. The magnitude of this ALT suggests more severe injury. There is also an element of cholestasis indicated by the marked increase in ALP and a minimal increase in bilirubin.

The hyponatremia is likely due to urinary sodium loss secondary to glucosuria (osmotic diuresis). Losses associated with diarrhea may have contributed. Additionally, cellular water may move from the intracellular compartment into the extracellular fluid compartment, diluting serum sodium (expect 1.6 mEq/L decrease in sodium for every 100 mg/dL increase in glucose). The hyperkalemia is probably due to a shift of potassium ions out of cells in exchange for hydrogen ions, which enter cells during metabolic acidosis. Another possibility is that the animal is becoming oliguric and retaining potassium.

Increased anion gap is due to the presence of "unmeasured" anions. In this dog, these likely include phosphates, as well as lactate, since the dog is markedly anemic. In addition, because this dog is diabetic, ketones may contribute to unmeasured anions. Since beta-hydroxybutyrate is not detected by routine urine dipstick methods, ketonuria may actually be present.

Summary

Further evaluation led to the findings of diabetes mellitus and hepatic lipidosis. The enlarged, fragile liver had led to a fractured liver. This latter injury likely contributed to the magnitude of the ALT increase.

Case 66

Signalment: 4-year-old DSH cat
History: Anorexia, weight loss, depression
Physical examination: Thin, icteric mucous membranes

Hematology		Reference interval
PCV (%)	29	24–45
NCC ($\times10^3/\mu L$)	13.7	5.5–19.5
NRBC ($\times10^3/\mu L$)	**0.1**	0
Segs ($\times10^3/\mu L$)	11.6	2.5–12.5
Bands ($\times10^3/\mu L$)	0.1	0–0.3
Monos ($\times10^3/\mu L$)	0.4	0–0.8
Lymphs ($\times10^3/\mu L$)	**0.7**	1.5–7
Eos ($\times10^3/\mu L$)	0.8	0–1.5
Platelets ($\times10^3/\mu L$)	304	200–500

Morphology: Many acanthocyte-like RBCs, occasional fragmented RBC.

Biochemical profile		Reference interval
Gluc (mg/dL)	67	67–124
BUN (mg/dL)	**14**	17–32
Creat (mg/dL)	1.2	0.9–2.1
Ca (mg/dL)	9.0	8.5–11
Phos (mg/dL)	5.1	3.3–7.8
TP (g/dL)	6.2	5.9–8.1
Alb (g/dL)	3.0	2.3–3.9
T. bili (mg/dL)	**6.3 (*108*)**	0–0.3 (*0–5.1 μmol/L*)
ALT (IU/L)	**332**	30–100
ALP (IU/L)	**2185**	11–210
Na (mEq/L)	149	146–160
K (mEq/L)	5.2	3.7–5.4
CL (mEq/L)	**109**	112–129
TCO_2 (mEq/L)	19	14–23

Interpretive discussion

Hematology

The leukogram shows a lymphopenia with a high normal concentration of mature neutrophils; this is interpreted as a stress or steroid leukogram. There are acanthocyte-like or spiculated cells present. These are commonly observed in cats with liver disease or hepatic lipidosis.

Biochemical profile

The mildly decreased BUN may be insignificant or may be due to decreased hepatic urea production or decreased protein intake. The combination of hyperbilirubinemia and increased ALT and ALP activities is characteristic of hepatic lipidosis in cats. The combination of the hepatocellular injury (indicated by increased ALT) and cholestasis (indicated by increased ALP) lead to failure of bilirubin clearance and hyperbilirubinemia. This degree of increase in ALP activity is unusual in cats, other than in association with hepatic lipidosis. Lipidosis is thought to occur as a result of massive fat mobilization from adipocytes in association with anorexia of several days' duration or acute diabetes mellitus.

Summary

The biochemical findings are characteristic of hepatic lipidosis, which was confirmed by liver aspiration cytology.

Case 67

Signalment: 5-year-old female alpaca in the late stage of gestation
History: Lethargy, anorexia
Physical examination: Thin, depressed

Hematology		Reference interval
PCV (%)	28	24–35
Hgb (g/dL)	12.7	11–19
RBC (×10⁶/μL)	12.1	8.8–15.4
MCV (fL)	23	21–30
MCHC (g/dL)	45.9	39.2–46.1
NCC (×10³/μL)	8.4	5.2–15.7
Segs (×10³/μL)	6.0	2.1–9.5
Monos (×10³/μL)	0.6	0–0.6
Lymphs (×10³/μL)	1.3	0.9–4.4
Eos (×10³/μL)	0.4	0–3.3
Platelets (×10³/μL)	2141	206–3600
TP (P) (g/dL)	**9.0**	5.4–7.2

Hemopathology: Few reactive lymphocytes, mild anisocytosis. Grossly lipemic plasma.

Biochemical profile		Reference interval
Gluc (mg/dL)	129	100–132
BUN (mg/dL)	14	12–33
Creat (mg/dL)	1.7	1.3–2.7
Ca (mg/dL)	8.9	8.0–10.4
Phos (mg/dL)	3.9	2.5–8.6
TP (g/dL)	6.3	5.3–7.6
Alb (g/dL)	3.6	2.6–4.7
Glob (g/dL)	2.7	2.7–2.9
T. bili (mg/dL)	0.1	0–0.2
Chol (mg/dL)	**364**	12–58
Trig (mg/dL)	**4330**	5–30
β-hydroxybutyrate (mmol/L)	**26.0**	0.2–1.1
AST (IU/L)	**474**	110–250
SDH (IU/L)	**17.6**	3–10
GGT (IU/L)	**76**	10–42
ALP (IU/L)	105	20–150
CK (IU/L)	45	40–500
Na (mEq/L)	146	142–156
K (mEq/L)	3.8	3.6–6.5
CL (mEq/L)	112	108–122
TCO_2 (mEq/L)	**13**	19–29
An. gap (mEq/L)	25	12–25
Grossly lipemic serum		

Urinalysis (catheter)			
Color	Light yellow	**Urine sediment**	
Transparency	Clear	WBCs/hpf	Rare
Specific gravity	1.006	RBCs/hpf	None seen
Protein	Negative	Epithelial cells/hpf	0–1
Glucose	Negative	Casts/lpf	0
Bilirubin	Negative	Crystals	0
Blood	Negative	Bacteria	0
pH	9.0		
Ketones	**1+**		

Interpretive discussion

Hematology

The plasma protein determined by refractometer is significantly higher than the total protein determined on the biochemistry panel. This is due to the marked lipemia of the sample. Lipemia occurs when triglyceride concentrations are increased. The refractometer estimates plasma proteins by the bending of light in relation to the concentration of solutes in the sample. Hyperlipidemia will cause an artifactual increase in the plasma protein measurement. Although hypercholesterolemia does not cause visible lipemia, if markedly increased it can artifactually increase the refractometric plasma protein measurement.

Biochemical profile

There is a marked increase in triglycerides and cholesterol, compatible with hyperlipidemia that may develop in sick camelids. In this case, negative energy balance accompanying late term pregnancy likely precipitated this condition. The glucose in this case is still normal.

Increased activity of AST in combination with a normal creatine kinase is compatible with hepatocellular injury rather than muscle origin of the AST. Increased activity of SDH also suggests hepatocellular damage while GGT is an indicator of cholestasis. Increased AST, SDH, GGT, triglycerides and cholesterol are common findings in camelids with hepatic lipidosis. Neither ALP nor bilirubin are increased and have been shown to be less reliable indicators of hepatic lipidosis in camelids.

The alpaca is ketotic as evidenced by the increase in serum β-hydroxybutyrate and the presence of ketones in the urine. The low TCO_2 indicates a decrease in bicarbonate and a metabolic acidosis. A blood gas profile is needed to completely assess acid/base status.

Urinalysis

The hyposthenuria is of unknown significance at this time. Camelids with hepatic lipidosis are at risk for developing renal failure secondary to accumulation of lipid in the renal parenchyma. Although her BUN and creatinine are normal, her renal function should be carefully monitored. The alkaline urine pH is normal for herbivores. However, this is somewhat surprising in the face of metabolic acidosis and ketonuria.

Summary

Increased activities of AST, SDH, and GGT along with hypertriglyceridemia and hypercholesterolemia are common findings in camelids with hepatic lipidosis. Ketosis and metabolic acidosis also can develop in these patients. Although not measured in this case, nonesterified fatty acids (NEFA) are expected to be increased as a result of mobilization of fat. Hepatic lipidosis can be precipitated by severe negative energy balance associated with late term pregnancy, stress, or anorexia. Fat is mobilized to supply fatty acids for energy production. However, the supply of fatty acids exceeds the ability to utilize them in the tricarboxylic acid (TCA) cycle. Fatty acids in the liver are incorporated into triglycerides and released as very-low-density lipoproteins (VLDLs), resulting in the hypertriglyceridemia. However, hepatic production of triglycerides exceeds the ability to export them as VLDL so triglycerides accumulate in the cells. Fatty acids also will be shunted into ketogenesis, resulting in the observed increase in β-hydroxybutyrate and ketonuria.

Contributor: Dr. M. Judith Radin

Case 68

Signalment: 7-year-old female border collie
History: Depression, anorexia
Physical examination: Ascites, dermatitis of face and genital area

Hematology		Reference interval
PCV (%)	**15**	37–55
MCV (fL)	**57**	60–72
Retics (×10³/µL)	**118**	<60
NCC (×10³/µL)	9.5	6–17
Segs (×10³/µL)	4.3	3–11.5
Bands (×10³/µL)	**2.2**	0–0.3
Metas (×10³/µL)	**0.6**	0
Monos (×10³/µL)	0.8	0.1–1.3
Lymphs (×10³/µL)	**0.7**	1–4.8
NRBC (×10³/µL)	**0.9**	0
Platelets (×10³/µL)	**20**	200–500

Hemopathology: Target cells, acanthocytes, schistocytes, toxic neutrophils, giant platelets.

Biochemical profile		Reference interval
Gluc (mg/dL)	**45**	65–122
BUN (mg/dL)	16	7–28
Creat (mg/dL)	1.0	0.9–1.7
Ca (mg/dL)	9.2	9.0–11.2
Phos (mg/dL)	3.8	2.8–6.1
TP (g/dL)	**4.5**	5.4–7.4
Alb (g/dL)	**1.7**	2.7–4.5
Glob (g/dL)	2.8	1.9–3.4
T. bili (mg/dL)	**3.3**	0–0.4
Chol (mg/dL)	**86**	130–370
ALP (IU/L)	**1391**	35–280
ALT (IU/L)	**239**	10–120
Na (mEq/L)	147	145–158
K (mEq/L)	**2.6**	4.1–5.5
CL (mEq/L)	122	106–127
TCO_2 (mEq/L)	**8.5**	14–27

Fluid analysis (abdominal)	
Color	Straw
Transparency	Clear
NCC (/µL)	1300
TP (g/dL)	1.5

Coagulation data		
PT (s)	**20**	6.5–9.0
aPTT (s)	**36**	12–16

Interpretive discussion

Hematology

PCV is decreased, indicating anemia. Reticulocytes are increased, indicating that the anemia is somewhat regenerative. MCV is decreased, particularly in light of increased reticulocytes, suggesting iron deficiency anemia secondary to chronic blood loss.

Inflammatory leukogram is present, as evidenced by the marked left shift and toxic change in neutrophils. In light of low normal number of segmented neutrophils, sepsis or endotoxemia may be present. Lymphopenia suggests a concurrent stress response.

The combination of thrombocytopenia, schistocytes, and prolonged PT and aPTT suggests disseminated intravascular coagulopathy (DIC). Alternatively, this degree of thrombocytopenia may be seen with immune-mediated destruction or ehrlichiosis.

Biochemical profile

Hypoglycemia may be due to sepsis (leukogram is suggestive of sepsis or endotoxemia), end-stage liver disease, insulinoma, or other type of neoplasia, such as a large hepatoma.

Hypoalbuminemia, in conjunction with low cholesterol, is indicative of GI disease (malabsorption, maldigestion, protein losing enteropathy) or end-stage liver disease. Another possible cause of low total protein is blood loss, since MCV indicates iron deficiency anemia. However, albumin is relatively lower than globulin.

Total bilirubin is increased. While the animal is anemic, and blood destruction is a possible cause, the MCV suggests blood loss. Therefore, the bilirubin is probably increased due to cholestasis or hepatocellular dysfunction. Increased alkaline phosphatase activity suggests cholestasis.

Cholesterol is decreased, likely due to end-stage liver disease (see hypoalbuminemia discussion).

Hypokalemia may be due to decreased intake. In face of acidosis, it indicates total body depletion of potassium.

Decreased total CO_2 indicates metabolic acidosis. The decrease is likely due to lactic acidosis in this patient, since the dog is not uremic and there is no evidence of diabetic ketoacidosis.

Abdominal fluid analysis

Transudate, likely due to liver disease and hypoalbuminemia.

Coagulation data

While prolonged PT and aPTT may be due to lack of synthesis of coagulation factors by the liver, another explanation is DIC, in light of the decreased platelets.

Summary

End-stage liver disease; cholestasis
DIC
Inflammation, possibly sepsis
Iron deficiency anemia

Dermatitis was determined to be necrolytic migratory erythema (superficial necrolytic dermatitis), which is associated with hyperglucagonemia, often seen with severe hepatic disease (hepatocutaneous syndrome).

Case 69

Signalment: 26-month-old female mixed-breed dog

History: Routine prespay CBC at 8 months of age revealed thrombocytopenia of 85,000/µL. Patient was 4Dx antibody and PCR negative for *Anaplasma platys, Ehrlichia canis,* and PCR negative for *Babesia canis* and *Babesia gibsoni.* Thrombocytopenia was persistent, ranging from 23-000 to 95,000/µL over the next several months. A tentative diagnosis of immune-mediated thrombocytopenia was made, and glucocorticoids were instituted (ranged from 0.5 to 1.0 mg/kg for approximately 18 months). Patient deteriorated rapidly 18 months following initial presentation. History at this time included lethargy and anorexia.

Physical examination: Marked muscle wasting, pendulous abdomen, palpable caudal liver

Hematology		Reference range
Packed cell volume (%)	**35**	36–54
RBC (×10⁶/µL)	**5.01**	5.5–8.5
Hgb (g/dL)	**11.4**	12–18
MCV (fL)	67	60–72
MCHC (g/dL)	34	34–38
NCC (10³/µL)	**24.8**	6.0–17.0
Segmented neutrophils (10³/µL)	**21.2**	3.0–11.5
Monocytes (10³/µL)	1.4	0.2–1.4
Lymphocytes (10³/µL)	2.0	1.0–4.8
Eosinophils (10³/µL)	0.2	0.1–1.2
Nucleated RBCs	0.2	0
Platelets (10³/µL)	31[a]	200–500
Plasma protein (g/dL)	6.6	6.0–8.0

[a]Platelet clumping seen on blood film.

Biochemical profile		Reference interval
Glucose (mg/dL)	91	75–130
Blood urea nitrogen (mg/dL)	**6**	7–25
Creatinine (mg/dL)	**0.4**	0.7–1.9
Calcium (mg/dL)	9.2	9.0–11.2
Phosphorus (mg/dL)	**2.4**	2.9–6.6
Total protein (g/dL)	5.4	5.4–8.2
Albumin (g/dL)	**1.7**	2.5–4.4
Globulin (g/dL)	3.7	2.3–5.2
Total bilirubin (mg/dL)	0.5	0.1–0.6
Cholesterol (mg/dL)	**306**	125–270
ALT (IU/L)	**1091**	10–118
ALP (IU/L)	**1152**	20–150
Sodium (mEq/L)	143	138–160
Potassium (mEq/L)	4.3	3.7–5.8
Bile acids (µmol/L)	**90**	0–25

Coagulation profile: aPTT and PT were within reference intervals.

Interpretive discussion

CBC

Slightly decreased PCV, RBC and hemoglobin indicate a mild anemia. Leukocytosis and neutrophilia, in the absence of lymphopenia, may be indicative of inflammation. Because of the long history of glucocorticoid therapy, it is surprising that the patient does not have a lymphopenia.

Chemistry

BUN is slightly decreased. When considered with the hypoalbuminemia and increased bile acids, this is likely associated with decreased liver function. The creatinine is decreased, which is compatible with muscle wasting in this patient. A mild hypophosphatemia is present, and may be due to increased glomerular filtration as a result of glucocorticoid administration.

Hypoalbuminemia is significant, and in this case is most likely due to liver dysfunction, considering increased bile acid concentration. Other considerations would be lack of intake of protein and loss through the kidney. A normal globulin makes protein losing enteropathy unlikely. A urine analysis was not performed.

Cholesterol is increased, which is likely due to glucocorticoid administration in this patient. While cholestasis may contribute to increased cholesterol, the bilirubin concentration is within the reference interval.

Increased ALT activity is indicative of hepatocellular damage.

The marked increase in ALP activity is not likely due to cholestasis, since the bilirubin is normal. The most likely cause is glucocorticoid induction in this patient.

Increased bile acids are indicative of liver disease. Considering the history of glucocorticoid administration, the increased ALT and ALP, the decreased albumin and BUN, it is very likely that this patient has a steroid hepatopathy with liver dysfunction, secondary to iatrogenic Cushing syndrome. The normal coagulation profile suggests that liver failure has not yet occurred.

An ACTH stimulation test to confirm iatrogenic Cushing syndrome was not performed. Adrenal glands of patients with iatrogenic Cushing syndrome do not respond (increase serum cortisol) to ACTH because their adrenal glands are atrophied.

Summary and outcome

One week later the patient had a syncopal episode and was cyanotic. She was rushed to the hospital, had recovered by time of admission, and was hospitalized for observation. The following morning, she ate, went for a walk, returned to her cage, and went into cardiac arrest. An autopsy revealed a pulmonary thromboembolism (Figures 1 and 2), pulmonary mineralization (Figure 3), steroid hepatopathy (Figure 4), and atrophied adrenal glands.

Thromboembolism has been reported in dogs and people with hyperadrenocorticism and iatrogenic Cushing disease due to a hypercoagulable state attributed to increased procoagulant factors and decreased fibrinolytic capacity. In healthy dogs treated with prednisone, a significant decrease in antithrombin was observed after 15 days of treatment.

Pulmonary mineralization has also been reported in dogs with hyperadrenocorticism and iatrogenic Cushing disease. Both pulmonary mineralization and pulmonary thromboemboli can result in hypoxemia, and pulmonary thromboemboli can result in death, as seen in this patient.

Prolonged glucocorticoid therapy can have significant side effects, including steroid hepatopathy, thromboembolism, and pulmonary mineralization, and should be avoided if possible. Some canine and human patients have chronic immune thrombocytopenia that is refractory to glucocorticoid therapy, and other treatment modalities should be tried, or conversely, if the platelet count does not drop below 30,000/μL one could opt to not treat, considering the serious side effects of glucocorticoids. While the cause of the chronic thrombocytopenia was not definitively diagnosed in this patient, immune thrombocytopenia is most likely.

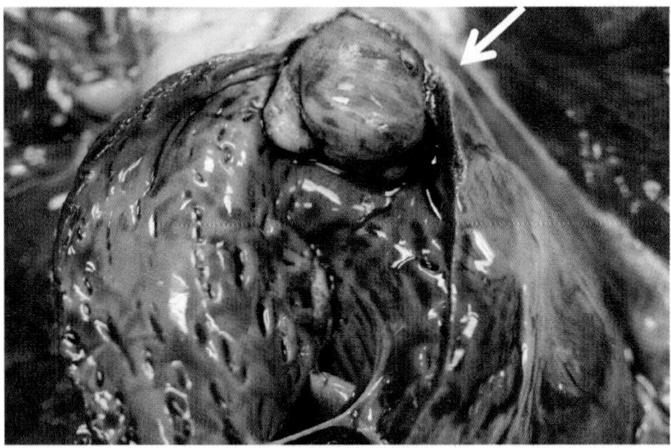

Figure 1 A large thrombus (arrow) obliterating the lumen of the pulmonary trunk. The inside of the right ventricle has been opened. Source: Photo courtesy Drs. Oscar Illanes and Elize Dorrestein.

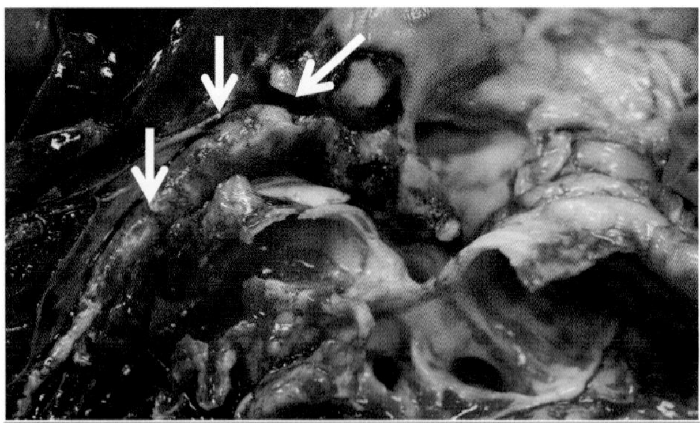

Figure 2 The thrombus extended into the lumen of the right and left pulmonary arteries (arrows). Source: Photo courtesy Drs. Oscar Illanes and Elize Dorrestein.

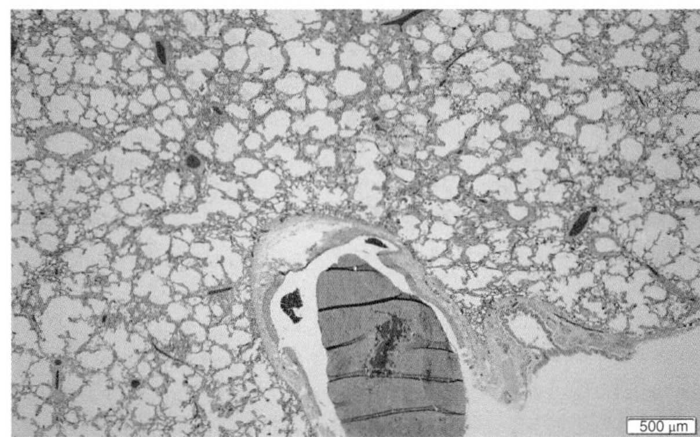

Figure 3 Histopathology of lung and clot. Mineralization is evident throughout. Source: Photo courtesy Drs. Oscar Illanes and Elize Dorrestein.

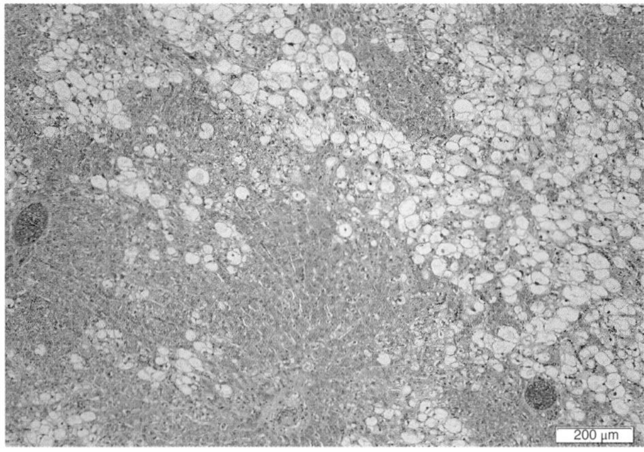

Figure 4 Histopathology of liver showing vacuolated hepatocytes containing glycogen as a result of steroid-induced hepatopathy. Source: Photo courtesy Drs. Oscar Illanes and Elize Dorrestein.

Contributor: Dr. Mary Anna Thrall

Case 70

Signalment: 5-year-old castrated male dog

History: Presented to the emergency department for investigation of hemorrhagic diarrhea.

The following laboratory results were attained **after** fluid therapy had been initiated.

Hematology		Reference interval
PCV (%)	**17**	37–55
RBC ($10^6/\mu L$)	**2.21**	5.40–8.40
Hemoglobin (g/dL)	**5.6**	12.0–18.0
HCT (%)	**16.6**	35.0–54.0
MCV (fL)	74.9	62.0–77.0
MCH (pg)	25.2	21.0–26.0
MCHC (g/dL)	33.7	32.0–37.0
RDW (%)	**13.8**	12.0–14.0
WBC ($\times 10^3/\mu L$)	**2.7**	8.0–14.5
Segmented neutrophils ($\times 10^3/\mu L$)	**2.3**	3.0–11.5
Lymphocytes ($\times 10^3/\mu L$)	**0.3**	1.0–4.8
Monocytes ($\times 10^3/\mu L$)	**0.00**	0.1–1.4
nRBC/100 WBC	15	
Absolute nRBC ($\times 10^3/\mu L$)	**0.4**	
Reticulocytes (%)	1.9	
Absolute reticulocytes ($\times 10^3/\mu L$)	**41.3**	
Platelets ($\times 10^3/\mu L$)	**46**	220–600
MPV (fL)	**17.8**	8.0–12.5
Total protein (refractometry g/dL)	**5.3**	6.0–7.8

Biochemical profile		Reference interval
Glucose (mg/dL)	**69**	80–115
Blood urea nitrogen (mg/dL)	**46**	8–22
Creatinine (mg/dL)	**3.62**	0.50–1.70
Calcium (mg/dL)	**7.5**	9.4–11.4
Phosphorus (mg/dL)	**12.4**	3.4–6.3
Magnesium (mg/dL)	**3.2**	1.7–2.2
Total protein (g/dL)	**4.2**	5.8–7.5
Albumin (g/dL)	**2.3**	2.6–4.2
Globulin (g/dL)	**1.9**	2.5–4.0
Total bilirubin (mg/dL)	**0.6**	0.0–0.4
Cholesterol (mg/dL)	**116**	150–240
ALT (IU/L)	**16 020**	0–60
AST (IU/L)	**10 110**	0–50
ALP (IU/L)	**435**	0–100
GGT (IU/L)	7	0–8
CK (IU/L)	**27 862**	0–200
Sodium (mEq/L)	147	140–153
Potassium (mEq/L)	5.3	3.8–5.5
Chloride (mEq/L)	**99**	107–115
Bicarbonate (mEq/L)	19.1	17.0–27.0
Anion gap (mEq/L)	**34.2**	7.4–19.8

Coagulation panel		Reference interval
PT (s)	**13.8**	5.0–8.5
PTT (s)	**18.1**	9.0–14.0

Interpretive discussion

Hematology

A severe, normocytic, normochromic, nonregenerative (<60-000 reticulocytes) anemia is present. Considering the hypoproteinemia, a preregenerative phase following acute blood loss cannot be excluded and should be considered given the history of hemorrhagic diarrhea. A truly non-regenerative anemia could also reflect decreased marrow production and is supported by the pancytopenia in this case. On initial inspection, there appears to be a significant increase in nucleated erythrocytes as indicated by the 15nRBC/100 WBC, but this does not take into consideration the leukopenia. If the anemia is preregenerative, the presence of nRBCs could be considered appropriate, however, if this is a true nonregenerative anemia, the response would be inappropriate and differentials such as endotoxemia, heatstroke, marrow disease, and altered splenic function should be considered.

The mild neutropenia could reflect overwhelming tissue utilization (inflammation) but we would typically expect to see a left shift or toxic neutrophils. One should also consider decreased marrow production, and given the hemorrhagic diarrhea, parvovirus remains a possibility, albeit less likely given the age of the animal. Another cause of neutropenia in this animal could be increased margination of neutrophils from the circulating pool as seen with acute endotoxemia. The leukopenia is also characterized by a lymphopenia that is due to stress (corticosteroid induced).

Causes in this animal for the thrombocytopenia include decreased production (marrow disease), increased consumption (hemorrhage/DIC), and sequestration (occurs with endotoxemia). Thrombocytopenia is too severe for hemorrhage alone. The moderately increased MPV could reflect bone marrow stimulation and release of macroplatelets.

Coagulation

Increased PT and PTT clotting times suggest abnormalities in both the extrinsic and intrinsic pathways or common pathway. Differentials to consider include DIC or a factor deficiency secondary to hepatic dysfunction (see below).

Chemistry

Hypoglycemia may be due to liver dysfunction, but sepsis should also be considered, particularly given the animal's clinical signs and neutropenia.

An azotemia is present and characterized by an increase in both BUN and creatinine. Concurrent hyperphosphatemia and hypermagnesemia support decreased GFR and renal insufficiency. A USG would be required to confirm a renal vs. prerenal (dehydration) component, however, it is important to note that a dilute USG following fluid therapy (as is the case here) does not confirm renal insufficiency.

Panhypoproteinemia could reflect a protein losing enteropathy, hemorrhage or severe hepatopathy with decrease protein synthesis, all of which are highly possible and may be contributing to this case.

The hypocalcemia is likely a consequence of hypoalbuminemia given that 40–50% of serum calcium is protein bound but hypocalcemia can also be seen with sepsis or renal disease.

Marked increased in ALT activity is indicative of hepatocellular injury. This is supported by the concurrent increase in AST, which may, however, also be due to muscle injury as evidenced by the increased CK. A moderate increase in ALP with GGT being within normal limits is suggestive of steroid isoenzyme induction rather than cholestasis although hyperbilirubinemia may support the latter. Furthermore, hypoglycemia, hyperbilirubinemia, hypoalbuminemia and hypocholesterolemia could reflect hepatic insufficiency.

A selective chloride loss is indicative of "secretional" metabolic alkalosis and vomiting is generally the most likely cause of this abnormality. The anion gap is increased reflecting an increase in unmeasured anions such as uremic acids and lactate. Given the complex acid-base disturbances, the bicarbonate/TCO_2 is as predicted.

Summary and outcome

Laboratory findings suggest a severe hepatopathy, enteropathy, consumptive coagulopathy, and anemia that could be preregenerative, azotemia of undetermined source and mixed metabolic acid-base disturbances (hypochloremic metabolic alkalosis and high-AG metabolic acidosis).

The dog was euthanized based on poor clinical condition and prognosis. Necropsy and histopathology indicated severe hepatocellular necrosis, acute necrohemorrhagic enterocolitis, gastric hemorrhage/mucosal necrosis, and dirofilariasis (single adult worm). Enteric cultures for clostridium and salmonella were negative. The clinical and laboratory findings and lesions are very typical of sago palm (Cycad palm) toxicity. All parts of plant are considered toxic; cycasin is the hepato/entero-toxin [1]. Liver failure can be seen 2–3 days postingestion. Although not definitively confirmed, the plant was found in the neighbor's unfenced yard.

Contributors: Drs. Alex Mau and Saundra Sample

Case 71

Signalment: 4-year-old dairy cow, 180 days in milk

History: Presented after being recumbent for 24 hours. One-month history of ulceration of the udder skin.

Physical examination: Unpigmented areas of the skin have extensive erythema and edema with exudative, ulcerative, and crusty lesions (Figure 1). Rectal temperature is 39.8 °C. Mucous membranes are jaundiced.

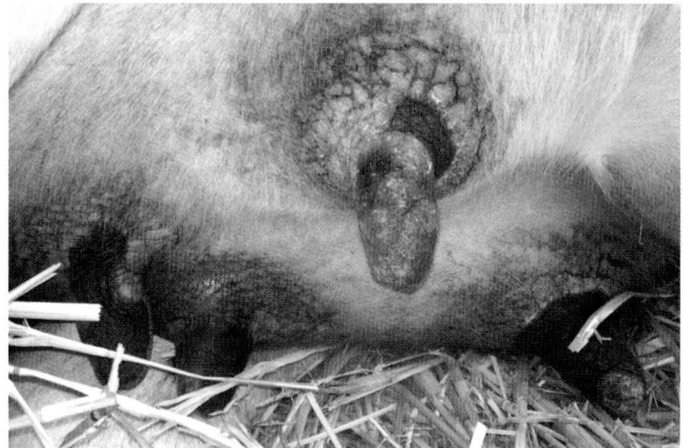

Figure 1 Photograph of the udder. Note the erythema, edema, and crusty lesions.

Hematology		Reference interval
PCV (%)	38	24–46
RBC (10^{12}/L)	8.1	5.0–10.0
Hemoglobin (g/L)	133	80–150
MCV (fL)	46	40.0–60.0
MCH (pg)	16	11–17
MCHC (g/L)	354	300–360
WBC ($\times 10^9$/L)	**13.5**	4.0–12.0
Segmented neutrophils ($\times 10^{12}$/L)	**5.5**	0.6–4.0
Band neutrophils ($\times 10^{12}$/L)	**3.8**	0.0–0.2
Lymphocytes ($\times 10^{12}$/L)	3.6	2.5–7.5
Monocytes ($\times 10^{12}$/L)	0.5	0.0–0.9
Platelets ($\times 10^9$/L)	322	100–600
Fibrinogen (d/L)	**12.0**	3.0–7.0

Biochemical profile		Reference interval
AST (IU/L)	**451**	60–150
GLDH (IU/L)	**684**	0–20
GGT (IU/L)	**1041**	0–36
CK (IU/L)	**3648**	50–400
Bilirubin (μmol/L)	**83**	2–18
Total protein (g/L)	**83**	58–80
Albumin (g/L)	31	22–36
Globulin (g/L)	**52**	24–40
Creatinine (μmol/L)	**67**	90–120
Calcium (mmol/L)	2.27	2.0–3.0
Phosphorus (mmol/L)	1.57	1.29–2.26
Magnesium (mmol/L)	1.06	0.70–1.20
BOHB (mmol/L)	0.3	0.0–0.9

Interpretive discussion

Hematology

Mild leukocytosis characterized by a mild neutrophilia and marked left-shift is indicative of active inflammation and supported by the hyperfibrinogenemia.

Chemistry

The mild to moderate increase in AST activity could reflect hepatocellular injury or muscle damage. Given the concurrent increase in CK, these changes are most likely due to muscle injury secondary to recumbency.

The marked increased GLDH enzyme activity indicates hepatocellular injury.

Markedly increased GGT activity is specific for cholestasis, most likely intrahepatic in origin. This is also supported by the hyperbilirubinemia, which could reflect hepatic or posthepatic causes, but not prehepatic, given the absence of hemolysis.

Hyperproteinemia is characterized by a mild-to-moderate hyperglobulinemia that is most likely due to increased gamma globulins, suggesting antigenic stimulation. The biochemistry was performed on serum, so an increased fibrinogen would not have affected the protein measurement.

Decreased creatinine concentration is typically not clinically significant but could reflect decreased muscle mass.

Summary and outcome

This animal had photosensitization secondary to severe acute hepatic necrosis and cholestasis. The cause of hepatic injury was uncertain but in cattle is most often secondary to oral hepatotoxins. Decreased hepatic function in this case leads to increased phylloerythrin escaping liver metabolism and being deposited in the skin, which, after being exposed to UV radiation, forms free radicals, leading to local tissue damage.

Contributor: Dr. Allan Kessell

Case 72

Signalment: Adult miniature horse mare
History: 10-day history of anorexia. Presented for investigation of colic.

Hematology		Reference range
Packed cell volume (%)	42	32–53
RBC ($\times 10^6/\mu L$)	8.99	6.0–9.0
Hgb (g/dL)	**15.5**	11.5–14.5
MCV (fL)	45.8	40–50
MCHC (g/dL)	37.6	37–41
NCC ($10^3/\mu L$)	7.0	5.0–11.0
Segmented neutrophils ($10^3/\mu L$)	3.9	2.7–6.7
Band neutrophils ($10^3/\mu L$)	**0.2**	0.0–0.1
Monocytes ($10^3/\mu L$)	0.3	0.0–0.8
Lymphocytes ($10^3/\mu L$)	2.6	1.5–5.5
Platelets ($10^3/\mu L$)	180	90–240
Plasma protein by refractometry (g/dL)	7.7	5.2–7.8
Fibrinogen (g/dL)	0.2	0.1–0.5

Hemopathology: Icteric plasma, moderate toxic neutrophils with Dohle bodies, foamy cytoplasmic basophilia, and rare toxic granulation.

Biochemical profile		Reference range
Glucose (mg/dL)	**149**	70–105
Blood urea nitrogen (mg/dL)	26	12–26
Creatinine (mg/dL)	**2.1**	1.2–2.0
Calcium (mg/dL)	**9.7**	11.3–13.4
Phosphorus (mg/dL)	**8.6**	2.7–5.0
Total protein (g/dL)	**5.8**	6.1–8.1
Albumin (g/dL)	**2.1**	3.0–4.1
Globulin (g/dL)	3.7	2.5–5.0
Total bilirubin (mg/dL)	**5.0**	0.0–2.0
ALP (IU/L)	**2409**	0–250
AST (IU/L)	**1490**	0–350
GGT (IU/L)	**246**	0–35
CK (IU/L)	**389**	0–350
Triglyceride (mg/dL)	**1961**	5–50
Sodium (mEq/L)	131	130–140
Potassium (mEq/L)	3.6	3.0–5.0
Chloride (mEq/L)	**92**	97–105
Bicarbonate (mEq/L)	**14.1**	23–33
Anion gap (mEq/L)	**28.5**	3–11

Blood gas (venous)		Reference range
pH	**7.34**	7.40–7.50
pCO_2 (mmHg)	**28**	40–50
Bicarbonate (mEq/L)	**16.8**	25–32
TCO_2 (mmol/L)	**15.8**	30–36
Base excess	**−9.2**	

Interpretive discussion

Hematology

The increase in hemoglobin concentration is discrepant with the other erythrocyte analytes (PCV, RBC) and probably due to artifact rather than a true or relative (dehydration) erythrocytosis. While not mentioned in the hematology profile, lipemia (see below) is most likely causing an erroneously high hemoglobin reading by the photometer in the hematology analyzer. This is also supported by difference between biochemical and refractometric measures of total protein, with lipemia falsely increasing the latter.

The presence of band neutrophils in combination with toxic change is indicative of inflammation with premature marrow release of immature forms. In the absence of a mature neutrophilia, the inflammation is likely to be acute or overwhelming. Endotoxemia is a possibility in this case and could be causing margination of mature neutrophils contributing to the low-normal value. With inflammation, an increase in fibrinogen is expected but not observed in this case, possibly due to the very acute nature of this process or decreased hepatic synthesis.

Chemistry and blood gas

In all mammals, a transient hyperglycemia can be induced by a corticosteroid or epinephrine response and is a possible cause in this case. Persistent hyperglycemia in equines can also be observed with pituitary pars intermedia dysfunction (**PPID**) which leads to insulin resistance from excess cortisol release.

A mild azotemia characterized by an increased creatinine and high normal urea is present and could be prerenal (dehydration) or renal. A urine specific gravity would be required to assess renal concentrating ability. It is also important to note that urea is a poor indicator of renal function in horses (compared to small animals) given their ability to excrete urea through the gastrointestinal tract. The concurrent hyperphosphatemia indicates decreased GFR and does not elucidate the mechanism of azotemia.

Hypocalcemia is likely a due to decreased protein binding (secondary to hypoalbuminemia) given 40–50% of circulating calcium is protein bound; measuring ionized calcium is warranted. Other differentials to consider in a horse include gastrointestinal disease (decreased absorption vs. increased loss), renal losses, or excessive sweating.

A hypoproteinemia with a component of hypoalbuminemia could reflect a protein losing nephropathy (PLN) or enteropathy, although the latter tends to lead to panhypoproteinemia. A completely urinalysis and assessment of proteinuria could aid in ruling in/out a PLN. Also, worth considering is loss through third spacing such as effusions, as well as decreased hepatic synthesis. Albumin is a negative acute phase protein and can also be decreased with inflammation.

Anorexia is a common cause of hyperbilirubinemia in horses. However, the concurrent increase in ALP and GGT activity suggest cholestasis, such as might be seen with cholangiohepatitis. The concurrent increase in AST activity may suggest hepatocellular injury but could also be due to muscle injury with increased CK supporting this (AST has a longer half-life than CK).

There is a hyperlipidemia characterized by a marked increase in triglycerides. In horses, this typically occurs in states of negative energy balance, where poor nutrition leads to lipolysis and subsequent production of VLDL. Predisposing factors include being a miniature horse, anorexia, obesity and other conditions leading to insulin resistance (PPID, pregnancy). Excessive VLDL production can lead to storage of triglycerides in hepatocytes and result in hepatic lipidosis, a possibility in this case given the evidence of hepatobiliary disease.

Hypochloremia is present and the corrected chloride is calculated to be 94.8 mEq/l, indicating a mild selective chloride loss. Differentials to consider include gastrointestinal disease (diarrhea, gastric reflux) and excessive sweating.

With a selective chloride loss, one would expect a metabolic alkalosis. This, however, is not the case as the decreased bicarbonate and increased anion gap reveals a titrational metabolic acidosis with increased concentration of unmeasured anions. In this case, uremic acids and lactate are the most likely contributors. Blood gases confirm a metabolic acidosis with a compensatory respiratory alkalosis (low pCO_2). It is also likely that the chloride was slightly falsely decreased due to hyperlipidemia. Since an indirect ion-selective electrode measuring system was used. For every 885 mg/dL increase in total lipid concentration, there is a decrease of 1 mEq/L in chloride [1].

Summary and outcome

Laboratory abnormalities in combination with signalment and history are consistent with equine hyperlipemia syndrome. Hepatic lipidosis, inflammation and lactic acidosis are likely in this case.

Investigation revealed free peritoneal fluid that was septic and suppurative. The horse unfortunately died and presented to the necropsy service, where it was revealed to have hepatic lipidosis, renal tubular lipidosis, pulmonary hemorrhage, lymphoplasmacytic enteritis, a portion of necrotic cecum, and evidence of an early pregnancy. Cultures revealed salmonellosis.

Contributors: Drs. Alex Mau and Saundra Sample

Case 73

Signalment: 10-year-old spayed female miniature schnauzer
History: Polydipsia, polyuria, weight loss, abdominal "cramping" for 1 month
Physical examination: Tense abdomen, thin with mild truncal alopecia and comedones on dorsal midline

Hematology		Reference interval
PCV (%)	48	37–55
NCC ($\times 10^3/\mu L$)	**34.4**	6–17
Segs ($\times 10^3/\mu L$)	**29.0**	3–11.5
Bands ($\times 10^3/\mu L$)	**2.0**	0–0.3
Monos ($\times 10^3/\mu L$)	**3.4**	0.1–1.3
Lymphs ($\times 10^3/\mu L$)	**0**	1–4.8
Platelets ($\times 10^3/\mu L$)	Adequate	200–500
TP[a] (g/dL)	**9.0**[a]	6–8

[a] Although dog fasted, plasma is markedly lipemic, so refractometric measurement of total protein may be falsely increased.

Biochemical profile		Reference interval
Gluc (mg/dL)	**353 *(19.4)***	65–122 *(3.7–6.8 mmol/L)*
BUN (mg/dL)	**35 *(12.5)***	7–28 *(6.1–11.4 mmol/L)*
Creat (mg/dL)	1.2	0.9–1.7
Ca (mg/dL)	11.0	9.0–11.2
Phos (mg/dL)	6.0	2.8–6.1
TP (g/dL)	6.0	5.4–7.4
Alb (g/dL)	2.7	2.7–4.5
Glob (g/dL)	3.3	1.9–3.4
T. bili (mg/dL)	**1.2 *(26.5)***	0–0.4 *(0–6.8 μmol/L)*
Chol (mg/dL)	**900 *(23.4)***	130–370 *(3.4–9.6 mmol/L)*
ALT (IU/L)	**987**	10–120
ALP (IU/L)	**1200**	35–280
Na (mEq/L)	**139**	145–158
K (mEq/L)	3.1	4.1–5.5
CL (mEq/L)	**100**	106–127
TCO_2 (mEq/L)	12.2	14–27
An. gap (mEq/L)	**30**	8–25
Lipase (IU/L)	**3500**	30–560

Urinalysis	
Color	Yellow
Transparency	Clear
Sp. gr.	1.035
Protein	Neg
Gluc	2+
Ketones	Neg
Bilirubin	+
Blood	Neg
pH	6.0

Endocrine data		Reference interval
ACTH stimulation		
Serum cortisol (μg/dL) (pre)	**4.5 *(124)***	1–4 *(25–110 nmol/L)*
Serum cortisol (μg/dL) (post)	14.6	<20
Low-dose dexamethasone suppression test		
Serum cortisol (μg/dL) (pre)	3.5	1–4
Serum cortisol (μg/dL) (8-h post)	1.5	<1.5

Interpretive discussion

Hematology

Lymphopenia is indicative of increased endogenous (stress or hyperadrenocorticism) or exogenous corticosteroids. Increased immature neutrophil concentration is indicative of inflammation. Neutrophilia may be due to inflammation or stress. In summary, an inflammatory and stress (steroid) leukogram is present.

Biochemical profile

Hyperglycemia is of the magnitude that diabetes mellitus should be suspected. Hyperglycemia may also be secondary to hyperadrenocorticism; therefore, adrenocorticotropic hormone (ACTH) stimulation and low-dose dexamethasone suppression (LDDS) tests are indicated.

BUN is increased, but creatinine is within the reference interval. Urine specific gravity indicates kidneys are capable of concentrating, thus the azotemia is prerenal, perhaps clue to dehydration. However, albumin is within reference interval. The PCV is normal, suggesting that GI bleeding is not the cause of the increased BUN.

Total bilirubin is increased suggesting cholestasis, because anemia is not present. Alkaline phosphatase activity is increased, which is also suggestive of cholestasis. Another consideration is hyperadrenocorticism, with an increase in the corticosteroid-induced alkaline phosphatase isoenzyme. Increased cholesterol of this magnitude is probably due to lipidemia, although some component of the increase could also be due to cholestasis. ALT activity is increased, which is indicative of hepatocellular damage.

Sodium and chloride concentrations are decreased. Sodium may be lost through thc kidncy, although this animal is capable of concentrating. Although it is not mentioned in the history, abdominal pain may have been associated with vomiting, which would result in electrolyte loss. Hyperglycemia results in increased serum osmolality with a shift of intracellular fluid to extracellular fluid in an attempt to decrease extracellular fluid solute concentration. Sodium can be expected to decrease by 1.6 mEq/l for every 100 mg/dl increase in glucose.

Total CO_2 is decreased, indicating metabolic acidosis. The anion gap is increased, indicating increased unmeasured anions are present. In this case, unmeasured anions might be ketones, although they are not present in the urine. Urine ketone tests that use the nitroprusside reaction do not detect β-hydroxybutyric acid; therefore, the presence of this ketone cannot be ruled out. Other possibilities include lactic acidosis.

Serum lipase activity is increased. In this patient, this increase could partially be due to decreased GFR, as indicated by azotemia. However, the inflammatory leukogram, increased bilirubin, increased alkaline phosphatase activity, hyperglycemia, and lipemia are also suggestive of pancreatitis. This magnitude of lipase increase is highly supportive of pancreatitis. Prerenal azotemia due to hemoconcentration and poor renal perfusion is a common complication of pancreatitis. Likewise, so is hepatocellular injury and cholestasis.

Urinalysis

Urine specific gravity of 1.035 indicates the dog is capable of concentrating, thus the increase in BUN is prerenal (perhaps dehydration). Glucosuria and bilirubinuria are to the expected in light of the serum concentrations.

Endocrine data

ACTH stimulation test: Baseline cortisol is slightly above normal. Normal animals stimulate to around 10–16 μg/dl. Low-dose dexamethasone suppression test: Baseline cortisol is normal. Dog suppressed marginally at 8 hours. The endocrine data are not supportive of hyper-adrenocorticism.

Summary

This dog has primary hyperlipidemia, which has been shown to be familial in miniature schnauzers [1], and pancreatitis with secondary diabetes mellitus. Dogs with hyperlipidemia are predisposed to development of pancreatitis. While diabetes mellitus may be transitory, treatment is indicated. Some abnormalities (hyperglycemia, stress leukogram, increased alkaline phosphatase activity, lipemia, history, and physical appearance) were suggestive of hyperadrenocorticism. This possibility was ruled out by the ACTH stimulation and LDDS test. Imaging revealed evidence of swelling in the area of the pancreas.

Case 74

Signalment: 9-year-old female spayed miniature schnauzer
History: Not eating, vomited a few times
Physical examination: Tense abdomen

Hematology		Reference interval
PCV (%)	**32.0**	37–55
MCV (fL)	68.0	60–72
NCC (×10³/μL)	**5.2**	6–17
Segs (×10³/μL)	**2.7**	3–11.5
Bands (×10³/μL)	**1.4**	0–0.3
Monos (×10³/μL)	0.2	0.1–1.3
Lymphs (×10³/μL)	**0.6**	1–4.8
Basophils (×10³/μL)	0.1	rare
Platelets (×10³/μL)	**111**	200–500

Hemopathology: Marked toxic neutrophils, giant platelets, hemolyzed and lipemic.

Biochemical profile		Reference interval
Gluc (mg/dL)	***226*** ***(12.4)***	65–122 *(3.5–6.7 mmol/L)*
BUN (mg/dL)	20	7–28
Creat (mg/dL)	1.2	0.9–1.7
Ca (mg/dL)	**8.2** ***(2.0)***	9.0–11.2 *(2.2–2.8 mmol/L)*
Phos (mg/dL)	5.1	2.8–6.1
TP (g/dL)	**5.0**	5.4–7.4
Alb (g/dL)	**1.8**	2.7–4.5
Glob (g/dL)	3.2	1.9–3.4
T. bili (mg/dL)	**1.4** ***(23.9)***	0–0.4 *(0.6–8.4 μmol/L)*
Chol (mg/dL)	**666** ***(17.3)***	130–370 *(3.4–9.6 mmol/L)*
ALT (IU/L)	33	10–120
AST (IU/L)	51	16–40
ALP (IU/L)	**1282**	35–280
GGT (IU/L)	5	0–6
Na (mEq/L)	152	145–158
K (mEq/L)	**3.7**	4.1–5.5
CL (mEq/L)	116	106–127
TCO_2 (mEq/L)	14	14–27
An. gap (mEq/L)	25	8–25
Amylase (IU/L)	**2421**	50–1250
Lipase (IU/L)	**2256**	30–560
Triglycerides (mg/dL)	**2884**	ND[a]

[a]Not determined.

Urinalysis		Urine sediment	
Color	Golden	WBCs/hpf	2–3
Transparency	Cloudy	RBCs/hpf	3–5
Sp. gr.	1.034	Epith cells/hpf	Negative
Protein	**2+**	Casts/lpf	2
Gluc	**4+**	Crystals	Negative
Bilirubin	**3+**	Bacteria	Negative
Blood	**2+**		
pH	8.0		
Ketones	Negative		

Coagulation data		Reference interval
PT (s)	9.3	7.5–10.5
aPTT (s)	**19.5**	10.5–16.5

Abdominal fluid analysis	
Color	Red
Supernatant	Light yellow
Refractometric protein (g/dL)	**7.2**
NCC (×10³/μL)	2.0
Triglyceride (mg/dL)	**257**
Chol (mg/dL)	**728**

Interpretive discussion

Hematology

The PCV is mildly decreased, no polychromasia was noted in the blood film, and the MCV is normal, indicating a mild nonregenerative anemia. Marked lipemia and hemolysis may have resulted in *in vitro* hemolysis, but this typically does not result in an important decrease in the PCV. There is a neutropenia with increased bands and marked numbers of toxic neutrophils. This suggests consumption as a result of severe inflammatory disease. Lymphopenia indicates a stress component. The thrombocytopenia is discussed with the coagulation data.

Biochemical profile

The serum glucose concentration is moderately increased. In this range, it is possible that this is a stress hyperglycemia but is more likely due to some metabolic or endocrine abnormality.

The BUN and serum creatinine concentrations are normal. The serum phosphorus is normal, but there is a mild decrease in serum total calcium concentration. Given the degree of hypoalbuminemia, it is wise to attempt to correct the total calcium for the hypoproteinemia. In this case, the corrected value is 9.9 mg/dl ($8.2 - 1.8 + 3.5$), which is normal.

The serum cholesterol concentration is markedly increased. While this may be associated with cholestasis, given the degree of increase in cholesterol one should also consider other metabolic abnormalities including hepatic disease, disorders of lipoprotein metabolism, or endocrinopathies. The serum triglyceride concentration is markedly increased, and further supports a diagnosis of a metabolic and/or endocrinologic disorder. Cholestasis is indicated by the increased total bilirubin and ALP activity. The serum ALT, AST, and GGT activities are normal or near normal, reducing the likelihood of hepatocellular injury,

The serum amylase and lipase activities are significantly increased, and in the absence of azotemia suggest acute pancreatitis. This is a frequent complication of severe prolonged hyperlipidemia. The concurrent findings of hyperlipidemia and pancreatitis in a miniature schnauzer should alert one to the potential diagnosis of a primary dyslipidemia.

Coagulation data

The coagulation profile includes a normal PT, but prolonged aPTT. While it is more common for the PT to become prolonged first when there is impaired coagulation factor synthesis by the liver, incipient DIC (note the thrombocytopenia) or heparinization of the patient may result in changes in the aPTT alone.

Abdominal fluid analysis

Abdominal fluid chemical analysis similarly indicates accumulation of excess lipids in the peritoneal cavity. It is likely that the increased total protein by refractometry is spuriously elevated by this lipid. The cell concentration suggests a modified transudate.

Urinalysis

The urine specific gravity indicates that the kidneys are capable of concentrating, and the number of leukocytes and erythrocytes are not significant. However, there is 2+ proteinuria, some occult blood, and some hyaline and fine granular casts. Thus, there may be mild tubular and/or glomerular disease. In addition, there is significant glucosuria, which is explained by the hyperglycemia. It would be useful to evaluate the UPC in order to determine the magnitude of the proteinuria. Given the hypoalbuminemia and hypercholesterolemia, one should consider, the possibility of nephrotic syndrome; there may be a protein losing glomerulopathy without azotemia.

Summary

Miniature schnauzer hyperlipidemia and acute pancreatitis.

Case 75

Signalment: 11-year-old castrated male cat
History: Polyuria and polydipsia for 2 months, anorexia and lethargy more recently
Physical examination: Presented in lateral recumbency, 10% dehydrated

Hematology		Reference interval
PCV (%)	40	24–45
Hgb (g/dL)	12.8	8–15
RBC ($\times 10^6$/dL)	8.64	5–11
MCV (fL)	46	39–50
MCHC (g/μL)	34	33–37
NCC ($\times 10^3$/μL)	18.7	5.5–19.5
Segs ($\times 10^3$/μL)	**15.0**	2.5–12.5
Bands ($\times 10^3$/μL)	**2.4**	0–0.3
Monos ($\times 10^3$/μL)	0.2	0–0.8
Lymphs ($\times 10^3$/μL)	**0.9**	1.5–7.0
Eos ($\times 10^3$/μL)	0.2	0–1.5
Platelets ($\times 10^3$/μL)	375	200–500
TP (P) (g/dL)	**11.7**	6–8

Hemopathology: Slightly toxic neutrophils, many echinocytes.

Biochemical profile		Reference interval
Gluc (mg/dL)	**766 *(42.7)***	67–124 *(3.7–6.8 mmol/L)*
BUN (mg/dL)	**127 *(45.3)***	17–32 *(6.1–11.4 mmol/L)*
Creat (mg/dL)	**6.4 *(566)***	0.9–2.1 *(78–186 μmol/L)*
Ca (mg/dL)	10.1	8.5–11
Phos (mg/dL)	**7.9 *(10.0)***	3.3–7.8 *(1.1–2.5 mmol/L)*
TP (g/dL)	**9.7**	5.9–8.1
Alb (g/dL)	**4.4**	2.3–3.9
Glob (g/dL)	**5.3**	2.9–4.4
T. bili (mg/dL)	0.3	0–0.3
Chol (mg/dL)	**388 *(10.1)***	60–220 *(1.6–5.7 mmol/L)*
ALT (IU/L)	**124**	30–100
AST (IU/L)	**354**	14–38
ALP (IU/L)	65	6–106
GGT (IU/L)	1	0–1
Na (mEq/L)	**172**	146–160
K (mEq/L)	5.1	3.7–5.4
CL (mEq/L)	**132**	112–129
TCO_2 (mEq/L)	**10.9**	14–23
An. gap (mEq/L)	**34**	10–27
Calc. osmolarity (mOsm/L)	**417**	290–310

Urinalysis (cystocentesis)			
Color	Yellow	**Urine sediment**	
Transparency	Cloudy	WBCs/hpf	**6–8**
Sp. gr.	1.034	RBCs/hpf	2–3
Protein	**2+**	Epith cells/hpf	1–3 transitional
Gluc	**2+**	Casts/lpf	0
Bilirubin	Negative	Crystals	0
Blood	**4+**	Bacteria	0
pH	5.0	Ketones	Negative
		Other	Small amt of fat

Interpretive discussion

Hematology

Leukogram abnormalities include neutrophilia, a left shift, lymphopenia, and slightly toxic neutrophils. This is an inflammatory leukogram indicating a tissue demand for neutrophils. The lymphopenia suggests concurrent increase in corticosteroid concentrations due to stress. Toxic neutrophils indicate a rapid rate of neutrophil production.

Echinocyte formation can be an artifact, but in this case, it may have resulted from the marked hyperosmolality and electrolyte abnormalities. These may have caused movement of water from the cytoplasm of erythrocytes to the plasma with resulting shrinkage and crenation of erythrocytes.

Biochemical profile

The serum glucose concentration is markedly increased. The most likely cause of hyperglycemia of this magnitude is diabetes mellitus. Severe, acute excitement with release of catecholamines can cause marked hyperglycemia in cats, but serum glucose concentration is seldom greater than 400 mg/dl in such cats. This cat is azotemic, and decreased renal excretion of glucose, secondary to decreased glomerular filtration rate, may have augmented the magnitude of the hyperglycemia. Moreover, the cat does not have an excitement leukogram (lymphocytosis).

Both BUN and serum creatinine concentrations are increased. Since the urine specific gravity suggests adequate renal concentrating ability (i.e., the specific gravity is greater than 1.030), this appears to be a prerenal azotemia. However, the marked hyperproteinemia and hypernatremia suggest severe dehydration, and an even higher urine specific gravity would be expected in this situation. It is, therefore, possible that this cat has some loss of urine concentration ability. Alternatively, osmotic diuresis due to glucosuria may have contributed to the lower-than-expected urine specific gravity. The hyperphosphatemia is a result of a decreased glomerular filtration rate. Maintenance of normal serum phosphorus concentrations depends on phosphorus excretion through the kidney.

Hyperproteinemia (both plasma and serum protein) with concurrent hyperalbuminemia and hyperglobulinemia is typical of dehydration. Contraction of plasma water volume results in proportional increases in concentrations of both albumin and globulin. Although other abnormalities can cause hyperglobulinemia, dehydration is the only cause of hyperalbuminemia. Diuresis secondary to glucosuria is common in diabetes mellitus and can result in dehydration.

The serum cholesterol concentration is increased. In this case, this abnormality is probably secondary to diabetes mellitus and related abnormalities in lipid metabolism.

Serum activities of both ALT and AST are increased. The increased serum ALT activity is due to hepatocyte injury and subsequent leakage of this enzyme. This injury was probably caused by fatty change that developed secondary to the metabolic abnormalities of diabetes mellitus. The increased serum AST activity may also be due to leakage of AST from injured hepatocytes, but the higher activity of AST as compared to ALT suggests that there is also an extrahepatic source. This source may be muscle and may have resulted from muscle injury secondary to hypoperfusion, since the cat is very dehydrated.

Hypernatremia and hyperchloremia are probably due to severe dehydration. Glucosuria causes diuresis resulting in Na and Cl loss through the kidneys in nondehydrated or mildly dehydrated, diabetic animals. This can lead to hyponatremia and hypochloremia. When such animals become severely dehydrated, however, diuresis no longer occurs, and hypernatremia and hyperchloremia develop. These changes, in combination with hyperglycemia and azotemia, result in severe hyperosmolality.

Decreased serum total CO_2 concentration probably represents a primary metabolic acidosis. Serum total CO_2 concentration may also decrease as a compensatory reaction in animals with primary respiratory alkalosis, but in animals with diabetes mellitus, metabolic acidosis is more likely to be the primary alteration. Increased serum concentrations of ketones are a common cause of acidosis in diabetic animals, but the absence of urine ketones suggests that this cat is probably not ketotic. Urine ketone tests that use the nitroprusside reaction do not detect β-hydroxybutyric acid, therefore, the presence of this ketone cannot be ruled out. Increased serum lactate concentration may be contributing to the acidosis in this cat. The cat is markedly dehydrated and is, therefore, probably experiencing tissue hypoxia that may lead to increased lactate production.

The anion gap is increased. In most diabetic animals, increased ketoacid concentration in the blood is the major cause of this abnormality. In this cat, which is apparently not ketotic, increased blood lactate concentration is probably contributing to this gap.

The calculated osmolarity is increased and, in combination with other laboratory changes, suggests this cat has diabetic nonketotic hyperosmolar syndrome (see summary).

Urinalysis

This cat has a proteinuria with a mild pyuria. It is possible that the protein exuded into the urine as part of the inflammatory process; however, the degree of proteinuria appears to be excessive compared to the degree of pyuria. Other causes of proteinuria such as glomerular and tubular disease should be considered in this case. Although glomerular disease has been associated with diabetes mellitus in humans, this has not been documented in animals.

The strongly positive reaction on the chemical test for blood in combination with normal numbers of erythrocytes suggests that the positive reaction is due to either free hemoglobin or myoglobin. It is unlikely that this represents a hematuria with subsequent lysis of erythrocytes since such lysis is unlikely in urine with a high specific gravity. Absence of anemia suggests a significant hemolytic problem is not occurring in this cat. Myoglobinuria is a possible explanation, and severe muscle hypoxia secondary to hypovolemia may have occurred in this cat. However, the serum AST activity, while increased, does not suggest such massive muscle injury.

Glucosuria is a result of the serum glucose concentration exceeding the renal threshold.

Summary

The clinical diagnosis was diabetic nonketotic hyperosmolar syndrome. This syndrome is characterized by marked hyperglycemia (blood glucose concentration >600 mg/dL), hyperosmolarity (>350 mOsm/L), and absence of ketosis in a diabetic animal. Such animals commonly have prerenal or renal azotemia. The hyperosmolarity results in dehydration of neurons and subsequent neurologic signs. This syndrome is associated with a high fatality rate.

After a brief, unsuccessful attempt to decrease serum glucose concentrations with insulin therapy and to improve the cat's electrolyte and fluid balance by administration of fluids, the owner elected euthanasia. Necropsy revealed severs islet cell degeneration and amyloidosis and severe hepatocytic vacuolar degeneration. A few mineralized casts were present in renal tubules, but the kidneys were otherwise normal, and the azotemia was probably prerenal in this case. The cause of the inflammatory leukogram was not determined.

Case 76

Signalment: 10-year-old male castrated feline DSH
History: Not eating well, lethargic
Physical examination: Slightly dehydrated

Hematology	Day 1	Reference interval
PCV (%)	38.0[a]	24–45
Hgb (g/dL)	12.8	8–15
RBC ($\times 10^6/\mu L$)	9.25	5–11
MCV (fL)	44.0	39–50
MCHC (g/dL)	35.0	33–37
Retics ($\times 10^3/\mu L$)	**80**	< 60
NCC ($\times 10^3/\mu L$)	12.9	5.5–19.5
Segs ($\times 10^3/\mu L$)	12.5	2.5–12.5
Lymphs ($\times 10^3/\mu L$)	**0.3**	1.5–7.0
Platelets ($\times 10^3/\mu L$)	Adequate	200–500
TP (P) (g/dL)	**9.0**	6–8

Hemopathology: Giant platelets, slight increase in polychromasia, slightly toxic neutrophils, **2+ Heinz bodies.**
[a]PCV was 27% on Day 5, and 17% on Day 7.

Biochemical profile	Day 1	Reference interval
Gluc (mg/dL)	**328 *(18.0)***	67–124 *(3.7–6.8 mmol/L)*
BUN (mg/dL)	29	17–32
Creat (mg/dL)	1.5	0.9–2.1
Ca (mg/dL)	9.4	8.5–11
Phos (mg/dL)	**1.9 *(0.6)***	3.3–7.8 *(1.1–2.5 mmol/L)*
TP (g/dL)	8.0	5.9–8.1
Alb (g/dL)	**4.3**	2.3–3.9
Glob (g/dL)	3.7	2.9–4.4
T. bili (mg/dL)	**2.1 *(35.9)***	0–0.3 *(0–5.1 mmol/L)*
Chol (mg/dL)	**512 *(13.3)***	60–220 *(1.6–5.7 mmol/L)*
ALT (IU/L)	**282**	30–100
ALP (IU/L)	99	6–106
Na (mEq/L)	**130**	146–160
K (mEq/L)	**2.2**	3.7–5.4
CL (mEq/L)	**74**	112–129
TCO_2 (mEq/L)	**10.5**	14–23
An. gap (mEq/L)	**47.7**	10–27
Lipase (IU/L)	**161**	3–125

Blood gas data (arterial)		Reference interval
pH	**7.280**	7.33–7.44
pCO_2 (mmHg)	**20.0**	35–42
pO_2 (mmHg)	85.5	73–92
HCO_3 (mEq/L)	**9.2**	16–22
Ionized Ca++ (mg/dL)	**4.64**	4.8–5.3

Urinalysis		Urine sediment	
Color	Yellow	WBCs/hpf	0–1
Transparency	Clear	RBCs/hpf	0–1
Sp. gr.	1.033	Epith cells/hpf	0–1
Protein	**1+**	Casts/lpf	**3–4 granular**
Gluc	**4+**	Crystals	Negative
Bilirubin	**1+**	Bacteria	Negative
Blood	**1+**	Other	
pH	6.0		
Ketones	**3+**		

Interpretive discussion

Hematology

The packed cell volume, hemoglobin, and total RBC count are normal, but given the degree of hemoconcentration represented by the hyperproteinemia, it is possible that the PCV is actually lower. There is a slight increase in polychromasia and mild reticulocytosis. The anemia is rapidly progressive over a 1-week period of time. The presence of 2+ Heinz bodies indicates significant oxidative damage to the red blood cells, and is commonly observed in cats with diabetic ketoacidosis; however, the owner should be questioned as to whether the cat has received acetaminophen or other oxidant drugs or chemicals. Another potential cause of hemolytic anemia in this patient is hypophosphatemia. There is a stress leukogram, as indicated by the high normal neutrophil count and lymphopenia.

Biochemical profile

The serum glucose concentration is moderately increased. While a glucose concentration of this magnitude may be encountered due to extreme excitement (sympathetic activation) or stress (glucocorticoid release), diabetes mellitus is more likely. Evidence against excitement-induced hyperglycemia is the lack of an excitement leukogram (lymphocytosis). The BUN and serum creatinine concentrations are normal.

The serum phosphorus concentration is decreased, and given the degree of hyperglycemia, one should consider diabetic ketoacidosis-induced urinary phosphate loss. The serum total calcium concentration is normal, reducing the possibility of an endocrine abnormality causing the change in serum phosphorus. The serum total protein concentration is at the upper end of the reference interval, and serum albumin is increased, indicating hemoconcentration due to dehydration.

The serum cholesterol concentration is moderately increased. While this may be associated with cholestasis, as indicated by the increased total bilirubin, the ALP activity is normal. Given the degree of increase in cholesterol, one should consider metabolic abnormalities including hepatic disease, disorders of lipoprotein metabolism, or endocrinopathies. If not due to cholestasis, then the increase in bilirubin may be due to hemolysis. The serum ALT activity is increased modestly, which indicates hepatocellular damage. ALP is not induced by steroids in cats, thus, hyperadrenocorticism is a possibility. Serum lipase activity is only slightly increased, possibly reducing the probability for concurrent pancreatitis; however, increased lipase activity is not a reliable marker for feline pancreatitis.

Serum Na, K, and Cl concentration are decreased significantly. One should consider typical causes for electrolyte depletion, including pathologic losses from the gastrointestinal and urinary systems, as well as a shift to third space. The marked hyperglycemia should initiate consideration of diabetic ketoacidosis with subsequent urinary electrolyte loss. There is a marked decrease in serum total CO, suggesting metabolic acidosis. The increase in the anion gap is likely due to the presence of ketones, which are unmeasured anions.

Blood gas data

The blood gas panel indicates a metabolic acidosis (decreased pH and HCO_3) with respiratory compensation (decreased pCO_2). Ionized calcium is marginally decreased.

Urinalysis

The urinary specific gravity is normal. However, with marked increases in the concentration of solutes, such as glucose, not pertinent to urinary concentration capacity, one might question the accuracy of this measure, and consider determining urinary osmolality to address urinary concentration capacity specifically. The presence of 1+ protein and coarse granular casts is consistent with renal tubular disease. The absence of more significant proteinuria speaks against the possibility of glomerular protein loss, but a urinary protein:creatinine ratio should be determined to confirm this. In either case, urinary tract inflammation is not a likely cause of the observed changes, as there is only a small amount of occult blood and no pyuria. The presence of significant amounts of glucose and ketones supports a diagnosis of diabetic ketoacidosis. The mild bilirubinuria is a result of the increased serum bilirubin and subsequent renal excretion.

Summary

Diabetic ketoacidosis; Heinz body anemia

Case 77

Signalment: 8-year-old castrated male Labrador retriever

History: Two months of decreased activity, progressing to muscle fasciculations and mild intermittent seizures. Referring DVM prescribed phenobarbital and prednisone 5 days previously.

Physical examination: Obese, reluctant to move. Normal body temperature, heart rate, respiratory rate. Normal chest radiographs and abdominal ultrasound.

Hematology		Reference interval
Packed cell volume (%)	40	37–55
Hemoglobin (g/dL)	14	12–18
RBC ($\times 10^6/\mu L$)	5.75	5.5–8.5
MCV (fL)	69	60–72
MCHC (g/dL)	35	34–38
Total nucleated cell count ($\times 10^3/\mu L$)	14.5	6–17
Segmented neutrophils ($\times 10^3/\mu L$)	**12.5**	3–11.5
Band neutrophils ($\times 10^3/\mu L$)	0	0–0.3
Monocytes ($\times 10^3/\mu L$)	1.3	0.1–1.3
Lymphocytes ($\times 10^3/\mu L$)	**0.7**	1–4.8
Eosinophils ($\times 10^3/\mu L$)	0	0.1–1.2
Platelets ($\times 10^3/\mu L$)	463	200–500
Plasma protein (g/dL)	7.0	6–8

Biochemical profile		Reference interval
Glucose (mg/dL)	**24**	65–122
Blood urea nitrogen (mg/dL)	16	7–28
Creatinine (mg/dL)	1.2	0.9–1.7
Calcium (mg/dL)	10.5	9.0–11.2
Phosphorus (mg/dL)	4.5	2.8–6.1
Total protein (g/dL)	6.8	5.4–7.4
Albumin (g/dL)	3.5	2.7–4.5
Globulin (g/dL)	3.3	1.9–3.4
Total bilirubin (mg/dL)	0.3	0–0.4
Cholesterol (mg/dL)	256	130–370
Alanine aminotransferase (IU/L)	110	10–120
Aspartate aminotransferase (IU/L)	32	16–40
Alkaline phosphatase (IU/L)	**602**	13–141
Gamma glutamyltransferase (IU/L)	**9**	0–6
Sodium (mEq/L)	151	145–158
Potassium (mEq/L)	4.1	4.1–5.5
Chloride (mEq/L)	116	106–127
Total CO_2 (mEq/L)	17	14–27
Anion gap	22	8–25
Other		
Serum insulin ($\mu U/mL$)	**46.2**	5–25

Interpretive discussion

Hematology

The only abnormalities are a mild mature neutrophilia and lymphopenia, consistent with a stress/steroid leukogram. This is not surprising given the history of prednisone administration.

Biochemical profile

Increased ALP and GGT activities are most likely due to steroid induction given the history of prednisone administration. There is no other evidence to support cholestasis or liver disease.

Hypoglycemia is pronounced. Appropriate sample handling procedures were followed, ruling-out artifactual hypoglycemia due to delayed removal of serum from the red cells, and episodic hypoglycemia fits the clinical signs. There is no evidence for sepsis (no inflammatory leukogram) or liver failure (BUN, cholesterol, albumin are normal).

Serum insulin concentration is increased at the same time this dog is hypoglycemic, which is an inappropriate response. Normally, feedback mechanisms result in low serum insulin concentrations when hypoglycemia exists. Uncontrolled insulin production from a neoplasm is most likely. The most common tumor associated with hypoglycemia in dogs is insulinoma, a neoplasm of pancreatic β-cells.

Summary

An exploratory laparotomy was performed and a small pancreatic mass was identified and removed. Small nodules were present in the liver, and regional lymph nodes were enlarged. Aspirates from an enlarged node were taken intraoperatively, and a metastatic endocrine tumor was diagnosed by cytology. Histopathology confirmed a β-cell carcinoma in the pancreas with metastases to liver and lymph node. It is important to measure serum insulin concentrations at the same time the dog is hypoglycemic, preferably when the blood glucose is <50 mg/dl. Under these conditions, a serum insulin concentration that is increased or in the upper half of the reference interval indicates a relative insulin excess, suggesting uncontrolled insulin production.

CASES

Case 78

Signalment: 6-day-old female Holstein
History: Scours
Physical examination: Severe dehydration

Hematology		Reference interval
PCV (%)	**58.0**	24–46
Hgb (g/dL)	**19.0**	8–15
RBC (×10^6/μL)	**17.1**	5.0–10.0
MCV (fL)	**34.0**	37–53
MCHC (g/dL)	33.0	33–38
NCC (×10^3/μL)	5.0	4.0–12.0
Segs (×10^3/μL)	3.2	0.6–4.0
Monos (×10^3/μL)	**1.7**	0–0.8
Lymphs (×10^3/μL)	**0.1**	2.5–7.5
Platelets (×10^3/μL)	288	200–800
Fibrinogen (mg/dL)	600	200–600
TP (P) (g/dL)	**10.9**	6–8

Hemopathology: Many acanthocytes and keratocytes, RBC fragments, hypochromic RBCs.

Biochemical profile		Reference interval
Gluc (mg/dL)	**31**	55–95
BUN (mg/dL)	**87**	7–20
Creat (mg/dL)	**4.6**	1.0–1.8
Ca (mg/dL)	**7.8**	8.2–9.9
Phos (mg/dL)	6.9	4.3–7.0
TP (g/dL)	**10.3**	6.3–7.6
Alb (g/dL)	**5.3**	2.5–4.3
Glob (g/dL)	**5.0**	2.6–5.0
T. bili (mg/dL)	**0.8**	0.1–0.4
CK (IU/L)	**352**	57–280
AST (IU/L)	**286**	40–130
GGT (IU/L)	14	10–26
SDH (IU/L)	17	8–23
Na (mEq/L)	**129**	136–147
K (mEq/L)	**6.7**	3.6–5.2
CL (mEq/L)	**91**	95–105
TCO_2 (mEq/L)	**17.0**	24–32
An. gap (mEq/L)	**27.7**	14–26

Blood gas data (venous)		Reference interval
pH	**7.140**	7.32–7.45
pCO_2 (mmHg)	**45.7**	34–44
HCO_3 (mEq/L)	**15.3**	23–31

Urinalysis			
Color	Yellow	**Urine sediment**	
Transparency	Clear	WBCs/hpf	0–1
Sp. gr.	**1.014**	RBCs/hpf	0–1
Protein	Negative	Epith cells/hpf	1–2
Gluc	Negative	Casts/lpf	Negative
Bilirubin	Negative	Crystals	Negative
Blood	Negative	Bacteria	Negative
pH	5.0		

Interpretive discussion

Hematology

There is a monocytosis and a lymphopenia that represent the effects of stress. The plasma protein concentration is increased, most probably due to dehydration. Erythrocyte indices reflect hemoconcentration as well, as evidenced by the increased RBC count, hemoglobin concentration, and PCV. The MCV is decreased, which may be due to an underlying iron-deficiency anemia of the newborn that is obscured by hemoconcentration. The presence of several erythrocyte morphologic abnormalities supports this. Iron deficiency is frequently associated not only with a microcytic anemia but also with oxidative damage to the erythrocytes, resulting in membrane abnormalities and fragmentation changes.

Biochemical profile

There is a profound hypoglycemia, which in a neonatal calf with diarrhea is most probably related to decreased food intake, as well as the possibility of sepsis. Sepsis is unlikely, considering the normal neutrophil concentration.

The BUN and serum creatinine concentrations are increased, but the origin of this azotemia cannot be discerned from this data alone. Refer to the discussion in the urinalysis section below.

Serum calcium is mildly decreased, possibly due to decreased milk intake. The serum total protein and albumin concentrations are increased, further reflecting hemoconcentration due to dehydration. The serum CK and AST activities are modestly increased, which may be related to muscle damage subsequent to prolonged recumbency or hypoperfusion. The total bilirubin is increased. Together with the increased AST activity, this may indicate hepatocellular damage. Alternatively, there may be cholestasis due to dehydration or prehepatic icterus due to increased destruction of oxidatively-damaged iron-deficient erythrocytes.

The serum sodium and chloride concentrations are decreased, reflecting decreased intake and/or increased loss from the body. *Escherichia coli*-associated diarrhea in neonatal calves commonly results from increased sodium chloride loss induced by the enterotoxin that promotes active secretion into the gut lumen. Increased water loss follows this osmotic gradient. Bicarbonate is also lost in the feces, and hypovolemia may lead to tissue hypoperfusion, lactic acidosis, and decreased bicarbonate concentration as well. Fecal potassium loss is typically increased, but concomitant metabolic acidosis results in exchange of intracellular potassium for extracellular protons and a redistributional hyperkalemia.

Blood gas data

There is a combined metabolic (decreased bicarbonate) and respiratory (increased pCO_2) acidosis. The metabolic acidosis results from bicarbonate loss in the diarrhea and from lactic acidosis due to tissue hypoperfusion. The increased anion gap reflects the accumulation of unmeasured anions such as lactate. The mild respiratory acidosis indicates pulmonary dysfunction. Early pneumonia or decreased pulmonary perfusion secondary to dehydration are possible explanations.

Urinalysis

The only significant abnormality is a urine specific gravity of 1.014. Six-day-old calves, unlike neonates of many other species, should have mature capacity to concentrate urine. Dehydration should stimulate antidiuretic hormone release from the hypothalamus, and increased water reclamation by the renal tubules. However, electrolyte loss in this type of hypotonic dehydration often leads to medullary solute depletion and a loss of the renal concentration gradient. Another alternative is that there is renal disease, due to renal hypoperfusion, sepsis, etc., resulting in both azotemia and loss of concentrating ability.

Summary

Secretory diarrhea and hypotonic dehydration in a neonatal calf.

CASES

Case 79

Signalment: 9-month-old bull
History: Anorexia, depression
Physical examination: Enlarged abdomen

Hematology		Reference interval
PCV (%)	**19**	24–46
MCV (fL)	**31**	37–53
NCC ($\times10^3/\mu L$)	**18.0**	4.0–12.0
Segs ($\times10^3/\mu L$)	**10.5**	0.6–4.0
Bands ($\times10^3/\mu L$)	**2.5**	0–0.1
Monos ($\times10^3/\mu L$)	1.0	0–0.8
Lymphs ($\times10^3/\mu L$)	3.5	2.5–7.5
Eos ($\times10^3/\mu L$)	0.5	0–2.4
Platelets ($\times10^3/\mu L$)	Adequate	200–800
Fibrinogen (mg/dL)	**1000**	200–600
Hemopathology: Numerous schistocytes, keratocytes.		

Biochemical profile		Reference interval
Gluc (mg/dL)	**618**	55–95
BUN (mg/dL)	**90**	7–20
Creat (mg/dL)	**6.1**	1.0–1.8
Ca (mg/dL)	**7.8**	8.2–9.9
Phos (mg/dL)	**14.1**	4.3–7.0
TP (g/dL)	**10.1**	6.3–7.6
Alb (g/dL)	**4.5**	2.5–4.3
Glob (g/dL)	**5.6**	2.6–5.0
T. bili (mg/dL)	**0.8**	0.1–0.4
CK (IU/L)	**1100**	57–280
AST (IU/L)	**350**	40–130
Na (mEq/L)	**130**	136–147
K (mEq/L)	**3.1**	3.6–5.2
CL (mEq/L)	**47**	95–105
TCO_2 (mEq/L)	**50**	24 32

Blood gas data (venous)		Reference interval
HCO_3 (mEq/L)	**49.3**	23–31
pH	7.412	7.32–7.45
pCO_2 (mmHg)	**80**	34–44

Interpretive discussion

Hematology

PCV is decreased, indicating anemia.

MCV is decreased, suggesting iron deficiency anemia secondary to chronic blood loss.

Neutrophilia, increased band neutrophils, and monocytosis are indicative of chronic inflammation.

Increased fibrinogen also suggests inflammation.

Keratocytes and schistocytes are commonly seen with iron deficiency anemia.

Biochemical profile

Glucose is markedly increased, perhaps a sympathoadrenal response that can be seen in severely ill cattle. Other possibilities include prior treatment with glucose-containing fluids, diabetes mellitus, or acute pancreatitis. Other lab data supports proximal duodenal obstruction, in which marked hyperglycemia is a consistent finding. This may be due to a combination of stress-induced hyperglycemia and poor peripheral perfusion, so that the glucose isn't used. Also, low K may result in decreased cell uptake of glucose.

BUN, creatinine, and phosphorus are increased. Urine specific gravity would help determine if renal or prerenal. Because of severe dehydration as indicated by increased albumin, at least a prerenal component is likely. Phosphorus may also be increased due to high GI obstruction, which is likely the diagnosis.

Calcium is slightly decreased. Phosphorus is excreted in the saliva of ruminants; with GI obstruction, elimination of phosphorus via the GI tract is decreased. Mild hypocalcemia has been reported with abomasal and forestomach disease.

Total protein and albumin are increased, indicating dehydration. Globulin is increased, which may be due to dehydration or antigenic stimulation.

Bilirubin is increased, which in this patient may be due to cholestasis or anorexia.

Serum creatine kinase activity is increased, probably indicative of myopathy. AST is mildly increased, either from myopathy or hepatocellular damage.

Marked hypochloremia is probably due to abomasal acid secretion into the lumen. Obstruction of abomasal outflow and distention exacerbates. Chloride is decreased more than would be expected with abomasal displacement or volvulus; this degree of hypochloremia is indicative of high GI obstruction. Potassium is likely decreased for the same reason.

Sodium is low and is perhaps being lost in urine. This may be due to hyperglycemia resulting in osmotic diuresis and thus increasing urinary losses of electrolytes.

Hyperosmolality may also be contributing to hyponatremia, as a result of cellular water moving into extracellular fluid compartment, diluting serum sodium (1.6 mEq/l decrease in Na for every 100 mg/dl increase in glucose)

Total CO_2 and HCO_3 are increased, indicating marked hypochloremic metabolic alkalosis. pH is in the high normal range as a result of compensatory respiratory acidosis (increased pCO_2). Remarkable hypochloremia and alkalosis indicated that there is obstruction of abomasal outflow, preventing re-exchange of chloride and bicarbonate.

Increased anion gap (36 mEq/L) also indicates increase in unmeasured anions. Most of the anions contributing to this are not truly "unmeasured," but are the increased phosphates and protein. Additionally, there may be increased lactate due to decreased tissue perfusion, or increased sulfates due to tissue breakdown.

Summary

This animal had a high GI obstruction (foreign body), thus explaining many of the abnormalities.

Azotemia was probably prerenal due to dehydration, although there are abnormalities in distal tubular transport that may be due to hypochloremia; osmotic diuresis may be also contributing to these abnormalities.

Inflammation is present, perhaps associated with the GI obstruction.

Iron deficiency anemia from chronic blood loss is present (perhaps abomasal ulcer, GI parasites).

Other tests that should be performed include urinalysis, especially specific gravity, and fecal occult blood.

CASES

Case 80

Signalment: 9-day-old female Holstein
History: Several days' duration of diarrhea, anorexia, extreme weakness
Physical examination: Hypothermic, 12% dehydrated

Hematology		Reference interval
PCV (%)	**51**	24–46
NCC ($\times 10^3/\mu L$)	**19.7**	4.0–12.0
Segs ($\times 10^3/\mu L$)	**11.4**	0.6–4.0
Monos ($\times 10^3/\mu L$)	**2.0**	0–0.8
Lymphs ($\times 10^3/\mu L$)	6.3	2.5–7.5
Platelets ($\times 10^3/\mu L$)	Adequate	200–800

Biochemical profile		Reference interval
Gluc (mg/dL)	**46**	55–95
BUN (mg/dL)	**63**	7–20
Great (mg/dL)	**3.7**	1.0–1.8
Ca (mg/dL)	**5.9**	8.2–9.9
Phos (mg/dL)	**14.5**	4.3–7.0
TP (g/dL)	**3.0**	6.3–7.6
Alb (g/dL)	**1.9**	2.5–4.3
Glob (g/dL)	**1.1**	2.6–5.0
T. bili (mg/dL)	0.2	0.1–0.4
CK (IU/L)	**7819**	57–280
AST (IU/L)	**177**	40–130
GGT (IU/L)	**28**	10–26
Na (mEq/L)	**158**	136–147
K (mEq/L)	**7.9**	3.6–5.2
CL (mEq/L)	**117**	95–105
TCO_2 (mEq/L)	**15**	24–32
An. gap (mEq/L)	**33.9**	14–26

Blood gas data (venous)		Reference interval
pH	**7.140**	7.32–7.45
pCO_2 (mmHg)	**45.7**	34–44
HCO_3 (mEq/L)	**15.3**	23–31

Interpretive discussion

Hematology

There is a neutrophilia and monocytosis, indicating an inflammatory leukogram. The PCV is increased, reflecting hemoconcentration due to dehydration.

Biochemical profile

There is a profound hypoglycemia, which in a neonatal calf with diarrhea is most probably related to decreased food intake, as well as the possibility of sepsis. Considering the increased neutrophil concentration, sepsis is unlikely.

The BUN and serum creatinine concentrations are increased, but the origin of this azotemia cannot be discerned without a urinalysis. However, given the other evidence of hemoconcentration, prerenal azotemia is the most likely cause. Although higher serum phosphorus concentrations are common in young animals, this degree of hyperphosphatemia is more likely related to decreased glomerular filtration rate. There is a marked hypocalcemia, but this may be due solely to the hypoalbuminemia; i.e., the ionized calcium concentration may be normal, but the protein-bound fraction is decreased.

There is marked hypoproteinemia, despite the severe degree of dehydration. This is due both to hypoalbuminemia and hypoglobulinemia. The former may be due to liver disease, inanition, or intestinal loss associated with the diarrhea. The latter is very likely due to lack of passive transfer, which would have subsequently predisposed this neonate to infections, resulting in diarrhea and sepsis.

The increased serum CK and AST activities may be due to muscle damage, to prolonged recumbency, or hypoperfusion. The very slight increase in GGT activity may be due to absorption of a small amount of colostrum, which is high in GGT activity in ruminants.

The increased serum sodium and chloride indicate that this calf is hypertonically dehydrated. One typically expects hypotonic dehydration to develop in a neonatal calf with scours, owing to electrolyte loss in the secretory diarrhea. Thus, it is more likely that this is not a secretory diarrhea but rather another infectious cause of diarrhea, with or without septicemia. Water loss in excess of solute may be compounded by reduced water consumption, increased insensible losses due to fever, and/or exudation (along with albumin) across a damaged intestinal mucosa. Although there may have been significant potassium loss in the diarrhea, redistributional hyperkalemia is commonly observed in cases like this owing to exchange of intracellular potassium for extracellular protons (H^+) in response to the metabolic acidosis. The respiratory acidosis suggests inadequate pulmonary perfusion.

Blood gas data

There is a combined metabolic (decreased bicarbonate) and respiratory (increased pCO_2) acidosis. The metabolic acidosis results from bicarbonate loss in the diarrhea and from lactic acidosis due to tissue hypoperfusion. The increased anion gap reflects the accumulation of unmeasured anions like lactate.

Summary

Nonsecretory diarrhea and hypertonic dehydration in a neonatal calf following failure of passive transfer.

Case 81

Signalment: 6-year-old male castrated Yorkshire terrier
History: Intermittent vomiting and diarrhea for past 7 weeks, seizured for a few minutes a few hours before presentation
Physical examination: Lethargic, weak, "bloated"

Hematology	8/8	8/17	Reference interval
Packed cell volume (%)	**28**	**22**	40–55
Hgb (g/dL)	**8.9**	**7.0**	13–20
RBC ($10^6/\mu L$)	**3.81**	**2.95**	5.5–8.5
MCV (fL)	73	73	62–73
MCHC (g/dL)	**32**	**32**	33–36
Total nucleated cell count ($\times 10^3/\mu L$)	**17.3**	**17.9**	4.5–15
Segmented neutrophils ($\times 10^3/\mu L$)	**14.4 (83%)**	**16.3**	2.6–11
Band neutrophils ($\times 10^3/\mu L$)	**0.3** (2%)		0–0.2
Monocytes ($\times 10^3/\mu L$)	0.3 (2%)	1.3	0.2–1.0
Lymphocytes ($\times 10^3/\mu L$)	1.9 (11%)	**0.2**	1–4.8
Eosinophils ($\times 10^3/\mu L$)		0.2	0.1–1.2
Platelets ($\times 10^3/\mu L$)	302	323	200–500
Plasma protein (g/dL)	**2.5**	**2.9**	6–8
Reticulocytes ($\times 10^3$)	**80** (2.1%)	**209** (7.1%)	60

Hemopathology: Slight polychromasia, slightly toxic neutrophils.

Biochemical profile	Slightly hemolyzed		Reference interval
Glucose (mg/dL)	123	99	75–130
Blood urea nitrogen (mg/dL)	8	9	7–28
Creatinine (mg/dL)	**0.5**	**0.4**	0.7–1.9
Calcium (mg/dL)	**4.4**	**5.1**	9.0–11.7
Phosphorus (mg/dL)	**1.7**	**1.5**	2.1–6.0
Magnesium (mg/dL)	**0.9**	**0.7**	1.8–2.5
Total protein (g/dL)	**2.1**	**2.3**	5.4–7.4
Albumin (g/dL)	**1.2**	**1.2**	2.7–4.5
Globulin (g/dL)	**0.9**	**1.1**	2.0–3.8
Total bilirubin (mg/dL)	0.1	0.1	0–0.3
Cholesterol (mg/dL)	**69**	**71**	130–300
Alanine aminotransferase (IU/L)	**600**	**274**	10–110
Aspartate aminotransferase (IU/L)	**540**	**163**	16–50
Alkaline phosphatase (IU/L)	**660**	**405**	20–142
Creatine kinase (IU/L)	**1343**	**356**	50–275
GGT (IU/L)	**77**	**108**	0–9
Sodium (mEq/L)	**136**	**140**	142–152
Potassium (mEq/L)	**2.9**	3.6	3.5–5.2
Chloride (mEq/L)	**106**	109	108–120
Bicarbonate (mEq/L)	17.6	20.6	16–25
Anion gap (mEq/L)	15	14	13–22
Calc. osmolality (mOsm/L)	**267**	275	284–304
Iron	100	140	75–280
TIBC	110	153	
Sat percent	91	92	
UIBC	<10	13	
Ionized calcium (mmol/L)	0.96	0.80	1.30–1.46

Coagulation		Reference interval
Protime (s)	17.5	7.5–10.5
aPTT (s)	52.9	10.5–16.5

Antithrombin 45% of normal pooled sera.

Interpretive discussion

Hematology

Regenerative anemia is present as evidenced by reticulocytosis. This may be due to blood loss or blood destruction. Hypomagnesemia has been reported to cause hemolytic anemia in humans. The total protein is not useful to differentiate hemolysis from loss in this case, as it is likely decreased due to other causes. Blood loss could be though the GI tract.

An inflammatory leukogram is present as evidenced by neutrophilia and increased bands on 8/8.

A stress leukogram is present on 8/17 as evidenced by mature neutrophilia and lymphopenia. A monocytosis may be a component of a stress leukogram.

Plasma protein by refractometry is markedly decreased (see biochemical profile interpretation).

Biochemical profile

Numerous biochemical profiles were performed over several weeks. The common abnormalities are marked hypoproteinemia, hypoalbuminemia, hypoglobulinemia, and hypocalcemia, Hypocholesterolemia is present in three of the profiles, as well. All but the first biochemical profile also showed increased ALT, AST, ALP, and CK. Sodium and potassium are decreased in the last three profiles, and serum magnesium is markedly decreased. Serum creatinine is also decreased on the last two profiles. These abnormalities are discussed below.

Panhypoproteinemia

The most likely differential for a decrease of this magnitude in both serum albumin and globulin, particularly in a dog with a history of diarrhea, is protein losing enteropathy. Other possible causes would be blood loss or loss of protein into the abdominal cavity due to inflammation. The PCV is not low enough to explain this degree of hypoproteinemia.

Hypocalcemia

While some of the hypocalcemia can be explained by hypoalbuminemia, this cannot account for this degree of hypocalcemia. When corrected for hypoalbuminemia, the calcium is still low. (For example, in the profile on 8/17, $5.1 - 1.2 + 3.5 = 7.4$.) The decreased ionized calcium further substantiates that both ionized and bound calcium are decreased.

There is probably no differential for this degree of hypocalcemia other than the hypocalcemia that may occur in patients with protein losing enteropathy, since primary hypoparathyroidism should result in increased phosphorus concentration. While hypocalcemia with protein losing enteropathy is usually because of hypoalbuminemia, decreased ionized calcium may also occur in these patients as a result of decreased GI calcium absorption and also because of decreased vitamin D absorption. Hypomagnesemia may also result in hypocalcemia by leading to decreased synthesis or release of PTH or by leading to decreased responsiveness to PTH by skeletal and renal tissue. Moreover, hypomagnesemia can cause decreased activation of vitamin D by kidneys.

The hypomagnesemia is severe and in this case is likely due to loss through the GI tract. Decreased vitamin D may result in decreased magnesium absorption.

(Other possible causes of hypomagnesemia include loss through the kidney or shifts of magnesium from extracellular to intracellular, but there is no evidence for renal disease. Other disorders associated with hypomagnesemia include diuresis, diabetic ketoacidosis, pancreatitis, sepsis, and primary hyperparathyroidism, but again, there is no history or evidence of these.)

Hypocholesterolemia is usually due to either decreased intake through the GI tract, or decreased production as a result of liver failure. In this patient, it is likely due to increased intake, secondary to protein losing enteropathy.

Increased ALT and AST in later profiles are indicative of hepatocellular damage, although the AST may be increased due to muscle damage, as CK is increased. ALT may be induced by steroids, as well.

Increased GGT and ALP may be due to cholestasis or induced by corticosteroids. The serum alkaline phosphatase and GGT were not increased in the initial biochemical profile performed by the referring veterinarian. Additional history revealed that the dog had been receiving injectable glucocorticosteroids, which are likely responsible for the increase in these enzymes. The dog likely has a steroid hepatopathy at this time.

Hyponatremia and hypokalemia are also likely due to losses through the GI tract.

The increase in aPTT and PT are likely due to decreased vitamin K absorption, as it is also a fat-soluble vitamin.

The decreased antithrombin III is likely due to concurrent albumin losses.

Additional tests needed

Parathyroid hormone assay, vitamin D assay.

Summary

The most likely diagnosis in this dog is protein losing enteropathy with resulting severe hypocalcemia and hypomagnesemia, and likely secondary hypoparathyroidism.

Outcome

PTH was low normal and vitamin D was decreased. Small bowel biopsy showed mixed inflammation, dilated crypts, necrosis, bacterial overgrowth, and mild lymphangiectasia. Dog had positive occult blood in feces. It was treated by changing diet (Eukanuba low-residue dry), Prednisone (1.3 mg/kg bid), Tums, and enrofloxacin (Baytril), and coconut oil (10–20 mL per day added to food).

Case 82

Signalment: 10-year-old spayed female mixed-breed dog
History: Chronic weight loss, chronic voluminous diarrhea, ravenous appetite
Physical examination: Bright and alert, thin with a 1/5 body condition score, 5% dehydrated

Hematology		Reference interval
Packed cell volume (%)	37	36–54
Plasma protein (g/dL)	**5.2**	5.4–7.2

Biochemical profile		Reference interval
Glucose (mg/dL)	94	77–126
Blood urea nitrogen (mg/dL)	17	5–20
Creatinine (mg/dL)	1.1	0.6–1.6
Calcium (mg/dL)	9.7	9.3–11.6
Phosphorus (mg/dL)	4.1	3.2–8.1
Total protein (g/dL)	5.3	5.1–7.1
Albumin (g/dL)	3.0	2.9–4.2
Globulin (g/dL)	2.3	2.2–2.9
Total bilirubin (mg/dL)	0.1	0.1–0.4
Cholesterol (mg/dL)	**49**	80–315
ALT (IU/L)	44	10–55
AST (IU/L)	23	12–40
ALP (IU/L)	66	15–120
Creatine kinase (IU/L)	81	50–400
Sodium (mEq/L)	145	143–153
Potassium (mEq/L)	4.1	4.1–5.4
Chloride (mEq/L)	112	109–120
TCO_2 (mEq/L)	22	16–25
Anion gap	15	15–25

Other data		
Bile acids–fasting (µmol/L)	1.0	<15.5
Bile acids–post prandial (µmol/L)	7	5–20
Folate (µg/L)	20.4	7.7–24.4
Cobalamine-B12 (ng/L)	**154**	251–908
Trypsin-like immunoreactivity (TLI)–fasting (µg/L)	**0.2**	5.7–45.2
Fecal float	Negative	

Interpretive discussion

The decrease in the plasma protein may be compatible with loss of protein or decreased protein production. On the biochemical profile, total protein, albumin and globulins are at the low end of the reference interval. Because the dog is dehydrated, it is possible that these values will decrease below the reference interval when the animal is rehydrated. Given the history of chronic diarrhea and the low body condition score, protein losing enteropathy or exocrine pancreatic insufficiency (EPI) are primary differential diagnoses.

The hypocholesterolemia can be the result of malabsorption, maldigestion, protein losing enteropathy, or liver failure. Given the normal liver enzymes and total bilirubin, there is no evidence of hepatocellular damage or cholestasis. However, liver enzymes do not measure liver function: fasting and postprandial bile acids were done to evaluate for hepatic insufficiency. Given the normal fasting and postprandial bile acids, decreased production of cholesterol secondary to hepatic insufficiency is unlikely.

The low normal total protein, albumin, and globulin in conjunction with hypocholesterolemia is compatible with protein losing enteropathy or EPI resulting in malabsorption and maldigestion, respectively. Both of these conditions are associated with diarrhea and weight loss. Differentiating these two conditions requires additional testing. The normal serum folate in conjunction with decreased cobalamnie-B12 is compatible with distal small intestinal disease or EPI. The low TLI is diagnostic for EPI.

Summary

This dog was diagnosed with exocrine pancreatic insufficiency (EPI), and she responded to dietary supplementation with pancreatic enzymes and cobalamine injections. The syndrome of EPI results from inadequate production and release of pancreatic enzymes into the intestinal tract. Maldigestion and malabsorption of nutrients results in diarrhea that is often voluminous. Steatorrhea and hypocholesterolemia are consequences of maldigestion and malabsorption of fats. Unlike patients with protein losing enteropathy, many patients with EPI maintain their serum protein within the reference interval. Intrinsic factor is required for absorption of dietary cobalamine/vitamin B12. Because the pancreas is the source of intrinsic factor in the dog, cobalamine deficiency may develop as a result of malabsorption secondary to EPI and is reflected in the low serum cobalamine levels seen in this patient. Pancreatic ascinar atrophy is the most common cause of EPI in younger dogs and is seen most commonly in the German shepherd breed. When pancreatic ascinar atrophy occurs in an older dog such as this patient, other causes of EPI such as pancreatitis or neoplasia should be explored.

Contributor: Dr. M. Judith Radin

Case 83

Signalment: 4-year-old male mixed-breed dog that weighs 31 kg

History: Anorexia and vomiting for 1 week

Physical examination: Dehydrated. Hypovolemic shock on presentation.

Hematology	Day 1	Day 3	Reference range
Packed cell volume (%)	47	**25**	36–54
RBC ($\times 10^6/\mu L$)	7.02	**3.91**	5.5–8.5
Hgb (g/dL)	16.5	**8.8**	12–18
MCV (fL)	68	69	60–72
MCHC (g/dL)	34.5	32.5	34–38
Reticulocytes ($10^3/\mu L$)	NP	11.7	0–60
NCC ($10^3/\mu L$)	**42.5**	**37.3**	6.0–17.0
Segmented neutrophils ($10^3/\mu L$)	**36.1**	**33.9**	3.0–11.5
Band neutrophils ($10^3/\mu L$)	**0.8**	0	0–0.3
Monocytes ($10^3/\mu L$)	**3.5**	**2.2**	0.2–1.4
Lymphocytes ($10^3/\mu L$)	1.7	**0.7**	1.0–4.8
Eosinophils ($10^3/\mu L$)	0.4	0.4	0.1–1.2
Platelets ($10^3/\mu L$)	229	**158**	200–500
Plasma protein by refractometry (g/dL)	**10.5**	**5.6**	6.0–8.0

Biochemical profile	Day 1	Day 3	Reference range
Glucose (mg/dL)	**120**	110	60–110
Blood urea nitrogen (mg/dL)	**78**	15	7–25
Creatinine (mg/dL)	**2.9**	1.0	0.3–1.4
Calcium (mg/dL)	**12.1**	9.0	8.6–11.3
Phosphorus (mg/dL)	**9.4**	**2.3**	2.9–6.6
Total protein (g/dL)	**9.8**	**5.2**	5.4–8.2
Albumin (g/dL)	4.4	2.5	2.5–4.4
Globulin (g/dL)	**5.4**	2.7	2.3–5.2
Total bilirubin (mg/dL)	0.3	0.3	0.1–0.6
ALT (IU/L)	56	10	10–118
ALP (IU/L)	65	51	20–150
Sodium (mEq/L)	**134**	**135**	138–160
Potassium (mEq/L)	**3.2**	**3.1**	3.7–5.8
Chloride (mEq/L)	**80**		108–120
Lactate (mmol/L)	**12.7**	**2.7**	**0.5–2.5**

Venous blood gases		Reference range
pH	**7.48**	7.31–7.46
pCO_2 mmHg	30	28–50
HCO_3 (mEq/L)	**32**	17–28

Abdominal surgery was performed on Day 1.

Interpretive discussion

CBC

The dog is anemic on Day 3, likely due to blood loss and rehydration. Considering that the dog was clinically dehydrated on presentation, the PCV on Day 1 is likely falsely increased.

An inflammatory leukogram is present, as indicated by the marked neutrophilia and presence of band neutrophils on Day 1. The monocytosis on Day 1 is also likely due to inflammation. A stress or corticosteroid leukogram is also present on Day 3, as indicated by the lymphopenia.

The platelets are slightly decreased on Day 3, possibly secondary to blood loss.

The plasma protein is markedly increased on Day 1, which should trigger measurement of albumin and globulin, and is compatible with marked dehydration.

Chemistry

A mild hyperglycemia is compatible with stress and increased cortisol.

Increased BUN and creatinine, indicating decreased glomerular filtration rate, resolved completely with fluids, indicating prerenal azotemia. The BUN is relatively more increased than the creatinine, suggesting prerenal azotemia. A urine analysis was not performed, but presumably the urine specific gravity would have indicated the ability to concentrate.

Hypercalcemia is mild and normalizes with fluid therapy. This may be due to dehydration (associated with a high-normal albumin) and decreased GFR; an ionized calcium would help determine if a true hypercalcemia is present.

The hyperphosphatemia is also due to decreased glomerular filtration, and corrects with fluid therapy. The calcium × phosphorus product is 114, suggesting the possibility of mineralization of the kidneys. However, the improvement of the azotemia following fluid therapy indicates that this has not occurred.

Marked hyperproteinemia is evident on Day 1. Albumin is at the high end of the reference interval, and hyperglobulinemia is present. This may be due to antigenic stimulation, but since it normalizes following fluid therapy, the hyperglobulinemia is likely due to dehydration. It is also possible that the protein decrease is due to blood loss.

Hyponatremia and hypokalemia are likely due to loss due to vomiting. Chloride is very low (corrected chloride is approximately 90), indicating a disproportionate loss of chloride. This is likely due to loss of gastric fluid in the vomitus consistent with a hypochloremic metabolic alkalosis.

Serum lactate is markedly increased, indicating severe lactic acidosis. The dog is alkalemic as indicated by the increased pH, and has a high blood bicarbonate, confirming metabolic alkalosis. This dog has a mixed acid-base status. In spite of the increased lactate, the dog has a metabolic alkalosis as a result of vomiting gastric fluid.

Summary

The presence of hypochloridemia and metabolic alkalosis in a vomiting dog suggests bowel obstruction and should trigger abdominal radiographs (Figure 1). The most common electrolyte and acid base abnormalities in dogs with gastrointestinal foreign bodies, regardless of the site or type of foreign body, are hypochloremia (51%), metabolic alkalosis (45%), hypokalemia (25%), and hyponatremia (20%). Hypochloremic, hypokalemic metabolic alkalosis is seen with both proximal and distal gastrointestinal foreign bodies.

Abdominal radiographs

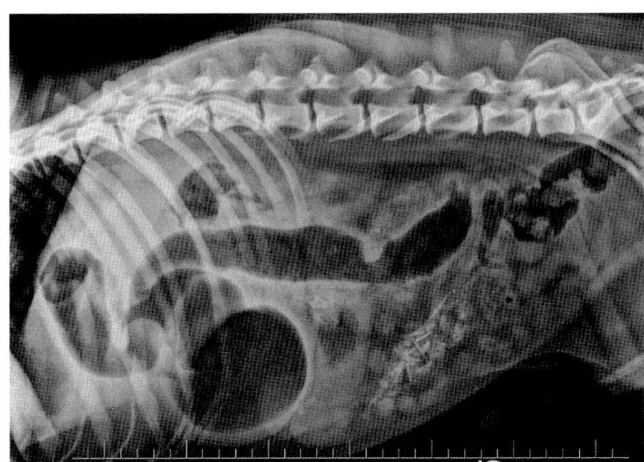

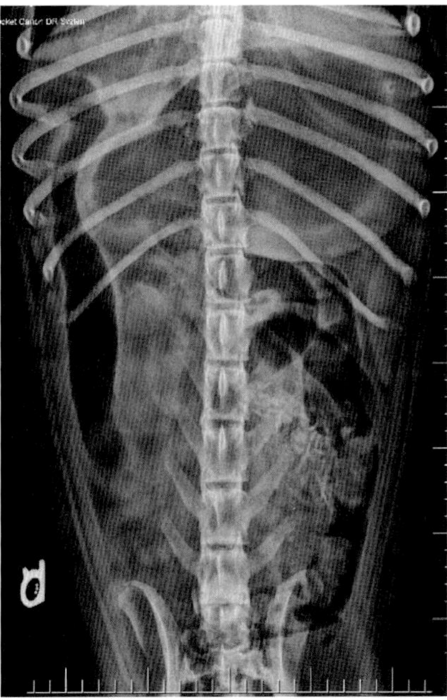

Figure 1 The stomach is distended with gas and fluid. There are two populations of small intestine with regard to diameter. The larger population includes the descending duodenum and some of the jejunum. The distended segments contain fluid and gas. In the lateral view there is also a region of distended small intestine in the caudal abdomen that contains bone shards accumulating against a rectangular object with a reticular gas pattern, this object is typical of a corncob. The images are diagnostic of a proximal small intestinal obstruction due to corncob ingestion.

Contributors: Drs. Mary Anna Thrall and Donald Thrall

CASES

Case 84

Signalment: 4-year-old neutered male dachshund
History: Anorexia and vomiting for 4 days
Physical examination: Dehydrated and lethargic

Hematology		Reference range
Packed cell volume (%)	**61**	40–55
RBC (×10⁶/μL)	**9.5**	5.5–8.5
Hgb (g/dL)	**21**	13–20
MCV (fL)	63	62–73
MCHC (g/dL)	34	33–36
NCC (10³/μL)	**24.4**	4.5–15
Segmented neutrophils (10³/μL)	**20.3** (83%)	2.6–11
Monocytes (10³/μL)	**3.7** (15%)	0.2–1.0
Lymphocytes (10³/μL)	**0.5** (2%)	1.0–4.8
Platelets (10³/μL)	413	200–500
Plasma protein by refractometry (g/dL)	**10.2**	6.0–8.0

Biochemical profile		Reference range
Glucose (mg/dL)	**141**	75–130
Blood urea nitrogen (mg/dL)	**138**	7–32
Creatinine (mg/dL)	**4.5**	0.4–1.5
Calcium (mg/dL)	9.7	9.2–11.7
Phosphorus (mg/dL)	**13.9**	2.1–6.0
Total protein (g/dL)	**9.1**	5.3–7.2
Albumin (g/dL)	**4.8**	2.5–4.0
Globulin (g/dL)	**4.3**	2.0–3.8
Total bilirubin (mg/dL)	**0.4**	0–0.3
Cholesterol (mg/dL)	**466**	130–250
ALT (IU/L)	48	10–110
ALP (IU/L)	**215**	20–142
Sodium (mEq/L)	**136**	142–152
Potassium (mEq/L)	**4.1**	3.5–5.2
Chloride (mEq/L)	**72**	108–120
Bicarbonate (mEq/L)	**26.4**	16–25
Anion gap (mEq/L)	**42**	13–22
Calculated osmolality (mOsm/kg)	**318**	284–304
Amylase (IU/L)	**2136**	50–1200
Lipase (IU/L)	**1138**	30–650

Urinalysis	
Specific gravity	1.022
pH	5

No other abnormalities.

Interpretive discussion

Hematology

Packed cell volume, hemoglobin, and red blood cell count are all increased. Considering the clinical evidence of dehydration and increased total protein, this is likely a relative erythrocytosis secondary to water loss as a result of vomiting. A leukocytosis is present due to neutrophilia and monocytosis. Considering the lymphopenia, the neutrophilia and monocytosis likely represent a stress leukogram. Plasma protein by refractometry is increased due to dehydration and there is a discrepancy of 1.1 g/dL between the refractometric estimate of total protein on the plasma and the biuret method on the clinical chemistry. While 0.2–0.4 g/dL discrepancy is expected, due to the presence of fibrinogen in the plasma, a discrepancy of approximately 0.7–0.9 g/dL remains in this patient, and can be explained by the increased serum urea and cholesterol, both of which contribute to the total solids measured by refractometry. Every 39 mg/dL in cholesterol accounts for an increase in the plasma protein refractometric reading by 0.14 g/dL [1]. Since the cholesterol in this patient is approximately 200 mg/dL over the upper limit of the reference range, cholesterol could be increasing the total protein estimate by approximately 0.5 g/dL. Moreover, azotemic patients may have refractometric total protein estimates of 0.5 g/dL or more over protein measured by the biuret assay, further explaining the marked discrepancy [2].

Chemistry

A mild hyperglycemia is compatible with stress and increased cortisol.

Increased BUN and creatinine, indicating decreased glomerular filtration rate, may be prerenal due to hydration, or renal. The urine specific gravity is 1.022, and while this might suggest renal impairment, the hyponatremia is likely interfering with concentrating ability due to medullary wash out (see below). The hyperphosphatemia is also due to decreased glomerular filtration.

Hyperproteinemia, hyperalbuminemia and hyperglobulinemia are present, likely due to dehydration, although an increase in immunoglobulins due to antigenic stimulation could be causing the hyperglobulinemia.

Bilirubin is very slightly increased, and since the dog is not anemic, this is either due to an intrahepatic cause, or cholestasis.

The cholesterol is markedly increased, and while cholesterol increases with cholestasis, this hypercholesterolemia is so marked that hypothyroidism and Cushing syndrome should be considered. Tests for endocrine function were not performed.

The ALP activity is increased, which in this case is also compatible with mild cholestasis, but could also be due to steroid induction.

Hyponatremia and hypokalemia are due to loss in vomitus. The hypokalemia may also be due to movement of potassium into cells, and hydrogen out of cells, in an attempt to correct the alkalosis. Chloride is very low, indicating a disproportionate loss of chloride when compared to sodium. This is likely due to loss of gastric fluid in the vomitus consistent with a hypochloremic metabolic alkalosis.

The bicarbonate is increased, indicating a metabolic alkalosis. Blood gas was not performed.

The anion gap is increased, indicating increased unmeasured anions. In this patient, the most likely cause of the increased anion gap is lactate, although acids due to azotemia may be contributing. Serum lactate was not performed.

Calculated osmolality is increased, in this case primarily due to increased urea.

Both amylase and lipase activity are increased, and while pancreatitis cannot be excluded, decreased glomerular filtration results in an increase in both serum amylase and lipase activity, because the enzymes are presumably eliminated through the kidney.

Urinalysis

The urine specific gravity is 1.022. Specific gravity should be at least greater than 1.035 in a dehydrated dog whose kidneys are concentrating maximally. However, the patient is hyponatremic, which is interfering with concentrating ability due to medullary washout. The urine is acidic, and in a dog with metabolic alkalosis this is indicative of paradoxical aciduria. The hypochloremia and hypovolemia stimulate aldosterone, which promotes sodium resorption by the kidney. Normally sodium is exchanged for potassium, but since potassium is depleted, it is exchanged for hydrogen, resulting in a paradoxic aciduria.

Summary and outcome

The presence of hypochloremia and metabolic alkalosis in a vomiting dog strongly suggests bowel obstruction, and should trigger abdominal radiographs. The most common electrolyte and acid base abnormalities in dogs with gastrointestinal foreign bodies, regardless of the site or type of foreign body, are hypochloremia (51%), metabolic alkalosis (45%), hypokalemia (25%), and hyponatremia (20%). Hypochloremic, hypokalemic metabolic alkalosis is seen with both proximal and distal gastrointestinal foreign bodies [3].

Unfortunately, abdominal radiographs were not performed in this patient, and an erroneous diagnosis of acute renal failure due to ethylene glycol toxicosis was made due to the presence of azotemia, relatively low urine specific gravity, and increased anion gap. The dog was euthanized, and at autopsy a peach pit (seed) was observed obstructing the intestine approximately 30 cm aboral to the pyloric sphincter. No histopathologic evidence of kidney disease or liver disease was seen, and no other gross lesions were observed. This case emphasizes the importance of suspecting an intestinal foreign body when hypochloremic metabolic alkalosis is observed.

Contributor: Dr. Mary Anna Thrall

Case 85

Signalment: 4-year-old spayed female German shepherd dog

History: Intermittent vomiting and voluminous diarrhea on and off since birth

Hematology		Reference interval
Packed cell volume (%)	38.0	37–55
Hemoglobin (g/dL)	12.0	12–18
RBC (10^6/μL)	5.51	5.5–8.5
MCV (fL)	69.0	60–72
TNCC (×10^3/μL)	8.5	6–17
Segmented neutrophils (×10^3/μL)	6.2	3–11.5
Monocytes (×10^3/μL)	0.6	0.1–1.3
Lymphocytes (×10^3/μL)	1.4	1–4.8
Eosinophils (×10^3/μL)	**0.3**	0–0.1
Platelets (×10^3/μL)	298	150–900
Plasma protein (g/dL)	**5.5**	6–8

Hemopathology: Clumped platelets.

Biochemical profile		Reference range
Glucose (mg/dL)	91	65–122
Blood urea nitrogen (mg/dL)	11	7–28
Creatinine (mg/dL)	1.3	0.9–1.7
Calcium (mg/dL)	9.0	9.0–11.2
Phosphorus (mg/dL)	3.3	2.8–6.1
Total protein (g/dL)	**5.1**	5.4–7.4
Albumin (g/dL)	**2.5**	2.7–4.5
Globulin (g/dL)	2.6	1.9–3.4
Total bilirubin (mg/d(g/dL))	0.3	0–0.4
Cholesterol (g/dL)	**125**	130–370
ALT (IU/L)	50	10–120
AST (IU/L)	34	16–40
ALP (IU/L)	235	35–280
GGT (IU/L)	5	0–6
Sodium (mEq/L)	148	145–158
Potassium (mEq/L)	**5.8**	4.1–5.5
Chloride (mEq/L)	119	106–127
Total CO_2 (mEq/L)	**13.1**	14–27
Anion gap (mEq/L)	21.7	8–25

Additional tests		Reference interval
Urine protein: creatinine ratio	0.2	<0.5
Cobalamin (vitamin B12) (ng/L)	**180**	252–908
Folate (μg/L)	**28.9**	7.7–24.2
TLI (μg/L)	**2.1**	5–35
Fecal alpha-1 protease inhibitor (μg/g feces)	**18.1**	0.23–5.67

Interpretive discussion

Hematology

A mild eosinophilia is usually associated with hypersensitivity reactions that may be secondary to allergic or parasitic disease, but mild eosinophilia can also be seen in this breed and in Rottweilers. In cases where there is a lack of a stress leukogram, Addison's disease should always be considered. A baseline cortisol or an ACTH stimulation test is recommended to rule in or out Addison's disease.

The plasma proteins are decreased, which may be due to decreased albumin (decreased production or loss) or decreased globulins. See chemistry section.

Chemistry

Glucose, phosphorus and renal parameters are within reference intervals.

Calcium is low normal and may be associated with the low albumin as approximately 40% of total calcium is albumin bound.

Total proteins and albumin are decreased with globulins within reference interval.

Decreases in albumin may be associated with decreased production by the liver or losses due to GIT or renal disease or third space shifting. Exudative skin disease is another less common possibility. Albumin may be decreased with severe or end stage liver disease, but this is not apparent on this sample. Liver enzymes are not necessarily increased in these cases as healthy functional hepatocytes are required to produce enzymes. The liver also produces BUN, glucose, and cholesterol. BUN and glucose are within reference intervals, making severe liver disease and decreased production less likely. Renal albumin loss can be excluded by the low urine protein:creatinine ratio.

GIT protein loss is evidenced by the increase in fecal $\alpha 1$-proteinase inhibitor (PI).

This is a protein that resists degradation by digestive and bacterial proteinases in feces and has nearly the same molecular mass as albumin and that is lost into the GI lumen at approximately the same rate as albumin and other plasma proteins. Both dogs and cats with gastrointestinal protein loss have an increased fecal α_1 PI concentration before protein loss is severe enough to notice hypoalbuminemia. α_1-PI of one individual sample of $\geq$15.0 µg/g feces is considered abnormal.

Liver enzymes are all within reference intervals, which suggests no overt liver abnormality. Normal serum bile acids would confirm normal hepatic function in most cases.

Cholesterol is decreased. Hypocholesterolemia can be associated with both liver failure and PLE, but elevations in $\alpha 1$-proteinase inhibitor can be used to differentiate these and should be normal in cases of liver disease.

The total CO_2 is mildly decreased suggesting a metabolic acidosis, which may be seen with diarrhea. This tends to be associated with increases in potassium. Anion gap is within reference interval in this case.

Other Tests

A decrease in vitamin B_{12} (cobalamin) with increased folate (because of bacterial overgrowth) in dogs suggests EPI, and TLI testing is indicated. Bacterial overgrowth increases serum folate concentrations because of bacterial synthesis of folate, and it decreases serum vitamin B_{12} concentrations because of bacterial binding of vitamin B_{12}.

Small intestinal bacterial overgrowth (SIBO) should always be considered with this combination of results. In this case the TLI is decreased, which is consistent with EPI (exocrine pancreatic insufficiency). Antibiotic responsive diarrhea (SIBO) is a relatively widespread secondary problem in dogs with EPI, and a common cause of cobalamin deficiency in dogs. Low B_{12} and high folate has a low sensitivity (5%) for detecting bacterial overgrowth but has high specificity (almost 100%).

Summary

This dog was diagnosed with exocrine pancreatic insufficiency (EPI) with concurrent antibiotic responsive diarrhea small intestinal bacterial overgrowth (SIBO). There was secondary gastrointestinal protein loss.

Contributor: Dr. dawn Seddon

CASES

Case 86

Signalment: 2-year-old border collie
History: Weight loss and diarrhea for 3 months
Physical examination: Emaciated and slightly weak. Pasty, light brown stools noted.

Hematology		Reference interval
Packed cell volume (%)	38.0	37–55
Hemoglobin (g/dL)	12.0	12–18
RBC ($10^6/\mu L$)	5.51	5.5–8.5
MCV (fL)	69.0	62–73
Total nucleated cell count ($\times 10^3/\mu L$)	8.3	6–17
Segmented neutrophils ($\times 10^3/\mu L$)	6.6	3–11.5
Monocytes ($\times 10^3/\mu L$)	0.6	0.1–1.3
Lymphocytes ($\times 10^3/\mu L$)	1.1	1–4.8
Platelets ($\times 10^3/\mu L$)	298	150–900
Plasma protein (g/dL)	**5.0**	6–8
Hemopathology: clumped platelets		

Biochemical profile		Reference interval
Glucose (mg/dL)	110	65–122
Blood urea nitrogen (mg/dL)	16	7–28
Creatinine (mg/dL)	**0.8**	0.9–1.7
Calcium (mg/dL)	10.1	9.0–11.2
Phosphorus (mg/dL)	3.5	2.8–6.1
Total protein (g/dL)	**5.2**	5.4–7.4
Albumin (g/dL)	**2.2**	2.7–4.5
Globulin (g/dL)	3.0	1.9–3.4
Total bilirubin (mg/dL)	0.3	0–0.4
Cholesterol (mg/dL)	**120**	130–370
ALT (alanine aminotransferase) (IU/L)	115	10–120
AST (aspartate aminotransferase) (IU/L)	30	16–40
ALP (alkaline phosphatase) (IU/L)	**320**	35–280
Sodium (mEq/L)	149	145–158
Potassium (mEq/L)	4.5	4.1–5.5
Chloride (mEq/L)	107	106–127

Urinalysis	
Urine specific gravity	1.036
Urine pH	6

Other tests		Reference interval
Serum cobalamin pmol/l	**89**	140–300
Serum folate nmol/l	**38**	11–30
Fecal examination for parasites: negative.		

Interpretive discussion

Hematology

RBC parameters are at the lower end of the reference range and could reflect the early stages of an anemia of chronic disease.

Chemistry

A mild decrease in creatinine typically indicates low muscle mass and is often of minimal clinical significance. However, in this case it is most likely due to emaciation.

The hypoproteinemia characterized by hypoalbuminemia and the concurrent low cholesterol is probably due to gastrointestinal losses. Animals with protein losing enteropathies (PLEs) commonly have panhypoproteinemia, but if there is inflammation present this could increase the globulins, making interpretation difficult. Hypoalbuminemia and hypocholesterolemia can also be observed with hepatic insufficiency, albeit there is no overt evidence of hepatic disease in this case (ALT within normal limits). Bile acids are indicated to exclude the possibility of liver dysfunction.

The mild increase in ALP activity could be associated with gastrointestinal disease and is a relatively nonspecific finding. Furthermore, in dogs this could reflect induction of the corticosteroid isoenzyme associated with chronic stress.

Urinalysis

A USG of 1.036 demonstrates adequate renal concentration ability, as there is no azotemia or dehydration.

Other

Decreased B12 (cobalamin) and increased folate can be seen associated with small intestinal bacterial overgrowth (SIBO, antibiotic responsive diarrhea), and EPI.

Low B12 is also associated with villous atrophy and/or distal small intestinal disease.

Summary

Clinicopathological abnormalities in conjunction with the history and clinical signs are suggestive of a SIBO. A definitive diagnosis of SIBO is often difficult, but additional diagnostic tests may include Canine Microbiota Dysbiosis Index, or response to Tylosin. Specific culture of feces, and PCR may also be helpful.

Biopsy may be required in hypoproteinemic patients for a definitive etiological diagnosis but marked hypoalbuminemia in this patient could lead to dehiscence of an intestine biopsy.

A Trypsin-Like Immunoreactivity (TLI) assay would be required to rule out/in exocrine pancreatic insufficiency, a very possible differential diagnosis in this case.

Contributor: Dr. dawn Seddon

Case 87

Signalment: 5-year-old Labrador retriever

History: Three months' duration of intermittent vomiting. No response to bland diet of chicken and rice for 4 weeks and cimetidine for 2 weeks.

Physical examination: Thin, no abnormalities found on abdominal palpation, and well hydrated

Hematology		Reference range
CBC within reference intervals		
Total protein (g/dL)	**4.8**	5.3–7.4

Biochemical profile		Reference range
Glucose (mg/dL)	110	65–122
Blood urea nitrogen (mg/dL)	16	7–28
Creatinine (mg/dL)	1.1	0.9–1.7
Calcium (mg/dL)	**11.5**	9.0–11.2
Ionized calcium (mg/dL)	**5.9**	4.5–5.6
Phosphorus (mg/dL)	3.5	2.8–6.1
Total protein (g/dL)	**4.2**	5.4–7.4
Albumin (g/dL)	**2.1**	2.7–4.5
Globulin (g/dL)	2.1	1.9–3.4
Total bilirubin (mg/dL)	**0.5**	0–0.4
Cholesterol (mg/dL)	**110**	130–370
ALT (alanine aminotransferase) (IU/L)	**145**	10–120
AST (aspartate aminotransferase) (IU/L)	30	16–40
ALP (alkaline phosphatase) (IU/L)	**300**	35–280
Sodium (mEq/L)	148	145–158
Potassium (mEq/L)	4.3	4.1–5.5
Chloride (mEq/L)	**105**	106–127
HCO_3 (mEq/L)	15.1	14–27

Urinalysis	
Urine specific gravity	1.019
Urine pH	6
Negative dipstick for glucose, proteins, ketones, blood.	
Fecal examination for parasites negative.	

Interpretive discussion

Hematology

Hypoproteinemia was the only observed abnormality on hematology and will be discussed in the chemistry section.

Chemistry

Mildly increased total calcium is significant with a lowered albumin as 40% of total calcium is protein bound. This is verified by the increased ionized calcium, which reflects a true hypercalcemia. The most common differential for a chronic hypercalcemia in a mature dog is hypercalcemia of malignancy.

Hypoproteinemia characterized by a hypoalbuminemia may suggest either decreased protein production, protein losing nephropathy (PLN) (e.g., amyloidosis and glomerulonephritis), or a protein losing enteropathy (PLE) (e.g., intestinal parasites, *Campylobacter*, *Salmonella*, *Giardia*, inflammatory bowel disease, neoplastic bowel disease, etc.). Third space shifting is another consideration. The simplest way to differentiate PLE/ third spacing from PLN is to do a dipstick examination on the urine looking for proteinuria, in this case a negative proteinuria makes PLN less likely. Additionally, cholesterol is usually increased with PLN. With a history of GI disease and chronic vomiting, PLE is the most likely differential and supported by the hypocholesterolemia, which is most likely due to GIT losses.

Mildly increased ALP, bilirubin and ALT can be seen in primary liver disease (e.g., cholangiohepatitis) and possibly gut disease. Differentials include hepatic neoplasia (lymphoma), chronic active hepatitis (Dobermans), bile duct obstruction (extrahepatic mass, choleliths), amyloidosis and idiopathic hepatic cirrhosis. Increased ALP activity may also be due to chronic stress and subsequent induction of the steroid isoenzyme.

The very mild hypochloremia may be insignificant, however, given the history of vomiting, this could be related to loss through stomach acid.

Urinalysis

Although the dipstick is negative for protein; with dilute urine (USG 1.019) one cannot rule this out completely and a protein: creatinine ratio may be indicated. A single low USG is not necessarily significant (especially in a well-hydrated animal) but is worth repeating this to see if reproducible. The low specific gravity is likely associated with increased calcium causing inhibition of ADH.

Summary

Clinical signs in conjunction with laboratory abnormalities is strongly suggestive of a protein losing enteropathy. Protein losing enteropathy (PLE) can be associated with variety of disorders such as idiopathic inflammatory gastroenteropathies, small intestinal bacterial overgrowth (SIBO)/antibiotic responsive diarrhea, intestinal neoplasia, chronic intussusception, infectious enteritis, lymphangiectasia, etc.

On further workup the dog was found to have intestinal lymphoma. Retrospectively the mildly increased total and ionized calcium were clinically significant.

Contributor: Dr. dawn Seddon

Case 88

Signalment: 8-year-old ovariohysterectomized female Labrador retriever that weighs 35 kg

History: Presented to referring veterinarian 2 weeks earlier for lameness in left shoulder, presumably due to osteoarthritis. She was treated with carprofen and tramadol. She became lethargic a few days after taking carprofen and was vocalizing in the night due to pain. Benadryl was prescribed to help her sleep. One day prior to presentation at referral clinic she vomited and had one episode of diarrhea, A few hours prior to presentation she began panting, continued vomiting, was ataxic and running into walls, and developed hematuria.

Physical examination: Obtunded on arrival at referral clinic. Pupils unresponsive to light, laterally recumbent, tachypneic, hypersalivating, and icteric mucous membranes. Approximately 5% dehydrated.

Hematology		Reference range
Packed cell volume (%)	**19**	36–54
RBC (×10⁶/μL)	**2.65**	5.5–8.5
Hgb (g/dL)	**6.0**	12–18
MCV (fL)	71.5	60–72
MCHC (g/dL)	32	32–36
Reticulocytes (10³/μL)	**71 (2.69%)**	0–60
RDW (%)	**14**	11.3–13.5
NCC (10³/μL)	13.8	6.0–17.0
Segmented neutrophils (10³/μL)	**4.5**	3.0–11.5
Band neutrophils (10³/μL)	**5.9**	0–0.3
Metamyelocytes (10³/μL)	**0.5**	0
Monocytes (10³/μL)	—	0.2–1.4
Lymphocytes (10³/μL)	**0.3**	1.0–4.8
NRBC (10³/μL)	**2.6**	
Platelets (10³/μL)	**23**	200–500

Hemopathology: A hazy pink background consistent with free hemoglobin is present on the blood film, indicating hemolysis. A severe decrease in RBC density is present, consistent with severe anemia. Numerous spherocytes are present in every field, with occasional ghost erythrocytes. No red cell agglutination is observed. A few eccentrocytes are present. Mild polychromasia is observed. More band neutrophils than segmented neutrophils are present. Neutrophils have moderate toxic change with vacuolated basophilic cytoplasm and Dohle bodies. Lymphocytes are reactive with increased amount of basophilic cytoplasm. Blood film examination confirms thrombocytopenia, although a few small platelet clumps are seen. Numerous large platelets are present.

		Reference range
Glucose (mg/dL) prior to biochemical profile	**10** (before glucose Rx)	60–110
	43 (after glucose Rx)	60–110

Biochemical profile (serum icteric and hemolyzed)		Reference range
Glucose (mg/dL)	85	60–110
Blood urea nitrogen (mg/dL)	**50**	7–25
Creatinine (mg/dL)	**2.2**	0.3–1.4
Calcium (mg/dL)	9.9	8.6–11.3
Phosphorus (mg/dL)	4.6	2.9–6.6
Mg (mg/dL)	2.1	1.9–2.5
Total protein (g/dL)	7.1	5.2–7.3
Albumin (g/dL)	**0.9**	3.0–3.9
Globulin (g/dL)	**6.2**	1.7–3.8
Total bilirubin (mg/dL)	**9.0**	0.1–0.6
Cholesterol (mg/dL)	189	100–250
ALT (IU/L)	**1997**	12–54
ALP (IU/L)	**483**	16–140
GGT (IU/L)	0	0–6
CK (IU/L)	**1740**	43–234
Sodium (mEq/L)	140	138–160
Potassium (mEq/L)	4.6	3.7–5.8
Na:K ratio	30.4	27.7–35.9
Chloride (mEq/L)	**103**	108–122
HCO_3 (mEq/L)	**13**	18–26
Anion gap (mEq/L)	**27.6**	11.2–19.9
Lactate (mmol/L)	**7.7**	0.4–3.0
Amylase (IU/L)	832	230–1330
Lipase	**978**	300–560

Venous blood gases		Reference range
pCO_2 (mmHg)	30	18–32
pO_2 (mmHg)	**18**	26–46
pH	7.38	7.30–7.48
HCO_3 (mmol/L)	**17.7**	20.7–29.2
TCO_2 (mmol/L)	**18.6**	21.8–30.6

Coagulation profile		Reference range
aPTT (s)	**21.6**	9–16
PT (s)	**>120**	7–11

Radiographs

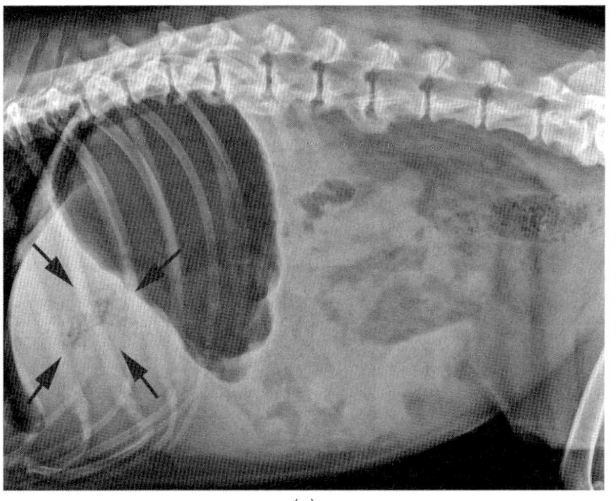

(a)

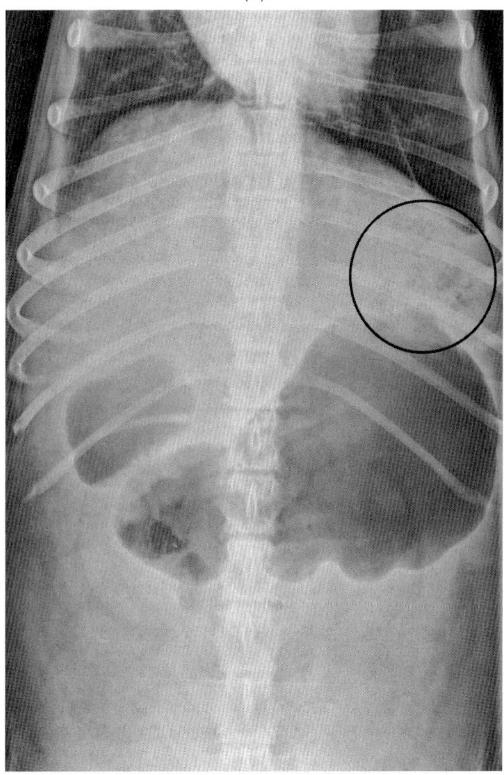

(b)

Figure 1 (a) Lateral radiograph of the abdomen. (b) Ventrodorsal radiograph of the cranial abdomen.

Abdominal fluid analysis	
Color	Dark red
Clarity	Hazy
PCV (%)	1
NCC (μL)	45 000
Total protein	NP

Description: Cells consist of 95% moderately degenerate neutrophils and 5% macrophages. Neutrophils occasionally contain one to two large rod-shaped bacteria (likely *Bacillus* or *Clostridium* sp.) within lysosomal vacuoles. Some macrophages contain hemosiderin and occasional rhomboid yellow crystals, consistent with hematoidin. No evidence of neoplasia is seen.

Interpretive discussion

Hematology

The PCV, RBC, and Hgb are all markedly decreased, with a normal MCV and MCHC, indicating a normocytic normochromic anemia. The reticulocyte concentration is slightly increased but is inadequate for this degree of anemia. It is possible that the anemia is too acute to have generated a bone marrow response yet (preregenerative anemia). Another possibility is that because the dog has severe inflammation, an anemia of inflammatory disease is superimposed on the original cause of anemia, resulting in a suppressed bone marrow response. The presence of spherocytes and ghost cells are diagnostic for immune-mediated hemolytic anemia (IMHA) with intravascular hemolysis. The presence of eccentrocytes suggests that oxidative damage may be playing a role in the hemolytic anemia. Increase in nucleated erythrocytes is compatible with a regenerative anemia and/or bone marrow damage, likely due to hypoxia or sepsis in this patient. The RDW is mildly increased as a result of increased variability in erythrocyte size.

The leukogram is markedly inflammatory as evidenced by the increase in band neutrophils. That immature neutrophils are more numerous than segmented neutrophils indicates an extreme tissue demand or overwhelming inflammation such as would be seen with bacterial peritonitis and/or sepsis (see abdominal fluid analysis). The toxic appearance of neutrophils is also indicative of inflammation since it results from rapid production and early release. A stress (cortisol) component is present as evidenced by lymphopenia. Reactive lymphocytes are likely a result of antigenic stimulation.

The patient is markedly thrombocytopenic. Large immature platelets indicate that the bone marrow is producing platelet Differentials for thrombocytopenia in a patient with IMHA are disseminated intravascular coagulopathy and immune-mediated thrombocytopenia. The thrombocytopenia in conjunction with prolonged aPTT and PT (see below) is very suggestive of disseminated intravascular coagulopathy (DIC).

Chemistry

Marked hypoglycemia on presentation is likely responsible for many of the clinical signs, including ataxia, blindness,

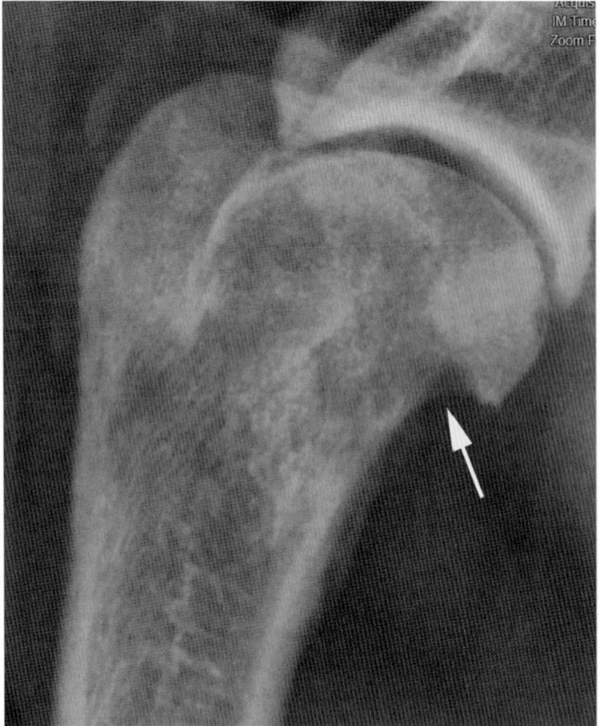

Figure 2 Lateral radiograph of the left shoulder.

and collapse, although increased blood ammonia concentrations could also account for these neurologic signs. Blood ammonia was not measured. Coma can occur at glucose concentrations at around 40–50 mg/dL, and neuronal death occurs at approximately 15 mg/dL. Differentials for severe hypoglycemia include insulinoma, administration of insulin, sepsis and liver failure. Insulin concentration was not measured in this patient. An insulinoma is less likely considering the history, as dogs with insulinomas usually have a longer history of intermittent weakness as a result of hypoglycemia. Sepsis is likely playing a role, considering the leukogram. Hypoglycemia secondary to sepsis is thought to be due to a combination of decreased caloric intake, hepatic dysfunction, and increased glucose consumption by bacteria, neutrophils, and peripheral tissues, the latter of which is attributable to inflammatory mediators. Liver necrosis in this patient (see summary) also likely contributed to the hypoglycemia, and although it does not typically result in this degree of hypoglycemia in dogs, hypoglycemia as severe as 10 and 37 mg/dL was reported in two human patients with liver failure [1].

The BUN and creatinine are increased, indicating decreased glomerular filtration rate. Urine specific gravity was not measured, thus it cannot be determined if the azotemia is prerenal due to dehydration or hypovolemia, or renal due to kidney dysfunction. Kidney dysfunction due to hemoglobinuria should be considered, since the patient has a hemolytic anemia.

The albumin is markedly decreased, and the globulin concentration is markedly increased. Part of the decrease in albumin could be due to inflammation, but hypoalbuminemia of this magnitude in the face of an increased globulin is likely due to either a lack of production by the liver or increased loss through the glomerulus. Since a urine analysis was not performed, it is not known if proteinuria is present.

Hyperglobulinemia of this magnitude should trigger protein electrophoresis to determine if the gammopathy is polyclonal or monoclonal. Based on other findings in this case, it was likely polyclonal and secondary to the bacterial infection and other causes of inflammation.

The serum bilirubin is markedly increased. Because the ALP activity is also increased, some of the increase is likely due to cholestasis. However, considering the increased ALT activity indicating marked hepatocellular damage, the increase in bilirubin could also be due to liver dysfunction. A third probability is increased erythrocyte destruction, since the dog has a hemolytic anemia.

CK is increased, indicating muscle damage.

Chloride is decreased below the reference interval, and sodium is at the lower end of the reference interval. In this case, sodium and chloride are likely being lost proportionally since the "corrected" chloride is in the reference interval (109.6 mEq/L). To correct the chloride to determine if chloride is being lost disproportionally to sodium, the following formula is used: *Corrected chloride = (normal sodium/measured sodium) ×measured chloride, where normal sodium is the midpoint of the reference range.*

The HCO_3 is decreased, evidence of a metabolic acidosis, likely due to increased lactate. The increased anion gap indicated an increase in unmeasured anions, and in this patient is also primarily due to the increase in lactate. Increase in lactate is probably due to hypovolemia and the hypoxia associated with immune-mediated hemolytic anemia [2].

The lipase activity is slightly increased, which might indicate pancreatitis. However, increases in lipase activity cannot be interpreted in animals that are azotemic, since the increase may be secondary to decreased glomerular filtration.

Venous blood gases

Venous pO_2 is below the reference interval, and although arterial pO_2 is needed to accurately determine hypoxia, this marked decrease in venous blood suggests that the patient is hypoxic.

HCO_3 and TCO_2 are decreased, indicating metabolic acidosis, even though the patient's pH is in the reference interval.

A high anion gap metabolic acidosis such as is seen in this patient is a result of bicarbonate being consumed in buffering the lactic acid, leaving the anion of lactic acid in its place. The HCO_3 is improved from the one on the biochemical profile. This could either be due to serum having been exposed to air, which could falsely decrease the profile $HC0_3$ (which is actually a measurement of TCO_2), or could be due to the blood gas sample having been taken after fluid therapy was instituted, reflecting true patient improvement.

Coagulation panel

Both the aPTT and PT are prolonged; considering the thrombocytopenia, this is likely due to DIC. D-dimer concentration to confirm DIC was not performed due to hemolysis. Although hemolysis is considered to be a contraindication for performing the test, hemolysis itself does not actually significantly interfere. Because hemolyzed samples are often a result of traumatic venipuncture, with concurrent tissue contamination of the sample, it is generally recommended that hemolyzed samples not be used, but this is not true for intravascular hemolysis [3].

Liver failure in this patient could also contribute to decreased coagulation protein production, resulting in increased aPTT and PT. While the hypoalbuminemia and hypoglycemia may be due to liver failure, urea is increased and cholesterol is within the reference interval, which would argue against liver failure.

Radiographs

Lateral and ventrodorsal radiographs of the abdomen were made (Figure 1). There is a loss of contrast in the abdomen consistent with fluid and/or inflammation. There are multiple small gas pockets in the left ventral aspect of the liver (arrows). This is most consistent with a hepatic abscess though an emphysematous hepatic mass cannot be ruled out. Emphysematous cholecystitis would not be considered due to the left sided nature of this lesion. The gas in the stomach is most likely due to aerophagia.

Upon an ultrasound examination, there was no mass associated with the region of gas pocketing, raising concern for hepatic necrosis rather than an abscess. Also, an entire liver lobe in the right cranioventral liver, likely the right medial lobe, was hypoechoic and consistent with infarction. There was no blood flow in this lobe using Doppler interrogation.

A lateral radiograph of the right shoulder was also acquired (Figure 1). There is mottled lysis of the medullary cavity and a smooth periosteal reaction on the proximal humerus. There is an area of cortex effacement on the proximocaudal aspect of the metaphysis (arrow). There is also a small area of lysis in the caudal humeral head. The borders of the lesion are indistinct. This is an aggressive lesion and, in this location, a primary bone tumor should be considered. However, an attempt should also be made to tie this lesion in with all of the other findings in this patient rather than concluding two separate disease entities.

Abdominal fluid analysis

Septic suppurative inflammation, previous hemorrhage. The presence of a single type of bacterium is more consistent with a ruptured abscess than a ruptured GI tract. *Clostridium* organisms are sometimes seen in liver abscesses. The bacterial peritonitis is likely responsible for the neutropenia, since all available neutrophils are being recruited into the abdominal cavity.

Summary and outcome

The patient was intubated on presentation and remained so throughout the diagnostic procedures. She had a continuous infusion of lactated Ringer's solution and dextrose. She also received numerous dextrose boluses (0.5 mL/kg).

Because of the severity of the clinical signs and the likelihood of a neoplasm in the humerus, the patient was humanely euthanized.

On autopsy, primary findings include icterus, numerous petechia, numerous portal vein thrombi that are occluding blood supply to the liver, and melena, all likely due to DIC. Marked hepatic and adrenal gland necrosis is present, as is peritonitis. Approximately 150 ml of dark red fluid is present in the abdominal cavity.

The pancreas is neoplastic, and although poorly differentiated, appears to be a very aggressive exocrine pancreatic carcinoma with metastasis to the left humerus, left femur, liver, intestine, and adrenal glands.

The kidneys show moderate hemoglobinuric nephrosis. Approximately 50% of the tubules have no epithelium.

The bone marrow shows a mild increase in immature hematopoietic cells.

Cerebral edema is diffuse, likely secondary to severe hypoglycemia, and was probably responsible for the neurologic signs. Unlike most other body tissues, the brain requires a continuous supply of glucose. Diminished neuronal glucose concentration leads to inadequate ATP production within the neurons, leading to vascular permeability, vasospasm, vascular dilation, edema and neuronal death from anoxia. A lack of brain glucose also results in glutamate and aspartate accumulation, which is thought to play a role in sodium and water influx and edema formation, and may also be directly responsible for neuronal dysfunction and death during hypoglycemia.

In summary, the pancreatic tumor and metastasis were responsible for most of the laboratory abnormalities and clinical signs seen in this patient, including lameness, liver necrosis, and DIC. The liver necrosis, secondary to both metastasis and lack of blood supply, likely led to bacterial overgrowth in the liver, with resultant septic peritonitis. Hypoglycemia secondary to sepsis or liver necrosis was responsible for brain edema, which resulted in neurologic signs. Immune-mediated hemolytic anemia was also likely triggered by the neoplasm or its associated inflammation, and the hemolytic anemia was responsible for hemoglobinuric nephrosis.

Contributors: Drs. Mary Anna Thrall and Donald Thrall

Case 89

Signalment: 11-month-old thoroughbred filly
History: Weak with depression and anorexia, watery diarrhea
Physical examination: Mildly dehydrated, pyrexic

Hematology		Reference range
Packed cell volume (%)	35	29–49
Hemoglobin (g/dL)	13.5	11.2–18.0
RBC ($10^6/\mu L$)	7.7	7.0–11.8
MCV (fL)	45.0	35–49
MCHC (g/dL)	38.6	36.1–39.6
NCC ($\times 10^3/\mu L$)	**3.0**	5.7–12.0
Segmented neutrophils ($\times 10^3/\mu L$)	**0.27**	2.9–6.9
Band neutrophils ($\times 10^3/\mu L$)	**0.39**	0.0–0.0
Metamyelocytes ($\times 10^3/\mu L$)	**0.06**	0.0–0.0
Monocytes ($\times 10^3/\mu L$)	**0.84**	0.2–0.7
Lymphocytes ($\times 10^3/\mu L$)	**1.44**	1.5–6.3
Platelets ($\times 10^3/\mu L$)	118	90–350
Plasma protein (g/dL)	**5.5**	6–8
Fibrinogen (g/dL)	0.38	0.15–0.5

Hemopathology: Neutrophils have moderate toxic changes.

Biochemical profile		Reference range
Glucose (mg/dL)	**65**	70–110
Blood urea nitrogen (mg/dL)	15	14–27
Creatinine (mg/dL)	1.2	1.1–2.0
Calcium (mg/dL)	**10.5**	11.0–13.7
Phosphorus (mg/dL)	**1.2**	1.9–4.1
Total protein (g/dL)	**5.2**	5.8–7.6
Albumin (g/dL)	**2.9**	3.2–4.0
Globulin (g/dL)	**2.3**	2.6–4.6
Total bilirubin (mg/dL)	**2.8**	0.6–2.1
AST (IU/L)	260	185–600
GGT (IU/L)	15	7–45
SDH (IU/L)	8	0–9
CK (IU/L)	**480**	130–470
Sodium (mEq/L)	**130**	133–145
Potassium (mEq/L)	2.2	2.2–4.6
Chloride (mEq/L)	**96**	100–111
TCO_2 (mEq/L)	**21.5**	24–34
Anion gap	**17.7**	5–15

Interpretive discussion

Hematology

The erythrogram is within reference intervals. Dehydration may mask anemia but these RBC parameters will most likely still be within range even taking this into account.

The leukogram shows a leukopenia, neutropenia, and toxic change with a significant left shift back to metamyelocytes, consistent with a significant (degenerative) left shift usually associated with severe inflammation. Neutropenia this low may predispose to sepsis if not already evident. Given the history of diarrhea, this leukogram is likely associated with GIT disease.

The leukogram is referred to by some as degenerative because there is a mature neutropenia that has immature neutrophils (band neutrophils and metamyelocytes) that exceed mature neutrophils. Prognostically this change is poor and suggests endotoxemia or overwhelming inflammation.

The lymphopenia is likely due to stress. Viral disease can also lower lymphocyte concentration.

Plasma protein is decreased. Serum proteins help to evaluate further – please see discussion under serum chemistry.

Plasma protein: fibrinogen ratio is 14.5. In horses a plasma protein fibrinogen ratio >15 is normal and can occur with dehydration, but <15 is suggestive of a true increase in fibrinogen concentration, which is consistent with inflammation.

Chemistry

Hypoglycemia can be due to decreased intake (history mentions anorexia) but can also be associated with sepsis, and given the leukogram, this remains a strong differential.

BUN and creatinine are both low normal and may be associated with decreased muscle mass or anorexia.

Apparent hypocalcemia is likely due to decreased albumin, as approximately 40% of total calcium is albumin bound. An ionized calcium is required to verify a low serum calcium. Decreased phosphorus can be due to decreased intake with anorexia.

Panhypoproteinemia may be due to a protein losing enteropathy (which is supported by the history), less likely a protein losing nephropathy (globulins are not normally decreased in these cases due to selective protein loss due to size), but can also be associated with third space shifting if there is a focus of inflammation such as a peritonitis or abscess.

Increased bilirubin with other liver parameters within the reference interval in horses may be due to anorexia, or can be associated with functional cholestasis, secondary to inflammatory mediators and cytokines due to extrahepatic disease.

Mild increases in CK are not an uncommon finding and can be seen with a struggling animal, difficult bleed, prior injections, etc. and are generally not considered to be clinically significant at this activity.

Decreased sodium and chloride are likely due to GIT loss with the history of diarrhea.

Total CO_2 equates with bicarbonate and is decreased below the reference interval and is consistent with a mild metabolic acidosis most likely secondary to the diarrhea.

Potassium is low normal and in the light of an acidosis suggests that the potassium may even be lower as acidosis tends to be associated with increased potassium. There may be total body loss of potassium due to the diarrhea.

The anion gap is mildly increased, and a calculated estimation of the unmeasured anions present that are commonly found in cases of diarrhea such as lactic acid.

Differentials related to causes of panhypoproteinemia in horses of this age include intestinal parasites, cryptosporidium, coccidiosis, salmonellosis, *Rhodococcus, Lawsonia,* larval cyathostominosis (small strongyles), eosinophilic enteritis, small intestinal adenomatous polyposis (rare), to name a few. Given the leukogram a differential such as *Salmonella* with an endotoxemia would be the most likely consideration in this case.

Summary

A fecal culture revealed growth of *Salmonella*. The horse was diagnosed with salmonellosis, endotoxemia and severe protein losing enteropathy.

Unfortunately, response to treatment was poor and the hypoproteinemia progressed; the horse deteriorated and was euthanized on humane grounds.

Contributor: Dr. dawn Seddon

CASES

Case 90

Signalment: 10-month-old stockhorse colt

History: This horse was kept in a small paddock with 15 other similarly aged horses. 10-day history of lethargy, inappetence, and weight loss. There is also moderate fecal staining of the perineum.

Now presenting with severe edema of the ventrum and all four limbs.

Hematology		Reference interval
PCV (%)	33	24–46
RBC (10^{12}/L)	7.1	6.5–12.5
Hemoglobin (g/L)	**106**	110–190
MCV (fL)	43	34.0–58.0
MCH (pg)	15	12–18
MCHC (g/L)	353	310–370
WBC (×10^9/L)	**34.5**	5.5–12.5
Segmented neutrophils (×10^9/L)	**31.0**	2.5–8.0
Lymphocytes (×10^9/L)	1.7	1.5–5.5
Monocytes (×10^9/L)	**1.3**	0.0–0.9
Eosinophils (×10^9/L)	0.3	0.0–0.8
Platelets (×10^9/L)	250	100–500
Fibrinogen (g/L)	4.0	1.0–4.0

Biochemical profile		Reference interval
Glucose (mmol/L)	6.0	3.5–6.5
Blood urea nitrogen (mmol/L)	6.4	3.6–8.9
Creatinine (μmol/L)	99	81–164
Calcium (mmol/L)	**2.28**	2.5–3.6
Phosphorus (mmol/L)	**0.62**	0.8–1.7
Total protein (g/L)	**28**	58–76
Albumin (g/L)	**9**	28–38
Globulin (g/L)	**19**	26–40
Total bilirubin (μmol/L)	13.4	4–100
AST (IU/L)	**135**	150–400
GLDH (IU/L)	0	0–20
GGT (IU/L)	**<1**	20–38
CK (IU/L)	**792**	50–400
Triglycerides (mmol/L)	0.28	0.2–2.6
Sodium (mmol/L)	**124**	132–152
Potassium (mmol/L)	3.5	2.8–5.0
Chloride (mmol/L)	**88**	98–110
Bicarbonate (mmol/L)	30	23.0–22.0
Anion gap (mmol/L)	9.5	8–20

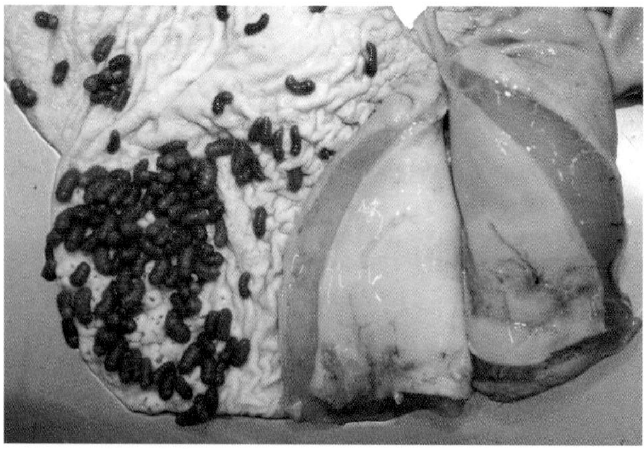

Figure 1 Photograph of the stomach. Note the parasitic botfly larvae (*Gasterophilus* spp.) attached to the gastric mucosa. There is marked edema of the submucosa.

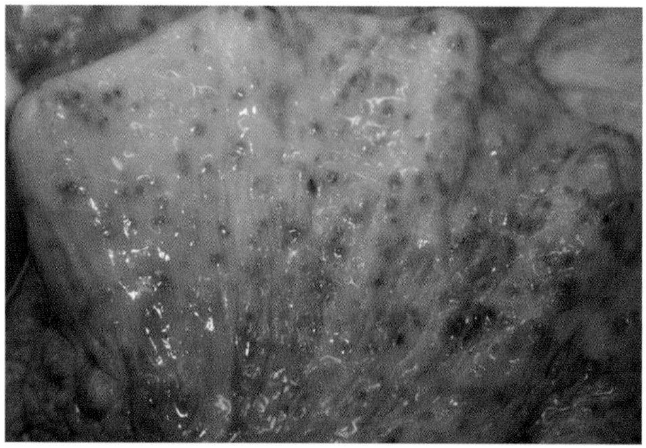

Figure 2 Photograph of the large colon. Notice the multiple red, nodular foci scattered throughout the mucosa.

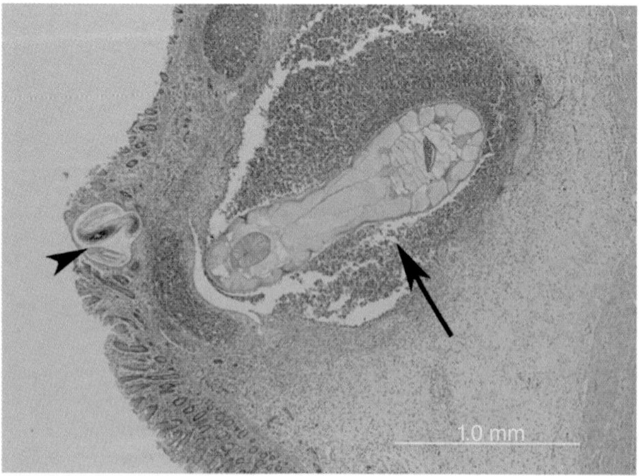

Figure 3 Histological section of the right ventral colon. A small strongyle is encysted within the colonic mucosa (arrowhead). The submucosa is edematous and contains a large strongyle surrounded by a lake of neutrophils (arrow).

Interpretive discussion

Hematology

The decreased Hgb in the absence of anemia is likely an artifact.

A marked mature neutrophilia with a mild monocytosis suggests a significant inflammatory focus. Note also the fibrinogen is at top end of the reference interval.

Chemistry

Given that 40–50% of serum calcium is protein bound, the hypocalcemia is probably due to the hypoalbuminemia. An ionized calcium measurement may help further characterize this, and other causes to consider include gastrointestinal losses or excessive sweating (particularly in horses).

Hypophosphatemia is most likely due to decreased gastrointestinal absorption or increased losses (diarrhea). Note the animal has evidence of diarrhea.

A panhypoproteinemia comprised of marked hypoalbuminemia and moderate hypoglobulinemia is strongly suggestive of gastrointestinal losses (protein losing enteropathy). In the absence of anemia or a history of hemorrhage, hypoproteinemia due to blood loss is unlikely. Third spacing, and loss of protein through effusions is also possible in this case. Inflammation is also present, and this may be contributing to the hypoalbuminemia (albumin is a negative acute phase protein).

A decreased AST and GGT is not likely to be clinically significant. Mildly increased CK activity may be an indication of muscle injury.

The corrected chloride is calculated at 101 mmol/l, indicating a proportional loss of sodium and chloride. In this case, this is likely due to gastrointestinal losses from diarrhea and is compatible with the concurrent panhypoproteinemia. Other causes to consider include excessive salivating, drinking, or sweating, although the latter is less likely given that potassium is within reference interval.

Summary

At postmortem, this animal had severe submucosal edema of the gastrointestinal tract secondary to marked hypoalbuminemia (Figure 1). The botfly larvae present in Figure 1 were an incidental finding and are typically of no clinical significance but provide evidence to support poor deworming procedures as an aggravating factor in this case. There were also low numbers of large strongyles within the proliferative arteritis that was found within the wall of the cranial mesenteric artery.

The cause of hypoproteinemia was a protein losing enteropathy that developed as a result of severe intestinal infection with small strongyles (nodules in Figure 2), and to a lesser extent, large strongyles. The histological section (Figure 3) demonstrates both small and large strongyles within the colonic wall and the associated neutrophilic inflammation present in the form of "microabscesses." The focus of inflammation evidenced by the inflammatory leukogram is likely the large intestine.

Further investigation showed that these animals had been wormed three times with Ivermectin, but each dose was given within the first 3 months of life, and none of the animals had been wormed in the previous 6 months. This, combined with the high stocking density, explains the finding of high numbers of both small and especially large strongyles, which have a longer and more complex life cycle.

Contributor: Dr. Allan Kessell

CASES

Case 91

Signalment: 5-year-old mini horse gelding
History: 2-day history of colic and fever; slight improvement with NSAIDs

Hematology	Day 1	Day 8	Reference interval
Packed cell volume (%)	32.9	30.7	30.6–42.1
Hemoglobin (g/dL)	13.0	12.1	11.4–16.9
RBC ($10^6/\mu L$)	7.85	7.37	6.41–10.12
MCV (fL)	41.9	41.7	38.7–52.3
MCH (pg)	16.6	16.4	15.0–19.4
MCHC (g/dL)	39.5	39.4	35.0–40.8
RDW (%)	27.2	26.5	21.6–27.6
NCC ($\times 10^3/\mu L$)	**1.84**	**4.18**	4.79–10.88
Segmented neutrophils ($\times 10^3/\mu L$)	**0.17**	**2.67**	3.4–6.27
Band neutrophils ($\times 10^3/\mu L$)	**0.24**	**0.08**	0.00–0.00
Monocytes ($\times 10^3/\mu L$)	0.06	0.21	0.00–0.48
Lymphocytes ($\times 10^3/\mu L$)	1.36	1.21	1.15–4.58
Platelets ($\times 10^3/\mu L$)	132	**92**	97–254
Total protein (refractometry g/dL)	**5.2**	**<2.5**	6.1–7.5
Fibrinogen (g/dL)	0.3	N/A	0.1–0.5

Hemopathology: Day 1 – moderate neutrophil toxicity, few reactive lymphocytes, marked erythrocyte echinocytes (possibly crenation). Day 8 – few reactive lymphocytes, mild neutrophil toxicity.

Biochemistry	Day 1	Day 3	Day 5	Day 8	Ref. int
Glucose (mg/dL)	**152**	77	104	93	77–107
BUN (mg/dL)	17	13	15	23	11–24
Creatinine (mg/dL)	1.2	0.9	1.0	1.0	0.9–1.7
Calcium (mg/dL)	**8.5**	**8.8**	**8.5**	**7.8**	11.2–12.8
Phosphorus (mg/dL)	2.4	2.9	3.2	4.2	1.8–4.0
Magnesium (mg/dL)	**1.4**	**1.0**	**1.1**	**1.1**	1.5–2.3
Total protein (g/dL)	**4.9**	**3.5**	**2.3**	**1.6**	5.7–7.5
Albumin (g/dL)	2.5	**1.6**	**1.1**	**0.7**	2.5–3.6
Globulin (g/dL)	2.4	**1.9**	**1.2**	**0.9**	2.4–4.1
Total bilirubin (mg/dL)	**4.9**	**3.5**	1.6	0.8	0.6–2.8
AST (IU/L)	217	**139**	**143**	280	203–415
GLDH (IU/L)	1	6	10	95	N/A
GGT (IU/L)	**9**	**6**	**6**	9	10–30
CK (IU/L)	140	108	145	281	112–444
Triglycerides (mg/dL)	**184**	**597**	**457**	**290**	14–62
Sodium (mEq/L)	126	**120**	**119**	**122**	132–141
Potassium (mEq/L)	2.7	2.9	3.0	2.9	2.7–4.3
Chloride (mEq/L)	**88**	**91**	**93**	**94**	96–105
Bicarbonate (mEq/L)	27	**22**	**23**	**23**	25–33
Anion gap (mmol/L)	14	10	**6**	**8**	8–15

Interpretive discussion

Hematology

On initial presentation, there is a leukopenia characterized by a marked neutropenia and degenerative left shift consistent with overwhelming and likely, acute inflammation. Underlying endotoxemia may lead to margination of neutrophils and contribute to lower circulating numbers. Over the duration of a week, the neutropenia becomes less severe and the left-shift becomes mild, suggesting improvement of the inflammation. Fibrinogen remains within reference intervals on Day 1 and likely reflects the acute nature of the inflammation. On Day 8, fibrinogen was unable to determined due to the low (<2.5 g/dL) total protein reading, resulting in inability to calculate precipitated fibrinogen.

Observed echinocytes on Day 1 are possibly an artifactual change or may be a result of electrolyte depletion.

The mild thrombocytopenia observed on Day 8 is likely insignificant.

Chemistry

A mild hyperglycemia is observed on presentation and could reflect stress, endotoxemia or the potential use of some sedatives, namely Xylazine.

The persistent hypocalcemia in this horse most likely reflects gastrointestinal disease (increases losses or decreased absorption) and is supported by the hypomagnesemia that can also be observed with GI disease. Given that 40–50% of serum calcium is protein bound, the hypoalbuminemia is also contributing to the hypocalcemia. Hypocalcemia and hypomagnesemia are observed with blister beetle (Cantharidin) toxicosis and this should be considered if this animal is from an endemic region. Additionally, hypomagnesemia can result in hypocalcemia since magnesium is necessary for parathyroid hormone release.

Throughout serial measurements, the panhypoproteinemia becomes progressively worse and may reflect a protein losing enteropathy, decreased synthesis or third spacing (effusions). As albumin is a negative acute phase protein, inflammation may also be contributing to the hypoalbuminemia. Much less likely is a protein losing nephropathy given the concurrent loss of globulins. This may be assessed with a urine protein measurement.

Hyperbilirubinemia in a horse is most likely due to anorexia. Decreased feed intake and negative energy balance is also supported by hypertriglyceridemia, which occurs because of lipolysis and VLDL formation. Improvements to both analytes are observed by Day 8 and could indicate return of appetite in this animal.

Decreased AST and GGT activity are likely clinically insignificant.

On Day 1, there is a proportional hyponatremia and hypochloremia, which could reflect losses through electrolyte-rich fluid such as diarrhea or sweat. By Day 3 calculation of corrected chloride (103.5 mEq/L) indicates a selective sodium loss that, given the panhypoproteinemia, is most likely due to a protein losing enteropathy or loss through diarrhea. Furthermore, there is likely loss of bicarbonate through the gastrointestinal tract leading to a secretional metabolic acidosis. A low anion gap is observed on Day 5 and is the result of hypoalbuminemia.

Summary

This patient tested negative for salmonella, *Clostridium, Lawsonia,* and *Neorickettsia risticii.* It was later discovered that a herd mate was diagnosed with coronavirus prior to this animal's presentation and fecal PCR confirmed infection in this patient. Equine Coronavirus has fecal-oral transmission route. Common clinical presentation of coronavirus in horses include lethargy, anorexia, fever and gastrointestinal signs.

Contributors: Drs. Alex Mau and Saundra Sample

Case 92

Signalment: 14-year-old female thoroughbred horse
History: Patient is 3 months pregnant and presented for investigation of a 5-day history of anorexia and diarrhea
Physical examination: Dehydrated, muddy mucous membranes with toxic line noted

Hematology		Reference range
Packed cell volume (%)	**54**	32–53
RBC (×10^6/μL)	12.68	6.80–12.90
Hgb (g/dL)	**22.5**	11.0–19.0
MCV (fL)	43	37–59
MCHC (g/dL)	**41.7**	31.0–38.6
NCC (10^3/μL)	6.99	5.40–14.30
Segmented neutrophils (10^3/μL)	5.45	2.26–8.85
Monocytes (10^3/μL)	0.21	0.00–1.00
Lymphocytes (10^3/μL)	**1.33**	1.50–7.70
Platelets (10^3/μL)	168	100–350
Plasma protein by refractometry (g/dL)	**9.9**	5.8–8.7
Fibrinogen (g/dL)	**0.5**	0.1–0.4

Hemopathology: Few reactive lymphocytes, mild neutrophil toxicity.

Biochemical profile		Reference range
Glucose (mg/dL)	**239**	77–109
Blood urea nitrogen (mg/dL)	**99**	11–24
Creatinine (mg/dL)	**5.8**	0.9–1.7
Calcium (mg/dL)	**7.0**	11.0–12.9
Phosphorus (mg/dL)	**8.6**	1.8–5.1
Magnesium	2.1	1.5–2.3
Total protein (g/dL)	**9.3**	5.8–7.6
Albumin (g/dL)	3.2	2.5–3.6
Globulin (g/dL)	**6.1**	2.4–4.8
Total bilirubin (mg/dL)	**3.2**	0.6–2.8
AST (IU/L)	373	203–415
GGT (IU/L)	13	10–30
CK (IU/L)	353	112–498
Triglyceride (mg/dL)	**753**	14–62
Sodium (mEq/L)	**112**	132–141
Potassium (mEq/L)	**2.1**	2.7–4.3
Chloride (mEq/L)	**73**	95–104
Bicarbonate (mEq/L)	**16**	25–33
Anion gap (mEq/L)	**25**	8–15

Interpretive discussion

Hematology

A transient/relative erythrocytosis is present and supported by the hyperproteinemia. In horses, increased PCV can also be seen with splenic contraction. The hemoglobin is disproportionately increased, possibly due to lipemia (see triglyceride concentration). Increased MCHC is not physiologically possible and considered an analyzer artifact, perhaps due to hypo-osmolality in this animal, or due to a possibly false increased hemoglobin, since the MCHC is calculated by dividing the hematocrit into the hemoglobin.

Mild neutrophil toxicity is suggestive of inflammation and correlates with the hyperfibrinogenemia. However, it is important to note in dehydrated animals, fibrinogen can be relatively elevated (as with total protein). In such cases a total protein: fibrinogen ratio may shed light on the cause of hyperfibrinogenemia. For this case it is calculated to be 19.9 which is not definitive for inflammation (ratio <15) [1]. Despite this, the concurrent presence of reactive lymphocytes and hyperglobulinemia mean that inflammation cannot be excluded.

There is a mild lymphopenia that may reflect a stress (corticosteroid)-induced response.

Chemistry

A transient hyperglycemia could be an epinephrine or corticosteroid response, the latter supported by the lymphopenia. If this were a persistent hyperglycemia, disease states resulting in insulin resistance should be considered such as equine metabolic syndrome and pars pituitary intermedia dysfunction (PPID).

A moderate azotemia and concurrent hyperphosphatemia are suggestive of decreased glomerular filtration rate. This may be due to renal dysfunction, although a prerenal (dehydration) component is likely present. A urine specific gravity would be required to fully assess renal concentrating ability.

Hypocalcemia is moderate to marked and is unlikely to be linked to decreased protein binding as albumin is within reference range. In horses, gastrointestinal disease resulting in decreased absorption or increased loss of calcium is most common. Also possible in horses is excessive sweating leading to loss of calcium and some electrolytes such as potassium and chloride. Less likely is hypocalcemia associated with pregnancy, given the relatively early stage in this animal.

A hyperproteinemia characterized by a hyperglobulinemia is present. While a component of dehydration is likely present (given the history and clinical signs), inflammation should be considered as a differential for the hyperglobulinemia.

In the absence of increased hepatobiliary enzyme activity, the hyperbilirubinemia is most likely due to anorexia. Decreased feed intake and pregnancy can lead to a negative energy balance, which is evidenced in this case by the hypertriglyceridemia, is a result of lipolysis and VLDL production. Although a simple negative energy balance may be responsible for this abnormality, co-contributing factors such as insulin resistance should be considered, particularly given the hyperglycemia.

There is a marked hyponatremia with a slightly more severe hypochloremia.

The Corrected Cl = (normal Na/measured Na) × measured Cl = 136/112 × 73 = 89 mEq/l indicating a selective chloride loss. This is most likely due to loss of chloride rich fluid through diarrhea but may also be from gastric reflux or excessive sweating.

Hypokalemia in this animal is likely multifactorial and caused by a combination of gastrointestinal losses, anorexia, renal losses (aldosterone mediated) and excessive sweating. The potassium concentration may be increased by a concurrent metabolic acidosis, which leads to potassium retention in exchange for H+ secretion.

Decreased serum bicarbonate and concurrent increase in anion gap is suggestive of a titrational metabolic acidosis due to production of increased unmeasured anions. In this case uremic acids and lactate are most likely, with ketones being unlikely given horses do not readily form ketones in negative energy balances.

Summary and outcome

Clinicopathological abnormalities are supportive of a severe gastrointestinal disease leading to electrolyte losses and acid base imbalanced. This patient was subsequently humanely euthanized and sent for necropsy. Postmortem findings indicated extensive granulomatous enteritis, colitis and renal tubular nephrosis. A fecal PCR detected *Neorickettsia risticii*, the causative agent of Potomac horse fever, also known as equine ehrlichial colitis. *N. risticii* is a Gram-negative obligate intracellular bacterium that is thought to be transmitted by ingestion of snails, trematodes, and various types of flies, such as dragonflies and caddisflies [2]. The onset of diarrhea is often accompanied by mild abdominal discomfort. Some horses develop severe signs of sepsis and dehydration. Clinical signs can be indistinguishable from those of *Salmonella* and other infectious causes of enterocolitis.

Contributors: Drs. Alex Mau and Saundra Sample

Case 93

Signalment: Friesian cow in calf
History: Off food with sudden drop in milk production
Physical examination: Acute weakness and dehydration

Hematology		Reference interval
Packed cell volume (%)	**51**	24–46
Hemoglobin (g/dL)	**17.5**	8–15
RBC ($10^6/\mu L$)	**10.7**	5.0–10.0
MCV (fL)	47	37–53
MCHC (g/dL)	34	34–38
NCC ($\times 10^3/\mu L$)	11.3	4.0–12.0
Segmented neutrophils ($\times 10^3/\mu L$)	**8.6**	0.6–4.0
Band neutrophils ($\times 10^3/\mu L$)	0	0–0.1
Monocytes ($\times 10^3/\mu L$)	0.3	0–0.8
Lymphocytes ($\times 10^3/\mu L$)	**2.3**	2.5–7.5
Eosinophils ($\times 10^3/\mu L$)	0.1	0–2.4
Platelets ($\times 10^3/\mu L$)	**506**	200–300
Fibrinogen (mg/dL)	**960**	200–600
Plasma protein (g/dL)	**9.4**	6–8

Morphology comment: Clumped platelets.

Biochemical profile		Reference interval
Glucose (mg/dL)	**127**	55–95
Creatinine (mg/dL)	**4.3**	1.0–1.8
Calcium (mg/dL)	**6.9**	8.2–9.9
Phosphorus (mg/dL)	**12.5**	4.3–7.0
Magnesium (mg/dL)	**3.2**	1.3–3.0
Total protein (g/dL)	**8.9**	6.3–7.6
Albumin (g/dL)	**5.1**	2.5–4.3
Globulin (g/dL)	3.8	2.6–5.0
Total bilirubin (mg/dL)	**1.2**	0.1–0.4
CK (IU/L)	**30,000**	57–280
AST (IU/L)	**850**	40–130
GGT (IU/L)	25	10–26
SDH (IU/L)	**31**	8–23
Sodium (mEq/L)	136	136–147
Potassium (mEq/L)	**3.1**	3.6–5.2
Chloride (mEq/L)	**64**	95–105
TCO_2 (mEq/L)	**48**	24–32
Anion gap (mEq/L)	**27.1**	14–26

Blood gases (arterial)		Reference interval
HCO_3 (mEq/L)	**51.5**	23–31
pH	**7.64**	7.32–7.45
pCO_2 (mmHg)	**57.6**	34–44

Interpretive discussion

Hematology

Increased PCV, hemoglobin, and RBC indicate polycythemia. Since this cow is 10% dehydrated, this is relative (transient) polycythemia secondary to dehydration, supported by the increased albumin.

While the mature neutrophilia and lymphopenia is a typical corticosteroid-mediated (stress) leukogram, the presence of hyperfibrinogenemia suggests inflammation. Fibrinous inflammation occurs more commonly in ruminants than in other species. When this occurs, mature neutrophilia (and, possibly, lymphopenia if the animal is stressed) may be the only change in the leukogram. Hyperfibrinogenemia, however, will indicate that inflammation is occurring.

Hyperfibrinogenemia may be the result of inflammation but can also be caused by dehydration. In order to negate the effect of dehydration, a plasma protein: fibrinogen ratio should be calculated in animals with high fibrinogen concentrations.

Since both plasma protein and fibrinogen should increase proportionately in dehydrated animals, their ratio should stay the same regardless of the degree of dehydration. In this case, the plasma protein: fibrinogen ratio is plasma TP/Fibrinogen = 9.4/0.96 = 9.79.

Note that the fibrinogen concentration has been converted from mg/dl to g/dl for this calculation. In ruminants, a plasma TP:fibrinogen ratio of $<10:1$ indicates a true increase in fibrinogen and suggests inflammation. In this case, therefore, it appears that inflammation is occurring.

Biochemical profile

The mild hyperglycemia is probably a result of stress and is commonly observed in cases of volvulus.

Increased serum creatinine indicates decreased GFR, but urine specific gravity must be known to determine if this is a renal or prerenal azotemia. As the cow is dehydrated, there is certainly a prerenal component.

The marked hypocalcemia is typical of a lactating ruminant that experiences anorexia and/or a gastrointestinal abnormality. This cow was probably producing a large amount of milk, and this required a steady intake of Ca. The GI problem in this cow has decreased the intake and/or absorption of Ca and the result is hypocalcemia.

At around this degree of hypocalcemia (<6.4 mg/dL) one typically observes clinical signs of "downer syndrome."

Marked hyperphosphatemia in ruminants is usually associated with gut stasis. Approximately 90% of phosphorus excreted by ruminants is excreted through saliva and then passes through the GI tract out of the body. With GI stasis, there is less production of saliva, and P that enters the GI tract does not readily leave the body (and is probably reabsorbed if the GI tract is capable of this). As in other species, P is also excreted through the kidneys of ruminants; therefore, decreased GFR is also playing a role in the hyperphosphatemia.

There is mild hypermagnesemia that is due to the decreased GFR.

A hyperproteinemia is present and characterized by a hyperalbuminemia and globulin within reference range. The increased albumin is due to dehydration. As 40% of total calcium is albumin bound, this makes the calcium relatively lower than measured.

Cholestasis and liver disease inconsistently cause mild to moderate hyperbilirubinemia in ruminants. Mild increases in bilirubin concentrations can occur in anorexic cattle. Hemolysis is a common cause of hyperbilirubinemia in ruminants, but the data in this cow do not suggest a hemolytic process (no anemia). Hyperbilirubinemia in this cow is probably a result of anorexia, but a liver component cannot be discounted. The increase is mild and is not the primary concern.

Increased CK and AST in this cow are the result of muscle injury. Only a mild increase in SDH suggests liver injury, which could be due to localized hypoxia as a result of recumbency. As the SDH increase is so mild, the liver is not the major source of AST in this case. It is likely that this cow is spending more time in a recumbent position than normal due to its illness, and that this is leading to hypoxic muscle injury.

Hypokalemia is the result of alkalosis and redistribution of K into cells. In alkalosis, H ions leave cells in an effort to balance the concentration of H ions inside and outside cells. As H ions leave cells, K ions enter cells and hypokalemia can result.

Severe hypochloremia in ruminants is usually the result of sequestration of Cl in the abomasum. In this case the change in chloride is disproportionate to the change in sodium. This can occur with any type of GI stasis but is most severe with abomasal volvulus and with high duodenal obstruction or a left displaced abomasum (LDA).

Increased serum bicarbonate concentration (increased TCO_2) can also result from abomasal sequestration of Cl. Secretion of Cl into the abomasum is accompanied by secretion of H ions (HCL). This also results in production of HCO_3 that passes into the blood.

CASES

Blood gas analysis

The increased pH indicates an alkalosis. The bicarbonate is increased (an alkaline change) and the pCO_2 is increased (an acid change). Since the bicarbonate has changed in the same way that the pH has changed (alkaline), this is the primary change. The correct description of this blood gas profile is, therefore, primary metabolic alkalosis with partial respiratory compensation. The term "partial" is used since the compensatory change in pCO_2 has not resulted in return of the pH to normal. The metabolic alkalosis is a result of the sequestration of H ions in the abomasum.

Summary

This cow has a left displaced abomasum resulting in blockage of outflow and sequestration of HCl in the abomasum. The electrolyte and acid-base changes as described above resulted.

Additional tests to consider

Serum levels of ketones (beta–hydroxybutyric acid or BHB) should be measured in this case of a lactating pregnant cow that is not eating and going down.

Depending on the level of BHB, the ketosis may be either primary or secondary.

If the cow is in poor body condition little fat is available to mobilize and thus in thin animals the ketone body increase may not be significant.

Measurement of NEFAS (Non-esterified fatty acids) gives an earlier indication of low energy reserves/ketone production.

Contributor: Dr. dawn Seddon

Case 94

Signalment: 3-year-old castrated male golden retriever
History: Lethargic, heat seeking
Physical examination: Obese, poor hair coat, tail-head alopecia

Hematology		Reference interval
PCV (%)	**34**	37–55
MCV (fL)	65	60–72
MCHC (g/dL)	35	34–38
Retics (×10³/μL)	**2**	<60
NCC (×10³/μL)	12.5	6–17
Segs (×10³/μL)	9.3	3–11.5
Monos (×10³/μL)	1.0	0.1–1.3
Lymphs (×10³/μL)	2.2	1–4.8
Platelets (×10³/μL)	Adequate	200–500
TP (P) (g/dL)	7.5	6–8

Hemopathology: Numerous leptocytes ("target cells") present.

Biochemical profile		Reference interval
Gluc (mg/dL)	105	65–122
BUN (mg/dL)	20	7–28
Creat (mg/dL)	1.2	0.9–1.7
Ca (mg/dL)	10.5	9.0–11.2
Phos (mg/dL)	4.0	2.8–6.1
TP (g/dL)	7.0	5.4–7.4
Alb (g/dL)	3.7	2.7–4.5
Glob (g/dL)	3.3	1.9–3.4
T. bili (mg/dL)	0.2	0–0.4
Chol (mg/dL)	**720 *(18.7)***	130–370 *(3.4–9.6 mmol/L)*
ALT (IU/L)	110	10–120
AST (IU/L)	35	16–40
ALP (IU/L)	220	35–280
Na (mEq/L)	**143**	145–158
K (mEq/L)	4.5	4.1–5.5
CL (mEq/L)	107	106–127
TCO_2 (mEq/L)	20	14–27

Endocrine data		Reference interval
TT4 (μg/dL)	1.6	1.4–4.0
Free T4 (ng/dL)	**0.24 *(3.0)***	1.2–3.4 *(15.4–4.8 pmol/L)*
Endogenous TSH (ng/mL) (immulite)	**0.5**	0.1–0.45

Interpretive discussion

Hematology

A mild nonregenerative, normocytic, normochromic anemia is the only abnormality in the CRC. "Target cells" are common and are not very diagnostically useful. They commonly present in animals with hypercholesterolemia.

Biochemical profile

The only abnormalities present are hypercholesterolemia and mild hyponatremia. Hypercholesterolemia is marked, and in conjunction with the history, physical examination, and mild anemia, is very suggestive of hypothyroidism. Mild hyponatremia has been reported in approximately 30% of dogs with hypothyroidism.

Endocrine data

Total T4 is within the reference interval. However, since many variables affect TT4, and this dog has clinical and laboratory findings that are suggestive of hypothyroidism a free T4 and endogenous TSH are indicated. The decreased FT4 and increased endogenous TSH are diagnostic for hypothyroidism.

Summary

Early primary hypothyroidism.

Case 95

Signalment: 13-year-old castrated male dog
History: Polyuria, frequent urination with small volumes
Physical examination: Overweight

Hematology		Reference interval
PCV (%)	**36.0**	37–55
Hgb (g/dL)	13.4	12–18
RBC (×10⁶/µL)	**5.26**	5.5–8.5
MCV (fL)	69.0	60–72
MCHC (g/dL)	37.0	34–38
NCC (×10³/µL)	**18.1**	6–17
Segs (×10³/µL)	**16.7**	3–11.5
Monos (×10³/µL)	1.3	0.1–1.3
Lymphs (×10³/µL)	**0.2**	1.0–4.8
Platelets (×10³/µL)	452	200–500
TP (P) (g/dL)	**8.2**	6–8

Hemopathology: Few Howell-Jolly bodies.

Biochemical profile		Reference interval
Gluc (mg/dL)	**806 *(44.3)***	65–122 *(3.5–6.7 mmol/L)*
BUN (mg/dL)	**81 *(28.9)***	7–28 *(2.5–10.0 mmol/L)*
Creat (mg/dL)	1.6	0.9–1.7
Ca (mg/dL)	**8.4 *(2.1)***	9.0–11.2 *(2.25–2.80 mmol/L)*
ionized Ca++ (mg/dL)	**3.56**	4.5–5.6
Phos (mg/dL)	**7.2 *(2.3)***	2.8–6.1 *(0.9–2.0 mmol/L)*
TP (g/dL)	6.0	5.4–7.4
Alb (g/dL)	3.3	2.7–4.5
Glob (g/dL)	2.7	1.9–3.4
T. bili (mg/dL)	**1.3 *(22.2)***	0–0.4 *(0–6.8 µmol/L)*
Chol (mg/dL)	**467 *(12.1)***	130–370 *(3.4–9.6 mmol/L)*
ALT (IU/L)	**1355**	0–120
AST (IU/L)	**341**	16–40
ALP (IU/L)	**4660**	35–280
GGT (IU/L)	**373**	0–6
CK (IU/L)	**266**	50–250
Na (mEq/L)	**144**	145–158
K (mEq/L)	**3.8**	4.1–5.5
CL (mEq/L)	**98**	106–127
TCO_2 (mEq/L)	18.5	14–27
An. gap (mEq/L)	**31.3**	8–25
Amylase (IU/L)	**1687**	50–1250
Lipase (IU/L)	**3746**	30–560

Urinalysis		Urine sediment	
Color	Yellow	WBCs/hpf	**50–100**
Transparency	Cloudy	RBCs/hpf	**>100**
Sp. gr.	**1.014**	Epith cells/hpf	Negative
Protein	**2+**	Casts/lpf	Negative
Gluc	**4+**	Crystals	Negative
Bilirubin	Negative	Bacteria	**3+ rods**
Blood	**4+**		
pH	5.0		
Ketones	Negative		

Coagulation data		Reference interval
PT (s)	7.5	7.5–10.5
aPTT (s)	**18.2**	10.5–16.5
FDPs (µg/mL)	**1:12**	<1:10

Endocrine data		Reference interval
Free T4 (ng/dL)	**<0.15**	1.2–3.4
Total T4 (µg/dL)	**0.85**	1.5–3.5
Endog TSH (ng/mL)	**0.05**	0.1–0.45

Interpretive discussion

Hematology

The PCV and total RBC count are marginally decreased, with no abnormalities in red blood cell size, hemoglobin content, or morphology. One should consider recent blood loss (particularly GI hemorrhage) even though plasma protein concentration is normal. Alternatively, there may be a mild normochromic, normocytic anemia associated with renal failure. The leukocyte count is increased, with a mature neutrophilia and lymphopenia. This is a stress leukogram, and may support the possibility of hyperadrenocorticism as part of the disease process.

Biochemical profile

The serum glucose concentration is markedly increased. This is well beyond the level encountered due to excitement (sympathetic activation) or stress (glucocorticoid release), and should immediately suggest diabetes mellitus.

The BUN is disproportionately increased relative to the mild increase in serum creatinine concentration. The BUN: creatinine ratio is 50.6, which should suggest gastrointestinal hemorrhage, leading to an increase in hepatic urea production. Nevertheless, some degree of azotemia (prerenal, renal, or postrenal) is probably also present (refer to discussion of urinalysis below). The serum phosphorus is moderately increased, and may be associated with the impaired glomerular filtration and the azotemia. Because the serum total calcium concentration is also decreased, one should consider dietary imbalance or renal disease as causes of secondary hyperparathyroidism. See discussion of ionized Ca below.

The serum total protein and albumin concentrations are normal. Unless there is a concomitant cause for hypoproteinemia, the absence of hyperproteinemia decreases the probability for hemoconcentration and prerenal azotemia due to dehydration.

The serum cholesterol is moderately increased. This may be related to cholestasis, as indicated by the moderate increase in serum to bilirubin concentration and serum ALP and GGT activities. However, the degree of increase in cholesterol is sufficient to warrant consideration of abnormalities in lipoprotein metabolism owing to hepatic disease or an endocrine abnormality. Likewise, the degree of increase in ALP and GGT activities suggests other means for their induction beyond cholestasis, such as hyperadrenocorticism. Marked increases in serum ALT and AST activities indicate hepatocellular damage, which may have contributed to the increases in ALP and GGT activities. The serum CK activity is essentially normal, and rules out the potential contribution of muscle damage to serum AST and ALT increases. Hepatic lipidosis associated with diabetes should be considered as a cause of hepatocellular injury and cholestasis.

A marginal increase in serum amylase and marked increase in serum lipase activities may indicate the presence of pancreatitis. However, concurrent azotemia may impair renal extraction of these enzymes from the serum, leading to increases in their activities.

Serum Na, K, and Cl concentrations are decreased. One should consider typical causes for electrolyte depletion, including pathologic losses from the gastrointestinal and urinary systems, as well as a shift to third space. The marked hyperglycemia should initiate consideration of diabetic ketoacidosis with subsequent urinary electrolyte loss. However, although the anion gap is increased, the serum total CO_2 is normal. It is possible that there are concurrent causes for metabolic acidosis (ketoacidosis) and metabolic alkalosis (vomiting and/or gastrointestinal stasis).

Urinalysis

The urinary specific gravity is in the isosthenuric range, despite azotemia and hyperphosphatemia. This may be the result of renal disease, or impaired concentrating ability due to electrolyte depletion and loss of the medullary concentration gradient. There is significant proteinuria, pyuria, hematuria, and bacteriuria, which most likely indicate a bacterial infection and inflammatory response in the urinary tract. In the absence of tubular casts or information regarding enzymuria or urinary fractional excretion of electrolytes, it is difficult to specify the anatomic location of this disorder. There is significant glucosuria corresponding to the marked hyperglycemia noted earlier. The absence of ketones on the dipstick speaks against the possibility of prominent ketoacidosis (and ketonuria) noted above. However, this test does not detect one of the ketones, β-hydroxybutyric acid. One can anticipate that detectable ketosis would develop if untreated.

Coagulation data

The coagulation profile indicates a slightly prolonged aPTT and mildly increased FDP concentration. This may be the result of liver disease (although one may expect a change in PT prior to one in the aPTT), or incipient DIC (although platelet concentration is usually decreased with DIC). If liver disease was severe enough to impair coagulation factor synthesis, one would first expect to see hypoalbuminemia and/or hypocholesterolemia. It is not possible to draw conclusions with these borderline abnormalities.

Endocrine data

Low free T4, low total T4, and low endogenous TSH are diagnostic for secondary hypothyroidism. Secondary hypothyroidism as a result of decreased endogenous TSH is commonly associated with diabetes mellitus.

Summary

Diabetes mellitus and secondary hypothyroidism.

Case 96

Signalment: 3-year-old MC English springer spaniel
History: Anorexia, occasional vomiting
Physical examination: Lethargic, thin, approximately 8% dehydrated

Hematology		Reference interval
PCV (%)	**32**	37–55
Hgb (g/dL)	**11.1**	12–18
RBC (×10⁶/μL)	**4.47**	5.5–8.5
MCV (fL)	72	60–72
MCHC (g/dL)	35	34–38
Retics (×10³/μL)	ND[a]	<60
NCC (×10³/μL)	9.8	6–17
Segs (×10³/μL)	5.6	3–11.5
Monos (×10³/μL)	0.8	0.1–1.3
Lymphs (×10³/μL)	2.2	1.0–4.8
Eos (×10³/μL)	1.2	0.1–1.2
Platelets (×10³/μL)	Adequate	200–500
TP (P) (g/dL)	**8.5**	6–8

[a]Not determined.

Biochemical profile		Reference interval
Gluc (mg/dL)	83	65–122
BUN (mg/dL)	**47 *(16.8)***	7–28 *(2.5–10.0 mmol/L)*
Creat (mg/dL)	1.6	0.9–1.7
Ca (mg/dL)	**13.8 *(3.45)***	9.0–11.2 *(2.25–2.80 mmol/L)*
Phos (mg/dL)	**6.2 *(2.0)***	2.8–6.1 *(0.9–2.0 mmol/L)*
TP (g/dL)	**7.5**	5.4–7.4
Alb (g/dL)	**5.0**	2.7–4.5
Glob (g/dL)	2.5	1.9–3.4
T. bili (mg/dL)	0.2	0–0.4
Chol (mg/dL)	135	130–370
ALT (IU/L)	49	10–120
AST (IU/L)	19	16–40
ALP (IU/L)	98	35–280
Na (mEq/L)	**132**	145–158
K (mEq/L)	5.5	4.1–5.5
CL (mEq/L)	**97**	106–127
TCO_2 (mEq/L)	**10**	14–27
An. gap (mEq/L)	**30**	8–25
Amylase (IU/L)	1300	50–1250
Lipase (IU/L)	570	30–560

Endocrine data		Reference interval
ACTH stimulation		
Serum cortisol (μg/dL) (pre)	**<0.1 *(<2.8)***	1–4 *(28–100 nmol/L)*
Serum cortisol (μg/dL) (post)	**<0.1 *(<2.8)***	<10.5 *(<290 nmol/L)*

Urinalysis	
Urine specific gravity	1.020

Interpretive discussion

Hematology

A mild anemia is present. Reticulocyte concentration was not determined, thus the degree of regeneration is unknown. Increased polychromasia is not mentioned, suggesting that the anemia is nonregenerative; however, the MCV is at the upper end of the reference interval, suggesting the presence of large immature erythrocytes. Considering the degree of dehydration, anemia is likely more severe than is apparent.

While the leukogram is normal, a patient that is ill and vomiting would be expected to have a stress leukogram. The absence of a stress leukogram should prompt consideration of hypoadrenocorticism.

Plasma protein is increased, probably as a result of dehydration.

Biochemical profile

Azotemia is evidenced by increased BUN, creatinine, and phosphorus concentrations. While azotemia may be prerenal, since the dog is dehydrated, one would expect the urine specific gravity to be greater than 1.030, if this were the case. However, the serum sodium concentration is decreased, and ability to concentrate is impaired by medullary washout of sodium. Refer to the discussion on sodium and potassium for further interpretation.

Hypercalcemia, in light of hyponatremia and hyperkalemia, is likely due to hypoadrenocorticism. The pathophysiology may be related to decreased glucocorticoids and subsequent increased GI calcium uptake, calcium retention by the kidney, as related to sodium loss, or increased albumin-bound calcium. Other causes of hypercalcemia, such as hypercalcemia of malignancy, primary hyperparathyroidism, and vitamin D toxicosis are much less likely in this patient.

Mild hyperproteinemia, due to hyperalbuminemia, is due to dehydration.

Hyponatremia and high normal potassium should cause suspicion of Addison's disease. While these electrolyte abnormalities are not marked, and result in a Na:K ratio of 24, they should prompt an ACTH stimulation test. Hyponatremia and hyperkalemia in this patient, on the other hand, could be a result of renal disease. Hypochloridemia is consistent with hyponatremia. Low total CO_2 is consistent with metabolic acidosis, and the anion gap is increased due to increased unmeasured anions, which in this dehydrated hypovolemic patient are probably lactic acids.

Mild increase in serum amylase and lipase activities are probably secondary to decreased glomerular filtration.

Endocrine data

The immeasurably low cortisol concentration with a "flat-line" response to ACTH confirms hypoadrenocorticism

Summary

Hypoadrenocorticism

Case 97

Signalment: 8-month-old intact male dog
History: Suddenly collapsed during grooming; bloody diarrhea
Physical examination: Extreme weakness, bradycardia, and cool extremities

Hematology		Reference interval
PCV (%)	42	37–55
Hgb (g/dL)	13.3	12–18
RBC ($\times 10^6/\mu L$)	6.6	5.5–8.5
MCV (fL)	64	60–72
MCHC (g/dL)	32	34–38
NCC ($\times 10^3/\mu L$)	12.0	6–17
Segs ($\times 10^3/\mu L$)	7.2	3–11.5
Monos ($\times 10^3/\mu L$)	0.6	0.1–0.3
Lymphs ($\times 10^3/\mu L$)	3.6	1–4.8
Eos ($\times 10^3/\mu L$)	0.6	0.1–1.2
Platelets ($\times 10^3/\mu L$)	410	200–500
TP (P) (g/dL)	6.9	6–8

Hemopathology: Normal.

Biochemical profile		Reference interval
Gluc (mg/dL)	87	65–122
BUN (mg/dL)	**63 *(22.5)***	7–28 *(2.5–10.0 mmol/L)*
Creat (mg/dL)	1.6	0.9–1.7
Ca (mg/dL)	10.3	9.0–11.2
Phos (mg/dL)	5.6	2.8–6.1
TP (g/dL)	6.8	5.7–7.4
Alb (g/dL)	3.9	2.7–4.5
Glob (g/dL)	2.9	1.9–3.4
T. bili (mg/dL)	0.3	0–0.4
Chol (mg/dL)	230	130–370
ALT (IU/L)	80	10–120
AST (IU/L)	32	16–40
ALP (IU/L)	90	35–280
Na (mEq/L)	**127**	145–158
K (mEq/L)	**7.5**	4.1–5.5
CL (mEq/L)	**99**	106–127
TCO_2 (mEq/L)	**12**	14–27
An. gap (mEq/L)	2.3	8–25

Urinalysis			
Color	Yellow	**Urine sediment**	
Transparency	Cloudy	WBCs/hpf	0–1
Sp. gr.	**1.019**	RBCs/hpf	2–3
Protein	Negative	Epith cells/hpf	1–2 transitional
Gluc	Negative	Casts/lpf	0
Bilirubin	Negative	Crystals	0
Blood	Negative	Bacteria	0
pH	6.0		

Endocrine data		Reference interval
ACTH stimulation:		
Serum cortisol (μg/dL) (pre)	1.1	1–4
Serum cortisol (μg/dL) (post)	**1.3 *(36)***	10–20 *(276–552 nmol/L)*

Interpretive discussion

Hematology

The CBC reveals no significant abnormalities.

Biochemical profile

This dog is azotemic. Since urine concentration is not adequate (i.e., it is not >1.030), this may be a renal azotemia, but prerenal azotemia with inadequate renal concentrating ability may occur in hypoadrenocorticism. The hypotension and dehydration that accompany hypoadrenocorticism may result in azotemia, whereas hyponatremia and solute diuresis may result in medullary washout that, in turn, limits renal concentrating ability. The result is azotemia with a urine specific gravity indicating inadequate renal concentrating ability.

Hyponatremia and hyperkalemia, in combination with the abnormal response to ACTH stimulation, confirms the diagnosis of hypoadrenocorticism (see discussion of the ACTH stimulation test below). While a Na:K ratio <23 : 1 is suggestive of hypoadrenocorticism, hyponatremia and hyperkalemia are not specific for this disease. Oliguric or anuric renal failure are common causes of hyponatremia and hyperkalemia and should be considered when these abnormalities are observed, but the response to ACTH stimulation should he adequate to distinguish these diseases.

Hypochloremia is common in animals with hypoadrenocorticism. In renal tubules, Cl is reabsorbed with Na in both the proximal tubule and the loop of Henle. After hyponatremia develops, the concentration of Na in the ultrafiltrate is decreased, and this, in turn, decreases the amount of Na available for reabsorption in these portions of the nephron. The decreased Na absorption results in decreased Cl absorption and hypochloremia.

Decreased serum total CO_2 concentration suggests metabolic acidosis. Metabolic acidosis is common in hypoadrenocorticism and results from decreased tissue perfusion secondary to hypotension and from decreased renal tubular excretion of H+ secondary to mineralocorticoid deficiency.

Urinalysis

Except for the evidence of inadequate urine concentrating ability (see the discussion of azotemia above), the urinalysis is normal.

Endocrine data

The inadequate response to ACTH stimulation in combination with hyponatremia and hyperkalemia confirms hypoadrenocorticism. Dogs with hypoadrenocorticism commonly have decreased basal plasma cortisol concentrations that fail to increase or increase only slightly after ACTH stimulation. If these values do increase after ACTH stimulation, they are usually well below normal post-ACTH stimulation values, especially in dogs with primary hypoadrenocorticism.

Summary

Hyponatremia, hyperkalemia, and a Na:K ratio of 17 : 1 strongly suggest hypoadrenocorticism. An inadequate response to ACTH stimulation confirms this disease. The azotemia with evidence of inadequate urine concentrating ability, while typical of primary renal failure, is more likely due to a combination of prerenal azotemia and decreased renal concentrating ability resulting from the effects of mineralocorticoid deficiency. It is typical of ill animals to have a stress leukogram (Iymphopenia); absence of stress leukogram in this ill animal is compatible with hypoadrenocorticism.

Case 98

Signalment: 6-year-old male canine
History: Lethargic, stopped eating
Physical examination: Depressed, weak pulse, apparent weakness

Hematology		Reference interval
PCV (%)	46.0	37–55
Hgb (g/dL)	16.2	12–18
PBC ($\times10^6/\mu L$)	7.10	5.5–8.5
MCV (fL)	65.0	60–72
MCHC (g/dL)	35.0	34–38
NCC ($\times10^3/\mu L$)	**20.4**	6–17
Segs ($\times10^3/\mu L$)	11.4	3–11.5
Monos ($\times10^3/\mu L$)	**1.8**	0.1–1.3
Lymphs ($\times10^3/\mu L$)	**5.5**	1–4.8
Eos ($\times10^3/\mu L$)	**1.6**	0.1–1.2
Platelets ($\times10^3/\mu L$)	574	200–500
TP (P) (g/dL)	**5.9**	6–8

Biochemical profile		Reference interval
Gluc (mg/dL)	**79**	65–122
BUN (mg/dL)	**95 *(33.9)***	7–28 *(2.5–10.0 mmol/L)*
Creat (mg/dL)	**3.8 *(334)***	0.9–1.7 *(80–150 μmol/L)*
Ca (mg/dL)	**14.3 *(3.57)***	9.0–11.2 *(2.25–2.80 mmol/L)*
Phos (mg/dL)	**9.9 *(3.2)***	*2.8–6.1 (0.9–2.0 mmol/L)*
TP (g/dL)	5.8	5.4–7.4
Alb (g/dL)	3.0	2.7–4.5
Glob (g/dL)	2.8	1.9–3.4
T. bili (mg/dl)	0.3	0–0.4
Chol (mg/dL)	130	130–370
ALT (IU/L)	62	10–120
AST (IU/L)	**108**	16–40
ALP (IU/L)	38	35–280
GGT (IU/L)	3	0–6
Na (mEq/L)	**124**	145–158
K (mEq/L)	**7.1**	4.1–5.5
CL (mEq/L)	**89**	106–127
TCO_2 (mEq/L)	**10.1**	14–27
An. gap (mEq/L)	**32**	8–25
Amylase (IU/L)	**1490**	50–1250
Lipase (IU/L)	130	30–560

Blood gas data (arterial)		Reference interval
pH	**7.213**	7.33–7.45
pO_2 (mmHg)	**101.0**	67–92
pCO_2 (mmHg)	27.6	24–39
HCO_3 (mEq/L)	**10.4**	14–24
Ionized Ca++ (mg/dL)	**6.40**	4.5–5.6

Urinalysis		Urine sediment	
Color	Yellow	WBCs/hpf	1–4
Transparency	Cloudy	RBCs/hpf	1–2
Sp. gr.	**1.018**	Epith cells/hpf	1–2
Protein	Negative	Casts/lpf	Negative
Gluc	Negative	Crystals	Negative
Bilirubin	Trace	Bacteria	Negative
Blood	Negative	Other	
pH	6.0		
UPC	0.93		

Endocrine data		Reference interval
ACTH stimulation		
Serum cortisol (μg/dL) (pre)	**0.04 *(1.1)***	1–4 *(28–110 nmol/L)*
Serum cortisol (μg/dL) (post)	**0.09 *(2.5)***	<20 *(<552 nmol/L)*

Interpretive discussion

Hematology

There are no erythrocyte abnormalities. There is a lymphocytosis, which should prompt brief consideration of lymphoma (note the hypercalcemia), or that could be explained by a corticosteroid deficiency. Whenever an ill animal does not have a stress leukogram, one should consider the possibility of hypoadrenocorticism.

Biochemical profile

The BUN, serum creatinine, and phosphorus concentrations are moderately increased. These findings indicate decreased glomerular filtration rate. However, one cannot differentiate the nature of the azotemia (prerenal, renal, or postrenal) based on these findings alone. Refer to the discussion of urinalysis results for further interpretation.

The serum total calcium concentration is moderately increased. The most common causes for this would be malignancy-associated hypercalcemia, hypoadrenocorticism, or renal failure. One might also consider primary hyperparathyroidism and vitamin D toxicosis.

The serum total protein, albumin, and globulin concentrations are normal. The absence of hemoconcentration decreases the probability for prerenal azotemia associated with dehydration.

There are no significant changes in indices of liver disease, with the exception of a mild increase in serum AST activity. This may be due to mild hepatocellular damage or muscle damage but is small enough that further consideration may not be necessary.

There are significant decrease in the serum concentrations of Na and Cl, as well as a significant increase in serum K concentration. The Na:K ratio is 17.5, which is strongly suggestive of hypoadrenocorticism. The presence of a metabolic acidosis (low total CO_2) is consistent with that possibility, and the anion gap may be increased owing to accumulation of unmeasured anions such as lactic acids or phosphates.

Blood gas data

The blood gas data indicate an uncompensated metabolic acidosis (decreased pH and HCO_3, normal pCO_2). The ionized calcium concentration is increased, further supporting a finding of hypercalcemia. One should consider the possibilities of either primary hypoadrenocorticism or renal disease resulting in a functional deficit in response to corticosteroids and calcium retention.

Urinalysis

The urinary specific gravity revels only marginal concentrating ability, which may result from either renal disease, or loss of the medullary concentration gradient due to electrolyte depletion. This is a common finding in hypoadrenocorticism that should prompt further diagnostics to rule out primary renal disease. The absence of nonregenerative anemia is evidence counter to chronic renal disease. The dipstick protein was negative, and the UPC is <1.0, supporting no significant urinary protein loss.

Endocrine data

The pre- and post-ACTH cortisol concentrations are both low, and there is an inadequate response. This confirms hypoadrenocorticism.

Summary

Hypoadrenocorticism with typical azotemia secondary to hypovolemia. While there is no biochemical evidence of hemoconcentration, hypovolemia is a consistent event in the pathogenesis of azotemia associated with hypoadrenocorticism.

Case 99

Signalment: 6-month-old FS Norwegian elkhound
History: Poor appetite, small, and has not grown well
Physical examination: Quiet, unhappy, thin dog

Hematology		Reference interval
PCV (%)	35.0	34–55
Hgb (g/dL)	11.8	11–18
RBC (10^6/μL)	5.6	5.5–8.5
MCV (fL)	63	60–72
MCHC (g/dL)	34	34–38
NCC (×10^3/μL)	7.7	6–17
Segs (×10^3/μL)	3.6	3–11.5
Bands (×10^3/μL)	0	0–0.3
Monos (×10^3/μL)	1.2	0.1–1.3
Lymphs (×10^3/μL)	2.4	1–4.8
Eos (×10^3/μL)	0.5	0.1–1.2
Platelets (×10^3/μL)	299	200–500
TP (P) (g/dL)	**8.5**	6–8

Biochemical profile		Reference interval
Gluc (mg/dL)	67	65–122
BUN (mg/dL)	**54**	7–28
Creat (mg/dL)	0.9	0.9–1.7
Ca (mg/dL)	**12.7**	9.0–11.2
Phos (mg/dL)	**10.2**	2.8–6.1
TP (g/dL)	**7.8**	5.4–7.4
Alb (g/dL)	**4.9**	2.7–4.5
Glob (g/dL)	2.9	1.9–3.4
T. bili (mg/dL)	0.2	0–0.4
Chol (mg/dL)	211	130–370
ALT (IU/L)	92	10–120
AST (IU/L)	22	16–40
ALP (IU/L)	155	35–280
Na (mEq/L)	**130**	145–158
K (mEq/L)	**7.7**	4.1–5.5
CL (mEq/L)	**98**	106–127
Na:K ratio	**17**	>25
TCO_2 (mEq/L)	**11**	14–27
An. gap (mEq/L)	**28.7**	8–25
Lipase (IU/L)	175	<500
Amylase	**1895**	220–800

Urine analysis	
Urine s.g. voided	**1.022**

Endocrine tests requested		Reference interval
ACTH stimulation		
Serum cortisol (μg/dL) (pre-basal)	0.4	1–4.5
Serum cortisol (μg/dL) (post)	0.5	5.5–20

Interpretive discussion

Hematology

The PCV, hemoglobin, and total RBC count are within reference limits but plasma protein is increased indicating dehydration. If the animal is dehydrated, it is likely that it is mildly anemic. There are no abnormalities in leukogram. Ill animals usually have a stress leukogram.

Biochemical profile

The most significant abnormalities are Na, K, Na:K ratio, and Cl. There are three possible differential diagnoses. The most likely differentials are Addison's disease or chronic renal failure, possibly with a ruptured urinary bladder third. Chronic renal failure is not as probable considering that the creatinine is normal and the animal is capable of concentrating urine. The BUN:Ct ratio is 50, therefore one should suspect dehydration or GI bleeding. Dehydration is determined to be present by increases in both albumin and total serum and plasma protein and can be further confirmed by physical examination. Creatinine will increase in dehydration due to decreased excretion; however, the BUN increases earlier because there will be decreased excretion and increased reabsorption from tubules. The slow transit time of glomerular filtrate through the tubules due to dehydration allows for increased reabsorption of BUN, hence it increases more than creatinine. The urine specific gravity would be expected to be >1.035 if the dog is dehydrated and has normal renal function. The inability to concentrate beyond 1.020 is likely attributable to medullary washout due to the low sodium. Ruptured urinary bladder is unlikely since the dog is urinating and there is no history of trauma. To confirm Addison's disease, one should perform an ACTH stimulation test following the determination of baseline cortisol concentrations.

Further support for Addisonian is: hypercalcemia. Hypercalcemia is seen in one third of dogs with hypoadrenocorticism. However, hypercalcemia can also be seen in a small percentage of dogs with renal failure. It would not be expected in a dog with ruptured bladder. The presence of hypercalcemia in this dog helps prioritize Addison's before renal failure, ruptured urinary bladder, and other differentials. Hyperphosphatemia is attributed to decreased glomerular filtration rate due to dehydration in this case.

The serum glucose concentration is at the low end of the reference interval. Hypoglycemia is sometimes seen in patients with hypoadrenocorticism, likely due to a lack of glucocorticoids as well as mineralocorticoids.

The decreased bicarbonate (TCO_2) is indicative of a metabolic acidosis. Amylase is increased and this is attributed due to decreased glomerular filtration rate. Amylase and lipase are excreted through the urine and any cause of decreased GFR may result in one or both enzymes being increased.

Urine specific gravity of 1.022 in a dog with dehydration indicates inadequate concentrating ability, which could be due to renal disease or medullary washout of sodium. The latter is more likely as azotemia is considered to be prerenal and medullary washout fits with Addison's and chronic hyponatremia. The two most important solutes that produce a concentration gradient in the medullary interstitium are UN and sodium. The decreased sodium in the medullary interstitium means glomerular filtrate (forming urine) can only be partially concentrated.

Special testing

ACTH stimulation confirmed hypoadrenocorticism. The basal sample is less than 1 μg/dL, which strongly implicates Addison's especially given a Na:K ratio of 17. The postsample of 0.5 is not an increase over basal and is therefore flatline, which confirms hypoadrenocorticism in this dog.

Summary

Hypoadrenocorticism (Addison's disease), with prerenal azotemia and probable medullary washout.

The most likely lesion is lymphyocytic adrenalitis, which destroys all three cortical zones of both adrenal glands. Regeneration will not occur therefore recommend treatment with glucocorticoids and mineralocorticoids for life. Dog was treated successfully, gained weight, and lived for 7 years.

Case 100

Signalment: 11-year-old spayed female beagle
History: Polyuria, polydipsia, polyphagia, and bilateral symmetrical alopecia for 5 months
Physical examination: "Pot-bellied," comedones in inguinal region, panting

Hematology		Reference interval
PCV (%)	50	37–55
NCC ($\times 10^3/\mu L$)	**22.6**	6–17
Segs ($\times 10^3/\mu L$)	**20.0**	3–11.5
Monos ($\times 10^3/\mu L$)	**2.3**	0.1–1.3
Lymphs ($\times 10^3/\mu L$)	**0**	1–4.8
Eos ($\times 10^3/\mu L$)	0	0.1–1.2
NRBC ($\times 10^3/\mu L$)	**0.3**	0
Platelets ($\times 10^3/\mu L$)	Adequate	200–500
TP (P) (g/dL)	7.6	6–8

Biochemical profile		Reference interval
Gluc (mg/dL)	**140 *(7.7)***	65–122 *(3.5–6.7 mmol/L)*
BUN (mg/dL)	**6 *(2.1)***	7–28 *(2.5–10.0 mmol/L)*
Creat (mg/dL)	1.0	0.9–1.7
Ca (mg/dL)	10.2	9.0–11.2
Phos (mg/dL)	**2.7 *(0.9)***	2.8–6.1 *(0.9–2.0)*
TP (g/dL)	7.2	5.4–7.4
Alb (g/dL)	4.1	2.7–4.5
Glob (g/dL)	3.1	1.9–3.4
T. bili (mg/dL)	0.2	0–0.4
Chol (mg/dL)	**460 *(12.0)***	130–370 *(3.4–9.6)*
ALT (IU/L)	**400**	10–120
ALP (IU/L)	**4500**	35–280
Na (mEq/L)	**159**	145–158
K (mEq/L)	**3.9**	4.1–5.5
CL (mEq/L)	127	106–127
TCO_2 (mEq/L)	20	14–27
An. gap (mEq/L)	16	8–25

Urinalysis	
Specific gravity	**1.005**

Endocrine data		Reference interval
ACTH stimulation		
Serum cortisol (μg/dL) (pre)	**12 *(331)***	1–4 *(28–110)*
Serum cortisol (μg/dL) (post)	15.5	<20
Low-dose dexamethasone suppression test		
Serum cortisol (μg/dL) (pre)	**9.0 *(248)***	1–4 *(28–110)*
Serum cortisol (μg/dL) (3 hr post)	**8.0 *(221)***	<1.5 *(41)*
Serum cortisol (μg/dL) (8 hr post)	**6.0 *(166)***	<1.5 *(41)*
High-dose dexamethasone suppression test		
Serum cortisol (μg/dL) (pre)	**10 *(276)***	1–4 *(28–110)*
Serum cortisol (μg/dL) (post)	**8 *(221)***	<1.5 *(41)*
Endogenous ACTH (pg/mL)	**10 *(2.2)***	20–100 *(4.4–22.0)*

Interpretive discussion

Hematology

Mature neutrophilia, monocytosis, and lymphopenia are typically seen with increased endogenous or exogenous corticosteroids. Increased concentration of nucleated RBCs is seen with a variety of conditions; in this case they are likely secondary to hyperadrenocorticism.

Biochemical profile

Mild hyperglycemia is consistent with increased endogenous or exogenous corticosteroids. Glucocorticoids increase gluconeogenesis and decrease peripheral utilization of glucose by antagonizing the effects of insulin.

The BUN concentration is below the reference interval. While decreased BUN may be associated with liver failure or inadequate protein intake, diuresis will also result in increased urinary loss of urea nitrogen. In this case, diuresis is probably stimulated by glucocorticoids.

Hypercholesterolemia is associated with numerous conditions, including hypothyroidism, diabetes mellitus, hyperadrenocorticism, and cholestasis. In this patient, the increase is probably due to hyperadrenocorticism.

Alanine aminotransferase activity is mildly increased, indicating glucocorticoid-induced increase in ALT production or hepatocellular damage. Hepatocellular damage is an important feature of steroid hepatopathy, which may be occurring in this dog. Alkaline phosphatase activity is markedly increased. While cholestasis may result in an increase of this magnitude, bilirubin is not increased, suggesting that the increase is likely due to corticosteroid induction of alkaline phosphatase. Activities of this magnitude are almost always related to steroid effect. Determination of steroid-induced alkaline phosphatase isoenzyme would be helpful.

Mild hypernatremia and hypokalemia are commonly seen in approximately 50% of dogs with hyperadrenocorticism.

Urinalysis

Urine specific gravity is low, and is likely due to hyperadrenocorticism. Glucocorticoids are thought to interfere with ADH receptors, resulting in isosthenuria or hyposthenuria, and polyuria and polydipsia.

Endocrine data

ACTH stimulation: The baseline cortisol concentration is well above normal and the post-stimulation cortisol concentration is within the reference interval. While most dogs with hyperadrenocorticism have normal basal cortisol concentrations, this increase is very suggestive of hyperadrenocorticism. While dogs with pituitary-dependent hyperplasia (PDH) have hyperplastic adrenals and dogs with functional adrenocortical tumors have the potential to respond to ACTH stimulation by increasing cortisol production and release, not all do so. Cortisol increases above the reference interval following ACTH stimulation in approximately 85% of dogs with pituitary-dependent disease, and in approximately 50% of dogs with adrenal tumors. In summary, while ACTH stimulation is a useful screening test for PDH and adrenal tumors, cortisol concentrations do not exceed the high end of the reference interval in many dogs. Thus, this dog may have pituitary-dependent disease or an adrenal tumor, based on the ACTH stimulation results.

Low- and high-dose dexamethasone suppression: Dexamethasone screening tests are diagnostically useful because in patients with pituitary-dependent disease, the abnormal pituitary is somewhat resistant to the negative feedback action of cortisol. Moreover, while dexamethasone may inhibit endogenous ACTH production in dogs with adrenal tumors, endogenous ACTH production is probably already maximally suppressed, and at any rate, these tumors usually autonomously secrete cortisol, independent of ACTH. In normal dogs, endogenous ACTH is suppressed by dexamethasone, resulting in a rapid decline in plasma cortisol concentrations, which remain suppressed for up to 48 hours. Thus, since this dog's cortisol concentration did not decrease, either pituitary-dependent disease resulting in adrenocortical hyperplasia, or adrenal neoplasia, is present.

Endogenous ACTH: Endogenous ACTH is below the reference interval in this dog, indicating that the dog has a functional adrenal tumor, rather than pituitary disease.

Summary

Hyperadrenocorticism due to functional adrenal tumor. On abdominal radiographs, a calcified mass cranial to the right kidney was observed. On ultrasound examination, a large right adrenal mass was seen. The left adrenal was not detectable. A CT scan of the brain was normal.

Case 101

Signalment: 4-year-old MC golden retriever
History: Polyuria, polydipsia for several months, on medication for flea allergy dermatitis
Physical examination: Exudative, erythematous plaques in inguinal area, "pot-bellied" appearance

Hematology		Reference interval
PCV (%)	**40**	37–55
NCC (×10³/μL)	**25.9**	6–17
Segs (×10³/μL)	**23.4**	3–11.5
Monos (×10³/μL)	**2.0**	0.1–1.3
Lymphs (×10³/μL)	**0.4**	1–4.8
Eos (×10³/μL)	0.1	0.1–1.2
Platelets (×10³/μL)	Adequate	200–500
TP (P) (g/dL)	7.5	6–8

Biochemical profile		Reference interval
Gluc (mg/dL)	**140 (7.7)**	65–112 *(3.5–6.7 mmol/L)*
BUN (mg/dL)	18	7–28
Creat (mg/dL)	1.2	0.9–1.7
Ca (mg/dL)	10.5	9.0–11.2
Phos (mg/dL)	4.0	2.8–6.1
TP (g/dL)	7.0	5.4–7.4
Alb (g/dL)	4.0	2.7–4.5
Glob (g/dL)	3.0	1.9–3.4
T. bili (mg/dL)	0.2	0–0.4
Chol (mg/dL)	350	130–370
ALT (IU/L)	110	10–120
AST (IU/L)	30	16–40
ALP (IU/L)	**5500**	35–280
GGT (IU/L)	**260**	0–6
Na (mEq/L)	**148**	145–158
K (mEq/L)	5.0	4.1–5.5
CL (mEq/L)	112	106–127
TCO_2 (mEq/L)	16	14–27
An. gap (mEq/L)	25	8–25

Urinalysis		Urine sediment	
Color	Yellow	WBCs/hpf	2
Transparency	Cloudy	RBCs/hpf	2
Sp. gr.	**1.002**	Epith cells/hpf	0
Protein	Negative	Casts/lpf	0
Gluc	Negative	Crystals	0
Bilirubin	Negative	Bacteria	4+
Blood	Negative		
pH	6.5		

Endocrine data		Reference interval
ACTH stimulation		
Serum cortisol (μg/dL) (pre)	1.2	1–4
Serum cortisol (μg/dL) (post)	1.2 *(33)*	>10.5; <20 *(>290; <550 nmol/L)*
Low-dose dexamethasone suppression test		
Serum cortisol (μg/dL) (pre)	2.0	1–4
Serum cortisol (μg/dL) (3 hr post)	**2.0 *(55)***	<1.5 *(<41 nmol/L)*
Serum cortisol (μg/dL) (8 hr post)	**1.7 *(47)***	<1.5 *(<41 nmol/L)*

Interpretive discussion

Hematology

Mature neutrophilia, monocytosis, and lymphopenia are indicative of a corticosteroid (stress) leukogram.

Biochemical profile

Mild hyperglycemia is consistent with increased endogenous or exogenous corticosteroids.

Alkaline phosphatase activity is markedly increased. While cholestasis may result in an increase of this magnitude, bilirubin is not increased, suggesting that the increase is likely due to corticosteroid induction of alkaline phosphatase. Determination of steroid-induced alkaline phosphatase isoenzyme would be helpful.

Gamma glutamyltransferase activity is also markedly increased, and with the lack of increase in ALT and AST activities, as well as bilirubin concentration, corticosteroid induction is likely.

The combination of mild hyperglycemia and increased ALP and GGT activities, with no other evidence of cholestasis, should trigger further endocrine testing.

Urinalysis

Low urine specific gravity (often hyposthenuria) is commonly seen in patients with hyperadrenocorticism. Glucocorticoids are thought to interfere with ADH receptors, resulting in isosthenuria or hyposthenuria, and polyuria and polydipsia. Bacteriuria without significant pyuria may also occur with hyperadrenocorticism.

Endocrine data

ACTH stimulation: Patients with iatrogenic hyperadrenocorticism have a "flat-line" response to ACTH stimulation (much like a patient with hypoadrenocorticism) due to feedback to the pituitary and secondary adrenal atrophy. While some corticosteroid drugs cross-react on the cortisol assay, the post-ACTH response will not be higher than the pre-ACTH response.

Low-dose dexamethasone suppression: LDDS is not helpful in diagnosing iatrogenic hyperadrenocorticism. The pituitary is already responding to feedback from iatrogenic corticosteroids, and adrenal glands are atrophied.

Summary

Iatrogenic Cushing disease that resulted from Vetalog injections for flea allergy dermatitis. Fleas were eliminated, and the dog was slowly withdrawn from corticosteroids by treating on alternate days with decreasing doses over several months.

Case 102

Signalment: 10-year-old spayed female Airedale
History: "Leaking" urine, polydipsia, limping
Physical examination: Ruptured anterior cruciate ligament, "pot-bellied," mild truncal alopecia

Hematology		Reference interval
PCV (%)	**58**	37–55
NCC ($\times 10^3/\mu L$)	**24.4**	6–17
Segs ($\times 10^3/\mu L$)	**21.5**	3–11.5
Monos ($\times 10^3/\mu L$)	**2.4**	0.1–1.3
Lymphs ($\times 10^3/\mu L$)	**0**	1–4.8
NRBC ($\times 10^3/\mu L$)	**0.5**	0
Platelets ($\times 10^3/\mu L$)	Adequate	200–500

Biochemical profile		Reference interval
Gluc (mg/dL)	**130 *(7.1)***	65–122 *(3.5–6.7 mmol/L)*
BUN (mg/dL)	18	7–28
Creat (mg/dL)	1.2	0.9–1.7
Ca (mg/dL)	10.2	9.0–11.2
Phos (mg/dL)	4.9	2.8–6.1
TP (g/dL)	5.7	5.7–7.4
Alb (g/dL)	2.7	2.7–4.5
Glob (g/dL)	3.0	1.9–3.4
T. bili	0.3	0–0.4
Chol (mg/dL)	350	130–370
ALT (IU/L)	65	10–120
AST (IU/L)	**60**	16–40
ALP (IU/L)	**4000**	35–280

Urinalysis	
Sp. gr.	**1.008**
Bacteria	Many

Endocrine data		Reference interval
ACTH stimulation		
Serum cortisol (μg/dL) (pre)	**8 *(221)***	1–4 *(28–110 nmol/L)*
Serum cortisol (μg/dL) (post)	**20 *(552)***	<20 *(<552 nmol/L)*
Low-dose dexamethasone suppression test		
Serum cortisol (μg/dL) (pre)	**6 *(166)***	1–4 *(28–110 nmol/L)*
Serum cortisol (μg/dL) (3 hr post)	0.9	<1.5
Serum cortisol (μg/dL) (8 hr post)	**1.7 *(47)***	<1.5 *(<41 nmol/L)*
High-dose dexamethasone suppression test		
Serum cortisol (μg/dL) (pre)	**9 *(248)***	1–4 *(28–110 nmol/L)*
Serum cortisol (μg/dL) (post)	**3 *(83)***	<1.5 *(<41 nmol/L)*
Endogenous ACTH (pg/mL)	**350 *(77)***	20–100 *(4.4–22.0 pmol/L)*

Interpretive discussion

Hematology

The PCV is mildly increased, with increased nucleated erythrocyte concentration. Possibilities for this combination might include hypoxia or other causes of increased erythropoietin concentration. Dogs with hyperadrenocorticism will sometimes have increased erythropoiesis. Additionally, corticosteroids may inhibit removal of NRBC by macrophages in spleen. Mature neutrophilia, monocytosis, and lymphopenia are indicative of a stress leukogram.

Biochemical profile

Mild hyperglycemia is consistent with a stress leukogram, and may be a result of increased endogenous or exogenous glucocorticoids.

Alkaline phosphatase is markedly increased, AST is mildly increased, and cholesterol is borderline high. No other abnormalities are present. Increased alkaline phosphatase activity and mild hypercholesterolemia may be secondary to cholestasis; however, serum bilirubin is not increased. Alkaline phosphatase activity may also increase secondary to steroid induction. This is most likely given the magnitude of increase. The slight increase in serum AST activity may be due to mild steroid hepatopathy or steroid induction.

Urinalysis

Urine specific gravity is quite low, and while it is not necessarily abnormal, it is consistent with decreased urinary concentrating ability in dogs with hyperadrenocorticism, related to decreased responsiveness to ADH. Bacteriuria without pyuria may be seen in dogs with hyperadrenocorticism.

Physical exam, history, stress leukogram, hyperglycemia, and increased serum alkaline phosphatase activity should trigger screening tests for hyperadrenocorticism.

Endocrine data

ACTH stimulation: Baseline cortisol is above normal and poststimulation is "borderline." Stimulation of above 20 is consistent with hyperadrenocorticism. Eighty-five percent of dogs with pituitary-dependent hyperplasia stimulate, as do approximately 50% of dogs with adrenal tumors. Thus, the ACTH stimulation is not diagnostic in this dog but is suspicious.

Low-dose dexamethasone suppression: Baseline cortisol is above normal. The dog suppressed at 3 hours, with escape from suppression at 8 hours. In normal dogs, endogenous ACTH is suppressed by dexamethasone, resulting in a rapid decline in plasma cortisol concentrations, which remain suppressed for up to 48 hours. Most dogs with adrenal tumors show no suppression at 3 or 8 hours. If a dog suppresses at 3 hours but does not remain suppressed at 8 hours, it is likely that the dog has PDH, rather than an adrenal tumor. This "escape" is thought to be due to rapid clearance of dexamethasone.

High-dose dexamethasone suppression: Baseline cortisol is above normal. The dog did not suppress to the range for normal dogs. Dogs with adrenal disease do not suppress, and most dogs with pituitary-dependent adrenal hyperplasia (PPH) do suppress. Very high-dose steroids will suppress ACTH production, and hence cortisol secretion, even with PPD. However, most dogs with pituitary macroadenomas do not suppress; an endogenous ACTH serum concentration is indicated.

Endogenous ACTH: Dogs with PDH have normal to increased endogenous ACTH, while dogs with adrenal tumors have decreased endogenous ACTH. Thus, this dog has pituitary-dependent disease.

Summary

A large pituitary macroadenoma was present in this dog. Note that multiple endocrine tests were required to make this diagnosis.

Case 103

Signalment: 8-year-old male castrated poodle
History: Hair loss, PU/PD
Physical examination: Hair loss along abdomen and legs, pendulous abdomen

Hematology		Reference interval
PCV (%)	42.0	37–55
Hgb (g/dL)	13.8	12–18
RBC ($10^6/\mu L$)	5.8	5.5–8.5
MCV (fL)	72.0	60–72
MCHC (g/dL)	33	34–38
NCC ($\times 10^3/\mu L$)	**23.4**	6–17
Segs ($\times 10^3/\mu L$)	**20.1**	3–11.5
Bands ($\times 10^3/\mu L$)	0	0–0.3
Monos ($\times 10^3/\mu L$)	2.7	0.1–1.3
Lymphs ($\times 10^3/\mu L$)	**0.6**	1–4.8
Eos ($\times 10^3/\mu L$)	0	0.1–1.2
Platelets ($\times 10^3/\mu L$)	455	200–500
TP (P) (g/dL)	6.5	6–8

Hemopathology: Few nucleated red blood cells noted.

Biochemical profile		Reference interval
Gluc (mg/dL)	**289**	65–122
BUN (mg/dL)	22	7–28
Creat (mg/dL)	0.8	0.9–1.7
Ca (mg/dL)	10.1	9.0–11.2
Phos (mg/dL)	5.2	2.8–6.1
TP (g/dL)	6.7	5.4–7.4
Alb (g/dL)	3.3	2.7–4.5
Glob (g/dL)	3.4	1.9–3.4
T. bili (mg/dL)	0.2	0–0.4
Chol (mg/dL)	**411**	130–370
ALT (IU/L)	**420**	10–120
AST (IU/L)	**122**	16–40
ALP (IU/L)	**6855**	35–280
Na (mEq/L)	146	145–158
K (mEq/L)	4.3	4.1–5.5
CL (mEq/L)	115	106–127
Na:K ratio	34	>25
TCO_2 (mEq/L)	20	14–27
An. gap (mEq/L)	15.3	8–25
Lipase (IU/L)	175	<500
Amylase	441	220–800

Urinalysis		Urine sediment	
Color	Yellow	WBCs/hpf	**20–30**
Transparency	Hazy	RBCs/hpf	**50–100**
Specific gravity	**1.008**	Epithelial cells/hpf	few
Protein	**2+**	Casts/lpf	neg
Glucose	**1+**		
Ketones	Neg		
Bilirubin	Neg	Crystals	Triple phosphate
Blood	**3+**	Bacteria	**1+**

Endocrine data	Cortisol (μg/dL)	Reference interval
Basal cortisol	**3.6**	1–4
ACTH stim	**28**	8–16
Basal cortisol	**4.1**	1–4
LDDS 8 hr post	**4.4**	<1.4
Basal cortisol		**3.8**
HDDS 4 hr	**4.6**	<1.4
HDDS 8 hr	**2.2**	<1.4
Endogenous ACTH pg/mL	**264**	10–80
Two weeks later		
Basal cortisol	**0.3**	1–4
ACTH stim	**0.4**	8–16

Interpretive discussion

Hematology

A few nucleated red blood cells are present in the absence of anemia. This may indicate a disruption in the endothelial barrier in centers of hematopoiesis, or is possibly a result of immunosuppression and lack of removal of nuclei by macrophages. Increased NRBCs can be seen with hemangiosarcoma, some leukemias, lead toxicity, hyperadrenocorticism (HAC) and DIC. The leukogram is characteristic of a stress or steroid response: mature neutrophilia, lymphopenia, eosinopenia, and monocytosis.

Biochemical profile

Marked increase in ALP with only mild increases in ALT and AST indicates possible cholestasis and/or hyperadrenocorticism. An ALP over 5000 IU/L without bilirubinemia and only mild increases in ALT and AST is most consistent with HAC. Further support for this diagnosis is history of alopecia and PU/PD coupled with dilute urine, cystitis and nucleated red blood cells. Over 90% of Cushingoid dogs will have mild to marked ALP. If ALP is not increased it is very unlikely that a dog has HAC. Cholesterol is increased, which in this dog could be cholestasis, hypothyroidism, or HAC. Increases in ALT and AST are attributed to glycogen (steroid) hepatopathy induced by hyperadrenocorticism. Hyperglycemia is moderate, which is consistent with hyperadrenocorticism.

The urine analysis has abundant evidence for infectious cystitis; numerous leukocytes and bacteria are present. Collection method is not specified, therefore inflammation could be present anywhere in the urogenital tract. Proteinuria may be due to the inflammatory response and increased capillary permeability. Absence of casts and no azotemia support cystitis over pyelonephritis. Dilute urine is likely a result of a failure to concentrate due to glucocorticoid interference with ADH, subsequent polyuria, and responsive polydipsia. Cystitis is fairly common in dogs with hyperadrenocorticism.

At this point, laboratory evaluation of the endocrine system should be done. Initially, a low-dose dexamethasone suppression (LDDS) test should be performed. If LLDS indicates hyperadrenocorticism, one should then perform an endogenous ACTH to distinguish pituitary-dependent hyperadrenocorticism (PD HAC) from an adrenal tumor.

Endocrine testing

In this patient, the ACTH stimulation was done, and although the basal cortisol is normal, the post-stim sample is >22 µg/dL, which is excessive and supports hyperadrenocorticism. One must now differentiate pituitary-dependent disease from an adrenal tumor. The basal concentration of cortisol in the LDDS is just above reference interval but the 8-hour value is well above 1.4 µg/dL, therefore there was failure to suppress and Cushing's disease is ruled in when all of the other data fit, as in this dog. (False-positive rate for LDDS, however, is as high as 50%, therefore all of the other lab and historical and physical exam results need to fit with HAC.) Unfortunately, a 4-hour sample was not collected, which could have proven helpful to distinguish pituitary and adrenal-dependent HAC. If the 4-hour sample exhibited suppression (<1.4) with the present value for the 8-hour sample of no suppression, it would have indicated a rebound, which is consistent with pituitary-dependent Cushing's disease, the more common cause of HAC. The HDDS is confusing or at least not very helpful. The basal cortisol is normal, the 4-hour sample clearly failed to suppress and the 8-hour sample is above 1.4, but it is almost 50% less than the basal and the 4-hour samples. The interpretation is the HDDS failed to suppress, indicating AT or PD HAC (suppression would indicate the dog had PD HAC). Although the endocrine testing to this point indicates an adrenal tumor is possible, adrenal tumors only account for 10–20% of dogs with HAC. Furthermore, there seemed to be some suppression by the HDDS but even using a decrease of cortisol by 50% from basal it still did not clearly suppress. Another way to define suppression is if the 8-hour sample is less than 50% of basal even if it is still greater than 1.4 µg/dL. In this dog the 8-hour sample is 57% of basal, and the 8-hour sample is 47% of the 4-hour sample. Because distinction of AT and PD is needed for treatment and the HDDS was equivocal, abdominal ultrasonography (US) and an endogenous ACTH concentration were performed. Abdominal US did not identify an adrenal tumor and the endogenous ACTH clearly indicates this dog has PD HAC.

Summary

The e ACTH is markedly increased, and therefore the dog has a pituitary neoplasm secreting ACTH. The dog was given mitotane. The ACTH stim 2 weeks postdiagnosis indicates a flatline response. The dog was clinically normal, and the electrolytes were normal, and therefore this indicated degeneration to necrosis of zona fasciculata by the mitotane. When dosed correctly the cortex will eventually regenerate. Under the stimulation of the ACTH-secreting pituitary tumor the adrenal cortex will regenerate and is the reason repeated ACTH stims will be required during maintenance therapy. The results of the ACTH stim are the same pattern seen with hypoadrenocorticism, spontaneous disease, or from mitotane or steroid therapy.

Case 104

Signalment: 6-year-old male dog
History: Change in temperament from docile to irritable. Severe constipation for several days.
Physical examination: No abnormalities detected

Hematology		Reference interval
PCV (%)	44	37–55
Hgb (g/dL)	14.5	12–18
RBC ($\times10^6/\mu L$)	6.7	5.5–8.5
MCV (fL)	66	60–72
MCHC (g/dL)	33	34–38
NCC ($\times10^3/\mu L$)	15.6	6–17
Segs ($\times10^3/\mu L$)	12.7	3–11.5
Monos ($\times10^3/\mu L$)	0.2	0.1–1.3
Lymphs ($\times10^3/\mu L$)	2.4	1–4.8
Eos ($\times10^3/\mu L$)	0.3	0.1–1.2
Platelets ($\times10^3/\mu L$)	440	200–500
TP (P) (g/dL)	6.8	6–8

Hemopathology: Normal.

Biochemical profile		Reference interval
Gluc (mg/dL)	80	65–122
BUN (mg/dL)	28	7–28
Creat (mg/dL)	1.5	0.9–1.7
Ca (mg/dL)	**14.3 *(3.57)***	9.0–11.2 *(2.25–2.80 mmol/L)*
Phos (mg/dL)	**1.7 *(0.5)***	2.8–6.1 *(0.9–2.0 mmol/L)*
TP (g/dL)	6.1	5.4–7.4
Alb (g/dL)	3.4	2.7–4.5
Glob (g/dL)	2.7	1.9–3.4
T. bili (mg/dL)	0.4	0–0.4
Chol (mg/dL)	235	130–370
ALT (IU/L)	100	10–120
AST (IU/L)	33	16–40
ALP (IU/L)	**285**	35–280
Na (mEq/L)	145	145–158
K (mEq/L)	5.3	4.1–5.5
CL (mEq/L)	115	106–127
TCO_2 (mEq/L)	21	14–27
An. gap (mEq/L)	14	8–25

Urinalysis (catheterized)		Urine sediment	
Color	Yellow	WBCs/hpf	0–2
Transparency	Clear	RBCs/hpf	0
Sp. gr.	**1.011**	Epith cells/hpf	0
Protein	Negative	Casts/lpf	0
Gluc	Negative	Crystals	0
Bilirubin	Negative	Bacteria	0
Blood	Negative		
pH	6.5		

Endocrine data		Reference interval
Intact parathormone	**22**	2–13 (pmol/L)
PTH-rp	Undetectable	<0.2 (pmol/L)

Interpretive discussion

Hematology

In light of normal results for other erythrocyte measurements, the decreased MCHC is marginal and not important.

The mild mature neutrophilia, in the absence of lymphopenia, suggests normal variability or very mild inflammation. This dog's irritability may have predisposed it to epinephrine release when the venipuncture was performed, although excitement leukograms are quite rare in dogs.

Biochemical profile

Hypercalcemia and hypophosphatemia can occur with primary hyperparathyroidism and pseudohyperparathyroidism (hypercalcemia of malignancy). In this case, the increased intact parathormone (iPTH) and normal parathormone-related protein (PTH-rp) concentrations are most suggestive of primary hyperparathyroidism (see discussion of hormone assays below). Other causes of hypercalcemia include vitamin D toxicosis, excessive bone resorption, and renal failure (5–10% of these cases in dogs), but serum phosphorus concentration is typically normal to increased in these cases.

The slightly increased serum alkaline phosphatase activity is not significant. There is no evidence suggesting either cholestasis or increased corticosteroid levels. Since this dog has an abnormality of calcium and phosphorus metabolism, it is possible that altered bone metabolism is occurring. Although the net effect in this animal is probably bone demineralization, increased osteoblastic activity, as part of effort to regenerate bone, may have resulted in this slight increase in activity.

Urinalysis

Low urine specific gravity may reflect this dog's hydration status and, therefore, may be normal in this patient. Hypercalcemia can, however, interfere with renal concentrating ability and can result in decreased urine specific gravity with subsequent polyuria and polydipsia. Nephrocalcinosis, other toxic effects of calcium on renal tubules, and interference with the action of antidiuretic hormone are possible mechanisms for decreased concentrating ability in hypercalcemic animals. The absence of polyuria and polydipsia in this dog suggests that calcium interference with renal concentrating ability is not a major factor.

Endocrine data

Increased intact parathormone (iPTH) concentration and undetectable PTH-related protein (PTH-rp) concentration indicate that this dog has primary hyperparathyroidism, rather than hypercalcemia of malignancy. The iPTH concentrations are increased due to overproduction of PTH by hyperplastic or neoplastic parathyroid glands. Parathormone-related protein is synthesized by malignant cells of neoplasms such as lymphoma and apocrine gland adenocarcinoma of the anal sac, but not by the parathyroid glands, and concentrations of PTH-rp are, therefore, not increased in animals with primary hyperparathyroidism.

Summary

The combination of hypercalcemia, hypophosphatemia, increased iPTH concentration, and undetectable PTH-rp concentration indicate primary hyperparathyroidism in this case. A mass in the neck region compatible in location with the parathyroid gland was found during a more thorough physical examination. Surgical removal and histopathologic examination revealed a parathyroid adenoma. This dog's clinical signs and serum calcium and phosphorus concentrations returned to normal after surgery. Irritability is unusual in hypercalcemic dogs; dullness is more common.

Case 105

Signalment: 11-year-old FS Australian cattle dog
History: Poor appetite
Physical examination: Quiet, adequate body condition

Hematology		Reference interval
PCV (%)	53	39–58
Hgb (g/dL)	19.7	13.8–20.3
RBC (10^6/μL)	7.67	5.7–8.0
MCV (fL)	75	61–75
MCHC (g/dL)	34.3	30.8–35.4
NCC (×103/μL)	6.91	4.4–11.6
Segs (×103/μL)	4.9	2.8–9.1
Bands (×103/μL)	0	0–0.3
Monos (×103/μL)	0.9	0.07–1.0
Lymphs (×103/μL)	2.4	0.6–3.3
Eos (×103/μL)	0.2	0–1.2
Platelets (×103/μL)	366	200–500
TP (P) (g/dL)	7.4	6.1–7.5

Biochemical profile		Reference interval
Gluc (mg/dL)	91	70–131
BUN (mg/dL)	14	6–26
Creat (mg/dL)	0.7	0.7–1.5
Ca (mg/dL)	**12.3**	9.3–11.5
Phos (mg/dL)	3.3	2.5–5.6
Magnesium (mg/dL)	2.0	1.8–2.5
TP (g/dL)	6.7	5.2–7.4
Alb (g/dL)	3.9	3–3.9
Glob (g/dL)	2.8	1.7–3.8
T. bili (mg/dL)	0.1	0–0.3
Chol (mg/dL)	274	124–344
ALS (IU/L)	72	12–54
ALP (IU/L)	62	16–140
GGT (IU/L)	5	0–6
CK (IU/L)	176	43–234
Na (mEq/L)	145	140–156
K (mEq/L)	4.4	4–5.3
CL (mEq/L)	111	108–122
Na:K ratio	32.6	>25
TCO_2 (mEq/L)	22	18–26
An. gap (mEq/L)	16.1	11.2–19
Lipase (IU/L)	210	12–147
Amylase	600	236–1337

Urine analysis	
Urine s.g. voided	1.007

Interpretive discussion

Hematology

Unremarkable; absence of a stress leukogram may prove informative.

Biochemical profile

Mild hypercalcemia is the only abnormality. The increased total serum calcium explains the dilute hyposthenuria, as hypercalcemia affects the function of ADH on tubules. Serum phosphorus is normal, which is somewhat helpful to shorten the list of differentials for hypercalcemia. Recommend rechecking calcium, total and ionized, and if both are increased pursue possible causes of hypercalcemia. The calcium is likely to be increased again given the urine specific gravity. The two most likely differentials are hypercalcemia of malignancy and primary hyperparathyroidism because the serum phosphorus is normal and there are no other significant biochemical abnormalities. Unlikely differentials are hypoadrenocorticism, renal failure, vitamin D toxicity, and granulomatous diseases, all of which usually have increased serum phosphorus and produce other biochemical disturbances. The only two diseases that produce hypercalcemia and hypophosphatemia in dogs are hypercalcemia of malignancy and primary hyperparathyroidism.

Summary and follow-up

Both total serum calcium and ionized calcium were increased on a recheck. On physical examination, no evidence of lymphoma or perirectal apocrine gland adenocarcinoma was found. Serum was sent for PTH and PTH-rp.

Endocrine data		Reference interval
PTH (pmol/L)	**35.5**	3–17
PTH-rp (pmol/L)	0	0–0.9
iCa	**1.65**	1.25–1.45

These results confirm hypercalcemia and rule in primary hyperparathyroidism.

The neck region was explored and a small mass was found in the region of one thyroid lobe. During surgery a STAT methodology to measure PTH pre- and postremoval of any mass was employed and the results were:

Additional endocrine data		Reference interval
PTH Sample 1, pre, Turbo intact PTH (pg/mL)	**98**	11.2–72.8
PTH Sample 2, post, Turbo intact PTH (pg/mL)	**9.0**	

The decrease in PTH in the second sample, after the parathyroid mass was removed is dramatic (less than 50% of previous sample) indicating that the offending lesion was removed.

Comment

The serum concentration of PTH was increased in this dog when it was hypercalcemic, which makes the diagnosis of primary hyperparathyroidism (HPTH) quite simple. However, increased PTH is only present in about 25% of dogs and the remaining dogs (75%) with primary HPTH will have a concentration of PTH within reference interval. Moreover, 45% of dogs with primary hyperparathyroidism will have serum PTH concentrations in the low to middle range. Increased concentrations of PTH are the exception in dogs, but if PTH is detectable in an animal that is hypercalcemic and not azotemic, then this combination is inappropriately abnormal because PTH should be decreased or undetectable in response to nonparathyroid-induced hypercalcemia. If PTH is within the reference interval, it is inappropriately high in the face of hypercalcemia, and therefore diagnostic for primary HPTH. It indicates the parathyroid gland is secreting PTH at a time when secretion should be suppressed. It is critical to measure PTH-rp concurrently as many dogs with hypercalcemia of malignancy will have measurable PTH.

Ultrasonography of the neck region is just as accurate at identifying a parathyroid mass as is measuring serum PTH and if positive will localize the side of the neck to look for the adenoma during surgery. More than one mass is possible, especially in keeshonds.

Case 106

Signalment: 1-year-old FS mixed-breed dog
History: Weight loss, poor appetite, and lethargy
Physical examination: Thin body condition, depressed attitude

Hematology		Reference interval
Packed cell volume (%)	**32**	39–58
Hemoglobin (g/dL)	**10.8**	13.8–20.3
RBC (10^6/μL)	**4.27**	5.7–8.01
MCV (fL)	74	61–75
MCHC (g/dL)	34	30.8–35.4
Total nucleated cell count (×10^3/μL)	10.2	4.4–11.6
Segmented neutrophils (×10^3/μL)	7.9	2.84–9.11
Band neutrophils (×10^3/μL)	0	0–0.3
Monocytes (×10^3/μL)	1.9	0.075–1.0
Lymphocytes (×10^3/μL)	**0.4**	0.59–3.3
Eosinophils (×10^3/μL)	0	0.03–1.2
Platelets (×10^3/μL)	386	190–468
Plasma protein (g/dL)	7.1	6.1–7.5

Biochemical profile		Reference interval
Gluc (mg/dL)	98	70–131
BUN (mg/dL)	**74**	6–26
Creat (mg/dL)	**3.7**	0.7–1.5
Ca (mg/dL)	**17.3**	9.3–11.5
Phos (mg/dL)	**7.3**	2.5–5.6
Magnesium (mg/dL)	**2.0**	**1.8–2.5**
TP (g/dL)	6.9	5.2–7.4
Alb (g/dL)	3.9	3–3.9
Glob (g/dL)	3.0	1.7–3.8
T. bili (mg/dL)	0.1	0–0.3
Chol (mg/dL)	254	124–344
ALS (IU/L)	**372**	12–54
AST (IU/L)	**388**	42–175
ALP (IU/L)	**662**	16–140
GGT (IU/L)	**15**	0–6
CK (IU/L)	111	43–234
Na (mEq/L)	141	140–156
K (mEq/L)	4.9	4–5.3
CL (mEq/L)	110	108–122
Na:K ratio	28.7	>25
TCO_2 (mEq/L)	**12**	18–26
An. gap (mEq/L)	**23.9**	11.2–19
Lipase (IU/L)	**510**	12–147
Amylase	**1724**	236–1337

Urinalysis cystocentesis		Urine sediment	
Color	Yellow	WBCs/hpf	0–3
Transparency	Clear	RBCs/hpf	**10–30**
Specific gravity	**1.010**	Epithelial cells/hpf	None
Protein	**1+**	Casts/lpf	Neg
Glucose		Crystals	None
Ketones	Neg		
Bilirubin	Neg		
Blood	**2+**		

Interpretive discussion

Hematology

There is a mild anemia. Although a reticulocyte count is not present, the indices are normocytic normochromic, which indicates it may be nonregenerative. The azotemia could explain this anemia if the azotemia is due to chronic renal disease. Anemia of inflammatory disease is another possible cause of the anemia in this dog. There is a stress leukogram as evidenced by the lymphopenia, eosinopenia, and monocytosis.

Biochemical profile

The dog has renal failure based on mild azotemia combined with isosthenuria. However, any time the serum calcium is increased the kidneys may not be able to concentrate urine adequately (interference with ADH) which in this case clouds the interpretation that primary renal disease is present. If this dog is dehydrated the azotemia may all or partially be due to prerenal and the dilute urine in the face of dehydration is caused by hypercalcemia. Hypercalcemia is severe, hyperphosphatemia is mild to moderate. The Ca × P product is 126, which indicates mineralization of soft tissues is occurring. Mineralization may have caused the renal failure or at least enhanced it. The diagnostic dilemma is to determine which came first, the renal failure or the hypercalcemia. It is often difficult to distinguish and there may be two diseases occurring, renal failure and a disease other than renal disease that caused hypercalcemia (e.g., a malignancy, vitamin D toxicity, etc.). In this dog it seems more likely the hypercalcemia came first or that there is a second disease causing hypercalcemia. This is based on mild hyperphosphatemia and marked hypercalcemia. Rules to help make this distinction are: the greater the serum P the more likely the primary disease is renal and the lower the serum P the more likely there is hypercalcemia of malignancy (HCM). The higher the serum calcium the more likely there is a malignancy and the lower the calcium the more likely renal disease is causing hypercalcemia. The greater the azotemia the more likely it is primary renal and the lower the azotemia the more likely the renal problems are caused by the mineralization or it is pre renal. The easiest way to distinguish is to either find the malignancy or identify the type of renal failure (chronic, acute, glomerular, pyelonephritis, etc.). In this dog it seems clear the primary disease is one that is causing hypercalcemia because the azotemia is mild, the hypercalcemia is severe and hyperphosphatemia is mild. This distinction can be more difficult in other cases. A reasonable plan is to search for cancer and give the dog fluids to see if the azotemia can be reversed. Measuring ionized calcium may also be diagnostically helpful. If the ionized calcium is within the reference interval, then primary renal failure is more likely, but if ionized calcium is increased, it could still be either primary renal or a malignancy.

The urine is not concentrated, which could be primary renal or secondary to hypercalcemia. There is some blood likely due to cystocentesis, which may also be responsible for the 1+ protein. The rest of the analysis is unremarkable.

The hepatic leakage enzymes are increased (ALT and AST) and the enzymes associated with cholestasis are increased (ALP, GGT). There are many possible causes of cholestasis in this dog, one of which is an infiltrative disease in the liver such as lymphoma, another possibility is pancreatitis. The increases in lipase and amylase are mild and seem more likely due to decreased GFR (azotemia) and therefore decreased excretion than pancreatitis. If the dog had pancreatitis it may have hypocalcemia, tender abdomen and be overweight with an acute onset of problems, none of which this dog has. The dog has a metabolic acidosis probably caused by dehydration and/or renal disease.

A reasonable plan is to search for lymphoma (palpate lymph nodes, search for an anterior thoracic mass, abdominal organ evaluation, etc.) and do a rectal and perirectal exam to evaluate if a carcinoma of the anal sacs is present. If a malignant tumor is found there is no need to perform PTH and PTH rp assays.

Summary

A mass was found in the pelvic vault, and aspirational cytology indicated it was a tumor of the anal sacs. These are invariably malignant, but repeated excisions and/or chemotherapy can extend a dog's life for months or years. These owners declined treatments. Intravenous and subcutaneous fluid therapy decreased the azotemia, but it did not return to normal. An autopsy was not performed so it is not known if or what type of renal disease was present and whether mineralization played a role. The anemia was due to anemia of chronic disease (cancer) and/or concurrent renal disease. The most common substance secreted by tumors is PTH-rp, which stimulates phosphaturia and results in hypophosphatemia, absolute or as in this dog relative for the degree of azotemia. Primary hyperparathyroidism could cause the hypercalcemia and phosphaturia, but rarely is there concurrent azotemia with primary hyperparathyroidism.

Case 107

Signalment: 9-year-old intact male dog
History: One seizure. Occasional tremors observed.
Physical examination: Physical abnormalities but had seizure during examination

Hematology		Reference interval
PCV (%)	44	37–55
Hgb (g/dL)	15.2	12–18
RBC (×10^6/μL)	7.1	5.5–8.5
MCV (fL)	62	60–72
MCHC (g/dL)	35	34–38
NCC (×10^3/μL)	**20.2**	6–17
Segs (×10^3/μL)	**17.2**	3–11.5
Monos (×10^3/μL)	**2.4**	0.1–1.3
Lymphs (×10^3/μL)	**0.6**	1–4.8
Platelets (×10^3/μL)	470	200–500
TP (P) (g/dL)	7.2	6–8

Hemopathology: Normal.

Biochemical profile		Reference interval
Gluc (mg/dL)	**138 *(7.6)***	65–122 *(3.5–6.7 mmol/L)*
BUN (mg/dL)	14	7–28
Creat (mg/dL)	**0.5**	0.9–1.7
Ca (mg/dL)	**4.0 *(1.0)***	9.0–11.2 *(2.25–2.80 mmol/L)*
Phos (mg/dL)	**7.0 *(2.3)***	2.8–6.1 *(0.9–2.9 mmol/L)*
TP (g/dL)	7.0	5.4–7.4
Alb (g/dL)	3.6	2.7–4.5
Glob (g/dL)	3.4	1.9–3.4
T. bili (mg/dL)	0.4	0–0.4
Chol (mg/dL)	161	130–370
ALT (IU/L)	38	10–120
AST (IU/L)	18	16–40
ALP (IU/L)	176	35–280
Na (mEq/L)	145	145–158
K (mEq/L)	4.4	4.1–5.5
CL (mEq/L)	**103**	106–127
TCO_2 (mEq/L)	22	14–27
An. gap (mEq/L)	24	8–25

Urinalysis		Urine sediment	
Color	Yellow	WBCs/hpf	0
Transparency	Clear	RBCs/hpf	0
Sp. gr.	1.032	Epith cells/hpf	0
Protein	Negative	Casts/lpf	0
Gluc	Negative	Crystals	0
Bilirubin	Trace	Bacteria	0
Blood	Negative		
pH	6.0		

Endocrine data		Reference interval
iPTH (pmol/L)	**2**	2–13

Interpretive discussion

Hematology

Mature neutrophilia, lymphopenia, and monocytosis are typical of a stress leukogram.

Biochemical profile

The serum glucose concentration is in the range typical for glucocorticoid-induced hyperglycemia. Stress is the most likely cause in this case, particularly in light of the leukogram.

Decreased serum creatinine concentration is meaningless in most cases. This abnormality can result from diuresis, but, if this is the cause, the BUN concentration is usually also decreased. The absence of a history of polyuria and the normal BUN concentration make diuresis unlikely in this case.

Hypocalcemia and hyperphosphatemia can occur in renal failure, pancreatitis with prerenal azotemia, eating a diet containing excessive phosphorus, or hypoparathyroidism. Hypoparathyroidism is most likely in this case. Normal BUN concentration and decreased serum creatinine concentration indicate that renal function is normal. Clinical signs are not typical of pancreatitis, and there is no evidence of a prerenal azotemia. This dog may be receiving a diet with excessive phosphorus, but this is very unlikely if the dog is receiving a commercial diet. Hypoalbuminemia is another cause of hypocalcemia, but the absence of hypoalbuminemia indicates that this is not a consideration. Vitamin D deficiency may also result in hypocalcemia, but hypophosphatemia rather than hyperphosphatemia is typical of such a deficiency. Hypoparathyroidism can be confirmed by measuring the serum intact parathormone concentration (see below).

Slight hypochloremia, in the absence of abnormalities in Na, K, or total CO_2, is probably insignificant.

Urinalysis

The urinalysis is normal.

Endocrine data

The serum intact parathyroid hormone (iPTH) concentration is at the low end of the reference interval. The normal response of the parathyroid glands to hypocalcemia is production of PTH. Low normal iPTH concentration in a hypocalcemic animal strongly suggests inability of the parathyroid glands to respond to hypocalcemia and, therefore, hypoparathyroidism. Other possible causes of hypocalcemia (discussed above) should result in high normal to increased iPTH concentrations.

Summary

The combination of hypocalcemia with low normal iPTH concentration indicate hypoparathyroidism. Other diseases can result in hypocalcemia and hyperphosphatemia, but iPTH concentration in these diseases is typically high normal to increased.

Case 108

Signalment: 17-week-old female mixed-breed dog
History: Vomiting, diarrhea, anorexia, weakness for few days
Physical examination: Dehydrated. Dog received fluids between Day 1 and Day 3.

Hematology	Day 1	Day 3	Day 5	Reference range
Packed cell volume (%)	42	41	**34**	36–54
RBC ($\times 10^6/\mu L$)	6.5	6.11	**5.45**	5.5–8.5
Hgb (g/dL)	13.8	13.1	**11.6**	12–18
MCV (fL)	65	65	65	60–72
MCHC (g/dL)	**32**	**33**	**33**	34–38
NCC ($10^3/\mu L$)	**28.3**	**19.7**	**17.6**	6.0–17.0
Segmented neutrophils ($10^3/\mu L$)	**14.7**	7.9	6.2	3.0–11.5
Monocytes ($10^3/\mu L$)	1.4	0.4	0.2	0.2–1.4
Lymphocytes ($10^3/\mu L$)	**9.6**	**9.3**	**9.0**	1.0–4.8
Eosinophils ($10^3/\mu L$)	**2.5**	**2.2**	**1.9**	0.1–1.2
Platelets ($10^3/\mu L$)	477	**520**	447	200–500
Plasma protein (g/dL)	6.3	6.2	**5.5**	6.0–8.0

Biochemical profile	Day 1	Day 3	Reference range
Glucose (mg/dL)	101	110	60–110
Blood urea nitrogen (mg/dL)	**125**	**29**	7–25
Creatinine (mg/dL)	**2.4**	0.6	0.3–1.4
Calcium (mg/dL)	**13.4**	**12.5**	8.6–11.3
Phosphorus (mg/dL)	**17.3**	**9.1**	2.9–6.6
Total protein (g/dL)	6.3	**5.0**	5.4–8.2
Albumin (g/dL)	3.0	2.7	2.5–4.4
Globulin (g/dL)	3.3	2.3	2.3–5.2
Total bilirubin (mg/dL)	0.3	0.3	0.1–0.6
Cholesterol (mg/dL)	259		130–300
ALT (IU/L)	38	34	10–118
ALP (IU/L)	**185**	**170**	20–150
Sodium (mEq/L)	**137**	**132**	138–160
Potassium (mEq/L)	**9.0**	**7.4**	3.7–5.8
Chloride (mEq/L)	**100**		108–120

Urine specific gravity: 1.022.

Interpretive discussion

Hematology

The dog is mildly anemic, which was masked by dehydration on Days 1 and 3. Considering the other laboratory findings, this is likely due to a lack of cortisol.

Neutrophilia in the absence of lymphopenia suggests inflammation. Although concurrent neutrophilia and lymphocytosis could be indicative of excitement, this is highly unlikely in a dog.

Eosinophilia may be due to hypersensitivity or parasites but with concurrent lymphocytosis, may be due to lack of cortisol.

Persistent lymphocytosis in this case is most likely due to a lack of cortisol considering hyponatremia and hyperkalemia, but other considerations would be recent vaccination considering the dog's age, tick-borne disease, especially ehrlichiosis, chronic lymphocytic leukemia, thymoma, and, less likely, excitement.

Monocytosis may be indicative of inflammation.

Chemistry

Increased BUN and creatinine, indicating decreased glomerular filtration rate, resolved almost completely with fluids, suggesting prerenal azotemia. The BUN is relatively more increased than the creatinine, suggesting prerenal azotemia due to dehydration or hypovolemia. A high-protein meal or blood loss into the intestine could also be contributing to an increase in BUN. The PCV is not decreased, suggesting no GI blood loss, although a decrease could be masked by dehydration.

While the urine specific gravity indicates an inability to concentrate (since the dog is azotemic), this is likely due to hyponatremia interfering with concentrating ability due to decreased medullary tonicity, rather than tubular disease, and/or hypercalcemia interfering with ADH receptors.

Hypercalcemia is moderate and decreases with fluid therapy. In this case, again considering Na and K, it is likely due to Addison disease. Approximately 30% of dogs with Addison disease are mildly hypercalcemic. Other considerations in this case would be vitamin D toxicosis (considering the hypercalcemia and hyperphosphatemia) and hypercalcemia of malignancy (considering the lymphocyte concentration). The hyperphosphatemia is also likely due to decreased glomerular filtration, although vitamin D toxicosis could be considered. Additionally, both calcium and phosphorus can be mildly increased in growing puppies. Since the phosphorus improves with fluid therapy, it is likely due to decreased GFR. The calcium × phosphorus product is greater than 200, suggesting the possibility of mineralization of the kidneys. However, the improvement of the azotemia following fluid therapy suggests that this has not occurred.

Mild hypoproteinemia is evident on Day 3, although both albumin and globulin are in the reference interval. The lack of hyperalbuminemia in the presence of dehydration on Day 1 suggests that the dog may be hypoalbuminemic. Hypoalbuminemia has been reported in dogs with Addison disease, likely due to GI protein loss resulting from a lack of cortisol, which is necessary to maintain GI mucosal health.

The ALP activity increase is not likely due to cholestasis, since the bilirubin is normal. Other possibilities include steroid induction (not likely since this dog appears to have hypoadrenocorticism based on Na and K) or bone isoenzyme, since this dog is still growing at 17 weeks of age.

Hyponatremia and hyperkalemia with a Na:K ratio of approximately 15 is extremely suggestive of hypoadrenocorticism. Other possibilities would include Na wasting through the GI tract or kidney. The animal may be acidotic, which could also cause a potassium increase. Other possibilities of potassium increase would be anuria, but this patient is urinating.

The hypochloridemia is likely related to the hyponatremia.

Summary

Primary hypoadrenocorticism resulting in a lack of both mineralocorticoids and glucocorticoids due to destruction of the adrenal gland is the most likely differential considering the hyponatremia and hyperkalemia, lymphocytosis, eosinophilia, and hypercalcemia. Vomiting is seen in approximately 85% of dogs with hypoadrenocorticism. The lack of aldosterone results in the electrolyte abnormalities, and the lack of cortisol results in the lymphocytosis. Only approximately 20% of dogs with Addison disease present with lymphocytosis. More typically, patients with Addison disease present with a lack of a stress leukogram (lack of lymphopenia), which is unusual, especially if vomiting, and the lack of a stress leukogram should always trigger consideration of hypoadrenocorticism. Other possible differentials would include pseudo-Addison disease such as is seen with *Trichuris* (whipworms) parasitism or renal disease, possibly secondary to hypercalcemia and kidney mineralization. The electrolyte abnormalities do not suggest the latter.

Additional tests

The hyponatremia and hyperkalemia triggered an ACTH stimulation test, which confirmed that the patient had Addison disease.

		Reference interval
Baseline serum cortisol (μg/dL)	**<0.5**	1–4
Post-ACTH stimulation serum cortisol (μg/dL)	**<0.5**	10–20

Other tests that could be performed include fecal examination for *Trichuris*, flow or PARR for chronic lymphocytic leukemia, PTH-rp for the possibility of hypercalcemia of malignancy, or vitamin D concentrations to exclude the possibility of vitamin D toxicosis.

The laboratory findings in this patient are very typical of primary hypoadrenocorticism. Ninety five percent of dogs with primary hypoadrenocorticism are hyperkalemic, and 86% are hyponatremic. Approximately 90% have increased BUN, 65% have increased creatinine, 80% have increased phosphorus, and 70% are unable to concentrate maximally. Approximately 30% are hypoproteinemic.

Animals do not recover from adrenal gland destruction without life-long therapy, which consists of a mineralocorticoid and glucocorticoid. This patient was treated with prednisone 0.2 mg/kg daily and deoxycorticosterone pivalate (Percortin, Novartis) 2.2 mg/kg IM every 25 days.

Contributor: Dr. Mary Anna Thrall

Case 109

Signalment: 5-month-old female Labrador retriever
History: Vomiting for approximately 1 week, anorexia, lethargy
Physical examination: Slightly dehydrated

Hematology		Reference range
Packed cell volume (%)	50	36–54
RBC ($\times 10^6/\mu L$)	8.05	5.5–8.5
Hgb (g/dL)	**18.5**	12–18
MCV (fL)	62	60–72
MCHC (g/dL)	34	34–38
NCC ($10^3/\mu L$)	13.0	6.0–17.0
Segmented neutrophils ($10^3/\mu L$)	5.4	3.0–11.5
Monocytes ($10^3/\mu L$)	**1.7**	0.2–1.4
Lymphocytes ($10^3/\mu L$)	**5.9**	1.0–4.8
Platelets ($10^3/\mu L$)	347	200–500
Plasma protein (g/dL)	NP	6.0–8.0

Biochemical profile		Reference range
Glucose (mg/dL)	93	60–110
Blood urea nitrogen (mg/dL)	**95**	7–25
Creatinine (mg/dL)	**2.3**	0.3–1.4
Calcium (mg/dL)	**13.5**	8.6–11.3
Phosphorus (mg/dL)	**13.0**	2.9–6.6
Total protein (g/dL)	5.8	5.4–8.2
Albumin (g/dL)	3.2	2.5–4.4
Globulin (g/dL)	2.6	2.3–5.2
Total bilirubin (mg/dL)	0.1	0.1–0.6
Cholesterol (mg/dL)	258	130–300
ALT (IU/L)	56	10–118
ALP (IU/L)	83	20–150
Sodium (mEq/L)	**123**	138–160
Potassium (mEq/L)	**6.8**	3.7–5.8
Chloride (mEq/L)	**98**	108–120

Urine specific gravity: 1.020.

Interpretive discussion

Hematology

The hemoglobin is slightly increased, with the RBC concentration and PCV at the upper end of the reference interval; this is likely due to dehydration.

Mild lymphocytosis in this patient is most likely due to a lack of cortisol, considering the hyponatremia and hyperkalemia (see below). Lymphocytosis in a vomiting dog should always trigger the suspicion of Addison disease, as dogs with adequate cortisol typically have a stress response (lymphopenia) when vomiting.

Monocytosis is very mild and may be indicative of mild inflammation.

Chemistry

Increased BUN and creatinine, indicating decreased glomerular filtration rate, may be renal or prerenal. The BUN is relatively more increased than the creatinine, suggesting prerenal azotemia due to dehydration or hypovolemia.

The urine specific gravity of 1.020 indicates an inability to maximally concentrate, since the dog is azotemic and dehydrated. In a patient with azotemia due to dehydration that has normal kidney function, one would expect a urine specific gravity of at least >1.035. However, inability to concentrate is likely due to hyponatremia causing a lack of tonicity in the medullary interstitium, and hypercalcemia interfering with ADH receptors. On the other hand, the calcium × phosphorus product is 175.5, and it is very possible that soft-tissue mineralization resulting in kidney dysfunction could be occurring.

Hypercalcemia is moderate, and considering hyponatremia and hyperkalemia, it is likely due to Addison disease.

Other considerations in this case would be vitamin D toxicosis (considering the hypercalcemia and hyperphosphatemia) and hypercalcemia of malignancy. The mechanism of hypercalcemia in adrenal insufficiency is not completely understood but is thought to be due to increased calcium mobilization from bone, increased intestinal absorption, and increased calcium reabsorption in the proximal tubule due to decreased glomerular filtration rate [1]. Glucocorticoid replacement results in calciuresis, and calcium concentrations rapidly normalize.

The hyperphosphatemia is also likely due to decreased glomerular filtration, although vitamin D toxicosis could be considered. Additionally, both calcium and phosphorus can be mildly increased in growing puppies.

Hyponatremia and hyperkalemia with a Na:K ratio of 18 is extremely suggestive of hypoadrenocorticism. Other possibilities would include Na wasting through the GI tract or kidney. The animal may be acidotic, which could also cause hyperkalemia. Other possibilities of hyperkalemia would be anuria, but this patient is urinating.

The hypochloremia is likely related to loss from vomiting and may be related to the hyponatremia.

Urine Analysis

The urine specific gravity of 1.020 in an azotemic dehydrated dog indicates an inability to concentrate maximally. In this case, it is likely due to hyponatremia, but renal disease, possibly due to mineralization, cannot be excluded. Additionally, hypercalcemia interferes with concentrating ability. The ability of the kidney to concentrate urine depends on two processes: (i) generation of hypertonicity in the medullary interstitium and (ii) antidiuretic hormone-mediated water and urea transport in the collecting duct. Hypercalcemia interferes with both of these processes [2].

Summary and outcome

Primary hypoadrenocorticism resulting in a lack of both mineralocorticoids and glucocorticoids due to destruction of the adrenal gland is the most likely differential considering the hyponatremia and hyperkalemia, lymphocytosis, and hypercalcemia. The primary differential is renal disease possibly caused by mineralization of the kidneys, considering the azotemia and low urine specific gravity,

The lack of a stress leukogram in a vomiting dog should always trigger suspicion of Addison disease.

The hyponatremia and hyperkalemia triggered an ACTH stimulation test, which confirmed that the patient had hypoadrenocorticism.

		Reference interval
Baseline serum cortisol (μg/dL)	**0.9**	1–4
Post ACTH stimulation serum cortisol (μg/dL)	**1.3**	10–20

In addition, abdominal radiographs and a barium series were performed, and were normal.

The azotemia resolved with therapy, indicating that kidney function was normal.

Contributor: Dr. Mary Anna Thrall

Case 110

Signalment: 10-year-old male neutered Labrador retriever
History: Presented for investigation of neurological signs
Clinical findings: Nystagmus, head tilt, and ataxia. No femoral pulse in the right pelvic limb and ultrasound confirmed an iliac artery thromboembolism. Ultrasound also revealed small adrenal glands and calcification of the kidneys and spleen.

Hematology		Reference interval
Total protein (refractometry g/dL)	**12.5**	6.5–8.1
Packed cell volume (%)	**36.0**	43–59
Hemoglobin (g/dL)	**11.5**	14.8–20.5
RBC ($10^6/\mu L$)	**5.51**	5.5–8.5
MCV (fL)	**63.0**	66–75
MCH (pg)	**20.0**	22–26
MCHC (g/dL)	**32.0**	33–36
RDW (%)	**15.0**	12–14
NCC ($\times 10^3/\mu L$)	9.1	4.6–10.7
Segmented neutrophils ($\times 10^3/\mu L$)	7.3	2.7–7.8
Monocytes ($\times 10^3/\mu L$)	0.4	0.1–0.8
Lymphocytes ($\times 10^3/\mu L$)	1.1	0.6–5.0
Platelets ($\times 10^3/\mu L$)	**414**	180–366

Hemopathology: Clumped platelets, mild polychromasia.

Biochemical profile		Reference interval
Glucose (mg/dL)	86	81–118
Blood urea nitrogen (mg/dL)	19	12–27
Creatinine (mg/dL)	1.5	0.6–1.5
Calcium (mg/dL)	10.7	9.5–10.8
Phosphorus (mg/dL)	4.5	2.7–5.4
Magnesium (mg/dL)	2.0	1.7–2.3
Iron (µg/dL)	**93**	109–250
Total protein (g/dL)	**7.5**	5.4–6.7
Albumin (g/dL)	3.2	2.8–3.6
Globulin (g/dL)	**4.3**	2.3–3.7
Total bilirubin (mg/dL)	0.3	0.1–0.3
Cholesterol (mg/dL)	**1347**	126–325
ALT (alanine aminotransferase) (IU/L)	21	21–68
AST (aspartate aminotransferase) (IU/L)	25	16–41
ALP (alkaline phosphatase) (IU/L)	30	10–92
CK (IU/L)	135	51–169
Triglycerides (mg/dL)	**1522**	20–79
Sodium (mEq/L)	**138**	139–151
Potassium (mEq/L)	**5.2**	3.9–5.1
Chloride (mEq/L)	111	106–115
Bicarbonate (mEq/L)	**12**	16–27
Na/K ratio	27	
Anion gap (mmol/L)	20	12–22

Venous blood gases (pertinent results)		Reference interval
pH	**7.27**	7.36–7.44
pCO_2 (mmHg)	29.1	24.5–41.0
HCO_3 (mmol/L)	**13.5**	16.0–25.0
Base excess (mmol/L)	**−11.3**	−5.1 to 1.9
Sodium (mmol/L)	146	143–150
Potassium (mmol/L)	**5.1**	3.0–4.7
Ionized calcium (mg/dL)	**6.1**	3.4–5.3
TCO_2 (mmol/L)	**14.4**	17.5–26.1
Osmol (mOsm/kg)	292	287–296

Urinalysis	
Urine specific gravity	**1.006**
Urine pH	7.1

Endocrine panel		Reference interval
Total thyroxine (TT4) (nmol/L)	**0**	11–60
Total triiodothyronine (TT3) (nmol/L)	**0.7**	0.8–2.1
Free T4 (pmol/L)	**0**	6–42
TSH (ng/mL)	**0.59**	0.00–0.58

Parathyroid hormone, parathyroid related hormone and baseline cortisol were within normal limits.

Interpretive discussion

Hematology

A mild, nonregenerative, microcytic, hypochromic anemia is present typical of iron-deficiency. Also contributing to this may be the mild, normocytic, normochromic anemia commonly observed in dogs with hypothyroidism (see below). The mild thrombocytosis in the face of platelet clumping is a reactive process and is a common observation in cases of iron deficiency and other conditions such as chronic inflammation and neoplasia.

Chemistry and blood gas

A decrease in serum iron is present (iron-deficiency/hypoferremia) and in an older dog is most commonly due to external blood loss (e.g., chronic gastrointestinal bleeding) and warrants testing for occult blood in feces. Less likely causes for this abnormality include iron sequestration due to inflammation or decreased intake, which is very uncommon in small animals.

Total protein concentration between the refractometer and biochemical analyzer is discrepant due to falsely increased total protein estimation by refractometry, in this case due to interference by cholesterol. However, hyperproteinemia is present characterized by a hyperglobulinemia and could be reflective of dehydration, inflammation, antigenic stimulation or much less likely, neoplasia (multiple myeloma).

This degree of marked hypercholesterolemia and hypertriglyceridemia are strongly suggestive of hypothyroidism (see below). Other causes of hypercholesterolemia include nephrotic syndrome and cholestasis, but there is no evidence of nephrotic syndrome (proteinuria) or cholestasis (ALP and total bilirubin are within normal limits), and this breed is not predisposed to familial disorders of lipid metabolism, making other differentials less likely.

A very mild hyponatremia and concurrent hyperkalemia is present. In isolation these values are likely to be insignificant, but this animal has a calculated Na/K ratio of 27 which is on the margin for suspicion of hypoadrenocorticism. The sodium concentrations measured by the biochemical analyzer and the blood gas machine are discrepant, and this is explained by the marked hypertriglyceridemia and hypercholesterolemia, which can result in pseudohyponatremia when indirect measures of potentiometry are used (as is the case with the Beckman biochemistry analyzer) [1]. Decreased serum bicarbonate and low pH reflects metabolic acidosis and could be due to consumption or loss; as the anion gap is not increased the latter is more likely. Loss of bicarbonate typically occurs through the gastrointestinal tract or kidneys. In this case, renal losses are more likely and could be due to aldosterone insufficiency, which leads to decreased excretion of H+ in the kidneys (increased retention) and subsequent decrease in serum bicarbonate [2].

There is a mild increase in ionized calcium as measured in the venous blood gases, and typical differentials to consider for this include paraneoplastic syndromes, hyperparathyroidism, and renal disease. Based on biochemistry and endocrinology results, there is no evidence of these.

Urinalysis

Hyposthenuria (USG <1.008) indicates the kidneys' ability to dilute urine. A possible cause in this case may be medullary washout secondary to hypoaldosteronism (not Addison's in this case.) Less likely are central and nephrogenic diabetes insipidus and there is no history of polydipsia.

Endocrine

A marked decrease in serum T4 and T3 and concurrent increase in TSH is strongly supportive of primary hypothyroidism. Despite the suspicions of hypoadrenocorticism this dog's baseline cortisol was within normal limits.

Summary

A diagnosis of primary hypothyroidism was confirmed, and the neurological signs were thought to be a manifestation of this disease. Neurological disease associated with hypothyroidism is rare and while the link between the two is not confirmed, some authors believe decreased mitochondrial ATPase activity in these cases leads to axonal degeneration, whilst some believe accumulation of mucopolysaccharides in the endoneurium and perineurium impede function [3, 4]. Further, hypothyroidism and the subsequent hypertriglyceridemia and hypercholesterolemia predisposes individuals to the development of emboli and atherosclerosis, which may explain the embolic event in this case.

The electrolytes derangements, hyposthenuria, hypobicarbonemia, and small adrenal glands raised concern for Addison's but was ultimately ruled due to a normal baseline cortisol. However, a case of mineralocorticoid deficiency preceding glucocorticoid deficiency in hypoadrenocorticism has been reported [5]. Despite the anion gap being within normal limits, the metabolic acidosis in this case was most likely due to lactate production secondary to ischemia, and a serum lactate would have been warranted in this case.

Contributors: Drs. Alex Mau and Clarissa Freemyer

Case 111

Signalment: 8-year-old neutered female miniature schnauzer
History: Vomiting, anorexia for 3 days, lethargy, polyuria and polydipsia for several weeks
Physical examination: Dehydrated, febrile

Hematology (plasma markedly lipemic)		Reference range
Packed cell volume (%)	**60**	36–54
RBC (×10^6/μL)	**11.1**	5.5–8.5
Hgb (g/dL)	**22**	12–18
MCV (fL)	64	60–72
MCHC (g/dL)	37	34–38
NCC (10^3/μL)	11.1	6.0–17.0
Segmented neutrophils (10^3/μL)	5.4	3.0–11.5
Band neutrophils (10^3/μL)	**3.0**	0–0.3
Monocytes (10^3/μL)	**2.0**	0.2–1.4
Lymphocytes (10^3/μL)	**0.5**	1.0–4.8
Platelets (10^3/μL)	**10**	200–500
Plasma protein (g/dL)	**9.3**	6.0–8.0

Biochemical profile (serum markedly lipemic)		Reference range
Glucose (mg/dL)	**450**	60–110
Blood urea nitrogen (mg/dL)	**70**	7–25
Creatinine (mg/dL)	**3.5**	0.3–1.4
Calcium (mg/dL)	9.4	8.6–11.3
Phosphorus (mg/dL)	**7.0**	2.9–6.6
Total protein (g/dL)	**8.9**	5.4–8.2
Albumin (g/dL)	**5.3**	2.5–4.4
Globulin (g/dL)	3.6	2.3–5.2
Total bilirubin (mg/dL)	**2.5**	0.1–0.6
Cholesterol (mg/dL)	**340**	100–250
Triglycerides(mg/dL)	**500**	20–112
ALT (IU/L)	**400**	10–118
ALP (IU/L)	**1200**	20–150
GGT (IU/L)	**17**	0–6
Sodium (mEq/L)	150	138–160
Potassium (mEq/L)	5.6	3.7–5.8
Chloride (mEq/L)	**102**	108–120
Total CO_2 (MEq/L)	**11**	14–27
Amylase (IU/L)	**4400**	50–1250
Lipase (IU/L)	**2200**	300–560
Pancreatic lipase immunoreactivity (μg/L)	**900**	0–200

Urine analysis		Reference interval
Color	Yellow	
Transparency	Hazy	
Urine sp. gr.	1.013	
pH	6.0	
Protein	**1+**	
Glucose	**2+**	
Ketones	Neg	
Sediment		
RBCs (hpf)	**6–10**	0–2
WBCs (hpf)	**15–20**	0–2
Bacteria	**Many Gram-negative rods**	0
Casts (lpf)	**3**	0
Protein:creatinine ratio	0.5	<1.0

Coagulation profile		Reference interval
aPTT (s)	14	10.5–16.5
PT (s)	9.0	24–39
FDPs	<10	<10

Interpretive discussion

Hematology

The PCV, hemoglobin and RBC concentration indicate erythrocytosis, likely relative, due to dehydration.

The increase in band neutrophils and monocytosis are indicative of an inflammatory leukogram, and the lymphopenia is indicative of a stress or cortisol leukogram.

Platelets are markedly decreased, and no comment regarding platelet clumping on the blood film was made. Causes of thrombocytopenia should include canine ehrlichiosis, immune-mediated thrombocytopenia and disseminated intravascular coagulopathy (DIC). The aPTT and PT were within the reference interval, and fibrin degradation products (FDPs) were also normal, which would exclude DIC as a differential (see below).

The plasma protein estimate by refractometry is increased, and considering the hyperalbuminemia in the biochemical profile, this is likely due to dehydration. Lipemia could also falsely. Increase the refractometric reading, but the plasma protein is only slightly higher than the serum protein analysis, and the difference can be accounted for by the presence of fibrinogen.

Chemistry

Hyperglycemia is of the magnitude that diabetes mellitus should be diagnosed. The increase in cortisol, as evidenced by the lymphopenia, could also be contributing slightly to the hyperglycemia. Fructosamine could be determined to further substantiate a diagnosis of diabetes mellitus but was not performed in this case.

Increased BUN and creatinine, indicating decreased glomerular filtration rate (GFR), is likely renal azotemia, considering the urine specific gravity. A prerenal component to the azotemia is also likely, considering that the dog is dehydrated. Phosphorus is slightly increased due to decreased GFR, and would probably be more increased if not for the polyuria.

Total protein and albumin are increased, likely due to dehydration.

Total bilirubin is increased, likely due to liver disease or cholestasis.

Cholesterol and triglyceride are both increased. Serum lipids are commonly increased in patients with diabetes, since fat is mobilized for energy. However, this patient has a long history of fasting lipemia, and considering the breed, this is likely familial hyperlipidemia that is commonly seen in miniature schnauzers. Triglycerides are increased in approximately 30% of miniature schnauzers, and the syndrome appears to worsen with age [1]. Cholesterol is increased in approximately 11% of miniature schnauzers, and is more likely to be increased in those that have marked hypertriglyceridemia. The disorder is thought to be familial, and may be due to decreased lipoprotein lipase activity, although the exact pathophysiology is still controversial.

The ALT activity is increased, indicating hepatocellular damage. Alkaline phosphatase and GGT activities are increased, suggesting cholestasis since the bilirubin is increased. Additionally, increased cortisol could be contributing to the increase in ALP and GGT activities. It is likely that the patient has hepatic lipidosis secondary to hyperlipidemia associated with diabetes mellitus and familial hyperlipidemia. Hepatic lipidosis could be responsible for both hepatocellular damage and cholestasis.

Chloride is slightly low and is likely being lost in the vomitus.

The total CO_2 is decreased, indicating metabolic acidosis.

By subtracting the sum of chloride and total CO_2 (major anions) from the sum of sodium and potassium (major cations) the anion gap in this patient is calculated to be 42.6 mEq/L (reference interval, 12–24). This increase in this patient is likely due to lactic acid or ketones, although the urine is negative for ketones. Urine test strips only measure for acetoacetate, and the major ketoacid in the blood is typically beta-hydroxybutyrate [2, 3]. Blood was not tested for ketones in this patient.

Amylase and lipase activity are both increased, and this increase is likely due to pancreatitis, although both amylase and lipase are commonly increased in patients that are azotemic, due to decreased clearance of the enzymes. Pancreatic lipase immunoreactivity is also increased, and this enzyme is not increased with azotemia [4], indicating that pancreatitis is quite likely. Although pancreatitis and hyperlipidemia are known to be associated with each other, and are speculated to be bi-directional (i.e., hyperlipidemia can cause pancreatitis, and pancreatitis can cause hyperlipidemia), recent studies have shown that only a small percentage of dogs develop hyperlipidemia secondary to pancreatitis, while a large percentage of dogs develop pancreatitis secondary to hyperlipidemia [5].

Urine Analysis

The urine specific gravity is only slightly above the isosthenuric range, and the glucose in the urine could be contributing to the urine specific gravity. In an azotemic, dehydrated dog with normal sodium concentration, this is very suggestive of renal azotemia. The urine contains glucose, as would be expected, since the serum glucose exceeds the renal threshold for glucose. The presence of protein in the urine is likely due to the inflammation secondary to the bacteriuria. The urine is negative for ketones, but the animal may be ketonemic since beta-hydroxybutyrate is not detected by the methodology used for urine (see above). The presence of bacteria and leukocytes in the urine is indicative of septic suppurative inflammation occurring somewhere in the urogenital tract. Considering the azotemia in this patient, pyelonephritis is likely. The erythrocytes may be present secondary to inflammation, or mild hematuria as a result of thrombocytopenia may be occurring.

Coagulation profile

The coagulation profile is normal, which excludes DIC as the cause of the thrombocytopenia.

Summary and outcome

Diagnoses in this patient include pancreatitis, diabetes mellitus, pyelonephritis, immune-mediated thrombocytopenia, and familial hyperlipidemia. It is likely that recurrent bouts of pancreatitis, likely caused by hyperlipidemia, resulted in diabetes mellitus. Diabetes mellitus probably predisposed to pyelonephritis, since glucosuria often results in cystitis that can ascend into the kidney. Therapy was instituted for the pyelonephritis and pancreatitis, the thrombocytopenia resolved, and the patient was treated with daily insulin and survived for 6 more years.

Contributor: Dr. Mary Anna Thrall

Case 112

Signalment: 25-year-old male gelding mule
History: Presented for investigation of decreasing body condition and inappetence
Note: Reference intervals are for an adult horse (not mule)

Hematology		Reference interval
Total protein (refractometry g/dL)	**8.2**	6.1–7.5
Total fibrinogen (g/dL)	0.3	0.1–0.5
RBC ($10^6/\mu L$)	**4.92**	6.41–10.12
Hemoglobin (g/dL)	**10.3**	11.4–16.9
HCT (%)	31.2	30.6–42.1
MCV (fL)	**63.4**	38.7–52.3
MCH (pg)	**20.9**	15.0–19.4
MCHC (g/dL)	**33.0**	35.0–40.8
RDW (%)	**21.0**	21.6–27.6
Total nucleated cell count ($\times10^3/\mu L$)	**65.73**	4.79–10.88
Segmented neutrophils ($\times10^3/\mu L$)	**6.57**	2.40–6.27
Band neutrophils ($\times10^3/\mu L$)	0.00	0.00–0.00
Lymphocytes ($\times10^3/\mu L$)	**58.17**	1.15–4.58
Monocytes ($\times10^3/\mu L$)	**0.99**	0.00–0.48
Platelets ($\times10^3/\mu L$)	185	97–254

Hemopathology: Mild anisocytosis, small to intermediate-size lymphocytes predominate.

Biochemical profile		Reference interval
Glucose (mg/dL)	96	77–107
Blood urea nitrogen (mg/dL)	13	11–24
Creatinine (mg/dL)	**0.7**	0.9–1.7
Sodium (mEq/L)	**129**	132–141
Potassium (mEq/L)	3.6	2.7–4.3
Chloride (mEq/L)	105	96–105
Bicarbonate (mEq/L)	29	25–33
Anion gap (mEq/L)	**−1**	8–15
Total protein (g/dL)	**8.0**	5.7–7.5
Albumin (g/dL)	2.5	2.5–3.6
Globulin (g/dL)	**5.5**	2.4–7.5
Calcium (mg/dL)	**25.4**	11.2–12.8
Phosphorus (mg/dL)	<1.0	1.8–4.0
Magnesium (mg/dL)	**2.6**	1.5–2.3
Triglycerides (mg/dL)	14	14–62
Total bilirubin (mg/dL)	**0.5**	0.6–2.8
AST (IU/L)	**667**	203–415
GGT (IU/L)	**57**	10–30
GLDH (IU/L)	2	No reference interval
CK (IU/L)	192	112–444

Endocrine panel		Reference interval
Parathyroid hormone (pmol/L)	**25.0**	0.6–11
Ionized calcium (mmol/L)	**4.19**	1.58–1.90
Parathyroid related protein (pmol/mL)	**0**	
TSH (ng/mL)	**0.59**	0.00–0.58

Urinalysis	
Urine specific gravity	1.004
pH	8.5
Sediment: moderate calcium carbonate	
Urine chemistry	
Creatinine (mg/dL)	17.6
Calcium (mg/dL)	13.2
Sodium (mEq/L)	23
Phosphorus (mg/dL)	<1.0

Interpretive discussion

Hematology

Interpretation of laboratory results is limited by the lack of well-established reference intervals for mules. The hemogram reveals a mild anemia that appears macrocytic (MCV) and hypochromic (MHCH) but these reference values are for an adult horse. Donkeys, and possibly mules, have a relative macrocytosis in comparison to horses. The subjective observation of anisocytosis is discrepant with the mild decrease in RDW, and erythrocyte morphology is possibly normal. Considering this, the anemia is suspected to be nonregenerative – possibly reflecting anemia of inflammation/chronic disease or an altered marrow microenvironment related to lymphoid neoplasia.

There is a marked leukocytosis comprised predominantly of small to medium sized lymphocytes. Assuming these lymphocytes have condensed chromatin and appear mature (rather than lymphoblastic), this is suggestive of late-stage lymphoma or chronic lymphocytic leukemia. Flow cytometry is recommended for immunophenotyping.

Chemistry and endocrinology

The mild decrease in creatinine likely reflects poor muscle mass.

The hyponatremia appears mild and unremarkable at first glance; however, chloride is observed moving in the opposite direction and in the upper end of the reference interval. The corrected chloride is calculated to be 111 mEq/l, indicating hyperchloremia. This discrepancy is normally associated with hypobicarbonemia (hyperchloremic/strong ion metabolic acidosis); however, bicarbonate concentrations are in the middle of the reference interval in this case and the anion gap is negative. A subtle acid-base disturbance is present in this animal, and given the negative anion gap, likely reflects increased concentrations of unmeasured cations (see below).

Hyperproteinemia characterized by hyperglobulinemia could be polyclonal (inflammation) or monoclonal (associated with B-cell lymphoid neoplasia) and a serum protein electrophoresis is recommended.

A marked hypercalcemia is present and in the presence of increased PTH and lack of evidence of PTH-rp, this is most consistent with primary hyperparathyroidism. Primary hyperparathyroidism additionally promotes hypermagnesemia and PTH-induced hypophosphatemia. The marked hypercalcemia and increase in ionized calcium (Ca2+) may be responsible for the unexpected anion gap.

A mild increase in AST activity in the absence of elevated CK is suggestive of hepatocellular injury. It is, however, possible that see persistent AST following muscle injury in which CK has returned to reference interval.

Donkeys can have increased GGT activity relative to horses, so it is uncertain whether this animal has a true increase in enzyme activity. This is coupled by the low total bilirubin, which makes cholestasis unlikely. Elevated GGT can be seen with gastrointestinal diseases in horses such as gastroenteritis.

Urine chemistry

By performing urine chemistry one can calculate the fraction excretion of analytes by the kidneys. Unfortunately, as the analyzer yielded results of <1 mg/dl for phosphate in both the serum and urine, a fraction excretion for this analyte could not be attained.

Fractional excretion of Calcium = (Urine Ca 13.2/plasma Ca 25.4) × (Plasma creatinine 0.7/urine creatinine 17.6) × 100 = 2%. This value is relatively low given the marked hypercalcemia and reflect renal retention of Ca, likely due to hyperparathyroidism.

Fractional excretion of Sodium = 0.7%. This value is high considering the hyponatremia any may reflect renal losses as a contributor to this.

Summary

This patient had been diagnosed with primary hyperparathyroidism a year prior to this presentation. Flow cytometry of peripheral blood was interpreted as B cell lymphoproliferative disease. Serum protein electrophoresis was reported as polyclonal.

Patient was euthanized, and the following abnormalities were identified:

- B cell small cell lymphoma/Leukemia with specific tissues affected including marrow, lymph nodes, liver, stomach, and intestines
- Pituitary pars intermedia adenoma
- Spindle cell sarcoma on the serosal surface of the large colon
- Chronic mild lymphocytic interstitial nephritis
- Cortical cyst in the right kidney
- Splenic lymphoid hyperplasia

Although masses were found adjacent to the thyroid, and the thyroid gland appeared enlarged, no parathyroid tissue was found in the cut sections of the thyroid and the adjacent masses were lymph nodes with the neoplastic lymphocytes. It is therefore uncertain what the source of PTH was, and there is minimal evidence in the literature to suggest PTH secretion with neoplastic conditions (as opposed to those that produce PTH-rp).

Contributor: Drs. Alex Mau and Saundra Sample

Case 113

Signalment: 14-year-old male Senegal parrot (*Poicephalus senegalus*)

History: Polyuria (marked amount of liquid in droppings) of 1-year duration

Physical examination: 136 g, poor body condition (BCS 3/9) based upon prominence of the keel bone, alert, agitated and polyureic

Hematology	Day 1	Reference range [1]
Packed cell volume (%)	42	36–48
Polychromasia	Moderate	
WBC ($10^3/\mu L$)	**25.1**	4.0–14.0
Heterophils ($10^3/\mu L$)	**21.3**	(2.1–10.0)
Heterophils (%)	**85**	55–75
Monocytes ($10^3/\mu L$)	0	(0–0.7)
Monocytes (%)	0	0–2
Lymphocytes ($10^3/\mu L$)	**1.5**	(1.7–10.0)
Lymphocytes (%)	**15**	25–45
Eosinophils ($10^3/\mu L$)	0	(0–0.4)
Eosinophils (%)	0	0–1
Basophils ($10^3/\mu L$)	0	(0–0.4)
Basophils (%)	0	0–1
Thrombocytes	Adequate	1–5/1000x field
Plasma protein (g/dL)	4.6	3.0–5.0

Normal leukocyte and thrombocyte morphology.

Biochemical profile		Reference range
Glucose (mg/dL)	**1064**	140–250
Blood urea nitrogen (mg/dL)	6	(<10)
Uric acid (mg/dL)	**15.1**	2.3–10
Calcium (mg/dL)	8.3	6.5–13.0
Phosphorus (mg/dL)	5.1	(5.0–7.0)
Total protein (g/dL)	**2.4**	3.0–4.5
Albumin (g/dL)	1.4	
Globulin (g/dL)	1.0	
Cholesterol (mg/dL)	**364**	(100–250)
AST (IU/L)	375	120–330
Creatine kinase (IU/L)	**960**	100–330
Sodium (mEq/L)	146	(130–160)
Potassium (mEq/L)	2.2	(2.0–4.0)
Chloride (mEq/L)	99.8	(111–120)
Bicarbonate (mEq/L)	21.1	(20–30)

Suggested decision levels when reference values are unavailable are in parentheses.

Interpretive discussion

Hematology

The bird has a normal packed cell volume with moderate numbers of polychromatic erythrocytes, which is suggestive of some erythrocyte regeneration. The moderate leukocytosis with normal heterophil morphology could be indicative of a moderate inflammatory response that may not involve an infectious etiology. However, the associated lymphopenia may make a stress leukogram more likely.

Chemistry

In general, the blood glucose concentration in normal birds ranges from 200 to 500 mg/dl: therefore, the plasma glucose concentration in this avian patient demonstrates a marked increase. Hyperglycemia occurs with diabetes mellitus, catecholamine release, and glucocorticosteroid excess, such as occurs with stress or administration of corticosteroids. Excess glucocorticosteroid result in a mild to moderate increase in the blood glucose concentration (≤600 mg/dL) in birds. Exertion, excitement, and extreme temperatures stimulate the release of catecholamines, which also results in a mild to moderate increase in the blood glucose concentration. Glucose concentrations of greater than 700 mg/dl are suggestive of diabetes mellitus in most birds. The pathophysiology of diabetes mellitus in birds varies among different species and may result from increased glucagon secretion or hypoinsulinemia. Birds with diabetes mellitus have polyuria and urinary glucose concentrations exceeding 1 mg/dl.

The normal plasma cholesterol concentrations of most avian species range between 100 and 250 mg/dl. Because cholesterol is eliminated in the form of bile acids, increases in the plasma cholesterol concentration may be associated with extrahepatic biliary obstruction, hepatic fibrosis, and bile duct hyperplasia. Hypercholesterolemia also can be associated with conditions other than liver disease, such as hypothyroidism, high-fat diets, lipemia, and during egg production. Postprandial increases in cholesterol may occur as well.

In general, a blood uric acid concentration greater than 13 mg/dl is suggestive of impaired renal function from a variety of causes, including nephrotoxins, urinary obstruction, nephritis, nephrocalcinosis, and nephropathy associated with hypovitaminosis A. Uric acid is not a sensitive test for renal disease in birds, because a significant loss (approximately 75%) of renal function is required to increase the blood concentrations of this analyte. Uric acid is also not a specific test for renal disease, because increases can occur after ingestion of a high-protein meal, during starvation, or with severe tissue necrosis. Blood uric acid can be used as an indicator of renal function in birds; however, it does not provide a diagnosis, nor do normal values guarantee an absence of renal disease. The blood urea nitrogen (BUN) concentration is slightly elevated. The normal blood urea nitrogen concentration of normal, noncarnivorous birds ranges between 0 and 5 mg/dl Urea is generally considered to have limited diagnostic value in the detection of renal disease in birds compared with that of uric acid. Unlike uric acid, which is generally excreted independently of hydration, BUN may be a sensitive test for prerenal azotemia in some avian species because it is eliminated by glomerular filtration, which depends on the hydration status of the bird. Therefore, the slightly increased BUN concentration may support a reduction of renal arterial perfusion in this bird. A urinalysis of the liquid component of this bird's droppings may have been useful in evaluation of the cause of the polyuria in this avian patient.

The normal plasma protein concentration in birds generally ranges from 2.5 to 4.5 g/dl with albumin representing 40–50% of the total plasma protein. The plasma albumin concentrations generally range from 0.8 to 2.0 g/dl in normal birds. Therefore, the total protein concentration in this bird may not be significantly decreased regardless of the published reference value. Avian albumin is difficult to measure accurately and results are likely often inaccurate as they may be below the sensitivity of the analyzer. Since albumin is subtracted from the total protein value to determine the globulin, globulin concentrations are also likely inaccurate. Both albumin and globulin are more accurately measured by protein electrophoresis.

The plasma creatine kinase (CK) activity is markedly increased, indicating skeletal muscle injury or exertion. The plasma aspartate aminotransferase (AST) activity is not significantly increased, which also supports skeletal muscle involvement. A much higher degree of AST activity would be expected with hepatocellular disease.

Summary

Because the bird's cachexia provided a grave prognosis, the owner elected for euthanasia rather than attempting treatment for diabetes mellitus. The body was submitted for necropsy. Significant necropsy findings included a moderate lymphoplasmacytic, heterophilic, multifocal, chronic-active cholangitis of the liver and moderate, multifocal, Islet cell vacuolar degeneration of the pancreas.

The vacuolar changes in the Islet cells within the pancreas are consistent with the metabolic disturbances resulting in marked increase in plasma glucose concentrations and the degenerative changes within the pancreas are suggestive of diabetes mellitus. Additionally, vascular degeneration within the liver and aorta was noted and appeared to be early atherosclerosis, which is relatively common in aged psittacines and can occur secondary to hypercholesterolemia and hyperlipidemia. This finding is often most prominent in the great vessels, although can occur in other arteries throughout the body. Diabetes mellitus and hypercholesterolemia predisposed this bird to atherosclerosis formation.

Contributor: Dr. Terry W. Campbell

Case 114

Signalment: Young adult neutered male cat
History: Anorexia, lethargy, and weight loss for several weeks
Physical examination: Dehydrated, febrile, mild abdominal effusion

Hematology		Reference range
Packed cell volume (%)	30	25–45
MCV (fL)	42	39–50
MCHC (g/dL)	32	32–36
Nucleated cells (μL ×10³)	12.5	5.5–19.5
Segmented neutrophils (μL ×10³)	8.5	2.5–12.5
Band neutrophils (μL ×10³)	**1.5**	0–0.3
Lymphocytes (μL ×10³)	**1.0**	1.5–7.0
Monocytes (μL ×10³)	**1.5**	0–0.8
Eosinophils (μL ×10³)	–	0–1.5
Nucleated RBCs (μL ×10³)	–	0
Platelets (μL ×10³)	200	150–700
Plasma protein (g/dL)	**10.8**	6.0–8.5

Biochemical profile		Reference range
Glucose (mg/dL)	100	67–124
Blood urea nitrogen (mg/dL)	**56**	17–32
Creatinine (mg/dL)	**2.3**	0.9–2.1
Calcium (mg/dL)	9.5	8.5–11
Phosphorus (mg/dL)	**8.0**	3.3–7.8
Total protein (g/dL)	**10.6**	5.9–8.1
Albumin (g/dL)	**4.8**	2.3–3.9
Globulin (g/dL)	**5.2**	2.9–4.4
Total bilirubin (mg/dL)	0.3	0–0.3
Cholesterol (mg/dL)	200	60–220
Alanine aminotransferase (IU/L)	**560**	30–100
Alkaline phosphatase (IU/L)	19	6–106

Urinalysis	
Color	Yellow
Transparency	Clear
Specific gravity	1.050

Dipstick and sediment normal.

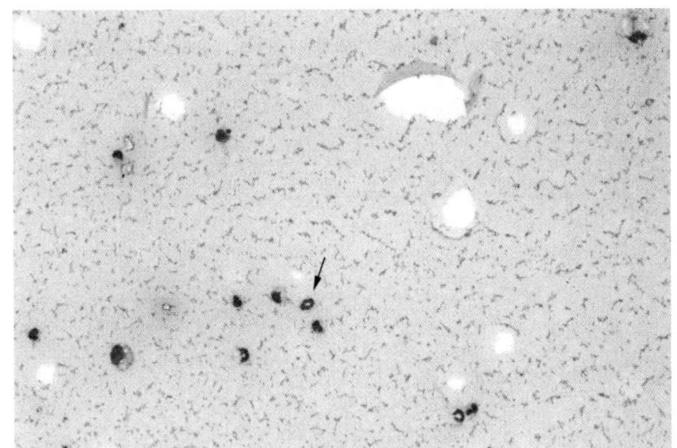

Figure 1 Direct film of abdominal fluid from cat. A few neutrophils (arrow) and macrophages are scattered throughout. Note the blue background and stippled appearance that are characteristic of a high-protein fluid. Protein has peeled off of the slide, leaving crescent-shaped structures and clear spaces.

Abdominal fluid analysis	
NCC (μL)	6000
Total protein (g/dL)	6.0

Cytology: A direct film of the fluid contains 60% segmented neutrophils that are nondegenerate, 30% lymphocytes, and 10% large mononuclear cells. No microorganisms are seen. The background is typical of a high-protein fluid (Figure 1).

Interpretive discussion

Hematology

The PCV is within the reference interval, but since the cat is dehydrated, he may actually have a mild anemia. The CBC should be repeated when the cat is rehydrated. An inflammatory leukogram is present as evidenced by the increased band neutrophils. The lymphopenia is due to a stress (cortisol mediated) response. The monocytosis may be due to either cortisol or inflammation.

Plasma protein estimate by refractometry is markedly increased, likely due to both dehydration and an increase in globulin (see below). The difference between the plasma protein and the serum protein is 0.2 g/dL, likely due to the presence of fibrinogen in plasma.

Biochemical profile

The BUN and creatinine are both increased. Considering that the urine specific gravity is 1.050, this is a prerenal azotemia, likely secondary to dehydration and hypovolemia. The hyperphosphatemia is also due to decreased glomerular filtration rate.

The albumin is increased, indicating dehydration. The globulin is also increased; a component of this increase is likely due to dehydration, but chronic antigenic stimulation is also likely a cause. A protein electrophoresis is indicated but was not performed.

Increase in ALT activity is indicative of hepatocellular damage.

Abdominal fluid analysis

The relatively low cell concentration and high-protein concentration are very suggestive of feline infectious peritonitis (FIP). The cell concentration of >3000 cells/µL puts the fluid in the exudate category. The differential count suggests mild mixed inflammation. The background protein seen in Figure 1 is very characteristic of FIP fluid.

Summary and outcome

A presumptive diagnosis of FIP was made in this cat, which was lost to follow-up.

Globulin concentration could be measured on the fluid; globulin concentration is consistently higher than albumin concentration in effusions caused by FIP.

FIP is a coronaviral disease that may affect cats of any age but is most common in cats that are 4–36 months of age. While some cats have a noneffusive form of FIP, the majority of cats have abdominal, or less commonly, pleural effusion. Most cats also have high serum globulin concentrations, usually a polyclonal gammopathy. The effusion has a very high-protein content that ranges from 3.5 to 9.8 g/dL and a relatively low cell concentration (<6000 cells/µL). The high-protein and globulin content in the effusion reflects that of the serum and results from leakage of proteins into the effusion due to serositis and vasculitis. The high-protein/Low cell concentration effusion is so characteristic of FIP that it suggests a presumptive diagnosis. Although the Rivalta test, a test to confirm the presence of protein in fluid, is commonly used to diagnose FIP effusions in Europe, it is rarely performed in the United States. Diseases other than FIP that produce positive Rivalta tests are lymphoma and bacterial peritonitis, which can usually be distinguished by cytologic evaluation of the fluid. Molecular tests can be used to help confirm a diagnosis of FIP, such as detection of viral RNA by serum or fluid reverse transcriptase polymerase chain reaction. The diagnostic gold standard is still histopathology for visualization of the classic lesions associated with FIP.

Contributor: Dr. Mary Anna Thrall

Case 115

Signalment: 11-year-old neutered male dachshund
History: Hematuria
Physical examination: No apparent abnormalities

Hematology	April[a]	September	Reference range
Packed cell volume (%)	42	**34**	37–55
RBC ($\times10^6/\mu L$)	6.29	6.12	5.5–8.5
Hgb (g/dL)	14.8	**12.1**	12–18
MCV (fL)	63	**54**	60–72
MCHC (g/dL)	**37**	34	32–36
Reticulocytes ($10^3/\mu L$)	NP	11.7	0–60
NCC ($10^3/\mu L$)	14.9	**23.1**	6.0–17.0
Segmented neutrophils ($10^3/\mu L$)	**12.7**	**18.5**	3.0–11.5
Band neutrophils ($10^3/\mu L$)	0	**0.5**	0–0.3
Monocytes ($10^3/\mu L$)	0.4	1.3	0.2–1.4
Lymphocytes ($10^3/\mu L$)	**0.9**	1.8	1.0–4.8
Eosinophils ($10^3/\mu L$)	0.4	0.7	0.1–1.2
Platelets ($10^3/\mu L$)	335	424	200–500
Plasma protein by refractometry (g/dL)	**8.1**	8.0	6.0–8.0

[a]Plasma lipemic.
An aPTT and PT were performed and were within the reference interval.

Biochemical profile (normal other than shown below)		Reference range
Alkaline phosphatase (IU/L)	**344**	20–150
Albumin (g/dL)	**2.3**	2.5–4.4

Urinalysis	April	June
Color	Yellow	Yellow-Brown
Turbidity	Hazy	Opaque
Specific gravity	1.026	1.022
pH	6.5	8
Protein	**1+** (30 mg/dL)	1+
Hb/blood	**4+**	4+
Sediment		
RBC/HPF	>**100**	>100
WBC/HPF	**5–10**	>20
Epithelial cells/HPF	**5–10 (clumps noted)**	2–5
Casts/lpf	**1 hyaline**	none
Crystals	none	struvite
Microorganisms	none seen	none seen

Radiographs

Radiographs were taken in June and September (Figures 1–2).

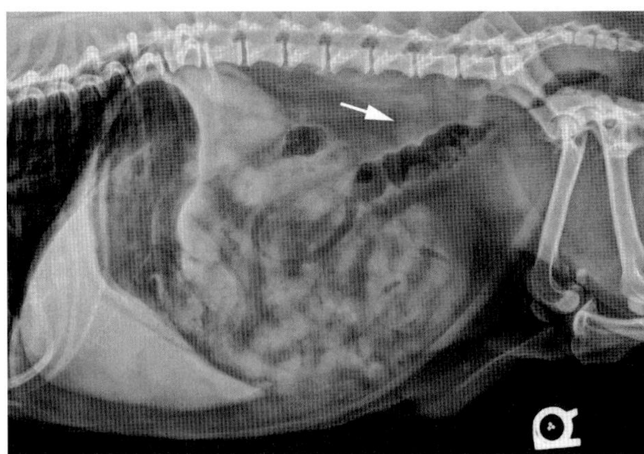

Figure 1 Abdominal radiograph made in June.

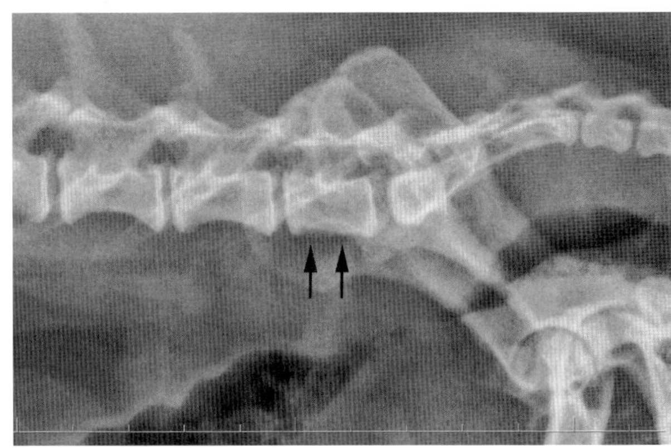

Figure 2 Close-up of the caudal aspect of the lumbar spine from June.

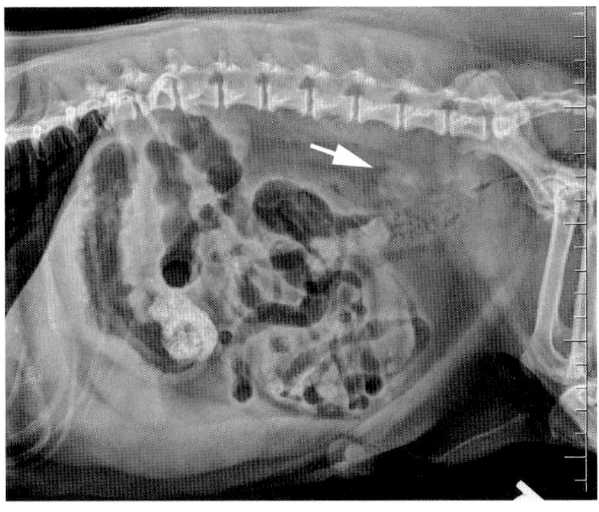

Figure 3 Abdominal radiograph made in September.

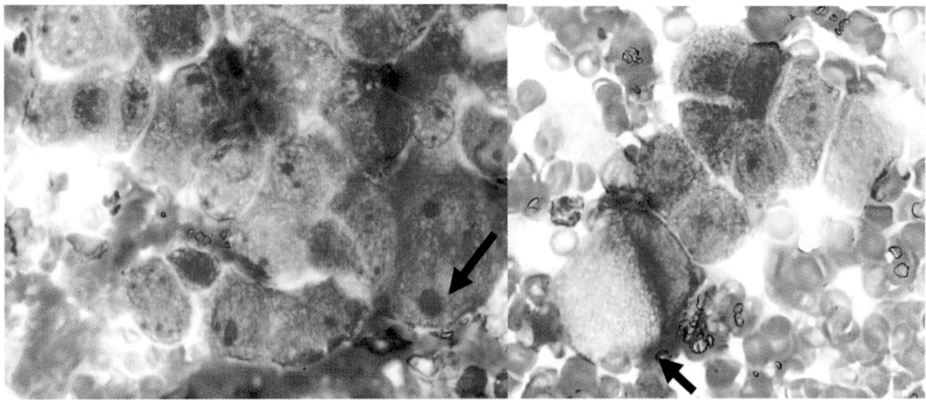

Figure 4 Traumatic catheterization of the bladder taken in June. Note the prominent nucleoli (arrows), anisocytosis, and anisokaryosis of the epithelial cells. The epithelial cell (arrow) in the image on the right contains eosinophilic amorphous material (glycosaminoglycans).

Cytology

A traumatic catheterization was performed due to the presence of clumps of epithelial cells in the urine sediment (Figure 2).

Interpretive discussion

Hematology

The patient became mildly anemic by September. The microcytosis suggests iron deficiency anemia secondary to chronic blood loss that may be associated with chronic hematuria or GI-tract blood loss due to a nonsteroidal anti-inflammatory drug (NSAID) he was given (see below). Serum iron was not measured. The increased MCHC in April is likely due to a falsely increased hemoglobin due to lipemia. A stress leukogram, characterized by a lymphopenia and mild neutrophilia, is present in June. The neutrophilia and increase in band neutrophils in September are indicative of an inflammatory leukogram.

The plasma protein by refractometry is slightly increased in June, and the increase may be false due to lipemia.

Chemistry

The increase in ALP activity is mild to moderate, and may be insignificant in an older dog. However, on imaging the liver was markedly enlarged, suggesting some type of hepatopathy with is likely resulting in the increased ALP activity. No further evaluation of the liver was made. The very mild albumin decrease could be due to inflammation or liver dysfunction, although there is no other laboratory evidence of liver dysfunction. Bile acids were not measured.

Urinalysis

Hematuria is evident, as reported in the history. The presence of leukocytes indicate inflammation somewhere in the urinary tract. Microorganisms were not seen, suggesting that the inflammation is not secondary to bacterial infection. One hyaline cast/lpf is likely not significant. The mild proteinuria is likely due to the presence of blood. The presence of clumps of epithelial cells in the urine triggered a traumatic catheterization (see cytology below).

Radiology

In the initial abdominal radiograph made in June, the prostate gland is enlarged and is displacing the urinary bladder cranially. There is a poorly defined mass effect just dorsal to the descending colon. In the closeup a very minimal smooth periosteal reaction is present on the ventral aspect of L7. Prostate gland enlargement is most commonly the result of benign hypertrophy but with the poorly defined mass effect in the territory of the sublumbar lymph nodes and the periosteal reaction on L7, neoplasia becomes the primary consideration. In the later abdominal radiograph, the mass effect is more obvious due to progressive enlargement of the sublumbar lymph nodes. The periosteal reaction on L7 is unchanged. The liver is also markedly enlarged. This could be due to vacuolar hepatopathy but other causes cannot be ruled out from survey radiographs.

Cytology

A traumatic catheterization was performed in June and was very cellular. Many clumps of epithelial cells were seen, and most of the cells exhibited criteria of malignancy, including large nucleoli, anisocytosis, and anisokaryosis. Some of the epithelial cells had round accumulations of eosinophilic granular material in the cytoplasm that is characteristic of glycosaminoglycans within urothelial cells (Figure 2).

Summary and outcome

A diagnosis of urothelial or prostatic carcinoma was made on the basis of cytology and imaging. Urothelial carcinomas and prostatic carcinomas are difficult to differentiate on cytology, and many carcinomas of the prostate arise from urethral transitional epithelial cells. The patient was treated palliatively with antibiotics, piroxicam (an NSAID), and famotidine (a histamine 2 blocker because of NSAID administration) and he clinically improved. He was lost to follow up after September.

Urothelial carcinoma (also called transitional cell carcinoma [TCC]) is the most commonly diagnosed cancer of the urinary tract of dogs. Hematuria is common, as was seen in this dog; other clinical signs include stranguria and difficulty urinating. Clinical signs are similar to those seen with a urinary tract infection. Diagnosis may be made by cytologic analysis of urine sediment, traumatic catheterization, prostatic wash and/or fine needle aspiration, although percutaneous sampling of TCC should be avoided because of possible seeding of the abdominal wall with neoplastic cells [1, 2]. Cytology of bladder epithelium can be difficult, since hyperplastic epithelial cells can appear neoplastic [3]. A sensitive PCR assay (CADET™ *BRAF* test, Antech) has been developed and is commercially available. This test detects a somatic gene mutation in the *BRAF* gene resulting from a substitution of T to A at nucleotide 1784, which in turn causes an amino acid substitution from valine to glutamic acid at codon 595. This test detects approximately 85% of uroepithelial and prostatic tumors in dogs, and requires only a small amount of urine, since tumor cells commonly exfoliate into urine [4].

Contributors: Drs. Mary Anna Thrall and Donald Thrall

CASES

Case 116

Signalment: 6-year-old female mastiff mix breed

History: Presented for the investigation of a large mass on the 5th digit of the left thoracic limb.

On presentation, the animal had a 5 to 6 cm diameter mass emanating from the 5th digit. The mass was well-circumscribed, unencapsulated, ulcerated and highly vascular. A dorsopalmar radiograph of the manus was made (Figure 1), and fine needle aspirates of the mass were taken and submitted for cytologic examination (Figures 2–4).

Interpretive Discussion

Radiology

Figure 1. There is a large mass in the 5th digit of the manus with abaxial deviation of the entire 5th digit due to the mass. There is nearly total effacement of the ungual process of the distal phalanx and visible lysis in the ungual crest. The keratinized nail is absent. The lesion extends into the medial aspect of the distal interphalangeal joint and there is active bone proliferation on the middle phalanx of this digit. There is also a very small amount of bone proliferation on the distal-lateral aspect of the proximal phalanx. Given the large mass and the extent of lysis, the findings are most consistent with a large soft tissue tumor with secondary bone effacement and a small amount of associated periosteal proliferation.

There is also a small amount of periosteal proliferation in the distal-lateral aspect of MCIII and on the distal-medial aspect of MCIV. The border of this new bone on MCIV is slightly irregular. These changes could be due to chronic pulling of interconnecting soft tissue as a result of altered weight bearing. However, that these sites represent metastatic sites cannot be ruled out. The irregular soft tissue mineralization association with digits 2 and 3 is most likely due to superficial debris.

Gross and radiographic changes are consistent with an expansile mass of the 5th digit with extensive ulceration of the overlaying epidermis and severe lysis/remodeling of the underlying bone.

Cytology

The preparations are highly cellular, but poorly preserved, composed of lysed neutrophils, keratinocytes of varying maturity and a population of atypical epithelial cells. Figures 2 and 3 depict many keratinocytes with angular borders surrounded by dense aggregates of degenerate neutrophils. Figure 4 demonstrates atypical epithelial cells surrounded by poorly preserved neutrophils. Atypical cells are large, have flattened cytoplasmic borders, moderate amounts of basophilic cytoplasm and a round, centrally placed nucleus with up to two distinct nucleoli. Clear cytoplasmic vacuoles frequently surround the nucleus.

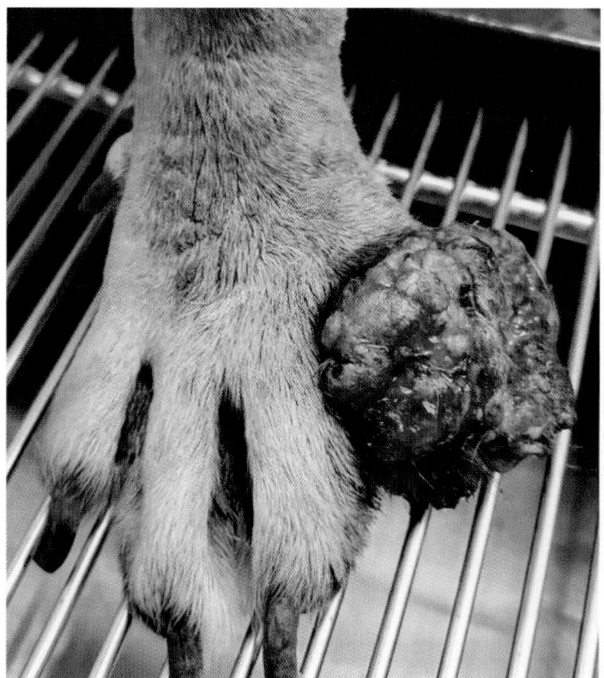

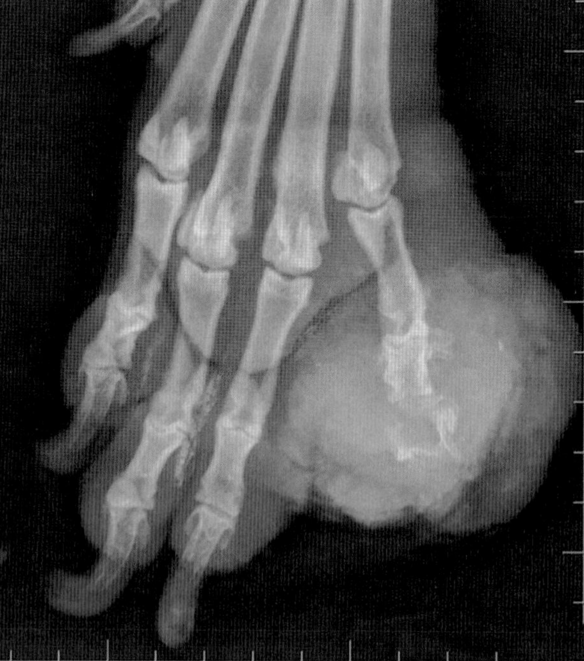

Figure 1 Gross image and radiograph of the left manus.

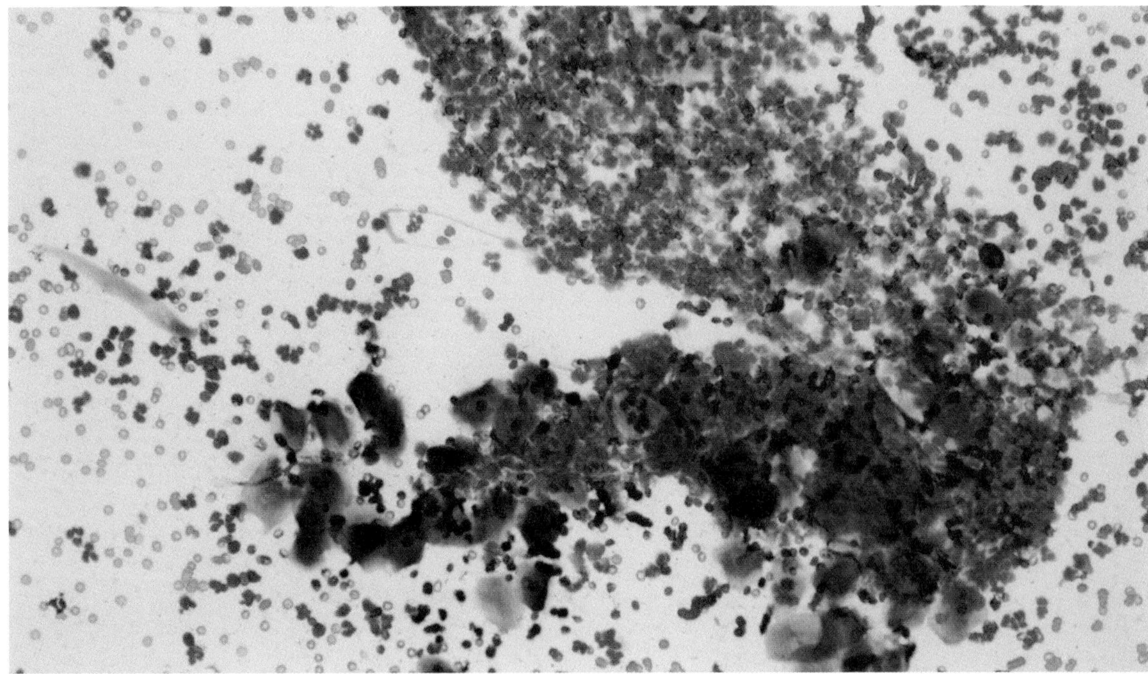

Figure 2 Fine needle aspirate of the digital mass. (Wright's stain, 10X objective) Image courtesy of Dr. Pedro Bittencourt

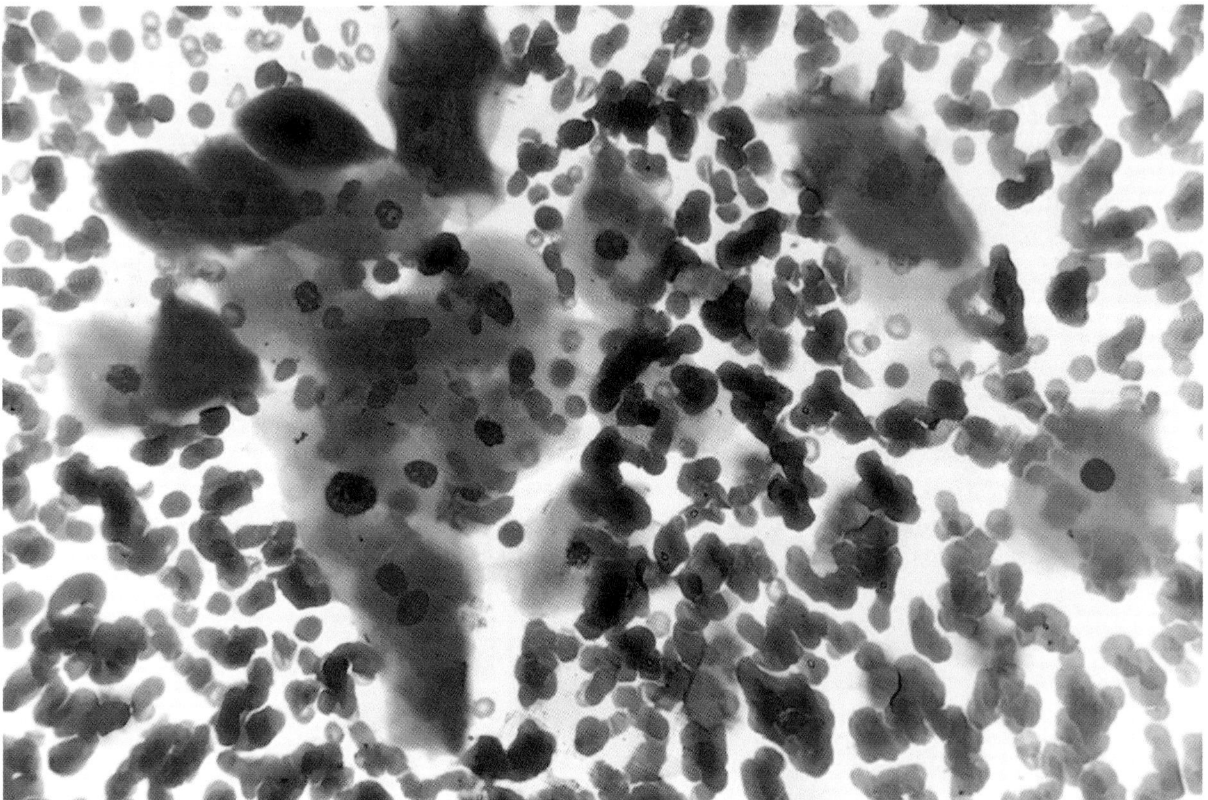

Figure 3 Fine needle aspirate of the digital mass. (Wright's stain, 40X objective) Image courtesy of Dr. Pedro Bittencourt

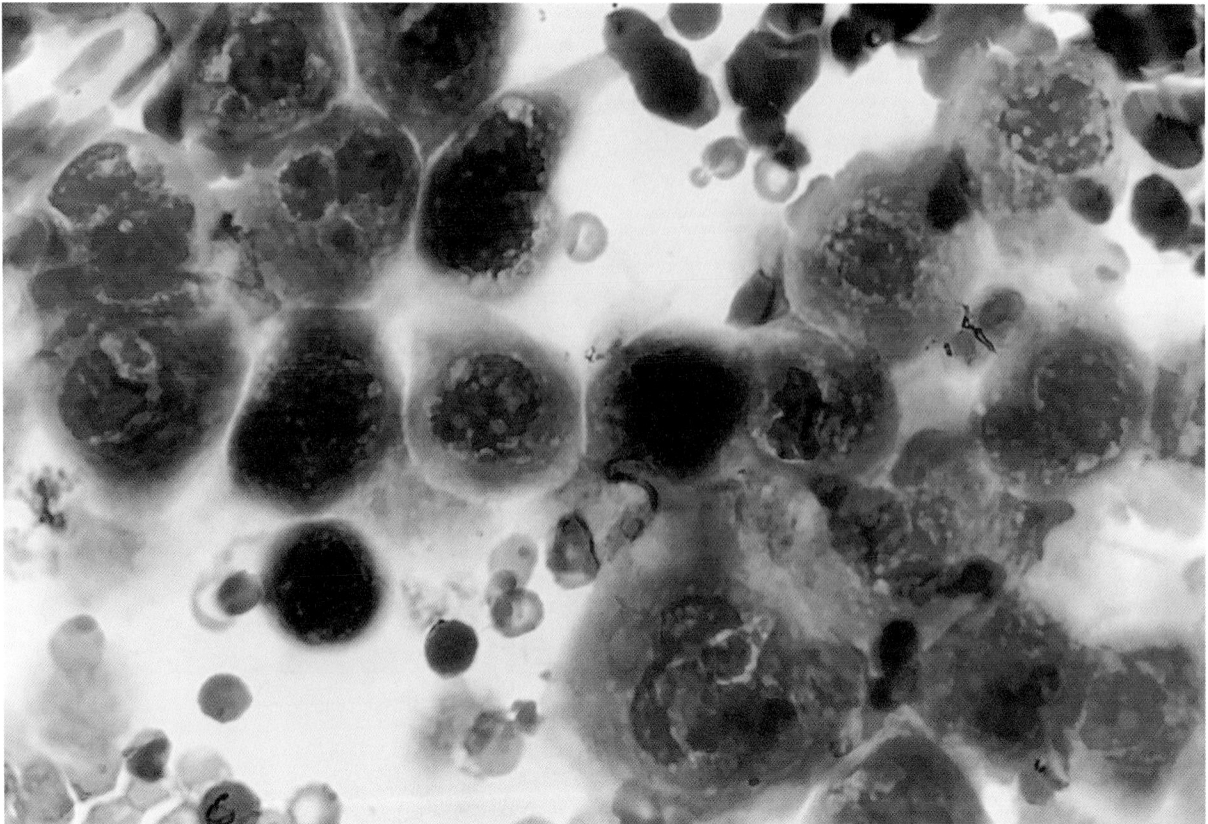

Figure 4 Fine needle aspirate of the digital mass. (Wright's stain 100X objective). Image courtesy of Dr. Pedro Bittencourt

Anisocytosis and anisokaryosis are moderate and multinucleate forms are present.

Interpretation of the atypical epithelial cells is difficult when concurrent inflammation is present as this could represent either a dysplastic or neoplastic change. The most likely diagnosis is a squamous cell carcinoma based on the criteria of malignancy present within the atypical epithelial cells and the perinuclear vacuoles, a common feature of SCC. Furthermore, suppurative inflammation is a common cytological feature of SCC and is likely a reaction to the keratin. Other conditions to consider include papilloma and much less likely, a non-neoplastic lesion such as an epithelial inclusion cyst. Ultimately, it was advised that this toe be amputated and submitted for histopathological analysis.

Histopathology

Extending from the surface epithelium and expanding the dermis, is an unencapsulated, infiltrative, moderately circumscribed neoplasm composed of inward papillary projections of epithelium supported by a thin fibrovascular stroma. Basal cells differentiate into hyperplastic, polygonal cells with distinct borders, abundant basophilic cytoplasm and a round to oval nucleus with stippled chromatin. Occasionally cells in the stratum spinosum have pale cytoplasm with eccentric nuclei (koilocytes). Neoplastic cells contain eosinophilic intranuclear inclusions (Figure 6, arrows) that measure up to 10 µm in diameter and commonly peripheralize the nucleus. The epidermis is multifocally ulcerated and contains varying combinations of neutrophils, cellular debris and mixed bacterial flora.

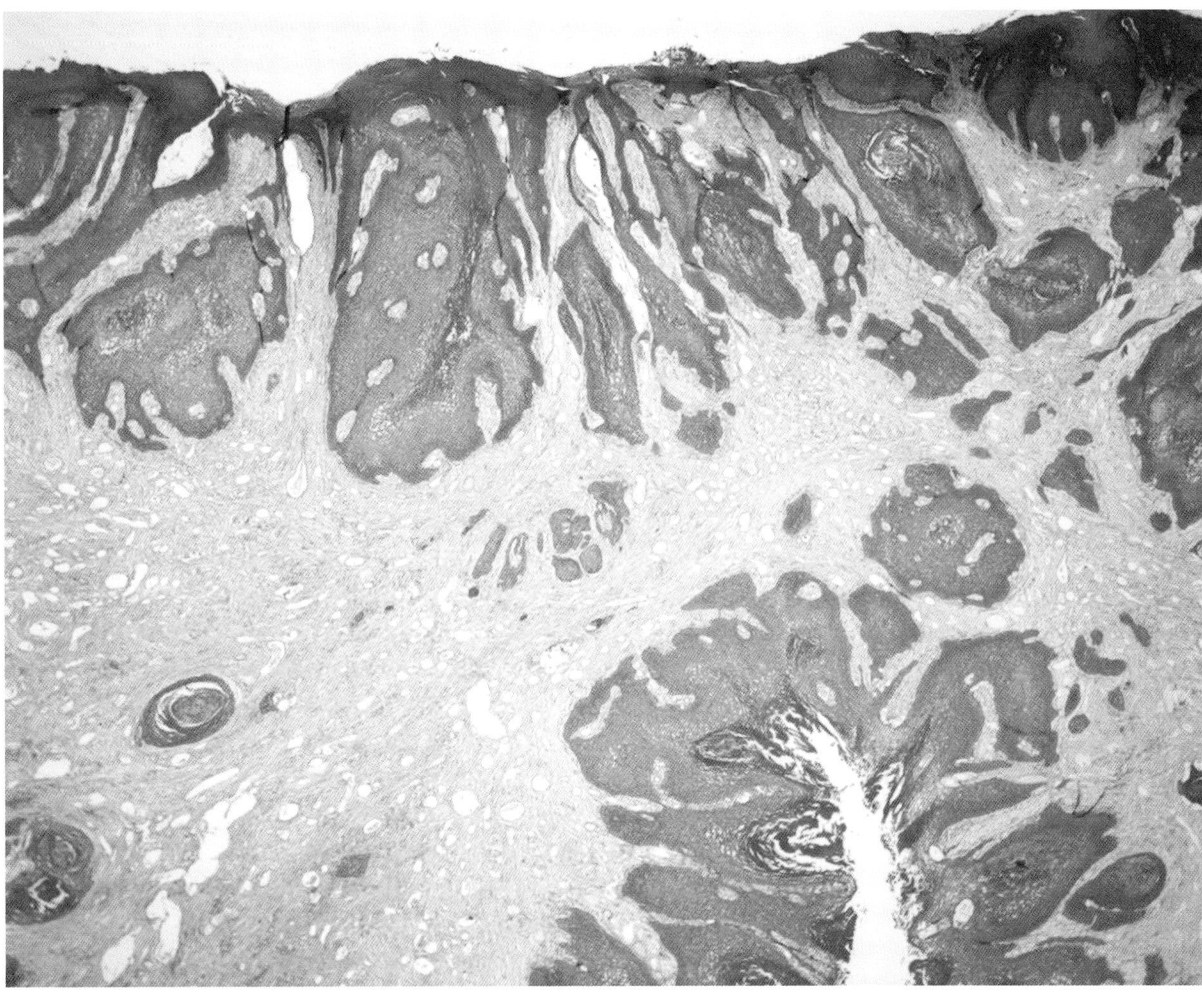

Figure 5 Histopathology of the digital mass. (H&E)

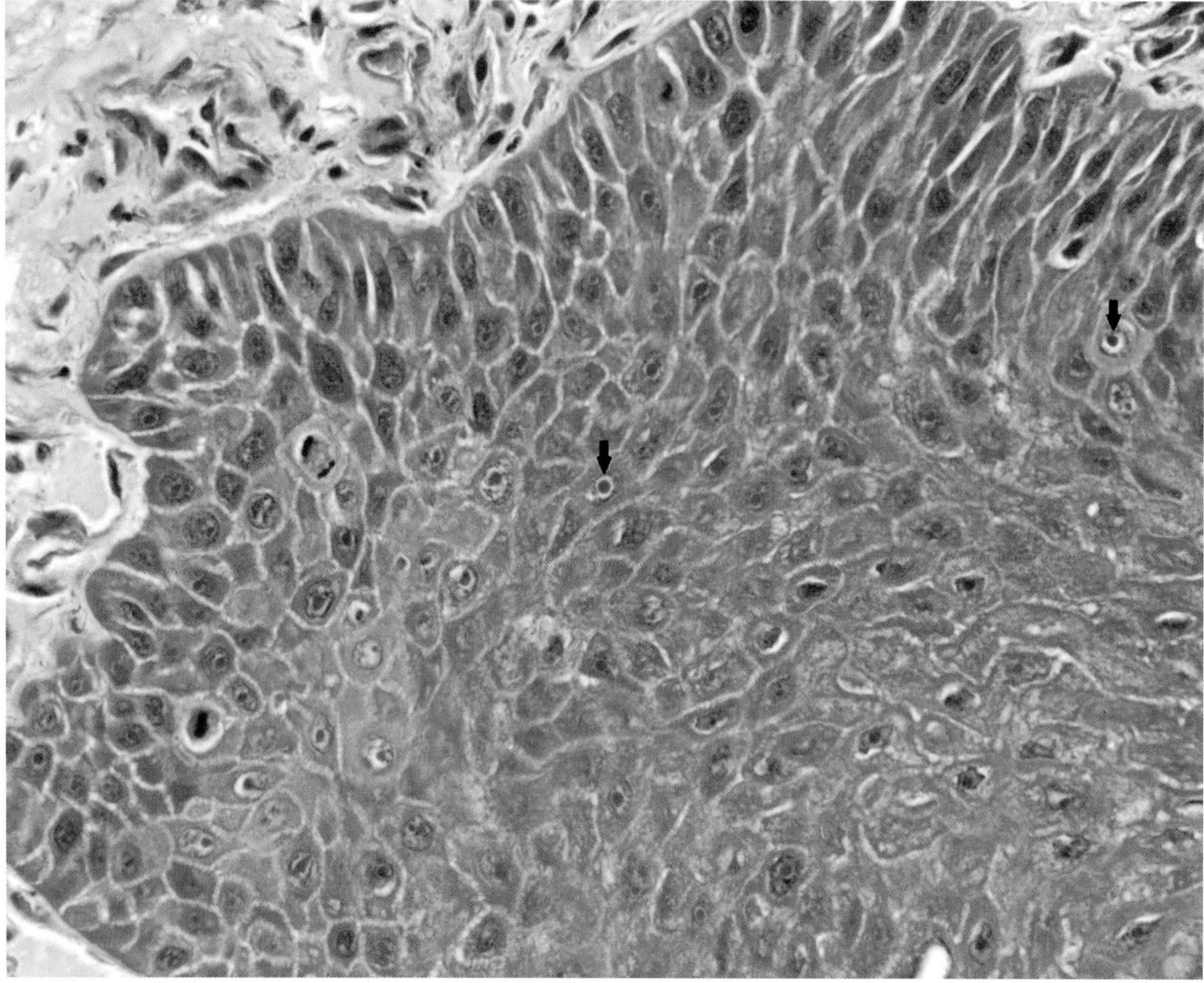

Figure 6 Histopathology of the digital mass. (H&E)

Summary and Outcome

Despite cytological findings, this neoplasm was ultimately diagnosed as an inverted canine viral papilloma. While most papillomas in dogs are exophytic (outwards growing), these neoplasms can occasionally grow inwards leading to inflammatory reactions secondary to exposure of the dermis to keratin. Subsequent inflammation and tissue reaction can lead to bone lysis and remodeling.

Contributors: Drs. Pompei Bolfa, Donald Thrall, Mary Anna Thrall, Pedro Bittencourt and Alex Mau

Case 117

Signalment: 24-year-old gelding horse
History: Chronic history of inappetence and pyrexia of unknown origin.

Hematology		Reference interval
Packed cell volume (%)	34	32–48
MCV (fL)	52	37–59
MCHC(g/dL)	31.6	31–39
Nucleated cells (×10³/μL)	8.66	5.4–14.30
Segmented neutrophils (×10³/μL)	**7.4**	3.0–6.0
Band neutrophils (×10³/μL)	0	0–0.1
Lymphocytes (×10³/μL)	**0.9**	1.5–5.0
Eosinophils (×10³/μL)	0.3	0–1.5
Nucleated RBCs (×10³/μL)	0.1	0
Platelets (×10³/μL)	109	100–400
Plasma protein (g/dL)	7.7	6.0–8.5
Fibrinogen (g/dL)	**1.1**	0.1–0.4

Hemopathology: Rare reactive lymphocyte and moderately toxic neutrophils with Dohle bodies and cytoplasmic basophilia.
Imaging: Thoracic ultrasound revealed a bilaterally nodular appearance to the lung.
Cytology: A fine needle aspirate of one of the lung-nodules was submitted for evaluation.

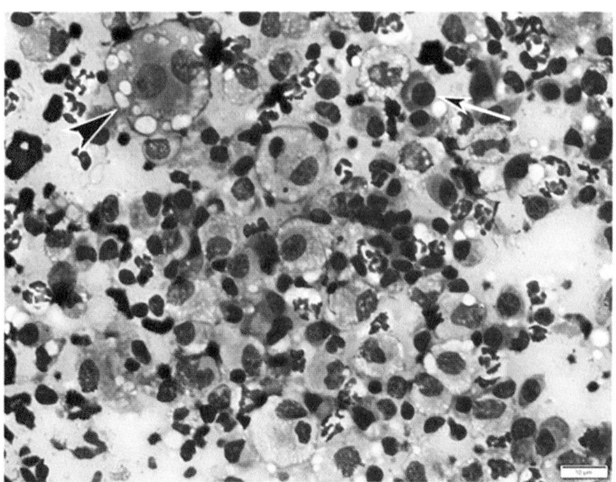

Figure 1 FNA of a pulmonary nodule. Wright stain. Source: Image courtesy of Dr. Pedro Bittencourt.

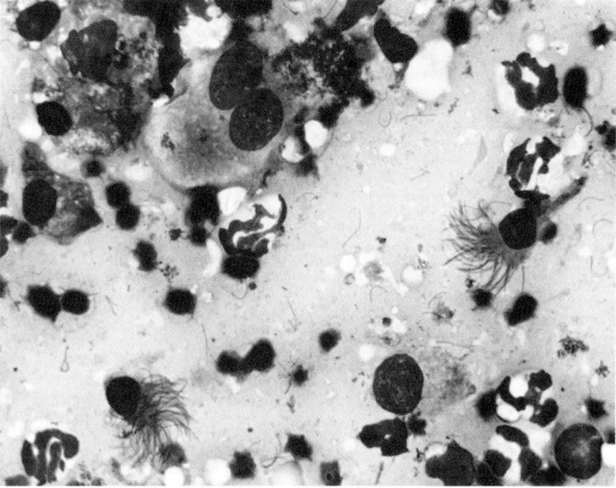

Figure 2 FNA of a pulmonary nodule. Wright stain. Source: Image courtesy of Dr. Pedro Bittencourt.

Interpretive discussion

Hematology

While only mild, the neutrophilia in combination with toxic change and hyperfibrinogenemia is indicative of active inflammation. The lymphopenia is an indication of a concurrent stress (cortisol) response.

Cytology

The cytological preparation consists of a mixed inflammatory population. Activated macrophages and neutrophils predominate. Occasional bi-nucleated macrophages (Figure 1 arrowhead) are present as are low number of plasma cells (Figure 1 arrow). Figure 2 demonstrates normal ciliated columnar respiratory epithelium amidst macrophages and neutrophils. This submission was interpreted as pyogranulomatous inflammation.

Outcome

The horse was started on broad spectrum antibiotics and treated concurrently with nonsteroidal anti-inflammatories but failed to improve. Humane euthanasia was elected, and the animal was subsequently submitted to the necropsy service.

Gross and histopathology

Histologically, most of the pulmonary parenchyma is effaced by multifocal to coalescing nodules composed of proliferating

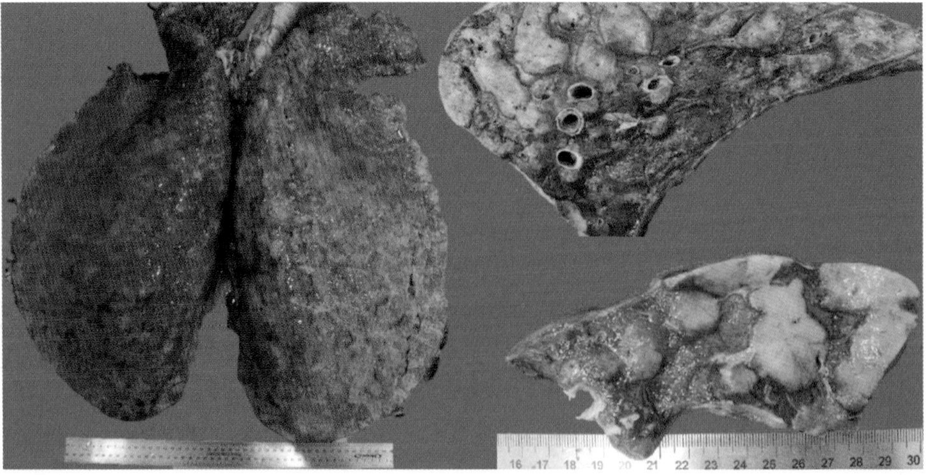

Figure 3 At the time of necropsy, the lungs were bilaterally enlarged and expanded by nodular, proliferative, and coalescing areas (from a few mm to more than 10 mm) that were hard in consistency and white to gray-tan. Tracheobronchial lymph nodes were mildly enlarged. Within the cortex of the left kidney was a white-gray multinodular area of similar appearance to the lung nodules.

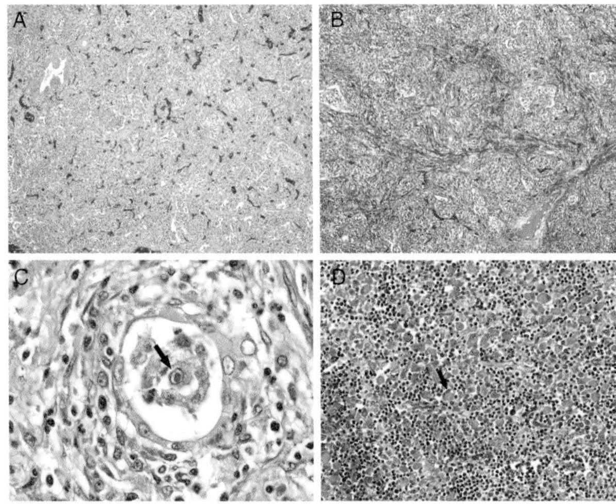

Figure 4 Histological sections of the lung (A–C) and tracheobronchial lymph node (D).

spindle cells (fibroblasts) (Figure 4A) embedded within a fibrillar eosinophilic (collagenous) stroma (stains blue on Masson's trichrome stain) (Figure 4B), and infiltrated by large numbers of lymphocytes and histiocytes, with fewer neutrophils. Occasionally, alveolar macrophages contained 3–4 μm diameter eosinophilic intranuclear inclusion bodies that peripheralized the chromatin (Cowdry Type A inclusions) (arrow in Figure 4C). The lymph node is expanded by an infiltrate of macrophages/histiocytes, some of which are multinucleated (arrow in Figure 4D).

Summary

Signalment, history, cytological and histological findings are consistent with a diagnosis of Equine multinodular fibrosis (EMPF). EMPF is a progressive fibrosing, interstitial lung condition associated with infection with Equine herpesvirus 5 (EHV-5). Grossly, this disease presents as multiple nodules of fibrosis within the lungs (Figure 3). Histologically, there is marked interstitial pulmonary fibrosis with airways containing neutrophils and macrophages. Occasionally in both cytological and histological specimens, macrophages may contain large eosinophilic intranuclear viral inclusion bodies.

Contributors: Drs. Pompei Bolfa, Pedro Bittencourt, and Alex Mau

Index

Note: Page numbers in "f" refer to Figures; those in "t" to Tables

Veterinary Hematology, Clinical Chemistry, and Cytology, Third Edition. Edited by Mary Anna Thrall, Glade Weiser, Robin W. Allison and Terry W. Campbell.

Companion website: www.wiley.com/go/thrall/veterinary